Small Animal

Gastroenterology

Donald R. Strombeck, D.V.M., Ph.D.

Professor, Department of Medicine
Clinician, Small Animal Medicine Service, VMTH

W. Grant Guilford, B.V. Sc., B.Phil.

Research Fellow, Department of Physiology
Clinician, Small Animal Medicine Service, VMTH
Diplomate, American College of Veterinary Internal Medicine

School of Veterinary Medicine
University of California
Davis, California

Small Animal

Gastroenterology

Second Edition

1990

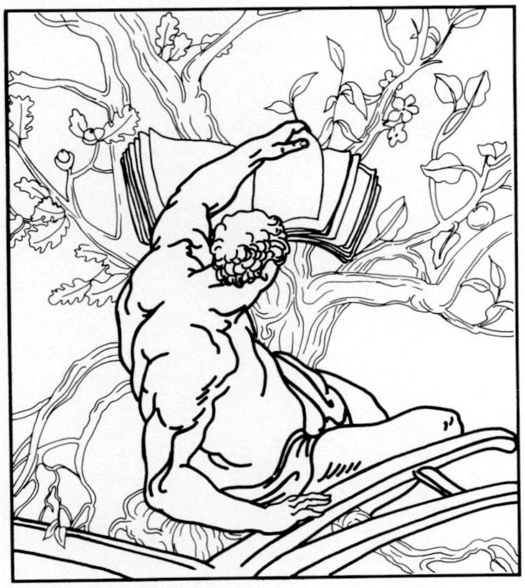

Stonegate Publishing Company
Davis, California

Small Animal Gastroenterology
Second Edition

ISBN 0-9619272-0-7

Stonegate Publishing, 633 Marina Circle, Davis, California 95616.

The author and publisher have exerted every effort to ensure that drug selection and dosage set forth in this text are in accord with current recommendations and practice at the time of publication. However, in view of ongoing research, changes in government regulations, and the constant flow of information related to drug therapy and drug reactions, the reader is urged to check the package insert for each drug for any changes in indications and dosage and for added warnings and precautions. This is particularly important when the recommended agent is a new or infrequently employed drug.

Dedicated to veterinarians who are committed to an excellence and who maintain a zeal for new knowledge.

Preface to the Second Edition

In the 10 years since the First Edition, knowledge of veterinary medicine and veterinary gastroenterology has expanded considerably. In the interim period we have seen such remarkable events as the birth of a highly virulent canine enteric parvovirus, witnessed the rise to prominence of immune-mediated gastrointestinal diseases, and observed the widespread application of diagnostic techniques such as endoscopy and ultrasound, once thought the exclusive purvey of the physician.

The Second Edition has been extensively rewritten to encompass these and other changes. The chapter on infectious diseases of the bowel has been expanded to include recently established pathogens such as canine parvovirus, feline immunodeficiency virus, *Campylobacter*, and *Clostridium perfringens*. In reflection of the newly found importance of inflammatory bowel disease and immune-mediated disorders of the liver, we have added a new chapter on gastrointestinal inflammation, and greatly expanded the chapters on the gastrointestinal immune system and inflammatory bowel disease.The chapter on gastrointestinal problems has been developed into a step-by-step description of the approach to approximately fifteen common gastrointestinal problems. The discussion of these problems is supported by tables listing useful diagnostic tests and prevalent causes. In view of the advances in diagnostic techniques, the chapters describing diagnostic techniques have been extensively rewritten, and a new chapter has been devoted to endoscopy.

The chapter on gastric-dilatation volvulus has been expanded in anticipation of heightened interest in this disease born of the advances in gastrointestinal reperfusion injury. Adverse reactions to food have received detailed discussion, prefaced by a plea for more appropriate use of terminology pertaining to food allergies and intolerances. The chapter on motility disorders has been expanded to encompass the diseases of irritable bowel syndrome, dysautonomia, and megacolon. The discussion of the liver has been broadened to describe the wealth of knowledge on etiopathogenesis of hepatitis, hepatic necrosis, and various hepatopathies. Also described is the greater understanding of identification, management, and prognosis for hepatitis and portasystematic shunts. And finally, the chapter on nutrition and gastrointestinal disease has been further developed in respect of the new-found realization of the importance of clinical nutrition to successful medical therapy.

Throughout this revision, we have had several aims. The first has been to provide the practitioner with a workable guide to the approach and treatment of gastrointestinal disease. The second has been to provide an extensive reference work on the physiology of the canine and feline gastrointestinal system and on the etiopathogenesis and pathophysiology of its diseases for those veterinarians with a penchant for deeper understanding of gastroenterology. Only from such knowledge can advances in the way we diagnose and treat gastrointestinal diseases develop. To some degree these two aims are contradictory. With exhaustive discussion of pathophysiology we run the risk of obscuring clinical details much to the frustration of the busy practitioner. To circumvent this problem we have, as mentioned, greatly expanded the chapter on the diagnostic evaluation of common gastrointestinal problems and, in addition, added a "clinical synopsis" to the description of those diseases in receipt of extensive discussion or which may have confusing diagnostic criteria. The "clinical synopsis" represents a collection of prominent clinical features along with a pragmatic suggestion as to therapy. Pragmatism does not sit well with medicine, and so it is our plea that clinicians take these therapeutic recommendations as guides for subsequent modification according to the particular needs of the patient under their care.

The third aim of the Second Edition is to provide an up-to-date information source on gastroenterology. To this end we have worked to bring this edition to completion within a year of conception . The fourth aim is to highlight areas where knowledge of small animal gastroenterology is lacking in the hope of stimulating research in those areas.

As with the First Edition, we hope this book will enable the clinicians to have a better understanding of the gastrointestinal problems that constitute an important part of small animal practice. Your critical suggestions are again invited.

Grant Guilford Donald R. Strombeck

Acknowledgements

In addition to the acknowledgements in the first edition, we wish to thank Veterinary Medical Teaching Hospital faculty, residents, and staff memebers who contributed in many different ways. Special thanks go to Quinton Rodgers and Hills Pet Products for providing the climate for our collaboration. Lorna McAdam deserves a special word of gratitude for her professional secretarial assistance.We are also especially appreciative of Andrea Hale's work in putting the book in final page form. Grant Guilford extends personal appreciation to the veterinarians who have trained, inspired, and encouraged him, most notably Drs Edward Kirk, Boyd Jones, Doug and Sandy Couper of New Zealand, CB Chastain, Brent Jones, Dudley McCaw, Dennis O'Brien of Missouri, and Gerald Ling and Donald Strombeck of Davis. He also wishes to affectionately thank his family, Patricia and Parry, for their constant support, and his wife, Sandy Forsyth, for her care, patience, and encouragement. Donald R. Strombeck wishes to affectionately acknowledge his wife, Elizabeth Strombeck, for her extensive contribution to this work and for her patience and encouragement.

Table of Contents

Chapter 1

Integration of Gastrointestinal Functions

INTRODUCTION

Functions basic to the gastrointestinal tract include those of motility, secretion, and absorption. Each function is regulated so that it integrates with a similar function in another part of the gastrointestinal tract; i.e., gastric motility is integrated by reflexes or hormones with colonic motility. Function of each type is regulated so that it integrates with the other types of functions; i.e., gastric secretion is integrated by reflexes or hormones with gastrointestinal motility. Absorption of electrolytes and nutrients, once thought to be unregulated, is influenced by many neural and endocrine/paracrine chemicals.

Function in the gastrointestinal tract is also integrated with that in other systems of the body. Gastrointestinal function changes in response to events in other systems and it is also determined by regulatory mechanisms that are located outside of the system. In the early nineteenth century William Beaumont described changes in gastric function caused by mental or psychological stimulation. Recent studies show how injection of many peptide hormones and other chemicals into parts of the brain stimulate or inhibit specific gastrointestinal functions. Many of the gastrointestinal peptide hormones are now identified as neurotransmitters in the nervous system (Table 1-1). Function in the gastrointestinal tract also causes changes in other systems. Cause-or-effect alterations in gastrointestinal function are either normal or abnormal. Since abnormal changes are often merely exaggerations of a normally well-regulated process, understanding the normal is important to understanding the pathogenesis of disease.

The importance of all or part of a system in the body is frequently determined by whether it is critical to life. Thus, a loss of a small part of the central nervous system or the cardiovascular system can result in death, whereas life can continue despite loss of the stomach or part of the small intestine. It is evident that the former two highly integrated systems cannot be altered without dire consequences. On the other hand, there have been few reservations about removing sections from any part of the gastrointestinal tract because no great changes were thought to occur in overall homeostasis. The dog is the most popularly used animal model for studying gastrointestinal function before new surgical procedures are performed on humans. This research has also generated most of the information on normal structure and function for small animal gastroenterology.

Table 1-1. Paracrine or Homonal Messengers Identified in Enteroendocrine Cells

5-hydroxytryptamine	Neurotensin
Glucagon/glicentin	Cholecystokinin
Somatostatin	Motilin
Substance P	Gastrin
Gastric inhibitory peptide	Peptide YY
Secretin	ß-endorphin/ß-lipotropin
	Pro-γ-melanocyte-stimulating Hormone

The gastrointestinal functions that begin in the posterior pharynx with the initiation of swallowing are reflex events, not under voluntary control. From that point on, the only conscious control is over the external anal sphincter. The functions of the pharynx and esophagus are entirely motor, in order to move food to the stomach; the actions are controlled by nerves that have their cell bodies in the brain stem. As food passes from the pharynx to the stomach, sphincters open and close the beginning and end of the esophagus. Nerves also control their function.

The movement of food into the stomach causes relaxation of the region near the entrance, which allows more food to enter without causing a great increase in intragastric pressure. Relaxation is a neurally mediated phenomenon. Motility increases in more caudal parts of the stomach in order to mix and empty its contents. This augmentation of motility, under the control of events occurring both inside and outside the stomach, is mediated by nerves and hormones. Events occurring in the small intestine influence gastric motility, with the primary objective of inhibiting motility and reducing the amount of chyme entering the small intestine. That prevents overloading of the digestive and absorptive capacities of the intestinal tract.

The stomach responds to a meal by secreting hydrochloric acid and protein digesting enzymes. The stimuli for secretion are quite specific, amino acids and gastric distention being the most important. The amount of gastric secretion is related directly to the volume of the diet and the amount of protein it contains. A prime mediator of secretion is the hormone gastrin, the release of which is subject to feedback control. Secretion is also dependent on the parasympathetic nerve supply to the stomach.

Chyme enters the small intestine at a programmed rate so that adjustments in pH can be made before the acidity and pepsin degrade pancreatic enzymes and mucosal cell structures. Chyme can be hyperosmolar, and regulation of its delivery to the intestine prevents excessive amounts from entering and osmotically drawing large amounts of extracellular fluid into the lumen. The stimuli of acidity and hyperosmolality reduce the rate of gastric emptying by reflex pathways that involve neural and endocrine messengers.

The pancreas and intestinal mucosa secrete enzyme and alkaline fluid into the intestine. Specific stimuli of acid pH, amino acids, and fatty acids cause the release of hormonal messengers from the intestinal mucosa, stimulating secretion of an alkaline and enzyme-rich pancreatic juice. The composition of this secretion is variable and reflects a purposeful response to the intestine's immediate needs, which may be either to neutralize acids or to digest proteins. The small intestine contains many different hormones that aid in the integration of all events during digestive periods.

The motility of the resting intestine changes when food enters. That is necessary to delay the food's passage so that processing can be complete. The motility change involves an increase in the strength and amplitude of rhythmic segmentation. The stimulus for this change is distention of the intestine by chyme. A neural reflex that is contained entirely within the wall of the intestine mediates the motility response. This motility is augmented by increased activity in parasympathetic fibers coming to the intestine from outside the gut. Some intestinal hormones can also increase motility. Intestinal motility can be inhibited in a few situations, often involving a pathological process.

Bile is added to chyme in the intestine at a rate that is determined by neural events in the vagi and by hormones released from the mucosa of the gut. These cause the gall bladder to contract. They also stimulate the liver to secrete bile acids, an important process since the pool of bile acids must circulate through the intestine and back to it via the liver two or three times during every meal.

Digestion of food is a chemical process; the amounts and kinds of both enzyme and substrate in the gut and the conditions under which the reaction must take place determine the rate of digestion. The process progresses to completion unless nutrients are sequestered by fiber, or secretion or motility in the intestine is abnormal. Absorption of nutrients is also an unregulated event, dependent on the surface area of the intestinal mucosa, the integrity of the mucosal epithelial cells, and the absence of disease in the lamina propria and lymphatics. Carbohydrate digestion and absorption is dependent on normal disaccharidase levels and a normal glucose transport mechanism in the epithelial cell. Lipid absorption requires normal lymphatic drainage and a surface area of the small intestine that has not been appreciably reduced.

The rate of blood flow to secreting organs dictates their rate of secretion, since the circulation must provide both fluid and electrolytes, needed to secrete a modified extracellular fluid, and the energy required for its formation. Rate of blood flow is also important in the intestine, where it influences the absorption of nutrients and electrolytes. Both neural events and hormones regulate the rate of splanchnic blood flow in response to a meal.

Hormones have a trophic effect on the mucosa of the alimentary tract; that is, they are required for mucosal growth and maintenance of normal size. These are important in maintaining the mucosa's secretory and absorptive functions.

A vast complicated system of microorganisms lives within the gastrointestinal tract. The host and this system live in harmony, but only as a result of the maintenance of normal functions in the alimentary canal. Overgrowth of the microflora is prevented by acid secretions of the stomach, by normal peristalsis, and by the inherent immune system of the gut. Gastrointestinal function is optimal with the intestinal microflora intact and properly ordered. When the balance within its ecology is upset, major clinical signs of disease appear.

CONTROL OF GASTROINTESTINAL FUNCTION

The components of the gastrointestinal tract have two basic functions. These are motility, which concerns smooth muscle primarily, and the transport of ions and organic molecules, which is accomplished by either secretion or absorption. These functions have been studied extensively in tissues removed from the body. Since such tissues can be studied so readily in *in vitro* preparations and appear to function spontaneously outside body, it is not surprising that the mechanisms were not thought to be very well regulated. Gastrointestinal motor function results from control exerted on the muscles by both primitive and sophisticated nervous systems and by the endocrines. Neural and endocrine control also regulate secretory and absorptive functions. Since both of those functions are dependent on changes in blood flow to the organ, control of microcirculation to the gut becomes important. Finally, the gross and microscopic structures of the tissues in the gastrointestinal tract depend for both growth and renewal on outside trophic influences.

MOTILITY AND FLUID TRANSPORT IN THE GASTROINTESTINAL TRACT

Basic Factors in Motility [1-5]

Most motility in the gastrointestinal tract is a function of smooth muscle. The only exception is in the esophagus. A combination of myogenic, neural, and hormonal factors regulate smooth muscle motility.

Myogenic factors are the chemical changes in smooth muscle that can cause contraction when the muscle has been completely stripped of its nervous regulation. Myogenic properties can be studied in an *in vitro* preparation by blocking all nerve transmission with tetrodotoxin. The myogenic factors are fundamental to function since tetrodotoxin-treated preparations exhibit both localized and propagated contractions. Thus, the factor that initiates the contraction can be propagated.

Spontaneous motor activity and autorhythmicity, which are features of myogenic activity, are run by slow waves, pacesetter potentials, basic electrical rhythm or electrical control activity, synonymous terms used to describe the regular periodic depolarizations that can be recorded (Figure 1-1). At the peak of each depolarization there is an increased excitability or an increased probability for a spike discharge, which triggers muscle contraction. The number of spikes that occur during the period of maximum depolarization determines the strength or amplitude of the contraction. Neural and humoral control over the smooth muscle influences the spikes and contractions. The periodicity of the slow wave or electrical control activity determines the rhythmic nature of the muscle contractions. Thus, this myogenic factor sets the basic pattern of the mechanical event.

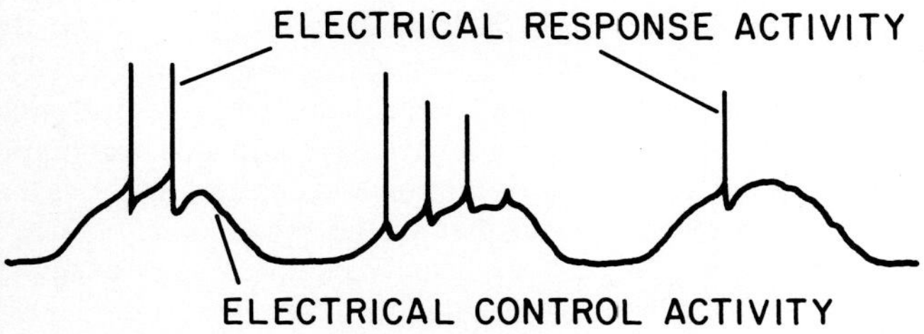

Figure 1-1. Schematic of electrical activity of smooth muscle in the gastrointestinal tract. A basic electrical control activity (slow waves)is always present that does not cause muscle contractions. Electrical response activity follows stimulation by a variety of means and results in muscle contractions.

Slow waves begin as a depolarization once believed to be generated in the longitudinal layer of small intestinal muscle. Slow waves appear to arise in the area between circular and longitudinal muscle, possibly from interstitial cells of Cajal, and activity spreads through the circular muscle, which is the most important muscle for both segmental and peristaltic contractions. Slow waves arise in circular smooth muscle in the colon. Slow waves are generated by changes in ion movements across the membranes of the smooth muscle cell. The nature of the mechanism is far from resolved, although it has been suggested that it results from either changes in sodium conductance (permeability changes for the ion) or from the modulating current produced by an oscillating electrogenic ion pump.

The local flow of current from one cell to another propagates slow waves. The factor that determines the amount of propagation is the degree of electrical coupling between muscle cells. Propagation occurs in the longitudinal muscle layer before spreading to the circular layer. The degree of electrical coupling may be influenced by hormones and by mechanical deformation of the muscle. This has an effect on contractile activity.

The rate of depolarization generating slow waves in smooth muscle differs between the parts of the gastrointestinal tract. Slow wave frequency is higher at the beginning of the small intestine than at the end. At each level there are short segments of muscle with a plateau of slow wave activity that determines the rate of rhythmic segmentation and peristaltic waves for that segment. The rates are less than in the adjacent segment at its oral end, but greater than in the segment at its caudal end. A number of chemicals influence slow waves. Tachygastria, an increase in slow wave activity, can be seen occasionally in normal dogs; the change could result from neural or humoral stimuli. Tachygastria is also produced by prostaglandins or norepinephrine, which may produce their effect by changing membrane permeability for ion movement.

By virtue of its myogenic properties, smooth muscle usually responds to being stretched by contracting, but if the muscle is actively contracting when stretched, it can respond by relaxing. Thus, stretch produced by distention can, on one hand, stimulate the strength of contractile motility (as in rhythmic segmentation and peristalsis), or it can cause relaxation (as in the fundus of the stomach or in the colon during filling). This latter phenomenon, called receptive relaxation, relies on these myogenic properties to assist the stomach and colon in receiving and holding large volumes without developing increased intraluminal pressure. Since smooth muscle cells can develop tension over a wide range of muscle length, contractile activity can be stimulated in the wall of the organ dilated with contents.

The contraction of smooth muscles occurs during the most excitable period, which is at the height of slow wave depolarization (Figure 1-1). Each contraction is accompanied by a period of rapid depolarization and repolarization. The electrical activity at this time has been called fast activity, action potentials, and electrical response activity but is now best known as spike potentials. The most important influences for its activity are neural and hormonal factors.

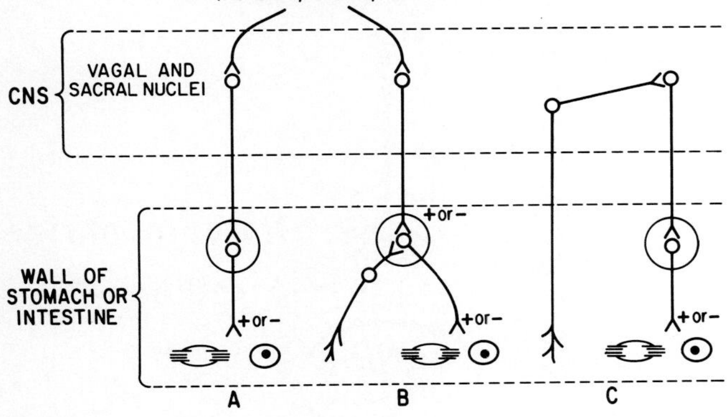

Figure 1-2. A) Schematic showing how control of function in muscle and secretory cells is augmented or inhibited directly by the central nervous system. B) Effect of the CNS to influence activity that is stimulated or inhibited by events within the alimentary tract. C) Events in the gastrointestinal tract regulate function by long pathways that synapse in the CNS.

Basic Factors in Fluid Transport

The secretions produced by various organs in the gastrointestinal tract differ in composition from the extracellular fluid from which they are derived. Energy-dependent transport processes are required for the production of different ion concentrations on opposing sides of the membranes. The basic ion-transport mechanisms have been studied *in vitro*. They all function under such conditions but do not show the optimum rates of transport found when they have neural and humoral regulation.

Neurologic Control of Motility and Fluid Transport

Regulation by Intrinsic Nervous System.[6,8] Control of motility and fluid transport, which is primarily due to secretion, is accomplished at the most rudimentary level by a primitive self-contained intrinsic nervous system. This system consists of subserous, myenteric, submucosal, and mucosal intrinsic plexuses, including their intercommunications. A simple reflex arc, illustrated in Figure 1-2, consists of: 1) a receptor that responds to chemical or mechanical stimuli in the lumen of the gastrointestinal tract; 2) a synapse; and 3) an efferent nerve fiber to a smooth muscle fiber or a secretory cell. Thus, this mechanism allows the gut to respond to events in the immediate vicinity. In general, stimulation of a local reflex arc elicits an excitatory response resulting in secretion or smooth-muscle contraction. The neurotransmitter for this pathway is acetylcholine, with a nicotinic receptor at the ganglionic synapse and a muscarinic type at the neuromuscular junction. Modification of function usually involves the use of drugs that act at one of these two synapses or directly on the end organ.

The intrinsic nervous system is always essential to gastrointestinal function. That is not always true for the extrinsic nerves. In some organs, removal of the control exerted by the extrinsic nervous system causes no significant changes in normal function. For example, a vagotomy changes motility and secretion in the small intestine very little. In other organs the extrinsic nerves are important for function. Vagotomy causes a loss in gastric motility, with resulting stasis. It also results in a marked decrease in gastric secretion. Without outside assistance, the intrinsic nervous system is unable to maintain an adequate level of function to prevent a loss of homeostasis.

Basic function in the ganglionic synapse can be modified by gastrointestinal endocrines and norepinephrine, the neurotransmitter for the sympathetic nervous system. Gastrin and cholecystokinin stimulate, and secretin inhibits, the release of acetylcholine and the contraction of smooth muscle in the gastroesophageal sphincter and intestines. Norepinephrine inhibits the release of acetylcholine in the ganglia.

Regulation by Extrinsic Nervous System.[6,9,10] The most important means of regulating function in the gastrointestinal tract is by the extrinsic nervous system and by hormones secreted in one part of the tract and acting on another part. The extrinsic nervous system consists of both efferent and afferent fibers in the vagal, sacral, and splanchnic nerves (Figure 1-3). The vagal and sacral nerves contain parasympathetic fibers that are the most important for regulating normal events. The splanchnics contain sympathetics that are less important in that a sympathectomy does not produce visible signs of disrupted function, whereas cutting the parasympathetic results in significant losses of function. In general, reflexes that receive stimuli in a proximal part of the bowel and produce a response in a more distal part are anticipatory in that they prepare the distal section for imminent events. For example, during the cephalic phase of gastric secretion, the stimulus to the animal of the presence of food before it arrives in the stomach results in a vagally mediated secretion of gastric juice that is rich in enzymes. The later presence of food in the stomach stimulates a gastroileal reflex that causes the ileum to evacuate its contents in anticipation of food that will be arriving soon. In contrast, reflexes that receive stimuli in a distal part of the bowel and produce a response in cranial parts are usually inhibitory. For example, chemical or mechanical stimulation of the duodenum causes inhibition of gastric motility by the enterogastric reflex.

Parasympathetic control. The efferent fibers in the vagal and sacral nerves are primarily excitatory and function to initiate and reinforce the motility and secretion that are necessary during the digestive period. They are all preganglionic in that they synapse on the ganglia of the intrinsic nervous system and, as is shown in Figure 1-2, they can modulate ongoing activity in the reflex arcs of the intrinsic system. The neurotransmitter in these pathways is acetylcholine; chemicals in the area of the synapse can modify its release, as shown in Figure 1-4. The nerves that carry these cholinergic fibers also contain nonadrenergic noncholinergic fibers that cause relaxation of smooth muscle when stimulated.[11] They are probably responsible for receptive relaxation in the fundus of the stomach. The neurotransmitter is most likely vasoactive intestinal peptide or in some cases adenosine triphosphate. Some postganglionic fibers in the colon are adrenergic, causing relaxation of smooth muscle when their parasympathetic innervation is stimulated. Nicotine stimulation of the ganglionic receptors produces relaxation, and this response is blocked by adrenergic antagonists. Thus, parasympathetic stimulation can elicit three types of chemical responses, with the main result being muscle contraction and stimulation of secretion.

Sympathetic control. Sympathetic nerve fibers leave the spinal cord through the ventral roots. Their preganglionic fibers

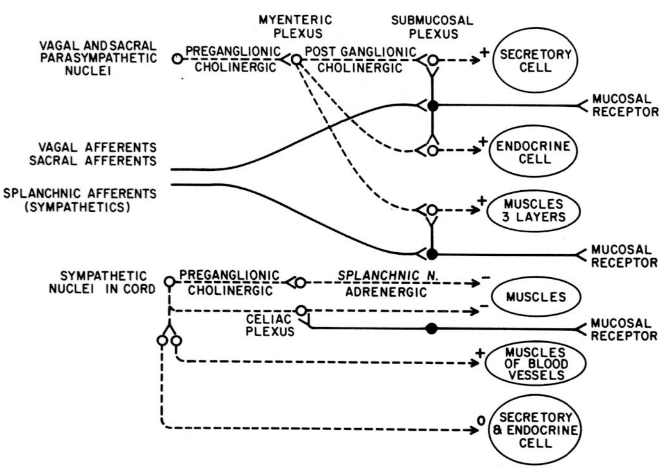

Figure 1-3. Role of autonomic nervous system in regulation of gastrointestinal function. Parasympathetics are mostly facilitatory, and sympathetics are inhibitory. Role of sympathetics is unimportant in normal function.

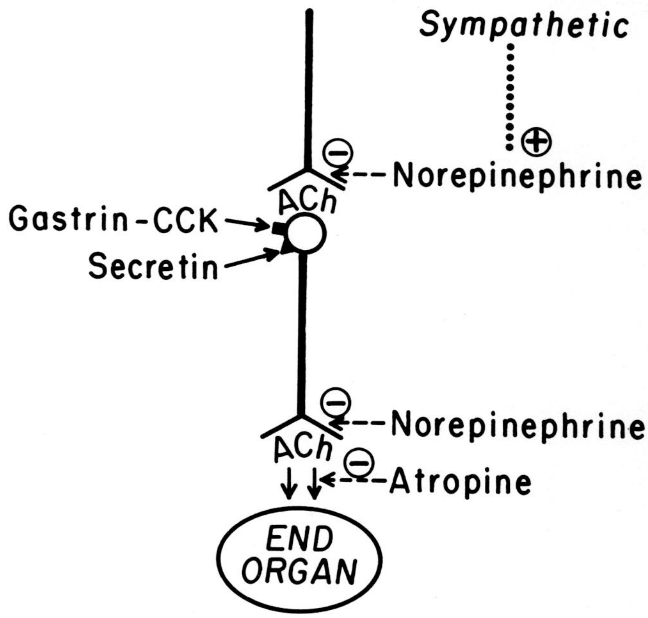

Figure 1-4. Diagram of ganglionic synapse and connection between nerve ending and structure innervated. Acetylcholine (Ach) release can be inhibited by norepinephrine, and its binding on receptor sites is blocked by atropine. The gastrin and secretin families of gut hormones possess receptors that can either augment or inhibit neural activity.

synapse in the celiac and mesenteric ganglia in regions that are remote from the walls of the bowel. Postganglionic fibers follow the arterial blood supply to the end organs and terminate on secretory cells, gastrointestinal smooth muscle, and blood vessel smooth muscle. Stimulation of these fibers usually reduces secretion, relaxes gastrointestinal smooth muscle, and causes blood vessel muscles to contract. Sympathetic fibers also terminate on ganglia, where their effect is to inhibit the release of acetylcholine, by this means blocking transmission through an excitatory pathway (Figure 1-4). The postganglionic neurotransmitter for sympathetic fibers is norepinephrine. This amine affects both smooth-muscle function and acetylcholine release but does not affect directly secretory function. Norepinephrine reduces rates of fluid secretion, though that response is secondary to the amine's effect in reducing blood flow. In summary, the overall effects of sympathetic activity are to reduce muscle activity and cell secretion, although it is questionable whether those effects are physiologically important in the normal animal. Increased sympathetic activity is important in the pathogenesis of the hypomotility that frequently follows trauma, surgery, and acute stress. In the extreme case, gastric dilatation or paralytic ileus develops.

Later chapters discuss a number of specific reflexes mediated by extrinsic nerves. They are all one of the general types discussed in this section and they illustrate the complex integration of each part of the gastrointestinal tract with other parts, and that of the entire system with all other systems in the body.

Neural Control of Hormone Release.[12] Gastrointestinal hormones act in a complex way in concert with the nervous system to regulate gastrointestinal function. Some of the hormones are released by a stimulus that acts through the nervous system. The best example of this is the vagally induced release of gastrin during feeding. This is a reflex over extrinsic nerves. An example of neurally released hormones over an intrinsic pathway is the release of gastrin from the gastric antrum in response to chemicals on the mucosal surface. Both of these neural pathways are cholinergic.

Chemical transmission in the neural regulation of the gastrointestinal tract occurs via a number of peptides as well as acetylcholine and norepinephrine (Table 1-2). All of the enteric neuropeptides are found in neurons elsewhere in the body, notably the brain. The peptides are grouped into families: a) substance P, b) vasoactive intestinal peptide, PHI, and secretin, c) opioids, d) bombesin, e) gastrin-CCK, and f) pancreatic polypeptide and NPY. Somatostatin and neurotensin are other neuropeptides or paracrines.

Substance P is an excitatory transmitter acting within the myenteric plexus on cholinergic neurons and also directly on smooth muscle during the peristaltic reflex. VIP is a neurotransmitter that stimulates pancreatic secretion, intestinal secretion, blood flow, and smooth muscle relaxation. Opioids released on neural stimulation after smooth muscle motility affect, the myenteric plexus and the muscle directly; the net effect is to delay transit. Opioid peptides also inhibit intestinal secretion. Bombesin is released during vagal stimulation and is the noncholinergic mediator of gastrin release. The effects of gastrin, CCK, pancreatic polypeptide, and somatostatin are summarized in Table 1-4.

Endocrine Control of Motility and Fluid Transport[7,13-15]

The mediators of gastrointestinal function are chemicals that bind to receptor sites and evoke a response. The chemicals released by neural reflexes are secreted instantly, in exact amounts, and at the point where they act. Endocrines are chemical mediators that are also released in exact amounts but perform their function at a point distant from release, with a physiological response that is less rapid. The actions of both the neurotransmitters and the endocrines produce specific responses. The gastrointestinal endocrines are produced by peptide-secreting cells, some of which are also amine-precursor-uptake decarboxylase (APUD) cells that originate in the neural crest of the embryo and migrate to sites in the gastric, intestinal, and pancreatic tissues. The hormones these produce are mostly polypeptides, many with structural and functional similarities. Some cells produce biogenic amines such as serotonin, which acts as a chemical messenger. A variety of stimuli, acting locally or remotely, release the hormones; each has receptor sites in all tissues of the gastrointestinal tract. Thus, to a greater or lesser degree, they have effects on all aspects of gastrointestinal function, with their most important effects on secretion. The variety and amounts of hormones described make the gastrointestinal system the largest and probably most complex endocrine organ in the body.

Release of Hormones by Intraluminal Events. Endocrines are released in response to specific chemical stimuli acting on the mucosa of the stomach and intestine. The receptors are highly specific in that they respond well to only certain stimuli. For example, gastrin release is mediated by amino acids of the sarcosine series (glycine, alanine, serine) that bathe the antral mucosa. Cholecystokinin is released by L-isomers only of tryptophan, phenylalanine, and valine, by fatty acids with carbon chains greater than 10, and to a slight extent by acid pH. Secretin is released by acid pH, with a threshold at 4.5, and the degree of acidity below pH 4.5 determines the amount released. Enteroglucagon release is stimulated by monosaccharides in the small intestine, and glucose is more effective than galactose and fructose. Present knowledge indicates that the stimuli are chemicals that act directly on the endocrine cell to stimulate hormone release, and the effect is not blocked by any known inhibitors of neural transmission. In general, calcium stimulates endocrine release when placed in the lumen of the gut. The

Acetylcholine	Somatostatin
Norepinephrine	VIP
5-Hydroxytryptamine	Enkephalin
Purine nucleotides	Substance P
Dopamine	Bombesin
Neurotensin	GABA
Cholecystokinin	Gastrin
Glycine	Histamine
Motilin	Thyrotropin-releasi Hormone
Angiotensin	Prostaglandins
Secretin	PHI
Galanin	GRP
Neuropeptide y	

Table 1-2 Neurotransmitter or Neuromodulatory Substances in Enteric Nervous System

mechanisms for release are unknown.

Release of Hormones by Hormones. The release of endocrines from peptide-secreting cells is not under feedback inhibition by blood levels of the endocrine. Other endocrines, however, stimulate and inhibit their release. Secretin and glucagon inhibit the release of gastrin, and catecholamines stimulate its release. Many of the important endocrines of the gut stimulate the release of insulin.

Release of Hormones by Neural Reflexes. Neural reflexes throughout the gastrointestinal tract release endocrines. This is the most important means of hormone release in the stomach. Elsewhere in the gut, the release of endocrines depends more on intraluminal chemicals. Vagotomy does not significantly alter normal digestive processes in the gastrointestinal tract caudal to the stomach. Gastrin is released from the antrum of the stomach by local neural reflexes in which mechanical distention stimulates a cholinergic pathway. The same mechanical stimulus in the fundus of the stomach triggers a neural reflex with a longer pathway, causing G-cells to release gastrin in the antrum. Chemical stimuli in the fundus stimulate gastrin release via the same pathway. Both of the antral and fundic receptors are also a part of long reflex arcs that synapse in the central nervous system and have afferent and efferent fibers in the vagi. In general, the physiological mechanisms for the release of gut hormones are among the last aspects to be understood adequately. The chemistry, localization, assay methods, and pharmacological effects of these endocrines have been investigated as the initial step. The mechanisms for gastrin release have been studied the most.

Neural and Endocrine Chemical Effects on Receptor Sites

Chemicals performing as neurotransmitters (the endocrine first messenger) bind to receptor sites on ganglionic synapses or on end organs, whether muscle fiber or secretory cell. There are separate sites for each class of chemically distinct substances (Figure 1-4). Thus, receptors are found for the neural transmitters already mentioned and for the endocrines. There are two main families of gut hormones: secretin and those structurally similar, and gastrin and its related peptides. There are separate sites for each family. Every neurally or chemically responsive tissue in the gastrointestinal tract has receptors for these two families of endocrines and for the neurotransmitters. The affinity of a receptor site is greatest for the chemical that produces its principal effect on that tissue. The substance exerting greatest affinity at its preferred site is a full agonist of function in that tissue. Other members of the same family of peptides have the ability to bind to the site, though usually with less affinity for it. Since their binding produces less than normal stimulation of function, they are only partial agonists of function. The number of peptide molecules binding at a receptor site is determined by its affinity for the site and by the number of similar molecules in the vicinity. If a partial agonist is present in high concentrations, the peptide will displace any full agonist present at lower levels, resulting in stimulation that is less than maximum. Affinity for a site is expressed as the rate at which the chemical associates and dissociates with the receptor. The interactions of two members of a peptide family can be illustrated with gastrin and its likeness, cholecystokinin. Gastrin causes maximum gastric acid secretion when it occupies its receptor sites on oxyntic cells. Cholecystokinin binds to the receptor with less affinity than gastrin, but if large amounts of the former are present, it will displace gastrin. In this case the resulting secretion is less than maximum, since cholecystokinin is only a partial agonist of secretion even though it is a stimulator of secretion. As stated earlier, there must also be a receptor for the secretin family of peptides, and when the receptor is occupied by secretin there is an inhibition of acid secretion. Gastric acid secretion requires interaction of activities at receptors for acetylcholine, gastrin, and histamine; these chemicals must interact with their respective sites before the secretion rate is optimum (Figure 1-5). Thus an interaction of a number of chemicals is required to produce a response. Selectively removing the effects of each of the chemicals involved illustrates the importance of the interaction of all these receptor sites. Acetylcholine levels can be reduced by vagotomy, and gastrin by antrectomy or by proglumide. The effect of histamine can be studied by competitively displacing it with a synthetic analog that has no stimulating properties. Any one of these procedures markedly inhibits gastric acid secretion in a stomach that feeding has stimulated to secrete. There are also receptor sites that regulate motility in the gastrointestinal tract. An example is shown in Figure 1-4, where the gastrin family of peptides are agonists of intestinal motility and secretin is an inhibitor. The interaction of these chemicals has important effects in the fed animal, which is not to imply that they disappear in the fasting state. Basal levels of the chemicals are present at all times. They contribute to a function that continues at low levels during the interdigestive period.

Endocrines Designed to Regulate Gastrointestinal Function

Gastrin; Cholecystokinin Family. The basic gastrin molecule consists of 17 amino acids, and the molecule of cholecystokinin is made up of 33 amino acids. The C-terminal 5 amino acids are identical in the two hormones (Table 1-3). Thus, that terminal is considered the hormones' active site. The

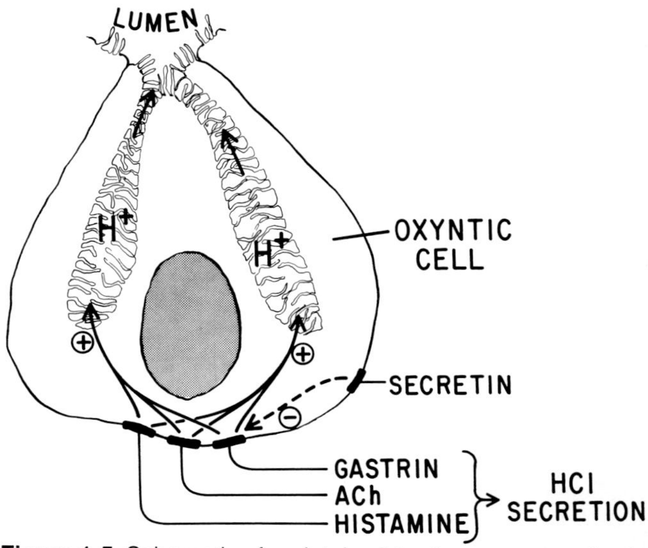

Figure 1-5. Schematic of parietal cell to show receptors for the secretagogues gastrin, acetylcholine (Ach), and histamine. All three are required to stimulate secretion. Also shows receptor for secretin, which inhibits secretion.

C-terminal tetrapeptide has about one-tenth the molar potency of the complete gastrin molecule in its ability to stimulate gastric acid secretion. Although they vary in potency, all forms of gastrin from the tetrapeptide to the heptadecapeptide are full agonists for gastric secretion. Pentagastrin, a pentapeptide, has considerably more activity. Cholecystokinin stimulates pancreatic enzyme secretion and contraction of the gall bladder. For it to be biologically active, the heptapeptide must possess a sulfated tyrosyl residue, and that is present in the seventh position from the C-terminus. The C-terminal octapeptide is five times as potent as the parent molecule, and the activity of the decapeptide is ten times as potent. Desulfation of the tyrosyl residue results in a loss of potency. The gastrin heptadecapeptide is found in a sulfated and nonsulfated form in its tyrosyl residue at position 6 from the C-terminus. They are gastrin II and I, respectively. Gastrin differs from cholecystokinin in that sulfation is not necessary for full biological activity. Moreover, the decapeptide of cholecystokinin becomes a full agonist of gastric acid secretion if its tyrosyl residue is desulfated. The sulfated tyrosyl is not as effective an agonist of gall bladder contraction and pancreatic secretion if it is in the 6-position from the C-terminus. The gastrin-cholecystokinin family contains another member, called caerulein, that is not found in mammals but occurs as a decapeptide in frog skin. The effects of this peptide on gastrointestinal function have revealed many of the function-structure relationships for members of the family.

Gastrin and cholecystokinin, like other gastrointestinal hormones, have receptors on all organs in the system. Thus, excitatory or inhibitory effects have been demonstrated for these hormones infused into experimental animals. The responses are due to the pharmacological effects of the hormone, and the question arises as to whether all the described effects are also physiological; that is, are they the same effects produced by the small amounts of hormones released under physiological conditions? In the dog and cat, gastrin concentrations increase from about 20 pmol/L to 70 pmol/L after a meal, and the changes in gastrointestinal function produced by those levels of gastrin are considered physiological (Table 1-4). Those changes in gastrin levels stimulate gastric secretion of acid and enzymes, motility of the antrum, insulin release, and splanchnic blood flow. Gastrin, being structurally similar to cholecystokinin, is a full agonist of pancreatic secretion of enzymes. Since, however, it is less potent than cholecystokinin in stimulating gall bladder contraction and secretion of bile by the liver, it is only a partial agonist of those functions. Cholecystokinin's major function is to stimulate pancreatic secretion, gall bladder contraction, and the secretion of bile by the liver. Its functions outside those organs are mainly on the stomach, where cholecystokinin is a partial agonist of acid secretion in the dog and a full agonist of acid secretion in the cat. Cholecystokinin stimulates the release of insulin and glucagon. The major effects of both gastrin and cholecystokinin on gut motility are to delay gastric emptying.

Table 1-3. Partial structure of gastrin (16 amino acids) and cholecystokinin (33 amino acids) showing end of peptides that possess biological activity.

Gastrin - 10 amino acids - Ala-TyrS-Gly-Trp-Met-Asp-Phe NH_2
Cholecystokinin - 26 amino acids - TyrS-Met-Gly-Trp-Met-Asp-Phe NH_2

The heptadecapeptide of gastrin has a half-life of three minutes. A larger peptide of gastrin, consisting of the 17 residue form joined with another 17 amino acids, has a half-life of nine minutes. The kidneys and intestines remove gastrin from the circulation. The liver removes fragments of gastrin molecules. The half-life of cholecystokinin is 2.6 minutes, and the kidney plays an important role in its removal and catabolism. With such a short half-life the hormone has to be taken up by other tissues in the body. It was thought that the liver is the most important organ in removal of gut endocrines from the portal circulation, but cholecystokinin, like intact gastrin, is not removed and catabolized by the liver. It seems logical that the liver would not remove these hormones, since they are secreted into the portal circulation and must make a pass through the circulation before they reach their target organ. If the liver removed them during the initial pass through, all their effects would be lost. Only if there were a portal type of circulation between the site of hormone release directly to the target organ would hormone inactivation by the liver be unimportant. It has been suggested that a portal system exists between the antrum and fundus of the stomach to transport gastrin directly to its site of action.

Cholecystokinin is found in lower vertebrates, whereas gastrin does not appear until the lower jaw and stomach have evolved. Thus, cholecystokinin can be considered an ancestor of gastrin in evolutionary terms.

Secretin, Glucagon Family. Secretin is similar in structure to glucagon, gastric inhibitory polypeptide (GIP), and vasoactive intestinal peptide (VIP), all of which are similar in function to varying degrees. The octapeptides at the N-terminus are identical in secretin and glucagon except for one amino acid. A total of 14 amino acids occupy the same positions in both hormones (secretin has 27 amino acids, and glucagon has 29). Secretin requires the complete sequence of the 27 amino acids to be biologically active. Secretin is basic because of its four arginine molecules, a histidine, and several glutamines. Secretin's molecular structure is unique in its unusual tertiary conformation, which must be maintained in order for it to possess biological activity.

In some respects, secretin has effects opposite to those of the members of the gastrin family, even though the hormone is designed to complement and potentiate the actions of cholecystokinin on pancreatic secretion. Secretin serves to mobilize the alkaline secretion of the pancreas in order to neutralize acid secretions entering the duodenum. Thus, it is not surprising that secretin has properties that inhibit gastric secretion. Another means of reducing the effects of acidity in the small intestine is to inhibit gastric motility, and secretin is capable of delaying gastric emptying. Other physiological functions of secretin, probably less important, are stimulation of pancreatic trypsin secretion, insulin release, biliary secretion, and inhibition of motility of the small intestine and resting pressure in the gastroesophageal sphincter.

Secretin has a short half-life (2.5 minutes) in dogs. Some can be removed by the liver, and the kidney can play an important role in its rate of disappearance. It is unlike vasoactive intestinal peptide, which the liver rapidly degrades.

Table 1-4. Summary of Biological Activities of Gastrointestinal Hormones

	Gastrin-Cholecystokinin Family		Secretin Family				Other Hormones		
	Gastrin	Cholecystokinin	Secretin	Glucagon	Gastric Inhibitory peptide	Vasoactive Intestinal peptide	Somatostatin	Pancreatic polypeptide	Prostaglandins
Esophagus									
Gastroesophageal sphincter	ss	I	I	I	I	I			
Stomach									
Acid secretion	S	sS	I	I	I	I	I	sS	I
Pepsin secretion	S	sS	SS	I	I	I	I		
Motility fundus	I	I	I		I				
Motility antrum	S	S	I	I	I	I		+	I
Emptying	I	I	I	I	I	I	I	+	I
Blood flow	S	S	I	I		S			S
Gastrin release			I	I	I	I	I		
Small intestine									
Fluid secretion	ss	ss	ss	S	s	S	I		S
Fluid absorption		si	si			I	I		I
Motility	ss	S	I	I	I	ss	I	+	S
Blood flow	S	S	I	S		S	I		S
Secretin release	S						I		
Pancreas									
Fluid secretion	ss	ss	S	I	–	sS	I	sS	I
Enzyme secretion	S	S	ss	I		S	I	I	–
Blood flow	S	S	S	S	–	S			I
Liver									
Bile secretion	ss	S	S	S		sS		–	
Gall bladder									
Motility	ss	S	ss	I		I	I	I	
Metabolic									
Insulin release	S	s	S	S	s	S	I		
Glycogenolysis				S	–	S		–	
Lipolysis			+	S	I	S			
Glucagon release	–	S	I	–	s		I		

S = full agonist for activity, sS = partial agonist for activity, ss = slight stimulation, I = inhibits activity, si = slight inhibition, – = no effect on activity. Responses are those seen with physiological blood levels of hormones.

Glucagon was first identified as a hormone secreted by the pancreas. Pancreatic glucagon is also produced in the gastric mucosa. Related but different glucagons found in the gastrointestinal mucosa are called enteroglucagons. Pancreatic glucagon is a peptide containing 29 amino acid residues, 14 of which are in the same position as in the secretin molecule. One of the enteroglucagons is the same size as pancreatic glucagon. Since glucagon is quite different from secretin in tertiary structure there is a major difference in their effects on the primary target organ of secretin, the pancreas. In contrast to secretin, glucagon inhibits pancreatic secretion. The major role of enteroglucagon is not established, but the conditions under which it is released may help in understanding its physiological significance. Glucose and long-chain triglycerides in the diet stimulate release of the hormone. Its blood level remains elevated for five hours after a meal. This is in contrast to the shorter peak activities of other gut hormones. The peak activity may be long because the highest levels of enteroglucagon occur in the ileum.[5] This is in contrast to gastric inhibitory polypeptide (GIP), found mainly in the cranial small bowel, which inhibits gastric motility. Enteroglucagon's high concentration in the intestine and its ability to inhibit gastric and intestinal motility may serve to delay transit of food in the entire gastrointestinal tract in response to a signal from the caudal small bowel. Enteroglucagon has glycogenolytic effects like those of glucagon. Since glucose stimulates enteroglucagon's release in the intestine, it is paradoxical that a hyperglycemic agent is released with the impending absorption of glucose. Since enteroglucagon is a signal for insulin release, its effect is modified by an antagonist of hyperglycemia. The catabolic sites of enteroglucagon are unknown.

Vasoactive intestinal peptide (VIP) is a hormone produced in the mucosa of the small intestine. It was named for the first properties found for it: production of vasodilation and hypotension. VIP is related structurally most closely to secretin in this group of four hormones. It consists of 28 amino acid residues that form a tertiary structure like that of secretin, consisting of a helix in one part and random coil in the other. The entire sequence is necessary for full biological activity.

VIP is a neurotransmitter released from nerve endings to a variety of gastrointestinal organs upon stimulation of extrinsic nerves. VIP is not released to the circulation, and its normally low and constant blood levels reflect spillover from synapses where the neurotransmitter is released. Many different stimuli promote VIP release. Some of its physiologic effects are evident on the gastroesophageal and other gastrointestinal sphincters, where VIP release following nerve stimulation results in sphincter relaxation and opening.

Other major effects of VIP are to inhibit motility in the stomach and gall bladder, to stimulate the release of glycogen stores and insulin, and, most importantly, to stimulate the secretion of fluid in the small intestine. This hormone has effects on other systems. In the respiratory system, VIP relaxes bronchi and dilates pulmonary vessels, whereas in the cardiovascular system it produces hypotension by dilating peripheral vessels. This hormone has been found also in endocrine)secreting tumors in humans. The clinical signs associated with such tumors illustrate the major biological effects of VIP, which are to cause a watery diarrhea and hypotension. Although those signs have been attributed to VIP, most such tumors also produce other hormones or vasoactive agents, suggesting that the clinical signs may not be due entirely to VIP. VIP is inactivated in the tissues where it is released. Some that escapes to the circulation is inactivated as it passes through the liver.

Gastric inhibitory polypeptide (GIP) is produced in the mucosa of the duodenum and jejunum. It consists of 43 amino acid residues and structurally resembles glucagon more closely than it does secretin and VIP. Since extracts of the small intestine inhibit gastric secretion, resection of a large part of the small intestine results in a hypersecretion of gastric juices. These effects are now known to be due to gastric inhibitory polypeptide.

GIP is released by glucose and fats in the small intestine, and its levels can be measured in the peripheral circulation. Therefore, GIP can affect different parts of the gastrointestinal tract. An important function of GIP is to inhibit the stomach's secretion of acid and pepsin. Secretin, a member of the same family, has these same properties, but GIP is much more potent as an inhibitor. GIP also inhibits gastric motility. Enterogastrone is the term used to describe a single humoral agent that affects gastric function in response to fats in the small intestine. It is apparent that enterogastrone is a response mediated by a number of hormones: the members of the secretin-glucagon family of gut hormones. Other major important functions of GIP involve carbohydrate metabolism. GIP is released by intraluminal glucose. GIP causes a release of insulin. This effect of the hormone is greater than that of hyperglycemia. Thus, GIP may be a primary signal for the pancreas to respond to a glucose load being absorbed from the small intestine. In the same context, it is suggested that cholecystokinin's release of insulin is an advance signal for the absorption of amino acids and fatty acids from the intestine. The catabolic sites of GIP are unknown, but it is apparent that the kidney but not the liver is important in removal of GIP from the portal circulation.

It is not known whether GIP is ever responsible for changes in function in pathological situations. It is secreted in a dose-related fashion to oral glucose and fats, and the insulin release is also a dose-related response. There may be some pathological entities in small animals in which inappropriate release of GIP causes an abnormal release of insulin, with subsequent effects on blood-sugar levels.

Somatostatin is a peptide hormone that was first shown to inhibit the release of growth hormone from the pituitary. The hormone consists of 28 amino acids and is found throughout the gastrointestinal tract, with the largest quantities found in the antrum, duodenum, and pancreas. Somatostatin functions as a paracrine in the gastrointestinal tract. Cells producing somatostatin have long cytoplasmic processes that terminate near gastric mucosal cells secreting hydrochloric acid or gastrin (Figure 1-6). In contrast to endocrine glands that release hormones to produce effects in distant tissues, paracrine cells release hormones for regulation of function in neighboring cells. Somatostatin has a physiologic role in regulating gastric acid secretion and release of insulin and glucagon. Somatostatin levels increase after feeding, especially with high protein and high fat meals.

Somatostatin inhibits secretion throughout the gastrointestinal tract. It also inhibits the normal occurrence of cyclic interdigestive migrating motility complexes. Somatostatin's major effect is to inhibit the release of most known gastrointestinal hormones. It is a potent inhibitor of secretin and CCK release. It is difficult to evaluate the effects of infusing pharmacologic doses of somatostatin on gastrointestinal function. Since somatostatin is a paracrine, the highest concentration of the hormone is at the target cell where the hormone is released. Circulating blood levels are much lower and do not indicate what concentrations must be released to be effective at the target cell. Somatostatin has a short effect; the hormone has a half-life of 1.8 minutes. Somatostatin is removed by the liver but is also degraded by peptidases near its site of release.

Pancreatic polypeptide consists of 36 amino acids and is produced in the pancreas. Release of the hormone is stimulated by high protein meals and to a lesser extent by fats in the duodenum. Cholinergic pathways mediate the reflex for pancreatic polypeptide release. Pancreatic polypeptide modulates

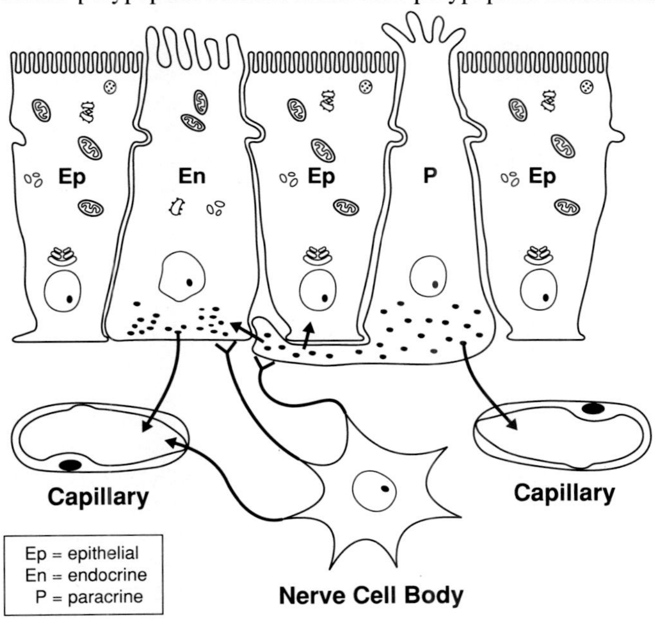

Figure 1-6. Schematic showing anatomic and functional relations of mucosal epithelial cells, endocrine cells, paracrine cells, neurons of intrinsic nervous system and mucosal capillaries. Endocrine secretion can be stimulated or inhibited by nerve activity and paracrine secretions. Nerve endings, endocrine and paracrine cells can all secrete chemical transmitters into capillaries.

the pancreatic responses to feeding. Its effects are largely inhibitory, but under some conditions the hormone can stimulate small amounts of secretion.

Neurotensin, a peptide hormone consisting of 39 amino acids, is produced in the ileal mucosa. Fats entering the small intestine stimulate neurotensin release. Pharmacologic levels inhibit gastric secretion and gastric emptying, but physiologic levels have only a slight effect to produce that inhibition. Thus, neurotensin is not likely an enterogastrone whose release is stimulated by fat entering the small intestine. A major function has not been defined for neurotensin.

Motilin is a peptide hormone consisting of 22 amino acids and produced in the cranial small intestine. Plasma motilin concentrations increase during interdigestive periods, and the increases coincide with the activity of the interdigestive myoelectric complex (IMC). Motilin is believed to initiate IMC activity. Other stimulants of motilin release include fats and acid pH in the duodenum. The physiologic importance of stimulation by these conditions is unknown. The major and maybe only significant biologic action of motilin is to increase motility during the intergastric period; the increase appears to be for smooth muscle throughout the gastrointestinal tract. Motilin has a short effect since its half-life is about 4.5 minutes. The kidneys are responsible for its clearance, but peptides with such a short half-life are removed by more than one vascular bed.

Peptide YY consists of 36 amino acids and is produced primarily in the ileum and colon. It is structurally similar to pancreatic polypeptide. Peptide YY inhibits gastrointestinal motility in the unfed state. The hormone inhibits gastric acid and pancreatic bicarbonate secretion; meals, and especially fats in the duodenum, stimulate the release of peptide YY. Release of unusual amounts of peptide YY could be evident in animals with malabsorption, resulting from increased amounts of fats reaching the ileum and colon. The effect would be an inhibition of gastric acid and pancreatic bicarbonate secretions.

Prostaglandins[17,18] Prostaglandins are hydroxy-fatty acids with many biologic effects in the gastrointestinal tract. They act as local regulators (secreted at one site and not transported by the circulation to act at another) since they are degraded where they are released and any escaping are almost totally inactivated by a single pass through the liver and lungs. Prostaglandins can be intracellular messengers; they are involved with secretion of fluid in the intestine.

Prostaglandins consist of 20 carbons which are hydroxylated at carbons 11 and 15. The E-type prostaglandins contain a hydroxyl group at carbon 9, and the F-type contain a ketone group at that point. The 20-carbon chain is folded back on itself, and carbons 8 through 12 form a closed 5-member ring (Figure 1-7). Prostaglandins are synthesized from dihomo-gamma-linolenic acid, eicosapentaenoic acid, or arachidonic acid. Prostaglandins that contain an unsaturated bond in the five-carbon ring are designated the A or B type, depending on the location of the bond.

Synthesis and storage of prostaglandins take place in the muscle and mucosa of the gastrointestinal tract, the pancreas, and the liver. Release from those tissues has been evoked by feeding, acetylcholine, vagal stimulation, gastrin, histamine, theophylline, and cyclic AMP. The prostaglandins released can be found in gastric juice. Glucagon stimulates the release of prostaglandins from the liver. Release of these fatty acids is

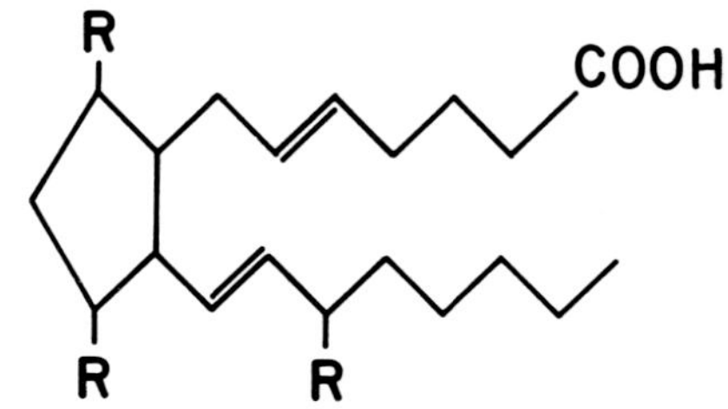

Figure 1-7. Structure of prostaglandins, which consists of a fatty acid chain of 20 carbons folded in the middle. R = oxy or hydroxy groups.

reduced by anti-inflammatory drugs such as aspirin and indomethacin. Their action is to inhibit the synthesis of prostaglandins, and the drug's anti-inflammatory and analgesic properties are due to their anti-prostaglandin properties. After formation, the prostaglandins are rapidly inactivated in the wall of the gastrointestinal tract, and by the liver, lungs, and blood. Inactivation is accomplished by a dehydrogenase and reductase in the tissues and by an isomerase in the blood. Prostaglandins have a wide range of biological activity on different tissues and are very potent in minute quantities. If they were not readily inactivated, they would exert their effect on other systems, particularly the cardiovascular.

Effects on Gastrointestinal Motility. Prostaglandins have varied effects on gastrointestinal motility. They stimulate contraction of longitudinal smooth muscle of the small and large intestine, and they can either stimulate or inhibit contractions of circular smooth muscle. The facilitatory response is due to stimulation via the intrinsic plexuses, while the inhibiting effect is the result of a direct action of prostaglandins on the muscle. In the dog, prostaglandins of the E-type inhibit motility in the gastric antrum and jejunum and augment ileal motility. The PGEs increase motility in both the jejunum and ileum. Their effects on large-bowel motility are not clear. Because prostaglandins stimulate secretion of fluid in the small intestine, it is difficult to determine their effects on the transit time of contents moving through the intestine; prostaglandins change the variables of intestinal secretion and motility (both determining transit). Prostaglandins may be involved in local regulation of gastrointestinal motility. A large number of different anti-inflammatory drugs are used in small-animal medicine, and those that inhibit prostaglandin synthesis may affect bowel function in some patients.

Effects on Gastrointestinal Secretion. Prostaglandins of the E and A type inhibit gastric secretion, a property that might make them the most useful type of agent in future treatment of ulcers caused by hypersecretion of acid.[18] They are effective when given parenterally or orally, inhibiting the stimulation of acid and pepsin secretion produced by histamine, gastrin, vagal activity, cholinergics, or food. These prostaglandins also prevent ulcer formation as produced experimentally by pylorus ligation, steroid administration, or constant infusion of stimulants to gastric secretion. Methyl analogs have been synthesized that, given orally, effectively inhibit gastric secretion.

Prostaglandins act directly on the oxyntic cell to inhibit acid secretion. They interfere with cyclic AMP's intracellular role of stimulating secretion. Cyclic AMP is the intracellular mediator for histamine's stimulation of acid secretion, and prostaglandins have direct effects on that adenine nucleotide, which is the likely basis for its inhibitory effects. Prostaglandins stimulate gastric bicarbonate and mucus secretion.

A commonly observed effect of prostaglandins is diarrhea. As mentioned earlier, altered intestinal motility may be a factor in its genesis. However, prostaglandins also stimulate secretion of fluid in the intestine. That follows intra-arterial infusion of all types of prostaglandins in the dog. The secretion is the result of profound changes in the circulation and is the direct effect of the prostaglandins on the epithelial cell. Prostaglandins increase mesenteric blood flow, and some of the secretion results from increased filtration of fluid from the capillary bed. They also inhibit sodium absorption and stimulate chloride secretion in isolated preparations of ileal mucosa. It is uncertain which of these factors is the more important in producing the secretion. Prostaglandins are an important cellular mediator in intestinal secretion caused by some enterotoxins. Increased intracellular prostaglandin levels are associated with increases for intracellular cyclic AMP and free calcium. Diarrhea can also be seen during estrus; it may be due to high circulating levels of prostaglandins released. Prostaglandins are also released from injured tissues and have been implicated in the pathogenesis of some chronic bowel diseases. If prostaglandins are the prime mediators of pathology in the intestinal tract, anti-inflammatory drugs to inhibit prostaglandin synthesis should control the clinical signs, but with a few exceptions that is not seen.

Pancreatic secretion of fluid and electrolytes is uninhibited by the E-type prostaglandins. There is no effect on enzyme secretion. These effects are accompanied by a decrease in blood flow.

The prostaglandins are potent vasoactive agents. The E and A types are hypotensive since they are vasodilators and cause gastric mucosal blood flow to increase. These effects on increasing blood flow may be the most important cytoprotective attribute of prostaglandins in the gastrointestinal tract. Intestinal blood flow is also augmented by prostaglandins that stimulate intestinal secretion. A physiological role for prostaglandins on blood flow is difficult to evaluate. Most experimental studies on prostaglandin's effects are based on its intra-arterial infusion. Since prostaglandins are rapidly inactivated by the tissues and blood in which they are released, the concentrations of prostaglandins at the sites where they are released under physiological conditions are not known.

Prostaglandins also contribute to the integrity of the gastric mucosal barrier. Protection of the barrier is due to prostaglandin's effect of increasing blood flow, inhibiting acid secretion, and stimulating secretion of bicarbonate and mucus. Inhibition of these effects by nonsteroidal inflammatory drugs often results in gastrointestinal erosions or ulcers.

Trophic Action of Gastrointestinal Hormones [19-21]

Gastrointestinal hormones influence the growth of the mucosa of the gut, which has one of the most rapid turnovers of any tissue in the body. These hormones also have trophic effects on the pancreas and liver. Numerous events engaged during the fed state stimulate growth of the gastrointestinal mucosa. Nongastrointestinal factors such as thyroxine and growth hormone also support growth. Animals subjected to a prolonged unfed state, such as starvation, lose more than half of their small intestinal weight while losing only one-third of their body weight. Absence of stimuli for hormone secretion results in gastrointestinal atrophy. The physical presence of food in the intestine also promotes growth. Food and intestinal motility combine to cause desquamation of villous cells, the loss of which stimulates proliferation of epithelial cells. Epithelial cells contain chalones that inhibit production of new cells; desquamation of mucosal cells results in loss of the inhibitory chalones, and replication increases to replace lost cells.

The growth-stimulating property of gastrin is the best understood. This hormone stimulates the synthesis of RNA, DNA, and proteins in the oxyntic glands, duodenal mucosa, and pancreatic exocrine tissue. Gastrin stimulates cell division in the stomach and duodenum, but has no trophic effects on the antral mucosa. The trophic effects of gastrin are best illustrated in animals fed by total parenteral nutrition, in which the fasting serum levels of gastrin decrease significantly. Tissues of the gastrointestinal tract and pancreas atrophy, which can be prevented by adding small physiological amounts of gastrin to the parenteral solutions. The trophic effects of gastrin are inhibited by secretin, but not by the histamine analogs that inhibit gastrin-stimulated secretion. Gastrin may also have a physiologically regulative trophic effect on colonic mucosa.

Cholecystokinin exerts a trophic effect on the pancreas in addition to its well-known ability to stimulate the synthesis of protein enzymes for export. The cholecystokinin effect on the pancreas is reflected by an increase in organ size and in DNA content. Cholecystokinin has no trophic action on gastric or duodenal mucosa. Large amounts of cholecystokinin compete with gastrin for receptor sites in the stomach and competitively inhibit the trophic effects of gastrin.

Secretin stimulates pancreatic growth but less so than CCK. Secretin inhibits gastric mucosal growth. It may act by blocking the action of gastrin.

Enteroglucagon may have a trophic effect on mucosa of the gastric oxyntic mass, small intestine, and colon. A close correlation is reported between hyperproliferation of small intestinal mucosa and enteroglucagon levels in humans with some intestinal diseases. Such a relationship has not been verified with studies showing a trophic effect during infusion of enteroglucagon.

Hormones inhibiting or stimulating release of trophic hormones have indirect trophic effects. Somatostatin inhibits and bombesin stimulates mucosal growth by their respective effects on gastrin release. Other hormones produced in gastrointestinal mucosa, such as epidermal growth factor, have trophic effects on the mucosa but it is uncertain whether such hormones have a physiologic role on growth.

The capacity to synthesize gastrointestinal hormones is dependent on the trophic effects of pituitary hormones. Removal of growth hormone by hypophysectomy decreases antral gastrin levels to one-fourth of normal, and subsequent injection of growth hormone increases this decrement significantly.

Smooth muscle as well as mucosa can be stimulated to grow. Smooth muscle thickness increases in the wall of hollow viscera or tubes in the gastrointestinal tract following chronic distension due to obstruction. Both longitudinal and circular muscles thicken; both hypertrophy and hyperplasia of smooth muscle cells cause the increase in size. Similar changes are seen for the intrinsic nervous sytem in these tissues. Whether any hormones stimulate the trophic changes is unknown. Gastrin can have such an effect on the smooth muscle of the pyloric sphincter. Administration of pentagastrin to pregnant bitches results in 25% to 30% of the pups being born with pyloric hypertrophy.[22] It is uncertain whether the changes are caused by cholecystokinin and secretin, which are released secondarily to the pentagastrin effects. These hormones also cause changes in the intrinsic nerves of the sphincter, which may affect sphincter growth and subsequent function after birth.

Trophic factors are important for the maintenance of normal liver size and for its regeneration following resection. Shunting the portal circulation around the liver results in a decrease in liver size. This result has suggested that hepatotrophic factors produced in the gastrointestinal tract and required by the liver are lost to the shunting blood flow. In part, portal hepatotrophic factors are interacting hormones generated by splanchnic organs and delivered directly to the liver. Some are also produced by the liver. Other important hepatotrophic factors are the maintenance of normal blood flow to the liver and the delivery of nutrients from the alimentary tract. All of these factors are interdependent, and exclusion of any one of them results in liver atrophy. Starvation, exclusion of the portal flow from the pancreas, or shunting of the mesenteric blood to the vena cava results in liver atrophy.

BLOOD FLOW AND DIGESTIVE FUNCTIONS[23-27]

Regulation of blood flow is as important to gastrointestinal function as regulation of motility, secretion, and absorption. Increasing blood flow to sustain augmented function is a response to stimulation of the organ's function. In some cases, it may be uncertain whether increased secretion of fluids is secondary to an increase in blood flow. Increased blood flow, whether cause or effect, is appropriate since motility and fluid-transport functions in the gastrointestinal tract are energy-dependent. During the unfed state total gastrointestinal blood flow is low, and after feeding it increases dramatically. During many physiological states and in some pathological ones, blood flow can be reduced to less than normal by shunting flow from the gastrointestinal system to other organs where optimum flow has a higher priority. In some situations blood can be shunted within the organ from one region to another. Thus, total blood flow can be diverted to and from the gastrointestinal tract, and it can be redistributed within an organ in the system. Figure 1-8 is a schematic of the circulation in the gastrointestinal tissues. The total flow of blood has a generally low priority in this system compared with the needs of other systems. Regulation of circulation in the gastrointestinal system is the result of neural and endocrine factors and the basic properties of the microcirculation.

The most primitive control of gastrointestinal blood flow can be studied in denervated organs lacking hormones. With the use of such preparations, it is possible to observe autoregulation of blood flow. This is the phenomenon of the maintenance of normal blood flow through the capillary beds despite wide variations in arterial inflow pressure. The mechanism for this ability to maintain homeostasis is in the inherent property of vascular smooth muscle to respond to pressure changes.

The responses cause a constriction of the resistance vessels when the arterial pressure increases and a vasodilation when the pressure decreases. Autoregulation operates over a wide range of arterial pressures from 70 mm Hg to 170 mm Hg to maintain the blood flow constant in gastrointestinal organs. Other inherent mechanisms maintain blood flow to the villi of the small intestine at the expense of the submucosa and muscle layers. Villous blood flow can be maintained at normal rates when arterial pressure falls to as low as 30 mm Hg. Autoregulation also plays an important role in preventing great increases in capillary blood pressure during portal hypertension. The response is a vasoconstriction of the resistance vessels so that arterial inflow is reduced. Autoregulation is an important mechanism that can override outside influences on intestinal blood flow. Neural and endocrine factors can change total blood flow. Most increase blood flow, although a few (mediated by the sympathetics and such hormones as vasopressin) reduce blood flow by their potent vasoconstrictive actions. If these influences prevailed, the intestinal mucosa would be deprived of nutrients that are necessary to maintain its integrity. Autoregulatory escape intervenes, so that adequate blood flow is maintained despite the vasoconstrictive influences. Blood flow to structures other than the mucosa is reduced, while mucosal flow actually increases. Thus, the overall effect is a redistribution of intestinal blood flow. Autoregulation is thought to be partially controlled by locally produced metabolic products. For example, increases in local blood carbon dioxide cause vasodilation, and decreases cause vasoconstriction. It is suggested that the metabolites increase when flow decreases, and their accumulation brings about a return to normal flow. Adenosine compounds and Krebs cycle intermediates have similar properties. This metabolic control of blood flow is more important in vascular beds outside the gastrointestinal tract.

The splanchnic bed of the dog contains 21% of the total

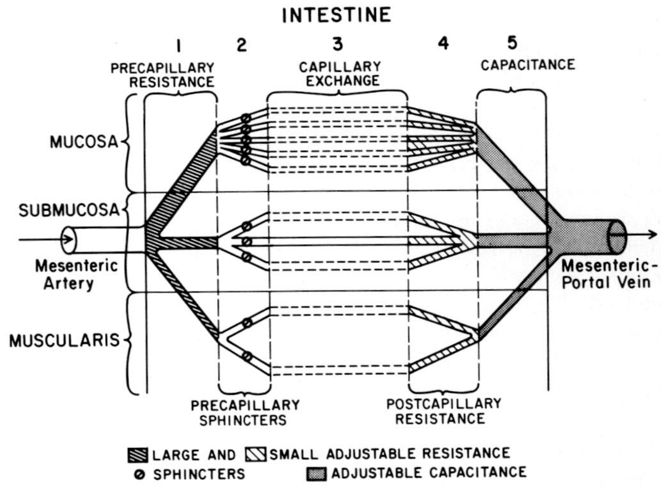

Figure 1-8. Schematic of blood flow in intestine. The major blood flow is through the mucosa. Hydrostatic pressure in capillaries is determined by resistance in arterioles and venules and by pressure in mesenteric veins. Hydrostatic pressure determines magnitude and direction of fluxes of fluid in capillaries. Precapillary sphincters determine whether blood flows through a capillary. Blood can be selectively shunted from the muscularis and submucosa into the mucosa at times when splanchnic circulation is reduced. The mucosa has the highest priority for maintenance of circulation. Some large shunt vessels are present whereby blood flow can bypass capillary beds.

blood volume. Neural influences are the most important to reduce splanchnic blood flow, and hormones are most important in its augmentation. The venous side of the splanchnic bed contains 14% of the total blood volume. It is a capacitance bed containing venous vessels that are more richly endowed with smooth muscle than are other systemic veins. An increase in the tone of these vessels reduces the capacity of the bed and shunts more blood into the arterial system. A decrease in venous tone results in splanchnic pooling of blood and a corresponding decrease in venous return to the heart, cardiac output, and arterial pressure. Thus, neural and hormonal influences can change the amount of blood in the splanchnic bed without changing its blood flow.

Neural regulation is due to splanchnic sympathetic nerves that cause vasoconstriction in both the arterial and venous vessels of the stomach, intestines, pancreas, and liver. This can reduce an organ's blood content by 40%. Activation of this sympathetic effect is physiological under some conditions such as exercise, and it is pathological in conditions such as shock. Stimulation of the parasympathetic system causes vasodilation and increased blood flow, but not directly. There are no known vasodilator fibers in the vagal and sacral efferent fibers. A local vasodilator reflex operates within the wall of the intestine. This neural pathway is noncholinergic and nonadrenergic, and it is suggested that serotonin is either the neurotransmitter or the chemical released to produce vasodilation.[28]

Gastrointestinal blood flow will double or triple during the functional hyperemia produced during digestive activity. This effect is produced by the gut endocrines gastrin, cholecystokinin, vasoactive intestinal peptide, and glucagon. Histamine is released during gastric secretion and contributes to the augmented blood flow. Crude secretin increases intestinal blood flow, but synthetic secretin has no effect on the circulation, which indicates that the crude hormone preparations used in older studies contained other agents with vasoactive properties. Hormones that increase gastrointestinal blood flow also tend to increase oxygen consumption. Acetylcholine also has a vasodilating effect when infused into the mesenteric artery. This effect is blocked by atropine. The vasodilating effects of gastrin and cholecystokinin are also blocked by atropine, which suggests that the effects of these hormones are mediated through cholinergic receptors. Glucagon's vasodilating effects are not altered by atropine. Postprandial vasodilation is not readily reduced by normal physiological events such as exercise, which is able to reduce the augmented gut blood flow by only 10% to 15%. Since blood flow doubles or even triples during digestive events, but infusions of pharmacological amounts of cholecystokinin or gastrin increase blood flow by only 50%, there must be other means of increasing it. Other gut hormones with vasodilating properties probably participate in functional hyperemia of the gut. Some of the prostaglandins have potent vasodilating effects on the splanchnic microcirculation. Some of the prostaglandins are more potent than the vasoactive peptides in augmenting blood flow, and they may have a physiologic role in the production of hyperemia. Serotonin may function in a similar manner. Most of the serotonin in the body is found in the gastrointestinal tract, but the reasons are unknown. It has been proposed that it participates in peristalsis and in postprandial hyperemia. It is thought that serotonin's acting as a vasoactive chemical is directly involved both in the previously described reflexly elicited vasodilation and as a neurotransmitter released on blood vessels following nerve stimulation. A number of pharmacologic agents increase splanchnic blood flow. They act on either the alpha adrenergic receptors, blocking transmission so as to produce vasoconstriction, or on the beta receptors to stimulate vasodilation. Epinephrine and isoproterenol are chemicals that act in this manner.

A naturally occurring substance, vasopressin, reduces splanchnic blood flow.[29] The effect of this peptide on blood flow has been studied in animals infused with pharmacological levels of the hormone. For this reason, there is some question whether the amount that is normally released has a physiological action in the gastrointestinal tract. Acute stress stimulates the release of vasopressin from the neurohypophysis, and it is generally thought that the amount of hormone released in situations such as hemorrhagic shock is sufficient to play an important role in the marked vasoconstriction of the splanchnic vascular bed that characterized the shock.

INTEGRATION IN THE FED AND UNFED STATES

In summary, the most important facilitatory influences on gastrointestinal motility are neurally mediated, whereas the major inhibitory factors are mediated by hormones (Table 1-5). Control by extrinsic nerves is indispensible for function in the esophagus and stomach, whereas most of the remainder of the gastrointestinal tract can function without regulation exercised by the extrinsic nerves. Secretion of gastric juices depends on both extrinsic neural regulation and regulation imposed by endocrines, whereas inhibition of gastric secretion is a function

Table 1-5: Neural and Endocrine Regulation of Normal Function in the Gastrointestinal Tract

		Facilitation	Inhibition
Esophagus	Gastroesophageal sphincter	N	N
Stomach	Acid secretion	N and E	E
	Pepsin secretion	N and E	E
	Motility fundus	N	N
	Motility antrum	N	E
	Emptying	N	E
	Gastrin release	N	E
	Blood flow	E	N
Small intestine	Fluid secretion	E	N
	Fluid absorption	N (?)	E (?)
	Motility	N	E
	Blood flow	E	N
Pancreas	Fluid secretion	E	-
	Enzyme secretion	E	-
	Blood flow	E	N
Liver	Bile secretion	E	N (?)
Gall bladder	Motility	N and E (?)	-

Summary of primary means of stimulating and inhibiting physiological activity in different parts of the gastrointestinal tract. N = facilitation or inhibition is primarily by neural means. E = effect is primarily by endocrines released from the gut. (?) = a major effect is unknown.

of the endocrine system alone. Facilitation of secretion in other parts of the system is largely mediated by the endocrines, and inhibitory mechanisms appear to play a minor role. Splanchnic blood flow is stimulated primarily by gut hormones and is inhibited under physiological situations by neural means. The trophic effects on gastrointestinal tissues are secondary to normal neural innervation and endocrine secretion and hence are responses rather than regulated changes.

This simplified overview is not to detract from recent reviews which have described how the gastrointestinal tract is far more complex than previously thought. The small intestine is an exquisitely designed sensory organ for monitoring activity at all levels;[30] that was hardly mentioned in this chapter. Also, ion transport which has been viewed as largely unregulated is now known to be affected by the nervous system in a very complex way.[31] The major work yet to be done in gastrointestinal physiology is to show how mechanisms learned from *in vitro* and unphysiologic studies are integrated and function in the normal animal.

The integration of gastrointestinal function described in this introduction is for animals in the fed state. The gastrointestinal tract also demonstrates important integrated functions in the unfed state, such as a coordinated pattern of motility that acts as an interdigestive housekeeper to clear the gastrointestinal tract of accumulating bacteria and debris.[32] Evidence for such motility was originally gained from electrical recordings showing caudal-moving bands of large amplitude action potentials starting in the duodenum and moving through the small intestine. The duration of a complex at each level of the bowel is 7.0 to 4.8 minutes. The length of each complex is 25 to 36 centimeters in the cranial small intestine and 6.0 to 12.0 centimeters in the caudal part. Two complexes can be in the intestine at any one time; 1.5 to 2.0 hours is required for a complex to travel from the duodenum to the ileum. Similar activity is seen in the gastroesophageal sphincter, stomach, and gall bladder. The cyclic activity in the colon migrates in both the cranial and caudal directions. During the active myoelectric and motor activity, small amounts of secretion are produced by the stomach, pancreas and biliary system. The fluid produced assists the motility in its housekeeping activity. Enteric neural mechanisms that are modulated by the central nervous system and by circulating hormones regulate the interdigestive motility and secretory activities. The activity ceases with feeding. Loss of the interdigestive housekeeping activity in unfed animals could be a basis for disease.

REFERENCES

1. Bass, P.: In vivo electrical activity of the small bowel. In, Handbook of Physiology. Section 6, Alimentary Canal, Vol. 4. Edited by C.F. Code. Washington, D.C., American Physiological Society, 2051-2074, 1968.
2. Bortoff, A.: Myogenic control of intestinal motility. Physiol. Rev. 56:418-434, 1976.
3. Duthie, H.L.: Electrical activity of gastrointestinal smooth muscle. Gut 15:669-681, 1974.
4. Szurszewski, J.H.: Electrical basis for gastrointestinal motility. In, Physiology of the Gastrointestinal Tract. Edited by L.R. Johnson, Raven Press, New York, 383-422, 1987.
5. Makhlouf, G.M.: Isolated smooth muscle cells of the gut. In, Physiology of the Gastrointestinal Tract. Edited by L.R. Johnson, Raven Press, New York, 555-569, 1987.
6. Kosterlitz, H.W.: Intrinsic and extrinsic nervous control of motility. In, Handbook of Physiology. Section 6, Alimentary Canal, Vol. 4. Edited by C.F. Code. American Physiological Society, Washington, D.C., 2147-2172, 1968.
7. Makhlouf, G.M.: The neuroendocrine design of the gut. Gastroenterology 67:159-184, 1974.
8. Wood, J.D.: Physiology of the enteric nervous system. In, Physiology of the Gastrointestinal Tract. Edited by L.R. Johnson, Raven Press, New York, 67-109, 1987.
9. Youmans, W.B.: Innervation of the gastrointestinal tract. In, Handbook of Physiology. Section 6: Alimentary Canal. Vol. 4. Edited by C.F. Code. Washington, D.C., American Physiological Society 1655-1664, 1968.
10. Roman, C., Gonella, J.: Extrinsic control of digestive tract motility. In, Physiology of the Gastrointestinal Tract. Edited by L.R. Johnson, Raven Press, New York, 507-533, 1987.
11. Cooke, A.R.: Control of gastric emptying and motility. Gastroenterology 68:804-816, 1975.
12. Dockray, G.J.: Physiology of enteric neuropeptides. In, Physiology of the Gastrointestinal Tract. Edited by L.R. Johnson, Raven Press, New York, 41-66, 1987.
13. Barrington, E.J.W. and Dockray, G.J.: Gastrointestinal hormones. J. Endocr. 69:299-325, 1976.
14. Rayford, P.L., Miller, T.A. and Thompson, J.C.: Secretin, cholecystokinin and newer gastrointestinal hormones. New Eng. J. Med. 294:1093-1101 and 1157-1164, 1976.
15. Walsh, J.H.: Gastrointestinal hormones. In, Physiology of the Gastrointestinal Tract. Edited by L.R. Johnson, Raven Press, New York, 181-253, 1987.
16. Taylor, T.V. and Torrance, B.: Is there an antral-body portal system in the stomach? Gut 16:781-784, 1975.
17. Waller, S.L.: Prostaglandins and the gastrointestinal tract. Gut 14:402-417, 1973.
18. Whittle, B.J.R., Vane, J.R.: Prostanoids as regulators of gastrointestinal function. In, Physiology of the Gastrointestinal Tract. Edited by L.R. Johnson, Raven Press, New York, 143-180, 1987.
19. Johnson, L.R.: The trophic action of gastrointestinal hormones. Gastroenterology 70:278-288, 1976.
20. Popper, H.: Implications of portal hepatotrophic factors in hepatology. Gastroenterology 66:1227-1230, 1974.
21. Johnson, L.R.: Regulation of gastrointestinal growth. In, Physiology of the Gastrointestinal Tract. Edited by L.R. Johnson, Raven Press, New York, 301-333, 1987.
22. Dodge, J.A. and Karim, A.A.: Induction of pyloric hypertrophy by pentagastrin. Gut 17:280-284, 1976.
23. Bynum, T.E. and Jacobsen, E.D.: Blood flow and gastrointestinal function. Gastroenterology 60:325-335, 1971.
24. Lundgren, O.: The circulation of the small bowel mucosa. Gut 15:1005-1013, 1974.
25. Bowen, J.C., Fang, W-F., Pawlik, W. and Jacobsen, E.D.: Gastrointestinal hormones and blood flow. In, Gastrointestinal Hormones. Edited by J.C. Thompson, Univ. of Texas Press, Austin 391-339, 1975.
26. Parks, D.A., Jacobson, E.D.: Mesenteric circulation. In, Physiology of the Gastrointestinal Tract. Edited by L.R. Johnson, Raven Press, New York, 1649-1670, 1987.
27. Granger, D.N., Kvietys, P.R., Perry, M.A. and Barrowman, J.A.: The microcirculation and intestinal transport. In, Physiology of the Gastrointestinal Tract. Edited by L.R. Johnson, Raven Press, New York, 1671-1697, 1987.
28. Biber, B.: Vasodilator mechanisms in the small intestine. Acta. Physiol. Scand. Suppl. 401, 1973.
29. Schapiro, H. and Britt, L.G.: The action of vasopressin on the gastrointestinal tract. Amer. J. Dig. Dis. 17:649-667, 1972.
30. Mei, N.: Intestinal chemosensitivity. Physiol. Rev. 65:211-237, 1985.
31. Hubel, K.A.: Intestinal nerves and ion transport: Stimuli, reflexes, and responses. Am. J. Physiol. 248:G261-G271, 1985.
32. Sarna, S.K.: Cyclic motor activity; migrating motor complex: 1985. Gastroenterology 89:894-913, 1985.

Chapter 2

Microflora of the Gastrointestinal Tract and Its Symbiotic Relationship with the Host

INTRODUCTION

The microflora of the gastrointestinal tract consists of hundreds of different species of bacteria. One part of the microflora (that in the colon) is the most complex ecosystem in the body. The numbers of bacteria in this region are 10^{10} to 10^{11} per gram. Bacterial numbers in the stomach and small intestine vary in the normal animal, depending on whether nutrients are present. The numbers and distribution of the intestinal flora are normally stable,[1-3] maintained in a symbiotic relationship with the animal. The vast reservoir of microorganisms in the gut poses a potential threat to the animal if they escape from the alimentary tract and multiply in other parts of the body. Despite a number of physiological mechanisms to control that threat, alternations can occur, resulting in disease.

The numbers and types of microorganisms vary with each part of the gastrointestinal tract. Each species has its own preferred niche. The numbers are maintained at a low level in the stomach and intestines. Many changes in normal gastrointestinal function cause the number of bacteria to increase in the cranial bowel. Such changes can also cause species of bacteria to colonize sites they do not normally occupy. Disruption of the normal flora permits colonization by foreign bacteria that are ingested. Diarrhea can develop from colonization by foreign microorganisms. Antibacterial agents can influence the number and distribution of bacteria in the intestines, which are determined by the type of diet. Diet and antibiotic therapy are therefore commonly used to control intestinal problems.

The intestinal microflora affects the metabolism of a host's nutrients, digestive enzymes, bile constituents, and steroids. It also has an impact on the structure and function of the intestinal mucosa. Thus, the intestinal microflora has important effects on the health of the host; conversely, the state of function and nutrition in the host determines the population of the microflora.

NORMAL MICROFLORA[3-8]

The numbers of microorganisms vary with each region of the gastrointestinal tract. The oral cavity is considered in this section, since it represents a major source of bacteria that populate the rest of the alimentary tract. The number of bacteria in the mouth is 10^7 per gram, as shown in Figure 2-1. The contents of the fasting stomach are practically sterile, containing only 10^1 to 10^2 organisms per gram of residual secretions. After a meal, the numbers increase to 10^4 to 10^5 per gram. After secretion of hydrochloric acid has reduced the pH to less than 3, the numbers decline to relatively few. Numbers in the empty small intestine are normally 10^1 to 10^2 per gram in the cranial part, increasing to 10^3 to 10^4 in the caudal part. When food is present, these counts increase by 10^2 to 10^3 bacteria per gram of intestinal contents. The number of bacteria in the colon is 10^{10} to 10^{11} per gram, a fairly constant number (as in the mouth). The numbers in each part are controlled by several different factors, discussed later.

The gastrointestinal tract contains a microflora consisting of large numbers of certain species of bacteria that are always found, making them the most important in the makeup of the normal resident population. The normal microflora is also made up of some species of bacteria that are always present, but in smaller numbers. Additionally, the gastrointestinal microflora always contains a small number of contaminants or transients from the mouth and from the diet. Most current knowledge

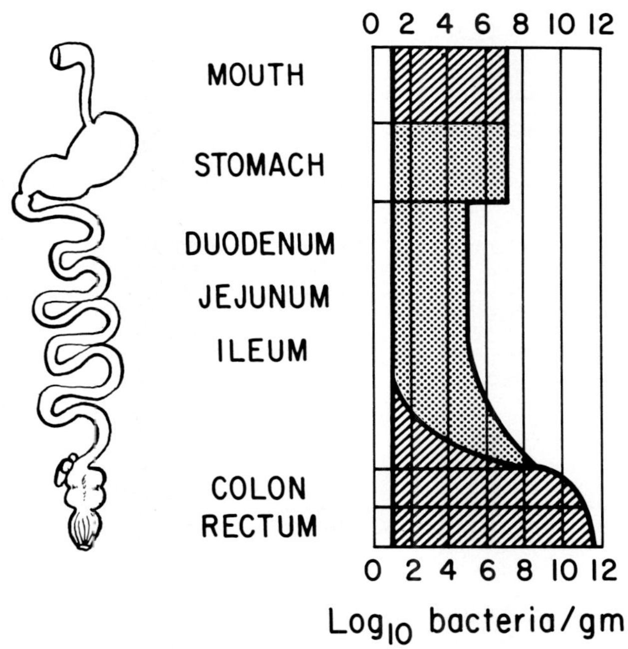

Figure 2-1. Numbers of bacteria in the alimentary tract. Diagonal bars indicate regions where bacteria are present at all times. Dotted area in the stomach and small intestine indicates the numbers of bacteria when nutrients are present. When this part of the gastrointestinal tract is empty the numbers of bacteria fall to 10^1 bacteria per gram.

about microflora of the gut is from studies on normal residents and transients that together make up the smallest part of the population; very little is known about the anaerobic organisms that make up the major part of the normal microflora. They exceed the aerobes by 1000 or more to 1. Until recently, it was not possible to study the anaerobes since no techniques were available for isolating, identifying, and quantitating those bacteria and investigating their properties. The great number of different bacteria in the normal microflora adds to the problem of gaining knowledge and an understanding of the entire ecosystem.

An important source of intestinal organisms is swallowed saliva. The predominant organisms in saliva are members of the *Bacteroides, Streptococcus, Lactobacillus*, and *Neisseria* genera (Table 2-1). Also frequently found are *Staphylococcus, Corynebacterium, Spirochaetes, Vibrios*, and yeasts. Bacteria in the stomach are transients deposited by saliva and food. Thus, all the typically oral organisms can be found in gastric contents after a meal. Organisms found in the fasting stomach are mostly acid-resistant species such as clostridia, streptococci, lactobacilli, Escherichia coli, and fungi. The cranial small intestine contains mostly gram-positive organisms, mainly clostridia, streptococci, lactobacilli, staphylococci and fungi. In the middle and caudal regions, the concentration of bacteria increases and the microflora begins to approach the composition of the flora in the colon. This level of the small intestine contains coliforms at concentrations of 10^5 per gram and enterococci at 10^4 per gram. Bacteroides and bifidobacteria are also found in low numbers throughout the small intestine. Clostridia in the small intestine are found in greater numbers in dogs than in humans.[9] The numbers of bacteria are dramatically increased in the large intestine at a point immediately across the ileocecal sphincter. In summary, all varieties of bacteria found in the mouth can be found in the colon, though their proportions differ. The predominant bacteria in the large intestine are anaerobes, with bacteroides and bifidobacteria found in the highest numbers. Enterobacteria, streptococci, and lactobacilli are found in large numbers. All other organisms exist in low concentrations.

REGULATION OF GASTROINTESTINAL MICROFLORA

The distribution and size of bacterial populations in the gut are determined by normal gastrointestinal function and by environmental factors within the lumen of the tract. The microflora is established shortly after birth[10] and remains relatively constant from then on, unless changes within the host alter normal physiologic function or changes in the host's environment dictate diet changes in the intraluminal environmental factors. These factors, dictated by the host's are interactions between members of the resident microflora. Physiologic regulation consists of those functions that are necessary to maintain each species of bacteria in its own niche and in proper numbers.

Table 2-1. Composition of Microflora of Alimentary Tract

Families	Genera		Mouth	Stomach	Small Intestine	Large Intestine
Pseudomonadaceae	Pseudomonas*	AE				+
Enterobacteriaceae	Escherichia coli*	FAN	--	10^1-10^3		10^7-10^8
	Klebsiella*	FAN		10^1-10^2	10^1-10^3	10^7-10^8
	Enterobacter (aerobacer)*	FAN		$10^{1.8}$	$10^{1.6}$	
	Proteus*	FAN				
Bacteroidaceae	Bacteroides*	AN	+	0	10^1	10^8-10^{10}
	Fusobacterium*	AN	+			
Neisseriaceae	Neisseria	FAN	+			+
	Veillonella	AN	+			$10^{5.9}$
Micrococcaceae	Staphylococcus*	FAN	+	$10^{0.4}$	$10^{0.4}$	$10^{4.7}$
Lactobacilliaceae	Streptococcus*	FAN	+	$<10^1$	10^1-10^3	10^8-10^9
	Lactobacillus*	FAN	+	$<10^1$-$10^{1.3}$	10^2	10^8-10^9
	Bifidobacterium*	AN	+		+	$10^{6.6}$
	Ruminococcus					+
Propionobacteriaceae	Eubacterium	AN	--			+
Corynebacteriaceae	Corynebacterium	FAN	+			$10^{8.7}$
Bacillaceae	Bacillus	AN				$10^{5.4}$
	Clostridium*	AN	--	$10^{0.3}$-10^3	$10^{0.1}$-10^4	10^7-$10^{9.1}$
Yeasts						10^5

*Clinically significant microorganisms
AE = Aerobe
FAN = facultative anaerobe

AN = Anaerobe
+ = Present
-- = Absent

Numbers are organisms per gram or milliliter of contents.
Data complied from references 4-8

This maintenance prevents the pathological effects produced by bacterial overgrowth of a normal resident or colonization of a part of the bowel either by a normal resident that does not belong at that site or by a transient organism that is pathogenic if it is able to colonize.

Physiologic Mechanisms of Regulation by Host

Secretion of Gastric Hydrochloric Acid.[3,9,11] Normal secretion of hydrochloric acid maintains a relatively sterile environment in the stomach. The bacteria that reach the stomach from the mouth are destroyed by hydrochloric acid. The normal flora of the small intestine, especially the cranial part, consists of transients from the mouth. When gastric secretion of acid is inhibited or reduced, the numbers of bacteria in the small intestine increase. Acid secretion is also important in preventing colonization or invasion by pathogenic bacteria. When secretion of acid is inhibited in the dog, the numbers of *E. coli* and clostridia increase. Thus, the fecal type of flora that prevails in the colon moves cranially in the small intestine from the ileum, where it is normally established at a reduced level. The achlorhydric stomach is usually heavily colonized with bacteria. The animal with gastritis is therefore susceptible to increased numbers of gastric bacteria. This patient is unable to produce a secretion of gastric juices with a pH less than 3 since back-diffusion of hydrogen ions is greatly accelerated. Procedures and situations such as feeding that neutralize gastric-acid secretion have a similar effect. The use of antacids or drugs such as anticholinergics and H_2-blockers can cause bacterial numbers to increase in the stomach and small intestine. It is questionable whether other secretions in the gastrointestinal tract have a primary function in controlling the total numbers of bacteria.

Normal Intestinal Motility.[3, 12-14] Normal peristalsis is necessary to maintain low concentrations of bacteria in the small intestine. It accomplishes this by moving the contents containing bacteria in an aboral direction, preventing any organisms from multiplying excessively within a given section of the intestine. Such motility provides a housekeeping function by cleaning out bacteria faster than they can multiply. The housekeeping motility is driven by electrical activity called the migrating myoelectrical complex (MMC), which moves slowly through the empty stomach and intestine at regular intervals. When drugs or disease disrupting MMC activity results in a loss of the housekeeping function, numbers of gastrointestinal bactria can increase.[15] In the absence of normal motility, intestinal microflora increase significantly and fecal organisms will appear in the cranial part of the small intestine.[16,17] Under these circumstances, bacteroides, bifidobacteria, and coliforms predominate. The rate of peristalsis is less in the ileum than in the duodenum and jejunum, probably one of the factors allowing establishment of a partial fecal flora in the ileum. The normal microflora is disrupted by diarrhea and will not return until normal motility is restored.[18]

Mucosal Barrier[5,19] The preceding section describes physiologic functions of the host that regulate the number and kind of bacteria within the lumen of the gastrointestinal tract and thereby prevent disease. Other factors, however, also prevent bacteria from producing pathology in the intestines; some achieve that without controlling numbers of bacteria in the lumen, by creating a barrier that prevents mucosal adherence and invasion by pathogenic bacteria. The barrier is a one-cell-thick epithelial layer with a protective surface coating of mucus, polysaccharides, and immunoglobulins. In addition, a population of nonpathogenic bacteria, normally adhered to the mucosal surface, form an integral part of the barrier against disease since they prevent colonization by pathogenic transient bacteria.

The epithelial cell is a physical barrier preventing invasion of microorganisms and the absorption of toxins. The surface of the cell is covered with a polysaccharide, glycocalyx, and over this is a layer of mucus secreted by goblet cells. The surface of the barrier also contains antibodies secreted by the mucosal cells after antibody synthesis by plasma cells. The antibodies are directed against specific organisms. The most important part of the barrier is the epithelial cell, with its glycocalyx. Another part of the barrier is a superficial layer of nonadhering mucus that entraps bacteria. Subsequently, the bacteria are cleared from the area as peristalsis moves the mucus caudally.

Few bacteria are capable of invading the epithelial cell.[5] *Shigella* and *Salmonella* are invasive species. Invasive strains of other microorganisms, such as *E. coli*, have also recently been recognized. With these few exceptions, the epithelial cell is an effective barrier that prevents the tremendous numbers of intestinal microorganisms from invading the host. To other pathogens, the mucosal cells form a true barrier against invasion. Pathogenicity of some noninvading organisms is related to their ability to attach to a cell's surface and elaborate an enterotoxin. Most of these organisms must penetrate the surface constituents and adhere to the cell surface before they can produce clinical signs of disease. Bacteria adhere to the mucosal surface by fimbriae that they possess, by agglutinins they secrete that act as an adhesive, and by adhesive properties of the bacterial capsule. Each of the normal bacteria attached to the intestinal mucosa has a preferred site on either the villus tips or in the crypts. In many cases, it is necessary for the normal flora to be displaced before a pathogen can adhere. Organisms that produce enterotoxins include some of the vibrios,[20] *E. coli*,[20] *Klebsiella*,[21] *Salmonella*,[22] and *Clostridium*.[23] Some of these groups of microorganisms consist of strains that produce specific adherence factors, which is why they are pathogenic.[24] Other strains are incapable of mucosal binding and are therefore nonpathogenic.[25] Enterotoxins must bind to sites on epithelial cells in order to cause diarrhea. It is possible that enterotoxins produced by the nonpathogenic strains are inactivated or destroyed in the lumen of the intestine by inhibitors or intestinal and bacterial proteases[25] and that binding is not possible. Enterotoxins are inhibited by normal contents of the intestine, although they are quite resistant to proteolytic destruction.[26]

Some other noninvading pathogens cause disease by producing a cytotoxin that damages and destroys normal intestinal epithelial cells. Acute enterocolitis is caused by a cytotoxin produced by *Clostridium difficile* that can overgrow when certain antibiotics suppress growth of members of the normal microflora.

The epithelial cell barrier is affected by the presence of normal numbers of bacteria.[27] Germ-free animals have cuboidal rather than columnar mucosal cells; the rate of cell turnover is slower in the germ-free than in the conventional animals. Germ-free animals have few inflammatory cells in their lamina propria. In contrast, intestinal bacterial numbers increased over normal, show many inflammatory cells and rapid turnover of epithelial cells that appear damaged. Therefore, the kinds and numbers of bacteria living in the intestinal lumen have profound affects on the mucosal surface and the barrier it provides.

Immunoglobulins synthesized by the host in the lamina propria are also important barriers to disease.[28] These are immunoglobulin-A (IgA), produced by plasma cells and secreted onto the surface of the mucosal cells. This secretory IgA is directed against specific organisms that can be pathogenic. Secretory IgA does not regulate the numbers of bacteria in the lumen of the intestine, nor is it thought to be directed against bacteria normally present on the mucosal surface.[25] The predominant members of the normal flora possess a low degree of immunogenicity.[29] The barrier produced by this local immunity is important primarily when pathogenic transients become a threat because normal physiologic function, e.g., peristalsis, is lost or the balance within the normal microflora is disrupted. One mechanism of action by the immune response is IgA's prevention of bacterial adhesion. Another mechanism is antibacterial in that the antibody causes destruction or inhibition of growth of bacteria that come in contact with the mucosal surface. This response is dependent on viable mucosal cells and is independent of complement.[25] It can be considered a type of cellular immunity.

Environmental Factors that Regulate Microflora

Bacterial Microflora Intraregulation.[3] The normal intestinal microflora in an animal is established during the first few weeks of life. Once established, it is difficult to change and is impossible to eradicate. There is some daily variation in the microflora of the stomach and intestines since those organs contain a population of transients that can change with eating habits. The population of the microflora is very stable since outsiders have difficulty in colonizing the gut. Stability is also reflected in the near-impossibility of changing the microflora intentionally. Even pathogens introduced orally are normally unable to colonize and cause disease.[30-32] Attempts have been made to convert a "putrefactive flora" to a "lactic flora" in patients with chronic diarrhea, but oral administration of large numbers of *Lactobacillus acidophilus* produces no changes in the distribution or number of any members of the normal microflora.[5,33] That has been attempted unsuccessfully also in the treatment of hepatic encephalopathy with the view that non-urease-producing organisms will replace organisms in the intestines that split urea to ammonia.[5] Newly introduced microorganisms are able to colonize with greater ease if they have been cultivated in an environment closely resembling the environment to which they are introduced.[25] In a totally strange environment the lag phase in their growth is prolonged, and they are mechanically eliminated before they can multiply and colonize; adaptation and colonization will require more than the short time taken for the normal passage of intestinal contents. Most human cultures believe the consumption of fermented milk products to be beneficial, attributing the effects to the consumption of lactobacillus organisms. To the contrary, the studies cited here and numerous others show that transient bacteria entering the oral cavity have great difficulty in colonizing. It should be recognized that this is of major importance to the host. A number of environmental factors are responsible for maintaining the size and distribution of the normal flora, and they are more important than local immune mechanisms for the prevention of disease.

The most important factor determining the numbers of any one species of bacteria in the gut is the makeup of the remainder of the population. Bacterial growth of any single species is much slower in the intestine of a conventional animal than in the germ-free intestine. (One study showed that when E. *coli* was the only bacteria present in the intestines of an animal, 95 isolates of anaerobic bacteria had to be added in order to reduce the very high numbers of *E. coli* to the low levels in the normal intestine.)[25]

The rate of growth of each species of bacteria is determined, directly or indirectly, by dietary nutrients.[34,35] As an example, consider when one of two organisms is able to digest insoluble polysaccharides and use the soluble carbohydrate products that are formed, and the second organism cannot split the polysaccharide but can use only the soluble products. Thus, both organisms depend on the organism that prepares the nutrients for use. The rate of growth of each, however, is determined by the organism that is able to use the products more readily, and that growth, in turn, affects the growth of the organism preparing the nutrients for use. Some bacteria may be able to use nutrients that others cannot use, which places them in a position where they do not have to compete. The predominating organisms of the large intestine are carbohydrate fermenters, which use ammonia as their major source of nitrogen.[36]

Bacterial growth rates are determined by the amount of available oxygen. Aerobes and facultative anaerobes consume any available oxygen, after which the aerobes are unable to grow, whereas the anaerobic bacteria can. Conditions in the large intestine are essentially anaerobic, and this is partly the reason that anaerobes there outnumber aerobes by 1000 to 1.

The growth of specific bacteria in the intestines is determined indirectly by some of the metabolic products formed. Some volatile fatty acids produced by bacteroides and coliforms act to inhibit the growth of other bacteria.[37] That is the basis for the resistance in some species to infection by salmonella and shigella given by mouth. Other bacteria can directly influence the concentrations of different populations in the microflora. The coliforms can release chemicals that kill related bacteria. These substances are called colicines, and when the populations of colicine-producing serotypes is great, there are fewer different strains in the microflora. When more transients are present, fewer colicines are produced and a greater variety of related strains is found.[38]

Dietary Influence on Intestinal Microflora.[39] Until recently, little was known about the anaerobic population of the gastrointestinal tract since culture methods were not adequate for yielding any useful information. Since the aerobes constitute only 0.1% of the normal fecal flora, measurement of their levels does not reflect the microecology in the animal's colon. The anaerobic 99.9% of the population has recently been investigated in relation to dietary influences. The results have been applied very crudely, at least at present, to the pathogenesis of little-understood diseases. Most of this work has been done on humans, where long-term retrospective studies are possible.

An early observation was made that colonic disease, including cancer, is greater in incidence in Americans than in Japanese.[40] In populations of the latter that came to the United States as adults and adopted the western diet, the rate of colonic problems increased, approaching that of American's. Gastric cancer, in contrast, is high in incidence among Japanese and comparatively low among Americans. These differences have been related to differences in the diet, and some of the disease processes are suggested to be the result of changes in gastrointestinal microflora that are determined by the diet. Thus a number of recent studies have been designed to investigate how diet influences microflora populations. The results are applicable also to an understanding of other gastroenterology problems that for years have been treated empirically with controlled diets, termed "bland" and "hypoallergenic." Most of the beneficial effects of these diets may indeed be due to changing intestinal microflora to populations more favorable to normal physiologic functioning of the alimentary tract.

Diet influences the intestinal microflora of animals,[11,33] although more is known about the effects in humans. In general, humans eating a western type of diet (higher in meat, fat and protein) have fecal levels of anaerobes that are higher and levels of aerobes that are lower than people on a largely vegetarian diet.[41] Anaerobes can produce carcinogens, and it remains to be seen how strong this relation is.[42] More recent experimental studies show that a high-protein diet causes an increase in numbers of anaerobic bacteroides that persists after return to a conventional diet.[43] Numbers of clostridia are lower on a high-protein diet. A low-protein diet causes coliforms to increase and bacteroides and bifidobacteria to decrease. Fungi increase and staphylococci decrease on a low-protein diet. There is some evidence that the fecal flora is not changed when a human adopts a vegetarian diet as an adult.[44]

A number of studies have produced conflicting reports on the effects of elemental no-residue diets on the composition of the fecal microflora. When nutrients were given that require no digestion and are completely absorbed in the upper small bowel, early reports indicated that fecal bacterial counts dropped precipitously,[45] whereas later studies reported no change in the numbers of most fecal bacteria with this type of diet.[40] Other studies indicate that an elemental diet does produce a decrease in the numbers of some aerobes.[5] The volume of feces is reduced when a no-residue diet is fed, and the feces consist primarily of desquamated epithelial cells, mucus, and microorganisms. The mucosal cells that slough in a normal continuous process provide the supply of nutrients for colonic bacterial growth.

Almost all studies to date have been performed on fecal samples in which bacterial numbers are based on units of fecal weight. Such a procedure does not reflect a reduction in total numbers accompanying reduced fecal output. The results of fecal studies do not reflect changes that occur in the colon, and even less in the small intestine. Very few studies have looked at the effect of diet on the normal microflora at different sites in the intestinal tract. There are dietary effects that change both the locations of colonization and the numbers of bacteria. Protein deficiency is associated with tropical sprue, which is characterized by increased total numbers of bacteria in the small intestine and by higher than normal concentrations of coliforms.[46] The diet in this case may cause the changes in the population of microorganisms, which in turn cause the pathology. It is also possible that the overgrowth of the microflora is an event secondary to the malnutrition. Whatever the case, this illustrates that diet has a profound effect, still little understood, on the microflora of the entire intestinal tract. Malnutrition in general has a profound effect on microbial contamination by a wide variety of organisms, which can be a feature of many chronic debilitating diseases. There is an overgrowth of yeast in some cases, and of anaerobes in others. The microflora varies in response to diet probably more in the small intestine than in the large intestine. In general, the specific requirements for the normal bacteria in the colon are for complex polysaccharides.[47] There is a general lack of proteolytic activity by the most predominant members, and they rely on ammonia for their nitrogen needs.

Dietary effects on the intestinal microflora can be demonstrated by different diets' changing the fecal activities of bacterial enzymes. These enzymes include β-glucuronidase, β-glucosidase, β-galactosidase, nitroreductase, azoreductase, 7α-dehydroxylase, and cholesterol dehydrogenase.[3,27] Increases in activities of these enzymes can increase the metabolites of nutrients and bile acids. For example, coprostanol and coprostanone, metabolites of cholestrol, can increase. The metabolites of bile acids can damage intestinal epithelial cells; some of the bacterial enzymes may also have that property. The bacterial enzymes can also convert food additives to chemicals capable of damaging the epithelium. Diets formulated from milk proteins and high in fiber produce significant changes in fecal bacterial enzyme activities, and these changes are associated with reduced incidence of some bowel problems. Clinical benefit is often seen with feeding milk-protein based diets. That benefit may not be associated with changes that can be demonstrated for fecal bacterial populations, but determination of fecal bacterial enzyme activity may show changes that are significant.

Endogenous and Exogenous Antibacterial Agents

Most of the luminal factors that regulate the growth of intestinal bacteria are related to the diet or are produced by the bacteria themselves. An additional endogenous substance that regulates their numbers is bile acids, which are inhibitory to many intestinal microorganisms.[48] Bile acids most likely regulate bacterial growth. The level of bile acids in the intestine is determined by the amount of fat in the diet; high-fat diets cause an increase in fecal concentration of bile acids. An increased amount of bile acids in the colon may be significant in causing chronic disease. Bile acids that are not absorbed and reach the region of greater bacterial populations are metabolized to form deconjugated bile acids and hydroxylated forms that interfere with fluid absorption and motility in the small and large intestines.[49] Some of the metabolic products of bile-acid degradation by bacteria are carcinogenic.

Antibiotics are the most important agents administered to animals for the purpose of eliminating, suppressing, or drastically altering the microflora.[5] Presurgical use of unabsorbed antibiotics has been advocated to "sterilize" the gastrointestinal tract. Combinations of neomycin or kanamycin with polymyxin or bacitracin have been recommended to minimize postsurgical infection, but controlled trials have shown no benefit over untreated presurgical preparation. More recent recommendations include the use of neomycin and metronidazole combinations. Since no single antibiotic is regularly effective against both aerobes and anaerobes, a combination of several drugs is used to suppress or eradicate both types of organisms. Unfortunately, fecal bacterial counts do not change with erythromycin, chloramphenicol, tetracycline, or probably most other antibiotics. Most bacteria have become resistant to neomycin. It can suppress some normal bacteria that are still sensitive, allowing the remaining flora to overgrow and cause an imbalance. In fact, some studies have shown that effective suppression of anaerobes without any effect on aerobes can cause coliforms to increase in parts of the gut from normal levels of 10^2 to levels of 10^7, resulting in death. That is an extreme example, but it shows what can happen if antibiotics are used indiscriminately in the alimentary tract.

CONTROL OF THE GASTROINTESTINAL MICROFLORA IN THE GASTROENTEROLOGY PATIENT

Many gastrointestinal-tract problems are thought to result from changes in the microflora of the gut. Changes in the intestinal microflora may involve normal flora that become pathogenic, or they may result from transient strains that are ingested with food and are able to colonize. Managing the problems associated with such changes requires an understanding of the fundamental concepts presented in this chapter.

More than 500 different varieties of bacteria are found in the gastrointestinal tract, and as a group they are not sensitive to any single antibacterial agent. Thus, any single antibiotic will suppress the numbers of only part of the microflora. The balance of the entire system is then upset, and other members of the normal flora will multiply and exceed normal numbers. Most antidiarrheal agents are formulated with a single antibacterial agent. The antibiotics used most often are directed against the aerobes, i.e., the coliforms, which constitute less than one out of every 1000 organisms found in the large intestine. It is therefore important to recognize that treatment directed against such a small part of the microflora has insignificant effects.

Drugs are used with the idea that they can sterilize the gut, or at least effectively reduce the numbers of bacteria. Antibiotics can reduce the numbers of some microorganisms in the gut, but after a week their numbers return to normal. Many bacteria are able to develop resistance to an antibiotic within 24 hours. Thus, it is important to realize that the very large concentrations of microorganisms in the colon (up to 10^{11} per gram of contents) cannot be suppressed by token amounts of antibacterial agents given orally.

If, indeed, gastrointestinal disease is related to changes in the microflora, it becomes important to consider factors determining the population of the microflora that can be controlled by the clinician and client. These factors have been listed in the preceding sections, and only a few of them can possibly be controlled.

Bacterial interactions have been shown to be important in determining the size and extent of the microflora population. Attempts have been made to put this factor to practical use. This goal is considered achievable by administering *Lactobacillus* cultures to patients with chronic bowel disease and hepatic encephalopathy. The concept here is to displace "bad" microorganisms with "good" ones. That result has not been realized, and it is now known that the resident microflora is very stable and difficult to displace. Cultures of nonpathogenic microorganisms offer little hope in modifying the microflora as it exists. In addition to internal environmental factors, external ones (such as stress) play a significant role in the development of gastrointestinal disease, which is accompanied by changes in the microflora. It is not known how stress changes the microflora and causes clinical signs to appear. In many cases it may be stress-induced changes in motility of the gut that produce a diarrhea: the changes in motility change the microflora, resulting in clinical signs. The normal population does not return until after normal function is regained.

The microflora of the gut is determined by the type of nutrients that the host consumes. The basis for this is just beginning to be understood. The beneficial effects of many different controlled diets in the treatment of chronic disease of the gut has been apparent for centuries. The response to these diets may reside in avoidance of an allergy-stimulating antigen. Controlled diets may also be beneficial because they result in a change in intestinal microflora to a population that is compatible with normal intestinal function.

The basis for chronic gastrointestinal disease will be understood better when more accurate means are developed for evaluating the intestinal microflora. Analyses of fecal samples for total numbers and types of bacteria yield useful information only when known pathogens, such as *Salmonella*, are present. Techniques must be developed to identify and quantitate microorganisms in the stomach and, more important, in the small intestine.

REFERENCES

1. Gorbach, S.L., Nahas, L., Lerner, P.I. and Weinstein, L.: Studies of intestinal microflora. Effects of diet, age and periodic sampling on numbers of fecal microorganisms in man. Gastroenterology 53:845-855, 1967.
2. Zubrzycki, L. and Spaulding, E.H.: Studies on the stability of norma fecal flora. J. Bact. 83:968-974, 1962.
3. Simon, G.L. and Gorbach, S.L.: Intestinal flora and gastrointestinal function. In, Physiology of the Gastrointestinal Tract. Edited by L.R. Johnson. Raven Press, New York, 1729-1747, 1987.
4. Broido, P.W., Gorbach, S.L. and Nyhus, L.M.: Microflora of the gastrointestinal tract and the surgical malabsorption syndromes. Surg. Gynecol. Obstet. 135:449-459, 1972.
5. Drasar, B.S. and Hill, M.J.: Human intestinal flora. Academic Press, London. 1974.
6. Gorbach, S.L.: Intestinal microflora. Gastroenterology 60:1110-1129, 1971.
7. Greenlee, H.B., Belbart, S.M., DeOrio, A.J., Francescatti, D.S., Paez, J. and Reinhardt, G.F.: The influence of gastric surgery on the intestinal flora. Amer. J. Clin. Nutr. 30:1826-1832, 1977.
8. Mitsuoka, T. and Kaneuchi, C.: Ecology of the bifidobacteria. Amer. J. Clin. Nutr. 30:1799-1810, 1977.
9. Broido, P.W., Gorbach, S.L., Condon, R.E. and Nyhus, L.M.: Upper intestinal microfloral control. Arch. Surg. 106:90-93, 1973.
10. Smith, W.H. and Crabb, W.E.: The faecal bacterial flora of animals and man; its development in the young. J. Path. Bact. 82:53-66, 1961.
11. Smith, H.W.: Observations on the flora of the alimentary tract of animals and factors affecting its composition. J. Path. Bact. 89:95-122, 1965.
12. Dixon, J.M.S. and Paulley, J.W.: Bacteriological and histological studies of the small intestine of rats treated with

mecamylamine. Gut 4:169-173.

13. Donaldson, R.M.: Role of indigenous enteric bacteria in intestinal function and disease. In, Handbook of Physiology, Sec. 6, Vol. 5. Alimentary Canal. Edited by C.F. Code. American Physiological Society, Washington D.C., 2807-2837.
14. Sumners, R.W. and Kent, T.H.: Effects of altered propulsion on rat small intestinal flora. Gastroenterology 59:740-744, 1970.
15. Scott, L.D. and Cahall, D.L.: Influence of the interdigestive myoelectric complex on enteric flora in the rat. Gastroenterology 82:737-745, 1982.
16. Drasar, B.S. and Shiner, M.: Studies on the intestinal flora. II. Bacterial flora of the small intestine in patients with gastrointestinal disorders. Gut 10:812-819, 1969.
17. Gorbach, S.L. and Tabaqchali, S.: Bacteria, bile, and the small bowel. Gut 10:963-972, 1969.
18. Gorbach, S.L., Neale, G., Levitan, R. and Hepner, G.W.: Alterations in intestinal microflora during experimental diarrhea. Gut 11:1-6, 1970.
19. Rowley, D.: Specific immune antibacterial mechanisms in the intestines of mice. Amer. J. Clin. Nutr. 27:1417-1423, 1974.
20. Formal, S.B., DuPont, H.L. and Hornick, R.B.: Enterotoxic diarrheal syndromes. Ann. Rev. Med. 24:103-110, 1973.
21. Klipstein, F.A. and Engert, R.F.: Purification and properties of *Klebsiella pneumoniae* heat stable enterotoxin. Infect. Immun. 13:373-381, 1976.
22. Koupal, L.R. and Deibel, R.H.: Assay, characterization, and localization of an enterotoxin produced by *Salmonella*. Infect. Immun. 11:14-22, 1975.
23. McDonel, J.L. and Duncan, C.L.: Histopathological effect of *Clostridium perfringens* enterotoxin in the rabbit ileum. Infect. Immun. 12:1214-1218, 1975.
24. Jones, G.W. and Rutter, J.M.: Contribution of the K88 antigen of *Escherichia coli* to enteropathogenicity; protection against disease by neutralizing the adhesive properties of K88 antigen. Amer. J. Clin. Nutr. 27:1441-1449, 1974.
25. Freter, R.: Interactions between mechanisms controlling the intestinal microflora. Amer. J. Nutr. 27:1409-1416, 1976.
26. Strombeck, D.R. and Harrold, D.: Comparison of the rate of absorption and proteolysis of (^{14}C) choleragen and (^{14}C) bovine serum albumin in the rat jejunum. Infect. Immun. 12:1450-1456, 1975.
27. Simon, G.L. and Gorbach, S.L.: Intestinal flora in health and disease. Gastroenterology 86:174-193, 1984.
28. Clancy, R. and Bienenstock, J.: Secretory immunoglobulins. Clinics Gastroenterology 5:229-249, 1976.
29. Carter, P.B. and Pollard, M.: Studies with *Lactobacillus casei in* gnotobiotic mice. In, Germ-Free Research. Edited by J.B. Heneghan. New York, Academic Press, 379-383, 1973.
30. Orcutt, R. and Schaedler, R.W.: Control of staphylococci in the gut of mice. In, Germ-Free Research. Edited by J.B. Heneghan. New York, Academic Press, 435-440, 1973.
31. Ralovich, B., Emody, L., Barna, K., Brasch, Gy., Marton, E. and Ternak, G.: Excretion of orally administered intestinal bacteria in humans. Abl. Bakt. Hyg., I. Abt. Orig. A 226:82-90, 1974.
32. Smith, H.W.: Survival of orally administered *E. coli* K12 in alimentary tract of man. Nature 255:500-502, 1975.
33. Dubos, R.: Man Adapting. Yale University Press, New Haven, 1965.
34. Wolin, M.J.: Metabolic interactions among intestinal microorganisms. Amer. J. Clin. Nutr. 27:1320-1328, 1974.
35. Zollner, N., Ruckdeschel, G. and Wolfram, G.: Verhalten der darmflora des menschen bei formeldiaten mit wechselndem kohlenhydratgehalt. Nutr. Metabol. 18:127-136, 1975.
36. Bryant, M.P.: Nutritional features and ecology of predominant anaerobic bacteria of the intestinal tract. Amer. J. Clin. Nutr. 27:1313-1319, 1974.
37. Meynell, G.G.: Antibacterial mechanisms of the mouse gut. II. The role of Eh and volatile fatty acids in the normal gut. Brit. J. Exp. Path. 44:209-210, 1963.
38. Branche, W.C., Young, V.M., Robinet, H.G. and Massey, E.D.: Effect of colicine production on Escherichia coli in the normal human intestine. Proc. Soc. Exp. Biol. Med. 114:198-201, 1963.
39. Hentges, D.J.: Does diet influence human fecal microflora composition? Nutr. Rev. 38:329-336, 1980.
40. Finegold, S.M., Atteberry, H.R. and Sutter, V.L.: Effect of diet on human fecal flora: comparison of Japanese and American diets. Amer. J. Clin. Nutr. 27:1456-1469, 1974.
41. Drasar, B.S. and Hill, M.J.: Intestinal bacteria and cancer. Amer. J. Clin. Nutr. 25:1399-1404, 1972.
42. Hill, M.J., Crowther, J.S., Drasar, B.S., Hawksworth, G., Aries, V. and Williams, R.E.: Bacteria and etiology of cancer of the large bowel. lancet 1:95-100, 1971.
43. Maier, B.R., Flynn, M.A., Burton, G.C., Tsutakawa, R.K. and Hentges, D.J.: Effects of a high-beef diet on bowel flora: a preliminary report. Amer. J. Clin. Nutr. 27:1470-1474, 1974.
44. Moore, W.E.C., Cato, E.P. and Holdeman, L.V.: Anaerobic bacteria of the gastrointestinal flora and their occurrence in clinical infections. J. Infect. Dis. 119:641-649, 1969.
45. Winitz, M., Adams, R.F., Seedman, D.A., Davis, P.N., Jayko, L.G. and Hamilton, J.A.: Studies in metabolic nutrition employing chemically defined diets. Amer. J. Clin. Nutr. 23:546-559, 1970.
46. Garcey, M. and Stone, D.E.: Microbial contamination of the gut: another feature of malnutrition. Amer. J. Clin. Nutr. 26:1170-1174, 1973.
47. Moore, W.E.C. and Holdeman, L.V.: Special problems associated with the isolation and identification of intestinal bacteria in fecal flora studies. Amer. J. Clin. Nutr. 27:1450-1455, 1974.
48. Floch, M.H., Binder, H.J., Filburn, B. and Gershengoren, W.: The effect of bile acids on intestinal microflora. Amer. J. Clin. Nutr. 25:1418-1426, 1972.
49. Midtvedt, T.: Microbial bile acid transformation. Amer. J. Clin. Nutr. 27:1341-1347, 1974.

Chapter 3

Gastrointestinal Immune System

INTRODUCTION

The concept of a gastrointestinal immune system functioning largely independent from the systemic immune system was first proposed in 1919 by Besredka,[1] following his demonstration that rabbits orally immunized with enteropathogenic bacteria were protected against dysentery regardless of the titers of serum antibody. In 1922, Davies[2] was able to demonstrate fecal antibodies against enteropathogenic bacteria before the development of serum antibodies. The significance of this observation was broadened in the 1960's when several laboratories showed that a unique immunoglobulin (IgA), with properties distinct from serum immunoglobulins, was the major gut immunoglobulin.[3] From these beginnings researchers have gone on to demonstrate that the gut mucosa contains the quantitatively most important B cell system of the body.[3]

In its broadest sense, the gastrointestinal immune system may be thought to include all the processes, both antigen-specific and antigen nonspecific, that protect the body against the deleterious effects of the material existent in the lumen of the intestinal tract. This material is both abundant and diverse. The intestinal milieu contains factors that are antigenic and non-antigenic, particulate and soluble, injurious and nutritious, persistent and transient, foreign and self. This antigenic variation and profusion necessitate a particularly versatile immune system that is sensitive to novel or injurious antigen but that is tolerant to persistent or benign antigen.

Effective gastrointestinal immunity is dependent on four interrelated processes (Figure 3-1). These are: exclusion from the mucosa of luminal materials; elimination of, or tolerance to, antigens that reach the mucosa; and regulation of the immune response.

The exclusion of antigenic material from the mucosa is the primary function of mucosal immune systems and the function to which they are most adapted. The processes of exclusion begin in the lumen. Large molecules are rendered non-antigenic by efficient digestion, and bacterial numbers are limited by interactions of flora, bactericidal gastrointestinal secretions, and rhythmical bowel motility. Exclusion is also dependent on an effective mucosal barrier. A single layer of epithelial cells separates the body from gastrointestinal content. The quantity and diversity of luminal material demands epithelial "permselectivity," allowing the body to receive adequate nutrition and to "sample" passing gastrointestinal antigens, but to prevent overwhelming exposure to deleterious antigens. Intestinal permeability, the components of the mucosal barrier, and the antigen-nonspecific factors controlling bacterial numbers are discussed in detail in other chapters. IgA secretion contributes to this mucosal exclusion. IgA secretion is initiated in the gut-associated lymphoid tissue and is an antigen-specific method of mucosal exclusion. It is a unique feature of mucosal immune systems, discussed in considerable detail in this chapter. Excluding antigen from the gut-associated lymphoid tissue contributes to antigen tolerance.

Once an antigen penetrates the gastrointestinal epithelium, it induces an immune response. Immune responses to food antigens and bowel bacteria are commonplace in healthy animals. The immune response results in either sensitivity or tolerance to the antigen. Antigen sensitivity results in antigen elimination. Elimination occurs through either antigen- nonspecific or antigen-specific mechanisms. The antigen-nonspecific mechanisms include the elimination of antigen by the mononuclear-phagocytic system, the inflammatory response, and the alternate complement cascade. Antigen-specific elimination is initiated and carried out by the gut-associated lym-

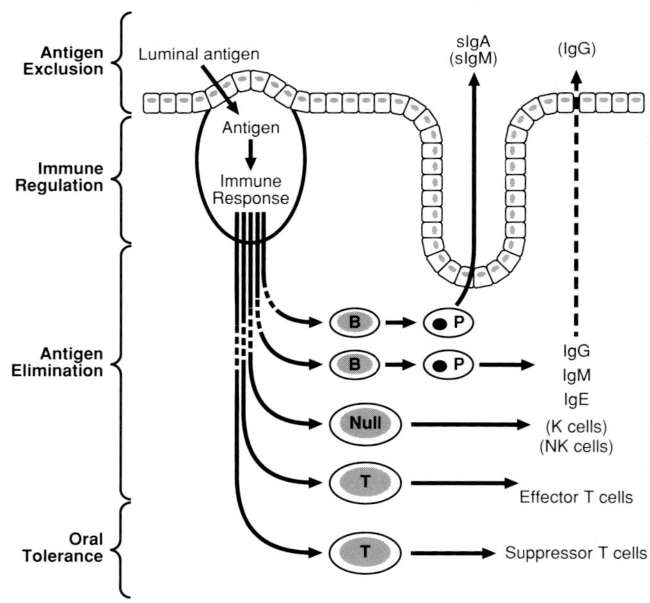

Figure 3-1. The Gastrointestinal Immune System. Effective gastrointestinal immunity is dependent on four interrelated processes: antigen exclusion; antigen elimination oral tolerance; and immune regulation. Modified from Figure 2 in reference 3.

phoid tissue. The mechanisms include secretion of IgG and IgE and activation of the cell-mediated immune response.

Oral tolerance is also initiated in the gut-associated lymphoid tissue. Tolerance, antigen-specific exclusion (IgA), and antigen-specific elimination involve intimate and complex interactions between phagocytes, T lymphocytes and B lymphocytes. These interactions result in the production of antibody, cytotoxic, helper, or suppressor cells, all with a high specificity for a certain antigen. A second unique feature of the gastrointestinal immune system is its propensity to mount immune responses dominated by T cell suppression (as well as IgA-mediated antigen exclusion) that ultimately render the immune system tolerant to ingested antigens and microbial flora. Tolerance to benign, persistent antigens avoids subjecting the mucosa and body to the harmful effects of prolonged, immune-mediated inflammation.

Antigen elimination and tolerance are not just local events. They result in systemic as well as local tolerance, and mucosal immunity at all mucosal surfaces of the body. These systemic manifestations of the gastrointestinal immune response relate to a third characteristic feature of the gastrointestinal immune system: the tendency of antigen-exposed lymphocytes to migrate from the gut lymphoid tissue and populate other lymphoid tissues and mucosal surfaces. This lymphocyte migration has lead to the concept of a mucosal immunological network.[4]

The regulation of the gastrointestinal immune system promotes and integrates mucosal exclusion, antigen elimination, and antigen tolerance into a remarkably effective system of mucosal defense that neatly balances the demands of protection with those of nutrition. Abnormalities in immune regulation are currently thought to contribute to a number of important digestive system diseases, including gluten enteropathy, food allergies, inflammatory bowel disease, lymphocytic cholangitis, and chronic hepatitis.

The majority of this chapter describes the mechanics, function, and consequences of the immune response in the gut-associated lymphoid tissue. Those aspects of the immune response unique to mucosal immune systems are given greatest emphasis. The mononuclear-phagocytic system, immunity to parasites, passive immunity, and the role of the immune system in producing gastrointestinal disease are also described.

THE MONONUCLEAR-PHAGOCYTIC SYSTEM

The mononuclear-phagocytic system is comprised of macrophages distributed throughout the body. The mononuclear-phagocytic system is distinct from the reticuloendothelial system because it excludes cells which *inadvertently* take up particulate matter such as epithelial and endothelial cells.[5] All of the cells of the mononuclear-phagocytic system originate from precursors in the bone marrow and reach the tissues in the circulatory system. These circulating, juvenile macrophages are called monocytes. Monocytes enter the tissues under the influence of various chemotactants. Some macrophages are found within connective tissues (histiocytes), and large numbers are located in lymph nodes, spleen, and bone marrow, and with gut-associated and bronchus-associated lymphoid tissue. Macrophages of particular importance to the gastrointestinal immune response are found in association with the gut-associated lymphoid tissue, in gastrointestinal lymph nodes, or lining the sinusoids of the liver (Kupffer cells). Within the gut-associated lymphoid tissue, macrophages are found immediately below the specialized epithelium of the lymphoid nodules and sparsely distributed throughout the lamina propria. In lymph nodes, macrophages congregate primarily in the medulla of the lymph node. Within the liver, macrophages form part of the fenestrated endothelial sheet that lines the sinusoids. The hepatic mononuclear-phagocytic system represents 75%-80% of the intravascular clearance capacity.[6]

Functions of the Mononuclear-Phagocytic System

Antigen Trapping. The functions of the mononuclear-phagocytic system are numerous. Together the phagocytes of the system represent an efficient and extensive antigen trapping net. In addition, they are intimately involved in the immune response and are able to secrete a wide variety of mediators important in the mediation of inflammation.

The macrophages of the mononuclear-phagocytic system are ideally situated to trap antigen carried to them in lymph or blood or passed to them by other cells. Ingestion of antigen by macrophages is a non-specific process that is facilitated by, but not dependent on, opsonins and antibody. Macrophages can function effectively even on first exposure to an antigen. After the development of antibody, however, the efficiency of macrophage ingestion of antigen is enhanced because macrophages possess receptors for both complement and antibody. In addition, following antibody production antigen trapping by lymph nodes is enhanced by the recruitment of dendritic cells. These macrophage-like cells possess numerous, long interdigitating cytoplasmic processes that, once coated by antibody, can absorb antigen onto their surface for presentation to lymphocytes. Dendritic cells have been identified in the Peyer's patches and lamina propria of the intestine, where they presumably have a similar role to the dendritic cells of the lymph nodes.[7] The phagocytic role of the mononuclear-phagocyte system is essential for homeostasis. It is responsible for the clearance from the body of tissue debris, aged or damaged cells, infective agents, and non-living antigens such as bacterial endotoxins, immune complexes, and products of intravascular hemostasis. Macrophages initiate tissue healing by the clean-up of cell debris and the stimulation of fibrosis.

Role in the Specific Immune Response. The mononuclear-phagocyte system is involved in the initiation, regulation, and effector arm of the immune response (Figure 3-2). The immune response is launched largely by the effective presentation of antigen to lymphocytes by macrophages. A subpopulation of macrophages conserves representative samples of ingested antigen on the macrophage cell surface, where it is presented, in association with class II major histocompatibility antigens (MHC II), to lymphocytes. The MHC II antigens are surface glycoproteins restricted to certain lymphocytes and antigen-presenting cells such as macrophages and dendritic cells. The MHC antigens are the product of the major histocompatibility gene complex. Their expression is thus under genetic control, providing a mechanism by which early immune system response can be genetically controlled. For instance, the murine response to cholera toxin is under the control of certain genes in the major histocompatibility complex.[8] These genes affect the expression of the MHC II antigens, which in turn influences

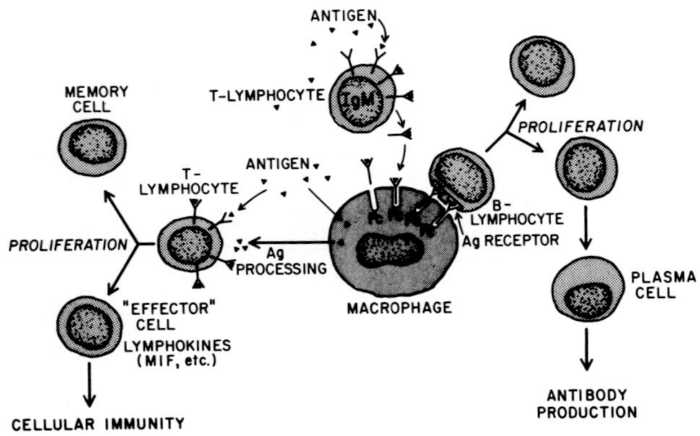

Figure 3-2. Schematic illustrating functions of macrophage in cellular and humoral immunity. Antigens are picked up by macrophages and processed before being transferred to lymphocytes for mediating an immune response. Antigens may also be picked up by immunoglobulin surface receptors of T lymphocytes and then transferred to macrophages. Attachment is by the Fc piece. The macrophage transfers the antigen to B lymphocytes, stimulating their proliferation and maturation into mature antibody-secreting plasma cells. Macrophages also process antigens and transfers them to T lymphocytes, which are subsequently stimulated to proliferate and form memory cells and effector cells that produce lymphokines, which are involved in cellular immunity. Figure 3-5 illustrates production of helper and cytotoxic cells in greater detail.

the immune system's ability to "read," and therefore respond to, the cholera toxin-MHC antigen complex. This process of antigen presentation is fundamental to the immune response. Without it, elimination of antigen is severely hampered. In contrast, tolerance still can develop if antigen evades the mononuclear-phagocyte system and reaches lymphocytes directly.[5] Macrophages' release of interleukin 1 and interferon plays an important role in immune regulation. As effector cells for the immune response, macrophages play a role in the destruction of virus-infected and tumor cells. They are particularly effective at cytotoxicity and microbial killing once stimulated by interferons.

Role in the Nonspecific Immune Response. Macrophages are important in the initiation, amplification, and regulation of inflammation. If restricted in duration, severity, and extent, the inflammatory response is beneficial and contributes to the repair of injury or elimination of infection. If protracted, flagrant, or extensive, the phagocyte inflammatory response can become detrimental to the host, as is exemplified by the macrophage's role in endotoxic shock and granulomatous enterocolitis. Macrophages influence the inflammatory response by secreting factors such as complement, proteases, platelet-activating factor, prostaglandins, leukotrienes, oxygen-derived free radicals, interleukin 1, and cachectin. Cachectin (tumor necrosis factor) is a polypeptide monokine released from stimulated macrophages. It has recently been recognized to have a wide range of biological effects in addition to mediating inflammation. These effects include the production of anorexia, weight loss, and fever, and the mediation of endotoxic shock.[9] Macrophages can initiate fever, neutrophil release, and hepatic synthesis of acute-phase proteins by releasing interleukin 1 (endogenous pyrogen); they can stimulate leukopoiesis by secreting colony stimulating factor. Sequestration of iron under the influence of interleukin 1 results in bacteriostasis and, if chronic, the anemia of chronic inflammation. The role of the macrophage in inflammation and tissue injury is more full discussed in the section on gastrointestinal inflammation.

Factors Affecting Function of the Monocyte-Phagocytic System

Many factors affect the function of the monocyte-phagocytic system. Its activity is dependent on an adequate supply of oxygen, glucose, and other sources of energy. It is enhanced by antibodies, interferons, and opsonins such as fibronectin and C-reactive protein. Fibronectin, a macrophage-produced protein, is an important nonspecific opsonin of particulate matter. If it is depleted, bacterial clearance by the mononuclear-phagocyte system, is severely hampered. C-reactive protein is an acute-phase protein released by the liver during acute inflammation. Infectious, neoplastic, and autoimmune diseases stimulate the monocyte-macrophage system, as do estrogens, small quantities of endotoxin, and various immunomodulators such as BCG. The function of the system is decreased by inadequate blood flow and by the acute phase protein serum amyloid A, released by the liver. Uptake of toxic products that damage the macrophages, such as asbestos, and the saturation of the system with overwhelming quantities of antigen eventually interfere with function. Shock, trauma, reduced hepatic mass, splenectomy, and corticosteroids also inhibit the system. It appears that trauma may adversely affect phagocytosis by changing the number or binding affinity of macrophage surface receptors for immunoglobulins, complement fragments, and fibronectin.[6] A similar change has been noticed in hemorrhage. The decrease in opsonization noted during hemorrhage compounds the decreased clearance that results from reduced blood flow to the mononuclear-phagocyte system. Hepatic vascular shunts markedly decrease phagocytic activity by reducing liver mass and blood flow.

In summary, a number of clinical situations can alter monocyte-phagocytic system function. Depression of activity can be expected during starvation, post-surgical periods, shock, trauma, and any condition reducing hepatic blood flow or delivery of nutrients to the liver. The more pronounced the phagocytic defect, the greater the mortality. In addition, many of the common clinical signs of disease such as anorexia, weight loss, fever, and anemia can result from the secretory products of the activated monocyte-phagocytic system.

STRUCTURE AND FUNCTION OF THE GASTROINTESTINAL LYMPHOID TISSUES

Components of the Gut-Associated Lymphoid Tissue

The gut-associated lymphoid tissue (GALT) is comprised of aggregated and non-aggregated lymphoid tissue within the gastrointestinal mucosa. The aggregated lymphoid tissues consist of lymphoid nodules and Peyer's patches. The non-aggregated lymphoid tissues includes luminal, intraepithelial, and lamina propria leukocytes. Some authors also include the mesenteric lymph nodes and the lymphoid tissue associated with ductal epithelium (DALT) as part of GALT. These lymphoid aggregates share anatomic proximity and some functions with GALT, but both tissues have important differences in structure and/or immune response compared to GALT. Therefore, for the purposes of this chapter, they are not included as components of GALT.

Lymphoid Nodules

Lymphoid nodules are present throughout the intestine and are the predominant type of aggregated lymphoid tissue in the large bowel of the dog. They are particularly numerous in the rectum.[10] Lymphoid nodules contain a single follicle of lymphoid cells, and range in size from approximately 0.5 to 3 mm. They occupy both the lamina propria and the submucosa.[10] The follicle-associated epithelium of the lymphoid nodules has not been as well studied as that which overlies the Peyer's patches, but the epithelia over both types of lymphoid tissue appear to be similar. M cells (see below) have been identified in the follicle-associated epithelium of lymphoid nodules in the guinea pig and are well described in the Peyer's patches of many species including the dog.[11] The structural organization and function of the isolated follicle in the lymphoid nodules also appears to be similar to that of the aggregated follicles in the Peyer's patches. B and T cells segregate within the nodule to the follicular and parafollicular areas, respectively. Helper cells constitute the major subset of T cells within the nodules.[12]

Peyer's Patches

Peyer's patches are differentiated from the isolated lymphoid nodules by their large size. They consist of a collection of lymphoid follicles (5-900 in humans) that are located in the lamina propria and submucosa of the small intestine. Peyer's patches are covered by a follicle-associated epithelium, are innervated by peptidergic neurons, and possess efferent, but not afferent, lymphatics that drain into the mesenteric lymph nodes. They can be recognized grossly in both the cat and the dog, and number approximately 20 in the dog.[13] In the duodenum of dogs they appear as umbilicated, whitish elevations measuring from a few millimeters to 4 cm in their longer diameter. In the jejunum and ileum they appear as dome-shaped elevations. For the last 20-25 cm of the canine ileum the lymphoid tissue presents a continuous strip. Occasionally pinpoint sized collections of lymphoid follicles resembling Peyer's patches are present in the colon and rectum of the dog.[13]

In some species, Peyer's patches are anatomically and perhaps functionally heterogeneous.[5] In the newborn sheep, Peyer's patches containing only B cells have been recognized in the ileocecal area. These Peyer's patches involute in early adulthood; it has been proposed that they are primary lymphoid organs that represent the Bursa-equivalent in this, and perhaps other, species. In contrast, jejunal Peyer's patches appear to be secondary lymphoid organs. They persist throughout life and contain up to 30%-40% T cells. Several days of antigen stimulation are necessary for the expansion and differentiation of the jejunal Peyer's patches, but antigen is not required for their initial formation.[14] Newborn animals require several days or weeks of antigen stimulation to produce a fully developed patch.

The primary functions of Peyer's patches, in animals other than the neonate, are to sample luminal antigen, present that antigen to subepithelial lymphocytes, initiate and regulate the immune response, and export resultant immunocompetent lymphocytes to the other mucosal lymphoid tissues of the body. Some studies have indicated that Peyer's patches are essential for the development of the mucosal immune response, whereas others have suggested that the whole mass of GALT, including the lymphoid nodules and diffuse lymphoid tissues of the lamina propria, can populate the mucosa with an effective mucosal immune system.[3] The immune response of GALT is discussed in detail later in this chapter.

Follicle-Associated Epithelium. The domed surface of Peyer's patches is covered by a specialized epithelium called the follicle-associated epithelium (Figure 3-3). This epithelium consists predominantly of cuboidal shaped, absorptive epithelial cells. Smaller numbers of goblet cells and M cells are interspersed between the absorptive cells. Lymphocytes are commonly observed between the epithelial cells, as is the occasional macrophage. The follicle-associated epithelium is derived from epithelial cell proliferation in the surrounding crypts. Up to 30 crypts may supply a single dome with cells. The number of goblet cells in the follicle-associated epithelium is reduced compared to that in the surrounding non-lymphoid epithelium, and it contains no IgA-transporting capacity.[15] This reduction is thought to create a mucus and IgA "break" that facilitates exposure of luminal antigen to the lymphoepithe-

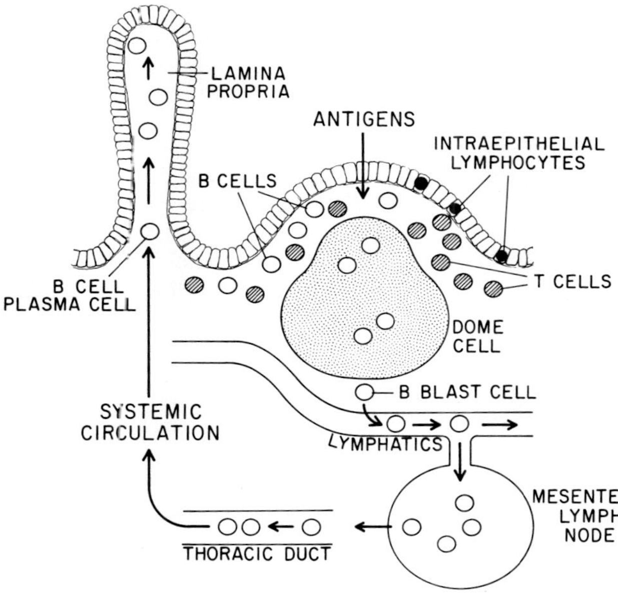

Figure 3-3. Diagram of development of local intestinal immunity. Antigens are absorbed by specialized epithelial cells in mucosa covering Peyer's patches. Intraepithelial lymphocytes interact with antigens entering the cells. Antigens stimulate maturation of B blast cells (In Peyer's patches) and initiate their migration through lymphatics to the systemic circulation. B blast cells mature to B lymphocytes and plasma cells and "home" to the lamina propria of intestinal mucosa.

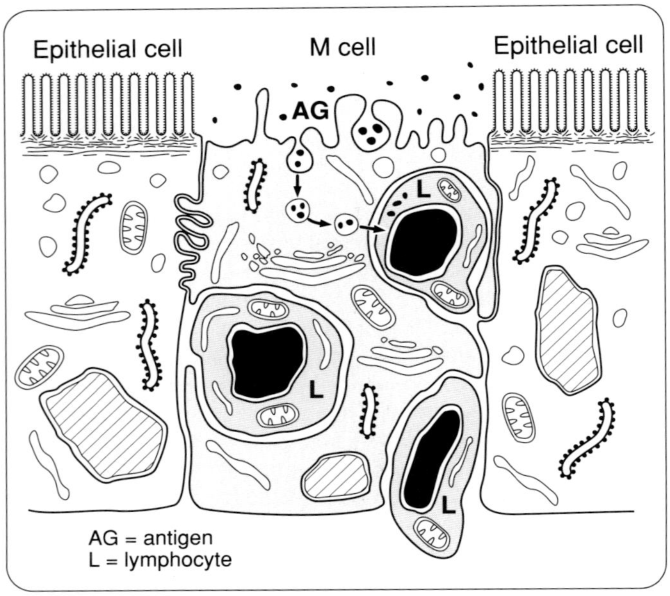

Figure 3-4. Schematic of M cell showing intraepithelial lymphocytes (L) migrating through the cell.

lium. Species and age differences exist in the percentage of M cells in the follicle-associated epithelium. In laboratory animals M cells account for 10%-50% of the follicle-associated epithelium. In newborn ruminants the follicle-associated epithelium has been reported to consist predominantly or exclusively of M cells.[11]

M Cells. M cells are specialized epithelial cells that are present in the follicle-associated epithelium of tonsillar, gut-associated, and bronchus-associated lymphoid tissue (Figure 3-4).[11,16] They can be identified with certainty only by electron microscopy. In light microscopy their presence is suggested by discontinuity of the intestinal brush border[11] especially following staining for brush border alkaline phosphatase.[15]

The term "M cell" has been used synonymously with "lymphoepithelial cell" and "follicle-associated epithelial cell." The name initially derived from the observation that the cells' apical surface contained microfolds rather than microvilli. When microvilli were also observed on the apical surface, the notation "M cell" was retained. Instead of designating "microfold cell," the term came to designate "membranous epithelial cell." This later term is descriptive of the mature M cell's attenuated rim of apical cytoplasm. This "membranous" cytoplasm surrounds one or more intrusive cells, which are usually lymphocytes, lymphoblasts, or macrophages. These cells indent the M cell cytoplasm to form a central hollow that brings the leukocytes cells within 0.3 μm of the lumen. The precursor cell and the site of differentiation of the M cell is unresolved. Some of the data suggest that M cells differentiate from mature absorptive cells on the domes of the lymphoid follicles. Other data suggest that at least some of the M cells develop directly from undifferentiated crypt cells and migrate onto the dome as they mature. It has been postulated that the differentiation and function of M cells is influenced by the underlying lymphoid follicle. M cells numbers in specific pathogen free mice can triple within seven days of exposure to a normal animal housing environment.[17]

It is unlikely that M cells have any digestive or nutrient absorptive function. Instead, it appears that M cells function to take up small quantities of intact luminal antigens by micropinocytosis and transport these antigens in vacuoles to the underlying macrophages and lymphoid tissues for participation in the immune response. The M cells attain this function very early in development and retain their transport capability throughout adulthood. In comparison, the absorptive enterocytes largely lose their ability to transport macromolecules soon after birth. The transported material includes particulate matter, proteins, and some microorganisms. The scant glycocalyx of the M cell appears to contain specific receptors for some pathogenic microorganisms. Some pathogens, such as certain types of mycobacteria, salmonella, chlamydia, reoviruses, rotaviruses, astroviruses, and coronaviruses, can utilize the M cells to access the body. In addition, macrophages can insert processes between M cells and are capable of phagocytosing organisms such as salmonella and giardia.[14]

Other bacteria, such as certain strains of E. *coli*, adhere to, but are not endocytosed, by the M cells. This adherence can precede the adherence of the bacterium to the absorptive enterocytes, and in such cases it is possible that the M cell plays an important role in the colonization of the bowel by the pathogen. The transport of macromolecules such as proteins by M cells raises the possibility that they may also play a role in allergic disease. M cells may also have the capability to transport material from the lamina propria into the bowel lumen, although the importance of this function is unknown. Lymphocytes from Peyer's patches have been observed to migrate through gaps in the apical cytoplasm of M cells. M cells may be a major route by which lymphocytes leave the mucosa to enter the bowel lumen.

Lymphoid Tissue. The lymphoid tissue of the Peyer's patch consists of three major areas: the follicle, which contains a germinal center; the dome overlying the follicle; and an interfollicular area (Figure 3-3).[4,16,18] Like the lymphoid nodules, the B and T cells are somewhat compartmentalized within these regions of the Peyer's patch. The follicle is composed primarily of B cells with an occasional T helper cell. The dome consists of a mixture of B cells, T cells, and macrophages, and the interfollicular area contains mainly T cells. Many of the B cells in the dome area appear to be of mature memory clones.[19] Some authors recognize a fourth area at the follicular rim composed largely of null cells and T cells with the suppressor/cytotoxic phenotype.[16,18] Overall, the adult Peyer's patch contains 40%-70% B lymphocytes and 11%-40% T cells.[16] The majority of B cells in the follicles of the Peyer's patch are precursors of IgA secreting plasma cells. Precursors of B cells for all immunoglobulin isotypes are, however, present. Post-capillary, high endothelial venules are seen at the interface between the T- and B-dependent areas of the follicles and are the sites for lymphocyte emigration from the vascular bed.[4]

Peyer's patches contain few plasma cells and do not appear to be important sources of immunoglobulin in vivo, although they can easily be induced to produce antibodies in vitro.[20] Likewise, lymphocytes from Peyer's patches do not appear able to undertake antibody-dependent cellular cytotoxicity or cell-mediated toxicity in the absence of previous sensitization, suggesting the absence of killer and natural killer cells. In contrast, T cells capable of cytotoxicity have been isolated from Peyer's patches.[18]

Luminal Leukocytes

Luminal leukocytes can be found in close association with the mucosa of normal animals.[21] In the rabbit appendix such cells contain approximately equal numbers of B and T cells along with some null cells and macrophages. Luminal leukocytes appear to migrate from the mucosa driven by luminal antigen. They have, as yet, not been demonstrated to back-migrate to the mucosa.[18] During infectious and inflammatory bowel diseases their numbers are increased and their ranks expanded by polymorphic cells. Luminal lymphocytes increase in number in Giardiasis and are often found closely associated with *Giardia* trophozoites.[22] The function and importance of these luminal leukocytes is unknown. Their presence in the feces has been utilized as a diagnostic indicator of intestinal inflammation.

Intraepithelial Leukocytes

The intraepithelial leukocytes reside between the intestinal epithelial cells. They are probably derived from the lamina propria and are particularly common in the follicle-associated epithelium. In the jejunum of healthy adult dogs the intraepithelial lymphocytes number approximately 11-15 per 100 epithelial cells. Their numbers are somewhat lower in preweaned puppies and in the ileum of adult dogs.[23] Their numbers increase up to five fold following exposure of the bowel to microbial antigen.[24] Disagreement exists over the subtype classification of intraepithelial lymphocytes. Such disagreement arises from variations in species studied, bowel sample location, methodology, interpretation of phenotypes, and presence or absence of disease. For instance, in inflammatory intestinal diseases polymorphic cells enter the intraepithelial compartment in greater numbers. In general, in the normal intestine the majority of the intraepithelial leukocytes are T lymphocytes, and most of these T cells are of the suppressor/cytotoxic phenotype.[4,12,18,24] It is still unclear to what extent this phenotypic majority reflects functional predominance.[15] An important subpopulation of intraepithelial lymphocytes consists of large granular lymphocytes of the natural killer type.[24,25] In some species, these may comprise more than 50% of the intraepithelial lymphocytes.[26] There is also evidence for the presence of mast cell precursors in the epithelium.[27] Very few B cells are found in the intraepithelial compartment.[28]

Intraepithelial lymphocytes are known to increase in numbers in human celiac disease and giardiasis, but their precise role in gastrointestinal immunity and disease is unknown. In wheat-sensitive enteropathy of Irish Setters, intraepithelial cell numbers increase from approximately 10 lymphocytes per 100 enterocytes to 19 lymphocytes per 100 enterocytes after susceptible dogs are challenged with gluten.[29] This increase in intraepithelial lymphocytes after gluten feeding occurs in all susceptible dogs, but it is only associated with accompanying pathological changes in villus height, brush border enzyme content, and bowel permeability if the dogs have been *reared* on a cereal-containing diet. Thus it appears likely that in spite of their increased numbers, intraepithelial lymphocytes do not mediate gluten toxicity in the wheat-sensitive enteropathy of Irish Setter dogs.[30]

The natural killer-like cells have cytotoxic activity against enterovirus infected cells. They are effective even in the absence of previous sensitization and may represent an important "front-line" defense.[25] Paradoxically, some coccidia and enterovirus species undergo development in the intraepithelial natural killer-like cells.[26] In addition, it is possible that intraepithelial lymphocytes return to the lamina propria and circulation after antigen priming,[18] thus serving a sentinel role.

Lamina Propria Leukocytes

Lamina Propria Lymphocytes. The lamina propria contains a wide variety of leukocytes. In contrast to the intraepithelial compartment, B cells are common in the lamina propria. In the species studied, including cats and dogs, IgA-producing B cells are the predominate B cell subtype.[31,32] In "normal" human mucosa, 70% to 90% of the B cells are IgA-producing cells, including plasma cells and their immediate precursors, compared with less than 5% in peripheral lymph nodes. Smaller numbers of IgG-, IgM-, and IgE-containing lymphocytes have also been identified. T cells with helper, suppressor, and cytotoxic functions are also present in the lamina propria. The majority of the T cells are of the helper subset.[12,20] The presence in the lamina propria of natural killer cells and killer cells capable of antibody-dependent cellular cytotoxicity is debated.[4] However, recent evidence supports the availability of a full complement of cytotoxic cells in the lamina propria.[18,33,34] The relative numbers of the B and T cell, and other leukocytes in the gut differ with antigenic stimulation, the age of the animal, and the sampling site in the intestine (both in luminal versus submucosal and oral versus aboral directions). In the dog, the greatest numbers of IgA-containing cells are found in the duodenum and become less numerous in more caudal parts, with the exception of a rise in number in the colonic lamina propria adjacent to the submucosa. Using an immunoperoxidase assay, the numbers of IgA-containing cells per counting zone (0.1 mm x 0.5 mm of a 6 μm section) in the dog have been reported to range from 68 ± 3.29 (in the apical lamina propria of the duodenum) to 4.21 ± 1.24 (in the apical lamina propria of the colon).[32,35] In human adults, B cells, T cells, and null cells have been reported to make up 25%, 50%, and 25% of the lamina propria lymphoid pool, respectively.[18] In calves the proportions of lymphoid subsets in the lamina propria is similar, with 28% and 45% expressing B and T cell phenotypes, respectively.[36] In diseased mucosa, the number of leukocytes in the lamina propria increases. The IgA isotype usually remains predominant, but the relative numeric increase is largest for the IgG-secreting cells.[3] The lamina propria lymphocytes are intimately involved in all aspects of the immune response, including antigen elimination, oral tolerance, and immune regulation. The lamina propria plasma cells are the source of the majority of the IgA for antigen-specific exclusion.

Macrophages, neutrophils, eosinophils, and mast cells are said to comprise less than 1% of lamina propria leukocytes in the normal human.[18] These lamina propria leukocytes are the cellular basis for gastrointestinal inflammation and serve a variety of other functions, including phagocytosis and antibody-dependent cellular cytotoxicity.

Lamina Propria Mast Cells. Two types of mast cell have been identified in the gut of rats, mice, sheep, and humans (those species in which suitable histochemical techniques have been applied).[37] They have been termed "mucosal" and "connective tissue" mast cells, in recognition of distinctive distributions. The mucosal mast cells are located primarily in the lamina propria, whereas the connective tissue mast cells are located in connective tissues throughout the body. In the bowel, such tissues include the submucosa, muscularis mucosa, and serosa. In rats, connective tissue mast cells predominate in the tongue, esophagus and non-glandular stomach, whereas mucosal mast cells predominate (up to 90%) in the glandular stomach and intestines.[38] It is likely that mast cell polymorphism also occurs in dogs and cats. Mast cells with properties reminiscent of rat mucosal mast cells have been identified in the gastrointestinal tract of the cat.[39]

Precursors of mucosal mast cells are present in Peyer's patches and mesenteric lymph nodes. It is probable that early in the immune response the Peyer's patch supplies the gastrointestinal mucosa with mucosal mast cells in a similar manner to which it supplies mucosal T and B cells.[40] It has recently been established that both types of mast cell are derived from a common lineage and that the cell's phenotypic expression is controlled by microenvironmental factors.[41]

Mucosal mast cells have important functions in the bowel, but the cells have been overlooked, until recent years, because of different staining properties to those of the conventional (connective tissue) mast cells. For instance, after standard formalin fixation, mucosal mast cells fail to stain with Toluidine blue and other stains that are commonly used to identify connective tissue mast cells.[14,42] Mucosal and connective tissue mast cells have different ultrastructure, biological behavior, and perhaps function.[42] Connective tissue mast cells are twice as large as mucosal mast cells, possess single-lobed nuclei, are long-lived, maintain relatively constant levels in tissues, and elaborate prostaglandins (among other mediators) in response to stimulation. In addition, they have many uniform-sized intracytoplasmic granules, have IgE only on their surfaces, and contain high concentrations of heparin and histamine. In contrast, mucosal mast cells are smaller (10 μm), possess unilobed or bilobed nuclei, are shorter lived, proliferate rapidly in response to interleukin 3, and elaborate leukotrienes to a greater degree after stimulation. Mucosal mast cells have fewer, variable-sized intracytoplasmic granules, possess cytoplasmic as well as surface IgE, possess a different type of protease, and contain chondroitin sulfate (not heparin) and only small amounts of histamine. Rat mucosal mast cells are resistant to certain secretagogues and anti-allergic compounds that influence connective tissue mast cells.[38] For instance, significant histamine release from mucosal mast cells will occur following challenge with substance P only, whereas connective tissue mast cells release histamine following challenge with substance P, somatostatin, vasoactive intestinal polypeptide, neurotensin, certain endorphins, and bradykinin. No secretory response by either cell type occurs on exposure to acetylcholine, bombesin, motilin, or pentagastrin. Theophylline and sodium cromoglycolate inhibit antigen-induced histamine secretion by connective tissue mast cells, but not by mucosal mast cells. Corticosteroids inhibit mast cell secretion and can dramatically reduce mast cell numbers in the intestine within 24 hours. Sulfasalazine may also inhibit mast cell secretion.[93] These findings may partly explain the efficacy of these drugs in the therapy of inflammatory bowel disease.

Mast cell discharge is now known to have many more stimuli than just IgE antibody-antigen complexes. The hormones and neuropeptides mentioned above are but some of these stimulating influences. Other known activators include the activated complement fragments C3a and C5a, certain products of macrophages (such as interleukin 1), certain classes of IgG, and a T cell lymphokine.[93] Whether the intestinal mast cell subtype responds to all of these secretagogues remains to be established.

Vagal stimulation also appears to facilitate histamine secretion; interestingly, mast cell secretion can be conditioned to an odor in the same way salivation can be conditioned to bell-ringing.[43] The nervous pathways involved in the conditioned mast cell response have not been determined, but substance P-containing nerves have been demonstrated, closely associated with the intestinal mast cells of rats.[93] These observations raise the possibility that the acute diarrhea manifested by many fearful dogs on presentation to, for instance, veterinary clinics, may result from a substance P mediated, conditioned discharge of the mucosal mast cell.

The functions of mast cells, in general, are complex and considerably more extensive than the mediation of immediate hypersensitivity. They have a role in delayed hypersensitivity, inflammation, smooth muscle contraction, cytotoxicity, angiogenesis, fibrosis, and immunoregulation.[93] How many of these functions are shared by *mucosal* mast cells, in particular, is largely speculative. Mast cell functions are initiated by the release of mediators, of which mast cells contain a wide array. Vasodilation, increased vascular permeability, and inflammation result from the release of directly or indirectly acting vasoactive and inflammatory mediators such as histamine, leukotrienes, platelet activating factor, proteases, and kallikreins.[5,93] The inflammatory properties of these factors are discussed in the section on intestinal inflammation. Certain leukotrienes released by mucosal mast cells, such as leukotriene C4, stimulate contraction of gastrointestinal smooth muscle. Kallikrein-like enzymes have been detected in the gastrointestinal mast cells of cats. A role for kallikrein in the absorption of nutrients and electrolytes has been proposed.[39] Kallikreins also act on kininogens to generate highly vasoactive kinins. Some of the mast cell mediators also have calming or healing effects. Thus, proteases released by canine mast cells are capable of degrading vasoactive intestinal peptide and substance P, two substances with potent effects on glandular secretion and smooth muscle tone.[44] Histamine activation of H_2-receptor-bearing suppressor lymphocytes has been widely demonstrated,[93] an interesting fact considering the suppressor-dominated functions of GALT. Histamine has been shown to induce fibroblast proliferation.[27] Serotonin release by mast cells is known to stimulate jejunal crypt cell renewal.[18]

The products of mast cell discharge may be involved in the pathogenesis of many gastrointestinal diseases. Increased numbers of mucosal mast cells have been noted in inflammatory bowel disease and celiac disease,[4,42] and increased mucosal concentrations of leukotrienes have been demonstrated in inflammatory bowel disease. Mast cell proliferation has been associated with intestinal fibrosis.[93] Mucosal mast cells also appear to be important in the elimination of helminth infections (see immune response to parasites discussed later), and they have a documented role in the pathogenesis of dietary allergies. In addition, release of chemotactic factors may result in the accumulation of eosinophils and neutrophils at sites of inflammation, resulting in the characteristic pathology of such disorders as eosinophilic gastroenteritis.

The recent revelations regarding the many functions of mast cells in addition to their traditional role in immediate hypersensitivity, and the discovery of the differences in mast cell subtype structure, function, and sensitivity to secretagogues and inhibitors of secretion, may prove to alter currently accepted roles of the mast cell in the pathogenesis of bowel disorders and may demand the development of a new range of pharmaceuticals effective in the modulation of mucosal mast cell function.

Duct-Associated Lymphoid Tissue

The duct-associated lymphoid tissue aggregates about glandular ducts. Such lymphoid tissue has been detected about the ducts of salivary tissue of some species, where its secretion of IgA is proposed to play an important role in the defense of the oral cavity.[45] Migration of IgA-bearing lymphocytes from GALT to salivary tissue has also been demonstrated.[46] In contrast to lymphoid nodules and Peyer's patches, M cells have not been demonstrated in DALT, and antigen is said to be exposed to the ductal lymphoid tissue by retrograde passage through the salivary ducts.[45] The significance of DALT in the dog and cat is unknown. Both IgA and IgM have been detected in the saliva of these species.[47,48] The parotid salivary glands of the dog appear to secrete saliva particularly rich in IgA (0.52 mg/ml).[47] Whether these salivary immunoglobulins are locally produced or derived from serum is uncertain. The latter possibility must be given serious consideration in view of the recent demonstration of selective serum IgA and IgM transport into the saliva of sheep by a process thought to be analogous to the way in which IgA is transported into bile.[49]

Mesenteric Lymph Nodes

Lymph nodes are secondary lymphoid organs whose position and structure are designed to facilitate antigen trapping and immune elimination. They are well organized tissues with a clearly defined capsule, cortex, medulla, and afferent and efferent lymphatics.[5] B lymphocytes are arranged into nodules in the cortex and are separated from the medulla by a T cell-rich, paracortical zone. In contrast to GALT, lymph nodes contain numerous plasma cells. These cells are located in the medulla. Lymph enters through the cortex of the node and is directed to the medulla along lymphatic sinuses. Antigen is trapped by mononuclear-phagocyte cells in the medulla or by dendritic cells in the cortex. The macrophages then migrate to the cortex and present the antigen to B and T cells for initiation of the immune response (see description of the mononuclear-phagocyte system).

The structure and function of the mesenteric lymph nodes is similar to that of the peripheral lymph nodes. They are located in the folds of peritoneum attaching the gastrointestinal tract to the body wall and are closely applied to the mesenteric vessels. In the dog, they average 6 x 2 x 0.5 cm. in size and vary in number. The mesenteric lymph nodes (inclusive of colic lymph nodes) drain the jejunum, ileum, cecum, and most of the colon (The duodenum and rectum are drained by the celiac and internal iliac lymph nodes, respectively).[10,23] Lymph leaving the mesenteric nodes enters the intestinal lymphatic trunks, the cisterna chyli, the thoracic duct, and ultimately the venous system.

Mesenteric lymph nodes are involved in the circulation of gut-associated lymphocytes. They are the first port-of-call for these migrant, gut-derived lymphocytes and may, in contrast to the Peyer's patch, provide an environment suitable for maturation of migrant, precursor, IgA-committed B cells into plasma cells. It has also been suggested that the mesenteric nodes amplify the GALT immune response by additional antigen presentation, resulting in further B cell proliferation.[15] Lymphocytes derived from the mesenteric lymph nodes show a tendency to "home" back to the mesenteric lymph nodes and intestinal lamina propria (and to a lesser extent the other mucosal surfaces).[18] Also in contrast to GALT, in response to antigen the mesenteric lymph nodes mount a very vigorous elimination response with little evidence of generation of tolerance. A component of this elimination response is the secretion of immunoglobulins other than IgA. The humoral secretions of the mesenteric lymph nodes contain a much greater proportion of IgG and IgE than do the secretions of GALT. Particularly vigorous immune responses result in hyperplasia of the abdominal lymph nodes. Mesenteric lymphadenopathy is an important diagnostic finding.

The Liver And Gastrointestinal Immunity

The liver serves an important role in gastrointestinal immunity, by virtue of its vast mononuclear-phagocyte system and by the secretion of IgA into bile. In the cat, the liver is a major source of intestinal IgA. IgA is the predominant immunoglobulin in feline bile, followed by IgM, and lastly IgG.[48,50,51] Disagreement exists over the quantity of IgA in canine bile.[5,52]

There are two sources of IgA in bile. The first is a hepatic "IgA pump." A proportion of dimeric IgA produced in the lamina propria of the bowel escapes secretion by the gastrointestinal epithelium and enters the lymphatic, portal, and systemic circulations. This dimeric IgA subsequently binds secretory component present on the surface of the hepatocyte and is transported through the hepatocyte and excreted into the bile.[53] The second source of biliary IgA appears to be local synthesis within the liver. Biliary IgA may have a role to play in local immunity of the biliary tree. In addition, the hepatic "IgA pump" is able to remove IgA-antigen complexes, a mechanism which offers a convenient method of ridding the circulation of food and bacterial antigen-antibody complexes generated in the intestine.[53]

IMMUNE RESPONSE OF THE GUT-ASSOCIATED LYMPHOID TISSUE[5]

The antigen-specific immune response of the gastrointestinal tract is initiated and, to some degree, regulated in the aggregated lymphoid tissues of GALT. The first steps in the initiation of the immune response are those of antigen uptake and presentation. Immunoresponsive cells subsequently undergo a closely regulated clonal expansion to produce precursors of antibody secreting cells and cells involved in cell-mediated immunity, immune memory, and immunoregulation. A peculiar feature of GALT is its predisposition to produce precursors of IgA-secreting plasma cells. Other characteristic features are its propensity to mount immune responses dominated by T cell suppression, and the rapid migration of immune response cells from aggregated lymphoid tissues to mucosal surfaces and lymphoid tissues throughout the body. In these positions the immune response cells are responsible for developing local, secretory immunity and ultimately rendering the entire immune system tolerant to mucosal antigens. This combination of immunity at the mucosal surface and oral tolerance provides effective defense against the complex antigenic environment of the mucosal surfaces.

Antigen Uptake and Presentation in GALT

Luminal antigen reaches GALT either after being "sampled" by the M cells of the Peyer's patches or lymphoid nodules or following invasion of the mucosal barrier. One consequence of a defective mucosal barrier is an alteration in the predominant route by which an antigen is exposed to the immune system. Antigen penetrating the mucosa through the absorptive epithelium bypasses the Peyer's patch and lymphoid nodules and is transported directly to either the mesenteric nodes, via the lymphatics, or the liver, via the mesenteric portal system. The route of exposure of antigen to the immune system may be important in determining the primacy of local versus systemic immunity or immunologic responsiveness versus tolerance.[18]

After penetrating the epithelium, the antigen is trapped by an antigen-presenting cell. In the Peyer's patch and lamina propria the most important antigen-presenting cell is the subepithelial, MHC II positive macrophage. Antigen presentation in both the Peyer's patch and lamina propria is supplemented by dendritic cells.[15] On occasion, B cells, endothelial cells, and epithelial cells can act as antigen-presenting cells following the expression of MHC II antigens on their surfaces. MHC II-positive endothelial cells have been identified in intestinal villi.[3] Epithelial cells may be of importance in the presentation of antigen in the bowel, because it appears that the natural killer-like cells of the intraepithelial lymphocyte compartment can induce or augment, through the release of lymphokines, the expression of MHC II antigens on adjoining epithelial cells, including the epithelial cells of the follicle-associated epithelium.[3,15,25] Mucosal expression of MHC II antigens is strikingly enhanced in many gastrointestinal diseases, suggesting that augmented presentation of antigen may play a role in their pathogenesis.[15] The antigen-presenting cells present the antigen to B cells and neighboring T cells, which together go on to generate the cell-mediated and humoral response.

Cell-Mediated Response of GALT[5]

Effective generation of effector T cells (and antibody) is dependent on the interaction of a T helper cell with an antigen-MHC II complex on the surface of an antigen-presenting cell. Secretion of interleukin 2 from T helper cells stimulates the clonal expansion of effector T cells primed by binding to an antigen-MHC 1 complex on the surface of an antigen-presenting cell (Figure 3-5). Several factors limit this proliferation, including the activity of concomitantly generated suppressor T cells. The stimulated T effector cells can differentiate into a number of populations, including memory cells and cytotoxic cells, and can synthesize numerous biologically active factors called lymphokines.

Cellular Cytotoxicity. Cytotoxic T cells can kill in a specific or nonspecific manner. In the antigen-specific mechanism, the T cell recognizes the inciting antigen in association with MHC 1 antigens on the target cell, adheres to, and perforates the target's membrane via insertion of a tubular structure that results from the polymerization of cytotoxic proteins called perforins. Stimulated cytotoxic T cells can also disrupt neighboring cells in a nonspecific manner by releasing soluble lymphotoxins into the local environment. The cytotoxicity of T cells is augmented by other types of cellular cytotoxicity. These include antibody-dependent cellular cytotoxicity and cell lysis by natural killer cells and activated macrophages.

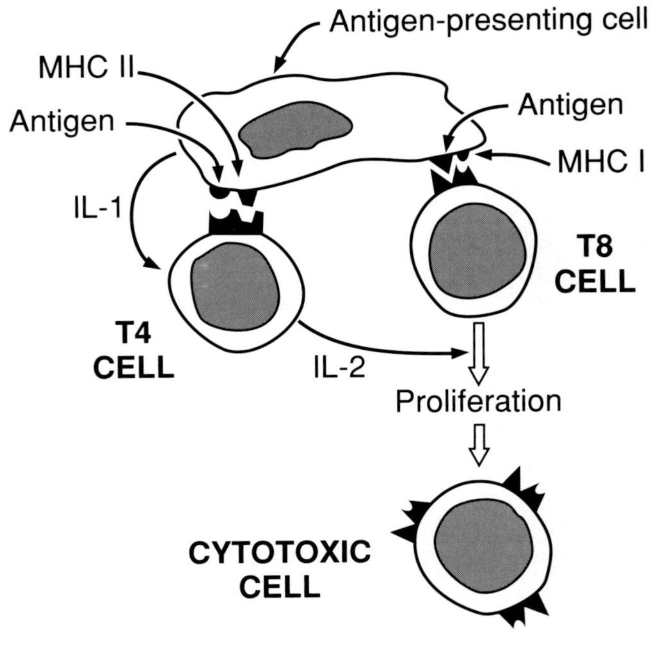

Figure 3-5. Schematic illustrating functions of macrophage in cellular and humoral immunity. T_4 and T_8 cells are helper and cytotoxic cells, respectively. From reference 5.

Antibody-dependent cellular cytotoxicity is mediated by leukocytes with receptors for immunoglobulin. These cells bind to antibody-coated cells and lyse them. Leukocytes capable of antibody-dependent cellular cytotoxicity include neutrophils, macrophages, eosinophils, and a population of non-B, non-T ("null") lymphocytes called killer cells. Antibody-dependent cellular cytotoxicity can enhance the cytotoxic capability of cells, such as the leukocytes of the inflammatory response. There is evidence to suggest that IgA is an effective antibody for this process.[15]

Natural killer cells are "null" lymphocytes that are similar to killer cells but may be functionally differentiated in that they do not require antibody for activity. They do have immunoglobulin receptors, however, and thus can participate in antibody-dependent cellular cytotoxicity. Natural killer cells have cytotoxicity against a wide range of cells including virus-infected, neoplastic and foreign cells. They are activated by interferon. Natural killer-like cells are a particularly important subpopulation of the bowel epithelium.

Macrophages may become cytotoxic when activated by T cell lymphokines, most notably interferon. They are cytotoxic to microorganisms and tumor cells. The lamina propria contains significant numbers of macrophages.

Cell-mediated cytotoxicity helps eliminate pathogens that penetrate the mucosal barrier and is critical to the destruction of neoplastic and, perhaps, dysplastic cells. Eosinophil-mediated, antibody-dependent cellular cytotoxicity is important in the elimination of helminths in the bowel lumen. Lysis of virus-infected cells by natural killer-like cells may be a particularly notable first-line defence of the bowel against enteroviruses.

Cell-mediated cytotoxicity, however, may also be important in the pathogenesis of bowel disorders. Chronic inflammation and immunoreactivity damage tissue by release of inflammatory products and by self-directed cytotoxicity. The self-directed cytotoxicity results from the nonspecific cytotoxicity of soluble mediators released by T cells and macrophages. In addition, on occasion cytotoxic cells will directly and specifically lyse self-tissue. The mechanisms for such autoimmunity are poorly understood but appear to be partly explained by the development of anti-epithelial cell antibodies, capable of arming cells for antibody-dependent cellular cytotoxicity, and by alterations of target cell, surface glycoproteins during the course of inflammation.[54,55] These specific and nonspecific mechanisms of tissue destruction are known to play an important role in the pathogenesis of inflammatory bowel disease.

Lymphokines. The activated T cell is capable of secreting a large number of lymphokines other than the cytotoxins. These lymphokines have immunoregulatory and inflammatory functions. One group of lymphokines is the interferons, which are responsible for an impressive array of immunoregulatory effects, including the activation of macrophages and the inhibition of macrophage migration, the inhibition of tumor cell growth, and the enhancement of both suppressor and cytotoxic T cell activities. Another important group of lymphokines is the interleukins. Interleukins 1 (a monokine) and 2 are particularly important in the generation of the early events of the immune response. Interleukin 3 encourages the maturation of immature T cells and the proliferation of mucosal mast cell populations. T cells regulate B cell immunoglobulin isotype, proliferation and differentiation through the release of isotype switch factor(s), and growth and differentiation factors, all of probable importance to the development of secretory (IgA) immunity.

Activated lymphocytes are responsible for the production of a macrophage chemotactic factor, a macrophage fusion factor, and a fibroblast stimulation factor, which contribute to the development of the granulomatous inflammation and fibrosis characteristic of some chronic bowel and liver diseases. T cells may be responsible for the villus atrophy and crypt hyperplasia that occurs in many enteropathies. Certainly, in experimental helminthiasis and giardiasis of rodents and intestinal allograft transplantation in dogs, such pathologic changes appear to be T cell mediated.[56] The mucosal mast cell is also capable of stimulating crypt cell division. The increased cellular turnover may help rid the body of pathogens adherent to the epithelium. The shortened villi reduce epithelial absorptive area, a process which, although resulting in nutrient malabsorption, may reduce additional mucosal ingress of pathological substances.

Suppressor Cells. Generation of suppressor T cell activity is an integral part of the immune response. The activity of suppressor cells is engendered in a similar manner to that of helper cells, but different antigenic epitopes vary in their ability to stimulate suppressor or helper activities. Suppressor T cells inhibit immune responses by releasing soluble suppressor factors. Some of these factors restrain antigen-specific responses, but others are antigen-nonspecific. Macrophages may also function as suppressor cells by releasing prostaglandin E_2. This eicosanoid inhibits lymphocyte proliferation and differentiation and restrains the secretion of interleukin 2 and the lymphokines involved in the accumulation and activation of macrophages, thus providing a possible mechanism by which granulomatous inflammation can be self-regulated. The role of prostaglandin E_2 in the bowel, however, is far from defined. Suppressor B cells have also been detected.

Cellular-dependent immune suppression is an integral part of immunoregulation and an important component of the phenomenon of "oral tolerance." It assumes particular importance in tissues such as the gastrointestinal tract in which the elimination of antigen, an important means of switching off the immune response, is often incomplete. Therefore, it is not surprising that one of the characteristic features of GALT is a predisposition to mount immune responses dominated by T cell suppression rather than T cell help. Recently, this function has been shown to involve the generation of suppressor T cell cascades which are capable of generating both cells and factors having widespread negative effects on the local and systemic immune systems, but which largely spare the secretion of IgA.[54,57] A failure to express adequate T cell suppression of GALT's elimination response to luminal antigens is currently thought to be important in the genesis of inflammatory bowel disease,[54] and may play a role in certain dietary allergies.[54] Defects of cell-mediated immune suppression have also been reported in human chronic active hepatitis and primary biliary cirrhosis.[12]

B Cell Differentiation and Immunoglobulin Isotype Regulation

In clear contrast to the systemic lymphoid tissues, most of the B cells in GALT bear the IgA immunoglobulin isotype and are committed to differentiate into clones of IgA-secreting plasma cells. This phenomenon appears due to the influence of T cells, specific for IgA responses, that act at multiple levels of B cell differentiation.[8,58] GALT contains regulatory T cells that induce the majority of the immature IgM-bearing B cells present in the aggregated lymphoid tissues to switch to immature, IgA-bearing, IgA-committed lymphocytes.[8,58] (IgM is the isotype normally present on immature, isotype-uncommitted B cells). These so-called "switch" T cells have been demonstrated in Peyer's patches but may also occur in lymphoid nodules and the lamina propria.[15,58] It is speculated that they induce isotype switching by release of a lymphokine that affects the course of DNA recombinations within the B lymphocyte. Recent evidence suggests that some of these switch cells may also contribute to the clonal expansion of IgA-committed B cells.[59]

A second proposal, to explain the predominance of IgA-committed B cells in GALT, suggests that the Peyer's patch (or lamina propria) provides a microenvironment in which antigen (such as lipopolysaccharide) can stimulate B cell proliferation but not differentiation. The proliferation leads to conventional, T cell-independent, sequential isotype switching from IgM to IgG to IgA due to repeated recombinations within the B cell genome, which eventually result in a disproportionate expression of the gene coding for IgA.[8,15,60]

It has been suggested that isotype switching and proliferation of gut B cells is not restricted to the aggregated tissues of GALT, but that it can also occur in the lamina propria. In addition, it has been proposed that in the lamina propria both of the aforementioned putative isotype switching pathways are active and contribute to isotype-switching and proliferation of poorly differentiated Peyer's patch derived B cells.[3,15]

Isotype-specific T cells whose primary function is regulation of the response of the is*otype-committed* B cells have also been identified in GALT.[8,58] The majority of these isotype-specific regulatory T cells provide help for those B cells committed to IgA production.[8,58] A small number of isotype-specific T cells regulate the response of those primitive B cells that either retain their surface IgM or go on to bear IgE or IgG.[4,8] These regulatory cells tend to suppress, rather than encourage, development of IgG-, IgM- or IgE-committed cells. In addition to helper and suppressor T cells, contrasuppressor T cells have been identified in GALT. While these cells have a role in the immunoregulation of GALT, recent work has shown no evidence of isotype specificity of the contrasuppressor T cells.[58] This finding suggests that, contrary to previous suggestions, IgA contrasuppression is not the primary reason for IgA dominance in GALT. Rather, IgA dominance results from both the "switch" cell conversion of early, isotype-uncommitted B cells to IgA-committed B cells and from preferential help of these IgA-committed B cells by IgA-specific regulatory T cells.[58]

When antigen is presented to the lymphoid tissues of GALT, the regulatory T cells bind to the MHC II-foreign antigen complex on the surface of the antigen-presenting cell and undergo clonal expansion (Figure 3-6). A helper, suppressor, and contrasuppressor response is generated. The suppressor response is essential to "oral tolerance." The helper response is required for an immune elimination response.

Under the influence of interleukin 1 secreted by the antigen-presenting cell, the helper regulatory cells begin secretion of stimulatory lymphokines (presumably interleukin 2 and B cell growth factor). The combined influence of interleukin 1 and the T helper-derived lymphokines encourages the proliferation of an antigen-specific clone of isotype-committed B cells that have been previously primed by binding to the foreign antigen. As the B cells divide, they are thought to be further influenced by other T cell lymphokines (B cell differentiation factors); the result is the terminal differentiation of the isotype-committed B cells into memory cells or plasma cells capable of secreting immunoglobulin specific for the inciting antigen. For these reasons, by far the majority of GALT-derived, isotype-committed B cells are stimulated to differentiate into plasma cells that produce IgA. The IgA is specific for the inciting antigen.

The sequence of events just described is not the only pathway for antibody production. For example, some antigens do not require the cooperation of T cells to achieve humoral immunity, but these are the exception rather than the rule. T-independent antigens tend to be large molecules with repeating antigenic determinants. One example, of relevance to the gastrointestinal tract, is lipopolysaccharide. Lipopolysaccharide from the cell wall of E. co*li* can function as a polyclonal activator of B cells. Thus, it can cause nonspecific B cell proliferation (perhaps important for the generation of B cells expressing IgA).

Little IgA secretion occurs in the Peyer's patch itself. Instead, the terminal differentiation of the IgA-committed B cells occurs later, either on route to, or at, distant lymphoid or mucosal sites. Several possibilities have been put forward to explain the lack of IgA secretion in the Peyer's patch. It has been proposed that the IgA-secreting precursors emigrate rapidly from GALT prior to their maturation to IgA-secreting cells.[3,19] An alternative explanation is provided by the discovery in the Peyer's patch of IgA-specific suppressor T cells.[61] Thus, terminal differentiation of IgA-committed B cells may occur only in tissues with an appropriate helper-to-suppressor T cell ratio.[18] It has been proposed, furthermore, that helper T cells responsible for elaboration of B cell differentiation factors are preferentially located in tissues other than GALT, for instance the mesenteric lymph nodes.[62]

Lymphocyte Migration and the Mucosal Immune Network

After interaction with antigen, lymphocytes leave the Peyer's patch and lymphoid nodule and begin a migration that carries them through intestinal lymphatics, mesenteric lymph nodes, spleen, thoracic duct, and blood vasculature and deposits them, three to six days later, in mucosal tissues throughout the body (Figure 3-3). The majority of lymphocytes derived from GALT or mesenteric nodes will return to the lamina propria of that segment of the gut that generated them, but a proportion will localize in respiratory, reproductive, salivary, and lacrimal mucosal tissues.[3,4] This migration has led to the concept of a mucosal immunologic network which, through inter-mucosa transfer of immunologically competent cells and humoral secretions, specifically protects the body surfaces against pathogenic organisms or materials capable of multiple portal entry.[4] The mucosal tissues probably also receive a minor contribution from peripheral lymph nodes and spleen facilitating integration between the systemic and mucosal immune systems.[3]

It has become apparent that a number of the cellular components of GALT are capable of this migration. The first recognized and best studied migratory cell is the B cell. Other migratory cells are T cells and perhaps mast cells. In addition, any epithelial surface bearing the receptors for secretory component (such as salivary gland and liver) may assimilate IgA produced in the bowel and transport it into that organ's secretions.

B Lymphocyte Migration. The majority of B cells activated by antigen and T cell lymphokines in GALT begin migration as undifferentiated, IgA-committed lymphocytes. A major subpopulation of these lymphocytes undergoes considerable differentiation as it migrates. When the lymphocytes reach the mesenteric lymph nodes, approximately one-half are IgA-containing lymphoblasts. In the thoracic duct, the proportion increases further. The B cells that enter the lamina propria from peripheral blood are heterogenous, comprising a variable number of IgM-, IgG-, and IgA-bearing lymphocytes, as well as the IgA-containing lymphoblasts.[3,15] Further antigen-driven, IgA-B cell proliferation of substantial magnitude, including isotype switching, apparently continues in the lamina propria and eventurally leads to a 70%-90% dominance of lamina propria lymphocytes by IgA-containing lymphoblasts or plasma cells.[3,15] There is evidence for mucosal migration of small number of IgM- and IgG-bearing lymphocytes.[4] The extent and significance of this migration is poorly defined.

The stimulus for this mucosal homing is unknown. Sug-

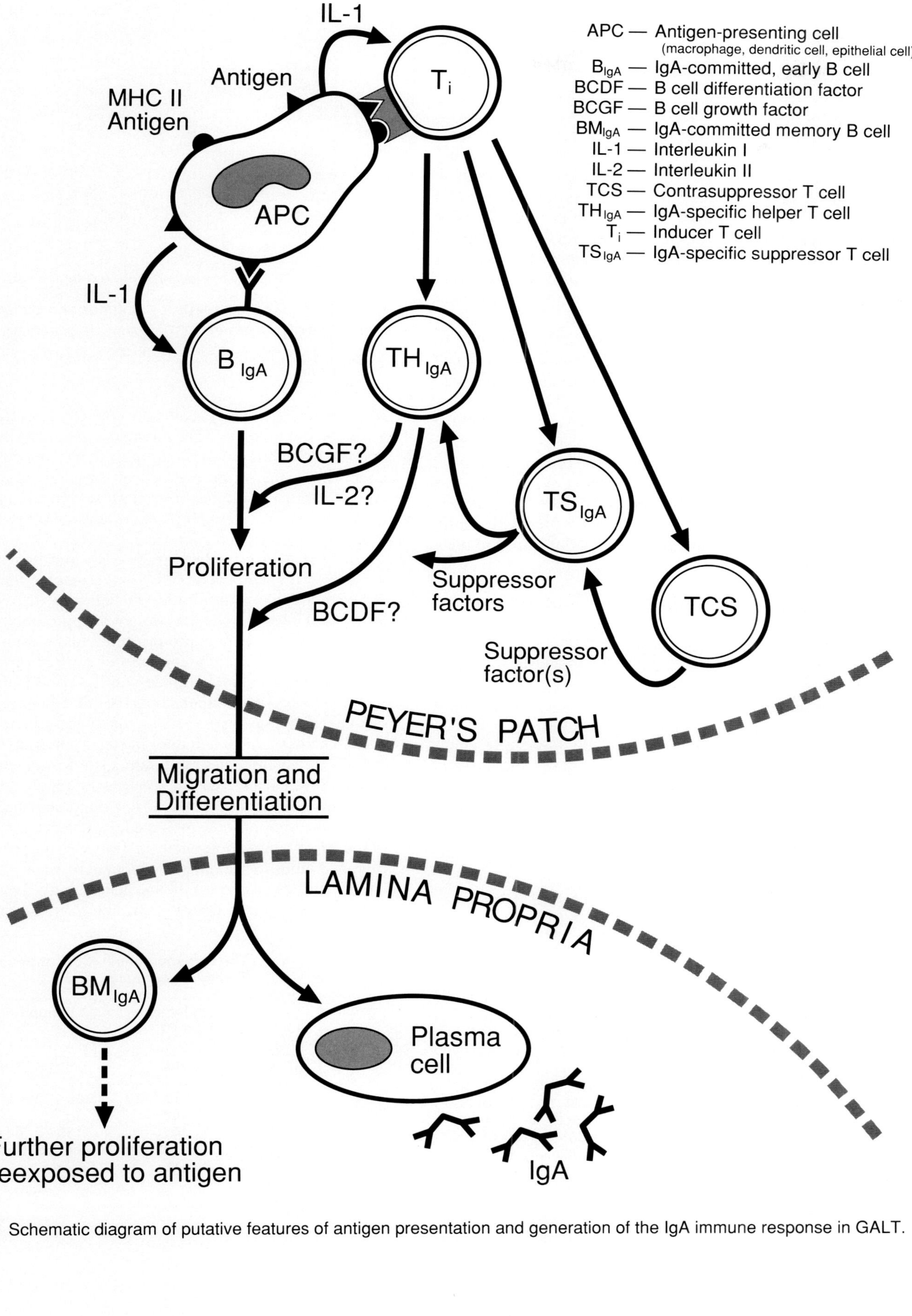

Figure 3-6. Schematic diagram of putative features of antigen presentation and generation of the IgA immune response in GALT.

gested factors have included receptor affinities for mucosal endothelial determinants, variations in blood flow, and epithelial chemotactic factors.[15] In contrast to earlier work, recent studies suggest that the homing of gut-derived lymphocytes to the lamina propria is largely antigen driven,[15] but this issue is far from resolved.

T Lymphocyte Migration. There is accumulating evidence that T lymphocytes migrate in a similar manner to B cells, albeit in smaller numbers. Reinjection of T lymphoblasts derived from mesenteric lymph nodes or thoracic duct results in their selective lodging in the bowel lamina propria and, unlike B cells, bowel epithelium.[4,14] The relative proportions of T suppressor and T helper subtypes is unknown, but members of both subsets appear to migrate. The migration of suppressor cells to lymphoid tissues throughout the body, in addition to mucosal surfaces, is considered important in the development of oral tolerance. The migration of helper subsets may be important for the proliferation and differentiation of B cells in the lamina propria. The homing of T cells to GALT and mesenteric nodes can be reduced by their prior incubation with vasointestinal polypeptide, an observation pertinent to the discussion of the neuroendocrine modulation of the immune system.[63]

Mast Cell Migration. The possibility of analogous mast cell migration has been proposed.[3,4] Some support for this hypothesis is provided by the observation that Peyer's patches, lamina propria, and mesenteric nodes all have significantly greater mucosal mast cell precursor populations than do bone marrow and spleen.[40]

IgA: Properties, Secretion, Assay and Function[3,5]

IgA Properties and Secretion. IgA is the predominant immunoglobulin in most, but not all, of the body secretions of cats and dogs(Table 3-1 and 3-2).[47,48] It is the second most abundant immunoglobulin in the serum of cats and the third most abundant in the serum of dogs (most studies).

IgA is a carbohydrate-rich immunoglobulin that is distinguished by its propensity to form dimers and to combine with an epithelial transmembrane protein called "secretory component." The IgA monomer has a structure like that of the other immunoglobulin monomers; it consists of two heavy chains linked together by disulfide bonds and two shorter light chains

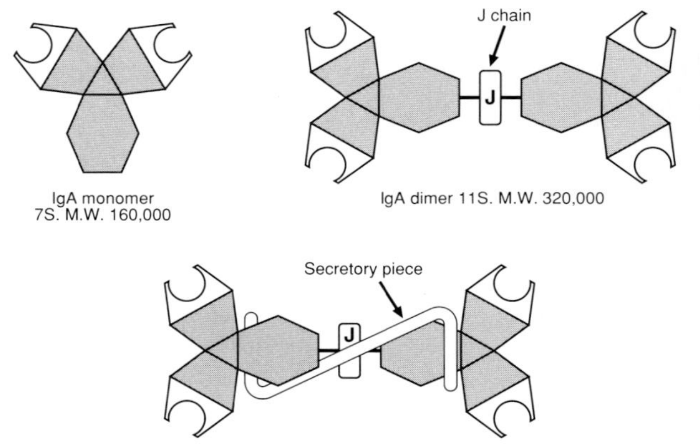

Figure 3-7. Structure of IgA monomer and dimer formed by interaction of monomers with J chain. Secretory piece is added before the dimer can attach to mucosal surface.(From Fig. 12-4. Reference 5).

attached to one end of each heavy chain by disulfide linkages, as shown in Figure 3-7. The molecular weight of the monomer is about 160,000 daltons. Monomeric IgA is found only in small quantities in the serum and is probably derived largely from IgA-secreting cells in the bone marrow.[64] In contrast to that in humans, almost all serum IgA in the dog and cat is dimeric, and most of this is derived from GALT.[31,65]

The major form of IgA produced by intestinal plasma cells is a dimer. It is composed of two immunoglobulin monomers linked by either a single joining (J) chain or perhaps by a J-chain dimer, and it has a molecular weight of approximately 320,000 daltons.[15] The J chain is produced by mucosal immunocytes, regardless of the immunoglobulin class they produce. However, J chain does not combine with IgG and is therefore not secreted by IgG plasma cells but is degraded intracellularly.[3] It is a 15,000 dalton peptide chain, that is disulfide-linked to the heavy chains of the IgA dimer. The incorporation of the J chain into the dimer furnishes the binding site for secretory component and is thus an essential prerequisite for secretion.[15]

The plasma cell releases the IgA dimer into the interstitium of the lamina propria. A small quantity enters the portal system or intestinal lymphatics, but the majority diffuses to the epithelium and binds to secretory component on the basal and basolateral surface of the epithelial cell (Figure 3-8). Secretory component is an 85,000-95,000 dalton glycoprotein that is

Table 3-1 The Immunoglobulin Concentrations of Feline Body Fluids

Specimen	Mean values and range of immunoglobulin levels (mg/dl)		
	IgG	IgA	IgM
Serum	1894 (1171-2258)	285 (203-582)	247 (60-390)
Colostrum	3570 (2750-4674)	254 (50-488)	110 (31-300)
Milk	189 (95-255)	13 (9-20)	20 (10-40)
Saliva	2 (0-6)	7 (3-20)	3 (0-12)
Nasal secretion	5 (0-39)	7 (3-29)	2 (0-15)
Tracheal fluid	20 (0-146)	42 (0-156)	11 (0-34)
Tear	2 (0-17)	14 (5-33)	4 (0-12)
Bile	11 (3-41)	46 (18-89)	54 (6-96)
Fecal fluid	3 (0-20)	35 (10-84)	34 (0-234)

From Reference 48.

Table 3-2 The Immunoglobulin Concentrations of Canine Body Fluids

Specimen	Mean values and range of immunoglobulin levels (mg/dl)		
	IgG	IgA	IgM
Serum	980 (520-1730	50 (20-120)	170 (70-270)
Colostrum	1200	285	15
Milk	10	130	15
Saliva	2 (0-5)	52 (17-125)	3 (1-7)
Bowel fluid	20	300	60

From Reference 47.

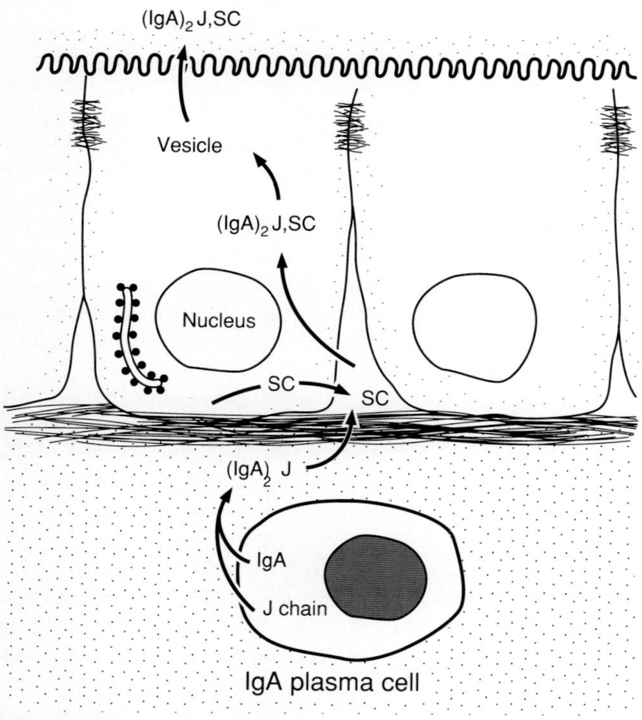

Figure 3-8. Schematic of secretion of IgA into the intestinal lumen. IgA = immunoglobulin A, J = joining chain, SC = secretory component.

synthesized by the epithelial cells of the intestine and some other tissues. In human small intestine it is produced primarily by the epithelial cells in the intestinal crypts, whereas in the colon it is generally also present in the surface epithelium.[3] Altered distribution and quantity of secretory component has been observed in a number of diseases in humans, the significance of which is unknown.[3] The synthesis of secretory component is independent of IgA synthesis. Thus, individuals with IgA deficiency can produce secretory component, and people with secretory component deficiency can produce IgA.[18] Deficient secretory component secretion has been proposed as a rare cause of failed secretory immunity and severe diarrhea in humans.[3] Secretory component occupies a transmembrane position and acts as a receptor for the J chain-containing IgA dimer. The binding stimulates pinocytosis by the epithelial cell, and the IgA-receptor complex is packaged into vesicles for transport to the apical epithelial surface. Here the vesicle fuses with the plasma membrane and the dimeric IgA-secretory-component-complex is released into the bowel lumen. This complex of secretory component, J chain and dimeric IgA is called secretory IgA (sIgA). It has a molecular weight of approximately 390,000 daltons. Secretory component stabilizes the dimeric IgA within the intestinal lumen. This appears to result from disulfide and non-covalent bridging of the secretory component to the IgA dimer and the resultant protection of the constant region of the IgA molecule from proteolysis by either bacteria or endogenous digestive enzymes.[5,15]

The secretion rate of IgA in humans has been estimated to be 0.78 g/meter of intestine/day. In the fasting dog, a rate of 0.25 g/meter/day has been suggested.[47] The canine vascular IgA pool has a daily turnover of 75%,[52] presumably due to a combination of hepatic catabolism and resecretion into the bowel via the liver and, perhaps, salivary tissue.

Regulation of IgA Secretion. The regulation of IgA secretion by IgA-committed lymphocytes is largely dependent on properties of the inciting antigen and on the cell-mediated immune response of GALT. Ingested antigen, permeable to the epithelium, incites a closely regulated immune response; this results in the generation of large numbers of mucosal plasma cells, that, for their short life-span of three to six days, secrete large quantities of secretory immunoglobulins. The secretory immune response continues while the antigen remains in the lumen and declines if the antigen is eliminated. The local humoral response is much more persistent and vigorous if antigen is presented locally rather than systemically. Regulation of the secretory immune response is also partly dependent upon non-immunologic mechanisms.[5,18] These regulatory influences include the genetic make-up of the host and non-specific immunosuppressive factors such as histamine (via H_2 receptors). The autonomic nervous system seems to facilitate gastrointestinal IgA secretion in coordination with the presence of swallowed antigens. In addition, substance P release has been reported to enhance IgA production by GALT; VIP decreases IgA secretion but increases IgM; somatostatin decreases IgA production;[66,67] and secretin appears to increase the luminal concentrations of both IgA and IgG.[18]

IgA Assay. In the serum of dogs, a wide range of IgA concentrations has been reported. These differences result largely from variations in the assay technique used and from discrepancies in the ages of dogs included in the reference population. Most laboratories utilize a single radial immunodiffusion technique. Important potential sources of assay-related discrepancy include the use of different forms of IgA as the standards and the utilization of disparate formulae to interpret the precipitation rings.[68] The time at which serum IgA concentrations reach adult levels is poorly defined, but by twelve months of age most dogs appear to have IgA concentrations within or approaching the adult range (Table 3-3).[69] Two recent reports suggest that by 16-17 weeks of age there is sufficient IgA in the serum of normal animals to allow differentiation between dogs with normal concentrations of IgA and those that are deficient.[69,70] A generous adult canine serum IgA reference range, which incorporates the extremes of the ranges of most publications, is 20-150 mg/dl. It is important, however, that whenever possible the clinician utilizes the reference range provided by his or her own laboratory and that he or she uses age-matched data.

Table 3-3 Serum IgA Concentrations (mg/dl) in Healthy Beagles

AGE	Mean IgA Concentration	95% Confidence Interval
4-6 months	36	18-56
12 months	63	24-166
24 months	58	34-147

From Reference 69

Table 3-4 Serum IgA Concentrations (mg/dl) in Healthy Cats

AGE	Environment	Mean	Range
Adults	Cattery	285	102-582
Adults	Cattery	175	35-500
Adults	SPF*	277	42-600
0.5-1.5 years	Household	71	25-188
1 year	SPF	33	30-50
14 weeks	SPF	22	12-30
12 weeks	SPF	123	30-254

*SPF = specific pathogen free
From References 48, 50, 84

The assay of serum IgA concentration in cats is affected by similar factors as those which affect that of the dog. By six to nine months of age the total serum protein and gamma globulin concentrations of cats rises to adult levels.[31] The environment of the cat has been shown to affect the serum IgA concentration (Table 3-4).[50]

Secretory IgA can be measured in intestinal content. Total immunoglobulin concentration in canine intestinal fluid was found to range from 110-810 mg/dl, with a mean of 380 mg/dl. On average, 80% (300 mg/dl) of this immunoglobulin was IgA, 15% (60 mg/dl) was IgM and 5% (20 mg/ml) was IgG. The concentration of IgA in canine feces ranges from 80-540 mg/dl with a mean of 300 mg/dl.[85] IgA also has been detected in the feces of cats and it appears that bile may make a significant contribution to intestinal IgA levels in this species.[48] After extraction from feces by centrifugation with an equal weight of PBS, feline fecal fluid had an average IgA concentration of 35 mg/dl with a range of 10-84 mg/dl.[48]

Because the serum IgA of the dog and cat is predominantly derived from intestinal plasma cell secretion, more so than humans, serum concentrations of IgA in general reflect the quantitative adequacy of the intestinal secretory IgA response. An obvious exception occurs, however, in the presence of defective intestinal epithelial transport of IgA. Rare cases of proposed secretory component deficiency in humans, in which normal serum levels of IgA were present but sIgA and secretory component were undetectable in saliva and intestinal fluid, have been reported.[3] Therefore, the measurement of sIgA in feces or intestinal secretions may be of occasional benefit. Another assessment of intestinal sIgA quantity can be made by immunohistochemical demonstration of immunoglobulin-containing cells in the lamina propria. Caution is necessary when interpreting the results of intestinal histochemistry, however, because IgA-bearing B cells are found in the blood, and presumably tissues, of many IgA-deficient humans;[71] this implies that the primary reason for selective IgA deficiency in some humans is a defect in the final maturation of B cells to plasma cells capable of secreting IgA. Both defective final maturation of plasma cells, or deficient epithelial transport of IgA could lead to a situation where the mucosa contains IgA-positive cells but the secretion of IgA into bowel lumen is defective.

IgA Function and Consequences of IgA Deficiency. Intestinal sIgA has been likened to an antiabsorptive "paint." Its primary function is to facilitate exclusion of specific bacterial, viral, and macromolecular antigens from the mucosa by preventing antigen-mucosal adherence. This blocking of mucosal adherence is not a specific function of IgA molecules, for immunoglobulins of the other classes share the ability. However, these other immunoglobulins, with the exception of secretory IgM (sIGM), cannot function in the intestinal lumen because they are unable to resist proteolytic degradation. Secretory IgA may also augment the nonspecific mechanisms of mucosal defense. It has been established, for example, that proteolysis of intestinal antigens is considerably greater in immunized animals than in nonimmunized controls, and it has been suggested that this enhancement results from interaction in the intestinal mucus coat of antigen-antibody complexes with pancreatic enzymes.[72]

Dimeric IgA in the lamina propria contributes to the elimination of mucosal antigen by facilitation of antibody-dependent macrophage cytotoxicity of bacteria[3,26] and by the rapid hepatic clearance of those IgA-antigen complexes that enter the vasculature and lymphatics.[25] However, IgA, in contrast to IgG, is not efficient at the fixation of complement and does not facilitate opsonization by tissue phagocytes. When IgA binds to antigen within the mucosa, it blocks the binding of IgG and therefore inhibits the phlogistic consequences of IgG-antigen complexes and IgG-facilitated phagocytosis.[26] The action of IgA in the mucosa may thus be likened to that of a "wet blanket" which suppresses the development of excessive gastrointestinal inflammation during mucosal antigen elimination.

Local humoral immunity is of known importance in some coronavirus infections, such as transmissible gastroenteritis of swine, in which serum IgG provides no protection. Some evidence suggests this is also true for canine coronavirus.[73] Local IgA production has been shown to occur in canine parvovirus infection, and IgA-deficient dogs appear more susceptible to parvovirus infection.[69] Specific IgA synthesized against macromolecules prevents damage by enterotoxins and prevents absorption of dietary antigens. When secretory IgA is deficient, there is an increase in the circulating levels of dietary and bacterial antigens and the appearance of abnormal immune-mediated responses from the prolonged activation of the systemic immune system.

The functions of IgA are further revealed by the disease associations of those people and animals deficient in IgA, although the accuracy of these conclusions is obscured to some degree by the increase in IgM secretion that commonly accompanies IgA deficiency, perhaps as a compensatory response. Selective IgA deficiency is the most common primary immunodeficiency in humans. Many of these IgA deficient people are asymptomatic, but predispositions to a number of diseases have been identified. Infectious gastrointestinal disease and malabsorption syndrome occur,[20,69] and cases of ulcerative colitis and regional enteritis associated with IgA deficiency also have been reported.[74] Disease associations in other body systems include upper respiratory infections, pneumonia, recurrent skin and urinary tract infections, allergies, and autoimmune diseases such as rheumatoid arthritis, SLE, and chronic active hepatitis.[75] In dogs, selective deficiencies of serum IgA levels have been reported in Beagles,[69] German Shepherds,[68] and Sharpeis.[70] Diseases associated with this deficiency are similar to those of humans and include increased incidence of parvovirus, chronic small intestinal disease, and respiratory and ear infections.[68-70]

Secretion and Function of IG Other Than IgA

The other classes of immunoglobulins are also present in the lamina propria. Some of this non-IgA immunoglobulin is produced in the lamina propria, although most comes from the plasma. To some degree, all classes of immunoglobulins that enter the gut can be derived from circulating levels. High blood levels of IgA that come from myelomas have been shown to enter the gut and become attached to the mucosa by molecules of secretory piece. While quantitatively small compared to the large quantities of IgA produced, these other immunoglobulin idiotypes are still important to the defense of the mucosa. Rather than a first line defense primarily directed at antigen exclusion (the major function of IgA), they become important when the epithelial barrier is broached. They defend the body by the processes of opsonization, complement fixation, and encouragement of an inflammatory response, all properties unshared by IgA. They also play an important role in the reaction to helminth parasites.

Immunoglobulin M. IgM is a 900,000 dalton, pentameric aggregate of the basic Y-shaped immunoglobulin molecule. The immunoglobulin monomers are bound by disulfide bonds, and two of the subunits are linked by a J chain. IgM is the predominant immunoglobulin produced in the systemic primary immune response. In addition, IgM can bind to secretory component and is excreted through epithelia via the same intracellular route as IgA.[3] IgM is found in large quantities in feline serum, bile, intestinal fluid, colostrum, and milk (Tables 3-1 and 3-2). In the dog, it reaches its highest concentrations in serum and intestinal fluid. In both species it has also been detected in most other body secretions; in most of these, it is the second most abundant immunoglobulin after IgA.

IgM is highly efficient at complement fixation, virus neutralization, opsonization, and agglutination of particulate antigen. Through these mechanisms it takes part in both antigen elimination and antigen exclusion in the gastrointestinal tract. In comparison to sIgA, however, sIgM is more rapidly degraded in the intestinal lumen.[15]

Immunoglobulin G. Immunoglobulin G is a monomeric immunoglobulin. It has a molecular weight of 180,000 daltons. IgG is the predominant immunoglobulin produced in an anamnestic systemic immune response. It does not bind to secretory component and so is not actively extruded into body secretions. Its small size relative to the other immunoglobulins, however, results in passive extravasation of small quantities of IgG into most of the body secretions (Tables 3-1 and 3-2). This leakage is markedly accelerated if inflammation or hypersensitivity responses increase vascular permeability.

IgG is the dominant antibody in serum and colostrum of both the dog and the cat. It will readily activate complement, facilitate antibody-dependent cellular cytotoxicity, and opsonize and agglutinate particulate antigen. The phlogistic properties of IgG result from the fixation of complement and the facilitation of phagocytosis. The complement cascade spawns a number of complement fragments that attract inflammatory cells and result in mast cell degranulation. Phagocytosis ultimately results in cell death and release of enumerable inflammatory mediators. Together these influences generate inflammation, with all its consequences.

An important function for IgG in the defense of the normal intestine is doubtful because of low luminal concentrations and rapid degradation. However, IgG may play an important role in diseases characterized by inflammation and increased permeability. Following prolonged gastrointestinal inflammation, IgG-containing cells increase dramatically in the lamina propria, and IgG antibodies to intestinal tissue may be demonstrated.[3,76] Two examples of diseases in which IgG does contribute to the disease process are helminthiasis and inflammatory bowel disease.

Immunoglobulin E. IgE is a monomeric immunoglobulin with a molecular weight of 196,000 daltons. Its existence in the cat is suspected but not convincingly established.[31,50] IgE possess a unique ability to bind to mast cells and basophils. It is found in very low concentrations in serum and can be detected in intestinal fluid and feces. It is rapidly degraded in the intestinal lumen.[15]

IgE-containing lymphocytes may be found in skin, mucous membranes, mesenteric nodes and spleen. It appears that, under appropriate stimuli, Peyer's patches may generate precursor IgE cells which migrate to the lymphoid tissues associated with the bowel.[3] The origin of gastrointestinal mucosal IgE is uncertain. The local synthesis of IgE by plasma cells in the lamina propria may contribute a small quantity of IgE to the mucosa. The possibility that some of the mucosal IgE might also be derived from IgE-containing mucosal mast cells must be considered.[15] It appears, however, that the major site of production of intestinal IgE, at least in the parasite-infected rat, is the mesenteric lymph nodes, which secrete the immunoglobulin into the lymphatics, from where it eventually reaches the mucosa via the blood stream.[18,77] IgE does not bind to secretory component, and so the small quantities of IgE found in intestinal secretions is presumed to derive from passive exudation from the vasculature and mucosa.

IgE is the antibody of anaphylaxis and immediate hypersensitivity. When antigen binds to the IgE molecules on mast cells and basophils in an appropriate manner, they are stimulated to degranulate. This results in the release of a large number of inflammatory mediators. Immediate hypersensitivities presumably enhance elimination of the inciting antigen from the mucosa, but the increased permeability that accompanies the response results in the increased absorption of unrelated macromolecules, and the severity of the reaction is an occasional cause of the signs of food allergy. IgE is also important in the defense against parasites. Luminal concentrations of IgE are known to increase in both parasitic infections and food allergies.[78]

Oral Tolerance[5,79]

Immunologic tolerance is a specific immune response to one or more antigenic determinants; it results in a reduced or absent humoral or cell-mediated elimination response to the inciting antigenic determinants. Tolerance manifests as nonreactivity, but it is important not to equate this with a total lack of an immune response. On the contrary, tolerance is an active, on-going arm of the "specific immune response," which instead of resulting in antigen elimination results in its tolerance. Like other forms of the specific immune response, tolerance will decline unless antigen is re-exposed. Tolerance is essential to life. It is the mechanism by which immunoreactivity to self-tissue is prevented. That is, autoimmunity results from a loss of tolerance.

Immunologic tolerance can develop if antigen is exposed to the immune system in too great an amount or too small an amount. It will occur if antigen evades antigen-presenting cells and comes in premature contact with lymphocytes, or if antigen is inadequately presented by the antigen-presenting cells. Similarly, exposure of antigen to animals with an immature immune system usually results in tolerance. In addition, some antigens contain antigenic determinants that, for poorly understood reasons, have an intrinsic ability to generate T suppressor rather than T helper responses. Furthermore, the ability to recognize an antigenic determinant, and therefore the ability to respond to antigens, is controlled by immune response genes through the expression of MHC antigens. Tolerance to "self" is now thought to result from active cellular suppression of the development of autoreactive lymphocyte clones.

Oral tolerance is immunologic tolerance that results from exposure of GALT to ingested antigens. It is characterized by tolerance to ingested luminal antigen at both the mucosal and systemic level. Thus, feeding of a tolerogenic antigen results in absent immunoreactivity to the antigen subsequently administered by a systemic route; it also results in a lack of mucosal immunoreactivity (with the exception of the production of secretory immunoglobulins, which is preserved during tolerance to some, but not all antigens).[8] Oral tolerance has been induced by many materials including haptens, bacteria, viruses, cellular antigens, and food and pollen proteins.[8,57,79] The mechanisms of tolerance to each of these categories of antigen may be slightly different.[79] Oral tolerance to soluble proteins can be induced by either a single large dose or by repeated feeding of smaller doses over several weeks. Small doses given over prolonged periods are usually more effective than the same total dose given once.[79] Unresponsiveness following oral exposure to soluble proteins affects IgG, IgM, and IgE humoral responses as well as the cell-mediated immune response.[8,79] Without re-exposure oral tolerance to soluble proteins can last from three to four months, whereas tolerance to bacteria, for instance streptococci, may be more short-lived.[79] Tolerance to intestinal bacterial flora also appears to be less complete than tolerance to many other antigens. Both humoral and cell-mediated immune responses to bacteria are dampened, but they are not eliminated. These findings, along with the observation that suppressor cells to bacterial-induced immune responses appear only after relatively vigorous mucosal stimulation by bacterial flora,[8] establish that the tolerogenic response to bacteria allows conservation of some immunoreactivity, perhaps to facilitate mucosal defence.

The mechanism of oral tolerance begins with effective antigen exclusion. As discussed above, antigen exclusion has both specific (IgA, IgM) and nonspecific (other components of the "mucosal barrier") aspects. In this regard, effective digestion is particularly important. Digestion can result in macromolecular fragments too small to be read by the immune system (i.e. non-antigenic), or it can reduce sensitizing proteins to fragments that, while retaining their antigenicity, induce tolerance rather than sensitization.[72] The secretion of IgA and IgM is a humoral immune response that contributes to tolerance more than to immunoreactivity. This results from the effectiveness with which these antibodies prevent antigen from entering the lamina propria, in other than closely regulated, suppressor-orientated sites such as the Peyer's patches. IgA also has a tolerogenic role within the lamina propria, where its function as a blocking antibody results in a "wet blanket" effect.

A profound suppressor response is responsible for the systemic hyporeactivity characterizing oral tolerance to non-invasive antigens. The majority of evidence suggests that this suppressor response is largely due to an antigen-specific suppressor T cell network generated by the Peyer's patch, the cells of which migrate to various lymphoid organs including the mesenteric lymph nodes, spleen, thymus, and peripheral lymph nodes.[8,57,79,80] The suppressor T cells release soluble suppressor factors; these induce accessory suppressor T cells to inhibit the effector T cells of the immune response.[57] In addition to suppressor T cells, tolerance to intestinal bacteria in some species generates suppressor macrophages.[8] Suppressor B cells are involved in the induction of tolerance to some antigens.[8,79] Suppressor B cells have been identified in Peyer's patches and mesenteric lymph nodes within a week of ingestion of haptens. Their production of IgG appears to produce suppression.[79] Antibody exerts a direct negative feedback on the production of more antibody when it binds to immunoglobulin receptors on B and suppressor T cells. In addition, antibody-antiantibody networks that suppress the immune response have been proposed. Circulating immune complexes also exert a negative feedback on the immune response and may contribute to systemic hyporeactivity.[57,79] IgA-antibody-antigen complexes, in particular, have been incriminated.[79] The liver may also play a role. Thus, there have been reports that portocaval shunting decreases tolerance induction via the oral route to certain antigens. It has been postulated that the Kupffer cells of the liver remove sensitizing antigen aggregates and allow tolerogenic protein fragments to reach peripheral tissue.[79]

Mucosal tolerance would appear necessary to prevent tissue injury from a continuous inflammatory response to persistent mucosal antigens. Systemic tolerance can be regarded as a defense against hypersensitivities and autoimmune diseases by inhibiting reactions to antigens that escape immune exclusion.[79] It is noteworthy from the therapeutic standpoint the short-term feeding of antigen to animals already parenterally sensitized to that antigen does not induce tolerance. In fact, ingestion of antigen in these circumstances may actually boost IgG and IgE titers.[79]

Immunity to Parasites[5,81]

Epidemiological evidence suggests that the gastrointestinal immune response is important in the elimination of many gastrointestinal parasites of the dog and cat. For instance, it is rare to see ascarid infections in animals older than one year; hookworm infections of adult dogs are usually subclinical, whereas those of puppies are often fatal; and coccidial infection rarely causes signs of gastrointestinal disease except in the very young. Unfortunately, however there is very limited experimental work to examine the extent to which the immune system explains these observations. Furthermore, the constituents of the immune response to parasites of small animals remain poorly elucidated.

Evidence, largely derived from other species, suggests that the immune reaction to parasites is a complex integration of specific and non-specific immune responses. The particular facets of the immune response that are important in a particular infection depend on a number of factors, including the species of host, the class of parasite, and whether the parasite resides

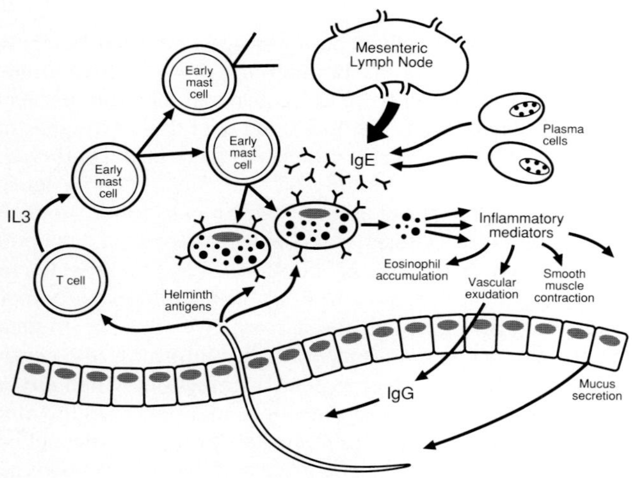

Figure 3-9. Schematic representation of the immune responses involved in the self-cure reaction against intestinal helminths.

extracellularly, intracellularly, or within the lumen of the bowel. As befits a well-adapted parasite, the immune response is often ineffective in eliminating the entire parasitic burden. Parasites have evolved a number of highly successful ways of avoiding the immune response of the host.

Nonspecific Resistance to Parasites. Nonimmunologic factors are important in the resistance to parasites. Interspecies and intraspecies competition limits parasite numbers and inhibits development. Genetic factors dictate whether an animal is susceptible to a parasitic infection and whether it will mount an immune-response to the parasite. The specific immune response to parasites often initiates nonspecific mechanisms of elimination. The best example of this interaction is the IgE-dependent mast cell degranulation that results in the so called "self-cure" response to helminth parasites. Another example is the T cell-mediated increase in epithelial cell turnover rate, which results in cryptal hyperplasia and villus atrophy in response to parasites such as giardia, hookworm, and roundworm. The villus atrophy and increased epithelial cell loss presumably inhibit attachment of the parasite but are also responsible for many of the clinical signs that accompany such diseases. Furthermore, both of the specific immune responses of T cell lymphokine release and IgE-mediated mast cell discharge stimulate increased mucus secretion. Copious secretion of mucus is reputed to interfere with the ability of parasites to attach to the mucosa.

Self-Cure Phenomenon. The self-cure phenomenon (Figure 3-9) to helminths has been best studied in *Haemonchus contortus* infections in sheep and *Nippostrongylus brasiliensis* infections in rats, but similar mechanisms are thought to result in the elimination of other helminth parasites. Helminth parasites secrete antigenic products into the mucosa that, in rodents at least, result in the migration of T cell precursors into the lamina propria, a response which appears essential for expulsion of the parasites. In response to the parasite, mucosal mast cells increase rapidly in number to peak at about five times the original level.[42] This proliferation is T cell-dependent and interleukin 3-induced. Concomitantly, with this mast cell response there is the development of an IgE-dominated humoral response. A prominent source of this IgE is the mesenteric lymph nodes. The IgE enters the lamina propria via the circulatory system and rapidly binds to the mucosal mast cells. Eventually, there is a combination of helminth antigen and mast cell-bound IgE that results in mast cell degranulation and the release of the mediators of goblet cell discharge and immediate hypersensitivity. These compounds promote smooth muscle contraction, increased vascular permeability, and, perhaps, reductions in intestinal fluid and water absorption. The result is vigorous intestinal contractions and profuse fluid and mucus exudation into the intestinal lumen. The exuded fluid is rich in IgG and may contain immunoreactive cells. The combination of processes results in dislodgement and expulsion of the majority of the worms.

Humoral Responses Other Than the Self-Cure Response. Parasite antigens are very adept at generating an IgE-mediated humoral response. However, even though IgE is the most significant humoral response to parasites, IgM, IgG, and IgA isotypes are also produced during parasitism. The humoral response is particularly effective against free-living tissue stages of parasites, but also affects intraluminal parasites via mediation of the immediate hypersensitivity response and perhaps by other poorly defined mechanisms.

In the lumen of the intestine, IgA is the immunoglobulin that comes in contact with parasites in the greatest concentration, but its function against these organisms remains uncertain. Animals infected with *Giardia* develop both a systemic IgG and a secretory IgA response against the parasite.[25] Humans with hypogammaglobulinemia (but not selective IgA deficiency) are predisposed to persistent giardiasis.[76] IgA is protective in coccidial infections.[27] A range of cell types, including lymphocytes, neutrophils and macrophages have receptors for IgA.[27] Adherence to trophozoites by neutrophils and phagocytosis of trophozoites by macrophages are increased in the presence of IgA and IgG,[88] and it appears that IgA can facilitate cytotoxicity against murine giardiasis.[27] These observations are of particular interest in light of the observation that lymphocytes and macrophages can be found in direct contact with *Giardia* trophozoites where they usually reside, i.e. in the intestinal lumen.

Within the tissues, antibodies protect the host by neutralizing proteolytic enzymes secreted by larvae to penetrate tissues, by blocking oral and excretory pores, and by inhibiting development. Probably the most important role of antibody in the tissues, however, is the mediation of antibody-dependent cellular cytotoxicity. This process appears to be of particular importance in the defense against helminth larvae in the tissues.

Cell-Mediated Response to Parasites. Sensitized T lymphocytes may successfully attack helminths or their larvae that are within the tissues. The blood eosinophilic response to parasites is usually greatest to parasites that have migratory forms in the tissues. The eosinophilia may be a result of an eosinophil-stimulating lymphokine released by sensitized T lymphocytes. The cell-mediated immune response incites a local immune response (granuloma) that inhibits parasitic growth or migration. In addition, cytotoxic T cells may be able to kill some larvae.

Evasion of the Immune Response by Parasites. Well adapted parasites have evolved a number of mechanisms to avoid the host immune response. These include mimicry of host antigens, antigenic variation, shedding of the glycocalyx, and immunosuppression of the host.[5]

Table 3-5 Neuropeptide Receptors on Immune Effector Cells

Neuropeptide	Receptor-Bearing Immune Cells
Bombesin	Phagocytes
Beta-endorphin	Lymphocytes, NK cells
Enkephalin	T lymphocytes, NK cells
Neurotensin	Mast cells, neutrophil
Somatostatin	Lymphocytes, monocytes, mast cells
Substance P	Lymphocytes, mast cells
VIP	Lymphocytes, NK cells

NEUROENDOCRINE REGULATION OF THE GASTROINTESTINAL IMMUNE RESPONSE

In recent years strong evidence has emerged to support neuroendocrine modulation of the immune system. This modulation appears to be most readily apparent in the gastrointestinal tract, where leukocytes are exposed to relatively high concentrations of neuropeptides.[66,82] The conditioned response of mast cell secretion, previously cited, is an appropriate example. Another is the ability to condition guinea pigs to develop an exudative peritoneal response to a skin scratch by previously pairing the skin scratch with intraperitoneal injections of a bacterial filtrate.[83]

The anatomical basis for such responses has come with the demonstration of peptidergic and noradrenergic innervation of mast cells and lymphoid tissues, including GALT, and with the demonstration of substance P, vasoactive intestinal peptide, and somatostatin receptors on leukocytes.[66,82] Functional studies have also suggested that leukocytes may possess receptors for bombesin, endorphins, enkephalins, and neurotensin.[82] The leukocytes containing neuropeptide receptors and the functions of those neuropeptides with the best-defined relationship to the bowel are shown in Tables 3-5 and 3-6.

It is also apparent that communication between the neuroendocrine system and the immune system is bidirectional.[66] Thus, there is good evidence to suggest that secretory products of the immune system can influence neural activity and that many mediators classically thought to have been synthesized by neuroendocrine tissue only are also elaborated by leukocytes. The latter include vasoactive intestinal peptide produced by neutrophils and mast cells, a somatostatin-like peptide secreted by basophils, and ACTH secreted by lymphocytes and macrophages.[66] The implications of these findings for homeostasis and gastrointestinal disease are obvious. The immune system may act as a sensory modality informing the central nervous system of problems, such as infection, which are not recognized by the classical sensory modalities.[86] On the other hand, the neuroendocrine-immune axis provides a mechanism (in addition to the less specific effects of steroid hormones and catecholamines) by which psychosomatic factors such as stress can influence disease processes. It is unlikely that "stress" initiates inflammation, but unconfirmed clinical suspicions suggest that such factors may influence the subsequent course and severity of the disease.[66] The release by neurons and leukocytes of inflammatory neuropeptides such as substance P and the influence of this and other neuropeptides on inflammation, mucus secretion, smooth muscle activity and vascular permeability may be important, for instance, in the pathogenesis of inflammatory bowel disease.

VACCINATION AGAINST GASTROINTESTINAL DISEASE

The humoral part of the mucosal immunologic defense system operates quite independently of the humoral system in the rest of the body. In general, the best-recognized means of protecting an animal against invasion by a microorganism is by parenteral administration of antigens prepared from the organism. However, parenteral injections do not stimulate gut

Table 3-6 Neuropeptides Shared by the Gastrointestinal and Immune Systems

Neuropeptide	Source	Target Cell	Effect
Somatostatin	Pancreas	Lymphocyte	Dec Proliferation
	APUD cell	Lymphocyte	Decreased IgA
	Basophil		
Substance P	C, A fibers	T cell	Inc proliferation
	Intestinal P cell	B cell	Increased IgA
	APUD cell	Monocyte	Chemotaxis
		Neutrophil	Inc phagocytosis
		Mast cell	Secretion
VIP	Cholinergic fibers	T cell	Dec proliferation
	VIP-ergic fibers	T cell	Altered migration
	APUD cell	NK cell	Alter cytotoxicity
	Neutrophil	B cell	Increased IgM
	Eosinophil	B cell	Decreased IgA

Modified from References 66 and 82.

plasma cells to produce IgA that will be secreted into the gut to prevent invasion at that site. Parenteral vaccination, will result in the production of circulating IgG antibodies that enter the gut in amounts that are proportionate to the serum IgG level.[87] The amounts of these antibodies secreted into the gut, however, are so small that they are rapidly degraded by proteases and can have only a minor influence on prevention of diseases.[88] The access of IgG to the gut lumen is greatly increased by the permeability breakdown subsequent to gastrointestinal inflammation. Thus, parenteral vaccination against enteric pathogens will limit the severity of disease, but is less effective at prevention.

The most effective means of stimulating the synthesis of secretory IgA is by oral administration of antigens.[89] Exposure of the mucosa to antigens produces effective and relative long-lasting immunity. This is illustrated by the long-lasting immunity produced after recovery from the disease. Recent studies have shown such to be the case with *Escherichia coli*.[90] The normal secretory IgA response following an infection is associated with the appearance of circulating humoral antibodies against the antigen.[91] The development of oral vaccines holds the most promise of producing long lasting immunity against enteric pathogens. The major problems to be solved in developing oral vaccines are to produce products that have lost their pathogenicity, have retained their antigenicity, and have not become so altered that they are readily degraded in the intestines. For example, heat inactivation of cholera enterotoxin causes a loss in its toxicity but changes the toxin from a protease-resistant molecule to one that is protease-susceptible.[92]

REFERENCES

1. Besredka, A.: De la vaccination contre les etats typhoides par la voie buccale. Ann Inst Pasteur 33:882, 1919.
2. Davies, A.: An investigation into the serological properties of dysentery stools. Lancet 2:1009, 1922.
3. Brandtzaeg, P., Valnes, K., Scott, H., Rognum, T.O., Bjerke, K. and Baklien, K.: The human gastrointestinal secretory immune system in health and disease. Scan J. Gastroenterology 20:(suppl 114) 17-38, 1985.
4. Bienenstock, J.: The Mucosal Immunologic Network. Ann. Allergy 53:535-540, 1984.
5. Tizard, I.: Veterinary Immunology. 3rd Ed. WB Saunders, Philadelphia, 1987.
6. Doran, J.E., Lundsgaard-Hansen, P.: Role of the reticuloendothelial system in the pathogenesis of organ damage. Brit. J. Hosp. Med. 39:221-225, 1988.
7. Pavli, P., Doe, W.F. and Hume, D.A.: Enrichment and characterization of dendritic cells from the lamina propria of murine intestine. Gastroenterology 94:A346, 1988.
8. Elson, C.O.: Induction and control of the gastrointestinal immune system. Scan J Gastroenterology 20:(suppl 114) 2-14, 1985.
9. Beutler, B and Cerami, A.: Cachectin: More than a tumor necrosis factor. New Eng. J. Med. 316:379-385, 1987.
10. Evans, H.E., Christensen, G.C.: The alimentary canal. In, Miller's Anatomy of the dog. WB Saunders Co, Philadelphia. 455-506, 1979.
11. Egberts, H.J.A., Brinkhoff, M.G.M., Mouwen, J.M.V.M., Van Dijk, J.E. and Koninkx, J.F.J.G.: Biology and pathology of the intestinal M cell. A review. Vet Quarterly 7:333-336, 1985.
12. Harty, R.F., Leibach, J.R.: Immune disorders of the gastrointestinal tract and liver. Medical Clinics of North America 69:675-703, 1985.
13. Stewart, T.H.M., Hetenyi, C., Rowsell, H. and Orizaga, M.: Ulcerative enterocolitis in dogs induced by drugs. J. Path. 131:363-378, 1980.
14. Bienenstock, J., Befus, D.: Gut- and bronchus-associated lymphoid tissue. Am J Anatomy 170:437-445, 1984.
15. Brandtzaeg, P., Bjerke, K., Kett, K., Kvale, D., Rognum, T.O., Scott, H., Sollid, L.M. and Valnes, K.: Production and secretion of immunoglobulins in the gastrointestinal tract. Ann. Allergy 59:21-39, 1987.
16. Wolf, J.L., Bye, W.A.: The membranous epithelial (M) cell and the mucosal immune system. Ann. Rev. Med. 35:95-112, 1984.
17. Smith, M.W., James, P.S. and Tivey, D.R.: M cell numbers after transfer of SPF mice to normal animal house environment. Am. J. Path. 128:385-389, 1987.
18. Hanauer, S.B., Kraft, S.C.: Intestinal immunology. In, Gastroenterology. Edited by J.E. Berk, W.S. Haubrich, M.H. Kalser, WB Saunders, Philadelphia; Chapter 99, 1607-1631, 1985.
19. Bjerke, K., Brandtzaeg, P.: Immunoglobulin- and J chain-producing cells associated with lymphoid follicles in the human appendix, colon and ileum, including Peyer's patches. Clin. Exp. Immunol. 64:432-441, 1986.
20. Dobbins, W.O.: Gut immunopathology a gastroenterologists view with emphasis on pathophysiology. Am. J. Physiol 242:G1-8, 1982.
21. Heatley, R.V., Bienenstock, J.: Luminal lymphoid cells in the rabbit intestine. Gastroenterology 82:268-275, 1982.
22. Owen, R.L., Nenamic, P.C., and Stevens, D.P.: Ultrastructural observations on giardiasis in a murine model. Gastroenterology 76:757-769, 1979.
23. Thomas, J., Anderson, N.V.: Interepithelial lymphocytes in the small intestinal mucosa of conventionally reared dogs. Am. J. Vet. Res. 42:200-203, 1982.
24. Carman, P.S., Ernst, P.B., Rosenthal, K.L., Clark, D.A., Befus, A.D. and Bienenstock, J.: Intraepithelial leukocytes contain a unique subpopulation of NK-like cytotoxic cells active in the defense of gut epithelium to enteric murine coronaviruses. J. Immunology 136:1548-1553, 1986.
25. Targan, S.R., Kagnoff, M.K., Brogon, M.D. and Shanahan, F.: Immunological mechanisms in intestinal diseases. Ann. Int. Med. 106:853-870, 1987.
26. Befus, A.D., Bienenstock, J.: Immunity to infectious agents in the gastrointestinal tract. J. Am. Vet. Med. Assoc. 181:1066-1068, 1982.
27. Befus, D., Lee, T.: Unique characteristics of local responses in host resistance to mucosal parasitic infections. Vet. Parasitology 20:175-194, 1986.
28. Van der Heijden, P.J., Stok, W.: Improved procedure for the isolation of functionally active lymphoid cells from the murine intestine. J. Immunological Methods 103:161-167, 1987.
29. Hall, E.J., Batt, R.M.: Challenge studies demonstrate gluten sensitivity of a naturally occurring enteropathy in Irish setter dogs. Gastroenterology 94:A167, 1988.
30. Hall, E.J., Batt, R.M.: Exclusion of dietary cereal from birth modulates subsequent sensitivity to gluten in a naturally occurring enteropathy of Irish setter dogs. Gastroenterology 94:A167, 1988.
31. Barlough, J.E., Jacobson, R.H. and Scott, F.W.: The immunoglobulins of the cat. Cornell Vet. 71:397-407, 1981.
32. Willard, M.D., Williams, J.F., Stowe, H.D. and Kutil, C.: Number and distribution of IgM cells and IgA cells in colonic tissue of conditioned sex-and breed-matched dogs. Am. J. Vet. Res. 43:688-692, 1982.
33. Gibson, P.R., van de Pol, E., Pullman, W. and Doe, W.F.: The role of mononuclear and LAK cell-mediated cytotoxicity in the pathogenesis of inflammatory bowel disease. Gastroenterology 94:A146, 1988.
34. Hogan, P.G., Hapel, A.J. and Doe, W.F.: Antibody-dependent-cellular-cytotoxicity of intestinal lamina propria mononuclear cells. Gastroenterology 94:A189, 1988.

35. Willard, M.D., Leid, R.W.: Nonuniform horizontal and vertical distributions of immunoglobulin A cells in canine intestines. Am. J. Vet. Res. 42:1573-1579, 1981.
36. Nagi, A.M., Babiuk, L.A.: Bovine gut-associated lymphoid tissue. Morphological and functional studies. J. Immunol. Methods 105:23-37, 1987.
37. Huntley, J.F., Newlands, G.F.J., Gibson, S., Fergusson, A. and Miller, H.R.P.: Histochemical demonstration of chymotrypsin like serine esterases in mucosal mast cells in four species including man. J. Clin. Pathol. 38:375-384, 1985.
38. Atkins, F.M.: Intestinal mucosal mast cells. Ann. Allergy 59:44-53, 1987.
39. Schachter, M., Longridge, D.J., Wheeler, G.D., Mehta, J.G. and Uchida, Y.: Immunocytochemical and enzyme histochemical localization of kallikrein-like enzymes in colon intestine, and stomach of rat and cat. J Histochemistry and Cytochemistry 34:927-934, 1986.
40. Kawanishi, H., Ihle, J.M.: In vitro induction and characterization of mast cells from murine Peyer's patches. Scand. J. Immunol. 25:109-120, 1987.
41. Kitamura, Y., Nakano, T. and Kanakura, Y.: Transdifferentiation between mast cell subpopulations. Dev. Growth Differ. 28:321-325, 1986.
42. Jarret, E.E.E., Haig, D.M.: Mucosal mast cells *in vivo* and *in vitro*. Immunology Today 5:115-118, 1984.
43. Russell, M., Dark, K.A., Cummins, R.W., Ellman, G., Callaway, E. and Peeke, H.V.S.: Learned histamine release. Science 225:733-734, 1984.
44. Caughey, G.H., Leidig, F., Viro, N.F. and Nadel, J.A.: Substance P and vasoactive intestinal peptide degradation by mast cell tryptase and chymase. J. Pharmacol. Exp. Ther. 244:133-137, 1988.
45. Hair, P.N.R., Schroeder, H.E.: Duct-associated lymphoid tissue (DALT) of minor salivary glands and mucosal immunity. Immunology 57:171-180, 1986.
46. Jackson, D.E., Lally, E.T., Nakamura, M.C. and Montgomery, P.C.: Migration of IgA-bearing lymphocytes into salivary glands. Cell Immunol. 63:203, 1981.
47. Heddle, R.J., Rowley, D.: Dog Immunoglobulins. I. Immunochemical characterization of dog serum, parotid saliva, colostrum, milk and small bowel fluid. Immunology 29:185-195, 1975.
48. Yamada, T., Tomoda, I. and Usui, K.: Immunoglobulin compositions of the feline body fluids. Jpn. J. Vet. Sci. 46:791-796, 1984.
49. Scicchitano, R., Sheldrake, R.F. and Husband, A.J.: Origin of immunoglobulins in respiratory tract secretion and saliva of sheep. Immunology 58:315-321, 1985.
50. Pedersen, N.C.: Basic and clinical immunology. In, Diseases of the Cat, Vol 1. Edited by J. Holzworth, WB Saunders, Philadelphia. 146-181, 1987.
51. Schultz, R.D., Scott, F.W., Duncan, J.R. and Gillespie, J.H.: Feline Immunoglobulins. Infection and Immunity 9:391-393, 1974.
52. Vaerman, J.P., Heremans, J.F.: The immunoglobulins of the dog - II. The Immunoglobulins of canine secretions. Immunochemistry 6:779-786, 1969.
53. Hodgson, H.J.F.: Gut-liver interactions in the IgA system. Scan. J. Gastroenterology 20:(suppl 114) 39-44, 1985.
54. Strober, W., James, S.P.: The immunologic basis of inflammatory bowel disease. J. Clin. Immunology 6:415-432, 1986.
55. Panzini, B., Fournier, D. and Podolsky, D.K.: Emergence of antigenic glycoprotein structures in ulcerative colitis detected through monoclonal antibodies. Abs 902 In: Proceedings of Digestive Diseases Week, pg A-226, 1988.
56. Ferguson, A., MacDonald, T.T.: Effects of local delayed hypersensitivity on the small intestine. Ciba Found. Symp. 46:305-319, 1977.
57. Gautam, S.C., Battisto, J.R.: Orally induced tolerance generates an efferently acting suppressor T cell and an acceptor T cell that together down-regulate contact sensitivity. J. Immunology 135:2975-2983, 1985.
58. Kawanishi, H., Kiely, J.: In vitro induction of a contrasuppressor immunoregulatory network by polyclonally activated T cells derived from murine Peyer's patches. Immunology 63:415-421, 1988.
59. Benson, E.B., Strober, W.: Regulation of IgA secretion by T cell clones derived from the human gastrointestinal tract. J. Immunology 140:1874-1882, 1988.
60. Gearhart, P.J., Cebra, J.J.: Differentiated B lymphocytes. Potential to express particular antibody variable and constant regions depends on site of lymphoid tissue and antigen load. J. Exp. Med. 149:216-227, 1979.
61. Hoover, R.G., Lynch, R.G.: Isotype-specific suppression of IgA: suppression of IgA responses in BALB/c mice by T cells. J. Immunology 130:521-523, 1983.
62. Kawanishi, H., Saltzman, L.E. and Strober, W.: Mechanisms regulating IgA class-specific immunoglobulin production in murine gut-associated lymphoid tissues. II. Terminal differentiation of postswitch sIgA-bearing Peyer's patch B cells. J. Exp. Med. 158:649-669, 1983.
63. Ottaway, C.A.: *In vitro* alteration of receptors for vasoactive intestinal peptide changes the *in vivo* localization of mouse T cells. J. Exp. Med. 160:1054-1069, 1984.
64. Mestecky, J., Czerkinsky, C., Russell, M.W., Brown, T.A., Prince, S.J., Moldoveanu, Z., Jackson, S., Michalek, S.M. and McGhee, J.R.: Induction and molecular properties of secretory and serum IgA antibodies specific for environmental antigens. Ann. Allergy 59:54-59, 1987.
65. Vaerman, J.P., Heremans, J.F.: Origin and molecular size of immunoglobulin-A in the mesenteric lymph of the dog. Immunology 18:27-38, 1970.
66. Shanahan, F., Anton, P.: Neuroendocrine modulation of the immune system. Possible implications for inflammatory bowel disease. Dig. Dis. Sci. 33:(March suppl) 41S-49S, 1988.
67. Stanisz, A.M., Befus, D. and Bienenstock, J.: Differential effects of vasoactive intestinal polypeptide, substance P, and somatostatin on immunoglobulin synthesis and proliferations by lymphocytes from Peyer's patches, mesenteric lymph nodes, and spleen. J. Immunology 136:152-156, 1986.
68. Whitbread, T.J., Batt, R.M. and Garthwaite, G.: Relative deficiency of serum IgA in the German shepherd dog: a breed abnormality. Res. Vet. Sci. 37:350-352, 1984.
69. Felsburg, P.J., Glickman, L.T. and Jezyk, P.F.: Selective IgA deficiency in the dog. Clin. Immunol. Immunopath. 36:297-305, 1985.
70. Moroff, S.D., Hurvitz, A.I., Peterson, M.E., Saunders, L. and Noone, K.: IgA deficiency in shar-pei dogs. Vet. Immuno. Immunopath. 13:181-188, 1986.
71. Lawton, A.R., Royal, S.A., Self, K.S. and Cooper, M.D.: IgA determinants on B-lymphocytes in patients with deficiency of circulating IgA. J. Lab. Clin. Med. 80:26-33, 1972.
72. Walker, W.A.: Pathophysiology of intestinal uptake and absorption of antigens in food allergy. Ann. Allergy 59:7-20, 1987.
73. Pollock, V.H., Zimmer, J.F.: Intestinal Immunity. Proceedings of the 8th Kal Kan symposium. 81-86, 1984.
74. Ammann, A.J., Hong, R.: Selective IgA deficiency: Presentation of 30 cases and a review of the literature. Medicine 50:223-236, 1971.
75. Guilford, W.G.: Primary immunodeficiency diseases of dogs and cats. Comp. Contin. Ed. Pract. Vet. 9:641-650, 1987.
76. Strober, W., James, S.P.: The immunopathogenesis of gastrointestinal and hepatobiliary disease. J. Am. Med. Assoc. 258:2962-2969, 1987.
77. Mayrhofer, G.: Sites of synthesis and localization of IgE in rats infested with *Nippostrongylus brasiliensis*. Ciba Found. Symp. 46:155-175, 1977.
78. Belut, D., Moneret-Vautrin, D.A., Nicolas, J.P. and Grillist, J.P.: IgE levels in intestinal juice. Dig. Dis. Sci. 25:323-332, 1980.
79. Tomasi, T.B.: Oral tolerance. Transplantation 29:353-356, 1980.
80. Mattingly, J.A., Waksman, B.H.: Immunologic suppression after oral administration of antigen. I. Specific suppressor cells formed in rat's Peyer's patches after oral administra-

tion of sheep erythrocytes and their systemic migration. J. Immunology 121:1878, 1978.
81. Zajac, A.M.: The role of gastrointestinal immunity in parasitic infections of small animals. Sem. Vet. Med. Surg. 2:274-281, 1987.
82. O'Dorisio, M.S.: Neuropeptides and gastrointestinal immunity. Am. J. Med. 81:(suppl 6B) 74-79, 1986.
83. Ader, R.: Psychoneuroimmunology. London, Academic Press, 1981.
84. Hiraga, C., Kanaki, T., Ichikawa, Y.: Immunobiological characteristics of germfree and specific pathogen-free cats. Lab. An. Sci. 31:391-396, 1981.
85. Reynolds, H.Y., Johnson, J.S.: Quantitation of canine immunoglobulins. J Immunology 105:698-703, 1970.
86. Blalock, J.E., Harbour-McMenamine D. and Smith, E.M.: Peptide hormones shared by neuroendocrine and immunologic systems. J. Immunol 135:858S-861S, 1985.
87. Pierce, N.F., Reynolds, H.Y.: Immunity to experimental cholera. II. Secretory and humoral antitoxin response to local and systemic toxoid administration. J. Infect. Dis. 131:383-389, 1975.
88. Parrott, D.M.V.: The gut as a lymphoid organ. Clinics in Gastroenterology 5:211-228, 1976.
89. Porter, P., Kenworthy, R., Noakes, D.E. and Allen, W.D.: Intestinal antibody secretion in the young pig in response to oral immunization with *Escherichia coli*. Immunology 27:841-853, 1975.
90. Lodinova, R., Wagner, V.: Development of fecal immunoglobulin and coproantibody in infants after artificial oral colonization with *E. coli* 083. Experientia 26:188, 1970.
91. Sack, R.B., Jacobs, B. and Mitra, R.: Antitoxin responses to infections with enterotoxigenic *Escherichia coli*. J. Infect. Dis. 129:1450-1456, 1975.
92. Strombeck, D.R., Harrold, D.: Comparison of the rate of absorption and proteolysis of (14C) choleragen and (14C) bovine serum albumin in the rat jejunum. Infect. Immun. 12:1450-1456, 1975.
93. Befus, D., Fujimaki, H., et al. Mast cell polymorphisms. Present concepts, future directions. Dig. Dis. and Sci. 33(Suppl):16s-22s, 1988.

Chapter 4

Gastrointestinal Inflammation

INTRODUCTION

Inflammation is the vascular and cellular response of tissue to injury. It is a protective mechanism by which phagocytes, immunoglobulins, complement, and other serum constituents are concentrated at the sites of tissue damage. Inflammation is usually an acute process concluded by elimination of the inciting cause and by tissue repair. If the inflammatory response fails to eliminate the cause, chronic inflammation will ensue and damage to the tissues may result. In this way the inflammation seen in disorders such as inflammatory bowel disease becomes detrimental to the host. Injurious processes that are capable of inciting inflammation are physical damage, infection, ischemia, toxins, neoplasia, and immune reactions including immediate, cytotoxic, immune complex, and delayed hypersensitivity reactions.

Vascular Changes During Inflammation[1-3]

Vasodilation and increased blood flow to perturbed tissues occur early in the inflammatory process. Increased vascular permeability and exudation of plasma, leukocytes, and red blood cells into the tissues accompany the vasodilation. Later in the inflammatory process blood flow tends to decline, platelets adhere to vessel walls, and intravascular clotting may ensue. Activated Hageman factor, contained in the exuded plasma, initiates the clotting cascade, the fibrinolytic cascade, and kallikrein synthesis. Kinins generated by kallikrein contribute to the vascular dilation and increased permeability. The results of these vascular changes are dilution of toxins by exuded fluid and isolation of microorganisms and damaged tissues by a defensive cordon of accumulated phagocytes, fibrin, and occasionally obstructed vasculature. The vascular changes are a result of various mediators, the most potent of which are the kinins, histamine, certain prostaglandins, and perhaps certain neuropeptides.

Chemotaxis and the Cellular Changes During Inflammation[4]

Chemotaxis is the process by which leukocytes move to damaged tissue along concentration gradients of chemotactic substances. It is at present an important area of research because chemotaxis is an early (perhaps inciting) event in the inflammatory process, one which determines the accumulating cell types and hence the microscopic classification of the inflammation. The more mobile leukocytes (neutrophils, eosinophils) enter the tissues first, followed later by monocytes. Some chemotactic substances attract most phagocytes, whereas others are specific for neutrophils, monocytes or eosinophils. In addition to chemoattraction, many of these substances stimulate other biological functions of the phagocyte, such as degranulation and phagocytosis. Neutrophils are attracted by complement fragments, immune complexes, eicosanoids, soluble bacterial products, oxygen-derived free radicals, kallikrein, certain lymphokines, and various tissue breakdown products including collagen and fibrin fragments. Of these products leukotriene B_4, 5-HETE, complement fragments C5a and C567, and N-formyl-methionyl-leucyl-phenylalanine (FMLP), are the most potent chemotactic products known. As a result of the wide variety of chemotactic products that attract neutrophils, most types of inflammation have some component of neutrophil infiltration. Eosinophils are attracted by complement fragments, histamine, certain leukotrienes, and the eosinophilic chemotactic factor of anaphylaxis (ECF-A). ECF-A is released by mast cells and basophils and is composed of two polypeptides, alanine-glycine-serine-glutamine and valine-glycine-serine-glutamine. Monocytes are attracted by complement fragments, certain bacterial peptides such as FMLP, some lymphokines, and collagen-breakdown products.

Once present in the tissues, the phagocytes adhere to and ingest foreign antigen and tissue debris. Serum opsonins such as fibronectin, C-reactive protein, antibody, and complement facilitate adherence, as does trapping of the antigen against exuded fibrin.

After ingestion the phagocytosed material in the phagolysosome is exposed to various toxic products and digestive enzymes. These include proteases, toxic proteins, and oxygen-derived free radicals. The latter are produced in great quantity by the respiratory burst of neutrophils.

INFLAMMATORY MEDIATORS

Eicosanoids[5-11]

Eicosanoids are derivatives of 20 carbon fatty acids. The most prevalent eicosanoids in mammalian systems appear to be those formed by the arachidonic acid cascade (Figure 4-1). Cell injury activates membrane phospholipases, in particular phospholipase A_2. The phospholipases initiate the arachidonic

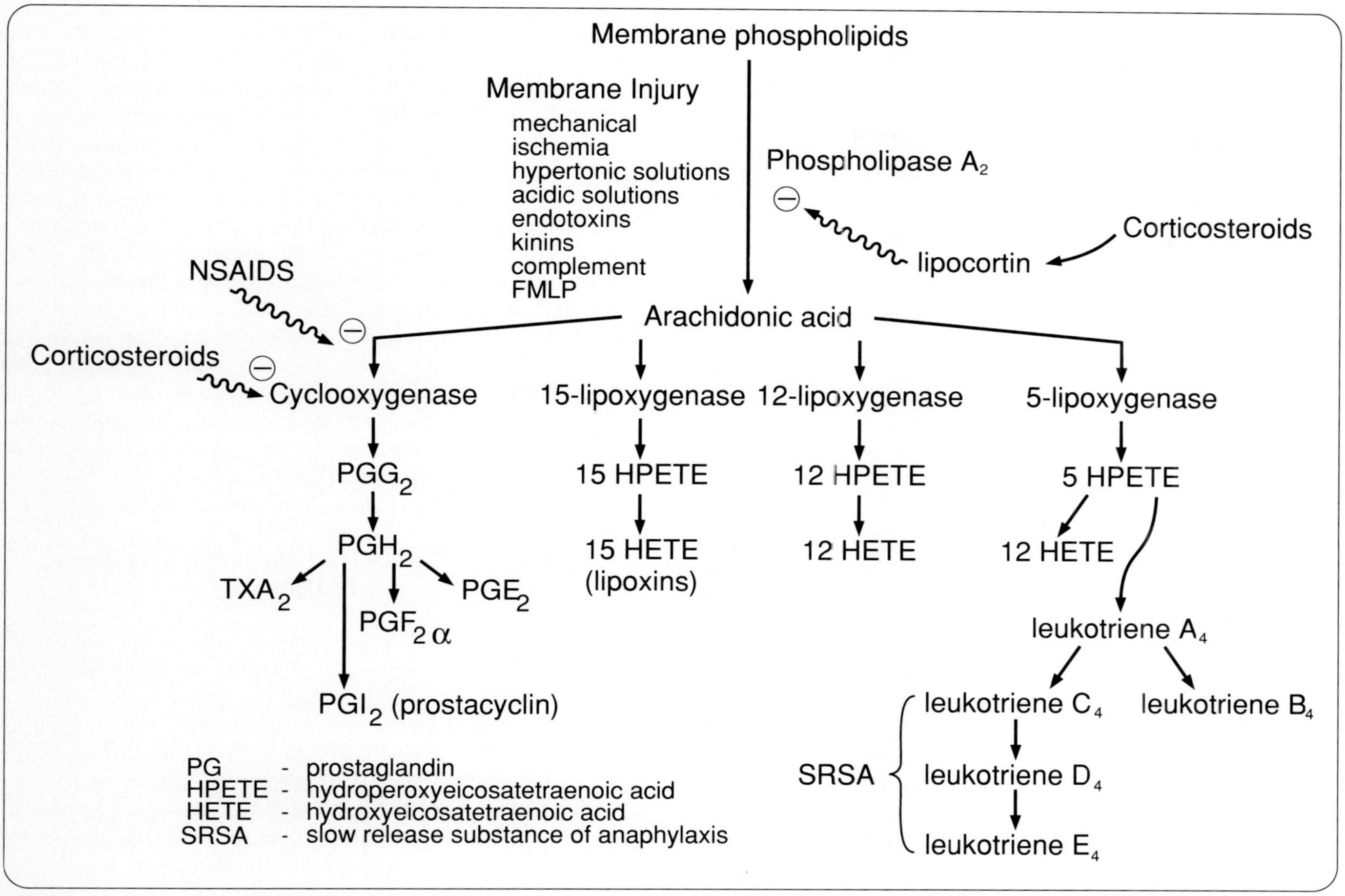

Figure 4-1 The arachidonic acid cascade.

acid cascade by releasing arachidonic acid from membrane phospholipids. In the gut, perturbations capable of releasing arachidonic acid include mechanical stimulation, ischemia, and exposure of bowel tissue (including resident leukocytes) to hypertonic solutions, acid or alkali, chyme, bile acids, bacterial endotoxins, FMLP, bradykinin, complement, and coagulation factors. Glucocorticoids inhibit arachidonic acid release by generating a membrane-bound protein called lipocortin. Once released into the cytoplasm, the arachidonic acid may be metabolized by either cyclooxygenases or lipoxygenases to various prostaglandins, hydroxyeicosatetraenoic acids (HETEs), or leukotrienes. Which of these pathways predominates depends on the concentration of these enzymes in the different tissues and the presence or absence of different inhibitors. For instance, non-steroidal antiinflammatory agents inhibit cyclooxygenase but not lipoxygenase channelling eicosanoid synthesis towards leukotrienes. In the bowel, prominent eicosanoid pathways recognized to date appear to be the synthesis of leukotriene B_4, prostaglandin E_2 (PGE_2), PGF_2 alpha, prostacyclin, thromboxane B_2, and HETE. The precise cellular origin of gastrointestinal eicosanoids has not been determined. Likely sites are leukocytes, platelets, and endothelial cells in the lamina propria. Their biotransformation is rapid. Half-lives range from seconds to minutes.

Leukotrienes

Leukotrienes are eicosanoids derived from the metabolism of arachidonic acid by lipoxygenases. The quantitatively most important leukotriene pathways in the gastrointestinal tract are those catalyzed by 5-lipoxygenase and 15-lipoxygenase. The principal arachidonic acid-derived product of 15-lipoxygenase is 15-hydroxyeicosatetraenoic acid, which has an important role in the modulation of 5-lipoxygenase. Enzyme activity of 5-lipoxygenase is prominent in leukocytes. The leukotriene products of 5-lipoxygenase (Figure 4-1) have potent inflammatory properties. The leukotriene precursors, 5-hydroperoxyeicosaetraenoic acid (5-HEPTE) and hydroxyeicosaetraenoic acid (5-HETE), impair net colonic fluid absorption; 5-HETE is also a chemotactic substance. Leukotriene B_4 attracts neutrophils and to a lesser extent eosinophils and monocytes. It may also increase vascular permeability and stimulate neutrophils to adhere to vascular endothelium. At high concentrations leukotriene B_4 stimulates neutrophil degranulation and superoxide generation. Leukotrienes C_4, D_4, and E_4 collectively comprise slow reacting substance of anaphylaxis. They cause a sustained contraction of certain smooth muscle, including that of the bowel. Leukotrienes C_4, D_4, and E_4 also cause vasodilation and increase vascular permeability of microvasculature. These leukotrienes cause these effects at much lower concentrations than histamine.

Leukotriene B_4 and HETEs are found in high concentrations in rectal mucosal samples taken from humans with ulcerative colitis. The severity of the inflammation positively correlates with the concentration of leukotriene B_4. Inhibitors of leukotriene synthesis have resulted in significant decreases in inflammation in various experimental colitis models. It is likely that these eicosanoids are important proinflammatory mediators in inflammatory bowel disease.

Prostaglandins

Prostaglandins (PG) are eicosanoids derived from the metabolism of arachidonic acid by cycloxygenase. Further metabolism of prostaglandin intermediates yields the prostacyclin (PGI_2), thromboxane (TxA_2), PGF_2 alpha, PGE_2, and PGD_2 prostaglandin series. In most tissues, prostacyclins are produced predominantly by vascular endothelium; platelets produce the thromboxanes; and most nucleated cells produce the PGE_2, PGF_2 alpha, and PGD_2 series. The prostaglandins have a wide range of biological activity. Tissue and species differences do occur. The individual prostaglandin series have different and often opposing effects. In vivo, the eicosanoids are released together, and complex interactions between them probably determine the net biological effect. In general, prostaglandins tend to serve a protective role in the gastrointestinal tract rather than being primary mediators that incite gastrointestinal inflammation. This is particularly clear in the stomach, where prostaglandins, especially PGE_2, have been shown to be "cytoprotective." The cytoprotection probably results from a number of beneficial effects, including stimulation of mucus and bicarbonate secretion, enhanced mucosal blood flow, decreased acid secretion, and enhanced epithelial proliferation and repair. Prostaglandins, particularly PGE_2, also appear to be largely protective in the intestine. PGE_2 can stimulate mucus secretion by the bowel, increase bowel mucosal blood flow (as can prostacyclin), maintain or enhance villus height after radiation damage, and protect the bowel against certain perturbations including alcohol-induced colitis, acetic-acid induced colitis, and clindamycin-induced colitis.[5] Futhermore, PGE_2 induces suppressor cell activity in peripheral blood lymphocytes and perhaps in bowel lymphocytes. The damage to the bowel that occurs following ingestion of non-steroidal antiinflammatory agents provides further, albeit indirect, evidence of prostaglandins' cytoprotection of the bowel.

While prostaglandins may not incite inflammation in the gastrointestinal tract, it is likely that in some situations they have a mild permissive effect on the inflammatory process and probably mediate some of its consequences, such as pain and diarrhea. Prostacyclin and PGE_2 alone do not increase vascular permeability, but they potentiate the increased macromolecular leakage that occurs due to other mediators. In some situations prostaglandins may induce diarrhea, abdominal "cramping," and perhaps nausea. Prostaglandin-mediated diarrhea probably results from increased secretion of fluid and electrolytes, in combination with altered contractility. PGF_2 alpha and thromboxane cause smooth muscle contraction, whereas prostacyclin causes smooth muscle relaxation. PGE_2 causes longitudinal smooth muscle contraction and circular smooth muscle relaxation. It has been suggested that PGE_2 is the mediator responsible for the decreased colonic segmenting contractions noted in humans with ulcerative colitis.[12] PGE_2 stimulates intestinal net secretion of chloride, potassium, sodium, and water. PGF_2 alpha also promotes secretion. Prostacyclin increases secretion of fluid and electrolytes in the large bowel but has variable effects in the small bowel. Increased synthesis of prostaglandins may mediate the intestinal secretion that occurs in a number of diarrheal diseases including certain immune-mediated diseases[13] and those due to enterotoxins from *E. coli*, and *Salmonella typhimurium*. Increased prostaglandin synthesis may also be involved in diarrhea due to excess thyroxine, excess vasoactive intestinal polypeptide, unconjugated bile acids, celiac disease, mastocytosis, neural crest tumors, and miscellaneous other disorders.[5] The role of prostaglandins in inflammatory bowel disease is unclear. Synthesis of prostaglandins, in particular PGE, PGF_2 alpha, prostacyclin, and thromboxane, increases during this disorder. This synthesis may alter local blood flow, influence smooth muscle contractility, and contribute to the diarrhea associated with the condition, but, based on the experimental evidence cited above, it is more likely to protect the mucosa than markedly exacerbate the inflammation.

N-Formyl-Methionyl-Leucyl-Phenylalanine (FMLP)

FMLP is a peptide derived from *E. coli*. Recent interest has been focused on FMLP because of the discovery that chemotactic peptides can breach the relatively impermeable mucosal barrier. This raises the possibility that they may be the inciting cause of inflammatory bowel disease (Figure 4-2). Neutrophils possess high and low affinity receptors for FMLP. FMLP bound to the high affinity receptors stimulates migration of the neutrophil. As the neutrophil approaches the area of inflammation, the concentration of the chemoattractant increases, and FMLP eventually binds to its low affinity receptor. The low affinity

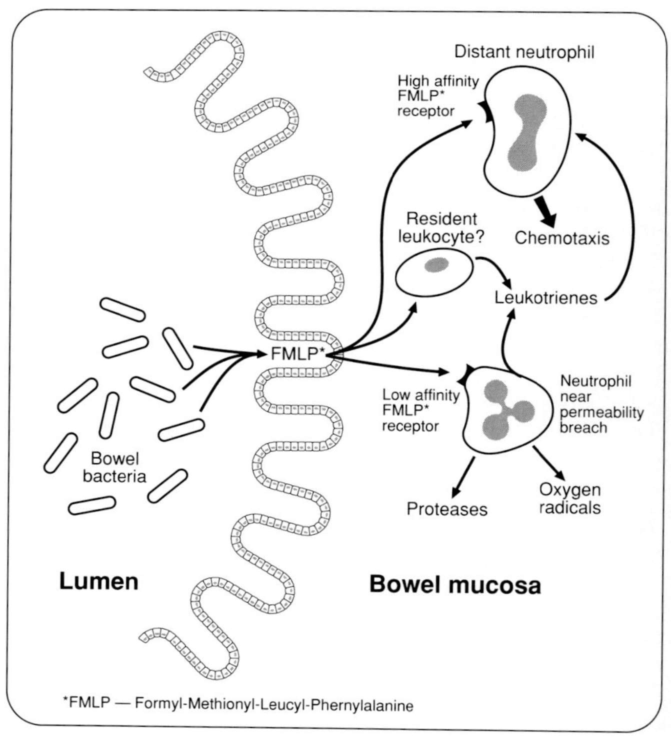

Figure 4-2 Chemotactic peptides and gastrointestinal inflammation.

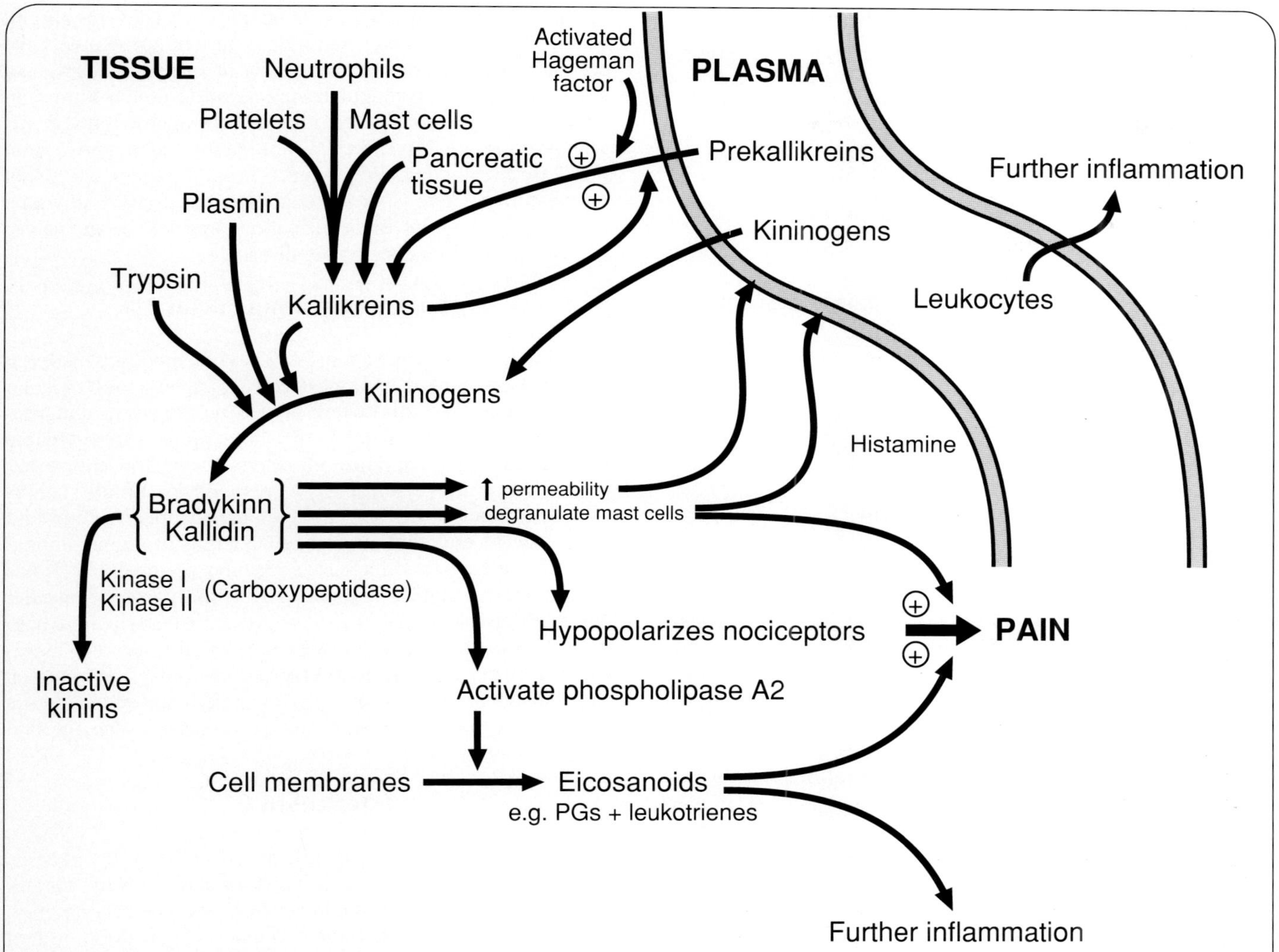

Figure 4-3 The Kinin System

receptor stimulates the neutrophil to phagocytose, degranulate, undergo the respiratory burst, and to elaborate eicosanoids. Neutrophils from patients with ulcerative colitis have increased responsiveness to FMLP.[14]

Histamine

Histamine (beta-imidazolyl-ethylamine) is released by degranulation of mast cells following a variety of stimuli (see chapter on GI immunology). The importance of histamine as a mediator of inflammation in the digestive system has not been established. Visceral mast cells contain less histamine than connective tissue mast cells. Histamine has a variety of effects on tissues. Some, but not all, of these effects are known to occur in the digestive system. Histamine dilates microvessels, increases vascular permeability, contracts gut smooth muscle, attracts eosinophils, stimulates gastric acid secretion, and contracts the hepatic veins of dogs. Histamine may have immunosuppressive activity, and it can induce fibroblast proliferation.

Serotonin[15]

The majority of serotonin (5-hydroxytryptamine) in the body is found in the enterochromaffin cells of the bowel and in platelets. Serotonin has been identified in the mast cells of rodents and cattle, but not of other species. Its importance as an inflammatory mediator is unknown. Release of serotonin from enterochromaffin cells is increased by mechanical stimulation, hypertonicity, acidity, norepinephrine, and vagal influences. Platelets release serotonin following aggregation. The effects of serotonin vary in different tissues and species. In most species studied, serotonin causes splanchnic vasoconstriction, has little influence on capillary permeability (except in rodents), and increases small intestinal motility, but decreases gastric and large bowel motility. In the dog, intravenous infusion of serotonin reduces gastric secretion of pepsin and acid, but increases the secretion of mucus. Serotonin also stimulates secretion of fluid in the intestines. In the rat stomach, there is some evidence that serotonin may be an important mediator of the phenomenon of adaptive mucosal cytoprotection.[16]

Figure 4-4 Consequences of kallikrein activation.

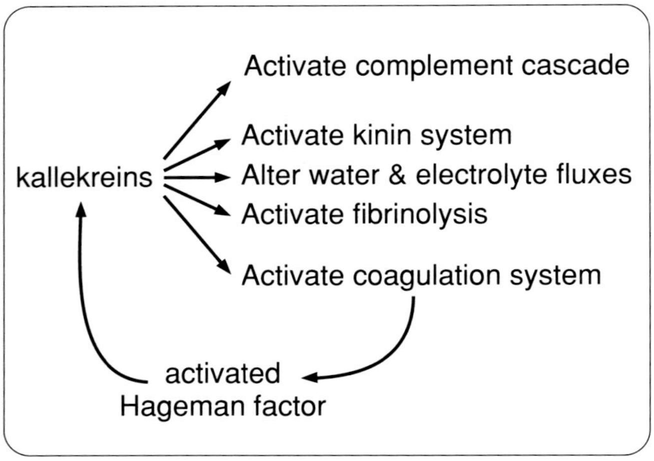

Kallikreins and Kinins[17]

Kinins are short-lived polypeptides derived from the action of kininogenases (serine proteases) on serum globulins called kininogens. Important kininogenases include kallikreins, trypsin, and plasmin. Kallikreins may be secreted by neutrophils, mast cells, basophils, and platelets (Figure 4-3). Kallikrein-like enzymes have been detected in the gastrointestinal mast cells of cats. A tissue kallikrein is found in high concentration in the pancreas, and kallikreins may be detected in salivary, pancreatic, and intestinal secretions. A plasma kallikrein is produced by the action of activated Hageman factor on plasma prekallikrein. Kallikrein in turn exerts a positive feedback on its own formation, stimulating coagulation by activating Hageman factor (Figure 4-4). In addition to their role in kinin generation and activation of coagulation, kallikreins may be involved in the activation of complement and in the physiology of water and electrolyte movement across membranes. Various plasma protease inhibitors, such as C1-esterase inhibitor, alpha-2-macroglobulin, and alpha-1-antitrypsin, inhibit the formation of kinins. The kinins are inactivated by kinases, one of which is otherwise known as angiotensin converting enzyme.

Two important kinins are bradykinin and kallidin. They are potent vasodilators and increase capillary permeability. They contract some bowel smooth muscle preparations and relax others. They stimulate pain responses if injected intraperitoneally or into various viscera. Kinins are chemotactic to leukocytes. Some of their effects may be mediated by kinin-stimulated release of eicosanoids and heparin. Kinins are likely to be important inflammatory mediators in the digestive system. They appear to play an important role in the local and systemic consequences of pancreatic inflammation. In the treatment of pancreatitis, the use of aprotinin (Trasylol), a protease inhibitor that blocks kallikrein and trypsin synthesis, has met with limited success.

Complement Fragments[18]

The complement system may be directly activated by many stimuli of relevance to the digestive system. These include IgG or IgM complexed with antigen, certain bacteria including some strains of *E. coli*, helminth cuticles, fungal cell walls, plasmin, kallikrein, and endotoxin. The consequences of complement activation include lysis of microorganisms and cells, promotion of coagulation, activation of the kinin and eicosanoid cascades, and the release of complement fragments with proinflammatory effects. Complement fragments C5a and C567 are chemotactic. Fragments C3a and C5a increase vessel permeability. There is strong evidence that immune complex formation and complement activation contribute to the pathogenesis of inflammatory bowel disease.[19]

Platelet Activating Factor[20]

Platelet activating factor (PAF) is a phospholipid mediator derived from leukocytes, mast cells, platelets, and vascular endothelium. PAF stimulates platelet aggregation and promotes the release by platelets of a large number of mediators including serotonin and thromboxane. At very low concentrations, PAF primes neutrophils to respond to stimuli such as complement and FMLP (see above). PAF stimulates neutrophil adherence to endothelial surfaces, leading to degranulation, vascular damage, and increased vascular permeability. It has been suggested that PAF produced by a mildly injured vascular endothelium may initiate a vicious cycle that leads to more neutrophil-mediated vascular injury.[20] Formation of PAF is increased in some experimental models of colitis.[21] It has been suggested that PAF is an important mediator of endotoxic shock. Infusion of PAF into rats causes gastric damage and hemoconcentration.[22]

Interleukin 1[23]

Interleukin 1 is a polypeptide product of a variety of cells. It is an important mediator of inflammation in many tissues and is probably also important in gastrointestinal inflammation (Figure 4-5). Interleukins induce formation of arachidonic acid metabolites and acute phase proteins, cause fever, and stimulate lymphocytes, neutrophilia, fibroblast proliferation and collagen synthesis. Interleukin 1 alters endothelial cell membranes, resulting in adherence of leukocytes, increased procoagulant activity, and the release of platelet-activating factor. It decreases plasma iron concentration, a change which may inhibit bacterial growth and free radical generation.

Colonic cells derived from humans and laboratory animals with ulcerative colitis synthesize greatly increased amounts of interleukin 1.[24,25] Interleukin 1 tissue concentrations correlate with colitis' severity in humans.[26]

Cachectin[23,27]

Otherwise known as tumor necrosis factor, this polypeptide is derived from activated macrophages. It has very similar properties to the interleukins, although it apparently does not share the latter's effects on the immune system. Cachectin induces interleukin. Along with interleukin, cachectin is responsible for the anorexia and fever that accompanies inflammatory disease. Cachectin induces fibroblast proliferation and the vascular changes described for interleukin 1.

Cachectin is induced by endotoxin and may be the prime mediator of endotoxic shock. When infused into mice or rats in quantities similar to those produced endogenously, cachectin

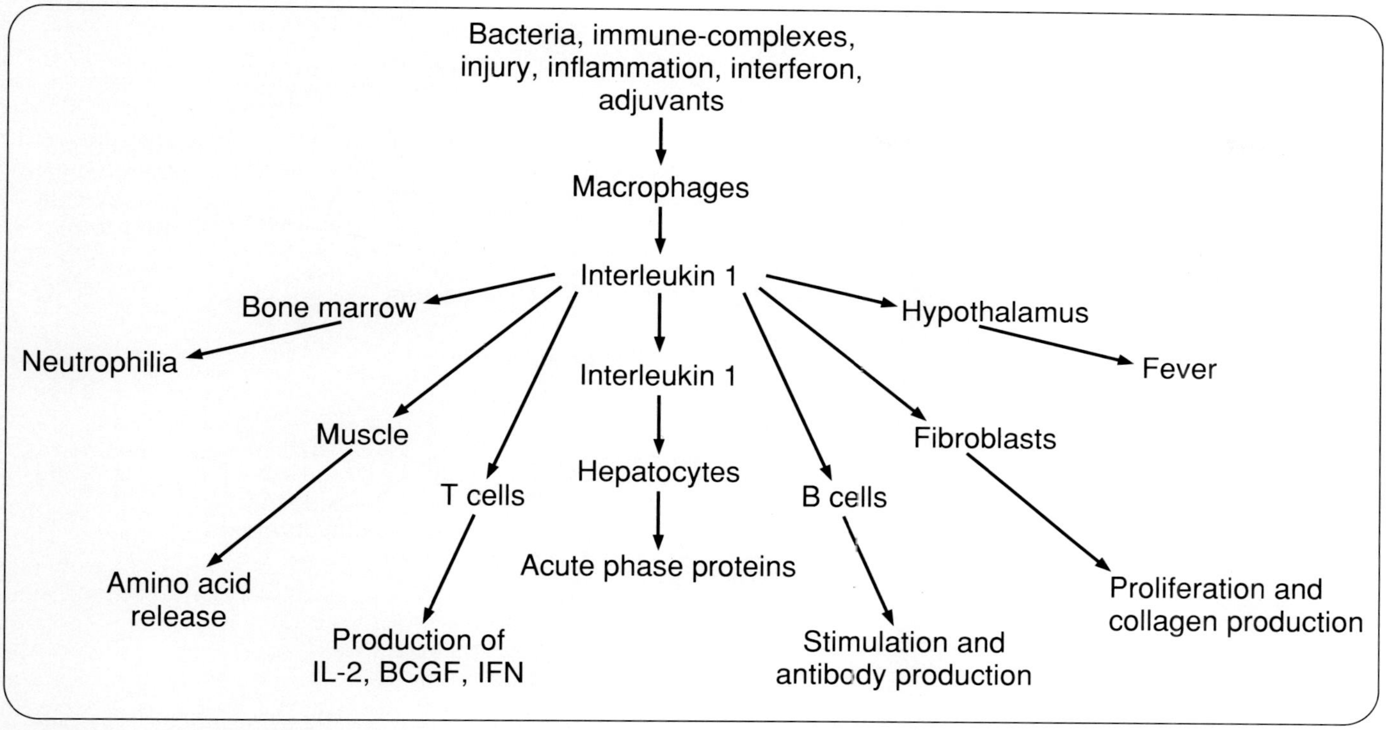

Figure 4-5. Biological activities of Interleukin 1. (From Figure 19-8, reference 1)

causes diarrhea, shock, and severe organ damage, including ischemic and hemorrhagic lesions of the gastrointestinal tract and pancreas. The hemorrhagic necrosis appears to occur due to vascular events such as procoagulation.

Neuropeptides[28]

The enteric nervous system releases several neuropeptides from unmyelinated afferent nerve endings. In addition to their function in the relay of sensory information and the control of gastrointestinal motility, some of these mediators are capable of causing vasodilation, plasma extravasation, and disordered smooth muscle contraction. Substance P is thought to be one of the most important mediators of this so-called "neurogenic inflammation." It is produced by enterochromaffin cells as well as sensory neurons. The secretion of substance P by sensory neurons is magnified by antidromic activation of their axon collaterals ("axon reflexes"). Chemical and physical irritation, including colonic distension,[29] can cause its release. The peptide results in vasodilation, plasma extravasation, pain, and smooth muscle contraction. Some of the vascular effects of substance P may be mediated by histamine. The concentration of substance P in biopsies of inflamed mucosa of humans with ulcerative colitis is significantly higher than its concentration in the non-inflamed mucosa of the same patients.[30] Recently, substance P and vasoactive intestinal polypeptide (VIP) have been shown to enhance the immunoreactivity of the gut-associated lymphoid tissue.[31,32]

VIP may also contribute to inflammation. By itself, it does not increase vascular permeability, but it does potentiate vascular leakage induced by other mediators.[10] VIP is a potent vasodilator,[33] it also stimulates pancreatic, intestinal, and salivary secretions. Their excessive release in "VIPomas" is associated with watery diarrhea. In contrast to these mediators of inflammation, another peptide hormone, somatostatin, appears to inhibit neurogenic inflammation.

The importance of neurogenic inflammation in the gastrointestinal system remains to be established. Species differences appear to exist, and there is some experimental evidence to suggest that neurogenic inflammation may vary in importance in different viscera and different regions of the bowel.

Oxygen-Derived Free Radicals[34-39]

Free radicals are molecules with unpaired electrons in one or more orbitals. They are unstable and highly reactive molecules with the propensity to oxidize other molecules. Oxygen-derived free radicals are radicals derived from the incomplete reduction of oxygen. The univalent reduction of oxygen yields superoxide anion. This reaction is catalyzed by several enzymes found in high concentration in the liver (xanthine oxidase), bowel mucosa (xanthine oxidase, aldehyde oxidase) and phagocytes (NADPH oxidase) (Figure 4-6). The high concentration of radical-generating enzymes in the digestive system and the large numbers of resident phagocytes in the bowel predispose the digestive system to free radical-mediated disease. Superoxide anion may also be generated by non-enzymatic autoxidation reactions, such as those with iron, and with certain flavins and quinones. Superoxide anion is a precursor for other oxygen-derived radicals, such as hydrogen peroxide and hydroxyl radical. Superoxide dismutase enzymes catalyze the dismutation of superoxide anion to hydrogen peroxide. The divalent reduction of oxygen by enzymes such as monoamine or diamine oxidase may also form hydrogen peroxide. In the presence of transition metals such as iron, superoxide anion and hydrogen peroxide can interact to produce the potent oxidizing

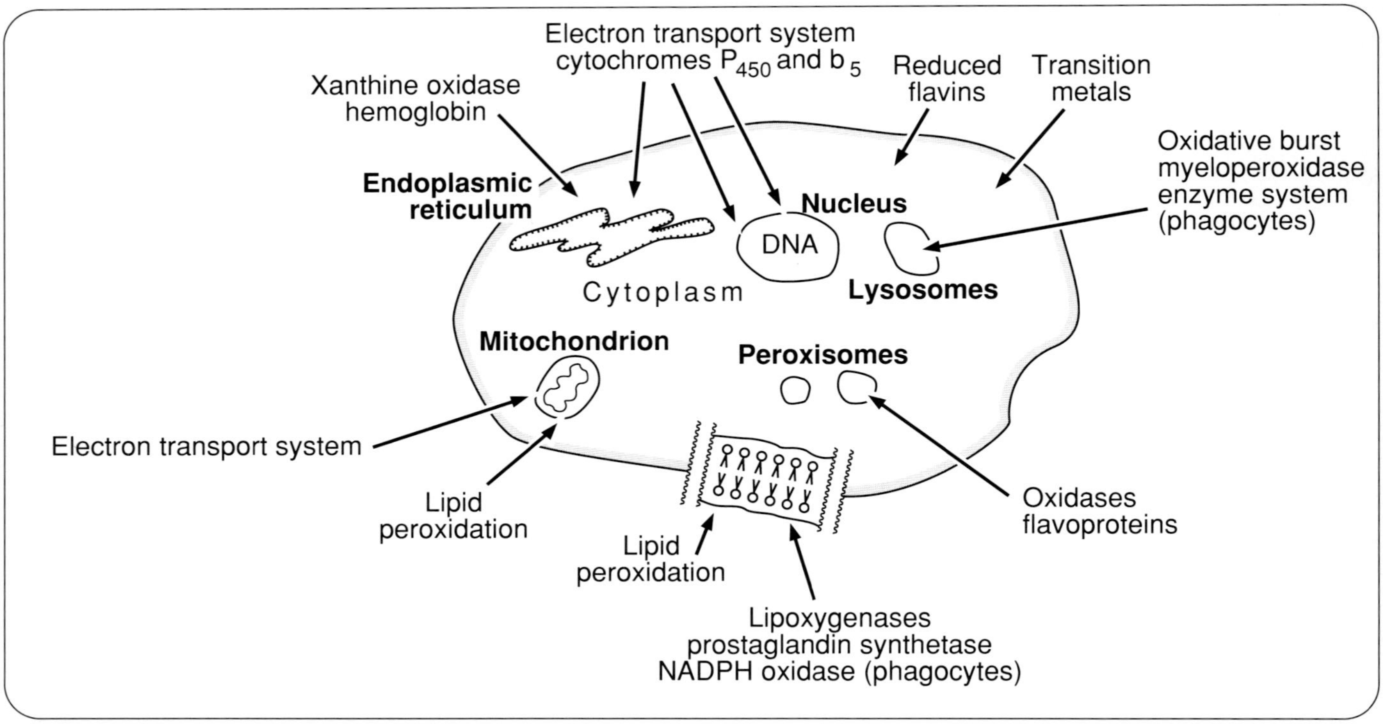

Figure 4-6. Cellular sources of free radicals. (From reference 36)

agent, hydroxyl radical. Hydrogen peroxide in the presence of chloride ion and certain peroxidases, such as neutrophil myeloperoxidase, leads to the production of hypochlorous acid. Hydroxyl radical and halogenated peroxides, such as hypochlorous acid, are thought to be the most toxic of the oxygen-derived free radicals.

Tissues employ a number of defenses against free radical attack (Figure 4-7). These include antioxidant micronutrients such as vitamin E, vitamin C, selenium, glutathione, and sulfur-containing amino acids. Important micronutrient interactions have been recognized. For instance, high levels of polyunsaturated fatty acids increase the requirements for antioxidants. An adequate level of vitamin C helps prevent depletion of vitamin E. The enzymes superoxide dismutase, catalase, and the selenium-dependent glutathione peroxidase and phospholipid glutathione peroxidase are also important defenses. Ceruloplasmin and ferritin, through copper sequestration, and iron sequestration and oxidation, also play a protective role. Mucin is known to scavenge hydroxyl radical and may play a role in the defense of the bowel epithelium. The bowel mucosa contains some of the highest concentrations of superoxide dismutase, catalase, glutathione, and vitamin E in the body.

Oxygen-derived free radical formation is only of pathological consequence if their rate of production exceeds their rate of inactivation. The small quantities of radicals produced during normal oxidative metabolism are easily dealt with by the antioxidant defenses. During inflammation, however, the rate of production of the radicals by phagocytes greatly increases, overwhelming the antioxidant defenses. An excess of free radicals may also result from a depletion of antioxidant protection. Antioxidants may be depleted by chronic inflammation or by absolute or relative dietary deficiencies. Whether derived from increased production or inadequate scavenging, an excess of oxygen-derived free radicals will cause considerable tissue damage, including lipid peroxidation and damage to DNA, carbohydrates, collagen, hyaluronic acid, enzymes, and transport proteins. Lipid peroxidation results in decreased membrane fluidity, altered permeability, and perhaps cell lysis. Damage to DNA carries the attendant likelihood of neoplasia. Free radicals and some of their products (hydroxy-alkenals) are also chemotactic. They enhance eicosanoid production and may stimulate the release of cytokines such as cachectin.[40]

Oxygen radicals may play an important role in the mucosal injury of ulcerative colitis and other inflammatory disorders of the bowel.[39] Sulfasalazine, and/or its active metabolite 5-aminosalicylate, is an oxyradical scavenger. This action may partly explain the successful deployment of this drug against ulcerative colitis. Sulfasalazine also inhibits cyclooxygenase.[8] Free radicals may be involved in the pathogenesis of acute gastric mucosal injury from chemicals such as aspirin.[41] Hydroxyl radicals degrades mucin, perhaps predisposing the epithelium to injury. Selenium deficiency has been associated with increased risk of esophageal cancer in humans, perhaps because of inadequate antioxidant protection. Radicals may mediate much of the liver damage resultant from certain toxicants such as carbon tetrachloride, acetaminophen, and endotoxin.[37,39,42] They also appear to be involved in the pathogenesis of pancreatitis,[39] and they play an important role in the tissue necrosis and inflammation resulting from gastrointestinal ischemic disorders.

Lactoferrin

Degranulating neutrophils release lactoferrin, which occurs in many gastrointestinal secretions. An antibacterial role has been attributed to this protein because of its ability to

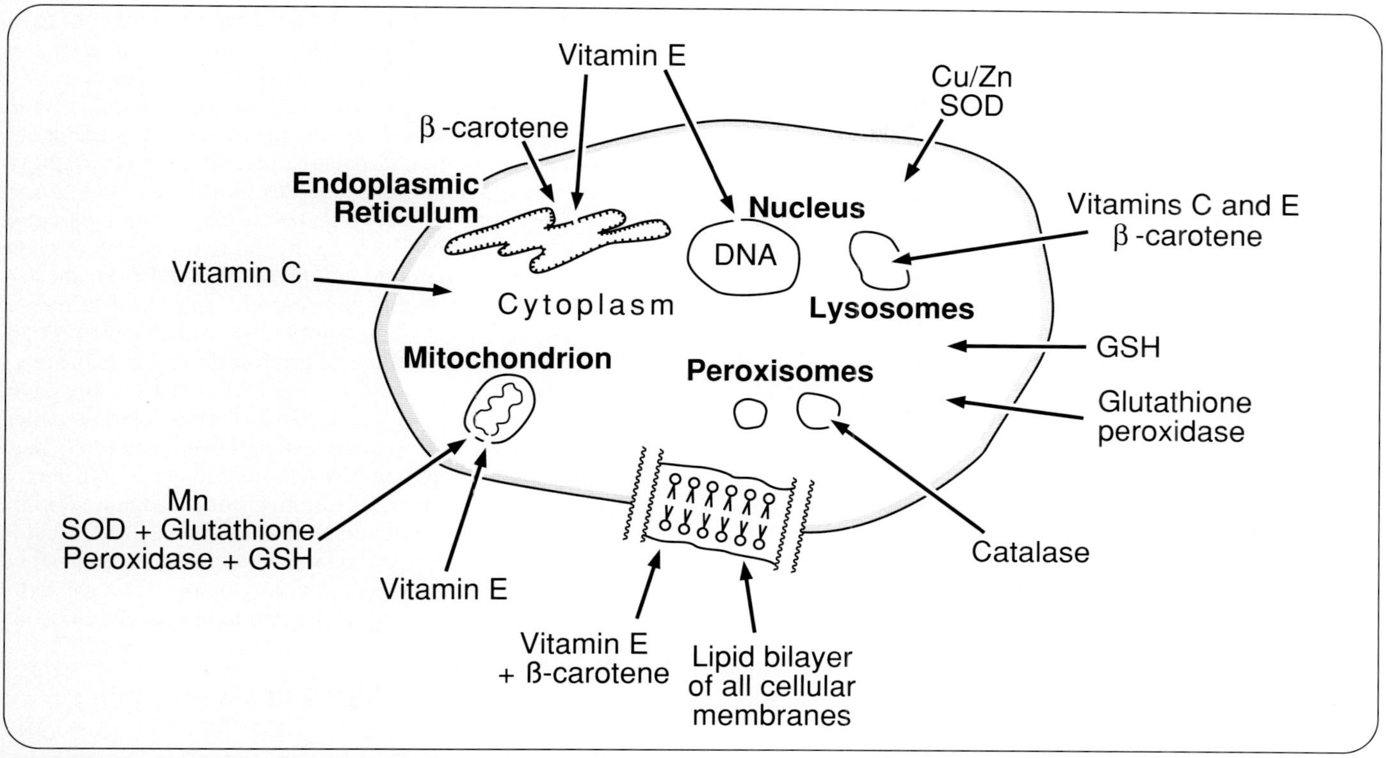

Figure 4-7. Antioxidant protection within the cell. (From reference 36)

deprive bacteria of iron. Recent observations have suggested that during inflammation, superoxide anion releases iron from lactoferrin. The increased concentration of iron amplifies the inflammatory process by facilitating the generation of hydroxyl radicals and by enhancing neutrophil adhesion to the endothelium.[20]

Proteases[10]

Phagocytes, in particular the neutrophil, release proteolytic enzymes into the tissues. These include kallikreins, plasminogen activator, elastase, collagenases, cathepsins, a serine protease, hyaluronidase, and lysozyme. Substrates of these enzymes include kinins, plasminogen, elastin, collagen, fibrin, proteoglycans, clotting and complement factors, immunoglobulins, and hyaluronic acid. These enzymes are thought to function in tissue defense and repair, but excessive release can damage healthy tissues and may activate the kinin, complement, and coagulation systems. The release of elastase by neutrophils is very destructive to vascular integrity.

CONSEQUENCES OF INFLAMMATION

Elimination of Microorganisms and Foreign Antigen

An important consequence of the inflammatory process is that phagocytes, which have been concentrated at the inflammatory focus by the chemotactic and vascular events described above, release the antibody, complement, and the multitude of toxic products and digestive enzymes that eliminate invasive microorganisms and other foreign antigen. As previously mentioned, an important consequence of the exudation of plasma at inflammatory sites is the dilution of toxins. Antigen not rapidly eliminated is walled off from the body by intravascular clotting, extravascular fibrin, the physical presence of amassed phagocytes, and ultimately by fibrous tissue.

Tissue Healing

Healing begins with the removal of debris by the processes of liquefaction and phagocytosis. Absorption, sloughing, or drainage remove the debris liquified by enzymatic digestion. Proliferation of fibrous tissue or regeneration then fill tissue defects at the inflammatory site. Macrophages are responsible for elimination of much of the debris from the inflammatory focus. They also stimulate fibrosis. The extent of tissue regeneration depends on both the extent of damage and the type of tissue destroyed. Hepatocytes have a remarkable capacity to regenerate, provided the reticulin framework of the lobule is intact. Bowel epithelium also regenerates readily provided denudation is not complete. Glandular epithelium, however, has less capacity for regeneration. Massive cellular destruction and chronic irritation result in the formation of considerable amounts of fibrous tissue. Hepatic cirrhosis, chronic pancreatitis, fibrosing gastritis, and fibrosing colitis are examples of such processes.

Tissue Damage

If the inciting cause is not expediently eliminated, damage to host tissues will occur. The tissue damage results from the chronic secretion by phagocytes of toxic products, and by concurrent elaboration of cytotoxic products by the immune response. The toxic agents most often incriminated in causing non-specific damage to host tissues are oxygen-derived free radicals, proteases (especially elastase), cytokines, and certain toxic proteins. Major basic protein released from eosinophils is toxic to epithelial surfaces.

Villous atrophy is a common morphological response to a variety of different pathological processes, one of which is inflammation. Villous atrophy results from villous contraction after a reduction in the quantity of villous epithelial cells. Acute inflammatory processes cause epithelial loss through rapid necrosis and/or sloughing of large expanses of epithelium. Chronic inflammation appears to cause epithelial loss by the secretion of T cell-derived lymphokines that cause premature loss of immature enterocytes from the villi. The consequence of villous atrophy is malabsorption. Severe tissue damage in the bowel can result in significant fluid, electrolyte, and protein loss. The consequences of inflammatory damage in the liver are discussed in the chapter on hepatic disease.

Altered Motility[28]

Gastrointestinal inflammation, even if restricted to the mucosa, can result in disordered bowel motility. The pathogenesis of the motility disturbances are not clear but probably result either from a direct effect of the mediators such as PGE_2 or leukotrienes on smooth muscle function or from an indirect effect of these mediators on the enteric nervous system. Direct projection of nerves between the mucosa, submucosa and muscle layers has been demonstrated. Communication from mucosa to muscularis may also occur via spinal reflex arcs. Localized or generalized ileus can develop due to pancreatitis, or cholecystitis. In ulcerative colitis in humans, there is a tendency for rhythmic segmentation to be reduced, resulting in a flaccid bowel with little resistance to the passage of luminal content and thus diarrhea. Hypermotility accompanies certain parasitic and bacterial disorders of the bowel and may help clear these undesirable agents from the bowel. On occasion, smooth muscle spasms may occur. This results in abdominal pain and may be the forerunner of intussusception.

Increased Bowel Permeability

Inflammation results in increased bowel permeability. The increased absorption of luminal antigens may perpetuate the inflammatory process by attracting more inflammatory cells and further activating of the immune system. The mechanisms by which inflammation increases permeability are probably multifactorial. Mucosal denudation is an obvious cause. Of interest is the recent in vitro demonstration that gamma interferon will increase epithelial tight junction permeability.[43] It is probable that many other inflammatory mediators increase bowel permeability. The consequences of increased permeability include fluid, electrolyte, protein and cell loss, as well as increased absorption of antigenic and toxic materials.

Systemic Consequences

Inflammatory processes in the gastrointestinal system can result in fever, nausea, anorexia, weight loss, and leukocytosis. These signs result from the release of certain mediators, such as interleukin 1 and cachectin, and from the absorption of toxic products. Signs pertaining to fluid, electrolyte, or albumin loss may be noted. Inflammation results in the generation of a number of mediators that can activate the complement cascade, the kinin system, and the coagulation cascade. This interaction becomes important in acute pancreatitis, where local inflammation can take on global consequences through the initiation of disseminated intravascular coagulation. Chronic inflammation is usually accompanied by a significant lymphocytic immune response. Soluble immune complexes derived from the humoral arm of the lymphocytic response may lead to distant manifestations of the inflammatory process. Three well-recognized systemic complications of gastrointestinal immune reactions are uveitis, polyarthritis, and dermatitis. On occasion, chronic inflammation is associated with amyloidosis. So-called "reactive amyloidosis" appears to result from ineffective degradation of the serum acute-phase proteins that occur in persistently elevated concentration during chronic inflammation. In the digestive system, amyloid is most commonly deposited in the liver of dogs and the pancreas of aged cats, but the intestinal tract is occasionally affected. Renal amyloidosis is occasionally observed in human patients with granulomatous enteritis.

REGULATION OF INFLAMMATION

Digestive system inflammation is prevented by maintaining an effective permeability barrier to luminal antigens. The high and low affinity receptor systems of phagocytes help ensure that these potentially destructive cells are attracted from a great distance but not activated until they reach the actual inflammatory site. Once initiated, inflammation is largely controlled by the elimination of the inciting cause. The predominance of non-complement mediated (IgA) humoral responses in the bowel further restricts inflammation. Scavengers restrict damage due to release of free radicals. Protease inhibitors such as alpha-1-antitrypsin and alpha-2-macroglobulin enter the areas of inflammation through the permeable vessel walls and block the activity of proteases, including those released from neutrophils and those that activate complement. A low molecular weight inhibitor, called antileukoprotease, has also been identified in human mucus and salivary secretions.[10] Proteases released by canine mast cells are capable of degrading vasoactive intestinal peptide and substance P. Proteases released by eosinophils partially reduce mast cell-mediated and basophil-mediated inflammation. Serum amyloid A is an acute phase protein which dampens the immune response to inflammation.

CATEGORIES OF INFLAMMATION[2,44,45]

Inflammatory processes are usually classified according to their longevity and the predominant exudate or cell type at the inflammatory focus. Two important factors determining the cell types present at the inflammatory site are the particular chemotactic factors produced by the inciting tissue insult and the duration of the inflammation. The categories of inflammation most frequently observed in the gastrointestinal tract are mucoid, fibrinous, hemorrhagic, suppurative, lymphocytic-plasmacytic, eosinophilic, and granulomatous. It is important to note that, like most biological processes, inflammation defies textbook classification. Intergrades of these classical descriptions are common.

Mucoid Inflammation

Mucoid inflammation is characterized grossly by mucus adherent to feces or mucosa, and microscopically by increased numbers of goblet cells. Mucoid inflammation is caused by chronic mild irritants. These include bacterial and viral infections of low virulence, parasitic disorders, and low grade immune-mediated processes such as mild chronic colitis.

Fibrinous (Pseudomembranous) Inflammation

Pseudomembranous inflammation is a type of fibrinous inflammation characterized by the formation of a dense, white or yellowish plaque on the mucosal surface. On occasion cylindrical fibrinous casts are passed in the feces, giving the initial impression that the patient has sloughed a segment of bowel. Causes of pseudomembranous inflammation include canine and feline parvovirus, *Salmonella, Clostridium difficle*, and perhaps *Bacteroides*, and *Fusobacterium* species. In the peritoneal cavity serous and fibrinous inflammation are important manifestations of peritoneal irritation. In the cat, feline infectious peritonitis is an important cause of fibrin exudation. Fibrous organization of peritoneal fibrin can lead to abdominal adhesions.

Hemorrhagic Inflammation

Hemorrhagic inflammation can result from diapedesis of red blood cells through highly permeable vasculature, or from hemorrhage through small vessels disrupted by inflammation, trauma, microorganisms, or toxic products. Causes include infection with highly virulent organisms such as *Salmonella, Clostridium perfringens, Neorickettsia helminthoeca*, canine hepatitis virus, leptospirosis, and parvovirus. Infection with *Prototheca* can cause a hemorrhagic colitis. Hemorrhagic colitis due to *Candida, Zygomycetes, Aspergillus*, and other opportunists has been reported in cats most commonly in association with panleukopenia. Other causes include poisoning by heavy metals such as arsenic and thallium, plants such as *Amanita* mushrooms, and various household products. Uremia, ischemic disorders such as shock and organ torsion, and immune-mediated disorders such as chronic colitis can also cause hemorrhagic inflammation. Severe pancreatic inflammation is commonly hemorrhagic in nature.

Suppurative (Purulent) Inflammation

Suppurative inflammation is characterized grossly by pus and microscopically by marked neutrophil infiltration or accumulation. Causes of suppurative inflammation in the liver include bacteremias and viral diseases such as canine hepatitis. Infections of bowel by bacteria such as *Salmonella*, coliforms, *Yersinia enterocolitica*, and certain anaerobic bacteria can result in suppuration. In liver, pancreas, and bowel, disorders resulting in ischemia or necrosis are eventually accompanied by neutrophilic infiltrates. Most suppurative processes are acute in nature.

Lymphocytic-Plasmacytic Inflammation

Lymphocytic-plasmacytic inflammation is said to result from "chronic antigenic stimulation." The inciting antigens, however, are poorly defined. In the bowel, the most important antigens are probably proteinaceous products absorbed from the lumen. On occasion, self-antigens probably initiate the inflammation (autoimmunity). In the liver, the inciting antigens are also unknown. The gross appearance of this inflammation is often unremarkable, and microscopic diagnosis is not without difficulty. The normal bowel has a small complement of lymphocytes, plasma cells, eosinophils, and histiocytes in the lamina propria along the proprial-submucosal junction. The majority of these lymphocytes and plasma cells are committed to IgA secretion (see Chapter 3). In the inflamed bowel the numbers of lymphocytes and plasma cells increase, and their distribution may widen to include the lamina propria of villi. Futhermore, the proportion of IgG versus IgA secreting plasma cells increases. Considerable experience is necessary to differentiate normal bowel from mild lymphocytic-plasmacytic enteritis. Lymphocytic-plasmacytic inflammation is prominent in the idiopathic disorders of lymphocytic-plasmacytic enteritis, chronic gastritis, chronic colitis, chronic hepatitis, and cholangiohepatitis. Lymphocytic infiltrates are common in gluten enteropathy, *Campylobacter* enterocolitis, and cryptosporidiosis. Bacterial overgrowth, giardiasis, and carcinomas are sometimes associated with mild infiltrations of these cell types.

Eosinophilic Inflammation

Small numbers of eosinophils are a normal finding in the lamina propria of the bowel, and mild eosinophilic infiltration is a common component of inflammatory processes with many causes, including immune-mediated diseases. Known causes of inflammation characterized by a predominance of eosinophils are parasitic and type 1 hypersensitivity disorders. On many occasions, the cause of the eosinophilic infiltration is not apparent. Examples include eosinophilic ulcers and hypereosinophilic syndrome in cats, oral eosinophilic granulomas in Siberian Huskies, and eosinophilic gastroenteritis. The eosinophil's release of proteases, radicals, PAF, leukotrienes, and various toxic proteins has a pro-inflammatory function. Diamine oxidase released by eosinophils degrades histamine.

Granulomatous Inflammation

Granulomatous inflammation is characterized by an accumulation of macrophages, some of which mesh to form multinucleated giant cells, and by the deposition of collagen about the irritant focus. The release of interleukin 1 and fibronectin from macrophages stimulates the collagen deposition. Granulomatous inflammation is a chronic process usually resulting from antigens of a fairly indestructible nature. Causes include phycomycosis, systemic mycoses, mycobacteria, tissue stages of parasites, and imbedded foreign materials. In cats granulomatous colitis due to FIP has been recognized. Idiopathic granulomatous inflammation occasionally occurs in the bowel and liver. A granulomatous colitis, characterized by accumulation of macrophages containing PAS-positive granules has been reported in Boxers and French Bulldogs.

Granulomas on occasion may be dominated by eosinophils rather than macrophages. So called eosinophilic granulomas have been reported in the oral cavity of dogs and cats and the stomach and intestine of dogs. Their cause is unknown.

Therapy of Inflammation

Inflammation is best treated by attention to the primary cause. When the cause of chronic inflammation is not apparent and infective causes are considered unlikely, antiinflammatory drugs such as prednisone are commonly employed. With the exception of 5-aminosalicylate, non-steroidal antiinflammatory drugs are *not* recommended for the treatment of gastrointestinal inflammation. There is good evidence that most non-steroidal antiinflammatory agents worsen bowel inflammation, possibly by increasing bowel permeability or interfering with suppressor T cell function. Furthermore they may lead to mucosal ulceration. It is likely that free radical scavengers and specific inhibitors of leukotrienes will eventually find application in the treatment of gastrointestinal inflammation. Therapy of gastrointestinal inflammation is described in more detail during the discussion of specific disorders.

REFERENCES

1. Tizard, I.: Veterinary Immunology. WB Saunders, Philadelphia, 267-280, 1987.
2. Jones, T.C., Hunt, R.D.: Veterinary Pathology. Lea & Febiger, Philadelphia, 175-213, 1983.
3. Thompson, R.G.: General Veterinary Pathology. WB Saunders Co, Philadelphia, 163-229, 1984.
4. Nast, C.C., LeDuc, L.E.: Chemotactic peptides. Mechanisms, functions, and possible role in inflammatory bowel disease. Dig. Dis. Sci. 33:50S-57S, 1988.
5. Hawkey, C.J., Rampton, D.S.: Prostaglandins and the gastrointestinal mucosa: Are they important in its function, disease, or treatment? Gastroenterology 89:1162-1188, 1985.
6. Eva Doran, J., Lundsgaard-Hansen, P.: Role of the reticuloendothelial system in the pathogenesis of organ damage. Br. J. Hosp. Med. 39:221-225, 1988.
7. Highland, R.L., Upson, D.W.: Simplified role of prostaglandins in the gastrointestinal tract. Comp. Contin. Ed. Pract. Vet. 8:188-194, 1986.
8. Goetzl, E.J., Burrall, B.A., Baud, L., Scriven, K.H., Levine, J.D. and Koo, C.H.: Generation and recognition of leukotriene mediators of hypersensitivity and inflammation. Dig. Dis. Sci. 33:36S-40S, 1988.
9. Schumert, R., Towner, J. and Zipser, R.D.: Role of eicosanoids in experimental colitis. Dig. Dis. Sci. 33:58S-64S, 1988.
10. Venge, P., Lindbom, A.: Inflammation. Almqvist & Wiksell International, Stockholm, 1985.
11. Rask-Madsen, J.: The role of eicosanoids in the gastrointestinal tract. Scand. J. Gastroenterology 22: 7S-19S, 1987.
12. Snape, W.J., Kao, H.W.: Role of inflammatory mediators in colonic smooth muscle function in ulcerative colitis. Dig. Dis. Sci. 33:65S-70S, 1988.
13. Karayalcin, S.S., Sturbaum, C.W., Dixon, M.U. and Powell, D.W.: Immune system-stimulated colonic secretion is mediated by the enteric nervous system. Gastroenterology 94:A217, 1988.
14. Anton, P.A., Targan, S.R. and Shanahan, F.: Neutrophil differences in FMLP-induced chemiluminescence and FMLP receptor number in patients with inflammatory bowel disease. Gastroenterology 94:A9, 1988.
15. Douglas, W.W.: Histamine and 5-hydroxytryptamine (serotonin) and their antagonists. In: The Pharmacological Basis of Therapeutics. Edited by Goodman Gilman, A., Goodman, L.S., Rall, T.W. Macmillan Pub Co, New York, 628-635, 1985.
16. Wallace, J.L., Gingras, G.R.: Mediation of adaptive cytoprotection by 5-Hydroxytryptamine? Gastroenterology 94:A485, 1988.
17. Douglas, W.W.: Polypeptides - angiotensin, plasma kinins, and others. In, The Pharmacological Basis of Therapeutics. Edited by Goodman Gilman, A., Goodman, L.S., Rall, T.W. Macmillan Pub Co, New York, 653-659, 1985.
18. Tizard, I.: Veterinary Immunology. WB Saunders, Philadelphia, 115-126, 1987.
19. Jewell, D.P., Patel, C.: Immunology of inflammatory bowel disease. Scand. J. Gastroenterology 20:119S-126S, 1985.
20. Jacob, H.S., Vercellotti, G.M.: Granulocyte-mediated endothelial injury: Oxidant damage amplified by lactoferrin and platelet activating factor. Upjohn symposium, Michigan, 57-62, 1987.
21. Boughton-Smith, N.K., Whittle, B.J.R.: Formation of the pro-Inflammatory mediatory, PAF-Acether in different models of colitis. Gastroenterology 94:A45, 1988.
22. Wallace, J.L., MacNaughton, W.K., Guarner, F., Rodriguez, R. and Malageleda, J.-R.: Role of leukotrienes as mediators of gastric damage and hemo-concentration induced by platelet-activating factor. Gastroenterology 94:A485, 1988.
23. Dinarello, C.A.: Interleukin-1. Dig. Dis. Sci. 33:25s-35s, 1988.
24. Ligumsky, M., Simon, P.L., Karmeli, F. and Rachmilewitz, D.: Interleukin-1 — Possible mediator of the inflammatory response in ulcerative colitis (UC). Gastroenterology 94:A263, 1988.
25. Rachmiliwitz, D., Simon, P.L., Sjogren, R., Fondacaro, J.D., Wasserman, M.A. and Boedeker, E.: Interleukin-1: A sensitive marker of colonic inflammation. Gastroenterology 94:A363, 1988.
26. Sartor, R.B., Chapman, E.J. and Schwab, J.H.: Increased interleukin-1 beta concentrations in resected inflammatory bowel disease (IBD) tissue. Gastroenterology 94:A399, 1988.
27. Beutler, B., Cerami, A.: Cachectin: More than a tumor necrosis factor. New Eng. J. Med. 316:379-385, 1987.
28. Mayer, E.A., Raybould, H. and Koelbel, C.: Neuropeptides, inflammation, and motility. Dig. Dis. Sci. 33:71s-77s, 1988.
29. Stapelfeldt, W.H., Go, V.L.W. and Szurszewski, J.H.: Colonic distension releases substance P in the guinea pig inferior mesenteric ganglion. Gastroenterology 94:A441, 1988.
30. Goldin, E., Karmeli, F. and Rachmilewitz, D.: Pathogenesis of diarrhea in ulcerative colitis — possible role of increased colonic substance P levels. Gastroenterology 94:A150, 1988.
31. Croitoru, K., Ernst, P.B., Bienenstock, J., Padol, R. and Stanisz, A.: The effect of substance P (SP) and vasoactive intestinal polypeptide (VIP) on murine intestinal natural killer activity. Gastroenterology 94:A80, 1988.
32. Hart, R., Wagner, F. and Duncygier, H.: Substance P enhances immune responses of the gut associated lymphoid tissue. Gastroenterology 94:A174, 1988.
33. Blank, M.A., Kimura, K. and Jaffe, B.M.: Vasoactive intestinal polypeptide (VIP) antagonist (N-AC0TYR[1], D-PHE[2]) - GRF(1-29) - NH_2: An inhibitor of vasodilatation in the feline colon. Gastroenterology 94:A39, 1988.
34. Grisham, M.B., Granger, D.N.: Neutrophil-mediated mucosal injury. Role of reactive oxygen metabolites. Dig. Dis. Sci. 33:6S-15S, 1988.
35. Hitt, M.E.: Oxygen derived free radicals - their pathophysiology and implications. Comp. Contin. Ed. Pract. Vet. 10:939-946, 1988.
36. Machlin, L.J., Bendich, A.: Free radical tissue damage: protective role of antioxidant nutrients. FASEB J. 1:441-445, 1987.
37. Cross, C.E., Halliwell, B., Borish, E.T., Pryor, W.A., Ames, B.N., Saul, R.L., McCord, J.M. and Harman, D.: Oxygen radicals and human disease. Ann, Intern. Med. 107:526-545, 1987.
38. VanSteenhouse, J.L.: Free radicals: relation to tissue damage

- a review. Vet Clin Path 16:29-35, 1987.

39. Parks, D.A., Bulkley, G.B. and Granger, D.N.: Role of oxygen-derived free radicals in digestive tract diseases. Surgery 94:415-422, 1983.
40. Clark, I.A., Thumwood, C.M., Chaudhri, G., Cowden, W.B. and Nunt, N.H.: Tumor necrosis factor and reactive oxygen species. In: Oxygen radicals and tissue injury. Edited by B. Halliwell. Upjohn symposium, Michigan, 122-129, 1987.
41. Phian, G., Regillo, B.A. and Szabo, S.: Free radicals and lipid peroxidation in ethanol- or aspirin-induced gastric mucosal injury. Dig. Dis. Sci. 32:1395-1401, 1987.
42. Mitchell, J.R.: Acetaminophen toxicity. New Eng. J. Med. 319:1601-1602, 1988.
43. Madara, J.L.: Gamma-interferon (Gamma-IFN) enhances intestinal epithelial permeability by altering tight junctions. Gastroenterology 94:A276, 1988.
44. Barker, I.K., Van Dreumel, A.A.: The alimentary system. In: Pathology of Domestic Animals. Edited by Jubb, K.V.F., Kennedy, P.C., Palmer, N. Academic Press, Inc, Orlando. 1-202, 1985.
45. Van Kruiningen, H.J.: Gastrointestinal system. In: Special Veterinary Pathology. Edited by Thomson, R.G. BC Decker Inc, Toronto, 133-227, 1988.

Chapter 5

Approach to Clinical Problems in Gastroenterology

INTRODUCTION

Diagnosis of medical problems begins with a thorough history and a complete physical examination. If therapy, prognosis, or communicability cannot be determined from the clinical examination, a diagnostic evaluation is required. The diagnostic workup should consist of an orderly series of procedures designed to determine the presence or absence of a particular class or cause of disease. The "problem-orientated approach" to diagnostics facilitates a systematic workup of complex cases. The sequence of diagnostic procedures depends to a large extent on logistical concerns such as cost as well as availability of staff and diagnostic equipment. The procedures selected early in the workup are designed to answer more general questions (such as the identity of the organ system(s) involved); they tend to be less invasive, less expensive, and have a higher diagnostic yield than procedures for identifying specific problems or diseases. At times tests designed to detect unlikely, but treatable, diseases are performed early in the workup simply because they diagnose diseases whose outcome the clinician can influence.

Ideally, the workup concludes with an accurate diagnosis. Unfortunately, because of financial constraints, limited knowledge about many canine and feline diseases, and restricted availability of refined diagnostic techniques, the diagnostic workup is often concluded before a specific disease entity is definitively diagnosed. This need not be of concern, provided the diagnostics have sufficiently defined the initial complaint to a point where appropriate therapy, accurate prognosis, and the likelihood of communicability to animals and humans have been determined.

PROBLEM-ORIENTATED APPROACH TO DIAGNOSIS

The "problem-orientated approach" formalizes problem solving into a logical sequence (Table 5-1). The first step is to gather information. The history, physical examination, and admission laboratory work establish the minimum data base. The second step is to identify and list the problems that constitute the presentation. These may be the owners' observations or may be abnormalities recognized by the veterinarian. The third step is to establish a list of diagnostic possibilities for *each* problem using, if required, the assistance of textbooks or colleagues. The fourth step is to design a plan to diagnose or treat *each* problem. The fifth step is to prioritize the problems according to their threat to the animal's health, their importance to the owner, and the logistics of your clinic, and then to institute the diagnostics. The sixth step is to update the problem list as the results of diagnostic procedures unfold. Updating is achieved by refining to a greater degree of specificity previously general problems and by adding new problems should they be uncovered. The diagnostic process ends when the problem is defined to the limits of the clinician's diagnostic capability and when follow-up indicates that therapeutics prescribed or advice given was effective. By using this system no problem is overlooked. Common themes may become apparent, and the problems may

Table 5-1 A Problem-Oriented Approach to Diagnosis and Treatment of Gastrointestinal Diseases

Step 1	**Information Gathering (establishing a Data Base)**
	a) History
	b) Physical examination
	c) Admission laboratory work
Step 2	**Identify and List All Problems**
Step 3	**Establish Rule-Outs for Each Problem**
Step 4	**Design a Plan to Diagnose Each Problem**
Step 5	**Prioritize the Work-up of Each Problem and Institute Diagnostics**
	a) Threat to health of patient
	b) Owners degree of concern
	c) Logistics and expense of work-up
Step 6	**Update the Problem List Until a Diagnosis is Reached or the Problem Sufficiently Refined**
	a) Institute therapy
	b) Advise of prognosis
	c) Educate client about the disease
Step 7	**Follow-up on Each Problem**
	a) Resolution of signs - end of problem
	b) Unsuccessful therapy - institute further diagnostics

Table 5-2 The Components of the Medical Interview

- Patient profile
- Owner's primary complaint
- Identification of clinical signs of disease
- Sequence, frequency, and progression of sign(s)
- Character of vomitus or diarrhea
- Severity of the signs
- Location of site of disease causing the sign(s)
- Aggravating or alleviating factors
- Review of body systems

eventually be recognized as manifestations of a single disease. Conversely, the clinician may identify two or more separate conditions that in combination result in the animal's signs.

History Taking

The history provides the most rapid and inexpensive progress towards a diagnosis. History taking has been referred to as the greatest of all of the medical arts. Along with the physical examination, it is the foundation on which all future diagnostic procedures are selected. The initial aims of the interview are formulation of a patient profile, definition of the owner's chief complaint, identification of clinical signs of disease, and acquisition of information pertaining to the clinical signs of the present illness (Table 5-2).

A patient profile that includes information about the patient's age, sex, breed, diet, environment, vaccinations, and medical history must be completed. Breed predispositions to many gastrointestinal diseases have been recognized (Table 5-3). It is extremely important that the history defines the owner's chief complaint. What concerns an owner about a pet may not necessarily be the clinical sign that most concerns the veterinarian. Failure to address the owner's primary concern, while pursuing clinical signs perceived as more serious by the veterinarian, is an important cause of owner dissatisfaction. The history should begin with general questions pertaining to this complaint and proceed to more specific interrogation as signs of disease are revealed.

Clinical problems in small animal gastroenterology present what are defined as primary and associated or secondary signs (Table 5-4). The important primary signs include dysphagia, regurgitation, vomition, bloat, borborygmus, diarrhea, dyschezia, melena, tenesmus, abdominal pain, flatulence, icterus, and ascites. Secondary signs include those which are not

Table 5-3 Suspected or Confirmed Breed Predispositions to Gastrointestinal Diseases

Abyssinian - megaesophagus due to myasthenia gravis
Airedale Terrier - pancreatic carcinoma
Basenji- lymphocytic/plasmacytic enteritis, hypertrophic gastritis
Beagle - chronic hepatitis, IgA deficiency
Bedlington Terrier - copper-induced hepatopathy
Boston Terrier - vascular compression of the esophagus, constipation
Boxers - gingival and circumanal neoplasia, mastocytoma, histiocytic colitis, chronic colitis
Brachycephalic breeds - gastric retention
Cocker Spaniel - gingival, oropharyngeal and circumanal neoplasia, chronic hepatitis, portasystemic shunts
Dachshund - colonic perforation
Doberman Pinscher - parvovirus, chronic hepatitis
English Bulldog - vascular compression of the esophagus, cleft palate, constipation, fecal incontinence
English Springer Spaniel - fucosidosis
Fox Terrier - circumanal neoplasia
French Bulldog - chronic colitis
German Shepherd - oropharyngeal neoplasia, exocrine pancreatic insufficiency, inflammatory bowel disease, stress-induced diarrhea, megaesophagus, vascular compression of the esophagus, sialocele, hepatic angiosarcoma, perianal fistula, bacterial overgrowth
German Short-haired Pointer - oropharyngeal neoplasia
Golden Retriever - oropharyngeal neoplasia
Great Dane - GDV, megaesophagus
Greyhound - megaesophagus
Irish Setter - wheat-sensitive enteropathy, megaesophagus, vascular compression of the esophagus, esophageal sarcoma, perianal fistula
Large-breed dogs - Gastric dilatation-volvulus
Lundenhund - protein-losing enteropathy
Manx cat - constipation, fecal incontinence
Miniature Schnauzer - hyperlipidemia, pancreatitis, megaesophagus, portasystemic shunts
Pointer - hepatic angiosarcoma, esophageal sarcoma, cleft palate
Poodle - sialocele
Rottweiler - parvovirus, gastric eosinophilic granuloma
Sharpei - IgA deficiency, food intolerances, inflammatory bowel disease, hiatal hernias
Shih Tzu - cleft palate
Siamese cat - megaesophagus, gastric retention, intestinal adenocarcinoma
Siberian Husky - oral eosinophilic granuloma
Small-breed dogs - hemorrhagic gastroenteritis
Swiss Sheepdog - cleft palate
Weimaraner - oropharyngeal neoplasia
West Highland White Terrier - copper-associated hepatopathy
Wirehaired Fox Terrier - megaesophagus
Yorkshire Terriers - portasystemic shunts

Table 5-4 Clinical Signs of Gastrointestinal Disease

Primary Signs	Secondary Signs
Dysphagia	Anorexia
Regurgitation	Fever
Vomition	Depression
Bloat	Cardiovascular signs
Borborygmus	Hypersalivation
Diarrhea	Shivering
Dyschezia	Behavioral changes
Melena	Perineal pruritis
Tenesmus	Polyphagia
Abdominal pain	Dehydration
Flatulence	
Icterus	
Ascites	

specific for a problem in any single system, such as anorexia, fever, depression, dehydration, polyphagia, weight loss, polydypsia, hypersalivation, shivering, evidence of shock, and perineal pruritus. The identification of all primary and secondary signs aids in determining the most likely site of the problem and assessing the severity of the animal's condition.

Historical information to be determined about each clinical sign is depicted in Table 5-2. It is important to determine when a sign became noticeable and which of a number of signs was noticed first. The frequency of occurrence of a given sign must also be noted. Additional information should be collected on the duration of a symptom and the intervals between periods of illness. The character of vomitus and bowel movements often provides useful information for differential diagnosis. The clinician should attempt to determine the anatomical location of the dysfunction. Identification of the site of a problem is of great value in deciding which procedures should be ordered first in a workup of the case. The severity of the sign or the limitation of function imposed by the disease should also be described. The severity of the process determines the necessity of supportive therapy and the appropriate amount of diagnostic effort. The owner should be queried to discover any factors that incite, aggravate, or alleviate the sign. Knowledge of aggravating or alleviating factors will not only help the clinician arrive at a diagnosis but often provide valuable clues toward outlining a successful management program. The history is concluded by screening other systems of the body with appropriate questions. The importance of this "systems review" cannot be overemphasized. The gastrointestinal system influences, and in turn is influenced by, other body systems. Even when the predominant clinical signs appear to result from gastrointestinal disease, asking questions pertaining only to the gastrointestinal tract, ignores the strong likelihood that a disease of another system may be causing secondary gastrointestinal dysfunction. Furthermore, it is not uncommon for animals to have more than one disease process affecting different body systems.

The Physical Examination

The objective of the physical examination is to recognize and describe gross deviations of physical appearance and behavior of the patient from those recognized as normal for the animal's age, sex, and breed. Information gathered from laboratory or radiologic procedures cannot make up for an incompletely conducted physical examination. The discussion below is limited to physical examination features directly pertinent to the gastrointestinal system, but the clinician should complete an examination of all body systems when presented with an animal manifesting signs of gastrointestinal disease.

Unrestrained Patient. The physical examination should begin by observing the unrestrained patient on the floor. The animal's size, weight, mentation, posture, respiratory rate, and behavior can be evaluated at this time while it is likely to be less excited. This is also a convenient time to give the patient food or water if swallowing or mastication is to be observed.

Oropharynx and Cervical Area. Physical examination for diagnosis of gastrointestinal signs includes examination of the oral and pharyngeal cavities. Complete examination of these structures often requires that the patient be anesthetized. Particular attention should be paid to the presence of foreign bodies which can become fixed in the oral cavity and pharynx. Examination of the tongue is assisted by dorsally directed digital pressure between the mandibular rami. Failure to recognize a string foreign body about the base of the tongue can seriously delay a diagnosis of obstruction due to a linear foreign body. The cervical region is examined for lymphadenopathy and masses that may be interfering with the movement of a bolus through the esophagus and for evidence of any dilated, flaccid, or air-filled enlargements in the area of the esophagus. In cats, careful palpation of the neck for thyroid nodules is recommended.

Abdominal Palpation. Abdominal palpation is an important part of the physical examination. Palpation is best accomplished by standing directly behind a patient made to stand on the examining table. Palpation must be systematic, and best sensitivity is afforded by alternating application and release of firm inward pressure on the abdomen by the fingers of both hands laid flat against the patient's abdomen. Raising the front end of the animal facilitates palpation of cranial abdominal organs. Sedation or anesthesia may be necessary for adequate examination.

The stomach of cats and dogs is usually difficult to palpate unless distended by ingesta. The intestines should feel soft, smooth, and should slide freely from between the examiner's hands. The ileocecal area of cats can often be palpated as a firmer knot-like structure in mid-cranial abdomen, and should not be confused with an abdominal mass. The colon can usually be defined because of its content of feces. Fecal material will normally indent or fragment when gently squeezed between the fingers, thus differentiating it from abdominal masses. The liver of healthy dogs is usually very difficult to palpate, whereas in the normal cat the liver can usually be felt. When examining tractable animals, standing in front of the patient and hooking the fingers behind the costochondral arch may facilitate palpation of the liver. Abdominal fluid may be detected by observation of a fluid wave that radiates from a site of percussion on one side of the abdomen to the other side of the abdomen.

Abdominal Auscultation. Examination of the gastrointestinal tract may include auscultation of the abdomen.[1] Most bowel sounds originate in the stomach; those that originate in the small intestine and colon are briefer. The colon generates sounds of high amplitude, short duration, and low frequency. Air increases the amplitude and frequency of sounds, especially in the stomach. On the other hand, fluid in the small intestine increases the number of sounds. Bowel sounds are caused by accumulated fluid and gas moving from one region to another. Peristaltic motility must be reduced for fluid and gas to accumulate. Thus, paradoxically, abnormal increases in bowel sounds are a reflection of a partial loss of intestinal motility rather than an augmentation of motility. Increased bowel sounds will result from agitation of abnormal accumulations of air and liquid in the stomach, as well as from faster movement of fluid and gas through the small intestine and colon as a result of decreased segmental contractility. If sounds are to be heard, sufficient motility must remain to produce movement of the accumulated fluid and gas. Few bowel sounds are heard when motility has disappeared, as in an ileus.[2] In general, auscultation of the abdomen is most useful for the detection of ileus. Failure to detect borborygmus after two to three minutes of auscultation suggests ileus. Auscultation of the abdomen will also occasionally reveal a vascular murmur that is produced by an intra-abdominal circulatory problem such as an arteriovenous shunt.

Rectal Examination. Examination of the abdominal cavity is not complete without a digital examination of the rectum. The rectal examination will provide a sample of stool for examination and will reveal abnormalities of the rectum, anus, prostate and pelvis. The importance of this procedure is obvious with signs of tenesmus or obstipation but is just as important in the evaluation of vomiting or diarrhea.

Admission Laboratory Work

For complex or refractory gastrointestinal cases the minimum data base is concluded with a complete blood count, a serum chemistry profile with electrolyte levels, a urinalysis, a fecal flotation, and a fecal direct smear. The admission laboratory work is conducted in order to evaluate the patient for systemic diseases that may result in signs of gastrointestinal disease, to identify any additional incidental problems in another system of the body, and to facilitate management decisions such as choice of fluid therapy.

HALITOSIS

Owners frequently complain about halitosis in dogs and less frequently cats. Common causes of halitosis are listed in Table 5-5. Important medical history includes the nature of the diet and whether the animal practices coprophagia. Highly proteinaceous diets are sometimes associated with halitosis, perhaps through the resultant excretion into the breath of odiferous products of protein fermentation such as ammonia, hydrogen sulfide, indoles, and skatoles. Remnants of food retained in the oral cavity and degraded by bacteria may be sufficient to cause disagreeable smells.

Physical examination must include careful inspection of ears, oral cavity, and lips. It is not uncommon for the smell of otitis externa to be mistaken for halitosis. Cheilitis is common in certain breeds, such as Cocker Spaniels, and can result in a surprisingly strong objectionable smell. The most common cause of halitosis is dental disease. Occasionally, other inflammatory or necrotizing oral or pharyngeal lesions such as neoplasia cause halitosis. The odor predominantly results from the breakdown of sulfur-containing amino acids derived from oral bacteria or cellular debris. Discharges from nasal lesions that drain caudally into the pharynx can also result in halitosis. Foreign bodies impacted in the nasal cavity, pharynx, oral cavity, or tonsillar crypts can cause halitosis either by inciting inflammation and necrosis or by their own fermentation, as in the case of food. The fermentation of retained food in a dilated or obstructed esophagus is an occasional cause of halitosis, as are protein malassimilation and systemic diseases such as uremia and liver failure.

Table 5-5 Causes of Halitosis

Dietary associated
- Food remnants
- Highly proteinaceous diets
- Coprophagia

Diseases of the lips
- Cheilitis

Oral cavity diseases
- Inflammatory or necrotizing oral lesions
- Foreign bodies

Pharyngeal diseases
- Inflammatory or necrotizing pharyngeal lesions
- Pharyngeal foreign bodies
- Tonsillar crypt foreign bodies

Nasal cavity & sinus disease
- Inflammatory diseases
- Necrotizing diseases

Dental disease
- Periodontitis
- Gingivitis
- Tooth root abscess
- Tartar

Esophageal diseases
- Megaesophagus
- Malassimilation

Systemic diseases
- Uremia
- Liver disease

Most cases of halitosis can be diagnosed by history and a thorough physical examination of the mouth, oral cavity, and pharynx. Occasionally, radiographs of the teeth, nasal cavity, pharynx, or esophagus are required. Examination of the pharynx with a dental mirror or endoscope and the nasal cavity with a rhinoscope is sometimes helpful. Management of halitosis depends on the primary cause but can include dietary manipulation and dental prophylaxis.

DROOLING & XEROSTOMIA

Drooling can result because of excessive production of saliva (ptyalism, hypersalivation, sialorrhea), or because of failure to swallow saliva produced in normal quantities (pseudoptyalism). Prominent causes of drooling are listed in Table 5-6. Drooling is a commonly observed response of the dog to imminent feeding and to high ambient temperature. In the cat drooling often accompanies purring.

Hypersalivation may be seen with inflammatory or painful oropharyngeal lesions. Important examples are foreign bodies and insect bites. Toxins responsible for excess salivation include those that irritate the oral cavity (caustics), thallium, metaldehyde, organophosphates, cresol, the secretions of various toads and newts, and certain plants such as *Amanita* mushrooms, nettles, and Dumb cane. Certain medications, especially in cats, can result in copious salivation. Examples include trimethoprim/sulfadiazine, piperazine, levamisole, bunamidine, cephalexin, and disinfectants. Any disease that results in nausea causes hypersalivation. Ptyalism is a characteristic clinical sign of portasystemic shunts in cats. Drooling has been reported with several diseases of the salivary gland, including infarction of the mandibular salivary gland and parotid salivary gland hyperplasia. Infectious disorders such as rabies, pseudorabies, botulism, and tetanus can result in drooling. Several dogs with gastroesophageal leiomyomas diagnosed at the University of California (UCD) VMTH have been observed to drool. The cause of the hypersalivation was not determined, but the drooling resolved after surgical removal of the leiomyoma.

Pseudoptyalism occurs when an animal is unable or unwilling to swallow saliva. Pseudoptyalism can result from conformational abnormalities of the mouth and lips (Saint Bernards), diseases causing oral deformity, disorders of the lips, or disorders of swallowing.

The diagnostic evaluation of drooling relies heavily on the history and physical examination (wear gloves if rabies is suspected). Careful observation of the patient often differentiates drooling due to nausea or swallowing difficulty from the other causes of hypersalivation. The differentiation of these categories of drooling is important because they have widely disparate diagnostic workups. Animals hypersalivating due to nausea will usually demonstrate other signs of nausea such as depression, lip licking, and retching. The appropriate workup to institute is that described for the evaluation of vomiting. Animals drooling due to swallowing disorders will often show evidence of inability to swallow food. These patients should be evaluated for dysphagia.

Consequence of persistent drooling include cheilitis and acne. Hypersalivation leads to increased aerophagia. The treatment of hypersalivation is varied because of the wide disparity of causes. Refractory hypersalivation can be treated by extreme measures such as excision of salivary glands or parasympathetic denervation.

Xerostomia, or dryness of the mouth, is uncommon. It is most often associated with feline dysautonomia. Xerostomia has also been reported following extensive radiation therapy of the head and neck and as a result of Sjogren's syndrome. The

Table 5-6 Causes of Drooling: Ptyalism and Pseudoptyalism

Physiological
- Imminent feeding
- Hyperthermia
- Purring

Toxicants/irritants
- Poisons (caustics, metaldehyde, organophosphates, cresol, others)
- Plants (Amanita mushrooms, nettles, dumb cane, philodendron, others)
- Insect/spider bites
- Secretions of toads & newts

Medications
- Antibiotics (trimethoprim/sulfadiazine, cephalexin)
- Anthelmintics (piperazine, levamisole, bunamidine)
- Disinfectants
- Others

Oropharyngeal diseases
- Inflammatory lesions
- Neoplasia
- Foreign bodies

Salivary gland diseases
- Parotid salivary gland hyperplasia
- Mandibular salivary gland infarction

Infectious disorders
- Rabies
- Pseudorabies
- Botulism
- Tetanus

Pseudoptyalism
- Conformational or innervation problems of the mouth and lips
- Deforming diseases of the mouth and lips
- Swallowing disorders

Miscellaneous
- Disorders causing nausea
- Portasystemic shunts (cats)
- Gastroesophageal leiomyoma

latter is an autoimmune disease of the lacrimal and salivary glands.

DYSPHAGIA, REGURGITATION, RETCHING, GAGGING, & VOMITING

Definitions and Differentiation

Dysphagia, regurgitation, and vomiting are considered primary clinical signs associated with problems in the pharynx, esophagus, stomach, and cranial small intestine. These primary signs are usually accompanied by secondary signs as listed in Table 5-7. Dysphagia and regurgitation are evaluated differently than vomiting. Therefore, it is of great importance that the clinician differentiates these problems during the clinical examination (Table 5-8). Failure to do so is a major cause of misdiagnosis of animals with signs of upper gastrointestinal disease. It is important to note, however, that patients may present with clinical signs of both regurgitation and vomiting. This mixed presentation is most commonly observed when chronic vomition leads to an esophagitis.

Dysphagia is defined as difficult or painful swallowing. Dysphagia may be further divided according to the anatomic area in which the swallowing dysfunction originates. Although regurgitation is the most prominent clinical sign of both oropharyngeal dysphagia and esophageal dysphagia, it is usually possible on a clinical basis to separate the two syndromes. Patients affected by oropharyngeal dysphagia make exaggerated swallowing movements and usually food will drop from the mouth within seconds of prehension. In contrast, esophageal dysphagia results in more delayed regurgitation and is usually not associated with exaggerated swallowing movements. More refined definition of dysphagia into disorders of the oral, pharyngeal, cricopharyngeal, esophageal, or gastroesophageal stage of swallowing requires barium swallows and fluoroscopy.

Regurgitation is defined as the retrograde expulsion of ingesta from the esophagus or pharynx. It most often results from esophageal disease. Regurgitation is a passive event with few prodromal signs. There is no abdominal effort, and no initiation of reflex neural pathways other than the gag reflex. Food is regurgitated from the esophagus and pharynx under the influence of gravitation. Retention of food in the pharynx can stimulate the gag reflex, with regurgitation following. There are usually no prodromal signs of nausea, although drooling because of inability to swallow saliva can on occasion give the impression of hypersalivation due to nausea. Regurgitated food is usually undigested and may take on a tubular shape if originating in the esophagus. The pH should not be acidic unless food has been first refluxed from the stomach. Regurgitated material from the esophagus is rarely bile stained, except for the infrequent occasions when regurgitation is preceded by esophagogastroduodenal reflux. Regurgitation may occur immediately after eating or may be delayed for several hours. Pharyngeal and cranial esophageal problems are typically characterized by immediate regurgitation, whereas esophageal disorders involving the lower cervical or intrathoracic segment are characterized by regurgitation that may be delayed for hours after eating.

Gagging is a reflexive contraction of the constrictor muscles of the pharynx resulting from stimulation of the pharyngeal mucosa. *Retching* is an involuntary and ineffectual attempt at vomiting. Retching is produced by contractions of the diaphragm and abdominal muscles, the same motor events that cause vomition. Retching should be differentiated from *expectoration*. The latter refers to the ejection of airway and laryngopharyngeal mucus or discharges. It is not uncommon for owners to confuse the forceful expectoration of airway fluid, such as commonly occurs with tracheobronchitis, with retching or vomiting. Differentiation is readily made by examination of the ejected material and by the presence or absence of nausea. Dogs with tracheobronchitis expectorate small quantities of white foam and do not show evidence of nausea.

Vomiting is the forceful, reflexive ejection of gastric content from the stomach following stimulation of a neural reflex that has synaptic centers in the brain stem. As described in Chapter 11, vomiting is accomplished by pronounced contraction of the muscles of the diaphragm and abdomen. It is always preceded by signs of *nausea* such as restlessness, depression, hypersalivation, lip licking, frequent swallowing, and retching. Low pH or presence of bile in the ejected material implies but does not prove vomiting. Material of alkaline pH may be vomit (gastroduodenal reflux), or it may have been regurgitated.

Table 5-7 Clinical signs that may be associated with loss of pharyngeal, esophageal, gastric, and/or small intestinal function. Primary signs usually comprise the owner's chief complaint. Occasionally, secondary signs represent chief complaints.

Primary Signs	
Vomiting	
Regurgitation	
Dysphagia	
Signs Usually Secondary	
Anorexia	Retching
Polyphagia	Malnutrition
Hypersalivation	Shivering
Esophageal colic	Pica
Dyspnea	Polydypsia
Cough	Melena
Abdominal pain	Dehydration
Bloat	

EATING DIFFICULTY

Eating difficulty may result from disorders of the jaw, oral cavity, tongue, pharynx, or esophagus. Eating difficulty should be differentiated from inappetence, a distinction which may escape the client. The diagnostic procedures employed in the evaluation of a patient experiencing eating difficulty depend on the tentative localization of the site of the disorder. This is determined by the history, the physical examination, and observation of the patient consuming a test meal. Together, these endeavors can usually differentiate disorders of prehension, mastication, or the oropharyngeal or esophageal phase of swallowing.

Table 5-8 Differentiation of Oropharyngeal Dysphagia, Esophageal Dysphagia, and Vomiting

	Oropharyngeal Dysphagia	Esophageal Dysphagia	Vomiting
• Abdominal Effort	None	None	Marked
• Signs of nausea	None	None	Present
• Time of food ejection	Immediate	Delayed, possibly for hours	Delayed, possibly for hours
• Character of food ejected	Undigested	Undigested	Can be partially digested, bile-stained, and with acid pH
• Number of swallowing attempts with single bolus	Multiple	Usually single	Single
• Visible evidence of bolus passing in the cervical esophagus	Not present	Present, maybe prolonged	Present
• Ability to drink	Poor	Variable	Normal
• Pain on swallowing	Possible	Possible	Absent
• Associated signs seen	Dyspnea, cough	Dyspnea, cough	Frequent retching
• Aggravating and alleviating factors frequently seen	Food consistency	Exercise, food consistency	Variable

Disorders of Prehension and Mastication

Animals with disorders of the oral cavity, tongue, or jaws have difficulty grasping and chewing food. The principal causes of prehension and mastication difficulty are listed in Table 5-9.

History of importance includes a review of the rabies vaccination record; inquiry as to any consumption of carrion that may result in botulism; and exposure to plants, electrical cord, insects, or caustic products that could produce stomatitis. Generalized weakness is supportive of myasthenia gravis or botulism.

Physical examination may reveal weak, ineffectual, or uncoordinated jaw movements. If the tongue is affected, animals have difficulty lapping water and soft foods, and the tongue may loll out of the mouth. An animal may place its head deeply into its water bowl to allow drinking. On occasion the patient will hold its head to one side to avoid painful lesions on one side of the mouth or jaw. Inability to open the mouth is commonly associated with disorders of the masticatory muscles such as masticatory muscle myositis (trismus), abnormalities of the temporomandibular joints, and retrobulbar abscess. Physical inability to close the mouth is most often due to the coronoid process' locking ventrally and laterally to the zygomatic arch, or due to temporomandibular dysplasia. Trigeminal nerve neuritis is characterized by an acute onset of transient, flaccid paralysis of the muscles that close the mouth, resulting in a slack jaw that dangles open. Neurological examination may reveal evidence of neuropathies of other cranial nerves, or CNS lesions. Oropharyngeal examination may disclose painful oropharyngeal lesions worthy of culture (rarely helpful) or biopsy. Signs of systemic disorders (uremia, sepsis, SLE) may be observed. The diagnostic procedures of utility for the evaluation of these disorders are listed in Table 5-10.

Oropharyngeal Dysphagia

Dysphagia may result from dysfunction of the tongue, pharynx, or esophagus. Important causes of dysphagia are listed in Table 5-11, and its differentiation from regurgitation or vomiting due to esophageal or gastric disease is described above. Animals with oropharyngeal dysphagia will usually prehend food readily but are unable to swallow the food normally. If concurrent dysfunction of the tongue is present, prehension and mastication, as well as swallowing, may be compromised. Affected animals may throw their heads back, or conversely ventroflex their necks, while swallowing. They may drool persistently because of incomplete swallowing of saliva, develop nasal discharges from entrance of food into the nasopharynx and nasal cavity, and cough from eventual aspiration of food retained in the pharynx by ineffectual pharyngeal contractions. Their gag reflex may be impaired. Useful diagnostic procedures are listed in Table 5-12 and include review of rabies vaccination record; neurological examination with particular attention to cranial nerves VII, IX, X, and XII; general anesthesia followed by a thorough oropharyngeal examination, including oropharyn-

Table 5-9 Causes of Difficult or Painful Prehension and Mastication

Stomatitis/Glossitis/Gingivitis
- Physical agents (electrical cord burns, trauma, insect bites)
- Caustic agents (petroleum products, alkalis, acids, thallium)
- Bacterial infections (Bacteroides melaninogenicus?)
- Viral infections (feline rhinotracheitis, calici, FELV, FIV)
- Fungal infections (Candida)
- Foreign bodies (fiberglass, imbedded plant material)
- Autoimmune diseases (SLE, pemphigus & pemphigoid diseases)
- Immune-mediated disorders (toxic epidermal necrolysis, idiopathic feline glossopharyngitis, eosinophilic granuloma)
- Immunodeficiencies
- Systemic disorders (uremia, sepsis)

Oral/Glossal Neoplasia
- Squamous cell carcinoma
- Fibrosarcoma
- Melanoma
- Rhabdomyosarcoma

Neurological Disorders
- Rabies
- Trigeminal paralysis
- Polyneuropathies
- Neuropathies of cranial nerves VII, IX, X, XII
- CNS lesions (cerebellar disorders, brain stem lesions, hydrocephalus)

Neuromuscular Junction Disorders
- Myasthenia gravis
- Botulism

Musculoskeletal Disorders
- Masticatory myositis (eosinophilic, plasmacytic/lymphocytic)
- Masticatory muscle myopathy
- Temporomandibular joint arthropathy
- Open-mouth jaw locking
- Renal secondary hyperparathyroidism
- Hyperparathyroidism
- Mandible fracture or subluxation
- Craniomandibular osteoarthropathy

Miscellaneous Disorders
- Retrobulbar abscess
- Salivary gland disorders
- Dental disorders (tooth root abscesses, fractured teeth)

geal palpation (use gloves); examination of the tongue, palate, tonsils, and tonsillar crypts, paying particular attention to the presence of masses or foreign bodies; examination of the nasopharynx with a retroflexed endoscope; pharyngeal radiographs; and barium swallow with liquid and barium coated food.

Esophageal Dysphagia

Dysphagia due to esophageal disease is usually characterized by the clinical sign of regurgitation. The workup of esophageal dysphagia is described below under the problem of regurgitation.

REGURGITATION

The differentiation of regurgitation from vomiting is described above. Regurgitation is usually a result of esophageal dysfunction, and less frequently pharyngeal disorders. Causes of regurgitation are listed in Table 5-13.

History. Rabies vaccination status should be assessed before examining any case of regurgitation. Exaggerated swallowing efforts in association with immediate regurgitation in a pup is indicative of cricopharyngeal achalasia. Regurgitation in young pups is most commonly a result of idiopathic megaesophagus, or a vascular anomaly such as persistent right aortic arch. If a dilated esophagus is recognized in a pup and a vascular ring anomaly is ruled out by a barium swallow, the probable diagnosis is idiopathic megaesophagus, and it is rarely justified to proceed with further diagnostics. In older dogs, however, the incidence of regurgitation due to secondary megaesophagus is much higher, and a more in depth workup is justified. A history of acute onset of regurgitation following bone or chew-toy ingestion raises the possibility of esophageal foreign body. Regurgitation beginning several weeks after a surgical procedure suggests esophageal stricture following gastroesophageal reflux. Regurgitation of solids but not liquids is suggestive of esophageal partial obstruction. The patient's environment determines the likelihood of toxicities causing esophagitis or vagal neuropathy and dictates the likelihood of access to carrion that may cause botulism. An associated cough may be indicative of concurrent aspiration pneumonia, or rarely, bronchoesophageal fistulation. The history is concluded by screening other systems of the body with appropriate questions to help detect systemic causes of swallowing dysfunction and identify incidental problems.

Physical Examination. A complete physical examination

Table 5-10
Diagnostic Procedures of Value for the Diagnosis of Difficult or Painful Prehension and Mastication

Procedure	Usefulness
Anesthesia oropharyngeal examination	Oropharyngeal lesions, foreign bodies
Neurological examination	Disorders of cranial nerves V, VII, IX, X, and XII, CNS lesions, polyneuropathies
Admission laboratory work	
Blood eosinophil count	Masticatory myositis
BUN level	Myositis, stomatitis
Calcium/phosphorus levels	Hyperparathyroidism
Serum tests	
ANA	SLE
Acetylcholine receptor antibody test	Myasthenia gravis
Fine needle aspiration	
Temporomandibular joints	Inflammatory/infectious arthritis
Masticatory muscles	Myositis
Mandibular or retropharyngeal lymph nodes	Neoplasia, lymphadenitis
Radiographs	
Teeth	Abscess
Temporornandibular joints	Arthropathy, subluxation
Maxilla and mandible	Osteoporosis, fracture, craniomandibular osteoarthropathy
Ultrasound	
Retropharyngeal area	Lymphadenopathy, foreign body, neoplasia
Biopsy	Oral lesions, myositis, myopathy, salivary gland disorders

should be performed. Particular attention is paid to examination of the oropharynx and neck to assist discovery of oropharyngeal foreign bodies or cervical masses. In some dogs, a dilated cervical esophagus may be visualized by forcibly compressing the animals thorax while briefly occluding its nostrils. If there is gas present in a flaccid esophagus, the result will be a ballooning dilation of the cervical part of the esophagus, visible to an observer carefully regarding the animal's left cervical area. Fermentation of food in a dilated esophagus may result in gurgling sounds and halitosis. Other physical examination findings that aid differential diagnosis of regurgitation include evidence of CNS disorders, lower motor neuron dysfunction (polyneuropathy), distemper, muscle weakness (myasthenia gravis, hypoadrenocorticism, botulism), muscle pain (polymyopathy), and skin or mucous membrane lesions (SLE). Dysautonomia, an important cause of regurgitation in the cat, has characteristic clinical signs including dilated pupils and dry mucous membranes.

Diagnostic Evaluation

The diagnostic procedures commonly employed for the evaluation of patients with regurgitation are listed in Table 5-12.

Admission laboratory work. Admission laboratory tests rarely help differentiate the causes of regurgitation. Exceptions include laboratory work suggestive of lead toxicity (basophilic stippling, nucleated RBC), SLE (anemia, lymphopenia, thrombocytopenia, acanthocytes, proteinuria, inflammatory joint taps), hypoadrenocorticism (eosinophilia, lymphocytosis, neutropenia, decreased sodium/potassium ratio), and Spirocerca lupi (ova).

Diagnostic Imaging. Survey radiographs of the pharynx, neck, and chest identify most cases of megaesophagus and many cases of pharyngeal and esophageal foreign body. They occasionally reveal a hiatal disorder. The detection of megaesophagus does not obviate the need for further diagnostics because megaesophagus in itself has a variety of possible causes (see Chapter 9). Swallowing studies using liquid barium followed by barium-coated food confirm obstructive disorders such as vascular anomalies, and they may detect esophageal diverticula. Fluoroscopy in association with the barium swallow is required to detect pharyngeal dysfunction, such as cricopharyngeal achalasia, and esophageal motility abnormalities. Ultrasonography is useful for the detection of masses causing esophageal compression in the pharynx and neck.

Endoscopy. Endoscopy and endoscopic biopsy may be required for the identification of some esophageal obstructive disorders such as esophageal neoplasia. Esophageal biopsy is commonly required for the diagnosis of esophagitis.

Miscellaneous Diagnostic Procedures. Various other diagnostic tests may be required. These include the tensilon test and the acetylcholine receptor antibody test (myasthenia gravis); toxicological analyses for lead, thallium, and pseudocholinesterase; serum CPK level (polymyositis); electrodiagnostics and nerve or muscle biopsy (neuropathies & myopathies); CSF taps or CAT scans (brain stem diseases); and the ACTH test (hypoadrenocorticism). Thoracotomy may be required for the definitive diagnosis of vascular ring anomalies and hiatal disorders.

Table 5-11 Causes of Oropharyngeal Dysphagia

Glossal Disorders
- Glossal neoplasia
- Neuropathies of cranial nerves VII, IX, XII
- Hydrocephalus, brain-stem lesions

Pharyngitis/Tonsillitis
- Physical agents (trauma, insect bites)
- Caustic agents (petroleum products, alkalis, acids, thallium)
- Infections (bacteria, infectious canine hepatitis, candida)
- Immune-mediated disorders (idiopathic feline glossopharyngitis, eosinophilic granuloma)
- Immunodeficiencies
- Systemic disorders (uremia, sepsis)
- Pharyngeal foreign bodies

Pharyngeal Neoplasia
- Squamous cell carcinoma, fibrosarcoma, melanoma, tonsillar carcinoma

Retropharyngeal Lymphadenopathy
- Neoplasia, lymphadenitis

Fractured Hyoid Bones

Pharyngeal Neuromuscular Disorders
- Rabies
- Neuropathies of cranial nerves VII, IX, X
- CNS lesions (cerebellar disorders, brain- stem lesions)
- Cricopharyngeal achalasia
- Cricopharyngeal/pharyngeal incoordination
- Myasthenia gravis
- Botulism

Palate Disorders
- Congenitally short or cleft palate

PERSISTENT VOMITING

The differentiation of vomiting from regurgitation is described above. The causes of vomiting are listed in Table 5-14.

History. The signalment of the animal helps rank the probability for possible causes. For instance, young animals are more likely to ingest foreign bodies. Linear foreign bodies are particularly common in cats. Uncastrated, young, male dogs are more likely to rove the neighborhood and be traumatized or ingest poisons or garbage. Pancreatitis is common in fat, small breed dogs. Knowledge of environment, diet, and any concurrent medication is helpful. Repeated access to trash, organophosphates, cleaners, mushrooms, or ornamental plants may be responsible for chronic vomiting.

Aggravation of vomiting by a certain diet raises the possibility of food intolerance or allergy. Almost any drug can cause vomiting as an idiosyncratic reaction.

The frequency and chronicity of the vomiting, the content of the vomitus, the animal's attitude and appetite, and the presence or absence of weight loss help determine the severity of the condition. Persistent vomiting of large volumes of liquid vomitus in spite of food restriction is highly suggestive of pyloric or upper intestinal obstruction. Vomiting of food greater than 12 hours after ingestion is pathognomonic for delayed gastric emptying. "Projectile" vomiting is traditionally ascribed to pyloric obstruction, but can occur from virtually any disorder causing violent vomiting. The history is concluded by screening other systems of the body with appropriate questions to help detect systemic causes of vomiting and identify incidental problems.

Physical Examination. A complete physical examination including abdominal palpation and digital rectal examination should be performed. Particular attention is paid to attitude, hydration, and cardiovascular status. The neurological examination should not be forgotten because persistent vomiting can result from CNS lesions. The physical examination may reveal the cause of the vomiting (e.g. obstructions), or yield findings that reduce the number of other possibilities (e.g. pain, jaundice, lymphadenopathy). Examination contributes to the assessment of the seriousness of the condition and dictates the volume of fluid deficit (if any). Rectal examination may detect melena, and in dogs with an intestinal obstruction it often reveals a dry, tacky mucosa.

Tabletop Assessment

Location of Site of the Disorder. By the conclusion of the clinical examination, the clinician should be able to differentiate expectoration, gagging, retching, regurgitation, and vomiting.

Assessment of Severity. The clinician should decide if the vomiting represents a serious departure from normality. Dogs and cats commonly vomit once or twice every few weeks. If the frequency of the vomiting increases beyond that accepted as normal for the particular animal, an abnormality is likely. Occasional flecks of fresh blood in vomitus are not of concern. Warning signs of serious disease include prolonged, frequent vomition; depression; anorexia; weight loss; weakness; dehydration; hyperpnea; pale, congested, or discolored mucous membranes; slow capillary refill; weak rapid pulse; fever; digested blood ("coffee grounds") in the vomitus; melena; delayed gastric emptying; abdominal organomegaly; pain, masses, or effusions; and continued vomiting while food is being withheld.

If the cause of the vomiting is not apparent following the clinical examination and warning signs of serious disease are present, the clinician is obligated to recommend supportive therapy and a diagnostic workup to expediently determine safe and effective therapy. In the absence of warning signs, therapeutic trials such as controlled diets or antacids are permissible, but unfortunately, many cases of chronic vomiting are refractory to symptomatic therapy.

Diagnostic Evaluation

The diagnostic procedures commonly employed for the evaluation of patients with chronic vomiting are listed in Table 5-15.

Table 5-12 Diagnostic Procedures of Value for the Diagnosis of Dysphagia and Regurgitation

Procedure	Usefulness
CBC	Pneumonia, immune-mediated disease, hypoadrenocorticism, lead toxicosis
Serum chemistry profile	Myositis, hypoadrenocorticism
CPK	Myositis
Urinalysis	Proteinuria supportive of SLE
Fecal	*Spirocerca lupi*
ANA	SLE
ACTH stimulation test	Hypoadrenocorticism
Distemper titers	Distemper
Acetylcholine receptor antibody test	Acquired myasthenia gravis
Oropharyngeal exam under anesthesia	Foreign body, inflammation, masses
Survey radiographs	Megaesophagus, mediastinitis, periesophageal masses, esophageal or pharyngeal foreign bodies, fractured hyoid bones
Swallowing study (fluoroscopy)	Megaesophagus, motility disorders, stricture, fistula, diverticula, hiatal disorders, periesophageal masses, esophageal masses, vascular ring anomalies, reflux esophagitis, cricopharyngeal achalasia
Gastrogram	Gastric disorders, pyloric obstruction
Ultrasound of retropharynx	Lymphadenopathy, foreign body, neoplasia
Endoscopic exam of nasopharynx	Pharyngeal masses, foreign bodies
Esophagoscopy & biopsy	Esophagitis, obstructive diseases
Esophageal manometry	Achalasia, esophageal neuromuscular diseases, gastroesophageal reflux
CSF tap	Brain-stem diseases, distemper
Evoked potentials	Brain-stem diseases
EEG	Hydrocephalus
CAT scan/MRI	Brain stem disease, hydrocephalus
Electromyography	Myopathy, polyneuropathy
Nerve conduction velocities	Polyneuropathy
Repetitive stimulation	Neuromuscular junction diseases
Tensilon test	Myasthenia gravis
Muscle biopsy	Polymyopathy, polymyositis
Nerve biopsy	Polyneuropathy
Toxicology	Plasma cholinesterase, lead, thallium
Exploratory surgery	Periesophageal masses, hiatal disorders

Admission Laboratory Data. A laboratory data base consisting of a CBC, serum chemistry panel, urinalysis, fecal flotation and occult blood should be gathered. A blood gas sample to determine acid base status can be useful. The data base identifies or provides clues for some causes of vomiting, identifies incidental problems in other body systems, and assists in the choice of fluid therapy.

Look for evidence of systemic diseases, such as kidney and liver insufficiency, toxemias (e.g. pyometra, peritonitis), diabetes mellitus, hypoadrenocorticism, and lead toxicity. If the data base points to any of these disorders, further diagnostic tests such as organ biopsy, liver function tests, ACTH stimulation

Table 5-13 Causes of Regurgitation

PHARYNGEAL DISORDERS

- **Pharyngeal obstructive disorders**
  - Foreign bodies
  - Pharyngeal tonsilar neoplasia
  - Retropharyngeal lymphadenopathy
- **Pharyngeal neuromuscular disorders**
  - Rabies
  - Botulism
  - Neuropathies of cranial nerves IX, X
  - CNS lesions (cerebellar disorders, brain-stem lesions)
  - Cricopharyngeal dysphagia
  - Myasthenia gravis
- **Palate disorders**
  - Congenitally short or cleft palate

ESOPHAGEAL DISORDERS

- **Esophagitis**
- **Esophageal obstructive disorders**
  - Foreign bodies
  - Stricture
  - Neoplasia
  - Vascular ring anomalies
  - Periesophageal masses
  - Granulomas *(Spirocerca lupi)*
- **Esophageal neuromuscular disorders**
  - Megaesophagus*
  - Motility abnormalities
- **Esophageal diverticula**
- **Hiatal disorders**

** Megaesophagus has a large number of possible causes. They are listed in Table 9-3*

tests, and lead levels may be required. The data base may confirm parasitism (physaloptera, salmon poisoning) and aid in the identification of eosinophilic gastritis and protein-losing gastropathies. Metabolic alkalosis and paradoxical aciduria are most common following persistent vomiting due to pyloric obstruction but can also occur from other causes of vomiting.

Perusal of the PCV, serum albumin, electrolyte panel, and blood gas data helps tailor the fluid (crystaloid, plasma, blood) and electrolytes (Na, K, Cl, HCO^3) administered.

Amylase/Lipase. On occasion the history (fat dog, high-fat diet) and the physical examination (anterior abdominal pain) strongly suggest pancreatitis. At other times the diagnosis is less readily apparent. Amylase and lipase tests are commonly used to confirm pancreatitis. Unfortunately, the accuracy of lipase and especially amylase is poor.

Survey Abdominal Radiographs. Gastrointestinal tract foreign bodies and intestinal obstruction are common causes of vomiting; they can occasionally be diagnosed by survey radiographs. Radiographs also assess gastric size, position, and content; detect gross abnormalities in liver and kidney size; and help detect abdominal fluid, abdominal masses, organ torsions, bowel perforation, peritonitis, and pancreatitis.

Abdominal Ultrasound. Abdominal ultrasound and radiographs are complementary examinations. In contrast to radiography, the ultrasound image is enhanced by ascitic fluid and compromised by aerophagia. Ultrasound is more sensitive for the detection of abdominal masses including intraorgan miliary masses (eg metastatic neoplasia), mural thickenings, lymphadenopathy, pancreatitis, and hepatic disorders.

Endoscopy. Endoscopy is a sensitive technique for the diagnosis of luminal and mucosal diseases that may cause vomiting. Endoscopy does not assess motility and it may miss mural lesions. Endoscopy and endoscopic biopsy may identify hypertrophic or atrophic gastritis, lymphocytic/plasmacytic or eosinophilic gastritis, gastric erosions, ulcers, granulomas, parasitism, neoplasia, or pyloric stenosis. Endoscopic examination and biopsy of the duodenum and colon may reveal intestinal disease. An important example is inflammatory bowel disease that, whether situated in the small intestine or colon, can cause vomiting.

Contrast Radiography. With the advent of endoscopy, the emphasis of gastrointestinal contrast radiography has moved towards procedures that assess gastrointestinal motility or detect intestinal obstructions. Double contrast gastrograms allow examination of the gastric mucosa and may be useful if an endoscope is unavailable. Liquid barium examinations may help detect gastric mural lesions missed by the endoscope and, if fluoroscopy is available, allow an appreciation of gastric motility. Administration of barium liquid will also detect gross obstructive disorders of the pylorus or intestine. Barium coated food gives a crude estimate of gastric emptying time. Gastric emptying usually begins within 30 minutes of ingestion. Inadequate gastric motility is inferred by delayed gastric emptying without associated endoscopic or surgical evidence of an outflow obstruction.

Fluoroscopy. Fluoroscopy allows definitive diagnosis of gastric and intestinal motility disorders. Enteroclysis is a very useful fluoroscopic contrast procedure for the diagnosis of small bowel partial obstructions. It also provides information about small bowel motility and mucosal topography.

Scintigraphy. More objective evidence of delayed gastric emptying can be obtained by use of scintigraphy. Causes of delayed gastric emptying are listed in Table 5-16.

Exploratory Celiotomy. Exploratory celiotomy may be required for the diagnosis of mural diseases of the gastrointestinal tract, mucosal lesions out of reach of the endoscope, gastrinomas, and low grade diseases of some organs such as chronic pancreatitis. Pyloric hypertrophy and large mass lesions of the gastric wall may be apparent on endoscopy, but definitive diagnosis may require full thickness biopsy.

Miscellaneous Diagnostic Evaluations. Various other tests may further aid in diagnosing some cases of vomiting. Microscopic examination of the vomitus may reveal Ollulanus tricuspis larvae (cats) or cytological evidence of inflammation, infection, or neoplasia. Unfortunately, cytological specimens are often distorted by the gastric acidity. CSF taps, CAT scans, or magnetic resonance imaging (MRI) may be required to detect animals' vomiting because of CNS lesions. The detection

Table 5-14 Causes of Vomiting

Adverse reactions to food
- Indiscretions
- Intolerances
- Allergies

Gastrointestinal inflammatory disorders
- Pharyngitis
- Gastritis (atrophic, hypertrophic, eosinophilic, others)
- Inflammatory bowel disease of small and large intestine
- Infectious enteritis (viral, bacterial, fungal)
- Hemorrhagic gastroenteritis
- Gastrointestinal neoplasia
- Gastroduodenal ulcers
- Lymphangiectasia

Gastrointestinal obstruction
- Foreign bodies
- Pyloric hypertrophy
- Mural thickenings (neoplasia, granulomas, strictures)
- Extraluminal compression (masses, adhesions)
- Intussusception
- Delayed gastric emptying
- Ileus
- Constipation

Gastrointestinal ischemic disorders
- Organ and mesenteric avulsion
- Infarction
- Organ torsions

Parasitism
- *Ollulanus tricuspis*
- Ascarids
- Physaloptera
- Salmon poisoning
- Heartworm (cats)

Disorders of other abdominal organs
- Hepatobiliary inflammation, hepatic neoplasia, bile duct obstruction, cholelithiasis, portasystemic shunts
- Pancreatitis, pancreatic adenocarcinoma
- Nephritis, nephrotic syndrome
- Peritonitis
- Metritis, pyometra

Systemic diseases
- Uremia
- Hepatic failure
- Sepsis and toxemias
- Congestive heart failure
- Metastatic neoplasia
- Acidosis
- Electrolyte imbalance (hypokalemia, hypercalcemia)

Endocrine Diseases
- Adrenocortical insufficiency
- Diabetic ketoacidosis
- Hyperthyroidism
- Gastrinomas

Neurologic diseases
- Dysautonomia
- Myenteric ganglionitis
- CNS tumors
- Meningitis
- Encephalitis
- Hydrocephalus
- Vestibular disturbances
- Visceral epilepsy?

Drugs, poisons, & chemical agents
- Apomorphine
- Thiacetarsamide
- Chemotherapeutics
- Narcotics
- Xylazine
- Digitalis
- Antiinflammatory drugs
- Insecticides
- Copper sulfate
- Lead
- Ethylene glycol
- Mycotoxins
- Household plants
- Others

Miscellaneous
- Pregnancy
- Atherosclerosis
- Anaphylaxis
- Pain, fear, other psychogenic

of an atropine-responsive bradycardia in a vomiting animal raises the likelihood that the vomiting is due to a CNS lesion's causing increased intracranial pressure. The entity of visceral epilepsy (vomiting due to a seizure focus in an area of the brain controlling visceral function) is an as yet unproven cause of vomiting. The basis for its diagnosis has been amelioration of the vomiting with phenobarbital, in the absence of demonstrable CNS disease. An ACTH test may be necessary for the diagnosis of hypoadrenocorticism. A small percentage of dogs with spontaneous hypoadrenocorticism and most dogs with iatrogenic hypoadrenocorticism have normal serum sodium and potassium levels, thus making the diagnosis difficult without the ACTH test. Elevated plasma gastrin levels support (but do not confirm) the diagnosis of gastrinoma. Gastric acid secretory testing may be useful for the diagnosis of achlorhydria or gastric hyperacidity.

CHRONIC DIARRHEA

Diarrhea is the primary sign of intestinal disease. Additional clinical signs are consistently present and occasionally become the principal ones for which the animal is presented for treatment. These secondary signs are listed in Table 5-17. In the following discussion, the term *"small bowel diarrhea"* is used to refer to diarrhea as a consequence of small intestine dysfunction resulting from diseases of the intestine itself, or from diseases of digestive organs such as the pancreas and liver that interfere with the ability of the small intestine to absorb food. The term *"large bowel diarrhea"* refers to diarrhea resulting from diseases of the cecum, colon, or rectum.

History. The patient's signalment, vaccination history, and the nature of its environment are determined. Young animals, for instance, are more prone to nutritional, microbial, and parasitic causes of diarrhea. Certain breed predispositions are apparent (Table 5-3). An animal with complete freedom in an unknown environment is more likely to develop infectious, toxic, and traumatic disorders. Diarrhea is often associated with environmental changes.

The animal's diet should be determined. Adverse reactions to food are a prominent cause of diarrhea, and the history is a rapid way to identify responsible nutrients. The nature of the diet most commonly determines the character of feces. If the diarrhea ceases when the animal is not fed, but starts again soon after feeding is reinstituted, an osmotic diarrhea is probable. Evaluation of the animal's weight in relation to caloric intake helps identify animals with problems in the absorption of nutrients.

The duration of the complaint and the frequency of normal and abnormal bowel movements are determined. The clinician

Table 5-15 Diagnostic Procedures of Value for the Differential Diagnosis of Chronic Vomiting

Procedure	Usefulness
Dietary trials	Adverse reactions to food
CBC	Sepsis, toxemia, eosinophilic gastritis, hypoadrenocorticism, lead toxicosis, blood loss, hydration
Serum chemistry profile	Hypoadrenocorticism, ketoacidosis, protein-losing gastropathy, uremia, liver disease, electrolyte levels
Urinalysis	Renal disease, liver disease, hydration ketoacidosis
Blood gas	Acid-base status
Fecal flotation	Physaloptera, ascarids, Nanophytes
Fecal occult blood	Neoplasia, ulcers
Vomitus microscopic examination	*Ollulanus tricuspis*, neoplasia
ACTH stimulation test	Hypoadrenocorticism
Liver function test	Liver disease
Serum amylase and lipase tests	Pancreatitis
Serum antibody/antigen tests	Heartworm, RMSF, histoplasmosis
Survey radiographs	Obstructions, foreign bodies, liver and kidney size, masses, pancreatitis, peritonitis
Ultrasonography	Masses, metastatic neoplasia, mural thickenings
Contrast radiography	Gastric disorders, pyloric obstruction, gastric emptying, intestinal obstruction
Fluoroscopy	Gastrointestinal motility disorders
Enteroclysis	Intestinal motility disorders, partial obstructions
Scintigraphy	Gastric emptying
Endoscopy	Luminal & mucosal gastric, duodenal, & large bowel disease
CSF tap	Brain-stem diseases, increased CSF pressure, meningoencephalitis
Evoked potentials	Brain-stem diseases
EEG	Hydrocephalus
CAT scan/MRI	Brain-stem disease, hydrocephalus
Toxicology	Plasma cholinesterase, lead, serum osmolality (ethylene glycol)
Gastric acid secretory testing	Achlorhydria, hyperacidity
Serum gastrin	Gastrinoma
Phenobarbital trial	Visceral epilepsy?
Exploratory celiotomy	Full-thickness biopsy, APUDomas, chronic pancreatitis

must establish if the client regularly observes the animal's bowel movements. Unobserved bowel movements are usually assumed to be normal. Diarrhea of several day's to a week's duration is likely to respond to symptomatic therapy, whereas diarrhea of greater than one to two weeks is likely to respond only once diagnostic effort has identified a cause and specific treatment has been instituted. At times, patients pass a normal bowel movement in the morning, but subsequent bowel movements during the day become soft or watery. This pattern may be repeated during the following days; it is a result of the patient's different levels of physical activity during the day and night. Inactivity promotes increased water resorption from feces, producing normal bowel movements, whereas increased activity encourages transit and exacerbates diarrhea. Alteration in activity is also one reason why some dogs presented with the complaint of diarrhea will have normal stools in the hospital but not at home. The frequency of bowel movements is increased in most cases of diarrhea. In small bowel diarrhea the frequency is usually two to four times per day, whereas in large bowel diarrhea the frequency is usually much higher, at approximately four to ten times per day. Tenesmus and dyschezia (painful defecation) are hallmarks of large bowel disease. Fecal incontinence is frequently a result of large bowel diseases and rarely of small bowel disorders. Clients sometimes fail to differentiate between the complaints of "fecal incontinence" and "diarrhea." The clinician should be careful to differentiate the two conditions, as they have some different causes and their workups and therapy are widely divergent.

The physical appearance of feces is of important diagnostic value. Fecal consistency can vary from formed feces that are merely soft at one end, as seen in mild diarrhea, to those that are watery and completely without form as severity increases. Both large and small bowel diarrhea can result in unformed feces, but defecation of large volumes of liquid feces is more characteristic of small bowel diarrhea. Fecal diameter may be reduced as a result of rectal strictures. The presence of excess mucus and fresh blood on the stool is suggestive of large bowel disease. A description of mucus must be explained to some clients.

Fecal color varies considerably with small bowel diarrhea. The primary determinate of fecal color is the extent of metabolism of the bile pigments. Rapid transit time is associated with the yellow and green colors of incompletely metabolized bilirubin. Melena refers to black, tarry feces resulting from upper gastrointestinal blood loss. Normal dogs and cats commonly have black feces, however, and it is important not to assume black feces are due to melena. Increased quantities of fecal fat impart a gray color to the feces. The stool may appear greasy and if enveloped in paper will cause an oily spot on the paper wrapping. Steatorrhea is an important observation; the abnormality has a number of different causes (Table 5-18).

The presence of undigested material in feces is noted. The discovery of sharp materials such as bone fragments may suggest a diagnosis of traumatic colitis. Foreign material such as food wrappings raises the likelihood of "garbage can enteritis." The passage of undigested particles of digestible foods is a result of maldigestion. The maldigestion most commonly results from pancreatic insufficiency or rapid transit time.

Fecal odor should be noted. Maldigestion and malabsorption often result in a characteristic sour odor. Steatorrhea can be associated with a rancid smell.

The history is concluded by screening other systems of the body with appropriate questions to help detect systemic causes of diarrhea and identify incidental problems.

Physical Examination. Attitude, behavior, and posture are examined while the animal is unrestrained. Abnormal posture raises the possibility of painful abdominal diseases. Dogs with painful diseases of the perianal area will sometimes carry their tail away from their perineum. Cats with hyperthyroidism will often appear hyperactive. Body weight, hydration status, and cardiovascular function should be assessed. Weight loss as a result of malassimilation may be apparent.

Abdominal palpation is an important part of the physical examination. On occasion, loops of bowel filled with fluid and gas can be palpated. Bowel infiltrated by inflammatory or neoplastic cells may feel thickened on palpation. Masses causing partial intestinal obstruction are accessible to palpation in most regions of the intestine. Detection of hepatomegaly raises the likelihood of hepatic or cardiac involvement in the diarrheic process. Absence of intestinal sounds following two to three minutes of abdominal auscultation is suggestive of ileus.

The perineal area should be carefully examined for evidence of perianal fistula and perineal hernias, both of which can cause clinical signs suggestive of large bowel disease. The rectal examination provides fecal material for inspection. Fecal impaction, rectal masses, rectal strictures, rectal foreign bodies, and anal diseases may be discerned.

Tabletop Assessment

At the conclusion of the clinical examination the clinician should be able to differentiate small bowel from large bowel diarrhea and to assess the severity of the patient's condition.

Differentiation of Small Bowel from Large Bowel Diarrhea. Because the workups of large bowel and small bowel diarrhea are different, it expedites diagnosis to tentatively localize the site of the intestinal dysfunction by use of a number of dissimilar, but not mutually exclusive, clinical features of small and large bowel diarrhea (Table 5-19). The different manifestations of disease in these two areas of the digestive tract reflect their different positions along the gastrointestinal tract and the different functions of the large and small bowel. The proximity of the large bowel to the formed fecal mass means that blood from the large intestinal mucosa is passed as a fresh coating on the feces (hematochezia), whereas blood from the upper gastrointestinal tract is passed digested and admixed with the feces (melena). The large bowel is primarily a storage organ; it contributes little to digestion and absorption of nutri-

Table 5-16 Causes of Deranged Gastric Emptying

DELAYED GASTRIC EMPTYING

- **Mechanical obstruction**
  - Pyloric foreign body
  - Gastric neoplasia or granulomatous disease
  - Pyloric hypertrophy
  - Antral mucosal hypertrophy
  - Antral polyps
  - Extrinsic compression of antrum or pylorus
- **Acid-base and electrolyte imbalances**
  - Hypokalemia
  - Acidosis
- **Increased sympathetic nervous system activity**
  - Nervousness
  - Stress
  - Pain
- **Decreased parasympathetic nervous system activity**
  - Feline dysautonomia
  - Anticholinergics
  - Vagal neuropathy (solids only)
- **Miscellaneous causes of deranged motility**
  - Inflammatory or ulcerative stomach or intestinal disease
  - Post-gastric dilatation volvulus
  - Gastric surgery
  - Gastric neoplasia
  - Uremia
  - Hepatic encephalopathy
  - Diabetic gastroparesis
  - Acute hyperglycemia
  - High-calorie parenteral nutrition
  - Tranquilizers
  - Idiopathic

ACCELERATED GASTRIC EMPTYING

- **Malabsorption syndromes**
- **Maldigestion syndromes**
- **Duodenal ulcers**
- **Gastrinomas**
- **Myenteric ganglionitis**
- **Vagal neuropathy (liquids only)**
- **Pyloroplasty**

ents. Therefore, disordered large bowel function is associated with frequent defecation and minimal weight loss. In contrast, the primary function of the small bowel is absorption of nutrients. Thus, small intestinal diseases are commonly associated with weight loss and less often with marked increases in fecal frequency.

Assessment of Severity. Intestinal disease can markedly affect fluid, electrolyte, and nutritional homeostasis. Warning signs of serious disease include prolonged periods of severe diarrhea; depression; anorexia; weight loss; weakness; dehydration; hyperpnea; pale, congested, or discolored mucous membranes; slow capillary refill; weak rapid pulse; fever; melena; and abdominal organomegaly, pain, masses, or effusions.

If the cause of the diarrhea is not apparent following the clinical examination and warning signs of serious disease are present, the clinician is obligated to recommend supportive therapy and a diagnostic workup to expediently determine safe and effective therapy. In the absence of warning signs, symptomatic therapy and treatment trials are permissible.

CHRONIC SMALL BOWEL DIARRHEA

The common causes of chronic small bowel diarrhea and the diagnostic procedures commonly employed for the evaluation of such patients are listed in Tables 5-20 and 5-21, respectively.

Admission Laboratory Work. For complex or refractory cases of diarrhea the minimum laboratory data base should include a complete blood count, a serum chemistry profile with electrolyte levels, a urinalysis, a fecal flotation for parasite ova, a direct smear of saline-admixed fresh feces for protozoa, and a Sudan stain of fresh feces for fat. In the cat, serological tests for FeLV, feline immunodeficiency virus, FIP, and thyroxine measurement may be warranted. The laboratory data base evaluates the patient for systemic diseases, such as infections, hyperthyroidism, and hepatic and renal insufficiency, that may result in signs of gastrointestinal disease; identifies any additional incidental problems in another system of the body; facilitates choice of fluid therapy; and aids in the identification of gastrointestinal problems, such as parasitism, eosinophilic gastroenteritis, protein-losing enteropathies, and steatorrhea. Eosinophilic gastroenteritis, hypoadrenocorticism, and some parasitic diseases are associated with a peripheral eosinophilia. Panhypoproteinemia characterizes protein-losing enteropathies, and the triad of lymphopenia, hypoalbuminemia, and hypoglobulinemia characterizes lymphangiectasia.

Tests of Pancreatic Function. Exocrine pancreatic insufficiency is a readily treatable cause of chronic diarrhea that should be ruled out early in the diagnostic workup. It is most common in the dog but is only occasionally diagnosed in the cat. If the patient is eating a diet of normal fat content and the Sudan stain for undigested fat is positive, pursue the diagnosis of pancreatitis by means of fecal digestion tests (cat and dog), or preferably the BT-PABA test (dog), or trypsin-like immunoreactivity test (dog). A less satisfactory approach to confirm the diagnosis is a treatment trial with a pancreatic enzyme supplement. Diarrhea due to many causes will appear to respond, or partially respond, to enzyme supplementation, resulting in overdiagnosis of exocrine pancreatic insufficiency and at times needless supplementation.

Survey Abdominal Radiographs. Partial obstructions due to foreign bodies, intussusceptions, or masses are occasional causes of diarrhea that in some instances can be diagnosed by survey radiographs. While not common causes, the serious consequences of misdiagnosing these disorders makes abdominal radiography a recommended part of the early workup. Furthermore, survey radiographs detect gross abnormalities in liver and kidney size and help detect abdominal fluid, abdominal masses, organ torsions, bowel perforation, peritonitis, and pancreatitis.

Abdominal Ultrasound. Abdominal ultrasound and radiographs are complementary examinations. Ultrasound is more sensitive for the detection of abdominal masses, intestinal mural thickenings, intussusceptions, and mesenteric lymphadenopathy. Ultrasound-guided percutaneous biopsy or aspiration of masses or abnormal organs is an effective diagnostic procedure.

Dietary Trial. Animals with no warning signs of serious disease (other than their chronic diarrhea), whose diarrhea remains undiagnosed after initial laboratory and imaging procedures, are further investigated with test diets. Test diets must be instituted before intestinal biopsies are taken, because certain diseases such as gluten-induced enteropathy, dietary allergies, and inflammatory bowel disease can be diagnosed only after evaluation of the response to a test diet. These diseases have similar biopsy findings, and it is the dietary response, or lack of, which allows their differentiation.

Place the animal on a controlled diet for at least two weeks. Use an easily digestible, simplified diet such as one part low-fat cottage cheese or Tofu to three parts boiled white rice. If signs resolve, slowly modify the basic diet until a tolerable, balanced diet is determined. If signs do not resolve, more extensive and invasive diagnostic procedures are then justified.

Endoscopy. Endoscopic biopsy is an effective technique for the diagnosis of intestinal mucosal diseases that are associated with morphologic changes. The procedure may identify intestinal inflammation of various causes or intestinal neoplasia. Aspiration of duodenal fluid for cytology can be used to

Table 5-17 Small and Large Intestinal Dysfunction Primary and Secondary Signs

Primary Sign: Diarrhea

Change in frequency, consistency, or volume of bowel movements

Secondary Signs

Abdominal distention	Melena
Abdominal pain	Polydipsia
Anal pruritus	Polyphagia
Borborygmus	Shivering
Dehydration	Tenesmus
Flatulence	Vomiting
Halitosis	Weight loss

Table 5-18 Causes of Steatorrhea

MALDIGESTION
- **Exocrine pancreatic insufficiency**
  - Pancreatic atrophy
  - Chronic pancreatitis
  - Pancreatic duct obstruction
- **Hepatobiliary disease**
  - Liver failure
  - Intrahepatic cholestasis
  - Extrahepatic cholestasis

MALABSORPTION
- **Inflammatory bowel diseases**
- **Neoplasia of the small intestine**
- **Stagnant loop syndrome (bacterial overgrowth)**
- **Lymphangiectasia**

MISCELLANEOUS
- **Hyperthyroidism**
- **Gastrinomas**
- **Dumping syndromes**
- **Unaccustomed high fat diet***

* *Dogs and cats can consume 40% and 64% fat diets (% dry matter), respectively, without gross steatorrhea, provided they are given sufficient time to accustomize themselves to the diet.*

diagnose giardiasis. Aspirated duodenal fluid may also be quantitatively cultured for the definitive diagnosis of bacterial overgrowth. Endoscopy, however, does not permit diagnosis of intestinal motility disorders, secretory diarrheas or brush border enzyme defects, and it is likely to miss lesions in the intestinal submucosa or muscularis. Furthermore, the restricted working length of many endoscopes compromises the ability of the endoscope to detect diseases primarily manifested in the jejunum. To be of value, endoscopic examination must be thorough; multiple biopsies of lesions at standardized areas of the gastrointestinal tract should be performed. If clinical signs suggest the possibility of an enterocolitis, colon biopsy may also be performed.

Tests for Malabsorption. Tests for malabsorption do not give a causal diagnosis, many are time-consuming, and they are all plagued to a greater or lesser degree by poor sensitivity and specificity. In the past, one of their major functions has been to provide the clinician with evidence that exploratory surgery and small intestinal biopsy are warranted. With the advent of the endoscope, the decision to biopsy the small intestine is less momentous. For these reasons, and because of the improved sensitivity of endoscopic biopsy (in comparison to malabsorption tests) for the detection of common morphologic mucosal diseases such as inflammatory bowel disease, many clinicians now perform endoscopy prior to instituting screening tests for malabsorption. If the clinician takes this approach, it should not be forgotten that endoscopic examination does not screen for the same spectra of diseases as do malabsorption tests. Endoscopy and endoscopic biopsy only permit diagnosis of intestinal diseases that have abnormal mucosal morphology. In contrast, malabsorption tests evaluate function; they identify abnormal carbohydrate or fat assimilation due to diseases such as motility disorders, bacterial overgrowth, or brush border enzyme deficiencies that need not, or do not, have morphologically recognizable abnormalities on bowel biopsy. Therefore, endoscopy should not be considered a replacement for tests of malabsorption.

Screening tests for malabsorption that have been used in the cat and dog include those that assess the absorption of xylose, hydrogen, fat, glucose, galactose, lactose, cobalamin, folate, vitamin A, and radio-labeled oleic acid. Screening tests of malassimilation include the indirect quantitative analysis of fecal fat, the Sudan stain for fecal fat, the radio-labeled-triglyceride (^{131}I-triolein), and the assessment of fecal- reducing substances and fecal pH. These tests vary considerably in their simplicity, availability, and reliability. The tests for carbohydrate malabsorption and fat malassimilation that are most commonly used at the UCD VMTH are the breath hydrogen analysis and the direct/indirect Sudan stain for fecal fat. We do not recommend use of the fat absorption test, which in our experience has often returned misleading results.

Tests for Bacterial Enteritis and Bacterial Overgrowth. Infection with known bacterial pathogens does not appear to be a common cause of chronic diarrhea. Intestinal colonization by a bacterial pathogen is most often secondary to events or processes that disrupt normal intestinal function. Disruption is caused by primary diseases such as intestinal lymphosarcoma, by stress such as caused by surgery, and iatrogenically as a result of antibiotic therapy. Bacterial enteritis can be seen as a cause of diarrhea in recently kenneled dogs. Overgrowth of the upper small intestine by normal bacterial flora is probably more common than chronic bacterial enteritis. Bacterial overgrowth can lead to biopsy changes resembling those found with inflammatory bowel disease.

If bacterial enteritis or enterocolitis is suspected, then the feces should be cultured for specific pathogens such as *Salmonella* species, *Campylobacter jejuni*, *Clostridia* species, and *Yersinia enterocolitica*. These bacteria can be cultured in small to moderate numbers from many normal dogs. Therefore, interpretation of culture results is made easier if the laboratory provides a comparative estimate of the number of the bacterial pathogen in relation to other bacterial flora. It is assumed that a heavy and relatively pure growth of a known pathogen or a member of the fecal flora is significant. Low numbers of pathogens amongst healthy mixed flora are more difficult to interpret.

A diagnosis of bacterial overgrowth of the small intestine cannot be made by fecal culture because very high numbers of bacteria are normally cultured from the feces, and those numbers do not reflect the numbers or composition of bacteria found in the small intestine. A definitive diagnosis of bacterial overgrowth can, however, be made by quantitative anaerobic and aerobic culture of duodenal fluid aspirated by endoscopy, suction capsule biopsy, or by needle at surgery. The breath hydrogen test provides firm supportive evidence for bacterial overgrowth, as does depressed serum vitamin B_{12} in association with an elevated serum folate level.

Whenever possible, treatment trials should be avoided for the diagnosis of chronic bacterial enteritis or bacterial overgrowth. Without attention to the underlying cause of bacterial

Table 5-19 Differentiation of Large and Small Bowel Diarrhea

Clinical Sign	Small Bowel	Large Bowel
Limitation of function	Weight loss usual, fecal incontinence rare	Weight loss unusual, fecal incontinence common
Quality of stool	Loose, no form, watery, possible fat droplets, undigested food, melena, color variable, malodorous	Loose to formed, mucus frequent, sometimes fresh blood, no undigested food color usually brown
Quantity of stool	Volume is always increased	Volume may be normal or increased
Frequency	Usually increased 2-4 times/day	Invariably increased 4-10 times/day
Exacerbating factors	Diet changes, high fat diets, poorly digestible diets	Stress and psychological factors may be important
Associated phenomena	Abdominal distention, flatus, borborygmus, halitosis, melena, polydipsia, polyphagia, vomiting, weight loss	Tenesmus, anal pruritus

overgrowth, and because of the rapid acquisition of antibiotic resistance by gastrointestinal bacterial pathogens, these conditions are often only at best temporarily responsive to treatment trials with broad-spectrum antibiotics. In addition, some drugs used for treatment trials, such as metronidazole, have well-recognized effects other than their antibacterial activity that seriously compromise interpretation of results. Diagnosis of bacterial overgrowth should be followed by further diagnostics to attempt to identify a predisposing cause.

Contrast Radiography. Liquid barium follow-through studies can identify some partial obstructions of the intestine. In general, however, this is a low-yield diagnostic procedure for the diagnosis of chronic diarrhea, especially if already preceded by ultrasonography.

Fluoroscopy allows definitive diagnosis of gastric and intestinal motility disorders. *Enteroclysis* is a very useful contrast procedure for the diagnosis of small bowel partial obstructions. It also provides information about mucosal morphology and small bowel motility. Persistent ileus can be caused by hypokalemia, hypoalbuminemia, or dysautonomia. Small intestinal hypermotility can result from mesenteric ganglionitis, carcinoid syndrome, and thyrotoxicosis.

Exploratory Celiotomy. Exploratory celiotomy optimizes visual inspection, palpation, and multiple biopsies of the abdominal organs. Biopsies should be taken even if the intestine looks normal. Many intestinal diseases need full thickness biopsy for definitive diagnosis, either because of location in the submucosa, myenteric plexus, or muscularis, or because of sparse or patchy incidence in the mucosa. Full thickness biopsy of the intestine is disadvantaged by the increased likelihood of wound dehiscence. The biopsy sites of debilitated and hypoalbuminemic animals are particularly likely to dehisce. In these patients, full thickness intestinal biopsy should be performed only after great circumspection and preferably in association with parenteral nutrition support. Exploratory celiotomy may also be required for the diagnosis of mucosal lesions out of reach of the endoscope and some "occult" diseases of other abdominal organs such as APUDomas.

Intestinal Biopsies. On most occasions, small intestinal biopsies, whether attained by endoscopy, guided suction biopsy capsules, or celiotomy, yield non-etiologic-specific pathology such as intestinal inflammation, villus atrophy and cellular infiltration. On occasion, a cause may be apparent, such as when infectious agents, neoplastic cells, or lymphangiectasia are evident. In some cases, such as eosinophilic gastroenteritis, the prominent cell type found suggests an immune-mediated problem. Diagnostic conclusions are most often dependent on the interpretation of the biopsy result in the light of previous diagnostic findings or the response to subsequent therapy. For example, a diagnosis of idiopathic inflammatory bowel disease is made only after a previous workup, including dietary trials, has ruled out obvious causes of intestinal inflammation and the clinical signs respond to immunosuppressive therapy. In some institutions, examination of small intestinal biopsy specimens by a dissecting microscope has been found useful to confirm villus atrophy, and subcellular fractionation techniques have been utilized to detect brush border enzyme deficiencies. When enterocolitis is suspected, or when biopsy of the small bowel is prohibited for any reason, such as anesthetic risk or expense, a biopsy of the colon is warranted. On some occasions, pathologic processes affect, to a lesser or greater extent, both the small intestine and colon.

Table 5-20 Causes of Small Bowel Diarrhea

Dietary	Hypermotility (myenteric ganglionitis)
Food poisoning	Ischemic diseases (mesenteric avulsion, infarction, torsions, strangulations)
Gluttony	Lymphangiectasia
Sudden change of diet	Hemorrhagic gastroenteritis
Intolerance	**Pancreatic disease**
Wheat-sensitive enteropathy	Chronic pancreatitis
Allergy	Pancreatic neoplasia
Stomach	Juvenile atrophy
Dumping syndromes	Obstruction of pancreatic ducts
Hyperacidity	**Liver disease**
Achlorhydria	Liver failure
Small intestinal disease	Intrahepatic cholestasis
Infectious enteritis (viral, fungal, invasive bacteria, Salmon poisoning, bacterial enterotoxins and endotoxins)	Bile duct obstruction
Parasitic enteritis (giardia, strongyloides, ascarids, hookworms)	**Kidney disease**
Inflammatory bowel disease (eosinophilic, plasmacytic/lymphocytic, other)	Uremia
Infiltrative neoplasia (lymphosarcoma, mastocytosis)	Nephrotic syndrome
Other infiltrative disease (fucosidosis, amyloidosis)	**Miscellaneous systemic disorders**
Partial intraluminal obstruction (neoplasia, strictures, fungal or eosinophilic granuloma, foreign body, intussusception)	Toxemias (pyometra, abscess, peritonitis)
Extraluminal obstructions (hernias, adhesions, masses)	Septicemias (leptospirosis)
Brush border enzyme defects	Congestive heart failure
Bacterial overgrowth	Immunodeficiencies (IgA deficiency)
Ileus (hypokalemia, hypoalbuminemia, enteritis, dysautonomia, other)	Autoimmune diseases (SLE)
	Hypoadrenocorticism
	Hyperthyroidism
	APUDomas (gastrinomas, VIPomas, carcinoid syndrome)
	Thyroid carcinoma
	Metastatic neoplasia
	Acrodermatitis
	Various toxins and drugs

Miscellaneous Diagnostic Evaluations. Various other diagnostic procedures may be useful for the diagnosis of some cases of chronic diarrhea. In animals with an exposure history, a histoplasmosis titer may be helpful. Percutaneous fine needle aspiration of thickened bowel loops can provide supportive evidence of inflammatory bowel disease, and the peroral string test or the IFA test on feces can be used to diagnose giardiasis. Absorption of chromium-labelled EDTA can confirm increased intestinal permeability. Diagnosis of protein-losing enteropathy can be assisted by ^{111}indium-labeled transferrin and ^{51}chromium-labeled albumin tests. Fecal occult blood tests may be required to confirm gastrointestinal blood loss. Measurements of fecal osmolality and fecal electrolyte concentrations in small animal patients require more investigation before they can be recommended. Assays of various hormones or their metabolites may be required to diagnose endocrinopathies such as the APUD tumors. Elevated plasma gastrin level supports (but doesn't confirm) the diagnosis of gastrinoma.

CHRONIC LARGE BOWEL DIARRHEA

The prevalent causes of chronic large bowel diarrhea and the diagnostic procedures commonly employed for the evaluation of such patients are listed in Tables 5-22 and 5-23, respectively.

Admission Laboratory Work. For refractory cases of large bowel diarrhea useful diagnostic procedures to complete the data base include a complete blood count, a serum chemistry profile with electrolyte levels, a urinalysis, a fecal flotation for parasite ova, a fecal direct smear for protozoa, a Romanowsky stained fecal smear, and rectal scraping. In cats, serum tests for FeLV, FIV, and FIP may be appropriate. The laboratory data base allows the clinician to evaluate the patient for systemic diseases, such as uremia, that may result in signs of colitis; identify any incidental problems in another system of the body; facilitate choice of fluid therapy; and aid in the identification of gastrointestinal problems, such as parasitic colitis and eosinophilic colitis.

Examination of two or three fecal samples for parasites is essential in all cases. False negative fecal examinations are not uncommon with lowly fecund parasites, such as *Trichuris vulpis*. Fecal smear or cytology of rectal scrapings may reveal inflammatory cells suggestive of colitis, spores of *Clostridium perfringens* supportive of *Clostridium perfringens* enterotoxin-associated diarrhea, or protozoal or *Histoplasma* organisms.

Treatment Trials. In view of the high incidence of chronic idiopathic colitis, many clinicians utilize treatment trials for

Table 5-21 Diagnostic Procedures for the Diagnosis of Chronic Small Bowel Diarrhea

Procedure	Usefulness
CBC	Sepsis, toxemia, eosinophilic gastroenteritis, hypoadrenocorticism, lymphangiectasia, PLE, lead toxicosis, hydration
Serum chemistry profile	Hypoadrenocorticism, uremia, protein-losing enteropathy, liver disease, electrolyte levels
Urinalysis	Renal disease, liver disease, hydration
Blood gas	Acid-base status
Fecal flotation	Ascarids, *Nanophytes*
Fecal direct smear and IFA	Giardiasis
Fecal Sudan stain	Steatorrhea
Fecal occult blood	Neoplasia, ulcers
Fecal digestion tests	Exocrine pancreatic insufficiency
Fecal culture	Bacterial enteritis
Peroral string test	Giardiasis
Trypsin-like immunoreactivity test	Exocrine pancreatic insufficiency
Serum antibody/antigen tests	FeLV, FIV, histoplasmosis
Serum thyroxine level	Hyperthyroidism
Serum vitamin B_{12}/folate test	Bacterial overgrowth
Breath hydrogen test	Bacterial overgrowth, carbohydrate malabsorption
Xylose absorption	Carbohydrate malabsorption
Fecal total fat excretion	Fat malabsorption
Survey radiographs	Intussusception, foreign bodies, liver and kidney size, masses, pancreatic abscess, peritonitis
Ultrasonography	Masses, metastatic neoplasia, mural thickenings
Dietary trials	Adverse reaction to food
Contrast radiography	Intestinal partial obstruction, gastric emptying
Fluoroscopy	Gastrointestinal motility disorders
Enteroclysis	Intestinal motility disorders, partial obstructions
Scintigraphy	Protein-losing enteropathy
Endoscopy	Luminal & mucosal gastroduodenal disease, giardiasis, bacterial overgrowth
Toxicology	Plasma cholinesterase, lead

this disorder early in the workup of patients with uncomplicated large bowel diarrhea. A tentative diagnosis of chronic idiopathic colitis can be made by a successful response to a treatment trial with a controlled diet with or without sulfasalazine. In endemic areas, treatment trials against whipworms are often instituted early in the workup, even if fecal flotation does not detect whipworm eggs.

Diagnostic Imaging. Survey abdominal films and ultrasound are rarely helpful. On occasions they may reveal rectal foreign bodies, bowel thickenings, cecal inversion, ileocolic intussusceptions, abdominal mass lesions, mesenteric lymphadenopathy, and prostatomegaly.

Barium or air enemas are of occasional value in the localization of large bowel disease. Their use, however, has been largely superceded by endoscopy.

Fecal Culture. The difficulties of interpretation of fecal cultures have been discussed above. Culture of feces for salmonella and campylobacter is especially indicated in animals with large bowel diarrhea that have been kenneled. A positive culture for *Clostridium perfringens* is particularly likely if clostridial spores were noted on fecal smears. If the histopathological picture is dominated by neutrophil infiltration and erosion or ulceration, bacterial colitis is a possibility and culture for enteric bacterial pathogens is warranted. If the histopathology shows pseudomembranous inflammation, culture for *Clostridium difficile* is indicated.

Endoscopy and Colon Biopsy. Rigid proctoscopy is preferred over flexible colonoscopy for the initial evaluation of large bowel disease. Rigid proctoscopy entails less risks, time, and cost than colonoscopy, yet it is able to diagnose the majority of large bowel diseases, because such diseases are commonly diffuse (e.g. colitis), and/or located within reach of a proctoscope (e.g. adenocarcinoma). Flexible colonoscopy should be performed if a diagnosis is not apparent using rigid proctoscopy, if the clinician perceives an increased likelihood of upper colonic disease (e.g. hematochezia without tenesmus), or if an evaluation of the extent of the disease is needed. Diseases identifiable by colonoscopy but not proctoscopy include cecal inversion, occult *Trichuris* infection, and ileocolic neoplasia.

The colon may be biopsied with a suction biopsy capsule (Quinton Instruments. Seattle, Washington); speculum biopsy forceps; or via pinch biopsies through a flexible endoscope. Full thickness colon biopsies should be avoided. As with small bowel biopsies, biopsy of the colon rarely reveals the cause of the diarrhea, but does allow a categorization of the disease process on which therapeutic and prognostic advice can be more soundly based.

Miscellaneous Diagnostic Tests. With reasonable frequency, colon biopsies show little or no inflammation in spite of persistent signs of large bowel disease. The further diagnosis of these signs is at present an enigma. It is probable that they represent a group of diseases that are somewhat analogous to irritable bowel syndrome in humans and may have a psychogenic component. Possible pathomechanisms include exposure to secretagogues, and deranged motility patterns. Increased fecal concentrations of unconjugated bile acids or hydroxylated fatty acids could be responsible for some of the cases. In the future, tests of bile acid absorption, or colonorectal manometry, may facilitate diagnosis. At present, diagnosis is largely made by treatment trials. Therapies used have included removing identifiable stressors; increasing dietary fiber; use of bile acid chelators such as cholestyramine (not in cats); and administration of narcotic analgesics (diphenoxylate or loperamide), anticholinergics, or tranquilizers.

TENESMUS

Tenesmus refers to persistent or prolonged straining that is usually ineffectual and often painful. The most prevalent causes of tenesmus are listed in Table 5-24. The diagnostic approach to tenesmus is similar to that described for large bowel diarrhea.

Clinical Examination. Clients often equate the clinical sign of straining with "constipation." In addition to history pertaining to the gastrointestinal tract, the clinician should obtain information concerning the normality, or otherwise, of urination. A description of the posture the patient adopts while straining may help localize the disorder. Female animals straining to urinate usually squat and hold their tail lower to the ground than those straining to defecate. Whether the tenesmus occurs before or after micturition or defecation can also aid differentiation. Obstructive disorders are more commonly associated with tenesmus before evacuation, whereas irritative disorders are often associated with persistent tenesmus after evacuation. In addition to physical examination of the large bowel, anus, and perineum, the clinician should carefully palpate the bladder, and closely examine the vagina or penis for evidence of pain, discharges, masses, or calculi.

Diagnostic Procedures. The diagnostic procedures are similar to those described for the evaluation of large bowel diarrhea. If the cause of the tenesmus is localized to genitourinary disease, various additional diagnostic procedures such as urinary catheterization, urinary tract contrast radiography, urethroscopy, cultures of urine or prostatic fluid, and biopsies of the urinary tact, uterus, or prostate may be required.

MELENA & HEMATOCHEZIA

Melena describes dark, tarry stools resulting from digested blood. Melena usually results from bleeding into the pharynx, esophagus, stomach, or upper small intestine. Life-threatening volumes of blood can accumulate within the gastrointestinal tract, with little or no visible signs of external blood loss. The first step in the diagnostic evaluation of melena is the objective confirmation of the problem. Subsequently diagnostic evaluations are selected to first localize the site of bleeding and then define the cause.

Hematochezia refers to the presence of red blood on the stool. The diagnostic evaluation of hematochezia is similar to that described above for the evaluation of large bowel diarrhea, but, particularly in the absence of other signs of large bowel disease, it should include coagulation tests. Important causes of gastrointestinal bleeding are listed in Table 5-25.

Confirmation of Melena. The classic appearance of melena is of coal-black, shiny, sticky, foul-smelling feces of tar-like consistency. On many occasions, however, feces will have some, but not all, of these classic features. For instance, there are a number of spurious reasons for black feces. Therefore, it can become important to confirm the presence of digested blood by use of tests for fecal blood, such as the orthotolidine (Hematest), and guaiac (Hemoccult) tablet tests. These tests are qualitative, only moderately sensitive, and can generate false positive results. Recently, a highly sensitive, quantitative fluorometric assay of fecal hemoglobin has been described.

Clinical Examination. The patient's age helps determine the likelihood of gastrointestinal neoplasia. The history should include inquiry as to the usage of non-steroidal antiinflammatory drugs or prednisone, evidence of bleeding tendency, and the likelihood of trauma (avulsions, infarction). Clinical manifestations of gastrointestinal bleeding depend on the extent and rapidity of the hemorrhage and range from mild weakness to collapse. Clinical signs usually pertain primarily to anemia and hypovolemia, but on occasion they may help localize the site of hemorrhage. Thus, concomitant regurgitation suggests esophageal or pharyngeal disease, cough raises the likelihood of hemoptysis, and jaundice and ascites imply liver disease. Hematemesis strongly suggests gastric or duodenal bleeding, but swallowed blood will also cause infrequent vomiting. The physical examination should include careful inspection of the nares and oropharynx for evidence of nasal or oropharyngeal sources of bleeding, and the skin of the abdomen and the mucous membranes for evidence of bleeding disorders. Fever occurs in 80% of humans with gastrointestinal hemorrhage of any cause. Gastrointestinal hemorrhage may precipitate hepatic encephalopathy in patients with liver disease.

Appearance of the Feces. Blackening of the stool occurs when enough hemoglobin is oxidized to hematin or other hematochromes. It is the duration of passage of blood that determines its color, not its level of origin. It has been estimated that blood must be retained in the intestinal tract of humans for at least eight hours for it to turn black. Black stools can result from lower small bowel or upper large bowel bleeding if transit time is sufficiently slow, such as can occur when bleeding occurs proximal to an obstructive neoplasm. In such cases, however, it is unusual for the stools to have a tarry appearance. Tarry stools result from bacterial breakdown of hemoglobin in the intestine. Melena will only appear tarry if there is a sufficiently large quantity of blood present. Fresh blood adherent to the feces is strongly suggestive of lower large bowel hemorrhage.

Diagnostic Procedures

The diagnostic procedures commonly employed for the evaluation of patients with melena are listed in Table 5-26.

Table 5-22 Causes of Large Bowel Diarrhea

Inflammatory large bowel disease

- Acute non-specific colitis
- Chronic colitis (plasmacytic/lymphocytic, eosinophilic, granulomatous, histiocytic)
- Infectious colitis (FIP, FeLV, histoplasmosis, *Entamoeba, Balantidium, Salmonella, campylobacter, Clostridium perfringens, Clostridium difficile, Prototheca.*)
- Parasites (*Trichuris*, *Giardia*, hookworms, Salmon poisoning, *Balantidium coli*, *Entamoeba histolytica*, *coccidia*)
- Pseudomembranous colitis (antibiotic-associated)

Obstructive large bowel disease

- Intraluminal obstruction (constipation, megacolon, neoplasia, strictures, foreign body, intussusception)
- Extraluminal obstructions (hernias, adhesions, masses)

Ischemic large bowel disease

- Trauma, infarction, torsion, strangulation, ileocolic intussusception, stress?

Neoplastic large bowel disease

- Adenocarcinoma
- Lymphosarcoma

Non-inflammatory large bowel disease

- Exposure to secretagogues (unconjugated bile acids, hydroxylated fatty acids)
- Motility abnormalities ("irritable bowel syndrome")
- Cecal inversion

Pancreatic disease

- Acute pancreatitis (segmental colitis)

Systemic disorders

- Toxemias (pyometra, abscess, peritonitis)
- Uremia
- Metastatic neoplasia
- Toxicities

Diet-related

- Food poisoning
- Intolerances or allergy?
- Foreign material (bones, hair, wrapping material)

Admission Laboratory Work. Along with the clinical examination the complete blood count helps determine the severity and chronicity of the condition. Microcytic, hypochromic anemias are common following prolonged gastrointestinal blood loss. The rapidity with which the hematocrit declines after hemorrhage is variable depending on such factors as hydration status and pre-existing anemia. Significant decline can occur within one to two hours. The platelet count usually declines little as a result of hemorrhage and in fact may rise as a result of increased platelet production. Leukocytosis and occasionally a leukemoid reaction can occur following hemorrhage. Reticulocytosis should be expected within two to four days.

The BUN:creatinine ratio rises after upper gastrointestinal hemorrhage due to the digestion and absorption of blood protein. Lower bowel hemorrhage has little effect on BUN, but will elevate blood ammonia. Slight hyperbilirubinemia is common in humans after gastrointestinal hemorrhage. The hyperbilirubinemia results from the breakdown of large quantities of heme. A fecal flotation for hookworm should not be neglected.

Tests Assisting Localization of Gastrointestinal Hemorrhage. In the absence of an endoscope, aspiration of esophageal or gastric content following the measured passage of a nasogastric tube may help localize the site of bleeding. The peroral string test has been successfully used for diagnostic purposes in the dog. One of the uses of this test in humans is the determination of the site of bleeding. To determine the level at which bleeding begins, the string is measured from the oral cavity to the proximal limit of the blood-stained string. Conversely, the level at which blood staining of the string is first detected is compared to the level at which bile staining of the string, or acidification of fluid absorbed into the string, is first detected.

In humans, endoscopy has an 80%-90% accuracy rate for the detection of upper gastrointestinal lesions resulting in bleeding, if performed early in the diagnostic workup. Radiography is usually of less value than endoscopy in localizing the site of the bleeding. Selective celiac arteriography may be required to determine the site of intestinal bleeding due to vascular anomalies. Such anomalies are difficult to recognize at endoscopy or surgery and are an important cause of gastrointestinal hemorrhage in older humans. Tests using ^{99m}Technetium-labelled red blood cells may be used to locate the site of bleeding. Miscellaneous other diagnostic procedures of value are listed in Table 5-26.

BORBORYGMUS & FLATULENCE

Borborygmus is a rumbling noise caused by the propulsion of gas through the gastrointestinal tract. Borborygmus and

Table 5-23 Diagnostic Procedures of Value for the Diagnosis of Chronic Large Bowel Diarrhea

Procedure	Usefulness
CBC	Sepsis, toxemia, eosinophilic colitis hydration
Serum chemistry profile	Uremia, electrolyte levels
Urinalysis	Renal disease, hydration
Fecal flotation	*Trichuris*
Fecal direct smear	Giardiasis, *Entamoeba*, *Balantidium coli*
Fecal cytology/rectal scrape	Bacterial colitis, inflammatory bowel disease, *Entamoeba*, *Balantidium coli*, clostridial spores, *Prototheca*, *histoplasmosis*
Fecal culture	*Salmonella*, *Campylobacter* enterocolitis, *Clostridia difficile*
Fecal clostridial enterotoxin levels	Clostridial enteritis
Serum antibody/antigen tests	FeLV, FIV, histoplasmosis, FIP
Survey radiographs	Ileocolic intussusception, foreign bodies, constipation
Barium enemas	Ileocolic intussusceptions, cecal inversion, masses
Ultrasonography	Pelvic masses, metastatic neoplasia, mural thickenings, ileocolic intussusceptions
Endoscopy	Colitis, neoplasia, foreign bodies, cecal inversion
Controlled diet trial	Adverse reaction to food, chronic colitis
Fiber trial	"Irritable bowel syndrome", bile acid malabsorption, perturbed flora, perturbed colonic secretion
Sulfasalazine trial	Chronic colitis
Cholestyramine trial (dogs)	Bile acid malabsorption
Panacur trial	Whipworms
Stress reduction	"Irritable bowel syndrome"
Manometry?	"Irritable bowel syndrome"
Exploratory celiotomy	Pelvic and pericolonic masses, biopsy

flatulence most commonly affect the dog. They usually result from dietary indiscretions, but on occasion in both species can herald more serious gastrointestinal disease.

The two most common sources of intestinal gas in dogs and cats are swallowed air and bacterial fermentation of nutrients such as carbohydrate and fiber. Additional sources are the chemical release of carbon dioxide from bicarbonates and diffusion of gas from the blood. The composition of intestinal gas is primarily nitrogen, oxygen, hydrogen, methane, and carbon dioxide, all of which have no odor. Odiferous potentially volatile substances such as ammonia, hydrogen sulfide, indole, skatole, mercaptans, volatile amines, and short chain fatty acids comprise less than 1% of intestinal gas. The transit time for gas is considerably shorter than that for liquids or solids. In humans, gas introduced into the stomach can be passed per rectum in as short a time as 15 minutes. Overdistension of the stomach or intestinal tract by gas can lead to considerable abdominal discomfort.

Excessive aerophagia can induce increased flatus and borborygmi. Diets high in legumes, such as soybean meal, also are associated with gaseousness. Legumes contain large quantities of indigestible oligosaccharides. Unabsorbed oligosaccharides are fermented by clostridia and other bacteria to produce hydrogen, carbon dioxide, and methane. Spoiled diets, and diets high in protein or containing onions, are particularly likely to yield odiferous gases. The type and abundance of bacterial flora also affect the composition and quantity of flatus. Milk products may cause gaseousness in some animals with lactase deficiency. Malassimilation can result in excessive intestinal gas.

The management of flatulence begins with a change to a highly digestible, low fiber diet, of moderate protein content. Reducing aerophagia by avoiding situations that provoke nervousness and by discouraging greedy eating, for instance by ensuring a dog does not have to compete for his food, may also be helpful. It is also likely that more air will be swallowed during the lapping of liquids than the eating of solid food. If dietary manipulation is not successful, consider investigation of the patient as for the evaluation of small bowel diarrhea.

ASCITES

Ascites is an abnormal accumulation of fluid within the peritoneal cavity. The fluid may be transudative, exudative, hemorrhagic, bilious, chylous, pseudochylous, or it may result from the accumulation of urine. Paracentesis classifies the abdominal fluid, markedly reducing the list of diagnostic possibilities and on occasion providing a diagnosis. The common causes of ascites and the diagnostic procedures commonly employed for the evaluation of such patients are listed in Tables 5-27 and 5-28, respectively. The following discussion of the workup of ascites assumes the results of a paracentesis are available.

Transudative Ascites

Transudates are colorless fluids, with a specific gravity of less than 1.017, a WBC count of less than 3000/μl (mainly mononuclear), and a protein content of less than 3 g/dl (usually less than 1.5 g/dl). Capillary permeability and plasma protein concentration influence the level of protein in the fluid. Pure transudates are due to hypoalbuminemia.

Hypoalbuminemia. Albumin maintains blood oncotic pressure. If the ascites is due solely to hypoalbuminemia, expect a plasma albumin concentration of 1 g/dl or less, with concurrent pleural effusions and edema. The most important causes of hypoalbuminemia of this severity are liver disease, glomerular disease, and protein-losing enteropathies. In view of these possibilities, appropriate workup for a patient with ascites and concomitant hypoalbuminemia includes evaluation of the liver by a serum chemistry profile, liver function test, and perhaps liver biopsy, and evaluation of the kidney by a serum chemistry profile, urinalysis, urine protein:creatinine ratio and, on occasion, renal biopsy. If the hypoalbuminemia can not be attributed to kidney or liver disease, and especially if it is associated with hypoglobulinemia and/or lymphopenia, consider a bowel biopsy to rule out protein-losing enteropathy. Transferrin labeled with ^{111}indium or ^{51}chromium labeled albumin scintigraphy can be used to confirm gastrointestinal protein loss. Scintigraphy is especially useful when mild hepatic disease has been detected and it is uncertain whether the hypoalbuminemia can be correctly attributed to liver dysfunction, or whether intestinal protein loss is the primary cause and intestinal biopsy is warranted.

Table 5-24 Causes of Tenesmus

Large bowel
- Constipation
- Colitis
- Neoplasia
- Miscellaneous large bowel diseases (Table 5-22)
- Rectal or anal foreign body

Perianal/perineal disorders
- Perineal hernia
- Perianal fistula
- Anal sac abscess
- Anal sac neoplasia

Genitourinary tract
- Cystitis or urethritis (esp FUS)
- Cystic or urethral calculi
- Prostatomegaly (neoplasia, hyperplasia, abscess)
- Genitourinary neoplasia
- Vaginal masses or foreign bodies
- Dystocia

Caudal abdominal cavity disorders
- Abdominal cavity masses
- Pelvic fractures
- Pelvic osteosarcoma

Ascites Due to Modified Transudates

Modified transudates are a common cause of ascites. They share some features of transudates and exudates and usually have a clear or serosanguinous appearance. The most important cause of ascitic modified transudates is portal hypertension. The portal hypertension can be posthepatic (heart disease), hepatic (cirrhosis), or prehepatic (organ torsion, local vascular compression from neoplasia). Posthepatic portal hypertension results in a transudate of relatively high protein concentration (often approaching the same concentration as the serum albumin) because the highly permeable hepatic sinusoids leak large quantities of plasma proteins when hypertensive. To identify congestive cardiac disease, use clinical signs, central venous pressure, chest radiographs, and cardiac and abdominal ultrasonography. The abdominal ultrasound may reveal dilated hepatic vessels and an enlarged spleen supportive of portal hypertension. Causes of prehepatic portal hypertension, such as abdominal carcinomatosis or mesothelioma, can be difficult to diagnose. Abdominal ultrasonography or exploratory laparotomy are commonly required. Care must be exercised not to confuse reactive mesothelial with neoplastic cells.

Exudative Ascites

Exudates have a cloudy appearance and variable color. They have a specific gravity of greater than 1.017, a protein content of greater than 3 g/dl, and a cell count of greater than 3000/μl (mainly neutrophils). Exudates are usually due to inflammatory processes such as FIP, septic or chemical peritonitis, or necrosis (torsions, large tumors). Diagnosis is based on culture and cytology of abdominal fluid, ultrasound, and exploratory laparotomy. In the case of FIP, the diagnosis is supported by a high FIP titer, a very high protein fluid (approaching the serum total protein concentration), and the presence of pyogranulomatous inflammation. Chemical peritonitis is commonly associated with clinical or laboratory evidence of acute pancreatitis.

Hemorrhagic Ascites

Hemorrhagic effusions are characterized by a PCV, total protein, and white blood cell count similar to peripheral blood. Observation of erythrophagocytosis, hemosiderin-laden macrophages, or the absence of platelets indicates pre-existing hemorrhage and rules out the possibility of misdiagnosed hemorrhagic effusion due to inadvertent puncture of the spleen, liver or a blood vessel during paracentesis. Consider trauma, coagulopathies, vascular disorders, or neoplasia as possible causes

Table 5-25 Causes of Melena

Swallowed blood
- Hemoptysis
- Nasal adenocarcinoma
- Oropharyngeal neoplasia

Esophagus
- Laceration
- Ulceration
- Neoplasia

Stomach
- Widespread erosions
- Ulcers (drugs, stress, uremia, liver failure, mastocytosis, gastrinoma)
- Severe gastritis
- Sharp foreign bodies
- Neoplasia (adenocarcinoma, leiomyosarcoma, lymphosarcoma)

Upper small intestine
- Duodenal ulcers (drugs, stress, uremia, liver failure, mastocytosis, gastrinoma)
- Severe duodenitis
- Neoplasia (mast cell neoplasia, lymphosarcoma, adenocarcinoma)
- Foreign bodies
- Hookworms

Lower small intestine & proximal colon
- Neoplasia
- Hookworms

Gastrointestinal blood vessels
- Laceration, varix, aneurysm, arteriovenous malformations,thrombosis, polyarteritis nodosa, SLE

Gastrointestinal ischemia
- Shock
- Volvulus
- Intussusception
- Mesenteric avulsion
- Gastrointestinal infarction

Liver (hemobilia)
- Hematoma that discharges into the biliary system
- Arteriobiliary fistula following penetrating trauma
- Hepatic cancer
- Liver failure

Pancreas
- Severe acute pancreatitis

Kidney
- Uremia

Hematologic disorders
- Thrombocytopenia
- Thrombocytopathy
- Clotting defects
- Von Willebrand's disease
- DIC
- Polycythemia

Drug Administration
- Non-steroidal antiinflammatory drugs
- Glucocorticoids

of hemorrhagic effusions. The disease of most concern in the middle-aged to older dog (especially German shepherds) is splenic hemangiosarcoma. Diagnostics of use include coagulation tests, ultrasound, and exploratory laparotomy.

Ascites Due to Accumulation of Urine

Animals with perforated urinary tracts can continue to urinate small amounts of urine and, if their bladders are intact, can urinate normally. They are usually uremic and azotemic. Urinary tract perforation can be diagnosed by a suitable history of trauma, in association with an ascitic fluid that has the appearance or smell of urine and has a higher BUN, creatinine and potassium level than the corresponding serum. BUN concentration can equalize rapidly in the abdominal fluid and blood following urine leakage. Differential potassium and creatinine concentrations appear to provide the most discrimination. Localization of the site of the leak may require an intravenous pyelogram, or exploratory surgery.

Bile Ascites

Rupture of the biliary tree is usually due to trauma or neoplasia. Bile is highly irritating and induces a chemical peritonitis. The ascitic fluid can be yellow-ocher in color and is usually exudative, containing many neutrophils. The diagnosis is confirmed by a highly positive bilirubin reaction on a urine dipstick immersed in ascitic fluid. Bilirubin crystals or bilirubin-laden macrophages may be observed in the ascitic fluid. Location of the leak requires scintigraphy or surgical exploration.

Chylous and Pseudochylous Ascites

Chylous ascites is due to accumulation of lymph in the abdominal cavity. Pseudochylous ascites is due to the accumulation of fluid with a high content of phospholipid-protein material. Chylous fluid appears white when the lymph contains a high concentration of triglyceride-rich chylomicrons. Pseudochyle appears white because of the high phospholipid-protein content. Chylous fluid can also be clear and water-like when its lipids are solubilized in a micellar solution. Such solutions are free of protein and the lipid content is demonstrated following staining with Sudan stain.

Chylous ascites usually results from rupture or leakage of abdominal lymphatics caused by trauma, lymphatic obstruction (congenital, neoplastic, adhesions), increased lymphatic flow, or increased lymphatic permeability. Pseudochylous effusions appear to be rare in the dog and cat. In humans, pseudochyle most commonly results from degenerating neoplastic, inflammatory, or mesothelial cells. Several tests can be used to differentiate chylous and pseudochylous effusions. Chyle forms

Table 5-26 Diagnostic Endeavors for the Evaluation of Apparent Upper Gastrointestinal Bleeding

• Clinical examination	
History	Trauma, drug usage
Physical examination	Nasal or oropharyngeal bleeding
Inspection of the stool	Location of site
• Admission laboratory work	
CBC	Severity & chronicity of blood loss; polycythemia
Reticulocyte count	Regenerative or non-regenerative anemia
Buffy coat	Mast cell neoplasia, lymphoma
Serum chemistry profile	Uremia, BUN: creatinine ratio, liver disease multiple myeloma
• Coagulation tests	
Platelet count	Thrombocytopenia
Bleeding time	Thrombocytopenia, thrombocytopathy
OSPT, APTT	Clotting defects
Von Willebrand's test	Von Willebrand's disease
Fibrin degradation products	DIC
• Procedures for localization and diagnosis of GI bleeding	
Nasogastric intubation	Localize site of hemorrhage
Peroral string test	Localize site of hemorrhage
Fecal flotation	Hookworms
Survey radiographs	GI masses, perforation
Ultrasound	GI mass lesions
Gastrogram	Gastric ulcers, masses
Scintigraphy	Localize site of bleeding
Arteriography	Aneurysm, thrombosis, arteriovenous malformations,
Rhinoscopy/nasal radiographs	Nasal adenocarcinoma
Pharyngoscopy	Pharyngeal neoplasia
Bronchoscopy/chest radiographs	Hemoptysis
Upper gastrointestinal endoscopy	Esophageal ulceration, esophageal neoplasia; gastric erosions, ulcers, neoplasia; severe gastritis; foreign bodies; varices; duodenal ulcers and neoplasms
Colonoscopy	Lower intestinal & proximal colonic neoplasia
Exploratory surgery	Miscellaneous diagnosis and therapy

a cream layer after standing, contains many lymphocytes, and has a cholesterol-to-triglyceride ratio less than 1. It will clear with ether and will not clear following centrifugation. Lipoprotein analysis should reveal chylomicrons.

Diagnostics useful for the evaluation of chylous effusions include thoracic radiographs to detect concurrent chylothorax, ultrasonography, lymphograms, and exploratory surgery.

ABDOMINAL PAIN

Etiopathogenesis

The causes of abdominal pain are listed in Table 5-29. Abdominal pain may arise from the parietal peritoneum or abdominal wall (somatic pain), the abdominal viscera (visceral pain), or extra-abdominal tissues such as with disc disease and certain thoracic diseases (referred pain). The site of origin of abdominal pain associated with some disorders, such as lead toxicosis and hypoadrenocorticism, is unknown.

Visceral pain may originate in the visceral peritoneum, mesentery, gastrointestinal tract, liver, pancreas, urinary system, spleen, or reproductive organs. It can result from distension of a hollow viscus; swelling of an organ; traction on a mesentery; or inflammation, ischemia, or perforation of an abdominal structure. These perturbations cause pain via stimulation of nociceptors by stretch or exposure to certain mediators such as kinins, prostaglandins, and substance P. In humans, visceral pain is reported to have a dull, gnawing, or cramping character and is usually poorly localized. In contrast, somatic pain is sharp, localized, and is aggravated by movement. These differing characteristics result from variations of the mode of transmission of the two different classes of pain. Visceral pain is transmitted by unmyelinated C nociceptive fibers. These fibers enter the sympathetic trunk and pass cranial or caudal in the trunk for variable distances before entering the rami communicans, to join the dorsal root of the spinal nerve and enter the spinal cord. There is thus extensive overlap of the spinal segments to which afferent fibers from one locale project. In contrast, transmission of somatic pain is by thinly myelinated,

A-delta fibers of spinal nerves. They project directly to their respective spinal cord segments with minimal overlap. The afferent pathway of nociception is complex and can be influenced by various inhibitory or facilitatory events at a number of different levels. The threshold for the sensation of painful stretch is lowered by the presence of kinins, and prostaglandins at the nociceptors. Thus, mild distension or stretching, such as might occur with minor organ congestion or normal bowel contraction, may produce considerable pain in abdominal organs in which inflammation exists.

Diagnostic Approach

The diagnosis of abdominal pain begins with the clinical examination. The clinical findings dictate the urgency of the patient's condition and the order and extent of subsequent diagnostics. A rapid, accurate decision as to whether celiotomy is required for diagnosis or treatment can be critical to patient survival.

History. The term "acute abdomen" is applied to painful abdominal disorders of acute onset. The animal with an acute abdomen is usually depressed, inappetant, and may have a hunched appearance. Other signs of abdominal disease, such as vomiting, diarrhea, and abdominal distension are often present. The animal may adopt postures of relief such as the "praying" position. Occasionally they "dog-sit" or lie on cold surfaces for abnormally prolonged periods. Animals may cry out when the owner lifts them, may be unwilling to move, or conversely may behave in a distressed and agitated manner, sometimes verging on hysteria.

The history may suggest the cause of the acute abdomen. Previous use of corticosteroids can lead to pancreatitis, colonic perforation, or gastric ulceration. Non-steroidal medications can cause gastrointestinal ulceration. A history of tenesmus suggests the possibility of prostatic, urinary tract, or colonic diseases. Trauma and toxicities are more likely in pets allowed to wander. Pancreatitis is common in obese, middle-aged dogs fed a high fat diet. Unvaccinated, young animals are more commonly afflicted with viral gastroenteritis. Gastrointestinal obstructions due to foreign bodies and intussusceptions are common in younger dogs. Large breed dogs are prone to organ torsions. Urinary obstruction is a common cause of abdominal pain in male cats. Schnauzers may develop abdominal pain in association with their hyperlipidemia syndrome. Chondrodysplastic breeds may suffer apparent abdominal pain from disc prolapse.

Abdominal pain developing several days after trauma raises the possibility of perforation of bowel, rupture of biliary or urinary tract, or necrosis of pieces of liver or spleen. Spasmodic pain is commonly due to contractions of a hollow viscus. Pain associated with defecation suggests large bowel, prostatic, or perianal disease. Post-prandial pain can occur with gastroin-

Table 5-27 Causes of Ascites

Transudative ascites

- Hypoalbuminemia (glomerulonephritis, liver failure, protein-losing enteropathy)

Modified transudates

- Prehepatic portal hypertension - vascular occlusion from torsions, strangulations (hernias), neoplasia (abdominal carcinomatosis, mesothelioma, metastatic neoplasia, others)
- Hepatic portal hypertension - cirrhosis, hepatic thrombosis, neoplasia, hepatic AV fistula, hepatic venous abnormalities
- Post-hepatic portal hypertension - congestive heart failure, obstruction of the caudal vena cava ("kinked" caudal vena cava, intraluminal obstructions, extra-luminal obstructions, GDV)

Exudative ascites

- Septic peritonitis (perforations of bowel; penetrating abdominal wounds; rupture of bowel, uterus, or abscess)
- Chemical peritonitis (pancreatitis, bile, urine)
- FIP
- Necrosis of neoplastic cells or organs
- Mesocestoides

Hemorrhagic ascites

- Trauma - ruptured liver or spleen, mesenteric avulsion
- Coagulopathies - warfarin toxicosis
- Vascular disorders - ruptured aneurysm
- Neoplasia - splenic hemangiosarcoma, ovarian neoplasia, hepatic neoplasia

Bile ascites

- Rupture of biliary tract - trauma, necrotizing cholecystitis

Chylous ascites

- Rupture of lymphatics - trauma, neoplasia
- Lymphatic hypertension - obstruction (congenital absence, neoplasia, cranial vena caval hypertension, increased lymph flow (hypoalbuminemia)
- Increased lymphatic permeability - perilymphatic inflammation (pancreatitis)

Pseudochylous ascites

- Neoplasia
- Others?

Table 5-28 Diagnostic Procedures of Value for the Diagnosis of Ascites

GENERAL	
CBC	
Hematocrit	Hemorrhage, hydration
Differential	Sepsis, toxemia
Lymphocyte count	Lymphangiectasia
Serum chemistry profile	
BUN/creatinine	Uremia
Liver enzymes, BUN, albumin	Liver disease
Albumin	Hypoalbuminemia
Globulin	Protein-losing enteropathy, FIP
Urinalysis	Renal disease, proteinuria
Fluid analysis	
Cell count	Characterize effusion
Protein concentration	Characterize effusion
Cytology	Inflammation, neoplasia
Anaerobic/aerobic culture	Septic peritonitis
BUN, creatinine, potassium level	Urinary tract perforation
Bile test	Biliary tract perforation
Amylase	Pancreatitis, intestinal perforation
Triglyceride:cholesterol ratio	Chyle
Lipoprotein analysis	Chyle
TRANSUDATIVE ASCITES	
Urine protein/creatinine ratio	Proteinuria
Liver function test	Liver failure
Scintigraphy	Protein-losing enteropathy,
Endoscopy	Protein-losing enteropathy
Thoracic radiography	Concomitant thoracic effusions
MODIFIED TRANSUDATE	
Thoracic radiography	Concomitant thoracic effusions, heart disease, diaphragmatic hernias
Abdominal ultrasonography	Masses, metastatic neoplasia, portal hypertension, liver disease, torsions
Cardiac ultrasonography	Heart disease
Portal pressures/CVP	Portal hypertension characterization
Portal venograms	Venous obstruction, shunts
Hepatic arteriograms	Hepatic AV fistula
Exploratory celiotomy	Neoplasia, torsions, strangulations
EXUDATIVE ASCITES	
Serum antibody tests	FIP
Serum amylase/lipase	Pancreatitis
Abdominal ultrasonography	Neoplasia, pancreatitis
Exploratory celiotomy	Necrotizing lesions, perforations
HEMORRHAGIC ASCITES	
PIVKA	Warfarin toxicosis
Clotting times	Warfarin toxicosis, clotting factor deficiencies
FDPs	DIC
Abdominal ultrasonography	Splenic neoplasia, other neoplasia, trauma
Exploratory celiotomy	Traumatic damage, neoplasia, vascular diseases
CHYLOUS ASCITES	
Lymphangiograms	Localize lymphatic obstruction, leakage
Exploratory celiotomy	Localize obstruction, leakage
BILE ASCITES	
Scintigraphy	Localize bile duct rupture
Exploratory celiotomy	Localize bile duct rupture

testinal tract, pancreatic, and biliary disorders. Important examples include pancreatitis, biliary carcinoma, and the "magenblase syndrome." The latter refers to abdominal pain due to gaseous gastric distension resulting from excessive aerophagia.

Physical Examination. Clinical signs of abdominal pain include a hunched stance and stilted gait. Abdominal palpation will usually evoke signs of pain. Rapid evaluation of the seriousness of the patient's condition is important. Hallmarks of severity and urgency include evidence of shock, hypothermia, tympany, hyperpnea, marked dehydration, weakness, and depression. In the presence of these signs rapid therapeutic intervention is essential. General features of the physical examination that deserve emphasis include oral, rectal, orthopedic, and neurological examinations. The mouth is examined for linear foreign bodies and discolorations of the mucous membranes such as jaundice. Rectal examination detects pelvic abnormalities, such as prostatomegaly, and may reveal melena. Diseases of the limbs and vertebral column can cause a hunched appearance and gait abnormalities that mimic abdominal pain. The clinician should examine the skin for oil or abrasion, and the claws of cats for shredding consistent with road trauma. The patient is checked for undescended testicles or vaginal discharge.

Abdominal palpation is performed in a careful and systematic manner. To begin, the clinician should run his or her fingertips through the hair of the entire abdomen. This facilitates detection of penetrating wounds (such as scabs from cat

Table 5-29 Causes of Acute Abdomen

Abdominal wall
- Strangulated hernias^{s}: inguinal, scrotal, abdominal, umbilical, diaphragmatic, hiatal, mesenteric
- Trauma^{s,m}
- Abdominal abscess^{s}

Peritoneum and mesentery
- Septic peritonitis^{s}: perforated viscus, penetrating wounds (foxtails)
- Bile peritonitis^{s}
- Urine peritonitis^{s}
- Mesenteric traction^{s,m}: large masses
- Mesenteric avulsion^{s}
- Adhesion^{s}

Gastrointestinal tract
- Gastroenteritis^{m}: viral, bacterial, toxic, hemorrhagic
- Gastric dilatation^{m,s}
- Gastric dilatation-volvulus^{s}
- Gastrointestinal gaseousness^{m}
- Gastroduodenal ulceration^{s,m}
- Anatomic gastrointestinal obstruction^{s}: foreign body, stricture, intussusception,
- Functional gastrointestinal obstruction^{m}: ileus
- Gastrointestinal perforation or dehiscence^{s}
- Intestinal volvulus^{s}
- Mesenteric artery thrombosis^{s}
- Colitis^{m}
- Irritable bowel syndrome?^{m}
- Cecal inversion^{s}
- Neoplasia^{s,m}

Liver
- Hepatitis^{m}
- Hepatopathy^{m}
- Neoplasia^{s,m}
- Bile duct obstruction^{s}: calculi, neoplasia, pancreatic abscess
- Biliary duct rupture^{s}
- Liver abscess^{s}

Pancreas
- Pancreatic abscess^{m,s}
- Pancreatitis^{m}
- Pancreatic neoplasia^{s}

Urinary system
- Acute nephrosis^{m}: ethylene glycol, aminoglycosides
- Acute nephritis and pyelonephritis^{m}
- Renal calculi^{s,m}
- Renal neoplasia^{s,m}
- Urethral obstruction^{s,m}: calculi, neoplasia, stricture
- Ureteral obstruction^{s}: calculi, neoplasia, stricture
- Urinary tract rupture^{s}

Spleen
- Torsion^{s}
- Neoplasia^{s}
- Trauma^{s,m}

Reproductive organs
- Uterine torsion or rupture^{s}
- Pyometra^{s,m}
- Ectopic pregnancy^{s}
- Ovarian or prostatic cysts^{s}
- Prostatic abscess^{s}
- Prostatic neoplasia^{s,m}
- Acute prostatitis^{m}
- Testicular torsion^{s}

Miscellaneous
- Abdominal hemorrhage^{m,s}
- Hypoadrenocorticism^{m}
- Mesenteric lymphadenopathy^{m}
- Heavy metal poisoning^{m}: lead, organophosphates
- Thoracic disease^{s,m} - referred pain
- Vertebral or disc disease^{s}

s - surgical therapy; m - medical therapy

Derived from reference 4.

bites) and swellings (hernias, hematomas). The clinician must differentiate abdominal pain from intractability. More significance is attributed to pain responses elicited in stoic animals and to pain that is localized, repeatable, and evident after minimal manipulation. Determination is made whether the painful area is superficial (skin or abdominal wall), located in the cranial or caudal abdomen, or originates from a specific viscus. Superficial pain restricted to a well defined area suggests somatic pain, perhaps of spinal cord, spinal nerve, or cauda equina origin. Cranial abdominal pain is common in pancreatitis. Generalized abdominal pain with board-like rigidity of the abdominal musculature suggests generalized peritonitis. Pain associated with acute tympany implies gas distension of stomach. Other palpable abnormalities, such as thickened bowel, abdominal masses, ascites, organomegaly, intussusception, and tympany, may reveal the cause of the acute abdomen or narrow the diagnostic possibilities. Abdominal auscultation may be a helpful adjunct. Failure to detect borborygmus after two to three minutes of auscultation suggests ileus.

Diagnostic Procedures

Diagnostic procedures of value for the evaluation of patients with abdominal pain are listed in Table 5-30. Diagnostics for urgent cases are usually limited to PCV, TP, urine specific gravity, reagent strip assessment of blood glucose and BUN, paracentesis, and abdominal radiographs or ultrasound. If available, serum electrolytes and blood gases are of value in tailoring fluid therapy. Diagnostics for more stable patients may be more extensive.

Admission Laboratory Work. The CBC, serum chemistry profile, urinalysis, and blood gas analysis provide informa-

Table 5-30 Diagnostic Procedures for the Evaluation of Abdominal Pain

CBC	Sepsis, toxemia, blood loss, hypoadrenocorticism
Serum chemistry profile	Uremia, liver disease, hyperlipidemia, electrolyte imbalance
Blood gas	Acid-base status
Urinalysis	Kidney, liver disease
Fecal flotation	Hookworms, Salmon poisoning, whipworms, liver flukes
Platelet count	DIC
OSPT, APTT, ACT	DIC
Fibrin degradation products	DIC
Lipase/amylase	Pancreatitis
Survey radiographs	Masses, perforation, organomegaly, calculi, foreign bodies, GDV obstructions, gaseousness
Ultrasound	Masses, fluid, biliary and urinary calculi, kidney & liver disease, uterine & prostatic disease, GI obstructions, torsions
Paracentesis	Fluid analysis (see Ascites)
Diagnostic peritoneal lavage	Fluid analysis (see Ascites)
Excretory urography	Renal and ureteral diseases
Gastrogram	Gastric ulcers, masses
Upper gastrointestinal contrast study	Obstruction, GI neoplasia
Scintigraphy	Biliary obstruction
Upper gastrointestinal endoscopy	Gastric ulcers, foreign bodies, neoplasia & severe gastritis; duodenal ulcers and neoplasms; inflammatory bowel disease
Colonoscopy	Colitis, colonic neoplasia, cecal inversion
Arteriography	Aneurysm, thrombosis
Exploratory celiotomy	Miscellaneous diagnosis and therapy

tion that greatly helps with differential diagnosis and case management. The laboratory data base may determine the organ(s) involved (liver, kidney, adrenal) and the type of disease process (inflammation, hemorrhage), and it may reinforce clinical assessment of severity (hypoglycemia, degenerative left shift, dehydration, acidosis, electrolyte imbalance). Lipase and amylase analysis aid detection of pancreatitis. Platelet number and tests of hemostasis may detect DIC. Fecal flotation may yield evidence of parasitism (hookworms, whipworms, *Nanophytes salmincola*). Toxicological analyses may be indicated depending on the likelihood of exposure.

Abdominal Radiographs. Abdominal radiographs may reveal free gas in the abdomen, suggestive of intestinal or body wall perforation. The free gas often accumulates between the diaphragm and the liver. Generalized loss of abdominal detail indicates abdominal effusion. Organomegaly, masses, calculi, obstructive disorders, foreign bodies, organ torsions, pancreatitis, and skeletal abnormalities may be apparent.

Abdominal Ultrasound. Abdominal ultrasound is a sensitive technique for the detection of abdominal masses, including intraorgan miliary masses (e.g. metastatic neoplasia), abdominal fluid, abscesses, cysts, mural thickenings, lymphadenopathy, biliary obstruction, biliary and urinary calculi, and pancreatic abscess. On occasion, portal hypertension or hydronephrosis may be apparent. Ultrasound-guided percutaneous biopsy or aspiration of organs, masses, cysts, or effusion may be appropriate.

Paracentesis. Paracentesis is indicated if abdominal fluid is detected during physical examination or diagnostic imaging. It provides fluid for culture, cytology, and chemical analysis, thus allowing the characterization of the effusion and markedly narrowing the diagnostic possibilities. Ultrasound guidance aids aspiration of localized collections of fluid.

Fluid Analysis. Fluid analysis may include visual inspection, cytology, gram stain, aerobic and anaerobic culture. Cell count, specific gravity, PCV, and concentration of total protein, potassium, creatinine, bilirubin, and amylase may also be determined. Fluid analysis may be suggestive of bowel perforation (mixed flora, vegetable matter neutrophils), organ torsion or neoplasia (modified transudates, anaplastic cells), urine leakage (higher BUN, creatinine or potassium in the abdominal fluid than in serum), bile peritonitis (bile positive), trauma (blood), or pancreatitis (non-septic exudate, high amylase). High amylase concentration in the abdominal fluid is not pathognomonic for pancreatitis; it can also occur following bowel perforation.

Diagnostic Peritoneal Lavage. Diagnostic peritoneal lavage (DPL) is indicated if paracentesis fails to yield abdominal fluid because of its paucity, flocculent nature, or because of loculation. DPL is very useful for the early detection of conditions such as abdominal hemorrhage, bowel dehiscence or perforation, pancreatitis, and neoplasia. Lavage of the abdomen with a large volume of fluid is utilized to improve the yield and sensitivity of the abdominal tap. Because DPL is more time

Table 5-31 Distinguishing Features of Hemolytic (Prehepatic) Jaundice

History	Acute onset. Blood transfusions.
Clinical signs	Primarily pertain to anemia: pale mucous membranes, mild jaundice.
CBC	Profound anemia. May be regenerative. Normal total protein. Spherocytes.
ALT	Normal to slightly increased
Serum alkaline phosphatase	Normal to slightly increased
Albumin	Normal to slightly decreased
BUN	Normal to high
Glucose	Normal
Cholesterol	Normal
Unconjugated:conjugated bilirubin	Not reliable test
Urine urobilinogen	Normal to increased
Clotting times	Usually not performed
Survey radiographs	Usually not performed
Ultrasound	Usually not performed
Scintigraphy	Usually not performed

consuming, dilutes abdominal effusions, and causes more patient discomfort, it should be performed only if paracentesis is unsuccessful. DPL does not detect retroperitoneal injury. Diagnostic criteria for DPL have been established to account for the dilution effects of the infused fluid. For instance, significant intra-abdominal hemorrhage is probable if the microhematocrit of the lavage fluid is greater than 2%. Peritonitis is likely if the neutrophil count is greater than 1500/µl.

Miscellaneous Tests. Various diagnostic tests pertaining to specific organ systems may be indicated. Examples include excretory urography, liver function tests, gastrointestinal contrast procedures, fine needle aspiration, or biopsy of abdominal masses. Endoscopy facilitates detection of upper gastrointestinal lesions, such as ulceration or neoplasia, and lower bowel lesions such as colitis, neoplasia, and cecal inversion. Arteriography may be required to demonstrate mesenteric thrombosus.

Exploratory Celiotomy. Abdominal surgery is required in some patients to establish the cause of the abdominal pain and in many patients for its treatment. The decision to operate may be based on a progressive and rapid worsening in a patient's condition, or on the diagnosis of a disease amenable to surgical therapy. Conditions generally warranting surgery are listed in Table 5-30. In some situations, rapid surgical intervention is clearly indicated. Against the need for urgency, the clinician must balance the benefit of adequate preoperative supportive care. Crystaloid fluid, blood, plasma, antibiotics, corticosteroids, or analgesic administration may be required. Concern regarding the effect of the narcotics on respiratory, pancreatic, and biliary function has limited their use for abdominal pain, although there is little firm evidence to suggest that they complicate recovery provided they are used at appropriate doses. Suitable analgesics for cats and dogs are butorphanol (0.2-0.6 mg/kg SQ q8 hr) and oxymorphone (0.05 mg/kg, SQ, q8 hr).

JAUNDICE

Etiopathogenesis

Jaundice is a syndrome of yellow discoloration of a patient resulting from hyperbilirubinemia and tissue deposition of bile pigment in the sclera, mucous membranes, and skin. Jaundice does not develop until serum bilirubin reaches 1.5-3.0 mg/dl. It is best visualized in the sclera. Jaundice may result either from increased production of bilirubin because of rapid hemolysis (pre-hepatic jaundice), or from failure to effectively excrete bilirubin due to liver disease (hepatic jaundice) or extra-hepatic biliary tract obstruction (post-hepatic jaundice). The first step in the evaluation of a patient with jaundice is to rule out hemolysis as the cause of the jaundice. If the pre-hepatic jaundice is excluded, the workup then focuses on differentiating hepatic from post-hepatic jaundice. The diagnostic evaluations of use in the differential diagnosis of jaundice, and the diagnostic features of prehepatic, hepatic and post-hepatic jaundice are shown in Tables 5-31, 5-32, and 5-33.

History. History compatible with hemolytic disorders includes acute onset of weakness and dyspnea. Recent blood

Table 5-32 Distinguishing Features of Hepatic Jaundice

History	Breed predispositions
Clinical signs	Primarily pertain to liver failure: mild to profound jaundice, non-pale mucous membranes, ascites, weakness, hepatomegaly.
CBC	Mild, non-regenerative anemia. Normal to low total protein
ALT	Slight to profound increase
Serum alkaline phosphatase	Slight to moderate increase
Albumin	Normal to profound decrease
BUN	Normal to low
Glucose	Normal to low
Cholesterol	Normal to low
Unconjugated:conjugated bilirubin	Not reliable test
Urine urobilinogen	Normal to increased
Prolonged clotting times	Not responsive to vitamin K
Survey radiographs	Hepatomegaly, microhepatica
Ultrasound	No evidence of bile duct dilation, or periductal masses.
Scintigraphy	No bile duct obstruction

transfusions raise the likelihood of hemolytic jaundice, as does travel to lands in which blood parasites such as babesia are present. Young, unvaccinated dogs are most commonly afflicted with canine hepatitis or leptospirosis as a cause of jaundice. Middle-aged, female Doberman Pinschers are predisposed to chronic hepatitis. Bedlingtons develop copper-associated hepatopathy. Anorectic, obese cats are prone to hepatic lipidosis. Inquiry is made into the likelihood of exposure to hepatotoxic drugs, chemicals, or plants. Examples include anticonvulsants, organic solvents, and *Amanita* mushrooms. Behavioral abnormality or depressed mentation is compatible with hepatic encephalopathy. Slowly progressive development of jaundice several days after a bout of vomiting raises the likelihood of post-hepatic jaundice's resulting from pancreatitis.

Physical Examination. Patients with hemolytic jaundice show clinical signs primarily suggestive of anemia. The animals may manifest weakness, dyspnea, pale mucous membranes, tachycardia, anemic murmurs, and red colored urine. Jaundice is usually only mild. Animals with hepatic jaundice may demonstrate any of a number of clinical signs pertaining to liver disease. These include ascites, weight loss, depression, anorexia, vomiting, polyuria/polydipsia, and behavioral abnormalities. Cranial abdominal pain can be caused by acute distension of the liver capsule or can signify pancreatitis and post-hepatic jaundice. Hepatomegaly occurs with acute hepatitis, acute hepatopathy, passive congestion (eg cardiac failure), infiltration with lipid or cells (e.g. neoplastic, macrophages, hematopoietic). Rectal examination may detect melena. In cats, fever and abdominal effusion are common with hepatic FIP. Peripheral lymphadenopathy raises the possibility of hepatic lymphosarcoma. Diagnostic effort is required to first localize the animal's disease process to the liver and then identify the probable cause.

Diagnostic Procedures

Complete Blood Count. In an icteric animal, the presence of a very low PCV in association with a normal total protein suggests hemolytic disease, not liver disease. On many occasions the anemia is strongly regenerative. In contrast, mild normocytic, normochromic, non-regenerative anemia is common in liver disease. On occasion, liver disease will result in gastrointestinal hemorrhage, and the PCV will decline precipitously. Unlike hemolysis, however, gastrointestinal hemorrhage is associated with the presence of melena and a concomitant reduction in total protein and elevation in the ratio of BUN to serum creatinine. Spherocytes are compatible with hemolytic jaundice.

If clinical signs and CBC findings are suggestive of hemolytic anemia, the clinician should pursue diseases such as immune-mediated hemolytic anemia, leptospirosis, hemobartonellosis, babesiosis, Heinz body anemias, and red blood cell enzyme defects.

Serum Chemistry Profile. Concomitant ALT elevation, hypoalbuminemia, hypoglycemia, low BUN, and low cholesterol is strongly suggestive of hepatic jaundice. A greater percent rise in concentration of serum ALT than ALP implies liver disease predominantly centered about the central vein (e.g. anoxic injury) or a necrotizing process. A greater percent rise of ALP than ALT implies predominantly periportal (cholestatic) liver disease, but drug administration or elevation of the bone ALP isoenzyme must be ruled out. Cholestasis may result from intrahepatic (infiltrative liver diseases) or extrahepatic causes.

Table 5-33 Distinguishing Features of Post-Hepatic Jaundice

History	Chronic process
Clinical signs	Moderate jaundice, pancreatitis, abdominal masses
CBC	Mild, non-regenerative anemia. Normal total protein
ALT	Slight to moderate increase
Serum alkaline phosphatase	Profound increase (especially dog)
Albumin	Normal to mild decrease
BUN	Normal
Glucose	Normal
Cholesterol	Normal to increased
Unconjugated:conjugated bilirubin	Not reliable test
Urine urobilinogen	Normal to decreased
Prolonged clotting times	Responsive to vitamin K
Survey radiographs	Normal liver size
Ultrasound	Evidence of bile duct dilation, or periductal masses
Scintigraphy	Evidence of failed excretion of bile

Hypoalbuminemia develops after 80% or more of liver function is lost. The liver converts ammonia to urea. Therefore, low BUN, especially with concurrent hypoalbuminemia and/or hypoglycemia is compatible with liver disease. Gastrointestinal hemorrhage may mask this change. Cholestasis may increase serum cholesterol, and decreases can occur with loss of hepatic mass.

Serum Bilirubin, Urine Bilirubin, and the Van den Bergh Test. Serum bilirubin is an insensitive indicator of liver disease in the dog (in comparison to the cat) because of the low renal threshold for bilirubin in the dog. In the dog elevations of urine bilirubin often precede elevations of serum bilirubin. Dog urine normally contains less than 1+ to 2+ bilirubin unless it is highly concentrated. Any bilirubin in cat urine is abnormal. A very high serum bilirubin (greater than 10 mg/dl) suggests intrahepatic cholestasis. The Van den Bergh test assesses the ratio of conjugated to unconjugated bilirubin and has been used to differentiate hemolytic from hepatic jaundice or post-hepatic jaundice. Objective investigation of this test has shown it to be unreliable, and its use provides no useful information.[3] The poor discrimination of the Van den Bergh test presumably results from a number of different phenomena, including poor accuracy of the chemical analyses commonly used, increased production of bilirubin from hemoglobin and non-hemoglobin sources during hepatobiliary diseases, secondary hepatic damage during hemolysis, and the rapid saturation during a hemolytic crisis of the transport mechanisms for the excretion of conjugated bilirubin, resulting in regurgitation of the conjugated bile back into the blood.

Urine Urobilinogen. The value of tests of urine urobilinogen is compromised by the many variables that affect the concentration of this bilirubin metabolite. Increased levels can occur in constipation, hemolysis or hepatocellular insufficiency. A negative urine urobilinogen test can result from low urine specific gravity, exposure of urine to light, antibiotic administration, rapid stool transit, acidic urine, malabsorption, and bile duct obstruction. Urine urobilinogen remains detectable in some dogs with bile duct obstruction, perhaps due to reduction of conjugated bilirubin within the obstructed biliary tree.

Liver Function Tests. The primary role of liver function tests is to identify hepatic insufficiency. Such tests do not assess prognosis and they rarely reveal a cause. They are usually unnecessary in the workup of jaundice because the clinical examination and admission laboratory work should be sufficient to differentiate hemolysis from liver disease. Hyperbilirubinemia due to hepatic disease is in itself evidence of an abnormal liver function, that of the ability of the liver to metabolize and excrete bilirubin.

Vitamin K Response Test. Steatorrhea resulting from bile duct obstruction causes impaired vitamin K absorption and eventually results in a prolonged prothrombin time that is correctable by the administration of vitamin K. If parenteral administration of vitamin K does not reduce the prothrombin time within 12 hours, parenchymal liver disease is probable.

Radiographs and Ultrasound. Radiographs and ultrasound give a crude indication of liver size. Small livers are compatible with cirrhosis, large livers with infiltrative or congestive diseases. Portal venograms may be used to diagnose portosystemic shunts. Ultrasound may reveal an obstructed biliary tree, biliary calculi, evidence of neoplasia, portal hypertension, and hepatic or perihepatic masses.

Nuclear Scintigraphy. Intrarectal technetium will bypass the liver of animals with portosystemic shunts. Intravenous technetium-disofenin complex is excreted through the biliary system and can be used for diagnosis of bile duct obstruction

Percutaneous Hepatic Fine Needle Aspiration. Fine needle aspiration of the liver is most useful in the cat where it can be used to differentiate hepatic lipidosis (aspirate fat) from hepatic lymphoma (aspirate anaplastic lymphoid cells) and FIP (aspirate macrophages and neutrophils).

Liver Biopsy. Liver biopsy is preferably performed percutaneously with ultrasound guidance. Biopsy enables classification of liver disease into broad categories such as inflammatory, immune-mediated, vacuolar, necrotizing, vascular, cholestatic, cirrhotic, or neoplastic. Biopsy only occasionally reveals a cause, but categorization of hepatic disease by biopsy helps determine therapy and prognosis.

Diagnostic Procedures to Determine the Prognosis of Liver Disease. Blood clotting abnormalities (especially prothrombin time), hypoglycemia, hypoalbuminemia, and extensive necrosis or fibrosis in multiple hepatic biopsies are suggestive of a poor prognosis.

REFERENCES

1. Politzer, J.P., Devroede, G., Vasseur, C., Gerard, J., and Thibault, R.: The genesis of bowel sounds: influence of viscus and gastrointestinal content. Gastroenterology 71:282-285, 1976.
2. Martin, D.C., Beckloff, G.L., Arnold, J.D., and Gitomer, S.: Bowel sound quantitation to evaluate drugs on gastrointestinal motor activity. J. Clin. Pharm. 11:42-45, 1971.
3. Rothuizen J. Hyperbilirubinemia in canine hepatobiliary disease. Thesis. University of Utrecht. 1985
4. Kirk, R.W., Bistro, S.I.. Hardback of veterinary procedures and emergency treatment. 4th Edition. W.B. Sanders, Philadelphia. 10-12, 1985.

Chapter 6

Procedure for the Evaluation of Pancreatic and Gastrointestinal Tract Diseases

INTRODUCTION

While discussing an orderly diagnostic approach to gastrointestinal problems, the previous chapter briefly referred to a large number of diagnostic procedures. The purpose of this chapter is to describe the most important of these procedures in more detail, with particular reference to their indications, limitations, complications, contraindications, and methodology.

LABORATORY EVALUATION OF VOMITUS

Vomitus should be evaluated for content and odor. Additional evaluations that are sometimes helpful include pH analysis, parasitology, cytology, virology, and toxicology. The content and pH of the "vomitus" help differentiate vomiting from regurgitation (Chapter 5).

Evidence for bile in vomitus makes pyloric obstruction unlikely. Small flecks of fresh blood in vomitus are common following prolonged vomiting. They result from capillary trauma; in and of themselves, they need not be of concern. The presence of "coffee grounds," however, is a warning sign of serious disease, and causes of upper gastrointestinal blood loss should be pursued (Chapter 5). Dogs and cats will occasionally vomit gastric or small intestinal parasites such as ascarids, *Physaloptera* species, cestodes, and *Capillaria* species.

Vomitus with an odor of feces can result from gastrointestinal obstruction, prolonged ileus, bacterial overgrowth, or coprophagia. "Vomited" food may smell of fermentation as a result of prolonged retention in the stomach or esophagus, or due to the ingestion of spoiled foods. Odiferous vomitus can also result from gastrointestinal necrosis.

Microscopic examination of vomitus will occasionally reveal the eggs of *Physaloptera* spp., the larvae or adult stages of *Ollulanus tricuspis*, spores of toxic fungi,[1] bacteria, and cellular remnants. Occasionally rafts of neoplastic cells will have sufficiently preserved morphology to allow diagnosis. The observation of large quantities of fecal-type bacteria in the stomach fluid is strongly suggestive of achlorhydria.

If poisoning is suspected, samples of vomitus can be submitted for toxicologic analysis. Examples of poisons which result in vomiting, and which may be diagnosed by analysis of vomitus, include alpha-naphthyl thiourea (ANTU), phosphorus, zinc phosphide, arsenic, herbicides, and fungicides.

GASTRIC SECRETORY TESTING

The most important gastric secretory function is the secretion of hydrochloric acid. Gastric acid secretion may become subnormal (hypochlorhydria), absent (achlorhydria), or increased, as seen with gastrin-secreting tumors and chronic renal or hepatic disease. The secretory activity of parietal cells cannot be quantified by gastric biopsy. This has led to the development of a number of tests for gastric acid secretion. The invasive nature, cost and limited indications of gastric secretory testing, however, have effectively barred the more laborious (and accurate) of these techniques from usage in clinical veterinary medicine. There may be a clinical role for some of the simpler tests of gastric acid secretion. Indications for these tests in veterinary medicine include the need to assess the response of patients with refractory gastroduodenal ulcers, reflux esophagitis, or gastrinomas to gastric antisecretory drugs; to differentiate between peptic ulcers and those due to gastric neoplasia; and to diagnose gastrinomas through an interpretation of serum gastrin results. Measurement of pepsin output does not provide a reliable assessment of canine gastric secretion.[2]

Gastric Aspiration and pH Determination

The simplest gastric acid secretory test is the aspiration of gastric fluid from a fasting patient by way of a nasogastric tube, or endoscope, and the determination of the pH. In one study of healthy dogs, the pH of gastric fluid during the fasting state was found to range from 0.9-2.5.[3] Post-prandial gastric pH was slightly higher (0.5-3.5) because of the buffering action of the food. In another study, the fasting gastric pH ranged from 0.8-8.0, with 70% of the dogs having a fasting gastric pH of less than 5.[2] If a strongly acidic fasting gastric pH is detected, it proves that the patient can secrete gastric acid. In a patient with refractory gastroduodenal ulcers, such an observation is sufficient reason to adjust the gastric antisecretory medication. The observation of a low gastric pH, however, does not rule out hypochlorhydria or gastric hypersecretory states because the rate of gastric acid secretion is not measured, the capacity of the gastric mucosa to respond further to secretagogues is not assessed, and pH in gastric fluid need not directly correlate to hydrogen ion "activity."[4]

In healthy dogs, basal gastric acid output is minimal during fasting. The bicarbonate in swallowed saliva and refluxed duodenal content has the potential to bring the pH of the gastric fluid towards neutrality. Thus, the acquisition of gastric fluid with a near-neutral pH, although unusual, cannot be taken as definitive evidence of achlorhydria. A near-neutral sample obtained after pentagastrin or histamine stimulation, however, is strongly suggestive of achlorhydria. Within 15 minutes of pentagastrin administration (6 μg/kg), 100% of healthy dogs had a pH of less than 2.[2] Similarly, a near-neutral pH in the presence of raised serum gastrin levels suggests the raised gastrin is a result of achlorhydria and not gastrinoma. Finally, in patients with gastric ulcers, the aspiration of a near-neutral gastric fluid pH after administration of a secretagogue strongly suggests that the gastric ulcer is neoplastic and not peptic in nature. This technique may aid therapeutic decisions in patients in which endoscopic appearance of the ulcer is suggestive of neoplasia but endoscopic biopsy of the ulcer is not definitive.

Radiotelemetric Determination of Gastrointestinal pH

A radiotelemetric technique for the measurement of gastrointestinal pH has been used in the dog.[3] The technique allows continuous, accurate measurement of pH, but is disadvantaged by the restricted availability of the equipment and by the occasional misdiagnosis of achlorhydria resulting from the immediate exit of the radiotelemetric capsule from the stomach into the duodenum.

Gastric Acid Output

Quantitative gastric acid secretory testing requires the placement of an indwelling tube in the pyloric antrum to allow the complete collection of gastric secretion during a defined time period. The technique may be performed by temporary pharyngostomy or by orogastric intubation using a specific anesthetic technique.[2]

Basal Gastric Acid Secretion. To estimate basal levels of acid output (BAO), gastric secretions are collected from the fasting stomach by continuous suction for four consecutive 15-minute collection periods. The samples are titrated with sodium hydroxide to pH 7 and the acidity expressed in mEq (mmol) of hydrogen ion produced per unit time. BAO is normally a fraction of 1 mEq of hydrogen ion per hour. The basal volume of gastric secretion is 0.37-2.95 ml/hour/kg$^{0.75}$. BAO analysis is of most use should the clinician wish to confirm a gastric hypersecretory state. The accuracy of this technique depends on appropriate tube placement, complete collection of gastric fluid, and minimal gastroduodenal reflux. Wide variations on repeated determinations from the same patient compromise the usefulness of this test. Increased BAO in humans is associated with stress, renal failure, duodenal ulcers, mastocytosis, increased intracranial pressure, and gastrinomas. In humans with gastrinomas, the BAO is usually 60% or more of the maximal acid secretory response to secretagogues. Similar findings have been reported with canine gastrinoma.[5]

Peak Acid Output. To determine peak acid output gastric acid secretion is quantified during consecutive 15-minute periods following administration of secretagogues such as histamine, betazole, or pentagastrin. The two consecutive 15-minute collections giving the highest acid output are chosen and their acid output doubled to give peak acid output (PAO) in mEq/hour. Alternatively, the acid outputs from the four consecutive samples are totalled. This is termed maximum acid output (MAO). Histamine stimulates maximum secretion when a single dose of 0.320 mg/kg of histamine base is given subcutaneously. In human gastric acid secretory testing, the following subcutaneous doses for the different histamine formulations are used: 0.04 mg/kg histamine acid phosphate, 2.75 mg/kg histamine hydrochloride, and 0.014 mg/kg histamine base. The secretion rate peaks during the second hour after injection (Figure 6-1). The mean maximum rate of secretion by dogs weighing 4.5 to 28 Kg is 14 to 40 mEq hydrogen ions/hr.[6] An almost linear positive correlation exists between parietal cell mass and maximal acid secretion.[6] H_1-receptor antagonists are given with histamine to minimize cardiovascular effects. The H_1-receptor antagonists do not interfere with gastric acid secretion.

Betazole (Histalog) is an analog of histamine that can be used to stimulate acid secretion without need for an antihistamine. The dose of betazole for maximum acid secretion is 30 mg/Kg body weight.[7] Much smaller doses (0.5 mg/kg SQ) are currently used during clinical testing in humans to minimize side effects.

Pentagastrin (Peptavlon) is a synthetic gastrin analogue. Pentagastrin (6 μg/kg SQ or IV) stimulates maximal acid output within 30-45 minutes in the dog. Reference values for peak hydrogen ion output after pentagastrin stimulation are 1.5-3.61 mEq/hour/kg$^{0.75}$.[2] Pentagastrin is the preferred secretagogue because of rapidity of action and less side effects.

The assessment of PAO or MAO can be used for the quantitative assessment of hypochlorhydria or gastric hypersecretion. Conditions associated with reduced gastric acid secretion in humans include gastritis, gastric carcinoma, and gastric polyps.

Serum Gastrin. Serum gastrin can be secreted by G cells in the pyloric antrum and duodenum or by neoplastic cells (gastrinomas), usually located in the pancreas. A radioimmunoassay kit for the measurement of human gastrin has been

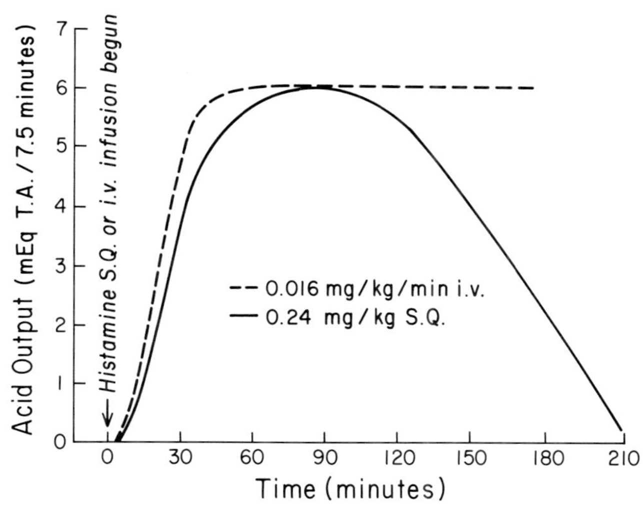

Figure 6-1. Gastric acid secretion following a single injection or continuous infusion of histamine (expressed as histamine base) in a large (30 kg) dog. Dogs weighing 5 to 10 kg have maximal secretory responses 35 to 85% as great when given the same doses. Total hourly secretion of titratable acid (T.A.) ranges from 15 mEq in 5 kg dogs to 40 mEq in 30 kg dogs.

Table 6-1 Possible Causes of Elevated Serum Gastrin Concentration

Achlorhydria
Gastric ulceration
Atrophic gastritis
Glucocorticoids
Antral G cell hyperplasia
Hypercalcemia
Antacids
Immunoproliferative small intestinal disease of Basenjis
Gastrinoma
Gastric antisecretory drugs
Pyloric stenosis
Gastric cancer
Renal failure
Gastric dilatation-volvulus

validated for use in the dog.[8] Serum for gastrin analysis should be collected in a cold tube, quickly separated from blood cells, and shipped frozen on dry ice. Normal fasting serum gastrin in the dog and cat have been reported to range from 23-190 pg/ml and 28-135 pg/ml, respectively.[2,5,8,9]

The serum gastrin level varies inversely with the concentration of hydrogen ions in the gastric lumen. In dogs and cats elevated serum gastrin has been reported in association with achlorhydria, atrophic gastritis, gastric dilatation-volvulus, pyloric stenosis, immunoproliferative small intestinal disease of Basenjis, renal failure, gastrinoma, antacids, gastric antisecretory drugs, and glucocorticoids.[10] Additional causes have been reported in humans (Table 6-1). Very high levels of gastrin (greater than 500 pg/ml) have been considered diagnostic of gastrinoma in the dog, although both human and veterinary experience indicates that levels of gastrin greater than 500 pg/ml can also occur with gastric hyposecretory states such as atrophic gastritis.[10,11] Therefore, in a patient with a markedly elevated serum gastrin, it would seem prudent to ensure that gastric pH is low before surgically exploring the patient for a suspected gastrinoma. In those dogs with moderately elevated gastrin levels in association with acidic gastric pH, various provocative tests of serum gastrin may be required to confirm gastrinoma (see APUDomas).

TESTS OF GASTROINTESTINAL NEUROMUSCULAR FUNCTION

At present, clinically applicable tests of gastrointestinal motor function in dogs and cats rely on the determination of gastric motility by way of fluoroscopy, or on the evaluation of gastric emptying by way of contrast radiography or scintigraphy. These radiographic techniques are discussed in the section on gastrointestinal radiography.

In the experimental setting, gastrointestinal motor function of animals has been accurately examined by implanting bipolar electrodes in the gastric or intestinal wall for the measurement of myoelectrical activity, and strain gauges for the measurement of mechanical activity. These techniques can detect gastric dysrhythmias and electromechanical dissociation.[12] Cutaneous devices for the recording of the "electrogastrogram" are also becoming available.[13]

Gastrointestinal manometry is extensively used in human medicine for the diagnosis of esophageal and large bowel motility disorders. The recent development of a peroral silicone pressure sensor device, which contains a series of pressure transducers encased in a 2.7 mm diameter flexible polyurethane sheath, now allows the accurate recording of gastric and small intestinal motility in clinical patients.[14] The value of manometric techniques in veterinary clinical gastroenterology remains to be established. The techniques have been successfully used on an experimental basis in dogs for the evaluation of lower esophageal sphincter tone, gastric pressure, and anal sphincter tone.[15,16]

EXAMINATION OF FECES[17-20]

Feces from every patient with a gastrointestinal problem should be evaluated for physical appearance and for parasites. In many cases it is important to examine the stool for signs of maldigestion, and in some cases it is useful to evaluate the feces for bacterial pathogens and occult blood.

Gross Examination

Physical Appearance. Diarrhea is defined as an increase in the volume or frequency of bowel movements, or a change in consistency of the feces. The content of water and fiber determines fecal volume. Normal feces contain 60% to 70% water; an increase of 10% can produce a watery diarrhea. Large volumes of normal feces can be due to excessive amounts of indigestible components. The volume of formed feces in a 30-lb dog exceeds 50 ml per day; the volume can be much greater than 50 ml when excessive fiber is fed. Normal feces are always completely formed. The last part of the feces passed should be as well formed as the first. Normal feces have indentations, produced by colonic contractions, and contain scant or no mucus, and no blood. The presence of fresh blood and mucus is suggestive of large bowel disease (Chapter 5). Normal feces can contain recognizable foods that are known to be indigestible, such as whole grains of corn. Indigestible materials such as grass and hair are also commonly present. Small amounts of ingested hair are of no concern, but larger amounts may be a cause of gastrointestinal irritation, gastric impaction, or constipation. Undigested particles of digestible foods suggest hurried passage or maldigestion. Steatorrhea is not grossly recognizable until fecal fat content is very high, reflecting an almost complete maldigestion or malabsorption. In acute exudative inflammation, animals may pass fibrinous casts of their bowel. Tapeworm proglottides are often noted in the feces of dogs and cats by their owners.

Color. The dark brown color of normal feces is imparted by bile pigments (stercobilin) that have been metabolized by intestinal bacteria. Complete absence of biliary secretions results in no fecal pigmentation, producing "acholic" or gray feces, an infrequent finding that is usually associated with jaundice. Brown coloration of feces also depends on adequate intestinal bacterial activity. Patients with diarrhea have reduced numbers of intestinal bacteria, and hurried passage of intestinal content. The result is incomplete metabolism of bile pigments, and altered fecal color to yellow, green or light brown. Antibiotics that reduce the number of intestinal bacterial flora also produce light-colored feces. The effect persists for only a few days, however, the longest time that the microflora can be suppressed with antibiotics. Diet also influences fecal color. Diets containing predominantly milk proteins produce light- colored feces. Diets containing predominantly meat proteins produce dark-colored feces because of the metabolism of heme pigments contained in the meat. Upper gastrointestinal hemorrhage results in black, tarry feces, termed melena (chapter 5). Excessive iron in feces causes a similar greenish-black appearance. Some drugs pigment feces. Charcoal, bismuth, and salicylates darken the feces, whereas antacids lighten them. Sulfobromophthalein (BSP) can color feces purple.

Odor. The odor of feces is produced by indole and skatol, products of bacterial activity on tryptophan; and by mercaptans, hydrogen sulfide, methyl sulfides, and related by-products of the sulfur-containing amino acids. The odor is greatest in feces produced from high-meat-protein diets. The odor is diminished on easily digestible high-carbohydrate or milk-protein diets. Any diet or antibiotic modifying the bacterial microflora can affect fecal odor. Feces from patients with maldigestion or malabsorption can smell acrid or sour. This odor is caused by short-chain fatty acids produced from bacterial fermentation of unabsorbed carbohydrates and fatty acids.

Microscopic Examination (Table 6-2)

Feces are examined microscopically for signs of malassimilation, for intestinal parasites, and for purposes of fecal cytology. Fecal examinations that are used to detect maldigestion or malabsorption are described in the section detailing tests of malassimilation.

Fecal and Rectal Scrape Cytology. Cytologic examination of feces or scrapings of rectal mucosa is indicated for the workup of patients presenting with evidence of large bowel diarrhea. To perform fecal cytology, a fleck of mucus or a sample of feces from the surface of the stool is smeared thinly on a slide and stained with hematology stains. To perform rectal scrapes, the gloved finger is used to manually abrade the rectal mucosa. The material adherent to the glove is transferred to a microscope slide by rolling the finger across the slide.

Large numbers of fecal neutrophils are suggestive of acute colonic inflammation, such as may occur with invasive bacterial infections, and should encourage culture of the stool, especially if concomitant fecal blood is detected.[21] In humans, large numbers of leukocytes in the stool are most commonly associated with invasion of the mucosa by *Shigella, E. coli, Entamoeba histolytica, Salmonella*, and *Campylobacter*. *Shigella, Campylobacte*r, and invasive *E. coli* cause the most severe purulent exudates. The presence of eosinophils in a fecal smear supports eosinophilic colitis, and the presence of a mixed leukocyte population can appear with inflammatory bowel disease.[22] On occasion, *Histoplasma* organisms may be noted in fecal macrophages or, more commonly, in macrophages from the rectal mucosa. A recent study comparing the results of rectal scrape cytology with colonoscopic examination and colon biopsy in dogs with chronic large bowel diarrhea found that rectal cytology was not able to differentiate rectal neoplasia, non-inflammatory colonic disease, and plasmacytic/lymphocytic colitis.[23]

Table 6-2 Microscopic Examination of Direct Smear of Feces

Parasites -	Ascarids, Hookworms, Whipworms, *Strongyloides, Giardia, Trichomonas, Coccidia, Entamoeba, Balantidium*
Fat - Triglycerides	Sudan III stain
Fatty acids	Acetic acid + Sudan III stain
Starch granules	Lugol's solution stain
Protein, muscle fibers	Cytology stains
Inflammatory cells (white blood cells)	Cytology stains
Microorganisms	*Staphylococcus* spp overgrowth *Clostridia* spp overgrowth *Clostridium perfringens* spores *Histoplasma, Campylobacter*

The presence of *Clostridium perfringens* endospores (Figure 6-2) in a fecal smear is highly suggestive of diarrhea due to *Clostridium perfringens* enterotoxin.[24] Such identification is difficult, however, because clostridial endospores can appear the same as other spores that may be found in fecal smears. Moreover, *Clostridium perfringens* does not sporulate as readily as many other organisms. Fecal smears occasionally identify overgrowth of normal microorganisms in the rectum. A gram stain helps determine the responsible bacteria, such as *Staphylococci* (gram-positive cocci) and *Clostridia* spp (gram positive bacilli). *Candida* may be visualized in its pseudomycelia and yeast forms. Overgrowth of the large bowel by a single bacterial species is an indication for fecal culture. Spirochetes are frequently seen in fecal smears of animals with diarrhea. These microorganisms are part of the normal microflora of the colon. During diarrheic episodes, they are dislodged from the colonic crypts, and can appear in large numbers in the feces. They appear to be nonpathogenic, and should not be confused with *Campylobacter*. *Campylobacter* are occasionally seen in direct

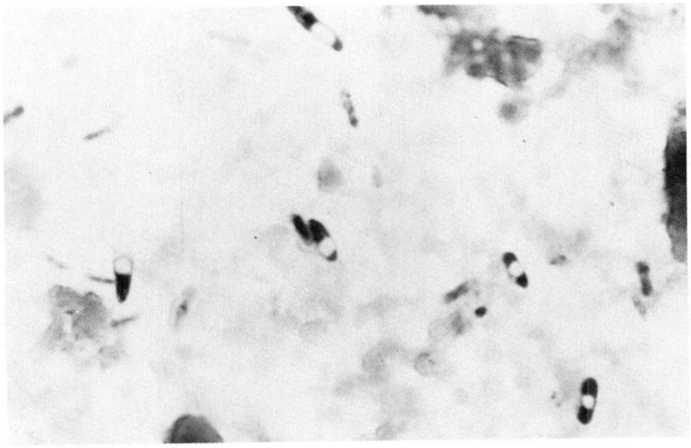

Figure 6-2 Clostridium perfringens spore. (in bacteria)

fecal smears. They have a characteristic "seagull-wing" appearance (Figure 6-3). Before *Campylobacter* is seen the organism must be in high concentrations; at least 10^6 organisms per gram of feces is necessary to see one per high power field. Identification is assisted by staining with Wright's or Wrights-Giemsa stain. Mushroom toxicity has been diagnosed by detecting fungal spores in feces or vomitus.[1]

Parasitology[25]

Microscopic evaluation of feces to identify intestinal parasites is indicated in all cases of diarrhea and may involve flotation, sedimentation, and direct smear techniques (Figure 6-4).

Direct Smears of Feces. Direct smears of feces readily identify the ova, oocysts, larvae, or trophozoites of some nematode and protozoal parasites. The direct smear is important in identifying *Strongyloides stercoralis* infection (because larvae rather than eggs are usually found in the stool) and *Trichomonas* and *Entamoeba* infections (because these protozoa have no form other than that of the trophozoite). Trophozoites are the active, feeding motile stage of protozoal parasites. The motility of trophozoites assists their identification in fecal smears, and is a useful, although by no means foolproof, technique for the diagnosis of protozoal disorders such as giardiasis.[26] Trophozoites are found only in fecal samples sufficiently fresh to maintain their warmth. As feces cool from body temperature, the trophozoites encyst. Direct smears of feces for trophozoites are, therefore, best examined immediately after collection. The fecal sample is placed on a warmed glass slide, and diluted with a few drops of saline to improve visualization of motile structures. Examine at 100x and 400x magnifications. The addition of a small drop of Lugol's iodine solution will enhance detection of parasitic forms, such as *Giardia* cysts. Confusing structures in feces that can resemble parasite cysts include plant cells, starch granules, and fungal spores. The primary limitations of the fecal smear are the small sample size and the lack of concentration of parasites.

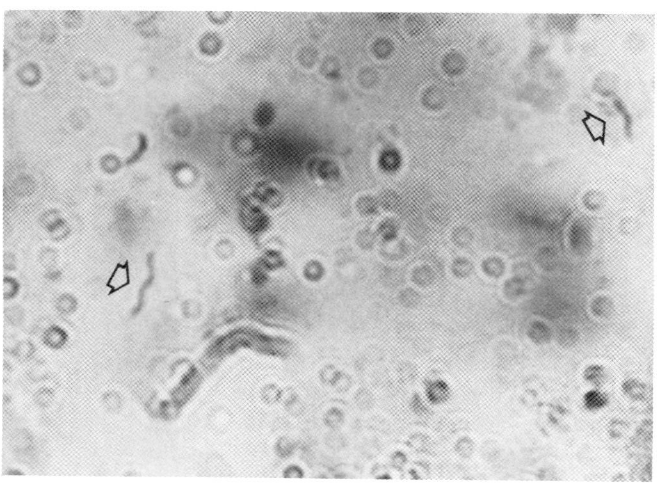

Figure 6-3 Campylobacter in fecal smear. (used with permission from Dr. Green, Reference 31.

Examination of air-dried smears of fresh feces that have been stained with hematology stains will occasionally identify *Giardia* and *Entamoeba* trophozoites. Trichrome stains are also effective for the diagnosis of giardiasis.[27,28] Acid-fast stains may identify *Cryptosporidia*.[29]

Fecal Flotations. Ova of nematode parasites and the cysts and oocysts of most protozoa are easier to find if they are concentrated by various flotation methods before microscopic examination. The principal of the procedure is the dispersion of ova and fecal material in saturated sugar or salt solutions, and their separation based on their differential density. Since most parasite ova have a lower density than these solutions, they will float to the surface of the solution, whereas the heavier fecal particulate matter will not float. The ova are collected on a coverslip in contact with the surface of the suspension. Separation of ova from fecal material can be hastened by centrifuging the suspension. Flotation solutions in use include 70% sodium dichromate, and saturated sugar, sodium chloride, sodium nitrite, magnesium sulfate, and zinc sulfate solutions. Saturated sugar solutions are not as dense as saturated salt solutions, and fluke eggs and some nematode eggs will not float in them. Sheather's sugar flotation is useful for the identification of *Toxoplasma* and *Cryptosporidia* oocysts.[29] The dichromate solution is yellow, making it easier to recognize the ova. Zinc sulfate flotation is an accurate test for the diagnosis of giardiasis.[26,28] Trematode, cestode, and *Trichuris* eggs may also float more reliably in this solution. Tapeworm ova are not found in microscopic examinations unless the proglottids containing the ova are broken. Multiple fecal examinations are at times necessary to identify whipworms.

Fecal Sedimentation. Fluke ova are best concentrated by sedimentation. Feces are dispersed in water, after which the mixture is strained and centrifuged. The supernatant is poured off, and a few drops of the sediment are examined microscopically for fluke ova. This technique, or variants thereof, is useful for the diagnosis of salmon poisoning in dogs and of *Eurytrema, Platynosomum*, and *Amphimerus* fluke infections in cats. The eggs of *Nanophyteus salmincola* will also float in many standard flotation media, however. Modified fecal sedimentation techniques, including the formalin-ether sedimentation technique,[30] have been described. *Diphyllobothrium latum* tapeworm ova must be carefully differentiated from fluke eggs.

Preservation of Feces for Parasitologic Examination. If delay until examination of the feces is expected, techniques can be used to preserve protozoal oocysts and helminth eggs. Small amounts of uncooled formed stool may be mixed with equal volumes of 10% formalin or, alternatively, with three times the amount of polyvinyl alcohol. Vials containing polyvinyl alcohol fixative are commercially available (Fekal FK10, Trend Scientific). Polyvinyl alcohol fixation can preserve fecal specimens for months and does not interfere with subsequent staining.

Immunoassay for Parasites. Giardiasis can be diagnosed by immunofluorescent assay for protozoal antigens in feces. The test shows promise for being highly sensitive and specific for *Giardia* species.

Fecal Culture

Indications. Routine cultures of feces from dogs and cats with diarrhea are not warranted, in view of the rarity with which

Figure 6-4. Parasites and parasitic ova found in the feces of small animals.

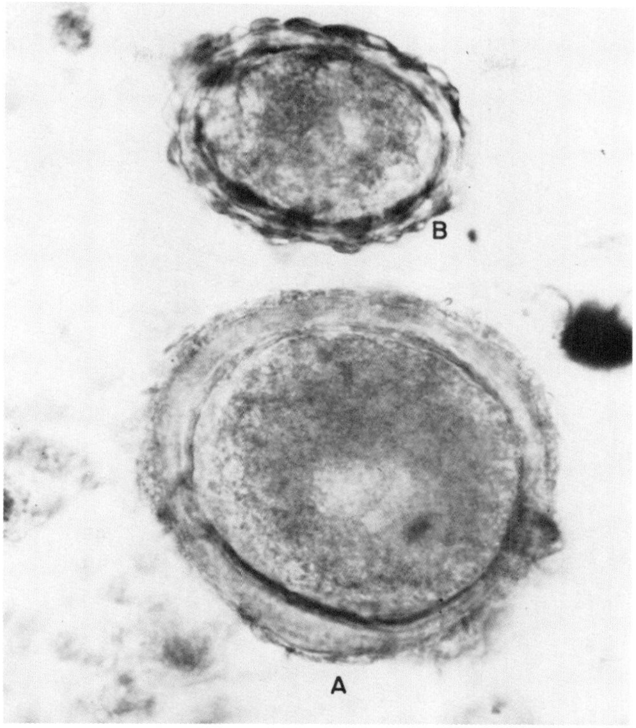

A. Toxocara canis ovum x 800
B. Ascaris lumbricoides ovum (spurious) x 800

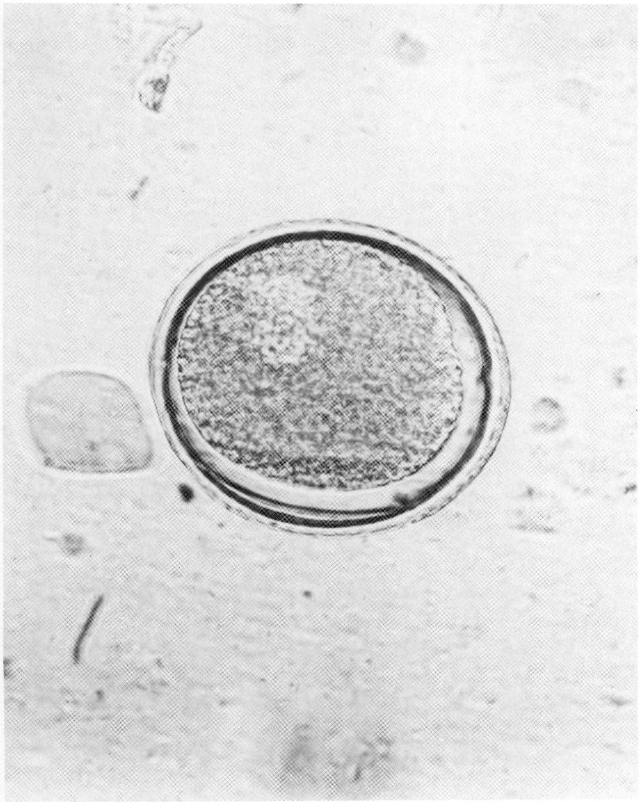

Toxocara cati (dog) ovum x 800

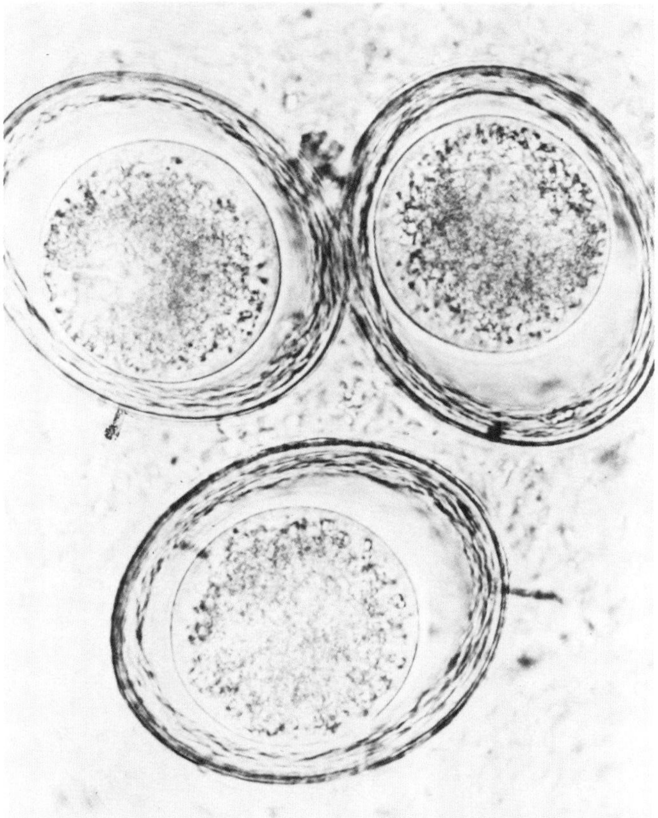

Toxascaris leonina (dog) x 800

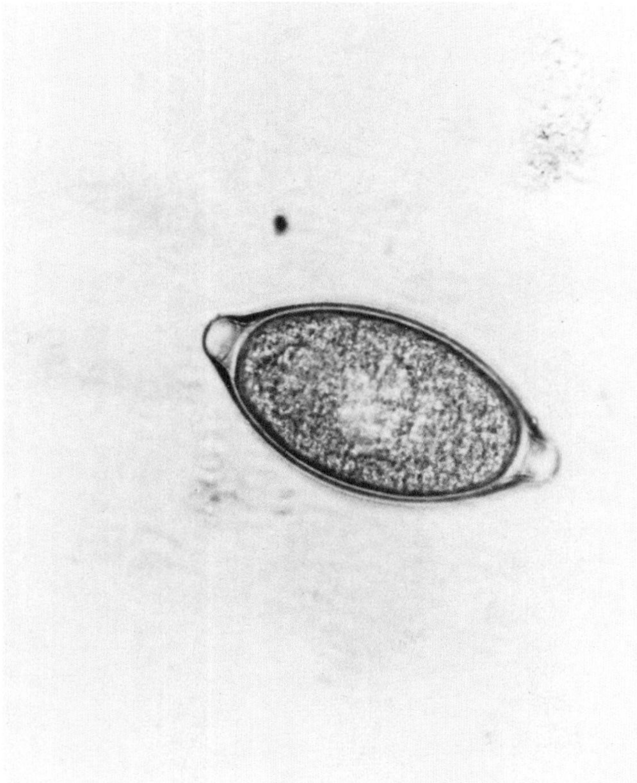

Trichuris vulpis (dog) x 800

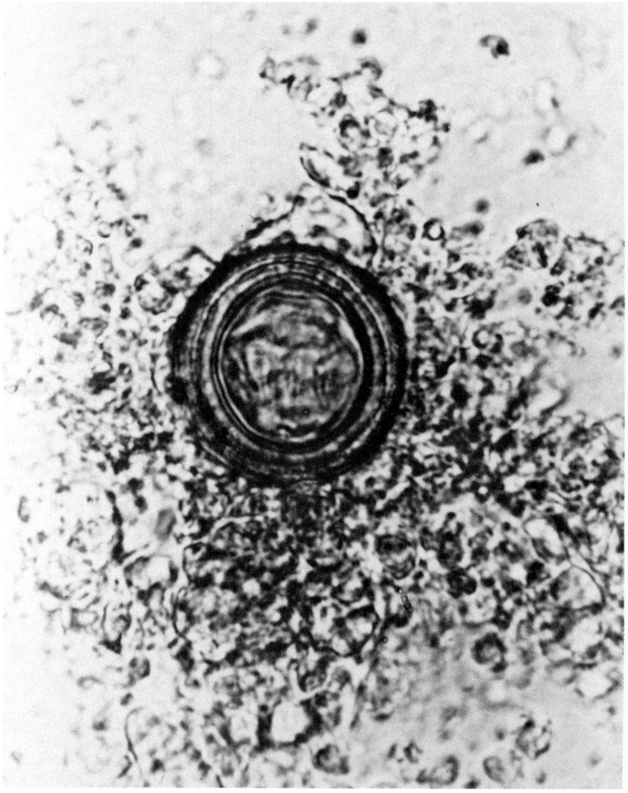

Taenia sp. (cat) ovum x 1300

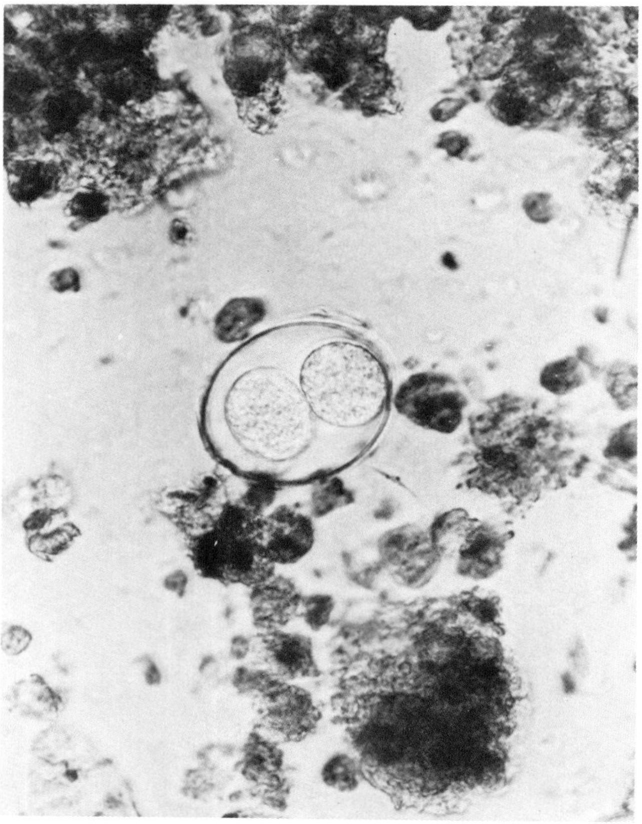

Cystoisospora (Isospora) felis (cat) oocyst x 800

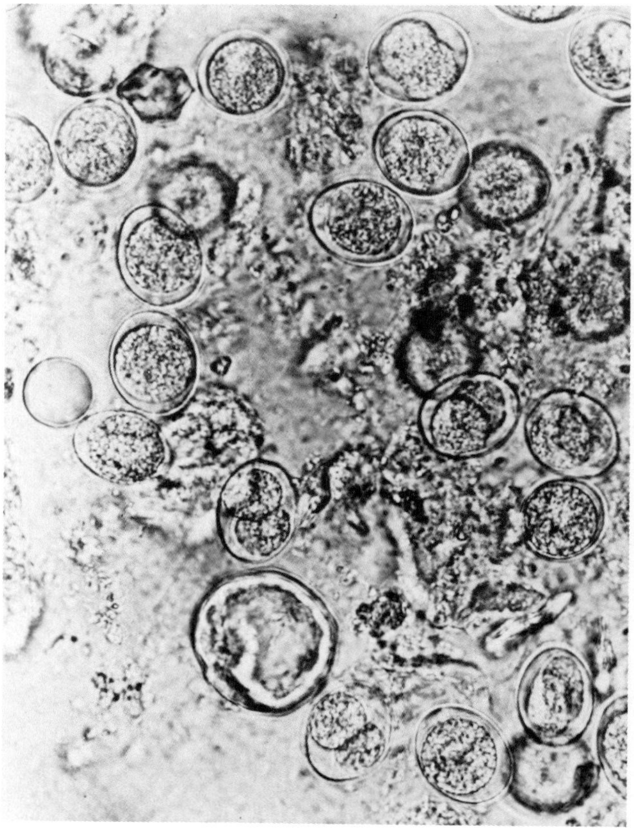

Cystoisospora (Isospora) ohioensis (dog) oocysts x 800

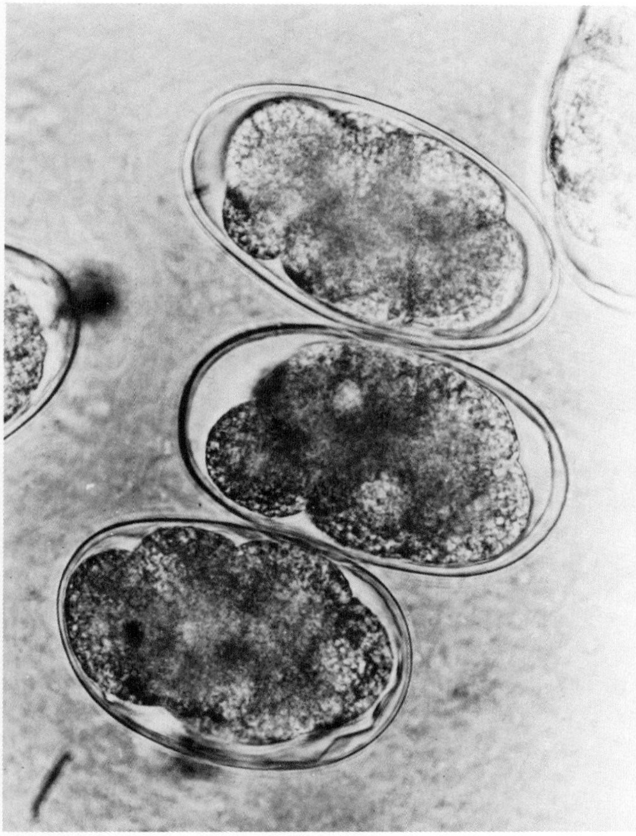

Ancylostoma caninum (dog) x 800

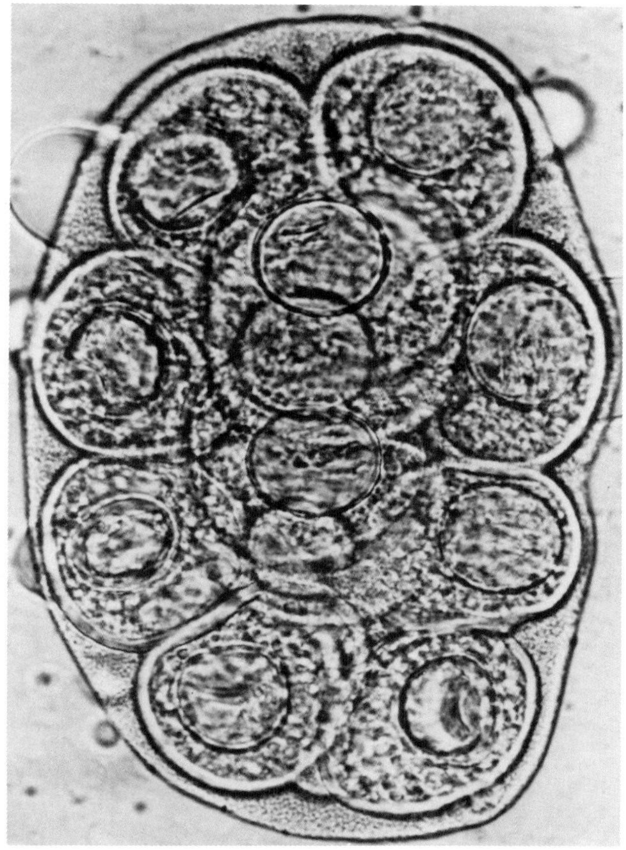

Dipylidium caninum (dog) egg packet x 300

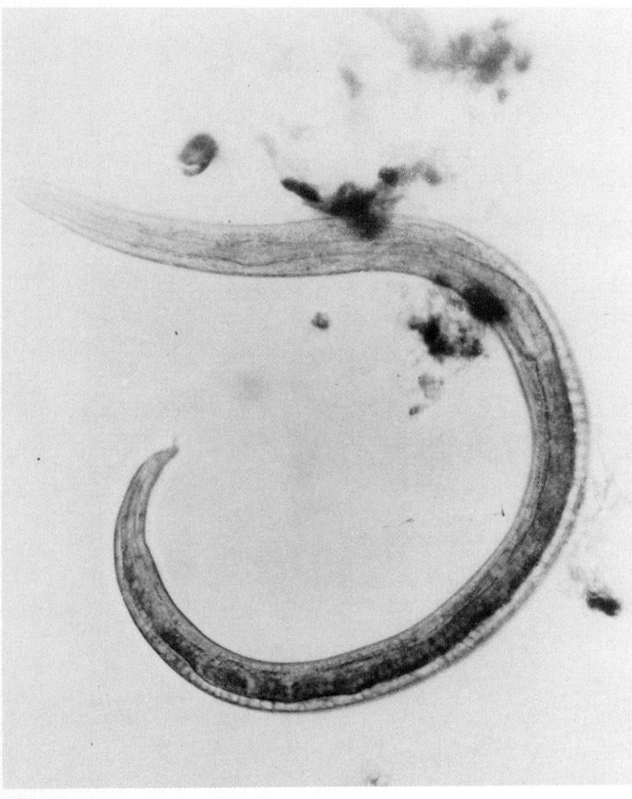

Aelurostrongylus abstrussus (cat) x 300

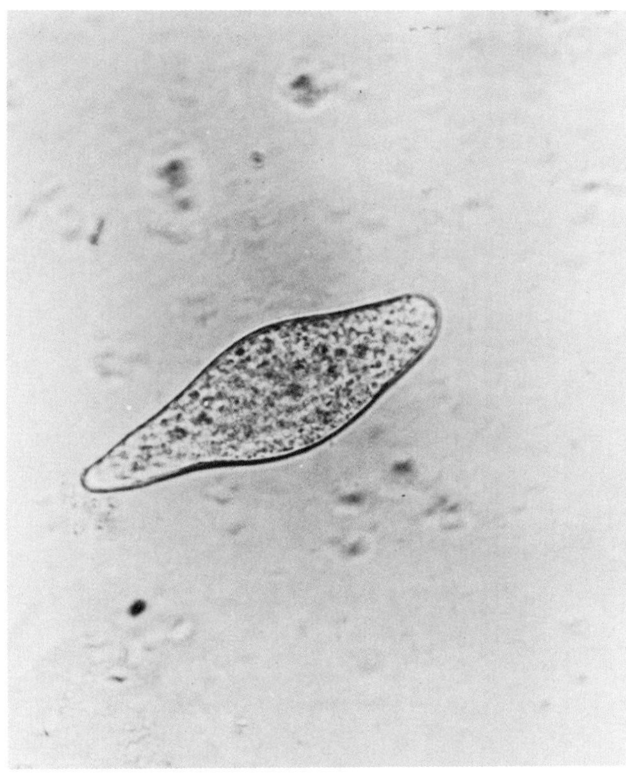

Demodex canis (dog) ovum x 800

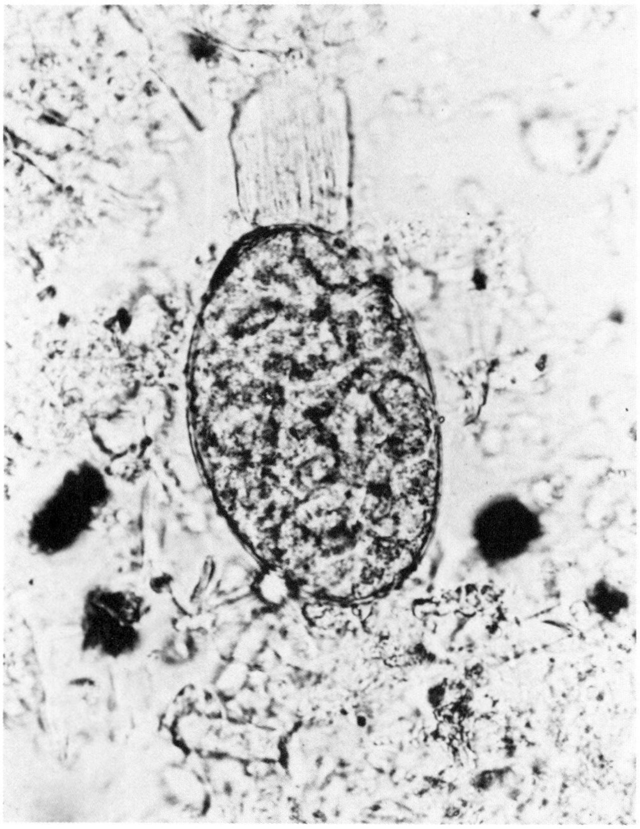

Nanophyetus salmincola (dog) ovum x 800

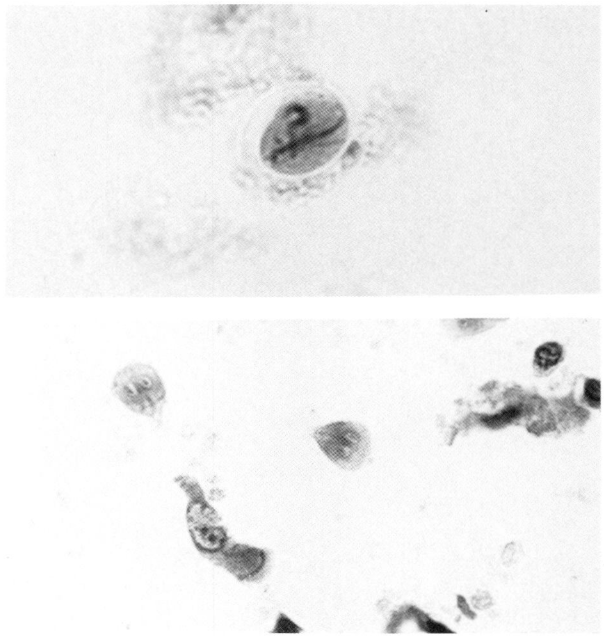

Giardia cyst and trophozoite

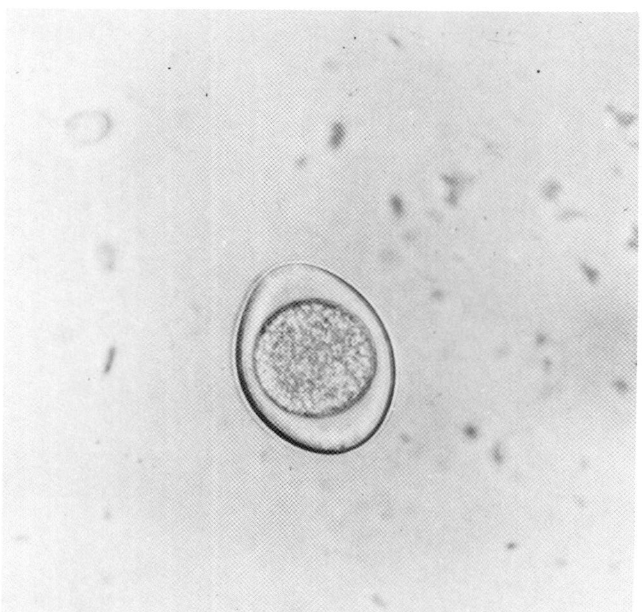

Cystoisospora (Isospora) felis (cats) sporulated oocyst x 800

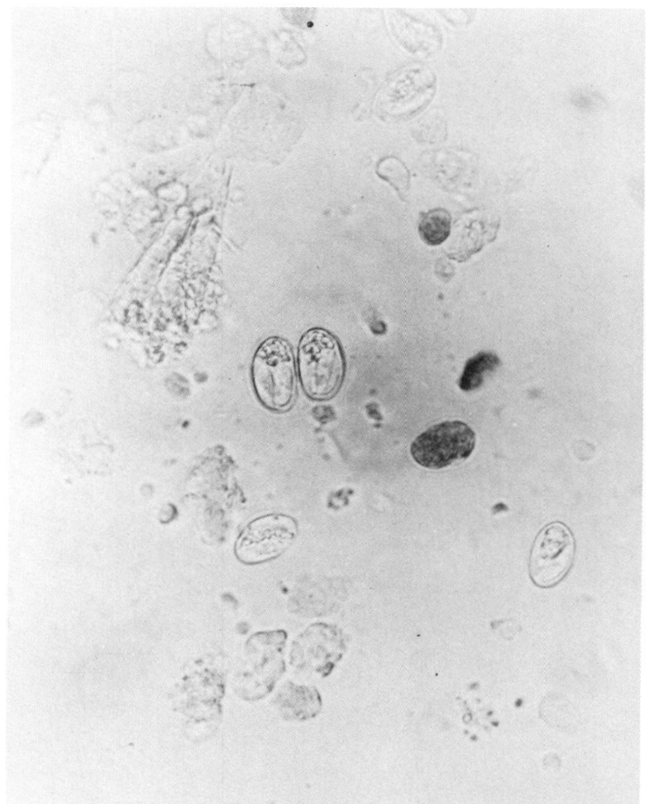

Sarcocystis sp. (dog) oocyst x 800

enteric pathogens are cultured, difficulties in the interpretation of culture results, the self-limiting nature of many bacterial infections, and the inappropriateness of antibiotic therapy for many bacterial-mediated diarrheas. Furthermore, isolation and identification of enteric pathogens is a labor intensive, expensive process that involves enrichment, plating, and identification steps performed sequentially over a three to four day period. There are occasions, however, when stool culture in animals with diarrhea is indicated (Table 6-3). These include a history of exposure to bacterial pathogens, outbreaks of diarrhea amongst more than one pet of a household, concern about a public health hazard or nosocomial infection, and clinical, cytological or biopsy evidence of bacterial-associated diarrhea. Clinical signs of infection with the currently known enteric bacterial pathogens are highly variable, but suspicion of infection should be aroused by dogs or cats that display an acute onset of a predominantly "large bowel" diarrhea. Clinical or laboratory evidence of sepsis should further heighten suspicion. Positive culture for *Clostridium perfringens* is particularly likely if clostridial spores are noted on fecal smears.[24] An assay for *Clostridium perfringens* enterotoxin has been successfully used to confirm *C. perfringens* enterotoxin-associated diarrhea.[24] If a biopsy of the colon is dominated by neutrophil infiltration, erosion and ulceration, bacterial colitis is a possibility. If the histopathology shows pseudomembranous inflammation, a culture for *Clostridium difficile* and an assay for its toxin may be rewarding. Quantitative culture of fecal bacteria has no clinical application. Quantitative culture of duodenal fluid is of value, however, and is discussed in the section on endoscopy. Culture of feces for fungal organisms such as *Histoplasma capsulatum* is less reliable than serodiagnosis or identification of fungal elements by biopsy or fecal cytology.

In summary, in certain circumstances, culture of the feces for specific enteric pathogens is warranted, and on some occasions, antibiotic therapy of a patient based on culture of an enteric pathogen is appropriate. On most occasions, however, the feces are cultured to identify patients that may be a public health risk.

Table 6-3 Indications for the Bacterial Culture of Feces in Cats or Dogs with Diarrhea

Historical findings
- onset after exposure to spoiled or contaminated food products
- onset after kenneling
- onset after show attendance
- onset after contact with an animal infected by a bacterial pathogen
- outbreak of diarrhea amongst more than one pet of a household

Physical exam findings
- acute onset of bloody diarrhea in association with evidence of sepsis (blood cultures also required)

Laboratory work
- evidence of sepsis (leukocytosis, leukopenia, hypoglycemia, etc)

Fecal smears
- large numbers of fecal neutrophils especially if with fecal blood
- bacterial overgrowth of the colon
- *Clostridium perfringens* spores
- Presence of "seagull-wing" bacteria

Colon Biopsy
- evidence of suppurative, or pseudomembranous inflammation.

Public health hazard
- young, elderly, or infirm humans in the household

Nosocomial infection hazard

Technique. Appropriate sample submission protocol and culture techniques vary widely for the different enteric pathogens. The clinician must advise the laboratory on which bacterial species to culture and must seek advice on the methods for collecting and submitting samples. Sterile, cotton-tipped applicators that are supplied with transport media or enrichment broth are suitable for the submission of fecal samples for culture of aerobic enteric pathogens.[31,32] When these swabs are used, it is preferable to sample the surface of a fresh stool including a portion of any mucus, exudate, or blood. Fecal samples for the culture of microaerophilic or anaerobic organisms should be very fresh. It is preferable to aspirate or remove the sample directly from the colon. Two to ten grams of solid feces or three to ten ml of liquid feces should be submitted in sterile airtight vials to the laboratory without delay.[31-33] If cotton-tipped swabs are used for the collection of these more fastidious bacteria, the swabs should be rubbed over the rectal mucosa and, once liberally coated with feces and exudate, placed immediately into transport media specifically suited for these organisms. Inadequate sample size is the most common error associated with fecal culture submission.[33] Feces should be submitted for culture early in the course of diarrhea, because as time progresses the numbers of pathogens decline, and their isolation becomes more difficult.

Interpretation. Because many normal flora can be opportunistic pathogens, and because many pathogens can be occasionally cultured from the feces of normal animals, the results of fecal cultures can be difficult to interpret. Furthermore, some pathogens such as certain *E. coli* can be diagnosed only by refined bacterial typing techniques. Interpretation of culture results is made easier if the laboratory provides a comparative estimate of the number of the bacterial pathogen in relation to other bacterial flora. It is assumed that a heavy and relatively pure growth of a known pathogen is significant. Light growths of pathogens amongst healthy mixed flora are more difficult to interpret.

Fecal Virology

Because of the self-limiting nature of many gastrointestinal viral infections, or the presence of characteristic clinical or laboratory features (as in parvovirus infections), virological studies of feces or vomitus are seldom utilized in small animal veterinary medicine. Identification of viral pathogens is indicated, however, when outbreaks of contagious diarrhea are being pursued in a kennel, cattery, or hospital situation, whereby identification of the viral agent may aid effective prophylactic procedures.

A number of procedures for the diagnosis of viral gastroenteritis from feces or vomitus have been proposed. These include virus isolation and identification in cell culture, immunofluorescence on cell culture, hemagglutination, ELISAs, and electron microscopy.[34,35] Fecal hemagglutination, ELISA and electron microscopy tests provide the most rapid diagnostic information and are preferred for clinical usage. The sensitivity and specificity of these tests for the diagnosis of viral gastroenteritis in dogs and cats have not been adequately examined. Improved detection of viruses by electron microscopy after ultracentrifuge preparation of specimens has been reported in humans and some farm animals.[36,37] Using convalescent serum to aggregate the fecal virus particles before examination may also improve the sensitivity of electron microscopy.[38] These latter techniques hold promise for the rapid, accurate diagnosis of viral gastroenteritis in small animal patients. A fecal ELISA test is available for the detection of rotaviruses (Rotaclone Test Kit - Cambridge Bioscience). Fecal hemagglutination tests and ELISA tests are widely utilized for the diagnosis of canine parvovirus.[39] The Parvo ELISA test is available in kit forms (e.g. Tech America, Diagnostics – Canine Parvovirus Test Kit). Limited experience with these tests suggests a low incidence of false positives, but a significant incidence of false negatives, probably as a result of the rapid decline in the number of viral particles excreted soon after the onset of clinical signs. No matter what technique is used, nor what virus is suspected, Submission of samples early in the diarrheic process greatly increases diagnostic yield.

Biochemical Evaluation

Fecal Water Percentage, Electrolyte Concentration, and Osmolality. The fecal water percentage provides an objective assessment of the severity of diarrhea. Fecal electrolyte concentration is used to diagnose congenital secretory diarrheas in human medicine. Fecal electrolyte concentration in association with the fecal osmolality is used to assist the differentiation of osmotic and secretory diarrheas. In osmotic diarrheas in humans, fecal osmolality is usually high, and a solute gap (Osmolality - (Na + K) x 2) of greater than 50 mOsmol per Kg of fecal fluid is detected. This concentration contrasts to that of secretory diarrheas, in which osmolality is lower and the osmolar gap within normal limits. The significance of a fecal osmolar gap, when fecal osmolality is greater than that of plasma, has been questioned.[40]

In spite of their utility for the diagnosis of secretory and osmotic diarrheas in other species, the value of fecal electrolyte and osmolality analysis in cats and dogs has yet to undergo objective evaluation. The osmolality, sodium concentration, and potassium concentration of the feces of 4 normal cats recently presented to the UCD VMTH ranged from 622-927 mOsm/Kg, 27-57 mEq/L, and 19-46 mEq/L, respectively. This preliminary data suggests that the fecal osmolar gap equation may not be of clinical relevance in the cat.

The percentage of stool weight present as water is determined by comparison of the wet weight of a stool sample with the weight of the same sample subjected to 48 hours of drying at 80 degrees Celsius in a vacuum oven. Fecal osmolality and electrolyte concentration are determined on an aliquot of stool water derived from the centrifugation of feces at approximately 10,000 x g for 15 minutes.

Fecal Blood. Feces may contain small amounts of blood not sufficient to produce melena. A variety of chemical tests can identify such "occult" gastrointestinal bleeding. The qualitative tests for occult blood are sufficiently simple and inexpensive to be suitable for inclusion in the routine data base. The significance of a positive occult blood test is that it raises the index of suspicion for inflammatory, ulcerative, or neoplastic gastrointestinal disease, as opposed to functional disorders. Occult blood tests may also be used for the differentiation of melena from pseudomelena.

Qualitative tests are based on blood's peroxidase activity, catalyzing the conversion of hydrogen peroxide to water and oxygen. Some chemicals can be oxidized during this reaction, forming colored products that are readily identified. The most sensitive peroxidase tests contain orthotoluidine (Hematest, Ames Co) or benzidine as the chemical oxidized to a colored product. To avoid false positive results, diets should not contain red meat for three days before testing. A less sensitive test to check for occult blood uses guaiac as the indicator chemical (Hemoccult kit, Smith Kline Corp.). This test requires less stringent prior dietary restriction because it is less sensitive than the others. The sensitivity of the guaiac test, however, is probably adequate to detect most bleeding lesions.

False positive occult blood tests can occur if the patient is consuming oral iron preparations, aspirin, cimetidine, or significant quantities of vegetable heme proteins or red meat. If in doubt as to the suitability of the diet for use during occult blood testing, a blended sample of the diet can be applied to the tablet to help determine if a false positive test is likely. Occult blood tests can remain positive for as long as a week after a single incidence of gastrointestinal hemorrhage.

A quantitative, fluorometric assay of fecal hemoglobin has recently been reported.[41] This assay allows the determination of the severity of gastrointestinal hemorrhage and has greater sensitivity and specificity than the peroxidase techniques.

MALASSIMILATION TESTS

Introduction

Malassimilation of nutrients can result from either maldigestion or malabsorption. The primary cause of maldigestion is exocrine pancreatic insufficiency, whereas the primary cause of malabsorption is small intestinal disease. Laboratory procedures have been developed to screen for malassimilation, maldigestion, or malabsorption. These tests have many limitations, not the least of which is the poor sensitivity of many of the procedures. As discussed in Chapter 5, this poor sensitivity and the now wide availability of endoscopy has led to a reduced reliance on malabsorption tests for the diagnosis of small intestinal disease. Endoscopy, however, should not be considered a replacement for malassimilation tests because the former detects morphologic disease only, whereas the latter may be considered tests of bowel function. Those tests that are most frequently used at the UCD VMTH are the Sudan stain of the feces as a screening test for malassimilation, the trypsin-like immunoreactivity test to detect exocrine pancreatic insufficiency, and the breath hydrogen test to detect carbohydrate malabsorption. Many other tests of small bowel and exocrine pancreatic function have been described and have application in some clinical situations.

Tests of Exocrine Pancreatic Function[42]

The primary indication for tests of exocrine pancreatic function is steatorrhea. The aim of the testing is to determine whether the steatorrhea results from pancreatic exocrine insufficiency, and by so doing identify which dogs require pancreatic enzyme replacement therapy and which do not.

Fecal Digestion Tests. Fecal digestion tests are a simple way to screen for maldigestion. There are several qualitative methods of identifying fecal protease activity. Homogenates of feces in buffered solutions can be incubated with strips of X-ray film (which have a gelatin coat) or with gelatin in test tubes. Digestion of the film coating or liquefaction of the gelatin in the test tube is suggestive of adequate fecal proteolytic activity. Unfortunately, not all types of X-ray film are digestible; gelatin digestion is difficult to evaluate with precision; and a high incidence of false positives have been reported in dogs.[19,43] Furthermore, fecal bacteria occasionally digest gelatin, falsely suggesting normal digestion even when a pancreatic enzyme deficiency exists.

Quantitative fecal digestion tests in humans have been based on the hydrolysis of synthetic chemicals that are split specifically by trypsin or chymotrypsin, releasing a compound that can be measured by spectrophotometric or titrametric methods.[44,45] Assay of chymotrypsin is preferred to assay of trypsin because less chymotrypsin is degraded during intestinal passage. A commercially available spectrophotometric test kit (Boehringher Mannheim, Monotest Chymotrypsin) for the assay of fecal chymotrypsin, which has been reported to have excellent accuracy for the diagnosis of human exocrine pancreatic insufficiency,[45] has also been shown to be useful in dogs.[46] Assays of fecal proteolytic activity using casein-based substrates also have application in dogs.[43,47,48] In cats, tests of pancreatic function are not commonly employed because of the apparent rarity of exocrine pancreatic disorders in this species. Recently, two fecal digestion tests of utility in the cat have been described. Fecal proteolytic activity was assayed colorimetrically using azocasein substrate, and by radial enzyme diffusion into agar gels containing casein substrate.[49]

Fecal proteolytic activity varies considerably from day to day in clinically normal dogs.[50] Thus, no matter what fecal digestion test is used, it is necessary to repeat the test on multiple stool samples collected over a three day period. Alternatively, an aliquot of feces collected over a three day period and stored at -20 degrees Celsius can be tested. If proteolytic activity is reduced in the feces, it is assumed that the secretion of proteolytic enzymes by the pancreas is deficient. Unfortunately, this interpretation need not be correct. Pancreatic enzymes are degraded by intestinal bacteria and by autodigestion, and if degradation proceeds at an excessive rate, or intestinal transit is delayed, all fecal proteolytic activity may be destroyed giving the false impression of inadequate small intestinal proteolytic activity. As little as 8% of trypsin activity remains in contents passing through the ileum.[51,52] Furthermore, increased fecal water may dilute the trypsin. Dietary changes introduce additional variability. Meat-based diets evoke a fivefold greater release of trypsin into the feces than do cereal-based diets. These difficulties compromise the reliability of fecal digestion tests, but they do not invalidate their use, provided one of the more quantitative assays are used and the veterinarian is prepared to assay more than one sample of feces. For example, an azocasein substrate test of the proteolytic activity of an aliquot of feces from a pooled three-day collection was recently reported to have a sensitivity of 95% and a specificity of 79% for exocrine pancreatic insuficiency.[48]

The BT-PABA Test. Direct measurement of pancreatic enzyme activity in the intestine is the gold standard for diagnosis of exocrine pancreatic insufficiency but requires intubation of the small intestine, stimulation of pancreatic secretion, and collection of intestinal contents.[53,54] These tests are technically difficult to conduct in dogs.[55] The BT-PABA test is a pancreatic-function test that indirectly measures the level of pancreatic enzyme activity in the small intestine.[56,57] It obviates the need to intubate the duodenum and stimulate pancreatic secretion. The BT-PABA test is indicated whenever steatorrhea is detected or fecal digestion tests are abnormal. Two versions of the test have been reported. In one version the PABA is recovered from the urine and in the second version the PABA is recovered from the plasma.

The urinary PABA test involves oral administration of a synthetic peptide made from n-benzyol-l-tyrosine and p-aminobenzoic acid (BT-PABA) (Figure 6-5). The peptide stimulates pancreatic enzyme secretion, is hydrolyzed by chymotrypsin, and releases free p-aminobenzoic acid (PABA), which is absorbed and excreted in the urine; most of the PABA appears within six hours of its administration, thus providing an indirect measure of the amount of chymotrypsin activity in the small intestine. BT-PABA is not hydrolyzed by any mammalian enzyme other than chymotrypsin,[58] although it is possible that certain bacteria such as some *Clostridia* may produce a peptidase with chymotrypsin-like activity. There is a significant correlation between the amount of PABA excreted and the amount of pancreatic enzyme activity measured directly in contents from the small intestine, as well as between PABA excretion and both pancreatic bicarbonate secretion and 72-hour fecal fat determinations.[59]

The technique is as follows. After an 18-hour fast the patient receives 0.25 ml (16.7 mg) of the BT-PABA/Kg of body weight by stomach tube, followed by 25-100 ml water. This dose results in excretion of exogenous PABA that is 25 to 30 times as great as endogenous PABA and other aromatic amines in the urine.[58] Dogs are confined for six hours in a cage, after which urine is collected by catheterization of the bladder and analyzed for PABA. The test cannot be instituted in dogs that have been treated with chloramphenicol, diuretics, sulfonamides, and pancreatic extracts within five days of the test, since those

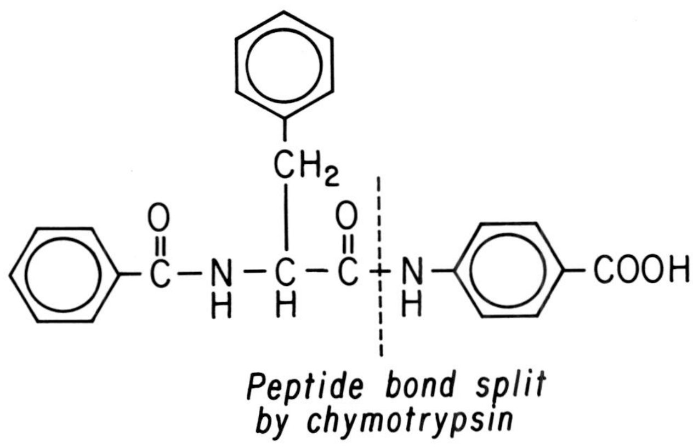

Figure 6-5. Chemical structure of compound used for pancreatic function test. Peptide bond at dashed line is split only by pancreatic chymotrypsin activity releasing para-aminobenzoic acid (compound on right).

will interfere with the validity of the results.[58] Dogs with evidence of renal insufficiency are also excluded, since the excretion of PABA depends on intact renal function.

In clinically normal dogs, six-hour PABA excretion of 63.1% ± 3.53 (mean ± SE) and 73.6 ± 13.7 (mean ± SD), have been reported.[57,58] PABA excretions of less than 46% are considered abnormal. Dogs with experimentally ligated pancreatic ducts excrete only 3.8% ± 0.6 (mean ± SE) of the administered dose.[58] This minimal PABA excretion represents the small concentration of measurable aromatic amines always found in the urine. Dogs require enzyme replacement therapy when their PABA excretion is less than 15.8% (actual PABA, less the 3.8% background level of aromatic amines).[57] Dogs with PABA excretions greater than 20% in six hours usually do not require pancreatic enzyme replacement therapy.[57] Dogs with PABA excretions of 20%-46% have intestinal pancreatic enzyme activity that is significantly less than normal and are described as partially deficient. In the dog, the urinary PABA test is a sensitive and specific test that quantifies the degree of exocrine pancreatic insufficiency and allows determination of whether enzyme replacement therapy is necessary.[57]

A similar test has measured plasma PABA concentrations rather than urinary excretion.[54,56] For convenience, this test can be performed concurrently with the xylose absorption test.[54] PABA is administered at 16.5 mg per 10 ml of water per kg of body weight. Peak plasma PABA concentrations (mean ± SE) in normal dogs, dogs with small intestinal disease, and dogs with exocrine pancreatic insufficiency (Figure 6-6) have been reported to be 31 ± 2.6, 25 ± 3.6, and 2.5 ± 0.8 μmol/L, respectively, in one study.[54] Another study yielded similar plasma PABA concentrations but showed a 20% overlap between dogs with exocrine pancreatic insufficiency and those with small intestinal disease.[48]

Plasma concentrations of PABA are reportedly lower in healthy cats than dogs. In cats the maximum mean PABA concentration reached 386.0 ± 134 μg/dl (mean ± SD).[60] In the same institution, the peak mean plasma concentration in dogs reached 670.4 ± 140.6 μg/dl.[61] In cats, the lower mean serum PABA concentration in association with wide variability, compromises the ability of the BT-PABA test to differentiate

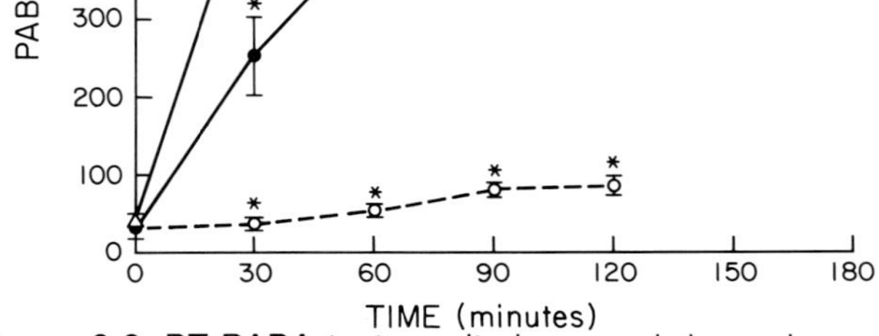

Figure 6-6. BT-PABA test results in normal dogs, dogs with small intestinal disease, and dogs with exocrine pancreatic insufficiency. *Significantly different (P<0.05) from healthy dogs.

cats with normal pancreatic exocrine function from those with abnormal function.[60,62]

Both the urinary and plasma recovery PABA tests are highly sensitive. The specificity of the plasma recovery PABA test appears to be less than that of the urinary recovery PABA test.[61] In both tests, some dogs with severe intestinal disease have reduced PABA absorptions when compared to normal dogs, but in 80% or more cases their PABA absorption is still clearly higher than that in dogs with exocrine pancreatic insufficiency.[48,54,63] There are two probable explanations for the slight overlap in PABA test results between dogs with exocrine pancreatic insufficiency and those with intestinal disease. Severe intestinal disease can induce a "functional" exocrine pancreatic insufficiency in some dogs.[54] The functional failure of pancreatic secretion possibly results from reduced release of pancreatic secretagogues due to a damaged duodenal mucsa.[54] Secondly, in dogs with exocrine pancreatic insufficiency, intestinal overgrowth of bacteria that are capable of metabolizing BT-PABA may lead to a "false" elevation of plasma PABA in the absence of pancreatic chymotrypsin. The most important limitation of the BT-PABA test is not its degree of accuracy, but its time-consuming nature.

Trypsin-like Immunoreactivity Test. The trypsin-like immunoreactivity (TLI) test is a highly sensitive and specific test for the diagnosis of canine exocrine pancreatic insufficiency.[48] Its application in feline exocrine pancreatic insufficiency and acute pancreatitis of the dog and cat remains to be established. The test involves the radioimmunoassay of trypsin-like proteins in the serum. In healthy dogs and dogs with exocrine pancreatic insufficiency, the trypsin-like immunoreactivity is primarily a measure of the small percentage (0.01-0.1%) of cationic pancreatic trypsinogen that diffuses into the blood stream. During pancreatitis, trypsin bound to alpha-1 protease inhibitor contributes to the trypsin-like immunoreactivity.[64] Serum trypsin-like immunoreactivity appears to depend primarily on pancreatic mass. Thus, as pancreatic mass declines, so does serum trypsin-like immunoreactivity. Acute pancreatitis can also elevate serum trypsin-like immunoreactivity.[64] Thus it is possible that some dogs with concurrent chronic pancreatitis and exocrine pancreatic insufficiency may have serum trypsin-like immunoreactivity in the normal range.[65] Post-prandial serum has higher trypsin-like immunoreactivity than preprandial serum.[65] Therefore, it is important to submit serum from dogs that have been fasted for a minimum of three hours and preferably twelve hours. The test is currently performed at the Kansas State University Veterinary Medical Teaching Hospital. Serum trypsin-like immunoreactivity is stable under most conditions and no special packing precautions are required for shipping. Normal values for the dog are 5-35 μg/L, with values below 2.5 μg/L considered diagnostic of exocrine pancreatic insufficiency.[48] Although the TLI test is believed to be the most definitive test available for use, there can be difficulty in evaluating the results for some dogs. A survey of 605 sera showed 10.7% had TLI values diagnostic of exocrine pancreatic insufficiency. A further 12% had values that were suspicious of the problem, however, making further testing necessary for confirming or ruling out exocrine pancreatic insufficiency.[144] That percentage reflects a large number of dogs with values less than 5.0 μg/L but greater than 2.5 μg/L.

The primary advantage of this test over the BT-PABA test is that it is less time consuming. Furthermore, it is not affected by intestinal disease and thus is more specific. Limitations of the TLI test include the aforementioned possibility of a false negative test in dogs with concurrent pancreatitis, as well as its inability to detect exocrine pancreatic insufficiency resulting from obstructive disorders of the pancreatic ducts.[48] The BT-PABA test is not influenced by pancreatitis and will detect exocrine pancreatic deficiency due to ductal obstruction. The two tests assay different proteolytic enzymes, and so it is theoretically possible that selective deficiencies of enterokinase or pancreatic enzymes, as have been reported in humans, could cause discordant results. The sensitivity of the two tests is essentially the same. One case has been described of a dog with clinical evidence of maldigestion, reduced pancreatic mass observed at laparotomy, low-normal intestinal chymotrypsin activity as judged by the serum PABA test, deficient trypsin activity as judged by the trypsin-like immunoreactivity test, and normal fecal proteolytic activity.[66]

Miscellaneous Tests. Additional tests of exocrine pancreatic function include the qualitative direct fecal fat test, the examination of the feces for starch granules and muscle fibers, and the radio-labeled triolein and cholesterol octanoate tests. These procedures are discussed below under malassimilation tests.

Tests of Fat Malassimilation

Qualitative Fecal Fat Test. The qualitative fecal fat test is a simple and useful screening test for fat malassimilation. In humans, the test has been shown to correlate very well with quantitative fecal fat assays.[67] In patients with fat malassimilation, the test is positive in 94%-100% of people excreting more than 10% of a dietary intake of 60 gm of fat. In patients with mild to moderate fat malassimilation (excreting 6%-10% of dietary fat), the test is positive in approximately 75% of the cases. In dogs with exocrine pancreatic insufficiency the qualitative fecal fat test was positive in 86% of cases.[63] Only 43% of these dogs had grossly recognizable steatorrhea. In another study of dogs with chronic diarrhea, a significant positive correlation between the quantitative and qualitative fat tests was observed in spite of the fact that only the "direct" qualitative fecal fat test was performed.[19] The qualitative test noted a trace of fecal fat once fecal fat excretion reached 0.64 ± 0.15 g/kg/day. In this study, steatorrhea was defined as fat excretion of greater than 0.3 g/kg/day.

For reliable results it is best to perform this test after feeding a diet containing a moderate fat content (approximately 8% as fed) for 24-48 hours. Repeating the test twice will also increase accuracy. False positive tests can be expected if the patient has suddenly been changed to an unaccustomed high fat diet, and false negative tests are likely if the diet contains little fat. It is important to perform the test on a fresh stool sample to lessen the chance of bacterial metabolism of fecal fat.

The qualitative fecal fat test is performed in two parts. The "direct" test detects undigested fecal triglycerides, whereas the "indirect" test detects "split" fats such as fatty acids. A comparison of the results of the direct and indirect tests helps to differentiate between fat malabsorption and maldigestion.

The direct fecal fat test is performed as follows. Place a drop of fresh feces on a slide. Mix feces well with a drop of Sudan III or IV, top with a coverslip, and examine microscopically under 10x magnification. Undigested fat appears as large, refractile, red-orange droplets. Dogs with normal fat digestion will have few if any fat droplets (less than 3 droplets per low-powered field) in their feces. To perform the indirect fat test, place 1-2 drops of glacial acetic acid (36%) on the edge of the coverslip of the slide just examined for undigested fat. Once the acetic acid has mixed with the stained feces, gently heat the slide until the first bubbles are seen under the coverslip, and then examine the specimen while it is still warm. Do not overheat. The acetic acid and heat convert fecal soaps into water-insoluble free fatty acids that aggregate into globules of sufficient size for visualization. Dogs with normal fat absorption will have less than 3 droplets of split fats per low power field. Maldigestion is most commonly associated with a positive test for triglyceride and split fat. A positive test for split fats in association with a negative test for triglyceride is suggestive of malabsorption.

Quantitative Fecal Fat Test. The quantitative fecal fat test is the most accurate test of fat malassimilation and is a sensitive test for small intestinal disease. A standard diet with a known amount of fat is fed for several days before collection of feces begins. All feces are collected for 72 hours, placed in a one-gallon container, and stored refrigerated. The amount of fat in a representative aliquot is determined by the van de kramer method, and the total fecal fat excreted is calculated. This test is very rarely used because of its time-consuming nature, inherent logistic difficulty, and failure to differentiate between malabsorption or maldigestion. It is tedious to collect all the feces, and unpleasant to store odiferous feces for a three day period. At times it is difficult to insure inappetant animals will eat sufficient fat. To circumvent some of these problems, some veterinarians collect the feces for only 24 hours. Normally, more than 90%-95% of dietary fat is absorbed. In one study of dogs with malassimilation, mean fat absorption was 83% (range 73-89%).[68] In another study of dogs with chronic diarrhea, steatorrhea was defined as a mean fecal fat excretion of greater than 0.3g/kg/day.[19] Dogs with exocrine pancreatic insufficiency generally have worse steatorrhea than dogs with small intestinal disease. Fat excretion has also been investigated in the cat.[69] Normal cats excrete 0.35 ± 0.23 g/kg/day, with greater than 3.5 g/day indicative of steatorrhea. Quantitative fat measurement may be useful for identifying suspected mild fat malassimilation when the qualitative fecal fat test fails to yield definitive results.

Plasma Tests of Lipid Malassimilation. The plasma turbidity test is a qualitative test that involves the administration of 3 or 6 ml/Kg of corn oil or Lipomul (The Upjohn Co, Kalamazoo, MI) to a fasting dog, followed by examination of plasma for lipemia two and three hours later. Clear plasma is said to identify animals with fat malassimilation. Unfortunately, this technique results in lipemia in only 50% of normal dogs.[70] A major source of the unpredictability in this test is variability in the rate of gastric emptying that results from the ingestion of the lipid bolus. Because of its subjective nature and inaccuracy, we do not recommend continued use of the plasma turbidity test. Other authors, using spectrophotometric analysis, also have observed a broad range of plasma turbidity in normal dogs.[71] Turbidity correlated poorly with the amount of lipids given. To improve the objectivity of the plasma turbidity test, a modification has been proposed in which serum triglycerides are measured before and after the administration of the corn oil. Plasma tests of lipid malassimilation are likely to be abnormal only if lipid malassimilation is marked, by which time steatorrhea can usually be identified on microscopic examination of feces for triglycerides and fatty acids. If fat malabsorption has been identified on fecal examinations, plasma tests of lipid malassimilation yield no additional useful information. Similarly, the use of vegetable oil, followed the next day by a vegetable oil/pancreatic enzyme mix, to diagnose pancreatic exocrine insufficiency cannot be recommended.

A pair of quantitative lipid-absorption tests that have been used to identify dogs with lipid malassimilation and to differentiate lipid maldigestion from malabsorption are the ^{131}I-triolein and the ^{131}I-oleic acid tests.[72] These absorption tests are in disuse because of their limited diagnostic accuracy and value and their cumbersome nature. Two other plasma tests of lipid malassimilation that have fallen out of favor for similar reasons are the vitamin A absorption test[73] and the serum carotene test.

In summary, plasma lipid malassimilation tests are currently of little value in the diagnostic evaluation of patients with chronic diarrhea due to the availability of more sensitive techniques for the detection of lipid malassimilation (qualitative and quantitative tests for fecal fat) and to more reliable ways to diagnose exocrine pancreatic insufficiency (trypsin-like immunoreactivity, BT-PABA, quantitative fecal digestion tests).

Breath Tests for Lipid Malassimilation. A variety of breath tests have been developed for the diagnosis of fat malassimilation. The most well established of these is the ^{14}C-triolein breath test.[74] ^{14}C-triolein is a triglyceride (glyceryl trioleate), in which the 1 acyl moiety is labeled with ^{14}C. The adequacy of the digestion of the triglyceride and absorption and metabolism of the labelled oleic acid can be determined from the amount of $^{14}CO_2$ excreted in the breath. This malassimilation test has been used in human medicine, but its value is limited by its qualitative nature, its failure to differentiate maldigestion from malabsorption, questionable sensitivity, the occurrence of false positives, and difficulties in interpretation when patients have various intercurrent diseases such as diabetes mellitus and pulmonary and liver disease. Subsequent administration of ^{14}C oleic acid to patients with abnormal ^{14}C-triolein tests helps determine if the fat malassimilation is due to maldigestion or malabsorption of fat. In the former, the absorption of this fatty acid is normal, whereas in the latter it is impaired. A test with similar applications and limitations is the cholesteryl octanoate breath test.[75] The usefulness of these tests in veterinary medicine would seem limited.

Carbohydrate Malassimilation Tests

Carbohydrate malassimilation tests are reasonably frequently used to screen for small intestinal mucosal disease, selective carbohydrate malabsorption due to brush border enzyme defects, and bacterial overgrowth.

Fecal Reducing Substances, pH, Osmolality, and Starch. Clinitest tablets (Ames) can be used to detect reducing substances, such as undigested carbohydrate, in feces. The fecal sample is first liquified by the addition of two volumes of water. Fifteen drops of the fecal solution are placed in a test tube, to which a Clinitest tablet is added. A positive test is indicated by the development of green-orange color. A positive test, especially in the presence of a low fecal pH and a high fecal osmolality, is indicative of carbohydrate malassimilation. The low pH and high osmolality are a result of the accumulation of unabsorbable, low molecular weight, acidic fermentation products of carbohydrate. The test must be performed on fresh feces, because colonic bacteria rapidly metabolize carbohydrate. For this reason, a negative test result is difficult to interpret. The value of this technique in the evaluation of dogs and cats with carbohydrate malabsorption is unknown. In preliminary work, the fecal reducing substances test was found to be positive in several dogs with carbohydrate malabsorption and negative in several healthy dogs on the same diet.[76]

Fecal smears can be stained with Lugol's solution to identify undigested starch granules (staining dark blue). These are found in increased numbers with pancreatic enzyme deficiency. This test is less sensitive than the qualitative assessment of fecal fat for the detection of maldigestion.

Xylose Absorption Test. Xylose is a five-carbon monosaccharide that has been widely used to evaluate intestinal absorption. Xylose is absorbed in the proximal small intestine by an incompletely understood mechanism. In some species xylose and glucose are transported by a common system that is sodium and ATP dependent. In other species, transport of xylose and glucose are independent, and the xylose is absorbed via facilitated or passive transport.[77] Xylose is transported from the intestinal mucosa by the portal circulation, with the lymphatics contributing little if any to its movement.

The xylose-absorption test is considered a test of carbohydrate malabsorption. Abnormal xylose tests are usually a result of morphological diseases of the intestine rather than functional diseases.[78] It primarily functions as a guide to the need for small intestinal biopsy. Its usefulness in this regard in veterinary medicine is compromised by its poor sensitivity and specificity. Endoscopy is a more specific and sensitive technique for the detection of morphologic mucosal disease, and 72-hour fecal fat excretion is a more sensitive screening test of generalized malassimilation disorders.

The xylose test is performed as follows. A 10% to 25% solution of D-xylose is given by stomach tube at a dose of 500 mg/Kg body weight to fasted patients. Water is used to flush the tube and reduce the concentration of a 25% solution. For xylose determinations, blood samples are obtained before the pentose is given and subsequently at one-hour intervals for five hours. There is too much variability in the 30-minute sample to make its determination useful. Laboratory determination of xylose levels involves heating the sample in acid solution and reacting the furfural formed with aniline to yield a colored compound. In healthy dogs, the mean blood level of D-xylose at 60 minutes is 63 mg/dl, with a standard deviation of ± 12. All values above 45 to 50 mg/dl at 60 minutes are normal (Figure 6-7). Plasma levels between 45 and 50 mg/dl are in the gray zone. Plasma xylose concentrations are not consistently reduced in dogs with chronic small intestinal disease (Figure 6-8). Approximately 10% of healthy dogs are in this range. In one report, values greater than 45 mg/dl at 90 minutes were considered normal.[68] Dogs with malabsorption in this study had blood xylose concentrations ranging from 13 to 43 mg/dl at 90 minutes. Xylose absorption testing, using current procedures, cannot be recommended for use in cats to investigate malabsorption because of the high degree of individual variability in xylose absorption and the insensitivity of the test in documenting feline intestinal disease.[60,62]

The rate of xylose absorption is determined by the amount

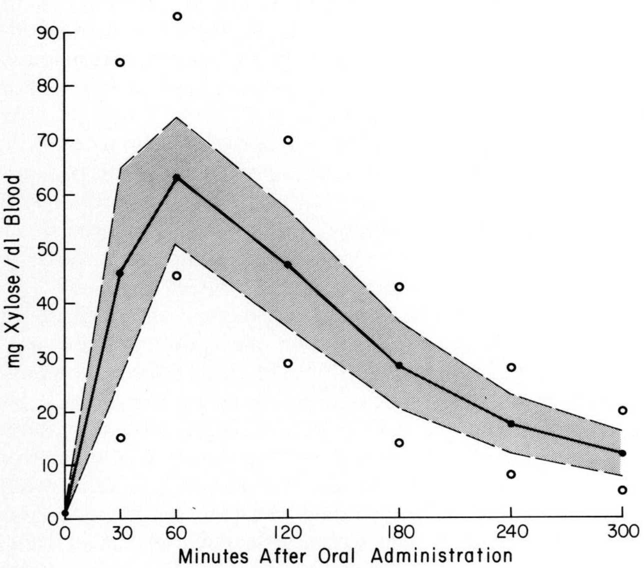

Figure 6-7. Xylose absorption test results in 32 normal dogs. Blood xylose concentrations from 0 to 5 hours after oral administration of 2 ml/Kg of a 25% xylose solution. Mean (solid line) ± standard error (dashed line) shows peak at 60 minutes. The highest and lowest individual values are represented by open circles. A one hour blood xylose test can be done with any value less than 45 mg/dl being abnormal.

administered, the rate of gastric emptying, the extent of bacterial metabolism of xylose, the size of the area for absorption in the small intestine, and the adequacy of intestinal circulation. Provided the amount of xylose used is standardized according to the patient's body weight and delayed gastric emptying is ruled out by history, radiographic procedures, and correct experimental technique (see below), abnormalities in the concentration of xylose appearing in the circulation can be confidently ascribed to reduced absorption or inadequate circulation. Reduced absorption may be a consequence of villus atrophy or bacterial overgrowth. Severe reduction of mucosal blood flow such as occurs in portal hypertension reduces xylose absorption. Lymphangiectasia occasionally interferes with absorption. Administration of a hypertonic solution delays gastric emptying and reduces absorption of D-xylose at 60 minutes. This can be a problem when a hypertonic, 25% xylose solution is used. However, residual gastric secretions and water used to flush the stomach tube usually dilute the xylose solution enough so that delayed gastric emptying is not a problem. Deceptively low serum xylose levels can result from sequestration of xylose in ascitic fluid, and falsely elevated xylose concentrations will result from renal insufficiency.[79] In humans, concomitant administration of several drugs, such as non-steroidal antiinflammatory drugs and neomycin, are thought to reduce xylose absorption.

Normally, very little xylose is metabolized either before or after absorption. Bacterial overgrowth, however, results in abnormally low blood xylose concentrations because of increased bacterial metabolism of xylose. When low xylose absorption due to bacterial overgrowth is suspected, antibiotic therapy can be instituted and the xylose-absorption test repeated in 48 hours. Figure 6-9 shows xylose-absorption tests for a dog before and after antibiotic therapy. Alternatively, other tests for the diagnosis of bacterial overgrowth can be instituted.

Oral Glucose-tolerance Test. The oral glucose-tolerance test is seldom performed. Absorption of glucose is a function of the absorptive area of the intestinal mucosa and the glucose transport mechanisms in the brush border of the epithelial cells. Extraintestinal variables, such as circulating glucagon and insulin, rapidly alter serum glucose concentrations. The oral glucose-tolerance test produces inconsistent results in dogs with consistent abnormalities in total fat excretion and xylose absorption. This test has no value in identifying animals with malabsorption problems.

Disaccharide Digestion and Absorption Tests. A test

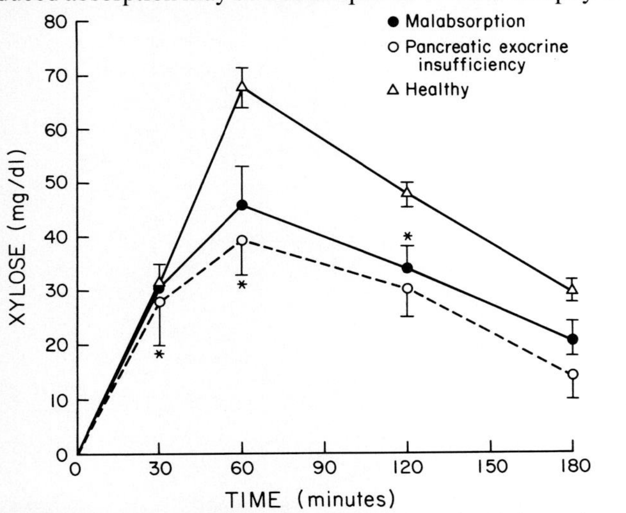

Figure 6-8. Xylose-absorption test results in normal dogs, dogs with small intestinal disease, and dogs with exocrine pancreatic insufficiency. *Significantly different (P<0.05) from healthy dogs.

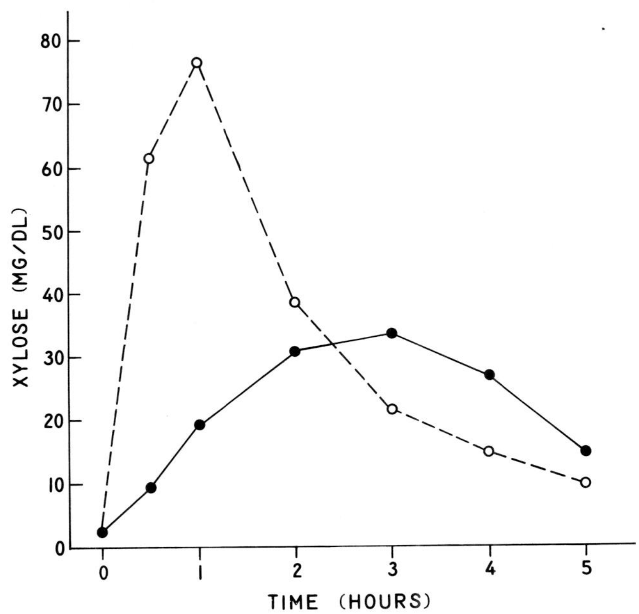

Figure 6-9. Results of xylose absorption testing in a dog with bacterial overgrowth of the small intestine. Initial xylose absorption test (solid line) was abnormal. After treatment with antibiotics a xylose absorption test was normal (dashed line).

employing one or more disaccharides can be used to evaluate brush border enzyme functions indirectly in patients with confirmed carbohydrate malabsorption. The disaccharides lactose, sucrose, and maltose require digestion by specific brush-border enzymes before absorption is possible. The monosaccharides released are glucose, galactose, and fructose. These tests are rarely conducted in small animal patients and are difficult to interpret because data are lacking on sufficient normal animals. Abnormal lactose absorption tests can be recorded from normal dogs.

After oral administration of 1 g of maltose, lactose, or sucrose/Kg body weight, blood glucose is measured at 30, 60, and 120 minutes. Normally blood glucose increases by greater than 30 mg/dl at 30 minutes. With a deficiency of one or more of the disaccharidases the increment is less than 10 mg/dl. A glucose-galactose absorption test is then conducted on the same patient by oral administration of the two monosaccharides followed by blood glucose determinations. When this test is normal and lactose tolerance is abnormal, there is a deficiency of lactase activity. The same controls are used to evaluate maltase and sucrase activity, employing the appropriate monosaccharides.

These tests are an indirect evaluation of brush-border enzyme activity. The interpretation is based on blood glucose levels, which can be influenced by a number of hormonal and metabolic factors that are not possible to control. The activity of brush-border disaccharidases can be directly assayed on biopsies of the small intestine.

Breath Hydrogen Test[80-83] The breath hydrogen test is a useful test for the diagnosis of both bacterial overgrowth and malassimilation of carbohydrate. It is more sensitive than the xylose absorption test for this purpose.[81] Fermentation of unabsorbed carbohydrate by intestinal bacteria generates hydrogen gas, some of which is absorbed by the blood stream and excreted from the lungs. There is a quantitative relationship between unabsorbed carbohydrate and pulmonary hydrogen excretion. The elevated breath hydrogen concentrations are first detected when the carbohydrate reaches large numbers of intestinal bacteria. In animals with a normal bowel transit time, carbohydrate malassimilation, and no bacterial overgrowth, the rise in breath hydrogen begins four to six hours after eating (Figure 6-10). If bacteria have overgrown the small bowel, increased breath hydrogen excretion is detected within one to two hours of eating (Figure 6-10). Preliminary data suggests that healthy fasted dogs have a breath hydrogen concentration of 0.9 ± 0.1 ppm (mean ± SE), and that a peak hydrogen concentration of 1.4 ± 0.2 ppm occurs eight hours after feeding of a highly digestible carbohydrate-based diet (d/d, Hill's Pet Products). Dogs with carbohydrate malabsorption due to exocrine pancreatic insufficiency have a fasting expired hydrogen concentration of 3.3 ± 0.9 ppm, which increases to a mean peak of 28.8 ± 2 ppm 6.5 hours after feeding. Dogs with chronic small intestinal disease have fasting expired hydrogen concentrations of 5.3 ± 1.3 ppm, which increases to a peak of 72.2 ± 18 ppm seven hours after feeding. In bacterial overgrowth or carbohydrate malabsorption, breath hydrogen usually increases to exceed 8 ppm.

A simple method is developed for collecting expired air. Using an anesthetic induction mask, a nonrebreathing valve, and a 1 liter latex bag, breath samples are collected each hour for eight hours after feeding a carbohydrate rich diet, such as a can of d/d (Hill's Pet Products). Allowing the patient to breath through the apparatus for 1 minute prior to attachment of the collection bag eliminates air in the dead space of the apparatus. An aliquot of expired air is withdrawn from the latex bag through a three-way sampling valve into a 35 cc. syringe. Syringes are capped by a three-way valve and can be stored at room temperature for at least twelve hours without significant loss of hydrogen (hydrogen is lost at the rate of approximately 5% per day from new syringes). Aliquots of the expired air are assayed for hydrogen by thermal conductivity gas chromatography or hydrogen-sensitive electrochemical cells.

The breath hydrogen test is a practical technique. Even though multiple samples are drawn, the sampling time is very brief and the sampling procedure very well tolerated by most dogs and cats. The assay of breath hydrogen is widely available at human hospitals, and the sampled breath is sufficiently stable for transport to local laboratories. Furthermore, the required equipment is minimally expensive and easily acquired by any practice. An important advantage of this test is its potential to differentiate between dogs with bacterial overgrowth and those with carbohydrate malabsorption. The most important disadvantage is that insufficient data is as yet available in the dog and cat to adequate assess the test's sensitivity, its specificity, or the importance of any confounding factors such as deranged intestinal transit times. Five to ten percent of humans with carbohydrate malassimilation do not produce excessive hydrogen gas,

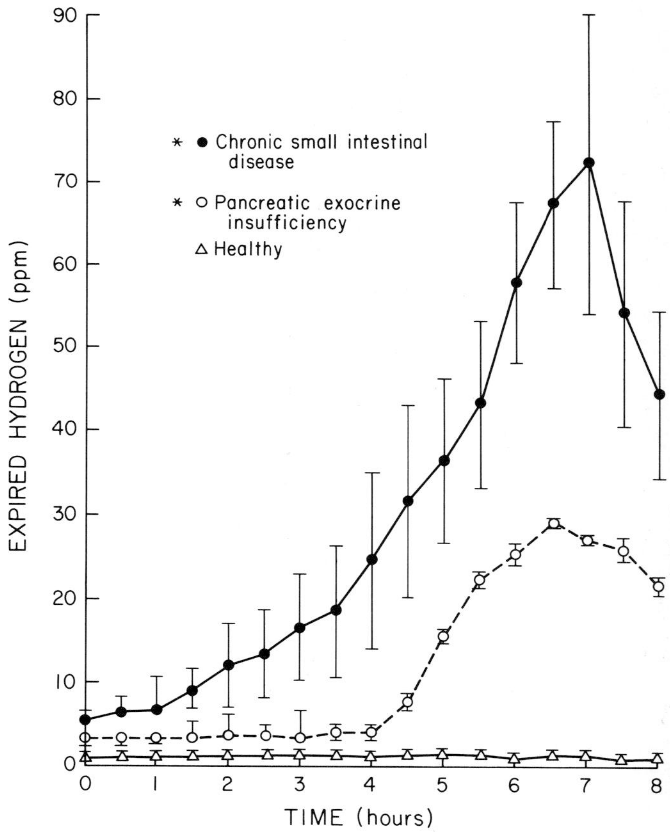

Figure 6-10. Breath hydrogen test results in healthy dogs, in dogs with pancreatic exocrine insufficiency (carbohydrate malassimilation and mild bacterial overgrowth), and in dogs with chronic small intestinal disease (carbohydrate malassimilation and marked bacterial overgrowth).

possibly because of an acidic colonic microclimate which reduces bacterial production of hydrogen.[84] These false negative results can be avoided by pretreatment of the patient with magnesium sulfate 70 mg/kg to alkalinize colonic content. Furthermore, hyperventilation and exercise immediately prior to the test can "wash out" breath hydrogen; accumulations of oral carbohydrate can artificially increase it.[85] The type of intestinal bacteria may also influence the amount of hydrogen excreted. Variations in the test diet markedly affect the breath hydrogen concentration because of differences in the digestibility of the carbohydrate and variable transit times. Other possible confounding factors include prior use of antibiotic therapy, and enemas. A recent study in humans found that breath hydrogen tests given after an oral glucose load in human patients had a sensitivity of 93% and a specificity of 78% for the diagnosis of bacterial overgrowth.[86] Breath hydrogen testing in dogs after an oral xylose load shows promise for having a high sensitivity and a high specificity (Figure 6-11).

Tests for Protein Malassimilation

Tests for protein malassimilation are rarely performed because specific defects of protein malassimilation in the absence of fat or carbohydrate malassimilation have not been recognized, and in patients with pancreatic or intestinal disease fat and carbohydrate malassimilation usually precedes protein malassimilation.

Fecal smears can be examined for undigested muscle fibers, which appear in larger numbers with protein maldigestion. Cytology stains help identify muscle fibers. The search for visual evidence of fecal protein is less rewarding than that for fat.

The fecal excretion of nitrogen can be measured by the macro-Kjeldahl method. The nitrogen measured is the residue of both endogenous and dietary protein. Elevations can indicate poor digestibility of the diet, pancreatic exocrine insufficiency, malabsorption, or protein-losing enteropathy (see scintigraphy). It has been suggested that measurement of breath hydrogen after the oral administration of glycoproteins may be useful for the detection of protein malabsorption, bacterial overgrowth, and protein-losing enteropathy.[87]

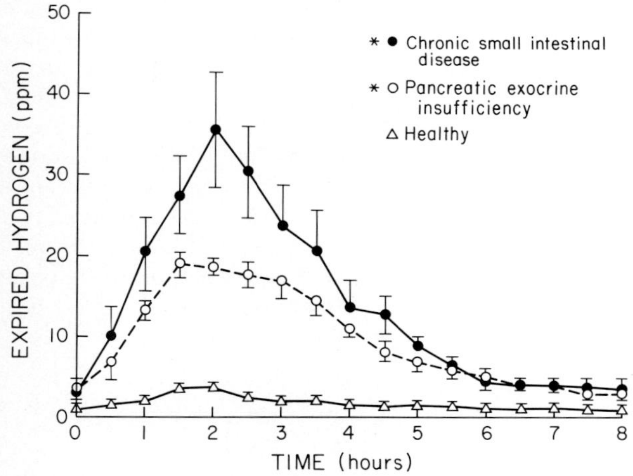

Figure 6-11. Breath-hydrogen test results in healthy dogs, in dogs with pancreatic exocrine insufficiency, and in dogs with chronic small intestinal disease after oral administration of xylose.

Miscellaneous Absorption Tests

Tests of Bile Acid Malabsorption. Tests of bile acid malabsorption may be indicated when secretory diarrhea of the large bowel is suspected, such as in some cases of canine large bowel diarrhea in which minimal or no inflammation is detected on biopsy. Various tests have been developed for the measurement of bile acid malabsorption in humans. These have included the bile acid breath test, a test utilizing a ^{75}Se-labeled cholyltaurine derivative, and the excretion of ^{14}C in stool after oral administration of ^{14}C-cholylglycine.[40] To date, no method has become universally accepted, however, and the most widely used technique remains a trial with the bile acid binding resin cholestyramine (Questran: Mead Johnson). A good response to cholestyramine suggests, but does not prove, that bile acid malabsorption is a cause of the diarrhea. For these purposes, cholestyramine is administered at 200-300 mg/kg. If a response is to be seen, it usually occurs within days. Cholestyramine should be used very judiciously in cats because it rapidly depletes them of taurine.

Urinary Indican.[88] Urine indican levels have been used to identify intestinal disorders ranging from enterotoxemias to abnormal bacterial numbers and species colonizing the small intestine. After bacteria that possess tryptophanase activity metabolize tryptophan, that amino acid produces indican. Theoretically, the amount of indican produced is a function of the level of tryptophan and the numbers of tryptophanase-positive bacteria in the small intestine. In practice, however, urinary indican has not proved useful for the identification of bacterial overgrowth. Marked indicanuria is found with gastrointestinal bleeding and protein-losing enteropathy.

Tests for Bacterial Overgrowth

A diagnosis of bacterial overgrowth of the small intestine cannot be made by fecal culture because bacteria cultured from the feces, even in heavy growth, need not be represented in the small bowel in significant numbers. A definitive diagnosis of bacterial overgrowth can, however, be made by quantitative anaerobic and aerobic culture of duodenal fluid aspirated by endoscopy, suction capsule biopsy, or by needle at surgery. The breath hydrogen test provides supportive evidence for bacterial overgrowth, as does a depressed serum vitamin B_{12} in association with an elevated serum folate level. Tests for bacterial overgrowth are indicated during the evaluation of most small bowel diarrheas. They are particularly likely to be rewarding if the patient is a German Shepherd or is manifesting steatorrhea. A test for pancreatic insufficiency should always precede a test for bacterial overgrowth because overgrowth of bacteria is a common consequence of maldigestion.

Culture of Duodenal Fluid. Quantitative culture of fluid from the duodenum or jejunum is the "gold standard" for the diagnosis of bacterial overgrowth. Intestinal fluid may be collected by syringe and a needle at surgery or by an aspiration tube inserted into the duodenum through the operating channel of an endoscope or through a peroral suction capsule (Quinton Instrument Company, Seattle, WA). A 2-5 ml volume of fluid is withdrawn and quantitatively cultured for anaerobic and aerobic bacteria. Bacterial colony counts greater than 100,000 per ml in the duodenal or jejunal fluid of fasted dogs are considered abnormal. A fecal type of microflora, coliforms and increased anaerobes, is a commonly found abnormality.

The Serum Cobalamin/Folate Test. Increased numbers of bacteria generate large quantities of folate which is absorbed in the upper small intestine. At the same time, the bacteria reduce the uptake of cobalamin (vitamin B_{12}) in the distal small intestine (Figure 6-12). A high serum folate concentration concurrent with a low serum cobalamin level is thus suggestive of bacterial overgrowth.[65,89] Preliminary experience with this test for the diagnosis of bacterial overgrowth in the dog has suggested reasonable specificity but poor sensitivity. Confounding factors include exocrine pancreatic insufficiency, which may reduce the absorption of cobalamin and increase the absorption of folate by various mechanisms; severe mucosal disease, which can reduce the absorption of either of these vitamins; low folate diets, which can rapidly reduce serum folate (unlikely); and therapeutic administration of vitamins, which can markedly elevate serum levels.[65,89] An inherited selective malabsorption of cobalamin has recently been reported in Giant Schnauzers. Various drugs, including phenytoin and sulfasalazine, interfere with folate absorption in humans.

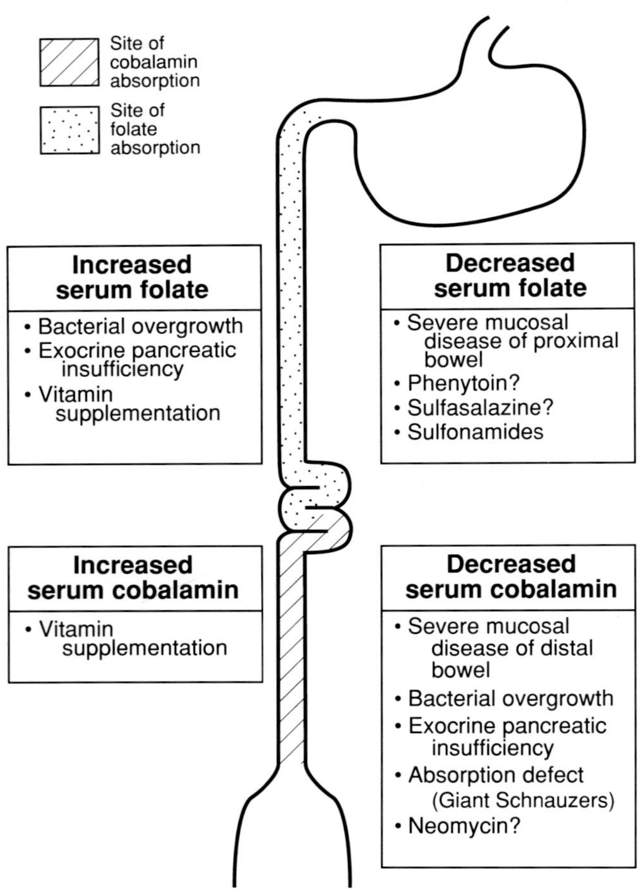

Figure 6-12. Schematic showing sites of B_{12} and folate absorption in the small intestine; also tabulated are the problems that can alter plasma levels of B_{12} and folate.

Neomycin can interfere with the absorption of cobalamin. Unlike other investigators,[89] we have found the serum levels of cobalamin and folate to be insensitive measures of intestinal mucosal diseases. Normal canine serum concentrations of cobalamin and folate determined by competitive-binding assay range from 300-800 ng/L and 7.5-17.5 µg/L, respectively.[65] The use of these vitamin assays in the cat has as yet to be validated.

The ^{14}C-D-xylose Breath Test. The ^{14}C-D-xylose breath test is a useful test for the diagnosis of bacterial overgrowth in man,[78] and control values have recently been established in the dog.[90] Small intestinal bacteria cleave the molecule and release the $^{14}CO_2$, which is assayed in the breath. This test may prove to be valuable in institutions with the capability to use radioisotopes.

Tests of Gastrointestinal Permeability

Gastrointestinal permeability is increased in many gastrointestinal diseases. Tests of gastrointestinal permeability have application for researchers studying these diseases. A technique for the quantitative assessment of intestinal permeability in dogs by measurement of the urinary excretion of ^{51}Cr-EDTA has recently been described.[91,92] Other techniques to examine permeability include the cellobiose/mannitol absorption test,[93] and absorption of phenol red, polyethyleneglycol and inulin.[94]

Peroral String Test

The peroral string test utilizes a 140 cm absorbent nylon yarn within a weighted gelatin capsule. The capsule is administered to the dog, and the free end of the yarn is tied to a piece of gauze tape which has been tied around the dog's mandible just cranial to the canine teeth. As the capsule passes by peristalsis into the duodenum, the yarn unwinds and soaks up gastrointestinal fluid, which is later analyzed once the yarn is retrieved from the dog's mouth.

The peroral string test (Entero-test, HDC Corp, Mountain View, CA) has been successfully used for the diagnosis of giardiasis in the dog.[95] In man it has also been used for the diagnosis of *Strongyloides stercoralis*, enteropathogenic bacteria, achlorhydria, and gastroesophageal reflux; for the acquisition of duodenal fluid for culture and cytology; and for the location of the site of gastrointestinal hemorrhage. To determine the level at which bleeding begins, the string is measured from the oral cavity to the proximal limit of the blood-stained string. Alternatively, the level at which blood staining of the string begins is compared to the level at which bile staining of the string, or acidification of fluid absorbed into the string, is first detected. The consequence of a dog's swallowing of the entire string has not been addressed. No ill effects have been observed in humans following this eventuality.

GASTROINTESTINAL IMAGING TECHNIQUES

Introduction

Veterinary gastrointestinal radiography has been the subject of several recent reviews.[96-106] The reader is directed to these publications for a detailed description of correct radiographic technique and interpretation. The bulk of this discussion is on the indications and limitations of gastrointestinal imaging techniques, with particular emphasis on newer techniques such as enteroclysis, ultrasound, and scintigraphy.

Imaging techniques are powerful tools for the investigation of gastrointestinal disease. Imaging techniques available to veterinary practitioners, either in their own practice or by referral to specialist hospitals, include radiography, fluoroscopy, ultrasonography, nuclear scintigraphy, computer-assisted tomography, and magnetic resonance imaging. Although some overlap occurs, each technique occupies a particular niche in the spectrum of application of diagnostic imaging modalities. Thus, gastrointestinal radiography is primarily suited to the detection of morphologic abnormalities that distort organ size or position; fluoroscopy is utilized to detect motility disorders; ultrasonography recognizes morphologic abnormalities resulting from altered tissue density as well organ size and position; scintigraphy examines the integrity of gastrointestinal physiologic functions such as gastric emptying, biliary excretion, and mucosal permeability; and computer-assisted tomography and magnetic resonance imaging are sensitive techniques for the diagnosis of morphologic abnormality.

Survey Radiographs

Survey pharyngeal, cervical, thoracic, and abdominal radiographs are indicated for the evaluation of many gastrointestinal problems. Their value in the workup of patients with regurgitation, chronic vomiting, diarrhea, and abdominal pain is discussed in Chapter 5. While it is not common for survey radiography to yield a definitive diagnosis, the procedure is still performed early in many diagnostic workups because it assists the clinician in tentatively ruling out disorders such as gastrointestinal obstruction, adynamic ileus, perforation, or peritonitis that have serious consequences if diagnosis is delayed. Furthermore, survey radiographs often provide valuable diagnostic clues, such as estimations of organ size and the presence or absence of masses or fluid, that help the clinician in reaching a diagnosis. A recent retrospective study of patients with suspected gastric disease determined that survey abdominal radiographs had a 25% diagnostic yield, whereas positive contrast studies had a 40% yield.[107]

Contrast Radiographic Examination

Indications, Contraindications, Complications. A major obstacle to effective gastrointestinal contrast radiography is the mistaken belief by many clinicians that there is one contrast procedure that provides adequate evaluation for the entire upper gastrointestinal tract. Unfortunately, this is not the case. For maximum diagnostic return from gastrointestinal radiography, the veterinarian must select from as many as nine different contrast techniques, each of which has different indications (Table 6-4).

Upper gastrointestinal contrast radiography and endoscopy are complementary procedures. Contrast procedures do not require anesthesia, and they provide a better estimation of luminal diameter (esophagus), mural masses, extramural compressive lesions, jejunal diseases, gastrointestinal motility, and gastric emptying. Endoscopy is more sensitive for the diagnosis of mucosal diseases of the upper gastrointestinal tract and offers the important advantage of definitive diagnosis through biopsy. In most cases of esophageal disease, barium swallows are performed before endoscopy. In most cases of suspected gastroduodenal disease, endoscopic examination should precede the contrast procedure.[107] In a recent prospective study in dogs, gastroscopy was found to be superior to double contrast gastrography for the diagnosis of gastric neoplasia, ulceration, and gastritis.[107] There is little place for the barium enema if endoscopy is available.

Contraindications for contrast radiography include inadequate preparation and rapid deterioration of a patient's condi-

Table 6-4 Indications for Contrast Radiology of the Gastrointestinal Tract

Liquid barium swallowing study
- Dysphagia
- Regurgitation
- Suspected morphologic disorders of the pharynx and esophagus
- Suspected motility disorders of the pharynx and esophagus

Barium-coated food swallowing study
- Dysphagia
- Regurgitation
- Suspected morphologic disorders of the pharynx and esophagus (especially partial obstructions)
- Suspected motility disorders of the pharynx and esophagus (especially subtle motility abnormalities)

Positive contrast gastrogram
- Chronic vomiting
- Suspected gastric foreign bodies
- Suspected mural gastric lesions
- Suspected extramural masses impinging on the stomach
- Suspected overt gastric mucosal disease
- Suspected pyloric obstruction
- Assist in locating stomach

Double contrast gastrogram
- Chronic vomiting
- Suspected radiolucent gastric foreign bodies
- Enhance detail of gastric mucosa

Upper GI contrast study with small bowel follow-through evaluation
- Chronic vomiting
- Chronic bloating
- Chronic diarrhea (rarely of value)
- Suspected intestinal foreign body
- Suspected intestinal obstruction
- Suspected herniation
- Assist localization of abdominal masses
- To assess gastrointestinal transit time

Barium Meal
- To assess gastric emptying time

Fluoroscopy
- Suspected gastrointestinal motility abnormality

Enteroclysis
- Chronic diarrhea
- Suspected intestinal partial obstruction
- Suspected intestinal motility abnormality

Air or barium enema
- Suspected large bowel mass
- Suspected ileocecal abnormalities
- Assist localization of pelvic and abdominal masses
- Assist localization of gastrointestinal gas accumulations

tion. Complications include aspiration of contrast material and barium peritonitis from gastrointestinal rupture. Aspiration of contrast material is particularly common in patients with megaesophagus. Animals with megaesophagus should never be placed back in their cages with an esophagus full of contrast material. The performance of a gastrogram delays upper gastrointestinal endoscopy by a minimum of 24 hours.

Contrast Procedures for the Evaluation of Swallowing. Contrast studies are done with barium as paste, liquid suspension, or mixed with food. The paste is a 70% w/w form containing a binding agent and can be administered with a syringe. It is used to outline the pharynx and cranial esophagus in animals with suspected pharyngoesophageal swallowing disorders. The suspension is used at a 30% w/v concentration for evaluating esophageal problems. Barium mixed with food is used for evaluating for both pharyngoesophageal and esophageal problems. Each of the three forms is given in small boluses and as frequently as necessary to satisfy that an accurate evaluation of pharyngoesophageal motility has been made and that obstruction is confirmed or ruled out.

If fluoroscopy is available, the passage of the barium contrast agents during swallowing can be observed. The study should include recording of three to six complete swallows of liquid barium suspension followed by a similar number of barium-coated food boluses.

If esophageal perforation is suspected, a water-soluble iodinated contrast material should be used. Such materials are less irritating to the periesophageal tissues. If the swallow does not identify a perforation, the study should be repeated with a liquid barium suspension because esophageal perforations may be missed with water-soluble agents.

Swallowing studies are done without giving patients any chemical restraint. If sedation is necessary, low-dose acetylpromazine has a minimal adverse affect on swallowing, but such a low dose is not likely to insure success in managing the patient.

Contrast Procedures for the Assessment of Gastric Morphology. Positive contrast gastrograms and double contrast gastrograms are the most useful contrast procedures for the assessment of gastrointestinal morphology. Positive contrast gastrograms utilize a large volume of dilute barium suspension (9-18 ml/kg) with the intent of causing mild gastric distension. This technique is particularly useful for the detection of poorly distensible mural lesions. In combination with fluoroscopy, it allows evaluation of gastric motility. Positive contrast gastrograms allow the visualization of some mucosal detail, but double-contrast gastrograms are the preferred technique for the radiographic evaluation of the gastric mucosa.[104] Double-contrast gastrograms may be performed after most of the barium from the positive contrast gastrogram has left the stomach, or alternatively by instilling into the stomach 2ml/kg of barium followed by sufficient air to ensure even gastric distension.

Contrast Procedures for the Assessment of Gastric Emptying. Gastric emptying time may be crudely assessed by contrast radiographic techniques. The gastric emptying of fluids and solids is dependent on markedly different physiologic mechanisms. The gastric emptying time of liquids has less clinical relevance. Normal gastric emptying times of liquids, using 10 ml/kg 60% w/v of barium suspension, have been reported to be 0.5-2 hours in dogs,[108] although another investigator, using a slightly different technique, has reported a range of 1-7 hours with a mean and standard error of 4 ± 0.2 hours.[107] Gastric emptying should begin within 45 minutes of administration of barium liquids.[107] Normal gastric emptying time of barium and food admixtures, using 7 ml/kg 60% w/v barium sulfate suspension mixed with 8 gm/kg of ground kibble has been reported to vary from 7-15 hours with a mean of 11 hours in mixed-breed dogs.[109] A similar study in beagles showed a barium-food mean gastric emptying time of 7 ± 0.74 hours.[110] The caloric density, nutrient composition, osmolality, and particle size of the test meal will affect emptying time and so must be standardized for consistent results. The emptying of 1 cm segments of radiopaque plastic tubing (0.2 cm diameter) that acts as indigestible solids has been successfully used as a simple, accurate, and inexpensive means of detecting abnormal gastric emptying in humans.[111] The markers are given with a meal and the time determined for their complete emptying. It is probable that this study also will have value in veterinary medicine.

Fear, pain, metabolic derangements, and certain tranquilizers will delay gastrointestinal transit times. If tranquilization is required, use acetylpromazine (0.05- 0.1 mg/kg SQ) for the dog. A tranquilization protocol that does not affect gastrointestinal motility yet provides safe and effective sedation has not been determined for the cat. Ketamine increases gastric motility and hastens transit time.[112]

More accurate techniques for the assessment of gastric emptying are available, but their use is restricted by their cumbersome nature or requirement for radionuclides. They include orogastric intubation methods and various scintigraphic techniques.

Contrast Procedures for the Evaluation of the Small Intestine. The contrast procedure of choice for the examination of small intestinal morphology is enteroclysis (see below). Crude assessment of morphology may be acquired by use of liquid barium "follow through" studies. In the absence of obstructive lesions, the rate of passage of contrast material through the gastrointestinal tract is a function of the frequency of peristaltic and segmental contractions of the stomach and intestine, the functional status of the pylorus, and the amount and viscosity of the contrast medium. As a result of these variables, gastrointestinal transit time is a poor measure of intestinal motility. Normal gastrointestinal transit and gastrointestinal emptying times using 10 ml/kg of 60% w/v liquid barium suspension in dogs have been reported to be 0.5-2 hours and 3-5 hours, respectively.[108] A transit time of greater than 4 hours is evidence of a transit defect in dogs. In the cat, transit is more rapid, ranging from 30-60 minutes.[112] As with gastric emptying, psychological factors and drugs can delay transit. The fluoroscopic inspection of the barium-filled gastrointestinal tract during the barium "follow through" study or enteroclysis provides the best assessment of intestinal motility.

Contrast Procedures for Examination of the Large Intestine. In the absence of an endoscope, barium enemas can be useful for the detection of morphologic abnormalities of the large bowel such as masses, strictures, ileocecal inversion, and ileocecal intussusception. Insufflation of the colon with air (15-20 ml/kg) through a balloon tipped catheter is a simple procedure to outline the large bowel and assist localization of colonic, of pelvic or abdominal masses and abdominal gas accumulations.

Fluoroscopy

Fluoroscopy, videofluorography, and cinefluorography are indicated for the diagnosis of gastric and intestinal motility disorders and the differentiation of swallowing disorders into oral, pharyngeal, cricopharyngeal, esophageal, and gastroesophageal phases. Only through fluoroscopy is it possible to assess the rate of gastrointestinal motility, the coordination of peristaltic movement, and the manner in which contrast medium is propelled through the gastrointestinal tract.[96,113] By the evaluation of esophageal motility, fluoroscopy helps determine the prognosis for patients with megaesophagus. Fluoroscopy can also be of value for various diagnostic and operative techniques, such as enteroclysis, balloon dilation of esophageal strictures, noninvasive suction biopsy of the small intestine, and fine needle aspiration of periesophageal thoracic masses.

Enteroclysis[113]

Enteroclysis entails the inflation of the small intestine with a dilute solution of barium through a tube placed directly into the duodenum under fluoroscopic guidance. The initial barium infusion is followed by an infusion of water. The result is a double contrast study of the distended small bowel. Enteroclysis is indicated for the diagnosis of suspected small bowel partial obstructions and for the further evaluation of patients with confirmed bacterial overgrowth. It also provides accurate information about mucosal morphology and small bowel motility. A uniform progression of barium through the gastrointestinal tract (as can be assessed with enteroclysis) is a more important indicator of normal gastrointestinal motility than is the exact transit time.[101,113]

The technique for enteroclysis follows food being withheld for two days and water for two hours prior to the procedure.[113] An enteroclysis solution containing 28% w/v barium sulfate is prepared by making a 3:5 (barium:water) dilution of the following suspension: Barium sulphate 750g, sodium citrate 15g, sodium carboxy-methylcellulose 10g, Tween-80 (polysorbate 80) 1ml, silicon antifoam emulsion 1.5ml, water (approx 800ml) to a volume of 1000ml. For smaller dogs, 21.5% W/V (2:5 barium:water) is preferred. Duodenal intubation is carried out under fluoroscopy using a 135 cm long, 14 french radiopaque polyvinyl catheter through which is inserted a lubricated flexible insertion guide wire. An infusion set, consisting of two disposable enema bags connected by a y-shaped connector and fitted with clamps to allow individual delivery of either water or barium suspension, is fitted to the duodenal tube. The patient is sedated and placed in left lateral recumbency. A mouth gag is positioned and the tube manuevered into the antrum and through the pylorus until the tip is positioned in the descending duodenum. The guide wire is removed, the tube taped in position, and the dog rotated to right lateral recumbency. The infusion bags are lifted to 60 cm above the table top and the barium suspension infused (giving an inward flow of 40-50cc per minute and an infusion time of 5-15 minutes). Infusion of barium suspension is stopped when filling of the cecum and colon begins (usually amounts to 20-25 cc per kg). Radiographs of the complete contrast-filled small intestine are made using high kVp (90-125) and low mAs settings. The bags are then lowered to 20-30 cms above the table and the water infused (at a rate of 60-100 cc per minute). Radiographs (double contrast) are taken of the successively distended bowel loops using the same technique listed above. Occasionally, compression radiographs are taken of particular areas. The water infusion forces the contrast column into the large bowel, leaving a thin layer of barium coating the intestinal mucosa. Between 20-40 cc of water per kg with an infusion time of 5-10 minutes results in full distension of the intestinal loops as well as a transient ileus (removing artefactual "strictures" due to peristalsis). The infusion of water is continued until a sufficient degree of transradiancy and distension has been achieved throughout the small bowel. Termination of infusion of water results in partial collapse of the bowel. The rectum is then intubated and rectal fluid drained. In the hands of experienced personnel, the total fluoroscopy time is 10 minutes, and the total procedural time is 40 minutes. Measurements of wall thickness, lumen width, and villus border height are assessed. The contrast column (before water) usually measures 12-13 mm in width in small dogs, and 13-16 mm in large dogs. Villus border width (mucosal barium margination) never exceeds 1 mm. Intestinal wall thickness measures 1-1.25 mm exclusive of the height of the villus border. Following full distension, the diameter of the intestinal lumen ranges from 15-18 mm in small dogs to 18-24 mm in larger dogs.[113]

Contraindications for enteroclysis include compromised cardiovascular or renal function or evidence of gastrointestinal perforation. To avoid aspiration, the procedure must be abandoned if excessive gastroduodenal reflux of barium occurs. Complications recorded in a series of 270 enteroclysis procedures on dogs include failure of intubation (5.5%), excessive reflux (3.3%), bowel perforation (0.4%), and vomiting (1.0%).[113] The rate of infusion of the barium suspension is the most important technical aspect of the study and must be adjusted to achieve forward movement of an uninterrupted column of barium through the small bowel. Too rapid infusion of the barium can result in an ileus producing barium-filled, amotile bowel loops that result in a non-diagnostic study.

Disadvantages of enteroclysis are the requirements for fluoroscopy and technical expertise. Advantages of enteroclysis over the upper gastrointestinal study are the shorter examination time, greater accuracy for the detection of morphologic disorders of the intestine, and better ability to assess small intestinal motility (during the barium infusion phase of the study). Enteroclysis has been successfully used in dogs to diagnose enteritis, villus atrophy, duodenal ulcers, intussusception, foreign bodies, strictures, and gastrointestinal neoplasia.[113] Our limited experience with the technique at UCD VMTH has been favorable.

Ultrasonography

Ultrasonography is a diagnostic technique which uses the reflection of high frequency sound waves from tissue interfaces to produce a visual image. Abdominal ultrasonography accurately depicts the size, shape, position, and spatial relationships of abdominal organs. Tissues of varying densities can be delineated, including those within an organ. Detailed information on ultrasonographic equipment, technique, and interpretation may be found elsewhere.[114-119]

Abdominal ultrasound and radiographs are complementary examinations. In contrast to radiography, the ultrasound image is enhanced by ascitic fluid and compromised by gas within any distensible viscus. Ultrasound is more sensitive than radiography for the detection of abdominal masses including intraorgan miliary masses (e.g. metastatic neoplasia), abdominal fluid, abscesses, cysts, mural thickenings, lymphadenopathy, pancreatitis, biliary obstruction, and radiolucent biliary and urinary calculi. On occasion, portal hypertension or hydronephrosis may be apparent. Furthermore, ultrasound-guided percutaneous biopsy or aspiration of organs, masses, cysts, or effusion is a safe and effective technique to obtain diagnostic material.[120,121] Additional advantages of ultrasonography are its non-invasive nature, the lack of ionizing radiation, and its ability to examine the entire abdominal cavity, not merely mucosal surfaces as is the case with endoscopy. Disadvantages of ultrasonography include the inability to penetrate bone or air, and the considerable financial investment and technical expertise required.

Ultrasonography is indicated for the evaluation of virtually any gastrointestinal or abdominal problem. Ultrasonography is very useful for the detection and characterization of experimental pancreatitis in the dog.[122] The normal pancreas cannot be visualized by ultrasonography but, during acute pancreatitis, the inflamed pancreas swells and often can be visualized. Experimental pancreatitis produces a uniform, poorly defined density in the left pancreatic lobe, dorsocaudal to the antrum and ventral and to the left of the portal vein. The ultrasound examination of the pancreas is enhanced by the introduction of fluid into the abdominal cavity, as is visualization of the liver.[123]

The ultrasonographic appearance of the stomach and intestines of the dog has recently been described.[124] In skilled hands, ultrasonography can detect mural thickenings of the gastric body, pylorus, and intestinal tract. Intussusceptions have a characteristic appearance. Ultrasound also provides information on gastrointestinal motility and in humans has been used to assess gastric emptying time.[125]

Endoscopic ultrasonography is carried out by endoscopes mounted with an ultrasound transducer at their tip, or alternatively by the passage of newly developed ultrasound probes through the operating channel of the endoscope. These instruments provide cross-sectional images of the gastrointestinal tract. They are particularly valuable for the detection of intramural lesions and evaluation of local lymph nodes. As such, they are beginning to occupy an important place in the early detection and staging of cancer.

Scintigraphy

Scintigraphy involves the administration of a radiopharmaceutical followed by scanning to determine the differential localization of the radionuclide within the tissues of the body. Nuclear imaging studies of the gastrointestinal tract are currently used in human medicine to investigate esophageal motility, gastroesophageal reflux, gastric emptying, and gastrointestinal transit time, and to detect gastrointestinal inflammation, bleeding, and protein loss. The most important applications of nuclear medicine in veterinary gastroenterology are the determination of gastric emptying time and the detection of hepatic vascular abnormalities, biliary obstruction, and gastrointestinal blood and protein loss.[126] Gastrointestinal nuclear scintigraphy has the ability to provide noninvasive, dynamic, quantitative information about organ function.[126] The most important limitations of scintigraphic techniques are their restricted availability and the necessity for several days of post-procedural hospitalization in a nuclear medicine facility until the patient has excreted sufficient radionuclide to be no longer a radiation hazard.

Scintigraphic Evaluation of Gastric Emptying. Gastric isotope scanning studies are indicated to confirm gastric emptying disorders and are especially useful after endoscopy has failed to reveal a physical obstruction to gastric outflow in a patient whose clinical history suggests delayed gastric emptying. Gastric isotope scanning has become the preferred technique for assessment of gastric emptying because of its noninvasive nature, fidelity to the physiologic process, and the ability to provide accurate quantitative or semiquantitative measurements of emptying of both liquids and solids.

Isotope scanning involves the ingestion by the patient of an intrinsically or extrinsically labeled liquid or solid meal. Gamma or scintillation counters determine the rate of emptying of the label; the counters are linked to computers to provide quantitative analysis of the scanning data. Isotopes that are most often used in humans include ^{113m}indium, ^{111}indium, ^{99m}Tc-labeled sulfur colloid attached to liver cubes, and ^{99m}Tc-labeled DTPA for liquid phase marking. An isotope in current use in the dog at the UCD VMTH is ^{99m}Tc disofennin, which after mixing with baby food and kibble provides a suitable solid phase marker.[127] Other isotopes reportedly useful for the examination of emptying time in the dog include ^{14}C polyethylene glycol, ^{57}Co cyanocobalamin, and ^{99m}Tc-DPTA.[128-130] Liquids are more easily labeled than solids, but the emptying of liquids has less clinical significance. Some investigators prefer double isotope labeling to allow individual assessment of both liquid and solid emptying.

Scintigraphy requires considerable expertise to minimize technical problems, such as straying of the label from the ingesta to gastric mucus or mucosa, and to correctly interpret the radionuclide data. Various presentations of the data have been proposed, including the time it takes for 50% emptying (suitable for liquids only), the percentage of label emptied over a set time period, the area under the emptying curve, and certain mathematical analyses of the emptying curve.[127,129,131] Gastroesophageal reflux of the label invalidates the study.

Scintigraphic Evaluation of Gastrointestinal Bleeding. Scintigraphy can aid in locating the site of gastrointestinal bleeding (see Chapter 5). In humans, various radionuclides have been utilized that vary in their sensitivity and half-life in the blood stream.[126] Agents with short half-lives are suitable for the detection of active but not recurrent bleeding. In dogs, the administration of ^{99m}Technetium-labelled red blood cells has been used to successfully locate the site of gastrointestinal bleeding.[132]

Scintigraphic Evaluation of Protein-losing Enteropathies. Tests for protein-losing enteropathy are indicated for the detection and localization of gastrointestinal protein loss. Until the advent of these tests, the diagnosis of protein-losing enteropathy was first made by excluding other causes of hypoalbuminemia, such as glomerular and liver disease, and then by acquiring a small intestinal biopsy. This "diagnosis by exclusion" runs the risk of hypoalbuminemia due to occult protein-losing enteropathies, such as lymphangiectasia, being wrongly ascribed to concomitant hepatopathies or glomerulonephropathies. Two scintigraphic techniques are available for the definitive diagnosis of protein-losing enteropathy. These are the ^{51}chromium-labeled albumin[133] and the ^{111}indium-labeled transferrin[134] tests.

NONINVASIVE BIOPSY OF THE ESOPHAGUS, STOMACH, AND INTESTINE[135,136]

A number of biopsy capsules and forceps have been designed to be passed through the mouth or through the rectum to obtain samples of gastrointestinal tissues. Unless passed alongside an endoscope, noninvasive biopsy instruments do not allow directed biopsies. Therefore, noninvasive biopsy is indicated only for the diagnosis of gastrointestinal diseases with a generalized rather than focal pattern. They are particularly useful if anesthesia is contraindicated, or if full-thickness biopsy is considered undesirable because of risk of debilitation. Multiple biopsies should be obtained from different sites to lessen the chance of missing pathological change. Noninvasive biopsy instruments acquire only mucosa, unlike full-thickness surgical biopsies, which also allow diagnosis of diseases located in the submucosa and muscularis. Suction biopsies are particularly desirable in the large bowel, where full thickness biopsies should be avoided. As discussed in Chapter 5, biopsies of the gastrointestinal tract rarely yield a causal diagnosis, but often allow a categorization of the disease process on which therapeutic and prognostic advice can be more soundly based. Biopsies of the gastrointestinal tract are contraindicated in patients with bleeding tendencies.

Suction biopsy instruments (Quinton Instruments, Seattle WA) (Figure 6-13) are the safest method for the acquisition of noninvasive biopsies. They may be used to obtain biopsies from the mucosa of the esophagus, stomach, small intestine, and large intestine. Noninvasive biopsy of the small intestine uses a single- or multiple-biopsy suction capsule (Quinton Instruments, Seattle WA) that is passed under fluoroscopic guidance into the duodenum.

Suction biopsy instruments possess a biopsy capsule at the end of a flexible insertion tube. The biopsy capsule contains a sliding, cylindrical knife and a biopsy port. The knife is connected by wire to a handpiece. The biopsy technique requires good coordination between operators, one of whom applies suction to the instrument via a large syringe, sucking a piece of mucosa into biopsy capsule (Figure 6-14). The second operator sections the aspirated tissue, applying traction to the biopsy knife by way of the handpiece. Cutting is best performed at suction pressures of 20-25 mm Hg. The biopsy capsule, containing the tissue sample, is removed from the lumen of the bowel, disassembled to retrieve the biopsy, and then reintroduced to obtain more samples. This device can be used to obtain tissue from the stomach and colon of the conscious animal with no need for sedation. The dog has a thicker mucosa than the human. As a result, suction biopsy capsules with large ports are best suited for biopsy of canine intestinal mucosa. Reasons for unsuccessful biopsy include equipment failure, the immersion of the biopsy capsule in fecal debris, and failure to aspirate air from the viscus being biopsied. The latter may result from failure to apply the biopsy port of the capsule to a mucosal surface or inability of the tightly stretched mucosa to be suctioned into the capsule.

Speculum forceps biopsy instruments are a less desirable way to obtain noninvasive biopsies. They are occasionally used to biopsy the large bowel. These instruments are particularly likely to cause perforation of the bowel but can be useful, especially if the bowel is poorly prepared, thus inactivating the suction biopsy instruments. One should never *depress* the bowel wall with the open jaws of the forceps and then biopsy. Instead, one should use the three-stage biopsy technique. This entails the following: Lightly grasp the mucosa with the biopsy jaws, gently pull the mucosa towards the center of the bowel lumen, and then severe the tissue (Figure 6-15). In most cases this technique allows the serosal and muscular layers of the bowel to slip out from the grasp of the biopsy instrument's jaws, avoiding perforation.

Biopsy specimens should be handled gently, should not be allowed to dry, and should be placed on some support such as a piece of cardboard or tongue depressor to minimize contrac-

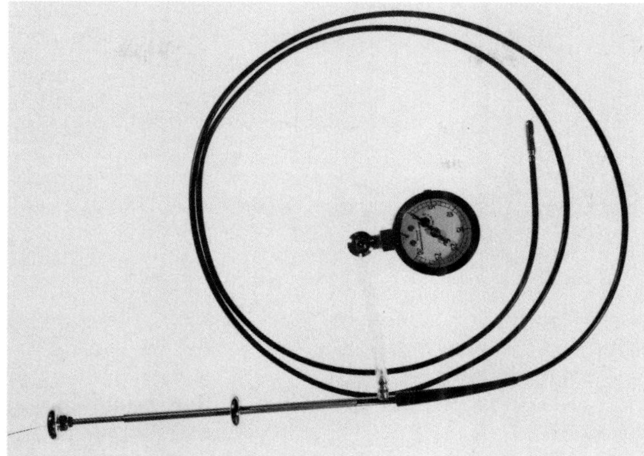

Figure 6-13. (above) Quinton biopsy instrument employing a Crosby capsule can be passed orally to obtain biopsies of the stomach and rectally to obtain biopsies of the colon (shorter cables are designed for colon biopsy). Closeup (below) shows the capsule with its port into which mucosal tissue is drawn in by vacuum and the knife with its wire that is drawn to cut a biopsy sample from the mucosa.

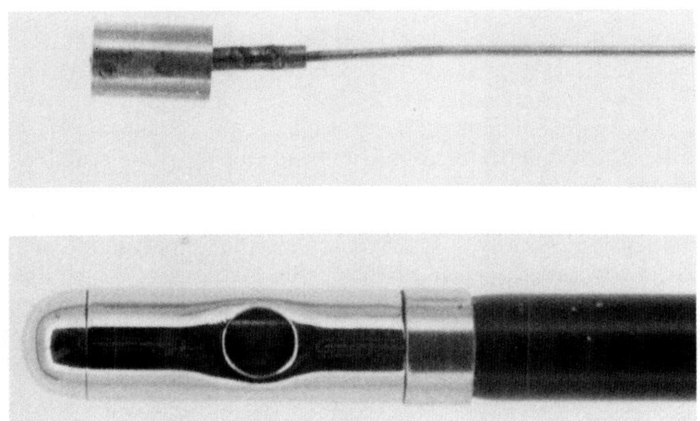

Figure 6-14. Drawing showing retrieval of mucosal biopsy with capsule biopsy instrument.

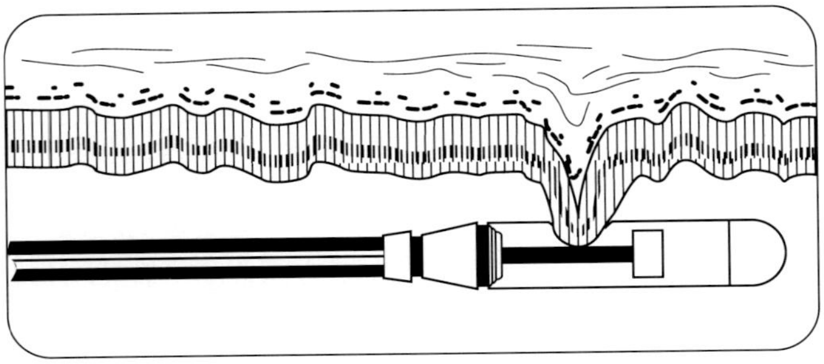

tion and preserve orientation. Always mount the mucosa upwards.

The most important complications of noninvasive biopsy are gastrointestinal perforation and hemorrhage. If perforation is suspected, it can usually be readily confirmed by the radiographic demonstration of free abdominal gas. If perforation is confirmed, immediate abdominal lavage and surgical repair of the defect are indicated. Significant hemorrhage from a gastrointestinal biopsy site is not common, but when it does occur it can be easily overlooked because of the reservoir capacity of the bowel. Therefore, it is prudent to observe patients closely after biopsy for clinical evidence of hemorrhage or for a rapidly declining PCV and total plasma protein. Most cases of biopsy-related gastrointestinal hemorrhage can be handled by the administration of fresh whole blood without the need for surgical intervention.

Evaluation of Brush Border Enzyme Activity

Unlike many other tissues of the body, serum concentrations of intestinal enzymes are not good markers of intestinal disease, because damaged and dying mucosal cells are sloughed into the lumen of the bowel with minimal resorption of their contents in an intact form.[137] Brush border enzyme activity can, however, be assayed on biopsy samples. The primary indication for brush border enzyme analysis is the diagnosis of congenital disaccharidase deficiencies that can result in carbohydrate malabsorption. The assay of brush border enzymes has also been proposed as an objective and sensitive measure of acquired small intestinal diseases.[138] For instance, in a series of dogs with bacterial overgrowth, pronounced brush border enzyme defects were observed consistently, whereas only a select few of the dogs had histologically recognizable lesions.

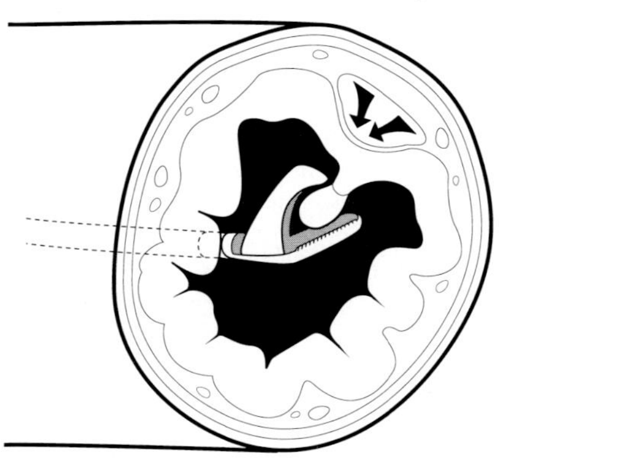

Figure 6-15. Biopsy of mucosa using forceps. Mucosa is pulled away from intestinal wall before mucosal tissue is severed.

The jejunum represents the greatest part of the digestive and absorptive area of the small intestine. The maltase activity in the jejunum is much greater than that of sucrase and lactase.[68] The ratio of maltase to sucrase to lactase is 10:2:0. Normal jejunal mucosal maltase, sucrase, and lactase activities in the dog are 38, 7.8, and 3.5 μmoles/g wet mucosa/minute (comparable to levels in human intestinal mucosa). Composition of the diet influences the levels of brush-border enzyme activity. The activities of these enzymes are decreased by enteritis or by any acute insult that damages the mucosal surface. Alterations in brush border enzyme activity have been reported in various canine intestinal diseases such as wheat-sensitive enteropathy of Irish Setters,[139] a sprue-like condition,[138] and bacterial overgrowth.[138]

PARACENTESIS AND DIAGNOSTIC PERITONEAL LAVAGE

Paracentesis

Paracentesis is indicated if abdominal fluid is detected during physical examination or diagnostic imaging. It provides fluid for culture, cytology, and chemical analysis, thus allowing the characterization of the effusion and markedly narrowing the diagnostic possibilities. Ultrasound guidance aids aspiration of localized collections of fluid.

The preferred site for paracentesis is the caudal abdomen. In male dogs a suitable site is just to the right of the prepuce. In bitches and cats an analogous site can be used. The advantage of such a caudal placement is the avoidance of the omentum, which frequently blocks the lumen of needles placed more cranially. The disadvantage of this site is its proximity to the bladder, which should always be emptied before the procedure. If this site does not yield fluid, up to three other quadrants may be penetrated. Suitable needles for paracentesis are 1-2 inch, 14-20 gauge. The needle is best inserted slowly to assist judgement of depth and lessen the likelihood of penetrating a viscus. Local anesthesia is usually not required.

Diagnostic Peritoneal Lavage

Diagnostic peritoneal lavage (DPL) is indicated if paracentesis fails to yield abdominal fluid, and yet there is a high likelihood of abdominal disease. Using an 18 gauge needle and an intravenous administration set, 20 ml/kg of warm sodium chloride or lactated Ringer's solution is infused into the abdomen. The needle is removed and the animal's abdomen gently manipulated. Altering the patient's body position also helps distribute the fluid. After several minutes, the abdominal tap is repeated and the abdominal fluid examined. Diagnostic criteria for DPL have been established to account for the dilution effects of the infused fluid. For instance, significant intra-abdominal hemorrhage is probable if the microhematocrit of the lavage fluid is greater than 2%. Peritonitis is likely if the neutrophil count is greater than 1500/μml.

EXPLORATORY CELIOTOMY

Abdominal surgery is required in some patients to establish the cause of the gastrointestinal disease, and in many patients for its treatment. The rapidity with which a clinician must resort to exploratory celiotomy for diagnosis is largely a reflection of the diagnostic equipment available. Celiotomy optimizes visual inspection and palpation of abdominal organs. Indications for celiotomy include rapid progressive decline in the condition of a patient with abdominal disease, and the need for multiple organ or full-thickness biopsies. Celiotomy is required for the diagnosis of intestinal lesions out of reach of the endoscope, gastrinomas, and low grade diseases of some organs such as chronic pancreatitis. Biopsies of the intestine should be taken even when it appears normal. Biopsy artifacts are reduced by placing the sample on a supporting surface before placement in formalin.[140]

Exploratory celiotomy is contraindicated if the diagnosis can be obtained by noninvasive means and/or if the patient is an unacceptable anesthetic risk. A major complication of full-thickness biopsy of the gastrointestinal tract is wound dehiscence. The biopsy sites of debilitated and hypoalbuminemic animals are particularly likely to dehisce. In these patients, full thickness intestinal biopsy should be performed only after great circumspection, and preferably in association with parenteral nutrition support. Proper technique is essential for an effective surgical evaluation of the abdomen and its contents. Detailed description of the correct approach to the exploratory celiotomy is available.[141-143]

REFERENCES

1. Wilson, R.B., Holladay, J.A.: Mushroom poisoning. Comp. Contin. Ed. Pract. Vet. 9:791-793, 1987.
2. Happe, R.P., De Bruijne, J.J.: Pentagastrin stimulated gastric secretion in the dog (orogastric aspiration technique). Res. Vet. Sci. 33:232-239, 1982.
3. Youngberg, C.A., Wlodyga, J., Schmaltz and Dressman, J.B.: Radiotelemetric determination of gastrointestinal pH in four healthy beagles. Am. J. Vet. Res. 46:1516-1521, 1985.
4. Walt, R.P.: Twenty four hour intrragastric acidity analysis for the future. Gut. 27:1-9, 1986.
5. Straus, E., Johnson, G.F., and Yalow, R.S.: Canine Zollinger Ellison syndrome. Gastroenterology 72:380-381, 1977.
6. Marks, I.N., Komarov, S.A. and Shay, H.: Maximal secretory response to histamine and its relation to parietal cell mass in the dog. Amer. J. Physiol. 199:579-588, 1960.
7. Ward, S., Gillespie, I.E., Passaro, E.P. and Grossman, M.I.: Comparison of histalog and histamine as stimulants for maximal gastric secretion in human subjects and in dogs. Gastroenterology 44:620-626, 1963.
8. Gabbert, N.H., Nachreiner, R.F., Holmes-Word, P. and Kivela, J.H.: Serum immunoreactive gastrin concentrations in the dog. Basal and postprandial values measured by radioimmunoassay. Am. J. Vet. Res. 45:2351-2353, 1984.
9. Middleton, D.J., Watson, A.D.: Duodenal ulceration associated with gastrin-secreting pancreatic tumor in a cat. JAVMA 183:461-462, 1983.
10. Breitschwerdt, E.B., Turj, J.R., Turnwald, G.H.: Hypergastrinemia in canine gastrointestinal disease. JAVMA 22:585-592, 1986.
11. Brooks, F.P.: Tests related to the stomach. In, Bockus Gastroenterology. Edited by Haubrich, W.S., Klaser, M.H., Roth, J.L., Schaffner, F. WB Saunders, Philadelphia 367- 377, 1985.
12. Graves, G.M., Becht, J.L. and Rawlings, C.A.: Metoclopramide reversal of decreased gastrointestinal myoelectric and contractile activity in a model of canine postoperative ileus. Vet. Surg. 18:27-33, 1989.
13. Bellahsene, B.E., Schirmer, B. and McCallum, R.: Validation of cutaneous EGG recordings by comparing with recordings from intragastric surgically implanted electrodes. Gastroenterology 92:1313, 1987.
14. Mathias, J.R., Sninsky, C.A., Millar, H.D.: Development of an improved multi-pressure sensor probe for recording muscle contraction in human intestine. Dig. Dis. Sci. 30:119, 1985.
15. Strombeck, D.R., Turner, W.D. and Harrold, D.: Eructation of gas through the gastroesophageal sphincter before and after gastric fundectomy in dogs. Am. J. Vet. Res. 49:87-89, 1988.
16. Strombeck, D.R., Harrold, D.: Anal sphincter pressure and the rectosphinteric reflex in the dog. Am. J. Vet. Res. 49:191-192, 1988.
17. Beeler, M.F. and Kao, Y.S.: Laboratory evaluation of pancreatic disorders. In, Clinical Diagnosis. Edited by I. Davidson and J.B. Henry. W.B. Saunders and Company, Philadelphia. 1974.
18. Beeler, M.F. and Kao, Y.S.: Examination of Feces. In, Clinical Diagnosis. Edited by I. Davidsohn and J.B. Henry, W.B. Saunders and Company, Philadelphia. 1974.
19. Burrows, C.F., Merrit, A.M. and Chiapella, A.M.: Determination of fecal fat and trypsin output in the evaluation of chronic canine diarrhea. JAVMA 174:62-66, 1979.
20. Drummey, G.D., Benson, J.A. and Jones, C.M.: Microscopic examination of the stool for steatorrhea. New Engl. J. Med. 264:85, 1961.
21. Siegel, D., Cohen, P.T., Neighbor, M., Larkin, H., Newman, M., Yajko, D. and Hadley, K.: Predictive value of stool examination in acute diarrhea. Arch. Pathol. Lab. Med. 111:715-718, 1987.
22. Pickering, L.K., DuPont, H.L., Olarte, J., Conklin, R. and Ericsson, C.: Fecal leukocytes in enteric infections. Am. J. Clin. Path. 68:562-565, 1977.
23. Hay, W.H., Chickering, W.R., Roth, L. and Leib, M.S.: Rectal cytology as a diagnostic aid in the evaluation of large bowel diarrhea in dogs. Abstract ACVIM Proceedings, 743, 1988.
24. Twedt, D.C., Jones, R.L., Collins, J.K. and Ogilive, G.: *Clostridium perfringens* enterotoxin associated with diarrhea in dogs. Abstract ACVIM Proceedings, 1046, 1989.
25. Georgi, J.R.: Parasitology for Veterinarians. WB Saunders, Philadelphia, 1974.
26. Zimmer, J.F., Burrington, D.B.: Comparison of four techniques of fecal examination for detecting canine giardiasis. J.A.A.H.A. 22:161-167, 1986.
27. Baker, D.G., Strombeck, D.R. and Gershwin, L.J.: Laboratory diagnosis of *Giardia duodenalis* infection in dogs. JAVMA 190:53-56, 1987.
28. Hahn, N.E., Glaser, C.A., Hird, D.W. and Hirsh, D.C.: Prevalence of Giardia in the feces of pups. JAVMA 192:1428-1429, 1988.
29. Current, W.L.: Cryptospoidiosis. JAVMA 187:1334-1338, 1985.
30. Bielsa, L.M., Greiner, E.C.: Liver flukes (*Platynosomum concinnum*) in cats. J.A.A.H.A. 16:269-274, 1985.
31. Green, C.E.: Enteric bacterial infections. In, Clinical Microbiology and Infectious Diseases of the Dog and Cat. WB Saunders, Philadelphia, 624-628, 1984.
32. Green, C.E.: Gastrointestinal, intra-abdominal, and hepatobiliary infections. In, Clinical Microbiology and Infectious Diseases of the Dog and Cat. Edited by C.E. Green. WB Saunders, Philadelphia, 247-268, 1984.
33. Shotts, E.B.: Laboratory diagnosis of bacterial infections. In, Clinical Microbiology and Infectious Diseases of the Dog and Cat. Edited by C.E. Green. WB Saunders, Philadelphia, 121-136, 1984.
34. Whitaker, H.S., Alderson, C.: The use of negative contrast electron microscopy for diagnosis of viral infections in animals. 23rd Ann Proc. Amer. Assoc. Vet. Lab. Diag. 321-350, 1980.
35. McGuire, S.J., Castro, A.E. and Stair, E.L.: Comparison of the

methods used in a diagnostic laboratory for the detection of canine parvovirus in dogs. 26th Ann. Proc. Amer. Assoc. Vet. Lab Diag. 345-364, 1984.

36. Hammond, G.W., Hazelton, P.R., Chuang, I. and Klisko, B.: Improved detection of viruses by electron microscopy after direct ultracentrifuge preparation of specimens. J. Clin. Microbiology 14:210-221, 1981.

37. Trampel, D.W., Kinden, D.A., Solorzano, R.F. and Stogsdill, P.L.: Parvovirus-like enteropathy in Missouri turkeys. Avian Diseases 27:49-54, 1984.

38. Ginsberg, H.S.: Reoviruses and epidemic acute gastroenteritis virus. In, Microbiology. Edited by B.D. Davis, R. Dulbecco, H.N. Eisen, H.S. Ginsberg, Harper and Row, Hagerstown. 1206-1216, 1980.

39. Guy, J.S.: Diagnosis of canine viral infections. Vet. Clin. No. Am. Small An. Pract. 16:1145-1156, 1986.

40. Fine, K.D., Krejs, G.J. and Fordtran, J.S.: Diarrhea. In, Gastrointestinal disease. Edited by Sleisenger, M.H., Fordtran, J.S. WB Saunders, Philadelphia. 290-316, 1989.

41. Boulay, J.P., Lipowitz, A.J., Klausner, J.S. and Ellefson, M.: Evaluation of a fluorometric method for the quantitative assay of fecal hemoglobin in the dog. Am. J. Vet. Res. 47:1293-1295, 1986.

42. Arvanitakis, C. and Cooke, A.R.: Diagnostic tests of exocrine pancreatic function and disease. Gastroenterology 74:932-948, 1978.

43. Westermack, E., Sandholm, M.: Fecal hydrolase activity as determined by radial enzyme diffusion: A new method for detecting pancreatic dysfunction in the dog. Res. Vet. Sci. 28:341-346, 1980.

44. Haverback, B.J., Dyce, B.J., Gutentag, P.J. and Montgomery, D.W.: Measurement of trypsin and chymotrypsin in stool. Gastroenterology 44:588-597, 1963.

45. Girella, E., Faggionato, P., Benetazzo, D. and Mastella, G.: The assay of chymotrypsin in stool as a simple and effective test of exocrine pancreatic activity in cystic fibrosis. Pancreas 3:254-262, 1988.

46. Reusch, C.: Photometrische chymotrypsinbestimmung im kot des hundes. Tierarztl Prax 14:147-152, 1986.

47. Williams, D.A.: The diagnosis of canine exocrine pancreatic insufficiency. Vet. Annual. 25:330-336, 1985.

48. Williams, D.A., Batt, R.M.: Sensitivity and specificity of radioimmunoassay of serum trypsin-like immunoreactivity for the diagnosis of canine exocrine pancreatic insufficiency. JAVMA 192:195-201, 1988.

49. Williams, D.A., Reed, S.D.: Comparison of two methods for evaluation of pancreatic function in cats by assay of fecal proteolytic activity.
ACVIM Proceedings, 1047, 1989.

50. Hill, F.W.G. and Kidder, D.E.: The estimation of daily faecal trypsin levels in dogs as an indicator of gross pancreatic exocrine insufficiency. J. Small An. Pract. 11:191-195, 1970.

51. Wormsley, K.G. and Goldberg, D.M.: The interrelationships of the pancreatic enzymes. Gut 13:398-412, 1972.

52. Chung, Y.C., Kim, Y.S., Shadchehr, A., Garrido, A., MacGregor, I.L. and Sleisenger, M.H.: A study of digestion and absorption of protein meal and trypsin in human distal ileum. Gastroenterology 72:1038, 1977.

53. Lundh, G.: Pancreatic exocrine function in neoplastic and inflammatory disease: a simple and reliable new test. Gastroenterology 42:275-280, 1962.

54. Batt, R.M., Mann, L.C.: Specificity of the BT-PABA test for diagnosis of exocrine pancreatic insufficiency in the dog. Vet. Rec. 108:303-307, 1981.

55. Sateri, H.: Investigations on the exocrine pancreatic function in dogs suffering from chronic exocrine pancreatic insufficiency. Acta. Vet. Scand. Suppl. 53:1-86, 1975.

56. Freudiger, U. and Bigler, B.: Die diagnose der chronischen exokrinen pankreasinsuffizienz mit dem PABA-test. Kleinteir-Praxis 22:45 84, 1977.

57. Strombeck, D.R.: New method for evaluation of chymotrypsin deficiency in dogs. JAVMA173:1319-1323, 1978.

58. Imondi, A.R., Stradley, R.P. and Wolgemuth, R.: Synthetic peptides in the diagnosis of exocrine pancreatic insufficiency in animals. Gut 13:726-731, 1972.

59. Arvanitakis, C. and Greenberger, N.J.: Diagnosis of pancreatic disease by a synthetic peptide. Lancet i:663-666, 1976.

60. Hawkins, E.C., Meric, S.M., Washabau, R.J. and Feldman, E.C.: Digestion of bentiromide and absorption of xylose in healthy cats and absorption of xylose in cats with infiltrative intestinal disease. Am. J. Vet. Res. 47:56744-569, 1986.

61. Strombeck, D.R., Harrold, D.: Evaluation of 60 minute blood p-aminobenzoic acid concentration in pancreatic function testing of dogs. JAVMA 180:419-421, 1982.

62. Sherding, R.G., Stradley, R.P., Rogers, W.A. and Johnson, S.E.: Bentiromide:xylose test in healthy cats. Am. J. Vet. Res. 43:2272-2273, 1982.

63. Zimmer, J.F., Todd, S.E.: Further evaluation of bentiromide in the diagnosis of canine exocrine pancreatic insufficiency. Cornell Vet. 75:426-440, 1985.

64. Williams, D.A., Moore, M.: Characterization of serum trypsin-like immunoreactivity in dogs with naturally occurring fatal acute pancreatitis and severe chronic renal failure. ACVIM Proceedings, 739, 1988.

65. Williams, D.A.: New tests of pancreatic and small intestinal function. Comp. Contin. Ed. Pract. Vet. 9:1167-1173, 1987.

66. Williams, D.A., Batt, R.M.: Exocrine pancreatic insufficiency diagnosed by radioimmunoassay of serum trypsin-like immunoreactivity in a dog with a normal BT-PABA test result. JAVHA 22:671-674, 1986.

67. Wright, T.L., Heyworth, M.F.: Maldigestion and malabsorption. In, Gastrointestinal Disease. Edited by M.H. Sleisenger, J.S. Fordtran. WB Saunders, Philadelphia, 263-282, 1989.

68. Hill, F.W.G. and Kelly, D.F.: Naturally occurring intestinal malabsorption in the dog. Am J. Dig. Dis. 19:649-665, 1974.

69. Lewis, L.D., Boulay, J.P. and Chow, F.H.C.: Fat excretion and assimilation by the cat. Feline Pract. 9:46-49, 1979.

70. Losinger, R.: Unpublished observations, 1989.

71. Brobst, D.F. and Funk, A.: Simplified test of fat absorption in dogs. JAVMA 161:1412-1417, 1972.

72. Kallfelz, F.A., Norrdin, R.W. and Neal, T.M.: Intestinal absorption of oleic acid 131I and triolein 131I in the differential diagnosis of malabsorption syndrome and pancreatic dysfunction in the dog. JAVMA 153:43-46, 1968.

73. Hayden, D.W., VanKruiningen, H.J.: Control values for investigating gastrointestinal function in the dog. JAVHA 12:31-36, 1976.

74. Butler, R.N., Gehling, N.J., Lawson, M.J. and Grant, A.K.: Clinical evaluation of the 14C triolein breath test: A critical analysis. Aust. NZ J. Med. 14:111, 1984.

75. Cole, S.G., Rossi, S. and Stern, A.: Cholesteryl octanoate breath test. Gastroenterology 93:1372-1380, 1987.

76. Chastain, C.B., Guilford, W.G.: Unpublished observations, 1987.

77. Heyman, M., Desjeux, J., Grasset, E., Dumontier, A. and Lestradet, H.: Relationship between transport of D-xylose and other monosaccharides in jejunal mucosa of children. Gastroenterology 80:758-762, 1981.

78. Craig, R.M., Atkinson, A.J.: D-Xylose testing: A review. Gastroenterology 95:223-231, 1988.

79. Krawitt, E.L. and Beeken, W.L.: Limitations of the usefulness of the d-xylose absorption test. Amer. J. Clin. Path. 63:261-263, 1975.

80. Washabau, R.J., Strombeck, D.R., Buffington, C.A. and Harrold. D.: Evaluation of intestinal carbohydrate malabsorption in the dog by pulmonary hydrogen gas excretion. Am. J. Vet. Res. 47:1402-1406, 1986.

81. Washabau, R.J., Strombeck, D.R., Buffington, C.A. and Harrold, D.: Use of pulmonary hydrogen gas excretion to detect carbohydrate malabsorption in dogs. JAVMA 189:674-679, 1986.

82. Washabau, R.J., Buffington, C.A. and Strombeck, D.R.: Evaluation and mangement of carbohydrate malassimilation. In, Current Veterinary Therapy. Edited by R.W. Kirk. WB Saunders, Philadelphia, 889-892, 1986.

83. Rumessen, J.J., Kokholm, G. and Gudmand-Hoyer, E.: Meth-

odological aspects of breath hydrogen analysis. Scand. J. Clin. Lab. Invest. 47:555-560, 1987.
84. Vogelsang, H., Ferenci, P., Frotz, S.: Acidic colonic microclimate - possible reason for false negative hydrogen breath tests. Gut 29:21-26, 1988.
85. Thompson, D.G., Binfield, P., De Belder, A., O'Brien, J., Warren, S. and Wilson, M.: Extra intestinal influences on exhaled breath hydrogen measurements during the investigation of gastrointestinal disease. Gut 26:1349-1352, 1985.
86. Kerlin, P., Wong, L.: Breath hydrogen testing in bacterial overgrowth of the small intestine. Gastroenterology 95:982-988, 1988.
87. Perman, J.A., Modler, S.: Glycoproteins as substrates for production of hydrogen and methane by colonic bacterial flora. Gastroenterology 83:388-393, 1982.
88. Aarbakke, J. and Schjonsby, H.: Value of urinary simple phenol and indican determinations in the diagnosis of the stagnant loop syndrome. Scand. J. Gastroenterology 11:409-414, 1976.
89. Batt, R.M., Morgan, J.O.: Role of serum folate and vitamin B12 concentrations in the differentiation of small intestinal abnormalities in the dog. Res. Vet. Sci. 32:17-22, 1982.
90. Dill-Macky, E., Williams, D.A.: Breath 14CO2 output following oral administration of ^{14}C-D-xylose to healthy dogs. Abstract ACVIM proceedings, pg 1044, 1989.
91. Hall, E.J., Batt, R.M. and Brown, A.: Assessment of intestinal permeability using 51chromium-labelled ethylenediamine-tetra-acetate. Gastroenterology 94:1422, 1987.
92. Marks, S.L., Williams, D.A.: Cumulative urinary recovery of orally administered 51Cr-EDTA in healthy dogs. Abstract ACVIM Proceedings. 1046, 1989.
93. Cobden, I., Rothwell, J. and Axon, A.T.R.: Intestinal permeability and screening tests for coeliac disease. Gut 21:512-518, 1980.
94. Ecknauer, R., Buck, B. and Breitig, D.: An experimental model for measuring intestinal permeability. Digestion 26:24-32, 1983.
95. Hall, E.J., Rutgers, H.C. and Batt, R.M.: Evaluation of the peroral string test in the diagnosis of canine giardiasis. J. Small An. Pract. 29:177-183, 1988.
96. Morgan, J.P., Silverman, S.: Techniques of veterinary radiography. Veterinary Radiology Asociates, Davis CA, 1982.
97. Aronson, E., Carrig, C.B. and Lattimer, J.C.: Radiology of the gastrointestinal system. In, Canine and Feline Gastroenterology. Edited by B.D. Jones, W.D. Liska. WB Saunders, Philadelphia. 380-486, 1986.
98. Burt, J.K.: Contrast radiology of the gastrointestinal tract. Proceedings of 8th Kal Kan Symposium 57-63, 1984.
99. Thrall, D.E., Lewis, R.E.: (2). Gastrointestinal radiography. In, Veterinary Gastroenterology. Edited by N.V. Anderson. Lea & Febiger, Philadelphia, 59-79, 1980.
100. Thrall, D.E.: Textbook of Veterinary Diagnostic Radiology. WB Saunders Co, Philadelphia, 1986.
101. Brawner, W.R., Bartels, J.E.: Contrast radiography of the digestive tract. Vet. Clin. No. Am. 13:599-626, 1983.
102. Allan, G.S.: Radiology of the digestive system. Aust. Vet. Pract. 17:25-34, 1987.
103. Kleine, L.J.: Interpreting radiographic signs of abdominal disease. Vet. Med. 80:73-86, 1985.
104. Evans, S.M.: Double versus single contrast gastrography in the dog and cat. Vet. Radiol. 24:6-10, 1983
105. Morgan, J.P.: The upper gastrointestinal examination in the cat: Normal radiographic appearance using positive contrast media. Vet. Radiol. 22:159-169, 1981
106. O'Brien, T.R.: Radiographic Diagnosis of Abdominal Disorders in the Dog and Cat. WB Saunders Co, Philadelphia, 1978.
107. Jakovljevic, S.: Gastric radiology and gastroscopy in the dog. Vet. Annual 28:172-182, 1988.
108. Miyabayashi, T., Morgan, J.P., Atilola, A.O. and Muhumuza, L.: Small intestinal emptying times in normal Beagle dogs. Vet. Radiol. 27:164-168, 1986.
109. Burns, J., Fox, S.: The use of barium meal to evaluate total gastric emptying time in the dog. Vet. Radiol. 27:169-172, 1986.
110. Miyabayashi, T. and Morgan, J.P.: Gastric emptying in the normal dog. Vet. Radiol. 25:187-191, 1984.
111. Feldman, M., Smith, H.J., Simon, T.R.: Gastric emptying of solid radiopaque markers: studies in healthy subjects and diabetic patients. Gastroenterology 87:895, 1984.
112. Hogan, P.M., Aronson, E.: Effect of sedation on transit time of feline gastrointestinal contrast studies. Vet. Radiol. 29:85-88, 1988.
113. Wolvekamp, W.T.C.: Enteroclysis. A new radiographic technique for evaluation of the small intestine of the dog. Iowa State University Press, Ames. 1989.
114. Nyland, T.G., Park, R.D., Lattimer, J.C.: Gray-scale ultrasonography of the canine abdomen. Vet. Radiol. 22:220-227, 1981.
115. Nyland, T.G., Bernard, W.V.: Application of abdominal ultrasound. Calif. Vet. 36:21-25, 1982.
116. Nyland, T.G., Park, R.D.: Hepatic ultrasonography in the dog. Vet. Radiol. 24:77-84, 1983.
117. Rantanen, N.W., Ewing, R.L.: Principles of ultrasound application in animals. Vet. Radiol. 22:196-203, 1981.
118. Lamb, C.R., Stowater, J.L. and Pipers, F.S.: The first twenty-one years of veterinary diagnostic ultrasound-a bibliography. Vet. Radiol. 29:37-45, 1988.
119. Wrigley, R.H., Konde, L.J., Park, R.D. and Lebel, J.L.: Ultrasonographic diagnosis of portacaval shunts in young dogs. JAVMA 191:421-424, 1987.
120. Hoppe, F.E., Hager, D.A., Poulos, P.W.: A comparison of manual and automatic ultrasound-guided biopsy techniques. Vet. Radiol 27:99-101, 1986.
121. Kerr, L.Y.: Ultrasound guided biopsy. Calif.Vet. 42:9-10, 1988.
122. Nyland, T.G., Mulvany, M.H. and Strombeck, D.R.: Ultrasonographic features of experimentally induced, acute pancreatitis in the dog. Vet. Radiol. 24:260-266, 1983.
123. Miles, K.G., Lattimer, J.C., Krause, G.F., Knapp, D.W. and Sayles, C.E.: The use of intraperitoneal fluid as a simple technique for enhancing sonographic visualization of the canine pancreas. Vet. Radiol. 29:258-263, 1988.
124. Pennick, D.G.: Submitted to Vet. Radiol. 1989.
125. Bateman, D.N., Whittingham, T.A.: Gastric emptying measurement by real-time ultrasound. In, Motility of the Digestive Tract. Edited by M. Weinbeck. Raven Press, New York, 1982.
126. Koblik, P.D., Hornof, W.J.: Gastrointestinal nuclear medicine. Vet. Radiol. 26:138-142, 1985.
127. Hornof, W.J., Koblik, P.D., Strombeck, D.R., Morgan, J.P. and Hansen, G.: Scintigraphic evaluation of solid-phase gastric emptying in the dog. Vet Radiol 1989.
128. Gue, M., Fioramonti, J. and Bueno, L.: A simple double radiolabeled technique to evaluate gastric emptying of canned food meal in dogs. Gastroenterol Clin. Biol. 12:425-430, 1988.
129. Van den Brom, W.E., Happe, R.P.: Gastric emptying of a radionuclide-labeled test meal in healthy dogs: A new mathematical analysis and reference values. Am. J. Vet. Res. 47:2170-2174, 1986.
130. Lawaetz, O., Olesen, H.P. and Andreasen, R.: Evaluation of gastric emptying by a simple isotope technique. Scand. J. Gastroenterology 16:737-748, 1981.
131. McCallum, R.W.: Motor function of the stomach in health and disease. In, Gastrointestinal Disease. Edited by M.H. Sleisenger, J.S. Fordtran. WB Saunders Co, Philadelphia 675-713, 1989.
132. Metcalf, M.R.: Scintigraphic gastrointestinal bleeding localization with 99mTc-labeled red blood cells. Vet. Radiol. 28:96-100, 1987.
133. Finco, D.R., Duncan, J.R., Schall, W.P., Hooper, B.E., Chandler, F.W. and Keating, K.A.: Chronic enteric disease and hypoproteinemia in nine dogs. JAVMA 163:262-271, 1973.
134. Berry, C.R., Koblik, P.D. and Guilford, W.G.: Unpublished observations, 1989.
135. Kasper, J.B., Chiapella, A.M.: Gastrointestinal biopsy techniques. In, Current Veterinary Therapy VII. Edited by R.W. Kirk. WB Saunders, Philadelphia, 962-969, 1980.
136. Bradley, R.L.: Digestive tract biopsy in dogs and cats. Mod.

Vet. Pract. 66:614-620, 1985.
137. Goldberg, D.M.: The enzymology of intestinal disease. Clin. Biochem. 20:63-72, 1987.
138. Batt, R.M.: New approaches to malabsorption in dogs. Comp. Contin. Ed. Pract. Vet. 8:783-794, 1986.
139. Batt, R.M., Carter, M.W. and McLean, L.: Wheat-sensitive enteropathy in Irish setter dogs: possible age-related brush border abnormalities. Res. Vet. Sci. 39:80-83, 1985.
140. Fenwick, B.W., Kruckenberg, S.: Comparison of methods used to collect canine intestinal tissues for histologic examination. Am. J. Vet. Res. 48:1276-1281, 1987.
141. Crowe, D.T.: The steps to arresting abdominal hemorrhage. Vet. Med. 83:676-677, 1988.
142. Crowe, D.T.: Dealing with visceral injuries of the cranial abdomen. Vet. Med. 83:682-699, 1988.
143. Crowe, D.T.: What to do with disorders of the caudal abdomen. Vet. Med. 83:700-709, 1988.
144. Animal Health Laboratories Network News. MAF Qual Animal Health Laboratory Network, Ministry of Agriculture and Fisheries, New Zealand. Vetscript. July, 1989.

Chapter 7

Gastrointestinal Endoscopy

INTRODUCTION

Endoscopy is the visual inspection of the viscera or cavities of the body by use of an optical instrument. In the decade since the first reviews of veterinary endoscopy,[1-6] the popularity of this procedure has increased considerably. The increase in favor of endoscopy reflects both the usefulness of endoscopy as a diagnostic and therapeutic modality and also the economic benefit from its use.

INDICATIONS & LIMITATIONS

General

Endoscopy is a relatively non-invasive, atraumatic technique that permits visual examination of gastrointestinal lesions and allows descriptive or photographic documentation of their severity and extent. Endoscopy provides biopsy, cytological, and fluid samples for laboratory evaluation. It allows therapeutic interventions such as foreign body retrieval, bougienage, and gastrostomy tube placement. It has a low morbidity and mortality but should only be used after routine workup has failed to reveal a diagnosis. Endoscopy is of most use for the diagnosis of esophageal, gastric, upper small intestinal, and colonorectal disorders with a mucosal or luminal location. Endoscopy detects morphologic but not functional disease. It will not detect abnormal gastrointestinal motility, gastrointestinal hypersecretory disorders, and subcellular defects such as brush border enzyme deficiencies. Furthermore, mid-small intestinal disease and mural lesions are difficult to assess with an endoscope. The clinical problems commonly evaluated by upper and lower gastrointestinal endoscopy are listed in Tables 7-1 and 7-2, respectively. The most frequent gastrointestinal endoscopic procedure at the UCD VMTH is the gastroduodenoscopy (Figure 7-1).

Endoscopy Versus Contrast Radiography

Upper gastrointestinal contrast radiography and endoscopy are complementary procedures. Contrast procedures do not require anesthesia, and they provide a better estimation of luminal diameter (esophagus), mural masses, extramural compressive lesions, jejunal diseases, gastrointestinal motility, and gastric emptying. Endoscopy is more sensitive for the diagnosis of mucosal diseases of the upper gastrointestinal tract and offers the important advantage of definitive diagnosis through biopsy.

The prime function of the esophagus is one of motility. Disordered motility from esophageal neuromuscular disease is the most common cause of esophageal dysfunction. Therefore, in most cases of suspected esophageal disease barium swallows, preferably with fluoroscopy, are performed before endoscopy.

The prime functions of the stomach are motility and secretion. However, most gastrointestinal disorders associated with overt evidence of upper gastrointestinal disease are a result of morphologic rather than functional disease. Furthermore, many functional disorders of gastric motility or secretion are a consequence of morphologic disease. Radiography is less sensitive than endoscopy for the detection of morphologic disease of the stomach in the dog;[7] it can localize morphologic disease but can rarely define its cause. Therefore, in most cases of suspected gastroduodenal disease endoscopic examination should precede contrast radiographic procedures. If morphologic disease is ruled out, radiographic procedures can then be used to assess motility, and gastric pH tests can be used to assess hydrochloric acid secretion. When endoscopy was used prior to contrast radiography for the diagnosis of suspected upper gastrointestinal disease in a series of human patients, only 5% of

Table 7-1 Principal Indications For Upper Gastrointestinal Endoscopy

Evaluation of dysphagia
Evaluation of regurgitation
Evaluation of chronic vomiting
Evaluation of hematemesis
Evaluation of melena
Evaluation of chronic diarrhea.
Retrieval of esophageal foreign bodies
Bougienage of esophageal strictures
Retrieval of select gastric foreign bodies
Placement of percutaneous gastrostomy tubes

Table 7-2 Principal Indications For Large Bowel Endoscopy

Persistent hematochezia	Chronic diarrhea
Persistent tenesmus	Fecal incontinence
Persistent mucoid stools	Dyschezia

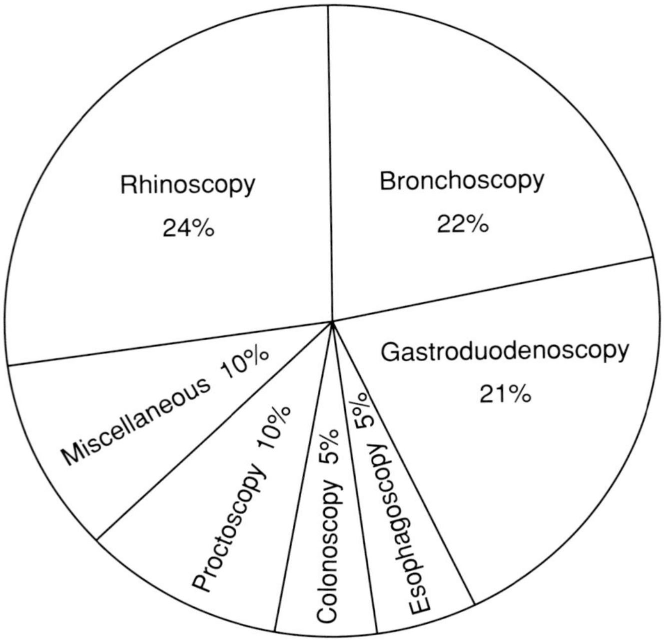

Figure 7-1. Graph of the frequency of the endoscopic procedures commonly performed at the UCD VMTH.

the persons subsequently required barium studies. In comparison, when contrast radiographs was the first procedure, 30% of the patients subsequently required endoscopy.[8]

Radiographic procedures are a poorly sensitive technique for the evaluation of the large bowel in comparison to endoscopy. Barium enemas do not reveal functional abnormalities or many mucosal changes and are limited to identifying marked mass lesions or stricture formation.

Proctoscopy Versus Colonoscopy

In the opinion of the authors, rigid proctoscopy is the technique of choice for the initial evaluation of previously untreated, uncomplicated large bowel disease. Rigid proctoscopy does not require anesthesia, and it entails less risks, time, and cost than colonoscopy, yet it is adequate to diagnose the majority of diffuse large bowel diseases. Furthermore, the majority of large bowel adenocarcinomas are located in the distal large bowel.[9] Colonoscopy should be performed prior to rigid proctoscopy following no response to therapy appropriate to colitis; with an increased likelihood of upper colonic disease (for instance persistent hematochezia without tenesmus); with suspected enterocolitis (concomitant endoscopic examination of both the small and large bowel is indicated in this situation); or with indications to effectively evaluate the extent disease (e.g. prior to surgical resection) or with the need to have a photographic record. Colonoscopy is indicated as a followup to rigid proctoscopy if a diagnosis is not apparent using rigid proctoscopy, or if the patient has not responded to prior therapy dictated by a previous proctoscopic examination.

CONTRAINDICATIONS

With the exception of animals unfit for anesthesia, there are few absolute contraindications to performing gastrointestinal endoscopy. The procedure is not appropriate if bowel perforation is suspected, because contamination of the surrounding tissues may increase as a result of the pressurization of the gastrointestinal tract by air insufflation. Endoscopy is discouraged in inadequately prepared animals and in animals with bleeding diatheses.

COMPLICATIONS

The principal complications of gastrointestinal endoscopy are shown in Table 7-3. Perforation of the gastrointestinal wall, with resultant mediastinitis, pleuritis, or peritonitis, can result from forceful insertion of the endoscope, especially during inadequate vision of the lumen, or more commonly from poor biopsy technique. If a perforation is suspected, immediate radiography usually confirms the diagnosis as large quantities of air rapidly escape the viscus to enter the surrounding body cavity. Small perforations are difficult to detect by endoscopy. Gastric-dilatation-volvulus can occur during preparation with oral lavage solutions or following endoscopic procedures, perhaps due to inadequate removal of insufflated air. Overdistention of the stomach with air during the procedure results in pronounced antral contractions, decreased tidal volume, compression of the caudal vena cava and a rapid drop in venous return and blood pressure (Figure 7-2). Unless rapidly recognized and corrected, this event is quickly fatal. Acute bradycardia, apparently due to vagovagal reflexes, can occur during endoscopy. This phenomenon most often occurs when the instrument enters the small intestine of small breeds; it is

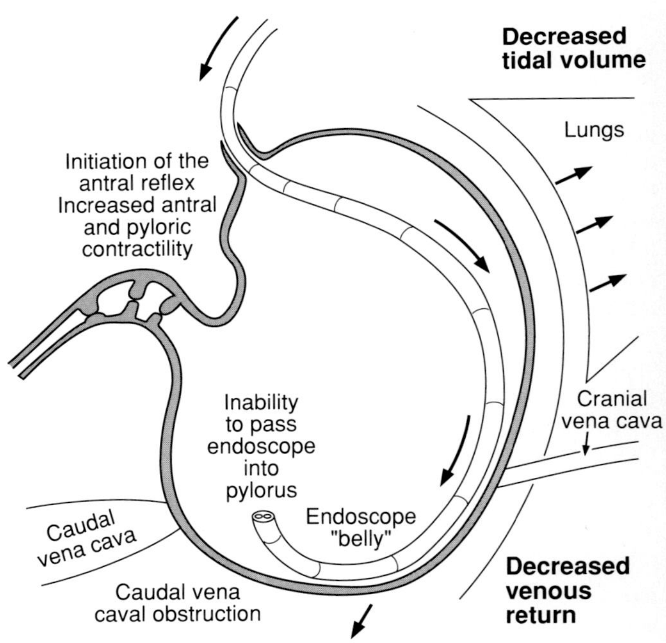

Figure 7-2. Schematic showing consequences of gastric overdistention.

perhaps caused by overdistention of the intestinal tract or by excessive traction on the mesentery. Rupture of major blood vessels can occur during removal of foreign bodies and during bougienage. Rarely, considerable hemorrhage can follow biopsy procedures. Poorly disinfected scopes can transmit enteropathogenic organisms. Following routine endoscopy, oropharyngeal or colonic organisms can be transiently cultured from the blood of 3%-8% of human patients.

EQUIPMENT

An appropriate selection of endoscopic equipment for a particular practice depends on the nature of the practice and requires an understanding of the range of equipment available and of the purposes for which that equipment is best suited.

Rigid Endoscopes

The rigid endoscopes now in common use consist of hollow plastic or metal insertion tubes with an accompanying light source, obturator, and insufflation bag (Figure 7-3). The plastic insertion tubes are disposable but can be reused. Most rigid endoscopes have a length of approximately 25 cm and an outside diameter of 20 mm. They are more durable, cheaper to purchase, and easier to use and clean than fiberoptic endoscopes. They are most commonly used for proctoscopy for which they are very effective. They allow visualization of the descending colon and rectum only. Rigid endoscopes are sometimes useful in the examination of the esophagus.

Fiberoptic Endoscopes

Flexible fiberoptic endoscopes consist of several components, the insertion tube, the hand piece, and the "umbilical cord." The insertion tube (Figure 7-4) is flexible and contains glass fiber bundles for both the transmittance and receiving of light. Fiberoptic bundles are fragile and can be damaged by inappropriate handling. Broken fiberoptic light-receiving bundles leave black specks in the field of vision. The insertion tube also has a biopsy and suction channel, an air and water channel, and deflection cables. The air/water channel is for insufflation of a viscus and cleaning the lens of debris. The distal tip of the insertion tube can be deviated by deflection knobs on the handpiece. The "umbilical cord" conveys light from the light source to the endoscope via fiberoptic bundles. Many types of fiberoptic endoscopes have been designed. Their suitability for different endoscopic procedures and for the diverse requirements of individual veterinary practices are discussed in the section on features of flexible endoscopes.

Video Endoscopes

The recently introduced video endoscope differs considerably from the fiberoptic endoscope. It has no fiberoptic bundles for receipt of light. Instead, a microelectronic chip (charge-coupled device), located on the distal tip of the instrument, receives the image, which wires transmit to the videoprocessor and monitor. This results in superior image resolution and a more robust scope. The image is integrated by the videoprocessor and projected onto a monitor. Video endoscopes have freeze frame capabilities for close examination of lesions, allow better permanent documentation of examinations, create an atmosphere of team participation, facilitate coordination of biopsy and retrieval procedures, are less fatiguing, and greatly facilitate teaching. At present, video endoscopes are not available in as small a diameter as fiberoptic scopes (smallest 9.5 mm), and a videosystem is more expensive than a fiberoptic system. The latter disadvantage may be defrayed by greater longevity.

Features and Characteristics of Flexible Endoscopes

Price. In general, the price of an endoscope reflects its quality. Savings can be made via purchase of used equipment or demonstration models.

Working Length. Most pediatric gastroscopes -- the most common scope used for upper GI exams in small animals -- have a 100-110 cm working length. This working length is adequate for the majority of gastrointestinal examinations in the small animal patient, with the exception of duodenoscopy of large breed dogs, for which endoscopes of 130 cm or greater are needed.

Insertion Tube Diameter. Gastrointestinal endoscopes range in diameter from 7.8-14 mm. The smaller diameter scopes are easier to insert, but they have diminished clarity and brightness due to smaller and fewer fiber bundles (other things being equal) and provide smaller biopsies. In general, for gastrointestinal endoscopy of dogs and cats the insertion tube diameter should be less than 10 mm. The smaller diameter endoscopes are very useful for feline duodenoscopy.

Biopsy Channel. Endoscopes designed for therapeutics (e.g. polypectomy) often have two operating channels. One operating channel suffices for veterinary endoscopy. Most gastrointestinal endoscopes have 2, 3 or 4 mm channels. The diameter of the biopsy channel and the length of the endoscope dictate the compatibility of through-the-scope accessories.

Tip Deflection. Most gastrointestinal endoscopes have four-way tip deflection. The maximum bending angle in each direction of deflection varies considerably with manufacturer and scope diameter. In general, gastrointestinal endoscopes should have at least 180-210 degree deflection in one direction and a minimum of 90-100 degree deflection in the other three directions. The greater the tip deflection, and the smaller the bending radius, the greater the maneuverability of the scope.

Direction of View. Forward viewing endoscopes are necessary for veterinary endoscopy. Side viewing scopes, utilized for certain catheterization techniques in humans, have not found an application in veterinary patients.

Angle of View. Most scopes have a field of view of 90-120 degrees. A wide angle of view facilitates orientation and panoramic examination, decreasing the likelihood of missing lesions due to tunnel vision.

Optics: The quality of an endoscope's optics is reflected in its depth of field, image resolution, image brightness, color rendition, evenness of illumination, image size, contrast range, and absence of artifacts such as flare. Acceptable depth of field for most purposes is 3-100 mm. Minimum visible distance greater than 3-5 mm compromises detailed examination of the mucosal surface. Image brightness is of particular importance in a large viscus. Without adequate brightness the stomach, for

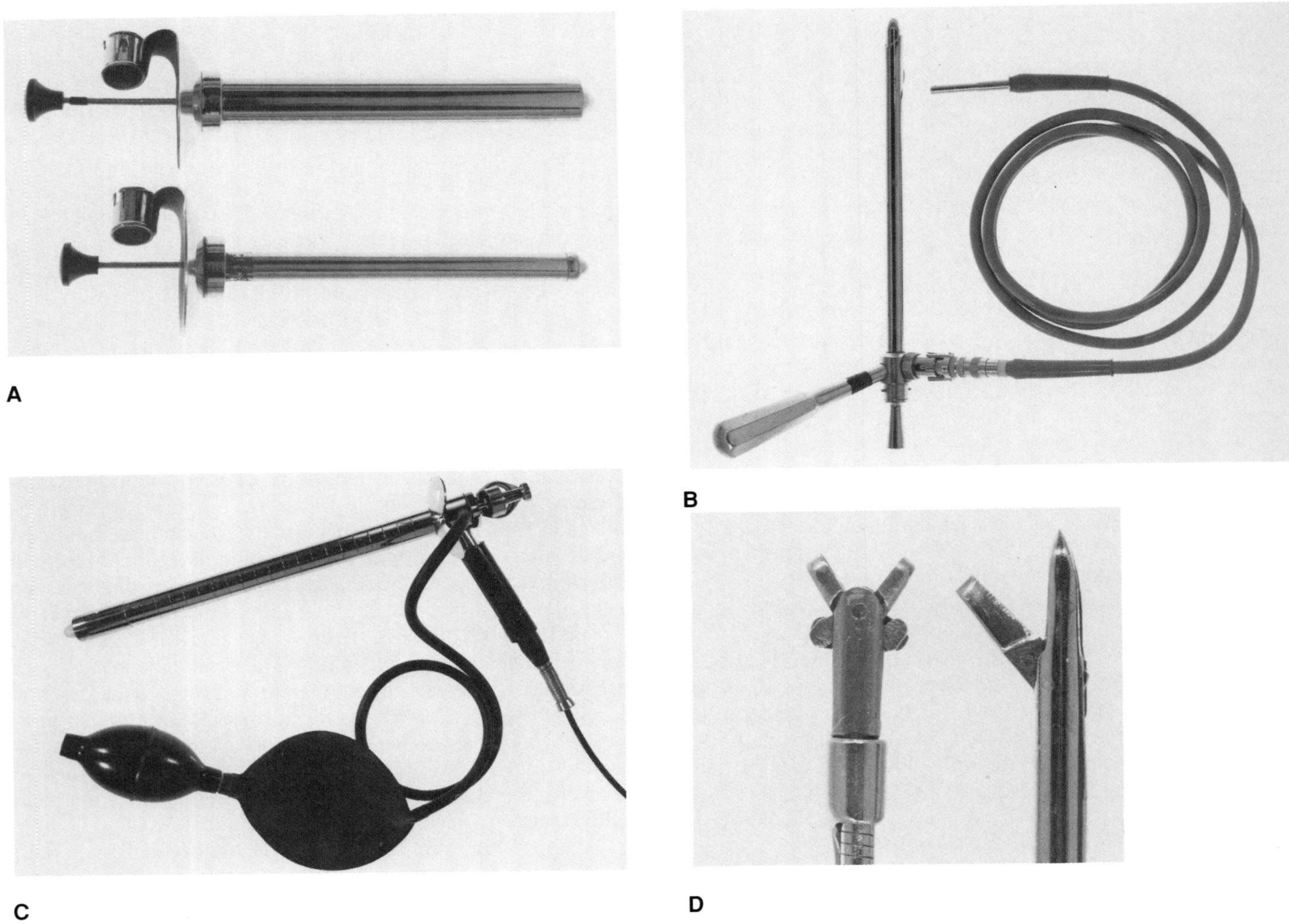

Figure 7-3. A) Rigid proctoscopes, B) Stortz rectal sigmoidoscope with cable to light source, C) Welch Allyn sigmoidoscope, D) Stortz biopsy forcep (left) and Wolf O'Connor biopsy forcep (right).

instance, may appear dark, prohibiting a panoramic examination. A wide contrast range allows vision in both shadowed and exposed areas of the bowel.

Handling. Endoscopes must be comfortable to hold in one hand, operating controls should be in easy reach; and biopsy channels must accept instruments easily, even while the tip is deflected.

Miscellaneous. The compatibility of an endoscope with any other endoscopy equipment owned by the practice is an advantage. The endoscope must be durable. Fully immersible endoscopes are easier to clean and may be more hardy.

Light and Vacuum Sources. Flexible endoscopes utilize halogen or xenon "cold" light sources of 150 to 300 watts. High light intensity is necessary for panoramic views of a large viscus and for photography. Fiberoptic and video endoscopes use continuous or strobed light sources, respectively. Videoprocessors integrate and project the video image. They can be used as a continuous light source for standard fiberoptic instruments. Light sources vary considerably in the sophistication with which they regulate illumination and in their efficiency at insufflation and flushing. A vacuum source is necessary for the aspiration of gastrointestinal fluid. Many varieties of pumps are available.

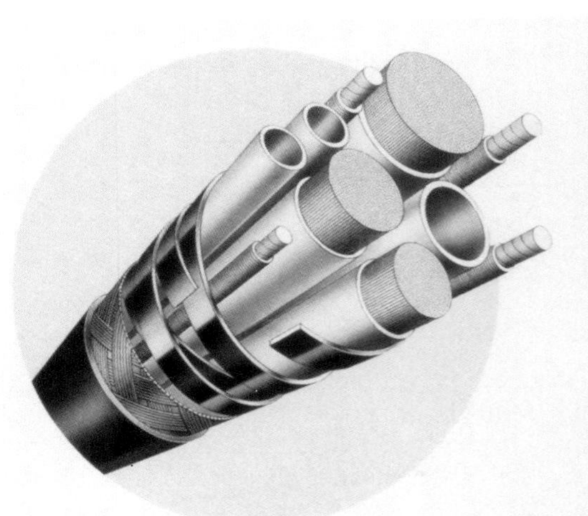

Figure 7-4. Cross-section of endoscope insertion tube showing glass bundles, channels, and deflection cables.

Endoscopic Accessories

Biopsy forceps, retrieval equipment, and cleaning accoutrements are essential endoscopic accessories. Useful but not essential accessories include cytology and culture brushes, mucus traps, polypectomy snares, endoscopic aspiration needles, balloon dilators or bougies, percutaneous endoscopic gastrostomy sets, camera equipment, videorecorders, adapters, procedure carts, endoscope storage cabinets, and endoscope washers.

Biopsy Equipment. The biopsy equipment should include two or three flexible pinch biopsy instruments. These instruments are flexible, through-the-endoscope forceps possessing at their distal end two opposing 2-3 mm cups with either smooth or serrated edges. Opening and closing is controlled by a handpiece at the proximal end of the instrument. Spiked models can facilitate biopsy in tubular lumens. Pinch biopsy equipment provides targeted biopsies.

The Quinton suction biopsy capsule (Quinton Instrument Co, Seattle WA) is the preferred instrument for non-targeted biopsy of the esophagus and descending colon. On occasion hand-held, speculum biopsy forceps with large diameter biopsy cups may be necessary for biopsy of the colon. A variety of types and sizes are available. They are the least desirable way to biopsy the colon.

Retrieval Equipment. Retrieval equipment should include through-the-endoscope equipment such as a basket retrieval instrument, a three- or four-prong grasper, and/or some form of jawed grasper, such as a rat tooth grasper. In addition it is helpful to attain some form of long, semi-rigid grasping instrument, such as are available in many hardware stores, for the removal of proximal esophageal foreign bodies.

Cytology Brushes. Shielded, through-the-endoscope cytology brushes are available for the attainment of targeted brush cytology specimens.

Balloon Dilators and Bougies. Suitable balloon dilators for gastrointestinal work have a 15-20 mm inflatable diameter with 6-8 cm lengths. Shorter lengths are inadequate for long strictures, as they may not extend past the margins of the lesion and therefore are difficult to keep in position during inflation. Rigid bougies are less desirable than balloon dilators because they produce less radial force and more shearing forces; however, they are still effective in many situations.

Cleaning Equipment. Cleaning equipment usually consists of cleaning brushes for passage through the operating channels of the scope and cleaning solutions such as glutaraldehyde. Gas sterilization is possible also. Manufacturers' recommendations should be followed closely.

ENDOSCOPIC TECHNIQUE

Patient Preparation

Gastroscopy. The patient should be starved for 12-24 hours, or longer if there is evidence of delayed gastric emptying. Retained gastric material interferes with visualization, may plug the endoscope, and may result in aspiration during recovery.

Colonoscopy. Adequate preparation is essential for effective evaluation and biopsy of the mucosa and for preservation of equipment. Considerable variation in technique is reported. A period of starvation is essential. Three days of starvation is ideal (where possible, begun at home), two days will often suffice, and one day is rarely adequate. The most effective cleansing of the entire colon, with the least attendant artifacts, is attained by the use of intestinal lavage solutions (CoLyte, Endlaw preps, NY; Golytely, Braintree Labs, MA). These solutions contain polyethylene glycol, which acts as an osmotic agent, and replacement electrolytes. They are administered in volumes of 20-30 ml/kg by stomach tube three to four times over a period of 12-24 hours prior to the procedure. Three to four hours should separate stomach tubings, and the last administration should be no less than four hours before premedication for anesthesia. Pretreatment with acetylpromazine facilitates ease of stomach tubing and reduces the likelihood of vomition. Metoclopramide administration prior to the stomach tubing may facilitate gastric emptying. Complications of intestinal lavage include vomition, aspiration of lavage solution, and gastric torsion. Lavage is contraindicated in intractable animals and should be used with extreme caution in animals with a known predisposition to stomach instability (e.g. Sharpeis, deep-chested dogs) and in dogs with delayed gastric emptying or swallowing dysfunction. Cheaper osmotic lavage solutions such as magnesium citrate, magnesium sulphate, and magnesium hydroxide should be avoided because of the risks of hypermagnesemia and volume contracture.

Enemas are less desirable for the preparation of the colon prior to colonoscopy. They are less effective at cleansing (especially proximally), and they can produce artificial mucosal erosions. In most animals, however, they are cheaper, easier and less time-consuming to administer. It is important to avoid additives in the enemas. Soap, especially if in high concentrations, can induce colitis in humans. Hypertonic sodium phosphate enemas (Fleet) and rectal administration of bisacodyl laxatives both alter proctoscopic and histologic appearance of the mucosa. Furthermore, hypertonic sodium phosphate enemas have been associated with fatal hyperphosphatemia and hypernatremia in cats. Large, cotton-tipped applicators (Scopettes, Birchwood, MN) can be used to swab out residual fecal material from the rectum.

Rigid Proctoscopy. One to two days of starvation and two to three warm water enemas usually provide adequate preparation for proctoscopy.

Anesthesia

Anesthesia is recommended for all endoscopic procedures, with the exception of proctoscopy with a rigid endoscope, in which sedation is usually adequate. Choice of anesthetic technique should be made with respect to the animal's general condition and presence or absence of intercurrent disease.

Anticholinergic premedication is an advantage to reduce bowel motility. Narcotic agents increase pyloric and cranial duodenal tone in humans, interfering with the easy passage of the scope.[10] Our clinical impression is that a similar phenomena occurs in dogs. Therefore, if the condition of the animal allows, these drugs are best avoided during gastrointestinal endoscopy.

Attention must be particularly given for signs of gastric overinflation, which include excessive abdominal distention, tachycardia, pale mucous membranes, and a precipitous drop in blood pressure, and for evidence of bradycardia suggestive of vagovagal reflexes.

A reliable gag *must* always be placed in the mouth to protect the endoscope.

General Endoscope Technique

Endoscope Handling. The endoscope is held in the left hand in such a manner that the controls can be comfortably manipulated (Figure 7-5). The right hand is used to advance and torque the scope. An assistant stabilizes the instrument in a particular position in the bowel and is necessary for efficient biopsy and retrieval procedures.

Endoscopes can be damaged by bites, collision with surfaces, inappropriate coiling, excessive insertion or torquing force, and repeated fluoroscopy. In general, endoscopes should not be coiled greater than 360 degrees, should not be forced into tight bends, and should not be forcefully inserted. Torque should be initiated by rotating the insertion tube (Figure 7-5). The hand piece should not be used to initiate torque, because its larger diameter allows the generation of sufficient rotational force to damage the endoscope.

On most occasions, the endoscope should be advanced only if the bowel lumen is in clear view. One exception to this is the "slide-by" technique. This entails the prior deflection of the tip of the endoscope in the perceived direction of a flexure, followed by the *gentle* sliding of the endoscope over the mucosa of the greater curvature of the flexure. The lumen is temporarily lost to view, and a tunnel view is not regained until the endoscope rounds the flexure.

Patient Positioning. For routine gastrointestinal endoscopy the patient is positioned in left lateral recumbency. In the case of upper gastrointestinal endoscopy this position facilitates examination of the pylorus. During large bowel endoscopy this position assists examination of the ileocecal region and encourages drainage of fluid to the descending colon, where it can be aspirated.

Description of the Mucosa. Written description of the mucosa should become part of the record of any animal undergoing endoscopy. Where appropriate, photographic records can also be kept. Consistent description of mucosal lesions is assisted by the preparation of endoscopy grading sheets for inclusion in the record. Grading sheets should include a description of the size and position of any lesions, such as masses or ulcers. In addition, each of the following parameters should be evaluated in a semi-quantitative fashion: degree of erythema, friability, granularity, erosions, mucus, and visibility of submucosal blood vessels. Of these parameters, increased mucosal erythema is least likely to correlate closely to presence of mucosal disease. The appearance of the mucosa varies considerably with degree of insufflation.

Esophagoscopy

Flexible endoscopes allow the most thorough examination of the esophagus, but rigid endoscopes, can be used and may have some advantages in the removal of sharp foreign bodies. The endoscope is directed through the upper esophageal sphincter and the esophagus insufflated with air until adequately distended to visualize the lumen. The tip of the endoscope is then slowly advanced to the gastroesophageal junction. The normal mucosa is pale and smooth. Slight reddening may be apparent at the gastroesophageal junction in normal animals.

Table 7-3 Most Common Complications of Gastrointestinal Endoscopy

Gastrointestinal perforation
Laceration of major blood vessels
Laceration of organs adjacent to the gastrointestinal tract
Decreased venous return due to gastric overdistension
Acute bradycardia
Gastric-dilatation volvulus
Mucosal hemorrhage
Transmission of enteropathogenic organisms
Bacteremias*

*Incidence uncertain in veterinary medicine

Submucosal vessels are usually not visible. The luminal diameter of the esophagus can be hard to judge by endoscopy. In the anesthetized animal the normal esophagus appears flaccid and may partially drape over thoracic vasculature. For these reasons, be wary of diagnosing megaesophagus based on endoscopic judgement only. When present, esophagitis may or may not be visually apparent. If it is apparent, erythema, erosions, and stricturing may be seen.

Because of its durable epithelium, biopsy of the esophagus is more difficult than the biopsy of other parts of the gastrointestinal tract. A suction biopsy instrument (such as the Quinton) is the safest and most effective method to biopsy the esophagus.

Gastroscopy

Following examination of the esophagus, the endoscope is gently advanced through the gastroesophageal sphincter into the stomach. The large size of the stomach requires a systematic approach be developed to gastroscopy; otherwise, lesions are overlooked. Particular care should be taken to observe the fundus, cardia, and lesser curvature, all areas of the stomach easily overlooked if the tip of the endoscope is single-mindedly passed to the pylorus. To observe the cardia and parts of the fundus and lesser curvature, it is necessary to retroflex the tip of the endoscope by up to 180 degrees and often to apply some torque to the insertion tube.

The normal stomach mucosa is bright pink to red and is lighter in color in the pyloric region. There should be no

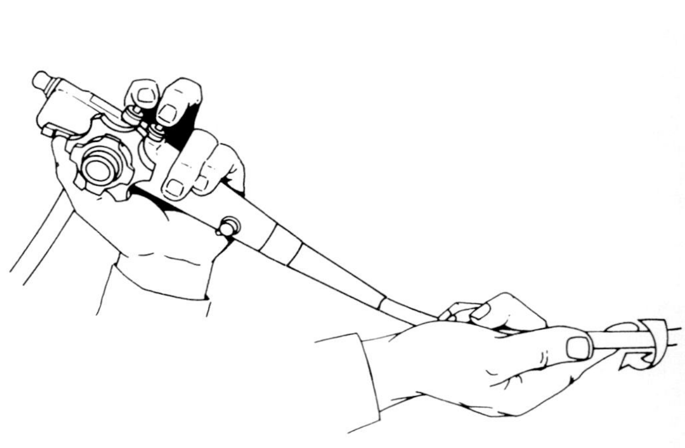

Figure 7-5. Scope handling. The endoscope should be held comfortably in the left hand. Torque should be applied from the insertion tube only.

evidence of erosions or friability, suggestive of gastritis, nor indication of submucosal vessels (with the exception of the cardia). The observation of submucosal vessels suggests a diagnosis of atrophic gastritis.

If fluid is retained in the stomach, it usually pools along the greater curvature. Large volumes of retained fluid should be aspirated to facilitate mucosal examination and to prevent future inhalation pneumonia.

The endoscopist should be cognizant of the readiness with which the stomach inflates and the rugal folds disappear. If the stomach does not inflate, consider the possibility that air is exiting the stomach via the esophagus (firmly occlude by digital pressure if necessary), that the equipment is not insufflating correctly, or that the stomach is unable to distend due to extramural compression or an intramural lesion. Prominent rugal folds are usually due to ineffective insufflation, but hypertrophic gastropathy must be considered. In the latter condition the folds often have an edematous appearance (thickened, prominent light reflectivity), the hypertrophy may be focal, and the folds may extend into the antrum (where it is unusual in normal dogs to find many rugae). In addition, there may be signs of mucosal erosions or ulcers.

The incisura angularis is an important landmark. It is a narrow shelf of tissue that divides the pyloric antrum from the lesser curvature of the gastric body. Its identification assists the location of the pyloric antrum, lesser curvature, and cardia. Once in the antrum, the tip of the endoscope is slowly advanced towards the pylorus. The pylorus of normal dogs has a wide variety of appearances. In general, it should have clean margins, should not be obscured by excessive folds, and usually demonstrates rhythmical opening and closing. Occasionally gastroduodenal reflux will be noticed. This is a normal occurrence in many dogs. A patient with a hypertrophic pylorus should have a history compatible with delayed gastric emptying, may have retained gastric ingesta, may have evidence of rugal hypertrophy and mucosal erosions (hypergastrinemia due to chronic distension), and has an enlarged, muscular-looking, protuberant pylorus with a small pyloric canal that is unable to accommodate the scope. The normal pylorus will usually yield to gentle pressure and allow entry of the tip of the endoscope into the duodenum. If not, metoclopramide (0.2 mg/kg IV) can be used to facilitate passage through the pylorus. Adroit manipulation of the endoscope is often necessary to penetrate the pylorus.

Duodenoscopy

After passage through the pylorus, the endoscope enters the short cranial duodenum and immediately encounters the cranial duodenal flexure. This is a very acute flexure that can be difficult to negotiate. It arises because of the rapid change of the cranial-and-to-the-right angulation of the pylorus and cranial duodenum to the caudal orientation of the descending duodenum. To negotiate this flexure, it is often necessary to maximally flex the endoscope tip, torque the insertion tube, and use a slide-by technique.

The duodenal mucosa has a pink, velvety appearance and a slightly more granular and friable nature than the stomach.

Colonoscopy

A digital examination of the anus should be carried out to detect anal lesions that are otherwise easily missed. The tip of the endoscope is then introduced with a gloved hand into the rectum. The large bowel is insufflated and once a luminal view is obtained the endoscope is steadily advanced towards the left colic flexure, which marks the junction between the descending and transverse colon. The flexure is usually rounded by a slide-by technique. Subsequently, the endoscope is further advanced towards the short, ascending colon. The flexure which unites the transverse and ascending colon, the right colic flexure, is sometimes not apparent, perhaps because cranial pressure of the endoscope forces the transverse colon cranially, a movement which tends to straighten the flexure. Once the ascending colon is entered it is generally possible to see the ileocecal valve and cecum. Skilled endoscopists can sometimes manoeuver their endoscopes into the distal ileum.

Careful examination of the ileocecal area is an integral part of the colonoscopic examination because that area has a significant frequency of disease, including intussusception, cecal inversion, parasitism, and neoplasia. The normal colonic mucosa is smooth and pink. Submucosal blood vessels should be clearly visible. There should be no evidence of erosions or ulcers, and the mucosa should not be obviously friable or bleed after gentle passage of the endoscope. There should be little mucus, and the colon should distend readily and evenly following insufflation.

Rigid Proctoscopy

The lubricated proctoscope is introduced through the anus with the obturator in place. The obturator is then removed; the glass viewing window, if present, is secured; and the colon is insufflated using the attached rubber bulb.

Completion of the Endoscopic Examination

After the endoscope reaches its full working length, it is slowly retracted. Biopsies, brush cytology, and aspiration of fluid are undertaken as indicated. All air should be aspirated from the gastric or colonic lumens before the endoscope is withdrawn. The animal should then be recovered from anesthesia and closely observed for the complications discussedbelow.

ANCILLARY ENDOSCOPIC TECHNIQUES

Brush Cytology

Brush cytology is a useful adjunct to endoscopic biopsy. It may improve diagnostic yield because superficial material, which otherwise may be lost during processing, is sampled. Thus, organisms such as protozoa that reside in the mucus of the gastrointestinal tract may occasionally be detected by brush cytology but not seen in biopsies. Furthermore, the brush ranges over a wider area than that examined by biopsy, and cytological specimens may be rapidly evaluated. Brush cytology has been shown to improve the diagnostic yield by up to 20% in some forms of gastrointestinal cancer in humans. A tentative diagnosis made by brush cytology should not be summarily dismissed if not supported by biopsy results. Instead, repeated biopsies may be prudent.

Aspiration of Duodenal Fluid

Aspiration kits (Harford Vet, Maryland), consisting of a stylet and sterilized plastic tubing, facilitate acquisition of duodenal fluid for culture and cytology.

Endoscopic Biopsy

Pinch Biopsy. Pinch biopsies are small (2-3 mm) biopsies that are attained by endoscopic guidance. In view of their small size, good technique is essential to acquire tissue samples of diagnostic value. The instrument must be sharp to avoid crushing artifacts. Where possible, the long axis of the biopsy instrument should be directed at a 90 degree angle to the mucosal surface to be biopsied. This lessens the likelihood of obtaining only villus tips, a common result if the biopsy forceps are directed parallel with the mucosal surface. In featureless lumens such as the small bowel, attaining a perpendicular orientation with the biopsy forceps is easier if the tip of the endoscope is extended until it encounters a flexure, or if the bowel is partially collapsed by the aspiration of the majority of luminal air. Over-distended stomachs are also harder to biopsy. It can be useful to obtain more than one pinch biopsy from the same site to increase the depth of the tissue sampled. This is particularly important when obtaining biopsies of masses because of the inflammatory reaction that commonly surrounds neoplasms. Biopsy of ulcerating lesions is best performed at their periphery to avoid the sampling of necrotic tissue. Because histologic anatomy varies within regions of the bowel, obtaining biopsies at consistent sites is likely to improve the ability of pathologists to differentiate normal from abnormal histology. For this reason, it has been suggested that as routine practice during upper gastrointestinal endoscopy, biopsies should be obtained from any visible lesions as well as from the duodenum, pylorus, angularis incisura, mid greater curvature, and cardia.[11] During lower gastrointestinal endoscopy, biopsies from visible lesions, cecum, ascending colon, orad transverse colon, orad descending colon, mid-descending colon, and aborad descending colon have been recommended. At each site a minimum of three to four biopsies are suggested.

Suction Biopsy. Using the Quinton suction biopsy instrument is a safe and effective technique for attaining mucosal tissue from the colon and esophagus. It is best suited for non-targeted biopsy of diffusely diseased tissue but, if the suction instrument is passed alongside the endoscope, targeted biopsies can occasionally be obtained. The biopsy technique is described in Chapter 6.

Speculum Forcep Biopsy. Occasionally, speculum forceps are used to biopsy the large bowel. They may be passed alongside or through proctoscopes. These instruments are particularly likely to perforate the bowel, but can be useful if the bowel is poorly prepared, thus inactivating the suction biopsy instruments. The technique is described in Chapter 6.

Handling of Biopsies. Endoscopic biopsy yields pieces of tissue which are small and easily damaged. They should be handled gently, should not be allowed to dry, and should be placed on some support such as a piece of coverslip paper to minimize contraction and preserve orientation.

Foreign Body Retrieval

Indications for Endoscopic Foreign Body Removal. Foreign bodies may be managed by conservative, endoscopic, or surgical means. Factors that influence this decision include the type of foreign object and its anatomic location, the clinical appearance of the animal, and the attentiveness with which the pet is observed by the owner.

All esophageal foreign bodies should be rapidly removed, because they cause pain and dysphagia and may result in esophageal stricture. Endoscopic removal is particularly desirable in view of the possible complications of esophageal surgery and thoracotomy. Timely endoscopic removal of all sharp objects from the stomach is recommended because of the risk of perforation of the stomach or, should the object leave the stomach, perforation of the intestine. To avoid gastrointestinal obstruction, the early endoscopic or surgical removal of foreign bodies judged too large to pass through the gastrointestinal tract is suggested. Foreign bodies suspected of containing lead, zinc (pennies), or caustic materials (batteries) must be removed from the gastrointestinal tract immediately.

Technique. Successful retrieval of foreign bodies requires considerable discretion, ingenuity, and technical prowess. Tightly wedged foreign bodies should *never* be forcibly removed. If a foreign object cannot be removed by firm traction under direct endoscopic vision, then surgical removal is indicated. Forceful removal bears a great risk of laceration of the viscus or adjacent vessels or organs. Furthermore, tightly wedged foreign bodies usually have caused significant mucosal pressure necrosis that requires surgical inspection to determine its mural extent.

Trial and error usually determines the best retrieval instrument for a particular retrieval; however, certain generalizations may be made. For instance, basket retrieval instruments are only useful in a lumen of sufficient diameter to allow their expansion. Pronged graspers are of little value in the retrieval of foreign bodies with smooth surfaces. If the surface is smooth but indentable, strong, jaw-tooth graspers are usually effective. Certain metals may be retrieved by magnetic extractors.

Useful retrieval techniques include entrapping the foreign body with suture material and then drawing the foreign body orally by traction on the suture material; pulling esophageal foreign bodies into a preplaced rigid tube in the esophagus, thus aiding atraumatic removal of sharp objects; pushing obstinate esophageal foreign bodies into the stomach, where they may be digested (e.g. bones), better manipulated to an appropriate orientation for removal, or more easily removed surgically; and placing a Foley catheter distal to the object and then using the inflated catheter to draw the foreign body out.

Bougienage

Endoscopy helps the clinician perform safe and effective esophageal bougienage. The endoscope allows visual assessment and biopsy of strictures before bougienage. This helps differentiate post-inflammatory strictures, extraesophageal compressions, and strictures resulting from neoplasia, thus facilitating the selection of an appropriate therapy. Furthermore, endoscopy simplifies the placement of the bougie directly into the orifice of the stricture and allows assessment of the effect of the procedure on the mucosal tissue and luminal diameter. Current evidence favors the use of balloon dilation. The technique is simple, relying on gradual inflation of the balloon under fluoroscopic (contrast media-filled balloon) or endoscopic visualization. Manometers can be purchased to estimate pressures applied, but are not essential.

Rigid bougies are used by systematically increasing the diameter of the bougie passed through the stricture. The stricture is dilated as widely as possible without the use of excessive force. The diameter of the largest bougie that is accommodated helps judge the success of the procedure. As an example, the comfortable passage of a 40 french diameter bougie through an esophageal stricture of a 20 kg dog would suggest adequate bougienage.

Complications of bougienage include perforation of friable esophageal tissues and the rupture of major periesophageal vessels entrapped by the inflammatory or neoplastic disease process that formed the stricture.

Percutaneous Placement of Gastrostomy Tubes

Percutaneous placement of a gastrostomy tubes is indicated for long-term (weeks to months) nutritional support of anorectic or dysphagic animals. Gastrostomy tubes are not recommended in vomiting animals. The tubes are better tolerated than pharyngostomy or nasogastric tubes and can be easily managed at home. They are of comparatively large diameter and thus allow the economic use of blended pet foods and the direct administration of medicines. Complications are rare, but include pressure necrosis of the gastric wall and peritonitis. Gastrostomy tubes may be difficult to place endoscopically in fat animals. The procedure necessitates a brief anesthesia. The patient is placed in right lateral recumbency. Two techniques are in use. The peroral technique utilizes the endoscope for the retrieval of percutaneously-placed suture material that is used to draw a gastrostomy tube, tipped by a catheter or plastic pipette, through the mouth, esophageal lumen, gastric lumen, gastric wall, and finally body wall. This technique is described in detail elsewhere.[12]

The percutaneous technique utilizes a series of trocars of increasing diameter, which are serially passed through the abdominal wall into the air-distended stomach (Wilson-Cook, PEG set). The largest trocar is of sufficient diameter for a Foley catheter to be passed directly into the stomach through the trocar. Once inserted, the Foley is inflated and used to fix the stomach against the body wall.

LAPAROSCOPY[13]

Indications and Limitations

Laparoscopy is a valuable technique for the visual inspection of the peritoneal cavity, but its use has declined somewhat with the advent of ultrasonography. The primary indication for laparoscopy is the biopsy of the liver and kidneys. Ultrasound-guided biopsy of these structures is less invasive and less time-consuming. Laparoscopy should not be considered a replacement for exploratory celiotomy, because it provides restricted visualization of the abdominal organs and has limited therapeutic capability.

Contraindications & Complications

Laparoscopy is contraindicated in patients with obesity, diaphragmatic hernias, and coagulopathies. Complications are not common but include abdominal hemorrhage from laceration of an organ or vessel; subcutaneous emphysema; air embolism; hypercapnia, if CO_2 is used as the distending gas; decreased cardiac output; infection at trocar sites; peritonitis, usually from penetration of bowel; pneumothorax; and biopsy-related morbidity.[14] Air embolism should be suspected if there is a sudden deterioration of the patient, or if "mill wheel" murmurs or the penetration of the spleen or a major vessel with the Verres needle are noticed.

Equipment

Equipment required is a cold light source, a Verres needle, a trocar, a source of gas for distension of the abdomen (nitrous oxide, CO_2, or nitrogen in declining order of preference), a method of recording intra-abdominal pressure, an optical system (usually composed of a lens and a series of fiber bundles encased in a metal tube), biopsy instruments, and warm sterile saline (Figure 7-6).

Technique

Laparoscopy can be performed under general anesthesia, or heavy sedation in association with local anesthesia. The patient is placed in left lateral recumbency to allow a right-lateral approach. This reduces the likelihood of damage to the spleen. The left-lateral approach should only be utilized if a left-sided lesion is suspected. The flank is surgically prepared and draped. A Verres needle is carefully inserted into the abdominal cavity. The mid-dorsal flank region is a suitable area for insertion. The clinician should ensure that the needle penetrates the peritoneum; otherwise, massive subcutaneous emphysema will ensue. Great care must be taken to avoid the penetration of abdominal organs. If the spleen is penetrated, fatal air embolism is likely. After the Verres needle is in place, the clinician should begin insufflation of the abdomen. Insufflation should be at a rate of less than 1 liter per minute and result in an intra-abdominal pressure of no greater than 20 mm of Hg higher pressures decrease cardiac output. Once the abdomen is tight to the touch, the skin is incised over the area of interest, the trocar is inserted into the laparoscope sleeve, and the trocar/sleeve is firmly driven through the body wall. Once the abdomen is penetrated, the trocar is removed, being careful not to lose insufflation, and the optical instrument is inserted. The entire assemblage is rotated cranially and caudally to view the entire extent of the visible abdomen. If the lens steams up, the optical system is withdrawn and warmed in warm sterile saline. Biopsy or aspiration instruments are inserted through separate trocars or, in the case of needle biopsy instruments, directly through the body wall.

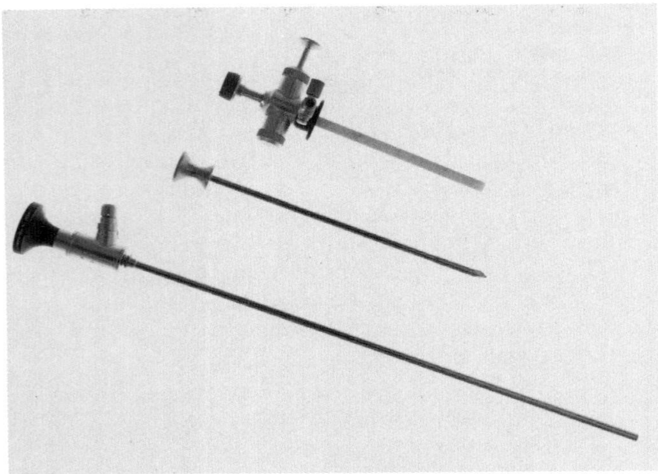

Figure 7-6. Laparoscopy equipment (Wolf) showing from top to bottom cannula passed though abdominal wall, trocar to aid in cannula passage, and laparoscope. Not shown is the light source and illuminating cable for the scope.

REFERENCES

1. Johnson, G.F., Twedt, D.C.: Endoscopy and laparoscopy in the diagnosis and management of neoplasia in small animals. Vet. Clin. N. Am. 7:77-92, 1977.
2. Johnson, G.F.: Gastroscopy. In, Veterinary Gastroenterology. Edited by N.V. Anderson. Lea and Febiger, Philadelphia, 84-88, 1980.
3. Johnson, G.F.: Duodenoscopy. In, Veterinary Gastroenterology. Edited by N.V. Anderson. Lea and Febiger, Philadelphia, 89-90, 1980.
4. Johnson, J.H.: Endoscopes. In, Veterinary Gastroenterology. Edited by N.V. Anderson. Lea and Febiger, Philadelphia, 77-79, 1980.
5. Happe, R.P., van der Gaag, I.: Endoscopic examination of esophagus, stomach, and duodenum in the dog. JAAHA 19:197-206, 1983.
6. O'Brien, J.A.: Esophagoscopy. In, Veterinary Gastroenterology. Edited by N.V. Anderson. Lea and Febiger, Philadelphia, 81-83, 1980.
7. Jakovljevic, S.: Gastric radiology and gastroscopy in the dog. Vet. Annual. 28:172-182, 1988.
8. Pariente, E.A., Kerlau, M. and Lanoe, J.L.: Fibroscopie ou radiographie oeso-gastroduodenale de premiere intention? Une evaluation pragmatique. Nouv. Press Med. 10:3477-3480, 1981. Cited in: Schuman, B.M.: Upper gastrointestinal endoscopy. In, Gastroenterology. Edited by J.E. Berk. WB Saunders, Philadelphia. 564-580, 1985.
9. Church, E.M., Mehlhaff, C.J. and Patnaik, A.K.: Colorectal adenocarcinoma in dogs: 78 cases (1973-1984). JAAMA 191(6):727-730, 1987.
10. Jaffe, J.H., Martin, W.R.: Opioid analgesics and antagonists. In, The Pharmacological Basis of Therapeutics. Edited by Gilman A. Goodman, L.S. Goodman, T.W. Rall. McMillam Publishing Company, New York, 502, 1985.
11. Leib, M.S., Roth, L.: Gastrointestinal endoscopy: Endoscopic and histologic correlation. Proc 7th ACVIM Forum, 784-786, 1989.
12. Mathews, K.A., Binnington, A.G.: Percutaneous incisionless placement of a gastrostomy tube utilizing a gastroscope; preliminary observations. JAAHA 22:601-610, 1986.
13. Rothuizen, J.: Laparoscopy in small animal medicine. Vet Quarterly 7:225-228, 1985.
14. Gilroy, B.A., Anson, L.W.: Fatal air embolism during anesthesia for laparoscopy in a dog. JAVMA 190:552-554, 1987.

Chapter 8

Pharynx and Esophagus - Normal Structure and Function

INTRODUCTION

Problems in gastroenterology frequently involve functions of the oral cavity concerned with the initial part of the eating process and functions that subsequently transport food to the stomach. The most important functions of the oral cavity are prehension and mastication of food. These functions, voluntary events under control of the cerebral cortex, are performed by muscles of the tongue and head. The act of swallowing is initiated by movements of these muscles to propel the bolus of food from the oral cavity to the oropharynx. Movement of the bolus from the pharynx to the stomach and through the remainder of the alimentary canal is almost entirely reflex. The normal structure and function required for this reflex must be understood if the pathological problems that frequently occur are to be adequately explained.

ANATOMY OF THE PHARYNX[1,2]

The pharynx is a funnel-shaped connection between the oral cavity and the esophagus, and between the nasal cavity and the larynx. Figure 8-1 shows a cross-section of the pharynx and its related structures. The pharynx is covered with mucous membranes, and its boundaries are defined by the root of the tongue ventrally, by the floor of the cranium and cervical flexor muscles dorsally, and by pharyngeal constrictor muscles laterally. The soft palate divides the rostral part of the pharynx into a dorsal cavity (the nasopharynx) and a ventral cavity (oropharynx). The common cavity caudal to the end of the soft palate is called the laryngopharynx. The pharynx has four important openings that open and close in an integrated fashion during swallowing and respiration. Openings connect the oropharynx with the oral cavity (aditus pharyngis), the nasal passages with the nasopharynx, the laryngopharynx with the larynx (aditus laryngis), and the laryngopharynx with the esophagus.

The muscles that form the lateral walls of the pharynx are primarily constrictors. These include the pterygopharyngeus and palatopharyngeus muscles, which constrict the rostral pharynx. The thyropharyngeus muscle and cricopharyngeus muscles respectively constrict the middle and caudal pharynges. The cricopharyngeus muscle and the caudal part of the thyropharyngeus muscle form the pharyngoesophageal sphincter. There is one muscle to dilate the pharynx, the stylopharyngeus muscle, which also acts to draw the pharynx forward. The pharyngeal muscles are striated and contract reflexly, not being under voluntary control. They are innervated by branches of the glossopharyngeal and vagus nerves.

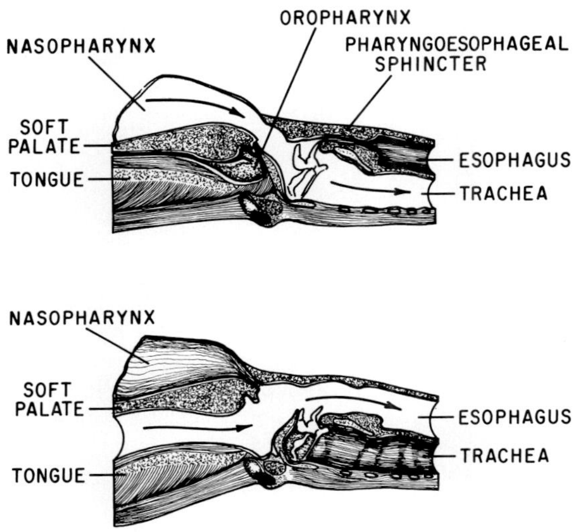

Figure 8-1. Drawing of sagittal section of pharynx, larynx, trachea, and esophagus. Upper drawing shows relative positions of structures during respiration. Lower drawing shows relative positions during swallowing.

Three sets of muscles control the function of the soft palate. The tensor veli palatini stretches the palate between the pterygoid bones. The levator veli palatini raises the caudal part of the soft palate, and the palatinus shortens the palate and curls the caudal border ventrally. These muscles are innervated by branches of the trigeminal nerves.

ANATOMY OF THE ESOPHAGUS[1,2]

The esophagus is divided into cervical, thoracic, and abdominal portions. The anatomical relations of the esophagus with other structures are shown in Figures 8-2 and 8-3. The cranial end of the esophagus begins at the level of the middle of the axis and the caudal border of the cricoid cartilage. The cervical esophagus lies ventral to the muscles on the left ventral border of the cervical spine. The trachea lies ventral and to the right of this part of the esophagus. The thoracic esophagus

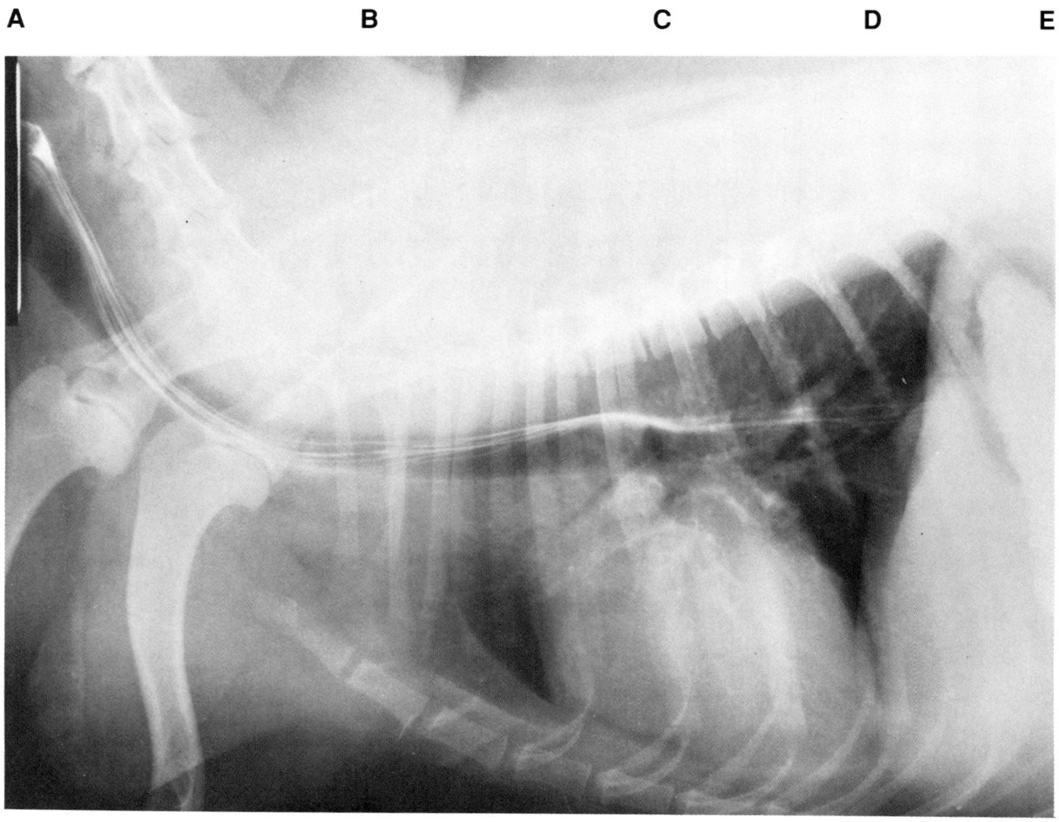

Figure 8-2. Lateral and dorsoventral radiographs of a dog after having swallowed a bolus of liquid positive-contrast medium. Transverse planes designated A,B,C,D, and E correspond to those with the same identification in the drawings of transverse sections shown in Figure 8-3.

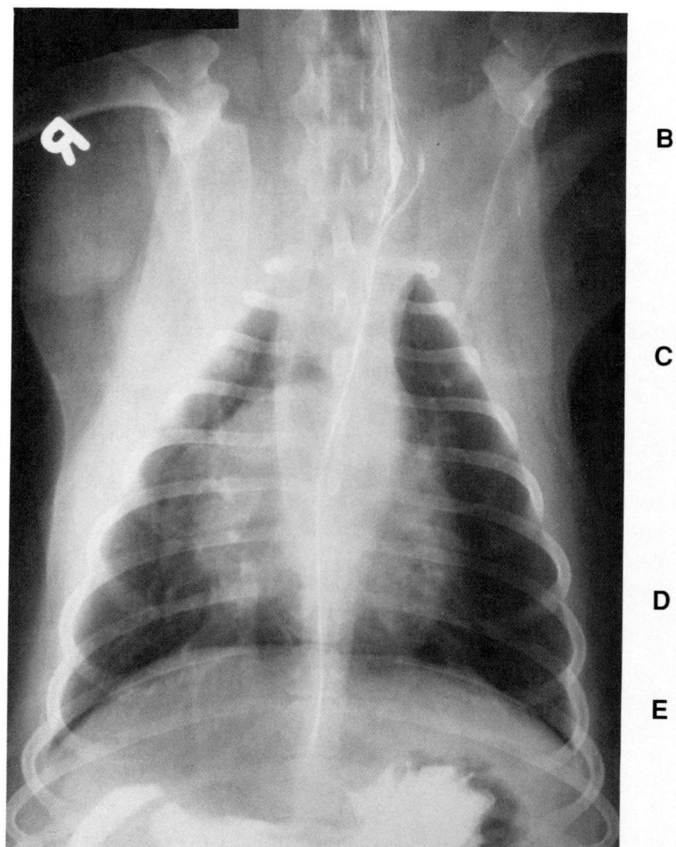

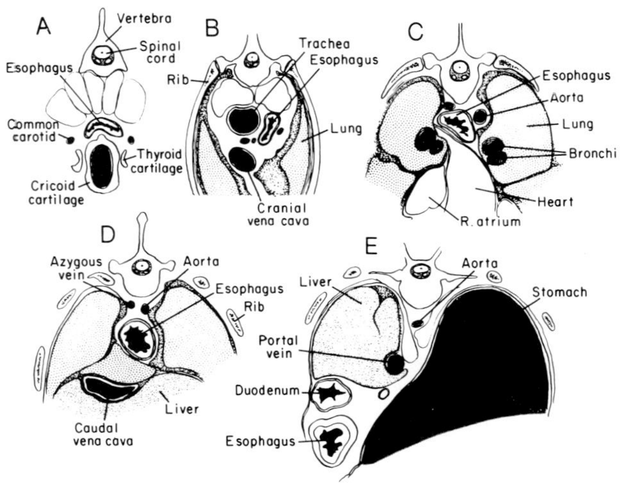

Figure 8-3. Topographic anatomy of the canine showing the relationship of the esophagus to adjacent structures at different transverse planes through the cervical, thoracic, and abdominal regions. The level of each plane corresponds to those bearing the same designations in the radiographs in Figure 8-2.

includes that portion of the esophagus from the thoracic inlet to the diaphragm. It begins on the left side of the trachea but lies dorsal to the trachea at its bifurcation at a site ventral to the fifth to sixth thoracic vertebrae. At this point it crosses the right face of the aortic arch and passes caudally in the median plane. There is a short segment of abdominal esophagus between the diaphragm and the stomach. The wall of the esophagus is thickest in the cervical and abdominal portions. The esophagus is least distensible at the points where it enters and leaves the thoracic cavity.

The esophagus consists of four layers: the adventitia, muscularis, submucosa, and mucosa. The thin fibrous adventitia covers the esophageal mucosa. The muscularis of the canine esophagus is composed of two oblique layers of striated muscle throughout its entire length. The muscularis of the cranial feline esophagus consists of striated muscle; the distal portion is composed of smooth muscle. The striated muscle of the feline esophagus consists of two layers that are oblique in the proximal portion and become spiral in the distal portion. They gradually form a distinct inner, circular layer and an outer, longitudinal layer. The muscle fiber transition from striated muscle to smooth muscle in the feline muscularis occurs gradually. The amount of smooth muscle increases distally until the final two to three cm. of the esophagus, where all of the muscle fibers are smooth. The submucosal layer contains mucus glands and loosely binds the mucosal and muscular layers together. This allows the relatively inelastic mucosal coat to be thrown into prominent longitudinal folds in the dog. Transverse folds constitute the serrated or herringbone pattern observed radiographically in the terminal thoracic esophagus of the cat. The mucosal layer has a stratified squamous epithelium that contains openings for the ducts of the esophageal mucus glands.[3] In the caudal half of the esophagus the mucosa is bounded by the muscularis mucosae.

Blood to the esophagus is supplied by the thyroid arteries in the cervical portion, by the bronchoesophageal artery in the cranial part of the thoracic portion, and by branches from the aorta, intercostals, and gastric artery in the remainder of the esophagus. Venous drainage of the esophagus occurs via satellite vessels of the arteries that supply it. The vagus nerve and its associated branches innervate the esophagus. The vagus nerve supplies somatic motor nerves to the esophageal striated muscle, autonomic nerves to the esophageal smooth muscle, and general visceral afferent nerves that form the esophageal sensory receptors. Sympathetic nerves, accompanying the vascular supply, also innervate the esophagus.

ANATOMY OF ESOPHAGEAL SPHINCTERS

Pharyngoesophageal Sphincter

The opening between the oropharynx and the esophagus remains closed except when a bolus of ingesta passes through. The cricopharyngeus muscles and the caudal part of the thyropharyngeus muscles maintain this closure. These muscles lie dorsal to the esophagus. Their origins are the lateral surface of the cricoid cartilage and the oblique line of the thyroid lamina. The two muscles insert on the median dorsal raphe. The pharyngoesophageal sphincter (PES) is formed dorsally and laterally by the two muscles and ventrally by the cricoid cartilage. The motor fibers to the cricopharyngeus and thyropharyngeus muscles are in the glossopharyngeal nerve and the pharyngeal branches of the vagus nerve.[4-6]

Gastroesophageal Junction and Sphincter

A number of sphincters, located strategically along the course of the gastrointestinal tract, maintain the movement of food unidirectionally in the normal aboral direction. The gastroesophageal sphincter (GES), the first of the most important ones, is located at the end of the esophagus. Physiological function in this sphincter, in conjunction with the anatomy of the gastroesophageal junction, prevents regurgitation of gastric contents into the esophagus.

The GES is a physiologic rather than an anatomic sphincter since it does not consist of a specialized large mass of muscle. In dogs, the GES consists of an outer layer of longitudinal striated muscle fibers that are continuous with longitudinal striated muscle in the esophagus and an inner layer of circular smooth muscle that merges with the circular striated muscle of the adjacent esophagus. The longitudinal muscle layer merges with the smooth muscle of the stomach about two millimeters caudal to the junction of gastric mucosa with esophageal stratified squamous epithelium. In cats the GES consists of only smooth muscle.[7]

The anatomical features of the gastroesophageal junction contribute to the prevention of reflux. These features include: 1) interdigitating rugal folds that converge near the gastroesophageal junction and continue into the terminal esophagus; 2) the right diaphragmatic crus, which serves as a muscular sling; 3) the oblique implantation of the distal esophagus into the stomach; 4) the muscular sling provided by the smooth muscle

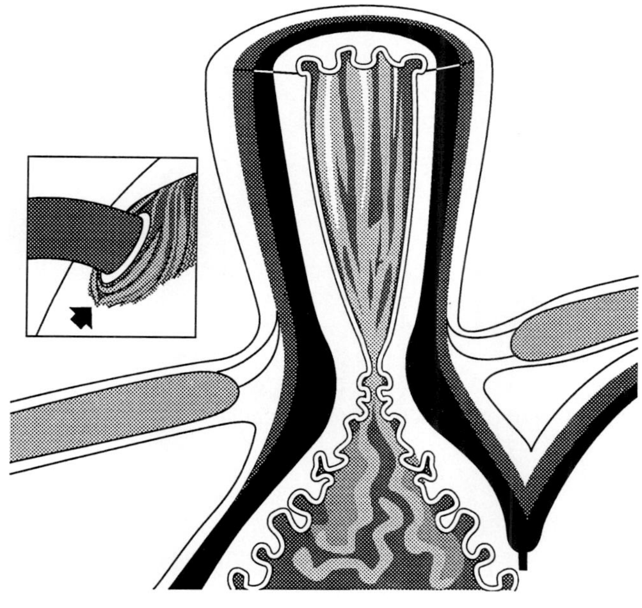

Figure 8-4. Competence of the GES junction to prevent reflux is maintained by rugal folds, muscular sling fibers, oblique angle of distal esophagus and stomach, and compression of intra-abdominal esophagus by stomach

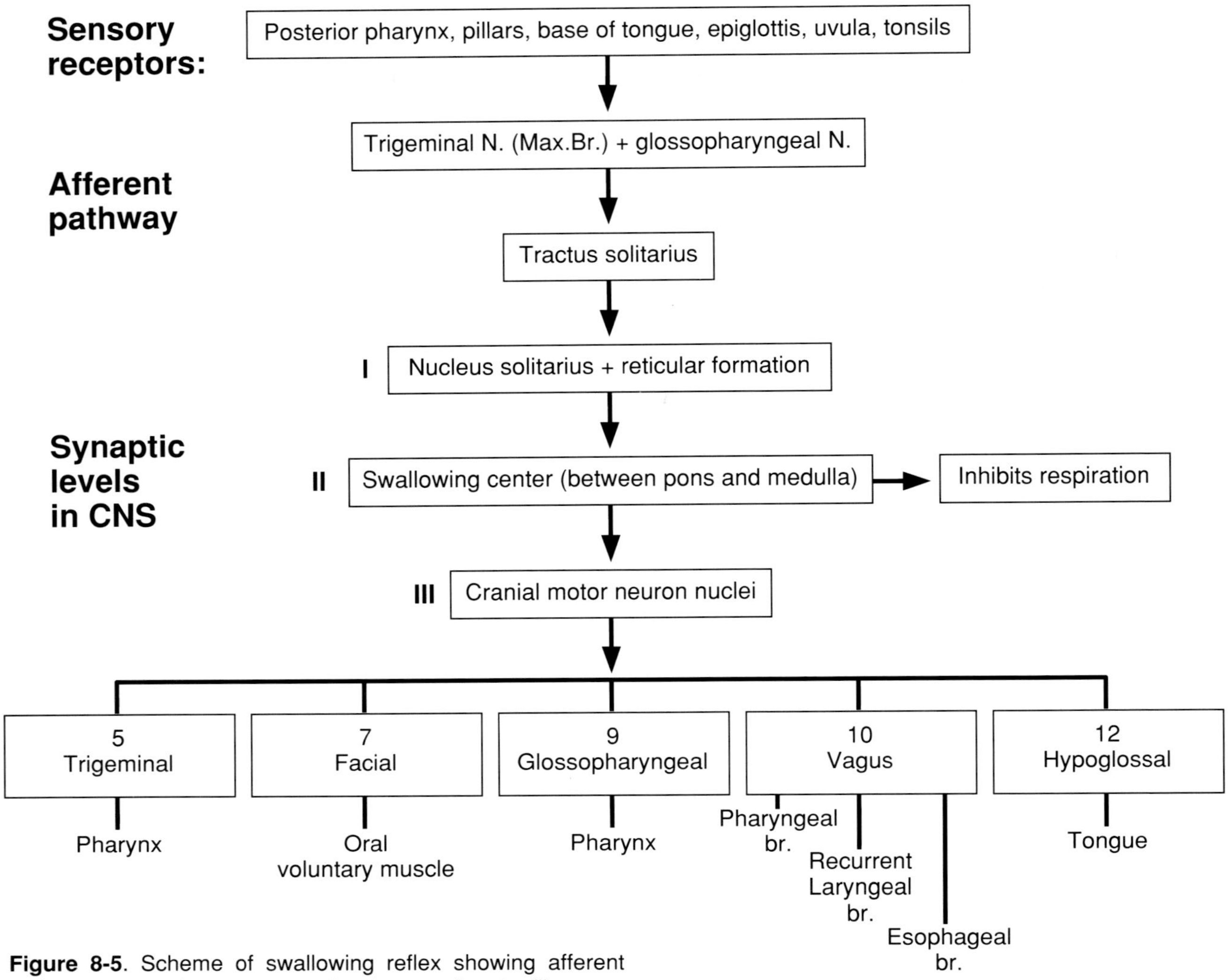

Figure 8-5. Scheme of swallowing reflex showing afferent pathways, central synapses, and pathways of motor fibers.

bundles of the lesser gastric curvature around the left side of the gastroesophageal junction; and 5) the compression exerted on the short intra-abdominal terminal esophagus by the positive intra-abdominal pressure (Figure 8-4).[8] A short segment of esophagus, including much of the GES, is normally found caudal to the diaphragm, thus being located within the abdominal cavity. This segment acts as a flutter valve when there are changes in abdominal and intragastric pressure.

Vagal fibers innervate the gastroesophageal junction and sphincter. The efferents to the striated fibers are somatic efferents from the nucleus ambiguus, and the efferents to the smooth muscle fibers are parasympathetics from the dorsal motor nucleus of the vagus. Both of these centers are in the brain stem. The smooth muscle is also innervated by an intrinsic nervous system that consists of the nerve plexuses of Auerbach and Meissner. Sympathetic fibers innervate the smooth muscle and may play a role in the regulation of sphincter function.[9]

PHYSIOLOGY OF SWALLOWING

Swallowing consists of a series of sequential, well-coordinated events that transport food and liquids from the mouth to the stomach. This process has been divided into three major phases: oropharyngeal, esophageal, and gastroesophageal. The oropharyngeal phase is further subdivided into oral, pharyngeal, and cricopharyngeal stages, with each stage related to the action of a particular group of structures. Following the prehension of food, the voluntary oral stage is initiated in which a bolus is formed in the oropharynx and is passed in an aboral direction to the base of the tongue. Pharyngeal contact by the bolus next stimulates a series of rapid pharyngeal peristaltic contractions that propel the bolus from the base of the tongue to the laryngopharynx. This is the second or pharyngeal stage of the oropharyngeal phase.

Pharyngeal Phase[10,11]

Since the pharyngeal phase of swallowing must move the bolus from the pharynx only into the esophagus, the other three major pharyngeal openings through which the bolus might pass must be closed. The pathway between the oral cavity and oropharynx is closed by muscles of the mouth and tongue. The orifice between the oropharynx and the nasopharynx is reflexly closed by elevating the soft palate and approximating the palatopharyngeal folds. That is accomplished by simultaneous contraction of the levator palati and palato-pharyngeal muscles. The opening to the trachea is protected by closure of the glottis and tipping of the epiglottis in such a manner as to divert food away from the glottis. To accomplish that, the larynx is drawn in a cranial direction by the thyroglossal and mylohyoid muscles. The epiglottis is pushed back over the laryngeal orifice by the tongue.

The movement of a bolus through the pharynx is accomplished by an orderly sequential contraction of the pharyngeal muscles, beginning in the rostral part of the pharynx and proceeding aborally. The reflex motor events that begin in the pharynx are initiated by the stimulation of numerous sensory receptors located in specific areas of the palate, pharynx, and epiglottis. The receptors' nerve fibers are found in the maxillary branch of the trigeminal nerve, in the glossopharyngeal nerve, and in the superior laryngeal nerve. The afferent pathways carrying the information from these receptors to the brain stem are shown in the reflex arc diagramed in Figure 8-5. Sequential firing in the nuclei of the cranial motor nerves evokes contraction of the buccal, tongue, pharyngeal, and esophageal muscles. The neural response produces the initial response in the rostral constrictors of the pharynx. The bolus is propelled aborally by the sequential contraction of constrictors of the remainder of the pharynx. Respiration is suspended during the pharyngeal phase of swallowing since the two events cannot occur simultaneously.

The sequential motor events in the pharynx are controlled by a central generator.[10] The entire sequence of pharyngeal swallowing is completed without peripheral feedback. Two functionally distinct central pattern generators are present for the pharyngeal and esophageal phases of swallowing. The sequential esophageal motor events are completed only with peripheral feedback. The presence of two central generators explains why most swallowing problems invoke either pharyngeal or esophageal abnormalities, not both.

The central pattern must be triggered by patterned sensory inputs over specific branches of the glossopharyngeal and vagal nerves. The sensory pattern determines which motor response is evoked; stimulation by the same modality, such as touch, on the same pharyngolaryngeal region can evoke different motor responses (i.e., vomiting, gagging, laryngeal adduction, or swallowing).[10]

Solid boluses are more effective than liquids in stimulating pharyngeal receptors for initiating swallowing. That water or saline may not be very effective in stimulating swallowing is evident on fluoroscopic studies in normal animals where multiple swallowing attempts may be necessary to stimulate deglutition. Oil does not stimulate swallowing; mineral oil given orally is often aspirated into the trachea without stimulating deglutition.

The smooth muscle in the muscularis mucosa may participate in a sensory function. The neural structures found in the intrinsic nervous system of the esophageal mucosa resemble sensory receptors in other tissues.[12] Motility in the muscularis mucosa may assist the sensory receptors in monitoring progression of a bolus and reinforcing the peristaltic wave carrying it to the stomach. Esophagitis disrupts motility in the esophagus of both the dog and cat; inflammation may cause that by disrupting function in the muscularis mucosa and sensory receptors.

Pharyngoesophageal Sphincter Function[10]

During a normal swallow, as contraction of the pharyngeal and palatine muscles closes the three openings from the pharynx into the mouth, nasopharynx, and larynx, the cricopharyngeus and thyropharyngeus muscles relax to open the oriface into the esophagus. These muscles remain contracted at all other times, maintaining closure of the pharyngoesophageal sphincter. With normal function in this sphincter, the thyropharyngeus and cricopharyngeus muscles relax at the proper time and remain relaxed long enough to allow the entire bolus of food to enter the esophagus. The sphincter closes promptly after passage of the bolus. The interval that the sphincter remains relaxed is determined by a central neural mechanism that senses the volume of the bolus propelled from the pharynx. During closure the sphincter shows phasic rather than tonic activity.[13] This generates a pressure in the sphincter that is higher than that on either side of the pharynx and esophagus. The high-pressure zone helps protect against esophagopharyngeal reflux and aspiration of intraesophageal contents. The pressure is highest during inspiration and predeglutition.[14] Conditions in the esophagus affect pressure within the pharyngoesophageal sphincter.[15,16] The pressure increases when the cervical esophagus is distended by liquid or its mucosal surface is bathed by acid solution. The reflux to increase PES pressure protects against regurgitation and tracheobronchial aspiration of fluid. Air, in contrast to fluid in the esophagus, causes PES pressure to fall; the reduction permits eructation of gas to be completed.[17] The response is to make the sphincter more competent in preventing reflux, and it is mediated by a neural reflex that has its afferent fibers in the recurrent laryngeal nerves.

Esophageal Phase[10,11,18]

The peristaltic wave generated in the pharynx is propagated through the esophagus and carries the bolus aborally to the GES. The esophagus is a flaccid tube at rest, offering little resistance to the passage of most substances. Hence, even a relatively weak peristaltic wave initiated by the cranial cervical esophagus can readily and rapidly propel a bolus of liquid throughout the length of the flaccid tube. A bolus of food encounters more resistance to passage, and therefore needs a more sustained wave of peristalsis. Esophageal speed of peristalsis in the dog is 80 to 100 cm/sec during water-induced swallows.[19] In the cat the transit rate of a bolus of food is slower than in the dog since striated skeletal muscle fibers contract rapidly, in contrast to smooth-muscle fibers. The speed of esophageal contractions is one to two cm/sec in sedated cats during liquid-stimulated swallows.[20] The rate in both species is slower in the caudal esophagus. Radiographic evaluation of esophageal function is accomplished with a positive-contrast medium in a liquid form or mixed with solid food. Inter- pretation of the results must be based on the difference in the handling of liquids and solids by the esophagus.

Regulation of Esophageal Phase of Swallowing.[10] The motor activity of the esophagus is a precisely coordinated series of sequential contractions of its striated muscle. They are produced by discharge from a group of neurons in the brain stem. The control of all phases of swallowing is shown in Figure 8-5, and reflex control of the esophageal phase is shown in Figure 8-6.

The striated muscles of the canine esophagus are innervated by efferent fibers in the vagus nerve. These fibers arise from lower motor neurons in the nucleus ambiguus. Efferent motor fibers from this nucleus are not parasym- pathetic even though they are carried in the vagus nerve. Like all other nerve fibers that innervate striated muscles, these fibers terminate on motor end plates in muscles. Upper motor neurons for the swallowing reflex are located in the swallowing center, in the medial part of the lateral reticular formation.[21] There are connections between this center and the center for respiration, since there must be important interactions between these functions. Respiration must be inhibited during deglutition. The pathway for afferent fibers to the swallowing center is in the tractus solitarius. This is the common central pathway for many peripheral afferents that reach the brain by way of the nerves shown in Figure 8-5. The nucleus tractus solitarius is important in the physiology of cardiovascular and respiratory function as well as for normal swallowing.[10] In some diseases of the esophagus, such as megaesophagus, some of the cardiovascular and respiratory reflexes (with afferent fibers in the vagi) cannot be evoked. Thus, some of these diseases are believed to be caused by a single central lesion, in this case in the nucleus tractus solitarius.

Smooth muscle of the esophagus is innervated by parasympathetic and sympathetic nerve fibers that control its motor function. Vagal parasympathetic fibers originate in the dorsal motor nucleus of the vagus in the brain stem. Long vagal preganglionic fibers synapse in the intrinsic plexuses located within layers of smooth muscle. Ganglionic neurons in the plexuses send out short postganglionic fibers that innervate smooth muscle. The only smooth muscle in the esophagus of the dog is the muscularis mucosae, and that contributes little if anything to the peristaltic movement of a bolus of food to the stomach. In contrast, the smooth-muscle structure of the esophagus in the cat depends on its intrinsic nervous system for motor function. Extrinsic parasympathetics are required for normal coordinated peristalsis.

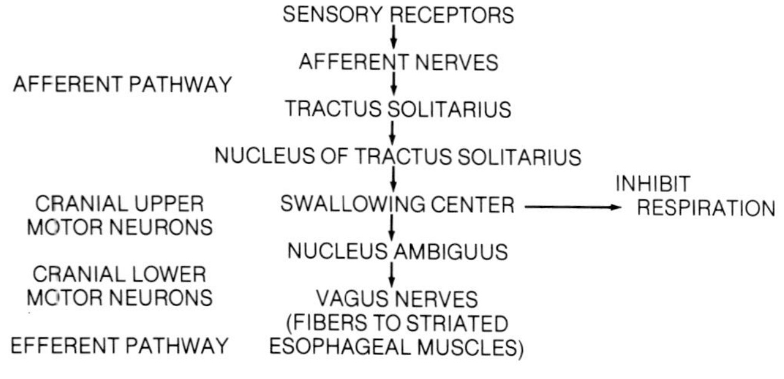

Figure 8-6. Neural pathway for the esophageal phase of swallowing in the dog. Sensory receptors are primarily in the pharynx. Motor fibers to esophageal muscles are somatic nerves in the vagus. Cats differ in that the caudal esophagus is made up of smooth fibers supplied by parasympathetic fibers in the vagus that have their origin in the dorsal motor nuclei of the vagus.

Function of the esophagus in the dog is controlled almost entirely by its extrinsic nervous innervation. If the vagi are sectioned in the cervical region, the distal part of the esophagus dilates, retains food, and has feeble simultaneous repetitive contractions during swallowing.[22] Cutting the vagi in the hilar region or cutting some of the multiple vagal esophageal branches results in similar dysfunction distal to the level of section. Thus, interruption of the efferent fibers paralyzes the esophagus. Denervation also produces the histologic changes of striated muscle atrophy that occur whenever this type of tissue loses its nerve supply.[23] Paralysis of the esophagus occurs also when the nucleus ambiguus is bilaterally destroyed in the dog, although not when the dorsal motor nucleus of the vagus is destroyed.[24] In contrast, cats that have the dorsal motor nucleus destroyed lose coordinated motor activity in the esophagus.[24] The difference reinforces the concept that the small amount of smooth muscle in the dog's esophagus does not contribute effectively to peristalsis, whereas the opposite is true in the caudal esophagus of the cat.

If a fistula is created in the lower cervical area of the esophagus to divert a swallowed bolus to the outside, peristalsis will be observed in the esophagus down to the fistula, but none will be evident in the distal part.[25] Therefore, the cervical esophagus relays information centrally that a bolus is passing by, and the reflex response is to continue the peristaltic movement. This primary peristaltic contraction does not fade away if a swallowed bolus is diverted from the esophagus in its thoracic part.[25] It was mentioned that esophageal sensory receptors maintaining the wave of peristalsis may not function normally in the presence of inflammation of the esophagus. In fact, it has been shown that experimental production of esophagitis in dogs results in severely disordered motor activity.[26] Similar findings are reported for cats with esophagitis.[27] The size of the bolus is also important for the development of the peristaltic wave that will progress through the entire length of the esophagus. Whereas the wave of peristalsis will always be complete as a bolus of food passes down a normal esophagus, peristaltic waves will sometimes be incomplete when a dog or cat swallows a liquid.

The importance of the afferent impulses transmitted from the esophagus is illustrated by what is termed "secondary peristalsis." Frequently, a large bolus of food becomes lodged in the esophagus, and the peristaltic wave that initially propelled its movement passes over it. The bolus would remain there unless a mechanism were present to move it on. This mechanism involves a reflex with connections in the central nervous system. Sensory receptors in the esophagus are stimulated by the lodged bolus, reflexly resulting in an efferent response that initiates a wave of peristalsis to move the bolus caudally. Secondary peristalsis begins in the esophagus cranial to the bolus and is indistinguishable from primary peristalsis in manometric evaluations.[28] In summary, esophageal motor activity of dogs is under complete control of the central nervous system and is dependent on afferent activity arising from within the esophagus.

Gastroesophageal Sphincter and Junction Function[10,19,29,30]

The gastroesophageal sphincter (GES) is important in ensuring unidirectional flow between the esophagus and stomach (Figure 8-7). The GES maintains a high-pressure zone between the esophagus and stomach. The GES relaxes and opens during swallowing. Fibers in the vagus reflexly mediate relaxation, which can be detected up to five seconds before a bolus reaches the sphincter. The relaxed sphincter opens when the bolus arrives. After the bolus passes through, the sphincter contracts and prevents reflux of gastric contents into the esophagus. The sphincter is not the only mechanism that prevents gastroesophageal reflux. For example, if the sphincter is replaced by a narrow stomach tube, a high-pressure zone persists between the esophagus and stomach, preventing gastroesophageal reflux.[31] Administration of pentagastrin further increases the pressure of this region.

The short segment of esophagus within the abdominal cavity is important in preventing gastroesophageal reflux. This segment acts as a flutter valve. When abdominal pressure increases, there is a potential for reflux caused by increasing pressure within the stomach. To prevent that, however, the increase in abdominal pressure is transmitted also to the intra-abdominal segment of esophagus; this causes the segment to close, and reflux does not occur since the pressure in the stomach is not greater than that which closes the segment. The pressure is normally greater in the lumen of the gastroesophageal sphincter than in the esophagus or stomach. When equal increments of pressure are added to both the sphincter (which is primarily in the abdominal cavity) and the stomach, the final pressure is still greater in the sphincter than in the stomach, and reflux does not occur. Increases in intra-abdominal pressure in cats results in comparable increases in both intragastric and GES pressures, so that GES pressure continues to exceed intragastric pressure.[32] If the intra-abdominal segment of esophagus, including the sphincter, moves into the thorax as a result of a hiatal hernia, the flutter valve function is lost, and an increase in intra-abdominal pressure results in gastroesophageal reflux.

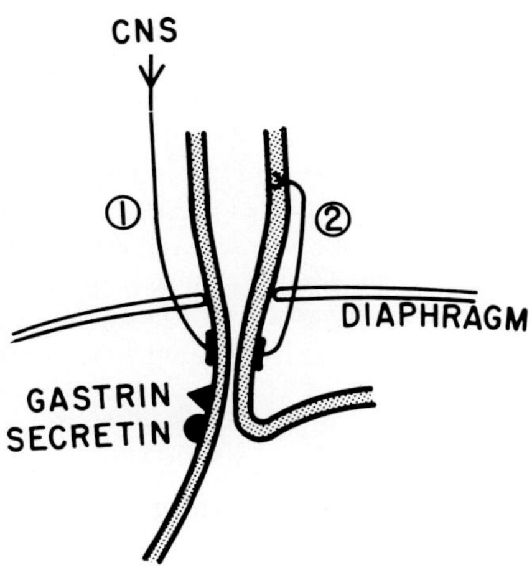

Figure 8-7. Diagram of gastroesophageal sphincter. Pressure in the sphincter is higher than in the esophagus at both the cranial and caudal ends. Pressure is maintained by vagal activity. During deglutition, vagal activity causes an immediate drop in pressure, via (1). When the bolus arrives at end of the esophagus, a neural reflex causes the sphincter to open (2). The sphincter also responds to gut hormones via receptors for gastrin and secretin families.

The angle at which the esophagus enters the stomach affects the ease with which gastric contents might reflux into the esophagus. The esophagus enters the empty stomach at an almost perpendicular angle. When the stomach is distended, however, the angle becomes very acute. Gastric distention results in compression of the esophagus by the fundus. This creates a valve whereby intragastric pressure maintains closure of the gastroesophageal junction (Figure 8-8). The oblique gastric muscle fibers at the junction contribute to the valve's competence. Contraction of these fibers accentuates the acuteness of the angle. However, removal of these "sling" fibers does not result in gastroesophageal reflux.

The diaphragm contributes to the competence of the gastroesophageal valve by helping maintain the oblique entry of the esophagus into the stomach, and by contraction of the crura of the diaphragm. Cutting the left crural fibers results in the development of reflux esophagitis in dogs. Mucosal folds in the cardia and the phrenoesophageal membrane are also thought to contribute to maintaining closure of the gastroesophageal valve. Many of the anatomic features of the gastroesophageal junction are important for normal function of the gastroesophageal sphincter, although the sphincter itself is controlled by the nervous system and, possibly, by peptide hormones.

Regulation of Function in Gastroesophageal Sphincter.[19,29,33,34] The dog's gastroesophageal sphincter consists of an outer layer of striated muscle and an inner layer of smooth muscle. The cat's gastroesophageal sphincter is composed entirely of smooth muscle. Striated muscle fibers are responsible for rapid closure of the sphincter, while smooth muscle fibers maintain closure. The sphincter opens and closes in response to neural activity associated with swallowing but can also function independently.

Normal GES pressure in dogs is maintained at approximately 50 mmHg by at least two excitatory neural influences. One is a vagal cholinergic mechanism that is blocked by vagotomy or by cooling of the vagus nerves, in which case GES

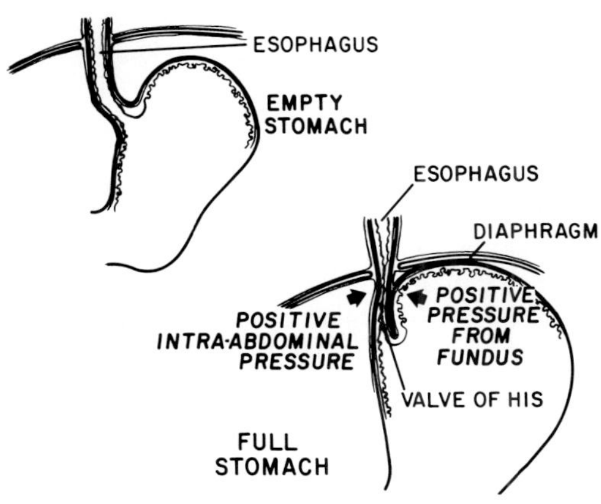

Figure 8-8. Schematic to show how filling of the stomach closes the gastroesophageal junction to form the valve of His.

pressure falls to 28 mmHg. The second influence is a nonvagal mechanism that uses both α-adrenergic and cholinergic (blocked by atropine) receptors. Both of the neural mechanisms contain a nicotinic ganglionic pathway. Atropine reduces GES pressure to 13 mmHg; the reduction greater than that caused by vagotomy alone supports the belief that there is a nonvagal as well as a vagal cholinergic control of GES pressure. Vagotomy also impairs relaxation and contraction with swallowing. The sphincter normally relaxes at the onset of swallowing as a result of impulses mediated by vagal nerve fibers. The vagally-mediated relaxation is lost with vagotomy. Blockers of cholinergic or adrenergic activity have no effect on the vagally mediated sphincter relaxation, an observation suggesting that a different neurotransmitter is involved.

Vagotomy does not cause the smooth muscle to become paralyzed, since it still contains intrinsic nervous elements that impart some function, as well as autonomous smooth muscle tone; hence, GES pressure maintains at 28 mmHg after vagotomy. The regulation from the remaining factors is much less effective than the control exerted by the central nervous system, however. The intrinsic properties of circular muscle from the sphincter have been studied in muscle-strip preparations. When graded tension is applied to these strips, resistance to stretch increases. The strips show a decrease in tension when they are stimulated electrically. Since the response is blocked by tetrodotoxin, it is thought to be mediated by the intrinsic nervous system that is still present. The intrinsic neural mechanisms in the smooth muscle can produce GES inhibition and contraction, and the myogenic mechanisms contribute to resting tone and may participate in GES relaxation and contraction. Although many peptide hormones and biogenic amines affect GES pressure, the extrinsic and intrinsic neural mechanisms are primarily responsible for basal GES tone.

Pressure in the GES is influenced by events in the stomach and esophagus. Increased intragastric pressure, whether produced by food, water, or abdominal compression, causes sphincter pressure to increase and remain above intragastric pressure. The increase in GES pressure is greater than the increases for both intragastric and intra-abdominal pressures.[35] This reflex protects against gastroesophageal reflux when intra-abdominal pressure is raised. Electrical stimulation of the central end of one vagus that has been cut causes an increase in pressure in the sphincter, suggesting that this response is dependent on sensory information from the stomach and sphincter that is transmitted via the vagus nerves. Part of the response is produced by the flutter valve action of the GES. Another reflex prevents against great increases in intragastric pressure, increases that could result in gastric rupture. Stimulation of intramural gastric nerves causes GES relaxation; presumably gastric distention stimulating those nerves permits venting of contents into the stomach and prevents gastric rupture.[36]

The GES is still able to open and close when all connections with the central nervous system are removed. The function is lost, however, when a circular cuff of muscle is removed from the esophagus just cranial to the sphincter, indicating that the caudal esophagus is controlling GES function. This esophageal-dependent control of sphincter function is lost when the most caudal parts of the esophagus are diseased. Esophagitis produced in experimental animals causes GES pressure to fall. The inflammation disrupts the reception of sensory information that maintains GES closure.[37] Distention of the caudal esophagus stimulates GES relaxation by a reflex mediated through the vagus.[38] Although the GES can still open and close without neural connections to the central nervous system, the regulation of that event is importantly controlled by the extrinsic nerves to the spincter.

The GES pressure of approximately 50 mmHg varies little from day to day in an unfed individual. Feeding increases the pressure by increments up to 20 mmHg; the response seems appropriate for preventing gastroesophageal reflux during times of maximum secretion of pepsin and hydrochloric acid, both of which can cause esophagitis. The GES has receptors for gastrin, histamine and acetylcholine.[39] Whereas the cholinergic mechanisms are primarily responsible for maintaining GES pressure in the unfed state, an interaction of events at gastrin, histamine, and cholinergic receptors is responsible for the increase in GES pressure after feeding.[40] Histamine mediates its effect at H_1-receptors rather than H_2-receptors because diphenhydramine but not cimetidine reduces the post-feeding GES pressure increment to unfed GES pressures. Peptide hormones (other than gastrin) released during feeding have been shown to increase GES pressure (Table 8-1). They include pancreatic polypeptide, motilin, and substance P.[41-43] It would be interesting to know whether GES pressure is reduced in dogs with pancreatic exocrine deficiency and a deficiency of pancreatic polypeptide. Motilin is released during the unfed state (fats may stimulate its release after feeding) and stimulates the interdigestive or migrating myoelectric complex that begins in the GES and increases GES pressure for short periods once every 1.5 to 2 hours.

A number of peptide hormones reduce GES pressure and are also released during the fed state. Despite the release of these inhibitory peptides the increment of approximately 20 mmHg is maintained. Under normal conditions they are probably unimportant for regulating GES pressure. In many cases the inhibitory effects of these hormones reflect a GES response to infusion of pharmacologic amounts of hormone. The effects are seen because gastrointestinal structures generally have receptors for all groups of peptide hormones. The structures show responses to peptide hormones with a primary action for the structure, but they can also exhibit responses (almost always smaller) to structurally similar peptides.

Secretin is a competitive inhibitor of the action of gastrin on the gastroesophageal sphincter. Secretin also inhibits the release of gastrin. Some experiments have shown that alkalinization of the stomach can increase sphincter pressure by reciprocal changes in secretion of the two hormones gastrin and secretin. Cholecystokinin and glucagon have an inhibitory

Table 8-1. Hormones and Chemicals with Effects on GES Pressure

Excitatory	Inhibitory
Gastrin	Cholecystokinin
Substance P	Secretin
Motilin	VIP
Histamine	Somatostatin
Met-enkephalin	Glucagon
Bombesin	Prostaglandins
Serotonin	Histamine
Cholinergics	Anticholinergics
α - adrenergics	ß-adrenergics
	Estrogens, progesterone

effect similar to that of secretin. Thus, gastroesophageal pressure is regulated by a number of gastrointestinal-tract hormones that compete for receptor sites. That finding is consistent with the hypothesis that any organ that can be shown to respond to one gastrointestinal hormone will respond to all of them.[44]

The GES pressure after feeding is determined by the type of food consumed. Protein meals increase GES pressure, presumably because protein is a potent stimulus for gastrin release and the histamine release necessary to sustain increased gastric acid secretion. High fat diets decrease GES pressure due to the lipid's effect of stimulating cholecystokinin's (and possibly other hormone's) release. Fat inhibits the gastrin-mediated increase in GES pressure. Other foods occasionally fed small animals can decrease GES pressure (Table 8-2). Food selection is important to successful management of animals with reduced GES pressure and reflux esophagitis.

In summary, normal anatomic relationships and regulation by vagus nerves and endocrines are necessary for optimum function of the gastroesophageal sphincter. The loss of some components does not result in sphincter incompetence. However, displacement of the sphincter into the thorax, cutting one crura of the diaphragm, or vagotomy causes substantial loss of function that can result in reflux esophagitis.

Drugs have an important effect on the gastroesophageal sphincter. Pre- and postoperative drugs including acepromazine, atropine, xylazine, and diazepam lower GES pressure in dogs.[45,46] Metoclopramide, meperidine, cisapride and bethanechol increase GES pressure in dogs.[40,45] The circular muscle of the sphincter is normally more sensitive to acetylcholine and norepinephrine than is other smooth muscle.[47] Catecholamines (epinephrine or norepinephrine) sometimes increase GES pressure and induce phasic contractions in the dog, but sometimes GES pressure is reduced.[40] Blocking these effects with either α-adrenergic of ß-adrenergic antagonists shows that stimulation of α-adrenergic receptors increases GES pressure and stimulation of ß-adrenergic receptors reduces GES pressure. Adrenergic neurons may contribute to the maintenance of GES pressure in cats.[9] Other chemicals such as serotonin increase GES pressure in dogs, and some such as domperidone cause strong and markedly phasic contractions.[40]

Because inflammation of the esophagus decreases GES pressure in cats,[48] as well as other species, inflammation can initiate a vicious cycle in which the esophagitis-induced decreased GES pressure increases the possibility of further reflux and perpetuation of the esophagitis. Drugs interfering with maintenance of normal GES pressure should not be used in the management of such cases.

Of the many neurotransmitters (many of which are peptide hormones) which reduce GES pressure, only vasoactive intestinal polypeptide (VIP) is believed to be the neurotransmitter released for relaxation and opening of the GES.[49,50] Sphincter muscle and its neural plexuses are associated with VIP-immunoreactive oval cells. An incompletely understood nonadrenergic and noncholinergic neural mechanism releases VIP, which appears to act directly on smooth muscle to inhibit motility.

Table 8-2. Foods Affecting GES Pressure

Increase	Decrease
Proteins	Fats Chocolate Citrus juices Tomato juice Spices (?)

The GES opens and closes under normal conditions only when a bolus travels through the esophagus to the stomach and when gas eructates from the stomach. Eructation of gas stimulates GES relaxation and opening via a neural pathway in the vagus which is not blocked by anticholinergic drugs.[51,52] The mechanism is probably the same as for GES opening during swallowing, namely a nonadrenergic, noncholinergic efferent neural pathway to release VIP. Relaxation of the cranial diaphragm, an event also seen with swallowing, accompanies the GES changes.[53,54] The sensory receptors for initiating eructation are not located in the gastric fundus nor in the gastric antrum.[55,56] Distention of the cardia by gas and not fluid is necessary for eructation; preventing such distention inhibits eructation.[57,58] As would be expected, changes in body position to maximize the opportunity for gas to accumulate in the cardia results in more frequent eructation.[59] During eructation the reflex changes also include relaxation and opening of the pharyngoesophageal sphincter.[60]

The GES transiently relaxes to permit eructation of gas at a frequency that is greater following a meal. Relaxations to vent gas from the stomach allow liquid contents to reflux into the esophagus. In normal dogs, over a three hour period there can be as many as 40 episodes of gastroesophageal reflux of acid.[61] The majority (77%) of refluxes are not associated with GES relaxation stimulated by swallowing. The acid reflux episodes correlated with gas eructation. In another study in dogs, when the gastric gas cap was dorsal to the esophagus at the onset of eructation, some ingesta invariably accompanied gas into the esophagus.[53] Ninety percent of the eructations were followed by a relatively slow (17 cm/sec) peristaltic wave that returned the refluxed material to the stomach. Similar patterns, but less frequent, of reflux are recorded in unfed dogs. The total time the esophagus is acidified is up to 3%; the time is determined by how rapidly and efficiently esophageal peristalsis clears the acid from the esophagus. The time of esophageal acidification is greater in the third hour than the first two hours after feeding. Thus, to a certain extent gastroesophageal reflux is a normal event.

Following birth, deglutition requires some months before maturation to the swallowing function evident in adults.[10] Studies show the sensory systems for swallowing to be well-developed in the fetus, but the maturation of the control of swallowing continues after birth. For example, stimulation of the superior laryngeal nerve in kittens up to a week old does not consistently evoke the pharyngeal phase of swallowing. Stimulation of the same nerve in puppies does not elicit a complete glottis closure; in fact, closure of the glottis is incomplete during swallowing in puppies up to six weeks old. Other studies show GES pressure to gradually increase in kittens so that by six weeks the pressure is one-half that of adults.[62] Similar maturation delays are found in pups.[17] It is evident that age-determined delays in maturation of swallowing must be considered when evaluating young pups and kittens for apparent swallowing abnormalities.

REFERENCES

1. Miller, M.E., Christensen, G.C., and Evans, H.E.: Anatomy of the dog. W.B. Saunders Co., Philadelphia. 1964.
2. Nickel, R., Schummer, A., Seiferle, E. and Sack, W.O.: The Viscera of Domestic Mammals. Springer-Verlag, New York. 1973.
3. Henk, W.G., Hoskins, J.D. and Abdelbaki, Y.Z.: Comparative morphology of esophageal mucosa and submucosa in dogs from 1 to 337 days of age. Am. J. Vet. Res. 47:2658-2665, 1986.
4. Lund, W.S.: A study of the cricopharyngeal sphincter in man and in the dog. Ann. R. Coll. Surg. Eng. 37:225-246, 1965.
5. Venker-van Haagen, A.J., Hartman, W. and Wolvekamp, W.Th.C.: Contributions of the glossopharyngeal nerve and the pharyngeal branch of the vagus nerve to the swallowing process in dogs. Am. J. Vet. Res. 47:1300-1307, 1986.
6. Suter, P.F. and Watrons, B.J.: Oropharyngeal dysphagias in the dog I. Vet. Radiol. 21:24-39, 1980.
7. Clerc, N.: Histological characteristics of the lower esophageal sphincter in the cat. Acta. Anat. 117:201-208, 1983.
8. Watrous, B.J. and Suter, P.F.: Normal swallowing in the dog: a cineradiographic study. Vet. Radiol. 20:99-109, 1979.
9. Behar, J., Kersein, M. and Biancani, P.: Neural control of the lower esophageal sphincter in the cat: studies on the excitatory pathways to the lower esophageal sphincter. Gastroenterology 82:680-688, 1982.
10. Miller, A.J.: Deglutition. Physiol. Rev. 62:129-184, 1982.
11. Doty, R.W.: Neural organization of deglutition. In, Handbook of Physiology, Section 6: Alimentary Canal, Vol. 4. C.F. Code, ed. Washington, D.C. American Physiological Society 1861-1902, 1968.
12. Christensen, J.: Origin of sensation in the esophagus. Am. J. Physiol. 246:G221-G225, 1984.
13. Levitt, M.N., Dedo, H.H., and Ogura, J.H.: The cricopharyngeus muscle, an electromyographic study in the dog. Laryngoscope 75:122-136, 1965.
14. Palmer, E.D.: Disorders of the cricopharyngeus muscle: A review. Gastroenterology 71:510-519, 1976.
15. Freiman, J.M. and Diamant, N.E.: Upper esophageal sphincter (UES) response to esophageal distension and acid, and its alteration with nerve blockade. Gastroenterology 70:970, 1976.
16. Frieman, J.M., El-Sharkawy, T.Y. and Diamant, N.E.: Effect of bilateral vagosympathetic nerve blockade on response of the dog upper esophageal sphincter (UES) to intraesophageal distention and acid. Gastroenterology 81:78-84, 1981.
17. Strombeck, D.R.: Unpublished Observations.
18. Code, C.F., and Schlegel, J.F.: Motor action of the esophagus and its sphincters. In, Handbook of Physiology, Section 6: Alimentary Canal, Vol. 4. C.F. Code, ed. Washington, D.C., American Physiological Society 1821-1839, 1968.
19. Gaynor, F., Hoffner, R.E., Nichols, M.F., Rosser, E., Moraff, H., Hahn, A.W. and MacCoy, D.M.: Physiologic features of the canine esophagus: effects of tranquilization on esophageal motility. Am. J. Vet. Res. 41:727-732, 1980.
20. Correnti, F.S., Little, A.G., Calleja, I.J. and Skinner, D.B.: Manometric evaluation of the feline esophagus. J. Surg. Res. 41:312-318, 1986.
21. Nakayama, S., Neya, T., Watanabe, K., and Tsuchiya, K.: Effects of electrical stimulation and local destruction of the medulla oblongata on swallowing movements in dogs. Rendic. Gastroenterology. 6:6-11, 1974.
22. Carveth, S.W., Schlegel, J.F., Code, C.F., and Ellis, F.H.: Esophageal motility after vagotomy, phrenicotomy, myotomy, and myomectomy in dogs. Surg. Gynecol. Obstet. 114:31-42, 1962.
23. Lynch, V.P., Schlegel, J.F., and Ellis, F.H.: Autotransplantation of the canine esophagus. Surg. Gynecol. Obstet. 138:396-400, 1974.
24. Higgs, B., Kerr, F.W.F., and Ellis, F.H.: The experimental production of esophageal achalasia by electrolytic lesions in the medulla. J. Thor. Cardio. Surg. 50:613-625, 1965.
25. Janssens, J., Valembois, P., Vantrappen, G., Hellemans, J., and Pelemans, W.: Is the primary peristaltic contractions of the canine esophagus bolus dependent? Gastroenterology 65:750-756, 1973.
26. Henderson, R.D., Mugashe, F., Jeejeebhoy, K.N., Cullen, J., Szczepanski, M., Boszko, A., and Marryatt, G.: The role of bile and acid in the production of esophagitis and the motor defect of esophagitis. Ann. Thorac. Surg. 14:465-473, 1972.
27. Liebermann-Meffert, D., Klaus, D., Vosmeer, S. and Allgower, M.: Effect of intraesophageal bile and acid (HCL) perfusion on the action of the lower esophageal sphincter. Scand. J. Gastroenterology 19(suppl92):237-241, 1984.
28. Janssens, J., Valembois, P., Hellemans, J., Vantrappen, G., and Pelemans, W.: Studies on the necessity of a bolus for the progression of secondary peristalsis in the canine esophagus. Gastroenterology 67:245-251, 1974.
29. Arimori, M., Code, C.F., Schlegel, J.F., and Sturm, R.E.: Electrical activity of the canine esophagus and gastroesophageal sphincter. Amer. J. Dig. Dis. 15:191-208, 1970.
30. Botha, G.S.M.: The Gastro-Oesophageal Junction: Clinical Applications to Oesophageal and Gastric Surgery. Boston, Little, Brown, 1962.
31. Moossa, A.R., Hall, A.W., Wood, R.A.B., Cooley, G.R., and Skinner, D.V.: Effect of pentagastrin (PG) infusions on gastroesophageal manometry and reflux status, before and after esophagogastrectomy. Abstract 80, Meeting Society for Surgery of the Alimentary Tract, Miami, 1976.
32. Boyle, J.T., Altschuler, S.M., Nixon, T.E., Pack, A.E. and Cohen, S.: Responses of feline gastroesophageal junction to changes in abdominal pressure. Am. J. Physiol 253:G315-G322, 1987.
33. Goyal, R.K. and Rattan, S.: Neurohumoral, hormonal, and drug receptors for the lower esophageal sphincter. Gastroenterology 74:598-619, 1978.
34. Pope, C.E.: Pathophysiology and diagnosis of reflux esophagitis. Gastroenterology 70:445-454, 1976.
35. Boyle, J.T., Altschuler, Nixon, T.E., Pack, A.I. and Cohen, S.: Responses of feline gastroesophageal junction to changes in abdominal pressure. Am. J. Physiol. 253:G315-G322, 1987.
36. Schulze-Delrieu, K.: Intrinsic reflexes between the esophagus and stomach. Gastroenterology 91:1568-1569, 1986.
37. Biancani, P., Barwick, K., Selling, J. and McCallum, R.: Effects of acute experimental esophagitis on mechanical properties of the lower esophageal sphincter. Gastroenterology 87:8-16, 1984.
38. Price, L.M., El-Sharkawy, T.Y., Mui, H.Y. and Diamant, N.E.: Effect of bilateral cervical vagotomy on balloon-induced lower esophageal sphincter relaxation in the dog. Gastroenterology 77:324-329, 1979.
39. Zwick, R., Bowes, K.L., Daniel, E.E. and Sarna, S.K.: Mechanism of action of pentagastrin on the lower esophageal sphincter. J. Clin. Invest. 57:1644-1651, 1976.
40. Strombeck, D.R. and Harrold, D.: Effect of gastrin, histamine, serotonin, and adrenergic amines on gastroesophageal sphincter pressure in the dog. Am. J. Vet. Res. 46:1684-1690, 1985.
41. Coltharp, W., Maher, J.W., Maher, M.S., Schlegel, J., Sandler, A. and McGuigan, J.E.: The effect of truncal vagotomy on the response of the canine lower esophageal sphincter to varying doses of pancreatic polypeptide. Surg. 103:620-623, 1988.
42. Meissner, A.J., Bowes, K.L., Zwick, R. and Daniel, E.E.: Effect of motilin on the lower oesophageal sphincter. Gut 17:925-932, 1976.
43. Reynolds, J.C., Ouyang, A. and Cohen, S.: A lower esophageal sphincter reflex involving substance P. Am. J. Physiol 246:G346-G354, 1984.
44. Grossman, M.E.: Gastrin and its activities. Nature (London) 228:1147-1150, 1970.
45. Strombeck, D.R. and Harrold, D.: Effects of atropine, acepromazine, meperidine, and xylazine on gastroesophageal sphincter pressure in the dog. Am. J. Vet. Res. 46:963-965, 1985.
46. Hall, J.A., Magne, M.L. and Twedt, D.C.: Effect of acepro-

mazine, diazepam, fentamyl-droperidol, and oxymorphone on gastroesophageal sphincter pressure in healthy dogs. Am. J. Vet. Res. 48:556-557, 1987.

47. Misiewicz, J.J.: Symposium on gastroesophageal reflux and its complications. Section 4, Pharmacology and Therapeutics. Gut 14:243-246, 1973.

48. Eastwood, G.L., Castell, D.O., and Higgs, R.H.: Experimental esophagitis in cats impairs lower esophageal sphincter pressure. Gastroenterology 69:146-153, 1975.

49. Behar, J., Field, S. and Marin, C.: Effect of glucagon, secretin, and vasoactive intestinal polypeptide on the feline lower esophageal sphincter: mechanisms of action. Gastroenterology 77:1001-1007, 1979.

50. Biancani, P., Walsh, J.H. and Behar, J.: Vasoactive intestinal polypeptide. A neurotransmitter for lower esophageal sphincter relaxation. J. Clin. Invest. 73:963-967, 1984.

51. Martin, C.J., Patrikios, J. and Dent, J.: Abolition of gas reflux and transient lower esophageal sphincter relaxation by vagal blockade in the dog. Gastroenterology 91:890-896, 1986.

52. Strombeck, D.R., Harrold, D. and Ferrier, W.: Eructation of gas through the gastroesophageal sphincter before and after truncal vagotomy in dogs. Am. J. Vet. Res. 48:207-210, 1987.

53. Heywood, L.H. and Wood, A.K.W.: A radiographic and electromyographic study of eructation in the dog. Abstracts 192, 1988.

54. Altschuler, S.M., Boyle, J.T., Nixon, T.E., Pack, A.I. and Cohen, S.: Simultaneous reflex inhibition of lower esophageal sphincter and crural diaphragm in cats. Am. J. Physiol. 249:G586-G591, 1985.

55. Strombeck, D.R., Turner, W.D. and Harrold, D.: Eructation of gas through the gastroesophageal sphincter before and after gastric fundectomy in dogs. Am. J. Vet. Res. 49:87-89, 1988.

56. Franzi, S.J., Martin, C.J., Dent, J. and Cox, M.R.: Localization of the gastric trigger zone that induces transient lower esophageal sphincter relaxation in the dog. Gastroenterology 95:865, 1988.

57. Menguy, R.: A modified fundoplication which preserves the ability to belch. Surg. 84:301-307, 1978.

58. Strombeck, D.R., Griffin, D.W. and Harrold, D.: Eructation of gas through the gastroesophageal sphincter before and after limiting distension of the gastric cardia or infusion of a ß-adrenergic amine in dogs. Am. J. Vet. Res. 50:751-753, 1989.

59. Little, A.F., Martin, C.J., Dent, J., Harris, A.J. and McMahan, S.J.: Postural suppression of transient lower esophageal relaxations and gastroesophageal reflux in the dog. Gastroenterology 90:1522, 1986.

60. Kahrilas, P.J., Dodds, W.J., Dent, J., Wyman, J.B., Hogan, W.J. and Arndorfer, R.C.: Upper esophageal sphincter function during belching. Gastroenterology 91:133-140, 1986.

61. Patrikos, J., Martin, C.J. and Dent, J.: Relationship of transient lower esophageal sphincter relaxation to postprandial gastroesophageal reflux and belching in dogs. Gastroenterology 90:545-551, 1986.

62. Hillemeier, C., Gryboski, J., McCallum, R. and Biancani, P.: Developmental characteristics of the lower esophageal sphincter in the kitten. Gastroenterology 89:760-766, 1985.

Chapter 9

Diseases of Swallowing

DIAGNOSIS

Clinical Signs

The clinical signs of swallowing disorders may be quite obvious or very subtle. The degree of pharyngeal or esophageal involvement, location of the problem, chronicity, and presence of secondary problems will influence the clinical signs. Clinical signs may be attributable to alimentary tract disease or to secondary complications, such as aspiration pneumonia, which may be mistaken for the primary problem.

Signs of swallowing diseases include regurgitation through the mouth or the nares, dysphagia, odynophagia, repeated swallowing movements, and copious salivation or drooling. A common misconception is that swallowing diseases cause regurgitation only immediately after eating: regurgitation may occur during and shortly after eating or may be delayed for several hours. Differentiating regurgitation from vomiting is important in distinguishing swallowing problems from lower gastrointestinal disease. Characteristics of vomiting include expulsion of digested and bile-stained food and retching with involuntary abdominal contractions. Gastric contents are highly acidic, and pH of vomited material may be tested. Vomiting involves the reflux of fluid into the stomach from the duodenum, however, and when rich in bicarbonate the fluid buffers the gastric acid. The vomited material may then have a neutral or near-neutral pH. Regurgitation involves less forceful casting-up of tubular, bile-free, undigested food. Regurgitation may involve only foam or liquid and, as stated previously, may or may not be directly related to ingestion of food. Mucoid secretions mixed with the undigested food usually have a pH 6.5 to 7.0. Copious salivation may also be a confusing sign. It may be a major sign of pharyngoesophageal problems, such as a foreign body, or it may be part of the prodromal signs preceding vomiting.

Signs of swallowing disorders may be attributable only to the respiratory system. Mucopurulent nasal discharge, dyspnea, or moist coughing will often accompany esophageal disease because of the high incidence of aspiration of ingesta. Dyspnea can be the major sign in dogs with a large filled esophagus compressing the lungs.

Weight loss in association with either anorexia or a voracious appetite may accompany esophageal disease. For example, anorexia and dysphagia usually occur with esophagitis or esophageal foreign bodies, and young animals with congenital megaesophagus might have a voracious appetite accompanied by regurgitation and weight loss. Other signs include cervical cellulitis or a draining fistulous tract secondary to esophageal perforation by a foreign body. Repeated attempts at swallowing accompanied by extension, flexion, or twisting of the head and neck are also hallmarks of swallowing disorders. All of these signs may be intermittent and prolonged, or acute and progressive, depending on the disease process. In summary, the major clinical signs of esophageal disease are regurgitation, dysphagia, coughing and dyspnea.

History

A complete and careful history is essential to recognizing regurgitation and indications that the workup should be for a swallowing problem. The primary complaint may be attributable to the primary pharyngoesophageal signs or to disease in other organs. Historical details should include the exact onset and course of the problems, the type of dysphagia, and its relationship to ingestion of food. Information regarding the animal's ability to retain liquids, soft food, or solid food may be helpful. If the animal shows signs in adulthood, the owner should be questioned regarding its possible exposure to caustic agents, foreign bodies, and traumatic incidents, previous neurologic problems, prior surgery, or anesthesia. Reports of concurrent muscle weakness or neurologic disorders should alert the clinician to an extraesophageal disease process that may underlie the esophageal disease. The clinical signs associated with congenital problems, such as vascular ring anomalies and cricopharyngeal achalasia, will be manifested in an animal that is still nursing or recently weaned to solid food. Acute onset of signs in either a young or older animal is often consistent with the presence of a foreign body. Chronic or slowly progressive regurgitation is more suggestive of gastroesophageal reflux or a developing esophageal stricture.

Physical Examination

Physical examination of patients with swallowing problems may be unrewarding but on occasion confirms the historical suspicion of pharyngoesophageal disease. In addition, the physical examination may reveal the cause of the disease (e.g., palpation of a cervical mass or esophageal foreign body); it provides valuable information with regard to the presence or absence of complications (such as pneumonia) and may aid in the formulation of a prognosis. Frequently, however, special diagnostic techniques are needed to identify pharyngoesophageal disease and to further evaluate any abnormalities noted on physical examination.

The physical condition of the animal may vary from normal to emaciated, depending on the severity of the disease process. Physical findings may explain any of the clinical signs discussed above. Examination of the oropharyngeal cavity usually reveals inflammation and foreign bodies. Useful information may be gained from observation and careful palpation of the cervical and thoracic inlet regions. A dilated cervical esophagus may be seen or palpated, especially when examined during respiration or when the animal's thorax is forcibly compressed while its nostrils are occluded. Auscultation of the cervical esophagus and thoracic inlet and thorax may be helpful. Coarse crackles (moist rales), associated with aspiration pneumonia or fluid movement in the dilated esophagus, may be detected. Watching the animal eat is often a valuable adjunct to physical examination. The type of dysphagia and regurgitation is easily observed.

The differentiation of various esophageal diseases depends on subtle differences in history and physical examination, especially in the character, duration, and time intervals between ingestion, dysphagia and regurgitation. Definitive diagnosis and differentiation of esophageal diseases depend on various diagnostic procedures including radiographic techniques (e.g., contrast studies and fluoroscopy), endoscopy, biopsy, and occasionally manometry, electromyography, and exploratory surgery.

Diagnostic Techniques

Radiology. Radiographic examination of the pharynx and esophagus is an essential procedure for both diagnosis and differential diagnosis of swallowing disorders. Cervical and thoracic survey films and static or dynamic contrast studies are used for that evaluation.

Survey radiographs in lateral and ventrodorsal projections are taken of the pharyngeal to cranial abdominal regions to examine the pharynx and entire esophagus. A right ventrodorsal oblique projection that reduces superimposition of the esophagus on the thoracic vertebrae may also be of value. A high mAs low kVp abdominal technique should be used to evaluate the cervical esophagus, whereas a high kVp-low mAs thoracic technique should be used to evaluate the thoracic soft tissue structures. Contrast studies are done with barium as paste, liquid suspension, or mixed with food. The paste is a 70% w/w form containing a binding agent and can be administered with a syringe. It is used to outline the pharynx and cranial esophagus in animals with suspected pharyngoesophageal swallowing disorders. The suspension is used at a 30% w/v concentration for evaluating esophageal problems. Barium mixed with food is used for evaluating both pharyngoesophageal and esophageal problems. Each of the three forms is given in small boluses and as frequently as necessary to satisfy that an accurate evaluation of pharyngoesophageal motility has been made and that obstruction is confirmed or ruled out.

If fluoroscopy is available, the passage of the barium contrast agents during swallowing can be observed. The study should include recording of three to six complete swallows of liquid barium suspension followed by a similar number of barium-coated food boluses.

If esophageal perforation is suspected, a water-soluble iodinated contrast material should be used. Such materials are less irritating to the periesophageal tissues. If the swallow does not identify a perforation, the study should be repeated with a liquid barium suspension because esophageal perforations may be missed with water-soluble agents.,

Swallowing studies are done without giving patients any chemical restraint. If sedation is necessary, low-dose acetylpromazine has a minimal adverse affect on swallowing, but such a low dose is not likely to ensure success in managing the patient.

Radiographic Interpretation.[1,2] The pharynx of normal animals is evident on radiographs because it is air-filled. The size of the air-filled space varies with disease. The size decreases with local inflammation or neoplasia, laryngeal edema, and elongation of the soft palate. Pharyngeal size increases with dysfunction of the pharynx or pharyngoesophageal sphincter, chronic respiratory (inspiratory) disease, and chronic, severe megaesophagus. Pharyngeal disease can also alter contrast to the pharyngeal region and may displace the larynx.

The normal esophagus is not visible on survey radiographs. An exception occurs following aerophagia due to excitement, nausea, dyspnea, or anesthesia. The presence of luminal air results in a radiolucency that allows visualization of part or all of the course of the esophagus and suggests some details of mucosal topography. Luminal air may also collect as a result of esophageal diseases, such as luminal obstructions or motility disturbances (megaesophagus). Several radiographic features aid differentiation between benign and pathologic accumulations of gas. Gas accumulations following aerophagia due to excitement or struggling are usually transient, and gas is often present in both the stomach and esophagus. Esophageal gas accumulation during anesthesia is usually generalized and uniform and outlines an esophagus of normal diameter and with normal mucosal borders.

Contrast media is not retained in the normal pharynx and cranial esophagus, and so radiographs taken immediately after swallowing contrast show the retention of virtually none. Observations made with fluoroscopy show the formation of a bolus in the pharynx, constriction of the pharynx, and propulsion of the bolus through the pharyngoesophageal sphincter and into the esophagus. Contrast materials are rapidly cleared from the normal esophagus by a series of brisk, aborally progressive peristaltic waves. Any persistent pooling of contrast material in the esophagus following administration should be regarded as abnormal. Pooling, as well as the mucosal pattern revealed, provides important diagnostic information. For example, pooling of contrast material at the level of the base of the heart suggests esophageal obstruction caused by a vascular ring abnormality. An irregular mucosal border is suggestive of an intramural lesion. Following administration of barium paste, the esophageal mucosa of a normal dog is outlined as a series of parallel longitudinal folds extending the entire length of the esophagus. At the thoracic inlet the esophagus may deviate ventrally and the mucosal pattern demonstrates some irregularity. This is a normal finding in the esophagus of young dogs and should not be diagnosed as an esophageal diverticulum. In cats, the barium-outlined mucosa of the cranial two-thirds of the esophagus appears as parallel longitudinal folds, whereas that of the caudal third of the esophagus has a characteristic irregular herringbone pattern that should not be misinterpreted as esophagitis.

The degree of dilatation revealed by the contrast medium and the amount of motility noted on fluoroscopy provide important prognostic information. Once severe esophageal dilatation is present, function is unlikely to be regained. Absence of motility is associated with a poor but not hopeless prognosis. It is important to realize that a hypomotile esophagus has sometimes been demonstrated in excited, dyspneic, or nauseated dogs and in young dogs with no signs of regurgitation. It is also a feature of esophagitis. Other radiographic features suggestive of the various types of esophageal disease are detailed along with the description of the disease.

Endoscopy. Endoscopy (esophagoscopy) with either rigid or flexible fiberoptic instruments is an increasingly important tool in the evaluation of esophageal diseases.

The advantage of endoscopy over the other methods of evaluating esophageal diseases is that one is able to visualize the esophagus and any of its lesions with a noninvasive procedure. Most endoscopes are equipped with an operating channel, which enables tissue specimens (biopsy, brush cytology, impression smears) to be obtained for a more definitive diagnosis. Most foreign bodies can be removed via endoscopy. The major disadvantage is that the procedure requires anesthesia.

Esophageal biopsy specimens may be obtained by three methods. The easiest method is to use alligator or biopsy forceps through either the rigid or the flexible endoscope. Surgical excisional biopsy may also be utilized. Another convenient method of esophageal biopsy is use of suction biopsy equipment.

Intraluminal esophageal manometry is a useful clinical and investigative method for the evaluation of esophageal pressure and motor function. It is currently being utilized extensively in human medicine and on research animals but is used on a limited basis in clinical veterinary medicine at this time.

OROPHARYNGEAL AND PHARYNGOESOPHAGEAL SPHINCTER DISEASES[1,3-5]

Swallowing problems can involve the oral, pharyngeal, and esophageal phases of deglutition. Structural or functional abnormalities can cause problems of the oropharyngeal component of swallowing.

Structural Abnormalities

Structural abnormalities are caused by pharyngeal swelling due to inflammation or edema, trauma and foreign bodies, intraluminal masses, and extraluminal masses (Table 9-1).[6] Clinical signs include salivation and the inability or reluctance to swallow saliva, painful swallowing and often refusal to drink or eat, retching, gagging, immediate regurgitation during attempts to eat, multiple chewing and attempts to swallow, nasal regurgitation, coughing and sometimes dyspnea. Animals making no attempts to drink or eat may show no signs other than depression and in some cases fever when a foreign body or trauma is the cause. Diagnosis is made on physical examination of the oropharyngeal and cranial cervical region; sometimes survey radiographs provide useful information. Foreign bodies such as bone fragments and needles are evident on radiographs. Evidence for gas shadows, swelling and loss of fascial lines may be seen in the retropharyngeal area. Such swelling reduces the size of the pharyngeal air space. Fractured hyoid bones can be seen in some cases of trauma resulting in dysphagia.

Table 9-1. Morphologic (Structural) Lesions causing oropharyngeal dysphagia

Pharyngeal edema:
pharyngitis, trauma, insect stings, snake bites, allergy, chemical or heat injury, impaired venous and lymphatic drainage

Trauma and foreign bodies:
bite wounds, gunshot wounds, fracture of hyoid bones, hematoma, surgical scars

Intraluminal masses (intrinsic):
elongated, inflamed soft palate; tonsillitis; cysts; sialoceles; neoplasms of epiglottis, tonsils, pharyngeal wall, or soft palate

Extraluminal masses (extrinsic):
retropharyngeal lymphadenopathy, retropharyngeal or pharyngeal wall abscesses, salivary gland enlargement, neoplasms, thyroid tumors, lymphosarcoma

Functional Abnormalities

Functional abnormalities are due to neuromuscular problems and result in oropharyngeal dysphagia and cricopharyngeal or pharyngoesophageal dysphagia. By definition, pharyngeal dysphagias result in swallowing disorders involving only the pharynx, and cricopharyngeal dysphagia involves only the pharyngoesophageal sphincter (PES). But many swallowing problems in the beginning of the alimentary tract involve the pharynx, PES, and cranial esophagus. That is not surprising, because the swallowing center has a generator for driving coordinated motility in the pharynx, PES, and cranial esophagus, and the swallowing center has a separate generator for coordinating motility in the esophagus.[7] The lesion would have to be unique for only part of the swallowing mechanism to be involved, i.e., only the pharynx or only the PES.

Oral Dysphagia

Oral dysphagia is an infrequent problem that makes it difficult for animals to drink water and prehend food. They lose motility of the tongue and must bury their muzzle in water and food to force enough into the pharynx, where they can be swallowed. Paresis of the tongue interferes with the ability to propel water and food into the pharynx. Tongue atrophy can be evident; loss of hypoglossal nerve function is responsible. Diagnosis is usually made by observing an animal attempt to drink or eat. Confirmation that pharyngeal and PES dysfunction are not problems can be confirmed by injecting liquids or placing food in the pharynx and observing whether contents in the pharynx can be swallowed. If necessary the same kind of evaluation can be made by radiographic observation of swallowing liquids and solids.

Pharyngeal Dysphagia

Pharyngeal dysphagia results from a loss of normal pharyngeal motility to constrict and propel pharyngeal contents through the PES. Also involved is loss of the ability to close the orifices where pharyngeal contents should not enter. Swallow-

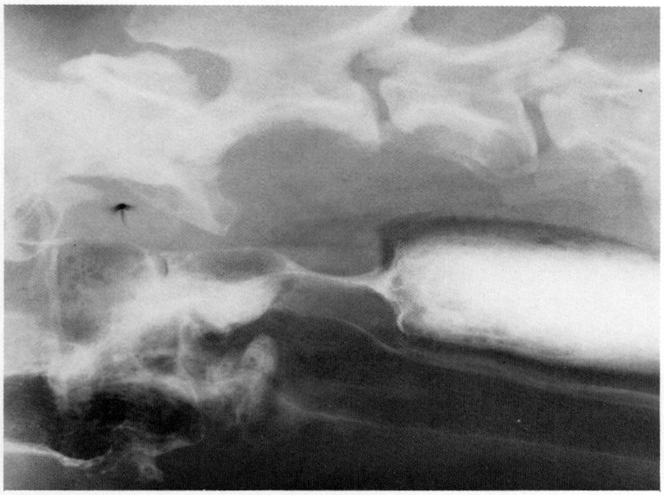

Figure 9-1. Lateral spot film made of pharyngoesophagael sphincter during a positive-contract study made under fluoroscopic control. During each inspiration the contrast medium was aspirated into the larnyx. Cough reflex was not evident; aspiration pneumonia was a problem.

ing is associated with closing of the nasopharyngeal and oropharyngeal orifices and moving of the glottis to close the entrance to the larynx. Clinical signs consistent with pharyngeal dysphagias are similar to signs seen with structural abnormalities, but anorexia and expression of pain during swallowing are not seen with dysphagias. Animals have usually lost weight and make great efforts to consume a meal. Signs of upper respiratory and lower respiratory problems are common, because pharyngeal dysphagia is almost invariably associated with a loss of coordination between swallowing and breathing; aspiration pneumonia is common (Figure 9-1). Clinical signs sometimes reflect a problem affecting muscles other than those of the pharynx. Atrophy of the temporal and masseter muscles, reflecting a neuromyopathy, may be seen.

The cause of most pharyngeal dysphagias is unknown. The cause is usually expected to be myopathy, neuropathy, or central nervous system disease involving nuclei of the glossopharyngeal and the pharyngeal branches of the vagus nerves. The cause may also involve sensory input for the pharyngeal phase of swallowing. Sensory input primarily comes from areas of the caudal pharynx. Disease of the efferent fibers, the tractus solitarius, or nuclei of the tractus solitarius could be responsible for pharyngeal dysphagia.

Confirmation of pharyngeal dysphagia is made only with radiographic studies observing animals swallowing liquids and food. Radiographic studies using contrast media and based only on events recorded on films cannot be relied upon in making a decision on pharyngeal dysphagia. Fluoroscopic confirmation of pharyngeal dysphagia is based on finding slow and incomplete constriction of the pharyngeal cavity, so that air and contrast persist throughout all swallowing attempts, incomplete rostral and dorsal movement of the larynx, and failure of the PES to open with each swallowing attempt because pharyngeal motility is unable to propel a bolus to the PES and cause it to open. Also seen is laryngeal aspiration of contrast medium and evidence of aspiration pneumonia. The laryngeal aspiration of fluid is not associated with the normally expected reflex gagging and coughing. That is not surprising, because some animals can retain food in the pharynx for two to twelve hours after eating. That the food does not stimulate one of many reflexes from sensory input from the pharynx suggests a defect in the afferent neural pathways.

Cricopharyngeal Dysphagia

Cricopharyngeal dysphagia is characterized by a failure of the PES to relax or a lack of coordination between PES relaxation and pharyngeal contraction. The problem is reported in dogs only; clinical signs appear most often at the time of or shortly after weaning, leading to the belief that the dysphagia is congenital. Other suggested causes include myositis, leading to atrophy and fibrosis; muscle hypertrophy or degeneration leading to cicatrization; neurogenic defects; and intoxications. Biopsy of cricopharyngeus muscle from most cases does not show any of these pathologic changes, however. Because most dogs with cricopharyngeal dysphagia show pharyngeal dysphagia and motility deficits of the most cranial part of the esophagus, a central nervous system lesion is likely. A loss of the normal coordination between swallowing and breathing also supports that likelihood. Dogs that can contract the pharynx and relax the PES but lack coordination between the two may have a loss or impairment of sensory input from the pharynx. A failure of complete development of part of the swallowing reflex may cause congenital cricopharyngeal dysphagia. The dysphagia sometimes appears in mature dogs of any age. The causes may be idiopathic, such as in the congenital cases, and they can include traumatic, inflammatory, and neoplastic causes. The dysphagias can also be a manifestation of generalized neuromuscular diseases such as polyneuropathies, polymyositis, muscular dystrophy, and myasthenia gravis.

Diagnosis of cricopharyngeal dysphagia is based on information from observations on an animal eating and drinking and from radiographic studies. The clinical signs do not permit a differentiation between pharyngeal dysphagia and cricopharyngeal dysphagia; the signs are the same for both. Physical examination is usually unremarkable; no unusual resistance or pressure is encountered in the PES. Usually the clinical signs are so pathognomonic of one or the other being the cause that a fluoroscopic examination of swallowing is part of the initial plan. Films taken with or without the dog's swallowing contrast can not be used to differentiate cricopharyngeal dysphagia from pharyngeal dysphagia. Fluoroscopic observations show a persistent or only intermittent inability for the PES to relax and open despite adequate bolus formation and adequate pharyngeal contractions for opening the PES (Figure 9-2). Such studies also show that no anatomic changes due to masses or inflammation are responsible for failure of transit through the PES. The pharynx shows retention of contrast in the pharynx and in many cases in the oropharynx, nasopharynx or larynx and trachea. Often affected dogs show retention of contrast in the cranial end of the cervical esophagus. Following repeated swallowing attempts, only small amounts of ingesta pass through the PES. In many cases swallowing liquids is almost as difficult as swallowing solid food.

Dysphagia with Multiple Dysfunctions

Most dogs with oropharyngeal, pharyngeal, and cricophar-

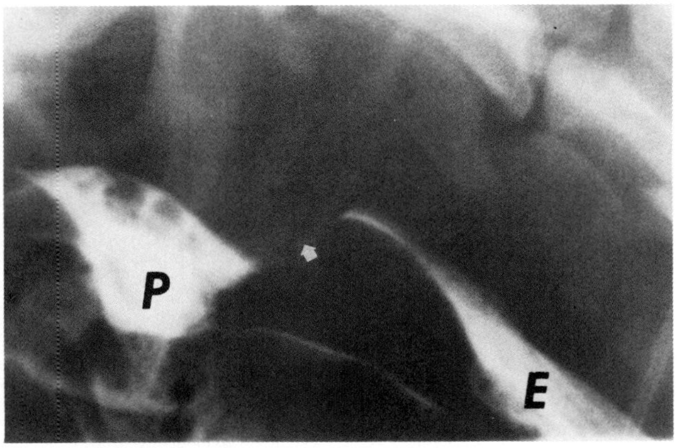

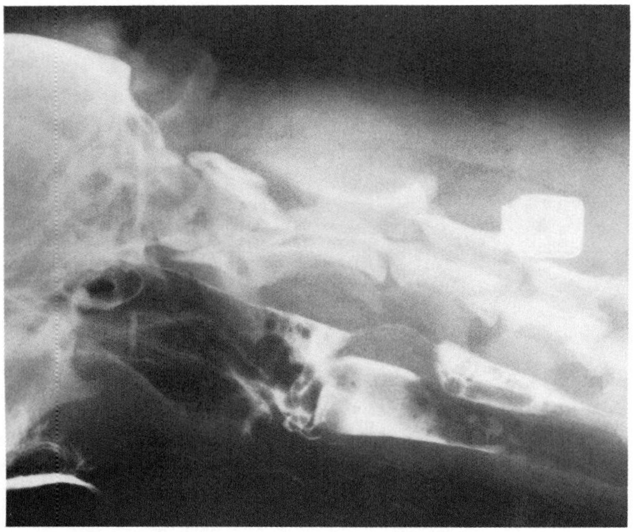

Figure 9-2. Dog with cricopharyngeal dysphagia. Lateral radiographs made when dog was swallowing a liquid positive-contrast medium. Radiograph above shows retention of contrast medium in the pharynx (P). Radiograph below shows same animal with aspiration of positive-contrast medium into upper airway. This illustrates that the normal integration of respiratory and swallowing was abnormal. Myotomy of the cricopharyngeus muscle (arrow) resulted in a remission of all clinical signs, but follow-up cinefluoroscopic studies revealed a persistent motility problem in the pharynx and cranial part of the cervical esophagus. E = Esophagus

yngeal dysphagias have a swallowing dysfunction with aspects of more than one of these dysphagias. The cricopharyngeal dysphagia has been commonly referred to as cricopharyngeal achalasia. The term *achalasia*, meaning failure of a sphincter to open, is used inappropriately because the dysfunction includes pharyngeal motility abnormalities and loss of coordinated motility during swallowing. The mixed dysphagias can represent loss of variable motor innervation in the glossopharyngeal and pharyngeal branches of the vagus nerves. The dysphagias may also represent disorders in the reception and processing of sensory input. Stimulation of the same areas in the pharynx can invoke swallowing, gagging, coughing, or vomiting. The pattern of the sensory input determines which response will follow. The pattern is also essential in determining whether a coordinated response is seen with stimulation of swallowing. Loss of a swallowing response or a coordinated swallowing response is often associated with loss of gagging and coughing responses. The clinical signs and radiographic findings of the mixed dysphagia are the same as those for specific dysphagias. With increased severity one additional radiographic finding can be observed, chalasia or failure of the PES to close. That PES dysfunction can often be identified on survey radiographs of the cranial cervical region (Figure 9-3).

Management

Management of dogs with oropharyngeal or pharyngeal dysphagia is supportive, with feeding procedures to provide caloric needs. Feeding can involve changing the consistency of foods to determine whether the diet is more easily swallowed as a liquid, solid, or solid in the form of chunks. If those attempts fail, feeding must occur by stomach, pharyngostomy, or gastrostomy tube. Diagnosis of specific neuromuscular diseases calls for specific forms of management. Cricopharyngeal dysphagia is managed by myotomy of the cricopharyngeus muscle. Complications of aspiration pneumonia are treated with antibiotics.

Prognosis is poor for oropharyngeal and pharyngeal dysphagias. Most dogs gradually worsen until they are unable to maintain nutritional homeostasis. Treatment of any form is usually unsuccessful. Occasionally a dog improves; improvement usually follows when the cause was traumatic. Myotomy of the cricopharyngeus muscle in such cases, where no cricopharyngeal dysfunction is demonstrated, invariably results in worsening and places the dog at greater risk for aspiration pneumonia. Prognosis is usually good for dogs with cricopharyngeal dysphagia. Success can be predicted for at least 70% of the cases. Most dogs affected young are treated successfully. Older dogs and ones with loss of coordination between pharyngeal and PES function are not as likely to respond well to surgery. On reevaluation of the dysphagia following cricopharyngeal myotomy, some dysfunction of pharyngeal and cranial esophageal motility is almost invariably seen. Such dysfunc-

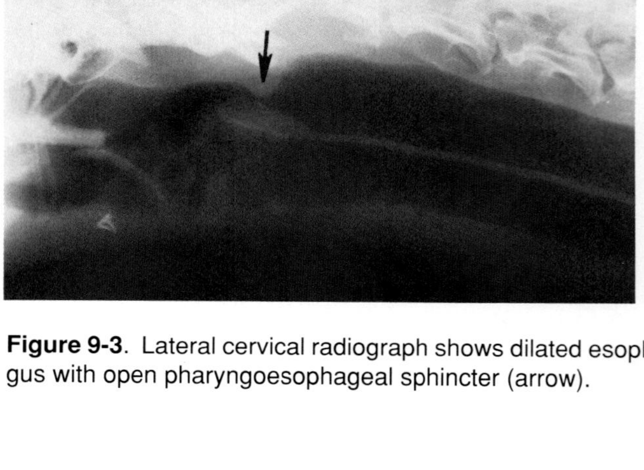

Figure 9-3. Lateral cervical radiograph shows dilated esophagus with open pharyngoesophageal sphincter (arrow).

tion persists and can be responsible for occasional signs of dysphagia.

ESOPHAGEAL MOTILITY DISORDERS

Diseases of the esophagus can be congenital and include a number of motility abnormalities; a form of idiopathic megaesophagus is the most common. Other congenital problems are vascular ring anomalies, hiatal hernias, diverticula, fistulae, atresia, and heterotopia of gastric mucosa in the esophagus. Esophageal diseases acquired after birth include idiopathic megaesophagus, megaesophagus with a known cause, and other motility disorders. Esophagitis, foreign bodies, strictures, periesophageal obstructing lesions, and neoplasia are also seen.

Megaesophagus[1,8-11]

Clinical Synopsis

Diagnostic Features

* Regurgitation
* Dilated esophagus observed by survey or contrast radiography
* Multitude of possible primary causes

Treatment

* Address primary cause if diagnosed
* Treat secondary pneumonia if present
* Feed high calorie, liquid diet from raised receptable

Megaesophagus is a descriptive term for esophageal dilatation, a manifestation of a number of distinct diseases of varied causes. Congenital idiopathic megaesophagus identifies a dilatation of unknown cause that manifests at or shortly after weaning. Adult onset idiopathic megaesophagus is a dilatation with onset after maturity. Secondary or acquired megaesophagus describes all other forms of esophageal dilatation where a cause can be identified.

Epidemiology. Esophageal dilatation is the most important cause of regurgitation in the dog and cat. It is seen with reasonable frequency in referral institutions. Seventy-nine and 125 dogs with generalized megaesophagus were presented to the University of Pennsylvania Veterinary Hospital and the University of California-Davis Veterinary Teaching Hospital, respectively, over eight year periods.[9,12] Over a period of eight years, fifty-three cases of canine megaesophagus were presented to the University of Missouri Veterinary Teaching Hospital, representing approximately one case per thousand of total visitations. The incidence of esophageal dilatation in the cat is generally thought to be lower than in the dog. However, the increased incidence of feline dysautonomia, a condition in which megaesophagus is common,[13] is likely to make megaesophagus an important clinical entity in cats.

Megaesophagus is seen most frequently in young dogs, making congenital idiopathic megaesophagus the most common form (Table 9-2). In one recent survey of fifty cases, however, only 36% were congenital.[8] In a similar number seen at the University of Missouri Veterinary Teaching Hospital, only one-third of the dogs were less than one year of age at presentation. These numbers are likely to be biased by the knowledge that acquired megaesophagus in a mature dog is more likely to be referred to a teaching hospital for evaluation and management than is suspected idiopathic megaesophagus in a very young pup.

Table - 9-2. Age Distribution of Dogs with Megaesophagus at Universities of Pennsylvania and California Reported as Percentage of Total Cases Recorded

	10 wk	1yr	2yr	7 yr	15yr
Pennsylvania	67%	13%	20%		
California	55%		10%	25%	10%

Breed Incidence of Megaesophagus in Dogs at Universities of Pennsylvania and California Reported as a Multiple of Normal Incidence (Equal to 1) if There Were no Breed Predeliction

	Great Dane	German Shepherd	Irish Setter
Pennsylvania	8	2	2
California	10	2	2

Idiopathic megaesophagus in very young dogs is known to be inherited in the Wirehaired Fox Terrier[14,15] and Miniature Schnauzer.[16] The inheritance mode in Wirehaired Fox Terriers is simple autosomal recessive,[14] whereas that in Miniature Schnauzer dogs is compatible with a simple autosomal dominant or a 60 per cent penetrance autosomal recessive pattern.[16] A breed predisposition exists for the German Shepherd, Great Dane, and Irish Setter.[9,12] The high incidence of idiopathic megaesophagus in these three breeds suggests a hereditary basis, as does the report of megaesophagus in litters of both German Shepherds[17] and Great Danes.[18] Numerous other breeds of dogs both, large and small, have been affected by the disease,[9,12,14,19] including a litter of Newfoundlands[20] and a litter of Greyhounds.[21] Breeding of dogs affected by idiopathic megaesophagus (or other close relatives) should be discouraged. There is some evidence that idiopathic esophageal dilatation may also be inherited in the cat[22] and that Siamese-related breeds are predisposed.[23] No breed dispositions are known for idiopathic megaesophagus in adult dogs or for any form of megaesophagus with a known cause.

Etiology and Pathophysiology of Idiopathic Megaesophagus. The cause, site of lesion and pathophysiology of idiopathic megaesophagus are unknown. The primary reasons suggested for the development of megaesophagus are abnormal function in the gastroesophageal sphincter (achalasia) or paralysis of esophageal muscle.

Achalasia. The term achalasia was once widely used in dogs for what is now collectively called megaesophagus. It was believed that the problem developed because failure of the gastroesophageal sphincter (GES) to open led to an accumulation of food and dilatation of the caudal esophagus. That theory was used to described the pathogenesis of achalasia in humans, and veterinarians considered the problem in dogs to be similar. The current belief is that canine megaesophagus does not develop for that reason and is different from achalasia in humans.[9,24-27]

Achalasia in humans results from an increased pressure in the GES. This pressure is associated with a reduced number of nerve cells in the intrinsic plexus of the sphincteric smooth muscle. Denervated smooth muscle can be supersensitive to the neurotransmitters that normally cause it to contract. Increased pressure in the GES of human beings with megaesophagus is suggested to be produced, at least in part, by circulating gastrin, since the intrinsically denervated smooth muscle is supersensitive to gastrin. The nerve cells also contain reduced amounts of vasoactive intestinal peptide, the neurotransmitter responsible for relaxation and opening of the GES.[28] In contrast, the sphincter smooth muscle from dogs with megaesophagus has a normal number of nerve cells in its intrinsic plexus. Dogs with normal intrinsic innervation could lose vagal innervation, explaining achalasia and subsequent megaesophagus. However, extrinsic parasympathetics only modulate GES function. Following extrinsic denervation, GES resting pressure decreases, and the sphincter can still open.[29] Thus, the sphincter offers less than normal resistance to the passage of a bolus.

GES in dogs with megaesophagus has been evaluated using both cineradiographic and manometric procedures; sphincter function was normal.[24] Dogs in that study had normal esophageal function in the most caudal part of the thoracic esophagus; the megaesophagus was confined to the cranial and middle parts of the thoracic esophagus. Studies of normal dogs indicate that neurogenic impulses, initiated as a bolus of food approaches the sphincter, are necessary to initiate sphincter relaxation. Removal of a segment of thoracic esophagus adjacent to the sphincter results in a loss of sphincter function. This experiment suggests that sphincter function is not likely to be normal in patients with generalized megaesophagus and provides an explanation for why the GES may not appear to open and close. If there is a normal segment of esophagus immediately cranial to the sphincter, however, the reflex is intact.[24] Distention of the normal esophageal segment evokes the GES relaxation; distention of a dilated segment results in no GES response. Achalasia has seldom been demonstrated by video fluoroscopic studies of megaesophagus at the VMTH at Davis (Figure 9-4). Dogs with generalized megaesophagus extending to the gastroesophageal sphincter cannot pass food through the sphincter until they are tilted in a vertical position. That finding has been used incorrectly to argue that the problem is achalasia. Once gravity moves the food, however, the GES offers no resistance to its passage. The GES does not appear to actively open, but it offers no resistance to passive dilation by the food.

Achalasia, or abnormality in GES opening and closing, has been seen in a few cases at the VMTH at Davis. Fluoroscopic studies showed a moderately dilated caudal thoracic esophagus with adequate, but not normal, motility for moving a bolus of food. When the food reached the GES, the sphincter did not open, and the bolus moved back and forth a number of times before the GES finally relaxed to allow passage of all or part of the bolus. The problem was blamed on a loss of coordination between esophageal and GES function and may represent a sensory deficit in the caudal esophagus. Achalasia has been described as important in the pathogenesis of idiopathic megaesophagus,[30] but there is little evidence for that idea's support. Manometric measurements of GES pressure before and during swallowing are necessary to identify an achalasia, an area of increased or persisting GES pressure.

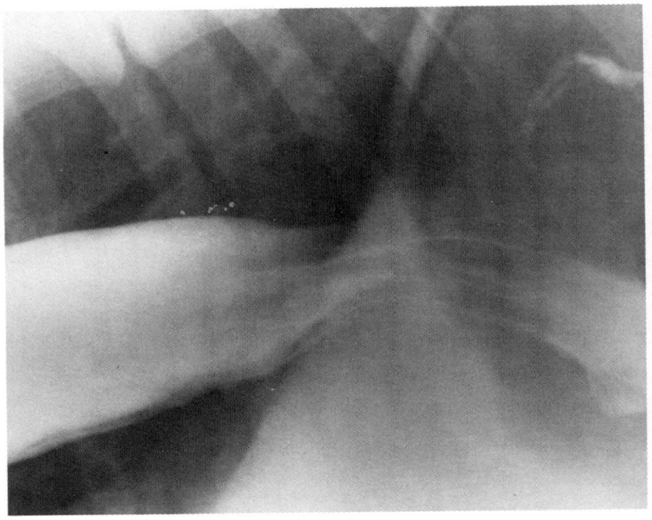

Figure 9-4. Megaesophagus in an 8-year-old German Shepherd. Lateral spot film made of gastroesophageal junction during a positive-contrast study made under fluoroscopic control. Figure illustrates normal function of the gastroesophageal sphincter that has been documented in dogs with megaesophagus.

Myoneural disease. Idiopathic megaesophagus has been described as a myoneural disease that affects the esophagus as well as the sphincter; pathology is suggested to be similar in humans and dogs. Megaesophagus in the two species cannot be compared, however, since the canine esophagus differs completely from the human esophagus in the anatomy of the middle and caudal thirds. The canine esophagus contains striated muscle throughout its length. This muscle is responsible for peristaltic movement of a bolus. A small layer of smooth muscle (the muscularis mucosae) is found, but it does not assist in producing peristaltic waves. The human esophagus contains only smooth muscle in its lower third and both striated and smooth muscle in its middle third. An important feature of achalasia in humans is degeneration of neurons in the intrinsic nerve plexus found within the esophageal smooth muscle. The result is esophageal paralysis. The numbers of neurons in the intrinsic plexus, controlling function in the muscularis mucosa, are not reduced in dogs with megaesophagus.[31] Thus, the esophageal lesions associated with megaesophagus reflect major differences between the species.

The abnormality in megaesophagus is loss of motor function. A defect in any part of the neural pathway for normal esophageal function or in the muscle and myoneural junction results in a loss of function. Megaesophagus can be produced experimentally in dogs by cutting the vagus nerves or by bilateral destruction of the nucleus ambiguus.[32] The motor unit is one part of the functional entity; it consists of cranial lower motor neurons in the nucleus ambiguus, efferent nerve fibers in the vagus, the myoneural junction, and striated muscle fibers. A defect in one part would cause paralysis of the esophagus. A defective motor unit should also result in denervation atrophy. Histologic studies have revealed, however, that the esophageal muscle of patients with megaesophagus is usually normal. Changes that are found are usually secondary to dilatation and esophagitis. Loss of motor unit function should also cause denervation potentials to appear on electromyograms of esophageal muscle.[33] Esophageal electromyograms, however, are normal in dogs with megaesophagus.[27,34] Stimulation of the vagus nerves in dogs with idiopathic megaesophagus results in contraction of the esophagus, indicating that at least some of the motor units are intact. If the motor unit can function in megaesophagus, the cranial lower motor neurons in the nucleus ambiguus must be normal. Serial sections of the brain stem from one dog with megaesophagus were reported to have fewer cell bodies in the nucleus ambiguus.[35] In contrast, unpublished data indicate that the number of neurons in the nucleus ambiguus is normal in dogs with megaesophagus.[36] Another study supports the proposal that the problem is primarily a neural defect.[25] No suggestions were made as to the site of the lesion. Physiologic and pathologic evaluation of dogs with idiopathic megaesophagus has not revealed any difference between congenital and acquired megaesophagus.[27]

If motor units are normal, the pathology must originate in either cranial upper motor neurons or in receptors or the afferent limb of the swallowing reflex. The afferent limb of the reflex consists of nerve fibers in the maxillary branch of the trigeminal nerve and the glossopharyngeal nerve. Their common pathway in the brain is the tractus solitarius, which leads to the nucleus solitarius. Other neurons connect the nucleus of the tractus solitarius with the swallowing center, which is located in the medial part of the lateral reticular formation.[37] The swallowing center contains the cranial upper motor neurons, and it sends fibers to both the respiratory inhibitory centers and the cranial lower motor neurons in the nucleus ambiguus. There is evidence that some of the respiratory reflexes mediated by afferent fibers in the vagus are abnormal in some dogs with megaesophagus.[27] That finding is consistent with the clinical evidence for impairment of respiratory reflexes found in the high frequency of aspiration pneumonia in dogs with megaesophagus.

Studies on other reflexes in dogs with congenital idiopathic megaesophagus provide additional support for a sensory defect.[38] Distention of the normal cranial esophagus or bathing that part of the esophagus with acid causes PES pressure to increase, which serves as a protective reflex. Distending the affected esophagus in dogs with idiopathic megaesophagus or bathing it with acid results in no PES pressure increase. In addition, vagal stimulation in dogs with megaesophagus shows a depressed cardiac response, suggesting a generalized neurologic dysfunction. GES smooth muscle function is not affected in that the migrating motility is not lost, although it may show some impairment.

The pathogenesis of the neurologic lesion in congenital idiopathic megaesophagus is completely unknown. Although there is evidence for its genetic transmission, karyotyping has not revealed any chromosomal abnormality in pups with the problem.[39] A delay in maturation of the esophageal neuromuscular system may cause congenital idiopathic megaesophagus; that explains why young dogs may improve with careful feeding management.[40]

Megaesophagus of unknown cause has also been reported in the cat.[22,41,42] The problems may be inherited,[22] and little is known of the site of the lesion(s) or of the pathogenesis.

Etiology and Pathophysiology of Secondary Megaesophagus. Numerous disease conditions have been associated with, or proposed as cause for, esophageal dilatation (Table 9-3). Any disruption of esophageal muscle or of the central, afferent or efferent pathways that control esophageal motility (Figure 8-5) could theoretically result in megaesophagus by interfering with the act of swallowing. Many such disruptions, either disease- or experimentally induced, have already been shown to cause megaesophagus. For instance, myositis and myopathy — associated with a variety of diseases, including SLE,[8,43] trypanosomiasis,[44] glycogen-storage disease,[45] polymyositis,[8,46] advanced dermatomyositis,[47] and cachexia[23] — have produced sufficient esophageal muscle damage to cause megaesophagus. Neuromuscular junction disease in botulism,[48,49] congenital or acquired myasthenia gravis,[8,50-52] and chronic anticholinesterase administration[53] have been shown to

Table 9-3. Diseases Associated with and Causes of Megaesophagus

Neuromuscular
Idiopathic megaesophagus(hereditary?)
Myasthenia gravis
SLE
Polymyositis and polymyopathy
Glycogen storage disease Type II
Dermatomyositis
Giant cell axonal neuropathy
Polyradiculoneuritis
Immune-mediated polyneuritis
Ganglioradiculitis
Dysautonomia
Spinal muscle atrophy
Bilateral vagal damage (surgical, traumatic, neoplastic)
Familial reflex myoclonus
Cervical vertebral instability with leukomalacia
Brain stem trauma, neoplasia or vascular accident
Botulism
Distemper
Esophageal Obstructive Diseases
Neoplasia
Vascular ring abnormalities
Extraesophageal compression
Strictures, granulomas, foreign bodies
Toxic
Lead
Thallium
Anticholinesterase
Acrylamide
Miscellaneous
Mediastinitis
Bronchoesophageal fistula
Cachexia
Pyloric stenosis
Gastric heterotopia
Addison's disease
Hypothyroidism
Pituitary dwarfism
Trypanosoma cruzi infection
Thymoma

produce esophageal dilatation. Various types of peripheral neuropathies, including polyradiculoneuritis,[8] ganglioradiculitis,[54] dysautonomia,[13] demyelinating neuropathies (such as thallium toxicosis),[55] and axonopathies such as canine giant axonal neuropathy,[56] spinal muscular atrophy,[57] and polyneuritis[23] have produced megaesophagus. Megaesophagus has also been associated with lead toxicity.[58] The suggested cause was a vagal polyneuropathy. Bilateral vagal damage due to trauma, neoplasia, or surgery may cause esophageal dilatation. Megaesophagus has been reported caudal to areas of mediastinitis subsequent to esophageal perforation from foreign bodies.[59] The dilatation was transient; the presumed cause was interference of vagal function by mediastinal cellulitis.[59] A similar finding was reported subsequent to a bronchoesophageal fistula in a dog.[60]

Central nervous system lesions have been established as causes of megaesophagus in dogs and cats. In dogs, both congenital[35] and experimental[32] lesions of the nucleus ambiguus were responsible. In cats, the lesions (experimental) were in the dorsal motor nucleus of the vagus[32,61] and the ventromedial nucleus of the hypothalamus.[62] The difference between the sites of the CNS lesions that cause megaesophagus in dogs and cats is a reflection of the difference in the proportion of the esophageal striated and smooth muscle between the species and therefore the respective importance of the somatic and autonomic nervous system in esophageal innervation. Other CNS diseases that have been associated with megaesophagus include cervical vertebral instability with leukomalacia or stroke, and choroid plexus carcinoma with hydrocephalus.[8] Distemper has been cited as a cause of megaesophagus in two dogs.[8,14] The pathogenesis probably relates to distemper-induced CNS lesions of the medulla or cranial nerve pathways. Familial reflex myoclonus of Labrador Retrievers has been associated with megaesophagus.[63] No pathogenesis was determined.

Hypothyroidism is often cited as a possible cause of megaesophagus. However, very few dogs with hypothyroidism appear to develop megaesophagus. One hypothyroid dog with megaesophagus regained normal esophageal function following thyroid medication.[64] Addison's disease can be associated with transient megaesophagus.[65-67] Esophageal asthenia presumably occurs for the same reasons as the skeletal muscle weakness characteristic of the disease. Some authors believe that any shock-like condition can result in megaesophagus.[68] Some canine pituitary dwarfs have a concurrent megaesophagus.[65]

Most obstructive esophageal diseases (neoplasia, granulomas, vascular rings, strictures, periesophageal masses, and foreign bodies) can lead to megaesophagus if they are of sufficiently chronic duration.[30] The pathogenesis probably relates to the physical overdilatation of the esophagus by accumulating ingesta cranial to the obstruction. Neoplastic invasion of the esophagus may cause motility disturbances,[69] which may contribute to the pathogenesis of the dilatation.

Thymomas are occasionally associated with myasthenia gravis and polymyositis in dogs and cats[70,71] and therefore have the potential to cause megaesophagus. Difficulty swallowing and retention of barium in the esophagus (caudal and cranial to the thymoma) were reported in two cats and several dogs with myasthenia gravis.

Megaesophagus in cats at the VMTH at Davis is seen at a rate of less than one case per 1000 cats seen. On the basis of anatomic similarities, megaesophagus in cats might be compared to achalasia in man. Both species have smooth muscle in all the muscle layers of the distal half to one-third of the esophagus. Histologic studies in feline megaesophagus, however, have shown a normal number of ganglion cells in the intrinsic plexuses.[72] Thus, the problem differs from that in man. Most of these cases are acquired with a recognized cause. A series of cats has been reported with esophageal dysfunction associated with abnormal gastric retention of food.[73] The clinical signs of persistent vomiting were corrected with a pyloromyotomy, and normal esophageal function returned. The cats had a reversible megaesophagus. It has been shown that esophagitis, as would be produced by chronic vomition, causes a loss of gastroesophageal sphincter competence.[74] Furthermore, an esophagitis causes deranged esophageal motility.[75] It is not unusual to see a loss of normal peristalsis, with some evidence for megaesophagus, when the esophageal mucosa has been traumatized chemically or mechanically. Megaesophagus associated with gastric heterotopia (gastric mucosa lining the esophagus) has also been reported in the cat.[76]

Clinical Signs. Clinical signs of megaesophagus include regurgitation, signs of pneumonia, enlargement of the esophagus in the cervical region, and poor body condition.[8,9,12,19,67] Not all dogs with megaesophagus regurgitate[14,19] although this is by far the most consistent clinical sign. The frequency of regurgitation varies greatly from once every two to three days to greater than ten times per day.[19] Regurgitation may be seen immediately after feeding or may occur up to 18 or more hours later. Regurgitation is delayed if the animal is inactive or if the esophageal dilation is marked.[23] Occasionally, however, regurgitation can occur during sleep.[30] Dogs with megaesophagus regurgitate both solids and fluids, in contrast to dogs with partial esophageal obstructions (caused by foreign bodies, strictures), in which fluids are often better tolerated.[30] If retained for prolonged periods, the regurgitated ingesta may ferment. Retained fermenting ingesta may cause halitosis and produce gurgling sounds detectable by the owner.[14] Profuse salivation may occur, presumably resulting from dysphagia. Such salivation may create the impression of nausea, more suggestive of nonesophageal disease. The poor body condition seen in some dogs is not a consistent finding. Up to half of the dogs in one study were presented in good body condition.[9]

Accumulation of food in the thoracic esophagus may produce respiratory distress, especially in the presence of aspiration pneumonia. Signs of aspiration pneumonia including mucopurulent nasal discharge, respiratory crackles, dyspnea, and pyrexia may be seen. Dogs with megaesophagus may die acutely due to intussusception of the stomach into the esophagus.[45]

Other clinical signs may reflect some of the causes of secondary rather than idiopathic megaesophagus. For instance, muscle pain and weakness may occur in dogs with megaesophagus associated with polymyositis.[46] Vomiting was the predominant sign in cats in which megaesophagus was secondary to pyloric dysfunction.[73] Weakness exacerbated by exercise occurs in both cats[51] and dogs[68] with megaesophagus associated with advanced myasthenia gravis and in dogs with megaesophagus due to polymyopathy.[77] Profound depression was the predominant clinical sign in a dog with megaesophagus associated with lead poisoning.[58] Ataxia and weakness were important signs in a group of dogs with megaesophagus and neuropathy.[56]

Physical examination of animals with megaesophagus is usually unremarkable. Weight loss or malnutrition is a variable finding. Some animals are able to maintain good nutritional homeostasis despite megaesophagus' involving the entire esophagus. Dilatation of the cervical esophagus is frequently evident on physical examination. The physical may provide clues suggestive of a systemic disease that underlies the regurgitation, such as muscle pain, weakness, ataxia, and dilated pupils.

Differential Diagnosis. Megaesophagus must be differentiated from other causes of dysphagia, regurgitation and vomiting, and aspiration pneumonia. A thorough diagnostic workup should be implemented to determine the cause of the megaesophagus. Treatment and prognosis depend on accurate diagnosis of the cause. The important differentials of regurgitation are shown in Table 5-13. At the beginning of the workup, it is essential to differentiate regurgitation from vomiting. The history may give a clue as to the cause of the regurgitation. Vascular ring abnormalities and cricopharyngeal dysphagia are more likely in younger dogs than in older dogs. A history of tolerance of fluids but not solids is more indicative of obstructive esophageal disease than megaesophagus. Regurgitation immediately after eating is suggestive of pharyngeal or early cervical esophageal disease.

Radiographic Evaluation.[1-2] The diagnosis of megaesophagus rests on radiographic procedures. Many cases can be identified without the introduction of a positive-contrast medium into the esophagus. The dilated esophagus may contain air, enabling the esophagus to be outlined with a negative-contract medium. The esophagus may also be found to contain fluid and food, which outline it with a positive-contrast medium. Examples of these findings are shown in Figures 9-5 and 9-6. In questionable cases, positive-contrast medium can be used to confirm a diagnosis of megaesophagus. That is necessary when air, present in the esophagus due to aerophagia in excited, nauseated, dyspneic, or anesthetized dogs, produces radiographic signs suggestive of megaesophagus.[78] Particular care is necessary in anesthetized animals because anesthesia causes a significant degree of esophageal dilatation.[79] In view of these difficulties, and in order to diagnose many of the obstructive esophageal diseases and functional esophageal diseases not associated with esophageal dilatation, it is often necessary to use contrast esophagrams, fluoroscopy and esophagoscopy. Such procedures may reveal obstructions, motility disturbances, or mucosal lesions unobserved on plain radiographs. Dilatation can involve the entire esophagus or be segmental in any part of the esophagus. The extent of esophageal involvement is often poorly correlated with the degree of clinical signs. In some animals, an esophagus that is dilated throughout its length shows few clinical signs, whereas in others a small dilatation in a short segment is associated with major regurgitation problems.

Evaluation for Specific Causes. Due to the varied nature of the possible causes of megaesophagus, the diagnostic approach must be very broad based. Useful tests are detailed in Table 5-12. Not all of these tests are necessary in the workup of every case but some are essential and all may be useful to confirm or rule out a suspected cause. Myasthenia gravis may be detected by the acetylcholine receptor antibody test or the repetitive stimulation or Tensilon tests. Esophageal dysfunction due to myasthenia gravis can precede the weakness characteristic of the disease; therefore, at least one of these tests must be undertaken to rule out myasthenia gravis before a diagnosis of idiopathic megaesophagus can be made. Botulism may be confirmed by mouse bioassay techniques. SLE may be detected by the presence of supportive systemic signs and positive LE and/or ANA tests. Neuropathies may be diagnosed by the presence of other peripheral nerve involvement and if necessary by nerve and muscle biopsies. Myositis and myopathy may be proven by EMG findings, serum chemistry results, and muscle biopsy. Lead, thallium, and anticholinesterase toxicities may be diagnosed by history, clinical signs, and toxicologic assays. Dysautonomia is usually obvious on physical examination but can be confirmed by various ocular response

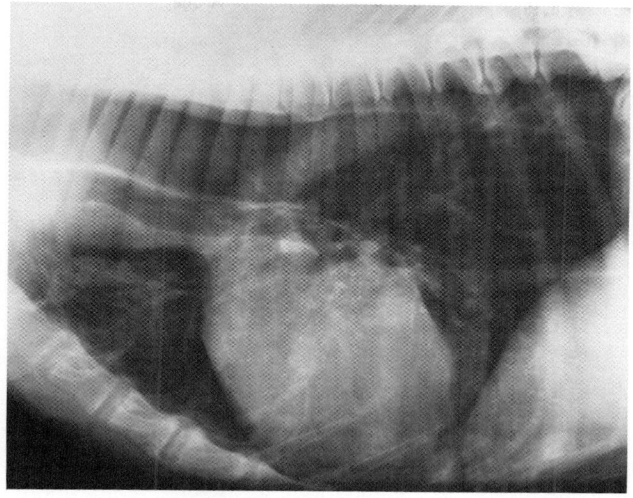

Figure 9-5. Megaesophagus, 4-year old Great Dane. Lateral thoracic radiograph shows dilated, air-filled esophagus. Accumulation of food and liquids in the dilated portion often produces signs of dyspnea and cough as the primary problems. This is produced by the ventral displacement and compression of the lungs and airways.

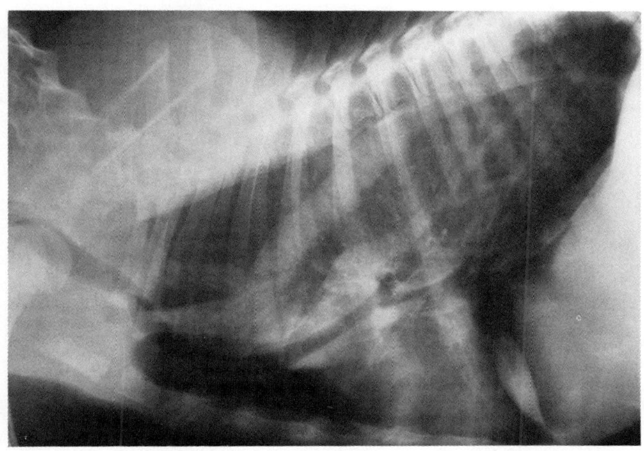

Figure 9-6. Lateral radiograph of pup with megaesophagus. Retention of fluid and food in dilated esophagus increases density of structure and enhances its radiographic appearance.

tests. Obstructive esophageal diseases and miscellaneous causes such as mediastinitis may be diagnosed by esophagoscopy and radiographic procedures. Idiopathic megaesophagus is a diagnosis of exclusion that can only be reached after an extensive workup.

Pathologic Evaluation. Muscle from the dilated esophagus is normal in histology. An exception occurs when chronic dilatation has caused secondary inflammatory changes. The esophageal mucosa will usually evidence esophagitis when food and liquids have been retained for more than a short time. Pathologic changes have not been demonstrated in either the vagus nerves or serial sections of the brain stem treated with both conventional and special stains.[39]

Treatment. When possible, treatment is aimed at the primary cause. Esophageal obstruction may be relieved by esophagoscopy, bougienage, or surgery.[68] SLE and immune-mediated polymyositis and polyneuritis may respond to immune suppression. Myasthenia gravis may be treated with prednisone or azathioprine and long-acting anticholinesterase agents such as neostigmine and pyridostigmine. Care is necessary when using prednisone and anticholinesterases concurrently, as exacerbation of weakness can result during the initial phases of this combination therapy. Removal of a thymoma may result in resolution of myasthenia gravis and clinical improvement in esophageal function. Toxic causes of megaesophagus may be treated by removal of the offending agent and/or use of specific antidotes. Megaesophagus secondary to pyloric stenosis may respond to pyloromyotomy.[73] Megaesophagus resulting from mediastinitis will improve with appropriate antibiotic therapy.

Therapy is entirely symptomatic for idiopathic megaesophagus and for most cases of megaesophagus due to neurologic diseases. Symptomatic treatment is also essential in cases of secondary megaesophagus for which specific treatment is indicated. Symptomatic treatment reduces the frequency and/or severity of the common complications of megaesophagus such as aspiration pneumonia, overdilatation of esophageal muscle by large amounts of retained ingesta, and esophagitis secondary to fermenting retained ingesta.

Successful management of megaesophagus requires special feeding practices. A high-caloric diet is selected and fed from an elevated source to enlist the aid of gravity in moving food through the paralyzed section of esophagus. Since a liquid meets less resistance that a semisolid, a semiliquid gruel is usually fed. If any peristaltic activity remains, it is able to propel a liquid bolus easier than a solid bolus. In fact, normal peristalsis in the cranial esophagus may be able to provide enough inertia to propel a liquid bolus through a paralyzed section, whereas a solid bolus would require a sustained peristaltic wave to transport it through the entire esophagus. An occasional animal will show fewer clinical signs when solid food is fed and fluids are restricted.

During client education, it is emphasized that the best management program for a particular patient may differ from that recommended for most animals with the problem, and that a number of different trials will reveal which method will be most successful. Some animals cannot maintain nutritional homeostasis, even with special feeding procedures. Feeding can be accomplished through a nasogastric or gastrostomy tube when necessary.

Many drugs have been used, but unsuccessfully, to improve esophageal function in dogs with idiopathic megaesophagus. Since the canine esophagus consists of striated muscle, drugs that only augment smooth muscle motility will not have any effect. Some of these drugs include cholinergics such as urecholine and bethanecol, anticholinergics such as atropine, and drugs such as metoclopramide acting on dopamine mechanisms. Calcium channel antagonists such as nifedipine have effects to inhibit smooth muscle contraction. They reduce GES pressure and would reduce motility in the cats' caudal esophagus but would have no effect in the dog's esophagus.[80] Calcium channel antagonists can also produce serious side effects. Although these drugs have no effect on esophageal striated muscle, they have been evaluated in dogs with idiopathic megaesophagus; there is no good evidence that any are of any value. Drug therapy may be of value in treating megaesophagus in the cat. Esophageal muscle is all smooth in the caudal esophagus of the cat. Dilatation of that part of the esophagus may improve with the metoclopramide. Even if the size of a megaesophagus is reduced, however, a loss of normal peristalsis may persist.

Reduction of GES pressure could benefit animals with megaesophagus associated with unusually high resting pressure or with failure of GES relaxation during swallowing. Reducing normal GES pressure may aid in sphincter opening when esophageal motility is weak and ineffective. In such cases a bolus of food approaching the GES is unable to generate enough pressure to open the GES. Anticholinergics are potent reducers of GES pressure to values less than a third of normal. One older study reports antispasmotics improved several pups with congenital idiopathic megaesophagus.[18] Newer drugs such as the calcium-channel blocker nifedipine are potent reducers of GES pressure. Whether they may be effective in dogs and cats is unknown. Esophagitis accompanying megaesophagus results in decreased GES pressure that may predispose the animal to gastroesophageal reflux which will worsen an esophagitis. If dogs with megaesophagus are at risk for reflux, anticholinergics will increase that risk further. Thus, if no benefits can be proven for using anticholinergics and if there is the possibility such drugs can worsen the problem, that therapy should not be used. Anticholinergics will reduce motility in the smooth muscle part of the feline esophagus. Their use in megaesophagus is likely to worsen the problem and handicap the ability of the esophagus to clear any refluxed material by returning it to the stomach. Combining anticholinergics with metoclopramide in an attempt to reduce GES pressure and improve esophageal function negates any effects of metoclopramide. Anticholinergics abolish the augmentation of smooth muscle motility by metoclopramide. Anticholinergics and metoclopramide have no effect on GES neural mechanisms for opening and closing. Noncholinergic, nonadrenergic nerves, releasing vasoactive intestinal peptide as the neurotransmitter, mediate GES relaxation and opening. Receptors in the caudal esophagus recognize the stimulus for opening. If megaesophagus affects that part of the esophagus, opening will be impaired, and no drugs can improve that situation.

The surgical treatment of idiopathic megaesophagus is a controversial subject. Some authors think that it is a worthwhile procedure,[81-83] whereas others, on the basis of pathophysiologic arguments and clinical experience, believe that it is of no value.[9,12,26] Surgical treatments for megaesophagus are based on the theory that achalasia exists for the gastroesophageal sphincter. As a consequence, a myotomy is recommended. At Pennsylvania, 40% of dogs with megaesophagus underwent surgery, and since the results were poorer than in untreated dogs, surgery is no longer recommended. From 1967 to 1975, 18% of the cases of canine megaesophagus at the VMTH in Davis were treated surgically, with poor results. All cases of megaesophagus that were managed surgically were also managed by elevating the food so that the dog had to eat in a semivertical position. If any improvement followed, it may have been due largely to the use of gravity to help move food to the stomach. There is no rationale for a myotomy unless radiographic studies reveal loss of coordinated GES function or a stricture at the gastroesophageal junction. As indicated earlier, gastroesophageal sphincter pressure is not abnormally high in dogs with megaesophagus.[24] Surgery would be indicated if manometric studies show GES pressure to be high and pressure reduction is not demonstrated during swallowing. Complications of myotomies on this sphincter have included gastroesophageal reflux and herniation of the stomach into the esophagus.

If surgery is undertaken, the modified short Heller's esophagomyotomy appears to be the procedure of choice, since it reduces GES pressure but still maintains enough GES competency to prevent esophageal reflex.[84] After surgery animals must still be fed from an elevated bowl.[85]

Megaesophagus in cats can be secondary to the esophagitis caused by chronic vomition. Treatment of the primary cause results in an improvement in the megaesophagus. That result has been reported in cats with megaesophagus secondary to pyloric stenosis.[73]

Prognosis. Esophageal paralysis usually persists in most dogs with megaesophagus despite any medical or surgical management. The prognosis depends on the cause and age at onset of clinical signs. Most clinicians believe that congenital idiopathic megaesophagus has a poor prognosis and that patients do not offer enough of a possibility of improvement to become acceptable pets.[8,9,12,19] Some clinicians give a more favorable prognosis.[16,23,86] There are at least two reasons for such differences of experience. First, when an affected pup is weaned early and solid dry food is fed, there is greater risk for accumulation and severe distention of the esophagus than if liquid or soft foods are fed. Severe distention distorts and damages the esophagus so that it may not regain its normal size and function. Such damage is seen in esophagi obstructed by persistent vascular rings; with severe distention, dilatation persists. Second, there is some evidence that megaesophagus in the very young dog may improve as the animal matures.[26,40,87] In one study, manometric evaluation of pups with megaesophagus was performed periodically until maturity.[40] The studies revealed that esophageal function improved with time. That may merely reflect normal maturation, however, rather than an improvement in the megaesophagus. Normal young dogs have incomplete function of the esophagus and as they mature the function improves. These suggestions support the recommendation that the earlier the condition is recognized and dietary management is begun, the better the prognosis.[23] The maturation of function seems to be necessary for Miniature Schnauzer pups with hereditary esophageal dysfunction that usually recover clinically and radiographically if they survive the first few weeks of life.[16]

Adult-onset idiopathic megaesophagus has a poor to hopeless prognosis. Secondary megaesophagus can have a good prognosis if the primary disease can be successfully treated. Dogs with megaesophagus recover esophageal function following successful treatment of primary diseases such as myasthenia gravis, polyradiculoneuritis, polymyositis, and SLE.[8,88] Megaesophagus secondary to Addison's disease, botulism, bronchoesophageal fistula, and mediastinitis has a favorable prognosis if treated early. Some dogs with idiopathic megaesophagus are reported to have recovered spontaneously. Generalizations are difficult to make on prognosis from case studies prepared by different groups of clinicians. Differing definitions of megaesophagus make it difficult to compare studies. Also the workup of some cases is more complete than for others. In some cases the diagnosis is based on survey radiographs, but with further studies the primary esophageal dysfunction appears to be a dysperistalsis rather than megaesophagus.

The prognosis of megaesophagus in cats with dysautonomia is poor. While up to 30 percent of cats with dysautonomia return to clinical normality, the presence of significant megaesophagus in an affected cat markedly worsens its changes of recovery.[13] Similarly, the prognosis of cats with megaesophagus associated with pyloric dysfunction is poorer than those with pyloric dysfunction alone.[73] Some cats with pyloric dysfunction-associated megaesophagus did, however, show improved clinical signs and reduced esophageal diameter after pyloromyotomy.[73]

The prognosis of megaesophagus associated with obstructive esophageal diseases is poor unless the correction of the obstruction precedes significant esophageal dilatation. Relief of the obstruction usually results in some clinical improvement, but the dilated esophagus rarely regains normal function.[89]

The prognosis of megaesophagus from any cause is adversely affected by evidence of concurrent inhalation pneumonia and debilitation and by the absence of any esophageal motility.

In summary, the prognosis of megaesophagus with few exceptions is guarded to poor.

Motility Disturbances

The motility of the esophagus can develop abnormalities with or without the appearance of megaesophagus; dysperistalsis is common to all. Their incidence is not known. It is undoubtedly greater than anticipated for two reasons. Motility disorders are seldom identified because fluoroscopic procedures are essential to their identification. Motility disorders can be caused by esophagitis, and since that problem can resolve, a number of such cases likely regain normal function before special radiographic studies are called for to evaluate the problem. Fluoroscopic studies are important also in dogs with megaesophagus because not all cases completely lose motility of the esophagus. The dilated segment of esophagus in some dogs will sometimes contract and develop a wave of peristalsis that moves its contents to the stomach. With our limited understanding it is not clear whether these should be identified and managed as motility abnormalities or as megaesophagus.

Etiology and Pathophysiology. Esophagitis frequently causes diffuse motility problems involving a large part of the esophagus. The esophagitis results from swallowing material that damages the mucosa. It is also seen after gastric contents are regurgitated but not expelled, remaining in the esophagus.

That can occur during surgical procedures in which the animal is positioned with its head down. Diffuse motility disorders are seen when esophagitis is experimentally produced in dogs.[75] Esophagitis in the cat also causes a loss of normal motility.[74] The inflammatory lesions causing motility deficits may involve only short segments of the esophagus. The lesion is caused most often by a foreign body that remains in a segment of the esophagus long enough to cause considerable damage. A frequent site for esophageal foreign bodies and subsequent motility disorders is the cervical esophagus adjacent to the thoracic inlet.

Diffuse esophageal motility disorders can develop spontaneously with no evidence for esophagitis. They may not be related to any other problem, but they often are. Anesthetic agents and concurrent infections in other organs have been associated with these motility disorders. Animals with esophageal motility disorders receive the same diagnostic workup recommended for those with megaesophagus.

The pathogenesis of motility disorders is not known. Esophagitis undoubtedly damages sensory receptors and may affect the peripheral part of the motor unit. Physiologic studies in normal dogs show that sensory information is relayed from the esophagus to the swallowing center in order to sustain the progression of a peristaltic wave. Loss of this reinforcement, provided by sensory receptors in the inflamed esophagus, is the most likely reason for the motility disorders seen with esophagitis. Damage to the striated muscle and its innervation more likely cause the motility disorders seen in short segments of esophagus following obstruction by a foreign body.

Damage to neurons in the central part of the swallowing reflex may cause diffuse motility disorders not related to an esophagitis. It is possible that neurons in the swallowing center are more sensitive than others to the effects of some drugs and toxins, accounting for the loss of normal function.

Clinical Evaluation. Regurgitation is the primary sign associated with segmental or diffuse motility disorders. Such regurgitation follows almost immediately after a bolus is swallowed. In contrast to pharynoesophageal disorders and megaesophagus, motility disorders frequently cause anorexia. The reluctance to eat may be due in part to painful spasms induced in the esophagus when a bolus is swallowed. Signs of esophageal colic can be correlated with fluoroscopic demonstration of spastic contractions of the esophagus around a bolus of food.

Motility disorders do not usually yield specific physical findings. Endoscopy is of no value in evaluating these problems.

Radiographic Evaluation. An esophageal motility disorder can be identified only through radiographic procedures (Figure 9-7). The patient must be studied while swallowing positive-contrast medium under fluoroscopic control. The motility disorders are often difficult to identify. Since some abnormal animals show normal esophageal function when the medium swallowed is a liquid, they should be reevaluated as they swallow boluses of food.

The most common motility disorder shows a diffuse loss of the normal peristaltic activity (dysperistalsis) that carries a bolus to the stomach. This activity is replaced by random and uncoordinated contractions. The abnormal esophageal motility results in retention of food throughout the diseased parts. The bolus can move as easily in the oral direction as in the caudal. Spasms of the esophagus around a bolus of food are seen in patients with esophageal colic. A motility defect may also involve only a few centimeters of the esophagus. These defects may be so subtle that they are difficult to identify by radiographic procedures.

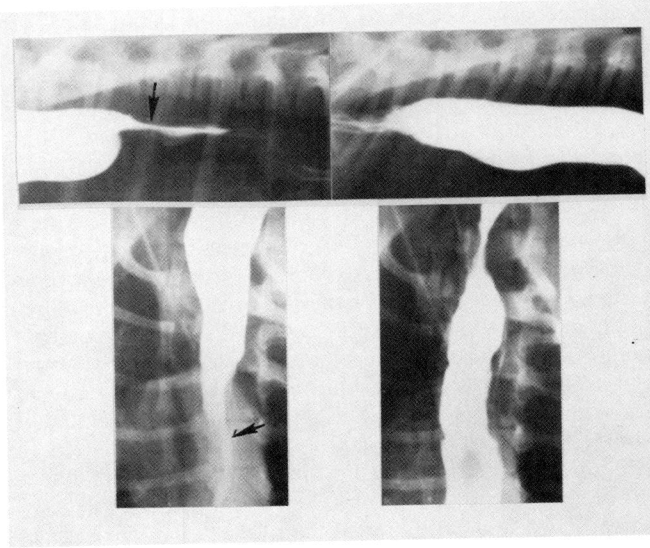

Figure 9-7. Esophageal motility disorders in an 18-month-old Toy Poodle. Lateral and ventrodorsal radiographs were made under fluoroscopic control at different intervals after oral administration of positive-contrast medium. Comparison of the views illustrates that segments of the esophagus appearing to have megaesophagus are able to generate peristalsis, and the esophagus appears to be of a normal size after the bolus moves caudally. In addition, segments that do not appear to have megaesophagus (arrows) are abnormally dilated when the bolus of contrast medium moves into the segment. This type of lesion can be segmental or diffuse. There is often poor correlation between severity of lesions and degree of clinical signs.

Pathologic Evaluation. Biopsy of the esophagus is used to identify esophagitis as the primary cause. The cause of other types of motility disorders are usually not revealed by biopsy or necropsy.

Diagnosis. Diagnosis of a diffuse esophageal motility disorder is based on clinical findings and radiographic evaluation. Both sources of information are important. Clinical findings are the most important source of information used to diagnose subtle motility disorders. A subtle motility abnormality can be seen in animals that show no clinical signs of esophageal disease. When such abnormalities are associated with clinical signs consistent with esophageal disease, however, a diagnosis can be made. Thus, no attempt should be made to correlate the degree of radiographic abnormalities with severity of clinical signs. The persistence of clinical signs typical of esophageal disease should be pursued in a manner analagous for megaesophagus.

Management and Prognosis. Esophagitis, when found, is treated as described later. The prognosis in dogs is good unless the inflammatory changes are severe or the problem has persisted for a long time. Esophagitis-related motility disorders are reversible in cats also. There is no specific treatment for motility disorders that are not caused by esophagitis. Management consists of maintaining nutritional homeostasis and treating any concurrent problems. The prognosis is unknown. Spontaneous recovery of esophageal function is possible up to six weeks after onset of the problem.

ESOPHAGEAL OBSTRUCTION

Obstruction of the esophagus is a relatively common problem in small animals because of their indiscriminate eating habits. Esophageal obstruction is an important problem because of the frequency of undesirable sequelae, such as permanent swallowing defects and life-threatening complications. Esophageal obstruction is important also since it is frequently a diagnostic challenge. Obstruction of the esophagus can result from intraluminal blockage, an intramural lesion that causes stenosis, or an extramural lesion that constricts the esophagus.

Intraluminal Obstruction

Etiology and Pathogenesis. Intraluminal obstruction of the esophagus is almost always caused by foreign bodies that become lodged during swallowing.[1,90,91] Herniation of the stomach into the esophagus occasionally causes this type of obstruction.[92] During vomition, it is common for the canine stomach to invaginate into the esophagus. The foreign bodies encountered most frequently are bones, although other objects are found occasionally, such as fabrics, stones, fishhooks, and large chunks of food. Dogs and cats are adapted to tear material and swallow it in relatively large pieces. Since the esophagus is quite distensible, esophageal retention with obstruction is less frequent than might be expected. Foreign bodies usually cause obstruction at points of least distensibility, such as the thoracic inlet, the base of the heart, and the diaphragmatic hiatus.

A foreign body usually becomes lodged in the esophagus because it has sharp points or edges that catch in the mucosal surface; the cranial esophagus is a common site. Smooth-surfaced objects become lodged only if they are large, or if there is insufficient lubrication. The lodged bolus stimulates secondary peristalsis. If the foreign body does not move, the pressure generated by peristalsis may cause necrotic ulcerative esophagitis. With subsequent esophageal perforation it is possible to see mediastinitis, pleuritis, and pneumonia. Foreign body obstruction is reported to be six times more common in dogs than in cats.[91] This species predilection appears to be related to the more discriminatory eating habits of cats. However, bones, threads with attached needles, and other small objects may cause pharyngeal or esophageal obstruction in the feline.

Clinical Evaluation. The history often provides important information pointing to consideration of an esophageal foreign body in making the differential diagnosis. Regurgitation is a usual primary sign. Patients with esophageal foreign bodies are usually anorectic, however, so that regurgitation may be infrequent. Complete anorexia can be seen with a fishhook in the esophagus even though it is not causing an obstruction. The anorexia is likely the result of esophageal pain. Clinical signs of pain are a frequent feature of esophageal foreign bodies and arise from the distention they produce and the esophageal spasms that result. These signs, similar to those observed in a dog with disc disease in the caudal thoracic spine, include a reluctance to move or be picked up. Hypersalivation is a common secondary sign, and if esophageal obstruction is complete, frequent regurgitation of saliva is also seen.

The client often knows that the animal has swallowed a foreign object, and radiographic procedures are indicated to identify the problem, but evidence suggesting an esophageal obstruction by a foreign body is often only indirect. This evidence comes from information that the animal has a habit of chewing foreign objects, has raided the garbage, or has freedom to run in an unknown environment. The client can usually provide information on the two most common esophageal foreign bodies, bones and fishhooks, when the animal's environment is known.

Physical examination of animals with esophageal obstruction is usually unremarkable. A foreign body causing esophageal inflammation and spasms of the esophagus can cause the animal to evidence pain when pressure is applied to the caudal part of the sternum, as demonstrated by picking up the animal with a hand under the sternum. Other physical findings are usually consistent with clinical findings. The examination should include careful attention to the base of the tongue and pharynx for linear foreign objects that may extend into the esophagus.

Radiographic Evaluation. Radiographic examination should include the entire esophagus. Radio-opaque foreign bodies are readily visualized. Radiolucent foreign bodies cannot be recognized on survey films but may cause accumulation of gas and fluid, and secondary dilatation, cranial to the obstruction. Positive-contrast medium is used to identify radiolucent objects. The contrast medium either surrounds and outlines the radiolucent foreign body or is absorbed and retained by it.

Perforation of the esophagus is suspected when inflammation is found in the adjacent mediastinal or pulmonary structures. Barium sulfate should not be used as a positive-contrast medium when esophageal perforation is suspected. This compound remains in mediastinal or pleural spaces into which it can leak, where it can promote granuloma formation. Esophagoscopy is superior to radiography in recognizing inflammation, punctures, and lacerations.

Diagnosis. The diagnosis of esophageal foreign bodies is usually confirmed with survey radiographs. A few cases require confirmation with radiographic procedures using positive-contrast medium or endoscopy.

Management. Treatment of esophageal foreign bodies consists of attempted removal with the aid of an endoscope.[93] If the object is cranial to the heart, it can be removed through the mouth. If the foreign body is located more caudally, an attempt can be made to push it into the stomach. If it is lodged, however, because peristalsis has been unable to move it past a point of resistance, and if necrosis of the esophagus has occurred, pushing it past the point of resistance can rupture the weakened tube. Care should thus be taken in removing such obstructing objects. In some cases, it may be necessary or preferable to remove a foreign body by esophagotomy. Patient care after removal of a foreign body should be directed at preventing the formation of strictures, as described later.

A flexible esophageal endoscope is passed into the esophagus to directly visualize the foreign body and to inspect for possible esophageal mucosal damage. Small foreign bodies are removed by passing flexible four-prong or basket grasping forceps through the endoscope, grasping the object, and pulling it retrograde out of the esophagus through the oral cavity. For large objects, rigid grasping forceps may be passed in conjunction with a flexible endoscope. Once the foreign body is grasped, it and the endoscope are pulled retrograde through the mouth. If flexible endoscopes are not available, rigid endoscopes are used. If the foreign body cannot be removed by these means, attempts can be made to push the object into the stomach. Once in the stomach, foreign bodies may be digested and excreted, or removed by gastrostomy. All manipulations of foreign bodies with the endoscopic equipment must be carefully performed in order to minimize further esophageal trauma and avoid laceration of thoracic vessels. Endoscopy cannot reveal foreign bodies that have penetrated the esophagus and migrated into the surrounding tissue.

Assessment of possible esophageal damage should follow removal of the foreign body from the esophageal lumen. The esophageal mucosa should be visualized throughout its entire length. The degree of mucosal damage is usually proportional to the duration of the foreign body entrapment. Erythema and mild ulceration are common endoscopic findings. Special attention should be given to any evidence of tears, lacerations, or perforation of the esophageal wall. Survey thoracic radiographs should be performed following foreign body removal to evaluate for the presence of pneumothorax or pneumomediastinum secondary to esophageal perforation. Minor tears, lacerations, and ulcerations will heal with esophageal rest. The use of pharyngostomy or gastrostomy tubes will allow the oral alimentation of an animal while resting the esophagus. Disadvantages to using pharyngostomy tubes are continuing irritation of the esophagus from the tube and the necessity of maintaining an open gastroesophageal sphincter, with the possible reflux of gastric contents.[94] Large defects in the esophageal wall with signs of concurrent mediastinitis or other thoracic cavity involvement require surgical exploration and repair.

Endoscopy was successful in removing esophageal foreign bodies in 86% of dogs and cats in one study; the recovery rate was 98%. Surgery to remove esophageal foreign bodies is successful in 82% to 85% of affected dogs and cats.[90,91,95] Thus, surgery is a good choice of treatment if an endoscopic procedure cannot be done or may be too traumatizing during foreign body removal.

Prognosis. At least one-third of animals with esophageal foreign bodies develop complications. Esophageal perforation from lacerations and esophageal necrosis can lead to mediastinitis or pneumonia. Trauma from foreign bodies with sharp points can include laceration of major blood vessels adjacent to the esophagus, resulting in severe hemorrhage. Septicemia can occur following esophageal laceration. The threat of this complication supports the use of antibiotics directed against transient bacteria that come into the esophagus from the mouth. Lacerations may also precipitate disseminated intravascular coagulation. Other complications may develop a week or more after successful removal of a foreign body. They include the formation of strictures or diverticula and local deficits in motility. Unusual chronic complications of esophageal foreign body impaction include esophagobronchial fistula formation, pericarditis, and persistent esophageal ulcers.

Intramural Obstruction

Etiology and Pathogenesis. Stricture of the esophagus produces stenosis when fibrosis develops in its wall. This differentiates strictures from the stenoses produced by masses, vessels, or fibrous bands that constrict the lumen of the esophagus from outside its wall. Strictures are usually acquired and can be found in any region of the esophagus. They can induce a stenosis severe enough for only liquids to pass.

The appearance of esophageal stricture is preceded by acute inflammatory changes, usually as a complication of reflux esophagitis, chemical trauma, or trauma from an esophageal foreign body. Inflammation or disruption of the epithelium without damage to the deeper structures usually does not stimulate the formation of cicatricial tissue. Erosions that extend through the lamina propria into the muscle layers, however, usually result in scar tissue. In severely damaged tissue, fibroblasts appear within 24 hours of the insult, and collagen fibers are formed within one week. The point to be emphasized is that even though stenotic changes begin early, symptoms usually do not appear until after fibrous tissue has reduced the diameter of the esophageal lumen.

If gastric juices reflux into the esophagus, they may cause esophagitis of sufficient severity to cause the formation of strictures.[96,97] Most of the cases seen in dogs at the VMTH in Davis have occurred two to three weeks after an ovariohysterectomy. Part of the cause may be that this surgery is usually performed with the animal in dorsal recumbency and tilted in a head-down position. It is postulated that gastric juices that have refluxed through a relaxed gastroesophageal sphincter digest the epithelial surface, resulting in inflammatory changes. The presence of pepsin augments epithelial erosion, and small amounts of bile and hydrochloric acid greatly increase the permeability of the esophageal mucosa.[98] It is not unusual to find bile mixed with the basal secretions of the fasting canine stomach. Postsurgical esophageal stricture formation, recognized more frequently now than twenty years ago, may be related to today's more frequent use of preanesthetic agents that decrease pressure in the gastroesophageal sphincter. Anticholinergics, narcotic analgesics, and diazepam are examples of drugs that affect the competence of the sphincter.[99-102]

Other causes of strictures include a number of drugs and any condition increasing exposure of the esophagus to gastric juices. They are described under esophagitis.

Clinical Evaluation. The clinical signs associated with esophageal stricture are similar to those seen with all other esophageal problems. Regurgitation is the predominant sign and is seen shortly after, if not during, eating. With chronic obstruction, regurgitation can be delayed. Liquids are tolerated better than solid food. Regurgitation usually appears abruptly and is then seen consistently. Anorexia and esophageal colic are usually not seen. Associated signs can include hypersalivation. In general, the signs are those of an animal that has developed an acute obstruction of the esophagus, but without the signs associated with acute inflammation caused by a foreign body or esophagitis.

Results of physical examination of the animal are usually unremarkable. Endoscopy provides the best means of identifying esophageal strictures. Endoscopy can substitute for radiographic procedures when there is good historical evidence suggesting that a stricture will be found.

Radiographic Evaluation. Radiographic procedures using positive contrast medium can be used to identify esophageal strictures. The stenosed area of the esophagus is the most difficult lesion to demonstrate radiographically. Other changes that may appear (and be more obvious to the radiologist) include dilation of the esophagus cranial to the stricture and a loss of normal motility that can extend throughout the entire esophagus. Radiography with passage of a radio-opaque tube to the stricture can be of aid in identifying the problem. Many strictures cannot be convincingly demonstrated without evaluation under fluoroscopic control. Even then, some strictures are difficult to identify. When fluoroscopy is not used, endoscopy must be used to recognize the stricture. Endoscopy should be done on all questionable cases.

Diagnosis. Identification of esophageal strictures is based on clinical findings that are supported most importantly with endoscopy. Radiographic procedures can be used but cannot identify all cases.

Management. Esophageal strictures can be corrected by dilation of the stenotic region. That can be accomplished by forcibly passing tubes of increasing diameter through the stenotic area. Such bougienage can be done with steel-stem or mercury-filled rubber esophageal dilators. Endotracheal tubes can be used as dilators for cervical strictures in small dogs and cats.[103] A Gruntzig balloon catheter can be used; the balloon is inflated after using fluoroscopic or endoscopic guidance to center it in the stricture.[104] The strictures often require repeated dilation, all of which must be done with the animal under general anesthesia. Strictures are more easily dilated when they have developed recently. Efforts should be made to dilate strictures, since the only other alternative is surgical resection of the stricture, a difficult procedure accompanied by many complications.

Following dilation, antibiotics effective against the normal microflora of the oral cavity should be given to prevent infection of the open lesion with these organisms. Corticosteroids should also be administered to prevent the reformation of fibrous tissue. Experimental work has shown that large doses of steroids administered with antibiotics for two to three weeks beginning at the time of esophageal injury prevent stenosis of the esophagus.[105] On the basis of those results, all cases of esophagitis or esophageal laceration that could result in stricture formation should be treated with steroids and antibiotics.

An important part of the treatment is placement of a feeding tube for one to two weeks after dilation of the stricture or after a severe laceration of the esophagus. Tube feeding rests the esophagus and allows it to heal. With pharyngostomy tubes the animal can eat on its own despite the tube. This procedure has greatly improved the results of treating strictures of the esophagus, although it not without some of its own problems. Pharyngostomy tubes are not tolerated well by most patients. The animals hypersalivate, gag, and attempt to vomit. Such signs may diminish after the tube has been in for 24 hours, however. If the tube is positioned with its tip in the stomach, gastric juices can reflux around the tube and cause esophagitis.

Prognosis. Dilation of esophageal strictures can be expected to produce good results when all measures to prevent stricture reformation are followed. The animals are able to eat any type of diet, with few if any clinical signs remaining. That is surprising, since radiographic reevaluation of these patients at two to four weeks following surgery usually reveals that abnormal motility and dilatations of the esophagus persist despite correction of the stenosis. A failure of the animal to improve should be investigated by examination for stricture reformation.

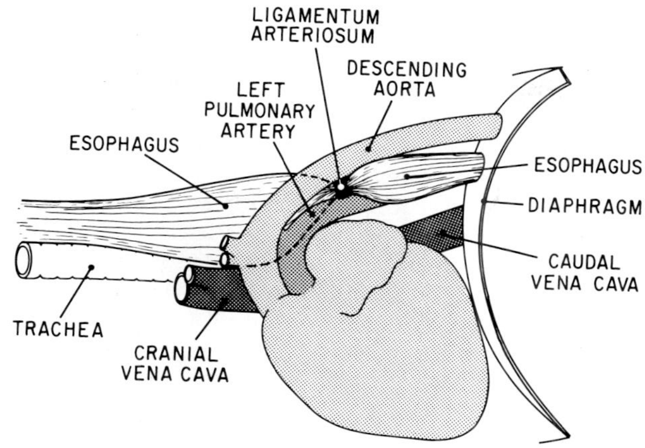

Figure 9-8. Drawing of thoracic structures in a pup with persistent right aortic arch that is constricting the esophagus and causing regurgitation.

Periesophageal Causes of Esophageal Obstruction

Stenosis of the esophagus can be caused by its compression from vascular anomalies, inflammatory or neoplastic masses, and degenerative diseases that cause enlargement of an organ adjacent to the esophagus.

Vascular Rings[1,106-109]

Etiology and Pathogenesis. Vascular rings caused by congenital anomalies of the aortic arches may constrict the esophagus and result in signs of obstruction. The aortic arch normally develops from the fourth left aortic arch and left dorsal aortic root in the embryo. The left sixth arch forms the ductus arteriosus, and the right fourth arch forms part of the right subclavian artery. In normal development, the arch of the aorta, the ductus arteriosus, and the pulmonary artery are positioned to the left of the esophagus, where the vessels offer no resistance to the movement of a bolus of food through the esophagus. When the embryonic aortic arches develop abnormally, vascular rings can constrict the esophagus.

The most common vascular ring is caused by persistence of the right fourth aortic arch (PRAA), which becomes the aorta. In this situation the esophagus is positioned between the right side of the aorta and pulmonary artery (Figure 9-8). These two vessels are connected by either the ductus arteriosus or ligamentum arteriosus, which crosses dorsal to the esophagus. Thus, the esophagus lies sandwiched between the vessels. The esophagus becomes constricted by a "ring," formed by the aorta on the right, the pulmonary trunk and base of heart ventrally, and the ligamentum arteriosum on the left.

A variation of this anomaly occurs with retention of both arches, in which case the right arch forms a functional aortic arch and the left arch forms a remnant. Another clinically significant anomaly results if the left subclavian artery originates from the right aortic arch. The final position of the vessel is such that it has to pass to the left and over the esophagus to follow its normal pathway, resulting in a constriction of the esophagus. Other varieties of esophageal abnormalities associated with vascular anomalies have been described.

Anomalies of the major vessels are common in canine anatomy specimens, with an incidence of 20%. Few of these are vascular ring anomalies, and only a fraction of those cause clinical signs of esophageal obstruction. The anomalies are inherited; the breed predilections for German Shepherds and Irish Setters are three times and ten times the predicted risk in a normal population, respectively. Boston Terriers are also at a higher than expected risk. Vascular rings are considerably less common in the cat, with persistent right aortic arch and constriction by ligamentum arteriosum being described.

Clinical Signs. The most common clinical sign in affected animals is an acute onset of regurgitation at the time of weaning to solid foods. In 90 percent of all dogs with PRAA, the condition is identified before the age of six months.[109] Although regurgitation usually occurs shortly after eating in the early stages of the disease, it may occur at variable times after eating as esophageal dilation progresses. Affected puppies are malnourished, weak, and demonstrate stunted growth. The food-filled esophagus may occasionally be palpated at the thoracic inlet. Coughing with respiratory distress is common and is indicative of a secondary aspiration pneumonia. In those patients, auscultation usually reveals coarse crackles.

Diagnosis. Patients with one of these anomalies typically develop signs that are similar to those of megaesophagus. Since the condition is congenital, the signs will be evident at a very young age. Vascular rings are diagnosed radiographically (Figure 9-9). Radiographs of the esophagus without contrast medium show a dilatation that contains food and air. After contrast medium is swallowed, the esophagus will appear to be dilated to various degrees cranial to a point over the base of the heart, where the esophagus appears constricted. Endoscopic evaluation of the esophagus will reveal an area that is constricted from without. Examination of the esophagus by fluoroscopy reveals a loss of motility in the cranial portion of the esophagus, proportional to the degree of dilation. Esophageal motility caudal to the stricture is usually normal.

Treatment. Treatment consists of surgical correction of the constricting bands forming the vascular ring. The prognosis for a complete recovery is poor. Only 9% of dogs are completely normal. A total of 40% do not survive long after surgery or are euthanatized. The other 50% continued to show occasional clinical signs. Complications are common because of the initial malnourished and debilitated condition of the animal and the high incidence of concurrent aspiration pneumonia. Permanent esophageal dilatation cranial to the constriction, as a result of irreversible degenerative changes in the esophagus itself, is common (Figure 9-9). A final possible sequela is an esophageal dilatation caudal to the vascular ring, a condition that probably occurs due to concurrent neuromuscular disease. Dogs with permanent esophageal disease following surgery should be managed with feeding procedures as described for patients with megaesophagus.

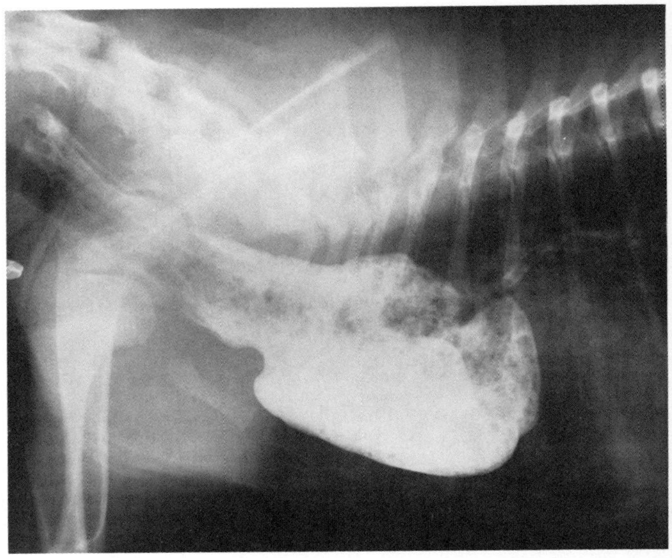

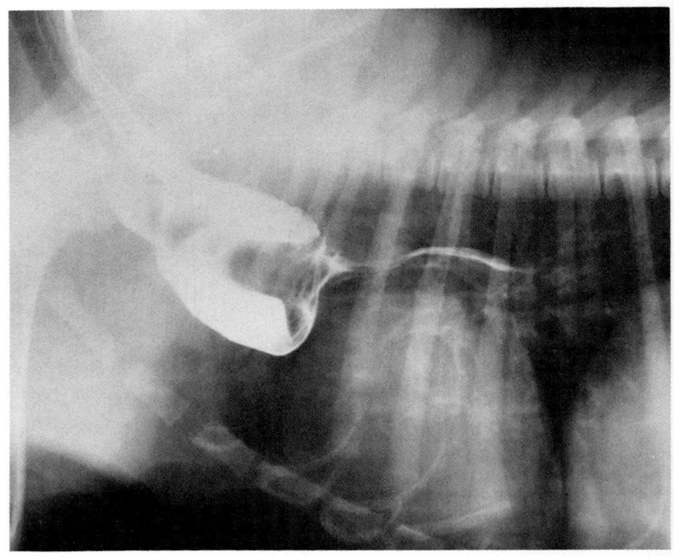

Figure 9-9. Persistent right aortic arch in 4-month-old Dalmation. Lateral radiograph (upper) was made following administration of contrast medium and shows dilated esophagus. The dilatation was caused by a stricture around the esophagus at the base of the heart. The stricture was surgically corrected and the dilatation was reexamined six weeks later. The later radiograph (lower) illustrates that the dilatation in the esophagus persists. The clinical signs of regurgitation persist in most dogs following surgical correction of vascular anomalies that constrict the esophagus.

Inflammatory, Neoplastic, and Degenerative Diseases[1]

Periesophageal structures can enlarge and cause clinical signs of esophageal dysfunction. For example, cardiac enlargement associated with congestive heart failure can compress the esophagus and cause signs of dysphagia or regurgitation. Bronchial lymph nodes can enlarge and cause partial obstruction. Mediastinal masses may also cause periesophageal obstruction (Figure 9-10). Tumors of the thoracic cavity, such as lymphosarcomas, thymomas, and heart-base tumors, are frequently associated with signs of esophageal obstruction. Neoplasms in the retropharyngeal and cervical area frequently compress the esophagus and produce clinical signs of obstruction.

Survey radiographs usually demonstrate a lesion; radiographic studies with contrast material invariably identify the

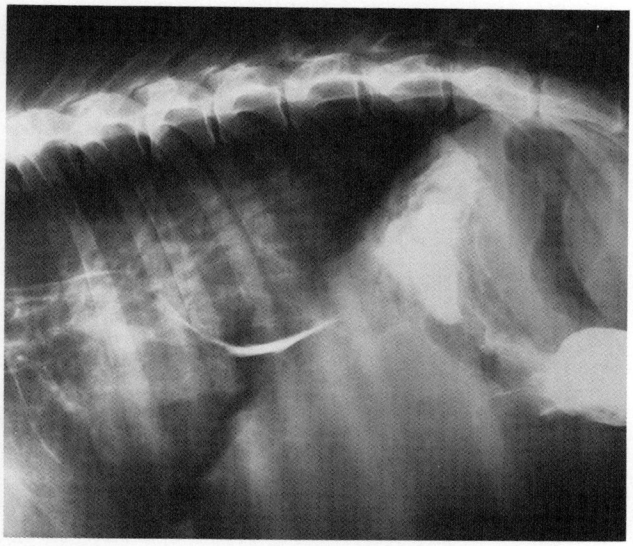

Figure 9-10. Mediastinal mass in 4-year-old Great Dane, lateral view. Clinical signs included dysphagia and regurgitation. The radiograph, made with the dog swallowing a positive-contrast medium, shows a ventral deviation of the esophagus that causes partial occlusion of the lumen. The mediastinal mass was caused by a migrating plant awn.

obstructive lesion. Esophagoscopy will reveal either luminal stenosis with no mucosal involvement, or stricture formation if the periesophageal mass has invaded the esophageal lumen. Treatment is directed toward the cause of the mass lesion.

ESOPHAGEAL DIVERTICULI

Esophageal diverticuli are sac-like dilatations in the esophageal wall that produce a pouch. These structures may be acquired or congenital and are rarely documented in small animals.[110] They are usually found in the lower cervical esophagus cranial to the thoracic inlet or in the thoracic esophagus just cranial to the diaphragm (epiphrenic location). Congenital diverticuli are thought to develop due to congenital weakness of the esophageal wall, abnormal separation of tracheal and esophageal embryonic buds, or eccentric vacuole formation in the esophagus.[1] Acquired forms are subdivided into pulsion and traction diverticula, on the basis of their etiopathogenesis.

Injuries to the esophagus have the potential of leading to diverticula or rupture because the esophagus lacks a serosa, its blood supply is poor, its muscle can be easily overdistended, and its movement is almost continuous.

Exaggerated intraluminal pressure in association with abnormal regional peristalsis or obstruction of normal peristalsis by a stenosis produces a pulsion diverticulum.[91] Pulsion diverticuli can form cranial to any stenosed or diseased esophageal segment and are found most often in the epiphrenic region.[108,110,111] Increased esophageal intraluminal pressure, along with food accumulation and deep esophageal inflammation, can lead to mucosal herniation. Histologically, the wall of a pulsion diverticulum generally consists of only esophageal epithelium and connective tissue. Many causes may initiate diverticulum formation, such as esophagitis, esophageal stenosis, foreign bodies, vascular ring anomalies, neuromuscular dysfunction with megaesophagus, and hiatal hernia.

Traction diverticuli have been reported in humans to follow a past inflammatory process involving the trachea, bronchi, or hilar lymph nodes. This inflammation leads to the production of fibrous tissue that later contracts, pulling out an area of the esophagus to form a pouch. Traction diverticuli are principally located in the cranial and midthoracic esophagus, where ample opportunity for adhesion formations exists.[1] The true incidence of traction diverticuli in veterinary medicine remains unknown. In contrast to a pulsion diverticulum, the traction diverticulum histologically consists of all four esophageal layers (adventitia, muscle, submucosa, and mucosa).

Diverticuli of either type should not be confused with esophageal redundancy seen at the thoracic inlet of normal young dogs and normal dogs of brachycephalic breeds. Contrast material or gas may accumulate in the pseudopouches, mimicking a pulsion diverticulum. Repeat radiography with the neck in an extended position removes any esophageal "slack" and results in the disappearance of a false diverticulum. Small diverticuli can be incidental findings and may be of little clinical significance. However, once a diverticulum is formed, it has the potential of progressing to esophageal impaction, chronic esophagitis with mucosal ulceration, and rupture of the diverticulum wall with resultant mediastinitis or esophagotracheal fistula formation.

Diverticuli that cause clinical signs are usually large and multilobulated and may be inflamed or filled with food, bone, or foreign bodies.[1] Typical signs are distress or gasping shortly after eating, post-prandial regurgitation, intermittent anorexia, fever, weight loss, thoracic or abdominal pain, and respiratory signs. Diverticuli can be identified on survey radiographs as either air- or food-filled masses in the area of the esophagus. Contrast procedures will demonstrate a focal portion of the esophageal lumen that fills partially or completely with contrast material. Esophagoscopy is a valuable tool for confirming the diagnosis while identifying associated complications such as ulceration and scarring.

Small diverticuli, without other esophageal lesions, may be treated conservatively by using a soft bland diet, feeding the animal in an upright position, and providing ample liquids to minimize food accumulation in the pouch. Large diverticuli require surgical excision and reconstruction of the esophageal wall, which warrants a less favorable prognosis. Any underlying cause must be treated appropriately.

ESOPHAGEAL NEOPLASIA

Primary malignant neoplasms involving the canine esophagus are rare but include squamous cell carcinoma, osteosarcoma, fibrosarcoma, and undifferentiated carcinomas.[112,113] Benign tumors are occasionally observed at necropsy and are usually leiomyomas.[113] Feline primary esophageal neoplasms are most frequently carcinomas.[114] Metastatic neoplasms to the esophagus are diagnosed more often than primary tumors but are still uncommon.[68] Reported metastatic tumors include bronchogenic carcinoma, gastric carcinoma, thyroid carcinoma, mammary adenocarcinoma, and squamous cell carcinoma.[113]

The most common primary esophageal neoplasias are

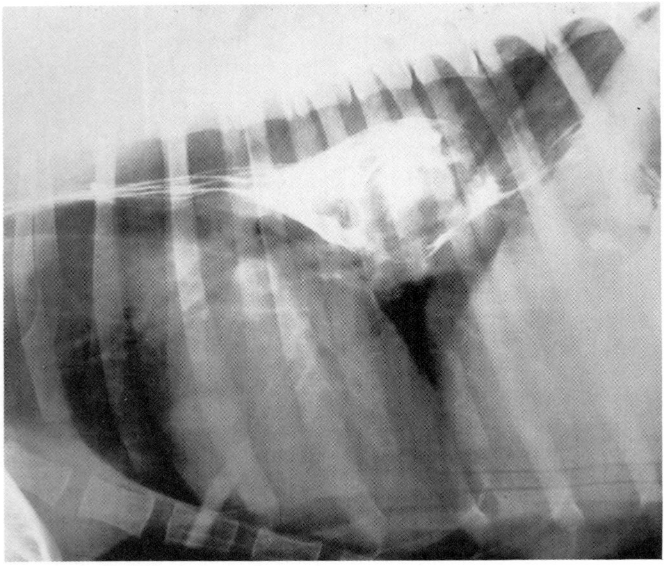

Figure 9-11. Lateral radiograph of dog with esophageal granuloma due to *Spirocera lupi.* Spondylitic lesions are also evident. Radiograph is courtesy of Dr. J.E. Bartels, School of Veterinary Medicine, Auburn University.

sarcomas. Fibrosarcomas of the esophagus, some of which undergo metaplastic transformation into osteogenic sarcomas, are often associated with the parasite *Spirocerca lupi*.[115] The malignant lesions are found in the thoracic esophagus, the site typically occupied by this parasite. The relationship, which appeared to be quite strong in one series of dogs in the USA, did not exist in a group of animals investigated in India, where no neoplasms are found in dogs with spirocercosis.

Adult *Spirocerca lupi* live in the wall of the esophagus. The parasite lays eggs that pass into the lumen of the esophagus and are subsequently eliminated from the body in feces. Eggs ingested by coprophagic beetles hatch, after which the larvae encyst in the beetle. This stage is infective for dogs. Alternately, the larvae can be ingested by rodents and birds, which act as transport hosts in which they reencyst. Canines are the definitive host. After ingestion of the beetle or transport host, the encysted larva is freed, invades the wall of the stomach, and migrates to the aorta by following the adventitia of arteries. The larvae concentrate in the thoracic aorta and migrate through small vessels to the esophagus, where they mature. Larvae that mistakenly migrate to other tissues become encysted. Larval migration and worm nodules in the esophagus can cause spondylitis in the adjacent bodies of vertebrae and aortic aneurysms as well as granulomatous lesions and neoplasia in the esophagus (Figure 9-11). Hypertrophic osteopathy has been reported in cases of esophageal fibrosarcoma with and without pulmonary metastasis.[116]

Clinical Signs. The predominant clinical signs in dogs with esophageal neoplasia include slowly progressive regurgitation, dysphagia, drooling, weight loss, and debilitation. Regurgitation may or may not be related to eating. Esophageal tumors usually occur in dogs and cats over six to eight years of age.

Diagnosis. Diagnosis may be aided by radiography; however, esophagoscopy and biopsy are required for a definitive diagnosis. The earliest and most consistent radiographic sign is the retention of intraluminal gas cranial to the tumor as a consequence of disturbed esophageal motility. Other abnormalities observed on survey films include a displacement of periesophageal structures and an increase in soft tissue or mineral density in the mediastinum. Positive contrast radiography is often required to delineate mural infiltration. Endoscopy will allow visualization of the mass and permit biopsy.

Treatment. Response to treatment and prognosis is dependent upon the cause for the neoplasia. Malignant tumors carry a poor prognosis; surgical intervention is often not practical. Radiation therapy may be palliative for radiosensitive tumors; however, radiation-induced esophagitis is a potential sequela. Treatment for *Spirocera lupi* infections has included the use of disophenol, diethylcarbamazine, and dithiazine iodide.[115] Fenbendazole and related compounds may be a useful adjunct, since they are effective against spirocerca larvae in extraintestinal tissue.

ESOPHAGEAL FISTULA

Fistula formation between the esophagus and airways may be due to congenital or acquired causes and is rarely reported in small animals. The fistula may be esophagotracheal, esophagobronchial, or esophagopulmonary. The esophagobronchial fistula is the most often reported esophageal fistula in the dog.[117,118] Congenital occurrence is thought to result from incomplete separation of the esophagus and airways during embryonic development.[1] The pathogenesis of acquired esophageal fistulas is poorly understood but usually includes a history of foreign body obstruction.

Clinical Signs. Clinical signs principally relate to respiratory dysfunction and include coughing, choking, regurgitation, and dysphagia. Coughing associated with drinking liquids is frequently observed in dogs with esophagobronchial fistulas but may not be present in all cases.[118] Anorexia, lethargy, weight loss, and pyrexia are also observed and are attributable to aspiration pneumonia with systemic infection. Crackles may be auscultated over consolidated lung regions on physical examination.

Diagnosis. Survey thoracic radiographs may demonstrate radiopaque foreign bodies, pulmonary consolidation, and pleural fluid accumulation. Contrast radiography will confirm the presence of esophageal perforation and locate the site of respiratory tract communication. Contrast esophagrams have been shown to be a reliable method for diagnosing esophagobronchial fistulas in dogs.[118] Esophagoscopy and bronchoscopy should be attempted but may prove futile in identifying the origin of the fistulous tract.

Treatment. Clinical management is aimed at surgical correction of the fistulous tract and its associated complications. Esophagotomy to remove foreign bodies and pneumonectomy of consolidated pulmonary tissues may be indicated. With thoracic cavity infection, appropriate bacteriologic cultures and antibiotic sensitivity testing should be performed. Those cases with limited esophageal trauma and minimal pulmonary pathology carry a favorable prognosis. A poor prognosis should be given to dogs with severe complications such as pneumonia, pulmonary abscesses, and significant pleural effusion.

HIATAL HERNIA

The esophageal hiatus is that diaphragmatic perforation that allows the esophagus to pass from the thoracic cavity into the abdominal cavity. The esophageal wall is secured to this hiatus by a phrenoesophageal membrane, which normally allows only minor cranial movement of the abdominal esophageal segment. Congenital or acquired lesions of the hiatus may allow hiatal hernia, periesophageal hiatal hernia, gastroesophageal intussusception, or diaphragmatic hernia to occur.[23,119]

Hiatal hernias allow for herniation of the abdominal esophagus, gastroesophageal junction, and stomach into the thoracic cavity and are uncommonly seen in the dog and cat. Gastroesophageal reflux usually accompanies hiatal hernia in dogs and cats, and reflux esophagitis is often an additional problem. Paraesophageal hiatal hernias are very rare and involve displacement of a portion of the stomach through a diaphragmatic deficit adjacent to the esophageal hiatus. Gastroesophageal intussusception describes the invagination of all or parts of the stomach into the thoracic esophagus. In severe cases, the spleen and pancreas may be herniated as well. Idiopathic megaesophagus or incompetency of the GES may predispose dogs to this disorder.[30,120] Although uncommon, gastroesophageal intussusception is most often seen in large breed dogs less than three months of age.[121]

Clinical Signs. Clinical signs associated with hiatal disorders include occasional or persistent regurgitation, vomiting, hypersalivation, and respiratory distress. Abdominal pain may be evident on palpation. Dehydration may lead to death in affected puppies. Survey radiographs frequently demonstrate esophageal dilatation with a well-circumscribed area of increased density in the caudal thoracic esophagus. Barium contrast procedures are usually necessary for diagnosis; in some cases fluoroscopy is necessary for confirming the diagnosis.

Treatment. Hiatal hernia is treated by surgical reduction of the esophageal hiatus, combined with a modified Nissen fundoplication.[119] The stomach can be anchored to the abdominal wall by a tube gastrostomy through the fundic wall. Fundoplication must only partially surround the intra-abdominal esophagus since more complete encircling prevents eructation of gas from the stomach and animals can bloat. Animals can be fed through the gastrostomy so that the esophagus can be rested. Surgery has been successful in only 25% of the cases reported. The newer combined surgical approaches appear to be more successful than only hiatal closure or some form of fundoplication. The prognosis must be guarded and will reflect the surgeon's skills and the level of understanding of anatomy and physiology of the diaphragm and gastroesophageal junction.

ESOPHAGITIS

Clinical Synopsis

Diagnostic Features

* Anorexia; painful swallow
* Excess salivation
* Regurgitation
* Evidence of esophagial inflammation on biopsy

Treatment

* No food for 48 hours
* Follow with high protein-low fat diet
* Sucralfate (as slurry) 1/2 - 1 g q 8 h PO for 7 days
* Cimetidine 5 mg/kg q 8 h PO for 14-21 days
* Metoclopramide 0.2 mg/kg just prior to feeding

Etiology

Inflammation of the esophagus may result from a variety of acute or chronic insults. Causes of esophagitis include the ingestion of chemical irritants, thermal insults, acute and persistent vomiting, foreign body obstruction, and gastroesophageal reflux. Infectious causes for esophageal inflammation are uncommon. Primary infectious esophagitis has been reported in immunocompromised patients and as a sequela to systemic phycomycosis in the dog.[122] Acute esophagitis with ulcerations has been observed in some cats with caliciviral upper respiratory infection.[123] The incidence of primary acute esophagitis is thought to be relatively low; however, this is most likely an underestimation because of the obscure clinical signs, limited use of endoscopy by the practicing veterinarian, and subtle radiographic findings associated with this disorder.

Gastroesophageal Reflux. Gastroesophageal reflux is a normal event in dogs and probably cats as well. Reflux is even more likely in young animals. The GES is incompetent at birth, and in cats and dogs GES pressure at six weeks is only one-half of that in adults.[39,124] Hence, regurgitation is common in young animals and is especially evident when human handling increases intra-abdominal pressure in recently fed individuals. Esophagitis does not follow unless the refluxed contents are not cleared in a relatively short time. In normal adult dogs, reflux occurs primarily during normally-occurring transient GES relaxation, which appears on an average of once an hour in both unfed and fed animals.[125] The pH of esophageal mucosa becomes acid for 5 to 30 seconds. Other studies have reported longer acidification times. Reflux with acidification also occurs with swallowing and belching. The transient refluxes are related to complete GES relaxation rather than low resting GES pressure.[126,127] After reflux, esophageal peristalsis removes acidic fluid refluxed from the stomach and brings swallowed saliva to the acidified regions of the esophagus so that bicarbonate rich saliva neutralizes the acid. Two determinants of whether esophagitis develops are the frequency of acid reflux and the length of time for restoring normal esophageal pH.

Activity in vagal nerves and intragastric pressure determine the frequency of gastroesophageal reflux. Vagotomy or vagal cooling abolishes transient GES relaxation and eructation in dogs; because atropine does not have that effect, noncholinergic fibers mediate the reflex.[128,129] Reflux in dogs is also associated with fundic contractions that appear to be a driving force for GES relaxation.[130] Fundic contractions increase intragastric pressure, and that change markedly reduces GES pressure in the cat and in humans.[131,132] Increasing intra-abdominal pressure raises GES pressure to maintain the antireflux barrier. Reducing resting GES pressure by any drug has not been shown to increase the frequency of gastroesophageal reflux. Lower than normal basal GES pressure does not increase frequency of reflux. The frequency is determined by how often GES pressure falls to that in the stomach.

The basis for transient GES relaxation is unknown, but in the dog, as in other species, there is a mechanism to meet a physiological need to overcome the competence of the gastroesophageal sphincter. This mechanism operates during vomition or the eructation of gastric gas. The competence of the sphincter is suppressed by movement of the intra-abdominal segment of esophagus and cardia into the thoracic cavity, followed by contraction of the diaphragm and abdominal muscles. In the dog, contraction of the striated longitudinal muscles of the esophagus accomplishes cranial translocation of the gastroesophageal sphincter. Thus, there are times when reflux could be expected in the normal dog. Since this physiologic sliding hernia is dependent on contraction of the longitudinal esophageal muscles, it follows that their denervation would eliminate the event. Dogs in experimental studies have been selectively vagotomized to paralyze the muscles of the caudal esophagus and abolish the physiologic means for the sliding hernia.[133] The success of the procedure in dogs has prompted the suggestion that it be considered for reflux esophagitis in humans. A conclusion that follows is that reflux occurs because of an exaggeration or persistence of this physiological response, which is normally invoked at irregular times for short periods.

The time for restoring normal esophageal pH is determined by how rapidly refluxed material is physically cleared and neutralized.[127] Primary esophageal peristalsis, stimulated by the swallowing of saliva, clears the refluxed volume. It is also cleared by secondary peristalsis, stimulated when the reflux distends the esophagus. It is not known whether acid pH stimulates secondary peristalsis; it is believed to stimulate esophageal contractions that do not clear the esophagus. The peristaltic reflexes depend on normal vagal innervation. Bicarbonate-rich saliva that has been swallowed and secretions of the esophageal submucosal glands neutralize refluxed acidic fluid. Peristalsis clears acid volume; saliva neutralizes acid and dilutes fluid; in addition, back diffusion across the esophageal mucosa causes hydrogen ions to disappear. Secretion of saliva, swallowing, and esophageal peristalsis are markedly reduced during sleep. Thus, the reduced clearing capacity at such times is associated with greater risk for esophagitis; frequency of transient GES relaxations increases at night in humans, which compounds the problem.[134]

Esophagitis and GES Function. Esophagitis develops when reflux is frequent and clearance is impaired. Increased reflux frequency accompanies increased times for transient GES pressure reductions. Basal GES tone is an inherent property of its smooth muscle. Esophagitis can cause that tone, and with it the antireflux barrier, to be lost.[135] Esophagitis can also disrupt the neural cholinergic and hormonal mechanisms for maintaining a high GES pressure. Reflux frequency can also increase with changes in the anatomic factors that contribute to the high pressure zone in the GES. These factors include a mucosal flap, flutter valve, acute esophagogastric angle, and compression by the gastric sling fibers to provide a one-way valve. The relation of the anatomy and physiology of the diaphragm to the esophagus also contributes to preventing reflux. Hiatal hernia disrupts this relationship, increasing the risk for reflux.

Persistant low GES pressure or increased intra-abdominal pressure does not by itself increase reflux frequency. An augmented gastric contraction rate and increased gastric volume can increase reflux frequency. Reflux is more likely with problems causing gastric retention; reflux can be demonstrated in many cases of gastric outflow obstruction. Conversely, reflux esophagitis can result in slower gastric emptying; there may be situations where it is unknown which problem developed first.[136]

Pathogenesis of Esophagitis. Gastric fluid refluxed into the esophagus can potentially damage the mucosa by its content of acid, pepsin, trypsin, bile acids, and lysolecithin. A combination of these constituents is necessary for the damage. Acid alone in the canine esophagus stimulates proliferation in the basal epithelium but no erosions or inflammation.[137] Acid combined with pepsin or bile acids causes severe ulcerative changes within an hour.[138] Bile acids alone increase the mucosal permeability for acid, small molecules, but it causes only minor if any morphologic changes within an hour. Bile acids must be in an acidic solution to produce damage, and there is some question whether any of the small amounts of bile acids in the stomach appear in the refluxed fluid.[139] Trypsin at pH 7.5 damages the esophageal mucosa more severely than bile acids or pepsin does.[140,141] Whether such conditions ever prevail is unknown. Recent studies in dogs show that the most severe esophagitis is caused by reflux during maximal gastric stimulation in the absence of duodenogastric reflux, which when present resulted in less severe changes.[142] Bile and acid perfusion of the esophagus in cats reduces GES pressure and swallowing pressure. Esophageal contractions are weak and uncoordinated; no peristaltic waves are evident. Abnormal motility persists for more than two days following the insult, although GES pressure can return earlier.[143]

Drugs and chemicals, as well as reflux or vomiting of gastric juices, cause esophagitis. Out of a small number of drugs evaluated in cats, a high percentage caused esophagitis (Table 9-4).[144] Drugs in tablet form pass through the esophagus easier than capsules. In humans, 65% of capsules taken without water lodge and dissolve in the esophagus; taken with water 9% lodge in the esophagus. Oral medications given to dogs and cats are more likely to remain in the esophagus because liquids are not taken with the medicine and the animal's body is not usually in a position for gravity to assist transit through the esophagus. Many of the drugs causing esophageal injury in humans are ones used in small animals.[145] Esophageal injury is due to drug-induced changes in mucosa pH, hyperosmolarity, or in many cases unknown means. In summary, oral medications cause esophageal injury, and since capsules and tablets are so easily retained in the esophagus, water should be routinely given by

Table 9-4. Drugs Causing Esophagitis in Cats

Acetylsalicylic acid	350 mg
Alprenol (ß-blocker)	50 mg
Ascorbic acid	–
Ferrosuccinate	75 mg
Ferrosulfate	100 mg
Doxycycline	100 mg
Emepronium bromide	50 mg
Potassium chloride	600 mg
Tetracycline	–

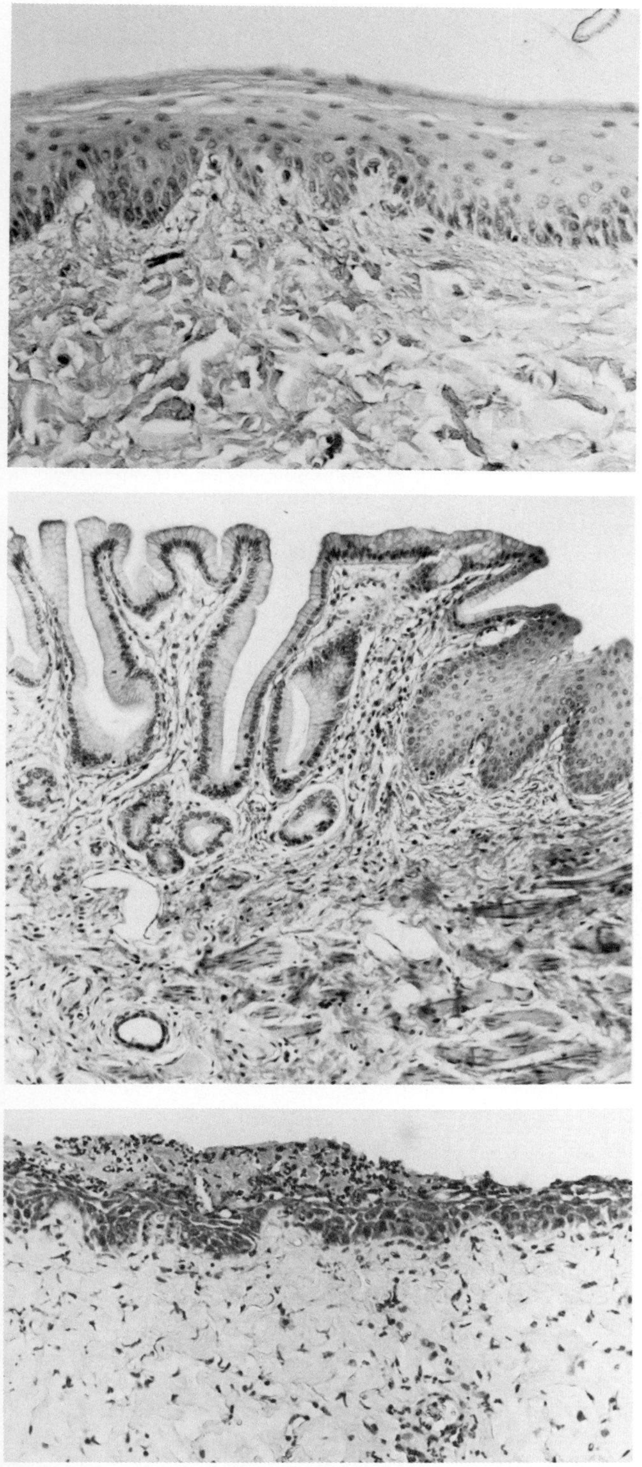

Figure 9-12. A. Biopsy of normal esophageal mucosa obtained with capsule.
B. Photomicrograph of junction of gastric and esophageal mucosa at the gastroesophageal junction from a normal dog.
C. Biopsy of esophagus at the gastroesophageal sphincter obtained with capsule. Shows an esophagitis characterized by infiltration by neurophils and necrosis of surface of epithelium. Typical changes caused by reflux of gastric contents into the esophagus.

syringe into an animal's oral cavity to minimize the risk of esophageal injury. This becomes more important when esophageal motility may not be normal because of esophagitis from vomiting, very young or old age, or a primary esophageal problem.

Clinical Signs. Mild esophagitis is often limited to mucosal damage and is usually self-limiting once the inciting process is removed. Clinical signs are mild or nonexistent, and the esophageal mucosa heals quickly without significant fibrosis. Deep esophagitis with involvement of the muscular layers is uncommon and can lead to severe complications such as persistent ulceration, stricture formation, and esophageal perforation.

The clinical signs associated with reflux esophagitis are subtle and difficult to evaluate. They can consist of esophageal discomfort leading to anorexia, weight loss, excessive salivation, and regurgitation of viscid saliva-like fluid that may contain blood. Many dogs with reflux esophagitis show milder signs that consist of intermittent or consistent vomiting of fluid during the night or early morning. The vomiting may be associated with a number of swallowing movements, where it appears that the animal is attempting to return a refluxed bolus to the stomach. Such dogs may or may not vomit, but in either case they usually eat when fed and show no more signs after eating. The food buffers acid in the stomach so that if any reflux continues it does not cause signs. Stimulation of receptors in the esophagus may initiate vomiting; it is generally believed that esophageal problems result in only regurgitation, however. Acid that bathes esophageal mucosa can also refluxly stimulate bronchospasm, which may cause an animal to be presented for respiratory signs. Conversely, respiratory signs of dyspnea and coughing can reflexly lower GES pressure, and that makes gastroesophageal reflux more likely. Physical examination is usually unremarkable.

Diagnosis. Radiographic procedures are sometimes useful in confirming a suspicion of esophagitis. Survey radiographs are usually unremarkable; severe cases may show signs of GES chalasia, hiatal hernia, or stricture formation. Contrast radiography using fluoroscopy may reveal gastroesophageal reflux and the effects of esophagitis to cause varying degrees of dilatation and dysperistalsis. Often, reflux esophagitis is considered only after evaluation has provided no evidence for gastroduodenal disease. When vomiting and other signs remain unexplained, a workup is conducted to evaluate for abnormalities using contrast fluoroscopic studies, biopsies of the caudal esophagus, and manometry of the GES. In humans, pH in the esophagus adjacent to the GES is monitored continuously. The number of episodes of reflux and the time and conditions prevailing are evaluated for a diagnosis of reflux esophagitis. In dogs, manometry and fluoroscopic studies are unreliable because their results can be normal most of the time, even in dogs with reflux esophagitis. Biopsy of the caudal esophageal mucosa is the most reliable procedure for identifying reflux esophagitis or esophagitis due to any other cause. An instrument that contains a capsule to retrieve suction biopsies makes that possible without general anesthesia. Biopsies are especially useful in identifying patients with esophagitis associated with grossly normal mucosa. Diagnosis is based on finding inflammatory changes when the problem is acute and on finding a thickening of the basal or germinative layer and elongation of the papilla when in chronic cases they approach the luminal

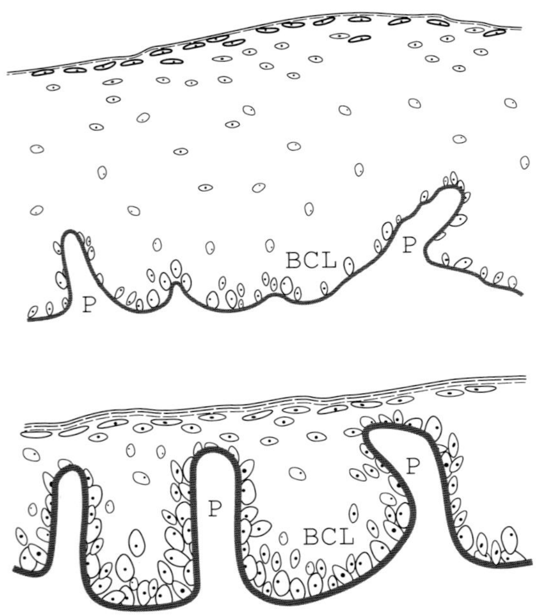

Figure 9-13. Drawing showing biopsy appearance of normal canine esophagus (above) and of dog with reflux esophagitis. Changes are seen for thickness of basal lamina(BCL) and for depth of papilla(P). Drawn from reference 142 figures.

surface (Figure 9-12 and 9-13).[142] Chronic inflammatory changes can include infiltration by eosinophils.[146] Biopsy of the esophagus is useful for ruling out heterotopic esophageal mucosa consisting of oxyntic, chief, and mucus- secreting cells.[147] That can be a cause for esophagitis and stricture.

Treatment. Esophagitis is treated initially by resting the esophagus; nothing except water is given by mouth. On resumption of feeding, foods are selected to maximize GES pressure and competence. A high-protein diet is fed. An increase in GES pressure follows and is believed to be the result of the gastrin released. A low-fat diet is fed because fats reduce GES pressure; that reduction is believed to be mediated by cholecystokinin. A number of other foods are known to reduce GES pressure, but the only one of importance in small animals is chocolate, which is sometimes seen to precipitate acute upper gastrointestinal signs when fed to dogs.

Medical management includes the use of antacids, which are given very often, hourly, in the acute phase. Antacids neutralize gastric acid, and that minimizes further damage when gastric juices reflux into the esophagus. Gastric acid's effects can also be reduced by cimetidine, an H_2 blocker, which greatly reduces acid secretion when given at a dose of 3 to 5 mg/lb every eight hours (Table 9-5). Ranitidine is more effective in inhibiting acid secretion when it is given at a dose of 0.2 mg/lb every twelve hours. Antacids are not given with cimetidine because absorption of cimetidine may be reduced. Drugs such as bethanechol, metoclopramide, and cisapride increase GES pressure in dogs and most likely in cats also. Metoclopramide is effective in dogs and can be used in the acute phase,[148] but it is not usually recommended in chronic cases since its pharmaceutical activity lasts for only 1.5-2.0 hours when given orally. Metoclopramide is of no value or even worsens reflux esophagitis in some children;[149] similar results are possible in some

Table 9-5. Drugs for Treatment of Esophagitis

Cimetidine	2-5 mg/lb	PO,IV,IM	Tid
Ranitidine	0.20 mg/lb	PO	Bid
Metoclopramide	0.05-0.15 mg/lb	PO,IV,SQ	QID
	0.005-0.05 mg/lb/hr	IV	Continuous

animals. Cisapride, when available, should be more useful in dogs.[150] Neither of these two drugs have any effect on striated esophageal muscle found throughout the canine esophagus, and so they are not indicated for any primary esophageal motility problems. They would have a beneficial effect on motility problems involving the caudal feline esophagus, which is composed of smooth muscle. Any anticholinergic or muscle relaxant is contraindicated. In addition to reducing GES pressure in both fed and unfed dogs and cats, they reduce motility in the caudal feline esophagus and impair the animal's ability to clear refluxed fluid back into the stomach. The use of prescription formulations containing an antiemetic and an anticholinergic could interfere with recovery of an animal with esophagitis. Anticholinergics also abolish any beneficial effects of metoclopramide on the GES.

Recommendation for management of the chronic once a day (in the morning) vomiter is to a) feed at bedtime (the buffering effect of a protein meal lasts for hours), b) give antacids at bedtime, or c) give an H_2 blocker at bedtime. The dog is fed again in the morning.

Acute esophageal lesions can be treated by colloidal bismuth suspensions, and they can be prevented by sucralfate.[151,152] Sucrose sulfate in sucralfate probably acts as a topical protectant. Other treatment of esophagitis is directed toward correcting the initiating cause and symptomatic therapy. Emesis should not be induced if caustic agents have been consumed. Unabsorbed acids may be neutralized with magnesium oxide solution (1:25 dilution with warm water) or milk of magnesia. A weak acid such as vinegar (1:4 diluted with water) or lemon juice administered orally is recommended following the ingestion of caustic alkalis.

A variety of different surgical procedures have been used in humans to treat reflux esophagitis; all have been performed experimentally on the dog. Surgical correction of hiatal hernias and prevention of reflux is accomplished in several ways. These include gastric fixation by gastropexy; restoration of the intra-abdominal segment of the esophagus; fundoplication, which creates an acute angle where the esophagus enters the stomach and "calibrates" or narrows the lumen of the tube at that point; and reduction of the size of the hiatus to prevent a reconstructed gastroesophageal junction from herniating into the chest.[119,153,154] One suggestion is to selectively vagotomize the caudal esophagus so that the normal physiologic sliding of the gastroesophageal sphincter into the thorax is no longer possible.[133]

REFERENCES

1. Suter, P.F.: Thoracic Radiography. P.F. Suter, Wettswill, Switzerland, 295-349, 1984.
2. Watrous, B.J.: Clinical presentation and diagnosis of dysphagia. Vet. Clin. N. Am. 13:437-459, 1983.
3. Watrous, B.J. and Suter, P.F.: Normal swallowing in the dog: A cineradiographic study. Vet. Radiol. 20:99-109, 1979.
4. Suter, P.F. and Watrous, B.J.: Oropharyngeal dysphagias in the dog: a cinefluorographic analysis of experimentally induced and spontaneously occurring swallowing disorders. I. Oral and pharyngeal stage dysphagias. Vet. Radiol. 24:11-24, 1983.
5. Watrous, B.J. and Suter, P.F.: Oropharyngeal dysphagias in the dog: a cinefluorographic analysis of experimentally induced and spontaneously occurring swallowing disorders. II. Cricopharyngeal stage and mixed oropharyngeal dysphagias. Vet. Radiol. 24:11-24, 1983.
6. White, R.A.S. and Lane, J.G.: Pharyngeal stick penetration injuries in the dog. J. Small An. Pract. 29:13-35, 1988.
7. Miller, A.J.: Deglutition. Physiol. Rev. 62:129-184, 1982.
8. Boudrieu, R.J. and Rogers, W.A.: Megaesophagus in the dog: A review of 50 cases. JAAHA 21:33-40, 1985.
9. Harvey, C.E., O'Brien, J.A., Durie, V.R., Miller D.J., and Veenema, R.: Megaesophagus in the dog: A clinical survey of 79 cases. JAVMA 165:443-446, 1974.
10. Strombeck, D.R.: Pathophysiology of esophageal motility disorders in the dog and cat, Vet. Clin. N Am. 8:229-244, 1984.
11. Leib, M.S.: Megaesophagus in the dog. In: Current Veterinary Therapy IX. Edited by R.W. Kirk. W.B. Saunders Co., Philadelphia, 848-851, 1986.
12. Strombeck, D.R.: Diseases In Swallowing. In, Small Animal Gastroenterology. Stonegate Publishing, Davis, Ca., 1979.
13. Sharp, N.J.H. and Nash, A.S.: Feline Dysautonomia. In, Current Vet Therapy IX. Edited by R.W. Kirk. W.B. Saunders Co., 802-804, 1986.
14. Osborne, C.A., Clifford, D.H., and Jessen, C.: Hereditary esophageal achalasia in dogs. JAVMA 151:572-581, 1967.
15. Strating, A. and Clifford, D.H.: Canine achalasia with special reference to hereditary. Southwest Vet. 19:135-137, 1966.
16. Cox, V.S., Wallace, L.J., Anderson, V.E. and Rushmer, R.A.: Hereditary esophageal dysfunction in the Miniature Schnauzer dog. Am. J. Vet. Res. 41:326-330, 1980.
17. Breshears, D.E.: Esophageal dilation in six-week-old male German Shepherd pups. VM/SAC 60:1034, 1965.
18. Palmer, C.S.: Achalasia or cardiospasms in Great Dane puppies. VM/SAC 63:574-578, 1968.
19. Leib, M.S.: Megaesophagus in the dog. Comp. Cont. Ed. Pract. Vet. 5:825-833, 1983.
20. Schwartz, A., Ravin, C.E., Greenspan, R.H., Schoemann, R.S. and Burt, J.K.: Congenital neuromuscular esophageal disease in a litter of Newfoundland puppies. J. Am. Vet. Radiol. Soc. 17:101, 1976.
21. Spy, G.M.: Megaesophagus in a litter of Greyhounds. Vet. Rec. 75:853-854, 1963.
22. Clifford, D.H., Soifer, F.K., Wilson, C.F., Waddell, E.D. and Guilloud, G.L.: Congenital achalasia of the esophagus in four cats of common ancestry. JAVMA 158:1554-1560, 1971.
23. Watrous, B.J.: Esophageal disease. In, Textbook of Veterinary Internal Medicine. Edited by S.J. Ettinger. W.B. Saunders Co., Philadelphia, 1191, 1983.
24. Diamant, N., Szczepanski, M., and Mui, H.: Manometric characteristics of idiopathic megaesophagus in the dog: An unsuitable animal model for achalasia in man. Gastroenterology 65:216-223, 1973.
25. Gray, G.W.: Acute experiments on neuroeffector function in canine esophageal achalasia. Am. J. Vet. Res. 35:1075-1081, 1974.
26. Sokolvsky, V.: Achalasia and paralysis of the canine esophagus. JAVMA 260:943-955, 1972.
27. Strombeck, D.R., and Troya, L.: Evaluation of lower motor neuron function in two dogs with megaesophagus. JAVMA 169:411-414, 1976.
28. Aggestrup, S., Uddman, R., Sundler, F., Fahrenkrug, J., Hakanson, R., Sorensen, H.R. and Hambraeus, G.: Lack of vasoactive intestinal polypeptide nerves in esophageal achalasia. Gastroenterology 84:924-927, 1983.
29. Arimori, M., Code, C.F., Schlege, J.F., and Sturm, R.E.: Electrical activity of the canine esophagus and gastroesophageal sphincter. Am. J. Dig. Dis. 15:191-208, 1970.
30. Hoffer, R.E.: Surgical esophageal disease. In: Pathophysiology In Small Animal Surgery. Edited by M.J. Bojrab. Lea & Febiger, Philadelphia, 90-100, 1981.
31. Clifford D.H. and Gyorkey, F.: Myenteric ganglial cells in dogs with and without achalasia of the esophagus. JAVMA 150:205-211, 1967.
32. Higgs, B., Kerr, F.W.F., and Ellis, F.H.: The experimental production of esophageal achalasia by electrolytic lesions in the medulla. J. Thor. Cardio. Surg. 50:613-625, 1965.
33. Pelemans, W., VanTrappen, G., Hellemans, J., Valembois, P., and Janssens, J.: Denervation potentials in the canine esophagus. In, Proc. Fourth International Symposium on Gastrointestinal Motility, Vancouver, Mitchell Press, 1974.
34. Rogers, W.A. Fenner, W.R. and Sherding, R.G.: Electromyographic and esophagomanometric findings in clinically normal dogs and in dogs with idiopathic megaesophagus. JAVMA 174:181-183, 1979.
35. Clifford, D.H., Pirsch, J.G., and Mauldin, M.L.: Comparison of motor nuclei of the vagus nerve in dogs with and without esophageal achalasia. Proc. Sco. Exp. Biol. and Med. 142:878-882, 1973.
36. Leipold, H.: Unpublished observations cited by Guffy, M.M. Esophageal Disorders. In, Veterinary Internal Medicine, Edited by S.J. Ettinger, W.B. Saunders Co., Philadelphia, 1975.
37. Nakayama, S., Neya, T., Watanabe, K., and Tsuchiya, K.: Effects of electrical stimulation and local destruction of the medulla oblongata on swallowing movements in dogs. Rendic. Gastroenterol. 6:6-11, 1974.
38. Tan, B.J.K. and Diamant, N.E.: Assessment of the neural defect in a dog with idiopathic megaesophagus. Dig. Dis. Sci. 32:76-85, 1987.
39. Strombeck, D.R.: Unpublished observations.
40. Diamant, N., Szczepanski, M., and Mui, H.: Idiopathic megaesophagus in the dog: Reasons for spontaneous improvement and a possible method of medical therapy. Can. Vet. J. 15:66-71, 1974.
41. Forbes, D.C. and Leishman, D.E.: Megaesophagus in a cat. Can. Vet. J. 26:354-356, 1985.
42. Crawley, A.J. and Gendreau, C.L.: Esophageal achalasia in a cat. Can. Vet. J. 10:195-197, 1969.
43. Krum, S.H., Cardinet, G.H., Anderson, B.C., and Holliday, T.A.: Polymyositis and polyarthritis associated with systemic lupus erythematosis in a dog. JAVMA 170:61-64, 1977.
44. Marsden, P.D. and Hagstrom, J.W.C.: Experimental *Trypanosoma cruzi* infection in beagle puppies. Trans. Royal Soc. Trop. Med. and Hyg. 62:816, 1968.
45. Walvort, H.C., VanNess, J.J., Stokhof, A.A. and Wolvekamp, W.T.C.: Canine glycogen storage disease type II: A clinical study of four affected Lapland dogs. JAAHA 20:279-286, 1984.
46. Kornegay, J.N., Gorgacz, E.J., Dawe, D.L., Bowen, J.M., White, N.A. and DeBuysscher, E.V.: Polymyositis in dogs. JAVMA 176:431-438, 1980.
47. Haupt, K.H., Prieur, D.J., Moore, M.P., Hargis, A.M., Hegreberg, G.A., Gavin, P.R. and Johnson, R.S.: Familial canine dermatomyositis: Clinical electrodiagnostic, and genetic studies. Am. J. Vet. Res. 46:1861-1869, 1985.
48. Darke, P.G.G., Roberts, T.A., Smart, J.L. and Bradshaw, P.R.: Suspected botulism in foxhounds. Vet. Rec. 99:98-100, 1976.
49. Van Nes, J.J.: Electrophysiological evidence of peripheral nerve dysfunction in six dogs with botulism type C. Res.

Vet. Sci. 40:372-376, 1986.
50. Knauer, C.M., Carbone, J.V., Brandborg, L.L. and Solverman, S.: Alimentary Tract and Liver. In: Current Medical Diagnosis and Treatment. Edited by M.A. Krupp, et. al. Lange Publ., Los Altos, 1985.
51. Mason, K.V.: A case of myasthenia gravis in a cat. J. Sm. An. Pract. 17:467-472, 1976.
52. Miller, L.M., Lennon, V.A., Lambert, E.H., Reed, S.M., Hegreberg, G.A., Miller, J.B. and Ott, R.L.: Congenital myasthenia gravis in 13 smooth Fox Terriers. JAVMA 182:694-702, 1983.
53. Harris, L.D., Ashworth, W.D. and Ingelfinger, F.J.: Esophageal aperistalsis and achalasia produced in dogs by prolonged cholinesterase inhibition. J. Clin. Invest. 39:1744-1751, 1960.
54. Cummings, J.F., deLahunta, A. and Mitchell, Jr. W.J.: Ganglioradiculitis in the dog. Acta Neurolpathologica 60:29, 1983.
55. Zook, B.C. and Gilmore, C.E.: Thallium poisoning in dogs. JAVMA 151:206-217, 1967.
56. Duncan, I.D. and Griffiths, I.R.: Canine giant axonal neuropathy; some aspects of its clinical, pathological and comparative features. J. Sm. An. Pract. 22:491-501, 1981.
57. Shell, L.G. Jortner, B.S. and Leib, M.S.: Spinal muscular atrophy in two Rottweiler littermates. JAVMA 190:878-880, 1987.
58. Zook, B.C.: The pathologic anatomy of lead poisoning in dogs. Vet. Pathol. 9:310-327, 1972.
59. O'Brien, J.A., Harvey, C.E. and Brodey, R.S.: The Esophagus. In, Veterinary Gastroenterology. Edited by N.V. Anderson. Lea & Febiger, Philadelphia, 372 1980.
60. Van Ee, R.T., Dodd, V.M., Pope, E.R. and Henrey, G.A.: Bronchoesophageal fistula and transient megaesophagus in a dog. JAVMA 188:874-875, 1986.
61. Cassella, R.R., Brown, Jr., A.L., Sayre, G.P. and Ellis, Jr., F.H.: Achalasia of the esophagus: Pathologic and etiologic considerations. Ann. Surg. 160:474-487, 1964.
62. Hara, T.: Experimental study on the pathogenesis of achalasia. Jap. J Smooth Muscle Res. 5:33, 1969.
63. Fox, J.G., Averill, D.R., Hallett, M. and Schunk, K.: Familial reflex myoclonus in Labrador Retrievers. Am. J. Vet. Res. 45:2367-2370, 1984.
64. Pidgeon, G.: Unpublished observations, 1987.
65. Chastain, C.B. and Ganjam, V.K.: Clinical Endocrinology of Companion Animals. Lea & Febiger, Philadelphia, 1986.
66. Feldman, E.C. and Tyrrell, J.B.: Hypoadrenocorticism. Vet. Clin. N. Am. 7:555-581, 1977.
67. Schaer, M., Riley, W.J., Buergelt, C.D., Bowen, D.J., Senior, D.F., Burrows, C.F. and Cambell, G.A.: Autoimmunity and Addison's disease in the dog. JAAHA 22:789-794, 1986.
68. Roudebush, P., Jones, B.D. and Vaughan, R.W.: Medical aspects of esophageal disease. In: Canine and Feline Gastroenterology. Edited by B.D. Jones. W.B. Saunders Co., Philadelphia, 54-80, 1986.
69. Ridgeway, R.L. and Suter, P.F.: Clinical and radiographic signs in primary and metastatic esophageal neoplasms of the dog. JAVMA 174:700-704, 1979.
70. Carpenter, J.L. and Holzworth, J.: Thymoma in 11 cats. JAVMA 181:248-251, 1982.
71. Darke, P.G.G., McCullagh, K.G. and Geldart, P.H.: Myasthenia gravis, thymoma and myositis in a dog. Vet. Rec. 97:392-394, 1975.
72. Clifford, D.H.: Myenteric ganglial cells of the esophagus in cats with achalasia of the esophagus. Am. J. Vet. Res. 34:1333-1335, 1973.
73. Pearson, H., Gaskell, C.J., Gibbs, C., and Waterman, A.: Pyloric and oesophageal dysfunction in the cat. J. Small An. Pract. 15:487-501, 1974.
74. Eastwood, G.L., Castell, D.O., and Higgs, R.H.: Experimental esophagitis in cats impairs lower esophageal sphincter pressure. Gastroenterology 69:146-153, 1975.
75. Henderson, R.D., Mugashe, F., Jeejeebhoy, K.N., Cullen, J., Szczepanski, M., Boszko, A., and Marryatt, G.: The role of bile and acid in the production of esophagitis and the motor defect of esophagitis. Ann. Thorac. Surg. 14:465-473, 1972.
76. Bishop, L.M., Kelly, D.F., Gibbs, C. and Pearson, R.A.: Megaloesophagus and associated gastric heterotopia in the cat. Vet. Pathol. 16:444-449, 1979.
77. Guilford, W.G.: Unpublished observations, 1986.
78. O'Brien, T.R.: Radiographic Diagnosis of Abdominal Disorders in the Dog and Cat. W.B. Saunders Co., Philadelphia, 1978.
79. Harvey, C.E. and O'Brien, J.A.: Esophageal disease and disorders. Scientific Presentations of the Annual Meeting. AAHA (2):155-161, 1975.
80. Cohen, S.: Esophageal motility disorders and their response to calcium channel antagonists. Gastroenterology 93:201-203, 1987.
81. Hofmeyer, C.F.B.: An evaluation of cardioplasty for achalasia of the esophagus in the dog. J. Sm. An. Pract. 7:281-287, 1966.
82. Hoffer, R.E.: Primary Esophageal Neuromuscular Diseases. In: Canine and Feline Gastroenterology. Edited by B.D. Jones. W.B. Saunders Co., Philadelphia, 89-100, 1986.
83. Hoffer, R.E. MacCoy, D.M., Quick, C.B., Barclay, S.M. and Rendano, V.T.: Management of acquired achalasia in dogs. JAVMA 175: 814-817, 1979.
84. Hoffer, R.E., MacCoy, D.M., Gaynor, F., Moraff, H., Aron, D., Quick, C.B. and Law, K.: Physiologic features of the canine esophagus: Effect of modified Heller's esophagomyotomy. Am. J. Vet. Res. 41:723, 1980.
85. Hofmeyr, C.F.B.: An evaluation of cardioplasty for achalasia of the oesophagus in the dog. J. Small An. Pract. 7:281-301, 1966.
86. Guffy, M.M.: Esophageal Disorders. In: Textbook of Veterinary Internal Medicine. Edited by S.J. Ettinger. W.B. Saunders Co., 1098-1124, 1975.
87. Kipnis, R.M.: Megaesophagus: Remission in two dogs. JAAHA 14:24-252, 1978.
88. Hendricks, J.C., Maggio-Price, L. and Dougherty, J.F.: Transient esophageal dysfunction mimicking megaesophagus in three dogs. JAVMA 185:90-92, 1984
89. Shires, P.K. and Lui, W.: Persistent right aortic arch in dogs: A long term follow-up after surgical correction. JAAHA 17:773-776, 1981.
90. Pearson, H.: Symposium on conditions of the canine esophagus. I. Foreign bodies in the oesophagus. J. Sm. An. Pract. 7:107-116, 1966.
91. Ryan, W.W. and Greene, R.W.: The conservative management of esophageal foreign bodies and their complications. A review of 66 cases in dogs and cats. JAAHA 11:243-249, 1975.
92. Pollack, S., and Rhodes, W.H.: Gastroesophageal intussusception in an Afghan hound: a case report. J. Am. Vet. Rad. Soc. 11:5-14, 1970.
93. Zimmer, J.F.: Canine esophageal foreign bodies: endoscopic, surgical, and medical management. JAAHA 20:669-677, 1984.
94. Lantz, G.C., Cantwell, H.D., VanVleet, J.F., Blakemore, J.C. and Newman, S.: Pharyngostomy tube induced esophagitis in the dog: An experimental study. JAAHA 19:207-212, 1983.
95. Knight, G.C.: Transthoracic oesophagotomy in dogs: a survey of 75 operations. Vet. Rec. 75:264-266, 1963.
96. Pearson, H., Darke, P.G.G., Gibbs, C., Kelly, D.F. and Orr, C.M.: Reflux esophagitis and stricture formation after anesthesia: A review of seven cases in dogs and cats. J. Sm. An. Pract. 19:507-519, 1978.
97. Harvey, H.J.: Iatrogenic esophageal stricture in the dog. JAVMA 166:1100-1102, 1975.
98. Safaie-Shirazi, S., DenBesten, L., and Zike, W.L.: Effect of bile salts on the ionic permeability of the esophageal mucosa and their role in the production of esophagitis. Gastroenterology 68:728-733, 1975.
99. Hall, A.W., Moosa, A.R., Clark, J., Cooley, G.R.,and Skinner, D.B.: The effects of premedication drugs on the lower oesophageal high pressure zone and reflux status of Rhesus monkeys and man. Gut 16:347-352, 1975.

100. Misiewicz, J.J.: Symposium on gastroesophageal reflux and its complications. Section 4, Pharmacology and Therapeutics. Gut, 14:243-246, 1973.
101. Pope, C.E.: Pathophysiology and diagnosis of reflux esophagitis. Gastroenterology 70:445-464, 1973.
102. Strombeck, D.R. and Harrold, D.: Effects of atropine, acepromazine, meperidine, and xylazine on gastroesophageal sphincter pressure in the dog. Am. J. Vet. Res. 46:963-965, 1985.
103. Harvey, C.E.: Conservative treatment of acquired esophageal stricture. In: Textbook of Small Animal Surgery. Edited by D.H. Slatter. W.B. Saunders, Co., Philadelphia, 1985, 661-662.
104. Sooy, T.E., Adams, W.M., Pitts, R.P. and Beck, K.A.: Balloon catheter dilatation of alimentary tract strictures in the dog and cat. Vet. Radiol. 28:131-137, 1987.
105. Pope, C.E.: Involvement of the esophagus by infections, systemic illnesses, and physical agents. In, Gastrointestinal Disease, Edited by M.H. Sleisenger, and J.S. Fordtran, W.B. Saunders Co., Philadelphia, 1973.
106. VanGundy, T.: Vascular ring anomalies. Comp. Contin. Educ. Pract. Vet. 11:36-48, 1989.
107. Leipold, H.W.: Nature and causes of congenital defects of dogs. Vet. Clin. N Am. 8:47-77, 1977.
108. Patterson, D.F.: Epidemiologic and genetic studies of congenital heart disease in the dog. Circ. Res. 23:171-202, 1968.
109. Patterson, D.F.: Canine congenital heart disease: Epidemiology and etiological hypothesis. J. Sm. An. Pract 12:263-287, 1971.
110. Pearson, H., Gibbs, C. and Kelly, D.F.: Oesophageal diverticulum formation in the dog. J. Sm. An. Pract. 19:341-355, 1978.
111. Lantz, G.C., Bojrab, M.J. and Jones, B.D.: Epiphrenic esophageal diverticulectomy. JAAHA 12:629-635, 1976.
112. McCaw, D., Pratt, M. and Walshaw, R.: Squamous cell carcinoma of the esophagus in a dog. JAAHA 16:561-563, 1980.
113. Ridgway, R.L. and Suter, P.F.: Clinical and radiographic signs in primary and metastatic esophageal neoplasms of the dog. JAVMA 174:700-704, 1979.
114. Vernon, F.F. and Roudebush, P.: Primary esophageal carcinoma in a cat. JAAHA 16:547-550, 1980.
115. Fox, S.M., Burns, J. and Hawkins, J.: Spirocercosis in dogs. Comp. Contin. Educ. Pract. Vet. 10:807-822, 1988.
116. Baily, W.S.: Parasites and cancer - sarcoma in dogs associated with Spirocheria lupi. Ann. N.Y. Acad. Sci. 180:890-923, 1963.
117. Caywood, D.D. and Feeney, D.A.: Acquired esophagobronchial fistula in a dog. JAAHA 18:590-594, 1982.
118. Park, R.D.: Bronchoesophageal fistula in the dog: Literature survey, case presentations, and radiographic manifestations. Comp. Cont. Ed. Pract. Vet. 6:669-677, 1984.
119. Ellison, G.W., Lewis, D.D., Phillips, L. and Tarvin, G.B. Esophageal hiatal hernia in small animals. JAAHA 23:391-399, 1987.
120. Pollock, S. and Rhodes, W.H.: Gastroesophageal intussusception in an Afghan Hound: A case report. J. Am. Vet. Rad. Soc. 11:5-14, 1970.
121. Rowland, M.G. and Robinson, M.: Gastroesophageal intussusception in an adult dog. J. Sm. An. Pract. 19:121-125, 1978.
122. Alder, P.L.: Phycomycosis in fifteen dogs and two cats. JAVMA 174:1217-1223, 1979.
123. O'Brien, T.R.: Radiographic diagnosis of abdominal disorders in the dog and cat: Radiographic interpretation - clinical signs - pathophysiology. W.B. Saunders, Philadelphia, 1978.
124. Hillemeier, C., Gryboski, J., McCallum, R. and Biancani, P.: Developmental characteristics of the lower esophageal sphincter in the kitten. Gastroenterology 89:760-766, 1985.
125. Patrikios, J., Martin, C.J. and Dent, J.: Relationship of transient lower esophageal sphincter relaxation to postprandial gastroesophageal reflux and belching in dogs. Gastroenterology 90:545-551, 1986.
126. Dodds, W.J., Dent, J., Hogan, W.J., Helm, J.F., Hauser, R., Patel, G.K. and Egide, M.S.: Mechanisms of gastroesophageal reflux in patients with reflux esophagitis. New Eng. J. Med. 307:1547-1552, 1982.
127. Dodds, W.J., Hogan, W.J., Helm, J.F. and Dent, J.: Pathogenesis of reflux esophagitis. Gastroenterology 81:376-394, 1981.
128. Strombeck, D.R., Harrold, D. and Ferrier, W.: Eructation of gas through the gastroesophageal sphincter before and after truncal vagotomy in dogs. Am. J. Vet. Res. 48:207-210, 1987.
129. Martin, C.J., Patrikios, J. and Dent, J.: Abolition of gas reflux and transient lower esophageal sphincter relaxation by vagal blockade in the dog. Gastroenterology 91:89-896, 1986.
130. Sarna, S.K., Gleysteen, J.J. and Ryan, R.P.: Fundic motor activity and its role in gastroesophageal reflux. Gastroenterology 91:1615, 1986.
131. Boyle, J.T., Altschuler, S.M., Nixon, T.E., Pack, A.I. and Cohen, S.: Responses of feline gastroesophageal junction to changes in abdominal pressure. Am. J. Physiol. 253:G315-G322, 1987.
132. Holloway, R.A., Hongo, M., Berger, K. and McCallum, R.W.: Gastric distention: A mechanism for postprandial gastroesophageal reflux. Gastroenterology 89:779-784, 1985.
133. Edwards, M.H.: Selective vagotomy of the canine oesophagus - a model for the treatment of hiatal hernia. Thorax 31:185-189, 1976.
134. Gill, R.C., Kellow, J.R. and Windgate, D.L.: Gastroesophageal reflux and the migrating motor complex. Gut 28:929-934, 1987.
135. Biancani, P., Barwick, K., Selling, J. and McCallum, R.: Effects of acute experimental esophagitis on mechanical properties of the lower esophageal sphincter. Gastroenterology 87:8-16, 1984.
136. Carvalho, P., Richter, H., Souza, G. and Nyhus, L.M.: Gastroesophageal reflux (GER) slows gastric emptying in dogs. Gastroenterology 94:A61, 1989.
137. DeBacker, A., Haentjens, P. and Willems, G.: Hydrochloric acid a trigger of cell proliferation in the esophagus of dogs. Dig. Dis. Sci. 30:884-890, 1985.
138. Salo, J.A., Lehto, V.-P. and Kivilaakso, E.: Morphological alterations in experimental esophagitis. Dig. Dis. Sci. 28:440-448, 1983.
139. Mittal, R.K., Reuben, A., Whitney, J.O. and McCallum, R.W.: Do bile acids reflux into the esophagus? Gastroenterology 92:371-375, 1987.
140. Lillemoe, K.D., Johnson, L.F. and Harmon, J.W.: Alkaline esophagitis: a comparison of the ability of components of gastroduodenal contents to injure the rabbit esophagus. Gastroenterology 85:621-628, 1983.
141. Salo, J.A. and Kivilaakso, E.: Contribution of trypsin and cholate to the pathogenesis of experimental alkaline reflux esophagitis. Scand. J. Gastroenterology 19:875-881, 1984.
142. Evander, A., Little, A.G., Riddle, R.H., Walther, B. and Skinner, D.B.: Composition of the refluxed material determines the degree of reflux esophagitis in the dog. Gastroenterology 93:280-286, 1987.
143. Liebermann-Meffert, D., Klaus, D., Vosmeer, S. and Allgower, M.: Effect of intraesophageal bile and acid (HCl) perfusion on the action of the lower esophageal sphincter. Scand. J. Gastroenterology 19(suppl 92):237-241, 1984.
144. Carlborg, B. and Densert, O.: Esophageal lesions caused by orally administered drugs. Eur. Surg. Res. 12:270-282, 1980.
145. Bonavina, L., DeMeester, T.R., McChesney, L., Schwizer, W., Albertucci, M. and Bailey, R.T.: Drug-induced esophageal strictures. Ann. Surg. 206:173-183, 1987.
146. Winter, H.S., Madara, J.L., Stafford, R.J., Grand, R.J., Quinlan, J-E. and Goldman, H.: Intraepithelial eosinophils: a new diagnostic criterion for reflux esophagitis. Gastroenterology 83:818-823, 1982.
147. Steadman, C., Kerlin, P., Teague, C. and Stephenson, P.: High esophageal stricture: a complication of "inlet patch" mu-

cosa. Gastroenterology 94:521-524, 1988.
148. Strombeck, D.R. and Harrold, D.: Effect of gastrin, histamine, serotonin, and adrenergic amines on gastroesophageal sphincter pressure in the dog. Am. J. Vet. Res. 46:1684-1690, 1985.
149. Machida, H.M., Forbes, D.A., Gall, D.G., and Scott, R.B.: Metoclopramide in gastroesophageal reflux in infancy. J. Pediatr. 112:483-487, 1988.
150. Strombeck, D.R., Turner, W.D. and Harrold, D.: Eructation of gas through the gastroesophageal sphincter before and after gastric fundectomy in dogs. Am. J. Vet. Res. 49:87-89, 1988.
151. Borkent, M.V. and Beker, J.A.: Treatment of ulcerative reflux oesophagitis with colloidal bismuth subcitrate in combination with cimetidine. Gut 29:385-389, 1988.
152. Katz, P.O., Geisinger, K.R., Hassan, M., Wu, W.C., Huang, D. and Castell, D.O.: Acid-induced esophagitis in cats is prevented by sucralfate but not synthetic prostaglandin E. Dig. Dis. Sci. 33:217-224, 1988.
153. Larrain, A., Csendes, A., and Pope, C.E.: Surgical correction of reflux. Gastroenterology 69:578-583, 1975.
154. Torrance, B.: Symposium on gastro-esophageal reflux and its complications: surgical treatment. Gut 14:249-253, 1973.

Chapter 10

Gastric Structure and Function

The stomach can be described as a receptacle located at the beginning of the gastrointestinal tract. It has several important functions. It serves as a reservoir that stores food temporarily and controls the rate of entry of ingesta into the small intestine. Motility in the stomach controls the rate of emptying and, like motility in the small and large intestine, moves contents in the aboral direction. The stomach participates in initial digestion of food by secreting acid and an important proteolytic enzyme. The gastric muscles are developed to help digestion by fashioning the organ into what has been described as a mixing and grinding unit.

STRUCTURE

Surface Anatomy[1-3]

The stomach is divided into five regions: cardia, fundus, body, antrum, and pylorus (Figure 10-1). The cardia is the point of entrance of the intra-abdominal segment of esophagus into the stomach. The fundus is a large blind outpocketing that is cranial, dorsal, and on the left side of the cardia. The body forms the large middle portion between the fundus and antrum. The antrum is the distal third of the stomach, with the pylorus as its most-terminal part. The boundaries between these regions are arbitrary; more properly, the stomach is better described as consisting of a proximal and a distal part. The proximal segment, concerned with adaptive changes necessary for the entrance and temporary storage of food, is important for the secretion of digestive juices. The distal part of the stomach functions to regulate the release of hydrochloric acid, to grind up food particles, and to empty the stomach. The distal part also includes the pylorus, an anatomical sphincter situated between the stomach and duodenum. The pylorus not only regulates the entry of solid food into the small bowel but also prevents the reflux of duodenal contents.

Topographic Anatomy

The stomach lies in a transverse plane, situated more on the left side than on the right side of the median plane (Figures 10-2 and 10-3). The greater curvature, the convex surface that forms the longest part of the stomach wall from the cardia to the pylorus, faces caudally, ventrally, and to the left. The lesser curvature is the shortest gastric surface between the cardia and pylorus, and it faces in the opposite direction, cranially, dorsally, and to the right. The concave surface of the lesser curvature forms an acute angle, the incisura angularis. This angle interferes with endoscopic visualization of the distal part of the stomach unless a flexible probe is passed around the bend formed by the angle. This angle is more pronounced in the

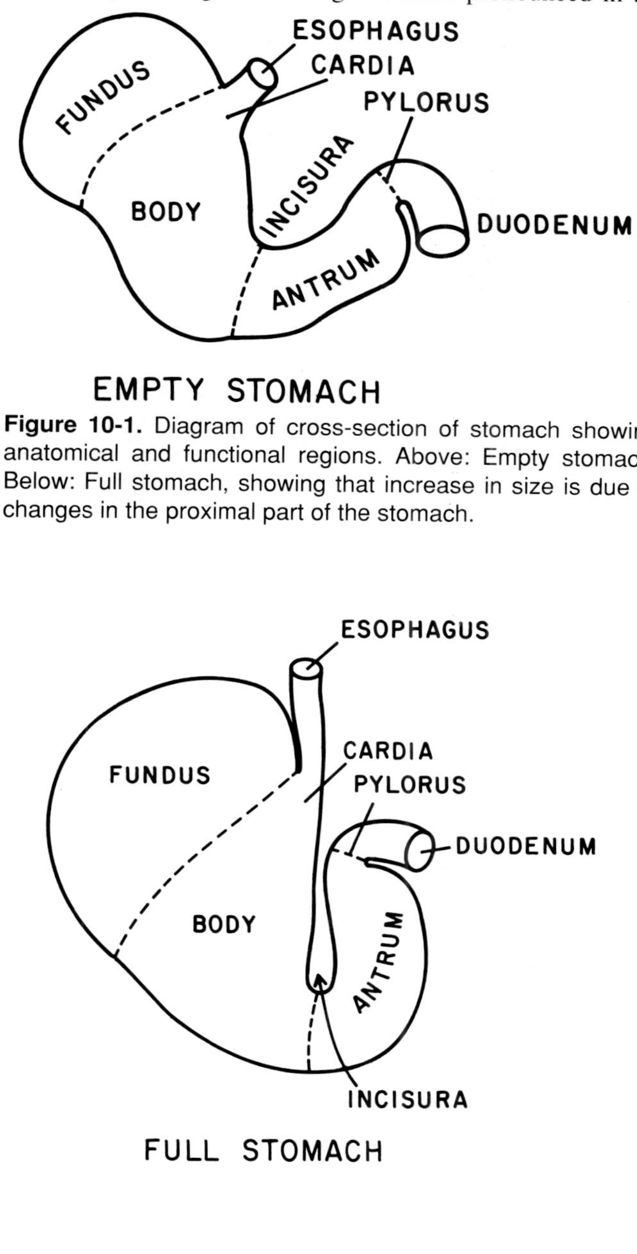

Figure 10-1. Diagram of cross-section of stomach showing anatomical and functional regions. Above: Empty stomach. Below: Full stomach, showing that increase in size is due to changes in the proximal part of the stomach.

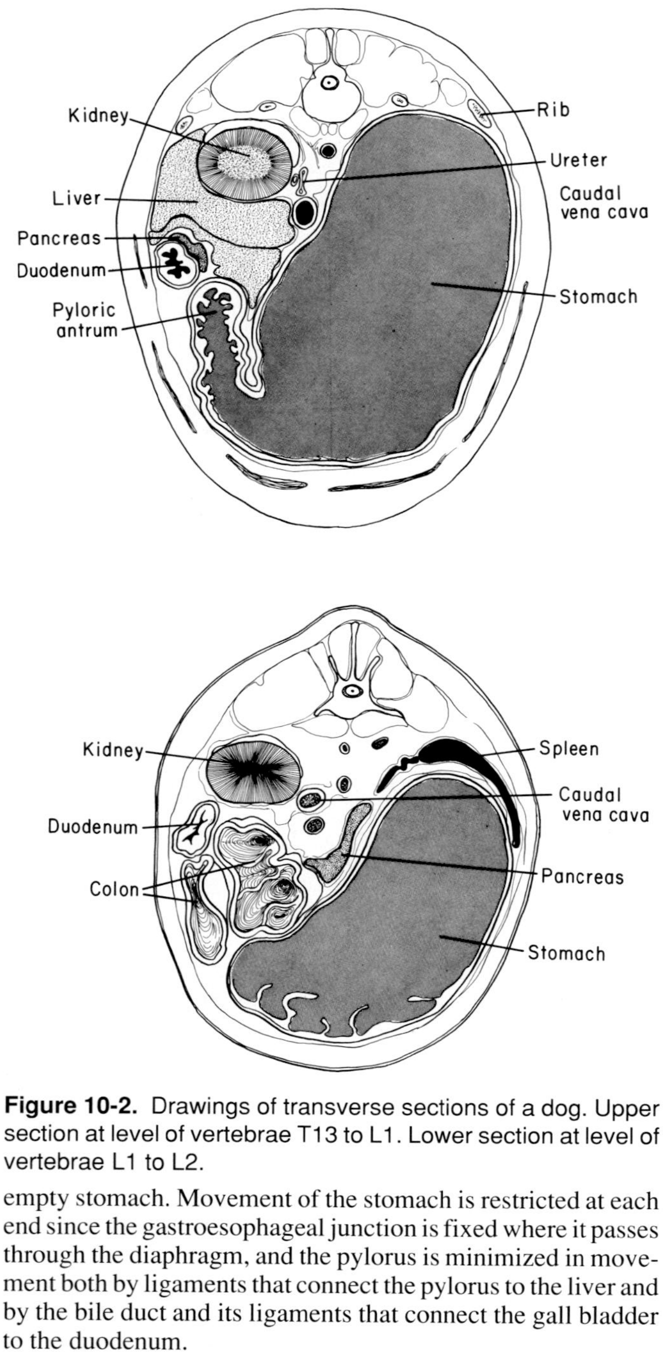

Figure 10-2. Drawings of transverse sections of a dog. Upper section at level of vertebrae T13 to L1. Lower section at level of vertebrae L1 to L2.

empty stomach. Movement of the stomach is restricted at each end since the gastroesophageal junction is fixed where it passes through the diaphragm, and the pylorus is minimized in movement both by ligaments that connect the pylorus to the liver and by the bile duct and its ligaments that connect the gall bladder to the duodenum.

The proximal half of the stomach, serving as a reservoir, expands rapidly during the ingestion of food. The fundus is filled first, accompanied by gastric distention in the caudodorsal direction. With subsequent filling, displacement of the stomach is caudoventral. The empty stomach is located cranial to the thoracic outlet. Thus, it is apparent that the empty organ is situated too far cranially to be palpated on physical examination. The full stomach is usually cranial to the costal margins and also not palpable.

The spatial relationships of the stomach to other organs in the abdominal cavity are important for understanding how inflammatory processes can extend from one structure to another. The parietal surface of the stomach is related to the liver and to the left and ventral abdominal wall (Figure 10-2). The visceral surface of the stomach, comprising less area, is related to the intestines, pancreas, and left kidney, structures located dorsally and to the right. The fundus lies under the vertebral ends of the eleventh and twelfth ribs. The pylorus lies at a point opposite the ventral part of the ninth rib and to the right of the median plane. It is related to the pancreas and to the portal fissure of the liver.

Circulation

Blood is supplied to the stomach by branches of the celiac trunk, the first visceral branch of the abdominal aorta. These branches are the hepatic and splenic arteries, giving rise to the right and left gastroepiploics, which run along the greater curvature and anastomose with one another. The lesser curvature contains the anastomosing branches of the right and left gastric arteries. The former is a branch of the hepatic trunk, and the latter is a branch of the celiac trunk. Venous drainage from the stomach occurs via any of the vessels that empty into the gastrosplenic vein from the left side and into the gastroduodenal vein from the right side. Venous blood flows through the portal circulation to the liver. Lymphatic drainage is through the hepatic lymph nodes after passing through the gastric and splenic lymph nodes.

Innervation

Nerves to and from the stomach are contained in the vagi and in nerves that follow the gastric branches of the celiac artery. Fibers in the vagi are predominantly afferents that are components of reflex pathways having connections in either the central nervous system or in another part of the alimentary tract. The vagi also carry parasympathetic fibers for motor and secretory activity in the stomach. The vagal trunks are dorsal and ventral to the esophagus as they pass through the diaphragm. The ventral vagus sends branches to the pylorus and to the liver in addition to the lesser curvature of the stomach. The dorsal branch sends fibers to the lesser curvature and the ventral wall of the stomach. The nerves that accompany the arteries contain sympathetic fibers and some afferents.

Gross Anatomy

The wall of the stomach consists of an outer thin serosal layer, a middle muscular layer, and an inner mucosal layer. The muscular layer consists of an outer layer of longitudinal fibers that are continuous with fibers in the esophagus. Longitudinal fibers are found primarily along the curvatures and the antrum. Inside these fibers is a layer of circular fibers that is complete for all the stomach except the fundus. This layer is the most complete and well developed of all the muscle in the stomach. It extends into the gastroesophageal junction and forms part of the sphincter. The circular layer in the antrum is well-developed, a necessary circumstance for the important motor requirements of the antral grinding mill.[4] Circular fibers from this layer form the pyloric sphincter. A distinct anatomical sphincter is formed, since there are a greater number of fibers that encircle the pylorus at that point. Circular fibers are bunched up in similar numbers at all points along the lesser curvature of the antrum and pylorus. Away from the pylorus and its smaller

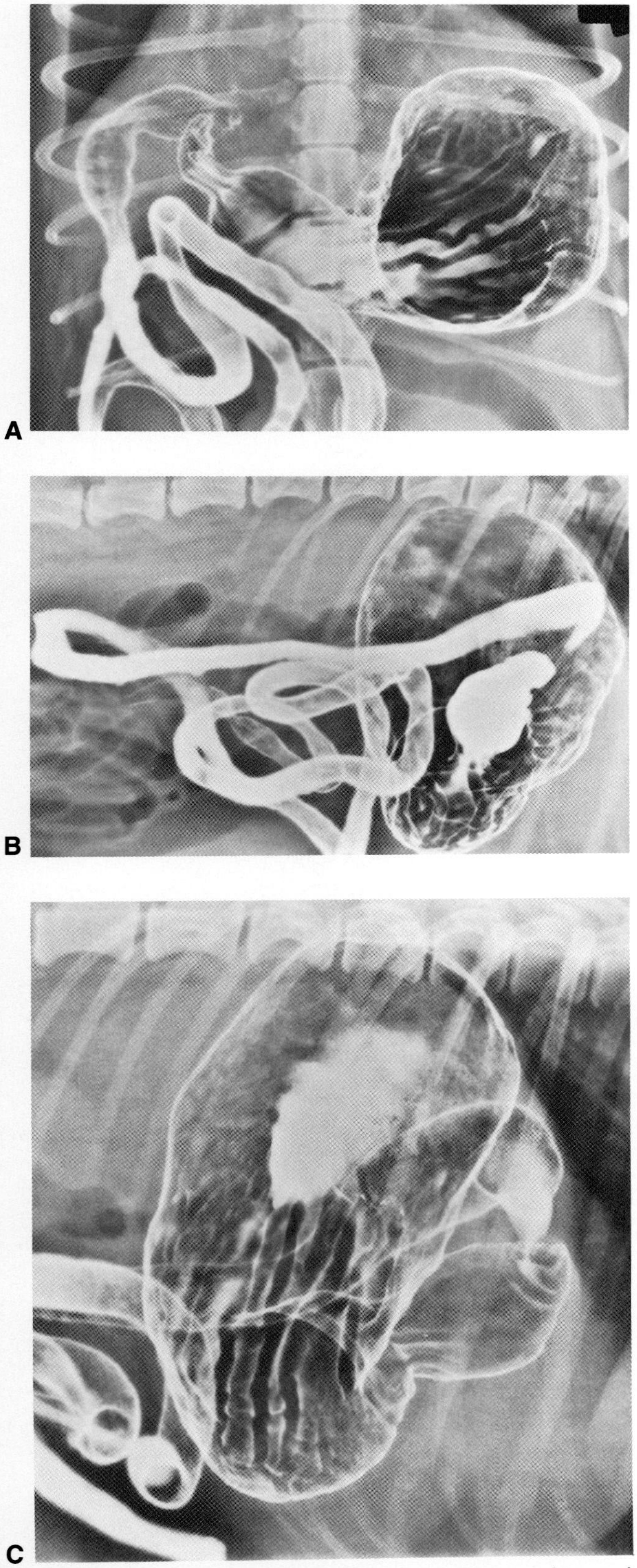

Figure 10-3 a, b, and c. Double contrast gastrogram of normal stomach, pylorus, and duodenum. A) Dorsoventral view. B) Lateral view with right side down. C) Lateral view with left side down. (Reproduced by permission of W. Th. C. Wolvekamp)

lumen, however, the fibers fan out over the larger lumen of the antrum as they cross to the greater curvature. This results in a layer of muscle that is thinner in the antrum than in the pylorus. This entire mass of muscle in the antrum and pylorus behaves as a functional unit despite the implication in their descriptive separation that they are individual units functioning dissimilarly[4] (as described later, pyloric circular muscle functions differently than pyloric longitudinal muscle). A connective-tissue septum separates the circular fibers of the pylorus from those of the duodenum. This septum is on the floor of a shallow groove that exaggerates the apparent thickness of the pyloric sphincter. A third layer of muscle fibers is found over the body of the stomach. The fibers run oblique to the other layers and are found between the circular layer and the submucosa. In the empty stomach, the mucosa and submucosa are thrown up into folds called gastric plicae or rugae. The muscularis mucosa, a thin layer of smooth muscle in the submucosa, facilitates the folding. The development of muscles in the stomach is not under special control; gastrin and possibly other hormones may have a trophic effect on the sphincter muscles.[5]

Microscopic Structure[6]

The inner surface of the stomach is lined with a single layer of columnar mucous cells, as shown in Figure 10-4. Thus, one cell, with its luminal and basal surfaces, makes up the barrier that keeps hydrochloric acid and digestive enzymes contained within the lumen, and it is also the primary structure that prevents the loss of abnormal amounts of extracellular fluid, plasma proteins, and erythrocytes into the stomach. A mucus that is secreted and remains on the surface of the mucosal cells contributes to the barrier. It protects proteins in the cell membrane against destruction by forming a barrier between the cell wall and proteolytic enzymes. Mucus is not in itself a barrier to the movement of hydrogen ions, but it becomes a barrier by the alkaline secretion it contains. Thus, it helps to restrict acid within the reservoir. The epithelium of the mucosa is invaginated to form pits that are also lined with mucous cells. At a short distance from the surface the epithelial lining of the pits changes, and specialized cells begin to appear. This transition marks the beginning of gastric glands, which secrete a variety of substances that either pass out into the stomach by way of the lumen (or pits) of the glands or are secreted in to the circulation.

Gastric Glands, Proximal Stomach. Gastric glands vary with the region of the stomach. In general, there is no sharp line of demarcation where cells of one type abruptly cease. The predominant glands in the cardiac region are mucous glands. They are branched tubular glands that have three to seven branches opening into each gastric pit. Although they have been termed cardiac glands, they are not limited to the cardiac region of the stomach, but are also found in the antrum.

The gastric glands in the proximal part of the stomach (fundus and body) are represented in Figure 10-4. These glands are branched and tubular. Several may open into the same pit. The gland is differentiated into an isthmus, neck, and base — from its most apical end (adjacent to the bottom of the pit) to the beginning of the gland (most distant from the lumen of the stomach). The cell types in these glands are oxyntic (parietal), chief, mucous, and endocrine.

Oxyntic Cells. Oxyntic cells, most abundant in the isthmus and neck, are responsible for the secretion of hydrochloric acid.

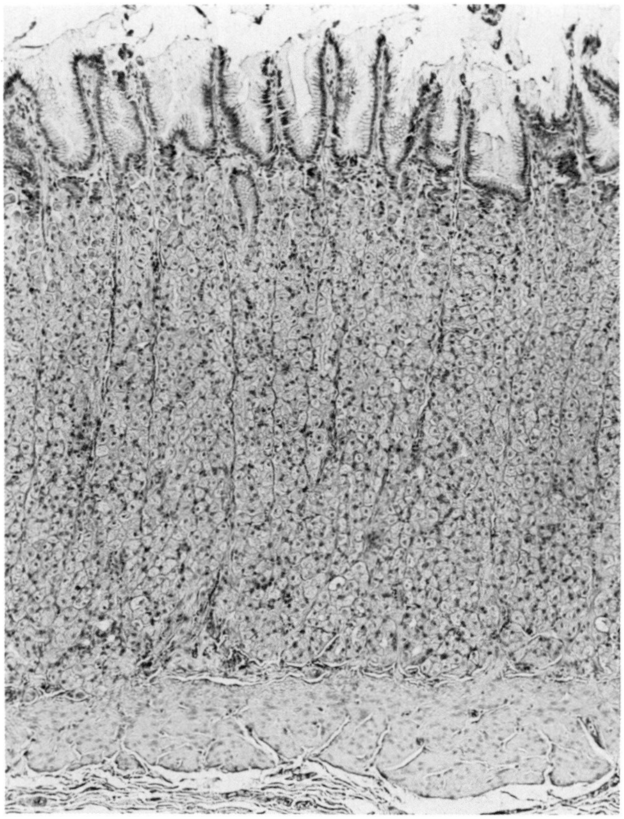

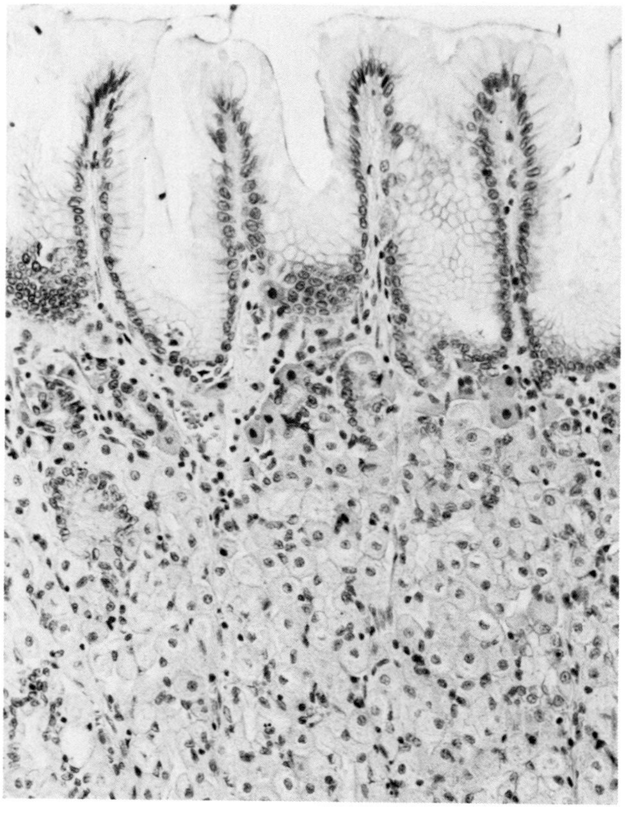

Figure 10-4a, b. Glands from body of normal canine stomach. Compare with Figure 10-4c for anatomic details.

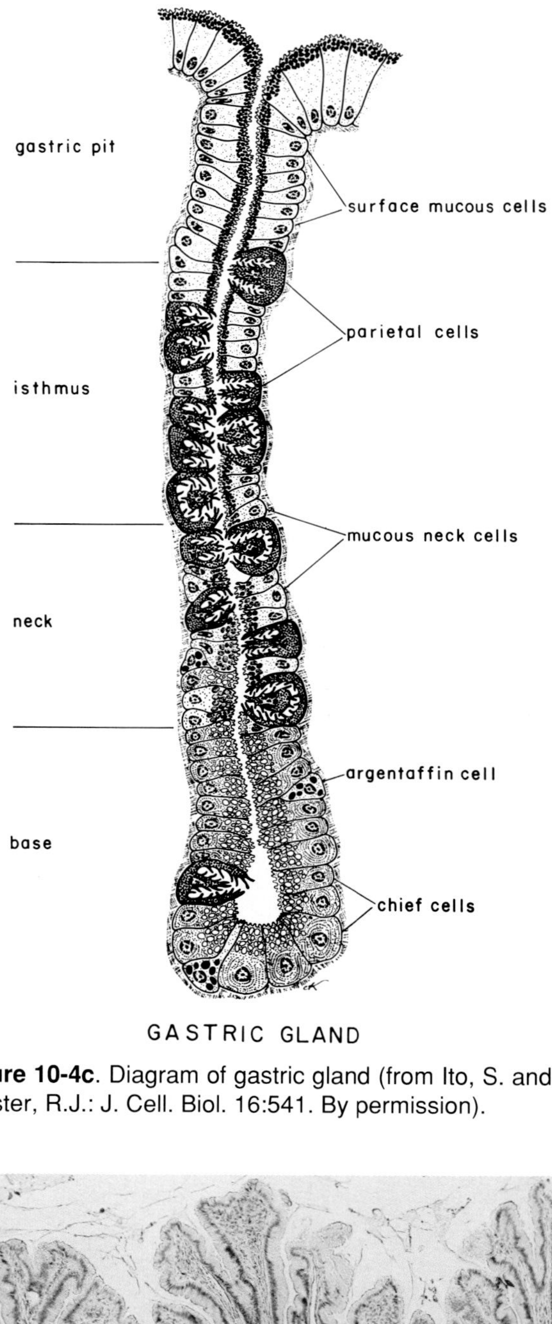

Figure 10-4c. Diagram of gastric gland (from Ito, S. and Winchester, R.J.: J. Cell. Biol. 16:541. By permission).

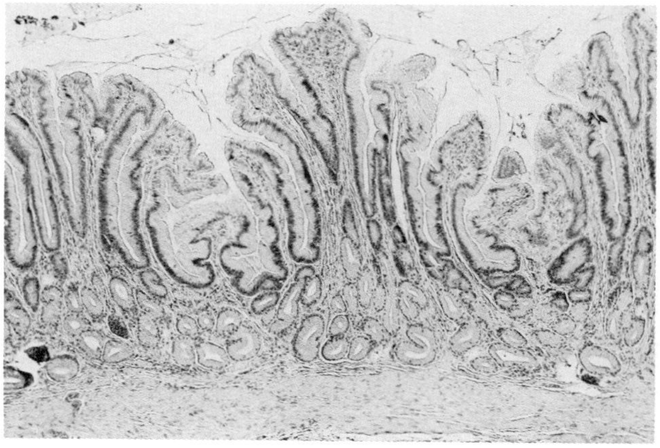

Figure 10-4d. Mucosa from normal gastric cardia.

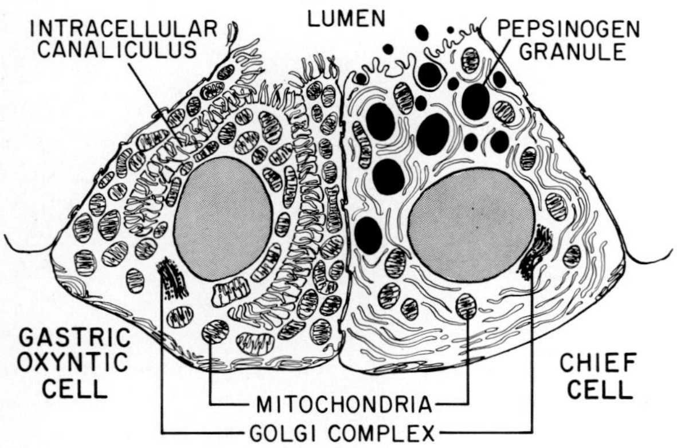

Figure 10-5a. Schematic drawing of gastric oxyntic and chief cells, which respectively secrete hydrochloric acid and pepsinogen.

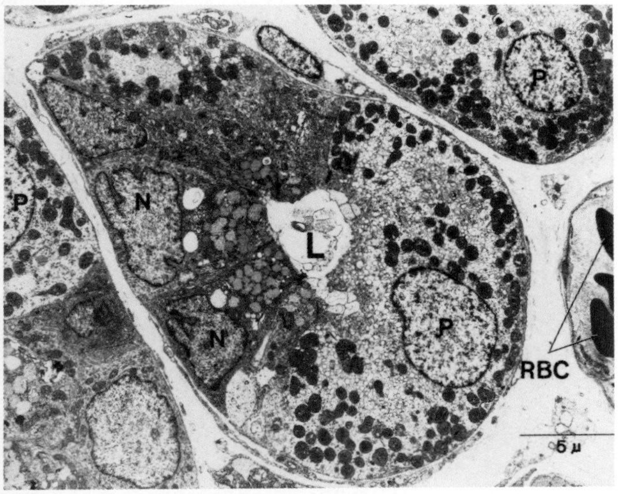

Figure 10-5b. EM of normal stomach. L = lumen of gastric gland, P = nucleus of parietal or oxyntic cell, N = nucleus of chief cell. X 2620.

Their structure is shown in Figure 10-5. They are large cells, oval or pyramid shaped, that stain deeply with eosin. A series of channels, seen with light microscopy, form an intracellular canaliculus produced by invaginations of the luminal cell surface. Some channels extend almost to the base of the cell. Electron microscopy reveals microvilli lining both the luminal border of the oxyntic cell and the network of canals traversing the cells. This modification of cell surfaces greatly magnifies the surface area, which is of obvious importance in absorptive epithelia. It is also important for maximizing the secretory capacity of a cell. The microvilli increase the capacity of the cell to secrete hydrochloric acid into the canaliculi that carry it to the lumen of the gland's duct. During active secretion of hydrochloric acid, the canaliculi increase in size.

Since the oxyntic cells' primary function is to transport ions, the remainder of the intracellular structures is designed to carry out this function. Ion-transporting cells contain many mitochondria, which are necessary to provide the energy for transport, especially when movement occurs across a membrane that maintains a large concentration gradient of the ion. Thus, the oxyntic cell contains many mitochondria. The Golgi complex is poorly developed since the oxyntic cell, unlike the pancreas, is not involved with the synthesis, packaging, and secretion of macromolecules. Smooth endoplasmic reticulum is present in an amount inversely proportional to the quantity of canaliculi. It was stated that the canaliculi are more prominent during secretion, and that state is associated with a manyfold increase in the surface area. The membrane of the endoplasmic reticulum may contribute to the formation of the expanded surface area during secretion.

Chief Cells. The chief cell, the primary cell type in the deepest part of the gland (in the base), is the source of pepsinogen (Figure 10-4). The cell appears basophilic in the basal part of the cell because of the abundant RNA in the rough endoplasmic reticulum. The apical part of the cell appears vacuolated since the zymogen granules stored there do not stain. The cell is designed for the synthesis, packaging, and transport of macromolecule. Thus, the cell is richly supplied with rough endoplasmic reticulum for protein synthesis and Golgi complex for packaging of pepsinogen for storage and transport. Since this process is less energy-dependent than is ion transport, there are fewer mitochondria than in the oxyntic cell. The luminal surface of the chief cell contains microvilli.

Mucous Neck Cells. Mucus-secreting cells are found in the gastric glands containing oxyntic and chief cells. Since they are morphologically dissimilar and stain differently from surface mucous cells, they are considered a distinct epithelial cell type. In contrast to the columnar epithelial shape of the surface mucous cells, these mucous neck cells in the gastric glands of the body are smaller and are deformed by adjacent oxyntic cells. The width of the cell is constricted at either the apical or basal end. The presence of mucus granules can make it difficult for conventional stains to differentiate these cells from the chief cells. The mucous neck cells are similar to surface mucous cells in intracellular structure. The mucus granules of the neck cells differ in size and density from the surface cells. The difference is reflected by different staining properties for the two types of mucus, indicating differences in structure and possible differences in function.

Endocrine Cells. Endocrine cells are found in the basal region of the gastric glands. They have a broad base, and the apex of the cell does not border on the lumen of the gland. This form is consistent with the view that they secrete their granules into the extracellular space and subsequently into the circulation instead of into the gland's lumen. Since many of the endocrine cells in the gastric glands of the fundus and body stain with silver, they have been called argentaffin cells. Their ability to stain with chromium salts results in their other designation, enterochromaffin cells. These cells contain biogenic amines, with serotonin the most abundant. Most of the serotonin in the body is found in the gastrointestinal tract. The physiological role of these rich stores is unknown. It was recently shown that these cells also produce polypeptide hormones that are important for gastrointestinal function.

Gastric Glands, Distal Stomach. The gastric glands of the antrum are different from those in the fundus and body. Their gastric pits, lined with surface mucous cells, are deeper and are equal to the length of the glands. These simple branched tubular glands are formed by mucous neck cells. No chief cells and only a few oxyntic cells are found. The glands contain endocrine cells that stain for biogenic amines and peptide hormones. Gastrin, the endocrine mediator of hydrochloric acid secretion, is synthesized and secreted by an endocrine cell (G-cell) in the gastric glands of the antrum.

Lamina Propria and Muscularis Mucosa. There is normally little lamina propria, the connective tissue between glands, in the gastric glands of the fundus and body, since the glands are so numerous and packed together. The muscularis mucosa lies directly beneath the mucosa. Defects in the mucosa down to this muscle layer are termed erosions, while a break extending through the muscle is an ulcer.

Epithelial Renewal. The epithelial cells of the gastric mucosa are rapidly renewed. The surface mucous cells are replaced by the migration of cells from the wall of the pits to the surface, a process that is completed in three days. The mucous neck cells do not migrate, and they are renewed in one week. Oxyntic and chief cells turn over more slowly. After an area of mucosa is removed or destroyed, the defect heals by the proliferation and migration of a thin layer of relatively undifferentiated surface mucous cells from the edges of the defect. Invagination of the new epithelium occurs, forming gastric pits and glands. The surface mucous cells lining the glands are transformed into mucous neck cells that are thought to differentiate to oxyntic and chief cells. The development and maintenance of gastric mucosa is dependent on the trophic effects of endocrines.[7]

FUNCTION

The functions of the stomach, in addition to being a reservoir, are: 1) motility to achieve mixing of food with gastric juices and evacuation of the contents; and 2) secretion of hydrochloric acid and digestive enzymes.

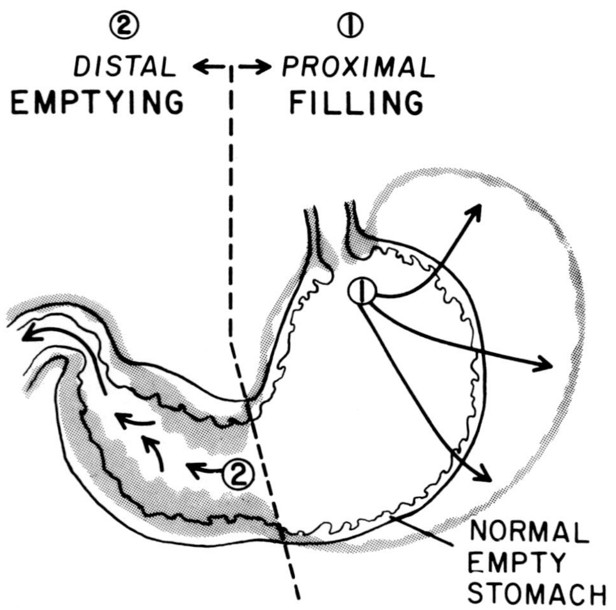

Figure 10-6. Schematic of stomach showing motor functions of each region. The proximal part is designed to adapt to entrance of food, and the distal part is concerned with vigorous motor activity to empty stomach.

Motility[1,4,8]

Proximal Stomach. Each area of the stomach has a different motor function (Figure 10-6). The fundus facilitates the reservoir function by adapting to the filling of the stomach with food. By what has been called receptive relaxation, the fundus shows decreased motor activity and a reduction in pressure during deglutition, and as a consequence this part of the stomach can be enlarged to accommodate the entrance of food. The fundus plays a major role in gastric motility and emptying. In the normal dog, increases in gastric volume are associated with intragastric pressures that remain below 10 cm of water. Removal of the fundus is followed by increases in pressure above that level, with comparable changes in gastric volume.[9] One effect of increased intragastric pressure is an increase in the rate of gastric emptying of liquids. The body of the stomach also adapts to changes in the volume of its contents by enlarging, subserving the reservoir function. During digestion, motility increases in the body of the stomach in order to mix the contents and move them in the proper direction.

Distal Stomach. Motility in the distal stomach of dogs is understood from a number of cineradiographic studies.[8] The motility patterns of the antrum serve its role as a grinding mill that actively churns gastric contents and propels them in the aboral direction. Motor activity is more frequent and more vigorous in the antrum than in other parts of the stomach. Peristaltic waves travel from the body of the stomach over the antrum, and when they reach the terminal antrum the final 3 to 4 cm of the dog's antrum contract vigorously and simultaneously. The pylorus is an integral part of the antrum, and part of its motor function is similar. The purposes of the pylorus are to delay gastric emptying of solids and to minimize the reflux of intestinal contents into the stomach.[4,8] As the antrum and pylorus begin to contract, the pylorus, having a narrower lumen, empties first, closing before the antrum has completed its contraction. It remains incompletely closed throughout the continuation of antral contraction, allowing nonliquid antral contents to be propelled forcibly in a retrograde direction. Closure of the pylorus is facilitated by a sliding movement of the loose pyloric antral mucosa into the pyloric opening to form a plug. The closure of the pylorus is usually incomplete, and a small amount of liquid antral contents is propelled into the duodenum with each contraction. The pylorus does not regulate the movement of liquid into the duodenum, although it has a major effect in regulating the rate of emptying solid food from the stomach.[10] This illustrates that the closure is not complete. The size of the mucosal plug can have an important effect on gastric emptying. The mucosa is attached loosely to the underlying structures and is normally freely movable. Hyperplasia of the gastric mucosa characterizes chronic gastritis. In some instances the mucosa that serves as the plug is thickened and becomes a factor in converting a patient with pyloric stenosis, showing few clinical signs, to a patient with signs of complete obstruction of the gastric outlet.

The pyloric ring is not a tonically contracted sphincter that opens occasionally to allow chyme to pass through. The pylorus is an integral part of the thickened wall of muscle around the antrum, and the pylorus and antrum function as a single muscle unit.

Although they function as a single unit, the pylorus has the properties to act differently. The pylorus has an outer layer of longitudinal muscle which can contract and cause the pylorus to open. It is not known what conditions cause that muscle to contract. The pylorus has an inner layer of circular muscle that contracts as a wave of peristalsis passes from the antrum through the pylorus. This layer of circular muscle also contracts independently of activity in the antrum. The canine pylorus shows phasic contractions at rates of one to fifteen per minute that maintain a zone of pressure about 11 mmHg higher than the stomach and duodenum.[11] The motility causing pyloric phasic contractions is independent of antral motility; regulation of their motilities is also different.[12]

Regulation of Motility[7,8,13-15]

The smooth muscle of the stomach can function without either its extrinsic or intrinsic innervation. With the loss of regulation by these nervous systems, there is a loss in coordinated activity, and any movements that are seen are not responses to a stimulus but, in general, only random movements, a fact that becomes evident with complete denervation.

A highly coordinated series of events that are neurally and hormonally regulated produce motor functions in the stomach. Understanding of the neural regulation requires knowledge of the physiology of gastric smooth muscle and of its intrinsic and extrinsic innervations. Gastric motility will be affected by alterations in function at any one of the levels of control.

Myogenic Properties of Gastric Muscle.[16] The basic properties of smooth-muscle function can be studied by measuring its electrical properties. An area of muscle, located at the junction of the fundus and middle third of the stomach and along the greater curvature, generates electrical potentials; it provides the first level of regulation of motor function in the stomach. The electrically active area is called a pacemaker, and the potentials it generates spread out over the stomach and end at the pylorus. The spreading potentials represent the electrical control activity, which has a rate of approximately 5 per minute in the dog. The electrical control activity is also called the pacesetter potential, or basic electrical rhythm. The basis of its generation is not known, but it has been likened to the pacemaker in the sinoatrial node for cardiac function. The potential is propagated by contacts between smooth-muscle cells arranged in a syncytium, and they also spread through the intrinsic nervous system that is distributed throughout the gastric muscles. Although the basic electrical rhythm is of myogenic origin, as demonstrated by its persistence after anatomic or pharmacologic denervation, it can be modified, as described later.

The basic electrical rhythm produces the slow electrical wave, a continuous activity. Fast-wave activity appears with gastric muscle contraction. The fast-wave or electrical response activity appears as spikes or action potentials in slow wave peaks (Figure 1-1). Slow waves determine the time of appearance and rate for fast wave activity and muscle contraction, so that the frequency of contractions is about 5 per minute. Thus, changes in the basic electrical rhythm influence action potentials and muscle contractions, affecting the mixing and evacuation of gastric contents.

Modification of Myogenic Properties.[17-19] A number of factors that affect gastric function influence the basic electrical activity. The extrinsic nervous system regulates this activity, for a truncal vagotomy causes the slow wave to become disorganized and to develop an abnormal shape. Addition of an electrical input also changes the activity; electrical stimulation can increase slow-wave activity, although not above 7 cycles per minute. Gastrointestinal hormones influence slow-wave activity. Frequency is increased by gastrin and decreased by secretin. In addition, fast-wave activity is augmented by gastrin and cholecystokinin and decreased by secretin. Temperature increases the frequency of slow waves. The frequency of fast waves increases after feeding. Gastric electrical activity can be absent for as long as six hours after surgery. Since the frequency of slow waves determines the rate of fast-wave activity and muscle contractions, many factors can modify basic electrical rhythm and change the strength and rate of gastric contractions and peristalsis.

In general, naturally occurring pathological problems delay gastric emptying more often than speeding it. The presence and the location of the pacesetter is important for normal emptying. Without the pacesetter, coordinated gastric motility is not possible. When another pacesetter is placed experimentally in the pylorus of a normal dog so that the electrical activity also spreads in an aboral direction, gastric emptying is slowed.[20]

Slow-wave activity generated by the pacemaker does not control the fundus or proximal third of the stomach. No pacesetter or action potentials are recorded from the fundus. Motility in the fundus is thus different and evident as tonic rather than phasic contractions. Tonic contractions initiate and sustain increased intragastric pressure for promoting emptying of liquids. Fundic tone can be inhibited for gastric filling.

Control of Motility by Extrinsic Nerves and Endocrines. The most important control of gastric motor activity is extrinsic. The autonomic nervous system and endocrines both play a part (Figure 10-7). Stimulation of vagal cholinergic fibers results in gastric contraction over most of the stomach. That is seen during feeding, and it can be demonstrated by inducing a hypoglycemia with insulin; the augmented motility is abolished by vagotomy. Some vagal fibers inhibit motility. Vagal activity is responsible for the receptive relaxation of the

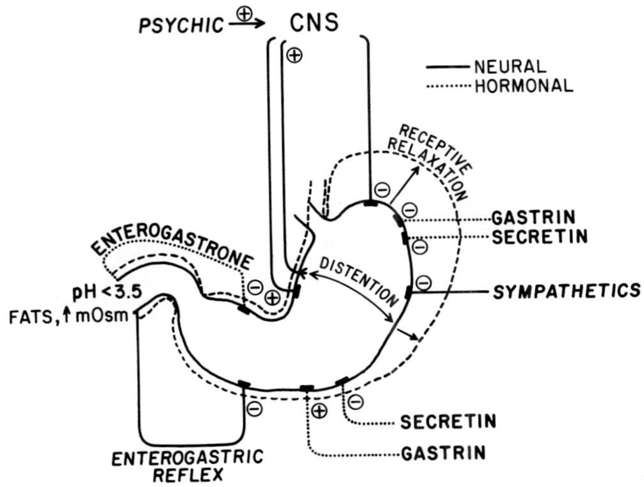

Figure 10-7. Neural and endocrine control of gastric motility. Both neural activity and endocrines cause relaxation (-) of proximal part of stomach. Distention of body of stomach stimulates (+) motility in antrum. The effect of reflexes and hormones from the duodenum is to inhibit gastric motility and emptying.

fundus that is stimulated during deglutition. Noncholinergic nonadrenergic nerves whose neurotransmitter is most likely vasoactive intestinal polypeptide (VIP) mediate the relaxation. The sympathetic innervation of the stomach is not recognized as having a major role in normal gastric motor function. Stimulation of these fibers inhibits gastric motor activity. Sympathetics may partially mediate the inhibition of antral motility under normal circumstances. Sympathetic activity is apparent in pathological situations. It is an important factor in the production of gastric atony, which can follow surgery or stressful situations.

Gastrin inhibits motility in the fundus and stimulates it elsewhere in the stomach. This has the effect of decreasing intragastric pressure and allowing the stomach to hold more in its reservoir part. The end result is that the gastric emptying of liquids and solids is delayed. Cholecystokinin has a similar effect, although weaker. Secretin glucagon, gastrointestinal inhibitory polypeptide, somatostatin, and VIP inhibit motility in all parts of the stomach.

Since the primary neural pathways are cholinergic and augment gastric motility, it follows that anticholinergic drugs inhibit gastric motility, and the cholinergics stimulate it. In the pathological situation, acid that enters a breech in the gastric mucosa can stimulate gastric motility. Acid can act directly on either the neurons in the intrinsic plexuses or the muscle. This effect of acid contributes to the spasms in the stomach that are associated with gastritis or gastric ulcerations.

Reflexes to Control Gastric Motility. The reflexes involved in stimulating gastric motility have receptors both within and outside the stomach. The primary factors that initiate and maintain motility after a meal are vagal activity and distention of the stomach. A cephalogastric reflex is present by which the sight, smell, and taste of food stimulate gastric antral motility and inhibit gastric fundic motility via vagal fibers. A gastro-gastric reflex, employing both the afferent and efferent pathways in the vagus, is present to stimulate gastric motility. The stimulus is gastric distention. Vagotomy abolishes both of those reflexes, and the stomach becomes atonic. Some recovery is observed with time, and the motor function that remains results from the inherent property of the muscle to respond to stretching. The driving force for mixing of food in the stomach and its evacuation is motor activity. The mechanisms designed to perform this function are not as well developed as those that control the rate of gastric emptying.

Regulation of Gastric Emptying[21,22] The balance between stimulators and inhibitors of gastric motility determines the rate of gastric emptying. The reflex mechanisms to reduce motility and delay emptying are more highly developed than those to facilitate motility. The stimulators and inhibitors of motility are both neural and endocrine. The neural inhibitory centers operate at higher levels in the central nervous system than do the excitatory centers, as shown by successive ablation of parts of the brain from high to low, resulting in a progressive increase in gastric motor activity. Neural reflexes with the afferents and efferents within the gastrointestinal tract inhibit gastric motility. The enterogastric reflexes, mechanisms to inhibit antral motility, are stimulated by events in the small intestine. Their receptors respond to stimuli that are mechanical (distention), physical (hypertonicity), and chemical (pH less than 3.5). Some pathways for these reflexes are in the vagi and operate by a nonadrenergic, noncholinergic mechanism.[23]

Gastrointestinal endocrines regulate gastric emptying. Acid in the duodenum, releases secretin, which inhibits motility in all parts of the stomach. Fats and proteins in the duodenum also delay gastric emptying. These nutrients are potent stimulators of cholecystokinin release, and this hormone, like secretin, slows gastric emptying since it inhibits motility in the fundus. These hormones' inhibitory response has been attributed to another distinct hormone, enterogastrone. The combined actions of a number of hormones most likely produce the inhibitory effects. All members of the secretin family can inhibit gastric motility and delay emptying. They are all released from the intestinal mucosa when chyme is present. Gastrin delays gastric emptying, since it is similar to cholecystokinin in reducing motility in the fundus. Fatty acids in the ileum also inhibit gastric emptying. A number of peptide hormones can be released from ileal mucosa but only peptide YY has properties to delay gastric emptying.[24]

Factors Determining Gastric Emptying. The emptying of gastric contents is a function of the driving force to generate intraluminal pressure and the resistance to movement of chyme, which is produced by contraction of the antrum and pylorus. The primary determinants of intragastric pressure are motility of the body and antrum and the degree of relaxation of the fundus. If the fundus is relaxed, the intragastric pressure is reduced and the rate of emptying will be minimal. If the fundus of the stomach is removed or possesses a high motility, the food entering will cause the intragastric pressure to increase, accelerating emptying. The role of the pylorus in regulating the emptying of the stomach has been controversial.[25,26] As a functional extension of the antrum, the pylorus opens and closes differently than other sphincters in the body. The sphincter never closes completely, since it always allows some chyme to pass. The pylorus does not regulate the emptying of liquids from the stomach, since permanent placement of a noncollapsible open tube through the sphincter does not increase the rate at which liquids leave the stomach of dogs and cats.[10]

The pylorus does have an important function in regulating the emptying of solid food. Gastric digestion and grinding in the antral mill must liquify solid food before it can pass through the normally small pyloric opening.

Particles must be less than two mm in size before they leave the stomach in dogs.[27-29] The pylorus does not completely close when a peristaltic wave operates to evacuate food from the stomach. Chyme rich in hydrochloric acid or fatty acids have the greatest effect to reduce pyloric diameter.[30] In unfed dogs with marked gastric contractions during phase III of gastric motility the pylorus may show little, if any, reduction in diameter. Thus, the pylorus can be relaxed and appear open, or it can show phasic or tonic activity. In either case, a higher pressure zone is maintained at 11 mmHg even though the pylorus shows a diameter of 20 mm at maximum relaxation.

Contraction of the pylorus is maintained by its intrinsic mechanical properties;[31] peptide hormones such as glucagon, secretin, and cholecystokinin induce contraction but are without any physiological relevance.[32] Histamine stimulates contraction following its release, mediated by its activity through the nonadrenergic noncholinergic neural pathway and its interaction with myogenic H_1 receptors.[33] Events in the duodenum stimulate pyloric contraction and reduction in pyloric diameter. Triglycerides, fatty acids, and acid pH stimulate pyloric tonic and phasic contractions to delay gastric emptying.[34] That stimulation may be mediated by cholinergic nerves from the duodenum to the pylorus; stimulation of such nerves induces pyloric tonic and phasic contractions.[11] That would be consistent with atropine's reducing phasic activity in the sphincter; also the vagally mediated paths to stimulate pyloric contraction are cholinergic.[35]

Relaxation of the pylorus is mediated by antral nerves with both nonadrenergic, noncholinergic and phentolamine-sensitive pathways. Stimulation of the antrum completely abolishes phasic activity and reduces tonic activity.[11] The relaxation may be coordinated with antral peristaltic activity to empty the stomach; in this case relaxation represents an opening of the pylorus.

Gastric emptying of solids is most importantly determined by motility in the antrum.[8] Factors regulating that motility are the same as those regulating phasic and tonic contractions in the pylorus. The neural events that occur with feeding stimulate antral motility. That motility would continue unimpeded escept that it is restrained by factors which demand a reduction in the gastric emptying rate. Neural mechanisms inhibit antral motility; truncal vagotomy markedly reduces the antral inhibition stimulated by fat in the duodenum. Inhibitors of neural transmission reduce the inhibition of gastric motility due to acid in the duodenum. Hormones such as secretin and cholecystolkinin inhibit antral motility and may play a role in delaying gastric emptying. Other possible inhibitors include gastrin, GIP, glucagon, VIP and somatostatin.

A variety of nutrients control gastric antral motility. Lipids in the proximal small intestine reduce antral motility; protein has a modest effect, and carbohydrates have no effect.[36] Carbohydrate and protein, but not fat, reduce gastric tone in the distal small intestine. The relaxation induced by intestinal nutrients is mediated by a nonadrenergic noncholinergic neural pathway in the vagus before vagal fibers enter the abdomen.[37] Acid and hyperosmolar chyme in the duodenum also inhibit antral motility.

In summary, fats are the most important nutrient determining gastric emptying. Fats reduce emptying by inhibiting antral and fundic motility and by stimulating pyloric tonic and phasic contractions. Energy density of a meal also influences empyting rates.[8] Isocaloric meals of fats, carbohydrates or fats all empty at the same rate. Each one controls emptying by stimulating duodenal receptors for fats, proteins or osmolality. Volume also determines emptying rates, with increased volumes emptying faster. Increasing fiber in the diet delays gastric emptying, probably because fibers such as pectin increase the diet's viscosity.[38]

Increases in resistance to flow through the duodenum could retard gastric emptying. No increase in duodenal resistance is found in dogs during stimulation of small intestinal mucosal osmoreceptors. Altered gastric and pyloric motility produces inhibition of gastric emptying.[39]

Motility must be coordinated between the stomach and duodenum to have a continuity for flow of chyme. Coordination may seem impossible because the pacesetter drives motility in the stomach with a frequency of 5 per minute, whereas a separate pacesetter drives motility in the duodenum at a frequency of 18 per minute. Some coordination is found in dogs. In the digestive state, contractions of the duodenal bulb and pylorus are inhibited when peristaltic waves travel across the antrum.[40] The duodenal bulb contracts when the waves arrive, but the timing between pyloric and duodenal contractions are imperfect. Different frequencies for their contractions can cause duodenal contracts before the pylorus is closed, resulting in to and fro movement of chyme. In the unfed state coordination of gastric and duodenal motility is optimal during phase III; strong antral contractions are regularly associated with inhibition of the duodenal bulb. Mechanisms for coordination are not known. Coordination of unfed and fed motor patterns in the stomach and duodenum is not mediated by intrinsic myoneural or luminal factors.[41]

Motility in the unfed state is driven by the interdigestive motor complex (IDMC), which is under control of the interdigestive myoelectric complex (IMC). Slowly moving peristaltic waves of the IDMC pass over the atrum and pylorus and into the duodenum at regular intervals. With the strongest waves of antral peristalsis, the pylorus relaxes to the greatest extent; that is in contrast to motility patterns during feeding. The pyloric relaxation shows maximum reduction in pressure and maximum pyloric diameter.[30,42] These changes are for gastric evacuation of residual particle material in the stomach after emptying of a meal. These changes allow foreign material or residue from a meal to leave the stomach; that is not possible during gastric emptying of a meal since the pylorus remains too constricted. The IDMC also intermittantly clears the stomach of bacteria, either survivors from those swallowed or organisms able to multiply in an acidic environment.

Duodenogastric Reflux. Reflux of duodenal contents through the pylorus and into the stomach is believed by some to be normal and by others to be pathologic and lead to gastritis.[43-44] Many of the studies on duodenogastric reflux have been on dogs. Normal unfed dogs reflux 0.15 ml duodenal contents per minute; in the fed state the reflux increases to about 1.0 ml per minute.[45-46] Segmental contractions of the duodenum produce reflux when the pylorus is open or forced open by the contractions.[47] The pylorus is an important determinant of antroduodenal resistance, but it has no major role in the control of duodenogastric reflux in unfed dogs.[48] Placing a tube in the pylorus to keep the sphincter open does not change the rate of duodenogastric reflux in unfed or fed dogs.[45] Antral motility may be the most important factor determining duodenogastric reflux, with reduced antral motility increasing that reflux.[49] Antral motility prevents reflux by generating a higher pressure in the antrum than the duodenum. Antral motility is also important for clearing reflux contents from the antrum. Drugs such as aspirin and indomethacin disrupt normal antral and pyloric motility, resulting in an increase in duodenogastric reflux.[50,51] In summary, duodenogastric reflux has been associated with clinical signs and gastritis in dogs, but the relationship between the two is not clear.[52]

Reflexes for Gastric Protection. Marked distention of the stomach stimulates spontaneous GES relaxations, relaxation of the body of the stomach, and contraction of the pylorus. These reflexes serve the storage function of the stomach by preventing the dumping of contents into the duodenum and by allowing for the stomach to accomodate a larger volume. The reflexes also permit venting of contents into the esophagus, which protects against gastric rupture. Stimulation of intramural gastric nerves results in relaxations of the GES and stomach, and distention of the stomach results in pyloric contraction believed to be mediated through cholinergic fibers, some possibly carried in the vagus.[53-55]

Gastric Secretion

Gastric secretions play an important role in the initiation of protein digestion, in intestinal absorption of calcium, iron, and vitamin B_{12}, and in the maintenance of the normal bacterial flora in the gastrointestinal tract. The secretions are a composite of macromolecular and electrolyte components.

Macromolecular Component of Gastric Secretion[56-58]

Enzymes. The macromolecular part of gastric secretions contains pepsinogen, which is an inactive precursor of the proteolytic enzyme pepsin. Hydrochloric acid converts the enzyme to its active form. That is accomplished by cleavage of small basic peptides from the pepsinogen molecule. The conversion becomes autocatalytic, since pepsin also converts pepsinogen. Pepsin degrades proteins by splitting peptides at the bond between an amino group of one amino acid and the carboxyl group of an aromatic amino acid. The products formed are primarily polypeptides. Pepsin has a pH optimum of 2.0. Its proteolytic activity ceases when chyme leaves the stomach, since the enzyme is irreversibly inactivated at neutral pH. Chief cells secrete a number of electrophoretically and immunologically distinct pepsinogens. These distinct pepsinogens have been studied more extensively in human gastric secretion than in the dog's. Pepsinogen is found in both the blood and urine of dogs, although the significance of this is unknown. The source of the enzyme in both the blood and gastric secretions is the chief cell. When the gastric mucosal barrier to hydrochloric acid is damaged, as would occur in a gastritis, the secretion of pepsinogen is increased.[59] That may be important in the development of gastric ulceration.

Other enzymes found in gastric secretions include ones exhibiting lipase, gelatinase, lysozyme, urease, neuraminidase, and carbonic anhydrase activity. None of these are known to be important in normal gastric activities.

Pepsinogen Secretion. Secretion of pepsinogen is stimulated by neurotransmitters, histamine and peptide hormones, and chemicals that alter intracellular levels of cyclic nucleotides and of calcium.

Vagal cholinergic pathways that act directly on chief cells stimulate pepsinogen secretion. Secretion follows stimulation of the vagi or follows the vagally mediated hypoglycemic response to insulin. Some secretion occurs via stimulation of local pathways. Atropine blocks the stimulation at a receptor that appears to be of the M-1 type, since it has a high affinity for pirenzepine.

Histamine stimulates pepsinogen secretion in the dog, suggesting histamine may have receptors (H_2) on chief cells. Histamine may stimulate pepsinogen secretion indirectly when acid stimulates a local cholinergic reflex in the gastric mucosa. Gastrin stimulates pepsinogen secretion indirectly. Gastrin stimulates histamine release, and both stimulate hydrochloric acid secretion. The histamine and acid are described above as stimulating pepsinogen secretion. Cholecystokinin (CCK) stimulates pepsinogen secretion by acting directly on chief cell receptors for CCK. The effect is not blocked by atropine, propanolol, or cimetidine. Since CCK is not a potent releasor of pepsinogen *in vivo*, it may have no physiological importance in regulating pepsinogen's secretion. Physiologic levels of secretin stimulate pepsinogen secretion. Vasoactive intestinal peptide, a member of the secretin family, has a function similar to secretin. Somatostatin inhibits pepsinogen secretion.

Intracellular cyclic AMP mediates pepsinogen secretion. Events that increase intracellular calcium levels also stimulate secretion. Physiologic and pathologic events that stimulate cyclic AMP levels or increase the entry of extracellular calcium into chief cells will stimulate pepsinogen secretion.

Pepsinogen secretion is not essential for digestion and absorption of a meal. Protein digestion by pancreatic enzymes in the small intestine is more important. Since pepsin is most active on collagen, its activity is more important for initiating digestion of meat rather than vegetable protein. The most important function of pepsin may be to release peptides that are more potent than intact proteins as stimulants of gastrin and CCK release. Thereby, pepsin activity contributes to the regulation of the overall process of digestion.

Intrinsic Factor. The stomach secretes a mucoprotein (called intrinsic factor) that is necessary to bind extrinsic factor, vitamin B_{12}, before the latter can be absorbed in the distal small intestine. Intrinsic factor has been identified in the cytoplasm of the oxyntic cell of cats. An intrinsic factor is described in pancreatic exocrine secretions of dogs.[60] Humans with atrophic gastritis frequently have a deficiency of intrinsic factor. Thus, a B_{12} deficiency anemia accompanies an achlorhydria. Neither pernicious anemia, as it is called, or a deficiency of hydrochloric acid secretion is recognized as a problem in cats or dogs. The amount of intrinsic factor that is secreted during resting conditions is great enough to bind all the B_{12} that must be absorbed, and the rate of secretion increases with that of hydrochloric acid secretion.

Mucin. Gastric juice contains mucus, which is a conglomerate of a variety of mucosubstances. They are macromolecules that contain significant amounts of carbohydrates. They all contain amino sugars. The most abundant mucosubstances are glycoproteins, some of which are molecules that determine blood groups. Mucopolysaccharides make up a smaller part of gastric mucus. The properties of mucus are largely those of polymers of amino sugars, which are water soluble and produce a viscous solution at low concentrations.

Properties of mucus such as gelation, adhesiveness, ability to form a film, and viscosity are determined by the chemical composition and structure of its components and by the three-dimensional structure of mucus.[61] The structure of mucus results from noncovalent bond formation between charged side-groups of adjacent components. High concentrations of hydrogen ions that lower the pH, as well as increasing ionic concentrations of electrolytes, exemplify events that interfere with the bonding, and thereby interrupt gel formation. Mucus secreted at a neutral pH is a gel and forms a continuous protective covering for the epithelial cell. Its function is to stabilize the microenvironment of the mucosal surface.

Although mucus is not digested by pepsin, it must be constantly synthesized and secreted to maintain the protective coating. The gel structure is necessary for its protective properties; as mentioned, acidity and increased ionic concentrations fragment mucus into its components. Mucus components are highly soluble because of their high carbohydrate concentration. Thus, they can be readily detached and lost from the gel on the mucosal surface. Protection of the gastric mucosa is directed

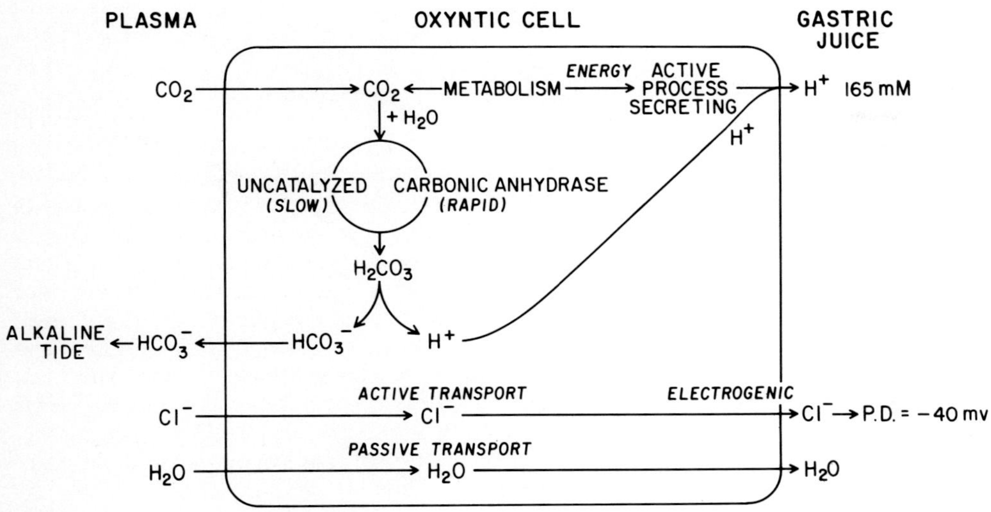

Figure 10-8. Schematic diagram showing the gastric oxyntic (parietal) cell's mechanisms to secrete hydrogen and chloride ions. Active transport of chloride ions creates electrical potential difference of 40 mv, with the luminal border negative.

against the effects of pepsin's acid and proteolytic digestion. Mucus protects against acid by virtue of its property to hold an alkaline fluid. Mucus can also protect cell membranes against the activity of pepsin. The forms with pepsin-inhibitory properties are sulfated. The major sulfated component of canine gastric juice is an acid mucopolysaccharide, chondroitin sulfate, produced by the chief cell, whereas the mucus gel contains mainly sulfated glycoproteins, produced by the crypt and surface epithelial cells.

Sulfated glycoproteins and mucopolysaccharides are present only in small quantities, yet they most likely have an important physiologic function since they inhibit pepsin activity. The sulfated polysaccharides in the mucus gel, layered over the epithelial surface, bind to protein constituents of the cell membrane and protect them against proteolytic degradation. Sulfation of the sugar in the mucus appears to be necessary for this binding. Amylopectin sulfate is a synthetic sulfated polysaccharide that binds to the gastric mucosal surface and to mucus at low pH. This sulfated sugar has been shown to accelerate the healing of gastric ulcers and to prevent the recurrence of duodenal ulcers in experimental animals.[62,63]

Mucus gel, lining the mucosal surface, acts as a fine meshwork that retards the passage of macromolecule but permits the movement of electrolytes and small molecules. The polysaccharides have a number of charged groups that provide them with the properties of an ion exchanger. The ion-exchange capacity controls the composition of the fluid in immediate contact with the mucosa. This selective permeability is extended to provide a barrier against microorganisms. Gastric mucin protects against infectious agents by aggregating microorganisms, interacting with bacterial enzymes to inhibit their activity, binding enterotoxins, and interacting with secretory immunoglobulins to protect the mucosa.[58,64]

Activity in cholinergic nerves stimulates gastric mucin secretion. Topical application of acetylcholine to canine gastric mucosa results in an increase in the mucous gel on the epithelial surface. Peptide hormones do not have an effect on mucin secretion in the stomach. Some prostaglandins stimulate release of mucin as part of their cytoprotective properties. Inflammation, toxins, and chemicals stimulate mucin release in pathologic situations.

Electrolyte Component, Gastric Secretions[65]

The primary electrolyte secreted by the gastric mucosa during stimulation is hydrochloric acid. However, the electrolyte composition of the gastric juices, whether in the stimulated or resting state, never reflects a secretion that contains only hydrogen and chloride ions. There are always significant quantities of sodium and potassium, the concentrations varying with the rate of acid secretion. The electrolytes also include small amounts of bicarbonate, phosphate, calcium, and magnesium.

Hydrogen-ion Secretion.[66-69] The oxyntic cell secretes hydrochloric acid. That has been verified by histochemical studies showing a pH below 2 in the canaliculi of oxyntic cells, and also by the morphological changes that occur in the canaliculi following stimulation of secretion. The mechanism for secreting hydrochloric acid is depicted in Figure 10-8. Hydrogen ions are transported across the barrier of one oxyntic cell from a concentration of $5 X 10^{-5}$ mEq/L in plasma to a concentration of 160 mEq/L in the primary secretion. This millionfold increase represents a large gradient for the ion to be transported against, which requires considerable energy.

The secretion of one liter of hydrochloric acid at a concentration of 160 mEq/L requires 1500 calories of energy. The hydrogen ion is secreted using energy derived from ATP and released membrane ATPase. Hydrogen ion secretion occurs via an ion exchange process involving potassium. The primary substrate for energy is glucose, which is oxidized through the hexose monophosphate shunt pathway. Oxygen is necessary to sustain optimum secretion, although the anaerobic metabolism of glucose supports some secretion.

Secreted hydrogen ions are derived from carbonic acid following the hydration of carbon dioxide to form carbonic acid, a conversion catalyzed by the enzyme carbonic anhydrase. A small amount of carbonic acid can be formed without aid of the enzyme, although not enough to sustain normal rates of acid secretion. Thus, large amounts of carbonic anhydrase are present in the oxyntic cell, and treatment with a carbonic anahydrase inhibitor reduces secretion of hydrogen ions. Bicarbonate is produced following the ionization of carbonic acid. Its intracellular level increases with transport of hydrogen ions from the oxyntic cell. Some of the excess bicarbonate diffuses to the extracellular fluid and into the plasma. The movement of a large amount of bicarbonate into the plasma is called the alkaline tide since it causes the pH of plasma to increase during gastric secretion of hydrochloric acid.

Chloride Secretion. Chloride is transported across the apical surface of the oxyntic cell via an energy-dependent mechanism. The net movement of chloride to the lumen of the gland exceeds that of hydrogen ions, so that the number of chloride ions on the mucosal surface exceeds that of hydrogen ions. This increment in chloride ions on the mucosal surface causes the region to be electrically negative with respect to the serosal side of the cell. Thus, a potential difference is generated that is of greatest magnitude in the body of the stomach, being -64 millivolts. The potential difference is -48 millivolts in the antrum and -11 millivolts in the duodenum. The chloride concentration is about 110 mEq/L in plasma and 165 mEq/L in gastric secretions. It takes less energy to secrete chloride and maintain this gradient than to maintain hydrogen-ion secretion. Chloride transport is inhibited by metabolic inhibitors, the effects of which cause the potential difference to fall toward zero. A variety of agents can increase the permeability of the mucosal barrier. If the barrier to chloride decreases, the back-diffusion of chloride causes the gradient to disappear and the potential difference to fall to zero.

Potassium Secretion. The concentration of potassium in gastric secretions is 10 to 20 mEq/L, which is greater than that in plasma (4.0 to 5.0 mEq/L). The concentration of potassium in gastric juice increases with increased rates of secretion, but after a prolonged period of secretion the levels fall, presumably because intracellular oxyntic cell potassium is depleted. Most potassium in gastric secretions is derived from cell rather than plasma potassium. Some gastric juice potassium is derived from desquamated cells. A special secretory mechanism is not necessary for potassium secretion. The hydrated forms of potassium ions are relatively small, and they have an electrochemical gradient allowing movement readily across membranes. The large potential difference across the mucosa, with the mucosal surface negative, is sufficient to cause passive

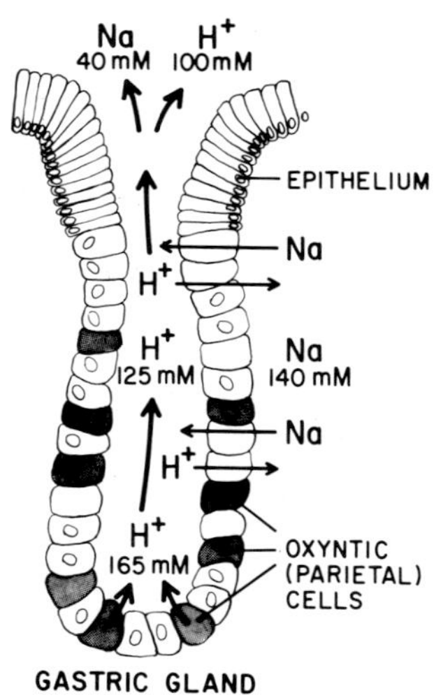

Figure 10-9. Diagram of gastric gland, showing hydrochloric acid secretion equilibrated with extracellular fluid as primary secretion moves out into lumen of stomach. Degree of equilibration is determined by rate of secretion and permeability of cells lining gastric gland.

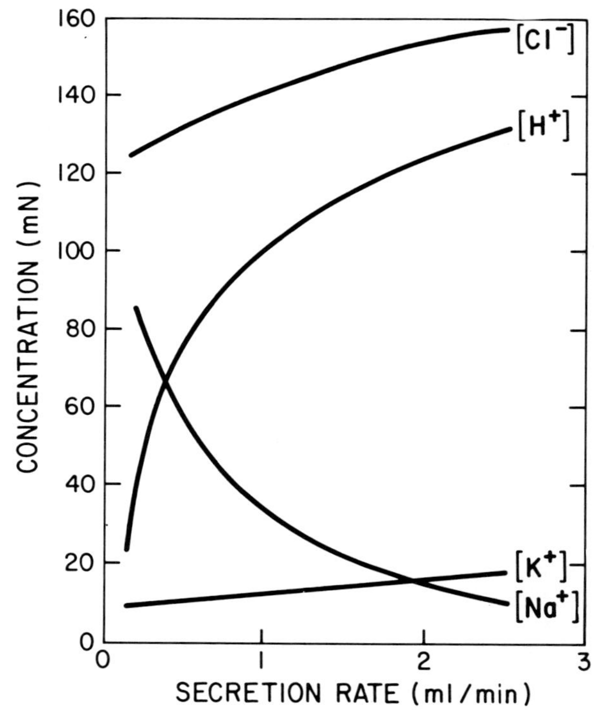

Figure 10-10. Graph showing that the electrolyte composition of gastric juice is a function of rate of secretion. As the rate increases, the juice comes to contain very little sodium. The concentration of potassium, however, is always greater than in the extracellular fluid.

movement of a large amount of positively charged potassium into the gastric secretions. Normal plasma potassium levels are necessary for hydrochloric acid secretion to be normal, but that appears to be related to the maintenance of normal structure and general functions in the oxyntic cells.

Sodium Secretion. Sodium concentrations in gastric juices vary inversely with those of hydrogen ions. Some sodium is added by the secretion of alkaline fluid from mucous surface cells. Sodium is also added by diffusion down the same kind of electrochemical gradient existing for potassium. During active secretion, oxyntic cells produce a 165mM hydrochloric acid solution. During movement through the ducts and gastric pits to the gastric lumen, ions and water diffuse in both directions across the epithelial cells. Sodium is the most abundant cation diffusing from interstitial fluid and with time the interstitial fluid, and gastric secretion equilibrate so that their compositions become more similar. The degree to which oxyntic cell secretions become like plasma is determined by how long gastric secretions remain in the ducts (Figure 10-9). At high rates of secretion the hydrochloric acid content is modified very little, and the final secretion may contain 120 to 150 mM hydrogen ion per liter (Figure 10-10). When the rate of secretion is very low, the composition of the final gastric fluid has had much more opportunity to be modified, and the hydrochloric acid concentration is very low.

Regulation of Acid Secretion

Gastric acid secretion is stimulated by neurotransmitters,

peptide hormones, histamine, and chemicals that alter intracellular levels of cyclic nucleotides and of calcium.

Activation of Oxyntic-Cell Secretion.[63-69] Three receptors for chemicals interact to stimulate the oxyntic cells' hydrochloric acid secretion (Figure 1-5). They are receptors for gastrin, histamine, and acetylcholine, all of which are necessary for optimum stimulation of secretion. Gastrin acts on its own receptor site but cannot stimulate the cell to secrete unless histamine and acetylcholine are available for binding to their own sites at the same time. Histamine occupies H_2-histamine receptor sites that are different from the H_1-histamine receptor sites, which are blocked by antihistamines. Analogs of histamine, such as cimetidine and ranitidine, can bind to the oxyntic cell's H_2-receptor sites, but they are unable to stimulate secretion of acid. Binding by these drugs prevents histamine binding and secretion of acid. These drugs are able to inhibit the secretory response to gastrin, food, cholinergics, and insulin. The receptor for acetylcholine interacts with any cholinergic agent to cause secretion. Blocking this receptor with atropine inhibits hydrochloric acid secretion. Atropine also inhibits the secretory response to both gastrin and histamine. Thus, it is apparent that selectively blocking any one of the three receptor sites markedly affects the response when any of the others is stimulated. Gastrin activity is blocked by proglumide, a selective antagonist of receptor binding by the gastrin-CCK family of peptide hormones. As already stated, all three of the receptor sites must be occupied by their agonists, and if one site is blocked, stimulation through the other receptors results in less than maximum response. Peptide hormones similar to gastrin can bind to gastrin receptors and stimulate some secretory activity. A hormone with no ability to stimulate acid secretion can remain bound and prevent interaction of gastrin with the receptor. The hormone becomes a competitive inhibitor of secretion. Cholecystokinin can bind to gastrin receptors and compete in this manner. The oxyntic cell has receptors for secretin, which is an inhibitor of acid secretion. Somatostatin also potently inhibits gastric acid secretion. Prostaglandins have a direct effect on the oxyntic cell and reduce secretion by inhibiting cyclic AMP formation. Local mucosal application of prostaglandins inhibits acid secretion.[70,71]

Gastrin, histamine, and acetylcholine are first messengers in the reflex to stimulate secretion, and they all act on cell membrane receptors. Their interaction stimulates intracellular events involving cyclic AMP and calcium that initiate acid secretion (Figure 10-11). An ATPase on the mucosal border mediates acid secretion. Drugs such as omeprazole block transport by that ATPase.[72]

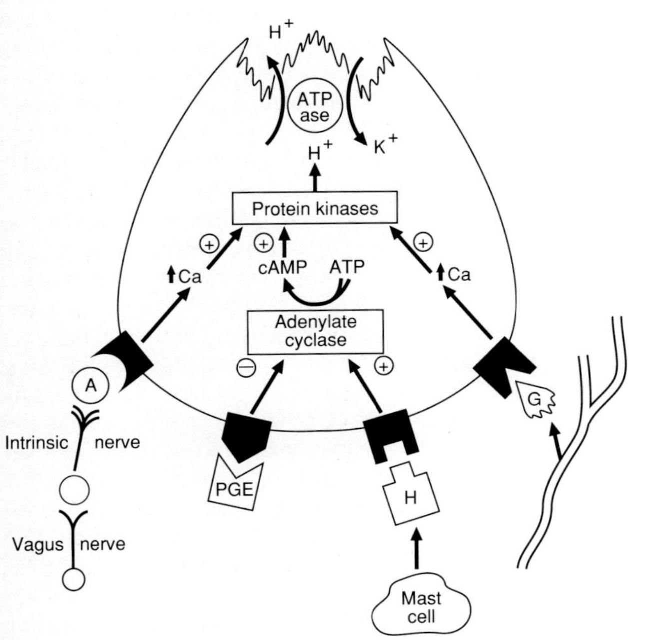

Figure 10-11. Schematic representation of oxyntic cell showing mechanisms for stimulating and inhibiting hydrogen ion secretion. A = acetylcholine, PGE = prostaglandins of the E series, H = histamine interacting on H_2 receptor, and G = gastrin.

Neural and Humoral Control of Gastric Secretion

Control of gastric secretion is a complex interaction of many neural and humoral factors that dictate secretion at controlled rates and at the proper time. Events occurring in parts of the gastrointestinal tract other than the stomach and in other systems of the body have an important role in regulating normal gastric secretion. The control is highly organized, so that secretion during interdigestive periods is minimal and the rate of secretion during a digestive period is programmed to the quantity and type of nutrients fed. In the resting state there is a continuous low level of vagal activity to the stomach, and gastrin is always present in the plasma. The background level of each is sufficient to stimulate the secretion of a small amount of gastric juice that is less than 1% of the maximum capacity for acid secretion in dogs. The rate of secretion oscillates in the resting state, as would be expected when excitatory and inhibitory influences are balanced. There is a small increase in secretion as the interdigestive myoelectric complexes pass through the stomach. The process of feeding stimulates secretion to rise over basal levels, and the increased rate is maintained until the stomach is empty. Mechanisms controlling acid secretion have their effect at three separate sequential times during the digestive process. The overall regulation of gastric secretion is diagrammed in Figure 10-12.

Cephalic Phase.[73,74] The anticipation, sight, taste, smell, and chewing of food stimulate the initial phase of gastric secretion. This is a reflex response mediated by higher cortical areas of the brain. The efferent or motor pathways to the stomach are in the vagus nerve. The fibers terminate on gastrin-secreting G-cells, oxyntic cells, and chief cells. Thus, activity in parasympathetic fibers to these cells stimulates the secretion of gastrin, hydrochloric acid, and pepsin. The vagally stimulated release of gastrin is somewhat resistant to inhibition with atropine. This neural mechanism is the major stimulus for the secretion of pepsin, plus small amounts of gastrin and hydrochloric acid.

As stated earlier, acetylcholine, gastrin, and histamine must all be present on their receptor sites for optimum secretion. This explains the synergism seen between vagal activity and gastrin levels. Removal of the former by vagotomy causes gastrin release and acid secretion to be only a fraction of that with the vagus intact, despite the fact that stimulation of the vagus normally produces only a small amount of hydrochloric acid secretion. Antrectomy to remove the source of G-cells also

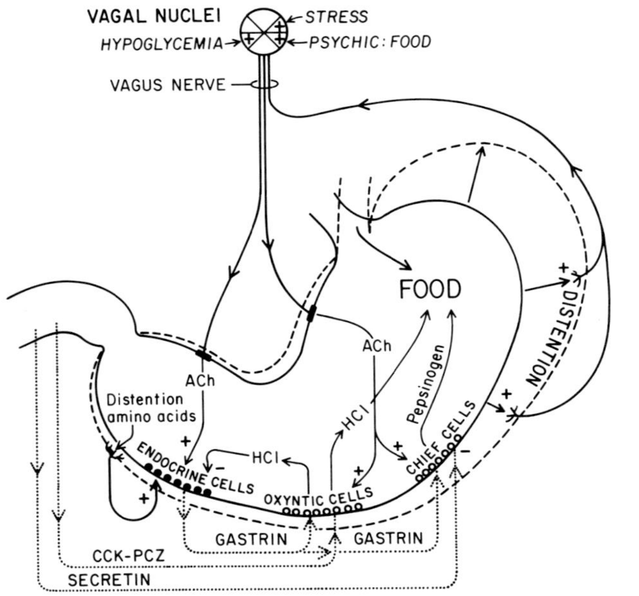

Figure 10-12. Diagram showing neural and endocrine control of gastric secretion of acid and pepsinogen. Illustrates cephalic, gastric, and intestinal phases. See text for description.

causes less vagally stimulated acid secretion than in the intact dog; the level is restored by the infusion of basal levels of gastrin.

Reduction of the gastrin-and histamine-stimulated response of the oxyntic cell by vagotomy does not reflect a decreased population of this cell type, for larger doses of the stimulants will produce a maximum response similar to that in intact dogs. This suggests that acetylcholine does not exert a trophic effect on oxyntic cells.

Intact vagal fibers, with their synthesis and release of acetylcholine, are necessary for the potential secretory capacity of the gastric chief cells to remain normal. Therefore, acetylcholine, like other hormones, exerts a trophic action on these mucosal cells. That action is illustrated by procedures in which the vagi are chronically stimulated, resulting in an increase in the capacity of the stomach to secrete pepsinogen.

Vagotomy lowers the basal level of secretion (that between meals), indicating that this secretion depends on a vagal activity that does not stop during the resting state. There are other CNS receptors that vagally stimulate gastric secretion. Central receptors respond to both hypoglycemia and decreased intracellular glucose levels, respectively produced by giving insulin and 2-deoxy-D-glucose. The response is vagally mediated gastric secretion of acid. In contrast, hyperglycemia suppresses serum gastrin levels and gastric-acid production.[75] A wide variety of peptide hormones are found in the brain. A large number of different peptides inhibit gastric secretion when infused into the cerebral ventricles of dogs stimulated by pentagastrin to secrete acid. Events mediated through the brain may be important in inhibiting as well as stimulating gastric acid secretion.[76]

Gastric Phase.[73] The most important determinants of gastric secretion are events that occur in the stomach. The most important factor in the gastric phase is the release of gastrin, which is stimulated by chemicals and by distention of the gastric mucosa. Neural pathways play a role in this release of gastrin and also stimulate acid secretion by less important means. The main (and possibly only) stimulus for gastrin release is mechanical distention of the antrum. The mechanism involved has been called the pyloropyloric reflex. Distention of the body of the stomach also causes gastrin release (the oxyntopyloric reflex). Also present is an oxyntooxyntic reflex, by which distention of the body of the stomach causes direct stimulation of the oxyntic cell. These reflexes have both long (vagovagal reflex) and short intramural neural pathways.

Chemicals can directly stimulate oxyntic cells to secrete, and it is now known that only L-isomers of amino acids are effective stimulants.[77] The chemicals act by a gastrin-independent local mechanism. The secretory response is sensitive to distention of the mucosa (which increases it) and to pH (which reduces it). Local anesthetics and anticholinergics reduce the response, which suggests a neural pathway, but a direct effect of the chemicals on the oxyntic cell nevertheless appears likely from the fact that secretion continues to a substantial degree. Amino acids given intravenously also stimulate gastric acid secretion by a cholinergic and gastrin-independent mechanism that is sensitive to gastric distention and pH.[78]

Secretion of hydrochloric acid is stimulated primarily by gastrin released from antral G-cells. This hormone is released by chemicals bathing the antral mucosa as well as by parasympathetic fibers that innervate the gland. Chemical stimulation is due to amino acids of the sarcosine series, primarily glycine, serine, and alanine; by proteins, especially liver, meat, and meat extracts; by acetic and propionic acids; by bile acids; and by neutralization of the antrum with antacids. (Acid secretion is 30% to 40% less when soy protein rather than meat protein is consumed.)[79] The mechanism for secretion contains a cholinergic pathway since acetylcholine on the mucosal surface stimulates release, and some mechanisms to stimulate gastrin release are inhibited by atropine. Local anesthesia on the antral mucosa abolishes the chemically stimulated secretion of acid that is assumed to be due to inhibition of gastrin release. Gastrin release in response to feeding in normal dogs is not inhibited by atropine, whereas acid secretion is. Atropine resistance of gastrin release can be explained by either a direct effect of chemicals on gastrin release, release of a peptide messenger to stimulate gastrin release, or the presence of a neurotransmitter other than acetylcholine. Catecholamines and calcium ions stimulate gastrin release in some species but not the dog.

Gastrin release is inhibited when the pH of the contents of the antrum is 3.0 or lower. At a low pH the most potent stimulators of gastrin release are ineffective. This control mechanism is important in regulating hydrochloric acid secretion. Cholinergic and noncholinergic neural pathways may mediate the inhibitory effect. Somatostatin may be important in this inhibition; it may block both gastrin release and acid secretion directly. Peptide hormones released during the intestinal phase of digestion and absorption may produce some of the inhibition. Such hormones with properties to inhibit acid secretion include secretin, gastric inhibitory peptide, enteroglucagon, and peptide YY. The stomach may have another mechanism for inhibiting acid secretion. Removal of the fundic mucosa in dogs re-moves an inhibitory mechanism of both secretion and gastrin release.[80]

Intestinal Phase.[73] Food in the small intestine stimulates hydrochloric acid secretion in the vagally innervated or denervated stomach. Stimulation is due to distention of the intestine and to amino acids and peptides. The response is mediated by a humoral agent called enterooxyntin to distinguish it from gastrin. It is biologically distinct from gastrin in being capable of augmenting the maximum secretory response to both gastrin and histamine. Enterooxyntin is not dependent on vagal innervation for its release from the intestinal mucosa. Gastrin is also found in small amounts in the small intestine, but it cannot augment secretory responses to exogenous gastrin. Cholecystokinin is also released, and since it is a competitive inhibitor of gastrin, being in the same family and a weaker agonist of acid secretion, the gastric response is less. Cholecystokinin stimulates submaximal gastric secretion, having an effect on both acid and pepsin. Its influence on secretion will depend on the background levels of gastrin.

In general, reflexes that arise from more aboral parts of the gastrointestinal tract are inhibitory. Thus, the major mechanisms in the intestine to control gastric secretion are inhibitory. They can be both neural and humoral.[81] The only neural reflex is a bulbofundic reflex that is stimulated by acid in the duodenum. Humoral agents that are released by the intestinal mucosa and inhibit gastric secretion belong to the secretin family, which includes gastrointestinal inhibitory polypeptide, vasoactive intestinal peptide, and glucagon. They all inhibit both hydrochloric acid and pepsinogen secretion, except that secretin stimulates pepsinogen secretion. The mechanism for secretin release is well-known, with receptors that respond primarily to acid in the duodenum. Fat in the intestine causes inhibition of gastric secretion by a humoral means, and the name enterogastrone has been applied to the phenomenon. Fats, amino acids, and oral glucose (to a lesser degree) stimulate the release of gastrointestinal polypeptide and probably vasoactive intestinal peptide. It is likely that the enterogastrone effect is mediated by a combination of these three of the four hormones in the secretin family, in concert with neurotensin and peptide YY. Gastrointestinal inhibitory polypeptide and vasoactive intestinal peptide inhibit the secretion of pepsin and also the secretion of acid stimulated by pentagastrin, histamine, and insulin. Neurotensin, a potent inhibitor of pentagastrin-stimulated acid secretion, is released by fat in the small intestine. It may be the most important mediator of the enterogastrone response. Fat in the intestine also inhibits gastrin release.[82] A number of other peptide hormones have some control over regulation of gastric secretion, although it is not known whether they are physiologically important. For example, bulbogastrone, a humoral factor distinct from secretin and cholecystokinin, is released by acid in the first part of the duodenum. Urogastrone, a substance found in the urine, is produced at an unknown site and inhibits the secretion of gastric juices. The small intestine performs other types of inhibitory actions on gastric secretion. Extensive resection of the small intestine results in hypersecretion of gastric acid. It is postulated that either an inhibitor of gastrin release has been removed or that an important function of the small intestine is to remove and degrade gastrin.[83]

Events in the colon can determine gastric functions. Infusion of the canine colon with liver extract, sodium oleate or hydrochloric acid inhibits gastric acid secretion.[84]

Bicarbonate Secretion[85]

The gastric mucosa secretes bicarbonate in addition to hydrochloric acid. The surface mucosal cells secrete bicarbonate derived from the bicarbonate produced in oxyntic cells during secretion of hydrogen ions. Bicarbonate is released to capillaries below the basement membranes of oxyntic cells. The capillaries continue to the area under mucosal surface cells, where the high blood bicarbonate diffuses out and into the mucosal cells; from there, the bicarbonate is secreted into the mucus layer on the surface. The capillaries have large pores which facilitate the diffusion of bicarbonate.

The amount of bicarbonate available for secretion is determined by the acid secretory activity of oxyntic cells, the blood bicarbonate concentration, and capillary blood flow in the tissue. Reduction in acid secretion can reduce bicarbonate secretion to the point that protection against acid in the stomach is inadequate. Acid placed in the stomach during histamine stimulation of acid secretion results in no gastric damage. Acid placed in the stomach during inhibition of acid secretion by cimetidine results in mucosal ulceration; insufficient bicarbonate is produced to maintain bicarbonate secretion into the surface mucus layer.

Prostaglandins stimulate bicarbonate secretion by gastric mucosal cells. Prostaglandins are more effective stimulants when applied to the mucosal surface than when injected intravenously. Cholinergic agents also stimulate secretion of bicarbonate. Anticholinergics such as atropine block both the prostaglandin and cholinergic-stimulated secretion. Drugs inhibiting prostaglandin synthesis, such as salicylates and ibuprofen, inhibit bicarbonate secretion in some species of animals. Peptide hormones such as pancreatic polypeptide, CCK, gastrin and neurotensin stimulate bicarbonate secretion; secretion is stimulated also by calcium and is inhibited by the carbonic anhydrase inhibitor acetazolamide, which reduces the formation of bicarbonate in oxyntic and other cells.

Acid bathing the mucosa stimulates gastric bicarbonate secretion. In one type of study the response is mediated by a humoral agent, not prostaglandins, that may be enteroglucagon. Other studies suggest prostaglandins mediate this response. Neural cholinergic pathways in the vagus nerve also stimulate gastric bicarbonate. Stimulation is primarily during the cephalic phase of secretion.

Gastric Blood Flow

When gastric secretion of fluid and electrolytes is stimulated, mucosal blood flow must increase in order to provide the constituents of the secretion and the energy to produce it. Most of the blood flow is directed to the mucosa at all times, increasing in parallel with increases in secretion. The blood supply to the gastrointestinal tract is designed so that blood flow can be shunted from one part to another under the influence of many neural and humoral factors. The control of gastric blood flow is described in the chapter on integration of function.

Gastric Mucosal Barrier[85-88]

The gastric mucosa is a barrier that separates and compartmentalizes the gastric juices and the interstitial fluid. The barrier has three physiological components: 1) It is a barrier to the movement of cellular elements of the blood, such as erythrocytes; 2) it acts to minimize losses from the blood into the gastric secretions of important macromolecules, such as plasma proteins; and 3) it is a highly specialized semipermeable membrane that controls the rate of movement of water and ions. Its restriction of hydrogen and sodium ions is very important if the stomach is to perform its digestive functions. The low permeability to hydrogen ions minimizes the rate at which they are able to leave the stomach, and the low permeability to movement of sodium ions aids in their restriction to the extracellular fluid.

The properties of the cell membranes determine the barrier to electrolytes. The mucosal surface is a mucus-covered cell membrane that consists of different proteins inserted into a lipid bilayer. The junction between cells has been called a tight junction since it appears on electron micrographs as an impermeable union that completely surrounds and cements one cell to another. Physiologic studies reveal that these junctions are in fact quite permeable to water and ions, more so than the cell membrane. Change in any aspect of the cell membrane changes its properties of selective permeability to ions. That can be evaluated in the gastric mucosa following measures to change the properties of the membrane. When a known amount of acid is placed in the stomach after such membrane alteration, the rate at which the composition of the acid changes is related directly to increases in permeability.

Integrity of the mucosal barrier is evaluated by its electrical potential difference and resistance between the luminal and basal sides of the cells. Both potential difference and the resistance fall with injury, but they also decrease with stimulation of acid secretion. Thus, evaluation of these parameters are of questionable value in assessing mucosal damage.

Injury and loss of surface mucosal cells is followed by mucosal reconstitution that is nearly complete within 30 minutes in most cases. The rapid reconstitution occurs when cells adjacent to lost cells migrate into the breech and cover the defect. Luminal pH of 3.0 or less inhibits reconstitution unless a very high concentration (48 mM) of bicarbonate is available on the basal side of the cell. Reconstitution requires calcium in the media; calcium may be necessary for microfilament function in the migration or for attachment of cells filling in the breech. Reconstitution is not influenced by prostaglandins.

The gastric mucosal barrier also consists of a surface mucus layer containing a bicarbonate-rich fluid. Secretion of the bicarbonate has been described from its sources in oxyntic cells and plasma bicarbonate. The bicarbonate from these sources contributes to bicarbonate in the gastric lumen, the mucus coating, the unstirred water layer, and the cytosol of surface cells. Hydrogen ions are neutralized in the lumen, but more importantly they are neutralized as the enter and back-diffuse through the mucus and unstirred layers. On breakdown of these barriers the intracellular bicarbonate protects against back-diffusion into surface cells. Hydrogen ions reacting with bicarbonate form carbonic acid, which must be converted to carbon dioxide and water for disposal. The enzyme carbonic anhydrase hastens that reaction; gastric surface cells have carbonic anhydrase activity equivalent to that in oxyntic cells.

Reduction of plasma bicarbonate concentrations compromises maintenance of the bicarbonate barrier. Luminal pH of gastric contents is less than 2.0 in normal fed animals. When systemic acidosis reduces blood pH to 7.0 or less, gastric ulcers develop even if the luminal pH increases to 3.5. Not enough bicarbonate is provided by the circulation to neutralize back-diffusing hydrogen ions. The bicarbonate barrier is also dependent on maintenance of normal mucosal blood flow. Hemorrhagic shock reduces mucosal blood flow, and when combined with bile acids bathing the mucosal surface, gastric ulceration follows. Drugs such as isoproterenol given to increase mucosal blood flow prevent ulceration by increasing delivery of bicarbonate to the mucosa. Thus, a combination of acidosis and reduced mucosal blood flow will invariably cause gastric ulceration.

In addition to holding bicarbonate-rich fluid, the layer of mucus protects the gastric surface by virtue of its physical properties. Mucus adheres tenaciously to underlying epithelial cells. Mucus also has a high viscosity, which prevents the shear and stress of gastric digestion from disrupting the integrity of the continuous mucus coat, and which determines a lubricating action for mucus. The mucus layer increases in thickness following a variety of stimuli. The increase may be more of a defensive response to an injurious agent than a physiologic response to neural or humoral stimuli. The mucus layer without bicarbonate does not inhibit diffusion of hydrogen ions, but it does retard the diffusion of pepsin. Mucus with debris from cell damage and disruption of the barrier forms a cap covering defects in the mucosa. That cap offers some protection, since its removal delays healing.

Prostaglandins have important cytoprotective effects on gastric mucosa.[89] At one time the protective effect was believed to operate directly on mucosal cells. The nonsteroidal, anti-inflammatory drugs (NSAID) cause gastric ulceration in dogs and possibly cats. However, inhibition of prostaglandin synthesis can be induced without causing gastric mucosal lesions. Thus, NSAID must cause ulceration by some other means. Prostaglandins are cytoprotective but by another means. They are protective by effects on mucosal circulation rather than the epithelial cells. Prostaglandins increase blood flow, and their cytoprotection may be due to increasing delivery of bicarbonate for protection against acid back-diffusion. The augmented blood flow also removes debris, chemicals, and damaging agents contributing to persistence of the injury. As described earlier, prostaglandins stimulate mucus and bicarbonate secretion.

Disruption of the Barrier

The mucus gel lining the surface cells is disrupted and lost by treatment with urea or n-acetylcysteine. Loss of the mucus layer allows pepsin and other proteolytic enzymes to digest membrane proteins. The rate of secretion of gastric mucus is reduced and its composition is changed by corticosteroids, ACTH, aspirin, phenylbutazone, and indomethacin. Those drugs are also factors in the development of ulcers, and it is suggested that the effect is due, at least in part, to their effect on mucus.[90] Alteration of membrane proteins, such as treatment with sulfhydryl reagents, can also cause enough changes that a marked loss of plasma proteins follows.

The lipids in the membranes are highly permeable to small lipid-soluble molecules. If such a compound is toxic after it enters the cell, disruption of the barrier can result. Aspirin is one compound that can break the barrier. At neutral pH, aspirin exists in an ionized form as a large polar molecule with a shell

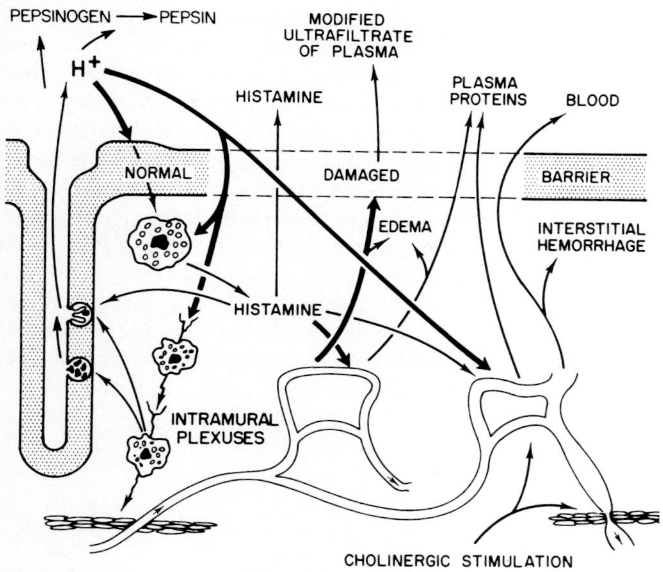

Figure 10-13. Pathophysiological consequences of the back-diffusion of acid through the broken mucosal barrier (from Davenport, H.W.: New Eng. J. Med. 276:1307, 1967. By permission).

of hydration. The ionized form moves across membranes at a slow rate through pathways for water-soluble molecules. Aspirin is an acid in the ionized form, and, once inside the cell, high concentrations damage cell structure and disrupt the barrier. High intra cellular concentrations follow aspirin crossing the membrane at a rapid rate. At the acid pH of gastric contents aspirin is un-ionized and lipid-soluble. This form of aspirin readily crosses lipid membranes. Intracellularly, where cytosolic pH is close to neutral, aspirin is ionized. The ionized form accumulates rapidly and is trapped inside since that form does not readily cross cell membranes. Adding a buffer to aspirin maintains most of it in an ionized form, so that absorption proceeds slowly.

Other organic acids that are undissociated at an acid pH behave like the salicylates, and, being lipid-soluble, they are readily absorbed and exert their toxic effect after being trapped inside the gastric mucosal cell. Thus, short-chain fatty acids such as acetic and propionic can break the barrier. Bile acids have a pK (or dissociation property) that is similar to that of the organic acids already mentioned. In addition, they are detergents, disrupting the lipid part of the cell membrane. Other detergents, such as digitonin, have a similar effect.

Enzymes that catalyze the degradation of the membrane lipids also disrupt the barrier. Phospholipase A can hydrolyze lecithin within the membrane, destroying it, but only if the enzyme is the one found in cobra venom. The phospholipase A from pancreatic secretion is not able to produce this effect, which makes questionable its role in the breaking of the barrier by the reflux of duodenal contents. Lysolecithin disrupts the barrier, however, and this compound is produced by the action of pancreatic phospholipase-A on lecithin during normal digestion in the duodenum. Reflux of lysolecithin from the duodenum may be important in clinical problems in which the integrity of the mucosal surface is altered. Tranquilizers have been shown to alter the barrier, and agents that affect the metabolism of mucosal cells also break the barrier. Examples of drugs that act in this manner are the carbonic anhydrase inhibitor acetazolamide, and sodium fluoride.

Hypertonicity of gastric contents causes mucosal permeability to increase. That has been shown with hypertonic solutions of glucose, sucrose, and urea. Some enteral diets are hypertonic and vomited when fed to some animals. They are often diluted when used to feed sick animals.

The integrity of the barrier is reflected by the rate of back-diffusion of hydrochloric acid. With increased back-diffusion of acid, a cascade of pathologic changes follow the increased amounts of acid entering mucosal cells and disrupting subepithelial structures and functions (Figure 10-13).

Back-diffusing hydrochloric acid stimulates neural plexuses in the intrinsic nervous system. This stimulates motility in gastric smooth muscles. The oxyntic and chief cells respond to stimulation of the plexuses with their respective secretions. Acid has direct effects, causing mast cells to release histamine. Histamine is a potent stimulator of the oxyntic cell to secrete hydrochloric acid. Thus, a positive feedback is set in motion, with the increased secretion of acid undergoing back-diffusion, stimulating further secretion. Histamine exerts its well-known effects on the microcirculation. It promotes vasodilation and increased capillary filtration, allowing an increase in the escape of plasma fluid through the broken mucosal barrier and into the lumen of the stomach. This fluid modifies the primary gastric secretions, and if large amounts escape into the lumen and are vomited, the pH of the vomitus will not be highly acidic. Histamine also increases capillary permeability, which results in the loss of increased amounts of plasma proteins. The barrier to plasma protein loss in the gastrointestinal tract is in the mucosal epithelial layer rather than the capillary wall. Capillaries in the stomach and intestine have large fenestrations that permit molecules the size of plasma proteins to move with little restriction in and out of the capillary bed. When the barrier is broken by sulfhydryl reagents placed in the stomach of the dog, the route of protein loss in the subsequent protein losing-gastropathy occurs through the intercellular spaces and the so-called tight junctions. Thus, the cell can remain a physiological barrier while escape is made possible by alterations in proteins that make up the cell-to-cell junctions.

It is apparent that blood flow to the gastric mucosa determines the metabolic status of the tissue, and that mucosal damage can change this flow, either increasing or decreasing it. Histamine and stimulation of the intrinsic nervous system cause vasodilation and increased blood flow, but histamine induces the triple response, with capillary stasis resulting, attended by a reduction in mucosal blood flow.

Augmentation of blood flow is a purposeful response in a number of ways. Reductions in gastric pH result in a decrease or loss of the mucus pH gradient that parallels the pH changes of gastric contents.[91] Treatment with prostaglandins to increase mucosal blood flow prevents the decrease in the mucus pH gradient. Without prostaglandin treatment and with reductions in intragastric pH to 1.0, the mucus pH gradient is lost but then is abruptly regained at high levels. These findings show that decreasing intraluminal pH gradually eliminates the mucus pH gradient. Once that is lost the back-diffusing hydrogen ions damage the epithelial cell so that ion permeability increases and bicarbonate freely diffuses out to restore the mucus pH gradient. The source of the bicarbonate in interstitial fluid is replenished by the circulation.

Reduced gastric blood flow contributes to barrier disruption. Ischemia would be thought to damage the barrier, yet a profound decrease in gastric blood flow does not cause a change in mucosal permeability to hydrogen and sodium ions. It does, however, reduce the delivery of bicarbonate for acid neutralization, and eventually ulceration appears.

A second type of barrier disruption occurs with the development of gastric erosions. In general, such disruption does not cause concomitant changes in the permeability to sodium and hydrogen ions. Erosions occur at focal points in the mucosa, destroying the barrier for blood elements. The pathogenesis of erosion formation is different from that of breaking the barrier for hydrogen ions. The bleeding that continues after normal ion permeability is restored in the model, as described above, may nevertheless develop in a similar manner in all gastric erosions. Hydrochloric acid must be present in the stomach for erosions to develop, and changes in mucosal blood flow are considered to play an important role.

Erosions in the gastric mucosa develop in clinical patients following any kind of physical or thermal trauma, shock, sepsis, or head injury. These erosions are usually not very apparent, becoming recognizable only when they extend through the muscularis mucosa to produce gastric ulcers. They are all termed stress erosions or ulcers since the underlying common factor in their development is a stress-induced change in mucosal blood flow. The change is a marked reduction of flow in the mucosal microcirculation. Hydrochloric acid is the other factor that must be present for the development of erosions. Stress can be produced in the experimental dog by blood loss or by endotoxins, and erosions develop if the stomach is exposed to isosmotic hydrochloric acid. The lesions do not develop, however, if a neutral solution is placed in the stomach. Erosions are not associated with increased back-diffusion of hydrogen ions or increased permeability for other cations. They are associated with a loss in the ability to deliver protective amounts of bicarbonate to the mucosa.

The vasoactive drugs norepinephrine and pitresin cause marked reduction in mucosal blood flow without altering cation permeability. Thus, endotoxic and hemorrhagic shock result in mucosal changes unaccompanied by the increased cation permeability and increased blood flow seen with chemical disruption of the barrier. The stresses that produce shock reduce mucosal blood flow by sympathetically mediated vasoconstriction in the vascular bed. Catecholamines are released and have the same effect. Serotonin, a vasoactive substance found in the mucosa, may be released and exacerbate the problem.

The pathogenesis of gastric erosions in the clinical case most likely involves a combination of all the factors discussed. Trauma patients with acid and bile salts in their stomachs are high risks for developing gastric erosions. Giving stressed patients drugs that affect the barrier increases the likelihood of their developing erosions. When the two prerequisites (presence of acid and decreased mucosal blood flow) are present, the pathogenesis of erosion is as follows. Focal ischemia occurs in places under the surface epithelium. The response of some of the cells is to empty out their mucus. It is usually the older cells that respond in this way when faced with ischemia at one border and hydrogen ions at the opposite side of the cell. When they have emptied their mucus contents, they represent a break in the barrier, with cation permeability resulting in a localized point. If the areas of all erosions are totaled, their sum is not great enough to give measurable evidence for an overall increase in cation permeability. The difference between an animal with a high rate of mucosal blood flow and one with a low rate is that the hydrogen ions cannot accumulate in subcellular spaces in the former but can in the latter, producing the erosion. This is a major difference between pathogenesis by the barrier breakers and by the erosion producers. As noted earlier, bile acids combined with reduced blood flow produce severe erosions, whereas neither can do so alone. Pretreating dogs with atropine before administering barrier-breaking chemicals reduces plasma protein loss in the stomach.[92] Pepsin secretion and acid secretion are stimulated by the same toxic agents, and the ameliorating effects of atropine pretreatment may be to reduce the secretion of enzyme and hydrochloric acid.

REFERENCES

1. Code, C. F. and Carlson H.C.: Motor activity of the stomach. In, Handbook of Physiology. Section 6: Alimentary Canal. Edited by C.F. Code. Washington, D.C., American Physiological Society, Vol. 4, 1903-1916, 1968.
2. Miller, M.E., Christensen, G.C. and Evans, H.E.: Anatomy of the dog, first edition. W.B. Saunders, Co., Philadelphia, PA, 1964.
3. Sisson, S. and Grossman, J.D.: Anatomy of domestic animals, 4th edition, W.B. Saunders Co., Philadelphia, PA, 1953.
4. Edwards, D.A.W. and Rowlands, E.N.: Physiology of the gastroduodenal junction. In, Handbook of Physiology. Section 6: Alimentary Canal, Edited by C.F. Code, Washington, D.C., American Physiological Society, Vol. 4, 1985-2000, 1968.
5. Dodge, J.A. and Karim, A.A.: Induction of pyloric hypertrophy by pentagastrin. Gut 17:280-284, 1976.
6. Ito, S.: Functional gastric morphology. In, Physiology of the Gastrointestinal Tract. Edited by L.R. Johnson. Raven Press, New York, 817-851, 1987.
7. Willems, G., Vansteenkiste, Y. and Limbosch, J.M.: Stimulating effect of gastrin on cell proliferation kinetics in canine fundic mucosa. Gastroenterology 62:583-589, 1972.
8. Meyer, J.H.: Motility of the stomach and gastroduodenal junction. In, Physiology of the Gastrointestinal Tract. Edited by L.R. Johnson. Raven Press, New York, 613-629, 1987.
9. Wilbur, B.G. and Kelly, K.A.: The effect of gastric fundectomy on canine gastric pacesetter potential, transmural pressure, and emptying. Gastroenterology 62:863, 1972.
10. Stemper, T.J. and Cooke, A.R.: Effect of a fixed pyloric opening on gastric emptying in the cat and dog. Am. J. Physiol. 230:813-817, 1976.
11. Allescher, H.D., Daniel, E.E., Dent, J., Fox, J.E.T. and Kostolanska, F.: Extrinsic and intrinsic neural control of pyloric sphincter pressure in the dog. J. Physiol. 401:17-38, 1988.
12. Golenhofen, K., Ludtke, F.E., Milenov, K. and Siewert, R.: Excitatory and inhibitory effects on canine pyloric muscle. In, Gastrointestinal Motility. Edited by J. Christensen. Raven Press, New York, 203-210, 1980
13. Daniel, E.E. and Irwin, J.: Electrical activity of gastric musculature. In, Handbook of Physiology, Section 6: Alimentary Canal. Edited by C.F. Code. Washington, D.C., American Physiological Society, Vol. 4, 1969-1984, 1967.
14. Duthi, H.L.: Electrical activity of gastrointestinal smooth muscle. Gut 15:669-681, 1974.
15. Thomas, J.E. and Baldwin, M.V.: Pathways and mechanisms of regulation of gastric motility. In: Handbook of Physiology, section 6: Alimentary Canal. edited by C.F. Code. Washington, DC, American Physiological Society, Vol. 4, 1937-1968, 1968.

16. Publicover, N.G. and Sanders, K.M.: Myogenic regulation in gastric smooth muscle. Am. J. Physiol. 248:G512-G520, 1985.
17. Kim, C.H., Azpiroz, F. and Malagelada, J-R.: Characteristics of spontaneous and drug-induced gastric dyerhythmias in a chronic canine model. Gastroenterology 90:421-427, 1986.
18. Gullikson, G.W., Okuda, H., Shimizu, M. and Bass, P.: Electrical arrhythmias in gastric antrum of the dog. Am. J. Physiol. 239:G59-G68, 1980.
19. Kim, C.H., Zinsmeister, A.R. and Malagelada, J-R.: Mechanisms of canine gastric dysrhythmia. Gastroenterology 92:993-999, 1987.
20. Sarna, S.K. Bowes, K.L. and Daniel, E.E.: Gastric pacemakers. Gastroenterology 70:226-231, 1976.
21. Kelly, K.: Gastric emptying of liquids and solids: rates of proximal and distal stomach. Am. J. Physiol. 239:G71-G76, 1980.
22. Hinder, R.A. and San-garde, B.A.: Individual and combined roles of the pylorus and the antrum in the canine gastric emptying of a liquid and a digestible solid. Gastroenterology 84:281-286, 1983.
23. DePonti, F., Azpiroz, F. and Malagelada, J-R.: Reflex gastric relaxation in response to distention of the duodenum. Am. J. Physiol. 252:G595-G601, 1987.
24. Pappas, T.N., Debas, H.T., Chang, A.M. and Taylor, I.L.: Peptide YY release by fatty acids is sufficient to inhibit gastric emptying in dogs.
25. Winans, C.S.: The fickle pylorus. Gastroenterology 70:622-623, 1976.
26. Weisbrodt, N.W.: The pylorus: keeper of the gate? Gastroenterology 82:995-996, 1982.
27. Meyer, J.H., Thomson, J.B., Cohen, M.B., Shadchehr, A. and Mandiola, S.A.: Sieving of sold food by the canine stomach and sieving after gastric surgery. Gastroenterology 76:804-813, 1979.
28. Ohashi, H. and Meyer, J.H.: Effect of peptic digestion on emptying of cooked liver in dogs. Gastroenterology 79:305-310, 1980.
29. Meyer, J.H., Dressman, J., Fink, A. and Amidon, G.: Effect of size and density on canine gastric emptying of nondigestible solids. Gastroenterology 89:805-813, 1985.
30. Ehrlein, H.J.: Motility of the pyloric sphincter studied by the inductograph method in conscious dogs. Am. J. Physiol. 254:G650-G657, 1988.
31. Biancani, P., Zabinski, M.P., Kerstein, M.D. and Behar, J.: Mechanical characteristics of the cat pylorus. Gastroenterology 78:301-309, 1980.
32. Phaosawasdi, K. and Fisher, R.S.: Hormonal effects on the pylorus. Am. J. Physiol. 243:G330-G335, 1982.
33. Biancani, P., Cilalzi, L.K. and McCallum, R.W.: Mechanism of histamine-induced excitation of the cat pylorus. J. Clin. Invest. 68:582-588, 1981.
34. Kumar, D., Ritman, E.L. and Malagelada, J-R.: Three-dimensional imaging of the stomach: role of pylorus in the emptying of liquids. Am. J. Physiol 253:G79-G85, 1987.
35. Mir, S.S., Telford, G.L., Mason, G.R. and Ormsbee, H.S.: Noncholinergic nonadrenergic inhibitory innervention of the canine pylorus. Gastroenterology 76:1443-1448, 1979.
36. Azpiroz, F. and Malagelada, J-R.: Intestinal control of gastric tone. Am. J. Physiol. 249:G501-G509, 1985.
37. Azpiroz, F. and Malagelada, J-R: Vagally mediated gastric relaxation induced by intestinal nutrients in the dog. Am. J. Physiol. 251:G726-G735, 1986.
38. Sandhu, K.S., El Samahi, M.M., Mena, I., Dooley, C.P. and Valenzuela, J.E.: Effect of pectin on gastric emptying and gastroduodenal motility in normal subjects. Gastroenterology 92:486-492, 1987.
39. Parr, N.J., Grime, J.S., Baxter, J.N., Critchley, M. and Mackie, C.R.: Small bowel resistances and the gastroduodenal brake. Gut 28:950-954, 1987.
40. Ehrlein, H.J. and Hiesinger, E.: Computer analysis of mechanical activity of gastroduodenal junction in unanesthetized dogs. Quart. J. Exp. Physiol. 67:17-29, 1982.
41. Tavaka, M., Hakim, N.S., Van Lier Ribbink, J. and Sarr, M.G.: Coordination of motility across the pylorus: role of myoneural and enteric continuity. Gastroenterology 95:891, 1988.
42. Defilippi, C.C. and Gomez, E.: Continuous recording of pyloric sphincter pressure in dogs. Dig. Dis. Sci. 30:669-674, 1985.
43. Heading, R.C.: Duodenogastric reflux. Gut 24:507-509, 1983.
44. Ritchie, W.P.: Alkaline reflux gastritis: a critical reappraisal. Gut 25:975-987, 1984.
45. Muller-Lissner, S.A., Schattenmann, G., Siewert, J.R. and Blum, A.L.: Effect of a transpyloric tube on gastric emptying and duodenogastric reflux in the dog. Digestion 28:176-180, 1983.
46. Muller-Lissner, S.A. and Blum, A.L.: To-and-fro movements across the canine pylorus. Scand. J. Gastroenterology 19(suppl 92):1-3, 1984.
47. Code, C.F., Steinbach, J.H., Schlegel, J.F., Amberg, J.R. and Hallenbeck, G.A.: Pyloric and duodenal motor contributions to duodenogastric reflux. Scand. J. Gastroenterology 19(Suppl 92):13-16, 1984.
48. Mearin, F., Azpiroz, F., Malagelada, J-R. and Zinsmeister, A.R.: Antroduodenal resistance to flow in the control of duodenogastric bile reflux during fasting. Gastroenterology 93:1026-1033, 1987.
49. Defilippi, C., Mamani, N. and Gomez, E.: Relationship between antropyloric and intestinal motility and duodenogastric reflux in fasting dogs. Dig. Dis. Sci. 32:171-176, 1987.
50. Pantoja, J.L., Defilippi, C., Valenzuela, J.E. and Csendes, A.: Nonsteroidal anti-inflammatory drugs: effect on pyloric sphincter and duodenogastric reflux. Dig. Dis. Sci. 24:217-220, 1979.
51. Dooley, C.P., Mello, W.D. and Valenzuela, J.E.: Effects of aspirin and prostaglandin E_2 on interdigestive motility complex and duodenogastric reflux in man. Dig. Dis. Sci. 30:513-521, 1985.
52. Happe, R.P. and van Den Brom, W.E.: Duodenogastric reflux in the dog, a clinicopathological study. Res. Vet. Sci. 33:280-286, 1982.
53. Schulze-Delrieu, K.: Intrinsic reflexes between the esophagus and stomach. Gastroenterology 91:1568-1569, 1986.
54. DePonti, F., Azpiroz, F. and Malagelada, J-R.: Reflex gastric relaxation in response to distention of the duodenum. Am. J. Physiol. 252:G595-G601, 1987.
55. Glise, H. and Abrahamsson, H.: Reflex vagal inhibition of gastric motility by intestinal nociceptive stimulation in the cat. Scand. J. Gastroenterology 15:769-774, 1980.
56. Hersey, S.J.: Pepsinogen secretion. In, Physiology of the Gastrointestinal Tract. Edited by L.R. Johnson. Raven Press, New York, p. 947-957, 1987.
57. Donaldson, R.M.: Intrinsic factor and the transport of cobalamin. In, Physiology of the Gastrointestinal Tract. Edited by L.R. Johnson. Raven Press, New York, 959-973, 1987.
58. Neutra, M.R. and Forstner, J.F.: Gastrointestinal mucus: synthesis, secretion and function. In, Physiology of the Gastrointestinal Tract. Edited by L.R. Johnson. Raven Press, New York, 975-1009, 1987.
59. Johnson, L.R.: Pepsin output from the damaged canine heidenhain pouch. Amer. J. Dig. Dis. 16:403-407, 1971.
60. Batt, R.M. and Horadagoda, N.U.: Role of gastric and pancreatic intrinsic factors in the physiologic absorption of Cobalamin in the dog. Gastroenterology 94:A1339, 1986.
61. Schrager, J.: The chemical composition and fuction of gastrointestinal mucus. Gut 11:450-456, 1970.
62. Kim, Y.S., Bella, A., Whitehead, J.S., Isaacs, R. and Remer, L.: Studies on the binding of amylopectin sulfate with gastrin mucin. Gastroenterology 69:138-145, 1975.
63. Zimmon, D.S. and Mazzola, V.: Amylopectin sulphate (SN-263) coats the gastric mucosal surface. Gut 14:847-849, 1973.
64. Strombeck, D.R. and Harrold, D.: Binding of cholera toxin to mucins and inhibition by gastric mucin. Infect. Immunity 10:1266-1272, 1974.
65. Hunt, J.N. and Wan, B.: Electrolytes of mammalian gastric juice. In, Handbook of Physiology, section 6: Alimentary

Canal. Edited by C.F. Code. Washington, DC, American Physiological Society, Vol. 2, 781-804, 1967.
66. Forte, J.G. and Wolosin, J.M.: HCL secretion by the gastric oxyntic cell. In, Physiology of the gastrointestinal Tract. Edited by L.R. Johnson, Raven Press, New York, 853-863, 1987.
67. Sachs, G.: The gastric proton pump: The H^+, K^+- ATPase. In, Physiology of the Gastrointestinal Tract. Edited by L.R. Johnson. Raven Press, New York, 865-881, 1987.
68. Soll, A.H. and Berglindh, T.: Physiology of isolated gastric glands and parietal cells: Receptors and effectors regulating function. In, Physiology of the Digestive Tract. Edited by L.R. Johnson. Raven Press, New York, 883-909, 1987.
69. Wolfe, M.M. and Soll, A.H.: The physiology of gastric acid secretion. New Eng J Med 26:1707-1715, 1988.
70. Nezamis, J.E., Robert A. and Stowe, D.F.: Inhibition by prostaglandin E of gastrin secretion in the dog. J. Physiol. (London) 218:369-383, 1971.
71. Robert, A.: Prostaglandins and the digestive system. In: Les Prostaglandins, INSERM Symposium, Paris. 297-315, 1973.
72. Konturek, S.J., Cieszkowski, M., Kwiecien, N., Konturek, J., Tasler, J. and Bilski, J.: Effects of omeprazole, a substituted benzimidazole, on gastrointestinal secretions, serum gastrin, and gastric mucosal blood flow in dogs. Gastroenterology 86:71-77, 1984.
73. Debas, H.T.: Peripheral regulation of gastric acid secretion. In, Physiology of the Gastrointestinal Tract. Edited by L.R. Johnson. Raven Press, New York, 931-945, 1987.
74. Tache, Y.: Central nervous sytem regulation of gastric acid secretion. In, Physiology of the Gastrointestinal Tract. Edited by L.R. Johnson. Raven Press, New York, 911-930, 1987.
75. MacGregor, I.L., Deveney, C., Way, L.W. and Meyer, J.H.: The effect of acute hyperglycemia on meal-stimulated gastric, biliary, and pancreatic secretion and serum gastrin. Gastroenterology 70:197-202, 1976.
76. Lenz, H.J., Klapdor, R., Hester, S.E., Webb, V.J., Galyean, R.F., Rivier, J.E. and Brown, M.R.: Inhibition of gastric acid secretion by brain peptides in the dog. Gastroenterology 91:905-912, 1986.
77. Konturek, S.J., Tasler, J., Obtulowiez, W. and Cieszkowski, M.: Comparison of amino acids bathing the oxyntic gland area in the stimulation of gastric secretion. Gastroenterology 70:66-69, 1975.
78. Konturek, S.J., Tasler, J., Cieszkowski, M. and Jaworek, J.: Comparison of intravenous amino acids in the stimulation of gastric secretion. Gastroenterology 75:817-824, 1978.
79. McArthur, K.E., Walsh, J.H. and Richardson, C.T.: Soy protein meals stimulate less gastric acid secretion and gastrin release than beef meals. Gastroenterology 95:920-926, 1988.
80. Soon-shiong, P. and Debas, H.T.: Fundic inhibition of acid secretion and gastrin release in the dog. Gastroenterology 79:867-872, 1980.
81. Pappas, T., Debas, H. and Taylor, I.: Enterogastrone-like effect of peptide PYY is vagally mediated in the dog. J. Clin. Invest. 77:49-53, 1986.
82. Rayford, P.L., Konturek, S.J. and Thompson, J.C.: Effect of duodenal fat on plasma levels of gastrin and secretin and on gastric acid responses to gastric and intestinal meals in dogs. Gastroenterology 75:773-777, 1978.
83. Wickbom, G., Landor, J.H., Bushkin, F.L. and McGuigan, J.E.: Changes in canine gastric acid output and serum gastrin levels following massive and intestinal resection. Gastroenterology 69:448-452, 1975.
84. Seal, A.M. and Debas, H.T.: Colonic inhibition of gastric acid secretion in the dog. Gastroenterology 79:823-826, 1980.
85. Flemstrom, G.: Gastric and duodenal mucosal bicarbonate secretion. In Physiology of the Gastrointestinal Tract. Edited by L.R. Johnson. Raven Press, New York, 1011-1029, 1987.
86. Silen, W.: Gastric mucosal defense and repair. In: Physiology of the Gastrointestinal Tract. Edited by L.R. Johnson. Raven Press, New York, 1055-1069, 1987.
87. Davenport, H.W.: Physiological structure of the gastric mucosa. In, Handbook of Physiology, Section 6: Alimentary Canal. Edited by C.F. Code. Washington, D.C., American Physiological Society, vol. 2, 759-779, 1967.
88. Moody, F.G., Cheung, L.Y., Simons, M.A. and Zalewsky, C.: Stress and the acute gastric mucosal lesion. Am. J. Dig. Dis. 21:148-154, 1976.
89. Miller, T.A.: Protective effects of prostaglandins against gastric mucosal damage: current knowledge and proposed mechanisms. Am. J. Physiol. 245:G601-G623, 1983.
90. Menguy, R.: Gastric mucus and the gastric mucous barrier. Amer. J. Surg. 117:806-812, 1969.
91. Patronella, C.K., Vanek, I. and Bowen, J.C.: In vivo measurement of gastric mucus pH in canines: effect of high luminal acidity and prostaglandin E_2. Gastroenterology 95:612-618, 1988.
92. Kauffman, G.L. and Davenport, H.W.: Effect of atropine in reducing plasma protein shedding by the canine oxyntic glandular mucosa induced by topical irrigation with histamine or cobra venom. Gastroenterology 69:198-199, 1975.

Chapter 11

Vomiting and Its Neural Control

Vomition is the most common cause of ejection of fluid and food from the alimentary tract through the oral cavity. Vomition is differentiated from regurgitation and gagging as described in Chapter 5 and this chapter.

MECHANICAL EVENTS DURING VOMITING[1-4]

Vomiting is a reflex act that includes anticipatory or prodromal signs. The animal senses initiation of the reflex and responds by depression and anxiety. Shivering, hiding, and seeking attention, which are often seen, can be followed by yawning and licking of the nose. Animals usually stand with their heads lowered, and hypersalivation begins. Salivation stimulates swallowing; repeated swallowing movements stimulate relaxation of the gastroesophageal sphincter in preparation for ejection of gastric contents. Retching movements begin, consisting of forceful contractions of the abdominal muscles and diaphragm, with the glottis closed and producing spasmodic respiratory movements.

Vomiting is associated with a number of motor events in the small intestine, stomach, and esophagus. An initial event is relaxation of intestinal motor activity so that motility is inhibited. That is followed by retrograde peristaltic contractions with the reverse peristalsis moving contents from the intestine into the stomach. The peristalsis is followed by a period of phasic contractions, which soon disappear, and all motility is inhibited. These reflex events in the small intestine are stimulated by chemicals such as apomorphine, that act on the chemoreceptor trigger zone and by hypertonic saline, which stimulates mucosal receptors in the small intestine. Anticholinergics inhibit the retrograde peristaltic contractions; these drugs do not interfere with any other responses in the vomiting reflex.

The reflex changes in the small intestine are followed by gastric antral contractions with no pattern and then by retrograde peristaltic contractions in the antrum. At the same time motility is inhibited in the body of the stomach, causing it to relax. The motility changes have been demonstrated with recordings of both mechanical and electrical activities in dogs.[3,5] Vagotomy, transecting nerves to the stomach and small intestine, abolishes all the gastrointestinal motor correlates of vomiting but none of the prodromal or somatomotor responses.

Coordinated with the gastric motor events is reflex relaxation of the gastroesophageal and pharyngoesophageal sphincters and of the entire esophagus. Activity in vagal nerve fibers mediates inhibition of motor activity in these structures. Anticholinergic drugs do not block the inhibitory response. To facilitate gastroesophageal sphincter relaxation, the intra-abdominal segment of the esophagus containing the gastroesophageal sphincter moves into the thoracic cavity via vagally-mediated contraction of the longitudinal muscles of the esophagus. This movement cancels the gastroesophageal sphincter's ability to prevent gastroesophageal reflux. Motility is inhibited in the circular muscles of the esophagus and the cricopharyngeal muscle fibers forming the pharyngoesophageal sphincter. As vomitus passes through the pharyngeal cavity, the orifice between it and the nasopharynx closes and the glottis closes, preventing pulmonary aspiration and nasal regurgitation. Thus, motility is inhibited throughout most of the esophagus and stomach.

The driving force for expulsion of gastric contents is contraction of the abdominal muscles and diaphragm. The force of this contraction generates enough inertia to propel the contents out from the flaccid stomach and through the esophagus and oral cavity. The small intestine and stomach do not develop pressure capable of ejecting contents from the alimentary tract.

NEURAL REFLEX OF VOMITING[1-4]

Vomiting is controlled by both the autonomic nervous system, with innervation to smooth muscle, and the central nervous system, with efferents to somatic muscles. Vomiting is still possible when autonomic control is removed, since the only influence of the control is to inhibit motility in most of the stomach and gastroesophageal sphincter and to augment motility in the antrum and cranial small intestine. Consequently, pharmacologic inhibition of the autonomic nervous system usually has little effect to inhibit vomiting. Denervation of the abdominal and diaphragmatic muscles, however, renders an animal incapable of vomiting.

Vomiting is a reflex act involving neural pathways that synapse in the medulla at the site of the vomiting center. This center contains a group of neurons associated anatomically with centers for the neural control of respiration, salivation, and swallowing. The act of vomiting is integrated with those other functions. For example, hypersalivation is a purposeful response preceding vomiting, and respiration must be inhibited during vomiting to prevent aspiration pneumonia. Stimulation of neurons in the vomiting center produces vomiting, and

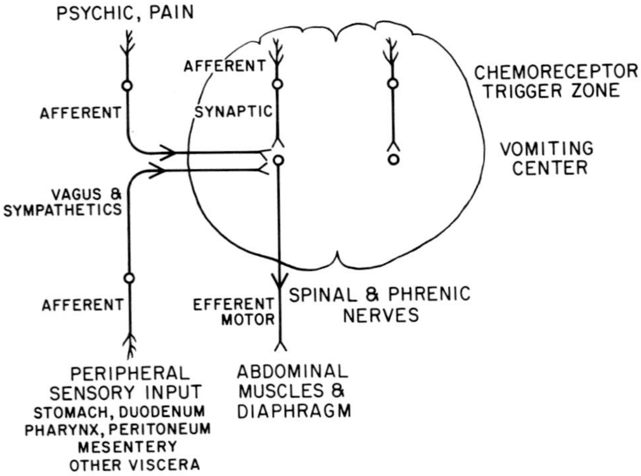

Figure 11-1. Diagrammatic cross-section of brain stem at level of the vomiting center. Afferent input is via three main pathways. Chemical interruption of the vomiting reflex is accomplished by using drugs that act at the chemoreceptor trigger zone or the vomiting center. The act of vomiting requires a normal efferent pathway in the spinal and phrenic nerves to the abdominal muscles and diaphragm.

destruction of the nuclei results in an animal that cannot vomit. The vomiting reflex is schematically represented in Figure 11-1.

Receptors and Afferent Pathways

A great number of different problems can cause vomiting (Table 5-14), which is initiated by the stimulation of receptors located throughout the body. Most of the receptors are found in the abdominal viscera. Important receptors are found in the duodenum, a structure that has been called the organ of nausea. Osmoreceptors regulate the rate at which gastric contents enter the duodenum. Rapid gastric emptying usually intensely stimulates those receptors and can cause vomiting. This normal response is to remove the stimulus, which could irritate and damage the intestinal mucosa. Acute distention or irritation of small intestinal mucosa can stimulate the vomiting reflex. Causes include acute erosions, chronic ulceration, inflammation, chemical irritation, and distention secondary to gas accumulation or obstruction. Distention of the small intestine induces vomiting more readily than distention of the stomach. Gastric foreign bodies may be long-standing and produce few clinical signs. Vomiting due to distention by obstruction is less frequent when the lesions are in the more terminal portion of the small intestine. Inflammation in other abdominal organs, such as the pancreas, also causes vomiting.

The afferent fibers for abdominal vomiting receptors are found in the vagal and sympathetic nerves. Most of the afferent fibers from the stomach and duodenum are in the vagi, and those from the remainder of the intestine are in the sympathetics.

Another type of receptor for vomiting is located on the floor of the fourth ventricle in an area known as the chemoreceptor trigger zone (Figure 11-1). It is located astride the opening of the spinal canal into the fourth ventricle. Bloodborne substances such as apomorphine and injected copper sulfate stimulate vomiting through those receptors. This center is important also for causing vomiting associated with motion sickness; many drugs, such as cardiac glycosides (Table 11-1); uremia; and possibly other metabolic diseases. A third type of reception that stimulates vomiting comes from higher centers in the central nervous system. The psychological basis for vomiting is well-established in humans. In some animals, acute stressful events can cause vomiting. Chronic stress, however, has not been proven to be a cause of persistent intermittent vomiting in animals. Stress-induced vomiting is a protective mechanism in wild animals against threats that can be escaped more easily on an empty stomach. Additionally, bitches that rear their pups under strictly defined conditions show vomiting that is considered physiological. The vomiting is described as epimeletic and is defined as care-giving behavior with the biological function of feeding the pups.[6] This behavior occurs regularly in wild animals, and there is some evidence that it can be acquired by male dogs that are quartered near pups and their nest-pen.

Table 11-1. **Emetic Agents and Their Site of Action to Stimulate Vomiting Reflex.**

Agents Acting on Chemoreceptor Trigger Zone	
Cardiac glycosides	Salicylates
Morphine, apomorphine, etc.	Serotonin
	Norepinephrine
	Histamine
Ergot alkaloids	Glutamate
Cancer chemotherapy agents	Gut peptide hormones i.e. gastrin, VIP

Vomiting Center of the Central Nervous System

Afferents from the abdominal viscera, floor of the fourth ventricle, and the higher CNS centers synapse with neurons in the vomiting center in the medulla. These neurons can be stimulated directly by certain drugs and chemicals; by toxins produced by bacteria (staphylococcal enterotoxin), uremia, hypoxia, and metabolic diseases; and by chronic disease processes via unidentified means. A tumor or inflammatory lesion in the brain stem will occasionally stimulate the vomiting center directly or through one of its afferents.

Efferent Pathways

The motor events in vomiting are mediated by activity in spinal and phrenic nerves that innervate abdominal and respiratory muscles. This innervation is essential for vomiting to occur. Activity in vagal parasympathetics (and other efferents and esophageal muscle) and splanchnic sympathetics is unessential for vomiting. These fibers mediate motility changes in the esophagus, esophageal sphincters, stomach, and duodenum during vomiting. Parasympathetic fibers to the salivary glands are responsible for hypersalivation, and some of the cranial nerves are responsible for the appropriate muscle activity in the pharynx.

PHARMACOLOGIC MANAGEMENT OF VOMITING[1-4]

Vomiting is treated with pharmacologic agents that act on one of three sites. The most effective drugs are those that inhibit neural transmission through the vomiting center (Table 11-2).[7] The phenothiazine antiemetics, drugs that are thought to act at this site, are the most consistently effective in controlling vomiting. Their antiemetic effects occur at drug levels much less than necessary to produce tranquilization. Because frequent complications with vomiting are dehydration and hypovolemia, the potential for aggravating a real or immanent hypotension should be considered in using tranquilizers. The phenothiazine antiemetics also inhibit neural activity through the chemoreceptor trigger zone and have some anticholinergic activity. Antiemetic drugs can act on the chemoreceptor trigger zone. Antihistamines inhibit vomiting by blocking at both the chemoreceptor trigger zone and the vestibular apparatus (Table 11-2). Dopaminergic antagonists such as metoclopramide also act at the chemoreceptor trigger zone to inhibit vomiting.

The cause of vomiting may influence the choice of drugs. Metoclopramide is more effective than phenothiazine antiemetics are in inhibiting vomiting from cisplatin therapy in normal dogs.[8] In clinical oncology cases, metoclopramide has not been as effective in preventing vomiting from chemotherapy drugs. Phenothiazine antiemetics are not proven to be an effective antiemetic in humans receiving chemotherapy for cancer.[9] Domperidone, a new dopaminergic antagonist, does not prevent retching from intragastric copper sulfate, but it prevents the gastrointestinal myoelectrical changes associated with vomiting.[10]

Antiemetic drugs can act on organs containing the receptors for stimuli that initiate the vomiting reflex. These drugs are effective only if they can inhibit the stimulation of the receptors. Contraction or spasm of smooth muscle in the stomach or intestines can stimulate receptors to initiate vomiting. Anticholinergics that relieve the spasms reduce the stimulus to vomit. Anticholinergics cannot effectively alter stimulation of the vomiting reflex by any other means. Drugs such as atropine are usually ineffective in controlling vomiting. Anticholinergic agents have no effect in preventing vomiting caused by gastritis or duodenitis due to either acid on gastric erosions or inflammation of the mucosa. Other agents to soothe irritated mucosal surfaces are commercially available. They include protectives, antacids, and nutrients. There is no evidence that they are effective except in a few cases of acute gastritis and duodenitis.

Table 11-2. Antiemetics Acting on Vomiting Center and Chemoreceptor Trigger Zone

Generic	Trade name
Vomiting Center and Chemoreceptor Trigger Zone	
Chlorpromazine	Thorazine
Prochlorperazine	Compazine
Thiethylperazine	Torecan
Haloperidon	Haldol
Chemoreceptor Trigger Zone	
Generic	**Trade name**
Diphenhydramine	Benadryl
Dimenhydrinate	Dramamine
Meclizine	Bonine
Trimethobenzamine	Tigan
Metoclopramide	Reglan
Fentanyl	Sublima

CAUSES OF VOMITING[1-4]

Causes of vomiting are listed in Table 5-14. The most frequent are abdominal problems that stimulate receptors in the gastrointestinal tract, liver, pancreas, urinary tract, internal genitalia, and mesentery. Inflammation of any of those organs can stimulate the vomiting reflex. Inflammation that stimulates receptors in the pharynx can also induce vomiting.

Interference with normal gastric emptying and obstruction of the intestinal tract results in vomiting. This reflex is in part stimulated by distention of the organ and irritation of its mucosa. The reflex is also stimulated by toxins absorbed from the gut above the site of obstruction that act on the central receptors to initiate vomiting. Phenothiazine antiemetics reduce vomiting caused by obstruction in the pylorus and small intestine, where anticholinergics have no effect.

Many systemic diseases can cause vomiting, including infectious diseases such as parvovirus infection, canine and feline distemper, infectious canine hepatitis, leptospirosis, salmon poisoning, and a host of others. Vomiting in these cases is stimulated primarily through central receptors. Congestive heart failure can produce vomiting when the effects of circulatory impairment result in altered gastrointestinal and hepatic function. Vomiting is often aggravated if the problem is managed with cardiac glycosides, which can stimulate vomiting through both central and peripheral receptors. Fluid and electrolyte imbalances are frequently a factor in the persistence of vomiting. Acidosis as seen in renal disease and diabetes is associated with vomiting. Depletion of body potassium contributes to a loss of normal gastrointestinal motility, often resulting in overgrowth of the normal bacterial microflora and the production of absorbable toxins. Thus, vomiting can be secondary to excessive loss of potassium. Hyponatremia and hypercalcemia can also cause vomiting.

Endocrine imbalances cause vomiting indirectly by metabolic changes and directly by altered hormone levels. Adrenocortical insufficiency results in hyponatremia and hyperkalemia; the altered ratio of these ions causes vomiting that is probably mediated through central receptors. Diabetes mellitus, producing a ketoacidosis with electrolyte imbalances, frequently causes vomiting. Administration of estrogens and changes in endogenous sex endocrine levels may also cause vomiting.

Diseases of the central nervous system can stimulate vomiting. Examples include increased intracranial pressure associated with tumors, infections, inflammation, hemorrhage, edema, and impaired circulation of the cerebrospinal fluid. Tumors in the brain stem can cause vomiting without increasing CSF pressure. Vestibular disturbances stimulate vomiting; the stimuli originates in the utricular maculae of the labyrinth and is transmitted by the auditory nerve of the vestibular nuclei to the uvula and nodulus of the cerebellum, and thence to the chemoreceptor trigger zone.

In addition to endogenous metabolites that act as toxins, many drugs, chemicals, and bacterial toxins stimulate the chemoreceptor trigger zone to cause vomiting. Some are listed in Table 11-1.

Psychogenic causes of vomiting may be important in some animals. Vomiting induced by pain can be due to a reflex through the thalamus. Such reflexes can be facilitated by a psychogenic factor originating from a higher CNS center. Trauma and shock frequently cause vomiting by stimulation through multiple afferent pathways.

DIFFERENTIATION OF VOMITING AND REGURGITATION

Regurgitation, like vomiting, is the ejection of previously swallowed material from the oral cavity. It differs in that a neural reflex is not needed to produce the event. Regurgitation is the movement of food or fluid from either the esophagus or stomach as the result of gravity or passive changes in intrathoracic or intra-abdominal pressure. That can be caused by changes in the animal's body position and can result also from increases in intra-abdominal pressure incidental to exercise, barking, strenuous abdominal breathing, etc. Regurgitation occurs because the esophagus is unable to move a bolus of food or liquids completely into the stomach. Regurgitation also occurs if the gastroesophageal sphincter is incompetent. In this case there is no sphincter to prevent the reflux of gastric contents into the esophagus, and either gravity or increases in intra-abdominal pressure can cause the contents to be lost through the oral cavity. Since reflux is not found very often in small animals, regurgitation of food is most likely to be from the esophagus, not the stomach. Regurgitation is a normal event in the very young animal, since the gastroesophageal sphincter is not developed sufficiently to be competent at birth.

Vomiting is always associated with antecedent events such as salivation, retching, shivering, etc., and the ejection of food is the result of repeated contractions of abdominal muscles, which can be seen by the observer. Regurgitation is not preceded by any associated signs, and it occurs as an almost immediate response to changes in body position, exercise, barking, etc. It is not produced by a pattern of repeated contractions of the abdominal muscles. The first step in assessment of a problem involving the ejection of swallowed food is to determine whether the animal is vomiting or regurgitating. That can usually be determined by obtaining a good history; observation of the animal at eating often gives more information than any subsequently conducted laboratory studies.

Sometimes it is difficult to differentiate vomiting from regurgitation, possibly because an animal exhibits both forms of behavior. It is possible that there may not be a very distinct difference between the physiology of vomiting and regurgitation. Clinical evidence for that is found in animals that show some prodromal signs of vomiting while they are regurgitating, as some studies prove when a problem such as megaesophagus is found. Experimental studies in dogs show that regurgitation with no evidence for vomiting is associated with propagation of retrograde peristaltic contractions.[3] Thus, regurgitation may not be merely a passive event but may be associated at times with prodromal signs such as salivation and physiological events such as reverse peristalsis in the antrum and intestine, both of which are responses in a neural reflex.

REFERENCES

1. Code, D.F., and Schlegel, J.F.: Motor action of the esophagus and its sphincters. In, Handbook of Physiology, Section 6: Alimentary canal, Edited by C.F. Code. Vol. 4, p. 13, 1821-1839. Washington, D.C., American Physiological Society, 1968.
2. Daniel, E.E. Pharmacology of the gastrointestinal tract. In, Handbook of Physiology, Section 6: Alimentary canal, Edited by C.F. Code. Vol. 4, 2267-2324. Washington, D.C., American Physiological Society, 1968.
3. Lang, I.M., Sarna, S.K. and Condon, R.E.: Gastrointestinal motor correlates of vomiting in the dog: Quantification and characterization as an independent phenomenon. Gastroenterology 90:40-47, 1986.
4. Thompson, D.G. and Malagelada, J.-R: Vomiting and the small intestine. Dig. Dis. Sci. 27:1121-1125, 1982.
5. Lang, I.M., Marvig, J., Srana, S.K. and Condon, R.E.: Gastrointestinal myoelectric correlates of vomiting in the dog. Am. J. Physiol. 251:G83-G838, 1986.
6. Korda, P. Epimeletic (care giving) Vomiting in dogs: a study of the determining factors. Acta Neurobiol. Exp. 34:277-300, 1974.
7. DeNovo, R.C.: Therapeutics of gastrointestinal diseases. In, Current Veterinary Therapy IX Small Animal Practice. Edited by R.W. Kirk. 862-872. W.B. Saunders, Philadelphia, 1986.
8. Gylys, J.A., Dorna, K.M. and Buyniski, J.P.: Antagonism of cisplatin induced emesis in the dog. Res. Comm. Chem. Pathol. Pharmacol. 23:61-68, 1979.
9. Laszlo, J.: Emesis as a critical problem in chemotherapy. New Eng. J. Med. 305:949-949, 1981.
10. Lee, K.Y., Park, H.J. and Chey, W.Y.: Studies on mechanism of retching and vomiting in dogs. Dig. Dis. Sci. 30:22-28, 1985.

mucosal lesions requires altered flow of mucosal blood.[26] Circulatory changes produce erosions found at points of mucosal ischemia. Any systemic problem that reduces gastric mucosal blood flow can contribute to ulceration, the most common causes being trauma and many severe diseases. In experimental animals, hypovolemia or endotoxic shock produces acute gastric lesions by reducing mucosal blood flow.[26]

Increased sympathetic nerve activity and humoral agents mediate reduction of mucosal blood flow. Stress-augmented nerve activity decreases gastric acid secretion in addition to reducing blood flow. Mucosal erosion and ulceration cannot develop without normal gastric acid secretion. Gastric lesions are probably produced only when reduced blood flow follows normal secretion of acid, or when acid secretion is stimulated after ischemia and before mucosal recovery.

Humoral agents can augment the effects of sympathetic activity to the point that ulcers result. Catecholamines produce gastric ulcers in dogs in part by reducing mucosal blood flow.[27] Catecholamines also stimulate histamine release, which stimulates acid secretion and contributes to erosions. Prior depletion of histamine makes it difficult to produce stress ulcers experimentally. Histamine produces ulcers in unstressed animals.[28] Serotonin, a vasoactive amine found in gastric mucosa, and vasopressin released during shock may play a role in reducing mucosal blood flow.

Sympathetic activity and humoral vasoconstrictors do not reduce blood flow uniformly throughout the different layers of the mucosa; instead, they produce focal areas of ischemia.[29] Autoregulation and shunting of blood attempts to maintain normal mucosal blood flow at the expense of flow in all other layers. Since some regions are unable to respond adequately to the neural and humoral influences, mucosal flow is reduced and the regions become ischemic. With normal mucosal blood flow, the back-diffusing hydrogen ions are removed instead of accumulating and damaging the mucosa. With ischemia, hydrogen ions back-diffuse in normal amounts, but their accumulation damages cells since circulation is reduced. Ischemia or low plasma bicarbonate reduces the delivery of bicarbonate to mucosal cells and the mucus protective layer. Loss of that bicarbonate results in an intracellular acidosis; that is magnified by an increased back-diffusion of hydrogen ions when less bicarbonate is secreted into the mucus layer. During acid secretion it is essential that circulation is normal so that bicarbonate formed in oxyntic cells during hydrogen secretion is available to be transported to surface mucosal cells for maintenance of the mucus buffering layer. Acid in the stomach without a normal circulation for that delivery results in mucosal ulceration (see Chapter 10).

Overall blood flow increases following gastric mucosal injury and is most likely a response to the injury rather than to the agent causing the injury.[30] Prostaglandin release stimulates the increased flow, an important response because the mucosal damage is likely to stimulate release of leukotrienes, which are potent vasoconstrictors. Any drugs reducing prostaglandin release without any effects on leukotriene synthesis are certain to cause mucosal ulceration.

Disseminated intravascular coagulation initiated by different problems can reduce gastric mucosal blood flow. Vascular thrombosis can result in ulceration of the mucosa. Ulceration can be severe and complicate the bleeding disorder, producing severe gastrointestinal hemorrhage. Gastric bleeding associated with low platelet numbers and low fibrinogen levels is suggestive of disseminated intravascular coagulation. Hepatic failure can contribute to gastric bleeding by causing disseminated intravascular coagulation and a deficiency of clotting factors. Hepatic disease can also increase the risk for bleeding by causing changes in capillaries. Most humans with cirrhosis develop capillary ectasia, an increase in capillary size that predisposes to bleeding.[31]

Infections cause stress ulceration by an unknown mechanism.[32] But infections can reduce mucosal circulation, increase acid and pepsin secretion, and reduce the effectiveness of the mucous barrier. Infected emboli may play a role, and the sepsis may initiate disseminated intravascular coagulation.

Gastric Mucosal Surface Factors.[33-35] *Mucus.* A thin layer of mucus gel covers the entire gastric mucosa. It is a viscous gel by virtue of its consisting of large glycoprotein polymers. Protection is maintained unless the coating is lost or is disrupted by proteolytic enzymes or sulfhydryl containing chemicals. The gel holds water in a very structured form and also contains bicarbonate, both of which minimize the movement of hydrogen ions into mucosal surface cells. In addition to pepsin, nonsteroidal inflammatory drugs and bile acids degrade the mucosal layer. Prostaglandins, acetylcholine and carbenoxolone stimulate mucus production; inhibitors are nonsteroidal inflammatory drugs, salicylates, cortisone, and ACTH. If the protective layer of mucus on the gastric mucosa is lost, ulcers can develop. Pepsin can digest the gastric mucosa when the mucous coating is lost. Sulfated gastric mucins are normally bound to the epithelial cells. An initial event during focal mucosal ischemia is complete disgorgement of mucous cells, leaving empty cells a vulnerable point for pepsin activity.[26] Sulfated glycopeptides bind pepsin, preventing ulcer formation in experimental animals.[36]

Bicarbonate Secretion.[33] Small amounts of bicarbonate are secreted into the mucus layer by mucosal surface cells and contribute to the cytoprotection. The bicarbonate secretion depends on adequate bicarbonate supplied from oxyntic cell metabolism and from plasma bicarbonate. Reduction of bicarbonate availability is possible with drugs such as carbonic anhydrase inhibitors (acetazolamide), anticholinergics, and nonsteroidal antiinflammatory agents; chemicals such as bile acids; and low plasma bicarbonate. Thus, acidosis creates a high risk for ulceration and is certainly involved in the pathogenesis of gastric lesions in dogs with shock or renal failure. Bicarbonate secretion is stimulated by calcium, some prostaglandins, and drugs such as sucralfate that stimulate prostaglandin secretion. As stated earlier, adequate mucosal circulation is essential to bicarbonate secretion sufficient to maintain the barrier.

Duodenal contents. Duodenal contents refluxed into the stomach and containing both bile and pancreatic juices produce gastritis and can cause ulceration.[34] Bile is more destructive than pancreatic juices. Duodenal reflux contributes to the pathogenesis of some stress-induced ulcers. Shock-induced gastric ulcers in dogs are associated with increased reflux of bile into the stomach.[35] Mucosal ulceration produced by drugs such as aspirin requires bile in the stomach.[36] Bile-duct ligation prevents aspirin-induced ulcer formation. Carbenoxolone and amylopectin sulfate[37] protect against the ulcerogenic effects of bile. Explanations for their effect are either binding and inactivation of bile, or inactivation of pepsin activity, which may be required for the ulcerative effect of bile. Gastric bile concentrations are greatest in the antrum, the region with the greatest incidence of gastric ulcers. Pepsinogen and gastrin[38] are released, exacerbating the pathology.

Bile acids increase the permeability of the mucosal barrier to hydrogen ions (but not to sodium ions) which contributes to breaking the barrier.[39] Bile acids damage the gastric mucosa after entering the cells. Diffusion into the cell is greatest at a low pH. The pKa of bile acids is around 4, so that the ionized form prevails at a higher gastric pH. At a pH lower than 4, bile acids are largely un-ionized, and, being lipid soluble, they can enter cells with ease. Bile acids are detergents that solubilize lipid cell membranes and can inhibit ion transport systems.

Bile damages the mucosal barrier so that diffusion increases for hydrogen and sodium ions in the canine stomach.[40] Bile causes dissolution of mucosal membrane lipids. Diversion of bile into the canine stomach causes histologic changes that include mucus depletion and epithelial cell degeneration within three months and mucosal atrophy at six months.[41] Reduction in acid secretion follows the degenerative and atrophic changes.

Duodenal contents also contain lysolecithin, which is produced by pancreatic phospholipase activity on lecithin in bile. Lysolecithin is a potent membrane-toxic phospholipid. Lysolecithin interacts with canine gastric mucosa at either acidic or pH neutral solutions and increases membrane permeability for hydrogen and sodium ions.[42] Lysolecithin does not enter membranes to cause damage but dissolves and removes membrane lecithin and possibly cholesterol to form intraluminal micelles.

Despite the studies showing damaging effects of bile and lysolecithin on gastric mucosa, it is not clear whether duodenogastric reflux can cause gastritis in dogs and cats. Dogs surgically altered to have chronic duodenogastric reflux do not develop any significant lesions in the antral mucosa.[43] With reflux of bile only, fundic mucosal changes are seen.[44] They include severe hyperemia and foveolar hyperplasia.[45] Isolated pancreatic juice reflux produces similar but milder changes. Surprisingly, diversion of bile from the duodenum of dogs results in changes predisposing to duodenal ulceration.[46] The changes include increased gastric acid secretion, increased plasma gastrin levels, reduced CCK levels and pancreatic enzyme secretion, and lower pH of duodenal contents. This suggests that bile is protective, probably because of its rich bicarbonate content. The gastroduodenal mucosa also secretes bicarbonate; the duodenal secretory capability is five times that for the stomach.[47] Constituents in bile and some hormones may be lacking to stimulate duodenal mucosal bicarbonate secretion in bile diverted dogs. Endogenous prostaglandins are important for stimulating duodenal bicarbonate secretion.[48] In summary, it appears that bile acids and lysolecithin can damage gastric mucosa but in the fundus primarily; the alkaline pH of refluxed fluid protects against that effect. Bile without acid does not damage gastric mucosa. When reflux excessively increases pH in the fasting stomach, the numbers of bacteria can increase.[49] It is not known how that might contribute to damage of the mucosa.

Gastroduodenal Reflux. Bile-stained vomitus, a frequent finding with gastritis, signifies gastroduodenal reflux of bile. As described in Chapter 10, some reflux of duodenal contents is normal in dogs and probably the cat also. The pylorus participates in the prevention of gastroduodenal reflux.[50] Its role is probably of lesser importance than other factors, however, since it is a functionally passive sphincter. Since the normal sphincter does not show tonic contractions in the fasting state, it remains open, providing no resistance to reflux. The lack of effect on gastric emptying of liquids when the pylorus is replaced by a plastic tube further illustrates the pylorus' passive nature.[51] Antral mucosa sliding into the pylorus contributes to sphincter competence, but that occurs only during meals. The length of the pyloric sphincter may be important in preventing reflux.

Prevention of reflux is the net effect of forces promoting gastric emptying and those in the duodenum promoting reflux. The gastric pacesetter potential slow wave (or electrical-control activity) has a frequency of five cycles per minute, and the slow waves pass over the antrum at the rate of 40 mm per second. The frequency of slow waves in the duodenum is eleven cycles per minute, with a speed of 200 mm per second. Propagations in both organs are always in the caudal direction. Stimulation of the distal duodenum, at rates exceeding the frequency of the inherent electrical-control activity, causes caudally-moving slow waves to increase to the imposed frequency. Waves moving cranially, which cause reflux of duodenal contents into the antrum are also initiated.[52] Slow wave activity can be modified (Chapter 1 and 10), and it is possible that disease can be a modifier to cause duodenal-gastric reflux in dogs with gastritis and vomiting bile. Anomalies of slow wave activity may be a factor in some cases of gastric ulcer formation. Inhibition of forces promoting gastric emptying include increased activity in some neural pathways which reduce antral motility; antral motility may be reduced to the extent that reflux readily occurs. Excessive secretion of gut hormones that inhibit antral motility would have the same effect. Anticholinergic drugs also reduce antral motility, which could contribute to gastroduodenal reflux.

Reflux of duodenal fluid is greater in fed than unfed animals, but the effects may be more important in unfed animals because no food is present to dilute or buffer the effects of duodenal fluid in the stomach. Fluid refluxing into the stomach of unfed animals is likely to remain until cleared by interdigestive migrating motility complexes (IDMC). Clearing of the stomach is due to phase III of the IDMC, strong peristaltic contractions of the antrum appearing once every 1.5 hours and lasting five to six minutes. Thus, duodenal contents can remain in the stomach for long periods of time. Drugs reducing antral motility (such as anticholinergics) can increase the amount of refluxed fluid and the time it remains in the stomach. Other drugs such as aspirin and even prostaglandins, with cytoprotective effects can disrupt IDMC so that phase III contractions become abnormal and the stomach is not cleared of refluxed fluid.[53] Cholecystectomy also increases duodenogastric reflux in dogs for unknown reasons; gastritis is associated with that reflux.[54]

Renal Disease

Gastric erosions and ulcers are common in patients with chronic renal disease. It has been thought that high gastric ammonia levels are responsible.[55] The ammonia is produced from urea following diffusion of urea from interstitial fluid into the stomach, where ureases convert it to ammonia. Urease sources are bacteria and gastric mucosal cells. The ammonia produced is suggested to reach levels that are toxic to the mucosal cells. Stomatitis accompanying uremia is proposed to have a similar pathogenesis.

Hypersecretion of gastric acid appears to be the most important factor in the pathogenesis of gastric lesions with renal disease. The stimulus for the hypersecretion is increased blood levels of gastrin. With chronic renal disease or following bilateral nephrectomy, gastrin is not effectively removed, leading to increased levels in the blood.[56] The kidney is an important site for degradation of peptide hormones, including gastrin. Impaired renal function leads to hypergastrinemia and hypersecretion of gastric acid. The increment of acid secretion is comparable to that produced by gastrin-secreting tumors, which are consistent producers of gastritis, upper gastrointestinal bleeding, and duodenal ulceration. Chronic renal disease can also produce hyperphosphatemia, due to decreased phosphate excretion. Secondary hyperparathyroidism develops and mobilizes calcium from bone, with calcium nephropathy developing. Calcium also precipitates in the stomach, where mineralization is a frequent finding in animals with chronic renal failure (Figure 12-3).

High concentrations of calcium ions do not remain in solution when present as a salt of phosphate. Higher concentrations of the salt are soluble at a lower pH. During secretion of hydrochloric acid, bicarbonate formed in the oxyntic cell diffuses into the interstitial fluid, making it more alkaline. With calcium phosphate in solution at a supersaturated level, the increase in pH causes precipitation, resulting in mineralization. Uremic gastropathy is a disease with lesions primarily in the mucosal lamina propria. The lesions can be attributed to anoxia caused by diffuse vascular injury and to altered oxyntic cell function. Eventually the gastric glands atrophy.[57]

Hepatic Disease

Acute and chronic hepatic disease can cause lesions in the gastric mucosa.[25,58] In acute hepatitis the gastric lesions are due primarily to bleeding disorders that are often complicated and difficult to resolve.[59] The mucosal lesions are secondary to reduced blood flow, usually the result of a thrombosis caused by disseminated intravascular coagulation. The liver is rich in thromboplastin, which is released during acute hepatitis and causes disseminated intravascular coagulation. Thromboplastin initiates the clotting cascade, causing widespread thrombosis and resultant gastric erosion and ulceration.

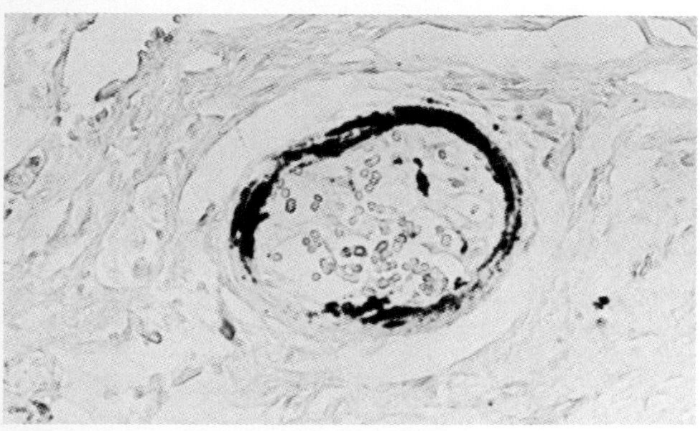

Figure 12-3. Photomicrograph of blood vessel in gastric submucosa from dog with uremic gastritis. Calcium stain outlines deposits in vessel wall.

The liver synthesizes most of the blood-clotting factors.[59] Acute hepatitis can result in factor deficiencies, especially of those with the shortest half-lives. Such could be a factor in hepatitis-induced disseminated intravascular coagulation. The liver also removes fibrin degradation products and some of the circulating anticoagulants.[59] The loss of these functions with hepatic disease may contribute to gastrointestinal bleeding.

Chronic liver disease can cause gastric lesions. They are produced both as the result of the liver's failure to remove gastrin and histamine in the portal circulation and from the effects of hepatic disease on blood flow through the stomach. Dogs with hepatic cirrhosis secrete more gastric hydrochloric acid after the portal circulation is partially shunted around the liver.[60] Blood levels of histamine and gastrin increase after the shunting, contributing to the effect. As described earlier, mucosal circulation is also abnormal because of changes in capillary size.

Mastocytosis

Histamine, produced by mast cells, is released in large quantities in systemic mastocytosis, producing gastric lesions. Although it has not been verified that acid hypersecretion occurs in small animals with mastocytosis, it has been shown that some humans with mastocytosis secrete excessive amounts of gastric hydrochloric acid. Histamine affects smooth muscle function in the same way as do other biogenic amines. Thus, some of the clinical signs in patients with mastocytosis are related to motility alterations as well as to mucosal lesions.

Infectious Diseases, Sepsis and Stress

Many physiologic and pathologic changes contribute to gastric lesions in animals with generalized infections and with sepsis. Some of the changes are responses to stress, while others are due to chemical changes from the infection or endotoxemia. In dogs, sepsis stimulates gastric acid secretion, which can be controlled with cimetidine.[61] Stress of any form stimulates catecholamine release, which causes splanchnic vasoconstriction. The body and fundus are especially vulnerable; they are susceptible to microcirculatory compromise leading to ischemia and hypoxia. The result is increased mucosal membrane permeability, increased hydrogen ion back-diffusion, histamine release, increased capillary permeability, edema, protein loss, and hemorrhage. Part of the animal's stress response is protective to gastric mucosa. Glucocorticoids are necessary for that cytoprotection; without glucocorticoid secretion neither cimetidine nor prostaglandins protect against aspirin damage to the mucosa.[62] Dogs with gastritis and vomiting because of either adrenocortical insufficiency or selective glucocorticoid deficiency should not respond to usual therapy for the upper gastrointestinal signs until glucocorticoids are given. The development of stress-induced lesions also involves changes in plasma levels of peptide and other hormones that stimulate or inhibit gastric acid secretion. Stress induced by hypothermia or restraint can change mucosal blood flow and stimulate gastric acid secretion and motility. In general, any form of stress that compromises mucosal blood flow predisposes to gastric ulceration; thus, many circulatory problems can be a cause. With severe ischemia, oxygen-derived free radicals appear to be important in the development of lesions. In cats with ischemia, treatment with allopurinol, superoxide dismutase, and dimethyl sulfoxide markedly reduces red blood cell loss across the gastric mucosa.[63] Superoxide radicals contribute to mucosal lesions as well as to capillary damage.[64]

Following injury, mucosal surface cells are replaced rapidly even when the luminal pH is very low (see Chapter 10).[65] A response to superficial damage of the gastric mucosa is rapid exfoliation of surface epithelial cells and the release of mucus and plasma. The cells, mucus, and fibrin from plasma fibrinogen form a cap over the site of damage. The cap is protective in that removal of the cap inhibits the rapid repair that is usually seen.[19] Antimicrobial immunologic defense mechanisms that protect the gastric mucosa also determine the rate of recovery from injury.[66] Antibiotics prevent gastric mucosal injury or hasten its recovery in some situations.

CLINICAL FINDINGS

Primary Sign

Vomiting. Vomiting, a consistent sign of acute gastritis, usually follows soon after drinking or eating. It is less frequent when the patient is given nothing to drink or to eat. The vomitus usually contains mucus, and it is often bile-stained. Small amounts of blood are often seen.

Secondary Signs

Anorexia and Depression. Acute gastritis usually causes complete anorexia and depression to varied degrees. **Pain**. Evidence of abdominal pain is variable. Abdominal pain is not pathognomonic for either gastritis or pancreatitis. Abdominal distention or assumption of a praying position is sometimes the manifestation of abdominal pain. **Borborygmus**. Abdominal sounds frequently increase, especially before the onset of vomiting. Abdominal sounds are dependent on motility in the stomach and large intestine. Few sounds are heard when acute gastritis has inhibited gastric motility. **Halitosis**. A frequent finding with acute gastritis is objectionable odors from the oral cavity that are intermittent and cannot be attributed to dental disease. **Shivering**. Distention and spasms of gastrointestinal smooth muscle are the most common cause of shivering. This sign, usually preceding vomiting, may cease when gastrointestinal motility is reduced to below normal. **Polydipsia**. Vomiting animals usually crave water, although little of the intake is retained. Such dogs often demand water from their caretakers. **Fever**. Elevated body temperature is infrequent with primary acute gastritis. Fevers are seen with gastritis due to one of the infectious diseases.

Physical Signs

Examination of the patient with acute gastritis usually yields unremarkable findings. It is imperative that the oral cavity and pharynx be examined, especially for foreign bodies and inflammatory lesions. The abdominal cavity should be thoroughly palpated, which is possible in most cases. The stomach is situated too far cranially to be palpated. The patient's fluid balance is estimated by skin turgor, pulse rate and character, and dryness of oral mucous membranes.

LABORATORY FINDINGS

Laboratory tests are called for if the causes appear to be extragastric. Determination of plasma lipase activity can assist in ruling out pancreatitis. Hepatic disease can be ruled out by measurements of blood chemistries including plasma alanine aminotransferase activity, sulfobromophthalein retention time, and blood ammonia concentration. Evaluation of acute renal disease requires urinalysis and determination of blood urea nitrogen. Hemograms are usually unremarkable, being of greatest value for identifying fluid imbalances that are not readily apparent. For example, the hematocrit and plasma proteins increase in dehydrated hypovolemic animals.

RADIOGRAPHIC FINDINGS

Radiographic procedures are used most often to rule out a foreign body as the cause of the gastritis. Radiographic evaluation of the stomach is unremarkable with gastritis. In addition, gastric ulceration is difficult to identify even with contrast studies. Obviously, radiopaque foreign bodies are readily iden-

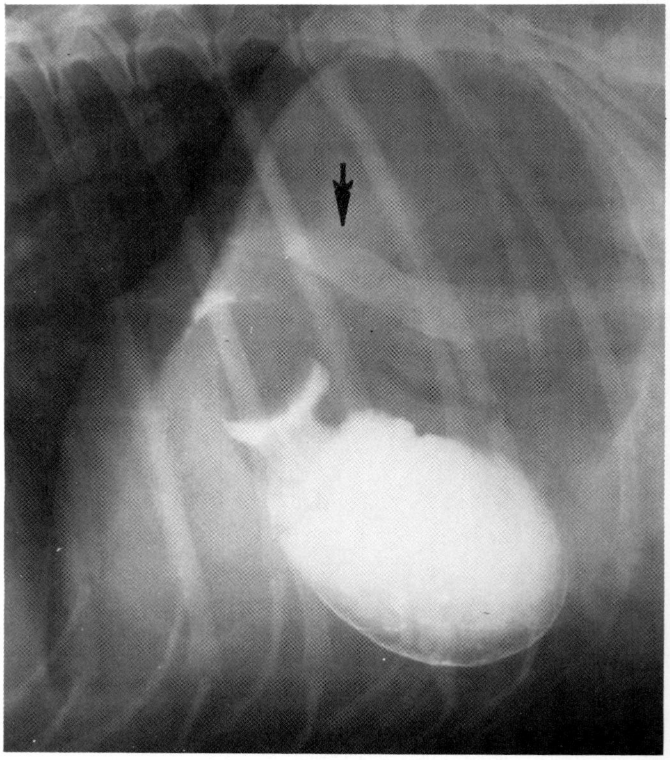

Figure 12-4a. Lateral radiograph of abdomen of Sheltie with clinical signs of intestinal obstruction. Positive contrast medium was given and appears in the caudal or distal part of the stomach. The pyloric antrum contains a filling defect that has a smooth circular outline, the shape of a ball. A minimal amount of the contrast is seen in the first part of the duodenum (arrows) which suggests that the gastric outlet obstruction is not complete. The dog was induced to vomit a rubber ball

tified. Radiolucent foreign bodies will usually be recognized only with either positive or negative contrast (Figure 12-4).

BIOPSY AND PATHOLOGY FINDINGS

The gastric mucosa is seldom biopsied in animals with acute gastritis. Changes are characterized by necrosis and hemorrhage (Figure 12-5).

DIAGNOSIS

The diagnosis of acute gastritis is suggested by the clinical findings. Recognition that acute gastritis is frequently seen compared with other causes of vomiting justifies treating the problem symptomatically, which is done most often. A complete remission of signs can be used to confirm the diagnosis. The laboratory aids are used for further evaluation of patients that do not respond to treatment or show clinical findings suggesting another problem.

A diagnosis of major gastric hemorrhage is sometimes difficult to confirm. Gastrointestinal hemorrhages are almost always in the stomach or large intestine. Gastric bleeding is manifested by bloody vomitus and melena. Colonic blood loss is recognized due to bloody feces. Sometimes it is difficult to identify the gastrointestinal tract as the site of major blood loss. Radiographic evaluation is of little value unless a major gastric ulcer can be identified. Endoscopy is of more help than other procedures in locating bleeding lesions. Gastroscopy is performed under anesthesia, and some of these patients are poor anesthetic risks.

MANAGEMENT OF ACUTE GASTRIC LESIONS

The treatment of acute gastric lesions is based on specific goals to correct specific problems. In general, the best treatment is none, including not feeding the patient, and most patients will recover. The theoretical goals in treating acute gastric lesions are to rest the organ; prevent infection; prevent vomiting; minimize pain; relieve gastric smooth-muscle spasm; neutralize the effects of hydrochloric acid, pepsin, and bile acids on the mucosa; protect the mucosa; minimize duodenogastric reflux of duodenal contents (if possible); control hemorrhage; replace fluid and blood losses; and treat inflammatory processes. Additional treatment includes correction of a primary contributing problem in another organ.

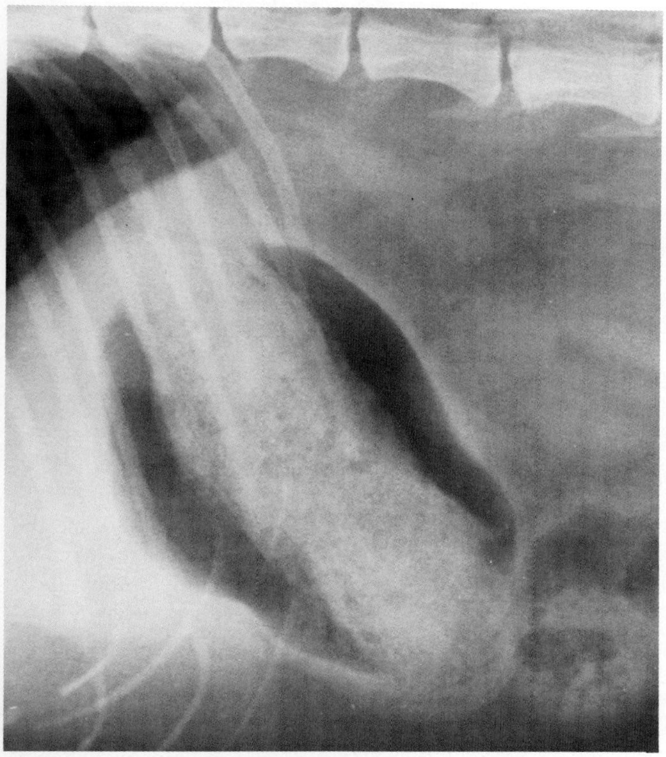

Figure 12-4b. Lateral radiograph of abdomen of 7-year-old cat. Stomach is in its normal position and contains an intraluminal mass. Radiographic density is that of fluid rather than bone or metal. Gastric wall is of normal thickness so there is probably no mural involvement. Most likely diagnosis is gastric foreign body, probably a hairball. This case shows the advantage of using air as a contrasting agent.

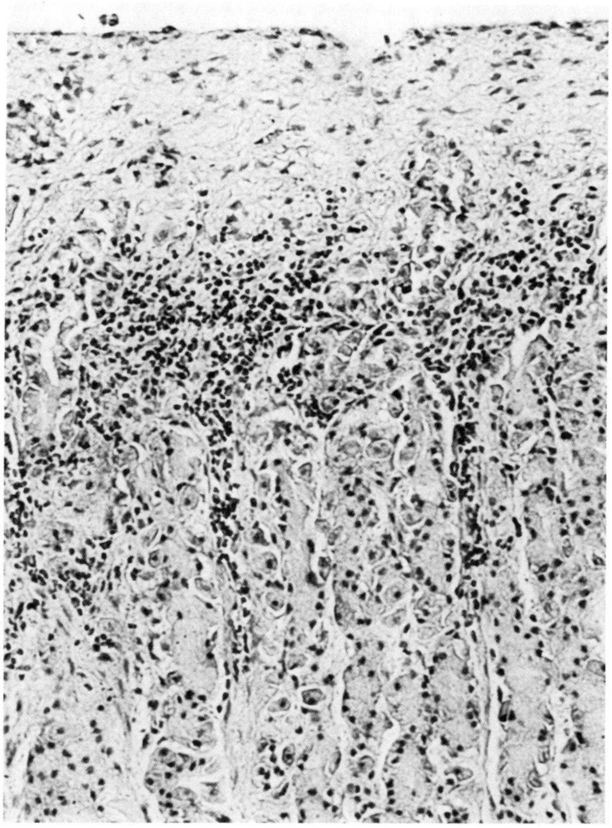

Figure 12-5. Photomicrograph of gastric mucosa from dog with signs of gastritis. Cells in luminal one-third are necrotic. Hemorrhage is evident in middle section, especially at border between necrotic cells and viable cells.

Dietary Management

The stomach has the function of serving as a reservoir for food, secreting digestive juices, and moving the contents in the aboral direction. The stomach with acute mucosal lesions must be relieved of those functions. That can only be accomplished by not feeding. Gastric distention by liquids or food stimulates motility, increasing abrasion of the mucosal surface. That accelerates mucosal cell exfoliation in the normal stomach, and the turnover rate is greater with gastritis. Gastric distention also stimulates secretion of hydrochloric acid by both neural and endocrine pathways, increasing the amount of acid available for back diffusion. That damages the gastric mucosa further. Gastric distention does not normally stimulate the vomiting reflex, but acute mucosal lesions cause the threshold to decrease, so that small increments for distention result in vomiting. Thus, in acute gastritis the reservoir function operates improperly since the animal vomits everything that is consumed. Hydrochloric acid secretion causes more pathology, and augmented motility causes abrasion and accelerated breakdown of mucosal surfaces. The most important treatment for acute mucosal lesions is to give nothing by the oral route. An exception is to provide ice cubes to lick, which usually alleviates the owner's concern over the animal's thirst.

On resumption of feeding, proper selection of foods minimizes the probability of relapse. The resting of the stomach is continued by feeding small meals frequently. Foods low in fiber are used since they are less abrasive on the mucosa. Nutrients with minimal ability to stimulate secretion of gastric juices are selected. Foods are selected which do not delay gastric emptying, since gastric retention can cause gastritis without any other factors involved. Nutrients are not to be fed in a form hypertonic with respect to extracellular fluid water.

Carbohydrates stimulate the secretion of gastric juices less than do other nutrients. Isotonicity is easier to maintain in the stomach when the form of carbohydrate fed is starch rather than mono- or disaccharides. An easily digested starch (such as rice) is used, rather than a sugar solution. Glucose solutions can be the first food given if they do not have more than twice the isotonicity of plasma (10% glucose). Feeding monosaccharides has the advantage of stimulating release of gastric inhibitory polypeptide, a hormone that inhibits the secretion of gastric acid. Disaccharides are not used, since many patients with gastritis also have an enteritis with loss of the enzymes (disaccharidases) that convert these sugars to monosaccharides. Protein intake should be resumed gradually since amino acids are the most potent stimulators of gastric acid secretion. This secretion is mediated by gastrin release, which also functions to delay gastric emptying, an undesirable effect. Since dietary fat also delays gastric emptying, it should not be fed. In summary, the diet should consist of easily digested carbohydrates and a small amount of a protein that is low in fat. When proteins are included in the diet, vegetable or milk protein may be better than meat protein. Acid secretion is 30% to 40% less in humans fed soy protein than in those fed beef protein.[67] In addition, soy protein causes gastrin release that is 65% to 75% less than with meat protein.

Table 12-5. Drugs Inhibiting Gastric Acid Secretion

Drug	Dosage for dogs (D) and cats (C)
Cimetidine (Tagamet)	5 to 10 mg/kg PO Tid or Qid (D,C) 10 mg/kg slow IV infusion over 30 min.
Ranitidine (Zantac)	1.1 to 4.4 mg/kg PO Bid (D)
Famotidine (Pepcid)	0.3 to 0.6 mg/kg PO Bid or Tid (D)*
Misoprostol (Cytotec)	Available in 100 μgm tablets* For humans
Omeprazole (Losec)	1 to 2 mg/kg PO (D)*

*Dose established in experimental dogs

Gastric Secretion of Acid[68,69]

Secretion of hydrochloric acid perpetuates acute mucosal lesions. Acid is also required for new lesions to develop. Acid secretion is minimized by giving nothing orally. Drugs can also inhibit gastric acid secretion (Table 12-5). Receptor antagonists can be given that block the interaction of secretagogues with their receptors. They include anticholinergics, H_2-receptor antagonists, and non-peptide gastrin antagonists. Other drugs such as prostaglandins and calcium channel antagonists act within oxyntic cells or on cell membranes to inhibit hydrogen ion secretion. A third type of drug, substituted benzimidazoles such as omeprazole, inhibits the ATPase mechanism for secreting hydrogen ions across the apical oxyntic cell membrane. All of these except the gastrin antagonists currently have the potential for being useful drugs. Proglumide, a gastrin antagonist, does not have sufficient potency to be useful.

Anticholinergics. Anticholinergic drugs can be used to block the neural mechanisms that stimulate secretion. It is questionable whether anticholinergics significantly reduce basal levels of acid secretion in the animal with acute gastritis. Cholinergic pathways are important for gastric acid secretion, but they carry no activity to stimulate secretion in the resting stomach. In gastritis, acid secretion is stimulated by back-diffusing acid that acts directly on intrinsic ganglia cells and on mast cells to release histamine, both of which stimulate the oxyntic cell. Anticholinergics have some effect in reducing basal secretion since they are able to interfere with function at acetylcholine receptors on the oxyntic cell. However, anticholinergics also have important effects on motility that delay gastric emptying. Retained gastric contents distend the gastric antrum and stimulate gastrin release, which stimulates acid secretion. Thus, anticholinergics can reduce acid secretion mediated by acetylcholine; at one time it was believed that they might cause increased gastrin release. Atropine reduces gastrin release in both intact and vagotomized dogs; however, background levels of gastrin remain three times higher in the vagotomized dogs.[70] Anticholinergics such as atropine reduce the acid output stimulated by food by only 30%; there may be little inhibition when 24 hour acid output is examined. Dogs with gastric retention and vagotomy secrete a much greater amount of hydrochloric acid than dogs with vagotomy and no retention.[71] Anticholinergics produce gastric retention by the same means as vagotomy. Acid hypersecretion caused by delayed gastric emptying interferes with recovery and can even cause gastritis in normal animals. In summary, anticholinergics are not used for reducing the basal low rate of gastric acid secretion in fasting animals, and they can have undesirable effects caused by the drug's action to delay gastric emptying, something that promotes acid secretion.

Two types of muscarinic cholinergic receptors are described. An agent like atropine and most other anticholinergics acts on both types so that both gastric motility and secretion are reduced. A selective muscarinic antagonist acting on only M_1 receptors, pirenzepine, inhibits gastric acid secretion without undesirable effects on gastric motility mediated by drugs acting on M_2 receptors. Pirenzepine is more potent than other anticholinergics in reducing stimulated acid secretion by 50% to 60%.

Prostaglandins. Some prostaglandins, primarily of the E series, have properties to inhibit gastric acid secretion. They also influence blood flow and motility in ways that can have undesirable side effects. Analogs of prostaglandins have been synthesized that inhibit gastric acid secretion in dogs and with minimum side effects.[72] These prostaglandins, given orally, may prove valuable in managing acute mucosal lesions. Prostaglandins inhibit acid secretion by reducing cyclic AMP production and thereby reducing the protein kinase activity essential to hydrogen ion generation. Cyclic AMP is reduced by inhibition of adenylate cyclase activity, an effect following interaction of prostaglandin with a membrane receptor. The use of prostaglandins provides a cytoprotective effect as well as inhibition of acid secretion. Prostaglandins also have atropic effect on gastric mucosa.[73] Misoprostol is an analog of prostaglandin that is available for human use in scored tablets of 100 µgm. Although the drug has been evaluated in research dogs, there is no information on its use in clinical cases. Side effects to be expected are diarrhea, which may be only transitory, and abortion in pregnant animals.

H_2-Receptor Antagonists. Many analogs of histamine have been synthesized and evaluated as inhibitors of gastric acid secretion.[68] They inhibit acid secretion by binding to H_2-histamine-receptor sites on the oxyntic cell and preventing interaction of the receptor with histamine.

Cimetidine was the first H_2-receptor antagonist used in dogs, shortly followed by ranitidine, and more recently a host of others. Cimetidine potently inhibits histamine-stimulated gastric acid secretion at doses of 3.0 mg/kg in dogs.[74] Inhibition peaks at 75% within 1.5 hours, and 50% inhibition of acid secretion lasts about two hours after an oral dose (Figure 12-6). The relatively short biologic effect results in the drug's usually being given three times a day. It is evident that cimetidine given at these doses results in only mild to moderate inhibition of acid secretion for a short part of any 24 hour period. The effects of the drug are gone after five hours. Ranitidine at a dose of 1.0 mg/kg inhibits acid secretion to a greater extent in dogs.[74] Inhibition peaks at about 90%, and 50% inhibition lasts four hours (Figure 12-6). The longer biologic effect leads to a recommendation that the drug be given only twice daily. At that schedule 50% acid secretion inhibition is in effect for only 8 out of 24 hours. Continuous infusion of ranitidine at a rate of 16.0 µg/kg per minute in dogs reduces acid secretion 70% to 80% and pepsin secretion 40%.[75] The degree of inhibition increases with meal size as the infusion rate remains constant. Based on a milligram per kilogram dog dosage, ranitidine is six to ten times more potent than cimetidine in inhibiting acid secretion stimulated by histamine, pentagastrin, or bethanechol. Both cimetidine and ranitidine are safe for use in dogs and cats. Earlier, reservations were expressed about their use, but no serious side effects have been documented.

Famotidine is a newer H_2-receptor antagonist that has been promoted as being more effective than both cimetidine and ranitidine. Studies on dogs show famotidine to be no more effective than ranitidine (Figure 12-7).[76,77] Little is known of any side effects for famotidine in small animals.

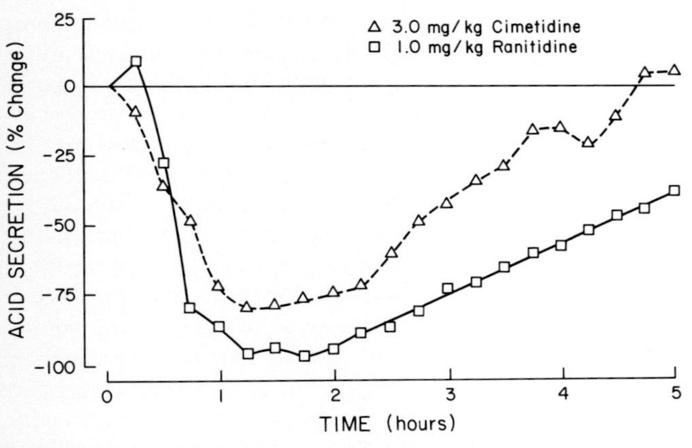

Figure 12-6. Graph of acid secretion in dogs during stimulation by histamine and inhibition by cimetidine or ranitidine.

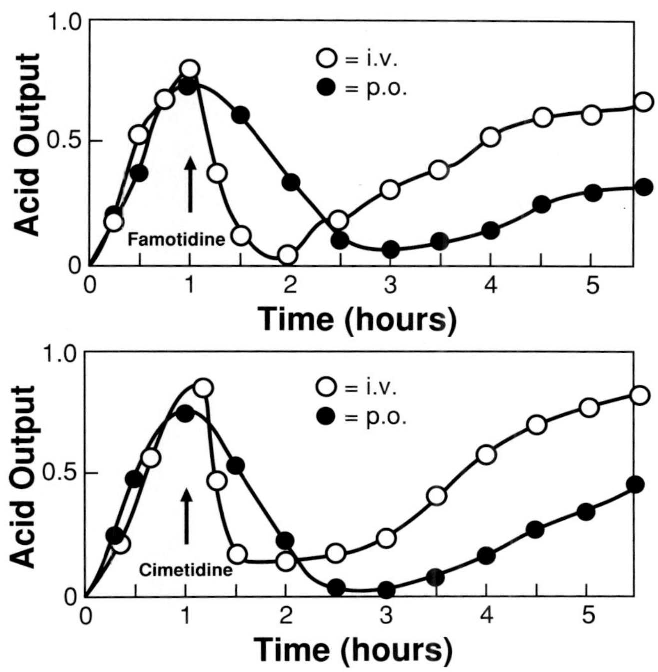

Figure 12-7. Graph of acid secretion in dogs during stimulation by histamine and inhibition by cimetidine or famotidine. Drugs were given orally (p.o.) or intravenously (i.v.).

Inhibition of acid secretion and control of gastric pH is difficult to achieve in critically ill humans.[78] That is likely to be similar in seriously ill dogs and cats.

Calcium Channel Blockers. Drugs are available to inhibit acid secretion by blocking the influx of calcium into oxyntic cells, an entry essential to secretion mediated by acetylcholine and gastrin. Current available drugs do not have sufficient potency for inhibition of acid secretion to make them useful.

ATPase Inhibitors. Omeprazole is a substituted benzimidazole that inhibits the proton pump at the apical border, reducing the exchange for hydrogen and potassium ions. Omeprazole inhibits secretion stimulated by any secretagogue, and in dogs its potency is five to ten times greater than that of cimetidine.[79] A single daily dose can result in virtual antacidity, which is accompanied by hypergastrinemia and gastrin cell hyperplasia. The drug does not affect other gastrointestinal secretion in dogs.[80] Omeprazole accumulates in oxyntic cell canaliculi into which hydrogen ions are secreted. The drug accumulates to higher levels at a low pH because it is a weak base with a pka greater than 1.0. Omeprazole does not accumulate in other cell organelles where the pH is about 5.0. When acid is not being secreted, the drug does not accumulate and is inactivated. The drug may prove to be useful in treating diseases where profound inhibition of acid secretion is desired. Such an inhibition predisposes to bacterial overgrowth. That would be a possibility in dogs, and possibly other species, because a single dose of omeprazole inhibits acid secretion for up to four days.[79]

Antacids. Gastric acid can be neutralized with antacids, which have been used for years in treating acute mucosal lesions. The use of antacids is indicated since acid is necessary for lesions to develop and to persist. Antacids must be given frequently since the acid neutralization is of short duration. Intermittent use of antacids causes total daily acid secretion to increase, for the following reason. Acid pH on the gastric antral mucosa inhibits the release of gastrin. Neutralization of gastric contents removes this inhibitory influence, and gastrin release increases. The result is greater acid secretion. This problem is circumvented by neutralizing acid continuously as it is formed. Antacids administered two or three times a day result in greater than normal rates of acid secretion. After the buffering capacity of the antacid is consumed, the secreted acid further damages the mucosa. Thus, antacids are given continuously or as often as necessary to neutralize all acid as it is being secreted. Continuous antacid therapy is not usual treatment for gastritis but is reserved for cases that fail to respond or that have serious gastric bleeding.

Antacids vary in the form of cations and anions they contain (Table 12-6). Each has a different buffering capacity and some unique side effects. The cation of antacids can be aluminum, calcium, or magnesium; in some there may be a combination. Calcium has effects to promote constipation, and magnesium causes feces to contain more water so that they can be unformed. Aluminum reduces gastric motility and thus delays emptying. Aluminum also interacts with dietary phosphorus, resulting in both increased fecal excretion and reduced intestinal absorption for phosphate.[81] Hypophosphatemia can follow, which stimulates bone demineralization. Hypercalcemia can appear in aluminum antacid use during chronic renal failure. Aluminum also accumulates when used with that problem. Administration of excess calcium antacids can result in diseases of calcium excess, most likely the formation of renal calculi. The excess calcium is also damaging to renal tissue. Administration of absorbable antacids such as sodium bicarbonate can result in alkalosis. This side effect is minimized in animals receiving fluids and possessing good renal function. Milk is not an antacid. Antacids have other side effects that should be recognized. They have the potential to predispose to bacterial overgrowth.

Table 12-6. Antacid Composition and Side Effects

Antacid	Composition		
	Aluminum*	Magnesium**	Calcium*
Amphojel	+		
Aludrox	+	+	
Basaljel	+		
Camalox	+	+	+
Gaviscon	+	+	
Gelusil	+	+	
Maalox	+	+	
Milk of Magnesia		+	
Riopan	-	-	-

* Aluminum and calcium have constipating effect

** Magnesium has a laxative effect

Control of Vomiting

Management of vomiting is sometimes indicated, and a number of antiemetics are available for use.[82] Most episodes of vomiting require no antiemetic therapy; spontaneous remission follows upon withholding food and water for 24 hours. Vomiting is not a serious problem when intravenous fluid administration can replace the lost fluids. Persistent vomiting requires antiemetic therapy, but such therapy is given with the understanding that it is merely controlling a sign and is not expected to treat the cause for the vomiting. The reflex act of vomiting (see Chapter 11) is mediated through neural activity in the chemoreceptor trigger zone (CRTZ) and/or the vomiting center in the brain stem. Antiemetic drugs act on transmission through these centers, and some may inhibit vomiting by also acting on peripheral sites. The vomiting reflex operates through neural pathways with dopaminergic, H_1-histaminic, and muscarinic cholinergic receptors. Drugs able to block these receptors usually have antiemetic properties.

The phenothiazine derivatives, such as chlorpromazine and prochlorperazine, are the most effective antiemetics for managing animals with gastrointestinal problems (Table 12-7). These antiemetics inhibit activity at all those types of receptors. Other phenothiazine antiemetics are less effective. These drugs are more commonly used as tranquilizers that also have hypotensive effects caused by alpha-adrenergic antagonism. Vomiting patients are hypovolemic and at risk for hypotension; phenothiazine antiemetics can precipitate that. These drugs also increase the risk for seizures; they are not used in patients with a history of seizures. Vomiting is inhibited in a dose-related effect by these drugs.

Metoclopramide is a derivative of procainamide and has

Table 12-7. Antimetic Drugs and Doses

Drug (site of action)	Dosage for Dogs (D) and Cats (C)
Triethylperazine (VC) (Torecan)	0.25 mg/kg Tid IM (D) 0.5 mg/kg Tid rectal (D) 0.125 mg/kg Tid IM (C)
Chlorpromazine (VC) (Thorazine)	0.5 mg/kg Tid IM (D,C) 1.0 mg/kg Tid rectal (D)
Prochlorperazine (VC) (Compazine)	0.1 mg/kg Qid IM (D,C)
Diphenhydramine (CRTZ) (Benadryl)	2.0 to 4.0 mg/kg Tid PO (D,C)
Dimenhydrinate (CRTZ) (Dramamine)	8 mg/kg Tid IM (D,C)
Trimethobenzamine (CRTZ) (Tigan)	3 mg/kg Tid IM (D)
Metoclopramide (CRTZ) (Reglan)	0.2 to 0.5 mg/kg TID PO, SC (D,C) 1 to 2 mg/kg daily slow IV (D,C)
Haloperidol (CRTZ) (Haldol)	0.02 to 0.1 mg/kg (D)
Fentanyl (CRTZ) (Sublimaze)	0.01 mg/kg (D)
Dexamethasone (?) (Azium)	0.1 mg/kg (D)

(VC) = vomiting center (CRTZ) = See text

inhibitory effects on dopamine receptors both at the CRTZ and peripheral receptors. The drug, acting on peripheral receptors, stimulates gastrointestinal motility. That motility is reflexly reduced during vomition, and its stimulation by metoclopramide may contribute to its antiemetic effects. Because it is effective at the CRTZ, metoclopramide does not inhibit vomiting mediated directly through the vomiting center, which is the type of vomiting seen most often with gastrointestinal problems. Metoclopramide also does not have a long effect; the drug's half-life is about 1.5 hours, and so it must be administered continuously or frequently. For these reasons metoclopramide is not the ideal or most effective antiemetic for dogs and cats.

The antihistamines diphenhydramine and dimenhydrinate inhibit some forms of vomiting mediated through the CRTZ by an action at H_1-receptors. These drugs are used to prevent motion sickness. Vomiting by some drugs is mediated through the CRTZ and can be inhibited with antihistamines. The H_2-receptor antagonists do not possess antiemetic properties.

A number of other dopamine antagonists act on the CRTZ to inhibit vomiting. Butyrophenones such as droperidol and haloperidol and diphenylbutylpiperidines such as pimozide and penfluridol are effective in blocking vomiting induced by chemicals such as narcotics. At higher doses the butyrophenones block vomiting also at the vomiting center. Pimozide is long-acting; it is able to prevent drug-induced vomiting in dogs for up to six days.

Opiate receptors are found in the vomiting center, and drugs binding to those receptors can inhibit vomiting. Morphine stimulates vomiting in dogs, but after one or two vomitions further vomiting is inhibited. A narcotic such as fentanyl penetrates the brain rapidly, and after binding to opiate receptors in the vomiting center it inhibits vomiting.

Anticholinergics are incorporated with antiemetics to produce products for treating gastroenteritis in animals. There are no studies demonstrating any antiemetic properties for anticholinergics, and since this class of drug reduces gastrointestinal motility there are few if any indications for their use.

Other drugs used as antiemetics include dexamethasone, which has an unpredictable effect by an unknown mechanism. Bismuth subsalicylate may be effective by an unknown mechanism. Cannabinoids (Nabilone, Eli Lilly) are less effective than the drugs described with antidopaminergic effects. Trimethobenzamide (Tigan, Beecham) is less effective than the other antiemetics. Domperidone (Motilium, Janssen), if available, is another dopamine antagonist that is effective as an antiemetic in the dog.[83]

The antiemetic drugs are effective in small animals with gastrointestinal problems. Continued vomiting despite antiemetic therapy should be reevaluated. Many such animals have a gastrointestinal obstruction. More effective antiemetic effects are necessary when animals are treated with some potent anticancer drugs. One such drug, cisplatin, is very predictable in causing vomition when given in doses of 3 mg per kg intravenously.[84] The drug induces vomiting within 90-120 minutes, and vomiting continues for five hours. Pretreatment with a large dose (3.0 mg/kg subcutaneously) of metoclopramide provides 99% protection against vomiting. Metoclopramide (1.0 mg/kg), chlorpromazine (1.0 mg/kg), or haloperidol (1.0 mg/kg) provide a 55%-60% protection against vomiting. In clinical cases treated with 1.6 mg cisplatin per kg, butorphanol pretreatment at 0.2 mg/kg subcutaneously and repeated in three hours limits vomiting to usually only one episode. Such treatment depresses some dogs for unacceptably long periods of time. Failures in preventing vomition can be managed by following the initial treatment with dexamethasone 0.1 mg/kg and metoclopramide 0.1 mg/kg. When butorphanol's effects are unacceptable, chlorpromazine can be given at a rate of 2.0 mg/kg, which can be repeated in three to four hours. A single episode of vomiting is seen, as with butorphanol. Metoclopramide at a dose of 0.2 mg/kg has no effect on vomiting, and doses of 1.0 mg/kg produce an unacceptable dementia.

Antibiotics

Microorganisms enter the stomach from the oral microflora and in the diet. In the empty stomach their numbers are reduced to virtually zero by the acid pH of the gastric secretions. With acute mucosal lesions, the back-diffusion of gastric acid makes it difficult to maintain the optimum low pH necessary to prevent bacterial growth. Moreover, the use of antacids or inhibitors of acid secretion increases gastric pH, so that bacterial growth is possible.[85] When the pH of gastric contents is less than 3.0, bacteria entering the stomach are destroyed within 15 minutes; some bactericidal activity remains up to pH 4.0. Bacterial numbers increase more than 100 times with reduced gastric acidity, whether the result of disease or of drugs' inhibiting or neutralizing hydrogen ion secretion. Thus, antibiotics may be indicated to prevent and treat for mucosal invasion by bacteria, which are thriving where they normally would not survive. With clinical evidence for disruption of the mucosal barrier, such as hematemesis or frequent persistent vomiting, antibiotic therapy is justified. Microorganisms readily cross the gastrointestinal mucosa when the barrier is broken. Bacteria can even invade through an intact mucosal barrier during a noninvasive procedure such as endoscopy, resulting in a transient bacteremia.[86] The stress produced by vomiting and dehydration reduces the capability of the monocyte phagocytic (reticuloendothelial) system to respond to bacterial invasion. This further justifies the rationale for using antibiotics to treat acute gastritis. The microflora of the oral cavity and the gastrointestinal tract contains both aerobic and anaerobic bacteria. Penicillins and metronidazole are effective agents against invasion by anaerobes, which make up the oral flora (see Chapter 16). Aminoglycosides or trimethoprim sulfa are useful against aerobic infection. Chloromycetin can be used against both aerobes and anaerobes but is less effective than a penicillin and the aminoglycosides. Antibiotic therapy is important when acute mucosal lesions perforate the gastric wall and bacteria contaminate the abdominal cavity. Abscessation can follow, caused by enteric anaerobes. Penicillin prevents their formation. Once formed, abscesses are difficult to treat medically. Antibiotics to treat acute gastric lesions are given parenterally by injection. Orally administered unabsorbed antibiotics are of no value.

Conditions of increased pH favoring greater bacterial numbers can persist for months after recovery from some forms of gastritis in animals and humans. Lipopolysaccharide, derived from pseudomonas organisms, and increased ambient temperature reduce gastric secretion in dogs. Any of these conditions could be responsible for overgrowth of the gastrointestinal microflora and clinical signs of diarrhea and vomiting.[86]

Locally Acting Protectives, Nonspecific

There is no evidence that many of the medications designed to nonspecifically protect the gastric mucosa are effective in hastening the recovery of acute mucosal lesions. Some drugs may beneficially bind microorganisms, toxins, and bile acids, but few of them coat the mucosal surface to provide a protective barrier against the contents of the stomach. Gastric protectives are usually vomited by animals with acute mucosal lesions, which is another reason they are seldom used.

Locally Acting Protectives, Specific

Sucralfate is the aluminum salt of a sulfated derivative of sucrose that is indicated for topical treatment of gastric and duodenal lesions.[88] The drug binds to proteins at the site of an ulcer and provides a protective barrier against the action of acid and pepsin. Sucralfate also inhibits pepsin activity and binds bile. Although it contains aluminum, sucralfate is not an antacid; it stimulates bicarbonate secretion via surface mucosal cells and also the release of prostaglandins. The latter contributes to increased rates for bicarbonate secretion, mucosal blood flow, and mucosal repair. Sucralfate also increases the viscosity of gastric mucus and improves its ability to impede hydrogen ion diffusion.[89] Sucralfate is given at a dose of 250 mg four times per day to a 15 kg animal. No toxic side effects are reported. As with many chemicals with the property of binding others, sucralfate interacts with drugs such as cimetidine, phenytoin, and tetracyline. Other drugs should not be given within two hours of giving sucralfate.

Colloidal bismuth subcitrate, where available, can be used for topical treatment of gastritis. The drug does not inhibit acid secretion but inhibits pepsin activity and interacts with exposed protein to coat ulcers. Colloidal bismuth also interacts with mucus to improve the barrier to hydrogen ion diffusion. The drug has antibacterial activity against campylobacter-like organisms and possibly others. Bismuth causes the feces to blacken, and some bismuth is absorbed from the intestine and excreted in the urine. Toxicity is possible with reduced renal function. Colloidal bismuth is very effective in the healing of ulcers in humans.

Other specific protective agents have been designed to interfere with the effects of bile and pepsin in causing acute mucosal lesions. Bile increases permeability to hydrogen-ion back-diffusion and readily produces ulcers in dogs. This is prevented by pretreatment with carbenoxolone sodium, a drug that protects the gastric mucosa.[90] Carbenoxolone has undesirable aldosterone-like properties that cause sodium retention and accelerated potassium wasting. A similar gastric mucosal protectant, lauryl glycyrrhizinic acid, is effective in the dog. Cholestyramine binds and inactivates bile acids, except that it is ineffective in treating mucosal lesions because binding does not occur at acid pH.

Drugs with antipepsin activity may be of value in treating acute mucosal lesions. They include sulfated mucopolysaccharides and glycoproteins, which bind to the mucosal surface, preventing the digestion of membrane by pepsin. Gastric mucin and synthetics such as amylopectin sulfate also have this protective property.[91]

Fluid Therapy

Fluid lost by vomiting is different from extracellular body fluid in that it contains less sodium, more potassium, more water, more hydrogen ions, and less bicarbonate. Thus, the remaining extracellular fluid changes in composition resulting in hypernatremia, hypokalemia, and alkalosis. Hyponatremia is common in anorectic patients that continue to drink large amounts of water and vomit. Some of the water consumed is absorbed from the stomach, and some of the body's electrolytes (including sodium) are lost in each vomitus. The net result is that absorbed water dilutes the reduced total body store of electrolytes. Thus, hyper- or hyponatremia can exist, identifiable by measuring the electrolytes. Most small-animal patients have access to water, making hyponatremia more likely than hypernatremia. When no measurements are made, sodium should be replaced by administering a balanced electrolyte solution. Vomiting causes potassium losses, and the total body stores of potassium are depleted in anorectic patients. The renal loss of potassium is also accelerated in dehydrated animals. Measurement of plasma electrolytes can show normokalemia, although hypokalemia is more usual. Normokalemia can be found with potassium depletion, especially if acidosis accompanies it. Potassium-depleted patients are treated with solutions containing potassium at a greater concentration than is present in body fluids. The loss of potassium by vomiting and urinary excretion is great enough that it cannot be replaced with a balanced electrolyte solution since the volumes required exceed the amount of fluids an animal can be given. Alkalosis is managed by correcting volume deficits to initiate a diuresis. This results in a renal excretion of excess bicarbonate. No acidifying agents are used. In summary, a balanced electrolyte solution is used unless there is laboratory evidence for hypernatremia or hyponatremia. Potassium can be added and administered slowly while monitoring for toxic effects. Volumes are given to correct volume deficits and initiate a diuresis.

Gastric Hemorrhage

Initial therapy for gastric hemorrhage is replacement of the blood losses. Stored whole blood is used unless it is determined that disseminated intravascular coagulation (DIC) is the basis for the bleeding. Activated clotting time, platelet numbers, and plasma fibrinogen level are determined for evaluation of DIC. Heparin is the treatment for a DIC that is not associated with hepatic failure. In these cases, blood transfusion worsens the DIC. DIC and a deficiency of clotting factors characterize bleeding caused by liver disease. The DIC is treated with heparin, but if the deficiency in clotting factors is not corrected the bleeding will worsen. The clotting factors are replaced by transfusing fresh whole blood with heparin added. Thrombocytopenia can also be corrected by this treatment. Thrombocytopenia that is not due to DIC but is caused by autoimmune disease is treated with corticosteroids or chemotherapy as used to treat some forms of cancer. Gastric hemorrhage resulting from ulcerations caused by thrombosis is difficult to treat.

Control of gastric bleeding is the second goal of treatment. The prognosis is poor when hemorrhage continues despite the use of inhibitors of acid secretion, antacids, antiemetics, antibiotics, complete rest, and management for DIC. Failure of this indirect therapy is indication for initiation of direct means to control bleeding.

Gastric lavage with ice water is used to control gastric hemorrhage in humans. The cold temperature promotes vasoconstriction, reducing blood flow and bleeding. The same is achieved to some extent by providing ice cubes to eat. Visceral cooling by intraperitoneal injection of cold saline also controls gastric bleeding in dogs.[92]

Vasoactive drugs are used to control gastric bleeding. The drugs are most effective when infused directly into the mesenteric artery through catheters positioned under fluoroscopic control. Vasopressin infusion is significantly more effective than conventional therapy in controlling bleeding, though it does not increase survival rates.[93] Vasopressin has side effects resulting from its cardiovascular and antidiuretic activity.

The potent vasoconstrictive properties of catecholamines have been used to control gastric bleeding. These drugs can produce mucosal ischemia and ulcer formation, but smaller amounts produce vasoconstriction without causing ischemia and tissue anoxia. Norepinephrine, given intragastrically (8 mg free base in 500 ml saline) or intraperitoneally (8 mg free base in 100 ml saline) to dogs with experimental gastric bleeding, can save animals that would otherwise die from exsanguination.[94] This treatment causes portal blood pressure to double for five minutes, after which it decreases to normal. Norepinephrine reduces portal blood flow to one-third of normal. Systolic and diastolic blood pressure change little. Systemic cardiovascular effects are minimal because catecholamines given intraperitoneally are rapidly removed from the portal circulation and metabolized by the liver.

If all medical management fails to control gastrointestinal bleeding, a partial or complete gastrectomy can be performed.

Steroids

Corticosteroids may contribute to the formation of chronic gastric ulcers by altering gastric mucin. Corticosteroids are commonly used to treat shock, with the view that they stabilize lysosomal membranes during endotoxic, cardiogenic, and hemorrhagic shock, and prevent the release of destructive lysosomal enzymes.[95] The beneficial effects attributed to corticosteroids in treating clinical cases of shock are poorly documented, however, even though many consider them essential for success. In humans under severe stress, steroids prevent ulceration of the gastric mucosa.[96] Steroids are administered when shock is first recognized and are continued for at least 48 hours. Corticosteroids are necessary to prostaglandins' maintaining cytoprotection for the gastric mucosa.[97] Animals with corticosteroid deficiency show signs of gastritis and vomiting; remission of signs is not seen until treatment includes corticosteroids.

REFERENCES

1. Davis, R.E. and Ivy, A.C.: Thermal irritation in gastric disease. Cancer 2:138-143, 1949.
2. Drasar, B.S. and Hill, M.J.: Human intestinal flora. Academic Press, London, 1974.
3. Broido, P.W., Gorbach, S.L., Condon, R.E. and Hyhus, L.M.: Upper intestinal microflora control. Arch. Surg. 106:90-93, 1973.
4. Smith, H.W.: Survival of orally administered *E. coli* K12 in alimentary tract of man. Nature 255:500-502, 1975.
5. Osborne, A.D. and Wilson, M.R.: Mycotic gastritis in a dog. Vet. Rec. 85:487-488, 1969.
6. Howard, E.B.: Acute mycotic gastritis in a dog. VM/SAC 61:549-552, 1966.
7. Henry, G.A., Long, P.H., Burns, J.L. and Charbonneau, D.L.: Gastric spirillosis in Beagles. Am. J. Vet. Res. 48:831-836, 1987.
8. Cheli, R., Perasso, A. and Giacosa, A.: Gastritis. Springer-Verlag, New York, 1987, p. 36-44.
9. Johnson, L.R.: Pepsin output from the damaged canine heidenhain pouch. Am. J. Dig. Dis. 16:403-407, 1971.
10. Cooke, A.R.: The role of the mucosal barrier in drug-induced gastric ulceration and erosions. Amer. J. Dig. Dis. 21:155-164, 1976.
11. Menguy, R.: Gastric mucus and the gastric mucous barrier. Am. J. Surg. 117:806-812, 1969.
12. Cheung, L.Y., Moody, F.G. and Reese, R.S.: Effect of aspirin, bile salt, and ethanol on canine gastric mucosal blood flow. Surgery 77:786-792, 1975.
13. Lichtenberger, L.M., Richards, J.E. and Hills, B.A.: Effect of 16, 16-dimethyl prostaglandin E_2 on the surface hydrophobicity of aspirin-treated canine gastric mucosa. Gastroenterology 88:308-314, 1985.
14. Urquhart, J.: Two cheers for NSAIDs. Gut 27:1287-1291, 1986.
15. Crawford, L.M. and Wilson, R.C.: Melaena associated with dexamethasone therapy in the dog. J. Sm. Anim. Pract. 23:91-97, 1982.
16. Thomas, N.W.: Piroxicam-associated gastric ulceration in a dog.
17. Gilmour, M.A. and Walshaw, R.: Naproxen-induced toxicosis in a dog. JAVMA 191:1431-1432, 1987.
18. Sorjonen, D.C., Dillon, A.R., Powers, R.D. and Spano, J.S.: Effects of dexamethasone and surgical hypotension on the stomach of dogs: clinical, endoscopic, and pathologic evaluations. Am. J. Vet. Res. 44:1233-1237, 1983.
19. Silen, W.: What is cytoprotection of the gastric mucosa? Gastroenterology 94:232-235, 1988.

20. Fromm, D.: Mechanisms involved in gastric mucosal resistance to injury. Ann. Rev. Med. 38:119-128, 1987.
21. Zinner, M.J., Turtinen, L. and Gurll, N.J.: The role of acid and ischemia in production of stress ulcers during canine hemorrhagic shock. Surgery 77:807-816, 1975.
22. McGuigan, J.E.: The endocrine ulcer concept. Am. J. Dig. Dis. 21:144-147, 1976.
23. Shaw, D.H.: Gastrinoma (Zollinger-Ellison syndrome) in the dog and cat. Can. Vet. J. 29:448-451, 1988.
24. Straus, E., Johnson, G.F. and Yalow, R.S.: Canine Zollinger-Ellison syndrome. Gastroenterology; 72:380-381, 1977.
25. Murray, M., Robinson, P.B., McKeating, F.J. and Lauder, I.M.: Peptic ulceration in the dog: A clinico-pathological study. Vet. Rec. 91:441-447, 1972.
26. Moody, F.G., Cheung, L.Y., Simons, M.A. and Zalewsky, C.: Stress and the acute gastric mucosal lesion. Am. J. Dig. Dis. 21:148-154, 1976.
27. Nicoloff, D.M., Peter, E.T., Leonard, A.S. and Wangensteen, O.H.: Catecholamines in ulcer provocations: Their possible role in stress ulcer formation. JAMA 191:383-385, 1965.
28. Ritchie, W.P., Breen, J.J. and Grigg, D.I.: Prevention of stress ulcer by reducing gastric tissue histamine. Surgery 62:596-600, 1967.
29. Lucas, C.E., Sufawa, C., Friend, W. and Walt, A.J. Therapeutic implications of disturbed gastric physiology in patients with stress ulcerations. Am. J. Surg. 123:25-34, 1972.
30. Gronbech, J.E., Matre, K., Stangeland, L., Svanes, K. and Varhaug, J.E.: Gastric mucosal repair in the cat: role of the hyperemic response to mucosal damage. Gastroenterology 95:311-320, 1988.
31. Quintero, E., Pique, J.M., Bombi, J.A., Bordas, J.M, Sentis, J., Elena, M., Bosch, J. and Rodes, J.: Gastric mucosal vascular ectasias causing bleeding in cirrhosis. Gastroenterology 93:1054-1061, 1987.
32. Douglass, H.O., Jr., Falk, G.A. and LeVeen, H.H.: Infection: A cause of acute peptic ulceration in hypersecreting animals. Surgery 68:827-830, 1970.
33. Rees, W.D.W.: Mucus-bicarbonate barrier — shield or sieve. Gut 28:1553-1556, 1987.
34. Lawson, H.H.: Effect of duodenal contents on the gastric mucosa under experimental conditions. Lancet 1:469-472, 1964.
35. DenBesten, L. and Hamza, K.N.: Effect of bile salts on ionic permeability of canine gastric mucosa during experimental shock. Gastroenterology 62:417-434, 1972.
36. Djahanguiri, B., Abtahi, F.S. and Hemmati, M.: Prevention of aspirin-induced gastric ulceration by bile duct or pylorus ligation in the rat. Gastroenterology 65:630-633, 1973.
37. Calcraft, B., Rhodes, J., Cross, S. and Hole, D.: Strengthening the gastric mucosa. Gut 14:423, 1973.
38. Nahrwold, D.L.: Bile as a gastric secretory stimulant. Surgery 71:157-160, 1972.
39. Black, R.B., Rhodes, J. and Hole, D.: Measurement of bile damage to the gastric mucosa. Am. J. Dig. Dis. 12:411-415, 1973.
40. Duane, W.C. and Wiegand, D.M.: Mechanisms by which bile salt disrupts the gastric mucosal barrier in the dog. J. Clin. Invest. 66:1044-1049, 1980.
41. Thomas, W.E.G.: Gastric morphological and functional changes produced by bile in the canine stomach. Eur. Surg. Res. 13:125-133, 1981.
42. Duane, W.C., McHale, A.P. and Sievert, C.E.: Lysolecithin-lipid interactions in disruption of the canine gastric mucosal barrier. Am. J. Physiol. 250:G275-G279, 1986.
43. Fontolliet, C., Mosimann, F., Diserens, H., Burri, B., Loup, P.W. and Mosimann, R.: Modifications of the gastric mucosal barrier induced by experimental duodenogastric reflux: an electron microscopic study. Scand. J. Gastroenterology 19(Suppl 92):75-77, 1984.
44. Diserens, H., Krstic, R., Burri, B., Mosimann, F. and Mosimann, R.: The gastric mucosa in experimental duodenogastric reflux. Scand. J. Gastroenterology 19(Suppl 92):133-135, 1984.
45. Burri, B., Mosimann, F., Diserens, H., Fontolliet, C., Mirkovitch, V., Felber, J-P., Jequier, E. and Mosimann, R.: A long-term study of different types of experimental alkaline reflux and the affects of its suppression in dogs. Scand. J. Gastroenterology 19(Suppl 92):81-86, 1984.
46. Rhodes, J., Davies, H.A., Wheeler, M.H., Psaila, J., Newcombe, R.G., Jones, J.M. and Bloom, S.: Bile diversion from the duodenum: its effect on gastric pancreatic function. Scand. J. Gastroenterology 19(Suppl 92):221-223, 1984.
47. Garner, A., Flemstrom, G. and Allen, A.: Current concepts of gastroduodenal mucosal protection. Scand. J. Gastroenterolgoy 19(Suppl 92):78-80, 1984.
48. Konturek, S.J., Tasler, J., Bilski, J., Kaminska, A. and Laskiewicz, J.: Role of prostaglandins in alkaline secretion from the gastroduodenal mucosa exposed to acid and taurocholate. Scand. J. Gastroenterology 19(Suppl 92):69-74, 1984.
49. Meshkinpour, H., Thrupp, L.D., Shiffler, P., Kitts, D. and Fisher, J.: Reflux gastritis syndrome. Arch Surg. 116:1148-1152, 1981.
50. Winans, C.S.: The fickle pylorus. Gastroenterology 70:622-623, 1976.
51. Stempter, T.J. and Cooke, A.R.: Effect of a fixed pyloric opening on gastric emptying in the cat and dog. Am. J. Physiol. 230:813-817, 1976.
52. Kelly, K.A., Schlegel, J.F., Steinbach, J.H. and Code, C.F.: Duodenal-gastric reflux caused by retrograde duodenal pacing. Mayo Clinic. Proc. 50:534, 1975.
53. Dooley, C.P., Mello, W.D. and Valenzuela, J.E.: Effects of aspirin and prostaglandin E_2 on interdigestive motility complex and duodenogastric reflux in man. Dig. Dis. Sci. 30:513-521, 1985.
54. Brough, W.A., Taylor, T.V. and Torrance, H.B.: The effect of cholecystectomy on duodenogastric reflux in dogs and humans. Scand. J. Gastroenterology 19(Suppl 92):242-244, 1984.
55. Merrill, J.P. and Hampers, C.L.: Uremia. New Eng. J. Med. 282:953-961, 1970.
56. Falcao, H.A., Wesdorp, R.I.C. and Fischer, J.E.: Gastrin levels and gastric acid secretion in anephric patients and in patients with chronic and acute renal failure. J. Surg. Res. 18:107-111, 1975.
57. Cheville, N.F.: Uremic gastropathy in the dog. Vet. Pathol. 16:292-309, 1979.
58. Kirk, A.P., Dooley, J.S. and Hunt, R.H.: Peptic ulceration in patients with chronic liver disease. Dig. Dis. Sci. 25:756-760, 1980.
59. Roberts, H.R. and Cederbaum, A.I.: The liver and blood coagulation physiology and pathology. Gastroenterology 63:297-320, 1972.
60. Hein, M.F., Silen, W., Skillman, J.J. and Harper, H.A.: The effect of portacaval shunting on gastric secretion in cirrhotic dogs. Gastroenterology 44:637-641, 1963.
61. Odonkor, P., Monat, C. and Himal, H.S.: Prevention of sepsis-induced gastric lesions in dogs by cimetidine via inhibition of gastric secretion and by prostaglandin via cytoprotection. Gastroenterology 80:375-379, 1981.
62. Szabo, S., Gallagher, G.T., Horner, H.C., Frankel, P.W., Underwood, R.H., Konturek, S.J., Brzozowski, T. and Trier, J.S.: Role of the adrenal cortex in gastric mucosal protection by prostaglandins, sulfhydryls, and cimetidine in the rat. Gastroenterology 85:1384-1390, 1983.
63. Perry, M.A., Wadhwa, S., Parks, D.A., Pickard, W. and Granger, D.N.: Role of oxygen radicals in ischemia-induced lesions in the cat stomach. Gastroenterology 90:362-367, 1986.
64. Itoh, M. and Guth, P.H.: Role of oxygen-derived free radicals in hemorrhagic shock-induced gastric lesions in the rat. Gastroenterology 88:1162-1167, 1985.
65. Gronbech, J.E., Grong, K., Varhaug, J.E., Lekven, J. and Svanes, K.: Gastric epithelial restitution at low luminal pH during influence of pentagastrin or cimetidine in the cat. Gastroenterology 93:753-764, 1987.
66. Valnes, K., Brandtzaeg, P., Elgjo, K. and Stave, R.: Specific and nonspecific humoral defense factors in the epithelium of normal and inflamed gastric mucosa. Gastroenterolgoy

86:402-412, 1984.

67. McArthur, K.E., Walsh, J.H. and Richardson, C.T.: Soy protein meals stimulate less gastric acid secretion and gastrin release than beef meals. Gastroenterology 95:920-926, 1988.

68. Wolfe, N.M. and Soll, A.H.: The physiology of gastric acid secretion. New Eng. J. Med. 319:1707-1715, 1988.

69. Feldman, M.: Inhibition of gastric acid secretion by selective and nonselective anticholinergics. Gastroenterology 86:361-366, 1984.

70. Hirschowitz, B.I., Gibson, R. and Molina, E.: Atropine suppresses gastrin release by food in intact and vagotomized dogs. Gastroenterology 81:838-843, 1981.

71. Klempa, I., Holle, F., Bruckner, W., Welsch, K.H., Handle, H. and von Wolff, A.: The effect of selective proximal vagotomy and pyloroplasty on gastric secretion and motility in the dog. Arch. Surg. 103:713-719, 1971.

72. Robert, A., Schultz, J.R., Nezamis, J.E. and Lancaster, C.: Gastric antisecretory and antiulcer properties of PGE2, 15-methyl PGE2, and 16, 16-Dimethyl PGE2. Gastroenterology, 70:359-370, 1976.

73. Reinhart, W.H., Muller, O. and Halter, F.: Influence of long-term 16, 16-dimethyl prostaglandin E_2 treatment on the rat gastrointestinal mucosa. Gastroenterology 85:1003-1010, 1983.

74. Daly, M.J., Humphray, J.M. and Stables, R.: Inhibition of gastric acid secretion in the dog by the H_2-receptor antagonists, ranitidine, cimetidine, and metiamide. Gut 21:408-412, 1980.

75. Frislid, K., Guldvog, I. and Berstad, A.: Kinetics of the inhibition of food-stimulated secretion by ranitidine in dogs. Eur. Surg. Res. 17:360-365, 1985.

76. Takagi, T., Takeda, M. and Maeno, H.: Effect of a new potent H_2-blocker,3-[[[2-[(diaminomethylene)amino]-4-thiazolyl]methyl]-thio]-N^2-sulfamoylpropionamidine (YM-11170) on gastric secretion induced by histamine and food in conscious dogs. Arch. Int. Pharmacodyn 256:49-58, 1982.

77. Katz, L.B., Tobia, A.J. and Shriver, D.A.: Effects of ORF 17583, other histamine H_2-receptor antagonists and omeprazole on gastric acid secretory states in rats and dogs. J. Pharmasol. Exp. Ther. 242:437-442, 1987.

78. Martin, L.F., Max, M.H. and Polk, H.C.: Failure of gastric pH control by antacids or cimetidine in the critically ill: a valid sign of sepsis. Surgery. 88:59-68, 1980.

79. Larsson, H., Carlsson, E., Junggren, U., Olbe, L., Sjostrand, S.E., Skanberg, I. and Sundell, G.: Inhibition of gastric acid secretion by omeprazole in the dog and rat. Gastroenterology 85:900-907, 1983.

80. Konturek, S.J., Cieszkowski, M., Kwiecien, N., Konturek, J., Tasler, J. and Bilski, J.: Effects of omeprazole, a substituted benzimidazole, on gastrointestinal secretions, serum gastrin, and gastric mucosal blood flow in dogs. Gastroenterology 86:71-77, 1984.

81. Spencer, H. and Lender, M.: Adverse effects of aluminum-containing antacids on mineral metabolism. Gastroenterology 76:603-606, 1979.

82. Willard, M.D.: Some newer approaches to the treatment of vomiting. JAVMA 184:590-592, 1984.

83. Lee, K.Y., Park, H.J. and Chey, W.Y.: Studies on mechanism of retching and vomiting in dogs. Dig. Dis. Sci. 30:22-28, 1985.

84. Gylys, J.S., Dorow, K.M. and Buyniski, J.P.: Antagonism of cisplatin induced emesis in the dog. Res. Commun. Chem. Pathol. Pharm. 23:61-68, 1979.

85. Howden, C.W. and Hunt, R.H.: Relationship between gastric secretion and infection. Gut 28:96-107, 1987.

86. LeFrock, J.L, Ellis, C.A., Turchik, J.B. and Weinstine, K.: Transient bacteremia associated with sigmoidoscopy. New Eng. J. Med. 289:467-469, 1973.

87. Guth, P.H.: Mucosal coating agents and other nonantisecretory agents, are they cytoprotective? Dig. Dis. Sci. 32:647-654, 1987.

88. Colin-Jones, D.G.: There is more to healing ulcers than suppressing acid. Gut 27:475-480, 1986.

89. Slomiany, B.L., Laszewicz, W. and Slomiany, A.: Effect of sucralfate on the viscosity of gastric mucus and the permeability to hydrogen ion. Digestion 33:146-151, 1986.

90. Morris, T.J., Calcraft, B.H., Rhodes, J., Hole, D. and Morton, M.S.: Effect of a deglycyrrhizinised liquorice compound on the gastric mucosal barrier of the dog. Digestion 11:355-363, 1974.

91. Zimmon, D.S. and Mazzola, V.: Amylopectin sulphate (SN-263) coats the gastric mucosal surface. Gut 14:847-849, 1973.

92. LeKagul, S., Smyth, N.P., Brooks, M.H. and Barry, K.G.: The control of upper gastrointestinal hemorrhage in the dog by intraperitioneal cooling. J. Surg. Res. 10:423-431, 1970.

93. Conn, H.O., Ramsby, G.R., Storer, E.H., Mutchnick, M.G., Joshi, P.H., Phillips, M.M., Cohen, G.A., Fields, G.N. and Petroski, D.: Intraarterial vasopressin in the treatment of upper gastrointestinal hemorrhage: A prospective, controlled clinical trial. Gastroenterology 68:211-221, 1975.

94. LeVeen, H.H., Falk, G., Diaz, C., Wynkoop, B-J., Piccone, V.A., Yarnoz, M.D., Langsam, A.A., Nelson, J.H., Pedowitz, W.J. and Belfasky, R.B.: Control of gastrointestinal bleeding. Am. J. Surg. 123:154-159, 1972.

95. Clermont, H.G., Williams, T.S. and Adams, J.T.: Steroid effect on the release of the lysosomal enzyme acid phosphatase in shock. Ann. Surg. 179:917-921.

96. Jama, R.H., Perlman, M.H. and Matsumoto, T.: Incidence of stress ulcer formation associated with steroid therapy in various shock states. Amer. J. Surg. 130:328-331, 1975.

97. Szabo, S.: Peptides, sulfhydryls, and glucocorticoids in gastric mucosal defense: coincidence or connection. Gastroenterology 87:228-229, 1984.

Chapter 13

Chronic Gastritis, Gastric Retention, Gastric Neoplasms, and Gastric Surgery

CHRONIC GASTRITIS

Clinical Synopsis

Diagnostic Features

* Persistent intermittent vomiting exacerbated by eating or drinking
* Physical examination usually unremarkable
* Laboratory data base may reveal systemic cause
* Gastric biopsy may have a variety of appearances but chronic changes such as infiltration with plasma cells and lymphocytes are usually present
* Recovery from primary chronic gastritis is usually slow and often requires therapy

Standard Treatment

* NPO or no food for 24-72 hours
* Parenteral fluid therapy as required
* Subsequently place on easily digestible, "bland" diet for 2-4 weeks
* Cimetidine (5 mg/kg PO q 8 h) or ranitidine (1 mg/kg PO q 12 h) for 1-2 weeks if concomitant gastric erosions observed
* Prednisone (1-2 mg/kg PO q 12 h for 1-2 weeks followed by decreasing doses over an additional 4-6 week period) if lymphocytic, plasmacytic, or eosinophilic infiltrates are heavy and remission not obtained by controlled diet.

Chronic gastritis can result from continued irritation by agents that cause acute gastric mucosal lesions. The incidence of chronic gastritis is unknown, although it is low in pathologic findings from biopsies and necropsies. Gastric biopsies are seldom obtained, however, and gastric tissue is usually not saved for histology when its gross appearance is normal. A study of clinically normal Beagles reported that 9% of dogs 8 to 20 months old had microscopic evidence of chronic gastritis.[1] In contrast, the dogs had no gross lesions of chronic gastritis. Animals that vomit occasionally are seldom evaluated for chronic gastritis. In fact, some animals presented with intermittent signs show advanced inflammatory changes that would be expected to produce more severe and more consistent signs. There is ample evidence that the incidence of chronic gastritis is greater than has been thought.

Etiology and Pathogenesis

The pathogenesis of chronic gastritis is seldom understood from retrospective studies since the lesions are not recognized early in their development.

An understanding of the pathogenesis of chronic gastritis in dogs is gained from experimental studies. Chronic gastritis can be produced experimentally by using a mucosal irritant to initiate an immune-mediated pathologic process. Chronic gastritis can also be simulated in dogs by intravenous injection of human gastric juices[2] or by subcutaneous injections of autologous or homologous gastric juice.[3] The chronic gastritis was accompanied by autoantibodies to gastric juice.[4] Cell-mediated immunity also appears to play a role in the pathogenic process. In humans a relationship is seen between chronic gastritis and a number of autoimmune diseases that include some forms of thyroiditis, diabetes, hypoadrenalism, myasthenia, and others.[5] Laboratory evaluations can demonstrate autoantibodies and cell-mediated immune responses to antigens in the gastric mucosa. A similar relationship may sometimes be found in animals.

Experimental Canine Model. An experimental model in dogs is produced by intradermal injections of homologous gastric juice in Freund's complete adjuvant.[6] The initial morphologic change, appearing within two weeks, is an infiltration of the superficial part of the lamina propria by chronic inflammatory cells, producing a superficial gastritis. Inflammatory cells infiltrate the mucosa containing the gastric glands (Figure 13-1) to a marked degree over the next two to four weeks. Fibrosis, with degeneration of oxyntic and chief cells, appears five to ten weeks after immunization. Paralleling the morphologic changes is a reduced ability to secrete hydrochloric acid. The pathologic changes are associated with the appearance of delayed or cell-mediated hypersensitivity. Within two weeks of immunization, the dogs show positive skin tests for gastric juice, and inhibition of leukocyte migration; a phenomenon of cell-mediated immunity is evident. Circulating auto-antibodies do not appear until three to six weeks after immunization. Thus, both humoral and cell-mediated immunity may play a role in the pathogenesis of the gastritis. Since the early morphologic changes are accompanied by the appearance of cell-mediated immunity, whereas humoral antibodies develop later, cell-mediated immunity is likely to be more important in the pathogenesis. All the pathologic changes are reversible on removal of the stimulus, and gastric morphology returns to normal. Cell-mediated immunity is produced against different

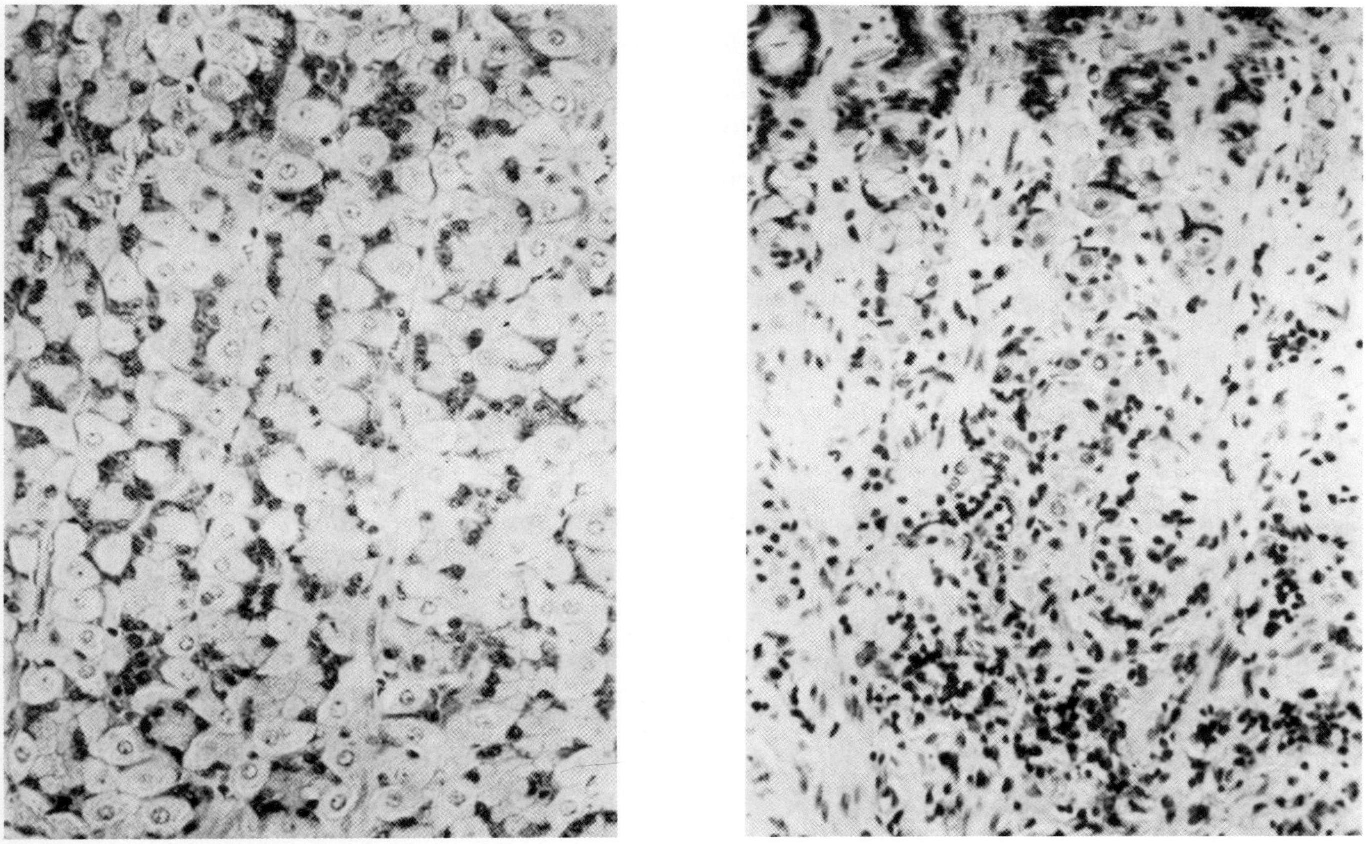

Figure 13-1. Left. Photomicrograph of gastric fundic mucosal biopsy from a normal untreated dog. Right. Photomicrograph of gastric fundic mucosal biopsy taken 3 weeks after immunization with autologous gastric juice. Reveals chronic inflammatory infiltrate and atrophy of gastric glands. (By permission K.J.E. Krohn, Clin. Exp. Immunol. 14:237-245, 1973).

antigens in gastric juice, including those in oxyntic cells and intrinsic factor.

Autoimmune gastritis is produced in other animals following thymectomy done shortly after birth.[7] Infiltration by T lymphocytes is seen early, and B lymphocytes are seen later. The inflammatory response can lead to glandular atrophy with the loss of oxyntic and chief cells; circulating antibodies to oxyntic cells can be demonstrated. In other cases the inflammatory response leads to mucosal hypertrophy. The delayed-type hypersensitivity reaction appears to be involved with the tissue damage. Self-tolerance breaks down so that the autoimmune disease can appear. The thymectomy causes the loss of self-tolerance, probably due to a loss of suppressor T lymphocytes that can inhibit the development of both cell-mediated and humoral immunity.

Chronic gastritis can be produced by injections of gastric juice alone (not in Freund's adjuvant), though it takes longer. Consequently, defects in the gastric mucosal barrier would allow gastric contents to be absorbed and stimulate the cell-mediated immune response. In this manner, chronic irritation could cause an immune mediated chronic gastritis. A pathogenesis based on the gastric absorption of antigens in gastric juices and mucosal cells indicates the importance of maintaining an animal with gastritis in complete remission. That is difficult in animals showing few clinical signs with the disease; there are few signs for monitoring the problem.

Protein-Losing Gastropathy. Excessive amounts of plasma proteins are lost through the mucosa with chronic gastritis. This phenomenon has been studied in experimental dogs, where there appears to be an immune-mediated factor in the pathogenesis of protein-losing gastropathy.[8] The gastric mucosal barrier is broken by the phospholipase enzyme in cobra venom, which degrades lecithin in cell membranes. Initial application of the toxin to the mucosal surface does not increase permeability to plasma proteins, whereas reapplication of the toxin four weeks later results in great amounts of plasma proteins leaking through the mucosa. The leakage is through the so-called tight junctions between epithelial cells. Four weeks are required for this response to develop, regardless of whether toxin reapplication is at weekly or bi-monthly intervals. The time required for appearance of the protein-losing gastropathy is consistent with the development of an immune response to mediate the effects. Supporting this theory are findings that venom-induced protein-losing gastropathy is less severe in dogs given corticosteroids, and protein loss does not appear in dogs treated with the immunosuppressive drug azathioprine.[8] Protein loss is reduced when the azathioprine is initiated after the gastropathy has developed. In humans with protein-losing enteropathy that is due to hypertrophic mucosal changes, the protein appears to leak through the tight junctions.[9] The protein loss is increased by pentagastrin and bethanechol and is reduced by anticholinergics, suggesting the pathway or mechanism for protein loss is affected by a cholinergic mechanism.

Arthus Reaction. The Arthus reaction is suggested to be involved in the formation of gastric ulcers.[10] In this reaction, excessive amounts of humoral antibodies are synthesized against an antigen, and then, on a subsequent encounter, they react with it. The excess antigen-antibody complexes initiate circulatory changes that result in congestion, edema, and hemorrhage. Morphologic changes in clinical cases of ulceration resemble those found in the Arthus reaction. Most antigens entering the stomach are dietary, which makes this a description of dietary allergy. The clinical signs of an allergy to certain foods include a usually rapid response, often characterized by acute vomiting and gastric mucosal changes. Signs can be less severe, however, consisting of discomfort and a vomition that does not immediately follow eating.

Infection. Chronic infection is sometimes suspected as a cause of chronic gastritis. Spiral organisms were identified in the stomach of animals over a century ago; since then a number of organisms have at one time or another been suspected as a cause of chronic gastric disease.[11] Campylobacter-like organisms are found in some humans with gastritis and peptic ulcer disease, and the lesions improve with elimination of the organism. Survival is possible in the stomach because the bacteria grow in crypts where the pH is not too low. No such organism has been found in dogs or cats, nor has it been shown that they can be infected. Recent studies report organisms resembling those of the genus *Spirillum* in the gastric glands and oxyntic cell canaliculi of normal Beagles.[12] Histologic changes were few and minimal. The organism closely resembled *Campylobacter* species and spirochetes. A number of other reports describe spirochetes in dogs. It is apparent that some spiral-shaped organisms are part of the normal gastric microflora, living in crypts of gastric glands. *Chlamydia* species have been identified in both clinically normal cats and cats with signs of gastric disease.[13] The significance of that organism with signs of disease is unknown. Bacteria in the stomach probably contribute to disease caused by other insults. Some gastric ulcers produced in experimental animals do not develop if pretreated with antibiotics.

Fungal agents are reported as a finding in the stomach of animals with chronic gastritis.[14] It is unknown whether fungi are primary and the cause, or whether they are opportunists that multiply when the normal defense mechanisms are compromised by chronic gastritis.

Parasites can be responsible for chronic gastritis and clinical signs in cats. *Ollulanus tricuspis*, a gastric nematode of cats, is distributed worldwide and is associated with anorexia, vomiting, and chronic gastritis.[15,16] Infection with the parasite is infrequently identified because routine parasitologic procedures and routine necropsy examinations usually fail to detect the parasite. The parasite's very small size and unusual life cycle precludes easy identification. Neither adult nor larval parasites are usually passed in feces. The organisms are vomited, and transmission is due to uninfected cats' eating the vomitus. Infected animals are identified by histology of the gastric mucosa, but that effort is unreliable because 50% of infected cats do not show the organism on three histologic sections. Dogs are also reported to be infected with *Ollulanus tricuspis*. Infection with the nematode *Gnathostoma* species is also described in cats.[17] The organism produces a granulomatous mass in the stomach wall that may or may not cause clinical signs. Fecal examinations can reveal parasitic ova.

Duodenogastric Reflux. Reflux of duodenal contents into the stomach is suggested to cause chronic gastritis.[18-20] As described in Chapter 10, bile and lysolecithin can damage mucosal surfaces. Bile by itself is not damaging to the gastric mucosa. Lysolecithin produced by pancreatic phospholipase activity on bile lecithin is capable of lysing cell membranes. Thus, duodenal fluid containing lysolecithin could damage the gastric mucosa, and such changes can be demonstrated in experimental dogs with duodenogastric reflux. Normal dogs show a low rate of duodenogastric reflux, and the rate increases following a meal.[21] Thus, if reflux is normal, chronic gastritis must be due to other causes. After eating, during a time when duodenal contents are rich in bile and pancreatic enzymes, there is a continuous to and fro movement of fluid across the pylorus.[22] Contractions of the pylorus control that movement and minimize reflux after eating. Performing a pylorectomy increases the rate of fluid refluxing into the stomach after eating. These surgical procedures reduce resistance across the pylorus, and they should increase the likelihood of gastritis, but that is not seen. The potential for damage by refluxed duodenal contents is determined by how much refluxes and how long the contents bathe the gastric mucosa. The amount refluxed is determined by pyloric resistance, duodenal muscle tone, and whether the fed or unfed state prevails.[23] Increased duodenal resistance caused by disease or augmented motility promotes reflux. Gastric emptying and gastric secretion of fluid determine the amount of refluxed fluid and the time that such fluid bathes the gastric mucosa. Emptying is determined most importantly by antral motility, reduction of which results in refluxed fluid's remaining in the stomach a longer period of time.[24] In the fed state contents remaining in the stomach buffer the refluxed contents, and gastric secretions dilute the refluxed fluid and reduce its damaging effects. Reduced gastric secretions, seen with achlorhydria, do not allow that. In the unfed state the stomach is emptied of refluxed fluid by strong antral contractions seen during the five minutes of phase III interdigestive motility complexes.[25] If that activity occurs only once an hour, the stomach could be damaged more by the reflux in the unfed state than by the greater amounts refluxed after feeding.

Duodenogastric reflux as described is normal in dogs and probably also in cats. Increased duodenogastric reflux may be a sign of preexisting gastric and intestinal disease rather than a cause of gastric disease. Normal amounts of duodenogastric refluxed fluid will impart a bile stain to vomited material and gastric mucosa. Dogs with histological signs of gastritis or enteritis, with gastric acid hyposecretion, and with delayed gastric emptying show duodenogastric reflux that may be increased or persistent. But all these conditions predispose to either greater reflux or reduced clearance of the refluxed fluid. Thus, it is not possible to determine whether abnormal amounts of duodenal fluid in the stomach are a cause or effect of chronic gastritis. Once chronic gastritis develops, it is likely that antral motility is abnormal in the fed state and that phase III motility is abnormal in the unfed state. Evaluation of duodenogastric reflux is difficult in clinical cases because intubation for collecting gastric juices stimulates reflux and because some bile is always present. In summary, increased duodengastric reflux is more likely a consequence rather than a cause of gastroduodenal disease.

Secretagogue Producing Tumors. Neoplasms producing histamine or peptide hormones able to stimulate gastric acid secretion are causes for chronic gastropathies.[26,27] Mast cells produce histamine, and mast cell-tumors release large amounts of histamine. The result is increased acid secretion that can cause gastric pathology and duodenal ulceration. The most important and often only signs of systemic mastocytosis relate to this acid hypersecretion. Thus, vomiting, anorexia, and abdominal discomfort are usually manifested. Since no therapy is effective in reducing the tumor mass, affected patients are managed with inhibitors of acid secretion. Other tumors can produce peptide hormones that stimulate gastric acid secretion and in some cases hypertrophy of the gastric mucosa. These tumors can produce biogenic amines, such as histamine and serotonin, as well as a number of different peptide hormones. Reports of animals with these tumors are very few. They present with clinical signs similar to animals with mast cell tumors. Management is with drugs to inhibit gastric acid secretion. Protection of the gastroduodenal mucosa is also dependent on bicarbonate secretion.[28,29] Therefore, correction of any systemic acidosis, maintenance of normal blood flow for bicarbonate delivery, and stimulation of bicarbonate secretion by the gastroduodenal mucosa are essential to ideal management. The analogs of prostaglandin E (misoprostol) improve mucosal blood flow and stimulate bicarbonate secretion as well as inhibiting acid secretion. Its affects to reduce acid secretion may not be sufficient to control the clinical signs; more potent drugs may be required.

Gastropathy with Hepatic and Renal Disease. Chronic lesions with or without ulceration develop in dogs and cats with chronic renal or hepatic disease. Some of the changes are due to increased plasma levels of histamine and gastrin and some are due to morphological changes in the microcirculation.[30,31] In addition to erosions and ulceration, chronic gastritis develops. Humans with chronic renal insufficiency have lesions of superficial gastritis over half the time.[5] Smaller numbers develop preatrophic or atrophic gastritis. See Chapter 12 for additional discussion.

Endocrine diseases are sometimes associated with chronic gastritis. Chronic gastritis with achlorhydria is described for humans with hypothyroidism; these may be two manifestations of related changes in an autoimmune disease.[32] Surprisingly, similar gastric changes are found in humans with hyperthyroidism.[5] A form of chronic gastritis in humans with diabetes mellitus shows achlorhydria and evidence for metaplasia of the mucosa. Chronic gastritis is also described in humans with hypoadrenalism. Adrenal steroids are necessary for prostaglandins to exert their cytoprotection in the gastric mucosa.

Drugs. Prolonged administration of some drugs can cause chronic gastropathies. Corticosteroids in addition to nonsteroidal inflammatory drugs are used very commonly and have potential for damaging gastric mucosa.[33,34] See Chapter 12 for additional discussion.

Pathophysiology

Chronic gastritis can affect all the major functions of the stomach. Inflammation can involve the stomach wall, with a loss of normal motility and reservoir function. Widespread inflammation of the mucosa can cause the secretory functions to be lost and can cause the mucosa to proliferate and interfere with gastric emptying.

Superficial Gastritis.[5] Chronic gastritis may begin in most cases with superficial gastritis. Grossly it is characterized by adherent mucus, patchy reddening, and edema sometimes associated with aphthae-like small erosions. Histology shows epithelial cells of variable diameter; microerosions may be seen. Mucous neck cells show degenerative changes; glandular cells are normal. Interstitial tissue between gastric pits (openings to the gastric glands) is infiltrated by inflammatory cells, with plasma cells prevailing. Some lymphocytes may be seen.

Atrophic Gastritis.[5] Chronic gastritis progresses to gastric atrophy, whose gross appearance includes as discoloration and thinning of the mucosa and also the appearance of blood vessels. Histology shows changes similar to those in superficial gastritis but more extensive and more severe. The gastric mucosal parenchyma is reduced, and inflammatory cells infiltrate into the deepest areas. In addition, glandular components are affected. The mucosal epithelium is generally flat, consisting of elongated cells that have oval-shaped nuclei. Metaplastic cells are frequent; many goblet or enterocyte-like cells appear. The gastric pits are shortened and tortuous, and special staining of surface mucosal cells shows abnormal mucus. Staining with PAS decreases, and acid mucopolysaccharides appear. Increased numbers of plasma cells can extend through the mucosa to and through the muscularis mucosa. Lymphocyte numbers also increase. The reduction in parenchymal thickness results from loss of glands and their cells. Residual glands are ectatic and their cells are deformed, showing vacuolar degeneration and sometimes substitution by metaplastic cells. Metaplasia is a change to the type of epithelium seen in the small intestine. Sometimes chronic gastritis is described as preatrophic or atrophic, depending on the extent of the pathology.

Chronic gastritis is mostly patchy or focal in humans; diffuse inflammation occurs in only one-third of affected patients. Pathologic changes, especially metaplasia, spread from the antrum to the fundus as a human ages. Biopsy is necessary for diagnosing chronic gastritis because there is a poor correlation between endoscopic appearances and histologic findings; superficial gastritis as well as chronic gastritis can appear normal grossly and abnormal gross appearances can be associated with normal biopsy findings. There is good agreement between gross and microscopic changes in cases of atrophic gastritis.

The gastric function of secreting gastric juices is lost with mucosal atrophy. Secretions of hydrochloric acid and pepsinogen are not essential for the assimilation of proteins, so that nutritional homeostasis does not suffer. Acid secretion is necessary for control of the bacterial microflora of the stomach and small intestine. The inability to secrete hydrochloric acid (achlorhydria) results in an increase in the bacterial population of the empty stomach and small intestine. This increase results in malabsorption and a loss of nutritional homeostasis. The effects of increased numbers of microorganisms in the stomach are not well known. The continuous presence of microorganisms in an organ where they do not normally survive, however, is a potential threat for infection. Microorganisms sometimes found deep within the stomach wall are more likely opportunists that invaded when conditions permitted rather than being pathogens that initiated the pathology. Gastric mucosal atrophy in humans results in a deficiency of intrinsic factors necessary for the absorption of vitamin B_{12}. Signs of deficiency appear as anemia. That condition has not been recognized in dogs with chronic gastritis. Since normal gastric acid secretion is required for absorption of calcium and iron, those elements could become deficient with mucosal atrophy.

Gastric Mucosal Hypertrophy and Hyperplasia. A response of the gastric mucosa to a chronic irritant can be hypertrophy and hyperplasia.[35] Hypertrophy is an increase in the size of mucosal constituents with little or no increase in cell numbers causing the thickening. Hyperplasia is mucosal thickening due to an increase in cell numbers. Hypertrophy is a frequent finding in endoscopic and radiographic examinations of the stomach. Hypertrophy can result from contraction of the muscularis mucosa and/or gastric muscle, which will cause folding of the gastric mucosa. Humans with such folding show normal thickness for the mucosa, and histology shows atrophic gastritis and often a normal mucosa.[5] Small animals have been reported to have chronic hypertrophic gastritis.[36,37] Hypertrophy or rugal enlargement is reported with hypertrophic pyloric gastropathy. In some cases the hypertrophy is caused by pathology in pyloric muscle with none reported for the mucosa. Hypertrophy may be an appropriate term to describe changes in pyloric and antral muscle but an inappropriate term for gastric mucosal changes. Mucosal hypertrophy does occur when interstitial edema or cystic formation increases mucosal thickness. Inflammation does not cause hypertrophic changes, but it does cause mucosal thickening as a result of increased amounts of connective tissue and the inflammation.

Hyperplasia is an increase in mucosal cell numbers that causes an increase in mucosal thickness.[38] The increase can be situated in the normal glandular epithelium. In some cases the hyperplasia affects metaplastic epithelium that has replaced the normal glandular epithelium. Increased numbers of mucous cells may contribute to the mucosal thickening, and retention of material in mucous cysts is sometimes found. Hyperplasia is accompanied by varying amounts of connective tissue and inflammatory cells.

Focal hyperplasia of the antral mucosa is not unusual; less common is widespread hypertrophy and hyperplasia. Most cases of hypertrophy and hyperplasia are found in small breed dogs (less than 10kg) such as the Lhasa Apso, Shih Tzu, and Miniature Poodle; older dogs predominate with the mean age 10 years old (range, 3 to 15 years). Males outnumber females two to one. In some cases the hypertrophy is associated with gastric ulceration. The specific causes of the mucosal changes are unknown. Chronic administration of salicylates can produce focal hypertrophy. Mucosal hypertrophy can be seen also with gastric-outlet obstruction, causing gastric retention. Gastric retention stimulates release of gastrin, a hormone that is trophic for gastric mucosa but only in the body of the stomach. The excessive gastrin could cause hyperplasia, but that is then a secondary problem; since it doesn't involve the antrum, it would not contribute to gastric retention. Hypertrophy or hyperplasia could be primary, however, causing gastric outlet obstruction as a secondary problem. Mucosal hyperplasia involving oxyntic and chief cells, seen in dogs with gastric retention due to pyloric stenosis, is presumably due to the retention. Cholecystokinin and acetylcholine, also trophic like gastrin for gastric mucosa, could be released in excess by chronic vagal activity.

Mucosal changes invariably include infiltration by inflammatory cells, lymphocytes, plasma cells, eosinophils, and variable numbers of neutrophils. In some cases these cells reflect an immune-mediated response that is causing the hypertrophic mucosal response. In others, these cells may infiltrate in response to an increased amount of antigens that diffuse through the defective mucosal barrier.

Hypertrophic gastritis in dogs has been compared to Menetrier's disease in humans.[39,40] Similarities include gross and morphologic features, protein-losing gastropathy, and infiltration of mucosa and submucosa with lymphocytes and plasma cells. The cause in either species is unknown. The pathogenesis of the problem in humans may involve an immune-mediated mechanism since the gastric mucosa contains an increased number of IgM-bearing cells.[41] Gastrin levels are normal in humans with Menetrier's disease.[42]

Gastric Retention and Outlet Obstruction. Chronic inflammatory disease of the stomach can involve all of its layers in a granulomatous process. The mucosa often appears uninvolved. Normal gastric motility is lost, and since the disease more often involves the antrum, gastric emptying ability is impaired. These patients show signs of gastric retention and gastric-outlet obstruction. By the time the impaired motility produces clinical signs, the changes are grossly evident and can be demonstrated radiographically.

Clinical Findings

Clinical signs include vomiting, diarrhea, weight loss, anorexia, depression, and anemia. Vomiting and weight loss are seen most commonly, although not consistently. Vomiting may be intermittent, not seen every day. Vomitus may consist of food or bile-stained liquid from the fasting stomach. Hematemesis is unusual, but melena is often seen with gastric bleeding. Since clinical signs are usually subtle early in the disease, many patients are not presented for treatment until the problem is in an advanced stage.

Physical findings are usually unremarkable. Evidence for anemia can be found. Rectal examination is done to evaluate feces for melena. Disruption of nutritional homeostasis is signified by weight loss and changes in skin and hair coat.

Laboratory Findings

Problems found in the hemogram are mostly reflections of complications of chronic gastritis, rather than a sign reflecting the pathogenesis of the primary problem. Eosinophilia that is not due to gastrointestinal or external parasites, skin disease, heartworms, pulmonary disease, or adrenocortical insufficiency is attributed to eosinophilic gastroenteritis until confirmed by biopsy or response to treatment. Leukocytosis and changes in the differential are induced by secondary infection and stress. Hypoproteinemia that is not due to renal disease can be attributed to protein-losing gastropathy. Anemia suggests gastric bleeding when it is associated with melena.

Blood chemistries are done to screen the patient for chronic renal, hepatic, pancreatic, and endocrine diseases, since one of these is more likely to be the cause of the clinical signs. Fractionation and quantitation of plasma proteins shows a loss of both albumin and globulins. Measurement of electrolytes and blood gases often identifies an alkalosis and hypokalemia.

Urinalysis is usually unremarkable. Although vomiting is not reported for some patients, low chlorides in the urine signify that vomiting is a problem.

Radiographic Findings

Radiographic studies using positive and negative contrast techniques are useful in identifying the site of a problem when chronic gastritis has produced gastric retention and outlet obstruction, thickening of the stomach wall, and, in some cases, gastric mucosal hypertrophy. Most gastric changes associated with chronic gastritis cannot be identified radiographically. Evaluation of gastric motility under fluoroscopic control shows loss of normal motility with advanced disease. Ultrasonography is useful in demonstrating focal or diffuse thickening of the gastric wall or pylorus.

Table 13-1a. Endoscopic Lesions Seen in Gastric Disease

Lesion	Cause
Hyperemia	Physiologic increased blood flow; inflammation; low intensity illumination
Paleness	Anemia; mucosal atrophy; excess illumination
Hyperreflectivity	Edema; excess illumination
Submucosal vessels (body & antrum)	Atrophic gastritis
Friability	Inflammation
Lack of mucosal pliancy	Infiltration
Petecchia/ecchymosis	Intramucosal hemorrhage
Bleeding	Mucosal or mucosal-submucosal disruption; coagulopathy
Erosions	Mucosal disruptions
Ulcers	Mucosal-submucosal disruption
Rugal hypertrophy	Failure to insufflate; hypertrophic gastritis; hypergastrinemia
Polyps	Epithelial hyperplasia; submucosal masses
Yellow nodules	Xanthomas
Pyloric stenosis	Neoplasia; hypertrophy
Altered luminal shape	Neoplasia; extrinsic compression; scarring from healed ulcer

Table 13-1b. Additional Endoscopic Lesions Seen in Duodenal Disease

Lesion	Cause
Increased mucosal granularity	Altered villus architecture
Cobblestoning	Ulcerations with intervening mucosal thickening
Patches of white villi	Lymphangiectasia

* A wide variety of lesions can be recognized by gastroscopy (Table 13-1a). For completeness, additional endoscopic lesions in duodenal disease are also listed.

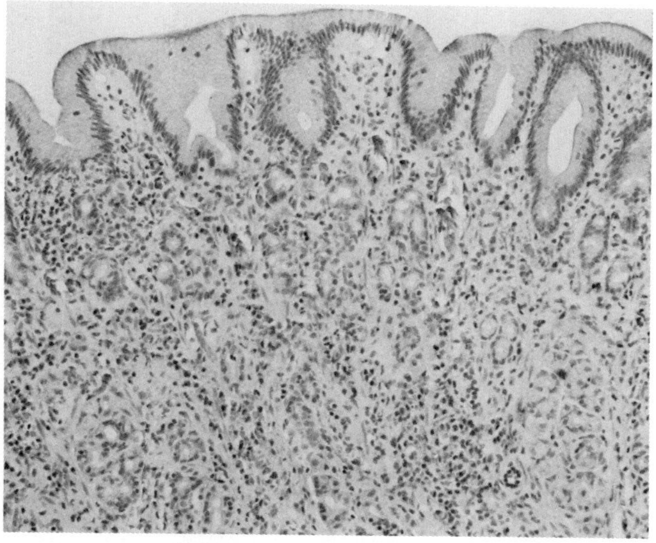

Figure 13-2a. Mild chronic gastritis. There is mild infiltration with mononuclear cells and a slight decrease in oxyntic and chief cell numbers.

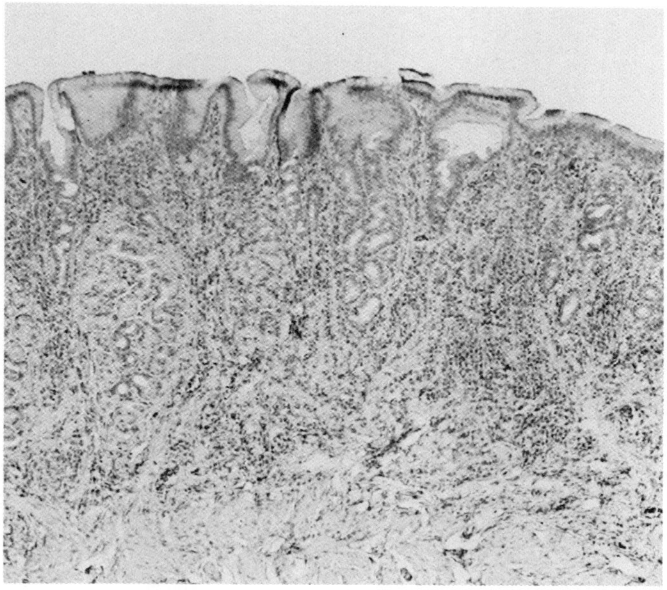

Figure 13-2b. Moderate chronic gastritis, typical of eosinophilic gastritis. Widespread infiltration of all regions of mucosa by mononuclear cells and eosinophils.

Endoscopy

Endoscopy is indicated for evaluating chronic gastritis. The mucosa may be grossly normal; in most cases some gross changes are seen (Table 13-1). Granulomatous lesions consisting of either focal or diffuse thickening of the stomach wall may be difficult to identify but are recognized on biopsy. Erosions and ulcers are identified more reliably with endoscopy than with radiographic studies. Endoscopy permits the retrieval of biopsies from sites suspected of being diseased with chronic focal gastritis.

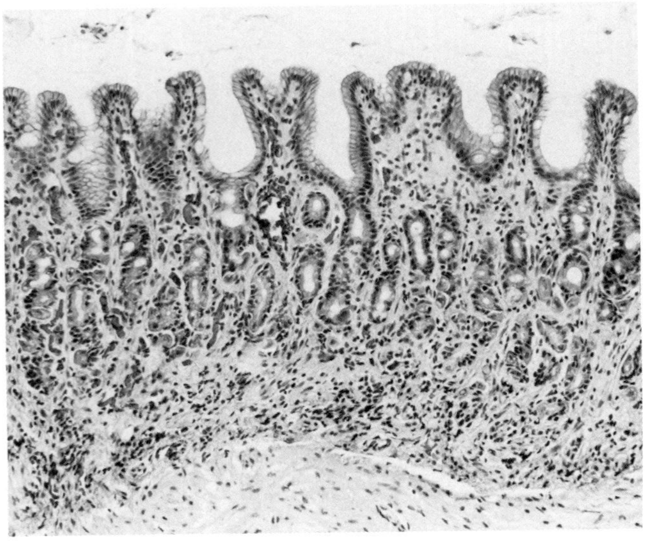

Figure 13-2c. Moderate atrophic gastritis. Tissue from body of stomach shows deepening of gastric pits with elongation of ridges to produce papillary effect, reduced numbers of oxyntic and chief cells, chronic inflammation throughout but especially in basal area where glandular cells have disappeared. Overall mucosal thickness is reduced.

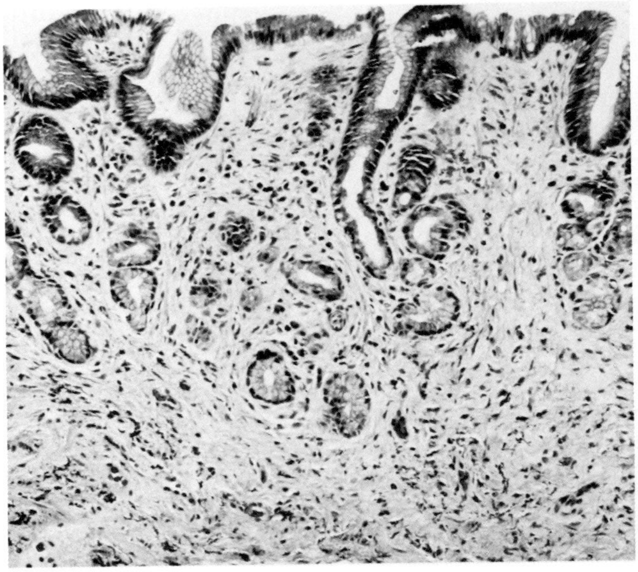

Figure 13-2e. Moderate gastric atrophy. Gastric pits are deepened. Oxyntic and chief cells are replaced almost entirely by goblet cells. Few glandular cells of any type remain.

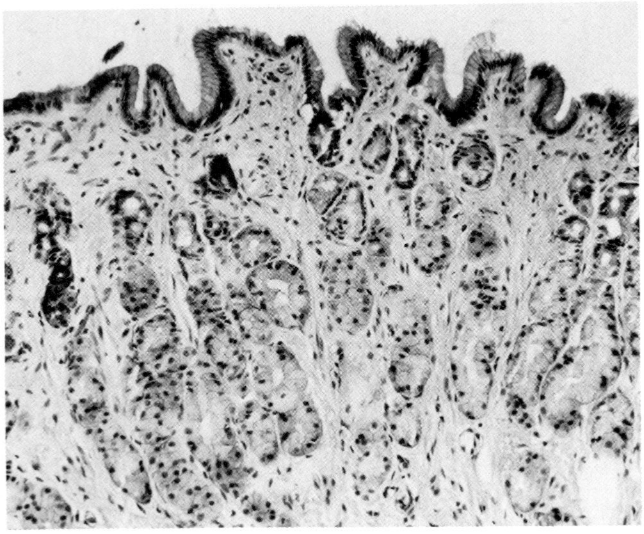

Figure 13-2d. Mild gastric atrophy. Glandular epithelium is slightly reduced with no replacement of oxyntic and chief cells by globlet cells. Little evidence of inflammation.

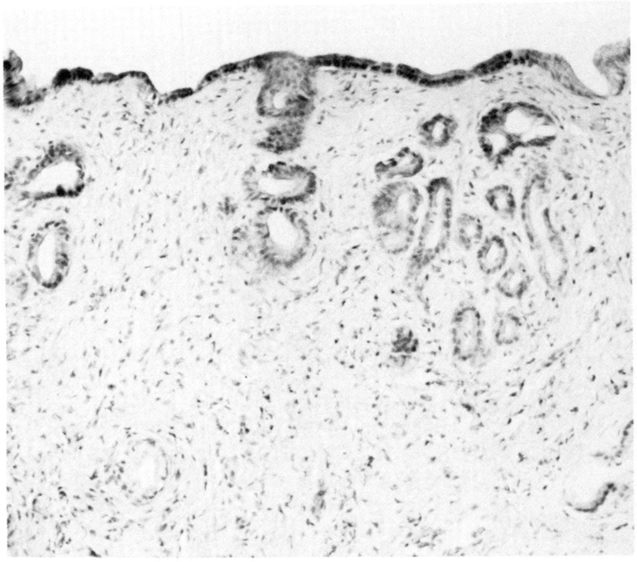

Figure 13-2f. Severe gastric atrophy. Reduced numbers of gastric glands. Deepening of one gastric pit. Evidence for intestinal metaplasia in epithelia of both surface and glands. The appearance of cells resembling intestinal epithelium with absorptive properties is associated with increased cell turnover. The accelerated rate of proliferation by mucous neck cells affects their differentiation to oxyntic and chief cells so that intestinal epithelial type cells are produced. Corticosteroid therapy may reverse this pathology. Little evidence for inflammation.

Biopsy and Pathology Findings

Histologic evaluation of gastric tissue is essential for a diagnosis of chronic gastritis. Most lesions involve the mucosa and submucosa, so that biopsy of the entire stomach wall is seldom required. Mucosal biopsies can be obtained with a suction biopsy capsule passed through the oral cavity and esophagus in unsedated animals. Biopsies with this technique identify diffuse lesions and are likely to miss focal lesions.

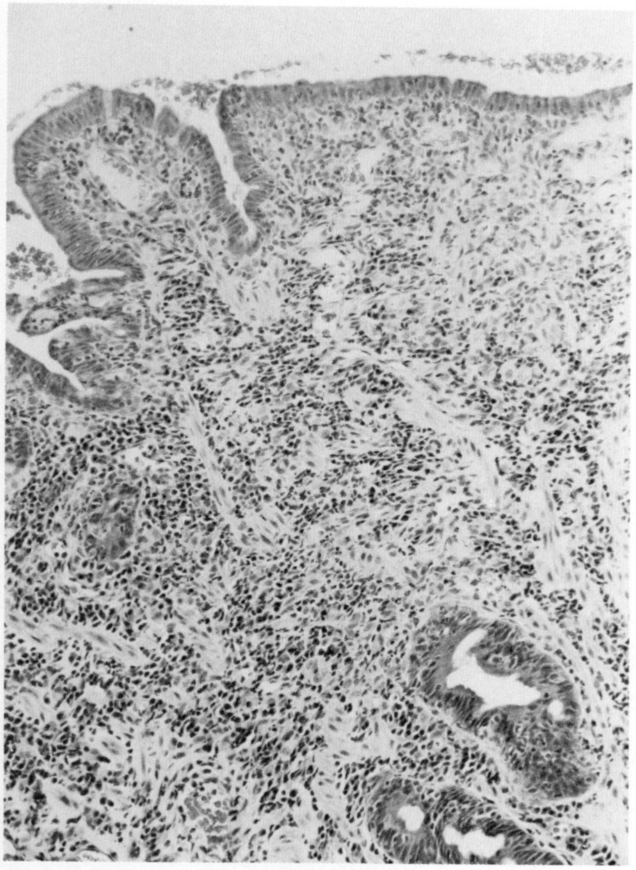

Figure 13-2g. Severe atrophic gastritis. There is diffuse infiltration by inflammatory cells that extends to submucosa. Intestinal glands have almost disappeared. Intestinal metaplasia evident by intestinal like epithelium replacing both surface and glandular epithelium.

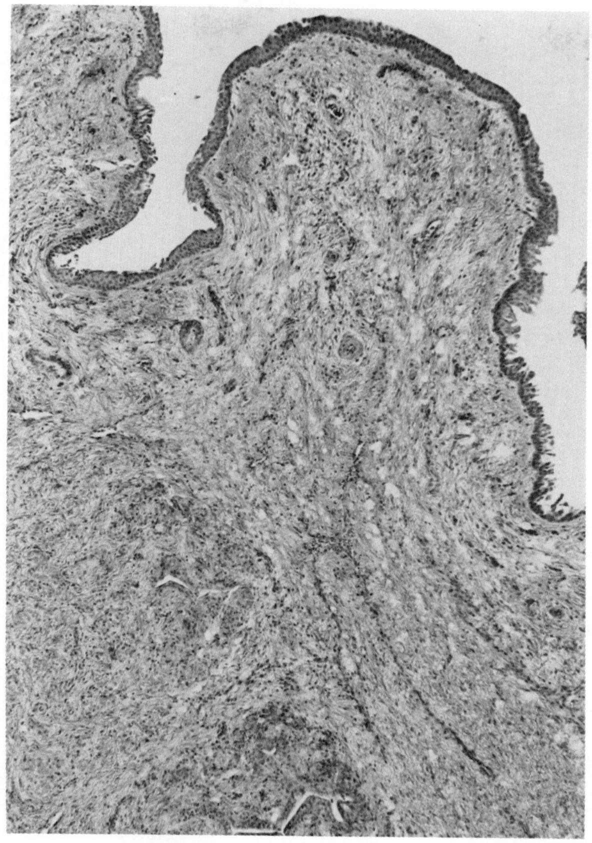

Figure 13-2h. Severe atrophic gastritis. Changes similar to and more severe than Figure 13-2g except for inflammation which is minimal.

Directed biopsies can be obtained via endoscopy to identify focal lesions. A full-thickness biopsy of the stomach wall during celiotomy is usually indicated for evaluating lesions that are demonstrated radiographically to increase the thickness of the wall.

Mild chronic gastritis may show leukocyte infiltration as the only change (Figure 13-2). That can be accompanied by edema and erosions. Restriction of the lesions to the mucosal surface produces a superficial chronic gastritis. With time, the surface epithelia can be destroyed and replaced by fibrous tissue, leaving the inner part of the mucosa relatively normal. With increased severity, bands of inflammatory cells can dissect and destroy the glandular mucosa, with subsequent replacement by fibrous tissue, producing an atrophic gastritis. Glandular epithelium can also respond by undergoing metaplasia, so that no normal secretory cells are seen. Mononuclear cells are the predominant cell type, with variable numbers of lymphocytes, plasma cells, and eosinophils. The appearance of lymphocytes and plasma cells supports an immune-mediated mechanism for the pathogenesis and signifies chronicity. These findings are not used to describe any specific disease or incriminate any etiology. The appearance of eosinophils is used to confirm eosinophilic gastritis. Neutrophils appear with necrosis. With increased severity, pathology can extend through the muscularis mucosa, producing ulcers. An inflammatory reaction surrounds the ulcer. Mucosal ulceration provides an avenue for microorganisms to invade the submucosa and muscle layers.

Chronic gastritis can develop into chronic granulomatous gastritis, with the lesions extending throughout all layers of the stomach. The lesions can involve only the submucosa and muscle layers, leaving the mucosa normal. Figure 13-3 is an example of one form, with the wall of the stomach greatly thickened and showing all forms of inflammatory cells, necrosis, edema, and fibrosis. Special stains did not identify any microorganism, although bacteria and fungi can sometimes be found. The pathology involved the antrum, pylorus, and beginning of the duodenum, producing signs of gastric retention and outlet obstruction.

Granulomatous gastritis can be characterized by a predominance of eosinophils. Three cases have been reported,[43] and two have been seen at the VMTH in Davis. The pathology section in Figure 13-3 characterizes the changes in the stomach of dogs with circulating eosinophilia of 15,000 to 30,000 cells/μl. Both dogs had single masses in the stomach, and one also had multiple masses in the spleen and small intestine. The

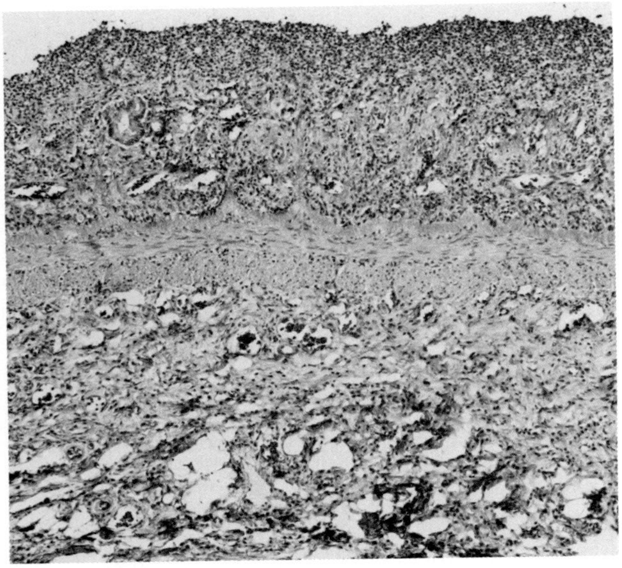

Figure 13-2i. Severe chronic histiocytic gastritis (cat). Total disruption of normal mucosal architecture by diffuse infiltration of large foamy histiocyte. Neutrophils predominate near luminal surface. Cells were not found in submucosa where edema is marked. Similar lesions were found in the pancreas. Remainder of findings were unremarkable. Cause was undetermined.

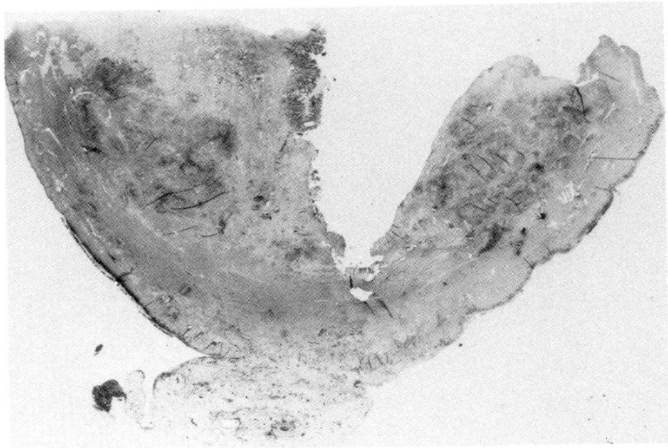

Figure 13-3a. Chronic granulomatous gastritis showing greatly thickened wall of stomach. The extent of the increased thickness is appreciated by the thickness of the mucosa that covers a small part of the luminal surface on the left center of section.

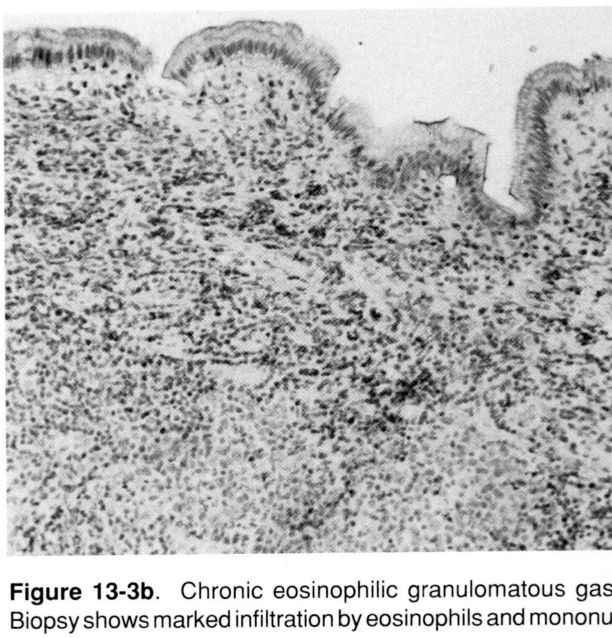

Figure 13-3b. Chronic eosinophilic granulomatous gastritis. Biopsy shows marked infiltration by eosinophils and mononuclear cells.

masses consisted of mixed inflammatory cells in the lamina propria, and primarily of eosinophils elsewhere. Evaluation of these tissues and bone marrow revealed the process to be nonneoplastic. Similar gastric lesions containing migrating nematode larvae are seen in humans.[44] They are also found, however, without any identifiable etiologic agent.

Mucosal hypertrophy and hyperplasia are associated with inflammation throughout the mucosa and submucosa (Figure 13-4). Lymphocytes and plasma cells predominate, and fibrous tissue is increased. Proliferation of epithelial cells produces the hyperplasia by increasing the surface area of the mucosa, thereby throwing it up into folds. Folding of the mucosa increases the submucosal size. Morphologic changes are not found to explain the protein-losing gastropathy or gastric bleeding associated with hyperplasia.

Management and Prognosis

Most important in the management of chronic gastritis is removal of the cause. That is rarely identified, however. The primary cause can be presumed to be some insult that enters the stomach regularly. Thus, potential causes are reduced by prescribing a controlled diet with the assumption that the cause is most likely in the diet. The most controlled diet needed to manage chronic gastritis consists of cottage cheese or tofu and boiled rice. In humans, soy protein stimulates gastric acid secretion less than meat protein; a similar effect may contribute to tofu's beneficial effects in dogs.[45] Adding linoleic acid to the diet may also be beneficial, since it increases prostaglandin secretion, which is cytoprotective for gastric mucosa.[46] The results of diet therapy are almost always evaluated only by clinical signs.

Response to treatment is evaluated by the disappearance of any of the primary and secondary clinical signs found before treatment began. In some cases the response is evaluated by changes in specific laboratory findings. Total circulating eosinophil counts return to normal in dogs with eosinophilic gastritis that are treated with a controlled diet. That consistent finding suggests a dietary antigen as the etiology. Eosinophil numbers can be monitored to determine the value of treatment, especially when new foods are introduced. Similarly, determinations of plasma protein can be used to follow the treatment of protein-losing gastropathy, which in the case of mucosal hypertrophy may respond to anticholinergics.[47]

Eosinophilic gastritis can be managed successfully with a controlled diet. The disease can also be treated with corticosteroids. Such drug therapy, without feeding a controlled diet, must be continued indefinitely; cures are not seen. Corticosteroids

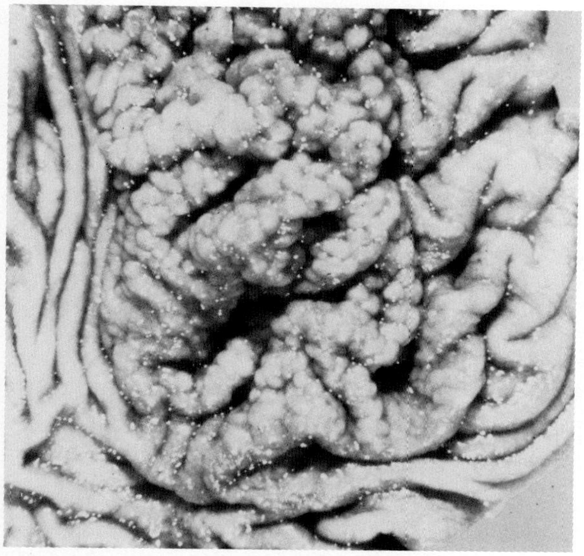

Figure 13-4a. Gastric mucosal hypertrophy. Numerous folds produced by hypertrophy can cause gastric outlet obstruction.

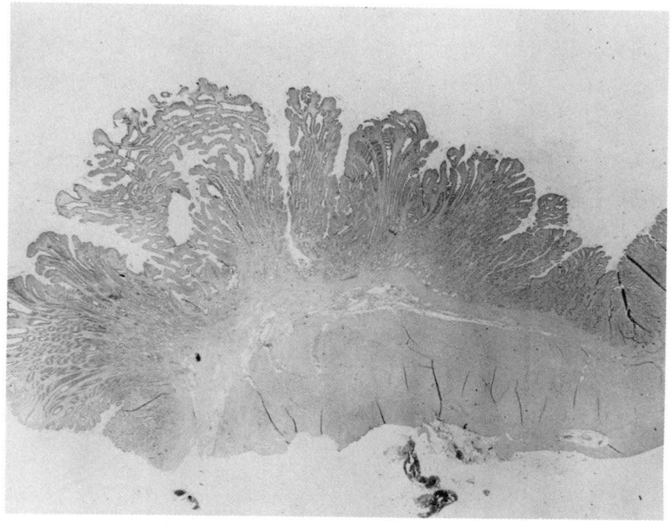

Figure 13-4b. Gastric mucosal hypertrophy. Cross section of stomach wall shows thickening that grossly resembled neoplastic process at surgery.

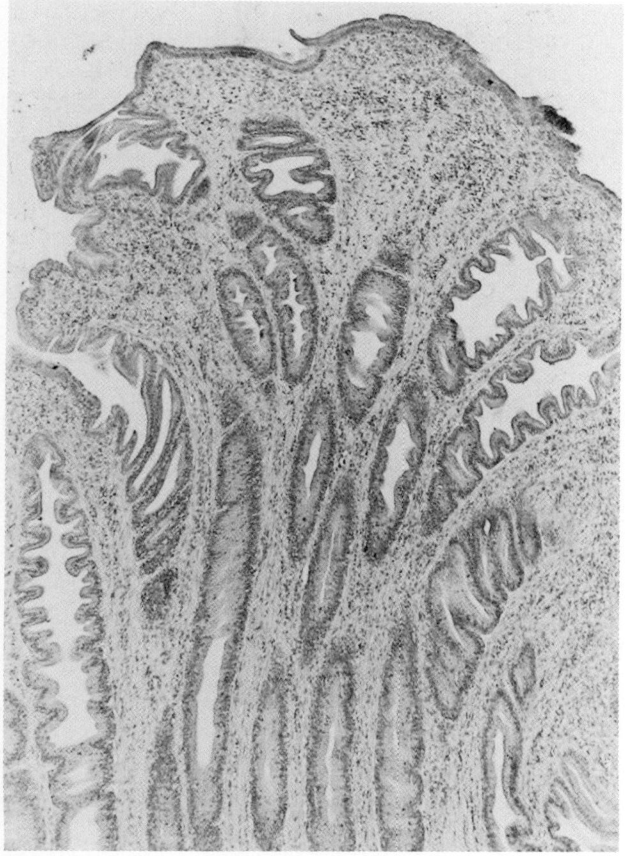

Figure 13-4c. Gastric mucosal hypertrophy. Microscopic of gross specimen in Figure 13-4a. Greatly thickened antral mucosa produced by marked hyperplasia of epithelial cells that typify intestinal metaplasia throughout section. Increased lamina propria contain fibrous connective tissue and moderate numbers of inflammatory cells. Lesions caused signs of gastric outlet obstruction which were successfully corrected by surgical excision.

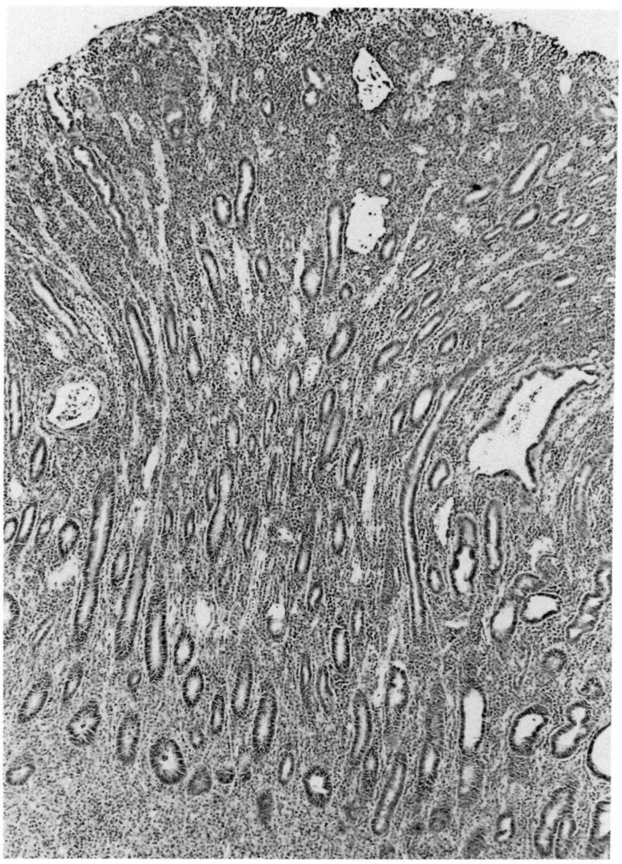

Figure 13-4d. Gastric mucosal hypertrophy. Changes in epithelium similar to Figure 13-4c except for marked infiltration by inflammatory cells.

are also indicated when biopsy findings include lymphocytes and plasma cells, suggesting an immune-mediated pathologic response. Gastric atrophy in humans has been treated with corticosteroids, although their value is not yet established. The drug can be used for gastric atrophy in small animals. Experimental studies show that gastric atrophy in the dog is reversible when the cause is removed, in which case drugs are not needed.

Corticosteroids are not recommended unless complete remission is not possible with a controlled diet. Animals with immune-mediated chronic gastritis have lost oral tolerance to some dietary constituents when they are found to improve with a controlled diet. A cure is not possible unless the oral tolerance is regained. That tolerance is developed by some supressor T lymphocytes; any drug reducing numbers or function of such cells prevents an animal from regaining oral tolerance.

Surgical resection is indicated for all tissue with granulomatous lesions. Resection has been successful in dogs with nonspecific and eosinophilic granulomatous gastritis. In three cases, remission was complete following surgery and a controlled diet. One to two years later, when the dogs were being fed conventional dog foods, the lesions reappeared in all three. Dietary control should be continued indefinitely following surgery. Surgical resection of the mucosa and pyloromyotomy may be indicated in dogs with mucosal hypertrophy and obstruction of the gastric outlet.

Antibiotics are of little value in treating a granulomatous lesion. They can be used for short periods where indications exist for acute gastritis. Antibiotics will not reduce the numbers of gastric bacteria increased by achlorhydria due to gastric atrophy. Unabsorbed antibiotics do not remain in the stomach long enough to be effective, and the gastric microflora is continuously renewed by oral microflora.

Antimicrobials may have beneficial effects in some animals with chronic gastritis. Colloidal bismuth is effective in reducing *Campylobacter* numbers in humans with chronic gastritis and ulceration. Such drugs could be effective in reducing the possibility of bacterial invasion by the normal microflora. Bacterial numbers are increased with atrophic gastritis, and that contributes to the greater risk for secondary infection.

Inhibition of gastric acid secretion may not be necessary with chronic gastritis and it may even be contraindicated. With atropic gastritis inhibition of gastric acid secretion is unnecessary, because achlorhydria or hypochlorhydria already exists. Drugs that reduce any remaining acid secretion allow bacteria to overgrow, resulting in new problems. If any antisecretory drugs are used, analogues of prostaglandins may be of greatest benefit because they are cytoprotective, primarily because they maintain normal mucosal blood flow.

Locally acting drugs used for acute gastritis can be used for treating chronic gastritis. See Chapter 12 for additional discussion.

GASTRIC RETENTION

Clinical Synopsis

Diagnostic Features

* Vomiting of food >8-12 hours after ingestion highly suggestive
* Abdominal distention and tympany may be present
* Gastric retention apparent on survey radiographs
* Abnormal gastric emptying studies
* Absence of documented outflow obstruction at surgery implies gastric motility disorder

Standard Treatment

* Attention to primary cause
* Metoclopramide 0.2 - 0.4 mg/kg PO administered one hour before meals

Abnormal retention of food in the stomach is caused by either gastric motility disorders or gastric-outlet obstruction, or a combination of both.

Etiology and Pathogenesis

Gastric-Motility Disorders. Acute stress produced by trauma and inflammatory diseases can reduce motility throughout the gastrointestinal tract. Reduction of gastric motility results in gastric retention. The effect is mediated through the sympathetic nervous system. Acute pancreatitis, peritonitis, gastritis, and gastric ulceration usually reduce gastrointestinal motility. Trauma and surgery of the abdomen and spine often cause gastric atony. Large losses of potassium through vomiting reduce motility, contributing to gastric retention. Motility does not return to normal until these deficits are replaced. Anticholinergics inhibit gastric motility and sometimes produce gastric retention. Acute gastric dilatation can lead to gastric hypomotility and retention that may not recover to normal. Uncorrected chronic obstruction of the gastric outlet can also lead to irreversible loss of gastric motility. Now it is known that more subtle abnormalities can contribute to abnormal gastric emptying times.

Intragastric pressure, which is regulated by gastric motility in the fundus, determines normal gastric emptying.[48] Loss of normal fundic motility results in gastric retention. With fluoroscopic evidence of fundic hypomotility, gastric retention may not be improved by surgical correction of gastric-outlet obstruction. Antral motility and the pyloric sphincter determine gastric emptying of solids.[48,49] The emptying of liquids is determined by fundic and antral motility, not by the pyloric sphincter.[49] Diseases disrupting antral motility result in gastric retention. They may be subtle problems that result in exaggeration of normal physiologic responses to change gastric motility. They can also be gastric diseases changing the stomach anatomically, such as chronic granulomatous disease and gastric neoplasms with involvement of gastric muscles.

Gastrointestinal motility is planned and coordinated by neural activity and by hormones (Table 13-2) to protect the small intestine as a first priority and the stomach as a second priority. Overdistention of the stomach results in reflux constriction of the pylorus and relaxation of the stomach, protecting the duodenum from movement of large volumes from the stomach into the small intestine.[50] Further distention of the stomach results in gastroesophageal sphincter relaxation, allowing contents to overflow from the stomach into the esophagus rather than into the small intestine, thereby protecting the stomach from rupture. Gastric relaxation is stimulated by a number of reflexes; all have an effect to delay gastric emptying.

Table 13-2. Hormones affecting gastric motility

Stimulates	
Entire stomach	motilin
Proximal stomach	neurotensin
Distal stomach	gastrin, CCK, bombesin
Inhibits	
Entire stomach	enkephalins, GIP, glucagon secretin, somatostatin, VIP
Proximal stomach	CCK, gastrin
Distal stomach	neurotensin

Distention of the esophagus, duodenum, or stomach stimulates gastric relaxation through neural inhibition of motility.[51] Fats in the duodenum or ileum decrease gastric motility, delaying emptying.[52,53] Stress, surgery, and inflammation or irritants anyplace in the abdomen can reduce gastric motility due to increased activity in vagal nonadrenergic inhibitory fibers.[54] Vagal denervation or anticholinergics remove a primary excitatory stimulus for gastric motility, delaying gastric emptying. H_2-receptor antagonists may also delay gastric emptying.[55]

Gastric emptying in the unfed state is achieved by gastric contractions during phase III of the interdigestive migrating motility complex (MMC).[25] That activity clears the stomach of particles greater than 2 mm in diameter that are not normally cleared during the fed state, primarily because of pyloric contractions. Gastric ulceration reduces antral motility, and it also disrupts the interdigestive MMC so that emptying is inhibited in the unfed state.[56]

Gastric emptying may be delayed by gastric dysrhythmias, which can be an abnormally fast rhythm (tachygastria), abnormally slow rhythm (bradygastria), or abnormally irregular rhythm (arrhythmia).[57,58] Tachygastria and arrhythmia originate from an ectopic pacemaker in the distal antrum; electrical activity is propagated from the antrum through the body of the stomach. The reversed direction of motor activity prevents normal gastric emptying. The contractions accompanying tachygastria are weak or absent. Dysrhythmias in dogs can be spontaneous or are induced by epinephrine, glucagon, or prostaglandins; abdominal discomfort, vomiting, and gastric stasis are noted in affected or treated animals.

Pyloric motility also determines gastric emptying.[59] Pyloric motility increases in fed dogs when fats in the duodenum stimulate phasic contractions.[53] Gastric distention has the same effect. Histamine, released to promote gastric acid secretion, stimulates pyloric contractions by acting at H_1-receptors on pyloric smooth muscle.[60] Diphenhydramine or phenylephrine block the response; anticholinergics have no effect. Nonadrenergic, noncholinergic nerve fibers and H_1-receptors on smooth muscle mediate the response. Opioids inhibit pyloric contractions and reduce pyloric pressure; they also initiate MMC activity. These two changes result in promotion of gastric emptying in unfed animals.[61,62] Opiates have different effects in the fed state, where they delay gastric emptying.

Food particle size and meal viscosity determines gastric emptying after feeding. Normal emptying occurs when gastric motility can reduce food particles to less than 2 mm in size. Larger particles remaining after a meal leaves the stomach are evacuated during interdigestive MMC phase III activity, which is also a time when the pylorus is relaxed. Particles greater than 5 mm in diameter leave the stomach at this time. Meals with a high viscosity leave the stomach more slowly than do meals with a low viscosity.

Procedures are currently available to evaluate patients for abnormalities in gastric emptying and gastric motility. Most of these abnormalities are subtle causes of clinical signs. Any of the problems or physiologic factors causing motility derangements may be found during one of the procedures to evaluate delayed gastric emptying.

Gastric-Outlet Obstruction. Intraluminal foreign bodies lodged in the pylorus produce gastric retention. The gastric outlet can be obstructed by polyps in the pyloric antrum and by hypertrophy or hyperplasia of antral mucosa.

Intramural problems of the antrum or pylorus most often cause gastric outlet obstruction. Causes include chronic granulomatous gastritis, stenosis from scar tissue formed following acute pancreatitis, gastric neoplasms, and pyloric stenosis.

Pyloric stenosis. Pyloric stenosis is a common cause of gastric-outlet obstruction. The incidence of pyloric stenosis in dogs at the VMTH at Davis is 6.5 cases per 10,000. It is recognized most often in young animals, with a breed tendency in the Boxer and Boston Terrier. The incidence in those breeds at the VMTH is 10 times higher than expected. Pyloric stenosis or dysfunction is also reported in cats, almost all of which were Siamese.[63-65] The pylorus did not appear abnormal; with no evidence of stenosis or muscular hypertrophy, the problem may have been a pyloric dysfunction rather than stenosis. Despite no evidence for abnormal gastric motility, gastric emptying time was abnormal, and that was corrected by pyloromyotomy or pyloroplasty.

Excessive secretion of gastrointestinal hormones may produce pyloric stenosis. Gastrin has potent trophic effects on gastric smooth muscle as well as on the mucosa of the gastric body. Gastrin injections in bitches during pregnancy cause more than one-fourth of the pups to be born with pyloric stenosis.[66] The pyloric circular muscle is hypertrophied and appears identical to changes seen in the spontaneous disease. Some changes are found also in ganglia cells of the intrinsic plexuses. Gastroduodenal ulcerations are found in some, probably resulting from gastrin-stimulated hypersecretion of hydrochloric acid. The pyloric-muscle hypertrophy could result from excessive release of secretin and cholecystokinin secondary to acid hypersecretion.[67] In human infants there is an increase in serum gastrin levels that persists after surgical correction of the stenosis.[68] Recent studies also show a marked loss in peptide hormone immunoreactivity in nerves within pyloric muscle.[69]

Pyloric stenosis, due to hypertrophy of the pyloric muscles, has been recognized more often in mature animals at the VMTH at Davis. Less than 30% of those cases recognized over a seven-year period were in animals under a year of age, with most of that 30% in animals six to twelve months old. Incidence was greatest (33%) in animals four to seven years old. The pathogenesis of adult onset of pyloric stenosis is unknown. The history often indicates some vomiting shortly after weaning, controlled with a few adjustments in the diet. Others have a long history of intermittent vomiting, although never severe enough to prompt the seeking of medical advice. This all suggests a problem, present at birth, that worsens with time. Mild gastric

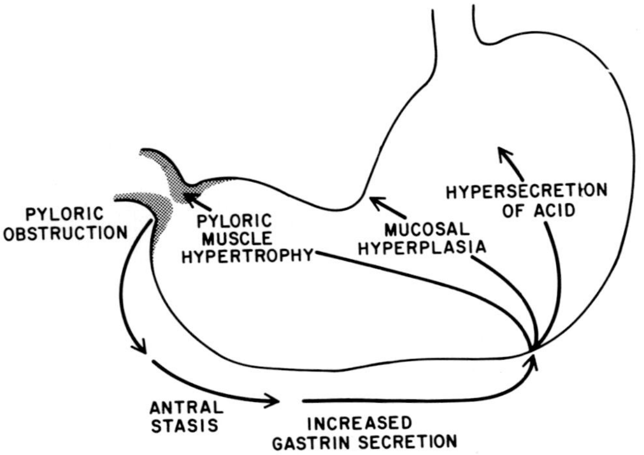

Figure 13-5. Schematic of stomach with effects of abnormal retention of contents. Chronic distention of antrum stimulates gastrin release, which has trophic effects on pyloric muscles and gastric mucosa. Gastrin is also the most potent stimulus for acid secretion. The events can progress to produce gastric-outlet obstruction.

retention can cause a mild gastric-outlet obstruction to worsen. Chronic distention of the stomach stimulates gastrin release. Gastrin's trophic effects on the mucosa of the gastric body cause hypertrophy, producing a larger mucosal plug that may contribute to blocking the pylorus (Figure 13-5). Normal mucosa forms a loose layer of tissue that slides into and partially closes the pyloric orifice, permitting only a small amount of liquid chyme to pass through with a peristaltic wave. Hypertrophied mucosa must sometimes be resected in treating pyloric stenosis. Mucosal hypertrophy develops over the years if hypertrophy of pyloric muscles is congenital, since pyloric stenosis is seen in dogs ten years old. Pyloric stenosis can cause gastric dilatation, with normal gastric motility irreversibly lost in some cases. Pyloric stenosis is not likely to be due to abnormal motility of pyloric muscle. In humans with the problem, manometric studies show no unusual motor activity of the pylorus.[70] In some cases constriction of the pyloric lumen is not found, suggesting that gastric retention may be due to failure of diastolic filling of the antrum, so that when contraction occurs, less is delivered through the pylorus. This justifies cutting a wide band of the muscles over the antrum and pylorus to correct the stenosis. Smooth muscle in the gastrointestinal tract cranial to a stricture undergoes hypertrophy. When that is evident in the gastric antrum, myotomy of antral muscles as well as the pylorus may be more beneficial than surgery on only the pylorus.

Pylorospasm: An entity? The term "pylorospasm" is suggested by some radiographic findings as appropriate for describing abnormal contraction of the pyloric muscle to close the sphincter. There is no other evidence that the sphincter can close to create a "pylorospasm".[70] During gastric emptying of a meal the pyloric sphincter does not function independently of the antrum.[70] Smooth muscle layers of the antrum and sphincter are continuous and contract as a unit on neural stimulation. Peristaltic waves traveling over the stomach cause the antrum to contract, followed by contraction of the pylorus. The pylorus does not relax to open the sphincter and allow food to pass. Furthermore, the pylorus never closes completely,[49] even with pyloric hypertrophic stenosis.[70] Identifying intermittent periods when positive contrast medium cannot be seen in the pyloric canal is not evidence that the pyloric spasm has occluded the lumen and is responsible for delayed gastric emptying. Phasic activity is normal in animals and is most apparent after feeding a high-fat meal, where phasic activity increases as duodenal and antral motility decreases. The purpose of the phasic activity is to delay gastric emptying. Pyloric phasic activity is inhibited by activation of non-adrenergic noncholinergic nerves in the antrum and is stimulated by intrinsic nerves from the duodenum and extrinsic vagal nerves. Atropine inhibits phasic contractions.[59] Radiographic observations of the pylorus opening and closing most likely represent pyloric phasic contractions. "Pylorospasm" as the phenomenon of phasic pyloric contraction is not abnormal. With clinical signs of gastric-outlet obstruction and radiologic evidence for "pylorospasm," pyloric stenosis should be ruled out, by surgery if necessary. "Pylorospasm" is often thought to respond to medical management with anticholinergics; most forms of gastric-outlet obstruction respond to changes in feeding practices, however, and anticholinergics may relieve vomiting. A response can be seen despite the adverse effects of anticholinergics in reducing gastric motility and delaying emptying.

Clinical Findings

The primary sign is vomition, frequently accompanied by bloat. Anorexia and depression are usually not seen with pyloric stenosis but are consistent with other types of gastric retention. Weight loss may or may not be a problem. Vomiting can occur immediately after eating, but it is more usual for food to be vomited at the time the stomach should be empty. Vomition of food consumed the previous day is diagnostic for gastric retention. The normal stomach empties completely within six to eight hours after a meal. The vomitus need not always contain food. Consequently, finding no food in the vomitus does not rule out gastric retention. The vomiting is described as sometimes being projectile. That term has been poorly defined but usually means an explosive type of vomiting, with little preceding in the way of salivation and retching. Food in the vomitus appears digested or undigested. Vomitus with a fecal odor is seen with both intestinal obstruction and gastric retention. Lipemia persisting more than twelve hours after feeding can be seen with gastric retention.

Radiographic Findings

Radiographic studies are the most important means of identifying gastric retention and gastric-outlet obstruction.[71,72] Survey films of the abdomen often show gastric retention of fluid and food at a time that it should be empty. Gastric motility is evaluated with a positive-contrast medium under fluoroscopic control. Gastric retention due to motility problems is identified by a loss of normal antral motility. A generalized loss of gastric motility is usual. Films taken sequentially during studies with positive-contrast medium show delayed entry of gastric contents into the duodenum (Figure 13-6) and a delay in complete evacuation of the stomach. In addition, pyloric constriction can sometimes be identified (Figure 13-7). Thickening of the gastric wall can sometimes be shown radiographically (Figure 13-9).

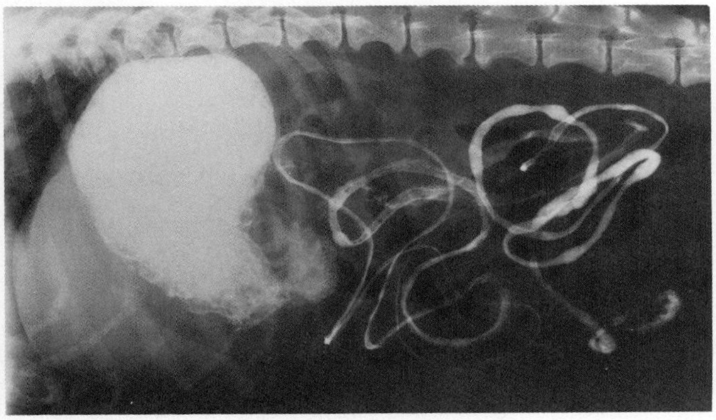

A

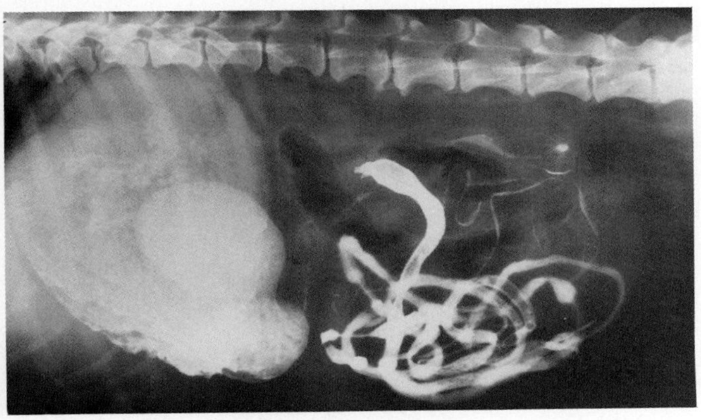

B

Figure 13-6. Lateral radiographs of abdomen of 11-year-old Dalmatian presented with clinical signs of postprandial vomiting and abdominal distention. At the time of the study the animal had received no drugs and had undergone no surgery. There was no history of an episode of acute dilation. The dog was not excited at the time of the study. Fluoroscopic control after the administration of positive-contrast medium revealed no gastric motility. Film taken at 15 minutes (A) shows that contrast that has left the stomach moves normally through the small bowel. The film taken at 2.5 hours (B) shows further distention of the stomach and diminution of the contrast's density. This results from gastric secretions accumulating in the stomach. Gastric retention of contents with subsequent distention is a potent stimulus for gastric secretion. Diagnosis in this case was chronic gastric atony.

Normal findings on radiographic studies with liquid positive-contrast medium do not rule out pyloric stenosis. Dogs with pyloric stenosis confirmed by surgery and biopsy can have a normal radiographic study of the stomach with liquid positive-contrast medium. The radiographic appearance of the pylorus can be normal (Figure 13-8). When gastric emptying problems cannot be confirmed with standard radiographic procedures, gastric emptying of food should be evaluated. Gastric emptying studies can be done by mixing barium with food and determining the time required for complete emptying of the stomach. The stomach is not completely emptied of food until five to fifteen hours after feeding, in contrast to the complete emptying of liquid contrast within two hours in dogs.[73] After feeding kibble the mean complete emptying time was 7.0 hours in one study and 10.9 hours in another study.[74,75]

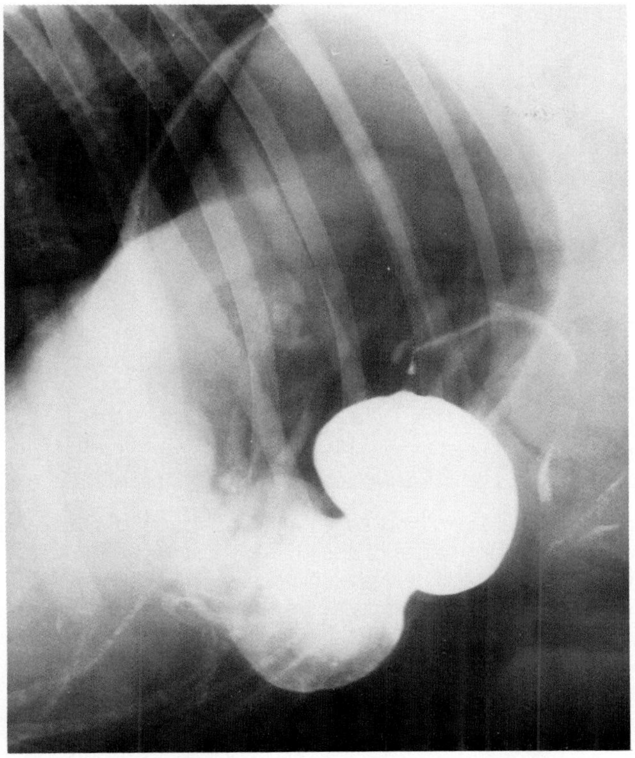

Figure 13-7. Lateral (right-side down) radiograph taken of dog with clinical signs of gastric-outlet obstruction. Liquid positive-contrast medium was administered, and radiograph was taken 60 minutes later. The distended antrum shows a wave of peristaltic contraction, and examination under fluoroscopic control showed gastric motility to be normal. A minimal amount of contrast is seen entering the duodenum. Subsequent radiographs showed persistence of these findings. It is essential to follow these abnormalities with a sequence of radiographs. A diagnosis of pyloric stenosis was confirmed during surgery. Treatment with pyloromyotomy corrected the problem.

Gastric retention of positive contrast medium mixed with food for eight to ten hours supports the clinical diagnosis of delayed gastric emptying. Gastric emptying studies are done also with scintigraphic techniques using radioactive tracers mixed with food. The emptying time for normal animals varies considerably because of differences in the foods used. Liquid diets empty faster, with a half-time of 1.0 to 1.5 hours in normal dogs.[76] Nearly complete emptying (95%) is seen in 2.5 hours. Dry cereal in another study had a half-time of 2.9 hours.[77] In yet another study, feeding a dry cereal showed a half-emptying time of 3.7 to 4.9 hours in mixed-breed dogs and Beagles, respectively.[78] Scintigraphic evaluation confirmed that a number of dogs with signs consistent with abnormal gastric retention and normal conventional positive contrast radiographic examinations had abnormal retention. Some of these dogs had pyloric problems that were corrected by surgery; some had inflammatory disease of the duodenum and in some cases the stomach, where a combination of surgical and medical management corrected the problem. Scintigraphic procedures are also available for identifying gastrointestinal bleeding.[79] Endoscopy is considered the most reliable procedure for that, however.

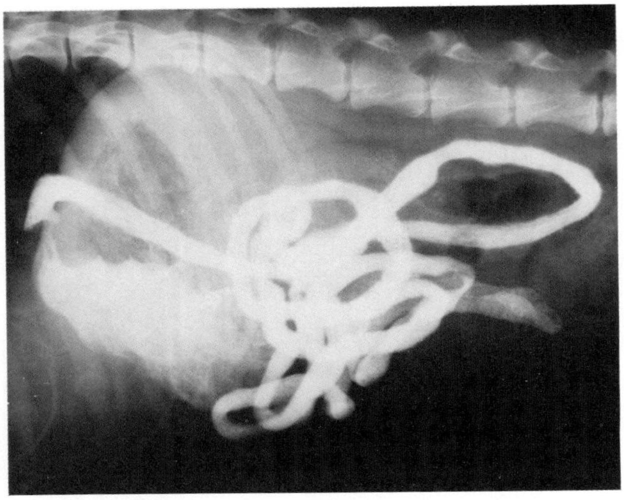

Figure 13-8. Lateral radiographs taken of 9-month-old Doberman showing clinical signs of gastric-outlet obstruction. Liquid positive-contrast medium was administered, and the 15-minute film shows considerable emptying into the small intestine. The wall of the pyloric canal is thickened and the lumen is narrow. The spot film shows magnification of the pyloric canal. Such cases should be examined under fluoroscopic control since a similar appearance is possible in normal dogs. During an exploratory laparotomy the pyloric muscles were hypertrophied and a pyloromyotomy was performed. Complete remission of clinical signs followed. Diagnosis was pyloric stenosis.

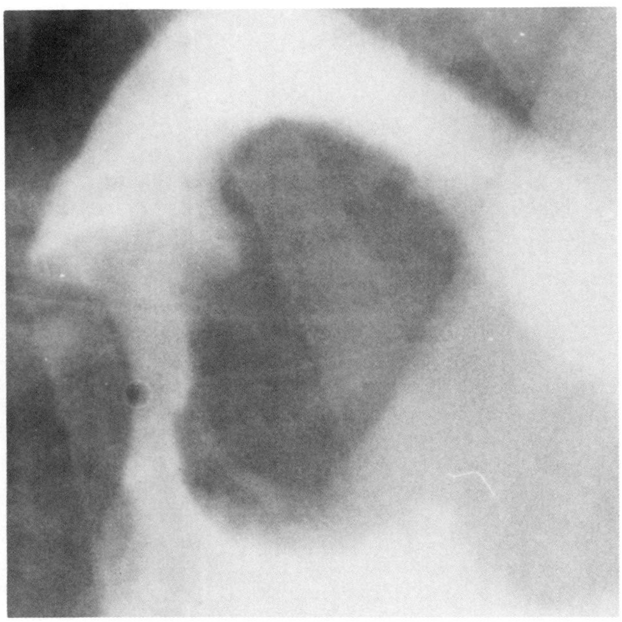

Diagnosis

Gastric retention and outlet obstruction is usually diagnosed with radiographic findings. If survey radiographs are normal but clinical signs are highly suspect for gastric retention or gastric-outlet obstruction, studies are done to evaluate gastric emptying of food. Moderate to considerable food remaining in the stomach after eight to ten hours is enough evidence to consider emptying delayed and obviates the need for such procedures. Gastric emptying studies using scintigraphy are evaluated using normal times established for that protocol. If abnormal gastric emptying is confirmed the problems is evaluated further by gastrotomy. Surgery is performed to ruleout pyloric obstruction, increase pyloric diameter and to obtain biopsies of the stomach and duodenum. In some cases the pylorus is grossly normal, and a diagnosis cannot be confirmed on histology of sphincter muscle or mucosa. Although many such patients respond to pyloric surgery, the diagnosis remains speculative. Biopsies of gastroduodenal mucosa showing inflammatory changes provide a diagnosis, and such animals usually respond to the combination of pyloric surgery and medical management of the inflammatory bowel disease. Endoscopy can also be used to evaluate delayed gastric emptying Biopsies of the gastroduodenal mucosa can be obtained during endoscopy, but pyloric stenosis due to muscular hypertrophy can be missed and another anesthesia is required if pyloric surgery is deemed necessary. Therefore, with abnormal gastric retention confirmed, it is recommended that celiotomy be done rather than facing the limitations of an endoscopic procedure. Neither celiotomy nor endoscopy is performed, however, before all esophageal problems and medical problems in other organs are ruled out.

Management

Correction of Gastric-Outlet Obstruction. Gastric outlet obstruction is managed surgically.[36,37,80] Granulomatous lesions are not successfully treated medically. All of the diseased tissue should be surgically resected. Pyloric stenosis is treated by pyloromyotomy or pyloroplasty. Myotomy of the pyloric ring should extend into the hypertrophied antral muscles to correct any inadequate filling of the antrum. Pyloroplasty can include an incision through the mucosa to obtain biopsies, resect hyperplastic or hypertrophic mucosa, or remove any polypoid masses in the mucosa. With extensive disease, the pylorus is sometimes resected and a gastroduodenostomy is performed. In all cases biopsies are obtained from pyloric tissue and gastroduodenal mucosa. The prognosis is good, except for some animals with malignancies that cause the gastric retention. None of these surgeries alters gastric emptying rates for food.[81-83] Following such surgeries the regulation of gastric emptying of food is preserved.[84] Removing only the antrum or the pylorus, not both, preserves the dog's ability to retain food in the stomach until particle size is less than 1.0 mm.[85] Thus, particles 5.0 mm or greater in size still empty during unfed phase III motor activity rather than with food in the fed state.[86] Duodenogastric reflux would appear to increase and cause chronic gastric following one of these surgeries on the pylorus. In fasting dogs that is not seen; neither Pyloroplasty nor pylorectomy increases the rate of duodenogastric reflux.[21] In the fed state pylorectomy but not pyloroplasty causes an increase in duodenogastric reflux. Temporary losses of gastrointestinal motility following these surgeries can be treated with beneficial results by metoclopramide.[87]

Medical management of chronic gastritis and duodenitis is described earlier. Although pyloric surgery can improve the abnormal retention in animals with these inflammatory diseases, satisfactory remission is not possible without appropriate use of controlled diets and medical management.

GASTRIC NEOPLASMS

Gastric-outlet obstruction and motility deficits are seen occasionally as a result of primary and metastatic neoplasms. Primary gastric neoplasms are diseases of older dogs, with the earliest age reported being five years and a mean age of nine to ten years.[88-93] Males are affected more frequently, representing 61% of the total reported. A higher risk was noted for rough collies and Staffordshire bull terriers in one study.[93] The incidence is low, at 3 cases per 10,000.

Etiology and Pathogenesis

Little is understood about the pathogenesis of gastric neoplasms in any species of animals. The incidence of gastric neoplasms is highest in humans, where the frequency can be correlated with the nature of the diet. The incidence of gastric neoplasms is greater in humans on a high-carbohydrate, high-fiber and low-protein, low-fat diet. This incidence may be related to the effects of the diet on gastric bacterial varieties and numbers or to additives the diet may contain. Predisposing gastric disease is related to the incidence of gastric neoplasms in humans. Gastric atrophy and reduced acid secretion predispose to tumor development. The secondary increase in gastric bacterial numbers may contribute to its pathogenesis. Increased bacterial activity may convert chemicals such as nitrates into carcinogens.

Clinical Findings

The clinical signs are the same as for chronic gastritis, gastric retention and gastric outlet obstruction. Consistent findings are vomiting, anorexia, and weight loss. Diarrhea and melena are often seen. Hematemesis is unusual. Anemia can result when blood loss is marked.

Radiographic and Endoscopic Findings

Radiographic studies with positive-contrast medium often identify gastric abnormalities that prove to be neoplasms (Figure 13-9). Gastric ulcerations identified radiographically are usually caused by gastric carcinomas. Radiographic results are often normal, however, in animals with gastric carcinomas that have metastasized to the lymph nodes, pancreas, and liver. Endoscopy may be of limited value in identifying gastric neoplasms, since lesions involving the wall of the stomach and covered with normal-appearing mucosa are difficult to recognize.

Biopsy and Pathology Findings

Primary gastric neoplasms are found equally in the pylorus and in the body of the stomach.[88,89,91] Most are diffuse and involve both regions. Few are found in the fundus. One study reported 11 adenocarcinomas and 3 adenomatous polyps. Another reported 14 carcinomas, 3 lymphosarcomas, 2 leiomyomas, and 1 leiomyosarcoma. The neoplasms found at Davis were 8 leiomyomas, 3 carcinomas, 1 fibroma, 1 sarcoma, and 1 lymphosarcoma (Figure 13-10). Carcinomas consisting of glands were termed adenocarcinomas, and those having marked infiltration of fibrous tissue were classified as scirrhous adenocarcinomas. One survey reported benign tumors accounting for 31% (8% epithelial and 23% mesenchymal in origin) and malignant tumors representing 68% (53% epithelial and 15% mesenchymal in origin).[92] Malignant tumors regularly spread initially to regional lymph nodes.

Diagnosis

Gastric neoplasms are diagnosed by biopsy. Surgically correctable granulomatous disease of the stomach grossly resembles and is often mistaken for a gastric neoplasm. Biopsy is required to distinguish between the two, a treatable and a highly untreatable disease.

Neoplasms in tissues outside the stomach can produce chronic gastric disease. Some tumors can produce secretagogues for gastric acid secretion; they are primarily mast cell tumors, which are not uncommon, and gastrin secreting tumors, which

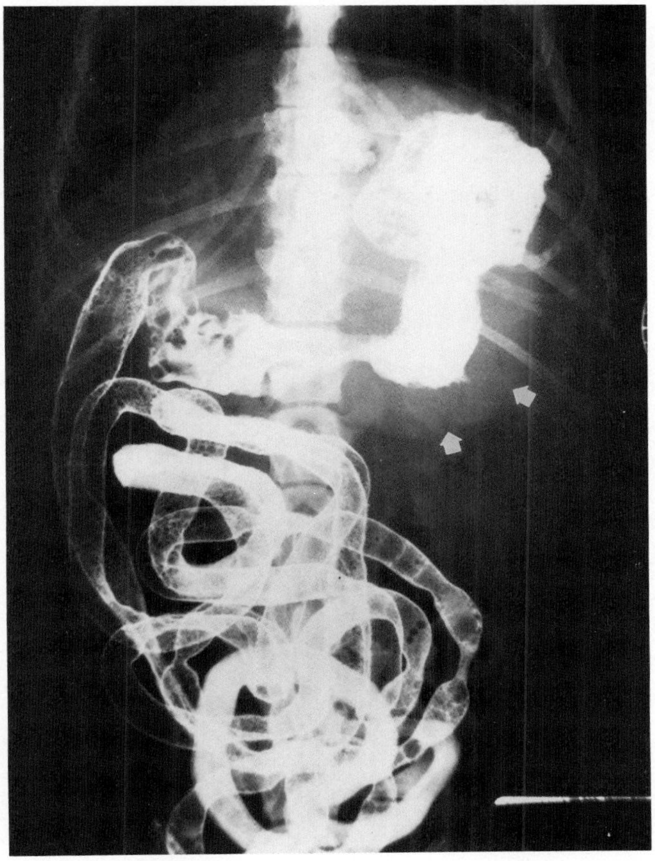

Figure 13-9. Dorsoventral radiograph of 9-year-old Keeshound with clinical signs of intermittent vomiting over a period of 6 to 8 months. Positive-contrast medium was administered, and the distal part of stomach shows a marked thickening of the wall (arrows). An ulcer crater evident in the thick part is suggestive of a tumor. There is an absence of any rugal pattern over the area involved. The narrowing of the body and antrum of the stomach was a consistent finding on several films, suggesting that it was not a wave of peristaltic contraction. Diagnosis of schirrhous carcinoma was made on histologic examination of biopsy tissue. The appearance of stomach is shown grossly in Figure 11-9a and microscopically in Figure 11-9b.

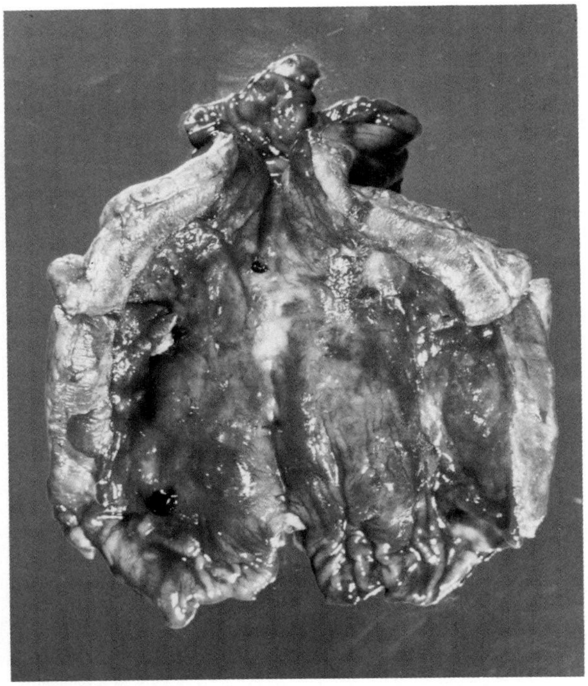

Figure 13-9a. Photograph of stomach removed from dog in Figure 11-9.

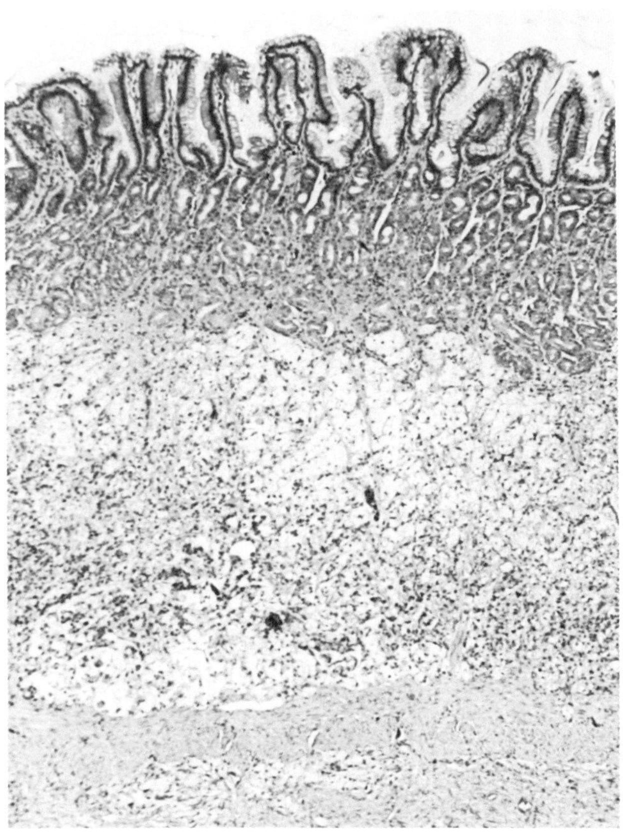

Figure 13-9b. Photomicrograph of stomach removed from dog in Figure 11-9. Entire submucosa and part of mucosa is infiltrated by adenocarcinoma cells. In other sections the muscles and entire mucosa were involved.

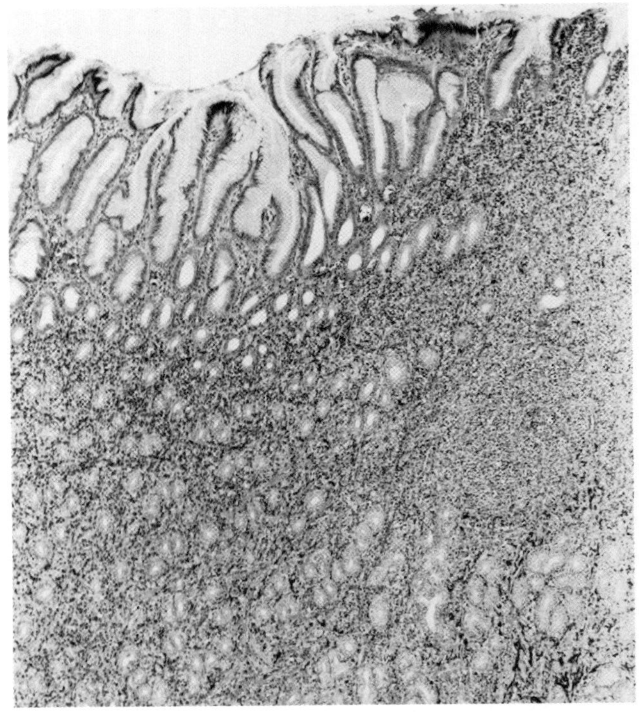

Figure 13-10. Photomicrograph of gastric biopsy from cat showing diffuse infiltration of lymphocytes, diagnostic for lymphosarcoma. Primary signs were anorexia and intermittent vomiting. No evidence was found for lymphosarcoma in any other tissues at necropsy.

are rare.[26,27] These tumors can be found also in the stomach. Mast cell tumors are diagnosed by finding unusual numbers of mast cells on a hemogram and by biopsy of the tumor mass or tissue containing metastatic cells. Gastrinomas are also diagnosed by biopsy of the tumor. Measuring the gastrin response to intravenous secretin or calcium gluconate also assists with the diagnosis.[27] Finding high gastrin levels without doing either one of these tests is not reliable for identifying gastrinomas. Hypergastrinemia can be caused by many different factors, making such gastrin measurements unreliable. Gastrin assay is available for the dog.[94]

Management

Gastric neoplasms are all treated by surgical resection. Lymphosarcoma can also be treated with chemotherapeutic agents. Tumors releasing secretagogues are managed by inhibiting gastric acid secretion.

EFFECTS OF GASTRIC SURGERY ON GASTRIC FUNCTION

A number of gastric problems are corrected by surgery, including pyloromyotomy, pyloroplasty, gastroduodenostomy and partial gastric resection. Postoperative management requires an understanding of the effects of surgery on gastric function. Surgery primarily affects gastric emptying.[95-97] Motility is altered by surgical interruption of gastric parasympathetic innervation and by muscle damage. It appears that damage must be extensive to alter gastric emptying, for that is not affected in dogs that have recovered from acute gastric dilatation.[98]

Motility

Gastrotomy. Surgical incision on the stomach during gastrotomy should be parallel to longitudinal muscle fibers in order to minimize the loss of normal motility.[99] Longitudinal muscles propagate the electrical control activity or pacemaker potential.[100] Transverse section of these muscles results in loss of the propagation of contractile activity. With good suturing techniques, normal motility is usually regained within two weeks. Propagation of contractile activity over the stomach can be permanently lost from poor technique, resulting in abnormal gastric emptying of solids. Gastric emptying of liquids is not affected unless surgery involves the fundus. Emptying of liquids is a function of intragastric pressure, which is determined by fundic motility. Postsurgical radiographic evaluation of gastric emptying with liquid positive-contrast medium shows a normal rate of emptying of the liquid in most cases, but that does not evaluate the rate of emptying of solids, which can be delayed.

Pyloric Surgery. Pyloromyotomy or pyloroplasty is used to treat gastric-outlet obstruction due to pyloric stenosis and to correct abnormal gastric retention. This surgery does not alter terminal antral contractions, and food is still triturated to small particles before leaving the stomach[81] Gastric emptying of solids remains normal. Pyloroplasty in normal dogs has little effect on emptying of solids and causes minor acceleration of emptying of liquids.[96,101]

The pylorus regulates or delays the emptying of solids until they become liquefied. Surgery on a stenotic pylorus rarely alters this function enough to cause clinical signs. Accelerated gastric emptying can produce the dumping syndrome, which appears when hyperosmolar gastric contents enter the duodenum too rapidly and precipitate a complex of clinical signs. Large fluxes of extracellular fluid rapidly enter the intestine, resulting in hypovolemia. Intestinal fluid accumulation and distention results in bloat. Hyperosmolar stimuli in the duodenum cause vomiting. Contributing to clinical signs are chemicals released from the intestinal mucosa in response to the hyperosmolar stimulus. They include biogenic amines such as serotonin, vasoactive peptides such as bradykinin, and some gastrointestinal peptide hormones. Pyloroplasty in dogs also doubles fecal fat excretion but without producing diarrhea.[102]

Antrectomy. Surgery to remove the antrum removes the part of the stomach that contracts with each peristaltic wave and retropulses food away from the pylorus.[103] Retropulsion acts to delay gastric emptying of solids. Although antral motility is required for normal gastric emptying, antrectomy is invariably combined with removal of the pylorus, with a net effect of accelerated gastric emptying of solids. Antrectomy alone in normal dogs has no effect on gastric emptying of solids or liquids.[96]

Pacemaker. Surgical procedures around the cardia can remove the center where electrical-control activity originates.[104] With its loss, a new center of activity arises in a region just distal to the site of resection. The new pacemaker beats more slowly, retarding gastric emptying.

Vagal Denervation. Surgical procedures should take care that the vagal nerves are not interrupted. Loss of vagal innervation to the proximal part of the stomach produces a persistent loss of motility in the fundus and body of the stomach and a transient loss of motility in the antrum (lasting three weeks).[97] Normal fundic motility is required for normal gastric emptying. Dogs with a loss of vagal innervation retain food almost completely for the first hour after feeding, after which emptying begins.[97] Pyloroplasty returns gastric emptying to normal after vagal denervation of the proximal stomach. Parasympathetic denervation of both the distal and proximal stomach produces more severe gastric retention.

Secretion

Gastric acid secretion can be affected by gastric surgery. Postsurgical gastric retention causing prolonged distention of the antrum stimulates gastrin-mediated acid secretion.[97] Mucosal ulceration seen following gastric retention is due in part to that increase. Little is known about either increases or reductions in secretion of gastric juices in clinical cases following surgery on the stomach. Reduced gastric acid secretion can be expected to cause increased numbers of intestinal bacterial.[105] Removal of the fundus in dogs results in increased gastric acid secretion and gastrin release.[106]

REFERENCES

1. Hottendorf, G. H. and Hirth, R.S.: Lesions of spontaneous subclinical disease in Beagle dogs. Vet Pathol. 11:240-258, 1974.
2. Brunschwig, A., vanProhaska, J., Clarke, T.H. and Kandel, E.V.: A secretory depressant in gastric juice of patients with pernicious anemia. J. Clin. Invest. 18:415-422, 1939.
3. Smith, W.O., Joel, W. and Wolf, S.: Experimental atrophic gastritis associated with inhibition of parietal cells. Trans. Assoc. Am. Phy. 71:306-311, 1958.
4. Hennes, A.R., Sevelius, H., Lewellyn, T., Joel, W., Woods, A.H. and Wolf, S.: Atrophic gastritis in dogs. Arch. Pathol. 73:281-287, 1962.
5. Cheli, R., Perasso, A. and Giacosa, A.: Gastritis. Springer-Verlag, New York, 1987.
6. Krohn, K.J.E. and Finlayson, N.D.C.: Inter-relations of humoral and cellular immune responses in experimental canine gastritis. Clin. Exp. Immunol. 14:237-245, 1973.
7. Fukuma, K., Sakaguchi, S., Kuribayashi, K., Chen, W-L., Morishita, R., Sekita, K., Uchino, H. and Masuda, T.: Immunologic and clinical studies on murine experimental autoimmune gastritis induced by neonatal thymectomy. Gastroenterology 94:274-283, 1988.
8. Davenport, H.W.: Prevention and suppression by azathioprine of venom-induced protein-losing gastropathy in dogs. Proc. Nat. Acad. Sci. (USA) 73:968-970, 1976.
9. Kelly, D.G., Miller, L.J., Malagelada, J-R., Hizenga, K.A. and Markowitz, H.: Giant hypertrophic gastropathy (Menetrier's Disease): pharmacologic effects on protein leakage and mucosal ultrastructure. Gastroenterology 93:581-589, 1982.
10. Siegal, J.: Gastrointestinal ulcer-Arthus reaction! Ann. Allergy 32:127-130, 1974.
11. Blaser, M.J.: Gastric campylobacter-like organisms, gastritis, and peptic ulcer disease. Gastroenterology 93:371-383, 1987.
12. Henry, G.A., Long, P.H., Burns, J.L.and Charboneau, D.L.: Gastric spirillosis in Beagles. Am. J. Vet. Res. 48:831-836, 1987.
13. Hargis, A.M., Prieur, D.J. and Gaillard, E.T.: Chlamydial infection of the gastric mucosa in twelve cats. Vet. Pathol.

20:170-178, 1983.
14. Barsanti, J.A., Attleberger, M.H. and Henderson, R.A.: Phycomycosis in a dog. JAVMA 167:293-297, 1975.
15. Hargis, A.M., Prieur, D.J. and Blanchard, J.L.: Prevalence, lesions, and differential diagnosis of *Ollulanus tricuspis* infection in cats. Vet. Pathol. 20:71-79, 1983.
16. Reindel, J.F., Trapp, A.L., Armstrong, P.J. and Stickle, R.L.: Recurrent plasmacytic stomatitis-pharyngitis in a cat with esophagitis, fibrosing gastritis, and gastric nematodiasis. JAVMA 190:65-67, 1987.
17. Kirkpatrick, C.E., Lok, J.B., Goldschmidt, M.H. and Mellman, S.L.: Gastric gnathostomiasis in a cat. JAVMA 190:1437-1439, 1987.
18. Happe, R.P. and Van Den Broyn, W.E.: Duodenogastric reflux in the dog, a clinicopathologic study. Res. Vet. Sci. 33:280-286, 1982.
19. Ritchie, W.P.: Alkaline reflux gastritis: a critical reappraisal. Gut 25:975-987, 1984.
20. Heading, R.C.: Duodenogastric reflux. Gut 24:507-509, 1983.
21. Muller-Lissner, S.A., Schattenmann, G., Siewert, J.R. and Blum, A.L.: Effect of a transpyloric tube on gastric emptying and duodenogastric reflux in the dog. Digestion 28:176-180, 1983.
22. Muller-Lissner, S.A. and Blum, A.L.: To-and-fro movements across the canine pylorus. Scand. J. Gastroenterology 19(suppl 92): 1-3, 1984.
23. Mearin, F., Azpiroz, F., Malagelada, J-R. and Zinsmeister, A.R.: Antroduodenal resistance to flow in the control of duodenogastric bile reflux during fasting. Gastroenterology 93:1026-1033, 1987.
24. Code, C.F., Steinbach, J.H., Schlegel, J.F., Amberg, J.R. and Hallenbeck, G.A.: Pyloric and duodenal motor contributions to duodenogastric reflux. Scand. J. Gastroenterology 19(Suppl 92):13-16, 1984.
25. Defilippi, C.C. and Gomez, E.: Continuous recording of pyloric sphincter pressure in dogs. Dig. Dis. Sci. 30:669-674, 1985.
26. Boosinger, T.R., Zerbe, C.A., Grabau, J.H. and Pletcher, J.M.: Multihormonal pancreatic endocrine tumor in a dog with duodenal ulcers and hypertrophic gastropathy. Vet. Pathol. 25:237-239, 1988.
27. Shaw, D.H.: Gastrinoma (Zollinger-Ellison syndrome) in the dog and cat. Can. Vet. J. 29:448-451, 1988.
28. Starlinger, M. and Schiessel, R.: Bicarbonate (HCO_3) delivery to the gastroduodenal mucosa by the blood: its importance for mucosal integrity. Gut 29:647-654, 1988.
29. Dayton, M.T. and Schlegel, J.: The effect of secretin on canine gastric mucosal HCO_3^- production. J. Surg. Res. 35:319-324, 1983.
30. Quintero, E., Pique, J.M., Bombi, J.A., Bordas, J.M., Sentis, J., Elena, M., Bosch, J. and Rodes, J.: Gastric mucosal vascular ectasias causing bleeding in cirrhosis. Gastroenterology 93:1054-1061, 1987.
31. Sarfeh, I.J. and Tarnawski, A.: Gastric mucosal vasculopathy in portal hypertension. Gastroenterology 93:1129-1131, 1987.
32. Seino, Y., Matsukura, S., Inoue, Y., Kadowaki, S., Mori, K. and Imura, H.: Hypogastrinemia in hypothroidism. Am. J. Dig. Dis. 23:189-191, 1978.
33. Crawford, L.M. and Wilson, R.C.: Melaena associated with dexamethasone therapy in the dog. J. Small Anim. Pract. 23:91-97, 1982.
34. Sorjonen, D.C., Dillon, A.R., Powers, R.D. and Spano, J.S.: Effects of dexamethasone and surgical hypotension on the stomach of dogs: Clinical, endoscopic, and pathologic evaluations. Am. J. Vet. Res. 44:1233-1237, 1983.
35. Jubb, K.V.F. and Kennedy, P.C.: Pathology of domestic animals. Vol. 2, Academic Press, New York, 1970.
36. Matthiesen, D.T. and Walter, M.C.: Surgical treatment of chronic hypertrophic pyloric gastropathy in 45 dogs. JAAHA 22:241-247, 1986.
37. Sikes, R.I., Birchard, S., Patnaik, A. and Bradley, R.: Chronic hypertrophic pyloric gastropathy: A review of 16 cases. JAAHA 22:99-104, 1986.
38. Clark, W.A.: Canine gastric hyperplasia. Vet. Annual 25:245-247, 1985.
39. Van der Gaag, I., Happe, R.P. and Wolvekamp, W. Th. C.: A Boxer dog with chronic hypertrophic gastritis resembling Menetrier's disease in man. Vet. Pathol. 13:172-185, 1976.
40. Van Kruiningen, H.J.: Giant hypertrophic gastritis of Basenji dogs. Vet. Pathol. 14:19-28, 1977.
41. Hansen, O.H., Jensen, K.B., Larsen, J.K. and Soltoft, J.: Gastric mucosal cell proliferation and immunoglobulin containing cells in Menetrier's disease. Digestion 16:293-298, 1977.
42. Isenberg, J.I.: Gastric secretory testing. In, Gastrointestinal Disease. Edited by M.H. Sleisenger and J.S. Fordtran, W.B. Saunders, Philadelphia, 1973.
43. Hayden, D.W. and Fleischman, R.W.: Scirrhous eosinophilic gastritis in dogs with gastric arteritis. Vet. Pathol. 14:441-448, 1977.
44. Raffin, S.: Granulomatous and infectious disease of the stomach. In, Gastrointestinal Disease, Edited by M.H. Sleisenger and J.S. Fordtran, W.B. Saunders Co., Philadelphia, 1973.
45. McArthur, K.E., Walsh, J.H. and Richardson, C.T.: Soy protein meals stimulate less gastric acid secretion and gastrin release than beef meals. Gastroenterology 95:920-926, 1988.
46. Grant, H.W., Palmer, K.R., Kelly, R.W., Wilson, R.H. and Misiewicz, J.J.: Dietary linoleic acid, gastric acid, and prostaglandin secretion. Gastroenterology 94:955-959, 1988.
47. Smith, R.L. and Powell, D.W. Prolonged treatment of Menetrier's disease with an oral anticholinergic drug. Gastroenterology 74:903-906, 1978.
48. Kelly, K.A.: Canine gastric motility and emptying: Electrical, neural, and hormonal controls. In, Proceedings Fourth International Symposium on Gastrointestinal Motility. Mitchell Press, Vancouver: 463-470, 1974.
49. Winans, C.S.: The fickle pylorus. Gastroenterology. 70:622-623, 1976.
50. Schulze-Delrieu, K.: Intrinsic reflexes between the esophagus and stomach. Gastroenterology 91:1568-1569, 1986.
51. DePonti, F., Azpiroz, F. and Malagelada, J-R.: Reflex gastric relaxation in response to distention of the duodenum. Am. J. Physiol. 252:G595-G601, 1987.
52. Welch, I.McL., Cunningham, K.M. and Reed, N.W.: Regulation of gastric emptying by ileal nutrients in humans. Gastroenterology 94:401-404, 1988.
53. Keinke, O. and Ehrlein, H-J.: Effect of oleic acid on canine gastroduodenal motility, pyloric diameter and gastric emptying. Q.J. Exp. Physiol. 68:675-686, 1983.
54. Glise, H. and Abrahamsson, H.: Reflex vagal inhibition of gastric motility by intestinal nociceptive stimulation in the cat. Scand. J. Gastroenterology 15:769-774, 1980.
55. Dubois, A. and Castell, D.O.: Histamine H_2-receptor involvement in the regulation of gastric emptying. Am. J. Physiol. 250:G244-G247, 1986.
56. Malbert, C-H., Hara, S. and Ruckenbusch, Y.: Early myoelectrical activity changes during gastric or duodenal ulceration in dogs. Dig. Dis. Sci. 32:737-742, 1987.
57. Kim, C.H., Zinsmeister, A.R. and Malagelada, J-R.: Mechanisms of canine gastric dysrhythmia. Gastroenterology 92:993-999, 1987.
58. Kim, C.H., Azpiroz, F. and Malagelada, J-R.: Characteristics of spontaneous and drug-induced gastric dysrhythmias in a chronic canine model. Gastroenterology 90:421-427, 1986.
59. Allescher, H-D., Daniel, E.E., Dent, J., Fox, J.E.T. and Kostolanska, F.: Extrinsic and intrinsic neural control of pyloric sphincter pressure in the dog. J. Physiol. 401:17-38, 1988.
60. Biancani, P., CiCalzi, L.K. and McCallum, R.W.: Mechanism of histamine-induced excitation of the cat pylorus. J. Clin. Invest. 68:582-588, 1981.
61. Allescher, H-D., Ahmad, S., Daniel, E.E., Dent, J., Kostolanska, F. and Fox, J.E.T.: Inhibitory opioid receptors in canine pylorus. Am. J. Physiol. 255:G352-G360, 1988.
62. Gue, M., Fioramonti, J., Honde, C., Pascaud, X., Junien, J.L.

and Bueno, L.: Opposite effects of K-opioid agonists on gastric emptying of liquids and solids in dogs. Gastroenterology 95:927-931, 1988.
63. Pearson, H., Gaskell, C.J., Gibbs, C. and Waterman, A.: Pyloric and oesophageal dysfunction in the cat. J. Small Anim. Pract. 15:487-501, 1974.
64. Twaddle, A.A.: Pyloric stenosis in three cats and its correction by pyloroplasty. N.Z. Vet. J. 18:15-17, 1970.
65. Twaddle, A.A.: Congenital pyloric stenosis in two kittens corrected by pyloroplasty. N.Z. Vet. J. 19:26-27, 1971.
66. Dodge, J.A. and Karim, A.A.: Induction of pyloric hypertrophy by pentagastrin. Gut 17:280-284, 1976.
67. Wattchow, D.A., Cass, D.T., Furness, J.B., Costa, M., O'Brien, P.E., Little, K.E. and Pitkin, J.: Abnormalities of peptide-containing nerve fibers in infantile hypertrophic pyloric stenosis. Gastroenterology 92:443-448, 1987.
68. Moazam, F., Rodgers, B.M., Talbert, J.L. and McGuigan, J.E.: Fasting and postprandial serum gastrin levels in infants with congenital hypertrophic pyloric stenosis. Ann. Surg. 188:623-625, 1978.
69. Bleicher, M.A., Shandling, B., Zingg, W., Karl, H.W.A. and Track, N.S.: Increased serum immunoreactive gastrin levels in idiopathic hypertrophic pyloric stenosis. Gut 19:794-797, 1978.
70. Edwards, D.A.W. and Rowlands, E.N.: Physiology of the gastroduodenal junction. In, Handbook of Physiology, Section 6, Alimentary Canal. Vol. 4, Edited by C.F. Code, Washington, DC, American Physiological Society, 1985-2000, 1968
71. Jakovljevic, S.: Gastric radiology and gastroscopy. Vet. Annual 28:172-182, 1988.
72. Evans, S.M.: Double versus single contrast gastrography in the dog and cat. Vet. Radiol. 24:6-10, 1983.
73. Miyabayashi, T., Morgan, J.P., Atilola, M.A.O. and Muhumuza, L.: Small intestinal emptying time in normal Beagle dogs. Vet. Radiol. 27:164-168, 1986.
74. Miyabayashi, T. and Morgan, J.P.: Gastric emptying in the normal dog. Vet. Radiol. 25:187-191, 1984.
75. Burns, J. and Fox, S.M.: The use of a barium meal to evaluate total gastric emptying time in the dog. Vet. Radiol. 27:169-172, 1986.
76. Van den Brom, W.E. and Happe, R.P.: Gastric emptying of a radionuclide-labeled test meal in healthy dogs: A new mathematical analysis and reference values. Am. J. Vet. Res. 47:2170-2174, 1986.
77. Burrows, C.F., Bright, R.M. and Spencer, C.F.: Influence of dietary composition on gastric emptying and motility in dogs: Potential involvement in acute gastric dilatation. Am. J. Vet. Res. 46:2609-2612, 1985.
78. Hornoff, W.J., Koblik, P.D., Strombeck, D.R., Morgan, J.P. and Hansen, G.: Scintigraphic evaluation of solid-phase gastric emptying in the dog. Vet. Radiol. In Press, 1989.
79. Metcalf, M.R.: Scintigraphic gastrointestinal bleeding localization with ^{99}mTc-labeled red blood cells. Vet. Radiol. 28:96-100, 1987.
80. Walter, M.C., Matthiesen, D.T. and Stone, E.A.: Pylorectomy and gastroduodenostomy in the dog: Technique and clinical results in 28 cases. JAVMA 187:909-914, 1985.
81. Meyer, J.H., Thomson, J.B., Cohen, M.B., Shadcheher, A. and Mandiola, S.A.: Sieving of solid food by the canine stomach and sieving after gastric surgery. Gastroenterology 76:804-813, 1979.
82. Fox, S.M. and Burns, J.: The effect of pyloric surgery on gastric emptying in the dog: Comparison of three techniques. JAAHA 22:783-788, 1986.
83. Papageorges, M.: Does pyloroplasty accelerate gastric emptying? JAAHA 23:248, 1987.
84. Ehrlein, H-J., Thoma, G., Keinke, O., Tsiamitas, C. and Schumpelick, V.: Effects of nutrients on gastrointestinal motility and gastric emptying after distal gastrectomy with Roux-Y gastrojejunostomy in dogs. Dig. Dis. Sci. 32:538-546, 1987.
85. Hinder, R.A. and San-Garde, B.A.: Individual and combined roles of the pylorus and the antrum in the canine gastric emptying of a liquid and a digestible solid. Gastroenterology 84:281-286, 1983.
86. Meyer, J.H., Dressman, J., Fink, A. and Amidon, G.: Effect of size and density on canine gastric emptying of nondigestible solids. Gastroenterology 89:805-813, 1985.
87. Stanton, M.E., Bright, R.M., Toal, R. and DeNovo, R.C.: The use of metaclopramide after Y-U pyloroplasty in dogs. Vet. Surg. 16:103, 1987.
88. Brodey, R.S. and Cohen, D.: An epizootiologic and clinicopathologic study of 95 cases of gastrointestinal neoplasms in the dog. Science Proceedings 101st annual meeting of American Veterinary Medical Association: 167-179, 1964.
89. Murray, M., Robinson, P.B., McKeating, F.J., Baker, G.J. and Lauder, I.M.: Primary gastric neoplasia in the dog: A clinicopathological study. Vet. Rec. 91:474-479, 1972.
90. Patnaik, A.K., Hurvitz, A.I. and Johnson, G.V.: Canine gastrointestinal neoplasms. Vet. Pathol. 14:547-555, 1977.
91. Sautter, J.H. and Hanlon, G.F.: Gastric neoplasms in the dog: A report of 20 cases. JAVMA 166:691-696, 1975.
92. Landes, C. and Sandersleben, J.V.: Primare Neoplasien und schleimhauthyperplasien in magen des hundes. Tierarztl. Prax. Suppl. 1:139-158, 1985.
93. Sullivan, M., Lee, R., Fisher, E.W., Nash, A.S. and McCandlish, I.A.P.: A study of 31 cases of gastric carcinoma in dogs. Vet. Rec. 120:79-83, 1987.
94. Gabbert, N.H., Nachreiner, R.F., Holmes-Wood, P., and Kivela, J.H.: Serum immunoreactive gastrin concentrations in the dog: basal and postprandial values measured by radioimmunoassay. Am. J. Vet. Res. 45:2351-2353, 1984.
95. Bueno, L., Fioramonti, J. and Ruckebusch, Y.: Postoperative intestinal motility in dogs and sheep. Am. J. Dig. Dis. 23:682-689, 1978.
96. Hinder, R.A. and Bremner, C.G.: Relative role of pyloroplasty size, truncal vagotomy, and milk meal volume in canine gastric emptying. Am. J. Dig. Dis. 23:210-216, 1978.
97. Klempa, I., Holle, F., Bruckner, W., Welsch, K.H., Handle, H. and Wolff, A.: The effect of selective proximal vagotomy and pyloroplasty on gastric secretion and motility in the dog. Arch. Surg. 102:713-719, 1971.
98. Van Sluijs, F.JU. and van den Brom, W.E.: Gastric emptying of a radionuclide-labeled test meal after surgical correction of gastric dilatation-volvulus in dogs. Am. J. Vet. Res. 50:433-435, 1988.
99. Cannon, W.B.: The mechanical factors of digestion. New York, Longmans, 1911.
100. Bedi, B.S., Kelly, K.A. and Holley, K.E.: Pathways of propagation of the canine gastric pacesetter potential. Gastroenterology 63:288-296, 1972.
101. Yamagishi, T. and Debas, H.T.: Control of gastric emptying. Interaction of the vagus and pyloric antrum. Ann. Surg. 187:91-94, 1978.
102. Wastell, C. and Ellis, H.: Effect of various pyloroplasties on fecal fat excretion in dogs and humans. Am. J. Dig. Dis. 23:45-50, 1978.
103. Dozois, R.R., Kelly, K.A. and Code, C.F.: Effect of distal antrectomy on gastric emptying of liquids and solids. Gastroenterology 61:675-681, 1971.
104. Kelly, K.A. and Code, C.F.: Canine gastric pacemaker. Am. J. Physiol. 220:112-118, 1971.
105. Greenlee, H.B., Gelbart, S.M., DeOrio, A.J., Francescatti, D.S., Paez, J. and Reinhardt, G.F.: The influence of gastric surgery on the itnestinal flora. Am. J. Clin. Nutr. 30:1826-1833, 1977.
106. Soon-Shiong, P. and Debas, H.T.: Fundic inhibition of acid secretion and gastrin release in the dog. Gastroenterology 79:867-872, 1980.

Chapter 14

Gastric Dilatation, Gastric Dilatation - Volvulus and Chronic Gastric Volvulus

GASTRIC DILATATION

Clinical Synopsis

Diagnostic features

* Clinical evidence of gastric over-distension
* Radiographs including a right lateral view that do NOT demonstrate any volvulus

Management

* Orogastric intubation and lavage
* Emetics

Incidence and Signalment

Over-distension of the stomach without concomitant volvulus occurs occasionally in dogs of all sizes and ages. It is most common in young dogs but is occasionally seen in adults.

Etiology and Pathogenesis

Gluttony is the most common cause of gastric dilatation. In most cases, over-dilatation is relieved by vomiting and eructation. In some cases, over-distention of the stomach results in gastric atony, and the dilatation becomes persistent. In this eventuality, fermentation of food by bacteria acquired from the oral cavity or food results in the generation of considerable amounts of gas, exacerbating the gastric distention.

Clinical Findings

The history often reveals access to trash or appetizing food. Gastric over-distension results in a clinical syndrome characterized by abdominal enlargement, depression, discomfort, and intermittent, largely ineffectual retching and vomiting. Palpation of the abdomen may reveal an enlarged and doughy stomach due to impacted ingesta. The dogs usually are hemodynamically stable and rarely show drum-tight, tympanic abdomens. In susceptible dogs, gastric dilatation can be complicated by gastric volvulus, resulting in progression of abdominal fullness to tympany and rapid deterioration of clinical condition.

Diagnosis

Diagnosis of gastric dilatation relies on an appropriate history and on observation of clinical signs. Radiographs, including a view taken of the patient in right lateral recumbency, are recommended to rule out the possibility of accompanying volvulus.

Management and Prognosis

Passing a stomach tube can relieve accumulated gas and fluid. If the dilatation is due to impacted ingesta, however, this procedure may not be successful. Use of an emetic agent such as apomorphine succeeds in relieving the distention. The dose can be titrated by placing an apomorphine tablet in the subconjunctival sac and removing it as soon as nausea and retching begin. Emetics should not be used if there is any suspicion of ingestion of caustic or sharp materials, if the animal appears hypovolemic, or is mentally depressed to the point where it is unlikely to be able to protect its airway. In some dogs gastric decompression may require gastric lavage with warmed water; anesthesia and tracheal intubation are required. On rare occasions, gastrostomy is necessary to remove impacted material. Most dogs can be successfully managed for gastric dilatation and they usually recover completely.

GASTRIC DILATATION-VOLVULUS

Clinical Synopsis

Diagnostic features

* Acute onset of abdominal tympany due to gastric dilatation
* Right lateral radiograph demonstrating gastric volvulus

Treatment

* Lactated Ringer's bolus 45 ml/kg over 15-30 min
* Gastric decompression by orogastric intubation or trocarization
* Maintenance lactated Ringer's (2-10 ml/kg/hr) supplemented by potassium chloride (20 mEq/L)
* Ranitidine (1-2 mg/kg q 8-12 hr IV,IM,PO) or cimetidine (4-5 mg/kg q 8 hr IV,IM,PO) for 5-7 days
* Trimethoprim sulfa 15 mg/kg q 12 hr SC or PO for 5-7 days

* Surgical correction (once patient is stable) followed by gastropexy to prevent recurrence
* When indicated (see text), supplemental therapy may include dextran 70, plasma, blood, sodium bicarbonate, parenteral antibiotics, corticosteroids, non-steroidal antiinflammatories, antiarrhythmics, heparin, metoclopramide, sucralfate, dopamine or dobutamine, enteral or parenteral nutrition.

Monitoring

* Close postoperative monitoring is essential for successful treatment
* Depending on dog's condition monitoring may include some or all of repeated physical examinations; serum electrolyte, blood gas, glucose, BUN, liver enzyme, and bilirubin concentrations; PCV/TP and/or CBC; urinalysis; blood pressure, CVP, and EKG; clotting times.

Incidence and Signalment

The incidence of acute gastric dilatation-volvulus (GDV) without spontaneous remission in the general canine population is relatively low. In a seven-year period at the VMTH at Davis, 13 cases of GDV were recorded per 10,000 patients. The incidence is higher in emergency clinics, however, and within the breeds with greatest predilection GDV is an important cause of morbidity and mortality. For instance, 3.3% of the Great Danes presented to one clinic were afflicted with GDV. Acute GDV is most common in large breed, deep-chested dogs such as the Great Dane, German Shepherd, Saint Bernard, Irish Setter, and Doberman Pinscher.[1] GDV has occasionally been reported in smaller breeds such as the Dachshund, the Basset, the English Bulldog, the Terrier, the Miniature Poodle, the Pekingese, and the cat. GDV can occur in dogs of any age. A range of two months to fifteen years with a mean of 5.2 ± 2.9 years was reported in one study.[1] No predisposition by sex has been established.

Predisposing Causes of Gastric Dilatation-Volvulus

Introduction. A singular cause of GDV has not been identified. More than likely, the disease results from an additive interaction between risk factors, which in combination eventually result in GDV (Figure 14-1). The determining factor precipitating GDV may be any one of the different factors; GDV may have any of a number of precipitating causes provided the appropriate foundation of predisposing causes is in place. Which predisposing causes are essential to the development of GDV and which are not remains to be established. It is important to note that some apparent risk factors may simply reflect techniques common in the management of large dogs rather than being true predisposing causes. Certainly, two events must occur before GDV will develop. There must be over-distension of the stomach with gas and fluid, and volvulus must occur. It is probable that either of these two events can precipitate GDV. That is, volvulus can cause dilatation, just as dilatation can cause volvulus.

Dilatation of the Stomach. Gastric over-distension can

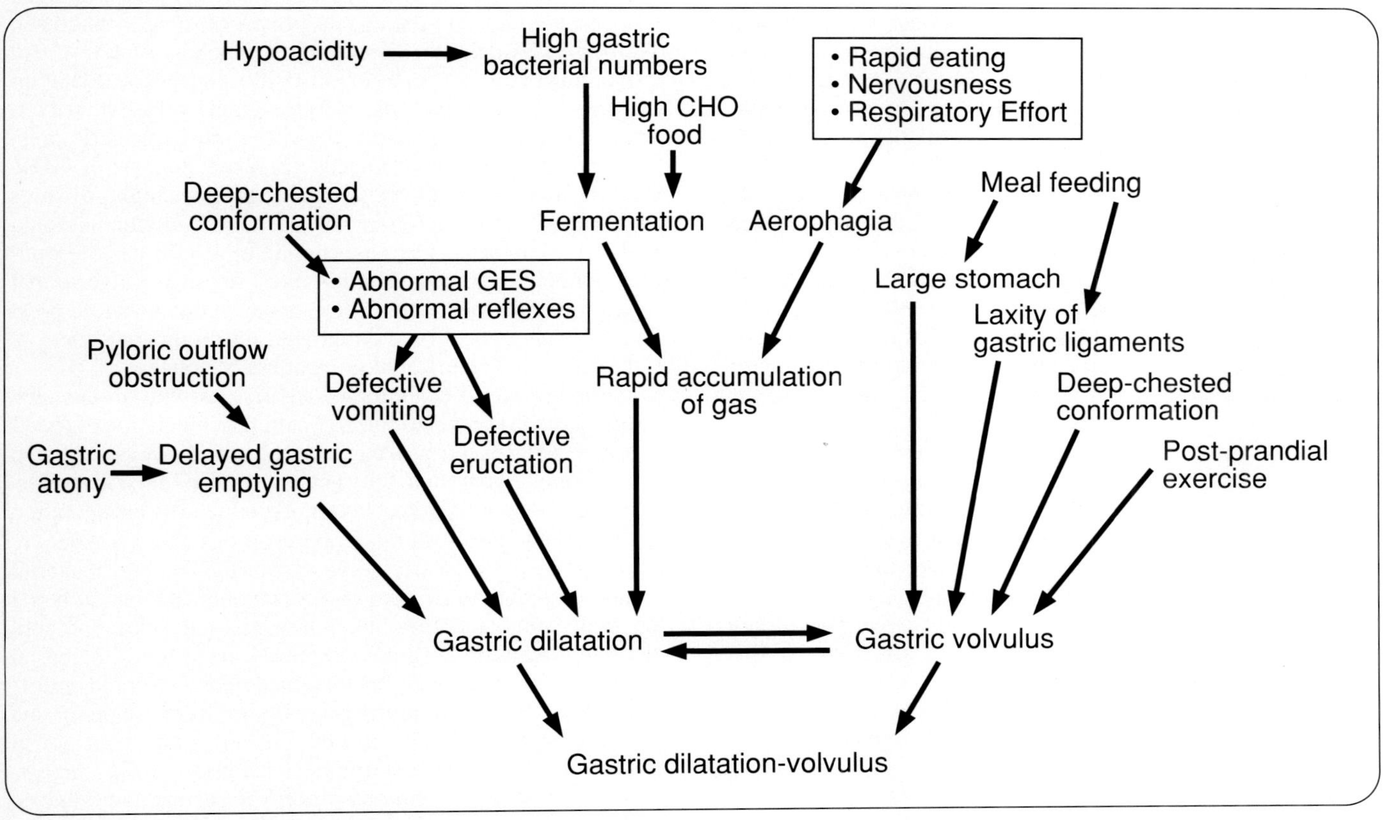

Figure 14-1. Schematic representation of the interaction of the predisposing causes of gastric dilatation-volvulus.

lead to volvulus and thus GDV. Dilatation causes the greater curvature of the stomach to move ventrally, causing the pylorus to move dorsally and to the left, becoming adjacent to the esophagus on the right. Gastric movement displaces the spleen by way of the gastrosplenic ligament. Once displaced, the spleen engorges and may inhibit spontaneous reversibility of the gastric torsion. Stomach dilatation can result from accumulation of gas, fluid, or food. Gastric gas is derived from aerophagia, fermentation, and acidification of bicarbonate. Gastric fluid is derived from ingesta and gastric secretions. Gastric secretion of plasma-like fluid is normally minimal. With GDV, however, extracellular fluid moves into the gastrointestinal tract. The influx of fluid is secondary to increased hydrostatic pressure from to venous obstruction and to increased mucosal permeability.

Gastric Volvulus. Gastric volvulus is usually considered a consequence of gastric dilatation. There is little evidence to refute the suggestion, however, that volvulus could precede dilatation.[2] Dogs with gastric volvulus without dilatation have been observed at the UCD VMTH[3] and have been reported by others.[4] These dogs commonly have a history of recurrent bouts of mild gastric distension; the syndrome is described as *chronic volvulus*. Gastric volvulus compromises gastric emptying of gas and ingesta and can progress to dilatation and GDV. The cause(s) of gastric volvulus is unknown.

Conformation. Deep-chested body conformation predisposes dogs to the development of GDV, perhaps through increasing the likelihood of volvulus, or by altering anatomic relationships at the gastroesophageal sphincter and thus impairing eructation.

Laxity of the Gastric Ligaments. Laxity of hepatoduodenal and hepatogastric ligaments may increase the likelihood of volvulus. Stomachs with apparently normal ligamentous attachments, however, can be readily displaced at surgery into a volvulus position. Thus it appears that there is sufficient laxity in normal hepatoduodenal and hepatogastric ligaments to permit rotational instability.

Post-Prandial Exercise. Vigorous exercise by dogs with a stomach distended by food or water may physically displace the stomach and increase the likelihood of volvulus.

Composition of Diet. GDV is a disease of domestication, since the incidence is greater in dogs fed commercial dog foods than in dogs fed natural diets. The composition of the diet influences the rate of gastric emptying and the amount of fermentable substrate. High-fat diets are retained in the stomach longer than low-fat diets. High-fat diets, having higher caloric density, require feeding smaller volumes than low-fat diets and they are likely to ferment less than low-fat diets. These benefits of a high-fat diet may be more important than the prolonged gastric food retention promoted by a high-fat diet. However, a direct causal relationship between the type of food eaten and the development of GDV has not been proven. GDV has been reported in dogs eating meat, soy, or cereal based diets, and in dogs fed free-choice or by single meals. Intake of dry food that swells once entering the stomach has been proposed as a cause of GDV. The in-hospital incidence of GDV at the UCD VMTH declined when dry food was dampened prior to feeding.

Intake of Large Volume of Ingesta. Rapid intake of a large volume of food or water causes gastric dilatation and may precipitate GDV. The stomachs of dogs fed commercial dry dog food once per day for two years become significantly larger than the stomachs of dogs fed commercial dry dog food three times per day, and than the stomachs of dogs fed meat and bone rations. Chronic intake of large volumes of the dry food because of the infrequent feeding leads to the gastric hypertrophy.[5] A similar phenomenon is well documented in laboratory rodents. Large volumes of food take longer to empty than smaller volumes of food, resulting in a more prolonged period in which food is available for fermentation. Damage to the stomach by over-dilation, resulting in deranged myoelectrical activity and impaired gastric emptying, has also been hypothesized.[5]

Increased Production or Intake of Gastric Gas. It is probable that abnormally rapid accumulation of gas in the stomach predisposes to GDV. GDV is associated with retention of gas in both the fed and unfed stomach. The gas has been suggested to be swallowed air, to be produced by bacterial activity on gastric contents, or to result from the reaction of gastric acid with secretions containing bicarbonate.

In several studies, gastric gas analyses revealed an elevated carbon dioxide concentration in comparison to atmospheric gas. In one study the carbon dioxide concentration reached 10%, and no concomitant rise of methane or hydrogen was detected.[6] The absence of methane and hydrogen weighed against significant bacterial fermentation, and the gastric gas was suggested to be swallowed air contaminated with carbon dioxide derived from the interaction of gastric bicarbonate and gastric acid. The gastric bicarbonate is thought to derive from saliva or from leakage of extracellular fluid. Air is swallowed during drinking and eating, the amounts increasing with rapid eating and gulping of liquids. Aerophagia may also occur in nervous, excited, or dyspneic animals. Significant aerophagia, as a result of greedy eating, and hyperventilation has been reported in association with a series of cases of GDV.[2] An association between respiratory difficulty and gastric dilatation was noted in one human study.[7] Aerophagia by itself, however, would be unlikely to produce the very high intragastric pressures recorded in the stomachs of some dogs with GDV. Swallowed air does not accumulate to produce high pressures but escapes by eructation in normal dogs. Aerophagia could explain most of the gastric gas accumulation if the gastroesophageal junction begins to function like a one-way valve so that eructation is not possible. The esophagus can generate pressures high enough to force swallowed air through the junction, and a one-way value would prevent eructation.

Another possible source of gastric gas with an elevated carbon dioxide concentration is bacterial fermentation of food.[8] Gas-producing bacteria, in particular clostridia, were suggested as the origin.[8] Short chain fatty acids were also found in the gas, supporting a bacterial role. Gas is not produced by fermentation in the normal empty stomach, because bacteria numbers are kept very low by gastric acidity.[9] During feeding, bacterial numbers increase to 10^5 per gram of contents, the sources being the oral cavity and the diet. Numerous species are found, including many organisms found in the fecal flora. Increased numbers of gas-producing bacteria in the stomach could predispose to GDV. Gas-producing clostridia were found in the gastric content of dogs with GDV in one study,[8] but not in another.[6] It has not been determined whether large dogs, predisposed to GDV, have a reduced capacity to secrete hydrochloric acid. Morphologic findings indicate that these dogs have normal numbers of oxyntic cells.

It is probable that the proportion of gas derived from aerophagia, bacterial fermentation, and gastric bicarbonate varies considerably among different dogs with GDV, depending on such factors as the dog's temperament, the type and quantity of food in the stomachs at the time of the volvulus, and the duration of the volvulus.

Defective Eructation or Vomiting. Impaired ability to relieve gastric dilatation by eructation or vomiting may predispose to GDV. These abnormalities could result from an abnormal gastroesophageal junction or from defects anywhere in the complex vagal reflexes that control these functions.

The correlation of GDV with animal size suggests that an anatomical factor may contribute to the problem. Many dogs of the larger breeds have relatively deep chests, altering anatomic relations between the stomach, esophagus, gastroesophageal junction, and diaphragm. Anatomic arrangements of this area are designed to prevent gastroesophageal reflux. The anti-reflux mechanisms include the oblique angle at which the esophagus enters the stomach, fundic pressure, the diaphragmatic cura, the intra-abdominal esophagus, and the gastroesophageal sphincter (GES) muscle. Any exaggeration of these anti-reflux mechanisms could prevent normal eructation of gastric gas. For instance, surgical wrapping of the gastric fundus around two-thirds of the intra-abdominal segment of esophagus (fundoplication) does not interfere with eating but does prevent vomiting, and gastric dilatation is a continuous problem.[10] The gastroesophageal junction remains patent, but a one-way valve is formed. Furthermore, elimination of the valve of His by fundectomy has helped two dogs with recurrent gastric dilatation treated at the VMTH at Davis.

Although dogs with GDV cannot eructate it is unlikely that GES dysfunction alone is an adequate explanation. Both humoral and neural regulation controls GES function; of the two the neural regulation is more important.[11,12] High levels of some hormones, such as gastrin, elevate GES pressure but it is uncertain whether gastrin is physiologically important to GES function.[13] Gastrin plasma levels increase after feeding and increasing GES pressure follows. The augmented GES pressure does not impair eructation because gas is eructated at the same frequency and at the same low intragastric pressures as in unfed dogs with much lower GES pressure.[14] Plasma gastrin levels are high in dogs with acute GDV and in dogs three to six months after recovery from GDV.[15] The significance of this observation is unknown, however. It may reflect a continuing gastric retention of contents, resulting in distention, an important stimulus for gastrin release. It is possible that affected dogs had high plasma gastrin levels before GDV. High plasma gastrin levels could also reflect a loss of normal vagal nerve activity. The dogs may also have had high GES pressures but that does not reflect an increased risk for GDV. The drugs metoclopramide and cisapride greatly increase GES pressure in dogs, but the dogs are able to eructate gas from the stomach at the same frequency and at the same low intragastric pressures as in dogs with very low GES pressure that is reduced by an anticholinergic.[16,17] In summary, GES function that determines sphincter pressure is not a determining factor in the dog's ability to eructate.

Failure of the dogs that develop GDV to vomit or eructate gas could be partly due to a loss of normal vagal innervation to the caudal esophagus. The intra-abdominal segment of esophagus is retracted into the thoracic cavity as part of the vomiting reflex. Vagal nerves that cause contraction of esophageal longitudinal muscles mediate this retraction. Selective vagotomy of the caudal canine esophagus abolishes the animal's ability to retract its intra-abdominal segment.[18]

Failure of eructation in dogs with GDV could also result from disruption of the neural reflex for eructation. Eructation is abolished by vagotomy; damage to the vagal nerves could cause loss of the ability to eructate.[17] There is no evidence that dogs affected with GDV have vagal nerve damage, however. Eructation is also abolished by anything limiting distention of the gastric cardia; eructation is stimulated by distention of the cardia.[14] Eructation is mediated by stimulation of receptors in the cardia and transmission of that information via vagal afferents to synapses in the brain. The motor response is a reduction in GES pressure to less than that in the stomach so gas can escape. Disease limiting cardia distention or affecting sensory reception and transmission of neural information will result in failure to eructate gas. Acute GDV from any cause may distend and damage the structures in the gastric cardia to a degree that eructation is impaired even after clinical recovery; such damage may explain why a dog with acute GDV is at greater risk than other dogs for repeated episodes of GDV. Failure of eructation could also result from an inability of the cardia to be further distended by gas. The stomach normally rotates during filling. With increasing distention the rotation around the gastroesophageal junction limits the freedom for the cardia to be distended by intragastric contents. The anatomy of the stomach in some breeds of dogs may cause such restricition to happen sooner than in dogs at low risk for GDV. Filling with gas markedly distends the GES-cardia area of the stomach when compared to filling the stomach with comparable amounts of fluid and food (Figure 14-2). Therefore, distention of the cardia, as a prerequisite for reduction in GES pressure, is caused readily by relatively small amounts of gas when compared with filling with similar amounts of a liquid. Two other factors determine eructation of gas. Body position determines the location of gas in the stomach and whether it is in the region where it can distend the cardia. Eructation is least frequent in dogs lying in a left lateral position; the frequency is up to twice as great in dogs lying in a supine or right lateral position; and the eructation frequency is five times greater in standing dogs.[19] Gastric motility should also be important to eructation. When

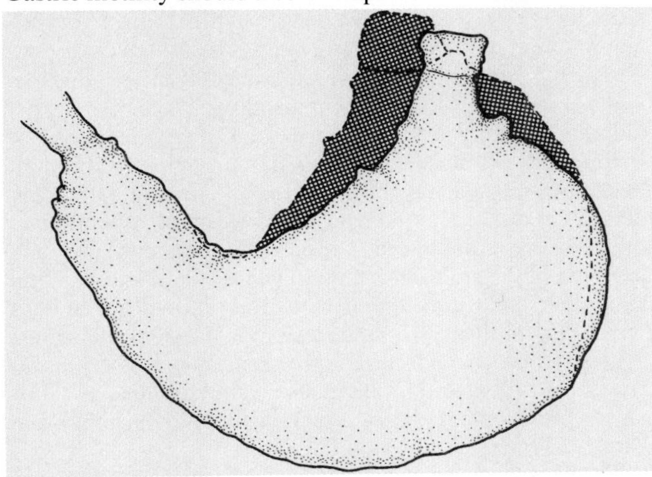

Figure 14-2. Comparison of distention of gastric cardia by saline (unshaded) with distention by saline and air (shaded).

body position determines that gas is not in the gastric cardia, gastric motility moves the gas to the cardia so that it can be eructated. Without such motility, gas eructation would not be evident in dogs lying in a left lateral position.

Delayed Gastric Emptying. Delayed gastric emptying due to pyloric disorders has been associated with GDV in a number of small breed dogs, implying that this delay is a risk factor for the disease. Once partial volvulus ensues, compression of the duodenum occurs and will inhibit gastric emptying. Gastric atony due to high sympathetic tone following trauma, spinal surgery, and major abdominal surgery has been associated with GDV. General anesthesia can cause gastric dilatation, a phenomenon which may also be mediated by the nervous system. Gastrin has a trophic effect on the gastric mucosa and in pharmacologic doses may inhibit gastric emptying. As noted above, high gastrin levels have been detected in the plasma of dogs affected with GDV. Whether these high gastrin levels are sufficient to inhibit pyloric outflow in GDV remains to be established. Although gastric emptying may be delayed during recovery from GDV, a recent study shows normal gastric emptying of a liquid meal in dogs that have recovered from an acute episode of GDV.[20] This finding suggests that delayed gastric emptying is not a preexisting problem causing EDV.

Pathophysiology - Gastric[21,22]

Gastric Pathology. The accumulation of gastric gas and fluid in GDV results in intragastric pressures that usually range from 9 to 62 mm Hg with a mean of 23 mm Hg.[23] Pressures as high as 80 mm Hg have been recorded.[24] Pressures of 30 mm Hg are sufficient to distend the stomach to a volume of approximately 3 liters in dogs of 20-30 kg body weight.[25] The degree of gastric volvulus in GDV varies from 90-360. These perturbations cause gastric pathology that ranges from mild edema and hemorrhage in one or more tissue layers, to full thickness necrosis and perforation. In spontaneous GDV, serosal hemorrhage, and mucosal hemorrhage and necrosis are frequently observed. Full thickness necrosis and perforation occasionally occur. Infarction and necrosis most often occur along the greater curvature proximate to the short gastric vessels. Avulsion of the short gastric vessels and the epiploic branch of the left gastroepiploic artery can occur. In experimental GDV of anesthetized dogs, pathologic changes in the stomach are also most common in the fundus and body. Mucosal necrosis and ulceration is less consistent in experimental models than in spontaneous GDV.[25-27] Prominent histological changes consist of submucosal edema and hemorrhage, acute myo-necrosis of the longitudinal muscle layer, and neutrophil infiltration, hemorrhage, and edema in the serosa.[25,28] The histopathologic changes are minimal at the end of 2.5 hours of experimental GDV, but are pronounced 4 hours after the deflation and derotation of the stomach (resuscitation).[25] Gross submucosal edema develops within minutes of resuscitation. Seven days after GDV, prominent histologic lesions in the stomach include subserosal fibrosis and chronic inflammation of the muscularis.[28] It is probable that the gastric pathology due to GDV results from a combination of ischemia, reperfusion injury, and gastric acid injury.

Pathomechanism of Gastric Ischemia and Edema. Experimental GDV causes an immediate 92% decline of gastric surface oxygen tension.[25] The very low surface oxygen tension strongly suggests profound gastric ischemia. The ischemia is likely to be particularly catastrophic for the gastric mucosa, which requires 80% of the total gastric blood flow in order to sustain its metabolic requirements. The origin of the gastric ischemia is probably multifactorial, resulting from gastric volvulus, dilatation, infarction and edema, reduced cardiac output, and perhaps from increased sympathetic tone.

Gastric volvulus (360 degrees) impairs gastric blood flow by obstructing gastric venous outflow.[74] Increased gastric pressure also reduces gastric blood flow. In the canine intestine, experimentally elevated pressures at or above 30-60 mm Hg result in a stepwise decrease in intestinal blood flow as the pressure increases.[30] At a pressure of 30 mm Hg, blood flow to the mucosa and muscularis is markedly impaired but that to the serosa and submucosa is maintained even at pressures as high as 90 mm Hg. It would seem likely that similar alterations in mucosal and muscularis blood flow would occur in the stomachs of dogs affected by GDV. Canine gastric mucosal blood flow may not be impaired until intragastric pressures reach 37 mm Hg.[31] In contrast, increased intragastric pressure at 8 mm Hg or above produces a graded decrease in mucosal and muscularis blood flow in the cat stomach, with the greatest decreases noted in the fundus and body.[32] The mechanism by which gastrointestinal distension selectively decreases blood flow in the mucosa has not been established. Simple compression of vascular beds by increasing wall pressure is one theory, whereas reflex alterations mediated by the enteric nervous system is another.

Infarction of microvasculature is a common complication of ischemia. The infarction is a result of neutrophil accumulation in the microvasculature or of thrombosis developing secondarily to vascular pooling in association with damage to vessel walls. Marginated neutrophils are common in the microvasculature of the tissues of dogs with experimental GDV.[25] In the same dogs, the gastric and splenic veins are noted on occasion to be thrombosed, and rare microthrombi are noted in the gastrointestinal tissues.

Gastric edema also reduces gastric blood flow. Increased tissue hydrostatic pressure, resulting from the interstitial edema, decreases capillary flow. The gastric edema develops after deflation, presumably as a result of increased capillary permeability and hydrostatic pressure. Increased capillary permeability is a complication of ischemia and is exacerbated by reperfusion injury of the endothelial cells. Increased capillary hydrostatic pressure is initially due to venous obstruction and after resuscitation is due to visceral hyperperfusion. The visceral hyperperfusion is a result of volume repletion in association with profound local vasodilation in the previously ischemic vascular beds. The transudation of fluid into the gastric wall may be compounded by decreases in oncotic pressure resulting from the administration of large volumes of intravenous fluids at the time of resuscitation.

Increased sympathetic tone resulting from acute stress is likely to further compromise gastric blood flow. Importantly, ischemia resulting from sympathetic activity, gastric edema, and gastric infarction is likely to persist long after surgical correction of the GDV, and may explain the not uncommon development of postoperative gastric necrosis.

Relationship of Gastric Acid to Gastric Ulceration. The presence of gastric acid is required for the development of gastric ulceration in models of gastric ischemia[33] and gastric dilatation.[34,35] Gastric acid is able to penetrate the mucosal barrier because reduced mucosal circulation compromises epithelial integrity. The reduced flow also allows hydrogen ions to accumulate, eventually leading to acid-induced mucosal necrosis and ulceration. A potential role for gastric acid in GDV-induced gastric ulceration is implied by the observation of a correlation between low plasma bicarbonate concentration and gastric ulceration following gastric dilatation.[27]

Pathomechanism of Disordered Gastric Motility. Disordered gastric motility and delayed gastric emptying have been reported following GDV. The disordered motility consists of intermittent gastric tachyarrhythmias, decreased electrical-mechanical coupling, and decreased contractile amplitude.[36] The disordered motility was transient (nine days) in experimental models but appeared more persistent during recovery from spontaneous GDV.[37] If GDV is not corrected within approximately four hours, the atony or deranged motility may become irreversible. The cause of the disordered motility appears to be gastric ischemia and over-distension. Acute myo-necrosis of the gastric longitudinal muscle layer is a consistent early lesion in experimental GDV. The proximity of the myo-necrosis to the cells of Cajal (the putative source of the basal electrical rhythm) suggests that this lesion may be one cause of the disordered motility. Direct ischemic damage to the myenteric plexus is another proposed cause of the gastric dysrhythmias.

Pathophysiology - Cardiovascular

Cardiovascular Dysfunction and Pathology. Experimental models of gastric dilatation and GDV produce immediate decreases in cardiac output (40%-89% decline), systemic mean arterial pressure (5%-50%), pulmonary artery mean blood pressure (20%), and wedge pressure (3 mm Hg) (Figure 14-3).[23-25,29,38,39] Coronary artery flow decreases (50%), as does myocardial oxygen consumption (50%).[24] Subendocardial necrosis and cardiac arrhythmias are associated with the cardiac ischemia. Total peripheral resistance and heart rate increase during GDV and decline during resuscitation.[25,38,39] Intra-abdominal caudal vena caval pressure increases in proportion to the intragastric pressure.[38-40] Portal pressure increases two to threefold.[29] Central venous pressure remains unchanged in some studies,[25,39] and declines in others.[38] GDV causes a rapid decrease in the surface oxygen tension of the duodenum (80% decline), jejunum (45%), liver (45%), and pancreas (45%).[25] The reduced surface oxygen tension implies a profound reduction in local blood flow. The severity of abdominal organ ischemia is variable in individual dogs, but is sufficient to cause damage to most tissues.

After deflation and derotation of the stomach the cardiac output improves transiently but does not return to normal.[23,24,38] If crystaloid fluid administration (90 ml/kg) accompanies the gastric deflation and derotation (resuscitation), the cardiac output rises transiently to 50% above baseline but within 1.5 hours declines again to below baseline. The surface oxygen tension of all abdominal organs except the liver returns to near-normal values after resuscitation. The surface oxygen tension of the liver remains low, however, suggesting that the oxygen demands of the liver outstrip oxygen delivery even after resuscitation of the GDV patient.

Pathomechanism of the Circulatory Changes. The distended stomach interferes with splanchnic circulation by directly compressing adjacent large veins and by compressing distant veins and vascular beds by way of increased intra-abdominal pressure. The dilated stomach occludes or partially occludes the caudal vena cava at a level that varies from the T12 to L4 vertebrae.[21,39] The caudal vena caval compression reduces venous return to the heart. Collateral flow through the ventral vertebral sinuses and azygous veins partially compensates for the reduced caudal vena caval flow.[41] Blood flow through the portal vein is also reduced. This appears to be due to gastric dilatation rather than gastric volvulus.[74] The liver becomes congested in 50% of dogs during experimental GDV, implying that in some dogs post-hepatic portal hypertension occurs, perhaps due to compression of the hepatic veins against the diaphragm by forward displacement of the liver.[25] Hypertension in the caudal vena cava and portal vein reduces splanchnic blood flow. Portal hypertension promotes the pooling of blood in the splanchnic viscera and the movement of plasma fluid into the gastrointestinal tract.

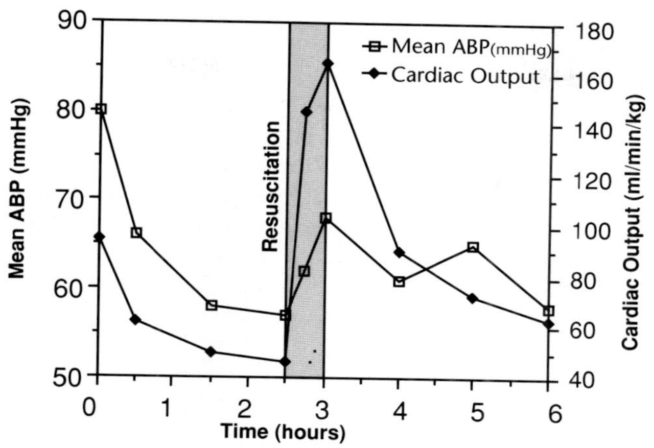

Figure 14-3. Mean arterial blood pressure and cardiac output before, during, and after acute GDV.

Experimentally elevated intra-abdominal pressure produces some, but not all, of the circulatory changes seen with elevated intragastric pressure, implying a potential contributory role for vascular bed compression due to raised intra-abdominal pressure in the pathogenesis of GDV. Increased intra-abdominal pressure, created by the inflation of a large volume intra-abdominal bag to pressures of 20-40 mm Hg, markedly decreases cardiac output and absolute blood flow to both abdominal and thoracic viscera.[40] At intra-abdominal pressures of 40 mm Hg, the blood flow to the abdominal organs (except the kidney and adrenal) decreases to 20%-40% of baseline. This decline in blood flow is greater than could be accounted for by the decline in cardiac output, suggesting a direct pressure effect on local abdominal organ blood flow. One important difference between this model and GDV is that overall venous return and systemic blood pressure did not appear to be impaired. Decreased venous return and blood pressure, as seen in GDV, would be expected to further reduce the visceral blood flow.

Decreased venous return is the primary cause of the reduced cardiac output and mean blood pressure during GDV. After gastric decompression, release of sequestered circulating cardiodepressant substances may reduce cardiac contractility.[42] Myocardial depressant factor is the best described cardioinhibitory factor. It is a polypeptide thought to originate from protease activation in the ischemic pancreas during shock. Together with endotoxin, it is thought to cause negative inotropy, splanchnic vasoconstriction, and reticuloendothelial system depression. Tachycardia, elevated total peripheral resistance, and perhaps in some dogs increased ventricular contractility[42] provide partial compensation for the reduced systemic blood flow and perfusion pressure. These compensatory responses are likely to be mediated by increased sympathetic tone in response to both decreased blood pressure,[42] and acute gastric distension,[43] and in response to release of cardiostimulatory substances such as catecholamines.[42] Increased contractility, however, raises myocardial oxygen demand; additionally, in association with decreased coronary blood flow resulting from the tachycardia and decreased aortic blood pressure, it causes myocardial ischemia and necrosis.[24] Persistently increased venous sympathetic tone probably perpetuates the vascular pooling that initially results from vascular obstruction during GDV. Cardiac arrhythmias develop as a result of cardiac ischemia and are probably exacerbated by increased sympathetic tone, raised serum catecholamine levels, and electrolyte and acid base disturbances.[24,44]

Pathomechanism of Shock.[45,46] Shock is defined as inadequate tissue perfusion. In GDV the cause of shock is multifactorial. It is initiated by hypovolemia secondary to vascular pooling and is compounded by varying degrees of endotoxic and septic shock. Decreased cardiac output, blood volume, and arterial pressure lead to inadequate organ perfusion. Prolonged poor tissue perfusion with resultant insufficient tissue oxygenation eventually leads to the development of irreversible shock, signaled by the failure of any treatment to restore blood pressure and cardiac output. Shock becomes irreversible when tissue hypoperfusion persists for several hours in hemorrhagic shock models. Irreversibility is directly related to the extent of the tissue oxygen debt; it is also related to the amount of endotoxin entering the circulation. Endotoxic and septic shock develop as a result of portal venous occlusion and loss of the mucosal barrier. Experimental obstruction of a dog's portal vein for as little as 30 minutes results in death within 24 hours. Endotoxin enters the circulation by way of the peritoneal surface or lymphatics. The restriction of portal blood flow prevents removal of the toxin by the reticuloendothelial system of the liver.[47]

Endotoxin release and tissue hypoxia in the splanchnic viscera both activate a series of interacting cascades. These include the arachidonic acid and complement cascades, and the fibrinolytic and kallikrein-kinin systems. Platelets, granulocytes and macrophages marginate and release a variety of vasoactive and cytotoxic substances that result in microvasculature injury and leakage. Complement and cytokines such as interleukin and cachectin appear to be very important mediators of endotoxic and gram negative sepsis. Tissue proteases produce peptides with myocardial depressant and vasoactive properties, such as myocardial depressant factor. In combination with acid-base and electrolyte derangements, the aforementioned mediators perpetuate the inadequate tissue blood flow and eventually precipitate vascular collapse and death.

Pathomechanism of Disseminated Intravascular Coagulation. Disseminated intravascular coagulation can complicate GDV.[48] Widespread activation of the coagulation cascade results from a combination of factors including vascular sludging, endothelial damage, platelet activation, acidosis, and endotoxin, kallikrein, and pancreatic protease activation of Hageman factor.

Pathophysiology - Respiratory

Acute gastric distention applies pressure on the diaphragm and thorax, restricting pulmonary function and reducing tidal volume. There is an increase in inspiratory and expiratory resistance and a marked decrease in lung compliance.[7] Compensation is made by increasing respiratory rate, but as dilation worsens normal minute volumes cannot be maintained. The result of respiratory impairment is decreased blood oxygen tension, with the fall greatest in the caudal vena cava.[38] The hypoxemia associated with the circulatory changes accelerates tissue death from hypoxia.

Pathophysiology - Clinical Pathological Changes

Packed Cell Volume, Total Protein, and Albumin. Packed cell volume (PCV) rises transiently immediately after initiation of experimental GDV[25] or raised intraabdominal pressure.[40] Blood volume, however, remains unchanged during the first 30 minutes of gastric dilatation.[49] The increased PCV thus appears to reflect a release of sequestered red blood cells, the origin of which is uncertain. Subsequently, loss of plasma fluid into the gut and abdominal cavity further raises PCV, and to a lesser extent total protein.[26] Total protein concentrations remain little changed during experimental GDV. If crystalloid fluids (90 ml/kg) are administered at resuscitation, mean PCV, total protein, and serum albumin concentrations are transiently reduced to approximately 20%, 2.8 gm/dl, and 1 gm/dl, respectively. In some dogs, anemia and hypoproteinemia develop in the postoperative period, presumably due to loss of plasma or blood from abdominal vessel rupture or gastrointestinal mucosal damage. Reduced PCV significantly decreases the oxygen carrying capacity of the blood, a detrimental effect partially offset by improved perfusion due to decreased blood viscosity. The PCV which produces an ideal balance between viscosity and oxygen carrying capacity in dogs is 30%-40%;[50] it is desirable to maintain the PCV above 20%.[45] Reductions of serum albumin to 1 gm/dl markedly reduce plasma oncotic pressure to the point where tissue edema is likely.

Potassium. Serum potassium content gradually increases during experimental GDV[25,26,51] and rises, rapidly but transiently, immediately after gastric decompression.[25,51] In some dogs, the postdecompression rise in serum potassium concentration is as great as 1 mEq/L within 15 minutes (Figure 14-4). Potassium is released from degenerating cells, where its concentration is 30 times that in extracellular fluid. During the first one to two minutes after decompression of the experimentally distended intestine, potassium concentration in the venous effluent rises rapidly by 1 mEq/L and then declines to normal levels.[30] Hyperkalemia is rarely detected in spontaneous GDV, probably because of its transient nature in many dogs. In contrast, hypokalemia is more commonly noted, particularly in the postoperative period.[1] The hypokalemia probably results

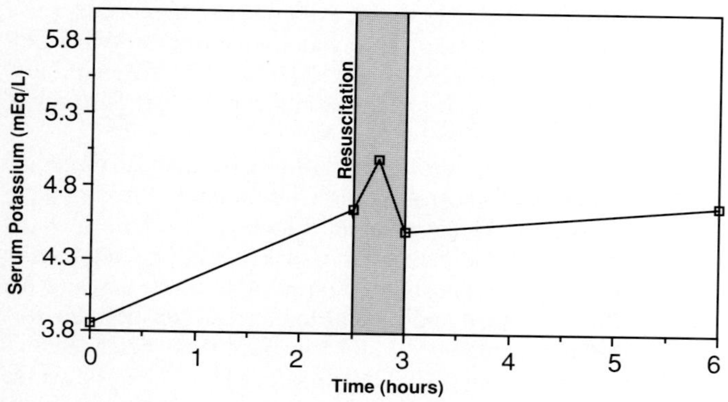

Figure 14-4. Mean serum potassium concentrations before, during, and after acute GDV.

from decreased intake in association with increased loss of potassium in vomitus, by sequestration into the dilated stomach, and resulting from metabolic alkalosis or hypovolemia-induced hyperaldostronemia.

Phosphorous. Serum phosphorus concentrations rise as much as threefold during experimental GDV.[25,26,51] Phosphorus is released from degenerating cells and by the breakdown of adenosine triphosphate during hypoxia. Decreased glomerular filtration may also contribute to the rise in serum phosphorus.

Sodium, Chloride, and Calcium. Serum levels of sodium and chloride remain little changed in experimental GDV, but occasionally they are increased or decreased in clinical cases. The variability is due to the opposing effects of hemoconcentration due to free water loss, and loss of electrolytes in vomitus or by sequestration into the dilated stomach. Serum calcium levels usually remain within the normal range.

Glucose. Serum glucose concentrations rise during experimental GDV.[26,51] and transiently decrease at the time of resuscitation.[25] The mean drop in glucose concentration in one study was 40 mg/dl. The glucose concentration of the worst-affected dogs dropped to 15-50 mg/dl. The cause of the decreased glucose may have been a combination of hemodilution, sudden tissue demand, and endotoxin release.

Creatine Phosphokinase. Serum creatine phosphokinase rises during experimental GDV.[26] The rise has been attributed to ischemic damage to caudal skeletal muscle mass.

Blood Gas and Acid-Base Changes. Metabolic acidosis develops during experimental GDV. Serum lactate concentrations[25,26] and base deficits[25,27] increase during GDV, resuscitation, and the ensuing shock. Blood pH and serum bicarbonate concentration decrease during experimental GDV, particularly at the point of resuscitation, or during ensuing shock.[25] Lactic acidosis develops as a consequence of anaerobic tissue metabolism. The worsened acid-base status during resuscitation presumably reflects washout of accumulated hydrogen ions. During the first one to two minutes after decompression of the experimentally distended intestine, pH in venous effluent decreases by 0.1 units.[30]

Venous PO_2 declines during experimental GDV and rapidly increases at resuscitation. Changes are closely correlated to cardiac output. During the latter stages of GDV, tissue oxygen uptake (cardiac index x AV oxygen content difference) increases by approximately 20%, while oxygen delivery (cardiac index x arterial oxygen content) decreases by approximately 50%. During resuscitation, the tissue oxygen uptake remains at 20% above baseline and the oxygen delivery increases by approximately 15%. Four hours after resuscitation, the tissue oxygen uptake is further increased to 30% above normal, whereas the oxygen delivery declines to approximately 50% of normal. Tissue oxygen uptake reflects the sum of all oxidative metabolic reactions. It can be rate-limited by circulation and increased by sepsis and various forms of tissue damage. Increased tissue oxygen uptake does not indicate an adequate circulatory supply of oxygen because increased requirements can outstrip supply.[46] Thus, it appears that at no stage during experimental GDV are increases in whole body tissue oxygen demands matched by adequate increase in oxygen delivery. Surface oxygen recordings suggest that much of this oxygen deficit may occur in the liver.

Pathophysiology - Abdominal Organs

Hepatic Pathophysiology

Mild to severe elevations in the serum concentration of ALT (SGPT) occur in spontaneous and experimental GDV.[25,26,52] The ALT activity in the serum of dogs with experimental GDV increases immediately after resuscitation, and within four hours can reach concentrations as high as 11,000 U/L (Figure 14-5).[25] This sudden rise in liver enzymes may be due to the flushing of pooled hepatic venous blood into the systemic circulation, or it may result from reperfusion-induced acute necrosis. The SAP concentration increases in most dogs to 200-300 U/L during experimental GDV, whereas the bilirubin changes little.[25]

Histologic examination of the liver of dogs subjected to experimental GDV shows minimal changes at the conclusion of 2.5 hours of GDV. Liver biopsies taken from many of the same dogs after four hours of reperfusion, however, show congestion, neutrophil infiltration, and moderate to severe hepatic necrosis.[25] Pathological examinations performed on spontaneous GDV presented to the UCD VMTH showed 70% to have gross or histologic evidence of hepatic pathology. Hepatic congestion, hemorrhage, and/or necrosis are the most frequently reported abnormalities in dogs dying acutely. Periportal or centrolobular cholestasis and fibrosis were observed in four dogs whose livers were biopsied after recovery from GDV. Hepatic volvulus in association with GDV has also been reported.[2]

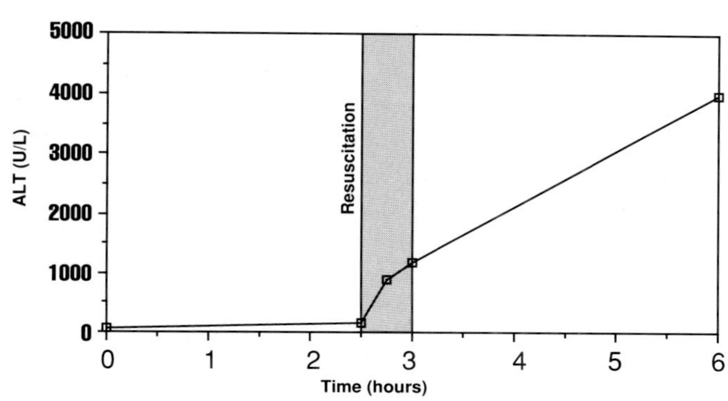

Figure 14-5. Mean serum concentrations of ALT before, during, and after acute GDV.

The hepatic pathology is probably caused by endotoxin absorption, venous occlusion, and ischemia-reperfusion injury to the hepatic vasculature and parenchyma. Support for the role of hypoxia in inducing the liver injury is provided by the low hepatic surface oxygen tension values, recorded during experimental GDV, that persisted after resuscitation.

Pancreatic Pathophysiology. Experimental GDV results in mild increases in the serum concentration of lipase and to a lesser extent amylase. These changes are associated with mild pancreatic edema but very little pancreatic necrosis.[25] Ischemia-induced, acute pancreatitis is thought to be relatively common in spontaneous GDV. Gross pathological evidence of mild to moderate pancreatitis is noted in 40% of dogs dying from GDV at the UCD VMTH.

Renal Pathophysiology. Slight increases in BUN and creatinine occur during experimental GDV.[25,26,51] Histopathologic changes are minimal, however, implying predominantly prerenal azotemia. Renal failure does occur in a significant number of cases of spontaneous GDV. In one series, renal failure was cited as a postoperative complication in 17% of dogs.[2]

Splenic Pathophysiology. Rotation of the stomach displaces the spleen by way of the gastrosplenic ligament. Splenic congestion develops as obstruction of splenic veins impairs splenic venous drainage. The spleen can also rotate clockwise or counterclockwise on its own pedicle. Splenic necrosis and thrombosis or avulsion of splenic vessels occasionally results.

Intestinal Pathophysiology. Experimental GDV causes extensive edema, hemorrhage, neutrophil infiltration and, in 50% of the dogs, necrosis of the longitudinal muscle layer of the duodenum and jejunum.[25] Changes in the serosa are similar. In some dogs, extensive epithelial sloughing also occurs. As was noted in the stomach and liver, the damage in the intestine is more severe after reperfusion than at the end of the GDV. The cause of the pathology in the muscularis is unclear, but may represent a neuronally-mediated response to gastric dilatation. The intestinal epithelial lesions are seen in the dogs with the lowest cardiac outputs, mean blood pressures, and surface oxygen tensions, implying that mucosal lesions result from intestinal hypoperfusion. The frequency of these lesions in spontaneous GDV is unknown.

Pathophysiology - Reperfusion Injury

The majority of the damage to transiently ischemic tissues occurs not during the period of ischemia, but rather when the ischemia is relieved and the tissues reperfused.[53] A number of investigators have demonstrated the central role of oxygen free radicals in the pathogenesis of the so-called "reperfusion injuries" of visceral tissues.[53-55] Oxygen-derived free radicals damage a wide variety of compounds and tissues, but the pathological process that has received most prominence is their ability to cause vascular damage by lipid peroxidation of cell membranes. The major sources of reperfusion-induced free radicals appear to be the tissue enzyme xanthine oxidase and neutrophil enzymes such as NADPH oxidase and myeloperoxidase. Xanthine oxidase is derived from the proteolysis of xanthine dehydrogenase by a calcium dependent enzyme. Xanthine dehydrogenase is present in high concentration in many tissues, including the liver and the mucosa of the gastrointestinal tract. Neutrophils rapidly accumulate in tissues subjected to ischemia and reperfusion. There is strong evidence to suggest that scavenging of free radicals, or pharmacological inhibition of free radical formation, will reduce the ischemia-reperfusion related tissue damage that occurs in the stomach and other portions of the digestive tract.[33,53-57]

Gastric-dilatation-volvulus results in ischemia of the stomach and associated visceral organs. Circulatory volume replacement and surgical correction of the dilation and volvulus results in reperfusion of the ischemic tissues. Thus, it would seem likely that the pathogenesis of GDV involves tissue damage due to reperfusion injury and, in particular, oxygen-derived free radicals. Experimental support for this concept, however, remains indirect. Tissue damage in GDV has been shown to be worse after four hours of reperfusion than at the end of ischemia.[25] Evidence of lipid peroxidation is noted in the liver, pancreas, and intestine of dogs subjected to experimental GDV.[29] Two studies, however, have failed to detect evidence of lipid peroxidative damage in gastric tissues.[2,29] Administration of allopurinol, a specific inhibitor of xanthine oxidase, to dogs subjected to experimental GDV has shown some promise, with a trend toward decreased lipid peroxidation being noted in one study,[29] and less gastric edema and hepatic necrosis observed in another study.[25] Furthermore, survival of dogs appeared to be improved following administration of a free-radical scavenger.[29] The recent observation that gradual reintroduction of oxygen reduces reperfusion injury in the cat stomach[33] may have future bearing on the decompression management of dogs with GDV.

Pathophysiology Summary

Gastric dilation and/or volvulus traps gastric ingesta and gas in the stomach. Further gas and fluid accumulate, eventually leading to extremely elevated intragastric pressure and gastric dilatation. Gastric blood flow is impeded, initially by the volvulus and raised intragastric pressure, and subsequently by gastric wall edema, thrombosis, and perhaps sympathetic-mediated vasoconstriction. Gastric ischemia, in association with gastric acid, leads to gastric ulceration, necrosis, and occasionally perforation and peritonitis. The gastric displacement malpositions the spleen, resulting in splenic congestion progressing at times to splenic thrombosis and necrosis.

The gastric dilatation reduces tidal volume, obstructs venous return, and compresses the splanchnic viscera, resulting in impaired respiration, acidosis, decreased cardiac output, poor perfusion of the visceral organs, vascular pooling and shock. Ischemia of the splanchnic viscera, probably exacerbated by endotoxin release, results in hepatic, pancreatic, and intestinal necrosis. Sepsis and DIC commonly result. If GDV is untreated, the visceral damage, shock, sepsis, peritonitis, and DIC are eventually fatal.

Resuscitation of dogs with GDV by sudden gastric deflation and derotation and by the rapid administration of large volumes of crystaloid fluids is a period of profound cardiovascular and metabolic stress, resulting from some or all of the events that include a transient decease in peripheral resistance, hyperkalemia, hypoglycemia, metabolic acidosis, hemodilution, liberation of cardiodepressant substances, and probably reperfusion injury and endotoxin release.

Surviving dogs may be affected by gastric motility abnormalities and hepatic cholestatic disorders.

CLINICAL FINDINGS

The clinical signs of GDV are characteristic. The most consistent historical findings are acute onset of depression in association with retching but not vomiting. Excessive salivation may be seen. Affected dogs are usually reluctant to stand and walk; some are in lateral recumbency or moribund. Abdominal tympany is usually evident and is easily confirmed by palpation. Cardiovascular failure is identified by rapid weak pulse, poor capillary refill time, and pale mucous membranes. Caudal venous distension may be apparent. Respirations are rapid, shallow, and dyspneic. Dehydration is usually not seen.

LABORATORY FINDINGS

Laboratory evaluation usually shows hemoconcentration. Metabolic acidosis and hypokalemia are common abnormalities, but metabolic alkalosis, respiratory acidosis, respiratory alkalosis, hyperkalemia, hypochloremia, and hypernatremia are also seen.[1] Mild increases in blood urea nitrogen and creatinine, slight to moderate increases in plasma lactate, ALT activity, creatine phosphokinase activity, and plasma phosphorus are often observed. Lipase and venous oxygen content are sometimes elevated.

RADIOGRAPHIC FINDINGS

Following fluid therapy and decompression, radiographs should be taken to determine whether gastric volvulus persists. The right lateral recumbent position provides the radiographic view of choice.[58] Residual gastric dilatation is readily identified radiographically by finding a large gas- and fluid-filled stomach (Figure 14-6). Volvulus is identified by finding a soft tissue fold that appears to compartmentalize the stomach, as illustrated in Figure 14-7. A key finding in the right lateral recumbent view is the observation of a gas-filled pylorus located dorsal to the fundus of the stomach.[59] Radiography may also identify splenic torsion, abdominal fluid suggestive of peritonitis or hemorrhage, free abdominal gas suggestive of perforation, and megaesophagus. The megaesophagus usually resolves spontaneously, but the other conditions require immediate surgery.

DIAGNOSIS

GDV is diagnosed on clinical findings and confirmed by successful gastric decompression and subsequent radiographic demonstration of gastric volvulus. Diagnostic evaluations such as a PCV/TP, a CBC, a venous blood gas analysis, an electrolyte panel, a serum chemistry analysis, a urinalysis, and cardiovascular monitoring should be instituted as soon as possible to help tailor therapy and identify likely complications of GDV.

TREATMENT

Management begins with rapid fluid therapy, followed by controlled decompression of the gastric dilatation. Supplemental therapy of possible benefit administered at or prior to decompression includes corticosteroids, non-steroidal antiinflammatory drugs, H_2-blockers, antibiotics, and perhaps oxy-

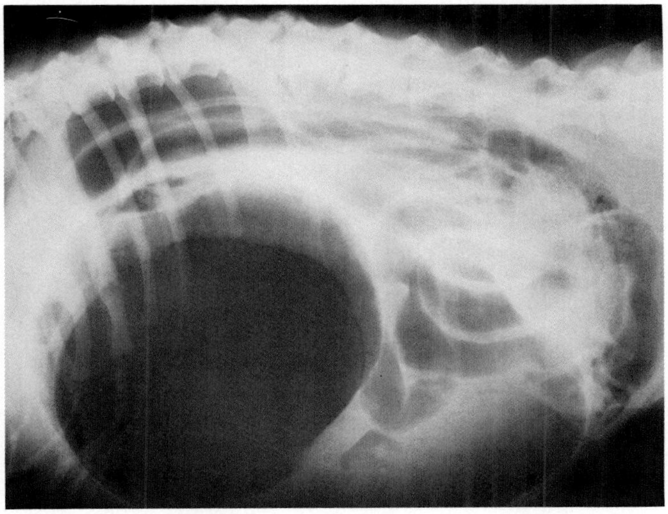

Figure 14-6. Lateral radiograph of 8-year-old Walker Hound presented with marked abdominal distension. The film shows gastric gaseous distention. The pylorus is situated in its proper location. There is no evidence of torsion.

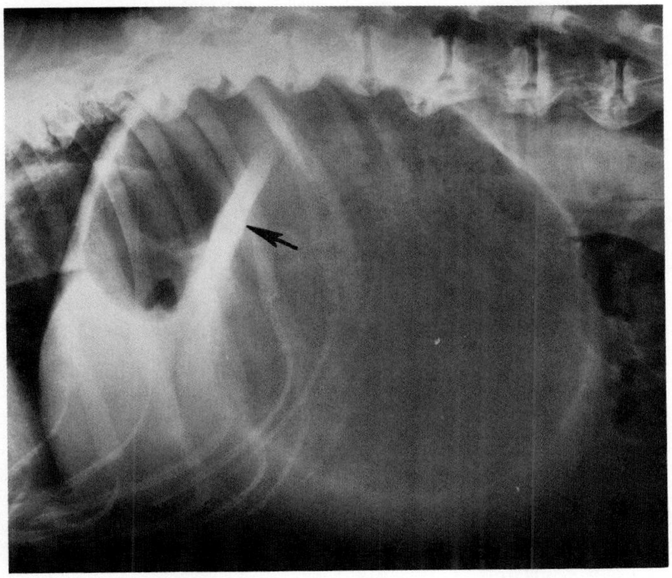

Figure 14-7. Lateral radiographs of abdomen of Saint Bernard presented with clinical signs of acute abdominal distention. The stomach is distended with gas. A pillar of column of soft tissue (arrows) suggests pyloric displacement. The esophagus is distended with contents, suggesting that the gastroesophageal junction is blocked. The spleen is not identified, because of rotation. The transverse colon is displaced caudally. No peritoneal fluid is evident. The spondylosis deformans has no significance for the current problem. Diagnosis is acute gastric dilation with rotation.

gen-derived free radical inhibitors or scavengers. After decompression of the stomach and stabilization of the clinical condition of the dog, the stomach is repositioned and gastropexy is performed. Subsequently, therapy may be required for various complications, including electrolyte imbalances, cardiac arrhythmias and disseminated intravascular coagulation.

Fluid Therapy. Intravenous fluid therapy should begin prior to gastric decompression[52] because of the risk of cardiovascular collapse, due to the sudden fall in total peripheral resistance and the release of sequestered cardioinhibitory factors that accompanies decompression. Those dogs exhibiting extreme respiratory compromise should be partially decompressed by way of a percutaneously placed needle while catheterization is in progress. Experimental data suggests that 45 ml/kg of a polyionic crystalloid fluid, such as lactated Ringer's solution, administered intravenously over a 15 minute period beginning just prior to decompression is sufficient to return the cardiac output to normal in dogs with transient GVD.[25] Rapid administration of larger volumes of crystaloid fluid (such as 90 ml/kg over 30 minutes) is associated with unacceptable hemodilution and little further improvement in cardiovascular function.[25] The alleviation of peripheral vasoconstriction and the restoration of acceptable pulse quality determines the end-point of volume replacement therapy for a particular dog. Central venous pressure assessment provides a further guide. Fluid is given until the central venous pressure increases. The cardiovascular and hydration status of the dog dictates the fluid administration rate required after initial volume replacement. A rate of 10 ml/kg/hour is usually appropriate for the immediate post-decompression period. After several hours, the rate can usually be reduced to between 2-5 ml/kg/hour.

The fluid of choice for initial volume replacement of dogs with GDV is a polyionic, isotonic crystalloid such as lactated Ringer's solution. The composition of fluid administered subsequently should be tailored to the dog's individual requirements as determined by repeated electrolyte, acid-base, glucose, and PCV/TP assessments. Supplemental potassium administration is commonly required. Initial infusion rates of potassium chloride as high as 0.5 mEq/kg/hr may be utilized. For subsequent maintenance, 20-30 mEq/liter of maintenance fluids is usually sufficient. Because acidosis is not a predictable finding in GDV, and because bicarbonate administration has the potential to cause significant adverse effects, bicarbonate should only be administered if blood gas data suggests a severe acidemia (pH below 7.2). The bicarbonate deficit may be determined from the following formula: body weight (kg) x 0.3 x (24 mEq/L - measured plasma bicarbonate). One half of this calculated deficit should be replaced over one hour and the acid-base status reassessed. During resuscitation some dogs become severely hypoglycemic. Supplementation of fluids with 5% dextrose may aid successful management.

Colloidal fluids such as plasma or dextran 70 are necessary if total protein levels decline below 3.5 gm/dl. Colloidal fluids will decrease fluid transudation from the vasculature and will support cardiac output for more prolonged periods than crystalloids. A suitable initial dose of plasma is 20 ml/kg administered over one to two hours. Dextran is usually administered at rates not exceeding 5ml/kg/hr and daily doses less than 20 ml/kg. A lack of response to colloids suggests that the shock is irreversible. If PCV declines are sufficient to cause clinical evidence of distress, whole blood therapy may be required.

Gastric Decompression. Decompression of the dilated stomach is achieved by passage of a stomach tube or by trocarization. Because of the cardiovascular changes and reperfusion injury that accompany decompression, sudden decompression is less desirable than a slower release of pressure. When a colt-size tube (1/4-inch inside diameter) can be passed, the contents of the stomach can be removed by lavage assisted by vacuum. This tube is too large to pass in some dogs without rupturing the gastroesophageal junction or stomach. In many dogs a relatively inflexible tube of smaller diameter can be passed and directed through the gastroesophageal junction under fluoroscopic control. Placement of the dog in a sitting position may facilitate passage of the tube. Inability to pass a stomach tube is not diagnostic for volvulus. Moreover, a stomach tube can be passed in some dogs that have volvulus. When time does not permit attempting to pass a stomach tube or a tube cannot be passed, decompression is achieved by trocarization of the stomach with a 16 to 18 gauge, 1.5 to 2 inch needle. Trocarization is rarely associated with peritonitis and can save the patient's life. Following partial decompression, attempts are again made to pass a large-bore stomach tube.

Decompression can be achieved by gastrostomy, which is performed caudal to the right costal arch under local anesthesia.[4,60] The introduction of decompression by gastrostomy (in association with effective stabilization prior to surgical correction of volvulus) reportedly reduced mortality at one institution from 68% to 33%. The gastrostomy fixes the stomach to the abdominal wall. Such fixation prevents a rotated stomach from returning to its normal position after gastric decompression.

Following gastric decompression, spontaneous repositioning of the stomach can occur. In many dogs, however, surgical correction of the volvulus is required. Controversy surrounds the most appropriate time to operate on dogs that have been decompressed but remain torsed. Because gastric blood flow is compromised by gastric volvulus,[29] and because full thickness gastric necrosis is not uncommon in GDV, it is our preference to operate on dogs with persistent gastric volvulus as soon as the dog's clinical condition and hemodynamic, electrolyte, and acid-base status have been stabilized by appropriate decompression and fluid therapy. This is usually accomplished within one to two hours of admission. Others prefer more prolonged periods of stabilization, and periods as long as 48 hours have been used without apparent adverse effect.[4] If gastric material is noted to contain digested blood (coffee-grounds), celiotomy should not be delayed longer than the initial stabilization period of one to two hours, because severe gastric ulceration is likely, and perforation may follow.[4] Similarly, if radiographic evidence of perforation and peritonitis are detected, surgery should not be delayed. During prolonged periods of stabilization, decompression can be maintained by nasogastric tubes, pharyngostomy tubes, or gastrostomy.

Anesthesia. Anesthetic regimens chosen should be minimally cardiovascular depressant. Balanced anesthesia, incorporating narcotics and muscle relaxants to lower the requirements for inhalation anesthetics, is the preferred technique but requires ventilatory support. In lieu of balanced anesthesia, mask induction with isoflurane is suitable. Isoflurane reportedly does not depress cardiovascular function during GDV. If premedication is required, low doses of meperidine (4 mg/kg SQ) or oxymorphone (0.02-0.05 mg/kg SQ) may be used. If intravenous induction is deemed necessary, low dose ketamine

(2.5 mg/kg IV) combined with valium (0.5 mg/kg IV) may be given, and the dogs maintained with minimal concentrations of inhalation agents. Nitrous oxide should be avoided to prevent exacerbation of gastric dilatation by accumulation of intragastric nitrous oxide.

Surgery. Surgical intervention in gastric dilatation volvulus has two roles. The first is therapeutic and the second preventative. For therapeutic purposes, residual gas, fluid, and ingesta are removed, the stomach is repositioned, and any areas of gastric necrosis are resected. Partial gastrectomy is required in 10% of dogs with GDV.[61] Recurrence rates of GDV treated without surgical gastropexy are as high as 80%.[62] Therefore, in order to prevent recurrence, all dogs presented with GDV should undergo surgical gastropexy.

Surgical methods for reducing the incidence of recurrence of GDV have included various gastropexy procedures, and procedures to accelerate gastric emptying. There is little evidence to support the continued use of procedures aimed at increasing gastric emptying, such as pyloromyotomy and pyloroplasty.[2,63] Appropriate fixation procedures are, however, very effective at reducing the frequency of recurrence. The techniques of choice are the circumcostal gastropexy, the muscular flap gastropexy, incisional gastropexy, and the tube gastrostomy.[4] The circumcostal, incisional, and muscular flap gastropexy techniques result in lower rates of recurrence (0-3.3%) than the tube gastrostomy (5-11%) techniques. Gastrostomy tube failure is a common occurrence following tube gastrostomy. It is usually due to rupture of the balloon of Foley-like catheters[2] and can result in peritonitis. Advantages of the tube gastrostomy include a short operation time, the ability to maintain gastric decompression post-operatively, and the ability to provide supplemental nutrition. Our preference is to place gastrostomy tubes only in critically ill dogs. In these patients, the benefits of shorter operation time, continued decompression, and enteral nutrition outweigh the disadvantages of this technique. The gastrostomy catheter is usually removed after five to seven days but may be kept longer if required. Splenectomy does not prevent recurrences but may be required for other reasons, such as splenic infarction.

Recurrence of acute gastric dilatation can occur in spite of the use of gastropexy. These techniques prevent gastric volvulus, but do not necessarily prevent gastric dilatation. It is likely that such recurrences could be treated by elimination of factors that contribute to the competence of the gastroesophageal junction. Possibilities include elimination of the intraabdominal esophagus and fundectomy to eliminate the valve of His. Gastroesophageal reflux, an undesirable complication, would develop with the former.

Corticosteroids. Corticosteroids are used routinely in managing shock. No controlled studies have shown that steroids increase long-term survival rates for animals in shock,[64] but the plethora of theoretical beneficial effects ascribed to glucocorticoids has resulted in their continued use. Beneficial effects of glucocorticoid administration particularly relevant to GDV include reduced absorption of intestinal endotoxin during intestinal ischemia, reduced leukocyte margination and diapedesis, decreased capillary permeability, and improved capillary flow. Administration of prednisolone succinate (6.6 mg/kg IV) 30 minutes prior to deflation of the dilated stomach tended to reduce the severity of gastric lesions in one experimental study of gastric dilatation.[27] A large number of adverse effects of corticosteroids have also been reported. Fortunately, the majority of these adverse effects result from long-term usage rather than the short-term, large dose therapy reportedly beneficial in shock. Adverse effects of corticosteroids of concern in GDV include promotion of acute pancreatitis and potentiation of sepsis. Doses commonly employed for the therapy of shock include prednisolone sodium succinate (30 mg/kg IV) and dexamethasone sodium phosphate (6-15 mg/kg IV).

Non-steroidal Antiinflammatory Drugs. Non-steroidal antiinflammatory drugs, such as flunixin meglumine, have shown beneficial effects in the treatment of endotoxic shock and other forms of shock.[65] The beneficial effects are off-set, however, by the rapidity (24 hours) with which flunixin can induce serious gastric ulceration in the dog when used alone,[65] and especially when used in conjunction with glucocorticoids.[66] Furthermore, non-steroidal antiinflammatory agents markedly potentiate ischemic renal damage resulting from hypotension. Flunixin meglumine usage should probably be restricted to a single injection, administered after volume replacement at the time of gastric decompression (the probable period of peak endotoxemia). Reportedly effective doses range from 0.25-1.1 mg/kg IV.

Antibiotics. The administration of antibiotics should be restricted to dogs demonstrating clinical or clinicopathological evidence of sepsis. The clinical signs initially include restlessness, fever, petechia, peripheral vasodilation, and worsening depression. Dogs with hemorrhagic diarrhea or gastric content suggesting mucosal necrosis are highly likely to develop sepsis. The laboratory findings include neutropenia, left shifted hemograms, thrombocytopenia, hypoalbuminemia, hypoglycemia, venous blood gas greater than 50 mm Hg (hyperdynamic shunting of blood), and positive blood cultures.

The source of bacteria causing sepsis in GDV is the gastrointestinal tract. Blood cultures are necessary to determine effective antibiotic therapy, because a wide variety of bacteria can gain access to the bloodstream from the bowel. Both anaerobic and aerobic bacteria may be absorbed, and no single antibiotic is usually effective against both. Ampicillin is an effective antibiotic against most, but not all anaerobes. Unfortunately, it decimates the anaerobic flora of the bowel, leading to overgrowth with more virulent gram negative organisms and increasing the risk of fatal sepsis. The resistance pattern of gram negative bacteria is highly variable, and further antibiotic resistance develops rapidly. Moreover, the aminoglycoside antibiotics, while effective against many gram negatives, are particularly nephrotoxic in the face of hypovolemia, common in GDV. If the clinician does not have the benefit of blood culture results, suitable antibiotics include trimethoprim-sulfa combinations or cephalosporins. If sepsis is felt to be fulminant or abdominal contamination has occurred, combination ampicillin, metronidazole, and gentamicin therapy may be utilized. The dose of gentamicin should be no greater than 2.2 mg/kg SQ q 8 hours. Amikacin (2.2 mg/kg SQ q 8 h) can be substituted for the gentamicin and at this dose may be less nephrotoxic than gentamicin.

Miscellaneous Pharmacological Therapy. Administration of H_2-blockers such as ranitidine (1-2 mg/kg q 8-12 hr IV, IM, PO) and cimetidine (4-5 mg/kg q 8 hr, IV, IM, PO) may ameliorate gastric ulceration. Ranitidine is preferred over cimetidine, because ranitidine is a more potent inhibitor of gastric secretion and does not depress hepatic microsomal mixed-function oxidase function. Sucralfate (0.5-1 gm q 8 hr PO) may facilitate healing of gastric ulcers.

Oxygen-derived free radical inhibitors and scavengers have been experimentally demonstrated to protect a number of organs against reperfusion injury, including those commonly affected by GDV such as liver, pancreas, heart, and gastrointestinal tract mucosa. Future research may clarify the role of these drugs in the therapy of GDV.

Lidocaine, administered at doses commonly employed to treat arrhythmias, has been shown to reduce gastric ulceration in experimental gastric dilatation, perhaps through its membrane stabilizing effects.[27]

Blood pressure support is best provided by adequate crystalloid and colloidal fluid therapy. If additional support is required, dopamine (5-10 µg/kg/min) or dobutamine (5-10 µg/kg/min) continuous infusions may be utilized. Over-dosage of these agents can induce tachycardia and cardiac arrhythmias.

Nutrition. Oral nutrition is begun after 24 to 48 hours. Small quantities of bland, easily digestible diets fed three to four times per day are usually selected. If vomiting ensues, feeding is stopped for a further 24 to 36 hours and tried again. Patients recovering from GDV should not be allowed to go without food for more than five days before enteral or parenteral nutrition is commenced.

Management of Complications

Monitoring. Complications are common during recovery from GDV, necessitating close monitoring. Complications reported in the post-decompression or post-operative period include electrolyte and acid base imbalances, anemia, vomiting, cardiac arrhythmias, shock, gastric wall necrosis, peritonitis, sepsis, paralytic ileus, pancreatitis, liver failure, renal failure, DIC, pulmonary thromboembolism, splenic hemorrhage, intussusception, intestinal volvulus, esophageal perforation and mediastinitis, bronchopneumonia, pneumothorax, and cerebral damage. Pneumothorax is most commonly associated with circumcostal gastropexy.

Physical examinations should be repeated frequently, paying particular attention to attitude, hydration status, body temperature, cardiovascular function, and mucous membrane appearance. In addition, depending on the condition of the dog, some or all of the following monitoring procedures may be useful. Repeated measures of body weight, PCV/TP, electrolyte and acid-base status help assess the adequacy of fluid therapy. Electrocardiograms and measurement of CVP and arterial blood pressure facilitate detection of serious arrhythmias and cardiovascular compromise. Repeated complete blood counts, venous oxygen content, and blood glucose concentration aid discovery of sepsis. Measurement of clotting times (APTT, OSPT, ACT), bleeding times, platelet count, and fibrinogen help reveal DIC. A serum chemistry profile and urinalysis help identify damage to liver and kidney. If peritonitis or abdominal hemorrhage is suspected, abdominocentesis may be performed.

Cardiac Arrhythmias. Cardiac arrhythmias occur in 40%-50% of dogs with GDV.[4,43,67] The cardiac arrhythmias associated with GDV usually begin between 12 and 36 hours after the onset of GDV but can exist at presentation or have an onset as delayed as 72 hours after presentation. They consist primarily of premature ventricular contractions, paroxysmal ventricular tachycardia, and ventricular tachycardia.[24,43,67] These cardiac arrhythmias are often resistant to therapy. Correction of acid-base and electrolyte abnormalities, especially total body potassium depletion, appears to improve the responsiveness of the arrhythmias. Thus, the first step in arrhythmia management is appropriate fluid therapy. Even in the face of normokalemia, it is advisable to provide supplemental potassium (20-30 mEq/L of maintenance fluids) to replete intracellular potassium.

Antiarrhythmic drugs should not be used indiscriminantly. Ventricular tachycardia with heart rates greater than 140-150 beats per minute requires therapy. Premature ventricular contractions need only be treated if they are multifocal, demonstrate the "R on T" phenomenon, or are associated with clinical evidence of hypoperfusion. Lidocaine hydrochloride is the usual therapy (2-4 mg/kg IV as a slow initial bolus, followed by a continuous infusion of 50-100 µg/kg/min for several days). If necessary, antiarrhythmic therapy can be supplemented and continued with procainamide hydrochloride (12-20 mg/kg IM q 6 h, followed by 12-20 mg/kg PO q 6 h). Procainamide may also be administered slowly IV (12-20 mg/kg over 15 -20 minutes), followed by a constant rate infusion of 10-40 µg/kg/min. If supraventricular arrhythmias are noted, quinidine sulfate may be useful (6-8 mg/kg IM q 6 h, or 6-16 mg/kg PO q 6 h).

Great care must be exercised in the use of the antiarrhythmic agents. Many GDV patients have significant hepatic and/or renal dysfunction. Lidocaine, procainamide, and quinidine are all metabolized by the liver and excreted by the kidneys. Therefore, the potential for toxicity is high. Although some of the toxicities of these drugs are reasonably characteristic (for instance the tremors and seizures of lidocaine overdosage), other signs of drug toxicity (such as vomiting, diarrhea, and, paradoxically, cardiac arrhythmias) may be wrongly attributed to complications of GDV and lead to continued or even increased dosage of the antiarrhythmics. Furthermore, lidocaine may detrimentally affect septic patients,[68] although it appears to reduce gastric mucosal injury following gastric dilatation.[27]

Gastrointestinal Motility Abnormalities and Vomiting. The gastric dysrhythmias resulting from GDV will usually resolve without therapy. Transient paralytic ileus occurs in as many as 30% of patients. Both ileus and delayed gastric emptying may be treated with metoclopramide (0.2-0.4 mg/kg q 6 hr IV, SC, PO) without significantly reducing eructation frequency.[16,69] Vomiting usually resolves spontaneously. If vomiting persists, metoclopramide and ranitidine or cimetidine may be beneficial.

Disseminated Intravascular Coagulation. Disseminated intravascular coagulation (DIC) occurred in approximately 10% of the dogs in one series.[2] DIC is treated with plasma in association with heparin (50-150 units/kg, SQ q 8 hr), administered in quantities sufficient to prolong the clotting time of the coagulation test being used to 1.5-2 times normal. If the underlying cause of the DIC has not been managed, therapy will be unsuccessful.

Recurrence of Gastric Dilatation or GDV. Without surgical fixation of the stomach, the GDV recurrence rate is as high as 80%.[62] Recurrence of GDV following appropriate surgical fixation, however, is relatively rare (less than 15%). Recurrent gastric dilation or dilatation in the absence of volvulus does on occasion develop. This complication usually resolves after gastric motility returns to normal, but on occasion it is recurrent and may be precipitated by aerophagia.[2]

Feeding three to four times a day instead of once may help prevent recurrence. Moistening of dry dog food, and restriction of exercise after consumption of large quantities of food or water, may also be helpful. Antifoaming agents have no value in preventing recurrence. Although no value has been demonstrated for any other drugs in clinical cases, ß-adrenergic drugs increase eructation frequenty in dogs and may be of value in some cases.[14]

Prognosis

The mortality associated with canine GDV is 30%-60%,[70] although more recent reports suggest more favorable results.[2] The mortality is as high as 63%-80% when partial gastrectomy is required.[2,61] In one study, the mortality rate was higher in patients presenting with clinically apparent compromised cardiovascular function and/or with depressed mentation. Thus, pulse rates greater than 180 per minute, weak or arrhythmic pulses, pale or cyanotic mucous membranes, and capillary refill times greater than 1 second at presentation were associated with mortalities greater than 55%.[2] Mortality was not found to be different in dogs decompressed early versus those whose compression was delayed. Most dogs that die in the postoperative period do so within the first four days.[4] The likelihood of recurrence of GDV following medical management is as high as 80%, but after appropriate surgical fixation the recurrence rate is low.

CHRONIC GASTRIC VOLVULUS

Clinical Synopsis

Diagnostic Features

* Historical reports of self-relieving mild to moderate gastric distension
* Absence of gastric tympany or evidence of shock
* Radiographic evidence of a torsed stomach

Treatment

* Gastropexy

Signalment and Incidence

Dogs with gastric volvulus but without concomitant gastric dilatation have been occasionally observed at the UCD VMTH and have been reported by others.[3,4,71-73] The disorder appears most common in deep-chested breeds. No age or sex predilection has been recognized.

Etiology and Pathogenesis

The cause of the gastric volvulus is unknown. The intermittent gastric dilatation is presumably a reflection of impaired ability to eructate, and, perhaps, delayed emptying of solids. Gastric emptying of liquids has been normal in the few dogs in which emptying studies have been performed.

Clinical Findings and Diagnosis

Dogs with chronic gastric volvulus usually have a history of recurrent bouts of mild gastric distension. The distension usually resolves spontaneously but on some occasions requires orogastric intubation. Vomiting, borborygmi, eructation, and weight loss have also been reported.[4] Physical examination is usually unremarkable. Diagnosis is dependent on radiographic or surgical demonstration of gastric volvulus in the absence of gastric dilatation. Laboratory tests are usually unremarkable.

Treatment and Prognosis

Resolution of the majority of clinical signs usually follows gastropexy. Prognosis is good.

REFERENCES

1. Muir, W.W.: (2). Acid base and electrolyte disturbances in dogs with gastric dilatation-volvulus. JAVMA 181:229-231, 1982.
2. Van Sluijs, F.J.: Gastric-dilatation volvulus in the dog. Thesis. Dept Small Animal Medicine and Surgery, University of Utrecht, 1987.
3. Strombeck, D.R.: Small Animal Gastroenterology. Stonegate Publishing. Davis, CA., 1979.
4. Leib, M.S., Monroe, W.E. and Martin, R.A.: Suspected chronic gastric volvulus in a dog with normal gastric emptying of liquids. JAVMA 191:699-700, 1987.
5. Van Kruiningen, H.J., Wojan, L.D., Stake, P.E. and Lord, P.F.: The influence of diet and feeding frequency on gastric function in the dog. J. Am. An. Hosp. Assoc. 23:145-152, 1987.
6. Caywood, D., Teaque, H.D., Jackson, D.A., Levitt, M.D. and Bond, J.H.Gastric analysis in the canine gastric dilation volvulus syndrome. JAAHA 13:459-462, 1977.
7. Byrne, J.J., Cahill, J.M.: Acute gastric dilatation. Am. J. Surg. 101:301-309, 1961.
8. Van Kruiningen, H.J., Gregoire, K. and Meuten, D.J.: Acute gastric dilatation: A review of comparative aspects, by species, and a study in dogs and monkeys. JAAHA 10:294-324, 1974.
9. Draser, B.S. and Hill, M.J.: Human intestinal flora. Academic Press, London, 1974.
10. Rasche, R. and Butterfield, W.C.: Bloating and the inability to vomit after the Belsey hiatal hernia repair. J. Thorac. Cardiovasc. Surg. 65:646-648, 1973.
11. Goyal, R.K., Rattan, S.: Neurohumoral, hormonal, and drug receptors for the lower esophageal sphincter. Gastroenterology 74:598-619, 1978.
12. Dodds, W.J., Hogan, W.J., Helm, J.F. and Dent, J.: Pathogenesis of reflux esophagitis. Gastroenterology 81:376-394, 1981.
13. Strombeck, D.R., Harrold, D.: Effect of gastrin, histamine, serotonin, and adrenergic amines on gastroesophageal sphincter pressure in the dog. Am. J. Vet. Res. 46:1684-1690, 1985.
14. Strombeck, D.R., Griffin, D.W. and Harrold, D.: Eructation of gas through the gastroesophageal sphincter before and after limiting distention of the gastric cardia or infusion of a ß-adrenergic amine in dogs. Am. J. Vet. Res. 50:751-753, 1989.
15. Leib, M.S., Wingfield, W.E., Twedt, D.C. and Bottoms, G.D.: Plasma gastrin immunoreactivity in dogs with acute gastric dilatation-volvulus. JAVMA 185:205-208, 1984.
16. Strombeck, D.R., Turner, W.D. and Harrold, D.: Eructation of gas through the gastroesophageal sphincter before and after gastric fundectomy in dogs. Am. J. Vet. Res. 49:87-89, 1988.

17. Strombeck, D.R., Harrold, D. and Ferrier, W.: Eructation of gas through the gastroesophageal sphincter before and after truncal vagotomy in dogs. Am. J. Vet. Res. 48:207-210, 1987.
18. Edwards, M.H.: Selective vagotomy of the canine esophagus-a model for the treatment of hiatal hernia. Thorax 311:185-189, 1976.
19. Little, A.F., Martin, C.J., Dent, J., Harris, A.J. and McMahan, S.J.: Postural suppression of transient lower esophageal relaxations and gastroesophageal reflux in the dog. Gastroenterology 90:1522, 1986.
20. VanSluijs, F.J. and vanden Brom, W.E.: Gastric emptying of a radionuclide-labeled test meal after surgical correction of gastric dilatation-volvulus in dogs. Am. J. Vet. Res. 50:433-435, 1988.
21. Wingfield, W.E., Cornelius, L.M. and DeYoung, D.W.: Pathophysiology of the gastric dilatation-torsion complex in the dog. J. Small An. Pract. 15:735-739, 1974.
22. Wingfield, W.E., Betts, C.W. and Rawlings, C.A.: Pathophysiology associated with gastric dilatation-volvulus in the dog. JAAHA 12:136-142, 1976.
23. Orton, E.C., Muir, W.W.: Hemodynamics in experimental gastric dilatation-volvulus in dogs. Am. J. Vet. Res. 44:1512-1515, 1983.
24. Horne, W.A., Gilmore, D.R., Dietze, A.E., et al.: Effects of gastric distention-volvulus on coronary blood flow and myocardial oxygen consumption in the dog. Am. J. Vet. Res. 46:98-104, 1985.
25. Guilford, W.G., Komtebedde, J., Haskins, S.C., et al.: Unpublished observations, 1989.
26. Merkley, D.F., Howard, D.R., Krehbiel, J.D., Eyster, G.E., Krahwinkel, D.J. and Sawyer, D.C.: Experimentally induced acute gastric dilatation in the dog: Clinicopathologic findings. JAAHA 12:149-153, 1976.
27. Pfeiffer, C.J., Keith, J.C. and April, M.: Topographic localization of gastric lesions and key role of plasma bicarbonate concentration in dogs with experimentally induced gastric dilatation. Am. J. Vet. Res. 48:262-267, 1987.
28. Wheaton, L.G., Thacker, H.L. and Caldwell, S.: Intravenous fluorescein as an indicator of gastric viability in gastric dilatation-volvulus. JAAHA 22:197-204, 1986.
29. Lantz, G.C., Badylak, S.F.: Reperfusion injury in experimental canine gastric dilatation-volvulus. Veterinary Surgery 18:70, 1989.
30. Boley, S.J., Girdhar, P.A., Warren. A.R., et al: Pathophysiologic effects of bowel distension on intestinal blood flow. Am. J. Surg. 117:228-234, 1969.
31. Durbin, R.P., Moody, F.G.: Water movement through a transporting epithelial membrane: the gastric mucosa. Symp. Soc. Exp. Biol. 19:299, 1965.
32. Varhaug, J.E., Svanes, K., Lysen, L.J., et al. The effect of intragastric pressure on gastric blood flow after partial devascularization of the stomach in cats. Eur. J. Surg. Res. 12:415-427, 1980.
33. Perry, M.A., Wadhwa, S.S.: Gradual reintroduction of oxygen reduces reperfusion injury in cat stomach. Am. J. Physiol. 254:G366-G372, 1988.
34. Bulkley, G., Goldman, H. and Silen, W.: Pressure injury to the gastric mucosa. Am. J. Surg. 117:193-203, 1969.
35. Alphin, R.S., Vokac, M.D. and Gregory, R.L.: Role of intragastric pressure, pH, and pepsin in gastric ulceration in the rat. Gastroenterology 73:495-500, 1977.
36. Hall, J.A., Solie, T.N., Seim, H.B. and Twedt, D.C.: Acute gastric dilatation alters gastric electromechanical activity in the dog. Gastroenterology 95:869, 1988.
37. Burrows, C.F., Stampley, A. and Ellison, G.: Gastric myoelectrical activity in spontaneous canine gastric dilatation volvulus. Abstract ACVIM Proceedings, 45, 1988.
38. Merkley, D.F., Howard, D.R., Eyster, G.E., Krahwinkel, D.J., Sawyer, D.C. and Krehbiel, J.D.: Experimentally induced acute gastric dilatation in the dog: Cardiopulmonary effects. JAAHA 12:143-148, 1976b.
39. Engler, H.S., Kennedy, T.E., Ellison, L.T. et al.: Hemodynamics of experimental acute gastric dilatation. Am. J. Surg. 113:194-197, 1967.
40. Caldwell, C.B., Ricotta, J.J.: Changes in visceral blood flow with elevated intraabdominal pressure. J. Surg. Res. 43:14-20, 1987.
41. Wingfield, W.E., Cornelius, L.M., Ackerman, N. and DeYoung, D.W.:Experimental acute gastric dilatation and torsion in the dog-2. venous angiographic alterations seen in gastric dilatation. J. Small An. Pract. 15:55-60, 1974.
42. Orton, C.E., Muir, W.W.: Isovolmetric indices and humoral cardioactive substance bioassay during clinical and experimentally induced gastric dilatation-volvulus in dogs. Am. J. Vet. Res. 44:1516-1520, 1983.
43. Longhurst, J.C., Spilker, H.L. and Ordway, G.A.: Cardiovascular reflexes elicited by passive gastric distension in anesthetized cats. Am. J. Physiol. 240:H539-H545, 1981.
44. Muir, W.W., Weisbrode, S.E.: Myocardial ischemia in dogs with gastric dilatation-volvulus. JAVMA 181:363-366, 1982.
45. Mitchell, A.R.: What is shock? J. Small An. Pract. 26:719-738, 1985.
46. Shoemaker, W.C.: Circulatory mechanisms of shock and their mediators. Critical Care Medicine 15:787-794, 1987.
47. Saba, T.M.: Reticuloendothelial systemic host defense after surgery and traumatic shock. Circulatory Shock 2:91-108, 1975.
48. Lees, G.E., Leighton, R.L. and Hart, R.: Management of gastric dilatation-volvulus and disseminated intravascular coagulation in a dog: A case report. JAAHA 13:463-469, 1977.
49. Williams, J.S.: Hemodynamic alterations in acute gastric dilatation in the dog. Surgical Forum 16:335-336, 1965.
50. Bryan-Brown, C.W.: Blood flow to organs: Parameters for function and survival in critical illness. Critical Care Medicine 16:170-178, 1988.
51. Wingfield, W.E., Cornelius, L.M. and DeYoung, D.W.: Experimental acute gastric dilatation and torsion in the dog-1. Changes in biochemical and acid-base parameters. J. Small An. Pract. 15:41-53, 1974.
52. Kirby, R.: Gastric dilatation-volvulus complex; Retrospective review of factors important to survival. Unpublished data, University of Pennsylvania, 1988.
53. Granger, D.N., Rutili, G., McCord, J.M.: Superoxide radicals in feline intestinal ischemia. Gastroenterology 81:22-29, 1981.
54. Parks, D.A., Granger, D.N.: Ischemia-reperfusion injury: a radical view. Hepatology 8:680-682, 1988
55. Sanfey, H., Buckley, G.B. and Cameron, J.L.: The role of oxygen-derived free radicals in the pathogenesis of acute pancreatitis. Ann. Surg. 200:405-413, 1984.
56. McCord, J.M.: Oxygen-derived free radicals in postischemic tissue injury. N. Eng. J. Med. 312:159-163, 1985.
57. Parks, D.A., Buckley, G.B., Granger, D.N., et al: Ischemic injury in the cat small intestine: Role of superoxide radicals. Gastroenterology 82:9-15, 1982.
58. Hathcock, J.T.: Radiographic view of choice for the diagnosis of gastric volvulus: The right lateral recumbent view. JAAHA 20:967-969, 1984.
59. Kneller, S.K.: Radiographic interpretation of the gastric dilatation-volvulus complex in the dog. JAAHA 12:154-157, 1976.
60. Pass, M.A. and Johnston, D.R.: Treatment of gastric dilatation-torsion in the dog. Gastric decompression by gastrotomy under local analgesia. J. Small An. Pract. 14:1131-142, 1973.
61. Matthieson, D.T.: Partial gastrectomy as treatment of gastric volvulus. Results in 30 dogs. Vet. Surgery 14:185-193, 1985.
62. Dann, J.R.: Medical and surgical treatment of canine acute gastric dilatation. JAAHA 12:17-22, 1976.
63. Greenfield, C.L., Walshaw, R. and Thomas, M.W.: Significance of the Heineke-Miknlicz pyloroplasty in the treatment of gastric dilatation-volvulus. Vet. Surg. 18:22-26, 1989.
64. Reichgott, M.J. and Melmon, K.L.: Should corticosteroids be used in shock. Med. Clin. N. Amer. 57:1211-1223, 1973.
65. Stegelmeier, B.L., Bottoms, G.D., Denicola, D.B. and Reed,

W.M.: Effects of flunixin meglumine in dogs following experimentally induced endotoxemia. Cornell Vet. 78:221-230, 1988.

66. Dowe, S.W., Rosychuk, R.A., McChesney, A.E., et al.: Adverse effects of flunixin meglumine administered with and without prednisone on the gastrointestinal tract of dogs. Abstract ACVIM Proceedings Pg 1045, 1989.
67. Muir, W.W., and Lipowitz, A.J.: Cardiac Dysrhythmias associated withgastric dilatation-volvulus in the dog. JAVMA 172:683-689, 1978.
68. Hardie, E.M., Rawlings, C.A., Shotts, E.B., et al.: Lidocaine treatment of dogs with Escherichia coli septicemia. Am. J. Vet. Res. 49:77-81, 1988.
69. Graves, G.M., Becht, J.L. and Rawlings CA. Metoclopramide reversal of decreased gastrointestinal myoelectric and contractile activity in a model of canine postoperative ileus. Vet. Surg. 18:27-33, 1989.
70. Wingfield, W.E., Betts, C.W. and Greene, R.W.: Operative techniques and recurrence rates associated with gastric volvulus in the dog. J. Small An. Pract. 16:427-432, 1975.
71. Leib, M.S., Blass, C.E.: Acute gastric dilatation in the dog: various clinical presentations. Comp. Contin. Educ. Pract. Vet. 4:677-682, 1984.
72. Boothe, H.W., Ackerman, N.: Partial gastric torsion in two dogs. JAAHA 12:27-30, 1976.
73. Frendin, J., Funkquist, B. and Stavenborn, M.: Gastric displacement in dogs without clinical signs of acute dilatation. J. Small An. Pract. 29:775-779, 1988.
74. Lantz, G.C., Bottoms, G.D., Carlton, W.W., et al.: The effect of 360 gastric volvulus on the blood supply of the nondistended normal dog stomach. Vet. Surgery 13:189-196, 1984.

Chapter 15

Small and Large Intestine, Normal Structure and Function

The alimentary tract caudal to the stomach is divided into the small and large intestines, which differ in function and in diameter of their lumen. In the dog and cat, the anatomic difference is small. The intestinal tract is designed primarily as an area for the digestion and absorption of food. Important motility functions aid in digestion and absorption processes and in moving the contents aborally. Integration of gastrointestinal functions is mediated by hormones and the nervous system.

The intestines contain the most complex ecosystem in the body, with a bacterial microflora consisting of many different members. The intestine possesses an immune system to protect the animal against invasion by bacterial opportunists or pathogens and against the absorption of antigenic substances.

Within the intestinal tract, function differs between the small and large intestines. The small intestine is concerned primarily with the absorption of nutrients and with continuously moving its contents in an aboral direction. The large intestine serves as a reservoir, holding its contents for longer periods, and it absorbs primarily fluids and electrolytes. Within the small intestine, function is regionalized further, as with the special ileal mechanisms for bile acid and cyanocobalamin absorption.

GROSS STRUCTURE[1-3]

Small Intestine (Figure 15-1)

The small intestine is divided arbitrarily into the duodenum, jejunum, and ileum. No definite anatomic dissimilarity permits a differentiation of one segment from another; the definite functional differences are not translated into differences in gross structure. The small intestine is 1.80 to 4.80 meters long in the dog and about 1.30 meters long in the cat.

The duodenum is the most cranial part of the small intestine. Beginning at the pylorus, it constitutes about 10% of the length of the entire small bowel. The first part begins at the right of the median plane and passes dorsally and to the right at the level of the ninth intercostal space. The duodenum is immobilized at this site by the hepatoduodenal ligament, connecting it to the liver, and by the mesentery containing the pancreas, to which it is closely related. The duodenum turns caudally at the cranial flexure and becomes the descending duodenum, which lies against the right dorsolateral abdominal wall and is not covered by the greater omentum. It is also related to the ventral caudal aspects of the right kidney. At the level of the fifth and sixth lumbar vertebrae, the duodenum forms the caudal flexure, which consists of the organ moving from right to left around the cecum and root of the mesentery. From this point forward, the duodenum passes as an ascending segment that lies between the cecum, ascending colon, and root of the mesentery, on the right, and the descending colon and left kidney, on the left. There are mesenteric attachments between the ascending duodenum and the colon in the duodenocolic fold. The transition from duodenum to jejunum occurs at the duodenojejunal flexure, located to the left of the root of the mesentery, from which the jejunum passes ventrally and caudally.

The jejunum and ileum account for approximately 90% of the total length of the small intestine. The jejunum is not fixed other than by long mesentery that contains vessels and nerves supplying the intestine. Thus, the jejunum is distributed throughout the abdominal cavity. It is displaced dorsally and to the right when the stomach becomes distended. The ventral and lateral surfaces of the jejunal mass are covered by omentum. The jejunum can be palpated throughout its length. Accomplishing that with some deep-chested breeds depends on elevating the cranial part of the animal. The ileum, the most caudal part of the small intestine, is the segment connected to the cecum by the ileocecal fold, supplied by vessels that pass to it from the cecum and colon. The ileum enters the proximal end of the ascending colon at the ileal orifice, located at the level of the first or second lumbar vertebra. A distinct anatomic sphincter is found, the ileocecal sphincter.

Large Intestine (Figures 15-1, 15-2)

The large intestine is relatively short in the dog and cat since its only purposes are to absorb salt and water and to serve as a reservoir, in contrast to the large colon of herbivores, required to digest and absorb polysaccharides. Together, the large intestine and rectum are 10% to 20% as long as the small intestine, amounting to 0.2 to 0.6 meter in the dog and 0.2 meter in the cat.

The cecum is 0.08 to 0.3 meter long in the dog and 0.02 to 0.04 meter long in the cat. The cecum is associated with the ileum and ascending colon and is related to the second to fourth lumbar vertebrae on the right side of the median plane. The cecum is related also to the ventral surface of the right kidney and the descending duodenum, which contains the pancreas in its mesentery.

The large intestine begins as a short segment designated as the ascending colon. It has the same spatial arrangement as the

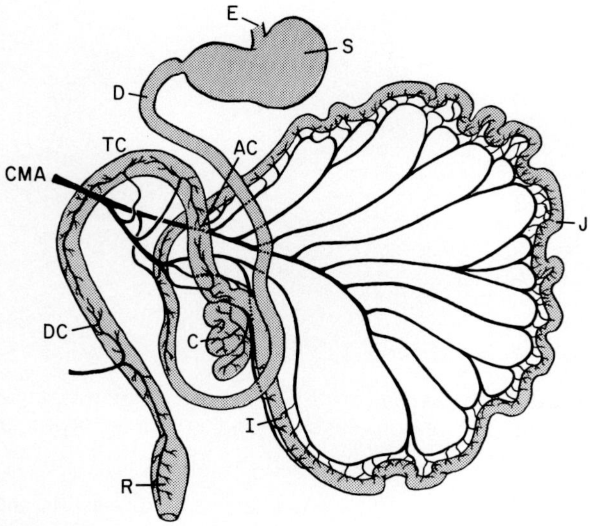

Figure 15-1. Anatomy of the small and large intestine. AC = ascending colon, C = cecum, CMA = cranial mesenteric artery, DC = descending colon, E = esophagus, I = ileum, J = jejunum, R = rectum, S = stomach, TC = transverse colon.

cecum. The next aborad part is a short segment of transverse colon. It exists as a flexure connecting the ascending colon to the most terminal part, the descending colon. The transverse colon passes around the root of the mesentery, caudally adjacent to the stomach, and from right to left at the level of the twelfth thoracic vertebra. The descending colon extends to the pelvic inlet, where the rectum begins. It lies to the left of the median plane and is related to the ascending duodenum by connections through the duodenocolic fold. The large intestine is palpable on physical examination. The cranial parts may not be reached in deep chested breeds.

Blood Supply and Lymphatics

The major blood supply to the small intestine is provided through the cranial mesenteric artery. The cranial part of the duodenum is supplied by branches of the celiac artery. Blood flow to the large intestine is via both the cranial and caudal mesenteric vessels. Mesenteric vessels to the small intestine form anastomosing arcades. If blood flow in a set of mesenteric vessels is obstructed, there is collateral flow through the vessels anastomosing with adjacent segments so that the tissue can survive.[4] Venous flow from the intestines is into the portal vein.

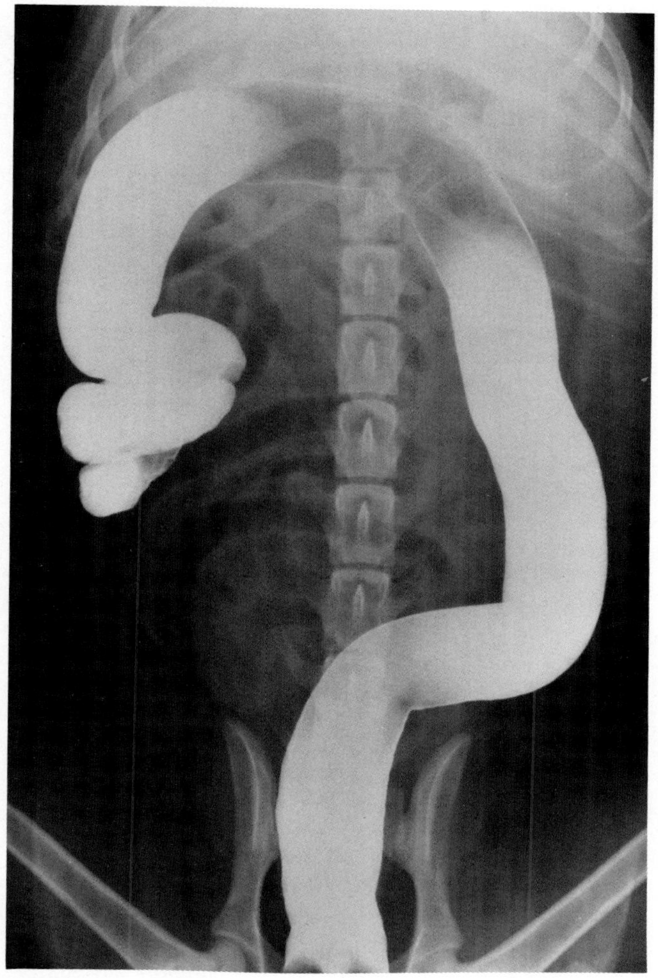

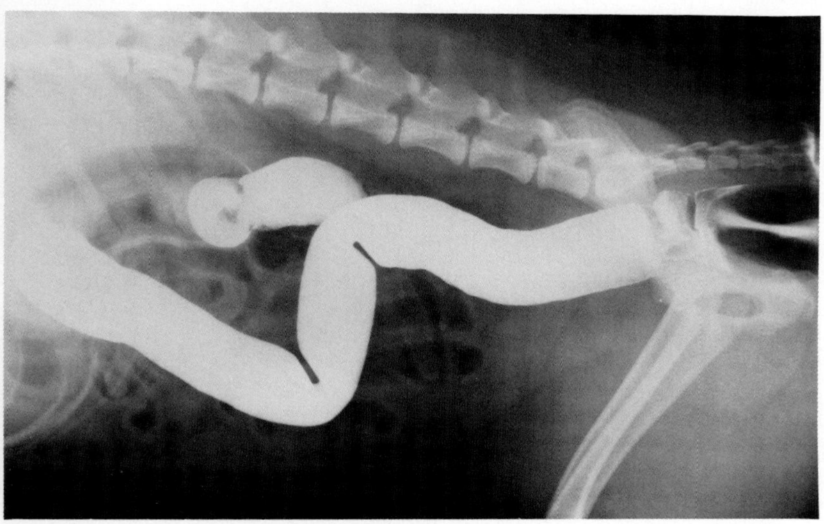

Figure 15-2a. Lateral and dorsoventral radiographs of a normal colon in a one-year-old Cocker Spaniel after a barium enema. The bowel was well prepared, since no filling defects are seen. Gas in the transverse colon will move with positioning. The lateral view shows a stricture in the caudal colon, a response due to the end of the enema tube. The cecum is filled and excess pressure is not exerted, so that no contrast has entered the small intestine. The location of the colon is normal, and the tendency toward a redundant colon is great.

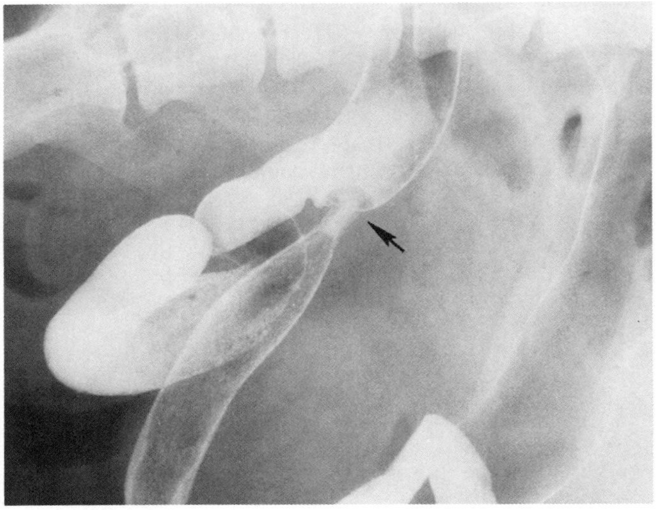

Figure 15-2b. Lateral radiograph of a dog following a barium enema, showing a normal ileocecal valve.

Lymphatic drainage is through one of the large number of lymph nodes that are scattered throughout the mesentery that contains the intestine.

Innervation

The efferent nerves to the intestines are parasympathetic and sympathetic fibers of the autonomic nervous system. The parasympathetics are important for regulation of normal function. The vagus supplies these fibers to the small intestine and to the first part of the large intestine. Parasympathetic fibers to the remainder of the large bowel arise from nuclei in the sacral cord and pass to the organ by way of pelvic nerves. Sympathetics play a minor role in normal intestinal function. They pass to the organ from a number of sympathetic ganglia, scattered throughout the abdominal cavity, that receive fibers from the paravertebral sympathetic trunk.

Function in the intestines depends on the reception and transmission of information regarding intraluminal events in the gut. Afferent fibers in both parasympathetic and sympathetic nerve trunks relay that information to central or peripheral synapses for evocation of the reflexes.

MICROSCOPIC STRUCTURE[5,6]

Small Intestine

The intestines are similar to the esophagus and stomach in possessing mucosal, submucosal, and muscle layers (Figure 15-3). The mucosal layer, involved with secretory and absorptive functions, provides a barrier between the outside environment and the interior of the body. A submucosal layer, interposed between the mucosal and muscularis layers, provides support and contains blood vessels, lymphatics, and nerves. The outer muscular layers provide motility to intestinal contents at a slow rate in the aborad direction.

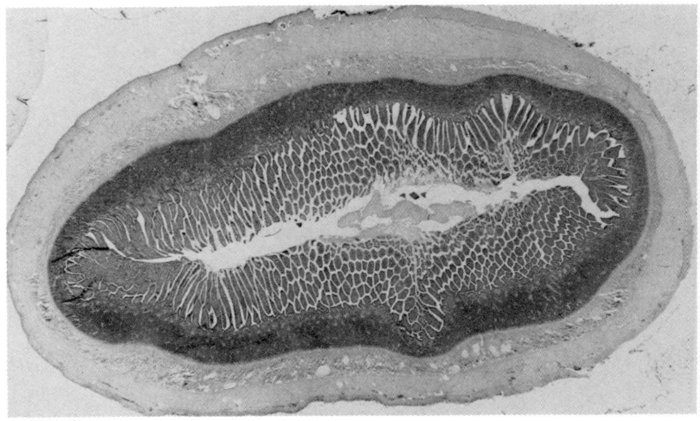

Figure 15-3. Cross-section of the small intestine, showing inner layers of mucosa and submucosa and two outer layers of smooth muscle.

Mucosa. The intestinal mucosa consists of a single layer of cells overlying a layer of loose connective tissue, vessels, and nerves. The structures beneath the surface cells form the lamina propria. The mucosa is thrown up into folds as illustrated in Figure 15-4. The surface mucosal cells are primarily epithelial cells, with a number of mucus-secreting goblet cells scattered throughout. Occasional argentaffin or enterochromaffin cells (endocrine-secreting) are found in the basal part of the epithelium

Epithelial Cell. The epithelial cells of the intestinal mucosa are basically the same in fine structure as the transporting epithelial cells of the tubules in the kidney, salivary ducts, and gallbladder. The luminal surface consists of a brush border made up of numerous microvilli (Figure 15-5). The surface of the brush border is covered with a polysaccharide, glycocalyx, synthesized by the cell and secreted onto its surface. The function of this carbohydrate layer is not known. It may function similarly to an ion exchange resin by attracting and concentrating substances at the cell surface in order to facilitate absorption. The glycocalyx may also trap and retain brush-border enzymes to enable digestion at the site of absorption on

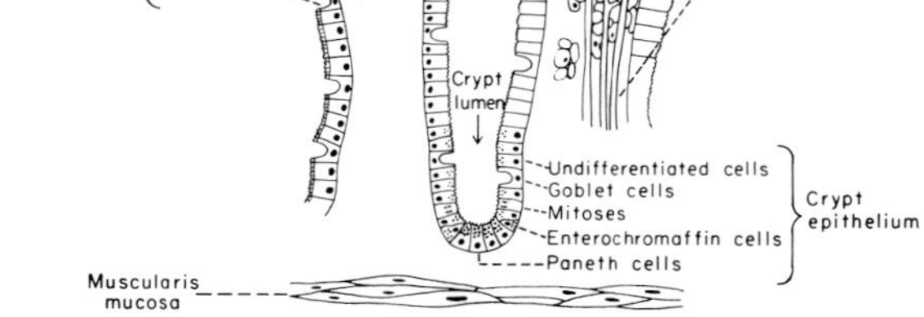

Figure 15-4a. Schematic diagram of two sectioned villi and a crypt to illustrate the histological organization of the small intestinal mucosa. By permission Trier, J.S., Handbook of Physiology, Sec. 6. Vol. III, Chap. 63, p. 1127.

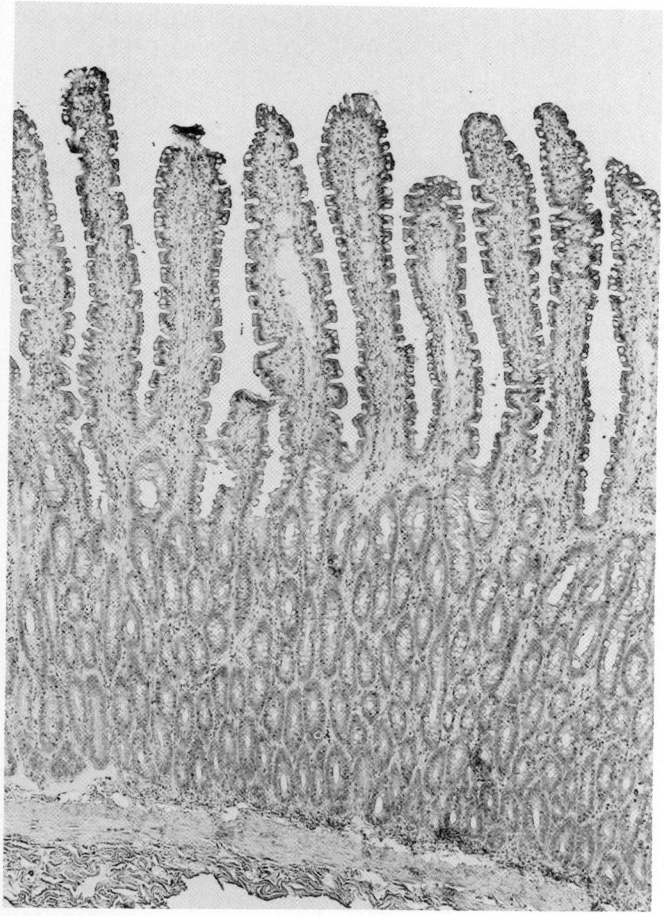

Figure 15-4b. Photomicrograph of canine jejunum

the cell surface. The glycocalyx may also protect the cell. Loss of the glycocalyx during bowel ischemia increases susceptibility of cells to destruction by proteases within the lumen.

The microvilli increase the area of mucosa available for digestion and absorption. Microvillous membranes possess

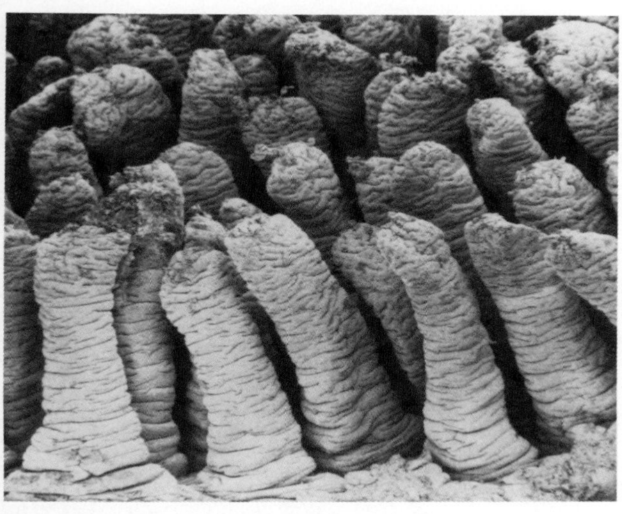

Figure 15-4c. Scanning electron micrograph of canine jejunum X 65.

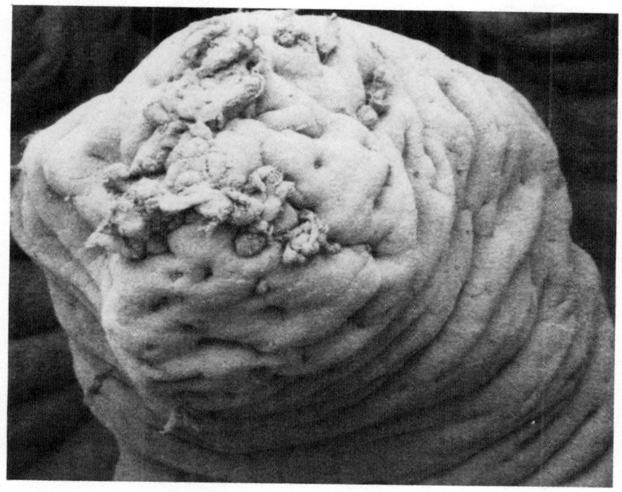

Figure 15-4d. Scanning electron micrograph of canine jejunum X 530. Mucous or goblet cells can be identified either as rounded protuberances if they contain numerous mucigen droplets, or a small depression if they have discharged their mucus. Debris at the very tip of the villus probably represents cells being shed into the lumen of the intestine.

special mechanisms for transporting monosaccharides and amino acids. They are also capable of absorbing material by pinocytosis. The brush border contains enzymes to digest disaccharides, oligosaccharides, and some small peptides. These enzymes exert most of their activity while remaining on the brush border or, at least, within the environment of the glycocalyx. Although electron micrographs do not make it apparent, the microvilli form a dynamic structure that is constantly changing morphologically in the living cell.

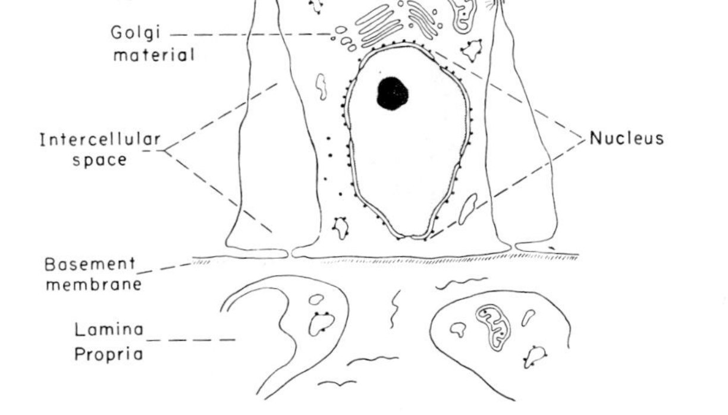

Figure 15-5a. Schematic diagram of an intestinal absorptive cell. By permission Trier, J.S., Handbook of Physiology Sec. 6, Vol III, Chap. 63, p. 1133.

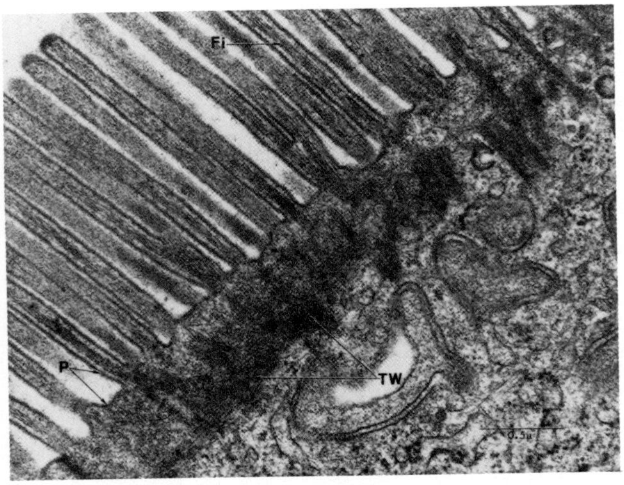

Figure 15-5b. Electron micrograph of canine duodenal epithelial cell showing microvilli. Fi = filaments of microvillus. TW = terminal web. P = plasmalemma X 25,700.

The epithelial cell is concerned also with the absorption and secretion of electrolytes and water. Sodium transport is more important than the transport of other electrolytes and is thought to involve membrane ATPase, an enzyme that histochemistry has shown to be located on cell membranes. Adenylate cyclase, an enzyme that generates the nucleotide cyclic AMP, is thought to be involved in secretion of fluid by the epithelial cell. This enzyme is found primarily on the membranes of the lateral and basal cell surfaces.

The brush border also contains proteins that bind a variety of substances to be absorbed, such as calcium, iron, and vitamin B_{12}.

All epithelial surface membranes are semipermeable, permitting diffusion of small monovalent ions. The surface area of cell membranes is mostly lipid, which permits lipid-soluble substances to diffuse across the membrane.

Intracellular design of the epithelial cell reflects its functions. Below the brush border a mesh of filaments forms the terminal web, with the function of providing skeletal support for the cell. The epithelial cell does not synthesize protein for export. Consequently, the structure that synthesizes protein, the rough endoplasmic reticulum, is found only in amounts necessary to meet the cell's own needs. The golgi apparatus is not well developed, since there is little need for the packaging of substances for export. Intracellular transport of nutrients is important, however, and is accomplished by an extensive system of canals provided by the smooth endoplasmic reticulum. Many mitochondria are found to provide the energy required for transport processes. Mitochondria are found most abundantly in the epithelial cells that have the major function of absorbing or secreting electrolytes and water. Intestinal epithelial cells possess many lysosomes, which contain large numbers of enzymes able to degrade the many substances absorbed. Lysosomes fuse with vesicles containing material absorbed by pinocytosis and release enzymes into a common vesicle known as a phagolysosome. A protective function of the cell is the degradation of foreign material to prevent it from making its way into the body.

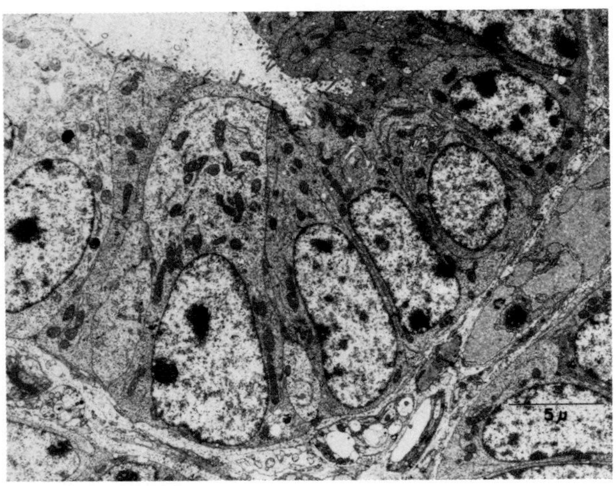

Figure 15-5c. Electron micrograph of canine duodenal epithelium X 2550.

Goblet Cells. Surface mucosal cells that secrete mucus are called goblet cells. They are interspersed between epithelial cells, increasing in relative numbers distally in the intestinal tract. The luminal border of the goblet cell contains few microvilli. The appearance of the cell is marked by engorgement with mucin, packaged in granules ready for release. The rough endoplasmic reticulum and the golgi apparatus are well-developed in order to synthesize and package mucin for export. Since energy needs are not great, few mitochondria are found.

Immature Crypt Cells. The epithelial cells on the villi differ from those in the crypts of Lieberkuhn. Cells of the villi are fully differentiated, so that they synthesize and secrete enzymes and perform absorptive functions. Mature villous cells develop from immature ones in the crypts by moving up the side of the villous in a sheet. During migration, the cells mature and acquire the highly developed function of the villous cell. Migration requires about two days. The cells are fully mature when the migration is one third to one-half completed. Cells in the crypts are morphologically immature. They have undeveloped brush borders, and the intracellular appearance resembles that of secretory cells more than absorptive cells. Secretion of intestinal fluid may be a normal function of crypt cells. The primary function of crypt cells is to replenish mature villus epithelial cells.

Endocrine-Paracrine-Secreting Cells.[7] Amine-precursor-uptake decarboxylase (APUD) and peptide-hormone-producing cells are found in the mucosal surface layer, interspersed between epithelial cells. As many as 15 types of endocrine-parocrine cells have been identified in the gastrointestinal tract. Most produce active peptides and some also biogenic amines. APUD cells synthesize and secrete biogenic amines (e.g., serotonin) and biologically active peptides (e.g., vasoactive intestinal peptide). The argentaffin cell is an APUD cell containing biogenic amines stored in abundance in secretory granules. APUD cells have a broad base that borders on the basement membrane and an apex that may not reach and border on the intestinal lumen. Thus, the cell is designed to secrete a product into the circulation rather than into the lumen of the gut. The peptide endocrines produced in many different cells were isolated and characterized before it was determined where they are produced. Some are true endocrine hormones released to the circulation, which carries the hormone to its target organ. Others, such as somatostatin, are paracrines; the hormone is

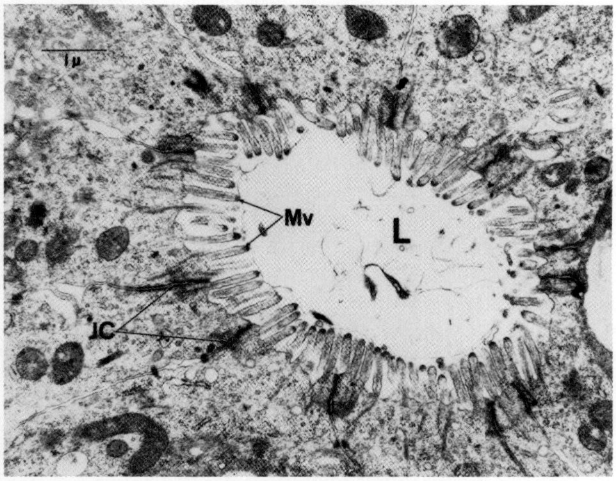

Figure 15-6. Electron micrograph of intestinal epithelial cells, showing the so-called tight junctions, which are in fact quite leaky to the movement of water and monovalent ions. L = lumen of intestinal gland, Mv = microvilli, JC = junctional complex. X 8770.

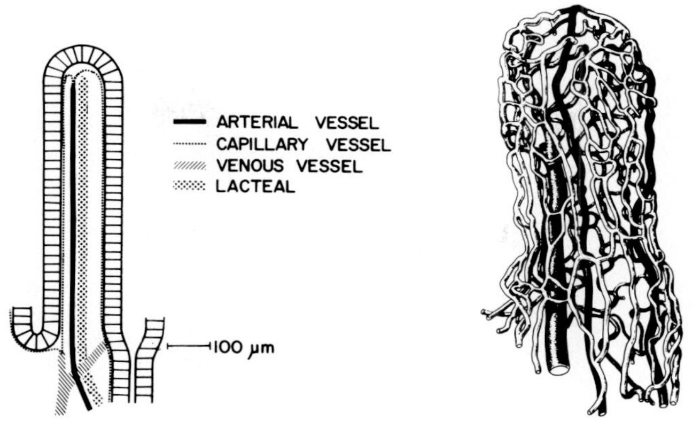

Figure 15-7. Schematic drawing of vascular network of villus. Arterial vessel (black) runs unbranched to tip of villus, where it arborizes into a capillary network that drains into a venous vessel (gray). By permission, D. Lundgren, Gut 15:1005, 1974.

released to act locally on an adjacent cell. The secretions of all the endo-paracrine cells are important in integrating functions within the alimentary canal.

Intercellular Association (Figure 15-6). The mucosal surface epithelium is remarkably competent in preventing particulate matter and large molecules from penetrating into the body from the gut. The mucosa is a semipermeable barrier to the movement of electrolytes. It prevents the loss of extracellular fluid into the lumen of the gut and regulates the rate of absorption of fluid from the gut. The semipermeable membrane consists of both the brush border and junctions between cells. These latter intercellular connections have been called tight junctions since, morphologically, they appear to form a tight barrier to the movement of fluid and ions. These junctions are not tight, however; they actually form the most permeable area of the mucosal surface. Thus, passive diffusional fluxes of ions and water across the mucosa are greatest through the so-called tight junctions.

The lateral basal-cell membranes transport sodium from inside the cell to the lateral intercellular space. Water follows osmotically, markedly dilating the space during active sodium transport. Hydrostatic pressure increases in the space, and fluid leaves, following pressure gradients. By this means fluid is transported from the lumen of the gut into the circulation. The leaky tight junctions permit diffusion of fluid from the dilated intercellular space back into the intestinal lumen. The junctions are less leaky in the ileum and large intestine, making absorption of fluid more efficient there, since there is less back-diffusion.

Basement Membrane. The basement membrane is a glycoprotein on which the mucosal cells abut. Although its morphological appearance does not support it, the basement membrane is readily permeable to the movement of macromolecules and some blood cells.

Mucosal Circulation.[8,9] Blood flow to the villus is provided by an arteriole that passes through the lamina propria to the end of the villus (Figure 15-7). It runs unbranched to the villus tip, where it arborizes, producing a fountain of vessels that form a dense subepithelial capillary network. Drainage from the capillaries is by veins that begin in the upper part of the villus in the dog and the lower part in the cat. The crypt epithelial cells are supplied by arterial vessels that are separate from those entering the villi. Control over the vascular beds is different in the two different regions, and blood flow can be increased selectively in one while decreased in the other. Capillaries in the intestinal lamina propria have many large fenestrations.[10] These pores enable a considerable amount of plasma proteins to move from the vessels into the interstitial space. This results in a serum albumin space that is three times that in most tissues of the body. That may be important in some abnormal situations that produce a diarrhea.[11] It also illustrates how a protein-losing enteropathy can easily occur when the one-cell epithelial barrier is defective. Fluid lost from the interstitium of the intestine is richer in plasma proteins than fluid from other tissues.

A lymphatic vessel, the lacteal, is situated in the lamina propria in the center of the villus. This is the avenue for absorption of most of the triglycerides, which are transported from the gut as chylomicrons.

Renewal of Mucosal Surface.[12-14] Mucosal epithelial cells normally desquamate from the tips of the villi and are replaced by cells migrating from the crypt cells. The number of cells on any one villus is determined by the rate of production of new cells and the rate of loss of mature cells. The rate of cell division is controlled by humoral factors.[15,16] Excessive amounts of any hormone with trophic effects, such as gastrin produce mucosal hyperplasia. The trophic effects depend on permissive effects of adrenal corticosteroids and possibly other hormones.

A number of factors cause cell turnover to increase and can lead to mucosal atrophy. Physical or chemical trauma increases cell loss; normal bacterial microflora cut the average cell life to half of what it would be if no microorganisms were present. Increased bacterial numbers cause villus atrophy. Protozoal infection increases epithelial cell turnover.[17] Dietary changes and changes in the composition of the microflora can speed mucosal cell loss. Drugs that interfere with cell division or the cells' metabolic functions prevent normal cell renewal, and the mucosa atrophies. Anticancer drugs and some antibiotics can have an antimetabolic effect. Since vitamin B_{12} and folic acid

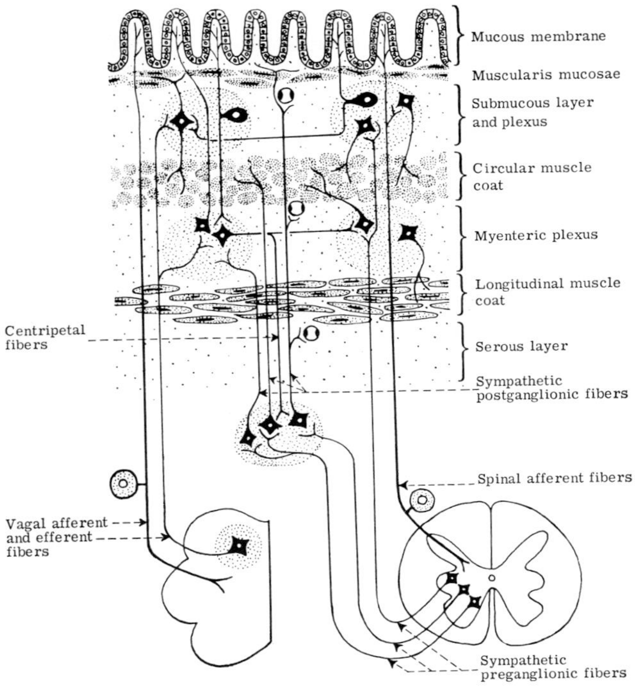

Figure 15-8. Schematic of extrinsic and intrinsic nerve fibers in the enteric plexus. (From Schofield, G.C., Handbook of Physiology Sec. 6, Vol. IV, Chap. 80, p. 1611. 1968. By permission).

are essential for cell renewal, a deficiency of either results in mucosal atrophy.

The balance between rates of renewal and loss determines villus size. Growth exceeding loss causes villus hypertrophy. When rate of loss exceeds growth, the villi atrophy. The migration time of crypt cells is considerably shorter when the villi are atrophied, which suggests that the villous cells are not completely mature.

Submucosa. The submucosa is separated from the mucosa by the muscularis mucosa. The submucosa contains blood vessels, lymphatics, and nerves in a loosely arranged bed of connective tissue. The submucosa also contains glands, although in the cat and dog the glands are restricted to the first few centimeters of the duodenum. The Brunner's glands are characterized by acini of cuboidal mucus-secreting cells that produce an alkaline watery mucoid fluid.

Muscularis.[18,19] The wall of the intestine contains an outer thinner layer of longitudinal smooth muscle and a thicker inner layer of circular muscle. The intestinal smooth muscle is similar in structure to that found elsewhere in the body. The muscle cells appear different from skeletal muscle cells since no myosin filaments are seen, even though myosin is present. The actin filaments are probably linked in series by aggregates of myosin that connect their ends. The smooth muscle cells have a definite sarcolemma, and there is intercellular continuity between the elements of adjacent cells. Intestinal smooth muscle has the property of propagating electrical activity through a number of its cells. Cell-to-cell transmission of this activity occurs through the nexus, which is a region of fusion of plasma membranes. This allows the layers of smooth muscle to function as a syncytium.

Neural Plexuses.[18,19] Neural control of intestinal function is mediated via nerves that synapse in a number of different ganglia in the wall of the intestine (Figure 15-8). The ganglia, with their afferent fibers, are organized into plexuses. One such center is located in the subserous plexus at the attachment of the mesentery. It is a point of transmission between the mesenteric nerve bundles and the plexuses that lie deep within the intestinal wall. The myenteric plexus, one of the internal plexuses, is located between the circular and longitudinal muscle layers. Another group of neural ganglia are found in the submucous plexuses scattered throughout the submucosa. Extensions of the submucous plexuses into the mucosa have been termed mucosal plexuses. There are communicating fibers between ganglia in the same layer of intestine and between those at different levels. Most of the fibers to and from the plexuses are afferents and parasympathetics. Some sympathetic fibers synapse on the ganglia and modulate neural activity.

Colonic Microscopic Structure

The surface of the mucosa of the colon is flat and contains no villi (Figure 15-9). Straight tubular glands extend from the surface through the entire thickness of the mucosa, reaching the muscularis mucosa. These glands, called crypts of Lieberkuhn, contain both mucous and epithelial cells near the surface and primarily mucous cells in the deepest parts of the gland. The surface is lined with mostly epithelial cells. Crypt cells multiply and differentiate as they migrate up the gland walls to replace surface epithelial cells. The tubular glands are packed close together, leaving room for only a minimal amount of lamina propria. The remainder of the wall of the colon is histologically similar to the wall of the small intestine.

FUNCTION

Motility,[20-23] Small Intestine

The small intestine contains smooth muscle that performs two basic functions. It mixes and slows the passage of contents through the tube, thus ensuring completeness of digestion and absorption. It functions also to move contents continuously in the aborad direction. The type of motility that slows the movement is rhythmic segmentation. This type of motility contributes to resistance in the intestinal conduit. The other type of motility, functioning to move the contents in the aborad direction, is called peristalsis. Several other types of movement have been described, such as pendulous movements and peristaltic rushes. Such phenomena result when the balance between segmentation and peristalsis is altered so that the contents move rapidly through more than a few centimeters of intestine. The movement of contents through the small intestine is thus the net effect of the braking action of segmentation and the accelerator effect of peristalsis. The mixing of intestinal contents is a function of both segmentation and longitudinal contractions.2[4]

Rhythmic Segmentation.[20,25] Rhythmic segmentation is a type of intestinal motility characterized by random contractions of the circular muscles. This motility is minimal when the intestine is empty, yet is able to maintain pressures 6mm Hg above atmosphere.[26] The strength of the contraction increases when stimulated by distention from food entering the intestine. The increase in activity is mediated by reflexes that have

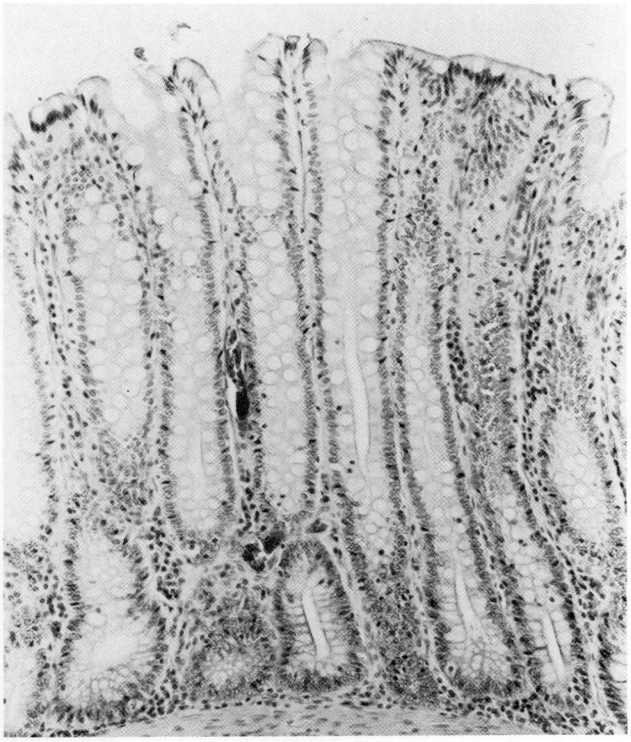

Figure 15-9a. Photomicrograph of normal canine colon.

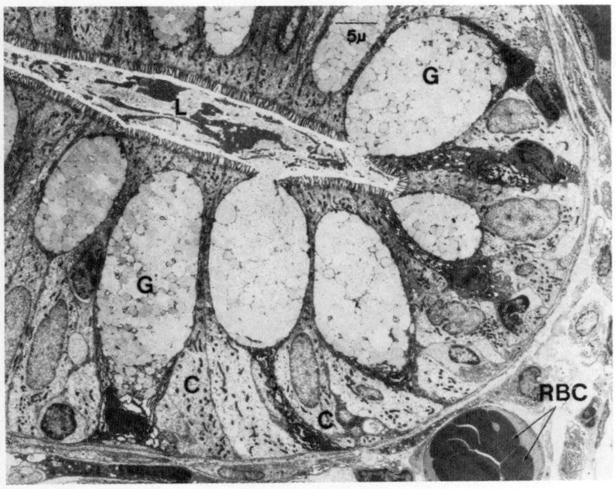

Figure 15-9b. Electron micrograph of normal canine colon. L = lumen of intestinal gland. G = goblet or mucus cell, C = columnar cell. X 1088.

pathways through the intrinsic plexuses (Figure 15-8). The locally initiated increased motility is augmented by incoming vagal-nerve activity that increases during the feeding state. Rhythmic segmentation performs two functions. One is to mix food with digestive enzymes and to bring nutrients into contact with mucosal absorptive surfaces. The other function is to increase resistance to the passage of nutrients through the intestine, giving digestion and absorption processes time for completion. The unstimulated intestine is a flaccid tube that offers little resistance to the flow of liquid contents through its lumen. Resistance to flow is increased by reducing the lumen of the tube, as illustrated in Figure 15-10. Thus, an intestine with strong contractions of rhythmic segmentation is one with considerable motility (hypermotile), while the flaccid bowel has little motility (hypomotile). The rate of the muscle contractions that produce rhythmic segmentation, fairly constant for each level in the small intestine, is determined by electrical-control activity, a basic property of muscle in the longitudinal layer. The rate is higher in the duodenum (18 to 19 contractions per minute) than in the ileum (8 to 10 per minute). Thus, motor activity decreases in the aborad direction.

The level of excitability, produced by activity over nerves to the muscles or by hormones determines the strength of these contractions. In general, animals with diarrhea have a decrease in the strength of normal segmentation, so that the bowel is in a flaccid (hypomotile) state, offering little resistance to the flow of contents through it. The rate of contractions, however, is not markedly affected.

Peristalsis.[20,21,25] Peristalsis is the second important type of motility. A peristaltic wave can be described as a ring of constriction that moves aborad over a short segment of intestine. In each very short section of intestine, peristaltic waves develop at the same frequency as rhythmic segmentation contractions, both rates being determined by the electrical-control activity. Therefore, the rate of generation of peristaltic waves is different in each level of the intestinal tract. The rate of development of peristaltic waves is greatest in the duodenum, and the decreasing rate in the aborad segments is responsible for the movement of the contents in the proper direction. Each wave is about 5 cm long in the duodenum and becomes shorter in the caudal small intestine. The length of each wave is determined by the length of intestine that has the same frequency of electrical-control activity.

Propulsive activity is found during both fed and unfed

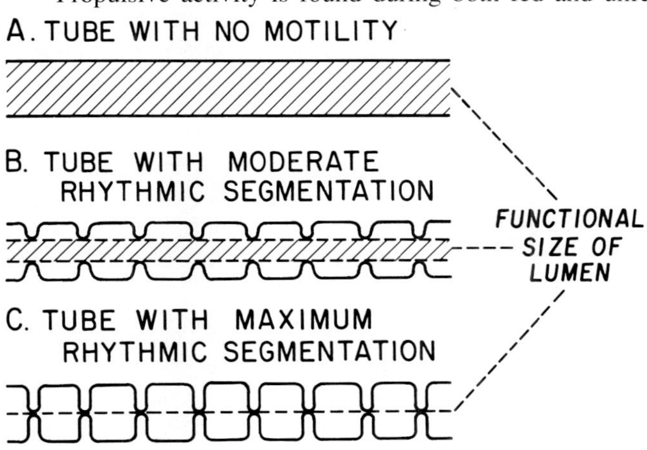

Figure 15-10. Schematic of intestine with varying degrees of resistance to flow of chyme. Rate of peristaltic flow in intestine is determined by resistance in tube. Flow is directly proportional to radius of tube:

$$\frac{\Delta P \pi r^4}{8Ln}$$

Resistance is inversely related to radius of tube:

$$R = \frac{\Delta P}{F} = \frac{8Ln}{\pi r^4}$$

Resistance to flow is produced by rhythmic segmentation stimulated by food, distending the intestine.

states. In the unfed state propulsive activity is periodic with intervals of no activity lasting an hour between propulsive waves. The peristaltic waves during unfed states constitute the interdigestive migrating motility complex (IDMC), which provides the interdigestive housekeeping activity for keeping the intestine cleared of bacteria and debris. Myoelectrical measurements show three different patterns that correspond to a phase I of no motility, a phase II of propulsive activity that is similar to peristaltic waves seen with feeding, and a phase III of maximum propulsive activity when the housekeeping function is operating. At any point in the intestine the hour of phase I inactivity is followed by first 15 to 40 minutes of phase II activity and then 4 to 8 minutes of phase III intense contractile activity. The interval between each cycle and the time for migration from the upper to lower small bowel is two to three hours. The IDMC cycle of activity is disrupted by feeding.

The migrating motility complex (MMC) changes from the cyclic pattern seen with the IDMC to the fed pattern of phase II contractions after consumption of a meal. The physical and chemical composition of the food determines the length of time before the IDMC pattern returns. Dogs fed milk develop the fed pattern for 2.5 to 4 hours. The type of nutrient is important in that isocaloric amounts of peptides, glucose, and medium-chain triglycerides cause fed patterns of 2.8, 4.8, and 7.5 hours, respectively. It is evident that propulsion of intestinal contents by the MMC is well regulated by events in the intestinal lumen. Propulsion is augmented both by food's stimulating a local reflex and by extrinsic nerve-fiber activity in the vagi. When segmentation and resistance to flow are reduced in the flaccid intestine, very little peristaltic activity is needed to propel liquid contents over a long span with relative ease. In animals with diarrhea, the rate of peristaltic activity need not be increased to contribute to the problem. A number of problems can induce frequent MMC, however, and that contributes to diarrhea. Intestinal parasites, intestinal bacterial overgrowth, bacterial infection, and ricinoleic acid stimulate MMC that can propel fluid rapidly through the unfed intestine.

Regulation of Motility[21,25]

Slow Wave or Electrical-control Activity. The frequency of rhythmic segmentation contractions and peristaltic waves is determined by the slow wave, electrical-control activity, or basic electrical rhythm, which is a property of the smooth muscle that has been stripped of all its nerves (Chapter 1). Slow waves are influenced by hormones, neural activity, feeding, and disease states. In the small intestine, however, hormones and neural activity have little effect on this activity. The generation of intestinal slow waves is not well understood but is most likely the result of membrane properties and changes in intracellular and extracellular electrolytes. Slow wave activity is known to be sensitive to low extracellular potassium levels,[27] and loss of normal intestinal motility is often associated with hypokalemia. In these cases, normal intestinal motility is not regained until potassium deficits are corrected. Slow wave activity also disappears during vomiting when retrograde intestinal contractions are seen.

Electrical-Response Activity. Slow wave activity governs the rate of the muscle contraction that causes segmentation or peristaltic movement; it does not initiate the contraction. Stimulation of the intestinal smooth muscle to contract comes from the electrical-response activity or spike potentials, which are generated by a number of different means. This activity is initiated by stimuli that arise from within the intestine or from without, such as by distention of the intestine with food and by psychic stimuli generated during the feeding process. The afferent impulses are carried to synapses in the intrinsic plexuses of the control nuclei of the vagus, where they initiate the stimulus for electrical response activity. In addition to activity in the extrinsic and intrinsic nerves, electrical-response activity is stimulated by hormones. The strength of smooth-muscle contractions is variable, being determined by the amount of neural or humoral stimulation. Thus, the rate of muscular contraction is normally constant and predetermined, whereas the strength of contractions in segmentation and peristalsis is variable, modulated by neural and humoral controls. Both contractions are phasic because they are determined by slow wave activity, which is phasic. Propagated waves of contraction only occur over short distances; then timing and velocity of propagation are determined by the slow wave in any segment of intestine.

Cholinergic Controls.[21] The intrinsic nervous system mediates stimulation of spike potentials. The release of acetylcholine at the ganglionic synapse and motor end plate stimulates motility, as shown in Figure 15-11. Following release, acetylcholine binds to muscarinic cholinergic receptors on the muscle. Muscle contraction is blocked by atropine, which also binds to the receptors. Nicotinic cholinergic receptors are found in the ganglia and in the muscle end plate. High levels of nicotine and hexamethonium block acetylcholine's effect at these sites. Parasympathetic fibers in the vagus and pelvic nerves mediate release of acetylcholine.

Adrenergic Control.[21,28] Adrenergic nerve activity stimulates release of a second type of neurotransmitter to alter intestinal motility. Alpha-adrenergic receptors are found on the post-ganglionic nerves of the myenteric plexus. The stimulation of adrenergic fibers to release norepinephrine inhibits activity in the cholinergic fibers to which it binds, thus inhibiting intestinal motility. Stimulation of vagal adrenergic fibers inhibits intestinal motility. Beta-adrenergic receptors are also found on intestinal smooth-muscle cells. Epinephrine acting on these sites inhibits intestinal motility. The adrenergic receptors do not play a role in the normal motor functions of the intestine.

Serotonergic Control.[20,21] Receptors for serotonin are found on intestinal smooth-muscle cells and on the intrinsic

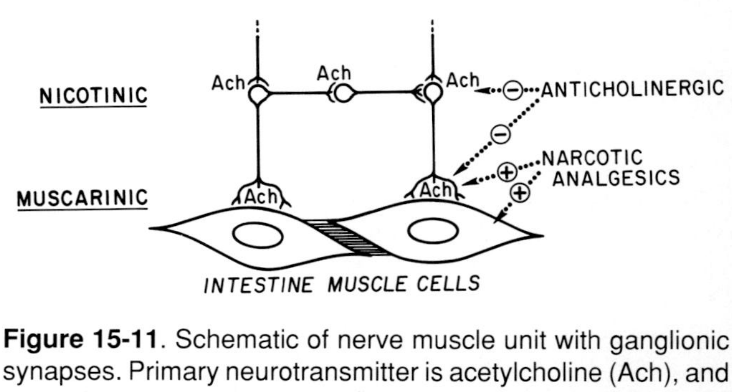

Figure 15-11. Schematic of nerve muscle unit with ganglionic synapses. Primary neurotransmitter is acetylcholine (Ach), and transmission is blocked (-) by anticholinergics. Two types of receptors are found, nicotinic and muscarinic. Narcotic analgesics stimulate smooth-muscle contraction by acting at the synapse and directly on the muscle.

nerves. This biogenic amine is thought to be an important neurotransmitter for peristalsis. Infusion of serotonin produces an initial tonic contraction of intestinal smooth muscle, followed by phasic contraction.[29] Serotonin is released from the intestine during stimulation by distention, which suggests that it plays a physiologic role. Large amounts of serotonin are released from some carcinoid tumors, causing diarrhea as a major clinical sign.[30] Inhibition of serotonin synthesis inhibits the diarrhea, suggesting that serotonin is a neurotransmitter for peristalsis. Serotonin also affects absorption and secretion of fluid in the intestine, however, which may be the basis for the diarrhea. There is no evidence that antiserotonin drugs reduce peristalsis and would be effective in treating diarrhea.

Control of Motility by Other Humoral Agents. Other chemicals affect smooth-muscle contractility, but it is uncertain whether they play a physiologic role in motor function of the intestines.[31] Some of the gut peptide hormones, such as cholecystokinin, stimulate muscle contraction (Table 1-4). Intestinal smooth muscle possesses receptors for these hormones, and their interaction is thought to be physiologically important. Other chemicals, such as histamine, have an effect on smooth-muscle contraction throughout the body. It has not been shown that histamine is either a neurotransmitter or plays a physiologic role. A number of basic peptides have properties similar to this property of histamine. Prostaglandins have potent effects to stimulate smooth muscle contraction, but it is not known whether they contribute to normal function. The circulating levels of prostaglandins are increased in some diseases with a diarrhea. In addition to their effects on motility, prostaglandins increase blood flow and stimulate the secretion of fluid in the intestine. Thus, it is difficult to determine whether diarrhea is caused by augmented intestinal propulsion or by secretion of intestinal fluid.

Other neurotransmitters are released by neural activity to the intestinal muscles. Some nerve activity is inhibitory, and the fibers are neither cholinergic nor adrenergic. These nerves have been designated as purinergic, and the neurotransmitter may be VIP or a purine metabolite such as ATP.[32] There is also evidence that postganglionic noncholinergic nerves stimulate intestinal contractions.

In summary, it is evident that a great number of chemicals can affect the contractility of intestinal smooth muscle. The most important neurotransmitter for normal function is acetylcholine, for which there are receptors on both neural elements and muscle fibers. The many other chemicals found in the intestine that have effects on smooth muscle function indicate how complex regulation of intestinal motility could be and probably is.

Long Intestinal Reflexes

Local events in the intestinal tract dictate patterns of motility within that region. Events in one part of the alimentary tract also influence motility in other regions, via long intestinal reflexes. The general purpose of these reflexes is to prepare the way for events that will soon follow. The gastrocolic reflex is a long reflex in which receptors in the stomach are stimulated to produce a motor response in the colon. The stimulus is food in the stomach; the response is an increase in the type of colon activity that evacuates the colon. The effect is mediated through a reflex with afferent fibers that synapse in the central nervous system and with efferents in parasympathetic fibers. The intestino-intestinal inhibitory reflex causes a loss of motility when a stimulus is applied to the intestine. The reflex is not readily apparent under normal conditions. Its effect can be mediated by sympathetic fibers that, when stimulated, can cause a loss of motility throughout the entire small intestine. Intrinsic neural pathways are responsible for some of these reflexes.[33] The stimulus can be acute distention of one part such as that produced by an intestinal obstruction. Trauma or extensive manipulation of the intestines during abdominal surgery can also stimulate the reflex. In association with electrolyte changes, this reflex produces the pathologic situation found in paralytic ileus. Experimental stimulation of the reflex by itself does not produce ileus, however.[34] When a segment of intestine loses motility and becomes a flaccid tube, fluid and gas accumulate. Since there are no restrictions to the rapid movement of fluid through hypomotile loops of intestine, diarrhea appears. For intestinal contents to move rapidly through the intestine, the conduit's resistance must decrease. Temporary loss of resistance is required for a peristaltic rush to occur. Thus, segmentation ceases as an essential part of mass peristaltic movements, and this cessation is mediated by long intestinal reflexes.

Small intestinal motility is coordinated after feeding so that solid particles and fluid move at the same rate unless the volume of fluid increases greatly, in which case fluid moves faster.[35] Nonnutrient components of the diet also influence the rate of transit. The addition of fiber in the form of bran, guar gum, or cellulose increases small intestinal transit time by 28%, 51% and 900%, respectively.[36]

Ileocecal Junction[37,38]

A well-defined anatomical sphincter is found surrounding the ileocecal orifice. It is not certain whether the muscles in this structure create a functional sphincter. Experimental studies show that ileal contents are rapidly evacuated into the colon during stimulation of the gastroileal reflex. This reflex, stimulated by food entering the stomach, serves to prepare the way for food that will soon enter the small intestine. It is not known whether this reflex functions to "open" the sphincter. The structure possesses all the requirements for a sphincter in that manometric measurements reveal that intraluminal pressure is higher in the sphincter than in adjacent structures.[39] The sphincteric pressure decreases in response to appropriate stimulation, which, in this case, is distention by contents in the ileum. The pressure in the sphincter increases when intraluminal pressure increases in the colon. Thus, the sphincter opens to allow contents to pass through in the proper direction, and it prevents the reflux of colonic contents into the ileum. Its most important function is to prevent colonic reflux, since that would contaminate the small intestine with a fecal type of bacterial flora.[40] Motility in the ileum is more important in controlling the movement of contents from the ileum to the colon than is the sphincter.[41]

The control of function in the ileocecal sphincter is not clearly understood. In general, increased vagal activity causes the sphincter muscles to contract, and anticholinergics block this response. Paradoxically, stimulation of sympathetics also causes contraction the sphincter. Catecholamines, acting on alpha-adrenergic receptors on muscle cells, appear to mediate the contraction. This action is in contrast to sympathetic effects on intestinal smooth muscle. It is not known how sphincter pressure decreases when the ileum is distended. Noncholinergic, nonadrenergic fibers promoting relaxation of the gastric fundus may similarly control ileocecal sphincter function. The therapeutic use of anticholinergics to treat diarrheas decreases the ability of the sphincter to generate and maintain a high pressure zone and prevent reflux of colonic contents. Drugs that increase motility in the sphincter, such as narcotic analgesics, reduce the possibility of reflux.

Structural and Functional Features of Colon

The structure and functions of the colon are essentially the same as those of the small intestine, with a few exceptions. The colon serves as a reservoir and completes the absorption of fluid and electrolytes. The reservoir function is similar to that of the stomach in that contents are retained and released slowly at the proper time. Food is not retained in the small intestine but is transported at a programmed rate. Although the colon is anatomically more similar to the small intestine, it is physiologically more like the stomach in that they both consist of two functionally distinct regions.

Motility, Colon[42,43]

The types of motor activity are similar in the large and small intestines. Rhythmic segmentation and propulsive movements are found in both. Segmentation retards the passage of and mixes colonic contents so that absorption is completed. The rate of segmentation is determined by the electrical-control or slow-wave activity of the colonic smooth muscle. The rate of slow-wave activity is less than five cycles per minute, consistent with the motor activity of the colon being at the lowest end of the gradient of slow-wave activity.

Three patterns of motility are recognized in the colon. The cranial colon shows antiperistalsis where over a period of two to eight minutes rings of contraction move cephalad rather than caudal at a frequency of contractions of about five per minute. The activity is followed by rest intervals of 10 to 15 minutes. The retrograde peristalsis mixes food and prevents its passage until absorption is complete. Colonic contents can be for relatively long periods of time in the cranial colon. The rings of contraction are equivalent to segmentation, which also retards the movement of contents. The middle of the colon shows coordinated peristalsis where tonic contraction rings move caudal. Colonic contents stimulate the contractions by distention; the contractions slow the passage of contents but also propel the contents toward the rectum. The caudal colon shows strong contractions that move caudally and empty the colon.

Occasionally colonic contents are seen to move rapidly over a relatively long distance; the phenomenon is called mass movements. Before peristalsis can move colonic contents in a mass movement, segmentation must disappear over the segment traversed. With segmentation eliminated, only small forces are needed to propel liquid contents.

Colonic motor functions are determined by slow waves or electrical-control activity. Besides determining the rate of contractions, slow waves are essential for spike potentials to initiate muscle contractions (Chapter 1). In contrast to the situation in the stomach and small intestine, wave activity is generated by the circular rather than the longitudinal muscle layer. Slow waves are generated at a site in a more caudal part of the most proximal one-third of colon. A pacemaker generates slow waves at a frequency of about six cycles per minute. The slow waves move cephalad toward the cranial end of the colon which has a slow wave frequency of 4.5 cycles per minute. Since frequency of slow waves determines the rate of muscle contractions, there is a reversed gradient of motor activity between the ileocecal valve and the colonic pacemaker. The reversed gradient moves contents in the cephalad direction. This type of gradient can be produced experimentally in the small intestine by surgically reversing a small section. This results in a segment of bowel with a functional obstruction, through which the intraluminal contents are not propelled. The reversed gradient exists over the cranial third of the colon. There is virtually no gradient for slow-wave activity over the caudal half except in the most caudal 10%.

The frequency of colonic slow-wave activity is influenced by electrolyte concentrations in interstitial fluid. Hyperkalemia reduces the frequency and amplitude of slow-wave activity. With hypokalemia also, the amplitude is reduced. Cholinergic agonists produce spike bursts on each wave of slow-wave activity. They prolong the duration of its activity but have no effect on its frequency. Serotonin and morphine have similar effects on the first two parameters, but they reduce the frequency.

Most observations on colonic motility are from studies in the cat. Similar studies in the dog show no major differences between the two species. When diarrhea develops as the result of natural disease or is produced by drugs, multiple pacemakers appear in the cranial part of the colon, and the integrated and reversed gradient is lost.

The colon possesses a second type of electrical activity, characterized by a prolonged burst of spikes or electrical-response activity. This is unrelated to the slow wave activity and its regular pattern of intermittent spike potentials. The prolonged bursts of spikes originate in the middle of the colon and progress in the caudal direction, and for this reason have been called the migrating spike burst. This activity is responsible for mass peristaltic movements. Migrating spike bursts are associated with prolonged and powerful contractions of the circular muscle layer.

The patterns of motility in the colon follow the electromyographic activity. The predominant activity in the cranial part is segmentation and retrograde peristalsis. Rings of contraction contribute to resistance in the tube, so that liquid contents entering the colon are unable to pass through rapidly. The retrograde peristalsis contributes to the reservoir function by retaining the contents so that water and electrolyte absorption can be thorough. There is virtually no gradient of electrical control activity in the caudal part of the colon. Segmentation is the dominant form of activity. It moves the contents back and forth over very short distances and slowly moves contents toward the rectum. The migrating spike burst, which is independent of slow-wave activity, stimulates mass movements, which in turn move the colonic contents rapidly over long distances. During mass movements the segmentation contractions disappear in the segment receiving the contents.

Both extracolonic and intracolonic factors regulate colonic motility. The primary intracolonic stimulus for motility in the normal animal is distention by contents entering from the ileum. Distention stimulates segmentation via reflexes mediated through nerves in the intrinsic nervous system, slowing the passage of contents through the colon. With a low-residue diet, the small quantities of bulk entering the colon may be insufficient to stimulate normal segmentation. When that causes diarrhea, fiber added to the diet gives favorable results.

Distention of the colon also stimulates propulsive activity. The amount of undigested matter in the colon determines the degree of distention in the normal state. The amount of residue is optimum in most diets, so that colonic contents are adequately processed before being defecated. Excessive residue, as in some commercial foods, results in more frequent bowel movements. Constipation can be a problem with a normal-residue diet when propulsive activity is insufficient to move colonic contents caudal at the proper rate. Added fiber frequently corrects the problem, with bowel movements returning to normal.

The extrinsic neural and humoral regulation of colonic motility is poorly understood. In general, parasympathetic activity stimulates segmentation motility, while sympathetic activity produces inhibition. Sympathetic denervation increases intraluminal colonic pressure. The primary inhibitory neural pathways are noncholinergic and nonadrenergic with inhibition mediated by a substance such as ATP, VIP or gamma-aminobutyric acid.

Reflexes coordinating colonic motility, especially movement of contents over relatively long distances, can be stimulated in one part of the colon and produce an effect in another. Regulation of the reflexes occur on three levels, via neural activity, through prevertebral ganglia, lumbosacral spinal centers, and centers in the brain. The reflexes through prevertebral ganglia are complicated in that the nerve processes contain a number of peptides and other chemicals that can act as neurotransmitters. They include VIP, enkephalins, substance P, somatostatin, CCK, and bombesin.

The effects of drugs on colonic function are not well understood. Cholinergic agents usually stimulate contraction of the right side of the colon and inhibit the motility in the distal colon, which together evacuate the colon. Anticholinergics have more unpredictable effects on colonic motility. Any depression of motility is slight and brief. Beta-adrenergic drugs inhibit motility. Morphine and prostaglandins stimulate colonic muscle contraction.

In summary, rhythmic segmentation, an important motor function of the colon, is stimulated by local events through the intrinsic nervous system. The extrinsic neural control is primarily inhibitory and is the important mechanism for reducing segmentation activity. It is only after resistance is removed from the colonic conduit that propulsive activity is able to move contents in the caudal direction. These concepts are important to understanding what type of drug to use for treating an animal with diarrhea. No drug should be used that can reduce segmentation motility even further. Thus, if anticholinergics can reduce segmentation, they should not be used. Drugs such as narcotic analgesics increase segmentation.

An old concept holds that diarrhea reflects a hypermotile state and that constipation results from a hypomotile state. Intraluminal pressure measurements of the colon show that just the opposite is true. The colon that possesses no segmentation type of motility is a flaccid tube in which intraluminal pressure is low. As a consequence there is no resistance to rapid flow through its lumen. This flow is, in large part, due to gravity, which is determined by body position. Gravitational effects are reduced when an animal is confined to a hospital cage. The clinician is presented with many chronic diarrheas that are not severe, but are frustrating, since response to cage rest is followed by relapse upon discharge from the hospital; bowel movements are normal in the hospital but become abnormal as soon as normal activity is resumed. Part of the cause for the favorable responses to the cage rest is undoubtedly reduction in the effects of gravity. With a mild food intolerance, cage rest may be the single change in management necessary for full compensation and the production of normal feces. With strong segmentation contractions, manometric pressure within the colonic lumen is great, and colonic transit is delayed, producing constipation.

Evaluation of Intestinal Motility[44]

Motility in the small and large intestine can be evaluated by determining the transit time, or the time it takes for a marker to pass through the intestines. Studies of intestinal motility have used a wide variety of markers in normal animals, abnormal animals, and animals treated with drugs. Transit times are usually estimated from the rate of barium movement in an upper GI study. In humans, barium studies suggest that small intestinal transit is more rapid in the diarrheic state, but that is not true if the barium is given with a test meal. A number of other techniques have shown that small-intestinal transit time is not altered in patients with diarrhea that arises from many different causes. In fact, it is possible to increase the rate of small-intestinal transit with some drugs, such as metoclopramide, without necessarily causing diarrhea. Diarrhea caused by increased secretion of intestinal fluid following administration of prostaglandins is not associated with a faster small intestinal transit. Clinical and experimental studies both show that rapid transit of contents through the colon is the consistent feature of diarrheas, rather than an alteration in small intestinal transit. Colonic transit increases with small-bowel problems when the reversed gradient is lost. Diarrhea is defined partly by changes in fecal weight, which is determined largely by colonic function. Fecal weights are greater after colonic resection, but not after small intestinal resection. In summary, transit times are difficult to measure, and the abnormalities most important in producing diarrhea are found in the large intestine.

Stress and emotions are recognized as being factors in the development of colonic problems based on abnormal motility. Psychogenic influences in humans can produce a chronic state that alternates between diarrhea and constipation. A similar type of problem has not been proven in small animals.

DIGESTION AND ABSORPTION

Digestion

The pancreas, intestinal mucosa, and biliary system contribute secretions for the intestinal digestion and absorption of a meal. The pancreas secretes enzymes that are important for the digestion of starch, proteins and lipids (Figure 15-12). Some enzymes are synthesized in an active form, including an alpha-amylase, lipase, ribonuclease, deoxyribonuclease, collagenase, and leucine aminopetidase. Enzymes synthesized as inactive

Starch	-	α -amylase
Lipids	-	lipase
		phospholipase
Proteins	-	trypsin
		chymotrypsin
		carboxypeptidase
		elastase
		collagenase
		leucine aminopeptidase
		ribonuclease
		deoxyribonuclease

Figure 15-12. Enzymes secreted by the pancreas, and the substrates they act on.

precursors are the proteases trypsin, chymotrypsin, carboxypeptidase and elastase, and the lipase phospholipase-A. The pancreas also secretes an alkaline fluid to provide a medium for optimum enzyme activity. Intestinal mucosal cells synthesize and secrete substances into the lumen of the gut and into the circulation. Secretions into the lumen consist of mucosal brush-border digestive enzymes (disaccharidases and peptidases), secretory immunoglobulins, and fluids resembling extracellular fluid. Small intestinal secretions are important since their loss causes major clinical signs of disease. The chemicals secreted into the circulation are peptide endocrines, biogenic amines, and possibly prostaglandins, all of which are suggested to participate in the regulation of gastrointestinal function. Bile acids are secreted by the liver and evacuated through the biliary system. They are required for normal lipid digestion and absorption.

Digestion of Carbohydrates.[45-48] Carbohydrate in the form of starch is usually the major constituent of diets for small animals. Some diets contain disaccharides, such as sucrose and lactose. Sucrose is not a usual dietary ingredient unless the animal is fed semimoist dog foods or human foods. Lactose is the major source of carbohydrate in animals that subsist on milk.

One component of starch is amylose, a straight-chain polymer of repeating units of glucose connected by alpha-1,4 bonds. Amylopectin, the major component of starch, has the same basic structure as amylose except that some chains of glucose are attached to others by alpha-1,6 linkages. Pancreatic alpha-amylase rapidly acts on starch at most alpha 1,4 bonds to hydrolyze it into smaller units (Figure 15-13). Very little glucose is produced. Amylase action produces maltose, a disaccharide of glucose, and maltotriose, a three-unit carbohydrate. These same carbohydrates are produced from amylopectin hydrolysis, which also produces alpha-limit dextrins that are composites of glucose, connected by both the alpha-1,4 and alpha-1,6 linkage. Oligosaccharides are also produced.

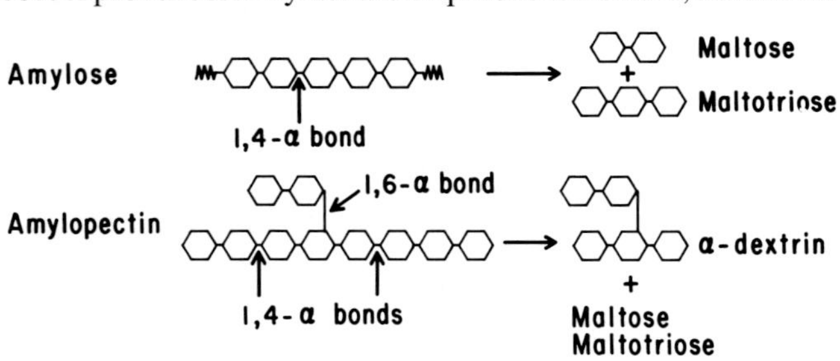

Figure 15-13. Schematic showing the sites of action of pancreatic amylase at the 1,4-α bonds of amylose and amylopectin to produce maltose, maltotriose, and α-dextrin. Amylase does not act at 1,6-α bonds.

Amylase is a protein that can be rapidly and irreversibly denatured by the low pH of acid chyme, but that possibility is prevented by pancreatic secretion of a bicarbonate-rich fluid. The level of carbohydrate in the diet determines the amount of amylase secreted. High-starch diets increase amylase secretion, and glucose substituted for starch further increases the amount secreted. This adaptation can be seen within four to five days of a diet change. The pancreas produces no known inhibitors of amylase.

Complete hydrolysis of carbohydrates to glucose is necessary for absorption. Final hydrolysis is achieved by brush-border enzymes of the mucosal epithelial cell. The enzymes are part of the outer membrane surface and may extend into the glycocalyx.[49] The enzymes are not released into the intestinal contents until the cell desquamates and degenerates. Thus, the enzymes are released without being secreted. Brush-border enzymes are designated by their activities, as maltase, sucrase, alpha-dextranase (isomaltase), and lactase.[50] There are at least two forms of each enzyme. Some maltases are not specific in activity; these hydrolyze sucrose and alpha-limit dextrins as well as maltose.

The levels of carbohydrate-digesting enzymes in the brush border vary with age, diet, and disease (Table 15-1). The concentrations of enzyme activity generally reflect an animal's needs. Young animals receiving lactose as the only source of carbohydrates have high levels of lactase. At weaning, lactase activity decreases, and concentrations of maltase and sucrase increase to reflect the carbohydrate composition of the diet. When a diet is changed, at least two days are required for the activity of these enzymes to adapt to new levels. This is the time the cells require to migrate from the crypts to the villus. The enzymes not only respond to dietary levels of carbohydrates but also respond to the amount of undigested carbohydrates in the lumen of the intestine. A decrease in the secretion of pancreatic enzymes causes an increase in the levels of brush-border enzymes in order to digest carbohydrates,[51] an adaptation expected with chronic pancreatic exocrine deficiency. Disaccharidase activity increases in intestinal contents following cholecystokinin-induced release of enzymes.[52] This is the only recognized means of stimulating enzyme release from the brush border.

Alteration of the mucosal brush border by disease results in a loss of its enzyme activity that often produces diarrhea. Enteritis due to infectious or toxic agents, overgrowth of the

Table 15-1. Brush Border Carbohydrase Activities in Dogs

Disaccharidase	Activity*
Maltase	0.238 ± 0.13
Sucrase	0.057 ± 0.02
Lactase	0.026 ± 0.01
Amyloglucosidase	0.049 ± 0.03

* Nanomoles of disaccharide hydrolyzed/mg protein/min
Data from reference 50

intestinal microflora, and bacterial enterotoxins result in a loss of enzyme activity.[53] Brush border enzyme activity is essential for completion of carbohydrate digestion and absorption, without which malabsorption appears and can cause diarrhea.

Bile salts that have been deconjugated by the large numbers of bacteria produce the damaging effects of bacterial overgrowth—distortion and denudation of microvilli. Following this type of insult, it takes two to seven days for enzyme levels to return to normal.[54]

Diarrhea of unknown etiology is often managed with a high-carbohydrate diet, primarily starch. With problems not involving the small intestine and not reducing disaccharidase activity, animals can adapt to greater amounts of carbohydrates and continue to digest nutrients completely. Levels of brush border disaccharidases decrease during fasting. Resumption of the feeding of carbohydrates should be gradual to allow enzyme activity to return.

Digestion of Proteins.[47,48,55-58] Proteins must be hydrolyzed to amino acids and peptides before absorption is possible. Protein digestion and absorption are completed in the cranial half of the small intestine. Consequently, the caudal half represents a large reserve of mucosal enzyme activity and absorptive surface. Digestion of proteins begins in the stomach, due to the action of pepsin, and is continued in the small intestine by pancreatic trypsin, chymotrypsin, elastase, and carboxypeptidase. The products of digestion are mostly small peptides (containing two to six amino acids) and a few amino acids. The pancreatic enzymes are more important than pepsin for protein digestion. Even when there is no pancreatic enzyme activity, half to two-thirds of the dietary protein is absorbed.

The most important pancreatic proteases are endopeptidases, which split bonds within the peptide chain (Figure 15-14). These include the trypsins, which break bonds at the site of a basic amino acid, and elastase, which acts at the site of a nonpolar amino acid. Trypsin is secreted as an inactive precursor, trypsinogen, which is prevented from being activated in the pancreas by pancreatic trypsin inhibitors. Enzymatically active trypsin is produced by the action of the intestinal enzyme enterokinase, which splits a hexapeptide from the amino-terminal end of trypsinogen. Once activated, trypsin rapidly activates more trypsin and also activates chymotrypsin, elastase, carboxypeptidase, and phospholipase. The carboxypeptidases split amino acids from either the carboxyl or the amino end.

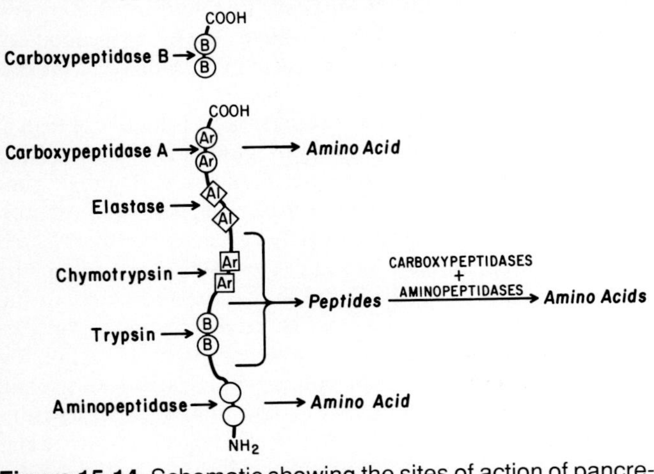

Figure 15-14. Schematic showing the sites of action of pancreatic proteases. B = basic amino acid. Ar = aromatic amino acid. Al = aliphatic amino acid.

The rates of secretion and disappearance of the proteases determine the level of protease activity in the intestine. The rate of synthesis and secretion of pancreatic proteases parallels the level of protein in the diet. Deficiencies in amino acids can result in decreased pancreatic proteases. Protease inhibitors added to the diet stimulate an increase in pancreatic proteases, as is seen by feeding a high-protein diet. A high-protein diet stimulates both the synthesis and transport of zymogen from the acinar cell to the duct. The level of activity of proteases in the intestine is also determined by the synthesis and secretion of adequate amounts of enterokinase. Duodenal mucosal disease can reduce the luminal activity of this protease-activating enzyme.

Protein digestion is completed at the brush border and within the epithelial cell. Small peptides can be completely hydrolyzed at the brush border. They can also be absorbed by the epithelial cell and hydrolyzed within. Small amounts of proteins can be absorbed unaltered and can be resistant to protease activity outside or inside the cell. Very little peptidase activity is found in the lumen of the intestine. About 80% is found within the cell in the cytoplasm in a soluble form. The remainder is bound to the brush border membranes. The intracellular peptidases are similar to those found in other organs of the body. The functions of the brush border and cytoplasmic enzymes are probably complementary. Large amounts of different peptidases are found, each with the ability to hydrolyze a number of different peptides. The rate of hydrolysis varies for each peptide, suggesting that each peptidase has some degree of specificity. The enzymes found, designated according to the activity they show, are called dipeptidases, tripeptidases, oligopeptidases, and leucylnaphthylamidase.

The regulation of epithelial-cell peptidase activity is not understood as well as that for the carbohydrates. High-protein diets increase brush border peptidase activity, but effects on intracellular peptidases are variable and depend on the type of protein.[59] Starvation decreases enzyme activity in the brush border but increases that in the cell.[60] Although brush border enzymes are lost with extensive mucosal disease, clinical signs of protein malabsorption seldom follow. Thus, the importance of brush border enzymes is questionable. If pancreatic enzymes can carry digestion to the level of small peptides, and if peptides can be absorbed and hydrolyzed within epithelial cells, the brush border enzymes are not needed. A deficiency of one mucosal peptidase, enterokinase, causes protein malabsorption. This enzyme is released to activate trypsin from trypsinogen.

Digestion of Lipids.[47,61-65] Digestion of lipids requires pancreatic lipase and bile acids. Lipase hydrolyses fatty acids from the outer ester bonds of triglyceride molecules (Figure 15-15), leaving a monoglyceride with the fatty acid esterified to the middle carbon. In that state, long-chain fatty acids and monoglycerides, normally relatively water-insoluble, become very soluble, following interaction with bile acids to form micelles. Lipase hydrolysis is necessary for absorption, since triglycerides and diglycerides are not solubilized by bile acids. The emulsification properties of bile acids increase the effectiveness of lipase by increasing the surface area of the oil-water interface. Bile acids also trap free fatty acids in emulsified fats, which ensures that resynthesis of triglycerides does not occur

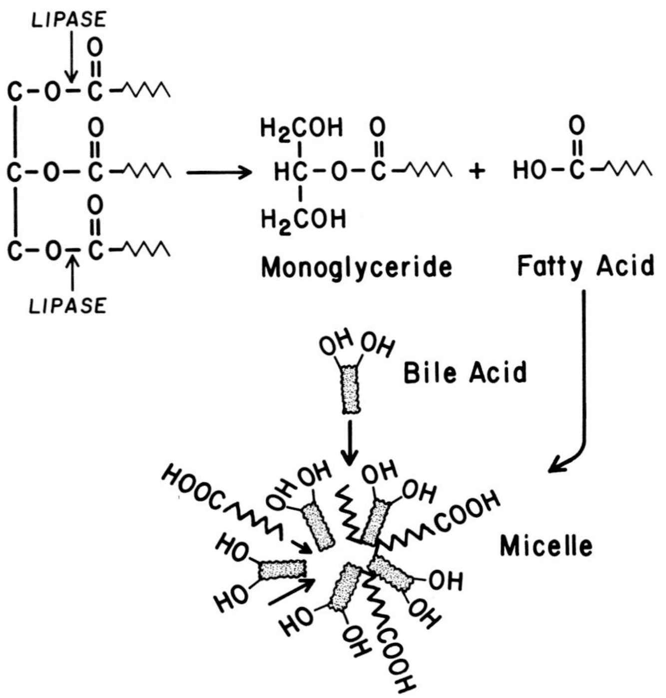

Figure 15-15. Schematic showing the digestion of triglycerides by pancreatic lipase and the formation of micelles. Lipase acts on the outer two ester bonds to form monoglycerides and fatty acids. Micelles are formed spontaneously when monoglycerides, fatty acids, and bile acids are present. Micelles are water-soluble since the polar groups of their constituents are on the surface of the sphere, with the hydrophobic part of the molecules in the interior.

before absorption. Like many enzymes, lipase catalyzes both directions of the chemical process, hydrolysis and esterification.

Pancreatic lipase is very unstable and is susceptible to rapid and irreversible inactivation. Lipase is secreted in its active form, but it requires bile salts and a lipase cofactor for full enzyme activity. Lipase has a pH optimum of 8.0, which bile acids reduce to 6.0, making the enzyme more effective at the pH of duodenal contents. A fat-rich diet increases pancreatic lipase secretion, with unsaturated fatty acids the most potent stimulus. High-protein diets also stimulate synthesis and secretion of lipase. High-carbohydrate diets decrease lipase production. No inhibitors of lipase have been found in animals.

The pancreas secretes phospholipases as precursors that require activation by trypsin. Calcium is necessary for optimum activity. Phospholipase A splits the fatty acid from the beta-position in lecithin, cephalin, phosphatidyl ethanolamine, and the plasminogens containing choline and ethanolamine. Removal of this fatty acid from lecithin produces a toxic compound, lysolecithin, which enters into cell membranes and results in lysis of the cell. Another phospholipase splits fatty acids from the A-position in lysolecithin. Lysolecithin, produced in the intestine by phospholipase activity on phospholipids in bile and the diet, does not damage mucosal epithelial cells. No natural inhibitors of phospholipase have been identified.

Bile acid molecules have polar and nonpolar regions. The nonpolar areas combine with monoglycerides and fatty acids to form micelles, small particles 40 to 50 Angstroms in diameter. The polar regions cover the surface of the micelle, with the nonpolar lipids and bile acids in the center (Figure 15-15). The lipid interior also contains fat-soluble vitamins and water-insoluble steroids, such as cholesterol. The formation of micelles is a physical-chemical reaction that proceeds spontaneously when the concentration of bile acids, monoglycerides, and fatty acids is optimum. A micellar solution is clear and waterlike, in contrast to an emulsion of fats. The smallest particle that can be produced by emulsification is about 100 times the diameter of a micelle. The formation of micelles increases the amount of fatty acids in solution by 1,000 times. Small emulsified fat particles pass through the lipid part of the membrane, but their diffusion coefficient is 1/8 that of micelles, which pass through the cell membrane much more readily.

The brush border contains enzymes with esterase activity for cholesterol and vitamin A esters, but the significance is unknown since there are pancreatic enzymes with this activity. The brush border also contains sphingomyelinase and phospholipase A activity.

Dietary fat levels vary in commercial pet foods, with canned preparations containing more fat than dry foods. All meat diets are also high in fat. Fat absorption is usually nearly complete, so that less than 5% of the dietary fat is excreted in the feces. The essential requirements for normal fat excretion are adequate bile and lipase secretions and normal surface area of the small intestinal mucosa. Surprisingly, the complete loss of either lipase activity or bile acids does not result in complete fat malabsorption. At least 50% of dietary fats can be absorbed in the absence of bile to form micelles. The same amount is absorbed with a loss of all pancreatic enzymes. Thus, while lipase and bile are not necessary for lipid absorption, they are essential for normal digestion and absorption. With progressive reductions in pancreatic enzyme activity, lipid malabsorption may be apparent before that of other nutrients. Lipid assimilation is slower than that of other nutrients and requires most of the small intestine. Inadequate lipase activity delays lipid digestion and presents more lipid to the terminal small intestine for digestion. The terminal jejunum and ileum do not have the capacity to absorb increased amounts of lipids.

Determinants of Intraluminal Enzyme Activity Adequate intraluminal pancreatic enzyme activity is required to satisfy digestive needs. With time, this activity disappears, though not before digestion is complete. The pH of the medium into which the enzymes are secreted, enzyme inhibitors, and the activity of bacterial proteases determine the rate of disappearance of enzyme activity. At a low pH trypsin is more stable than amylase or lipase but is rapidly degraded by pepsin. Both trypsin and chymotrypsin activities diminish during their transit through the intestines, with trypsin disappearing more rapidly. Some of the loss of activity may be due to inhibitors found in pancreatic secretions. Although these inhibitors reduce the activity of most proteases found in the intestine, most of the inhibitors are rapidly degraded. Bacterial lysosomal proteases destroy inhibitors that are resistant to tryptic digestion by pancreatic proteases. Disappearance of intestinal pancreatic enzyme activity is due primarily to digestion by proteases from the pancreas, bacteria, and mucosal cell lysosomes. Bacterial overgrowth of the small intestine causes a faster enzyme destruction, resulting in maldigestion and malabsorption. Effects of colonic bacteria to inactivate digestive enzymes are apparent in fecal digestion tests where aged fecal samples show no proteolytic activity, but a fresh sample repeated on the same individual shows normal proteolytic activity.

As would be expected, the synthesis and secretion of pancreatic enzymes are reduced in a patient having chronic pancreatitis or recovering from acute pancreatitis.

Secretion

Fluid and Electrolyte Secretion, Pancreatic.[66,67] Both the acinar cells and the cells lining the ducts derive the fluid and electrolyte component of pancreatic secretion from extracellular fluid. At low rates of secretion, pancreatic juice is similar to plasma in electrolyte composition. The bicarbonate content is a little higher than in plasma, and chloride content is lower. The concentration of sodium is 10 to 12 mEq/L greater in pancreatic secretion than in plasma, the result of a lower protein content in pancreatic juice since the osmolality is the same for both fluids. Upon stimulation of fluid secretion, the concentration of bicarbonate increases and that of chloride decreases, with their sum remaining fairly constant at any rate of secretion (Figure 15-16). Bicarbonate can increase to 150 mEq/L, in which case it makes up almost the total anions in the secretion. Other electrolytes in pancreatic secretion are small amounts of calcium and magnesium at lower concentrations than in plasma. Thus, the pancreas responds to stimulation with an isosmotic secretion that is like plasma, except that it is rich in bicarbonate.

The final electrolyte composition of pancreatic juice is produced by one of three physiological mechanisms, which are possible in any secreting gland that is made up of acinar cells and a transporting duct system. The composition of the final secretion results from: 1) an admixture of different secretions produced by each of the cell types, which may secrete at different rates; 2) a single cell type varying the composition of its secretion; or 3) a secretion by the acinar cells of a plasma-like fluid that is altered as it passes through the ducts by both selective addition and removal of ions.

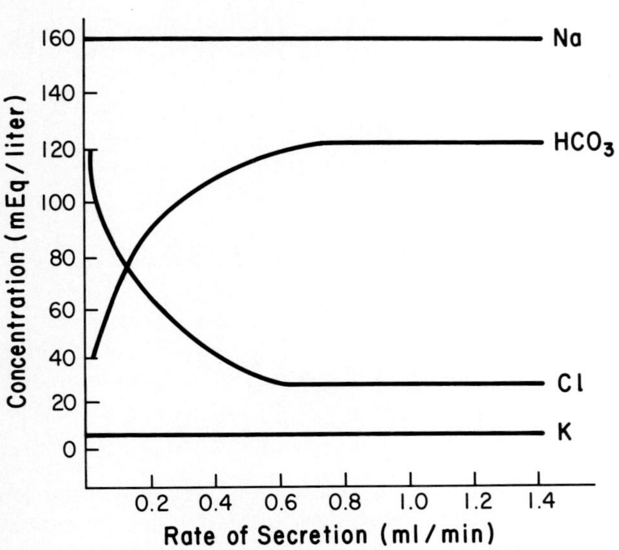

Figure 15-16. Graph showing the ionic composition of pancreatic secretions at different rates. The bicarbonate content increases when the pancreas is stimulated to secrete. The chloride concentration varies inversely with that of bicarbonate.

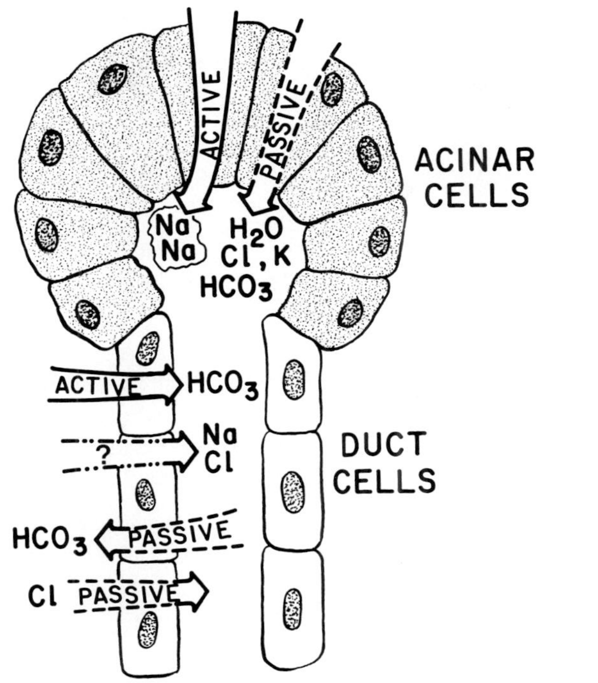

Figure 15-17. Schematic of pancreatic acinar cell and secretory duct. Active secretion of sodium by the acinar cells and bicarbonate by the duct cells produces the final secretion. Passive movement of ions through the semipermeable membranes of the ducts modifies the secretion.

The fluid secreted by acinar cells is like extracellular fluid in ionic composition. It is produced by the active transport of sodium ions across the acinar cell (Figure 15-17). The movement of water that accompanies it carries all the other ions passively by "solvent drag." This activity maintains zero concentration gradients for all ions across the acinar cell, and thus electrical neutrality. As this primary secretion of fluid passes through the ducts, it is modified by the addition of duct cell secretions. The ducts actively secrete bicarbonate into the fluid and cause the stimulated secretion to be bicarbonate rich. Sodium is also secreted by a process that may be active. The ducts are permeable to both bicarbonate and chloride, however, so that the ions can readily diffuse across the duct epithelium, and pancreatic secretions can equilibrate with interstitial fluid. At low rates of secretion when little bicarbonate and fluid are secreted, less fluid moves more slowly through a duct that is permeable to anions. Under these conditions chloride and bicarbonate readily diffuse across duct membranes and equilibrate with the interstitial fluids; the final product of secretion becomes more like plasma. At high rates of secretion after stimulation by secretin, large amounts of bicarbonate are secreted, and, since the fluid moves through the ducts rapidly, little bicarbonate diffuses across the permeable membranes to equilibrate with the plasma and interstitial fluid. In this case the final product of secretion is rich in bicarbonate.

Epithelial cells that produce and transport bicarbonate contain large amounts of carbonic anhydrase. In the pancreas this enzyme is found only in the ductal epithelium, where it catalyzes the reversible reactions in which carbon dioxide is hydrated to form carbonic acid (Figure 15-18). Inhibitors of

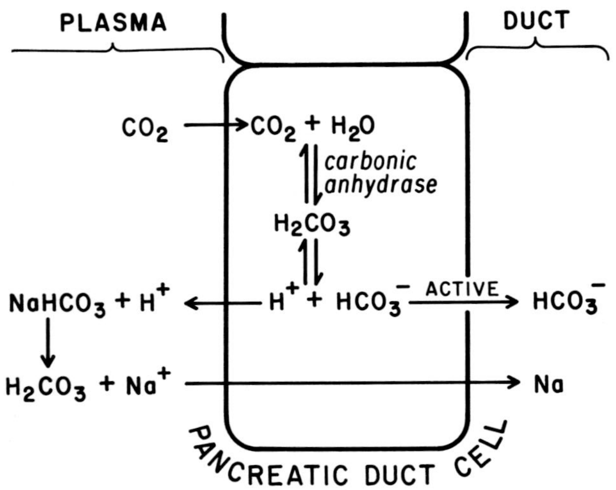

Figure 15-18. Diagram of a pancreatic duct cell that forms bicarbonate from carbonic acid and secretes it via an active process into the duct. The reaction requires the catalytic enzyme carbonic anhydrase to provide a sufficient amount of bicarbonate for secretion.

carbonic anhydrase have been used to study pancreatic secretion. They have a general effect of inhibiting the production and transport of bicarbonate. It has been shown, however, that in the pancreas one carbonic anhydrase inhibitor, acetazolamide, interferes with both chloride and enzyme secretion as well as with bicarbonate secretion. Even though the use of this commonly used carbonic anhydrase inhibitor interferes with the transport of more than one substance, those studies indicate the need for carbonic anhydrase to produce carbonic acid. Other studies have shown that if carbonic dioxide is not present in the bathing medium of *in vitro* pancreatic tissue, very little bicarbonate is produced. Thus, some of the bicarbonate is derived from plasma carbon dioxide as well as from plasma bicarbonate. In clinical cases, the pancreas' secretion of bicarbonate is increased by metabolic alkalosis and impaired by metabolic or respiratory acidosis.

The volume and bicarbonate concentration of pancreatic juice changes with pancreatic disease. The volume of secretion is reduced in humans with most types of pancreatic disease except in those recovering from acute pancreatitis, in which case secretion rates are abnormally high although the total output of bicarbonate is normal. The capacity to secrete bicarbonate is reduced in chronic pancreatitis, pancreatic atrophy, and pancreatic carcinomas. In humans with chronic pancreatitis, the capacity to secrete bicarbonate is reduced more than is the capacity to secrete enzymes. In humans recovering from acute pancreatitis, enzyme secretion is reduced while volume and bicarbonate secretions are normal or increased. Similar changes are found in small animals with pancreatic disease.[68]

Calcium and magnesium, normally at a lower concentration in pancreatic juice than in plasma, are part of the secretion of the acinar cell, with the amount secreted in proportion to the amount of amylase secreted.

Control of Pancreatic Secretion.[69-72] The autonomic nervous system and a number of endocrines control pancreatic secretion (Figure 15-19). It is stimulated, and in some cases inhibited, by events that occur in the initial stages of feeding as well as by the well-known events that occur when food enters the intestine. The regulation of pancreatic secretion has been divided into cephalic, gastric, and intestinal phases.

The cephalic phase is the initial step, and its effects are mediated primarily though the autonomic nervous system. This phase is stimulated by such psychological factors as the anticipation of food, which is reinforced by the oral events in eating. The motor pathway is in parasympathetic fibers in the vagi; the pancreatic response is a small volume of secretion, rich in enzymes. Stimulation of the cephalic phase initiates the synthesis of new enzymes in preparation for the food that will soon enter the intestine and require their activity for digestion. The pancreas does not contain a large store of enzymes, and production must begin early in order to supply some of the needs necessary to digest a meal. Vagal impulses have a little effect in stimulating the secretion of water and electrolytes. One component of the cephalic phase is controlled by a pathway that is partly neural and partly humoral. Stimulation of the cephalic phase causes the vagally-mediated release of gastrin from the gastric mucosa. Gastrin, a peptide hormone structurally similar to cholecystokinin (CCK), stimulates pancreatic secretion. Thus, this hormone participates in stimulation of the small volume and enzyme-rich secretion in the cephalic phase.

The gastric phase of pancreatic secretion, stimulated by events in the stomach, is mediated both neurally and humorally. One entirely neural pathway is a vagovagal reflex (gastropancreatic reflex), in which stimulation of the body of the stomach sends information to the brain via vagal afferents, and, after central synaptic transmission, a motor response is sent to the pancreas via vagal parasympathetics. Vagotomy abolishes the reflex. The second component of the gastric phase involves a humoral response mediated by gastrin, a hormone released by

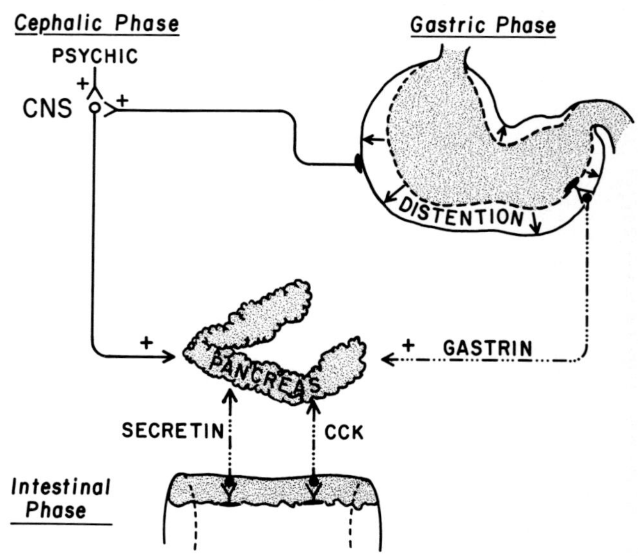

Figure 15-19. Diagram of regulation of pancreatic secretion. The cephalic phase primarily stimulates the secretion of enzymes by a cholinergic neural pathway. Distention and food in the stomach stimulates a neural pathway through the CNS and the release of gastrin to cause the pancreas to secrete enzymes. When acid chyme enters the intestine, secretion and CCK are released to stimulate the pancreas.

chemical and mechanical stimulation of the antrum of the stomach. These stimuli evoke a local cholinergic pathway and release gastrin. That response is well documented, but it is less certain whether stimulation of the antrum initiates another vagovagal reflex to either directly stimulate the pancreas via nerve fibers or indirectly stimulate the organ via gastrin release. The response of the pancreas to either direct neural or indirect gastrin stimulation is, again, a small volume of enzyme-rich juice.

The intestinal phase of pancreatic secretion, stimulated by events in the small intestine, is hormonally mediated. There may be short neural pathways in the wall of the intestine that are involved in the release of the hormones. The hormones synthesized primarily to stimulate pancreatic secretion are CCK and secretin. Less potent stimulators of pancreatic secretion are gastrin and vasoactive intestinal peptide (VIP). All four hormones are synthesized and released from the intestinal mucosa even though the primary site of gastrin production is in the antrum of the stomach. Intraluminal ionized calcium appears to be a universal stimulant of hormone release. Classically, it has been considered that acid pH releases secretin and that digestive products release CCK. Acid pH in the duodenum is the single important factor that stimulates the release of secretin. Below pH 3.0, the amount of bicarbonate that is secreted is independent of the pH of the chyme entering the duodenum. Between pH 3.0 and 4.5, the amount of bicarbonate secreted is proportional to the pH of chyme in the duodenum. The secretory response is also a function of both the rate of entry of titrable acid into the intestine and the length of small intestine that is acidified. The threshold below which the release of secretin is stimulated is pH 4.5. The amount of secretin in the duodenal mucosa follows a gradient that decreases aborally. Fatty acids also stimulate the release of secretin and bicarbonate secretion. The half life of secretin is less than three minutes and the kidney is the major site of its degradation.[73,74]

The amino acid L isomers of tryptophan, phenylalanine, valine, and possibly methionine stimulate the release of CCK. Acid pH and fatty acids of the aliphatic series, with carbon chains greater than 10, also release CCK. Fatty acids such as oleate are a potent stimulator of CCK release and pancreatic enzyme secretion, even moreso than amino acids. Acid pH is a weak stimulus of CCK release. The release of duodenal gastrin is stimulated by neural or alkaline pH and inhibited by acid pH. Both D and L isomers of amino acids of the sarcosine series (glycine, alanine, serine, etc.) also release duodenal gastrin. Short-chain aliphatic alcohols and fatty acids (C2 and C3) are weak stimulators of gastrin release. The physiological effect of VIP on pancreatic secretion most closely resembles that of secretin but with less potency. Vagal stimulation is the normal stimulus for VIP release.

The effects of these hormones are selective stimulation, on one hand, of the secretion of a large volume of fluid rich in bicarbonate and, on the other, of a secretion rich in enzymes. Secretin and VIP primarily stimulate fluid secretion. Other hormones similar to VIP, glucagon and gastric inhibitory peptide (GIP), have variable effects. The amino acid sequences of these peptides are similar; the terminal three amino acids at the end of the peptide, which are essential for physiological activity, are the same for secretin and VIP. Secretin is the hormone designed for maximum stimulation. VIP has about 20% of the potency of secretin. Since these structurally similar hormones stimulate secretion, they both bind to the receptor site on pancreatic secretory cells. When bound to the cell, VIP prevents the binding of secretin, thus competitively inhibiting the action of secretin. Glucose in the lumen of the intestine also inhibits the maximum secretory response to the infusion of secretin. Glucose in the small intestine causes the release of glucagon, and the blunting of the secretin response may be the competitive inhibition of secretin by glucagon. Small doses of glucagon inhibit the pancreatic secretion stimulated by secretin and CCK, but have no effect on basal secretion.

Gastrin and CCK constitute another family of gastrointestinal hormones. All forms of gastrin and CCK have the same five amino acids at the terminal end that are essential for activity. Thus, it is expected that their functions will overlap. Gastrin stimulates pancreatic secretion as well as gastric secretion. Although CCK's major function is to stimulate the pancreas, it also stimulates gastric secretion. Thus, CCK is a partial agonist of gastric secretion and a full agonist of pancreatic secretion. When CCK is infused in a dog stimulated to maximum gastric secretion, the rate of secretion falls. This illustrates how structurally similar CCK, a partial agonist for gastric secretion, competitively displaces gastrin from the receptor sites on the parietal cells; the weaker stimulus is unable to promote the maximum secretory capacity of the cells. On the other hand, at low levels of gastrin-stimulated gastric secretion CCK acts as a partial agonist and will augment secretion by binding to any free receptor sites.

Each end organ in the digestive tract has two receptor sites, one for the gastrin family of hormones and one for the secretin family. Pairs of hormones within a family may interact by augmenting (CCK on low rates of gastric secretion) or by inhibiting, either competitively (VIP on secretin-stimulated pancreatic secretion) or noncompetitively, the primary action of one member of the pair. There also is some potentiation between hormones bound to the two receptor sites. For example, CCK augments the low fluid and bicarbonate response of the pancreas stimulated by small amounts of secretin. Gastrin and cholinergic stimuli have the same effect. Secretin and VIP have a similar effect of potentiating low rates of enzyme secretion stimulated by CCK.

The pancreas is a rich source of somatostatin and pancreatic polypeptide. Plasma levels of both increase after feeding, and the hormones are potent inhibitors of pancreatic secretion. Somatostatin and VIP inhibit pancreatic enzyme and bicarbonate secretions following either neural- or hormone-mediated stimulation. Since the hormones are released from cells in the pancreas to act on other cells in the pancreas, the concentrations of these hormones on their target cell would be much greater than in plasma. Peptide YY, found in highest concentration in the ileum and colon, is another inhibitor of pancreatic secretion. Fatty acids are potent inhibitors of peptide YY release, especially in the distal small intestine. Cholinergic mechanisms are involved with vagally-mediated pancreatic secretion and the release of many humoral agents. Anticholinergic drugs inhibit vagally-mediated secretion and the release of intestinal hormones that stimulate secretion, but they have no effect on the action of the hormone on the secretory cell. Acid or food products in the intestine stimulate receptors for neural pathways to the hormone cells in the mucosa. Anticholinergics (such as atropine) usually block hormone release, and local anesthetics applied to the mucosa also prevent their release. Thus, anticholinergics can inhibit pancreatic secretion by acting both directly on the vagally-mediated pathways of stimulation and indirectly on the neurally mediated release of hormones that stimulate secretion.

Blood flow increases within an organ that is actively secreting digestive juices. The increased flow is necessary not only to meet the metabolic requirements for transport but also to provide the fluid and electrolytes in the secretion. Pancreatic blood flow increases when either the vagal parasympathetics or the hormones CCK and secretin stimulate the organ. The vagal effects may be the result of kallikrein-induced kinin formation, similar to the events that occur in the salivary glands during neural stimulation. It is also possible that vagal vasodilator fibers exist to produce the effect. All of the hormones discussed in this section have vasodilator properties, and in the case of VIP the property is very potent, as the name of the hormone implies. VIP can cause vasodilation to the point that a large volume of fluid is secreted into the intestinal tract. This occurs in some pathological situations caused by a VIP-secreting tumor.

The sympathetic nervous system does not play a role in the control of normal pancreatic function. Cutting the sympathetics to the pancreas increases secretion, and stimulation causes vasoconstriction and a concomitant decrease in secretory rates. The sympathetic nerves have an important effect on the pancreas whenever they are intensely stimulated, such as during shock. The pancreas releases proteases and toxic peptides into the circulation during shock and during acute pancreatitis. Pancreatic ischemia as a result of intense sympathetic activity is either the cause or is a severe complication contributing to the problem.

Intraluminal Digestion. Factors that determine how chemical reactions proceed dictate the hydrolysis of carbohydrates, proteins, and lipids into subunits that can be absorbed. Most of these reactions are catalyzed by enzymes with activities that are optimum at a certain pH and at a specific temperature. The optimum pH for enzymes acting in the small intestine is in the range of 7 to 8, normally provided by pancreatic secretion of bicarbonate. That may not be the case, however, in several situations. When acid contents from the stomach rapidly enter the duodenum at a rate exceeding the capacity of pancreatic secretions to neutralize them, the intestinal medium is at a pH in which the pancreatic enzymes are inactive. This situation can result from gastric surgery, which may lead to an increase in the rate of stomach emptying. Inadequate neutralization of gastric chyme is also a problem in an animal with pancreatic insufficiency that reduces the ability to secrete bicarbonate. In this case, pH cannot be maintained close to optimum levels until the secretion of intestinal fluid buffers the acid chyme entering from the stomach. Buffering may not happen until after the enzymes have been inactivated or after the nutrients have passed their major absorptive sites. Some of the enzymes require specific ions that act as cofactors. Deficiencies of cofactors have not been recognized as a cause of clinical problems. In general, isotonic conditions should prevail for maximum activity. As in any enzymatic reactions, the amount of enzyme and the amount of substrate determine the amount of products from hydrolytic activity. All of the chemical reactions proceed at a given rate, varying with the conditions described, and so the nutrients must remain in the intestine for a given time before digestion is complete.

Starch digestion and absorption was at one time thought to be more complete than that for protein and lipids. Starch assimilation, however, can be incomplete even when a low starch diet is fed.[75] The source of dietary starch is one factor determining variability in assimilation (Figure 15-20). Sources of starch such as rice are digested more completely than other sources of starch.[76] Digestibility also varies between different strains of one grain, and processing has an additional important effect (Table 15-2).[77] Commercially prepared diets contain modified food starches added for nonnutrient purposes, and they may be digested less efficiently.[78] Protein digestion is not as important as carbohydrate digestion because the protein content of the diet is much less, and peptides are absorbed as efficiently as amino acids. Since digestion of lipids is slower, a delay in intestinal transit is more important for optimum fat assimilation than for the other nutrients. In general, absorption, not digestion, is the rate-limiting step in the assimilation of nutrients in the alimentary canal.

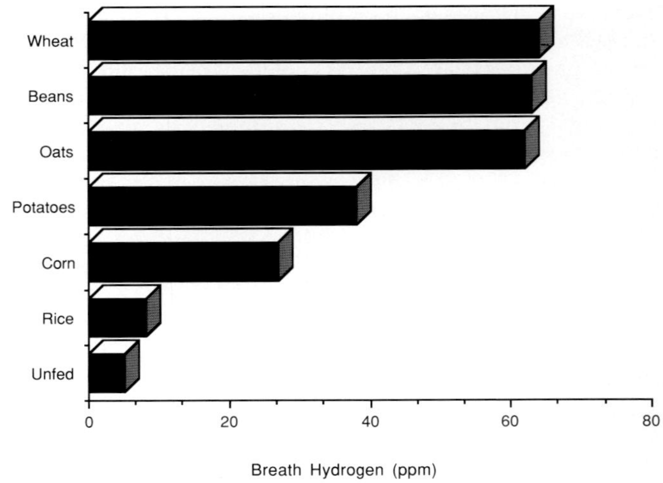

Figure 15-20a. Breath hydrogen concentration (humans) after ingestion of 100 gm of carbohydrate in various forms. Adapted from reference 76.

Intestinal Secretion of Fluid and Electrolytes.[79-81] Under certain normal and abnormal conditions, fluid and electrolytes are secreted in the small and large intestine. Abnormal secretion of fluid by the small and large intestine is a significant cause of diarrhea. Understanding the pathophysiology and management of diarrhea due to hypersecretion of intestinal fluid depends on knowledge of how the normal mechanisms operate, since they are suggested to be functioning at an uncontrolled rate.

Under normal conditions, fluid is secreted into the intestine

Table 15-2. Factors Affecting Starch Digestibility

Food Form	Fiber (Type)
Particle size	Antinutrients
Starch source	Phytate
Amylose content	Lectins
Amylopectin content	Tannins
Degree of gelatinization	Saponins
Cooking process	Enzyme inhibitors
Starch-nutrient interactions	

Adapted from reference 77

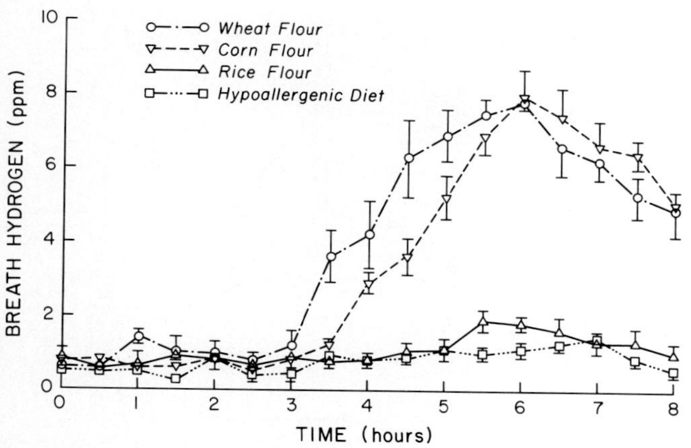

Figure 15-20b. Breath hydrogen concentration (dogs) after ingestion of various forms of carbohydrate added to a hypoallergenic diet. Adapted from reference 130.

upon the delivery of hypertonic contents into that segment. The contents of the intestine also become hypertonic as digestion proceeds in order to reduce large molecules to their subunits. This greatly increases the number of osmotically active particles, generating a force to draw fluid into the lumen.

The mucosa of the small intestine is the membrane most permeable to water and ion movement of any body surface facing the external environment. This is the site for greatest potential loss of fluid from the body. Within the small intestine the mucosa of the duodenum is the most permeable. The jejunum is ten times as permeable to water movement as is the stomach. Measurable rates of flux for sodium in the stomach are virtually zero compared with the high flux rates in the small intestine. The mucosa becomes less permeable in the caudal direction, making the ileum least permeable. The large intestine is relatively impermeable to fluid and sodium movement. Fluid moves across the mucosa through cells and through tight junctions between cells. Tight junctions are more permeable to fluid and ion movement than cell membranes. Fluid moves across the mucosa by diffusion, and chemicals that plug channels in the tight junctions dramatically reduce passive diffusional fluxes across the cell. As much as eight to ten liters of fluid move in and out of the intestine daily in a 20-kg animal. The diffusional fluxes in and out are equal, so that during fasting the intestine remains empty. With the extracellular fluid volume representing 25% of the body weight, the diffusional fluxes account for the daily movement of a volume double that of the total extracellular fluid volume. While large bidirectional fluxes of fluid are a normal feature of an epithelial surface, it is apparent that any shift in the forces that maintain the balance can cause large movements of extracellular fluid into the intestinal tract, which is essentially outside of the body. A number of factors determine the permeability of the mucosa as well as regulate the fluxes.

The number and size of a membrane's pores determine its permeability. The pores for water, ions, and polar molecules are suggested to be water-filled pores. The pores for lipid-soluble substances are thought to be in the lipid layers of the membrane. The overall permeability of the epithelial surface is a composite of properties of all its cell membranes. This includes characteristics of the cell's basal and apical surfaces and its intercellular junctions. Permeability to passive movement of water and ions is in the so-called tight junction. The chemical environment immediately adjacent to the membrane also determines the passive movement of water and ions. The lipid surface of the cell membrane causes a layer of water to be oriented along its surface; the water is so structured that ions are excluded. Physical chemical forces produce this barrier, the "unstirred" water layer, which makes a membrane less permeable to water and ion movement. The concept of different types of pores is a simplified functional concept that has no anatomic counterpart.

Figure 15-21 depicts the direction and magnitude of the passive diffusional fluxes across the intestinal mucosa. Fluid is also shown moving from the intestine into the circulation, representing the absorption of all other fluid entering the intestinal tract each day. This fluid is contributed by the diet and secretions of salivary, gastric, pancreatic, and intestinal juices, constituting 2 to 2.5 liters of fluid the intestine in a 20-kg animal must absorb. Active energy-dependent transport processes absorb this fluid at constant rates unless the mucosa is damaged. Another flux, shown in Figure 15-21, represents secretion of fluid into the intestine.

Factors that determine magnitude of fluxes when permeability of membranes is normal:

A&B
1. Capillary and interstitial fluid
   a. Hydrostatic pressure
   b. Colloid osmotic pressure
2. Intestinal lumen contents
   a. Osmotic pressure

C
1. Active transport of sodium
2. Active transport of sugars and amino acids

D
1. Activation of latent secretory process by enterotoxins

CAPILLARIES INTESTINE

H_2O + Na

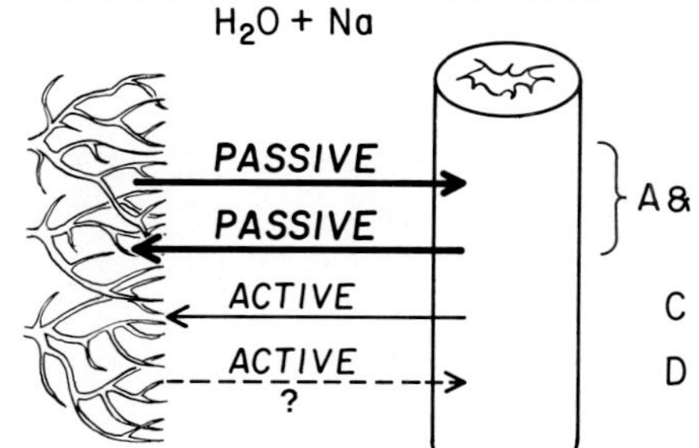

FLUID AND ELECTROLYTE FLUXES

Figure 15-21. Diagram depicting direction and magnitude of passive and active movement of fluid across the intestinal mucosa. The passive fluxes account for the movements of fluid volumes that are four times the volume of fluxes absorbed by the active processes. The passive fluxes are determined by the balance of physical forces on either side of the mucosal surface. The direction and magnitude of the passive fluxes are determined by the osmolality of intestinal contents, the plasma and interstitial fluid oncotic pressures, and the hydrostatic pressures in the capillary and interstitial fluids. The secretory flux is not evident in the normal state and the basis of its generation is not known.

Secretions of intestinal fluid are similar in composition to secretions of extracellular fluid. Osmolality and sodium concentration are the same as those of extracellular fluid. The concentration of bicarbonate is low in secretions from the cranial small intestine and high in secretions from the caudal part. This difference results in a pH as low as 6.3 cranially and as high as 7.8 in the ileum. The mechanism for modification of bicarbonate is unknown. The primary secretion of intestinal fluid may be similar in composition to extracellular fluid, which is then modified by the appropriate secretion and absorption of hydrogen and bicarbonate ions. Experimental studies supporting that scheme show that fluid secreted at low rates is modified maximally, so that bicarbonate levels are very low in the cranial small intestine and very high in the caudal part.[82] However, in fluid secreted at maximal rates the concentration of bicarbonate in each region changes and approaches bicarbonate levels in plasma.

The concentration of potassium in intestinal secretions is 10 to 15 mEq/L, which also differs from the concentration in extracellular fluid. Losses of small-intestinal secretions deplete total-body potassium. Potassium levels are high in intestinal secretions because of the permeability of epithelial membranes for potassium and because of the electrical potential gradient across the mucosa. The potential is created by the differential transport of ions in the transport processes.

The mechanisms for intestinal-fluid secretion and their regulation are incompletely understood. The secretion of fluid is suggested to be due to an active secretory mechanism in the epithelial cell. In addition, however, fluid can move into the intestine as a result of changes in the forces that determine the passive fluxes. The secretion of intestinal fluid is undoubtedly an effect of both active and passive secretory processes.

Many different neurohumoral chemicals, endogenous substances such as bile acids, and a number of bacterial toxins stimulate secretion of fluid in the intestine. Although there are variations between the effects of each on different species of animals and on different sites in the intestine, a general scheme can be described for the transport mechanisms they affect (Figure 15-22). Common to all of the stimulants is a property for increasing intracellular calcium by promoting either calcium entry into cells or calcium release from intracellular stores. The increased calcium stimulates prostaglandin formation following increased phospholipase and cyclooxygenase activities. Phosphatidylinositol formation, in addition to promoting prostaglandin formation, can increase membrane permeability for calcium, mobilize calcium from intracellular stores by inosital triphosphate formed from phosphatidylinositol, and activate protein kinases that may be involved with ion transport.

Prostaglandins stimulate cyclic AMP formation that promotes cellular uptake of chloride by a sodium and potassium dependent process. The increase in uptake may be caused by increased permeability of the cells' basolateral membranes. Prostaglandins also decrease the resistance of brush border or apical membranes so that the membranes become more permeable to chloride movement.

Increased intracellular calcium has the general effects of reducing absorption of sodium and chloride, increasing chloride secretion by increasing apical membrane permeability for chloride, and increasing efflux of potassium from cells. Some of these effects are not associated with changes in prostaglandins or cyclic AMP. Intracellular calcium concentrations also determine calcium-calmodulin levels, which regulate absorption of sodium and chloride and secretion of potassium but not chloride.

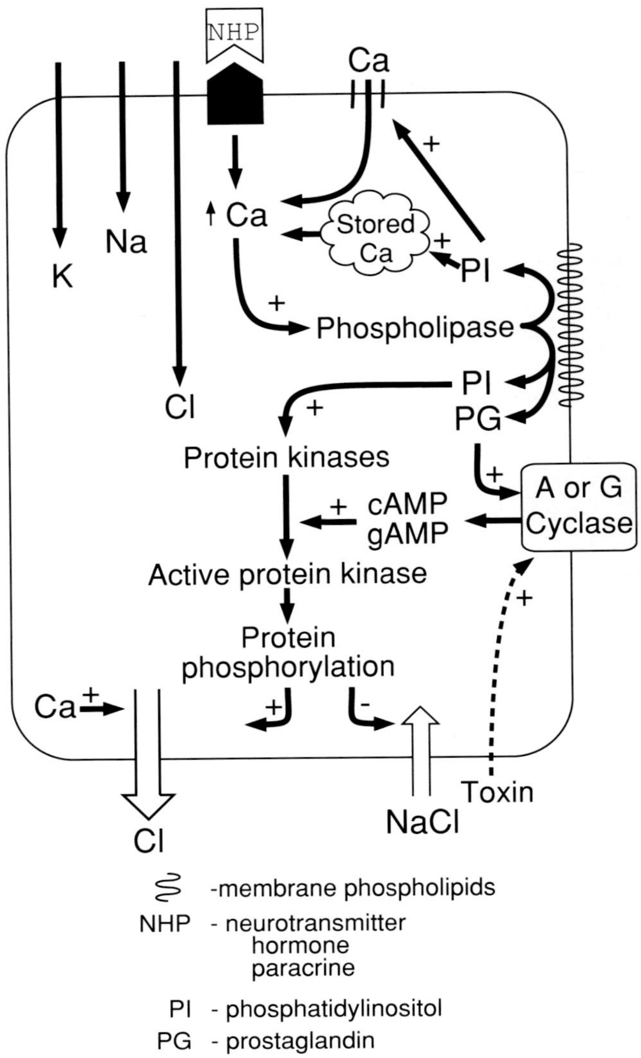

Figure 15-22. Schematic drawing showing mechanisms for secretion of fluid in the small intestine.

Secretion of intestinal fluid stimulated by bacterial enterotoxins has been studied to gain most of the understanding of secretory mechanisms. Toxins stimulate normal cellular mechanisms to secrete abnormal amounts of fluid. Following exposure, enterotoxins bind to brush border surfaces and secretion of fluid begins within 15 to 60 minutes. The initiation of secretion is associated with activation of the enzyme adenylate cyclase, which is located on the basal cell membranes. Some heat-stable enterotoxins stimulate the brush-border enzyme guanylate cyclase to increase intracellular cyclic GMP levels. Adenylate cyclase activity increases intracellular cyclic AMP levels, which, associated with the concurrent secretion of fluid, suggests that cyclic AMP stimulates a secretory mechanism. The secreted fluid is chloride-rich in the cranial small intestine and bicarbonate-rich in the caudal small intestine. The mechanism of toxin action is suggested to result in the secretion of anions and the inhibition of sodium absorption. This conclusion is based on studies of *in vitro* preparations of intestinal mucosa in which electrical parameters and ion fluxes were measured. Inhibition of phosphodiesterase activity also increases intracellular concentrations of cyclic AMP. Theophylline inhibits this enzyme and produces the same changes in ion fluxes and electrical parameters as enterotoxins in the *in vitro* preparation. However, when this drug is placed in the intestine it does not duplicate the massive secretory effects of enterotoxin in the *in vivo* animal models. The movement of ions in *in vitro* tissues represents micro amounts, and it has not been shown that these small changes in ion movements across an isolated sheet of cells represent what happens to cause massive secretion in *in vivo* loops in the intact animal.

During secretion passive ion fluxes across the membranes change in both directions. The permeability changes seen with enterotoxin-induced secretion are for ions only, since the permeability for small nonelectrolytes does not change. No significant structural alterations are evident by light or electron microscopy. Thus, unexplained permeability changes contribute to secretion in addition to changes in activity of biochemical mechanisms for anion secretion. The best-understood active ion-transport process in the intestine, that for glucose-dependent sodium transport, is not affected by enterotoxins.

Physical forces that determine passive movement across the intestinal mucosa influence the secretion of intestinal fluid. The bidirectional fluxes of fluid are dependent on Starling forces on the basal side of the epithelial cell. Effective intracapillary hydrostatic pressure is an important determinant of fluid secretion. Intra-arterial infusion of hormonal vasodilators, such as vasoactive intestinal peptide, glucagon, and prostaglandins, increases capillary pressure and produces secretion of fluid approximating that seen with enterotoxins.[83,84] Interstitial space changes disrupt the balance of the forces that maintain a steady state in the bidirectional fluxes between blood and intestinal lumen. Bacterial enterotoxin changes the gel-like structure in this space, so that increased amounts of plasma proteins escape into the interstitial space.[11] Toxin also changes the amount of structured water within the tissue, altering diffusion fluxes across the mucosa.[85] These physical and chemical changes in mucosal tissues that produce secretion may regulate normal secretion as well as represent a pathologic mechanism.

Intestinal fluid is secreted as a normal response to hypertonic solutions within the intestine. The osmotic stimulus draws interstitial fluid into the lumen. It also causes release of vasoactive peptides and biogenic amines, increasing capillary blood flow. These events can be exaggerated in pathological situations.

The regulation of normal intestinal secretion is poorly understood and probably involves an interaction of numerous factors. Relatively large volumes of secretion are normally produced during assimilation of a meal. Stimulation of that secretion is due to intraluminal factors, including bile acids and fatty acids that result from digestion, humoral factors (Table 15-3), and local paracrine/neural factors. To some degree the secretion of intestinal fluid may not actually be regulated but rather results from properties of the normal mucosa and the balance between physical, chemical, and electrical properties of the mucosa and the contents of the intestinal lumen.

Secretory Immunoglobulins.[86,87] The mucosa secretes immunoglobulins, which adhere to and protect the brush border surface (Chapter 3). The predominant immunoglobulin is of the IgA type, with some of the others also secreted. Plasma cells that have been transformed from sensitized B-lymphocytes synthesize IgA. Following secretion into the lamina propria, IgA is transported through the epithelial cell and transferred to the surface of the brush border. It is attached to the brush border surface by a peptide, called secretory piece, that epithelial cells synthesize.

Mucus Secretion.[88-90] Goblet cells secrete mucus in a gelatinous form. Secreted mucus spreads out and fuses with secretions of neighboring cells to form a continuous protective layer over the mucosal surface. This layer protects and stabilizes the microenvironment of the mucosa. The mucus layer traps microorganisms in the lumen of the small intestine. Peristalsis moves the layer caudal, reducing the numbers of bacteria in the small intestine. This also prevents colonization by foreign bacteria that are normally only transient. Mucus acts as a lubricant, and the amount secreted increases in the regions of the intestine where the contents are normally more solidified. Some mucins bind bacterial enterotoxins and inhibit their effects.[91] The mucosa responds to a toxin's presence by secreting copious amounts of mucus, a purposeful response in view of mucin's toxin-inactivating properties.

Mucus consists of a number of different substances or fluids with a high viscosity and contains significant amounts of bound carbohydrates, especially amino sugars. Glycoprotein, one type of mucin, consists of a core of protein with chains of carbohydrates attached. Chains consisting of neutral oligosaccharides produce neutral glycoproteins. Chains of sialic acid produce acid glycoproteins. Mucopolysaccharides are polymers of monosaccharides, of which some are amino sugars. They are neutral unless they contain uronic acid or sulfate esters, which give them acid properties. The mucopolysaccharides can be linked to a peptide or protein.

Secretion by Endocrine Cells. The hormones secreted by intestinal endocrine cells include peptides, such as secretin, cholecystokinin, enteroglucagon, vasoactive intestinal peptide, gastrin, and gastric inhibitory peptide; lipids, such as prostaglandins; and vasoactive amines, such as histamine, serotonin, kinins, etc. The physiological role of these chemicals is discussed in Chapter 1.

Absorption in Small and Large Intestines

Fluid and nutrients entering the small intestine are efficiently absorbed, allowing less than 5% to pass into the large intestine. Mechanisms are present to absorb digested nutrients, vitamins, and electrolytes. Small-intestinal absorption of water

Table 15-3. Chemicals stimulating intestinal secretion

Acetylcholine	VIP
Adenosine	Glucagon
ATP	Histamine
Bombesin	Neurotensin
Bradykinin	Motilin
Calcitonin	Prostaglandins
Cholecystokinin	Secretin
Gastrin	Serotonin
GIP	Substance P

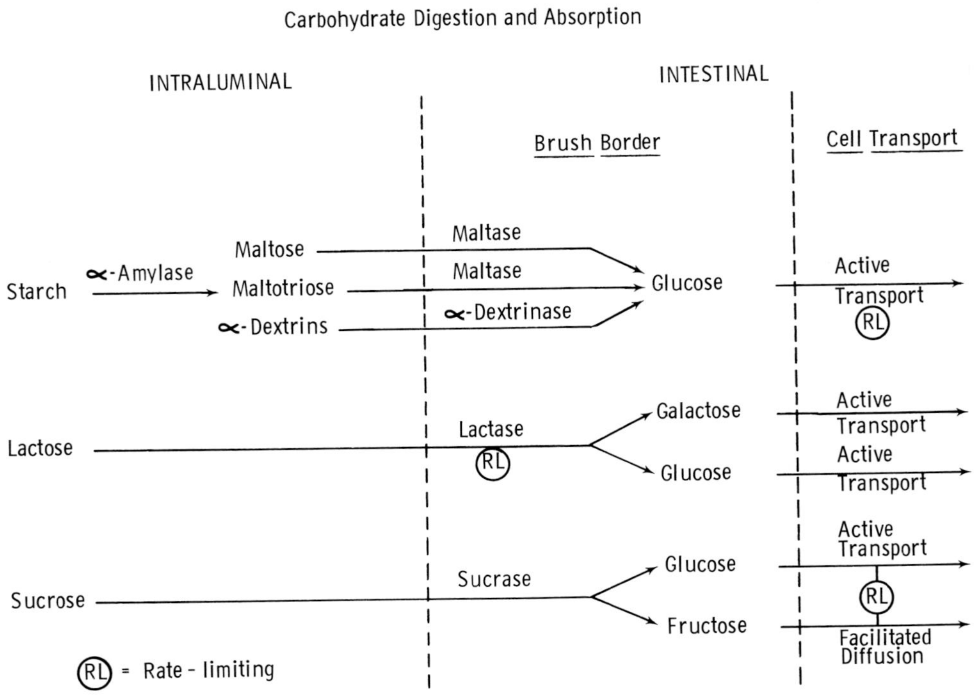

Figure 15-23. Digestion of carbohydrates by brush-border enzymes and mode of absorption of monosaccharides into the epithelial cell.

is largely a function of glucose and sodium absorption. Digested nutrients are absorbed in the small intestine. Some that pass into the large intestine can be fermented to products which can be absorbed. Fluid is absorbed in both the small and large intestines; with malabsorption of fluid in the small intestine, the colon has a reserve capacity for accommodating and absorbing additional fluid.

Absorption of Carbohydrates.[48,92-94] Carbohydrates must be in the form of a monosaccharide before absorption is possible (Figure 15-23). Monosaccharides are water-soluble molecules that are too large to move readily across cell membranes through the transport channels for water-soluble substances. The sugars glucose and galactose require a special mechanism to enter the epithelial cell. They bind to a brush border protein, which is suggested to function as a carrier that can translocate across the membrane and carry glucose to its intracellular surface, where it is released into the cytoplasm. Sodium ions determine the activity of this carrier, as is well documented in *in vitro* preparations. It has not been verified in the intact animal, since a glucose solution in the small intestine is absorbed readily whether sodium is added or not. When a sodium-free glucose solution is administered, however, it is likely that the passive serosal-to-lumen flux of sodium through the leaky tight junctions is large enough to provide a ready source of sodium for facilitating glucose absorption. Thus, sodium determines the absorption of glucose, but this mechanism is also a means for sodium absorption. Glucose transport is an energy-dependent process. The mechanism is able to move glucose up a concentration gradient, so that glucose can be absorbed from the intestine when intraluminal concentrations fall at the end of the absorptive process. Most of the glucose is delivered to the circulation in intact form. Some can be used for energy in the epithelial cell, resulting in the delivery to the circulation of metabolic intermediates such as lactate.

The electrochemical gradient for sodium determines hexose transport across the brush border. Sodium interacts with the transporting protein and enters the epithelial cell because of the gradient that results when low intracellular sodium levels and a negative electrical field attract a positively-charged ion. Glucose interacts with the sodium transport and is carried into the cell with sodium. The energy driving the sodium and glucose entry across the brush border is a derivative of ATP consumed by an ATPase on the basolateral cell membranes. Sodium and potassium stimulate the ATPase to transport sodium from the cell and, in exchange, to move potassium into the cell. Potassium does not accumulate excessively because it leaks from the cell continuously. The transport of sodium from the cell by the ATPase maintains very low intracellular concentrations of sodium, providing the chemical gradient for sodium to move from the lumen and across the brush border. A process of facilitated diffusion transports glucose from cells across basolateral membranes. The mechanism is not dependent on cotransport with sodium or any other ion, and an ATPase is not involved.

The carrier-mediated membrane transport of sugars is specific for glucose and galactose. The grouping at carbon-2 of a monosaccharide is most important in determining whether the sugar can be transported. If the hydroxyl at that site is altered to form the epimere of glucose or if it is substituted, the transport process is lost. Also important for the binding between sugar and carrier are the configurations at carbons 3, 4, and 6. Substitutions can be made on carbon-1 with the least effect on transport.

The other common monosaccharide in the diet, fructose, is a product of sucrose hydrolysis. Fructose moves across the brush border by diffusion, which is suggested to be facilitated by a special mechanism. Since the process is not energy-dependent, fructose cannot be absorbed against a gradient. The rate of fructose absorption is only 60% to 70% that of glucose. Fruc-

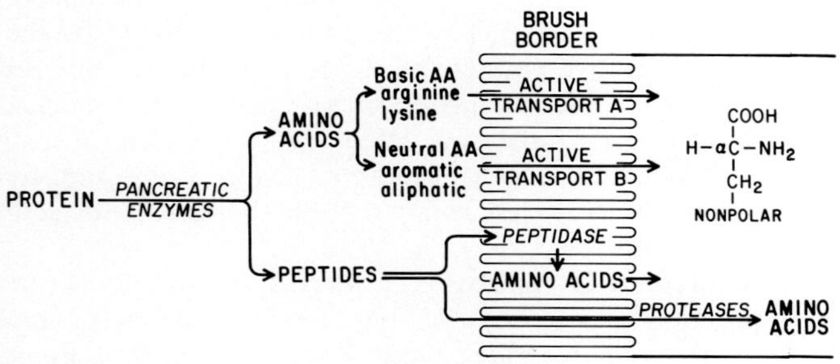

Figure 15-24. Diagram of digestion and absorption of dietary protein. Peptide absorption and the intracellular digestion route absorb protein more efficiently. Amino acid absorption is carried out by two different active transport processes, one for basic and one for neutral amino acids.

tose can be converted to glucose in the mucosal epithelial cell.

In a normal meal, most of the glucose is absorbed in the cranial half of the jejunum. Since glucose can be absorbed throughout the entire length of small intestine, the caudal half represents a reserve absorptive area. When mucosal disease develops, more than half of the area must be lost before sugar malabsorption becomes a problem.

Protein Absorption.[48,58,94,95] The absorption of proteins involves mechanisms for the absorption of amino acids and for the absorption of peptides and proteins. Amino acids are transported across the brush border membranes after combining with a carrier in the same manner as that for glucose. Sodium is required for this interaction. The amino acids are transported through the cytoplasm and actively extruded into the lateral intercellular space. The process requires energy, and amino acids are moved up a concentration gradient so that all the amino acids in the intestinal lumen can be effectively absorbed. Glucose and galactose compete with amino acids for transport. It is thought that the competition is for energy rather than for binding to a carrier common for their transport. Amino acids, with the exception of glutamine, are not metabolized during absorption.

There are different mechanisms for transporting different types of amino acids. The L-isomers are actively transported, whereas the D-isomers are absorbed by passive diffusion. Active transport is facilitated when the alpha-carbon is bonded to: 1) a free carboxyl group; 2) a free amino group; 3) a nonpolar R-group; or 4) a hydrogen (Figure 15-24). The neutral amino acids containing one amino and one carboxyl group are transported by active sodium-dependent carrier mechanisms that operate very rapidly and efficiently. Dibasic amino acids, such as lysine, arginine, ornithine, and cystine, are transported by an active and partially sodium-dependent mechanism. These amino acids are absorbed rapidly, although only 10% as fast as are the neutral ones. A third mechanism transports glycine and the amino acids proline and hydroxyproline. This mechanism is active and may be sodium-dependent, but the rate of transport is slow. A fourth carrier system is necessary for transport of the dicarboxylic acids, glutamic acid and aspartic acid. This mechanism operates rapidly, is probably active, and is partially sodium-dependent.

Special mechanisms at the basolateral membrane transport amino acids from epithelial cells. Transport is via a sodium-independent process that has no special energy requirements. The sodium gradient, which is established and maintained by an ATPase at the basolateral membrane, promotes amino acid uptake at the brush border. Thus, the mechanism is similar to that for hexose transport, where an energy-dependent process maintains sodium at very low intracellular levels.

Glutamine and glutamate are important sources of energy for intestinal epithelial cells. These amino acids can be removed from the circulation as well as being absorbed from the intestine. For uptake from the circulation the basolateral membrane has a sodium-dependent mechanism similar to that for other amino acids transported across the brush border.

The carrier mechanisms for the absorption of amino acids are identical in the intestine and proximal tubule of the kidneys. An occasional animal is born without one of these mechanisms. In humans, a deficiency of the mechanism to absorb neutral amino acids results in a clinical syndrome called Hartnup's disease. Deficiency develops for seven of the eight essential amino acids since they are not properly absorbed. That has not been recognized clinically in small animals, probably because they do not survive long after birth. The carrier mechanism to absorb dibasic amino acids is sometimes deficient in animals. Lysine is the only essential amino acid absorbed by this carrier, but that amino acid is also absorbed by passive diffusion and as a part of absorbed peptides, so no nutritional deficiency is apparent. Since this transport mechanism also recovers amino acids from the glomerular filtrate as it passes through the proximal tubule, a deficiency results in cystinuria from the failure of cystine reabsorption. This deficiency leads to the formation of cystine stones, which are seen occasionally in small animals.

Peptides are absorbed via mechanisms other than those for the amino acids. They are absorbed by the intestinal mucosa to provide an important means for protein assimilation. Peptides larger than three amino acids are not absorbed. Those of two and three amino acids are transported across the brush border by a sodium-independent mechanism. A proton gradient where the peptides are transported by a membrane carrier that carries hydrogen ions into the cell may drive peptide transport.[96] The observation of negative electrical potential inside the cell supports the idea that such a gradient exists. The proton gradient is thought to be established and maintained by an ATPase-driven transport of hydrogen ions across the basolateral membranes.

Absorption of amino acids is frequently more rapid from a solution of di- or tripeptides than from an equivalent solution of amino acids. There is little competition between amino acids for a common carrier when the dietary nitrogen is absorbed largely in the form of peptides. There is also no competition for absorption between amino acids and peptides, although there is between peptides. The specificity of the mechanisms for uptake does not appear to be great, since very dissimilar peptides inhibit each other's uptake. There may be more than one type of carrier with a specificity that is greater for one type of peptide. Peptides must have an unaltered amino and carboxyl terminal in order to have normal affinity for transport. They must contain L-isomers of amino acids to be absorbed. Peptides that are relatively nonpolar are absorbed more readily; once inside epithelial cells, peptides are hydrolyzed to amino acids.

Peptides are readily absorbed in the cranial part of the jejunum. There is evidence that peptide absorption is equally efficient in the ileum of some species but poor in others. Amino acids are absorbed throughout the small intestine, although more readily from the cranial part. The absorption of dietary protein, like that of carbohydrates, is essentially completed in the first half of the small intestine. The remainder of the small intestine represents a reserve.

Since protein malnutrition does not develop with a deficiency of the amino acid transport systems, peptide absorption must be an important means for absorption of protein. When gluten-induced enteropathy reduces the mucosal surface area, the number of amino acid carriers is reduced. The absorption of peptides, however, is not reduced as severely as that of amino acids. The same reduction in mucosal surface area is evident in patients with chronic overgrowth of the intestinal microflora. Villous changes can be seen with pancreatic enzyme deficiencies that cause secondary bacterial overgrowth. The differential absorption rate of amino acids and peptides has therapeutic implications. Elemental diets are frequently used to treat chronic intestinal mucosal disease and enzyme deficiencies. These diets contain amino acids as their nitrogen source. Since it is evident that peptides are absorbed more readily than amino acids, peptides are a better source of nitrogen in elemental diets fed to patients with mucosal disease or enzyme deficiency. Peptides are absorbed more readily than amino acids in animals with no pancreatic enzymes.[97] Thus, elemental diets containing oligopeptides are nutritionally and economically more advantageous than diets containing a mixture of amino acids.

Proteins can be absorbed intact from the small intestine.[98] They bind to brush border receptors and are absorbed by pinocytosis. Once inside the cell, cytoplasmic and lysosomal proteases degrade most proteins to amino acid. Some proteins are not degraded and leave the cell to enter the portal circulation, as has been shown to be the case with serum albumin placed in the small intestine. Following absorption, these foreign antigens can sensitize the animal. This causes immune reactions at a time of reexposure to and absorption of the antigen. A great number of foreign proteins are absorbed and

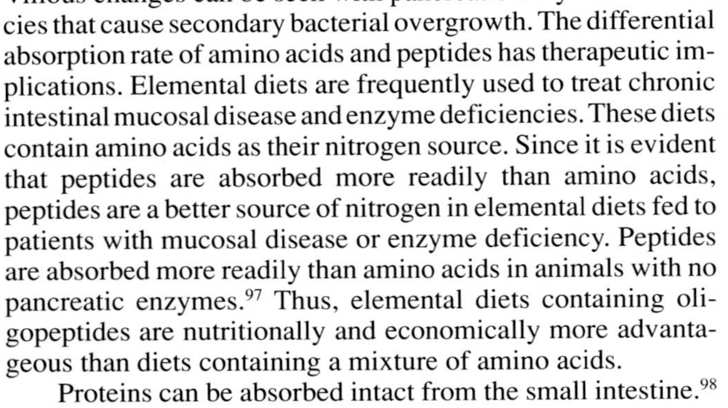

Figure 15-25. Diagram of absorption of dietary fat in the intestine. Micelles enter the brush-border membranes, where they break up and release their constituents. Fatty acids and monoglycerides enter the cell, and bile acids return to the lumen of the intestine. The components entering the cell are reesterified by triglycerides, after which they are formed into chylomicrons by the addition of a lipoprotein coating that also contains lipids. After transport from the cell the chylomicrons enter the lymphatics. Bile acids are absorbed by the ileum and recycled for use twice each meal.

remain immunologically competent after passage through the mucosal epithelial cell. They are normally removed by the monocyte phagocytic system of the liver. Failure of this removal results in the production of many antibodies against antigens absorbed from the gut. Bacterial enterotoxins can also be absorbed intact. They are quite resistant to digestion by cytoplasmic proteases but are susceptible to digestion by acid lysosomal proteases.[99]

Absorption of Lipids.[65,100-102] For fat absorption to be normal, micelles are formed. They contain bile acids, fatty acids, and monoglycerides, with a small amount of lipid-soluble vitamins and cholesterol. The intact micelle moves from the lumen of the gut into the lipid part of the brush-border membrane (Figure 15-25). This movement is due to passive diffusion. Within the membrane the micelle breaks up and bile acids move back out of the membrane into the lumen of the intestine. The free fatty acids and monoglycerides released from the micelle diffuse either into the cell or back into the lumen of the gut. After movement into the cell the endoplasmic reticulum rapidly esterifies them to form triglycerides. This process traps lipid digestion products in the cell, since triglycerides cannot back-diffuse across the cell membrane. The removal of fatty acids and monoglycerides by reesterification maintains a gradient of high levels outside the cell and low levels inside, which is the force for passive movement into the cell. Triglycerides are absorbed incompletely only if their fatty acid composition is unusual (containing a high percentage of saturated or long-chain fatty acids).

The length of the carbon chain in fatty acids determines its mode and pathway of absorption. Fatty acids with carbon chains of 10 or less are sufficiently polar to have some degree of water solubility. When triglycerides containing short-chain fatty acids are hydrolyzed, the water-soluble products are absorbed through the brush-border membranes without being incorporated into micelles. Short-chain fatty acids diffuse rapidly into the cell, and, if not reesterified, they are transported from the intestine by the portal circulation. Triglycerides that contain medium- or short-chain fatty acids are absorbed to some degree without being hydrolyzed. Thus, less lipase activity is required for their assimilation. As described, the barrier to absorption through the cell membrane consists of the lipid membrane with the unstirred layer of water attracted to it. The lipid layer is a barrier to movement of polar fatty substances such as medium- and short-chain fatty acids, while the unstirred water layer is a barrier to movement of long-chain fatty acids, which are relatively nonpolar.

Monoglycerides and fatty acids are resynthesized to triglycerides inside the cell. They are formed by the direct acylation of monoglycerides, which accounts for about 80% of the lipids that appear in the chylomicrons. The other 20% of triglycerides transported from the cell are formed from glycerol synthesized through the glycerophosphate and dihydroxyacetone phosphate pathways. That is important when little monoglyceride remains to provide a framework for direct acylation. Glycerol released during the intraluminal hydrolysis of triglycerides is water-soluble and enters the cell much more rapidly than the monoglycerides and fatty acids. There, it is metabolized for energy or it can enter the circulation. Either way, it is lost for the resynthesis of triglycerides, since not all the units needed for resynthesis are present within the cell at the same time. Long-chain fatty acids in epithelial cells promote the synthesis of triglycerides. The enzymes catalyzing this action are concentrated in the cranial small intestine, where most fat absorption takes place. These enzymes are found in the endoplasmic reticulum. Increasing the fat content of the diet augments their activity. The enzymes require adrenocorticosteroid hormones to maintain their levels of activity. Adrenal insufficiency can cause malabsorption of fat, the result of a decreased ability to esterify fats in the cell. The levels of reesterifying enzymes are reduced during starvation. This situation illustrates the importance of using low-fat diets when feeding is resumed after a long fast. Lipases are found in the cell, and their action is primarily on triglycerides made up of medium-chain fatty acids. These lipids are preferentially hydrolyzed and not resynthesized, so their components are transferred to the portal circulation.

In contrast to the relatively rapid absorption and appearance of triglycerides in the lymph, cholesterol, which enters the cell in the micelle, distributes throughout the cell and leaves slowly, with a half-life of about 12 hours. Half of the cholesterol that enters the cell is lost when normal desquamation occurs. Cholesterol can also be synthesized by the cell, with the rate unaffected by fasting or feeding. Bile, however, inhibits cholesterologenesis. Dietary cholesterol can be esterified with fatty acids. Some cholesterol ester hydrolases are present that break this bond, and others are found that promote synthesis of the ester. Cholesterol is absorbed more readily into the cell when it is not esterified. Most of the cholesterol that leaves the cell to enter the lymph is esterified.

Lipids are transported from the intestine within chylomicrons, which consist of a core of triglyceride, cholesterol ester, and free cholesterol surrounded by a coating of phospholipid, cholesterol, and protein. Chylomicrons are produced only after a meal. The chylomicrons are formed in the endoplasmic reticulum and can be stored in the golgi apparatus. They are subsequently released into the intercellular spaces by exocytosis. During fasting periods, smaller fat-containing particles are found in the mucosal cell and lymph. Designated as very low-density lipoproteins, they contain triglycerides and cholesterol. During fat absorption these particles take up more triglyceride and expand to form the larger chylomicrons. Synthesis of a protein to produce beta-lipoproteins is essential for chylomicrons to leave the epithelial cell. If synthesis of this protein is deficient or depressed, triglycerides accumulate in the cell, with fat malabsorption following. A deficiency of this lipoprotein is recognized in some humans. A reduction in protein synthesis is a feature of other mucosal diseases, such as gluten-induced enteropathy. In this case, the deficiency results in a decreased esterification of triglycerides, as well as reduced lipid transport from the cell. Any drugs that inhibit protein synthesis have this effect. Diets rich in triglycerides that contain medium-chain fatty acids bypass both of these defects, since the shorter-chain fatty acids need not be reesterified or incorporated into chylomicrons and are transported into the portal circulation.

Lipids are digested and absorbed primarily by chemical processes instead of regulated physiologic functions. Lipase activity is normally in great excess, so the rate of digestion is not a rate-limiting step in fat assimilation. Micelle formation has been suggested to be rate-limiting, but lipase activity and bile acids are normally abundant so that micelles can be readily formed. Under some circumstances solubilization of lipolytic products by micelles may be reduced, giving micellar formation the appearance of being a rate-limiting step. Uptake across the brush border is probably the most important step determining lipid assimilation in the jejunum. The unstirred water layer is the major barrier for uptake of large molecular structures such as micelles, and the lipid membrane is the major barrier against diffusion by smaller molecules. Limits may also exist for intracellular reesterification of lipids and their incorporation into chylomicrons. Reesterification usually is not limiting for lipid assimilation. Chylomicron formation can be limiting for fat assimilation in the ileum. The ileum is not prepared to absorb large amounts of lipids. When dietary fats are excessive and escape assimilation in the jejunum, the ileum may not be able to synthesize lipoproteins fast enough for their transport from the epithelial cell. Thus, the rate-limiting step for fat assimilation is not the same for different regions of the small intestine. The size of the surface area of the mucosa becomes important when it is reduced by disease, and under such circumstances surface area size becomes a rate-limiting step. Disease of the epithelial cell is seldom recognized as a factor unless the total number of cells is reduced.

Following absorption, chylomicrons are transported through lymphatics, and their obstruction can cause malabsorption. Lymphangiectasia, caused by obstruction, usually results from occlusion of lymph channels by granulomatous processes. Management of lymphangiectasia includes feeding triglycerides containing medium to short-chain fatty acids, which are absorbed through the portal circulation.

Bile acids are essential for micellar formation. An enterohepatic circulation sustains levels of bile acids in the intestine.[103] The recirculation of bile acid involves release of bile into the intestine from the gall bladder and biliary system, absorption from the small intestine, and uptake from the blood by the liver, followed by resecretion into the biliary system. This process must be efficient and rapid, since the entire pool of bile acids in the body is small and must be recycled two or three times during a single meal. Most bile acids are absorbed in the ileum by an active energy-requiring and sodium-dependent mechanism.

Bile acids are transported up a concentration gradient, a process that is inhibited by the same drugs that inhibit sodium transport. A loss of this function of the ileum results in bile-acid deficiency and fat malabsorption, since the synthesis of new bile acids by the liver cannot increase enough to supply the animal's needs. Some absorption of bile acids occurs via passive diffusion, depending on the species of animal and the type of bile acid. If the pKa of a bile acid is low, it is in its ionized form at neutral pHs. Taurocholate has a low pKa and is quite lipid insoluble because it is ionized. Consequently, it does not readily cross lipid-cell membranes by diffusion. Little taurocholate is absorbed from the jejunum of the dog.[104] Bacteria can deconjugate bile acids in the intestine, removing the amino acid; the products formed have a pKa that is greater than that of the conjugated form. Thus, the unconjugated bile acid is un-ionized near neutral pH, is lipid-soluble, and can cross cell membranes readily. Bacterial overgrowth of the intestinal microflora can deconjugate an excessive amount of bile acids. This activity results in rapid absorption of bile acids from the intestine, which leads to a bile acid deficiency and malabsorption of lipids. In summary, the absorption of fats depends upon adequate concentrations of bile acids in the intestine. This is influenced by reabsorption of bile acids in the ileum and by a minimum amount of deconjugation, which is achieved by control of the bacterial numbers in the intestine.

Gastric functions determine lipid assimilation. Gastric motility is essential for trituration of food in order to release nutrients sequestered within particles. Reducing gastric motility by vagotomy and antrectomy in dogs impairs particle size reduction, and less dietary fat is absorbed from a solid but not a liquid diet.[105] The nature of the diet also determines lipid assimilation. Fat assimilation is 97% complete in dogs fed a meat-base diet with a fat content of 35% of dry matter. When fed a cereal-based diet with a fat content of 11% of dry matter, fat assimilation is only 90% complete. Less fat is digested and absorbed when dogs are fed a cereal diet with a poorer digestibility.[106] Differences in lipid assimilation also develop when the relative amounts of saturated to unsaturated fats increase; then lipid absorption increases.[107]

Fiber Regulation of Assimilation.[108] Dietary factors other than carbohydrate, protein, and lipid content affect overall digestion and absorption of all nutrients. Diets that delay gastric emptying enhance assimilation. High-fat diets as described earlier slow gastric emptying; fibers such as pectin and guar gum have the same effect by increasing viscosity of gastric contents. Similar effects are suggested for small intestinal transit time, but no reliable conclusions can be made. Dietary fiber reduces activities of pancreatic digestive enzymes. Fiber that binds and increases fecal excretion of bile acids can reduce fat assimilation. Absorption of all nutrients is reduced by fiber that maintains luminal contents at such a high viscosity that contact is reduced between nutrients and the brush border. The mucosal surface area determines overall absorptive capacities. Fiber in the diet reduces villus numbers and surface area; feeding cereal-based high fiber diets does not result in the optimum mucosal area for absorption that is found with meat-based low residue diets.

Fiber is an important undigestable component of cell walls in unrefined foods. That fiber as well as fiber added to refined foods limits the digestibility of refined foods. Cell-wall fiber prevents release of carbohydrates, proteins, and lipids until digestion of the fiber by colonic bacteria. Evaluation of digestibility of carbohydrates is made by the glycemic response, the degree of hyperglycemia that the carbohydrate produces after feeding. In addition to the type of food, the form of the food ingested determines the glycemic response. For example, consuming whole rice results in flattened glucose and insulin responses, whereas consuming ground rice results in plasma increases for both glucose and insulin.

Increasing dietary fiber increases fecal excretion of nitrogen. The effect is caused primarily by an increase in growth for colonic bacteria. The increased bacterial mass is promoted by an increase in flow of unassimilated nutrients (fiber, carbohydrate, protein and lipids) from the small intestine. The nitrogen entering the colon sustains bacterial growth but the amount escaping assimilation in the small intestine is not sufficient to result in a nitrogen imbalance. Relatively small amounts escape digestion and absorption because of additional fiber in the diet.

High dietary fiber, either as part of natural foods in the diet or as fiber added to the diet, increases fecal fat. Fat in a higher fiber cereal-based diet is not as completely assimilated as fat in lower fiber meat-based diets. Both lipid digestion and absorption are impaired. In addition, as described earlier, fiber promotes fecal losses for bile acids; reduced bile acid availability results in greater lipid malassimilation.

Colonic Digestion and Absorption.[109,110] Digestion and absorption are important to normal colonic physiology. Colonic bacteria metabolize carbohydrates, proteins and lipids to produce a number of products that are excreted or absorbed. Bacteria metabolize carbohydrates to short-chain fatty acids (acetic, propionic, and butyric acids) and gases (hydrogen, methane, and carbon dioxide). Colonic mucosal cells metabolize some butyrate; the liver clears the remaining butyrate and propionate. Peripheral tissues take up and metabolize acetate. The carbohydrates entering the colon include non-starch polysaccharides (dietary fiber), starch (which can amount to 10% to 20% of total dietary starch), and small amounts of sugars (such as lactose) and oligosaccharides (such as raffinose and stachyose). Dietary fiber is metabolized or fermented to different degrees, depending on its source and structure. Lignification of cell walls reduces fermentation, as for example with bran. Increases in water solubility enhance digestibility. Other factors determining digestibility of polysaccharides include particle size, molecular structure, effect of food processing, the type of gut microflora, and transit time.

Unassimilated starch may represent the most important substrate for bacterial fermentation in the colon. Starch can escape digestion for a number of reasons. It may appear in the diet as ungelatinized starch granules, or because the diet contains alpha-amylase inhibitors, or because of reduced availability in complexes with other foods such as fat or protein, or because the starch is not released from unmilled grains. Fermentation of polysaccharides allows the colon to salvage carbohydrates escaping assimilation in the small intestine. That salvage may not significantly add to the animal's nutritional needs, but it does remove substances that contribute to increased fecal volume that in some cases results in diarrhea. The absorption of short-chain fatty acids promotes sodium and water absorption. Loss of that substrate could inhibit sodium absorption to the degree that diarrhea follows.

Absorption of Water and Electrolytes.[111-115] The absorption of water in the small and large intestine is a passive process that follows the transport of solutes across the cell. The net movement of fluid from the mucosal to the serosal border of the cell can be conceived of as the difference between the two

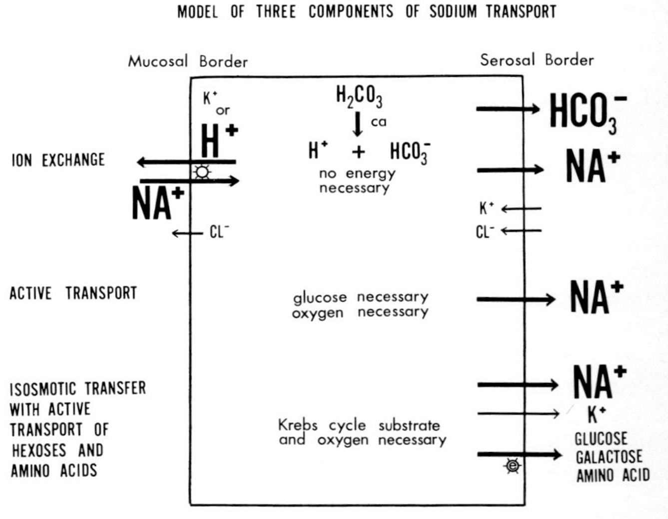

Figure 15-26. Schematic of intestinal epithelial cell, showing the three mechanisms for the nonpassive movement of sodium from the lumen of the gut into the circulation.

bidirectional fluxes found across the cell. This movement of fluid, dependent on energy, is determined by the transport of nonelectrolyte solutes and sodium. A number of different factors, such as the leakiness of the membrane and regulation of the circulation, influence the efficiency of transport.

Solute-mediated Fluid Transfer. The absorption of fluid is related directly to the absorption of a solute. The absorption of fluid in the jejunum largely results from the transport of sodium that can be coupled to the transport of a monosaccharide or amino acid. Sodium is the essential solute for fluid absorption in the distal ileum and the colon. During glucose absorption, movement across the brush border depends on an interaction between an actively transported monosaccharide and sodium (Figure 15-26). Glucose and glutamine supply energy. Some actively transported hexoses are not metabolized by epithelial cells. Galactose is actively transported with sodium, but galactose is not metabolized, and so transport ceases until the cell is provided with sources of energy.

Fructose is not coupled with sodium during its transport by a special carrier into epithelial cells. When fructose is the only sugar present, sodium still influxes into the cell but the flux is less than with glucose. Fructose uptake carries water passively by solvent drag, where the osmotic force generated by movement of solute particles moves the water. Fructose also supports sodium transport by another mechanism, because it can be converted to glucose and become source of energy. Thus, during hexose transport sodium can enter the cell through more than one process. In one, sodium is coupled with an actively transported sugar, and in another, it requires no accompanying nonelectrolyte. After feeding, the cotransport with hexoses and amino acids is responsible for 56% of the sodium absorbed by mucosal cells.

Nonelectrolyte-dependent sodium entry into epithelial cells provides a second important means for fluid absorption. Sodium can couple with chloride and move across brush borders by diffusion. Sodium moves down an electrochemical gradient through membranes that are semipermeabile to sodium diffusion. After feeding, this flux is responsible for absorption of 37% of the total sodium; in the unfed state it represents 85% of the total sodium absorbed.

A third and minor mechanism for fluid absorption is a sodium-hydrogen ion exchange. The exchange operates in association with an exchange mechanism for chloride and bicarbonate ions. The cation exchanges are responsible for 10% to 15% of the sodium that enters mucosal cells. In the jejunum sodium-hydrogen ion exchange causes luminal fluid to be slightly acid (Figure 15-26). On the other hand, secretions in the ileum and colon are slightly alkaline since there is a very active bicarbonate-chloride exchange process. The secretion of large amounts of bicarbonate in these regions negates the effect of hydrogen ions secreted by the sodium-hydrogen ion exchange process. If, however, chloride is replaced by a large anion, such as sulfate, that the bicarbonate cannot exchange with, ileal contents become acid from the ongoing sodium-hydrogen exchange. Carbonic anhydrase inhibitors reduce net sodium absorption in the ileum, which illustrates the importance of the exchange mechanism to the transport of sodium in this region of the intestine.

During the absorption of glucose or galactose, large intracellular concentrations can be produced. Glucose leaves the cell across the basal borders via facilitated diffusion, following the concentration gradient created by high levels inside the cell and low levels outside. Water moves with the glucose due to osmotic attraction. Ions in the water are carried along. This movement of ions across the cell is called solvent drag. The sugar osmotically drags the solvent, and the ions within the solvent are not selectively separated out.

In contrast to the passive movement of glucose, sodium is transported from the cell by a special mechanism. The basal lateral membranes contain transport mechanisms that actively move sodium from a low concentration in the cell to a high one in the intercellular space. Water follows osmotically into the space, causing it to enlarge, a change that is morphologically evident in mucosa that is actively transporting fluid. Hydrostatic pressure increases in the intercellular space. The fluid flows out into the interstitial space and is carried away by the microcirculation. The membrane transport mechanism is specific for sodium and requires energy supplied by glucose. This area of the cell membrane is a rich source of Na-K-dependent ATPase, an enzyme stimulated by sodium and potassium. The enzyme splits ATP and releases high levels of energy. In most species this enzyme is inhibited by cardiac glycosides, chemicals that also inhibit active sodium transport. Hence, the ATPase is either the sodium pump or provides energy for it. An electrical charge is generated across some tissues when its cells actively transport sodium. The electrical charge occurs when the transport does not involve a cation- or anion-exchange process or a tightly coupled accompaniment of an anion. The electrical charge results from a transport of sodium that is not associated with an equal and simultaneous movement of anions. The result is a slight excess of positive sodium ions on the serosal border and a slight excess of anions left behind on the luminal border, creating a measurable potential difference across the cell.

The leakiness of the tight junctions determines whether the epithelial surface maintains gradients for both ion concentrations and electrical potentials across cell membranes. These junctions are very leaky in the duodenum and jejunum, and fluid that is transported into the intercellular space is able to diffuse freely, through the leaky junctions between cells, back into the lumen of the gut. Thus, any differences in ion concentrations between the two sides of the cell become equalized. This equalization is unimportant in the jejunum since the primary force for the absorption of fluid there is glucose and amino acid transport. The direction of glucose movement is always toward the serosal side of the cell, so the flow to move sodium by solvent drag is always in that direction.

The glucose- and amino acid-mediated absorption of sodium is most important in the jejunum. In the distal ileum and colon, absorption of sodium is not coupled to transport of other solutes. The cell-to-cell junctions in these tissues are tight and relatively nonleaky, allowing the tissues to create high concentrations of sodium on the serosal side of the cell from low luminal levels. If the junctions were leaky, it would make the absorption of sodium a very inefficient process, since much of it would leak back before it had a chance to leave the intercellular space.

Apical membranes of colonic epithelial cells are less permeable than those of the small intestine to the entry of sodium. In the colon, sodium entry is the rate-limiting step for absorption. Sodium entry is driven by an electrochemical gradient, where sodium moves by diffusion from a high concentration in the lumen to a very low concentration intracellularly.

The colonic epithelial cell generates a greater electrical potential difference across its membranes than small intestinal cells do, and that electrical activity also promotes diffusion across apical membranes. Entry across those membranes occurs through pores; movement through the pores is inhibited by amiloride and high luminal sodium concentrations and is promoted by aldosterone and high luminal anion concentrations. An ATPase driven by sodium and potassium, with their exchange promoted across the basolateral membrane, transports sodium from colonic epithelial cells. Glucocorticoids and mineralocorticoids stimulate the transport. Sodium does not leak back into the cell, because the basolateral membranes are highly impermeable to sodium diffusion. The permeability is greater for potassium, which allows its diffusion from the cell.

About 2.7 liters of fluid must be absorbed each day in a 20-kg animal. Half of this is absorbed in the jejunum, and 75% of the remaining 1,350 ml is absorbed in the ileum. About 350 ml remains to enter the colon, where almost 90% is absorbed.

The movements of potassium, bicarbonate, and chloride as described can be summarized. Potassium movements are entirely passive throughout the small intestine. Their movement follows concentration and electrical gradients. Thus, some potassium will move from the lumen to the cell when concentrations in the lumen are high. Most of the potassium is absorbed by solvent drag, in the jejunum as a result of glucose and amino acid transport, and in the ileum as a result of sodium transport. Regardless of whether there is net absorption of potassium or whether the fluxes are in steady state, the concentration of the ion is higher in intestinal contents than in plasma water. The electrical potential difference, with the lumen negative, attracts potassium, a cation with a positive charge that is attracted to a negatively charged site. Thus, loss of fluid from any site in the gastrointestinal tract is accompanied by a greater potassium loss than water loss, leaving the animal more depleted in potassium than in water. The potential difference across the small intestine is small, so that the levels of potassium are not excessively greater in small intestinal secretion than in body fluids. The potential difference across the large intestine is greater than in the small intestine; it can be as great as 30 to 50 millivolts. This greater potential causes the secretion of large amounts of potassium into the colon. The secretion of potassium can produce concentrations that approach 100 mEq/L. Since the potential difference cannot account for an amount that great, the entire amount secreted requires an additional mechanism. Either sodium and water absorption is more complete at a site that is relatively impermeable to potassium and distal to the location for high potassium permeability, or a mechanism exists for active secretion of potassium. The active component may be represented by ATPase activity, driven by sodium and potassium at the basolateral membrane; that activity would lead to their loading of cells with potassium and would promote diffusion across the apical border. The active component may also be an apical membrane potassium conductance regulated by intracellular cyclic AMP and calcium levels, with increases in conductance promoting potassium secretion.

The anions chloride and bicarbonate are passively absorbed in the jejunum by solvent drag, created by glucose and amino acid absorption. The chloride for the bicarbonate-exchange mechanism is present in the jejunum, but its effects are dwarfed by the large amount of fluid and ions moved via solvent drag. The mechanism is not apparent in the fed state. Chloride and bicarbonate are not absorbed by passive forces via solvent drag in the ileum. Thus, the effects of the chloride-bicarbonate exchange mechanism are evident in the ileal contents, which are high in bicarbonate and low in chloride. The low concentration of bicarbonate in the jejunum does not imply that the ion is actively transported from a region of low concentration to one of high concentration, fulfilling the criteria for active transport. Bicarbonate is low in the jejunum, since hydrogen ions secreted in the exchange process react with bicarbonate to form carbonic acid and the evolution of carbon dioxide. Bicarbonate is lost in the carbon dioxide that is absorbed. The chloride-bicarbonate exchange process operates in the colon so that the colonic contents are normally alkaline.

In summary, the fluid entering the colon from the ileum contains sodium at a level the same as that in plasma water. Thus, the colon normally absorbs up to 40 mEq sodium in the 20-kg animal, in addition to 300 ml water. An equivalent amount of chloride is absorbed. Bicarbonate and potassium are secreted. The large electrical potential difference is the result of an active sodium-transport process through a tissue that has a relatively impermeable tight junction. The anion movements are the result of the exchange mechanism, and potassium secretion is passive.

Regulation of Fluid Absorption. The absorption of fluid, just like that of secretion, is influenced by forces determined by the circulation (Figure 15-21). The colloid osmotic pressure of the plasma and interstitial fluid, hydrostatic pressure in the capillaries and interstitial fluid, and osmotic forces in the lumen of the intestine determine the absorption of fluid and electrolytes. In the normal state the fluid entering the small intestine is isosmotic, so that osmolality is not a factor affecting absorption. Changes in pressure in the lumen of the gut have no effect on the absorption of fluid unless the pressure is so great that circulation of the tissue is compromised. Increases up to a pressure of 40 cm of water have no effect. Most of the changes that can occur to alter the physical forces are found on the serosal side of the cell. Small changes in pressure on the cell's serosal side markedly affect fluid absorption. Increases of less than 5 cm of water decrease absorption, and greater increases can result in secretion of fluid. That result can be readily demonstrated in *in vitro* preparations of intestinal mucosa.[116] It can also be shown in dogs by infusing large amounts of saline to increase hydrostatic pressure in the microcirculation of the mucosa. Such a procedure depresses the absorption of fluid.[117] Obstructing either lymphatic or venous drainage can also produce hydrostatic pressure increases. Lymphangiectasia is recognized in clinical cases, and the diarrhea that results is due in part to an impairment of fluid absorption. With increased venous pressure, there is a good capacity for compensation before absorption is severely impaired. The colloid osmotic pressure falls in the interstitial fluid as the hydrostatic pressure increases, and this response has a dilutional effect, which ends in promoting fluxes of fluid into the capillary and lymphatics.[118] Portal hypertension increases interstitial hydrostatic pressure, as seen in problems that range from cardiac disease to hepatic disease. In an attempt to reduce the intracapillary pressure there is a reflex change in arteriolar resistance in the microcirculation, but the net effect of increased pressure remains, and the absorption of fluid is inhibited. As would be expected, an increased plasma colloid osmotic pressure increases the absorption of fluid from the intestine. The epithelium is a leaky membrane that permits ready movement of fluids in either direction in response to osmotic gradients.

Fluid absorption is probably not affected by osmotic forces in clinical cases unless measurable changes in colloid osmotic pressure can be demonstrated. Dogs made acutely hypoalbuminemic by plasmapheresis develop diarrhea.[119] Diarrhea can begin when albumin is at or below 2.0 gm per deciliter. Plasma proteins are lost at an excessive rate in many animals with gastrointestinal problems. Reductions in plasma oncotic pressure follow and may contribute to difficulties in management of a diarrhea.

It is evident that blood flow has an effect on the absorption of many substances from the lumen of the intestine.[112] When blood flow is reduced below a normal resting rate, the absorption of most substances decreases. When the rate is increased, the absorption increases for lipid solutes and small un-ionized water-soluble solutes. The absorption of larger solutes is unaffected by blood flow. The mucosal absorption of solutes is a function of their rate of transfer across the epithelial surface and the rate of removal from the lamina propria by the circulation. The absorption of solutes that can pass across the barrier with relative ease will be very dependent on blood flow. The rate-limiting process is the crossing of the barrier by substances that require a special mechanism to cross the cell. Blood flow is not an important factor in determining their rate of absorption. The clinical importance of circulation on absorption relates mostly to states in which interstitial hydrostatic pressure is increased or colloid osmotic pressure is decreased, in which case fluid absorption is affected regardless of the solute that moves it.

Absorptive mechanisms in epithelial cells operate at fixed rates once they are stimulated with a goal of complete absorption for a solute. Epithelial cell absorption may be regulated by neural and endocrine/ paraendocrine mechanisms.[120] Chemicals released following stimulation of neural pathways, endocrines, and paracrines can influence epithelial cell function (Table 15-4). Studies done mostly on isolated tissues or cells show that many different chemicals have an effect on epithelial cell transport. The importance of any one chemical is not known. The knowledge that these chemicals can affect transport holds promise; drugs that alter electrolyte transport may be developed as a management for diarrhea.

Absorption of Iron.[121,122] The absorption of iron is regulated, which is important since iron has no avenue of excretion from the body. The amount in the diet is almost always adequate. Since the rate of iron absorption is small, it is currently recommended that 10 mg of iron be consumed with each 1,000 calories of food in order to maintain normal iron stores. In general, only 50% of the iron is released from food during its digestion. The percentage is less for cereals and vegetables, and greater for most digested animal proteins.

After digestion releases the iron, the absorption rate remains optimum as long as the iron remains in solution. The ferrous form of iron is absorbed better than the ferric form. Chelation with a large mucopolysaccharide secreted in the stomach and with ascorbate, citrate, some hexoses, and certain amino acids maintains iron in a soluble form. The iron remains in this form until the complex comes in contact with the brush-border membrane. Iron that fails to be chelated is changed at the higher pH of the small intestine and precipitates as ferric hydroxide. Bile, possibly as a result of its ascorbate content, facilitates iron absorption. Acid secretion in the stomach is important for maintaining iron as soluble as possible, especially the ferric form. Acid assists in the formation of soluble iron chelates of ascorbic acid. Not all forms of iron are effectively prepared by acid for optimal absorption. The iron in egg is not effectively released by acid in the stomach. Acid reduces rather than enhances the absorption of iron in hemoglobin, since acid renders heme insoluble. Heme is absorbed intact by the small intestinal mucosa, however, after which iron is released within the cell. Phosphates and carbonates form salts with iron that are relatively insoluble. Pancreatic bicarbonate reduces iron absorption; pancreatic exocrine deficiency promotes iron uptake.

Iron is absorbed mainly in the duodenum and the first part of the jejunum. The transport of iron from the cell to the circulation requires a special system, found in this cranial region of the gut. This system is the rate-limiting step in the absorptive process. Less iron is able to enter the mucosal cell at more caudal sites, since less survives in soluble form as the pH of gut contents increases. Ferrous iron is transported across the

Table 15-4. Chemicals Stimulating Intestinal Absorption

Aldosterone	Insulin
Angiotensin	Neuropeptide Y
Catecholamines	Somatostatin
Enkephalins	Vasopressin
Glucocorticoid	

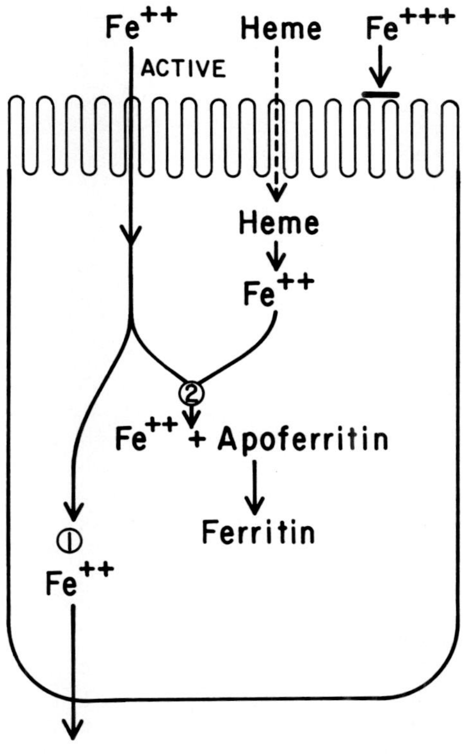

Figure 15-27. Diagram to show the absorption of iron in the small intestine. Only the ferrous form enters the cell, and that is due to an active transport mechanism. Iron passes through the cell and is absorbed unless apoferritin is present to sequester it. The amount of apoferritin in the cell determines the regulation of absorption.

brush-border by an active ATP energy-requiring process (Figure 15-27). It is either stored in a ferrous iron pool or transported out of the cell. The cell synthesizes a number of iron-binding proteins, and ferrous iron entering the cell is bound to it to form a complex, the most well-known being ferritin. If no binding protein is present, the ferrous iron is transported across the serosal border and, upon reaching the circulation, binds to a plasma-transporting protein called transferritin.

Events that take place in the immature epithelial cells before they migrate out of the crypt determine the rate of absorption of iron by villous epithelial cells. If stores of iron are low in the body, little plasma ferrous iron enters the crypt cells, and as a result, there is little stimulation to synthesize iron-binding proteins. When the cell migrates to the villus, there is little or no protein for bind iron entering the cell. Consequently, most of the iron is transferred to the circulation. On the other hand, with a large store of iron in the body, iron entering crypt cells stimulates iron-binding protein synthesis. This subsequently results in the binding of most of the absorbed ferrous iron in cells at the villus site. The iron is not released to the circulation, and it is lost into the lumen of the gut when the cell desquamates. The release of iron from heme in the cell is also regulated. Excessive ferrous iron in the absorptive cell inhibits the enzyme that hydrolyses heme, and no additional iron is released.

Absorption of Calcium.[123,124] Calcium absorption, like iron absorption, is dependent on digestive processes in the stomach and small intestine. Special mechanisms are present to absorb calcium; mechanisms that are more sophisticated than those for iron absorption regulate calcium absorption. Iron and calcium are both divalent cations less readily absorbed than a monovalent cation such as sodium. Since calcium is the most abundant cation in the body, there must be special mechanisms to ensure that adequate amounts are absorbed. In contrast, the needs for iron are small, and its absorptive mechanism is designed to prevent iron overload by limiting the rate of absorption instead of facilitating it.

Calcium absorption is directly related to the amount that is soluble and ionized in the small intestine. Many calcium salts, such as those of phosphate and carbonate, are quite insoluble at neutral pH. Digestion of foods at the acid pH of the stomach increases the amount of soluble calcium. Amino acids such as arginine, lysine, and tryptophan enhance calcium absorption, as do the antibiotics penicillin, neomycin, and chloramphenicol. Calcium absorption is depressed by corticosteroids, thyroid hormone, estrogens, excessive unabsorbed fatty acids, diets rich in oxalates or organic phosphates, excessive antacid administration, and achlorhydria. The type of organic phosphate is hexaphosphoinositol, which is found in bran.

The net absorption of calcium is the difference between the flux of calcium from the lumen to the blood and the flux in the opposite direction. The lumen-to-plasma flux is highest in the duodenum, which enables this part of the small intestine to be the most efficient in absorbing calcium. The plasma-to-lumen flux of calcium is about the same in the duodenum and ileum. When calcium is not present in the lumen, the secretory (plasma-to-lumen) flux becomes apparent. In the duodenum, this is reabsorbed. It is not reabsorbed in the ileum, however, and the net secretion of calcium represents a calcium loss from the body that is continuous when dietary calcium is low. Even though the control mechanisms are activated to absorb and conserve calcium more efficiently, there is still a negative calcium balance.[125] The nature of the calcium-transport mechanisms in the intestinal mucosa is not well understood. In the duodenum, calcium is transported by a carrier-mediated energy-dependent process. Hormones and vitamin D can regulate the efficiency of this transport system. Since this mechanism is located only in the duodenum, through which chyme passes fairly rapidly, it is the limiting factor in the overall absorption of calcium. Most of the calcium is absorbed in the remainder of the small intestine by passive or facilitated diffusion.

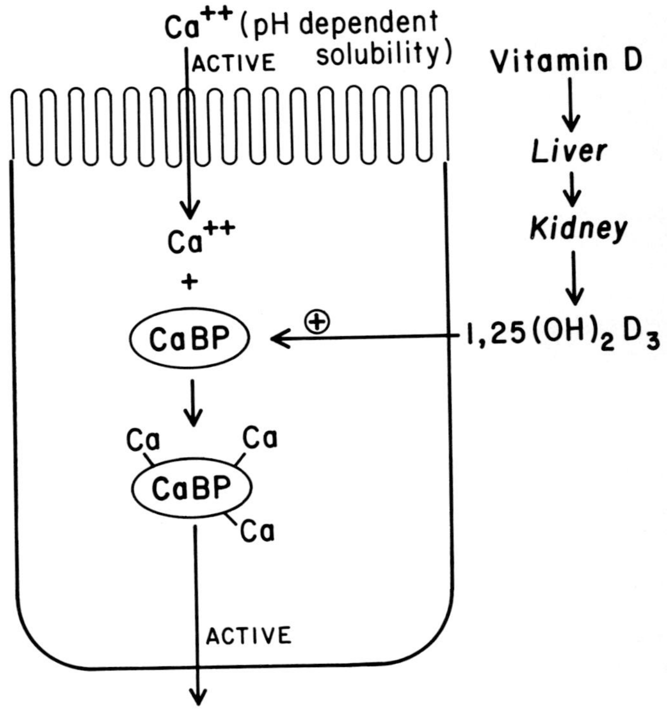

Figure 15-28. Diagram to show the absorption of calcium in the small intestine. Calcium absorption is regulated by vitamin D absorption and metabolism.

Vitamins and hormones regulate calcium absorption (Figure 15-28). Vitamin D is not biologically active on calcium absorption until after it has been hydroxylated, first in the liver, forming 25-hydroxycholecalciferol, and later in the renal cortex, forming 1,25-dihydroxycholecalciferol, which is the active chemical that regulates intestinal absorption of calcium. The kidney can also convert the hydroxylated form produced in the liver to 21,25-dihydroxy-cholecalciferol, an inactive form. Levels of serum calcium and parathyroid hormone determine whether the form produced will be inactive or active. Reductions in serum calcium cause release of parathormone, which stimulates synthesis and release of the active form. Thus, this arm of the regulation of intestinal calcium depends on normal renal function, normal parathyroid function, and absorption of vitamin D. Serum levels of phosphate determine the secretion of 1,25-dihyroxycholecalciferol. Low phosphate levels stimulate its synthesis and release, causing an increased absorption of phosphate in the intestine and probably in the renal tubule. Parathormone is primarily a regulator of calcium ions, but it causes an increased absorption of intestinal phosphate by the vitamin-D derivative, increasing serum levels. Thyrocalcitonin has no effect on the absorption of calcium from the intestine.

The effect of 1,25-dihydroxycholecalciferol is to stimulate the synthesis of a calcium-binding protein in the intestinal epithelial cell. Synthesis occurs primarily in the duodenal mucosa, where an active transport process is involved. It is suggested that the binding protein functions as a carrier.

Cushing's syndrome or prolonged administration of corticosteroids can cause bone demineralization. Corticosteroids cause decreased calcium absorption in the intestine. It is not known whether this effect is one directly on the mucosal cell or whether the steroids interfere with vitamin-D metabolism. A failure to absorb calcium properly from the intestine cannot be critically evaluated by measuring serum calcium levels. Bone changes become apparent, however, alerting the clinician to a problem. Calcium malabsorption is a possibility when there is fat malabsorption for any reason and when chronic renal disease has progressed to the extent that the metabolism of vitamin D to its active form is no longer adequate to meet the animal's needs.

Absorption of Magnesium. Magnesium is an important divalent cation necessary for the functioning of enzyme systems in the body. Little is known about its metabolism. There are no known special mechanisms for absorption of this ion, which occurs primarily in the cranial part of the jejunum. Magnesium salts are relatively water-soluble, and malabsorption does not engender clinical signs until it becomes a very severe problem.

Absorption of Vitamins.[126,127] Fat-soluble vitamins are absorbed with dietary lipids, and no deficiencies are seen unless fat malabsorption occurs. Water-soluble vitamins are absorbed by processes of simple diffusion, with several exceptions. The assimilation of vitamin B_{12} and folic acid by the intestinal mucosa is important clinically and involves processes that are more complicated.

Vitamin B_{12} Absorption. It is estimated that a year's supply of vitamin B_{12} is stored in the body, so its malabsorption must persist for some time before signs of deficiency appear. Vitamin B_{12} is necessary for the production of normal erythrocytes. A deficiency causes megaloblastic erythropoiesis. The source of all vitamin B_{12} to small animals is in the diet. Intestinal bacteria synthesize the vitamin, but only in the colon, where it cannot be absorbed. Dietary vitamin B_{12} is found only in animal protein or in food in which it has been synthesized by contaminating microorganisms. The vitamin is released from food during digestion in the stomach, after which it binds to a glycoprotein, called intrinsic factor, that the stomach secretes. Recent studies report its presence in pancreatic secretions of dogs.[128] The amount of B_{12} normally present in the diet is less than 5 micrograms per day. Binding to intrinsic factor is necessary for absorption of 20% of this intake. The complex of vitamin B_{12} and intrinsic factor passes through the small intestine to the ileum. The intrinsic factor not only resists proteolytic destruction of B_{12} by bacterial or pancreatic enzymes but also minimizes the utilization of B_{12} by bacteria within the lumen. The mucosa of the ileum contains receptor sites on the surface of the microvilli that bind the complex. After the binding the B_{12} is released and crosses the cell membrane by an active transport process. The vitamin is transported through the cell and released to the circulation, where it binds to one of two carrier proteins, transcobalamin. There is a definite rate-limiting step in the absorption of B_{12}, but it is not known whether it is in its attachment to the ileum or in the transport mechanism. Bile's vitamin B_{12} content is high and most of the vitamin is reabsorbed in the ileum. Loss of the ileal function to absorb vitamin B_{12}, represents a means for continued loss of the vitamin from the body.

There are clinical situations of reduced absorption of vitamin B_{12}. A deficiency of intrinsic factor, causing B_{12} malabsorption, is possible. Intrinsic-factor deficiency develops in humans with atrophic gastritis, but that has not been reported as a problem in small animals. It can be a problem in animals with partial gastrectomy or possibly with pancreatic diseases. Abnormalities in the small intestine influence vitamin B_{12} absorption. Increased numbers of intestinal bacteria consume vitamin B_{12}; microflora can increase to the point where they use most of the vitamin, leaving little for absorption in the ileum.[129] Such overgrowth occurs in regions of the small intestine cranial to a partial obstruction. In humans, intestinal parasites can consume B_{12} to the point of creating a deficiency. That situation has not been recognized in small animals. A deficiency of pancreatic secretions can also impair vitamin B_{12} absorption. The malabsorption that follows the enzyme deficiency is accompanied by an overgrowth of the microflora of the intestine, which use B_{12} and leave less for absorption. Malabsorption also lowers the pH of the intestinal contents through the bacterial flora's fermentation of unabsorbed oligosacharides. Pancreatic disease results in a deficiency of pancreatic bicarbonate secretion, augmenting the acidity of intestinal contents. Mucosal binding of the B_{12}-intrinsic factor complex is inhibited at a pH of less than 6.5. Malabsorption can also reduce calcium concentrations by precipitation of calcium with fatty acids. Calcium must be present for normal binding of the B_{12}-intrinsic factor complex to the ileal mucosa. Lastly, severe chronic disease of the ileum can result in vitamin B_{12} deficiency. Ileitis or regional enteritis is not uncommon in humans but has seldom been reported in small animals. Vitamin B_{12} absorption tests are conducted in humans but are rarely done in animals. In general, vitamin B_{12} deficiency is seldom recognized in animals.

Absorption of Folic Acid. Folic acid has a much shorter biological half-life than does vitamin B_{12}, so a deficiency can be seen within a month after intake ceases. Folates are necessary for synthetic reactions that involve methionine, purines, and pyrimidines. Deficiency results in megaloblastic changes in the bone marrow. Folic acid (pteroylglutamic acid) consists of three components. A pteridine ring and para-aminobenzoic acid (making up pteroic acid) are connected to glutamic acid. The natural form of folate in the diet consists of folic acid with a number of additional moieties of glutamic acid. The monoglutamate form is found in plasma. The diet contains up to 300 micrograms of folate per 100 calories, and the vitamin is widely distributed in foods. Folate is absorbed from the cranial part of the small intestine, and the capacity for absorption is in excess of the daily needs. The epithelial cell absorbs the natural form, polyglutamates, after which a lysosomal glutamyl peptidase reduces the glutamyl peptide chain to a mono- or diglutamate. The reduced form of these products is subsequently methylated in the cell to form methyltetrahydrofolate. The nature of the mechanism for transport of folate is unknown. Interference with the intracellular metabolic transformations inhibits its absorption.

Occasionally, a small-animal patient is seen that has a chronic bowel problem and evidence for a megaloblastic anemia. The important site of folate absorption is in the jejunum, pathology of which can cause a deficiency of absorption. Resection of a large part of small intestine and gluten-induced enteropathy lead to folate malabsorption in humans. Extensive intramural disease of the intestinal mucosa produces the same results. Bacteria produce folate that can be absorbed and supply the body's needs. Bacteria also consume folate, to the extent that low plasma folate deficiencies can develop with bacterial overgrowth of the jejunum.[129] Drugs are known to interfere with folate absorption. Diphenylhydantoin is the only one of these that is frequently used in small-animal medicine. In summary, megaloblastic anemia associated with chronic gastrotintestinal disease should be considered as a possible result of a deficiency of folate absorption.

REFERENCES

1. Miller, M.E., Christensen, G.C. and Evans, H.E.: Anatomy of the Dog. WB Saunders Co., Philadelphia, 1964.
2. Nickel, R., Schummer, A., Seiferle, E. and Sack, W.O.: The viscera of the domestic animals. Springer-Verlag, New York, 1973.
3. Dyce, K.M., Sack, W.O. and Wensing, C.J.G.: Textbook of Veterinary Anatomy. W.B. Saunders, Philadelphia, 1987.
4. Bonakdarpour, A., Ming, S., Lynch, P.R., Essa, N. and Reichle, F.: Superior mesenteric artery occlusion in dogs: A model to produce the spectrum of intestinal ischemia. J. Surg. Res. 19:251-257, 1975.
5. Creamer, B.: Intestinal structure in relation to absorption. In, Biomembranes, Vol. 4A, Intestinal Absorption, edited by D.H. Smyth, Plenum Press, New York, 1-42, 1974.
6. Madera, J.L. and Trier, J.S.: Functional morphology of the mucosa of the small intestine. In: Physiology of the Gastrointestinal Tract. Edited by L.R. Johnson. Raven Press, New York, 1209-1249, 1987.
7. Solcia, E., Capella, C., Buffa, R., Uselline, L., Fiocca, R. and Sessa, F.: Endocrine cells of the digestive system. In: Physiology of the Gastrointestinal Tract. Edited by L.R. Johnson. Raven Press, New York, 111-130, 1987.
8. Lundgren, O.: The circulation of the small bowel mucosa. Gut 15:1005-1013, 1974.
9. Granger, D.N., Kvietys, P.R., Perry, M.A. and Barrowman, J.A.: The microcirculation and intestinal transport. In: Physiology of the Gastrointestinal Tract. Edited by L.R. Johnson. Raven Press, New York, 1671-1697, 1987.
10. Casley-Smith, J.R.: Endothelial fenestrae in intestinal villi: Differences between the arterial and venous ends of capillaries. Microvasc. Res. 3:49-68, 1971.
11. Strombeck, D.R.: Effect of Vibrio cholera toxin on vascular and extravascular spaces of rat intestine. Proc. Soc. Exp. Biol. Med. 141:70-75, 1972.
12. Eastwood, G.L.: Gastrointestinal epithelial renewal. Gastroenterology 72:962-975, 1977.
13. Lipkin, M.: Proliferation and differentiation of normal and diseased gastrointestinal cells. In: Physiology of the Gastrointestinal Tract. Edited by L.R. Johnson, Raven Press, New York, 255-285, 1987.
14. Johnson, L.R.: Regulation of gastrointestinal growth. In: Physiology of the Gastrointestinal Tract. Edited by L.R. Johnson, Raven Press, New York, 301-333, 1987.
15. Barrowman, J.A.: The trophic action of gastrointestinal hormones. Digestion 12:92-104, 1975.
16. Hughes, C.A., Bates, T. and Dowling, R.H.: Cholecystokinin and secretin prevent the intestinal mucosal hypoplasia of total parenteral nutrition in the dog. Gastroenterology 75:34-41, 1978.
17. MacDonald, T.T. and Ferguson, A.: Small intestinal epithelial cell kinetics and protozoal infection in mice. Gastroenterology 74:496-500, 1978.
18. Schofield, G.C.: Anatomy of muscular and neural tissues in the alimentary canal. In: Handbook of Physiology, Sect. 6, Alimentary Canal, edited by C.F. Code, Washington, D.C., Am. Physiol. Soc., Vol. 4, 1579-1627, 1968.
19. Gabella, G.: Structure of muscles and nerves in the gastrointestinal tract. In: Physiology of the Gastrointestinal Tract. Edited by L.R. Johnson, Raven Press, New York, 335-381, 1987.
20. Hightower, N.C.: Motor action of the small bowel. In: Handbook of Physiology, Sect. 6, Alimentary Canal, edited by C.F. Code, Washington DC, Am. Physiol. Soc., Vol. 4, 2001-2024, 1968.
21. Weisbrodt, N.W.: Motility of the small intestine. In: Physiology of the Gastrointestinal Tract. Edited by L.R. Johnson, Raven Press, New York, 631-663, 1987.
22. Ehrlein, H.J., Schemann, M. and Siegle, M-L: Motor patterns of small intestine determined by closely spaced extraluminal transducers and videofluoroscopy. Am. J. Physiol. 353:G359-G267, 1987.
23. Schemann, M. and Ehrlein, H-J: Postprandial patterns of canine jejunal motility and transit of luminal content. Gastroenterology 90:991-1000, 1986.
24. Melville, J., Macagno, E. and Christensen, J.: Longitudinal contractions in the duodenum: Their fluid-mechanical function. Am. J. Physiol. 228:1887-1892, 1975.
25. Bortoff, A.: Myogenic control of intestinal motility. Physiol. Rev. 56:418-434, 1976.
26. Tasaka, K. and Farrar, J.T.: Intraluminal pressure of the small intestine of the unanesthetized dog. Pflug. Arch. 364:35-44, 1976.
27. Job, D.D., Bloomquist, W.E. and Bridgeforth, J.: Correlations between electrolyte content and spontaneous electrical activity in intestinal muscle. Am. J. Physiol. 226:1502-1509, 1974.
28. Celander, O.: Are there any centrally controlled sympathetic inhibitory fibers to the musculature of the intestine? Acta. Physiol. Scand. 47:299-309, 1959.
29. Burks, T.F., Jaquette, D.L. and Grubb, M.N.: Motility responses of dog and monkey isolated perfused intestine to morphine, 5-hydroxytryptamine and cholinergic stimulants. Comp. Gen. Pharmacol. 5:213-216, 1974.
30. Sjoerdsma, A., Lovenberg, W., Engelman, K., Carpenter, W.T., Wyatt, R.J. and Gessa, G.L.: Serotonin now: Clinical implications of inhibiting its synthesis with para-chlorophenylalanine. Ann. Internal Med. 73:607-629, 1970.
31. Schemann, M. and Ehrlein, H-J: Effects of neurohormonal agents on jejunal contraction spread and transit in the fed dog. Gastroenterology 90:1950-1955, 1986.
32. Burnstock, G.: Purinergic nerves. Pharmacol. Rev. 24:509-581, 1972.
33. Frantzides, C.T., Sarna, S.K., Matsumoto, T., Lang, I.M. and Condon, R.E.: An intrinsic neural pathway for long intestino-intestinal inhibitory reflexes. Gastroenterology 92:594-603, 1987.
34. Mishra, N.K., Appert, H.E. and Howard, J.M.: Studies of paralytic ileus. Effects of intraperitoneal injury on motility of the canine small intestine. Am. J. Surg. 129:559-563, 1975.
35. Williams, N.S., Meyer, J.H., Jehn, D., Miller, J. and Fink, A.S.: Canine intestinal transit and digestion of radiolabeled liver particles. Gastroenterology 86:1451-1459, 1984.
36. Bueno, L., Praddaude, F., Fioramonti, J. and Ruckebusch, Y.: Effect of dietary fiber on gastrointestinal motility and jejunal transit time in dogs. Gastroenterology 80:701-707, 1981.
37. Quigley, E.M.M., Phillips, S.F., Cranley, B., Taylor, B.M. and Dent, J.: Tone of canine ileocolonic junction: topography and response to phasic contractions. Am. J. Physiol 249:G350-G357, 1985.
38. Spiller, R.C., Brown, M.L., Phillips, S.F. and Azpiroz, F.: Scintigraphic measurements of canine ileocolonic transit. Gastroenterology 91:1213-1220, 1986.
39. Kelley, M.L., Jr., Gordon, E.A. and DeWeese, J.A.: Pressure responses of canine ileocolonic junctional zone to intestinal distention. Am. J. Physiol. 211:614-618, 1966.
40. Kumar, D., Phillips, S.F. and Brown, M.L.: Reflux from ileum

to colon in the dog. Dig. Dis. Sci. 33:345-352, 1988.
41. Holgate, A.M. and Read, N.W.: Effect of ileal infusion of intralipid on gastrointestinal transit, ileal flow rate, and carbohydrate absorption in humans after ingestion of a liquid meal. Gastroenterology 88:1005-1011, 1985.
42. Christensen, J.: Motility of the colon. In: Physiology of the Gastrointestinal Tract. Edited by L.R. Johnson, Raven Press, New York, 665-693, 1987.
43. Connell, A.M.: Motor action of the large bowel. In: Handbook of Physiology, Sect. 6, Alimentary Canal, edited by C.F. Code, Washington, DC, Am. Physiol. Soc., Vol. 4, 2075-2091, 1968.
44. Waller, S.L.: Differential measurement of small and large bowel transit times in constipation and diarrhea: A new approach. Gut 16:372-378, 1975.
45. Gray, G.M.: Carbohydrate digestion and absorption. Gastroenterology 58:96-107, 1970.
46. Semenza, G.: Pancreatic amylase: In: Handbook of Physiology, Sect. 6, Alimentary Canal, edited by C.F. code, Washington D.C., Am. Physiol. Soc. Vol 5, 2637-2645, 1968.
47. Wormsley, K.G. and Goldberg, D.M.: The interrelationships of the pancreatic enzymes. Gut 13:398-412, 1972.
48. Alpers, D.H.: Digestion and absorption of carbohydrates and protines. In: Physiology of the Gastrointestinal Tract. Edited by L.R. Johnson, Raven Press, New York, 1469-1487, 1987.
49. Johnson, C.F.: Disaccharidase localization in hamster intestine brush borders. Science 155:1670-1672, 1967.
50. Noon, K.F., Rogul, M., Brendle, J.J. and Keefe, T.J.: Detection and definition of canine intestinal carbohydrases using a standardized method. Am. J. Vet. Res. 38:1063-1067, 1977.
51. Caspary, W.F., Winckler, K., Lankish, P.G. and Creutzfeldt, W.: Influence of exocrine and endocrine pancreatic function on intestinal brush border enzymatic activities. Gut 16:89-92, 1975.
52. Dyck, W.P., Bonnett, D., Lasatter, J., Stinson, C. and Hall, F.F.: Hormonal stimulation of intestinal disaccharidase release in the dog. Gastroenterology 66:533-538, 1974.
53. Newcomer, A.D.: Disaccharidase deficiencies. Mayo Clin. Proc. 48:648-652, 1973.
54. Gracey, M., Houghton, M. and Thomas, J.: Deoxycholate depresses small intestinal enzyme activity. Gut 16:53-56, 1975.
55. Gray, G.M. and Cooper, H.L.: Protein digestion and absorption. Gastroenterology 61:535-544, 1971.
56. Keller, P.J.: Pancreatic proteolytic enzymes. In: Handbook of Physiology, Sect. 6, Alimentary Canal, edited by C.F. Code, Washington, DC, Am. Physiol. Soc., Vol. 5, 2605-2628, 1968.
57. Kim, Y.S. and Freeman, H.J.: Digestion and absorption of proteins. Ann. Rev. Med. 29:99-116, 1978.
58. Wiseman, G.: Absorption of protein digestion products. In: Biomembranes, Vol. 4A, Intestinal Absorption, edited by D.H. Smyth, Plenum Press, New York, 363-481, 1974.
59. Nicholson, J.A., McCarthy, D.M. and Kim, Y.S.: The responses of rat intestinal brush border and cytosol peptide hydrolase activities to variation in dietary protein content. J. Clin. Invest. 54:890-898, 1974.
60. Kim, Y.S., McCarthy, D.M., Lane, W. and Fong, W.: Alterations in the levels of peptide hydrolases and other enzymes in the brush border and cytosol fractions of rat small intestinal mucosa during starvation and refeeding. Biochem. Biophys. Acta. 321:262-273, 1973.
61. Desnuelle, P.: Pancreatic lipase. In: Handbook of Physiology, Sect. 6, Alimentary Canal, edited by C.F. Code, Washington, DC, Am. Physiol. Soc., Vol. 5, 2629-2636, 1968.
62. Hofmann, A.F. and Borgstrom, B.: The physico-chemical state of lipids in intestinal content during their digestion and absorption. Fed. Proc. 21:43-50, 1962.
63. Hofmann, A.F. and Small, D.M.: Detergent properties of bile salts: Correlation with physiological function. Ann. Rev. Med. 18:333-376, 1967.
64. Mattson, F.H. and Volpenhein, R.A.: The digestion and absorption of triglycerides. J. Biol. Chem. 239:2772-2777, 1964.
65. Shiau, Y-F.: Lipid digestion and absorption. In: Physiology of the Gastrointestinal Tract. Edited by L.R. Johnson, Raven Press, New York, 1527-1556, 1987.
66. Janowitz, H.D.: Pancreatic secretion of fluid and electrolytes. In: Handbook of Physiology, Sect. 6, Alimentary Canal, edited by C.F. Code, Washington, DC, Am. Physiol. Soc. Vol. 2, 925-933, 1968.
67. Schulz, I.: Electrolyte and fluid secretion in the exocrine pancreas. In: Physiology of the Gastrointestinal Tract. Edited by L.R. Johnson, Raven Press, New York, 1147-1171, 1987.
68. Strombeck, D.R., Wheeldon, R. and Harrold, D.: Model of chronic pancreatitis in the dog. Am. J. Vet. Res. 45:131-136, 1984.
69. Harper, A.A.: The control of pancreatic secretion. Gut 13:308-317, 1972.
70. Rayford, P.L., Miller, T.A. and Thompson, J.C.: Secretin, cholecystokinin and newer gastrointestinal hormones. New Eng. J. Med. 295:1093-1101 and 1157-1164, 1976.
71. Singh, M. and Webster, P.D.: Neurohormonal control of pancreatic secretion - a review. Gastroenterology 74:294-309, 1978.
72. Solomon, T.E.: Control of exocrine pancreatic secretion. In: Physiology of the Gastrointestinal Tract. Edited by L.R. Johnson, Raven Press, New York, 1173-1207, 1987.
73. Curtis, P.J., Fender, H.R., Rayford, P.L. and Thompson, J.C.: Disappearance half-time of endogenous and exogenous secretin in dogs. Gut 17:595-599, 1976.
74. Curtis, P.J., Fender, H.R., Rayford, P.L. and Thompson, J.C.: Catabolism of secretin by the liver and kidney. Surgery 80:259-265, 1976.
75. Flourie, B., Leblond, A., Florent, Ch., Rantureau, M., Bisalli, A. and Rambaud, J-C.: Starch malabsorption and breath gas excretion in healthy humans consuming low- and high-starch diets. Gastroenterology 95:356-363, 1988.
76. Levitt, M.D., Hirsh, P., Fetzer, C.A., Sheahan, M. and Levine, A.S.: H_2 excretion after ingestion of complex carbohydrates. Gastroenterology 92:383-389, 1987.
77. Jenkins, D.J.A., Jenkins, A.L., Wolever, T.M.S., Thompson, L.H. and Rao, A.V.: Simple and complex carbohydrates. Nutr Rev 44:44-49, 1986.
78. Warzburg, O.B.: Nutritional aspects and safety of modified food starches. Nutr. Rev. 44:74-79, 1986.
79. Hendrix, T.R. and Bayless, T.M.: Digestion:Intestinal secretion. Ann. Rev. Physiol. 32:139-164, 1970.
80. Banwell, J.G. and Sherr, H.: Effect of bacterial enterotoxins on the gastrointestinal tract. Gastroenterology 65:467-497, 1973.
81. Donowitz, M. and Welsh, M.J.: Regulation of mammalian small intestinal electrolyte secretion. In: Physiology of the Gastrointestinal Tract. Edited by L.R. Johnson, Raven Press, New York, 1351-1388, 1987.
82. Strombeck, D.R.: The production of intestinal fluid by cholera toxin in the rat. Proc. Soc. Exp. Biol. Med. 140:297-303, 1972.
83. Barbezat, G.O. and Grossman, M.I.: Intestinal secretion: Stimulation by peptides. Science 174:422-424, 1971.
84. Pierce, N.F., Carpenter, C.C.J., Elliott, H.L. and Greenough, W.B.: Effects of prostaglandins, theophylline, and cholera exotoxin upon transmucosal water and electrolyte movement in the canine jejunum. Gastroenterology 60:22-32, 1971
85. Udall, J.N., Alverez, L.A., Nichols, B.L. and Hazelwood, C.F.: The effects of cholera enterotoxin on intestinal tissue water as measured by nuclear magnetic resonance (NMR) spectroscopy. Physiol. Chem. Physics 7:533-539, 1975.
86. Brown, W.R.: Relationships between immunoglobulins and the intestinal epithelium. Gastroenterology 75:129-138, 1978.
87. Kagnoff, M.F.: Immunology of the digestive system. In: Physiology of the Gastrointestinal Tract. Edited by L.R. Johnson, Raven Press, New York, 1699-1728, 1987.
88. Horowitz, M.I.: Mucopolysaccharides and glycoproteins of the alimentary tract. In: Handbook of Physiology, Sec. 6, Alimentary Canal, edited by C.F. Code, Washington, DC, Am. Physiol. Soc., Vol. 2, 1063-1085, 1967.

89. Schrager, J.: The chemical composition and function of gastrointestinal mucus. Gut 11:450-456, 1970.
90. Neutra, M.R. and Forstner, J.F.: Gastrointestinal mucus: synthesis, secretion, and function. In: Physiology of the Gastrointestinal Tract. Edited by L.R. Johnson, Raven Press, New York, 975-1009, 1987.
91. Strombeck, D.R. and Harrold, D.: Binding of cholera toxin to mucins and inhibition by gastric mucin. Infect. Immun. 10:1266-1272, 1974.
92. Crane, R.K.: Absorption of sugars. In: Handbook of Physiology, Sect. 6, Alimentary Canal, edited by C.F. Code, Washington, DC, Am. Physiol. Soc., Vol. 4, 1323-1351, 1967.
93. Crane, R.K.: Intestinal absorption of glucose. In: Biomembranes, Vol. 4A, Intestinal Absorption, edited by D.H. Smyth, Plenum Press, New York, 541-553, 1974.
94. Hopfer, U.: Membrane transport mechanisms for hexoses and amino acids in the small intestine. In: Physiology of the Gastrointestinal Tract. Edited by L.R. Johnson, Raven Press, New York, 1499-1526, 1987.
95. Walker, W.A. and Isselbacher, K.J.: Uptake and transport of macromolecules by the intestine. Possible role in clinical disorders. Gastroenterology 67:531-550, 1974.
96. Ganapathy, V. and Leibach, F.H.: Is intestinal peptide transport energized by a proton gradient? Am. J. Physiol. 249:G153-G160, 1985.
97. Imondi, A.R. and Stradley, R.P.: Utilization of enzymatically hydrolyzed soybean protein and crystalline amino acid diets by rats with exocrine pancreatic insufficiency. J. Nutr. 104:793-801, 1974.
98. Gardner, M.L.G.: Gastrointestinal absorption of intact proteins. Ann. Rev. Nutr. 8:329-350, 1988.
99. Strombeck, D.R. and Harrold, D.: Comparison of the rate of absorption and proteolysis of (14C) choleragen and (14C) bovine serum albumin in the rat jejunum. Infect. Immun. 12:1450-1456, 1975.
100. Borgstrom, B.: Fat digestion and absorption. In: Biomembranes, Vol. 4B, Intestinal Absorption, edited by D.H. Smyth, Plenum Press, London, 556-620, 1974.
101. Brindley, D.N.: The intracellular phase of fat absorption. In: Biomembranes, Vol. 4B, Intestinal Absorption, edited by D.H. Smyth, Plenum Press, London, 621-671, 1974.
102. Jackson, M.J.: Transport of short chain fatty acids. In: Biomembranes, Vol. 4B, Intestinal Absorption, edited by D.H. Smyth, Plenum Press, London, 673-709, 1974.
103. Erlinger, S.: Physiology of bile secretion and enterohepatic circulation. In: Physiology of the Gastrointestinal Tract. Edited by L.R. Johnson, Raven Press, New York, 1557-1580, 1987.
104. Playoust, M.R., Lack, L. and Weiner, I.M.: Effect of intestinal resection on bile salt absorption in dogs. Am. J. Physiol. 208:363-369, 1965.
105. Doty, J.E. and Meyer, J.H.: Vagotomy and antrectomy impairs canine fat absorption from solid but not liquid dietary sources. Gastroenterology 94:50-56, 1988.
106. Merritt, A.M., Burrows, C.F., Cowgill, L. and Streett, W.: Fecal fat and trypsin in dogs fed a meat-base or cereal-base diet. JAVMA 174:59-61, 1979.
107. Thomson, A.B.R., Keelan, M., Clandinin, M.T. and Walker, K.: Dietary fat selectively alters transport properties of rat jejunum. J. Clin. Invest. 77:279-288, 1986.
108. Vahouny, G.V.: Effects of dietary fiber on digestion and absorption. In: Physiology of the Gastrointestinal Tract. Edited by L.R. Johnson, Raven Press, New York, 1623-1648, 1987.
109. Cummings, J.H., Englyst, H.N. and Wiggins, H.S.: The role of carbohydrates in lower gut function. Nutr Rev 44:50-54, 1986.
110. Herschel, D.A., Argenzio, R.A., Southworth, M., Stevens, C.E.: Absorption of volatile fatty acid, Na, and H_2O by the colon of the dog. Am. J. Vet. Res. 42:1118-1124, 1981.
111. Edmonds, C.J.: Salts and water. In: Biomembranes, Vol. 4A, Intestinal Absorption, edited by D.H. Smyth, Plenum Press, New York, 711-759, 1974.
112. Svanvik, J.: Mucosal blood circulation and its influence on passive absorption in the small intestine. Acta. Physiol. Scand. Suppl. 385:1-44, 1973.
113. Wright, E.M.: The passive permeability of the small intestine. In: Biomembranes, Vol. 4A, Intestinal Absorption, edited by D.H. Smyth, Plenum Press, New York, 159-198, 1974.
114. Powell, D.W.: Intestinal water and electrolyte transport. In: Physiology of the Gastrointestinal Tract. Edited by L.R. Johnson, Raven Press, New York, 1267-1305, 1987.
115. Armstrong, W.M.: Cellular mechanisms of ion transport in the small intestine. In: Physiology of the Gastrointestinal Tract. Edited by L.R. Johnson, Raven Press, New York, 1251-1265, 1987.
116. Hakim, A.A. and Lifson, N.: Effects of pressure on water and solute transport by dog intestinal mucosa in vitro. Am. J. Physiol. 216:276-284, 1969.
117. Mailman, D. and Jordan, K.: The effect of saline and hyperoncotic dextran infusion on canine ileal salt and water absorption and regional blood flow. J. Physiol. 252:97-113, 1975.
118. Johnson, P.C. and Richardson, D.R.: The influence of venous pressure on filtration forces in the intestine. Microvas. Res. 7:296-306, 1974.
119. Starling, E.H.: On the absorption of fluids from the connective tissue spaces. J. Physiol. 19:312-326, 1986
120. Cooke, H.J.: Neural and humoral regulation of small intestinal electrolyte transport. In: Physiology of the Gastrointestinal Tract. Edited by L.R. Johnson, Raven Press, New York, 1307-1350, 1987.
121. Callender, S.T.: Iron absorption. In: Biomembranes, Vol. 4B, Intestinal Absorption, edited by D.H. Smyth, Plenum Press, London, 761-791, 1974.
122. Conrad, M.E.: Iron absorption. In: Physiology of the Gastrointestinal Tract. Edited by L.R. Johnson, Raven Press, New York, 1437-1453, 1987.
123. Harrison, H.E. and Harrison, H.C.: Calcium. In: Biomembranes, Vol. 4B, Intestinal Absorption, edited by D.H. Smyth, Plenum Press, London 793-846, 1975.
124. Bronner, F.: Calcium absorption. In: Physiology of the Gastrointestinal Tract. Edited by L.R. Johnson, Raven Press, New York, 1419-1435, 1987.
125. Younoszai, M.K. and Schedl, H.P.: Intestinal calcium transport; comparison of duodenum and ileum in vivo in the rat. Gastroenterology 62:565-571, 1972.
126. Matthews, D.M.: Absorption of water-soluble vitamins. In: Biomembranes, Vol. 4B, Intestinal Absorption. edited by D.H. Smyth, Plenum Press, London, 847-915, 1974.
127. Rose, R.C.: Intestinal absorption of water-soluble vitamins. In: Physiology of the Gastrointestinal Tract. Edited by L.R. Johnson, Raven Press, New York, 1581-1596, 1987.
128. Batt, R.M. and Horadagoda, N.U.: Role of gastric and pancreatic intrinsic factors in the physiologic absorption of cobalamin in the dog. Gastroenterology 90:1339, 1986.
129. Batt, R.M. and Morgan, J.O.: Role of serum folate and vitamin B_{12} concentrations in the differentiation of small intestinal abnormalities in the dog. Res. Vet. Sci. 32:17-22, 1982.
130. Washabau, R.J., Strombeck, D.R., Buffington, C.A. and Harrold, D.: Evaluation of intestinal carbohydrate malabsorption in the dog by pulmonary hydrogen gas excretion. Am. J. Vet. Res. 47:1402-1406, 1986.

Chapter 16

Classification, Pathophysiology, and Symptomatic Treatment of Diarrheal Diseases

DIARRHEA AND THE SIGNS OF INTESTINAL DISEASE

Diarrhea is the most consistent manifestation of intestinal disease. Diarrhea is defined as a change in the frequency, consistency, or volume of bowel movements (Table 16-1). Stool weight and frequency are easy to measure, but an objective method for the quantification of stool consistency has yet to be developed. Increased stool frequency can result from diseases that cause tenesmus or from derangements that cause larger fecal volume. Larger fecal volume is usually due to a greater content of fecal water or to greater amounts of undigested and unabsorbed nutrients such as fiber. In normal animals, the fiber content of the diet determines stool volume. Fecal water content will increase when an intestinal problem causes increased secretion or decreased absorption of fluid. The consistency (fluidity) of bowel movements is primarily determined by fecal water content but is also influenced by the physical and chemical properties of the stool matrix. Water content is 60% to 80% in normal bowel movements and 70% to 90% in unformed and watery feces. Thus, small changes in fecal water content transform normal bowel movements to liquid feces.

About 2.5 liters of fluid enter the duodenal lumen each day in a 20-Kg animal. The sources of the fluid are shown in Table 16-2. The amount absorbed in each region is shown in Table 16-3. The greatest volume of luminal fluid is absorbed in the proximal small intestine, but the efficiency of the absorptive process increases in the more caudal regions of the bowel. For instance, the jejunum absorbs approximately four times as much fluid volume as the large intestine, but it is only half as efficient (Table 16-3). The colon has a capacity to absorb more than three times the water it normally absorbs. Thus, the volume of fluid entering the colon from the ileum must be large to exceed the colon's reserve absorptive capacity and cause diarrhea. In contrast, only minor abnormalities affecting either the colon's reservoir function or its absorptive capacity have profound effects on fecal properties. For example, a decrease in colonic water absorption from 300 ml to 290 ml, changing the volume of the stool from 50 to 60 ml, represents a 20% increase in fecal water and will cause diarrhea even though colonic absorption has been reduced only slightly.

The problem of diarrhea should be differentiated from the problem of fecal incontinence. Fecal incontinence is the inability to retain feces until defecation is appropriate. Diarrhea challenges the continence mechanisms, but animals with diarrhea need not develop fecal incontinence. Similarly, animals with fecal incontinence need not have diarrhea.

Diarrhea is only one of many signs suggestive of intestinal disease. Bowel movements may show other abnormalities, such as the appearance of blood, mucus, malassimilated nutrients, and melena. Colonic and rectal problems are often associated with tenesmus or dyschezia. The production and accumulation of abnormal amounts of gas can produce abdominal

Diarrhea Definition: Character of the bowel movement changes so that the following are increased:

Frequency

Fluidity or loose consistency
water content in normal bowel movement = 60% to 80%

Volume
determinants are water percentage and nondigestible content

Table 16-1. Definition of diarrhea. Frequency can increase with either formed or watery bowel movements. There is little difference in water content between formed and loose stools. Thus, small changes in the amount of water absorbed can easily cause a diarrhea. Both water content and fiber content determine the volume of the stool.

Dog - 45 Lbs (20 Kg) Daily Volume and Sources of Fluid Entering Gut

Diet - 600 ml
Saliva - 300 ml
Gastric - 600 ml
Bile - 300 ml
Pancreatic - 600 ml
Small Intestine - 300 ml

Total 2,700 ml

Table 16-2. Sources and amounts of fluid that enter the alimentary canal each 24 hours in a normal medium size dog.

Dog - 45 Lbs (20 Kg) Daily Volume of Fluid Absorbed From Gut

Jejunum	1,350 ml (50% of 2,700 ml)
Ileum	1,000 ml (75% of 1,350 ml)
Colon	315 ml (90% of 350 ml)

Table 16-3. Regional absorption of fluid in the intestinal tract shows the absolute amounts absorbed in each part. It also illustrates that the absorptive processes are more efficient in the caudal intestine. Greater than 98% of all the fluid entering the intestine is normally absorbed. Absorption in the jejunum is mainly secondary to glucose absorption, whereas in the caudal intestine is dependent on sodium transport.

distention, borborygmus, eructation, flatus, discomfort, and pain. Halitosis is often recognized. Marked distention of the intestine by gas or a foreign body can cause intermittent episodes of partial paresis. Salivation, shivering, and hiding are seen consistently when smooth muscles of the intestine are stretched or in spasms. Appetite varies from complete anorexia to polyphagia. Water consumption frequently increases. Weight loss appears with disrupted nutritional homeostasis. Thus, diseases of the intestinal tract can have a number of manifestations in addition to or in lieu of diarrhea. Furthermore, many clients do not closely observe their pet's bowel movements, or they may consider important abnormalities to be of no significance. Therefore, the absence of diarrhea from the clinical history does not preclude intestinal disease. The diagnostic approaches to diarrhea and the other manifestations of intestinal disease are outlined in Chapter 5.

CLASSIFICATION OF DIARRHEAL DISEASES

Diseases resulting in diarrhea can be classified by duration, anatomical site, pathophysiology, pathologic appearance and, when possible, by cause. Classifying diarrheal disorders as acute or chronic and large or small bowel diseases helps the clinician to determine appropriate diagnostic and therapeutic regimens. Classification according to pathophysiology helps the clinician grasp the underlying similarities of many diarrheal diseases of widely disparate cause, which in turn suggests common therapeutic approaches. A scheme to describe the pathophysiology of diarrhea is found in Table 16-4. Classification according to pathologic appearance usefully groups disorders that are likely to have similar pathophysiology and may, in some cases, have similar cause. Categorization according to cause is the most useful classification system for the clinician, but, unfortunately, the causes of many diarrheal diseases are unknown.

PATHOPHYSIOLOGY OF DIARRHEA[1]

Introduction

Diarrhea can result from a number of different pathophysiologic processes (Table 16-5). Accumulation of osmotically active particles in the intestinal tract, breakdown in the permeability barrier of the intestine, stimulation of intestinal secretory mechanisms, and alteration in intestinal motility can all result in diarrhea. Of these pathomechanisms, osmotic diarrheal diseases and diarrhea resulting from deranged permeability are thought to be the most common causes of diarrhea in dogs and cats. It is important to note that more than one pathophysiologic process may be simultaneously operative in many patients with diarrhea.

Osmotic Diarrhea

Pathophysiology of Osmotic Diarrhea. The number of osmotically active particles in the feces determines fecal water content. Increases in unabsorbed solutes increase fecal water (Table 16-6) and can lead to osmotic diarrhea. The proximal small bowel is highly permeable to water and NaCl. When hyperosmolar chyme enters the duodenum, water flows across the duodenal mucosa and rapidly reduces the osmolality of the fluid to that of plasma. Sodium diffuses down a concentration gradient from the plasma into the diluted intestinal fluid. The passage of sodium into the intestinal fluid continues to draw more water into the intestinal lumen, in spite of the rapid equilibration of plasma and duodenal osmolality. The ileum and large bowel have low permeability to water and sodium and active transport systems for the absorption of NaCl against

Pathogenesis of Diarrhea

1. High Volume Input to Colon with Normal Colonic Absorption
2. Normal Volume Input to Colon with Decreased Colonic Absorption
3. Abnormal Small and Large Intestine
4. Normal Volume Input to Colon with Normal Colonic Absorption

Table 16-4a. General concepts of pathophysiology of diarrhea. Situation numbers 1 and 3 reflect diseases of the small intestine. Situation numbers 2, 3, and 4 reflect diseases of the large intestine. Number 4 occurs when the pathology involves the most caudal part of the large intestine or the rectum.

Pathogenesis of Diarrhea

Small Intestine:

1. Decreased Absorption of Fluid and Electrolytes
2. Incomplete Absorption of Nutrients (Fats and Carbohydrates)
3. Increased Secretion of Fluid and Electrolytes

Large Intestine:

Decreased Absorption of Fluid and Electrolytes

Table 16-4b. Changes in the small and large intestine which can cause diarrhea.

Pathogenesis of Diarrheas

I. Osmotic Diarrheas
- A. Dietary overload
- B. Malabsorption
  - 1. Pancreatic enzyme deficiency
    - a. Absence of acinar tissue
      - congenital - juvenile atrophy
      - acquired - chronic relapsing pancreatitis
        - pancreatic interstitial fibrosis
    - b. Obstruction of pancreatic ducts - neoplasms
  - 2. Bile deficiency
    - a. Extrahepatic biliary obstruction
    - b. Intraheptic disease
    - c. Chronic ileitis
    - d. Intestinal stasis syndrome
  - 3. Duodenal mucosal disease
    - a. Loss of regulation of secretin and PCZ release
    - b. Loss of enterokinase secretin
    - c. Loss of regulation of gastric emptying by enterogastrone and enterogastric reflex-duodenal overload and lowered pH
  - 4. Small intestinal mucosal disease
    - a. Loss of brush border enzymes
    - b. Loss of transport mechanisms
    - c. Absence of lipid transport lipoproteins
  - 5. Small intestinal intramural disease
    - a. Physical obstacles to absorption
      - i. Cellular infiltration of lamina propria
      - ii. Fluid accumulation in lamina propria
    - b. i. Loss of villus circulation
      - ii. Loss of lymphatic circulation
      - iii. Systemic circulatory disease

II. Abnormal electrolyte and water transport with normal mucosal permeability
- A. Secretion stimulated by bacterial enterotoxins and endotoxins
- B. Inhibition of absorption by unconjugated bile acids
- C. Inhibition of absorption by hydroxylated fatty acids
- D. Secretion stimulated by endocrines

III. Diarrheas caused by abnormal mucosal permeability
- A. Abnormal permeability to fluid and electrolytes (increased)
  - 1. Invasive bacteria
  - 2. Secondary to malabsorption or enterotoxins
- B. Abnormal permeability to plasma proteins - protein losing enteropathy
  - 1. Abnormal metabolism or turnover of mucosal cells
  - 2. Mucosal ulceration by viral, bacterial or parasitic agents
    - a. Congenital absence - lymphangiectasia
    - b. Obstruction by inflammation, neoplasia or fibrosis
    - c. Obstruction secondary to circulatory disease
- C. Abnormal permeability to fluid and electrolytes (decreased)

IV. Diarrheas as a result of changes in intestinal transit time
- A. Transit too slow - stagnant loop syndrome, ileus
- B. Transit too fast
  - 1. Absence of segmentation with normal peristalsis
  - 2. Spasms

Table 16-5. Pathophysiology of diarrheas. Outline of types of changes in the gastrointestinal that result in diarrhea.

steep electrochemical gradients. As a result, NaCl and water are absorbed as the intestinal fluid traverses the ileum and colon. Because of the presence of the non-absorbable solute, however, the intestinal fluid volume does not return to normal, and diarrhea results.

Causes of Osmotic Diarrhea. Osmotic diarrhea can result from overeating, the ingestion of excessive amounts of poorly absorbed ions, maldigestion, or malabsorption. Overeating causes diarrhea due to overload of the intestinal tract with poorly absorbable nutrients, usually carbohydrates or divalent and trivalent ions such as phosphate or sulfate. The diarrhea can result from overeating a regularly fed diet, or it can be a consequence of a sudden change to a new diet containing a nutrient not previously fed in large amounts. After several days have elapsed, adaption to the diet due to an increase in secretion of pancreatic and intestinal digestive enzymes may resolve the diarrhea. The rationale for making dietary changes gradually is based on the need for such adaptation to a new diet. Many laxatives, for instance, contain poorly absorbable ions such as magnesium, sulfate, or phosphate and will induce diarrhea if ingested in excessive quantities.

Increased rate of delivery of food from the stomach to the small intestine can cause osmotic overload. Maldigestion results in the accumulation of nutrients inadequately prepared for absorption. These accumulated molecules lead to osmotic and secretory diarrhea. Ineffective absorption of adequately digested nutrients (malabsorption) can also lead to osmotic diarrhea.

Clinical Appearance of Osmotic Diarrhea. Clinically, osmotic diarrhea is characterized by the resolution of diarrhea when food is withheld for 24-48 hours. Cessation of diarrhea following starvation is not pathognomonic for osmotic diarrhea, however. For instance, diarrhea resulting from secretagogues contained in the food or induced by the digestive process (such as bile acids) will also cease when feeding is stopped. Analysis of fecal electrolytes from patients with osmotic diarrhea should show an osmolar gap, but, as discussed in Chapter 6, fecal osmolar gaps must be interpreted with caution in the dog and cat until additional validation of the technique is performed.

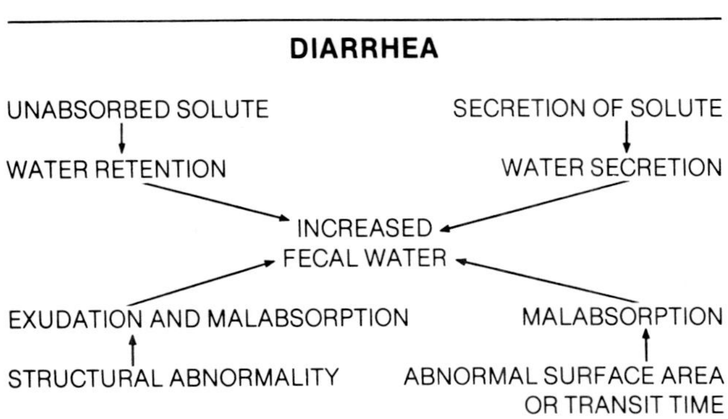

Table 16-6. Pathogenesis of increased fecal water to cause diarrhea. The increment in fecal water results from an increased number of osmotically active particles that are either not absorbed or enter the intestine at an increased rate due to changes in mucosal permeability or activation of an ion secreting mechanism.

Secretory Diarrhea

Pathophysiology of Secretory Diarrhea.[2] The intestine is capable of secreting vast quantities of fluid. The enterocytes in the intestinal crypts are thought to be the predominant source of this fluid, whereas those on the villi tips are the primary site of fluid absorption. In normal intestine, the magnitude of intestinal fluid and ion absorption exceeds that of intestinal secretion. In abnormal intestine, secretion can exceed resorption resulting in secretory diarrhea. Net intestinal ion secretion can result from either the stimulation of secretion to a greater than normal level (active secretion) or from an inhibition of intestinal absorption (passive secretion). Current evidence suggests that many mediators of active intestinal ion secretion also simultaneously inhibit intestinal ion absorption.[3] It is difficult to ascertain which of these processes dominates the activity of individual secretagogues. The intracellular second messages that are generated by secretagogues include cAMP, cGMP, calmodulin, calcium, and phospholipids.[1] These second messengers go on to stimulate active chloride secretion and may inhibit sodium absorption. Some secretagogues increase secretion by virtue of increasing the leakiness of the intestinal tight junctions.

As a result of intestinal secretion, the intestinal lumen will contain increased quantities of monovalent ions and water. It is important to note that secretory diarrhea is often present in association with a mucosa that has normal histologic features and that permeability and many transport processes, such as that for glucose absorption, may still be intact.

Causes of Secretory Diarrhea. A large number and variety of secretory agents and disease processes influence intestinal secretion (Table 16-7). These include various neuropeptides of the enteric nervous system, cholinergic agonists, gastrointestinal hormones, bacterial enterotoxins, deconjugated bile acids, and hydroxy fatty acids (see Chapter 15).

Enterotoxigenic bacteria attach to the mucosal surface without penetrating and produce secretory diarrhea by releasing an enterotoxin. The enterotoxin binds to the epithelial cell and stimulates the formation of second messengers such as cyclic AMP. Cyclic AMP in turn stimulates increased secretion of chloride and decreased absorption of sodium. Many organisms produce enterotoxins, including *Escherichia coli, Clostridium perfringens, Campylobacter* species, *Salmonella typhimurium, Staphylococcus aureus, Klebsiella pneumoniae*, and *Yersinia enterocolitica*. The importance of enterotoxigenic organisms in producing disease in small animals is unknown. Enterotoxigenic diarrhea is discussed in more detail in Chapter 17.

Table 16-7 Putative Causes of Secretory Diarrhea

- Enterotoxins
- APUD neoplasms
- Laxatives (castor oil, dioctyl sodium sulfosuccinate, Bisacodyl)
- Cardiac glycosides
- Bile acid malabsorption
- Fatty acid malabsorption
- Congenital defects
- Intestinal inflammation
- Intestinal lymphoma
- Giardiasis
- Hyperthyroidism
- Malignant carcinoid syndrome?
- Medullary carcinoma of the thyroid
- Mechanical irritation
- Circulatory defects

Any disease process, such as coronavirus infection, that preferentially damages the villi tips can reduce intestinal absorption. Decreased small intestine absorption of deconjugated, dihydroxy bile acids such as deoxycholic and chenodeoxycholic acid by the small intestine stimulate colonic secretion of fluid. The deconjugated bile acids cause secretion, at least partly, by increasing the leakiness of the tight junctions. Hydroxylated fatty acids are capable of inciting diarrhea in both the large and small intestine. The pathomechanism may be partly due to increased transcellular permeability and hence passive secretion. Vasoactive intestinal polypeptide and serotonin are responsible for profuse secretory diarrhea in humans with pancreatic cholera and the carcinoid syndrome, respectively. Prostaglandin E_2, substance P, HETE, HPETE, and bradykinin can be increased in inflamed tissues and are capable of stimulating intestinal secretion. Cardiac glycosides increase intestinal secretion, as do certain laxatives such as bisacodyl. Elevated venous pressure, lymphatic obstruction, hypoalbuminemia, and increases in epithelial permeability all alter fluid dynamics in the mucosa and can result in decreased absorption and a passive secretory diarrhea.

Clinical Appearance of Secretory Diarrhea. Secretory diarrhea is characterized clinically by the absence of a fecal osmolar gap, persistence of the diarrhea during fasting (not all types of secretory diarrhea), and the absence of inflammatory cells, blood, or fat in the feces. The secretory diarrheas that cease when the patient fasts include those due to fatty acid and bile acid malabsorption. It is not uncommon for patients to present with secretory diarrhea in association with osmotic diarrhea, blurring the clinical differentiation of these two conditions.

Diarrhea Resulting from Increased Permeability

Structure of the Intestinal Permeability Barrier. The mucosa of the small and large intestine forms a semipermeable barrier that controls the transmucosal movement of fluid and electrolytes and restricts the absorption or loss of larger molecules. Important epithelial components of the barrier include the mucus layer, the glycocalyx, the epithelial cells, and the tight junctions situated at the apical borders of the epithelial cells. The tight junctions appear to have a very important role in the maintenance of intestinal epithelial permeability. At the tight junctions, the lateral plasma membranes of adjacent cells come into close apposition with each other, forming a series of punctate membrane fusions linked by strands of what appear to be proteins. Tight junction morphology correlates with the permeability characteristics of the membrane. Thus, the paracellular permeability decreases as the junctional strand count increases.[4] Moreover, recent evidence suggests that tight junction permeability can be regulated by a perijunctional ring of actin and myosin, raising the possibility that transjunctional mucosal permeability can be finely regulated on a minute-by-

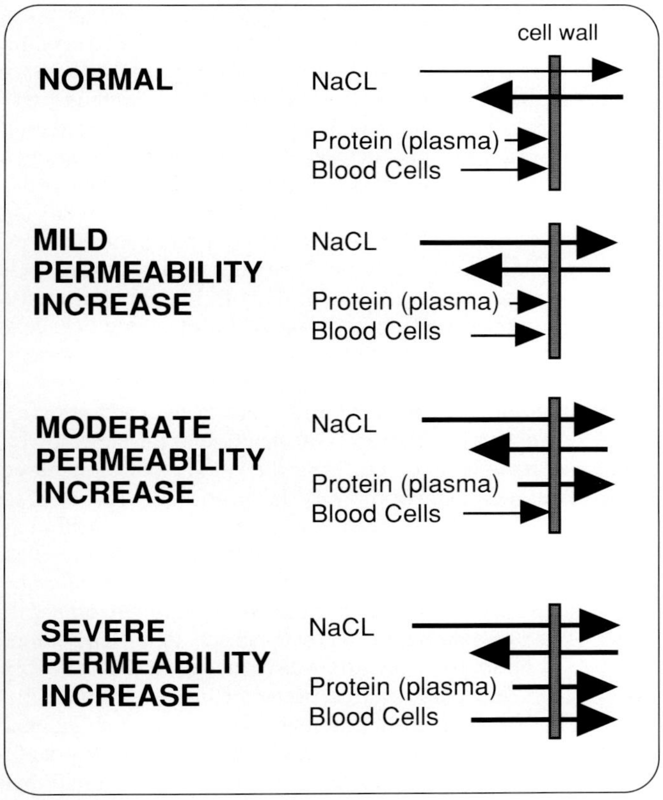

Figure 16-1. Effects of permeability changes on fluid and macromolecule loss into intestine.

minute basis.[5] The suggested importance of tight junctions in regulating intestinal permeability is compatible with recent concepts of intestinal absorption and secretion, in which the absorptive cell is believed to concentrate Na and Cl in the basolateral space, from whence it diffuses into the lamina propria. The tight junction is thus in a position to regulate the back leakage of fluid and electrolytes from the basolateral space into the lumen of the intestine. "Tight" junctions in the upper small intestine are known to be permeable to fluid, electrolytes, and other small solutes. The result is a predominance of passive fluid fluxes across the small intestine. In contrast, the tight junctions of the colon are impermeable to fluid and electrolytes, allowing the active transport of electrolytes against concentration gradients.

The capillaries and lymphatics of the mucosa have important functions in the maintenance of normal permeability. One of these functions is the conservation of plasma protein and another is the removal of absorbed fluid, preventing increased mucosal interstitial hydrostatic pressure. Additional components of the intestinal permeability barrier include the cellular and humoral immune system in the lamina propria and the mononuclear-phagocyte system in the liver. Defects in these systems permit an excessive amount of macromolecules to enter the body.

Pathophysiology of Diarrhea Resulting from Increased Intestinal Permeability

The intestinal permeability barrier has a number of different functions. One of these functions is to act as a semipermeable membrane that retains electrolytes absorbed by active or facilitated diffusion against concentration gradients. The effective retention of these electrolytes creates an osmotic gradient by which water can be absorbed from the intestinal lumen. If intestinal permeability increases, absorbed electrolytes flow back into the bowel, no concentration gradient develops; and fecal water concentration will increase. Therefore, mild increases in permeability result in reduced absorption of ions and water and lead to a net intestinal fluid loss. Mild permeability increases are thus sometimes referred to as a cause of "passive" secretory diarrhea.

If the epithelial permeability barrier becomes further deranged, plasma proteins such as albumin that reside in the interstitium of the lamina propria may be lost into the lumen of the bowel. If the permeability failure extends to involve the mucosal blood vessels, additional plasma proteins and eventually red blood cells may be lost (Figure 16-1). The loss of red blood cells requires a greater than 10,000 fold increase in pore size.

Another function of the mucosal permeability barrier is to prevent the unrestrained absorption of macromolecules from the lumen, thus helping maintain oral tolerance (Chapter 3). The barrier to the absorption of macromolecules includes not only the physical barrier provided by the epithelial cell, which possesses some ability to degrade proteins, but also the cellular and humoral immune system in the lamina propria and the mononuclear-phagocyte system in the liver. Defects in any one of the three permit an excessive amount of macromolecules to enter the body. As discussed in Chapter 3, the permeability to macromolecules is an age-related phenomenon, with intestinal "closure" occurring in most domestic species within several days of birth, but in carnivores being delayed for as long as ten-twelve days.[6] Furthermore, closure is never complete; adult animals absorb up to 2% of dietary protein intact, presumably largely through the intestinal M cells.

Causes of Increased Intestinal Permeability. Abnormalities that increase intestinal epithelial permeability include epithelial erosion or ulceration, mucosal inflammation, cellular infiltration of the lamina propria by neoplastic cells, and circulatory diseases that result in ischemia or lymphatic hypertension.

The most obvious cause of increased epithelial permeability is destruction of the enterocyte. The resultant intestinal erosions or ulcerations freely ooze interstitial fluid or blood. Gastrointestinal erosions and ulcerations may result from a wide variety of conditions including severe mucosal inflammation, intestinal neoplasia, mucosal ischemia, invasive infectious agents, toxins, antiinflammatory medications, uremia, mastocytosis, hepatic insufficiency, gastrinomas, stress, and perhaps inadequate mucosal bicarbonate or mucus secretion.[7]

Mucosal inflammation is known to increase intestinal epithelial permeability. The latter is a well recognized complication of chronic inflammatory bowel disease, gluten-induced enteropathy, and soy and milk protein intolerance. The pathomechanisms of the increased epithelial permeability are unclear, but proposals include epithelial denudation or, in less severe cases, the development of a less differentiated epithelium as a result of increased cell turnover.[8] Furthermore, gamma interferon increases epithelial tight junction permeability, as does increased mucosal fibrinolytic activity.

Circulatory disorders result in increased permeability due to increased hydrostatic pressure, which increases pore size. Additional factors known to increase mucosal epithelial permeability include exposure of the mucosa to bile salts, lysolecithin, and hyperosmolar solutions, and treatment with nonsteroidal antiinflammatory agents[9] and cytotoxic drugs such as 5-fluorouracil.[6,10,11] Surgical trauma to the intestine, intestinal ischemia, protein malnutrition, systemic anaphylaxis, and parasite infections also increase epithelial permeability.[6]

The permeability of intestinal capillaries is increased by a variety of pathologic interventions, including ischemia, exposure to *Escherichia coli* endotoxin, histamine, and bradykinin.[12] The majority of these conditions increase capillary permeability by increasing the diameter of large-size capillary pores resulting in increased protein leakage into the interstitium.

Clinical Appearance of Diarrhea Resulting from Increased Permeability. Diarrhea resulting from permeability disorders does not completely abate when food is withheld. Severe increases in permeability are characterized by melena, hematochezia, hypoproteinemia, and sometimes by evidence of gastrointestinal inflammation such as tenesmus or increased fecal leukocyte concentration.

Diarrhea Resulting from Deranged Motility

Pathophysiology of Deranged Motility. Disordered intestinal motility contributes to the pathogenesis of many diarrheal diseases and may be the primary pathomechanism in some cases (Table 16-8). It can be difficult to establish whether a motility abnormality is the cause of diarrhea or simply a secondary consequence of a primary disease process, such as inflammation.

Motility changes that speed intestinal transit cause diarrhea; these changes result in decreased intestinal fluid absorption, presumably due to decreased contact time between the enterocyte and the luminal content. Two motility abnormalities, decreased segmental contractions and increased peristaltic contractions can result in accelerated intestinal passage. The most common cause is decreased frequency of segmental contractions, which reduces the resistance of the intestinal tract to the flow of ingesta. Increased frequency of peristaltic contractions was initially thought to be a very important cause of diarrhea, but it now appears that few cases of diarrhea result from increased peristaltic activity. In contrast, reduced or deranged peristaltic activity may lead to diarrhea by predisposing the intestinal tract to bacterial overgrowth.

Causes of Deranged Intestinal Motility. Deranged intestinal motility in association with diarrhea has been documented in hookworm infections of dogs,[13] canine dysautonomia, a small percentage of cases of feline dysautonomia, canine pseudoobstruction syndrome, and feline colitis (Table 16-8). In parasite infections, violent intestinal contractions have been reported as part of the "self-cure" response resulting from mast cell degranulation. In a dog with myenteric ganglionitis, the transit time of barium from the stomach to the colon was very rapid (three minutes), strongly suggesting a motility defect, perhaps decreased segmental contractions.[14]

With colitis, deranged motility due to the inflammatory process compromises the reservoir function of the large bowel. In cats and, to a lesser extent, dogs the cranial half of the large intestine has a gradient of motility that is normally reversed, so that propulsive activity retains contents until absorption is nearly complete. That gradient is lost during colitis[15] and perhaps with other causes of diarrhea. Colonic inflammation also decreases segmentation motility contributing to an accelerated transit of material through the cranial colon. The pathogenesis of the motility disturbances is not clear but probably results either from a direct effect of the mediators such as PGE_2, or leukotrienes on smooth muscle function or from an indirect effect of these mediators on the enteric nervous system.

The importance of irritable bowel syndrome in animals has yet to be established (see Chapter 25).

Clinical Appearance of Diarrhea Resulting from Motility Disturbance. In view of the difficulty in definitively diagnosing motility derangements as the cause of diarrhea, there is no well recognized clinical picture associated with motility diarrheas. Humans suspected of having "motility" diarrhea reportedly have voluminous diarrhea that persists during fed times, as well as a fecal electrolyte pattern with no osmolar gap during the unfed state, and a slight osmolar gap with mild steatorrhea following eating.[3] Hypomotility in association with bacterial overgrowth may generate the clinical-laboratory features characteristic of bacterial overgrowth.

Table 16-8. Diarrheal Diseases in Which Deranged Motility May Play a Role

Irritable bowel syndrome
APUD tumors
Hyperthyroidism
Bile acid malabsorption
Myenteric ganglionitis
Dysautonomia
Infectious gastroenteritis
Gastrointestinal parasitism
Gastrointestinal neoplasia
Pseudoobstruction syndrome
Colitis
Bacterial overgrowth

CAUSES OF ACUTE GASTROINTESTINAL DISEASES

The acute onset of diarrhea with or without vomiting is a very common problem that has an extensive number of possible causes many of which are infectious, parasitic, or toxic in nature (Figure 16-2). The specific cause of acute diarrhea in an individual animal is seldom identified, however, because the transient nature of the clinical signs precludes extensive diagnostic evaluation.

Acute diarrhea often occurs as a result of a dietary change. This may be due to a transient maldigestion as a result of the provision of insufficient time for pancreatic secretion and intestinal brush border activity to acustomize to the dominant nutrients in the new diet. Alternatively, the diarrhea may result from a food intolerance or allergy.

Animals with an acute onset of vomiting and diarrhea are frequently suspected of inadvertent or malicious poisoning. The likelihood of toxicity is considerably greater in an animal with access to an unknown environment rather than an animal restricted to its own property. However, even within the closeted environment of the indoor pet, the list of potential toxins that can result in acute gastrointestinal upset is extensive.[16-18] Acute vomiting and diarrhea due to poisoning should be of particular suspicion in patients with concurrent clinical signs of other body systems. For instance, generalized parasympathetic over activity manifest as hypersalivation, vomiting, diarrhea, and pinpoint pupils, is suggestive of organophosphate or carbamate toxicity. Table 16-9 lists "cross-referenced" associations of the clinical signs from different body systems that may help determine the toxin involved.

Acute diarrhea can also be produced by infectious agents. Examples of viruses causing diarrhea are canine distemper virus, affecting a number of organ systems, and feline panleukopenia virus, affecting only the gastrointestinal tract. Rickettsial agents cause diarrhea in poisoning from ingesting salmon. Enteric bacterial pathogens such as *Salmonella, Clostridium perfringens, Campylobacter*, and *Yersinia enterocolitica* may cause diarrhea. They do not appear to be frequent causes of diarrhea and much of their importance lies in their zoonotic potential. Parasites such as ascarids, hookworms, whipworms, *Cryptosporidia*, and coccidia may also cause diarrhea.

DIAGNOSTIC APPROACH TO ACUTE GASTROINTESTINAL DISEASES

The approach to the diagnosis of acute gastrointestinal diseases should be by the problem-orientated approach. The diagnostic approaches to the common manifestations of acute gastrointestinal diseases, such as the problems of vomiting, diarrhea, and acute abdomen are described in Chapter 5. The diagnostic evaluation of most patients with acute gastrointestinal problems is largely restricted to a history and physical examination. Unless warning signs of serious disease are present, any further diagnostic endeavors are usually delayed until the response to a therapeutic trial have been evaluated.

The patient's signalment, vaccination history, anthelmintic history, and the nature of the environment is determined. Young animals are more prone to nutritional, microbial, and parasitic, causes of diarrhea. Certain breed predispositions are apparent (Table 5-3). A dog or cat recently placed in a boarding kennel is likely to have an infectious cause for gastroenteritis. An animal with complete freedom in an unknown environment is more likely to develop infectious, toxic, and traumatic disorders. Diarrhea is often associated with environmental changes. The animal's diet should be determined. Adverse reactions to food are a prominent cause of diarrhea and the history is a rapid way to identify responsible nutrients. Ingestion of salmon or trout in endemic areas raises the likelihood of salmon poisoning. Evidence of multisystemic disease increases the index of suspicion for distemper or toxicities (see Table 16-9).

Particularly important parts of the physical examination are the assessment of the animal's attitude, cardiovascular status and degree of dehydration; oral examination; abdominal palpation; and rectal examination. Fever in association with acute gastrointestinal disease is suggestive of severe mucosal breakdown such as can occur with enteroinvasive organisms.

The clinical examination rarely definitively determines the cause of acute vomiting or diarrhea but usually likely possibili-

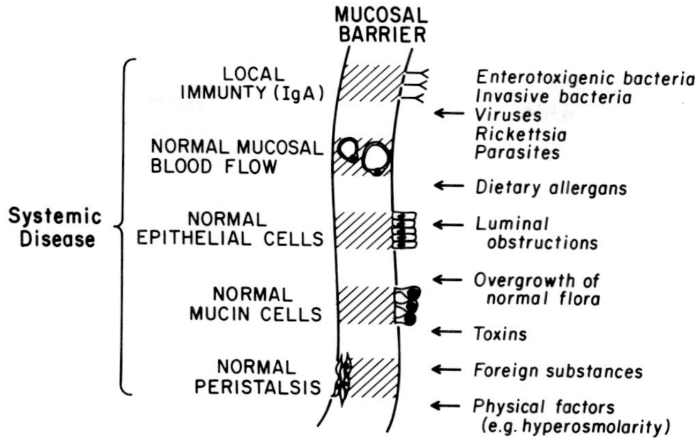

Figure 16-2. Diagram of causes of acute diarrhea and factors in the intestinal mucosa to prevent pathology and clinical signs from developing.

Table 16-9. Toxicities That Can Cause Vomiting and Diarrhea Categorized According to Likely Concurrent Clinical Signs

Vomiting and/or diarrhea with stomatitis
Acids and alkalis
Aldehydes
Caustic products
Detergents
Dieffenbachia
Mercury
Paraquat
Petroleum distillates
Phenols
Philodendron
Thallium

Vomiting and/or diarrhea with cardiac arrhythmias
Foxgloves
Lily of the valley
Oleander
Organophosphates
Thallium
Yew (Taxus sp)

Vomiting and/or diarrhea with hepatotoxicity
Aflatoxins
Amanita Sp mushrooms
Blue-green algae
Phosphorus

Vomiting and/or diarrhea with respiratory toxicity
ANTU
Organophosphates
Paraquat

Vomiting and/or diarrhea with nephrotoxicity
Amanita Sp mushroom
Amaryllis bulbs
Arsenic
Azalea
Castor bean
Daffodil bulbs
English Ivy
Horse chestnut
Iris bulbs
Jasmine
Mock orange
Organophosphates
Phosphorus
Rhododendron
Mercury
Nightshades
Lead
Paraquat
Phenols
Thallium

Vomiting and/or diarrhea with CNS signs
Ethylene glycol
Lead
Organochlorines
Organophosphates
Phenols
Mercury
Metaldehyde

Vomiting and/or diarrhea with generalized parasympathetic
Amanita Sp mushrooms
Carbamates
Organophosphates

ties are unearthed. Moreover, the physical examination is the prime guide to the severity of the patients condition. Gastrointestinal disease can markedly affect fluid, electrolyte, and nutritional homeostasis. Warning signs of serious disease include depression, anorexia, weight loss, weakness, dehydration, hyperpnea, pale, congested, or discolored mucous membranes, slow capillary refill, weak rapid pulse, fever, melena, and abdominal organomegaly, pain, masses, or effusions.

By the conclusion of the clinical examination the veterinarian should be able to locate the site of the disorder (e.g. large or small bowel diarrhea) and assess the degree of severity. If the cause of the diarrhea is not apparent following the clinical examination, and warning signs of serious disease are present, the clinician is obligated to recommend supportive therapy, and a diagnostic workup to expediently determine safe and effective therapy. In the absence of warning signs, symptomatic therapy and treatment trials are permissible. Toxicological analyses may be indicated depending on the likelihood of exposure.

LABORATORY FINDINGS & DIAGNOSIS OF ACUTE GASTROINTESTINAL DISEASES

A useful diagnostic evaluation in patient's with acute diarrhea is the examination of a direct smear of the feces. Fecal smears will occasionally reveal parasitic ova and protozoa; with staining, inflammatory cells may be recognized and are suggestive of an enterocolitis. Only heavy parasitic infestations are identified on direct smears. Examination for intestinal parasites by fecal flotation and sedimentation may be performed but even these concentration techniques have questionable reliability with watery diarrheic feces.

If bacterial pathogens are suspected (See Chapter 5 & 6) feces may be cultured, with the primary aim of identifying a bacteria with public health significance. It is not feasible at present to routinely identify enteropathogenic *E. coli* that may be of public health significance. Serotyping and various other refined subtyping procedures are required for the identification of enteropathogenic *E. coli* because this family has both pathogenic and benign strains. The serotyping systems are generally based on recognition of somatic (O), flagella (H), and capsular (K) antigens. Over 150 somatic (O) antigens and more than 40 flagellar (H) antigens have been recognized. Tests of feces for clostridial or coliform enterotoxins may also be of value in select cases as may virus identification procedures.

Little useful information is gained from additional laboratory examinations unless the history and physical examination reveal evidence of gastrointestinal obstruction, systemic problems or serious disease. If, such problems are identified a hemogram, blood chemistry panel, urinalysis, blood gas analysis, and/or survey abdominal radiographs may be required. These diagnostic procedures provide information that greatly helps differential diagnosis and case management.

Gastrointestinal biopsy is rarely of use in identifying the cause or pathogenesis of acute diarrhea. Enterotoxin stimulates epithelial cells to secrete fluid without changing their appearance. After 24 hours secondary changes may begin to appear but these are non-specific. Invasion by a pathogen produces an enteritis that cannot be differentiated from an enteritis caused by secondary invasion by a member of the normal microflora, although the ulcerative and suppurative nature of the process does raise the index of suspicion for bacterial infection rather than idiopathic inflammatory bowel disease. Causal organisms are seldom identified. An exception, is invasion of the mucosa by fungal agents (Figure 16-3), or protozoa. Postmortem changes in the intestine are rapid, being accelerated by the bacteria and proteases in the intestinal lumen. Consequently, even at necropsy it is often difficult to determine how the mucosa appeared at the time of death.

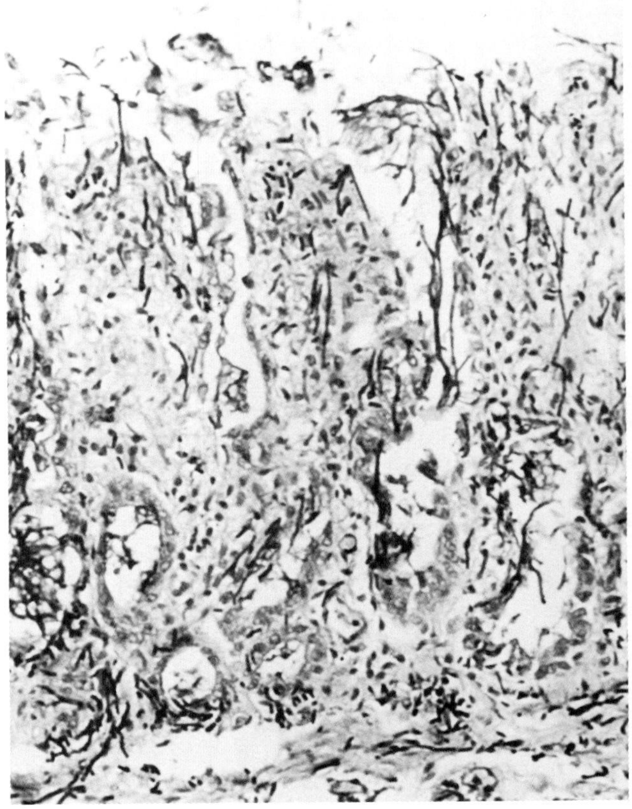

Figure 16-3. Jejunum from cat stained with PAS to show mycotic organisms causing enteritis. Branching septate hyphae are typical of aspergillosis. Animal was immunosuppressed as shown by severe hypoplasia of lymphoid tissues and bone marrow; the cause is unknown.

SYMPTOMATIC THERAPY OF ACUTE DIARRHEA

As with any medical problem, the therapy of a patient with acute diarrhea is best based on a knowledge of cause. Unfortunately, however, the causes of diarrheal diseases are often never ascertained, either because of the elusive nature of the disease process or because minimal diagnostic effort is expended in view of financial constraints or anticipated brevity of the diarrhea. As a result, the symptomatic therapy of diarrhea is commonplace in veterinary practice. Symptomatic therapy is also of importance in the adjunctive supportive treatment of patients with diarrhea in whom the primary cause is known.

The most critical aspects of the symptomatic treatment of

acute diarrhea are bowel rest and the maintenance of fluid and electrolyte homeostasis. Of additional concern in some patients is the prevention or elimination of septicemia. Furthermore, the patient may be treated symptomatically with agents that alter the motility of the gut, or act as protectives.

The symptomatic treatment of diarrhea is still largely empirical. Many methods are used that are honored by time but not science. Most animals recover from diarrhea whether or not they are treated. The high incidence of spontaneous remission reinforces the mistaken belief that certain inappropriate therapies, such as anticholinergic agents and oral aminoglycosides, are effective. In many cases it is more appropriate to conclude that the patient recovered *in spite* of the therapy.

Fluid Therapy

The administration of fluids, of sufficient volume and appropriate composition to correct preexisting fluid, electrolyte, and acid-base derangements and to satisfy ongoing requirements, is the single most important consideration in the therapy of any patient with diarrhea.

Decisions must be made with regard the route of administration, the quantity of fluid to be delivered, the composition of the fluid, and the rate of delivery. These considerations are addressed in detail in the chapter on fluid electrolyte therapy.

The intravenous route is the preferred route of fluid administration for dehydrated animals in all but intractable patients. Inability to place an intravenous catheter in a hypovolemic atient is an indication for a cut down procedure or for intramedullary administration of fluid, not an indication for subcutaneous fluids. The composition of the fluid administered is best judged by the serum electrolyte, total protein, and glucose concentration, and by the hematocrit. Choices include lactated Ringer's solution and 0.45% or 0.9% sodium chloride with added potassium chloride; sodium bicarbonate, or dextrose; dextrans; plasma; and blood. In most patients with diarrhea, an appropriate replacement fluid is lactated Ringer's solution supplemented with an additional 10-15 mEq of potassium chloride per liter. The volume administered is dependent on the patients body weight and estimated degree of dehydration (5-12%). The rate of administration should be sufficiently rapid to replace the patient's fluid deficit in as short a time as the patient's cardiovascular, respiratory, and renal systems will permit. For most patients with uncomplicated diarrheal disease, replacement of preexisting fluid losses can be achieved within six-twelve hours. Additional fluid is required to replace the patient's maintenance requirements (50-70 ml/kg/day) and ongoing additional losses. The latter are estimated from the volume of diarrhea or vomitus passed by the patient.

Harmful Effects of Antibiotics

- Overgrowth of fungi and minor organisms of normal flora
- Diarrhea due to neomycin, tetracycline, ampicillin
- Produces resistant bacteria
- Increases susceptibility to infection by pathogen
- Prolongs carrier state in salmonellosis
- Interferes with nutrition
- Systemic toxicity of aminoglycosides

Table 16-10. Harmful effects of antibiotics that can be used to treat diarrhea

Cooperative patients that are not markedly dehydrated may be treated with glucose-containing oral rehydration solutions (Enterolyte; Beecham). Even in secretory diarrheas it appears that the sodium-organic solute (glucose or neutral amino acid) absorption mechanism is still active.[1]

It is important to emphasize that the fluid, electrolyte, and acid-base derangements occurring in patients with gastrointestinal diseases are quite variable, and in all cases fluid therapy must be tailored to the particular fluid requirements of the individual patient.

Antibiotics[19-23]

Adverse Effects of Antibiotic Administration. Antibiotics have a number of predictable adverse effects on the gastrointestinal tract (Table 16-10) and if injudiciously used will complicate recovery from diarrhea.[24]

In the large intestine, antibiotic administration results in a slight, transient reduction of the total numbers of bacteria. Within one to two days, bacterial numbers return to their previous level in spite of continued administration of the antibacterial agent. While the total numbers of bacteria in the large bowel are little affected by antibiotics, fecal bacterial composition can be markedly altered. Bacteria that develop resistance to antibiotics slowly, such as the gram positive anaerobes, may be depressed for prolonged periods of time following the administration of antibiotics with efficiency against anaerobic bacteria. In contrast, coliform numbers can usually be significantly lowered only on a transient basis, because they rapidly develop antibiotic resistance. Antibiotic resistance possessed by one group of coliforms can be readily transferred to another within 24 to 48 hours. Within several days, the numbers of coliforms return to normal and, in the presence of a depressed anaerobic population, these potentially more virulent gram negative organisms may proliferate in excessive numbers, predisposing the animal to sepsis. For example, in guinea pigs, erythromycin suppresses anaerobes and causes intestinal coliforms to increase from 10^2 bacteria per gram of feces to 10^7 per gram, resulting in death within ten to fourteen days. Overgrowth by yeasts and fungi may also occur following prolonged antibiotic administration.[25]

The animal with diarrhea is particularly vulnerable to the adverse effects of antibiotics on the composition of bacterial flora. Dogs with diarrhea have a decreased number of Lactobacilli and increased numbers of *Bacteroides* and members of the *Enterobacteriaceae*.[26] The concentration of colonic anaerobes is reduced in the feces during diarrhea because these organisms normally require stasis, and the low oxygen environment it provides, for their growth.[27] Pathological processes such as malassimilation markedly alter the intestinal milieu, leading to derangements in the composition of bacteria. In this situation, a pathogenic opportunist such as *Salmonella* can colonize the bowel, whereas it may have been previously excluded by the resistance of the normal flora. Use of antibiotics further deranges the normal flora while not inhibiting the growth of bacteria such as *Salmonella*, further predisposing the animal to colonization by pathogens. Normal intestinal function does not

Table 16-11. Circumstances in Which Antibiotic Usage for the Treatment of Diarrhea has Justification

Acute hemorrhagic diarrhea
Culture of a known pathogen
Bacterial overgrowth
Evidence of sepsis
Presence of profound neutropenia (<1000/ul)

return until the microbial population of the gut returns to normal. Thus, a goal of treatment is to use no medication that interferes with renewal of the normal microflora.

Additional adverse effects of antibiotics include the prolongation of the carrier state in salmonellosis, and the production of various side effects including anorexia, vomiting, and iatrogenic diarrhea that can confuse the clinical picture and delay recovery. Gastrointestinal upset is most commonly seen in dogs and cats as a result of treatment with neomycin, tetracycline, erythromycin, metronidazole, or chloramphenicol. In humans, the diarrhea from neomycin administration is due to a malabsorption syndrome associated with only a mild morphologic defect. The malabsorption may result from precipitation of bile salts in the small intestine or from alteration of microbial flora in favor of species such as *Bacteroides* and *Clostridia* that secrete amidases capable of deconjugating bile salts.[28] Neomycin also appears to interfere with pancreatic lipase activity and decrease bile acid resorption.[29] The diarrhea resulting from tetracyclines results from changes in the intestinal microflora and possibly from of an irritative effect.

Aminoglycosides have well recognized renal toxicity, vestibular toxicity, and ototoxicity. The renal toxicity of aminoglycosides is enhanced by youth, dehydration, overdosage, and concurrent administration of certain drugs such as some cephalosporins and nonsteroidal antiinflammatory drugs. These predisposing conditions occur frequently in diarrheal diseases. Oral aminoglycosides are administered in quantities that far exceed the recommended parenteral doses. In normal animals the aminoglycoside is not absorbed, and no systemic toxicity results. In animals with a disrupted intestinal mucosal barrier, however, the absorption of oral aminoglycosides can be increased. In particular, toxic systemic levels can result if repeated oral administration is continued in an animal with decreased glomerular filtration from renal disease or dehydration.[29] Oral aminoglycoside preparations should never be given to dehydrated patients with evidence of a disrupted mucosal barrier.

The indiscriminate usage of antibiotics in small animal patients has serious public health implications. R-factor transfer of antibiotic resistance has been demonstrated in the dog, and there is good reason to believe antibiotic resistant bacteria could be transferred from pet to owner, leading to the possibility of antibiotic-nonresponsive gastrointestinal infections in humans.[28,30]

Indications for Antibiotic Therapy. Antibiotic usage for the treatment of diarrhea is justified only in a select group of circumstances (Table 16-11). The most frequent indication is suspicion that the bacteria have invaded the intestinal mucosa, from whence they could be a potential cause of bacteremia or septicemia. Evidence of mucosal invasion includes hemorrhagic diarrhea and evidence of sepsis such as fever, depression, degenerative left-shifted leukograms, or positive blood cultures. The presence of occasional streaks of fresh blood on the stool is not an indication for antibiotic therapy.

Antibiotic therapy is aimed at eliminating bacteria that have penetrated the mucosa, are circulating in the blood stream, or have distributed to other organs such as the liver. It is not aimed at "sterilizing" the bowel, a virtually impossible task. Therefore, under these circumstances parenteral administration of antibiotics is by far the most suitable initial route of administration. Subsequent antibiotics may be administered orally, but the antibiotic should be capable of systemic distribution.

Antibiotic usage can be considered if a known pathogen is cultured from the feces of the patient or if firm evidence of a bacterial pathogen is obtained by fecal smears, assays for fecal enterotoxins, or intestinal biopsy. Even in the face of a positive fecal culture, if the animal is not showing evidence of sepsis, the provision of antibiotic therapy may not result in more rapid recovery than the provision of supportive care alone. Animals have a large variety of natural defenses against bacterial pathogens, not the least of which is floral resistance. Thus, most bacterial enteritis conditions will resolve without the requirement for antibiotic intervention. Factors that enter into the decision of whether to treat with antibiotics include the type of bacteria cultured, the nature of the clinical signs, and the likelihood of a public health risk from the particular bacteria cultured.

Antibiotic usage is justified in the therapy of dogs with bacterial overgrowth of the small intestine (Chapter 17). Prophylactic antibiotic therapy is appropriate if an animal presents with a profound neutropenia, a common complication of parvovirus infection. Routine usage of antibiotics in non-hemorrhagic diarrhea is not warranted, in view of the rarity with which enteric pathogens are cultured, the self-limiting nature of many bacterial infections, and the potential adverse effects of antibiotic therapy.

Choice of Antibiotic. Bactericidal antibiotics capable of parenteral administration are recommended in the initial treatment of patients with acute, severe hemorrhagic diarrhea or of patients whose bacterial-mediated diarrheal process is complicated by vomiting. Non-absorbable oral antibiotics should not be used because of the potential for toxicity if the mucosal barrier is disrupted and because the aim of antibiotic therapy is to kill invading bacteria, not "sterilize" the bowel lumen.

The antibiotic should be chosen with consideration as to the spectrum of activity and the concentration of the antibiotic achieved within the bowel lumen, two factors which are prime determinants of the disruptive nature of the antibiotics on normal flora (Table 16-12). Ampicillin, and, to a lesser extent, amoxicillin are broad spectrum antibiotics that are highly disruptive of normal flora. These antibiotics should thus be avoided for the treatment of gram negative bacterial pathogens and should not be used in neutropenic animals because they predispose to gram negative intestinal overgrowth. Colonization of the gastrointestinal tract with gram negative pathogens often precedes bacteremia.[31]

A more suitable antibiotic in these situations is a trimethoprim sulfa combination, as these drugs have broad spectrum activity against aerobics and *invading* anaerobic bacteria but minimally disrupt intestinal flora. Trimethoprim-sulfa may not adequately inhibit some aerobes such as *Pseudomonas*, however, and if used for prolonged periods of time at high doses may delay bone marrow recovery.

Comparison of Antimicrobial Drugs Effect on Normal Flora

Drug	Effects on Normal Flora	Bactericidal Activity
Penicillin G	Minimal	Very good
Ampicillin	Major	Very good
Amoxicillin	Major	Very good
Trimethoprim-sulfa	Minimal	Very good
Metronidazole	Minimal to moderate	Very good
Fluoroquinolones	Minimal	Very good
Gentamicin	Minimal	Very good
Lincomycin	Major	Little
Chloramphenicol	Minimal	None
Tetracycline	Minimal	None
Erythromycin	Minimal-moderate	None
Vancomycin	? Minimal	Very good
Clindamycin	Moderate	Moderate

Table 16-12a. Comparison of effects of antimicrobial drugs that are effective against intestinal bacteria. Penicillin remains the drug of choice to treat against bacteria that may invade from the bowel.

On occasion it may be advantageous to use ampicillin or amoxicillin precisely because of their effectiveness against anaerobic flora in the intestinal lumen. For instance, these drugs are indicated in the treatment of patients with clostridial overgrowths, such as are seen in intestinal obstruction. There is some suggestion that orally administered ampicillin may be more effective than orally administered amoxicillin in this regard, because ampicillin is less completely absorbed than amoxicillin and so attains higher luminal concentrations.

Metronidazole is an antimicrobial drug with a very broad spectrum activity against anaerobic bacteria including *Bacteroides fragilis*, a beta lactamase-producing bacterium that is often resistant to penicillins. The importance of *Bacteroides fragilis* infections in small animal enteric disease is unknown, and the primary role of metronidazole is in the treatment of inflammatory bowel disease.

Tylosin is an antibacterial agent similar to erythromycin and whose use in small animals is virtually confined to the therapy of inflammatory bowel disease. Both metronidazole and tetracycline antibiotics have found a role in the therapy of bacterial overgrowth. Not uncommon side effects of tetracyclines are anorexia, vomiting, and diarrhea. These signs are particularly common in cats. Doxycycline is a unique antibiotic in that it is excreted directly through the mucosa of the gastrointestinal tract. It has been recommended for the treatment of coliform diarrheas in humans and has a broad spectrum of activity that includes anaerobes. The drug is excreted in the feces as an inactive conjugate or chelate and for this reason has minimal affect on the intestinal microflora.

Lincomycin and erythromycin have limited value in the treatment of diarrheal disease because of disruptive effects on microflora, needless expense, and, particularly in the case of erythromycin, a high incidence of drug-induced vomiting. Erythromycin is primarily indicated for the treatment of *Campylobacter*.[27] Chloramphenicol is considered the drug of choice by some for the therapy of *Salmonella*.[27]

Clindamycin is highly effective against many gram positive aerobes and most species of anaerobes, including *Bacteroides fragilis*. Clindamycin inhibits growth of sensitive organisms for up to two weeks after its discontinuation. It is associated with a high incidence of diarrhea in humans and in some patients has caused pseudomembranous colitis.

Cephalosporins (first generation) are increasingly used for veterinary patients. They are very effective against *Klebsiella* infections and have application in the treatment of sepsis and intestinal overgrowth by *Staphylococci*, and *Proteus* species. Their gram negative and anaerobic spectrum is limited.

Another class of antibiotics that is likely to be of prime importance in the treatment of enteric infections is the fluoroquinolones. Fluoroquinolones are derivatives of nalidixic acid. Fluoroquinolones such as norfloxacin (Noroxin; Merk, Sharp, & Dome) have reportedly been very effective in reducing the aerobic bacterial flora of the stool, generally without causing resistant organisms to appear or affecting the anaerobic flora.[31] The prime advantages of these drugs are a potent gram negative spectrum in combination with a very slow acquisition of resistance, perhaps through inhibition of plasmid transfer.[31] They have been found to be effective in the therapy of a variety of

Table 16-12b. Doses of antibiotics of potential use in the treatment of bacterial-mediated diarrheas in small animals.

DRUG	DOSE	Comment
Ampicillin	10-20mg/kg q 6-8 hr IV, SQ, IM, PO	Anaerobic infections Sepsis (use with aminoglycoside)
Cephalothin sodium	22-44 mg/kg q 6-8 hr IM, IV	Sepsis ?
Erythromycin	10 mg/kg q 8 hr PO	Campylobacter only
Gentamicin	2.2 mg/kg q 8 hr SQ, IV, IM	Sepsis only
Chloramphenicol	20-50 mg/kg q 8 hr PO, IV, IM, SQ	Minimize use; care in cats
Tetracyclines	20 mg/kg q 8 hr PO	Bacterial overgrowth
Trimethoprim-sulfa	15 mg/kg q 12 hr PO, IV, IM	General first choice in dogs, care in cats
Metronidazole	10-15 mg/kg q 8-12 hr PO	IBD, anaerobes
Norfloxacin	3-7 mg/kg q 12 hr PO	Gram negative pathogens;

intestinal pathogens in humans, including *Campylobacter*. A superior effect to trimethoprim-sulfa combinations has not been convincingly demonstrated. Fluoroquinolones are also particularly useful in the prophylactic therapy of neutropenic patients. Side effects are rare, but the drugs may produce cartilage erosions in young animals.

Animals with fecal cultures positive for bacterial pathogens may be treated according to the sensitivity pattern of the cultured bacterium; however, the in vivo response to the antibiotic often does not reflect the in vitro sensitivity pattern. An alternative approach is to use antibiotics considered by various authorities as "first choice therapeutics" for the particular pathogen (Chapter 18). These recommendations have been made on an empirical basis and should be followed only after careful assessment of the safety of the particular antibiotic in the individual under treatment.

Animals with positive blood cultures should be treated according to the sensitivity pattern of the cultured bacterium. If blood culture results are unavailable from a patient with suspected sepsis and the animal's condition is adjudged critical, combinations of parenteral penicillins and amikacin (2.2 mg/kg q 8 hr SQ or IV) or gentamicin (2.2 mg/kg q 8 hr SQ or IV) can be used. Both of these aminoglycosides should be used only after rehydration of the patient, and the duration of administration should be limited to five days. The popularity of kanamycin for the treatment of gram negative sepsis has declined with the realization of its limited spectrum of activity compared to that of the other aminoglycosides.[29] Antibiotics of any form are seldom required for longer than five days in the treatment of acute diarrhea, and forty eight hours is often sufficient. The effectiveness of selected antibiotics against gastrointestinal bacteria is shown in Table 16-12.

Probiotics such as *Lactobacillus acidophilus* cultures have no proven benefits in the therapy of diarrhea.[32]

Motility Modifiers

When resistance to flow is minimal in the flaccid intestine, very little peristaltic activity is needed to propel liquid contents over a long span with relative ease. Peristaltic activity is not increased with diarrhea, and it need not contribute to the problem.

The theoretical goals of treating diarrhea are to decrease the driving force for moving intestinal contents aborally and to increase resistance to their flow. Thus, attempts are made to decrease the driving force by inhibiting peristalsis and to increase the resistance to flow by stimulating rhythmic segmentation. Pharmaceutical agents cannot usually completely abolish peristalsis, however. As long as some peristaltic activity is present, no matter how weak, it can propel liquid contents through a flaccid tube. In some situations, peristalsis can be completely inhibited, but when that happens there is also a complete loss of segmentation. The result is ileus, and the paralyzed section of intestine is unable to move any contents through, resulting in a functional obstruction. Drugs used to decrease propulsive activity in the intestine do not abolish peristalsis, and they always reduce segmentation. Thus, the first goal is difficult to attain with drugs. The second goal, increasing the resistance to flow, is achieved with drugs that stimulate rhythmic segmentation.

Opioids stimulate rhythmic segmentation and are the only effective drugs for increasing resistance to flow.[33-37] They include morphine, meperidine, paregoric, diphenoxylate, and loperamide. Suggested doses of a selected number of these opioids are listed in Table 16-13. Opioids increase the amplitude of rhythmic segmentation and decrease the propulsive contractions (Table 16-14).[38] The opioids directly affect the intestinal smooth muscle[39,40] (Figure 15-11), producing both tonic and phasic contractions of the circular muscle; they also act centrally and on synapses to augment segmentation. Opioids either have no effect on longitudinal intestinal muscle in the dog, or they cause relaxation.[41,42] The net effect of narcotic analgesics is to inhibit the flow of intestinal contents. Additional effects are to delay emptying of the stomach and increase tone in the ileocecal valve and anal sphincter.[38] Some opioids, in particular loperamide and to a lesser extent diphenoxylate, also increase fluid and water absorption possibly by a calcium channel blocking effect[43] or by inhibition of the intrinsic calcium binding protein calmodulin.[1,43] Loperamide also inhibits the activity of certain secretagogues, including E. coli enterotoxin, VIP, bile acids, and prostaglandin E_2. Loperamide may have a faster onset of action than diphenoxylate. It is available as a liquid, which facilitates its usage in small patients. We have used loperamide without clinical evidence of toxicity in cats.

The major disadvantage to using these drugs is that they are narcotics, and most produce depression of the central nervous system if used in inappropriate doses. Atropine is added to diphenoxylate to minimize its abuse as a narcotic in humans (Table 16-15). The atropine in this preparation (Lomotil) has no pharmacologic effect on the gastrointestinal tract. It should be understood, of course, that opioids are only effective adjunct therapy, and should not be expected to cure primary problems due to an infectious agent. There is good reason to believe that opioids are contraindicated in diarrhea resulting from infection with invasive bacteria.[44] In these cases, diarrhea forms an important protective role that probably hastens the elimination of the organism. Slowing intestinal transit may prolong the residence time of the bacteria in the bowel, leading to greater opportunity for proliferation of the organism, invasion of the mucosa, and the absorption of toxic products. It is our preference not to use these drugs in patients with suspected enteroinvasive disease, except on occasions when intravenous fluid therapy cannot keep up with diarrheal fluid loss.

Acetylcholine has a stimulatory effect on intestinal peristalsis and segmental contractions of both circular and longitudinal smooth muscle of the intestine. Anticholinergics reduce the physiological effects of acetylcholine, and motility is reduced in both circular and longitudinal smooth muscle.[38] Peristalsis is reduced, but there is also a major reduction of resistance to flow in the intestinal tract (Table 16-16). Gastric secretions (including that of protein exudation induced by histamine) are reduced, but intestinal secretions are little affected. Pharmacologists recognize that anticholinergic drugs are "contrary to the mode of action of useful antidiarrheal agents."[4] Furthermore, they have been found to be disappointing agents when used for that purpose. The Food and Drug Administration (FDA) has recently restricted the claims that can be made for them and has questioned their effectiveness (Table 16-15). Anticholinergics are not innocuous drugs. Their use can precipitate ileus by further reducing the decreased amounts of motility found with diarrhea.

In summary, opioids remain the drugs preferred for the

Table 16-13. Suggested Doses of Opioids for the Treatment of Diarrhea*

DRUG	DOSE
Camphorated opium (Paregoric)	0.05-0.06 mg/kg PO q 8 hr (D,C)
Diphenoxylate (Lomotil)	0.05 - 0.1 mg/kg PO q 8 hr (D)
Loperamide (Imodium)	0.08 mg/kg PO q 8 hr (D,C)

(D) = dog, (C) = cat

* Most opioids are not licensed for use in the dog or cat

symptomatic treatment of diarrhea.[33,38,45-47] Evaluation of all motility modifiers has led to the classification of the FDA shown in Table 16-15, which is based on a review by the National Academy of Sciences-National Research Council and/or other information.

Locally Acting Drugs[38,48]

Long before either antibiotics or motility modifiers were available for the treatment of diarrhea, a wide variety of intestinal protectives and adsorbents were used. As with the many pharmaceuticals that have been used empirically for centuries, no controlled studies have been conducted to prove their effectiveness. A number of those substances are classified as protective because of their adsorbent properties.

Bismuth subcarbonate and magnesium trisilicate adsorb gases, toxins, and bacteria. As an additional property they supposedly coat over and protect the ulcerated mucosal surface, although there is no evidence that either of these two compounds has any such ability. Aluminum hydroxide, used as an antacid, also has adsorptive properties.

Activated charcoal has been used for many years to adsorb toxic substances. It is still incorporated into universal-type antidotes for treating the ingestion of toxic substances. It has also been used to bind gas in the intestine in managing excessive flatus, although it is questionable whether activated charcoal significantly reduces the content of intestinal gas. It is also thought to bind bacterial toxins. There have been no controlled studies to evaluate its efficacy. The drug is messy to use and is better administered as a powder than a tablet. The primary

Table 16-14. Opioids - Pharmacologic Actions

Stomach

1. Contracts antrum
2. Decreases antral propulsion

Net Effect - Delays Gastric Emptying

Small and Large Intestine

1. Increases tone and segmentation
2. Decreases propulsion
3. Contracts ileocecal and anal sphincters

Net Effect - Increases Transit Time

Table 16-15. FDA Classification of Effectiveness of Drugs as Adjunctive Therapy in Treatment of Acute Enterocolitis, Functional Gastrointestinal Disorders and Diarrhea.[a]

EFFECTIVE

Diban[b] - powdered opium, atropine
Donnagel-PG[b] - powdered opium, atropine, hyoscyamine, kaolin, pectin
Lomotil[c] - diphenoxylate, atropine
Parapectolin[d] - Paregoric, pectin, kaolin
Imodium[e] - Loperamide

PROBABLY EFFECTIVE

Pathilon[f] - Tridihexethyl chloride
Pro-Banthine[c] - propantheline bromide

POSSIBLY EFFECTIVE

Darbazine (Combid)[g] - prochlorperazine maleate, isopropamide iodide
Bentyl[h] - dicyclomine hydrochloride
Cantil[h] - mepenzolate bromide
Librax[i] - chlordiazepoxide hydrochloride, clidinium bromide
Quarzan[i] - clidinium bromide

[a]From literature in advertisements, drug inserts and PDR
[b]Robins Co., Richmond, VA
[c]Searle Co., Chicago, IL
[d]Rorer, Wm. H., Fort Washington, PA
[e]Ortho Pharm, Raritan, NJ
[f]Lederle Lab, Pearl River, NY
[g]Smith, Kline and French, Philadelphia, PA
[h]Merrell-National Lab, Cincinnati, OH
[i]Roche Lab, Nutley, NJ

Table 16-16. Pharmacological Effects of Anticholinergics on the Bowel

Decrease tone and propulsion
Decrease motility caused by opiates and serotonin
High doses decrease motility due to emotional stimuli
Some tone and movement are resistent to anticholinergics
May promote ileus
Decrease gastrointestinal secretions

The net effect is to reduce motility. The intestine in an animal with diarrhea is already hypomotile.

indication remains the treatment of toxicosis. The recommended dose is 0.7-1.4 grams/kg administered once.[48]

Kaolin, hydrated aluminum silicate, used to treat diarrhea, acts by binding toxins and bacteria. When used to treat colitis, it is doubtful whether any appreciable binding activity remains by the time it reaches the colon. Kaolin is indicated for treatment of intestinal fermentation, but, again, there is no documentation as to its usefulness. It may improve the consistency of the stool through its adsorbent properties, but it is unlikely to shorten the course of the diarrhea. It may also act as a coagulant in the intestine and thus may reduce gastrointestinal hemorrhage.[27] Kaolin may reduce the absorption of some antibiotics from the bowel. Its routine use in diarrheal diseases is not encouraged.

Pectin is a common part of diarrhea medications. It is a carbohydrate, polygalacturonic acid, found in apples and rinds of citrus fruits. The action of pectin is unknown, but it is suspected to be an adsorbent with protective properties. Paradoxically, administration of excess pectin causes normal dogs to develop diarrhea.

Bismuth subsalicylate is an effective agent for the treatment of enterotoxigenic diarrhea. In humans, the diarrhea, nausea, and abdominal pain associated with infective diarrhea are thought to be reduced. The salicylate moiety is thought to decrease intestinal secretion by interfering with prostaglandin production and by a more direct, but undefined, inhibitory effect on the generation of cAMP by the enterotoxin. Salicylate intoxication can result from over dosage of this drug, particularly in cats. A safe dose of bismuth subsalicylate (Pepto-Bismol) in dogs and cats is 0.25 ml/kg q 4-6 hr.[49] Doses greater than 7 ml/kg /day could produce toxicity.[49] It is a useful and practical therapy for acute nonspecific diarrhea. Palatability of Pepto-Bismol may be improved by refrigeration. Another useful product for the therapy of non-specific acute diarrhea is a combination of bismuth subsalicylate with paregoric (Corrective mixture; Beecham Laboratories). This product combines the antisecretory effects of the salicylate with the improved intestinal motility of an opioid. The dose is 0.25 ml/kg PO initially, followed by half the original dose q 4 hr.[23] The administration of this mixture is at present confined to dogs.

Astringents have been used in treating diarrhea. Tannic acid, the best example, acts by precipitating proteins on the mucosal surface, forming a protective coating presumably without entering and damaging the cell. This activity decreases cell permeability and has a constipating effect. Tannic acid also forms insoluble complexes with heavy-metal ions, alkaloids, and glycosides that could contribute to diarrhea. Tannic acid is now known to be hepatotoxic, causing severe centrolobular necrosis when appreciable amounts are absorbed.

Antacids have been used to treat diarrhea. All aluminum antacid compounds cause constipation, which in the case of aluminum hydroxide is not due to its astringent effects, since the concentrations used are too low. Aluminum hydroxide inhibits motility in the stomach, delaying gastric emptying.[50] Part of its constipating effects may be due to a very slow delivery of solutes to the intestinal mucosa, permitting more complete absorption. Aluminum antacids also adsorb many substances, including tetracycline and atropine given orally. Aluminum antacids bind phosphates and have been used to treat hyperphosphatemia. Part of aluminum's constipating effects are due to their precipitation of poorly absorbed soluble anions, which can cause an osmotic diarrhea.

Calcium antacids are also constipating and have been used occasionally to treat chronic diarrhea. They may have absorptive properties, and they form insoluble salts with anions such as phosphate. It is not known whether high concentrations of calcium have any effects on intestinal motility. Excessive administration of calcium to treat a chronic diarrhea can produce hypercalcemia and renal hypercalcuria, which can progress to nephrocalcinosis and renal failure. In contrast to calcium, magnesium salts are cathartic since they are soluble and poorly absorbed. Magnesium may also be cathartic, due to direct effects on smooth-muscle function. Both calcium and magnesium ions will reduce the absorption of oral tetracycline.

Barium sulfate has been used empirically to treat chronic diarrhea. The use is based on observations that diarrhea sometimes improves after barium sulfate has been given to conduct gastrointestinal radiographic studies. There have been no controlled studies to evaluate the usefulness of barium sulfate for treating diarrhea. Barium ions stimulate the release of acetylcholine from nerve synapses in intrinsic ganglia, and when a soluble barium salt is given orally it intensely stimulates all types of muscles in the body. Soluble barium salts cause vomiting, severe diarrhea, and colic. If barium sulfate is effective in treating diarrhea and acts via those neurogenic actions, it is possible that very minute amounts of barium ions are absorbed and stimulate acetylcholine release. That would have to be in amounts that augment segmentation and do not stimulate simultaneous contraction of the entire length of the intestine, causing a diarrhea.

Future Therapeutics

Alpha-2-adrenergic receptors are present on enterocytes and are involved in enterocyte fluid and electrolyte transport.[57] Alpha-2-receptor agonists enhance absorption and inhibit secretion of electrolytes in the small intestine. Clonidine is an example of an alpha-2-agonist that has been used successfully to treat experimental secretory diarrheas in rats and diabetic diarrhea and secretory diarrhea in humans due to bronchogenic adenocarcinoma.[43] The role of these agents in diarrhea therapy has yet to be defined, and their use may be limited by their sedative and hypotensive properties. Lidamidine is an alpha-2-agonist structurally similar to clonidine, but it has less such side effects.

Intestinal inflammation promotes the formation of prostaglandins of the E and F type, kinins, and lipoxygenase products (5-HPETE, 5-HETE); all are substances with a potent secretory effect on intestinal epithelium, and diarrhea follows. Prostaglandins stimulate chloride secretion and inhibit sodium absorption. Nonsteroidal antiinflammatory drugs that inhibit prostaglandin synthesis should be beneficial in managing some secretory types of diarrhea. Prostaglandins are also cytoprotective in the gastrointestinal tract, and inhibitors of prostaglandin synthesis can produce erosion and ulceration of the mucosal epithelium. With no proven benefit for nonsteroidal antiinflammatory drugs, and because of their risk for producing damage, inhibitors of prostaglandin synthesis should not be used for treating acute diarrhea due to any cause.

Lipoxygenase products and not prostaglandins are the mediators for inflammation in chronic colitis and possibly chronic inflammatory bowel disease. Drugs that inhibit leukotreine formation, such as 5-aminosalicylic acid and sulfasalazine, are effective in managing chronic colitis. Sulfasalazine, which inhibits both prostaglandin and leukotreine synthesis, is effective whereas nonsteroidal antiinflammatory drugs such as indomethacin and aspirin, which inhibit only prostaglandin synthesis, are ineffective. Prostaglandins and leukotreines may also contribute to diarrhea due to their effect of stimulating intestinal motility.

Somatostatin is a potent inhibitor of intestinal motility, splanchnic blood flow, enteric hormone release, and pancreatic, gastric, and intestinal secretion. A potent somatostatin analog (Sandoz Pharmaceuticals) is now available and may be useful for the therapy of diarrhea resulting from endocrine tumors. In humans somatostatin or somatostatin analogs have been successful in treating diarrhea from a number of different causes including VIPomas, carcinoid tumors, intestinal resection, and cryptosporidiosis.[43]

Calcium appears to have a role in regulating active intestinal ion secretion and has important effects on intestinal motility. Calcium channel blockers have shown promise in the treatment of diarrhea mediated by experimental infusion of substance P in dogs and of *Escherichia coli* enterotoxin-stimulated diarrhea in mice.[43] Nifedipine has shown some beneficial effects in the therapy of irritable bowel syndrome in humans.

Loperamide has properties to block calcium channels; the drug inhibits intestinal secretion that is stimulated by agents which increase membrane permeability for calcium.[43] Loperamide may also stimulate sodium chloride absorption by mucosa cells. Calmodulin antagonists also have properties to inhibit intestinal secretion of fluid stimulated by VIP, cholera toxin, *E. coli* enterotoxin, cyclic AMP, and PGE_2. Phenothiazines have an antidiarrheal action, which in part appears to be related to potent inhibition of calmodulin. Chlorpromazine is reported by some, but not by others, to reduce diarrhea in humans with secretory diarrhea due to cholera.

Enkephalins (opiates) may reduce diarrhea by a number of mechanisms.[43] Opiates may inhibit the release of secretory agents from enteric nerves. Opiates can act in the CNS to stimulate the peripheral release of adrenergic agents. They can stimulate intestinal sodium chloride absorption via delta receptors and inhibit motility via mu receptors.

Lithium salts change intestinal fluid and electrolyte movements in some unknown way to reduce some forms of diarrhea in humans.[43] Constipation and water retention are well-described side effects of oral lithium therapy.

Other interesting antidiarrheal agents include berberine, an alkaloid from the plant *Berberis aristata*, organic acids such as nicotonic acid and glutamic acid, and chloride channel blockers such as some anthracene derivatives.[43]

Dietary Management

The primary goal in treating acute diarrhea is to rest the gastrointestinal tract. Thus, for at least 24 hours no food should be fed, and thereafter the type of food and the manner in which it is fed become important. There are a number of reasons for not feeding the patient. When inflammation is present, the loss of mucosal cells is accelerated. Food in the intestine augments that rate of loss by its abrasive action. Thus, the goal is to minimize any possible physical damage to the mucosa. A second reason for not feeding the patient is to minimize the changes for colonization by foreign bacteria. Whenever diarrhea is a problem from any cause, the populations of normal microflora are markedly disrupted. Any transients that enter the intestine can colonize when the normal flora is upset. Transients enter from the flora of the oral cavity and in the diet. Their further entry is minimized by not feeding the animal until the intestinal microflora has a chance to recover. A third reason for withholding food is to reduce the chances that dietary antigens will be absorbed intact, which can sensitize the animal to subsequent contact with the same diet. It is not unusual to see an animal show repeated episodes of an intestinal problem following an acute attack of diarrhea. Such patients are unable to tolerate foods that had been previously fed. It is possible that many such animals absorb antigens from their normal diet during the first attack and thereafter can be managed only with special diets. A fourth reason to be in no hurry to feed such patients is that the small intestinal mucosa loses its brush border enzymes during the diarrhea. The loss of disaccharidases causes the most problems if the animals are fed. They are not able to digest any disaccharides, such as lactose or sucrose, and they have lost the ability to hydrolyze the small polymers of glucose that is necessary before the monosaccharide can be absorbed. Small polypeptides can be readily absorbed and are hydrolyzed within the cell, so that a brush border alteration affects protein digestion and absorption much less. In summary, there are important reasons to fast the patient completely for at least 24 hours.

The return to feeding should follow a number of important principles. The diet selected should be given in small amounts at frequent intervals so that osmotic overload is not a problem. The diet should contain nutrients that are easily digested and absorbed. Thus, the diet should consist of proteins and carbohydrates with minimum fat. The diet should be hypoallergenic, to minimize sensitization during the recovery phase. Since most antigens are proteins, the type and amount of protein to incorporate should be carefully considered. The diet should be low-residue to minimize physical abrasion of the mucosal surface. That also decreases the amount of polysaccharides made available for growth of bacteria in the colon, which may benefit the patient.[52] The diet should be one that allows the most rapid return of the microflora to normal. The presence of undigested and unabsorbed nutrients in the distal small intestine permits an increased number of bacteria to exist and thrive. Thus, the goal of the diet is to provide nutrients that are readily and completely assimilated. The food used should be processed, to reduce the numbers of viable transient bacteria. They are minimized by feeding canned products or cooked diets formulated by the owner. The final goal in formulating a diet is to provide one acceptable to the patient. That is frequently the most difficult to achieve. Poorly accepted diets are less of a problem for short-term use following an acute diarrhea than when they must be fed for extended periods.

The diet is formulated to contain a single source of each nutrient type used. The most controlled diet that can be fed consists of a single nutrient. A single source of carbohydrates, such as rice or potatoes, meets that requirement and has the advantage of being nonantigenic. One disadvantage is its poor palatability. In addition, few animals are normally fed high-carbohydrate diets and therefore do not have sufficient enzymes for their complete digestion. Several days are needed to adapt to such a diet by increased enzyme synthesis. Initially, a carbohydrate diet is not assimilated as efficiently as a protein diet.

Table 16-17. Formulation of a Controlled Diet

To one cup dry white rice (7-8 oz, 190-200 g) add two cups of water. Bring to boil and then simmer for 15 minutes.
Cool and add 4 oz. cottage cheese or tofu. The mixture contains 820 calories and maintains a 25 lb. dog.

The diet can be formulated with a single source of protein, a nutrient that is readily digested and absorbed. The disadvantages of protein include its antigenicity in sensitized animals and its ability to sensitize where absorption is possible through an abnormal mucosal barrier. Many proteins are high in phosphate, and excessive amounts of this poorly absorbed anion, osmotically retain water, to cause diarrhea. Proteins are usually included in controlled diets to enhance palatability and acceptance. The sources of proteins are usually meat, eggs, soy beans, and milk. The meat selected can be lean beef, lamb, or chicken. Lamb is frequently used when the patient is suspected of being sensitized to beef or poultry. Since most small animal patients have never eaten lamb, the possibility of an allergy is remote. Cooked eggs can be fed as the single source of protein. Soy bean protein is fed as tofu. Milk protein is usually fed as cottage cheese or yogurt. Those products contain some lactose, which may not be adequately assimilated during recovery from diarrhea. Buttermilk contains as much lactose as whole milk, and yogurt contains three-fourths as much. On the basis of protein content, cottage cheese has 10 to 15% of the lactose of whole milk. Cottage cheese or tofu as the source of protein results in remission of diarrhea more consistently than any other protein.

The initial diet is a combination of a single source of protein and a single source of carbohydrate. The amount of protein in the diet should not exceed half of the total amount, and that can be reduced in large breeds of dogs. Table 16-17 shows the most controlled diet that uses cottage cheese as a source of protein. The diet is fed three to four times a day in the beginning, although in total amounts that are less than the patient's caloric needs. No changes are made in the diet until the character of the bowel movement is determined to be normal and examinations are made for intestinal parasites.

The patient is reexamined a week to ten days after the initial visit, at which time samples of the bowel movements are brought in and examined. It is quite helpful if the client has maintained a record of the animal's progress, including amounts and kinds of food eaten, water consumption, activity, character and frequency of bowel movements, appetite, and associated signs such as intermittent halitosis, flatulence, borborygmus, and abnormal behavior. Such information is frequently useful in deciding whether the controlled diet should be continued. If the patient has responded well, the diet can be gradually changed to regular foods. No one brand of the common commercial pet foods is better than others in producing normal bowel movements. When a particular brand results in a diarrhea, changing brands is usually an incorrect approach to the problem since most commercial pet foods contain the same ingredients. If the stated analysis of contents does reveal a specific difference, however, a change may be justified. Even then, however, a commercial product that produces normal bowel movements can change as ingredients are changed according to fluctuations in the prices of raw materials. Some commercial diets have fixed formulas and contain a minimum of different ingredients, which permits them to be used as controlled diets for the management of diarrhea. Some Science diets and IAMs diets can be used that way.

The animal's environment must be controlled during treatment. An animal's dietary intake cannot be controlled when it is free to roam. Attempts to treat diarrhea often fail because the animal's environment is not controlled.

Management of acute diarrhea in cats is also based on feeding controlled diets. The diet can consist of chicken or turkey as the only constituent. In some case control of the diet can be less rigid, and a prescription diet can be fed. Diarrhea is often associated with the feeding of dry cat foods, in which case the cat's diet may have to be changed permanently. It is mandatory that a cat's environment be controlled in recovery. The client should be aware that a recurring problem may be a sign of one of the chronic virus infections.

Any controlled diet is fed three to four times a day in the beginning. In acute diarrheas, the patient can usually be weaned back to the normal diet within seven to ten days.

REFERENCES

1. Ooms, L. and Degryse, A.: Pathogenesis and pharmacology of diarrhea. Vet. Res. Commun. 10:355-397, 1986.
2. Ewe, K.: Intestinal transport in constipation and diarrhea. Pharmacology 36:73S-84S, 1988.
3. Fine, K.D., Krejs, G.J. and Fordtran, J.S. Diarrhea. Edited by Sleisenger, M.H., Fordtran, J.S. 4th Edition. WB Saunders Co, Philadelphia, 290-316, 1989.
4. Madara, J.L. and Trier, J.S.: Functional morphology of the mucosa of the small intestine. In, Physiology of the Gastrointestinal Tract. 2nd Edition. Edited by Johnson, L.R. Raven Press, New York, 1209-1249, 1987.
5. Madara, J.L., Moore, R. and Carlson, S.: Alteration of intestinal tight junction structure and permeability by cytoskeletal contraction. Am. J. Phsiol. 253:C854-C861, 1987.
6. Vellenga, L., Mouwen, J.M.V.N., van Dijk, J.E. and Breukink, H.J.: Biological and pathological aspects of the mammalian small intestinal permeabilty to macromolecules. Vet. Quarterly 7:322-332, 1985.
7. Moreland, K.J.: Ulcer disease of the upper gastrointestinal tract in small animals: Pathophysiology, diagnosis, and management. Comp. Contin. Ed. Pract. Vet. 10:1265-1280, 1988.
8. Ramage, J.K., Hunt, R.H. and Perdue, M.H.: Changes in intestinal permeability and epithelial differentiation during inflammation in the rat. Gut 29:57-61,1988.
9. Bjarnason, I., Williams, P. and So, A.: Intestinal permeability and inflammation in rheumatoid arthritis: Effects of nonsteroidal anti-inflammatory drugs. The Lancet. 1171-1174, Nov 24, 1984
10. Ecknauer, R., Buck, B. and Breitig, D.: An experimental model for measuring intestinal permeability. Digestion 26:24-32, 1983.
11. Siber, G.R., Mayer and Levin, M.J.: Increased gastrointestinal absorption of large molecules in patients after 5-fluorouracil therapy for metastatic colon carcinoma. Cancer Res. 40:3430-3436, 1980.
12. Granger, D.N., Kvietys, P.R., Perry, M.A. and Barrowman, J.A.: The microcirculation and intestinal transport. In, Physiology of the Gastrointestinal Tract. 2nd Edition. Edited by Johnson, L.R. Raven Press, New York, 1671-1697, 1987.
13. Burrows, C.F., Greiner, E.C., Tooker, J. and Springfels, S.: Hookworm infection disrupts canine jejunal myoelectric activity. Abstract ACVIM Proceedings, 741, 1988.

14. Willard, M.D., Mullaney, T., Karasek, S. and Yamini, B.: Diarrhea associated with myenteric ganglionitis in a dog. JAVMA 193:346-348, 1988.
15. MacPherson, B.R., Shearin, N.L. and Pfeiffer, C.J.: Experimental diffuse colitis in cats: observations on motor changes. J. Surg. Res. 25:42-49, 1978.
16. Osweiller, G.D.: A brief guide to clinical signs of toxicosis in small animals. In, Current Veterinary Therapy IX. Edited by Kirk, R.W. WB Saunders Philadelphia, 132-135, 1986.
17. Osweiller, G.D.: Household and commercial products. In, Current Veterinary Therapy IX. Edited by Kirk, R.W. WB Saunders Philadelphia, 193-196, 1986.
18. Ruhr, L.P. Ornamental toxic plants. Current Veterinary Therapy IX. Edited by Kirk, R.W. WB Saunders, Philadelphia, 216-220, 1985.
19. Drasar, B.S. and Hill, J.: Human intestinal flora. Academic Press, London, 1974.
20. Goodman, J.S.: Infections by anaerobic bacteria of the bowel. Adv. Int. Med. 21:129-147, 1976.
21. Kikuchi, T., Oikawa, T., Inoue, K., Sakai, M., Hara, N., Sunagawa, K. and Ichihashi, Y.: The effect of antibiotics against the intestinal bacterial flora. In, Germ Free Research, Edited by J.B. Heneghan, Academic Press, New York, 355-359, 1973.
22. Nichols, R.L. and Condon, R.E.: Role of the endogenous gastrointestinal microflora in postoperative wound sepsis. Surg. Annual 7:279-293, 1975.
23. DeNovo, R.C.: Therapeutics of gastrointestinal diseases. In, Current veterinary Therapy IX. Edited by Kirk, R.W. WB Saunders, Philadelphia, 862-872, 1986
24. Leight, D.A. and Simmons, K.: Effect of clindamycin and lincomycin therapy on fecal flora. J. Clin. Path. 31:439-443, 1978.
25. Hirsch, D.C.: Microflora, mucosa, and immunity. In, Veterinary Gastroenterology. Edited by Anderson, N.V. 199-219, 1980.
26. Ishikawa, H., Baba, E. and Matsumoto, H.: Studies on bacterial flora of the alimentary tract of dogs. III. Fecal flora in clinical and experimental cases of diarrhea. Jap. J. Vet. Sci. 44:343-347, 1982.
27. Greene, C.E.: Gastrointestinal, intra-abdominal,and hepatobiliary infections. In, Clinical Microbiology and Infectious Diseases of the Dog and Cat. WB Saunders, Philadelphia. 247-268, 1984.
28. Powers, T.E., Mercer, H.D.: Antimicrobial drugs. In, Veterinary Gastroenterology Edited by Anderson, N.V. 311-334, 1980.
29. Sande, M.A., Mandell, G.L.: Antimicrobal agents: The aminoglycosides. In, The Pharmacologic Basis of Therapeutics. 7th edition. Edited by Goodman, Gilman, A., Goodman, L.S., Rall, T.W. and Murad, F. Macmillan Publishing Co, New York, 1150-1169, 1985.
30. English, P.B., Prescott, C.W.: Antimicrobial therapy in the dog. I Related to body system or organ infected. J. Sm. An. Pract. 24:277-292, 1983.
31. Wolfson, J.S., Hooper, D.C.: Norfloxacin: A new targeted fluoroquinolone antimicrobial agent. Ann. Int. Med. 108:238-251, 1988.
32. de Dios Pozo-Olando, J., Warram, J.H., Gomez, R.G. and Cavazos, M.G.: Effect of a lactobacilli preparation on traveler's diarrhea. Gastroenterology 74:829-830, 1978.
33. Connell, A.M.: The motility of the pelvic colon: Part II. Paradoxical motility in diarrhea and constipation. Gut 3:342-348, 1962.
34. Ludwick, J.R., Wiley, J.N. and Bass, P.: Extraluminal contractile force and electrical activity of reversed canine duodenum. Gastroenterology 54:41-51, 1968.
35. Plant, O.H. and Miller, G.H.: Effects of morphine and some other opium alkaloids on the muscular activity of the alimentary canal: I. Action on the small intestine in unanesthetized dogs and man. J. Pharmacol. Exp. There. 27:361-383, 1926.
36. Templeton, R.D. and Alder, H.F.: The influence of morphine on transportation in the colon of the dog. Am. J. Physiol. 131:428-431, 1940.
37. Vaughan Williams, E.M. and Streeten, D.H.P.: The action of morphine, pethidine, and amidone upon the intestinal motility of conscious dogs. Brit. J. Pharmacol. Chem. Therapeut. 5:584-603, 1950.
38. Goodman, L.A. and Gilman, A.: The Pharmacological Basis of Therapeutics. MacMillan Co., New York, 1975.
39. Burks, T.F.: Vascularly perfused isolated intestine. In, Proc. 4th Int. Symp.: Gastrointestinal motility, Mitchell, Vancouver, 305-312, 1974.
40. Stewart, J.J., Weisbrodt, N.W. and Burks, T.F.: Central and peripheral actions of morphine on intestinal transit. J. Pharmacol. Exp. Therapeut. 205:547-555, 1978.
41. Bass, P. and Wiley, J.N.: Electrical and extraluminal contractile force activity of the dog. Am. J. Dig. Dis. 10:183-200, 1965.
42. Rinaldo, J.A., Jr., Orinion, E.A., Simpelo, R.V., Check, F.E. and Beauregard, W.: Differential response of longitudinal and circular muscles of intact canine colon to morphine and bethanecol. Gastroenterology 60:438-444, 1971.
43. Fedorak, R.N. and Field, M.: Antidiarrheal therapy. Prospects for new agents. Dig. Dis. Sci. 32:195-205, 1987.
44. DuPont, H.L. and Hornick, R.B.: Adverse effect of Lomotil therapy in shigellosis. JAMA 226:1525-1528, 1973.
45. Bass, P., Kennedy, J.A., Wiley, J.N., Villarreal, J. and Butler, D.E.: CI-750, A novel antidiarrheal agent. J. Pharmacol. Exp. Therapeut. 186:183-198, 1973.
46. Burks, T.F.: Gastrointestinal pharmacology. Ann. Rev. Pharmacol. Toxicol. 16:15-31, 1976.
47. Tijtgat, G.N., Meuwissen, S.G.M. and Hubregtse, K.: Loperamide in the symptomatic control of chronic diarrhea. Ann. Clin. Res., 7:325-330, 1975.
48. Wilcke, J.R.: The use of Adsorbents to treat gastrointestinal problems in small animals. Seminars Vet. Med. Surg. 2:266-273, 1987.
49. Papich, M.G., Davis, C.A. and Davis, L.E.: Absorption of salicylate from an antidiarrheal preparation in dogs and cats. JAAHA 23:221-226, 1987.
50. Hurwitz, A., Robinson, R.G., Vats, T.S., Whittier, F.C. and Herrin, W.F.: Effects of antacids on the gastric emptying. Gastroenterology 71:268-273, 1976.
51. Dijoseph, J.F., Taylor, J.A., Mir, G.N. and Rorer, W.H.: Alpha-2 receptors in the gastrointestinal system: A new therapeutic approach. Life Sci. 35:1031-1042, 1984. Disorders during treatment with an elemental diet. Gastroenterology 72:397-401, 1977.

Chapter 17

Maldigestion, Malabsorption, Bacterial Overgrowth, and Protein-Losing Enteropathy

MALASSIMILATION[1]

Definitions

Malassimilation is the defective transport of one or more nutrients from the intestinal lumen to the body fluids, whether due to faulty digestion (maldigestion) or faulty mucosal transport (malabsorption). The term malabsorption is sometimes used interchangeably with malassimilation, but for the sake of clarity "malabsorption" is used here to refer exclusively to deranged intestinal absorption of nutrients including that resulting from brush border enzyme defects.

Clinical Signs

No matter what the cause, malassimilation of nutrients results in a characteristic group of clinical signs suggestive of "small bowel" diarrhea (Chapter 5). Particularly in the early stages of the syndrome, weight loss is often more noticeable than abnormalities of the stool. The fecal changes are variable, ranging from formed stools of greater than normal size to watery diarrhea. Undigested food and fat may be evident. A sour odor is sometimes apparent from the fermentation of carbohydrates in the colon. The defecation frequency is usually mildly to moderately increased, and borborygmus may be heard. When malassimilation is longstanding, nutritional deficiency is manifested by skin and hair-coat changes, anemia, and hypoproteinemia. Physical findings are usually unremarkable except for the signs of malnutrition.

Etiopathogenesis

Theoretically, clinical evidence of malassimilation could follow defective digestion and absorption of any of the major classes of nutrients (Figure 17-1). In reality, however, the clinical signs of the syndrome are predominantly a reflection of the malassimilation of carbohydrate. Malassimilation of protein is rarely clinically evident because the amount of protein in normal diets is usually small, and protein digestion and absorption are highly efficient. Malassimilation of fat is usually clinically unremarkable because the fat content is low for most pet foods; the fat content is not the important source of calories. Malassimilation of fat results in an increase in the quantity of deconjugated bile acids and hydroxylated fatty acids in the colon. These products can cause diarrhea by a number of pathologic effects on colonic mucosa and colonic motility. The

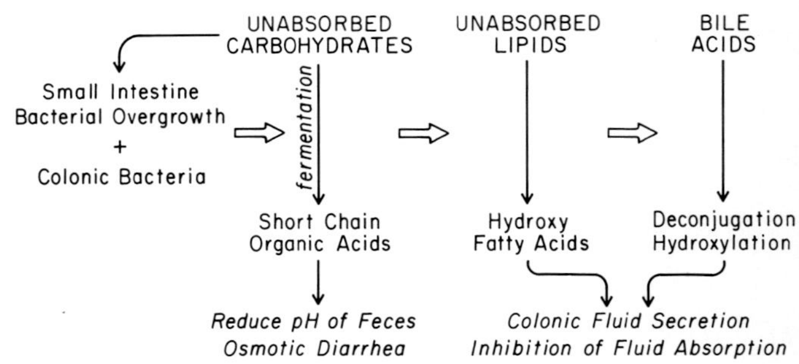

Figure 17-1. Diagram to show the mechanisms whereby unabsorbed nutrients cause diarrhea. Carbohydrates which are not absorbed cause overgrowth of the normal small intestinal flora. This in conjunction with the vast normal microflora of the colon results in alterations of carbohydrates, lipids, and bile acids to cause diarrhea.

steatorrhea caused by fat malassimilation may be associated with formed feces, however. In contrast, malassimilation of carbohydrate results in clinically apparent diarrhea, predominantly through osmotic mechanisms.

Maldigestion and malabsorption have a variety of causes. The approach to the differential diagnosis of malassimilation is described in Chapter 5, and additional details on the individual causes of malassimilation (including therapeutic information) may be found in the Chapters devoted to the discussion of pancreatic, hepatic, and intestinal disorders.

MALDIGESTION

Maldigestion can result from exocrine pancreatic insufficiency, inadequate bile secretion, deranged gastric emptying, and small intestinal mucosal disease. The most common cause of maldigestion is exocrine pancreatic insufficiency.

The secretions of the exocrine pancreas act on lipids, proteins, and carbohydrates (Figure 17-2), and their deficiency causes profound maldigestion and malassimilation of nutrients with resultant diarrhea. The concentration of each enzyme in pancreatic secretions parallels the level of each nutrient in the diet.[2] Animals fed a low-protein diet have low levels of trypsinogen and chymotrypsinogen in their pancreatic secretions. These levels increase when a high-protein diet is fed, but the adaptation requires several days. The capacity of the pancreas

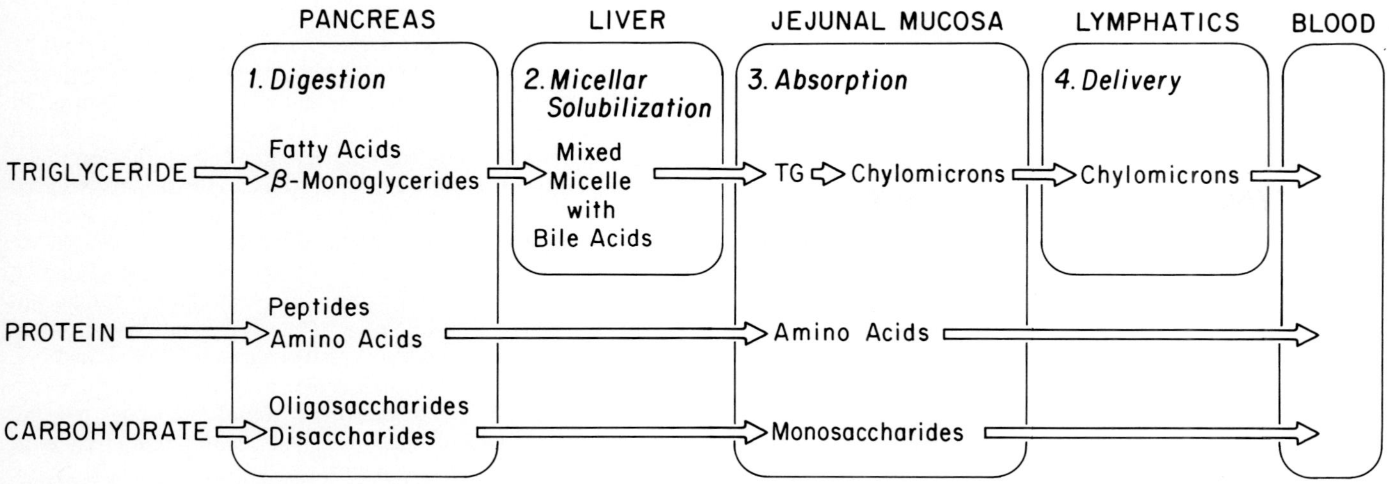

Figure 17-2. Comparison of fat, protein, and carbohydrate digestion and absorption.

to secrete amylase is determined by the carbohydrate content of the diet. Levels of pancreatic lipase parallel both the fat and protein content of the diet.

EXOCRINE PANCREATIC INSUFFICIENCY

Clinical Synopsis

Diagnostic features

* "Small bowel" type diarrhea with weight loss
* Steatorrhea
* Abnormal BT-PABA or trypsin-like immunoreactivity test
* Fecal digestion tests may be abnormal
* Abnormal breath hydrogen test
* Xylose absorption test often normal

Standard treatment

* Low fat diet, fed "little and often"
* Enzyme powder replacement therapy: 2 teaspoons/20 kg body weight preincubated with meals
* Cimetidine (5-10 mg/kg q 8 h PO) in refractory cases
* Antibiotics if evidence of concomitant bacterial overgrowth

Follow up

* Life long therapy required if disorder due to morphologic pancreatic disease

Exocrine pancreatic insufficiency can result from pancreatic disease, or from functional pancreatic insufficiency (Table 17-1). The latter disorder results from any disease process that interferes with the regulation of pancreatic secretion or with the activity of pancreatic enzymes in the lumen of the bowel.

Pancreatic Disease[3,4]

Chronic relapsing pancreatitis and juvenile pancreatic atrophy are the most common causes of deficient exocrine pancreatic secretion. The epidemiology and etiopathogenesis of these conditions are discussed in the chapter on pancreatic disease. Less frequent causes of exocrine pancreatic insufficiency are inflammatory processes or neoplasia that occlude the pancreatic ducts. Pancreatic insufficiency is most frequent in the dog, but also occurs in the cat but very seldom.[5] These diseases result in a deficiency of all the components of pancreatic secretion, including the entire spectrum of pancreatic enzymes and the bicarbonate-rich pancreatic fluid. Isolated deficiencies of only one of the pancreatic enzymes have been identified in humans, and it is possible that the same problems occur in small animals but have not been recognized.

Functional Exocrine Pancreatic Insufficiency[1]

Functional exocrine pancreatic insufficiency may be defined as exocrine pancreatic insufficiency without morphologic pancreatic disease. The condition can result from diseases of the intestinal mucosa, deranged gastric emptying, inappropriate luminal conditions for pancreatic enzyme activity, protein-calorie malnutrition, or excessively rapid degradation of the enzymes.

Duodenal Mucosal Disease. Mucosal disease of the small intestine, especially the duodenum, can occasionally result in deficient pancreatic secretion in spite of a histologically normal pancreas.[6] The mucosa of the small intestine produces the hormones cholecystokinin and secretin, which are released to stimulate pancreatic secretion. The mucosa also contains receptors for the neural reflex that releases these hormones. The duodenal mucosa possesses the highest concentration of receptors and endocrine-secreting cells but, to a lesser extent, pancreatic secretion can also be stimulated by hormones released from the jejunum. Chronic mucosal disease reduces the capacity to secrete hormones in response to stimulation by chemicals in chyme, resulting in functional pancreatic insufficiency. Duodenal mucosal function is affected by chronic dietary allergy since this part of the small intestine is subjected to the greatest stimulation by the offending antigen, at a place where no significant degradation of antigen has occurred. Mucosal damage in gluten-induced enteropathies is greatest in the duodenum, with a gradient of decreasing severity from cranial to caudal small intestine. With some mucosal diseases, the quantity of pancreatic enzymes released are normal, but their secretion is delayed until after most of the food has passed the

Table 17-1. Causes of Deficiency of Pancreatic Enzyme Activity in the Intestine

- I. Inappropriate secretion by pancreas
    - Reduced pancreatic synthesis
        - Pancreatic atrophy
        - Congenital enzyme deficiency
    - Reduced secretion by normal pancreas
        - Duodenal mucosal disease
            - Altered neural regulation
            - Altered humoral regulation
    - Delayed secretion by normal pancreas
        - Duodenal mucosal disease
- II. Decreased activation of enzymes
    - Duodenal mucosal disease
        - Enterokinase deficiency
    - Bile acid deficiency
        - Decreased activation of lipase
        - Decreased activation of trypsinogen by enterokinase
- III. Intestinal factors to reduce enzyme activity
    - pH too acid for optimum activity
        - Increased rate of gastric emptying
            - Duodenal mucosal disease
                - Altered enterogastrone mediate reflex
                - Altered enterogastric reflex
            - Overeating
        - Reduced rate of pancreatic secretion
        - Deficiency of bicarbonate secretion
    - Increased rate of proteolytic degradation of enzymes
        - Bacterial proteases
            - Overgrowth of microflora due to
                - Stasis
                - Obstruction
                - Hypomotility

duodenal papilla. Thus, the timing of secretion is too late to allow effective admixture of pancreatic enzymes with the chyme, and part of the diet is inadequately digested.

Small-intestine mucosal disease affects intestinal digestion by altering gastric emptying. Optimum digestion depends on regulation of the delivery of nutrients from the stomach to the intestine. The enterogastrone and enterogastrone reflex, stimulated by chyme, are mediated by hormones released from the mucosa to inhibit gastric motility. The enterogastric reflex is also stimulated by chyme on mucosa receptors, and its inhibitory effects are mediated by neural pathways. Function in one or both of these reflexes is probably impaired in chronic pancreatic exocrine deficiency, which accelerates gastric emptying. The chyme entering the duodenum is not buffered properly when bicarbonate secretion is deficient, which is one aspect of pancreatic deficiency. The acid chyme with pepsin activity damages the duodenal mucosa, thereby perpetuating the problem.

Mucosal disease also reduces synthesis and release of the enzyme enterokinase, which activates trypsin from trypsinogen.[7] Activation of trypsin is essential to the activation of all pancreatic proteases. Congenital deficiency of this enzyme can occur in humans, but it has not been reported in small animals.

Unsuitable Luminal Conditions. Functional exocrine pancreatic insufficiency can also result from inappropriate conditions in the lumen of the intestine. The properties of chyme in the intestine determine the activity of digestive enzymes.[2] Pancreatic enzymes have a broad pH range, but digestive activity is much lower at either end of the range. Pancreatic lipase and amylase are destroyed by very acid pH. Trypsin is more resistant to low pH, but if pepsin is still active after entering the small intestine it rapidly degrades trypsin. Pepsin is irreversibly inactivated and denatured at the neutral pH produced by normal pancreatic secretions. Thus, acidic duodenal content can result in maldigestion due to enzyme inactivation. Acidic duodenal pH may also inhibit bile acid functions. Acidic duodenal content can result from faster gastric emptying or reduced bicarbonate secretion by the pancreas or biliary system. The specific activity of the small amounts of enzymes secreted by the diseased pancreas will be suboptimal if the accompanying reduced secretion of alkaline fluid is insufficient to neutralize acid chyme entering the duodenum. Humans with exocrine pancreatic insufficiency do not have a more acidic duodenal pH in the unfed or fed states than do normal subjects, however.[8] The importance of excessive duodenal acidity in canine exocrine pancreatic insufficiency remains to be established.

Enzymatic digestion of any nutrient proceeds at a fixed rate under a given set of conditions. The rate does not increase with increased availability of substrate. Thus, an animal with a partial pancreatic exocrine deficiency being fed small meals two or three times a day is more likely to completely digest the smaller amounts of chyme leaving the stomach than if one large meal is fed. The rate of gastric emptying increases with the size of the meal, compounding the enzyme inadequacies.

Increased Degradation of Digestive Enzymes.[2] Functional exocrine pancreatic insufficiency can also result from accelerated degradation of pancreatic enzymes. Digestive enzymes lose their activity during transit in the intestinal tract, so that only a fraction of the original activity remains in the colon. The life span of an enzyme's activity is determined by a number of different factors. Enzymes are proteins, and are subject to degradation by proteolytic enzymes, such as activated pancreatic proteases, mucosal cell proteases released from desquamated villous cells, and bacterial proteases. The rate of pancreatic enzyme destruction is likely to be increased as a result of bacterial overgrowth. Bacteria multiply with any malassimilaton, using the abundant supply of unabsorbed nutrients.[35] Bacterial overgrowth is common in exocrine pancreatic insufficiency of the dog, and can be associated with biochemical and mild morphological mucosal changes.[9]

Diarrhea in dogs with exocrine pancreatic insufficiency often responds to antibiotics. The beneficial effect is most likely from reduction of an overgrown flora and inhibition of the destruction of small amounts of remaining enzymes.[10] Small amounts of pancreatic enzymes are absorbed and recycled through the pancreas.[11] The amounts that disappear in this manner are probably insignificant, yet this is an additional means by which pancreatic enzyme activity can be lost.

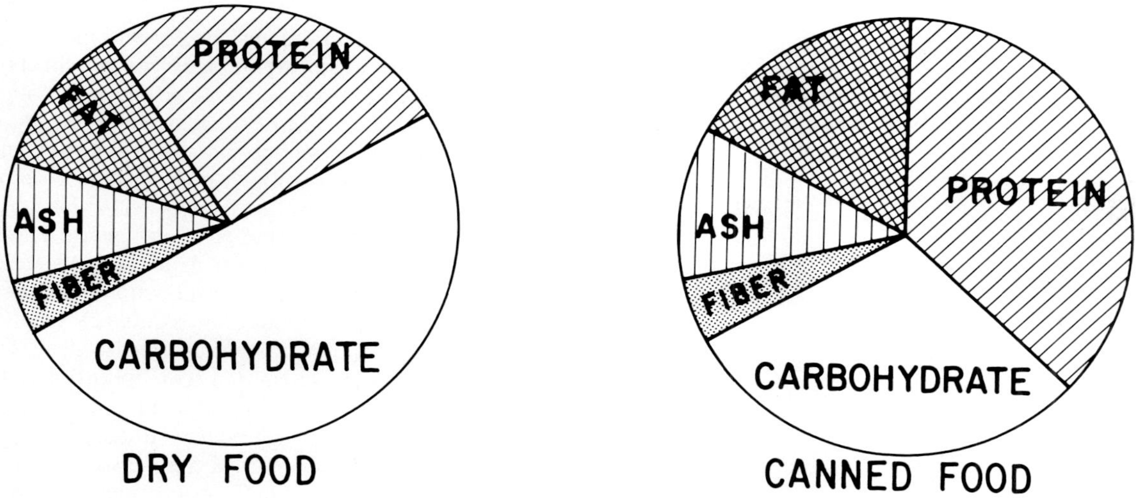

Figure 17-3. Nutrient composition of typical commercial dog foods on dry weight basis.

Effects of Exocrine Pancreatic Insufficiency on Assimilation of a Meal

Pancreatic enzymes are required for nutritional homeostasis and survival. With a complete loss of enzymes, however, some digestion and absorption of nutrients still proceeds. Pancreatic enzymes are most important for optimum fat and carbohydrate assimilation to be normal. Dietary proteins are almost completely digested and absorbed in the normal animal even if fed in excess. Fats and some carbohydrates, in contrast, are always incompletely absorbed. With normal fat intake, about 5% of dietary fat is found in the feces. That would be unremarkable if lipids were the most abundant nutrient in the diet, but their levels are relatively low (Figure 17-3).

Complete loss of pancreatic enzymes in experimental dogs results in marked and rapid weight loss and variable changes in the appearance of the feces.[12] Fecal volume is always increased but fecal consistency is variable. The most important changes are shown in Table 17-2. Both fecal wet weight and dry weight triple, indicating no change in relative fecal water content. Chymotrypsin activity disappears, as shown by a drop to background levels of PABA in urine. Loss of lipase activity causes a ninefold increase in total fecal fat excretion. The increase in fecal dry weight is not due primarily to the increased excretion of fat, since it accounts for only 15% of the increase. Thus, undigested protein and nitrogen-free extract, with some electrolytes, account for most of the increased fecal volume.

Pancreatic lipase is not essential for digestion and absorption of lipids, since 30% to 70% of dietary fat is absorbed without any lipase activity to digest triglycerides.[13] The percentage is not improved by adding bile acids.

Clinical signs of malabsorption appear when fecal fat content exceeds 8% to 10% of oral intake. Steatorrhea is reflected not in the percentage of fat excreted but the total amount excreted. Thus, steatorrhea is determined by the amount of fat in a diet.

Chronic diarrhea is frequently managed with controlled diets that are invariably low in fat. Animals with pancreatic enzyme deficiency and steatorrhea often improve on a low-fat diet. Protein aids in the assimilation of fats.[14] Proteins are like bile acids in having amphipathic properties to emulsify fats. Emulsification reduces particle size and improves absorption. The rate-limiting steps in fat digestion and absorption are not digestion by enzymes but micelle formation and the fixed capacity of the small intestine to absorb them. Micelles, formed to reduce particle size following lipid digestion, contain primarily monoglycerides, fatty acids, and bile acids. Micelles are minute particles in comparison with the size of an emulsified fat particle. The small size of micelles enables them to rapidly cross the mucosal membranes and be absorbed. Without micelle formation, emulsified dietary fats are still absorbed although a greatly expanded surface of intestinal mucosa would be required for absorption to be normal. With pancreatic enzyme deficiency, lecithin is not hydrolyzed, retaining its property to inhibit the absorption of fatty acids.[15]

Diarrhea associated with steatorrhea results from the increased quantities of fatty acids and bile acids that reach the lower small intestine and colon as a result of lipid malabsorption. The pathophysiological effects of malabsorbed bile acids and fatty acids are amplified by bacterial deconjugation of the bile acids and dehydroxylation of the fatty acids. The effects of these products on the bowel are discussed in detail in the section on bacterial overgrowth. The fatty acids in the colon are derived from malabsorbed fatty acids or from intact triglyceride that is hydrolyzed by colonic bacteria.[16] These long-chain fatty acids are poorly absorbed from the colon and increase the fecal water content by increasing epithelial permeability, stimulating active anion secretion and, to a lesser extent, altering colonic motility, and osmotic activity (Figure 17-4). The increased quantities of bile acids in the colon result from sequestration of bile acids in the malassimilated lipid. Bacterial deconjugation of dihydroxylated bile acids such as deoxycholic and chenodeoxycholic acid generates bile acids with virtually the same secretagogue properties and pathomechanisms as hydroxylated fatty acids. (Figure 17-5).[17] Deconjugated bile acids cause morphological changes in absorptive cells that include reduced size and loss of microvilli.[18] They cooperate with fatty acids to stimulate secretion of fluid and electrolytes. Bile acids and fatty acids increase the permeability of the colon, enhancing oxalate absorption.[19] Abnormal absorption of oxalates can lead to nephrolithiasis.

Table 17-2. Effects of ligation of pancreatic ducts of dogs on 24-hour fecal wet and dry weight. 24-hour fecal fat excretion, and urinary excretion of p-aminobenzoic acid 6 hours after oral administration as the sodium salt of n-benzyol-l-tyrosyl-p-aminobenzoic acid.

	Fecal wet wt. (g/10 Kg BW)	Fecal dry wt. (g/10 Kg BW)	Fecal fat (g/10 Kg BW)	Urine PABA (% of oral dose)
Normal dogs	158 ± 9[1]	47 ± 3	1.7 ± 0.3	77 ± 6
Pancreatic-duct-ligated	482 ± 27[2]	141 ± 8[3]	15 ± 1.2	2.4 ± 0.1

[1]Mean ± SE
[2]Percentage of fecal water is unchanged by duct ligation
[3]Increase represents 81 g carbohydrates, protein, and electrolytes, and 13.5 g fats

Carbohydrates are the most important nutrient that fails to be absorbed with pancreatic enzyme deficiency. Carbohydrate malabsorption plays an important role in the diarrhea, weight loss, and excessive intestinal gas that are consistent features of the disease.[20] Undigested carbohydrate accounts for most of the increased fecal volume. Carbohydrates are relatively abundant in commercial pet foods (Figure 17-3). Digestion and absorption of carbohydrates is an efficient process requiring only small amounts of pancreatic amylase. Carbohydrate must be hydrolyzed to monosaccharides by brush-border oilgosaccharidases before absorption is possible, however. These mucosal cell carbohydrate-digesting enzymes are relatively more important to the digestion of carbohydrates than are those from the pancreas. Dogs with pancreatic enzyme deficiency adapt by increasing the content of certain brush-border oligosaccharidases. The adaptation, however, is not sufficient to completely compensate for the pancreatic amylase deficiency. Unabsorbed carbohydrates lead to osmotic diarrhea and bacterial overgrowth of the small intestine with all its attendant consequences. The colon cannot absorb monosaccharides. Unabsorbed carbohydrate is fermented by intestinal bacteria, and the fermentation products, including short-chain fatty acids (proprionate, butyrate), CO_2, H_2, and methane, are rapidly absorbed from the small and large intestine. This absorption of fermentation products from the bowel reduces the severity of the diarrhea. The short-chain fatty acids are responsible for the acidic fecal pH characteristic of carbohydrate malabsorption.

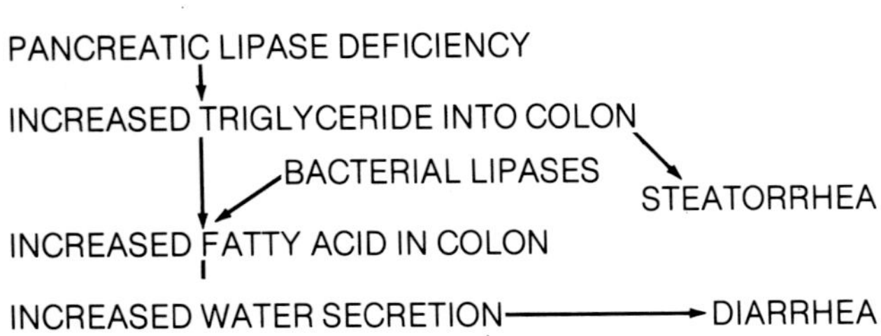

Figure 17-4. Scheme of mechanism of action of unabsorbed dietary lipids to cause both steatorrhea and diarrhea.

Dietary proteins depend the least on pancreatic enzymes for thier absorption to be complete. The protein content of most diets is relatively low, so needs for protease activity are not great. The contribution of the pancreatic proteases to protein digestion may be less important than what has been classically thought. Protein digestion begins in the stomach, under the action of pepsin, and is continued by pancreatic proteases. The products formed are amino acids and peptides. Absorption of both is by special transport mechanisms in the mucosal brush-border membranes. The mucosal cell contains proteases that degrade absorbed peptides to amino acids before they are absorbed into the portal circulation. In fact, the complete digestion of proteins to amino acids followed by their absorption is less efficient protein assimilation than the absorption of incompletely digested peptides by mucosal cells followed by their final digestion within the cell. In other words, protein assimilation is more rapid and complete if digestion before absorption is partial rather than complete.[21] Protein malabsorption, a late feature of pancreatic enzyme deficiency, is to some degree a complication of the malabsorption of other nutrients.

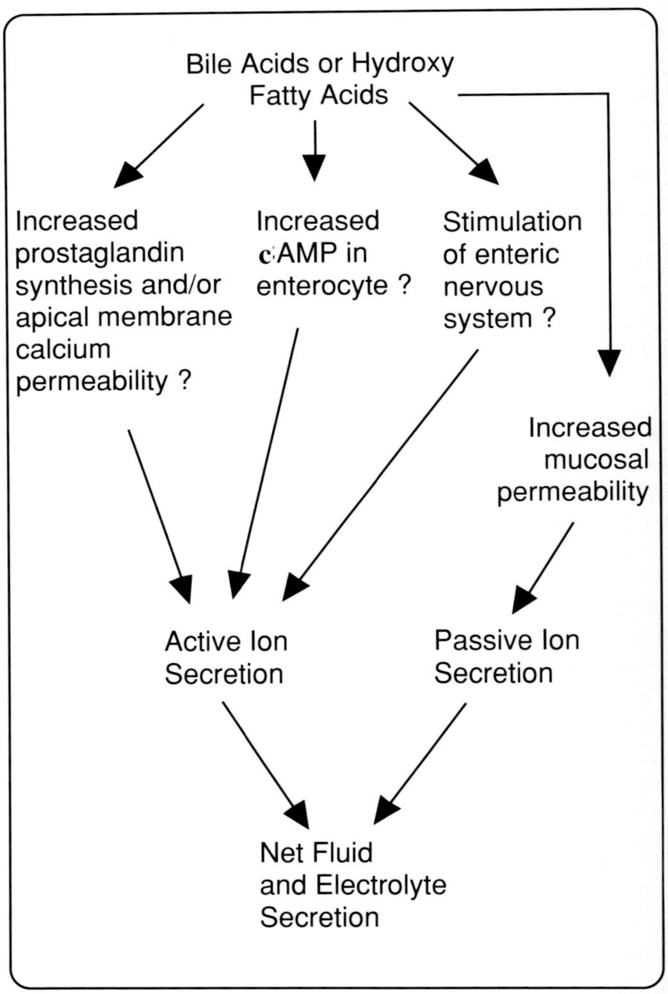

Figure 17-5. The influence of bile acids and hydroxy fatty acids on intestinal permeability, motility and secretion (modified from reference 17, Binder and Sandle).

For example, unabsorbed triglycerides sequester proteins and prevent their absorption. Increased intestinal bacteria secondary to malabsorption consume dietary nitrogen. The effects are protein malabsorption and protein deficiency. The absorption and final digestion of protein is dependent also on normal mucosal cells and brush border enzymes and transport mechanisms. The digestion and absorption of proteins is an efficient process that is completed in the cranial part of the small intestine.

A substantial reserve of pancreatic enzymes is available to perform the digestive functions of the animal. The adequacy of the pancreatic reserve depends on the composition of the diet. Thus, an animal with a partial enzyme deficiency may have steatorrhea and diarrhea on a diet with moderate amounts of fat, but the same animal placed on a low-fat diet has sufficient pancreatic reserve to cope with the lower level of dietary fat and no longer develops steatorrhea. When levels of enzyme activity are reduced to 10 to 15% of normal, no pancreatic reserve remains and maldigestion becomes clinically overt on any diet.[22-24]

Diagnosis of Exocrine Pancreatic Insufficiency

The approach to the diagnosis of maldigestion is described in Chapter 5. Exocrine pancreatic insufficiency has no consistent abnormalities on physical examination other than weight loss or the inability to gain weight, but the presentation of a young German Shepherd with the history of chronic diarrhea suggestive of malassimilation should raise the level of suspicion for pancreatic atrophy. Admission laboratory work is usually unremarkable. Screening tests for fat malassimilation such as the direct-indirect Sudan stain for fecal fat are usually abnormal, and quantification of fecal fat excretion will confirm steatorrhea. These tests for fecal-fat excretion provide poor discrimination between maldigestion and malabsorption. Fecal digestion tests are unreliable.

Therefore, once steatorrhea is confirmed, a diagnostic test to differentiate maldigestion from malabsorption should be performed. The most accurate tests are the trypsin-like immunoreactivity and the BT-PABA assay. Normal dogs excrete in the urine more than 70% of the orally administered PABA in a six-hour period. Dogs with pancreatic enzyme deficiency excrete less than 15% of the orally administered PABA in six hours.[24] Plasma determinations of PABA show peak levels less than 150 μg/dl in dogs with pancreatic exocrine insufficiency (Figure 6-6).[25,26] Peak levels are greater than 350 μg/dl in normal dogs. Concentrations of serum trypsin-like immunoreactivity in normal dogs are usually greater than 5.5 μg/L and in dogs with exocrine pancreatic insufficiency are less than 2.0 μg/L.[27] If fecal digestion tests are utilized they must be performed on fresh feces and must be repeated on three different samples from 3 different days. The absorption of xylose may be reduced in exocrine pancreatic insufficiency (Figure 6-8), because of bacterial overgrowth in the small intestine. The clinician should be careful not to assume a low xylose is due to intestinal disease. Breath hydrogen tests are also usually abnormal in exocrine pancreatic insufficiency, and allow tentative differentiation of carbohydrate malabsorption and bacterial overgrowth (Figure 6-10).[20] Recognition of the later condition is helpful in the decision as to whether to use antibiotics along with the enzyme supplements. Another way to recognize concomitant bacterial overgrowth and exocrine pancreatic insufficiency is to submit serum for assay of cobalamin and folate in association with the trypsin-like immunoreactivity. Qualitative lipid-absorption tests are too inconsistent to be of value, and are not recommended in the work up of diarrhea.

Diagnosis of exocrine pancreatic insufficiency is more difficult in cats. The canine trypsin-like immunoreactivity test has not been validated for the cat and the BT-PABA test is unreliable. Cats with exocrine pancreatic insufficiency usually have positive Sudan stains for fecal fat, however, and recently a fecal digestion test of utility in the cat has been described.[28]

The possibility of diarrhea due to functional exocrine pancreatic insufficiency should be considered if the patient's history or work up reveals evidence of excessive undigested fecal fat in association with a disease process, such as protein-calorie malnutrition, hyperacidity syndrome, duodenitis, or bacterial overgrowth. Functional exocrine pancreatic insufficiency should also be suspected if the trypsin-like immunoreactivity test is normal in the face of firm evidence of maldigestion such as a strongly positive direct fecal fat, or abnormal BT-PABA test. Such discordance suggests that a mucosal or luminal abnormality is resulting in the maldigestion and not an absolute deficiency of pancreatic enzymes. The serum concentration of trypsin-like immunoreactivity assesses pancreatic production of trypsinogen, but not the specific activity of trypsin within the bowel. The BT-PABA test, in contrast, assesses the activity of chymotrypsin in the bowel lumen. In other words, the trypsin-like immunoreactivity test detects a subset of maldigestion patients whose maldigestion is most often due to a morphologic pancreatic abnormality, whereas the BT-PABA test detects not only morphologic pancreatic disease but also functional causes of maldigestion (Figure 6-6). Other reasons for discordance between the trypsin-like immunoreactivity and BT-PABA test include obstructed pancreatic ducts, a selective deficiency of chymotrypsin or trypsin, and failure of a severely damaged intestinal mucosa to absorb free PABA. Functional pancreatic insufficiency is difficult to definitively diagnose, requiring a combination of findings including conclusive confirmation of maldigestion in association with a grossly and histologically normal pancreas. If severe mucosal disease is thought to be the cause of a reduced BT-PABA test due to functional pancreatic insufficency, the "strength" of the diagnosis is improved by the subsequent oral administration of free PABA. The administration of the free PABA is performed to rule out the unlikely possibility that the poor absorption of PABA derived from the BT-PABA is due to failed intestinal transport of PABA and not failed pancreatic digestion of the BT to PABA chemical bond.

Management of Exocrine Pancreatic Insufficiency

The treatment of functional exocrine pancreatic insufficiency is directed at the primary cause of the functional defect. The treatment of exocrine pancreatic insufficiency due to pancreatic disease centers on the provision of replacement pancreatic enzymes. The products preferred for replacement therapy are pancreatic enzyme concentrates, either in powder form or in crushed non-enteric-coated tablets (Table 17-3).[12] Uncoated enzyme tablets are not effective unless crushed. Enzyme powder is mixed in food at a level of 5.34 g (2 teaspoons) powder per each 20 Kg body weight. Increasing the

Table 17-3. Effects of therapy on 24-hour fecal wet and dry weight, 24-hour fecal fat excretion, and urinary excretion of p-aminobenzoic acid (PABA) 6 hours after oral administration as the sodium salt of n-benzoyl-l-tyrosyl-p-aminobenzoic acid in pancreatic-duct-ligated dogs weighing 20 Kg.

Pancreatic-duct-ligated dogs	**Fecal wet wt. (g/10 Kg BW)**	**Fecal dry wt. g/10 Kg BW)**	**Fecal fat g/10 Kg BW)**	**Urine PABA (%of oral dose)**
No Treatment	482 ± 27[1]	141 ± 8	15 ± 1.2	2.4 ± 0.1
One tsp. enzyme[2]	289 ± 37	85 ± 8	6 ± 2	39 ± 7
Two tsp. enzyme	235 ± 27[3]	72 ± 6[3]	4 ± 0.3	56 ± 2
Four tsp. enzyme	282 ± 10	90 ± 3	4 ± 0.5	65 ± 3
Two tsp. enzyme +				
a. 150 mg cimetidine	320 ± 21	98 ± 4	4 ± 0.2	43 ± 9
b. 300 mg cimetidine	230 ± 12	72 ± 3	2 ± 0.2[4]	58 ± 2
c. 30-min preincubation	235 ± 28	73 ± 7	3 ± 0.2	60 ± 6
d. 1 tsp. $NaHCO_3$	290 ± 2	85 ± 2	5 ± 1	54 ± 6
e. 4 tsp. $NAHCO_3$	287 ± 10	87 ± 3	4 ± 0.2	59 ± 2
f. 300 mg neomycin	274 ± 7	82 ± 3	3 ± 0.5	59 ± 6
g. 325 mg bile acids	288 ± 15	89 ± 5	4 ± 0.5	45 ± 7
Enzyme tablets	335 ± 10	108 ± 3[5]	5 ± 0.5	27 ± 6[5]
Enzyme tablets crushed	262 ± 12	81 ± .1	4 ± 0.3	—

[1]Mean ± SE.
[2]Viokase-V, A.H. Robins.
[3]All other treatments added to 2 tsp. enzyme do not improve results.
[4]Significantly less than treatment with enzyme only.
[5]Significantly different than equivalent amount of enzyme powder.

dose does not improve digestion any further. Enteric coated tablets should be avoided as the dissolution of their protective enteric coatings by the alkaline pH of intestinal contents is unpredictable.[12] The bicarbonate secretion needed to remove the enteric coating is reduced in pancreatic disease. As a result, the enteric coat is not removed until the tablet has reached the terminal parts of the small intestine. It is possible that pH sensitive microspheres of pancreatic enzymes (Pancrease) may be effective in enzyme replacement therapy in dogs.[29]

A considerable amount of pancreatic enzyme activity is lost in the stomach, with the rate of loss determined by the duration of exposure of the enzyme supplement to acidic gastric contents.[30] To minimize this problem, excess quantities of enzymes are usually premixed with the food and incubated at room temperature for 30 to 60 minutes before feeding. The product description of the different commercial preparations states the amounts of proteins, carbohydrates, and fats that a given amount of enzyme will digest. That is digestion in vitro, however, and one can expect that digestion by a given amount of enzyme will be less in the animal. Neither bicarbonate buffering or preincubation of the enzyme supplements appear to be necessary for adequate digestion.[12] The buffering effects of bicarbonate are short, and a subsequent acid rebound causes more acid to be secreted. Other forms of antacids with possible longer lasting effects are no better. Bile acids, which theoretically improve digestion by pancreatic enzymes, did not add to the beneficial effects of enzymes alone.

Cimetidine improves the response of dogs to enzyme-replacement therapy for exocrine pancreatic insufficiency.[12] The beneficial effect of the drug has been reported to be marked in some cases.[31] The mode of action of the cimetidine is thought primarily to be due to the reduced gastroduodenal acidity, which in turn decreases the amount of enzyme supplement destroyed in the stomach, and improves bile acid and pancreatic enzyme function in the duodenum. Cimetidine administration decreases pancreatic bicarbonate secretion in normal dogs but increases amylase secretion.[32] Its usage is controversial in humans.[33,34] Part of the explanation for the minimal beneficial effects of cimetidine in human patients is provided by the observation that duodenal pH of fasting or post-prandial human patients with pancreatic insufficiency is similar to that of normal subjects, implying a compensatory role for extrapancreatic sources of bicarbonate.[8] Cimetidine is best used as an adjunctive therapy for dogs that have not responded to enzyme supplementation alone.

Since malabsorption due to any cause often results in overgrowth of the normal bacterial flora, refractory patients may be treated with antibiotics. Diarrhea in dogs with exocrine pancreatic insufficiency often transiently improves in response to antibiotics. In some patients, antibiotics may be highly advantageous adjunctive therapy.[9]

No combination of therapy returns fecal dry weight or fecal wet weight to normal.[12] Only enzyme replacement combined with 300 mg cimetidine or 300 mg neomycin returns fecal fat excretion to normal. Thus, although weight gain and normal-appearing feces are achieved, enzyme replacement cannot result in a completely normal animal. Breath hydrogen also continues to be abnormal.[20]

Lipids are the first nutrients to escape absorption in maldigestion, which suggests that a low fat diet may add to the benefits of enzymes. Fats containing medium-chain fatty acids can be fed because they are more easily assimilated. Feeding a low fat diet requires the diet to be high in carbohydrates in order to provide the calories for the patient to gain weight. Excessive amounts of starches should be avoided, however, because dogs with pancreatic exocrine insufficiency malassimilate carbohydrates as well as fats.[20] Some affected dogs do not respond well to enzymes added to a low-fat diet. Such dogs may respond better to a diet where a substantial part of the calories is provided by fats; thus, a low-fat diet is not fed. In some patients it may be beneficial to feed commercial oligosaccharides prepared from digests of starch. An animal treated for enzyme deficiency maintains nutritional homeostasis with greater ease when fed three times a day. Diets high in fiber should probably be avoided because various types of fiber, including pectin and wheat bran will inhibit the activity of pancreatic enzymes, in particular lipase. Several pathomechanisms for the influence of fiber on exocrine pancreatic function have been proposed. Certain types of fiber increase duodenal juice viscosity and decrease duodenal pH. Fiber can adsorb enzyme reducing its availability.[35] Furthermore, wheat bran has been shown to decrease pancreatic lipase secretion in dogs.[36]

Some dogs will become hypersensitive to commercial concentrates of pancreatic enzymes prepared from hog pancreas. This rare complication, should be considered when abnormal bowel movements continue. Pancreatic enzymes derived from beef pancreas should be tried. A food intolerance can accompany the enzyme deficiency, in which case a properly controlled diet becomes part of the management.

The prognosis is favorable.

DEFICIENT BILE SECRETION[37,38]

Introduction

Efficient digestion and absorption of dietary lipids is dependent on adequate secretion of bile. One important components of bile is bile acids. The most important function of bile acids or their salts is the formation of micelles for the transport of lipid to the epithelial membrane of the enterocyte. Bile acids also contribute to the emulsification process, and have both stimulatory and inhibitory effects on pancreatic lipase. Bile salts reduce the pH optimum of pancreatic lipase activity from 8.0 to 6.0., but, in the absence of colipase, bile salt micelles inhibit the lipolytic activity of lipase. Bile is also necessary for activation of trypsinogen by enterokinase.[39]

Bile acid deficiency interferes less with lipid absorption than does deficiency of pancreatic enzymes.[22] Fecal fat lost in bowel movements is less than half as great with an absence of bile as with an absence of pancreatic enzymes.

Some of these differences are related to there being only a lipid maldigestion with bile deficiency, whereas with pancreatic deficiency there is bacterial overgrowth and a maldigestion of all nutrients, resulting in more secondary effects that contribute to lipid malabsorption.Other substances are amphipaths and can function like bile to emulsify lipids. Lipid solutions are stabilized in emulsions by dietary proteins, which explains why lipid absorption is still quite efficient despite the absence of bile.[14]

Causes of Deficient Bile Secretion

Bile acid deficiency can result when: 1) bile acids are not synthesized and secreted by the liver; 2) bile is not discharged into the duodenum because of bile-duct obstruction; 3) bile is altered within the intestine so that it loses its detergent properties; or 4) bile acids are lost form the body faster than they are synthesized. The most important cause of clinically significant bile acid deficiency is extrahepatic bile duct obstruction. Partial obstruction can be caused by cholecystitis and calculi, both of which are seldom recognized. Complete obstruction of the bile duct is most frequently caused by neoplasms of the pancreas, lymph nodes, or intestine. Bile duct obstruction can also be a complication of acute pancreatitis, perforated gastric or duodenal ulcer, and abscesses. Occasionally, intestinal parasites enter and obstruct the lumen of the duct. Complete obstruction of the biliary tract results in icterus and steatorrhea. In addition the feces appear gray or putty-colored due to the absence of bile pigments.

When bile acid secretion is reduced the only signs are an early steatorrhea with bowel movements remaining formed. With complete obstruction, fecal fat increases and in addition the feces appear unpigmented, being gray or putty-colored. Fecal color is due mainly to products of bile pigment metabolism. Bilirubin secreted in bile is metabolized by intestinal bacteria to form stercobilinogen (urobilinogen), which is further oxidized to the brown pigment of feces, stercobilin (urobilin). Only small amounts of bile are needed to produce brown feces. Thus, complete bile duct obstruction is required in order to produce gray feces. Bowel movement color also varies with the diet. Where milk proteins are the only source of nitrogen, light-colored feces are produced. Antibiotics given orally can drastically alter the microflora that metabolizes bile pigments, so that the feces appear lighter in color. With a large volume of watery diarrhea there is a reduction in bacterial numbers, which is associated with less time for metabolism of bile pigments; both changes contribute to lighter colored feces. If bile obstruction is complete, with acholic stools resulting, other evidence of the problem would have been seen much earlier, i.e., icterus.

Hepatic parenchymal disease can reduce bile acid secretion, but rarely to the extent where clinically obvious steatorrhea develops. With hepatic disease the liver loses its capacity to extract bile acids from the portal circulation and resecrete them. Thus, the total-body pool of bile acids may be normal but the reduced enterohepatic circulation makes less available for release into the intestine. Intrahepatic biliary obstructions usually do not produce a complete bile acid deficiency. Reduced bile acid secretion predisposes an animal to steatorrhea. This may not manifest until the animal is placed on a high fat diet.

Bile acids must remain conjugated in order to participate effectively in micelle formation.[38] The pKa of conjugated bile acids makes them ionized and water-soluble at the pH of intestinal contents. At that pH they readily form micelles. Intestinal bacteria deconjugate and metabolize bile acids, which increases their pKa so that they are un-ionized and lipid-soluble at a neutral pH, thus losing their ability to form micelles. Being lipid-soluble, they can be absorbed readily from the cranial small intestine and be lost for further micelle formation. Thus bile acid deficiency develops with bacterial overgrowth of the small intestine.

Intestinal bile acid concentration is determined by the adequacy of bile enterohepatic circulation. The bile acid pool is so small that it passes through the enterohepatic circulation two or three times during a single meal. Hepatic disease causes deficient uptake of bile acids from the portal circulation, resulting in elevated peripheral blood concentration of bile acids but less resecretion of the bile acid into the biliary tract. Biliary obstruction decreases the discharge of bile into the duodenum. Failure of adequate ileal reabsorption of bile acids also results in a deficiency, since hepatic synthesis of new bile acids is unable to replace losses in the feces. Surgical removal of the ileum, chronic disease of the ileum, or specific malabsorption of bile acids results in increased excretion of bile acids in the feces. The excess bile acids are actively metabolized by colonic bacteria, producing compounds that affect colonic morphology and transport processes and contribute to diarrhea.

Diagnosis and Therapy of Deficient Bile Secretion

A diagnosis of maldigestion of lipids due to deficient bile secretion is rarely made, because the clinical signs of the primary disorder usually overshadow the more subtle signs of the maldigestion. Thus, animals with obstructions of their biliary tracts will present with icterus or hyperbilirubinemia. Patients with liver disease of sufficient severity to cause significant bile acid deficiency will usually have clinical-laboratory evidence of liver disease. Patients with bile acid malabsorption usually have copious watery diarrhea due to the secretory effects of the bile acids on the colonic mucosa.

The therapy of bile acid deficiency is usually directed at the primary cause of the disorder. Feeding a low-fat diet can be an important adjunctive measure.

DUODENAL MUCOSAL DISEASE AND MALDIGESTION[1]

Mucosal disease of the small intestine, results in maldigestion as well as malabsorption. The mucosal disease causes maldigestion partially through decreased pancreatic enzyme secretion and activation as discussed above, but also through interference with the control of gastric emptying and bile secretion.

Optimum digestion depends on regulation of the delivery of nutrients from the stomach to the intestine. The rate of gastric emptying is partially controlled by hormones released from the duodenal mucosa, and partially by the enterogastric reflex. Function in one or both of these feedback systems can be impaired in chronic mucosal diseases. The result is accelerated gastric emptying, and inadequate buffering of chyme. The dumping of ingesta into the duodenum overwhelms pancreatic reserves and maldigestion can result. The acid chyme with pepsin activity damages the duodenal mucosa, thereby perpetuating the problem.

Duodenal mucosal disease also results in impaired bile secretion. Normal duodenal mucosa secretes cholecystokinin in response to chyme. Cholecystokinin stimulates release of gallbladder bile, which is essential for efficient fat digestion. Bile acid deficiency also affects protein digestion since activation of trypsinogen by enterokinase is reduced.[39]

DERANGED GASTRIC FUNCTION AND MALASSIMILATION

Gastric secretions are not essential for digestion, but they do facilitate the process. Pepsin and hydrochloric acid begin protein digestion in the stomach, but are not mandatory for effective protein digestion. Deficiency of hydrochloric acid can result in malassimilation as a result of bacterial overgrowth. Hydrochloric acid solubilizes ferric iron to make it available for chelation with substances that enhance its absorption.

Ordered antral segmental contractility is necessary to grind and emulsify food material. Rapid gastric emptying can result in duodenal ulceration, and intestinal overload that results in maldigestion and osmotic diarrhea. Humans with rapid gastric emptying can experience post-prandial abdominal pain, nausea, vomiting, diarrhea, and weakness. The symptoms constitute the so-called "dumping syndrome". The most common causes are gastric surgical procedures such as vagotomy with pyloroplasty, gastroenterotomy, and partial gastrectomy. The signs usually occur within 10-30 minutes of meals but can be delayed by up to several hours. The pathogenesis, relates to massive fluid shifts from the duodenal interstitium into the hyperosmolar lumen. This problem is minimized by feeding two to three smaller meals a day instead of one.

MALABSORPTION

Clinical Synopsis

Diagnostic features

* "Small bowel" type diarrhea with weight loss
* Steatorrhea
* Normal digestion tests (TLI, BT-PABA, fecal digestion tests)
* Abnormal breath hydrogen test
* Xylose absorption test often normal

Standard treatment

* Depends to a large extent on cause
* Low fat diets with easily assimilated carbohydrate and protein

Follow up

* Depends on cause

Causes of Malabsorption

Malabsorption of nutrients can result from a variety of causes including defects in mucosal transport systems, reduced mucosal surface area, reduced brush border enzymes, disease involving the lamina propria, and circulatory problems (see Chapter 16). The most common cause of chronic malabsorption in the dog and cat is inflammatory bowel disease.

Loss of Brush Border Enzymes. Brush border enzymes are lost secondarily to acute or chronic mucosal disease.[40] Severe infectious enteritis results in a loss of disaccharidases that continues until new epithelial cells move up from the crypts. Toxic agents and some drugs (e.g., neomycin and kanamycin) have a similar effect. Disaccharidases are reduced by at least 50% in chronic clinical entities of dogs such as

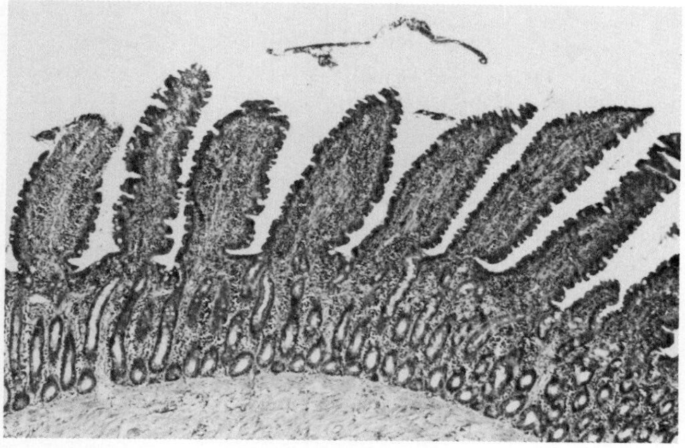

Figure 17-6. Plasmacytic enteritis. Moderate infiltration of lamina propria by primarily plasma cells with a few neutrophils and eosinophils. Increased villous thickness results in reduced numbers. Increased number of cells in crypts. Normal villous length and crypt depth. Changes produced diarrhea and weight loss. Compare with Figure 14-4, normal intestinal mucosa.

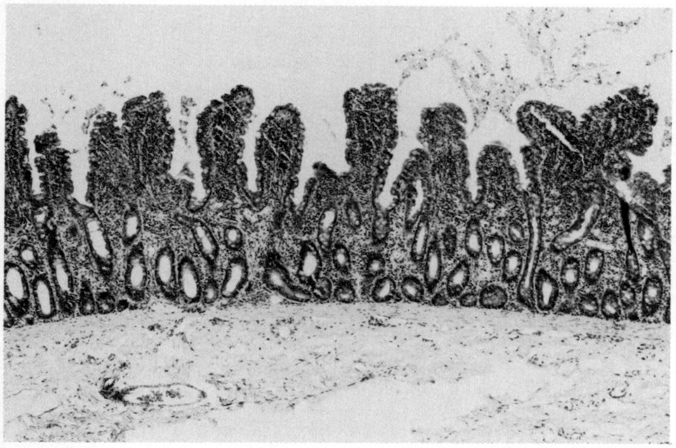

Figure 17-7. Chronic enteritis. Changes characterized by moderate villous atrophy and fusion of villi. Marked infiltration by plasma cells, lymphocytes, and eosinophils. Crypt depth is normal with increased mitotic activity and increased numbers of goblet cells in crypt glands. Crypts are of greater length than villi.

eosinophilic enteritis, neutrophilic enteritis with villus atrophy, histiocytic enteritis with villus atrophy, lymphosarcoma with villus atrophy, and villus atrophy associated with no particular cellular infiltration.[40] Reductions are seen also with lymphangiectasia.[40] Jejunal levels of maltase are normally greater than levels of lactase and sucrase, but in chronic enteropathies maltase activity is reduced more severely than are lactase and sucrase activities. Disaccharidase activity is lost in any problem that causes overgrowth of the microflora, such as intestinal obstruction and malabsorption of nutrients. Nutritional deficiency causes a loss of the disaccharidases. More specifically, chronic iron deficiency in growing dogs reduces the activity of all three disaccharidases to less than half.[41] Parasite infestation also can reduce maltase levels.[42] A congenital absence of brush border enzymes has been recognized in humans but has not been identified in small animals.[43] Lactase is the enzyme found

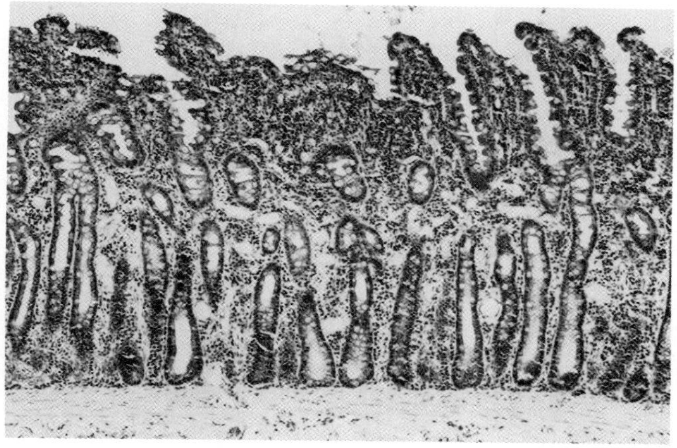

Figure 17-8. Chronic enteritis. Changes similar to Figure 17-5b except cellular infiltration is less, crypts are widely dilated and proliferation of crypt epithelium is more active.

deficient most frequently.

Mucosal disease also results in a loss of brush border peptidases. These losses are not critical, since peptides are digested more efficiently than oligosaccharides and some dipeptides can be absorbed intact. Any nitrogen deficiency associated with chronic enteropathies is more likely to be a result of anorexia, plasma protein exudation, and consumption of protein by increased numbers of bowel bacteria resulting from concomitant carbohydrate malabsorption.[44]

It is generally thought that all the fluid that enters the colon as the result of a disaccharidase deficiency is the result of osmotic attraction by the unabsorbed carbohydrate. When 40 to 80% of the dietary lactose is not digested and enters the colon, only 10% is excreted in the feces. The difference is metabolized by colonic bacteria, and the metabolites are absorbed, reducing the severity of the diarrhea. Osmotic attraction of water by unabsorbed carbohydrate may not be the only pathomechanism for the diarrhea associated with carbohydrate malabsorption. In some patients the amount of water entering the colon is three times the amount osmotically attracted by the unabsorbed carbohydrate.[45]

Careful attention must be paid to the composition of the diet offered to animals with brush border defects. Sufficient amounts of maltase may remain to digest a normal intake of starch, but the profound reduction of maltase that has been documented in many enteropathies illustrates that care should be taken to avoid excess carbohydrate. Animals with chronic enteric problems do not tolerate milk, which suggests that lactase levels are low. Diarrhea is often managed with diets containing cottage cheese, which contains, on the basis of a gram of lactose per gram of protein, about 10% of the lactose of whole milk. Yogurt, frequently used to treat diarrhea, contains almost as much lactose as whole milk.

Loss of Mucosal Absorptive Area. A reduction in the mucosal surface area is an important cause of malabsorption. The number of absorptive epithelial cells on the villi are reduced by both acute and chronic conditions. Bacterial toxins and metabolites, bile acid metabolites, parasites, and certain antigens can produce mucosal changes severe enough to cause malabsorption. Some changes are due to direct toxic effects on the intestinal mucosa, and others are mediated by the host's

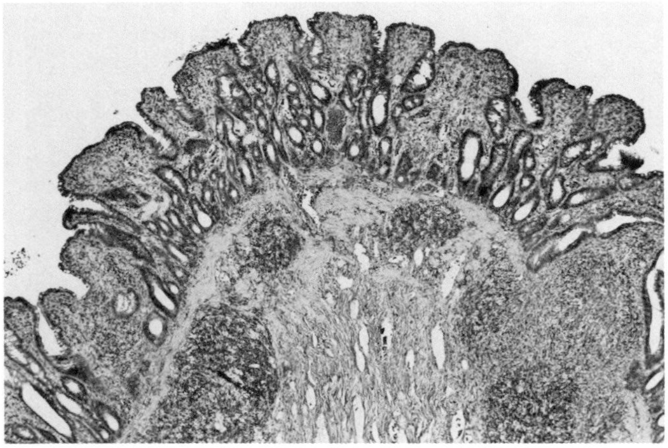

Figure 17-9. Chronic enteritis with subtotal villous atrophy. Villi are broad, very short, and infiltrated with inflammatory cells (primarily mononuclear). Crypts are dilated with epithelium actively proliferating. Crypt depth is normal. Submucosa is infiltrated with foci of inflammatory cells.

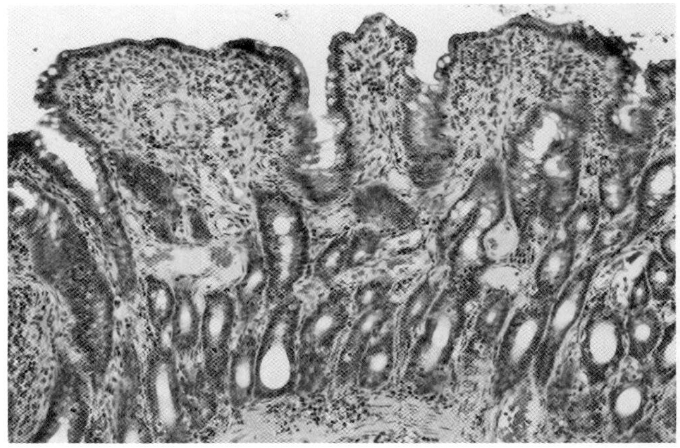

Figure 17-10. Higher magnification of Figure 17-9. Surface epithelium is cuboidal. With maintenance of normal amounts of crypt epithelium, recovery of near normal villous structure is possible.

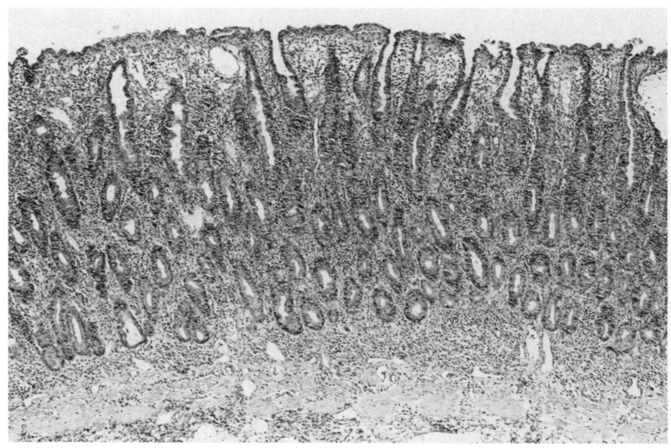

Figure 17-11. Chronic enteritis. total villous atrophy and surface epithelium is effaced. Marked infiltration of crypts by inflammatory cells, primarily mononuclear. Crypt mucosa is normal depth and amount of crypt epithelium is relatively normal. Villus renewal is possible with removal of cause. Total villous atrophy makes section to appear like colonic mucosa.

immune response. The mucosal crypts frequently hypertrophy, and the villi atrophy. The atrophied mucosa contains fewer mature epithelial cells that have the ability to produce brush border enzymes; thus, the capacity to digest oligosaccharides and proteins is reduced. The microvilli are also usually abnormal, further reducing absorptive capacity.

Acute enteritis causes villus loss and atrophy. The villi are blunted and atrophied by immune-mediated mechanisms following antigenic stimulation and by chronic infectious processes, malignancy, parasitism, and toxicities (Figure 17-6 to 17-11). Malabsorption results from a decrease in the total number of transport mechanisms that are specifically required for the absorption of glucose and sodium. The size of the surface area is also important for the absorption of some substances that are transported passively such as lipids. Most of the small intestine is required to absorb the required 95% of dietary lipid. Only moderate villus blunting and atrophy is needed to reduce the surface area by one half and cause a steatorrhea. Villus atrophy confined to the ileum, resulting in a primary bile acid malabsorption and chronic watery diarrhea, has been reported in humans.[46]

Loss of Transport Mechanisms. The mucosal surface area may be normal but lack specific transport mechanisms for a particular nutrient. A congenital absence of special transport mechanisms for hexoses, amino acids, or certain vitamins and minerals results in their deficiency.[47] Such defects have been identified in humans and animals.

Loss of Intracellular Mechanisms. Intracellular defects are uncommon causes of malabsorption. Malabsorption from mucosal disease, is usually caused by abnormalities at the rate-limiting steps of absorption which occur for most nutrients at the mucosal surface. After sugars enter the cell no special mechanisms are required for their transport into the circulation. Sugars also do not require metabolic transformation to leave the cell. Proteins require digestion if they enter the cell as peptides, but intracellular digestion is not rate-limiting, and is not significantly affected by most mucosal diseases. Lipids require metabolic transformation before they can leave mucosal cells but, as with proteins, the rate-limiting step in lipid assimilation is diffusion across the brush border.[48] Lipids require reesterification by endoplasmic-reticulum enzymes. This is followed by chylomicron formation, which is dependent on the synthesis of a beta lipoprotein. A deficiency of this lipoprotein causes the triglycerides to accumulate in the epithelial cell.[49] This problem is recognized in man but has not been reported in animals. Antibiotics that inhibit protein synthesis could have an effect on the production of this lipoprotein. The transport of chylomicrons from the cell is by a special mechanism that involves the microtubule system. Drugs, such as colchicine, that affect microtubular formation inhibit the transport of lipids from the cell.

Disease of Lamina Propria. The structure of the lamina propria is important for optimum absorption of fluid and nutrients. This part of the mucosa contains a loose array of blood vessels and connective tissue. The vessels lie immediately adjacent to the basal border of the mucosal cells, making the

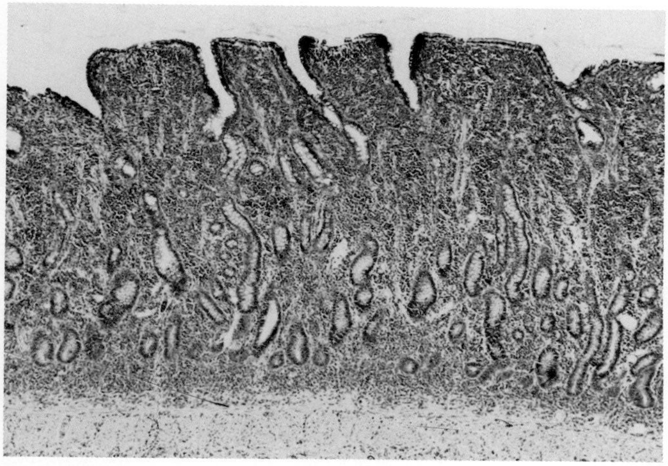

12

Figure 17-12 to 17-14. Diffuse infiltration by lymphoma cells uniformly produces villous atrophy (reducing absorptive area), often markedly increases thickness of crypt layer, and causes columnar epithelial absorptive cells to become cuboidal or squamous

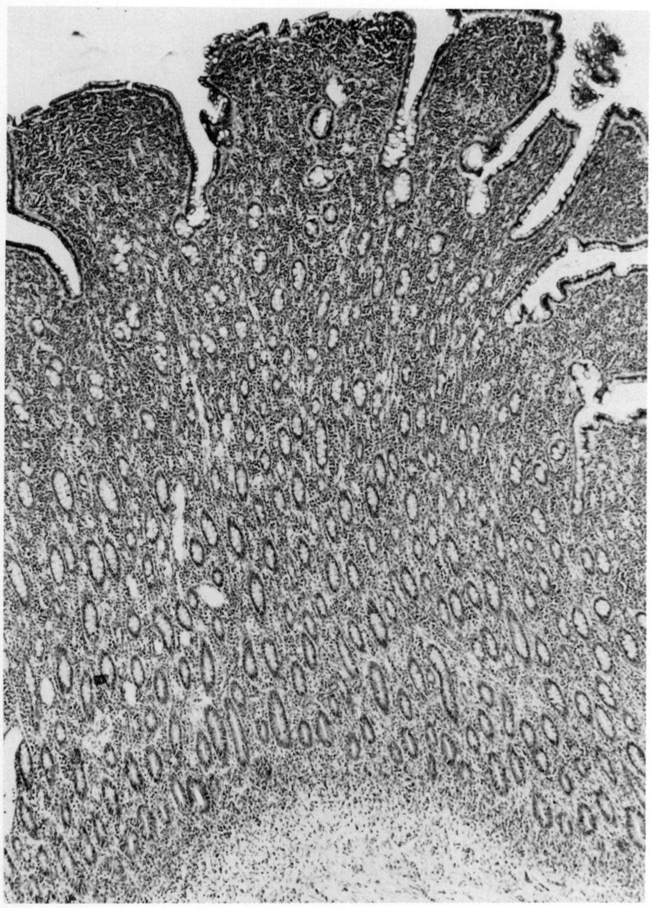

13

path short for absorbed particles to enter the circulation. Pathology in the lamina propria affecting absorption includes cellular infiltration, fibrosis, and accumulation of fluid. The types of cells infiltrating the lamina propria include lymphocytes, plasma cells, histiocytes, macrophages, eosinophils, neutrophils, mast

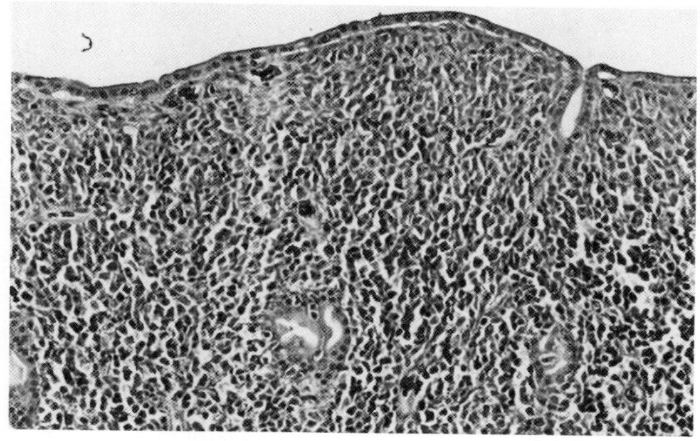

14

cells, and basophils. Signs of inflammation may be evident, or the lamina propria may be extensively infiltrated with neoplastic lymphocytes without evidence of inflammation (Figure 17-12 to 17-14). A case of fucosidosis, a lysosomal storage disease of English Springer Spaniels, has been reported in which malabsorption was due infiltration of the lamina propria with vacuolated macrophages.[50] Infiltrating cells create a barrier between the normal-appearing mucosal surface and the capillaries, interfering with normal diffusion of absorbed fluid and solutes. Thus, malabsorption is produced by an obstacle placed in the pathway of absorption. It is evident that this is only part of the problem, since the surface area of the mucosa is greatly reduced. Intestinal lymphomas cause the most severe type of cellular infiltration.

Circulatory Disease. Lymphatic disorders interfere with the absorption of chylomicrons, plasma proteins, and lymphocytes. Instead of being absorbed they accumulate in the lamina propria and are readily lost into the lumen of the intestine. Absorption of nutrients by capillaries is influenced by the physical forces that draw fluid into the circulation. Increased capillary hydrostatic pressure as a result of hepatic cirrhosis or congestive heart failure can result in malabsorption. A decreased plasma protein concentration reduces colloid osmotic pressure, so that forces are inadequate to draw absorbed fluid into the capillaries.

Consequences of Malabsorption

The consequences of malabsorption are similar to that described for maldigestion. When malabsorption is longstanding, nutritional deficiency manifests by skin and hair-coat changes, anemia, hypoproteinemia, and calcium deficiency. The accumulation of osmotically-active carbohydrates and fatty acids in the colon results in osmotic diarrhea. Fat malabsorption results in malabsorption of fat soluble vitamins. Probable vitamin K deficient bleeding has been reported in two cats with malabsorption syndrome due to lymphocytic-plasmacytic enteritis.[51] Fat malabsorption also results in a secretory diarrhea through the action of hydroxylated fatty acids or deconjugated bile acids on the colonic mucosa.

Malabsorption can result in bacterial overgrowth. Alternatively, bacterial overgrowth can result in malabsorption. Circulatory disorders, particularly lymphangiectasia can result in significant loss of protein from the bowel.

Malabsorption causes increased absorption of dietary

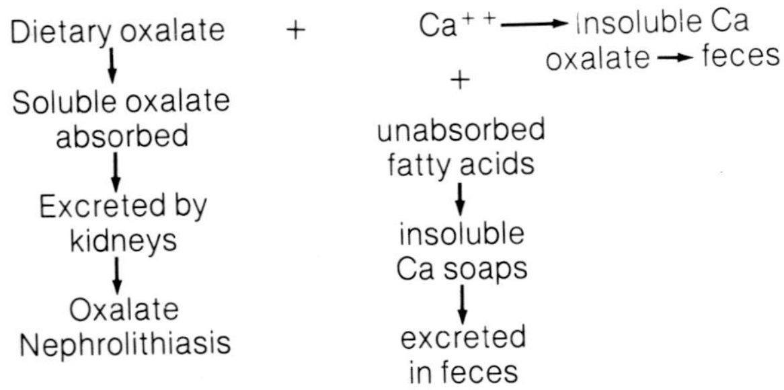

Figure 17-15. Schematic showing how unabsorbed fatty acids bind calcium and allow the absorption of dietary oxalate to cause oxalate nephrolithiasis. Dietary oxalate is normally bound to calcium to form insoluble Ca oxalate which is excreted in the feces. When excess fatty acids are present they react with the calcium leaving none to bind oxalate. In this case oxalate is freely absorbed.

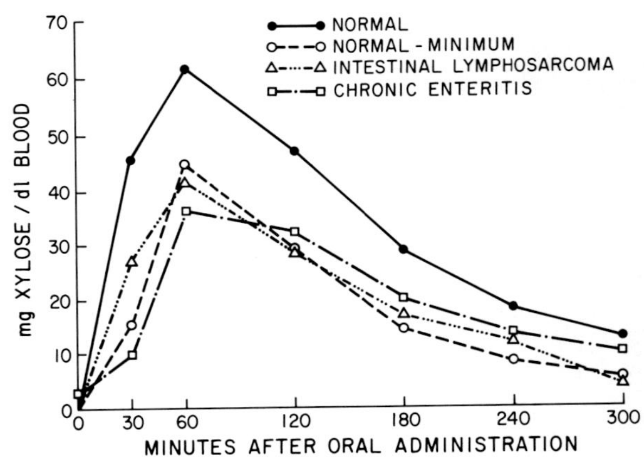

Figure 17-16. Graph showing xylose absorption in a dog with intestinal lymphosarcoma and in a dog with chronic enteritis. Mean xylose absorption in normal dogs is shown with minimum normal values. Note that only the 60 minute determination identifies abnormalities.

oxalate (Figure 17-15). The absorption of oxalate is normally limited by precipitation with calcium as an insoluble salt. Fat malabsorption results in chelation of dietary calcium with unabsorbed fatty acids, and less calcium is available for precipitation with oxalate. Consequently, oxalate remains in a soluble form that can be absorbed. Oxalate is absorbed in the colon,[52] and this is facilitated by the effects of bile acids and fatty acids in increasing the permeability of the colonic mucosa.[19] The manifestation of increased oxalate absorption is an appearance of oxalate crystals in the urine. That may be an incidental finding in an apparently normal animal. With absorption of large amounts, it is possible to see nephrolithiasis and acute nephritis. Chronic hyperoxaluria can be treated with oral calcium and aluminum salts.[53]

Laboratory Findings and Diagnosis of Malabsorption

The approach to the diagnosis of malabsorption is described in Chapter 5. Fecal fat tests are usually the most reliable screening tests for malabsorption from generalized mucosal disease. Plasma turbidity lipid-absorption tests are too unreliable to be recommended for screening test for malassimilation. The breath hydrogen test is a suitable screening test for carbohydrate malabsorption whether the malabsorption results from disaccharidase deficiencies or generalized mucosal disease. The xylose-absorption test is sometimes used to detect malabsorption due to generalized mucosal disease but the sensitivity of the test is poor. Normal xylose absorption depends on a number of factors including normal mucosal surface area and an absence of any obstacles in the pathway of absorption through the mucosa (Chapter 6). Figure 17-16 shows a xylose absorption curve from animals with malabsorption caused by villus atrophy. The histology of the intestinal mucosa from the cases (Figure 17-17 and 17-18) illustrates the reduction in surface area. The xylose-absorption test is influenced by the number of bacteria in the small intestine. Bacteria are able to utilize xylose, and an overgrowth of bacteria can produce results like those when there is a malabsorption. Thus, if bacterial overgrowth is suspected in the small intestine, antibiotics should be given before the test is conducted. The abnormal xylose-absorption test indicates that intestinal mucosa disease is a problem, and a definitive diagnosis requires biopsy and, in some cases, evaluation with a test diet.

Tests are available to determine an animal's ability to digest disaccharides as well as to absorb the monosaccharides formed. These tests are primarily indicated to evaluate the activity of brush border disaccharidases. The test used most commonly in humans is the oral lactose-tolerance test. These tests have not been sufficiently validated in the dog and cat (Chapter 6). A positive result does not distinguish between secondary disaccharidase deficiency and mucosal disease. Moreover, these two changes usually appear together.

Some types of malabsorption develop as the result of longstanding adverse reactions to food. These entities cannot be diagnosed by any laboratory procedure. For example, gluten-induced enteropathy causes mucosal changes that lead to a state of malabsorption, and the diagnosis can only be made by observing responses to the feeding of a controlled diet.

Small animal patients with malabsorption seldom have radiographically identifiable changes in the small intestine. Positive-contrast radiographic studies are occasionally performed to rule out adynamic ileus or mechanical obstructions (Figure 17-19). These changes result in bacterial overgrowth and malabsorption. Contrast studies of the intestinal tract occasionally identify mucosal morphology abnormalities, but do not differentiate the causes. The radiographic appearance of the intestinal mucosa in an animal with advanced lymphosarcoma can resemble that of an animal with allergic enteritis. Enteroclysis is a superior technique for the detection of intestinal mucosal disease and partial obstructions than the barium follow-through study.

Biopsy of the intestine is often the only means of characterizing changes of the intestinal mucosa. In many cases no definitive diagnosis is possible, although there is usually sufficient biopsy information to direct the course of treatment and offer a prognosis. Many changes are nonspecific and show a reduction in surface area and infiltration by immunocytes. That is seen, for example, in gluten-induced enteropathy, where a diagnosis can be made only from results of feeding test diets. In

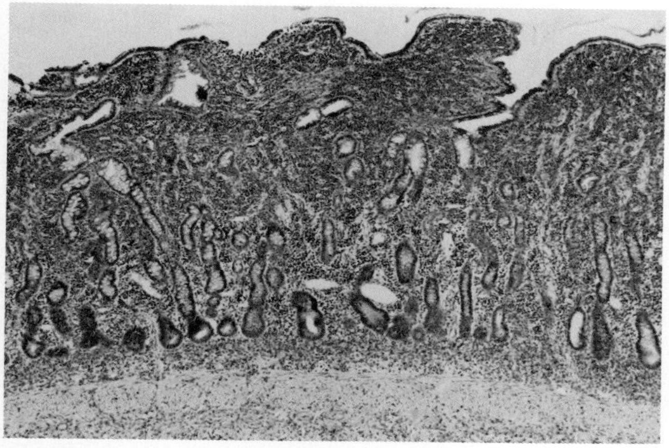

Figure 17-17. Intestinal lymphosarcoma. Diffuse infiltration of entire mucosa causing malabsorption of xylose as shown in Figure 17-16.

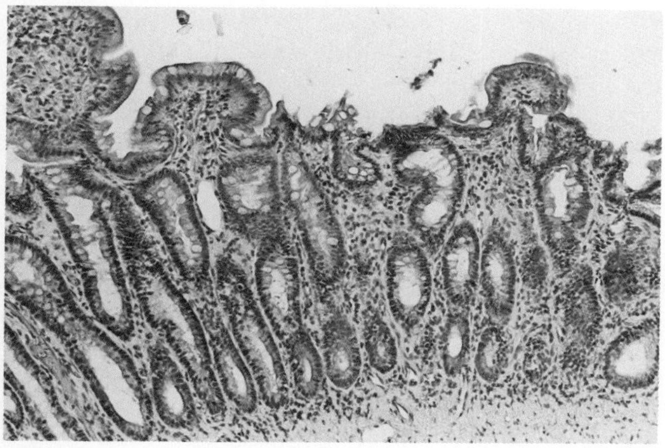

Figure 17-18. Chronic enteritis. Subtotal villous atrophy. Hyperplasia of crypt epithelium. Changes produced malabsorption of xylose shown in Figure 17-16.

general, assessments of the biopsy include evaluation of: 1) the size of the absorptive surface area; 2) the degree of cellular infiltration; and 3) the circulation in the mucosa. Those assessments are used to evaluate the contribution of the mucosal disease to the malabsorption and how the problem is to be best managed.

When biopsy is done early in the disease, normal findings are usually reported. The normal appearing mucosa does not reflect subtle pathological changes, however. Early consistent changes include loss of brush border enzyme activities, increased mucosa permeability to ion movement, and increased number of intraepithelial leukocytes. Changes in enzyme activities and permeability are functional rather than morphologic and may be identified with functional but not morphologic evaluation. In some cases the disease may result in morphologic changes that are most severe when the animal is in the fed state rather than when no nutrients are in the intestine. In such cases, withholding all food for 24 hours in preparation for biopsy may allow enough time for the lesions to change so they cannot be recognized. Increased intraepithelial leukocytes may provide an early and reliable clue for an immune-mediated pathologic process.

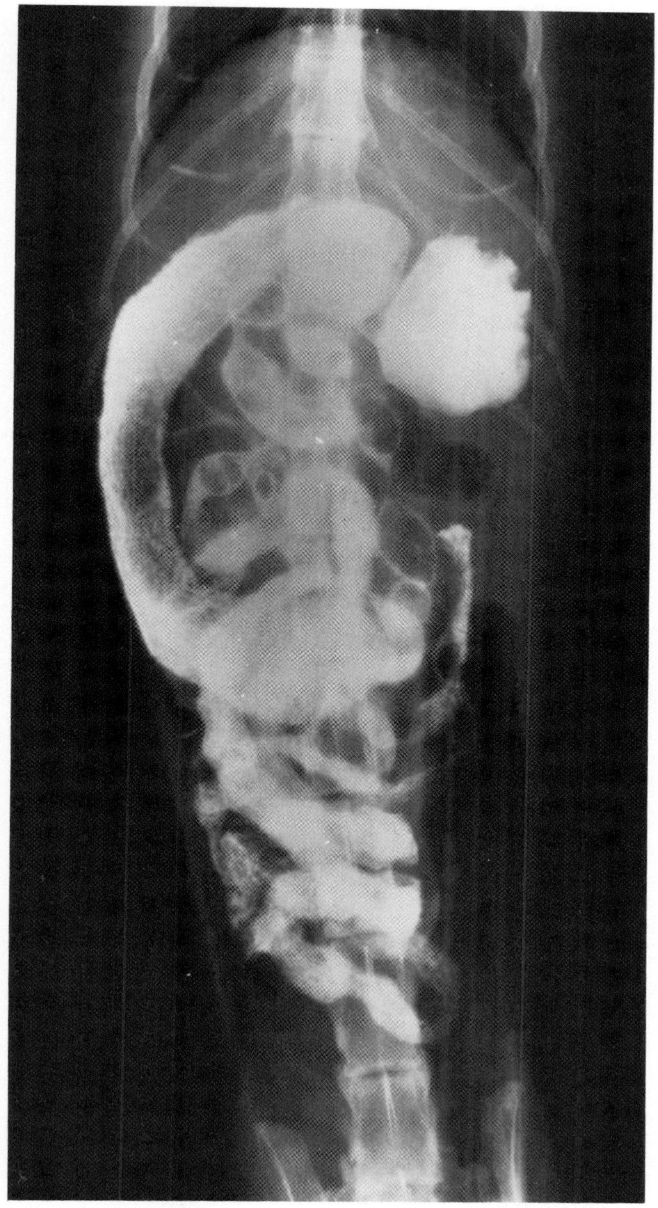

Figure 17-19. Dorsoventral radiograph of 10-year-old cat with clinical signs of anorexia, diarrhea and intermittent vomiting. Positive contrast medium outlines a dilated loop of small intestine cranial to a site of partial obstruction caused by an annular lesion. Biopsy of the resected lesion revealed an adenocarcinoma. Intestinal stasis in the dilated loop results in bacterial overgrowth which causes a number of changes that lead to the diarrhea.

Management of Malabsorption

The management of malabsorption is dependent on the primary cause. Readers are directed to the chapters on infectious and parasitic intestinal diseases, inflammatory bowel disease, intestinal obstruction, adverse reactions to food, and gastrointestinal neoplasia. The management of bacterial overgrowth and protein-losing enteropathies is discussed later in this chapter.

Bile acid malabsorption can respond favorably to binding and inactivating compounds. Cholestyramine is a resin-binding agent used to treat diarrhea caused by bile acid excess in the colon. Aluminum hydroxide is also effective in binding bile acids[54] as are various types of fiber such as that from plantago seed, and some vegetables such as celery, corn, lettuce, potatoes, and string beans. Digestion of vegetables by colonic bacteria, however, releases bound bile acids, permitting them to stimulate secretion. The effectiveness for the different types of fiber for the binding of bile acids varies considerably.

BACTERIAL OVERGROWTH OF THE SMALL INTESTINE[55-57]

Clinical Synopsis

Diagnostic features

* Intermittent "small bowel" type diarrhea with or without weight loss
* Steatorrhea
* Normal trypsin-like immunoreactivity test
* Abnormal breath hydrogen test
* Abnormal serum vitamin B_{12}-folate test
* Greater than 10^5 bacteria per ml of duodenal fluid

Standard treatment

* Correct primary cause if apparent
* Tetracyclines 20 mg/kg q 8 hr for repeated 10-14 day courses

Follow up

* Repeated antibiotic therapy during clinical exacerbations

Introduction

The incidence in dogs and cats of bacterial overgrowth of the small intestine is unknown. German Shepherds may be predisposed, an association perhaps related to the relatively low IgA concentration in this breed.[58] Small intestinal bacterial overgrowth has a wide variety of causes that result in a self-perpetuating syndrome of considerable pathophysiologic complexity. Overgrowth of the intestine has profound effects on the intestinal function. Many bacteria such as some *E. coli* and *Clostridia* synthesize and secrete enterotoxins that stimulate the secretion of intestinal fluid. Large numbers of many other bacteria cause morphological and functional changes in the mucosa that result in malassimilation. Malassimilation in turn provides more nutrients for continued bacterial growth. Bacterial overgrowth results in deconjugation of bile acids and the hydroxylation of dietary fatty acids, producing metabolites that are toxic to epithelial cells and stimulate secretion of intestinal fluid. Overgrowth of the microflora also results in lipid malabsorption because of deconjugation of bile acids and acceleration of pancreatic enzyme degradation. Long-chain fatty acids are unabsorbed and stimulate intestinal secretion.

Etiology

Bacterial overgrowth has many causes but the most important pathomechanisms are loss of normal intestinal motility, mechanical gastrointestinal obstruction, malassimilation, and depressed local immunity. Malassimilation causes bacterial overgrowth as a secondary event by providing for abundant bacterial growth with unabsorbed nutrients. Malnutrition also results in increased bacterial numbers in the small intestine. Intestinal stasis can be produced by partial constriction of the small or large intestine due to carcinomas, leiomyomas, inflammatory processes, or foreign bodies. Intestinal stasis is also caused by reductions in normal intestinal motility such as seen in adynamic ileus. Overgrowth of intestinal bacterial is predictable in the involved segments. Motility abnormalities in turn have many causes. Derangements in the normal bacterial population of the small intestine may also result from disordered peristalsis, gastric hypoacidity, compositional changes in the bacterial flora, deficient bile secretion, and defects in the secretory immune system.

Pathophysiology

When loops of small intestine retain their contents and become "stagnant," the numbers and kinds of bacteria increase, approaching the population and composition found in the colon or oral cavity.[59] Thus, where there are normally fewer than 10^5 organisms per gram of contents, 10^8 to 10^{10} organisms per gram are found. The numbers of anaerobes and coliforms are normally very low. During stasis, anaerobic numbers increase and colonic anaerobes such as *Bacteroides* appear. The numbers of *Lactobacilli, Enterobacter, coliforms*, and *Clostridia* also increase with Clostridia becoming the most common anaerobe. These bacteria produce morphological and functional mucosal changes that affect nutrition.

Morphologic Changes.[60] Bacterial overgrowth often does not cause any morphologic changes recognizable by light microscopy in the mucosa. Mucosal changes that are occasionally seen include hypertrophy of the crypt epithelium and atrophy with blunting of the villi.[61] These changes may be caused by immune-mediated mechanisms that are dependent on T lymphocytes. Bacterial endotoxins and possibly enterotoxins contribute to the changes.[62] It is questionable whether toxins contribute to the mucosal changes in chronic disease because immunity against toxins can quickly develop. It is more likely that lymphokines and activated cells of the immune response are responsible for the morphological changes seen in chronic bacterial overgrowth. Inflammatory changes, including lymphocytic-plasmacytic or neutrophil infiltration are sometimes evident in the lamina propria. The light microscopy changes are occasionally patchy.[57] Ultrastructural changes are invariably present even in cases where little or no light-microscope changes are evident.[63]

Biochemical Changes. Bacterial overgrowth causes abnormalities in the levels of brush border enzymes. The nature of the brush border abnormalities are dependent on the number and type of bacteria predominating in the colonized bowel with anaerobic bacteria producing a relatively more pronounced biochemical lesion than aerobic bacteria.[59] The activities of the disaccharidases maltase, sucrase, and lactase, or the peptidase leucyl-2-naphthylamidase were little affected in a series of 10

German Shepherds with predominantly aerobic bacterial overgrowth. The activity of intestinal gamma-glutamyltransferase activity was increased and that of alkaline phosphatase was reduced. Indirect evidence for enhanced lysosomal fragility and mitochondrial disruption was also detected.[64] Anaerobic overgrowth is associated with a marked reduction in brush border density, indicative of damage to the glycocalyx, but no change in brush border enzyme activities.[59]

The mechanisms by which bacterial overgrowth cause these biochemical abnormalities are undetermined, but they may be mediated by bacterial cytotoxins, deconjugated bile acids, or hydroxylated fatty acids. Additional biochemical or functional abnormalities that have been reported include deficiencies in the uptake of carbohydrates and amino acids, enteric blood loss, protein-losing enteropathy, and decreased enterokinase concentration.[56,57] All of the biochemical lesions reported to date are potentially reversible. The significance of these biochemical abnormalities remains to be established.[64]

Effects of Deconjugated Bile Acids on Small Intestinal Structure and Function.[65,66] Bile acids inhibit the growth of anaerobes in the normal ileum, but are not present at high enough levels to prevent bacterial overgrowth when suitable luminal conditions such as carbohydrate malabsorption occur.[67] *Bacteroides, Clostridia, Lactobacilli*, and cocci, but not coliforms, are able to deconjugate bile acids by hydrolyzing the glycine and taurine conjugates of cholic, chenodeoxycholic, and deoxycholic acids. Conjugation of bile acids to one of the two amino acids produces a molecule that is ionized, water soluble, and able to form micelles with monoglycerides and fatty acids. Since they are not easily absorbed, they remain in the intestines until they reach the ileum, where absorption takes place. Deconjugation to remove taurine or glycine renders bile acid molecules insoluble in water and soluble in lipids. Then they are not able to remain in solution and form micelles, and, being lipid-soluble, they can cross cell membranes at any site in the small intestine. Instead of absorption being delayed until they reach the ileum, deconjugated bile acids are absorbed at any site in the small intestine. This results in an increase in the amount of unconjugated bile acids in the plasma, where their levels can be ten times normal. The plasma levels of conjugated forms are normal, but the taurine conjugates are drastically reduced in comparison with the glycine forms. The deficiency of conjugated bile acids results in steatorrhea. The problem is reversed by using antibiotics to correct the overgrowth or by feeding conjugated bile acids.[68]

Dehydroxylation of bile acids by intestinal bacteria involves the removal of a hydroxyl group from the steroid nucleus.[66] By this means cholic acid, a trihydroxy bile acid, is converted to the dihydroxy bile acid deoxycholic acid. The latter form, being more lipid-soluble, enters the mucosal cell with greater ease, stimulating the secretion of fluid.

As discussed above, deconjugated bile acids such as deoxycholate have pronounced influences on fluid and electrolyte absorption in the intestine, particularly the colon. This effect appears to be mediated by all bile acids, but the nonpolar compounds are more effective since they enter the cells more readily. Consequently, the effect produced is greatest with deconjugated bile acids and with the dihydroxy bile acids. In the small intestine, deconjugated bile acids have some additional effects including the inhibition of absorption of monosaccharides,[69] and interference with the activity of all brush border enzymes and some mucosal cell lysosomal enzymes.[70] Thus, the effects of excess unconjugated bile acids extend to the absorption of all nutrients.

Functional Changes Caused by Lipids.[16] Bacterial overgrowth affects lipid assimilation. Bacteria produce many short-chain fatty acids from their action on different dietary constituents.[71] The products include acetic, propionic, and butyric acids. They are absorbed very rapidly in the small intestine and, in fact, accelerate the absorption of fluid. Thus they do not cause diarrhea. Medium- and long-chain fatty acids produced from the hydrolysis of triglycerides inhibit the absorption of fluid in both the small and large intestine. The length of the fatty acid chain determines the potential for stimulating fluid accumulation. Fatty acids with a chain length greater than seven carbons have an inhibitory effect on absorption that increases with increasing chain length.[72] Hexanoic acid, which contains six carbons, does not inhibit absorption unless present at high concentrations. Fatty acids are hydroxylated by intestinal bacteria, producing hydroxy fatty acids. Some of these, such as hydroxystearic acid and ricinoleic (12-hydroxyoleic) acid, are potent inhibitors of absorption and stimulators of fluid secretion. Any long-chain fatty acid has similar effects on intestinal fluid movement, with the effects augmented by hydroxylation. An unsaturated double bond is not necessary for the effects. There is also no requirement for an intact carboxyl group, since conjugation with taurine does not change the effects of fatty acids on fluid transport. It has been suggested that fatty acids produce the effect by activation of adenylate cyclase, as has been reported for the mechanism of action of the bacterial enterotoxins to produce secretion. However, the changes caused by fatty acids do not appear to be identical with those produced by enterotoxins. Fatty acids alter the absorption of glucose, xylose, bile acids, L-leucine, L-lysine, and folic acid, and they increase the mucosal permeability to inulin.[1]

Morphologic studies reveal that fatty acids cause structural changes that are characterized by villus shortening and damage, increased cell exfoliation, and brush border damage.[73] The changes are suggested to be due to the detergent properties of the fatty acids, which being amphophilic substances are able to solubilize components of the cell membrane and ultimately destroy the brush border of the intestinal absorptive cells.[73] Thus, fatty acids that are not absorbed cause changes at any level of the intestinal tract. Their effects are related to the concentration of fatty acids in the lumen, and when overgrowth of bacteria interferes with fat absorption there is increased conversion of fatty acids to their hydroxylated varieties, which have more potent effects on fluid transport.

Castor oil has been used as a safe and effective cathartic for centuries. The active ingredient is ricinoleic acid, which is an 18-carbon hydroxylated and monounsaturated fatty acid. It effectively inhibits fluid absorption and stimulates secretion. Castor oil also increases basic electrical rhythm, augmenting propulsion of contents. It has been questioned whether it causes catharsis by that means, since ricinoleic acid and its nonhydroxylated form, oleic acid, inhibit small-intestinal motor activity in the dog for as long as 45 minutes.[74] In vitro studies also show that ricinoleic acid, in addition to a number of detergents, inhibits motility in intestinal smooth muscle.[75] It is suggested that this effect in dogs, however, is indirect, being mediated by the release of cholecystokinin. For a cathartic, which stimulates fluid secretion, to be maximally effective it is necessary that motor function of the intestinal tract be reduced so that there is no resistance to the movement of fluid. Other surfactants have the same effects on the mucosal cell to secrete fluid and to inhibit smooth-muscle motility. They include dioctyl sodium sulfosuccinate (DSS), sodium dodecyl (lauryl) sulfate, polysorbate 80, sodium deoxycholate, and chenodeoxycholate.[75] Their effects are due also to their detergent effect on cell membranes.

Deconjugated bile acids and unabsorbed fatty acids frequently act synergistically to stimulate intestinal secretion of fluid. The magnitude of their single or combined effects is related to their concentrations in intestinal contents. Their effects in the small intestine are influenced also by levels of conjugated bile acids. The toxic effects of deoxycholate and oleic acid are eliminated by taurocholate, so that intestinal secretion stimulated by the former is converted to absorption when the latter is added to an intestine containing deoxycholate and oleic acid.[76]

Fatty acids should be regarded as mediators of diarrhea in both maldigestion and malabsorption. Triglycerides that enter the colon intact in animals with pancreatic enzyme and bile acid deficiency are hydrolyzed by bacterial lipases in the colon. This produces fatty acids, which act as mediators of diarrhea.

Effect of Bacterial Overgrowth on Absorption of Other Nutrients

Carbohydrate Assimilation. Bacteria metabolize carbohydrate in the small intestine to form small intermediates that are rapidly absorbed. As a result caloric deficiency or diarrhea does not result from the influence of small intestinal bacteria on carbohydrate. This is in contrast to maldigestion and malabsorption of oligosaccharides due to a brush-border enzyme deficiency, in which abnormal amounts of sugars are delivered to the colon and diarrhea is to a large degree the result of an increased volume of contents entering the colon from the small bowel.[45]

Protein Assimilation. Protein metabolism and nitrogen balance may be profoundly affected by bacterial overgrowth. Protein is relatively low in most diets and increased numbers of bacteria metabolizing protein create a deficiency of nitrogen available for absorption. The nitrogen content of the feces is increased with overgrowth, but it is not known to what extent that is due to decreased absorption of peptides and amino acids and to what degree abnormal loss of plasma proteins contributes to the loss. Unabsorbed peptides and amino acids are metabolized by intestinal bacteria. Many are deaminated, and the ammonia formed is absorbed and converted to urea, so that this nitrogen is lost to the animal. The effects of bacterial overgrowth on nitrogen balance can be severe enough to produce wasting and hypoproteinemia.

Unabsorbed tryptophan is converted by bacteria to form a decarboxylated product, tryptamine. This is a biogenic amine that has many biological effects, but it is metabolized by the intestinal mucosal to indole-3 acetic acid, which is absorbed and excreted in the urine. Tryptophan can be metabolized also by tryptophanase-producing bacteria, especially coliforms, forming indole, which is converted to indican and excreted in the urine.[77] It has been suggested that the level of indican in the urine reflects the number of bacteria in the small intestine and can therefore be used to diagnose such entities as "enterotoxemia." It has been shown, however, that there is no correlation between the amount of indican excreted in the urine and the number of bacteria in the small intestine.[78] There is some correlation between urinary indican levels and plasma protein loss into the intestines, but urine indican levels are not an accurate technique for the evaluation of malassimilation, intestinal bacterial numbers, or enterotoxemia.

Vitamin Assimilation. Intestinal bacteria use dietary vitamins for their growth and survival. The organisms compete with the animal for vitamin B_{12}. Considerable vitamin B_{12} is stored in the liver, and months are required for depletion. Folate is produced and absorbed in excessive amounts with bacterial overgrowth. Changes in the serum levels of these vitamins are used as a diagnostic test for bacterial overgrowth

Clinical Findings & Diagnosis of Bacterial Overgrowth

Bacterial overgrowth in dogs results in chronic intermittent diarrhea, with or without weight loss. Additional clinical signs are similar to those of malassimilation or can reflect the primary cause of the bacterial overgrowth. For instance, vomiting is to be expected in patients with gastrointestinal obstruction. Steatorrhea is common but tests for maldigestion are usually normal. Bacterial overgrowth in people is occasionally asymptomatic.[57] Procedures of value in the diagnosis of bacterial overgrowth are described in Chapters 5 & 6.

A diagnosis of bacterial overgrowth of the small intestine cannot be made by fecal culture because bacteria cultured from the feces, even in heavy growth do not represent bacterial kinds and numbers in the small bowel. A definitive diagnosis of bacterial overgrowth can, however, be made by quantitative anaerobic and aerobic culture of duodenal fluid aspirated by endoscopy or at surgery. Affected dogs have greater than 10^5 colony forming units per ml of duodenal fluid.[79] The breath hydrogen test provides firm supportive evidence for bacterial overgrowth as does a positive serum vitamin B_{12}/folate test. In our hands, the serum vitamin B_{12}/folate test appears reasonably specific but poorly sensitive. Treatment trials are fraught with difficulty for the diagnosis of bacterial overgrowth, and should be avoided whenever possible (see Chapter 5 & 6).

Management of Bacterial Overgrowth

Successful long term management of bacterial overgrowth is dependent on correction of the primary cause. For instance, surgical resection of mechanical obstructions or administration of pancreatic enzyme replacements may be required. Antibiotic administration in animals with a treatable primary cause for their bacterial overgrowth, such as exocrine pancreatic insufficiency, is best restricted to courses as short as 5 days. Such short courses are aimed at the initial control of bacterial levels, and rely on treatment of the primary cause to maintain low bacterial numbers thereafter. If a cause cannot be determined, long term administration of antibiotics is often required. The choice of the antibiotic is empirical and the most effective administration schedules remain to be defined. Many bacterial species with a variety of antibiotic sensitivities are often present, and the interactions between these species are undetermined. Antibiotics that have proven useful include tetracyclines, metronidazole, chloramphenicol, ampicillin, and tylosin. Tetracyclines used at 20 mg/ kg q 8 hr for repeated 10-14 day courses during clinical exacerbations of the disease is a reasonable initial therapeutic choice.[57]

Supportive therapy for the patient with bacterial overgrowth is the same as that for patients with malassimilation. Careful nutritional support is of prime importance and vitamin supplementation, in particular vitamin B_{12}, is indicated. The prognosis is dependent on the cause of the condition and the severity of the patient's clinical condition. The prognosis for idiopathic bacterial overgrowth is guarded.

PROTEIN-LOSING ENTEROPATHY[80-83]

The mucosa of the small and large intestines forms a semipermeable barrier that controls the transmucosal movement of fluid and electrolytes and restricts that of larger molecules, whether in the intestinal lumen or on the capillary side of the cell.

The intestinal mucosa is a tenuous barrier to the loss of plasma proteins from the body.[84] Plasma proteins normally turn over with half-lives that vary from 8 to 10 days. Albumin is synthesized by the liver, and this function accounts for about 25% of all protein the liver produces. The liver is able to double the rate of synthesis if it is stimulated by excessive losses and if the required nutrients are provided. The most important site of alubmin degradation is unknown. Degradation by the liver and intestine each accounts for about 10% of the total.[85] The rate of catabolism is constant at other sites unless renal or intestinal losses are accelerated, causing overall catabolism to decrease. Disease makes the intestine and the kidneys important sites of protein loss.

Hypoproteinemia involving all but the immunoglobulins can reflect decreased synthesis as a result of severe malnutrition, hepatic disease, and some chronic diseases. The immunoglobulins appear to be found in the beta-globulins as well as the gamma-globulins, making it sometimes difficult to evaluate the electrophoretic pattern of plasma proteins in deciding whether the most likely problem is decreased synthesis. That problem does not develop with acute disease processes. The half-life of plasma proteins in small animals is probably greater than 10 days, and protein synthesis would have to nearly cease for hypoproteinemia to become significant in that length of time.

Protein loss into the bowel is a common and potentially serious complication of several gastrointestinal diseases of widely disparate cause. The most common protein-losing enteropathies are shown in Table 17-4. In most of these diseases protein loss into the bowel is but one of the pathophysiologic processes operative in the disease. The protein loss is often accompanied by other pathophysiologic derangements such as the malassimilation of carbohydrate or fat, gastrointestinal inflammation, mucosal ulceration, or bacterial overgrowth. The term "protein-losing enteropathies" is clinically useful, because it refers to a restricted group of enteropathies with characteristic clinical-laboratory features, and similar nutritional obligations.

The unifying feature of these disorders is hypoproteinemia due to loss of plasma proteins into the bowel lumen. The source of the proteins is either the mucosal vasculature or the mucosal interstitial space. Normally, one-third to one-half of plasma proteins are found inside the vascular compartment, with the remainder in extravascular spaces. Capillaries in intestinal mucosa have large fenestrations that readily permit macromolecules to move into the interstitial space. In addition, the gel in the interstitial space is porous enough to accommodate large amounts of plasma proteins. Alteration of the mucosal epithelial barrier by disease results in loss of plasma proteins into the intestinal lumen. When plasma proteins are lost into the intestinal tract, both albumin and globulins are lost at an equal rate. The resultant hypoalbuminemia and hypoglobulinemia (panhypoproteinemia) helps differentiate protein-losing enteropathies from the hypoproteinemia of glomerular and hepatic disease which on most occasions is restricted to a hypoalbuminemia.

Causes of Protein-Losing Enteropathy

Plasma proteins are lost into the lumen of the intestine during acute inflammatory processes caused by infections and parasites. Recovery is usually rapid, so that losses cease and hypoproteinemia does not become apparent. The most important protein-losing gastroenteropathies are associated with

Table 17-4. Causes of Protein-Losing Gastroenteropathies

- Acute inflammatory diseases
  - Acute infections
  - Toxins
  - Parasites
  - Mechanical irritation (foreign body)
  - Acute gastrointestinal ulceration
- Chronic inflammatory diseases
  - Chronic gastric ulceration
  - Chronic gastritis
  - Chronic inflammatory bowel diseases
    - Small intestine enteritis
    - Large intestine colitis
- Immune-mediated diseases
  - Gluten-induced enteropathy
  - Food allergies
  - Eosinophilic gastroenteritis
- Circulatory diseases
  - Lymphatic disease
    - Lymphangiectasia
    - Neoplastic obstruction
    - Obstruction by granulomatous lesions
  - Congestive heart failure
- Intestinal-motility disorders, bacterial overgrowth
  - Neoplasms
    - Gastric carcinomas, ulceration
    - Small-intestinal carcinomas, stricture formation
- Diseases of other systems
  - Systemic lupus erythematosus

chronic inflammatory diseases and circulatory diseases such as lymphangiectasia (Table 17-4). The circulatory diseases usually cause more severe hypoproteinemia than chronic inflammatory diseases.

Pathophysiology of Protein-Losing Enteropathy

Inflammatory Disease. Protein can be lost into the intestines without evidence of any morphological damage to the mucosa. Permeability is increased in the tight junctions, and the protein loss appears to be by that route.[86] The pathogenesis of the increased permeability is not well understood. Protein-losing gastroenteropathy can be produced in experimental animals by X-irradiation or intraperitoneal injection of 5-fluorouracil. Increases in the fibrinolytic activity of intestinal tissue are found in experimental and naturally occurring protein-losing gastroenteropathies.[87] Protein loss is reduced in both situations by an antiplasmin agent, trans-4-aminomethyl cyclohexane carboxylic acid, suggesting that fibrinolytic activity of the enzyme plasmin plays an important role in enhancing mucosal permeability to protein movement.

In addition to the loss of protein through a leaky barrier in chronic inflammatory disease, an increased degradation of plasma protein is likely by inflammatory cells in the lamina propria and by proteases within epithelial cells. When plasma proteins are lost by protein-losing gastroenteropathy due to inflammation, there are almost invariably clinical signs of gastrointestinal disease that lead one to seek the problem in the alimentary tract. Occult hypoproteinemia is a more frequent problem when the protein-losing gastroenteropathy is caused by a circulatory problem.

Lymphangiectasia

Clinical Synopsis

Diagnostic features

* Mild "small bowel" type diarrhea in many but not all cases
* Panhypoproteinemia and lymphopenia
* Hypocholesterolemia and hypocalcemia
* Steatorrhea
* Normal digestion tests
* Variable absorption tests

Standard treatment

* Low fat - high calorie controlled diet
* MCT oil 1-2 ml/kg per day
* Prednisone 1-2 mg/kg q 12 h PO for 1-2 weeks; tapered to alternate day therapy over several months as described for lymphocytic-plasmacytic enteritis

Follow up

* Life-long dietary therapy
* Monitor body weight and serum albumin
* Adjust diet accordingly

Lymphangiectasia.[81-83] Intestinal lymphangiectasia is an idiopathic abnormality of the lymphatics that results in protein loss into the bowel as a result of lymphatic hypertension.[81] It is characterized by a ballooning dilation of the lacteals in the villi. The disorder is a prominent feature of the Lundehund enteropathy descibed in the inflammatory bowel disease chapter, and dilated lacteals are also occasionally seen in association with lymphocytic-plasmacytic enteritis of other breeds.

Lymphangiectasia may be present at birth or it may be acquired later in life. In congenital lymphangiectasia, total lymph flow is reduced because the numbers of lymphatic vessels are insufficient to remove interstitial fluid. The stasis that appears in adult animals is usually caused by obstructive lesions developing throughout the lymphatics. A not uncommon cause of the obstruction is granulomatous lesions within and around the lymphatics.[88,89] Occasionally lipogranulomas will appear in other organs such as the liver.[90] It has been suggested that acquired lymphangiectasia develops in dogs with a congenitally compromised lymphatic system.[91] It is hypothesized that intermittent postprandial lymphatic hypertension causes lipids to diffuse from lymph vessels into the interstitium. Lipids are foreign and irritating to interstitial structures. Macrophages accumulate to phagocytize and remove the lipids and eventually form granulomas. Clinical signs of lymphangiectasia appear when lymph flow is reduced further by the encroaching granulomas. Lymphangiectasia in association with chylothorax has been occasionally seen at the VMTH and has been reported by others.[92] This association raises the likelihood of a more widespread lymphatic defect. Lymphatic stasis can also arise from venous hypertension at the site where lymphatics enter the venous circulation. Lymphangiectasia can be produced experimentally by complete occlusion of all mesenteric lymphatics, but experimental obstruction of the thoracic duct failed to produce the disease.[93,94] Limited investigations for infectious agents have been unsuccessful.[89]

Lymphatic stasis results in lymphatic hypertension, which causes interstitial fluid to leak out into the abdominal cavity and into the lumen of the intestine. The protein-rich fluid passes into the intestine by a paracellular route through widened tight junctions.[95] When protein losses are faster than hepatic synthesis, hypoproteinemia develops. The hypoproteinemia of lymphangiectasia is caused by a loss of all plasma proteins. Electrophoretic separation of plasma proteins cannot be used to differentiate lymphangiectasia from inflammatory causes of protein loss. Lymphangiectasia can on occasion be differentiated from other causes of protein-losing problems on the basis of numbers of lymphocytes in the hemogram. Lymphatic obstruction causes a loss of lymphocytes into the intestine. Lymphocytes leave the intestine by way of the lymphatics and are transformed into lymphoblasts, which, after passing through lymph nodes and the circulation return to the lamina propria of the intestine, where they are transformed into plasma cells. Lymphangiectasia prevents the lymphocytes from leaving their site in the intestine, and they are lost into the lumen. Thus, the animal with lymphangiectasia has a lymphopenia in addition to the hypoproteinemia. The loss of a large number of long-living lymphocytes leaves the animal with a deficiency in the ability to mount a cellularly based immune response. The lymphocyte numbers represent one criterion that can be used to help differentiate lymphangiectasia from other causes of protein-losing gastroenteropathy. Lymphopenia is a common hematological finding in "stressed" animals, however, and so the detection of lymphopenia should only be considered suggestive of lymphang-

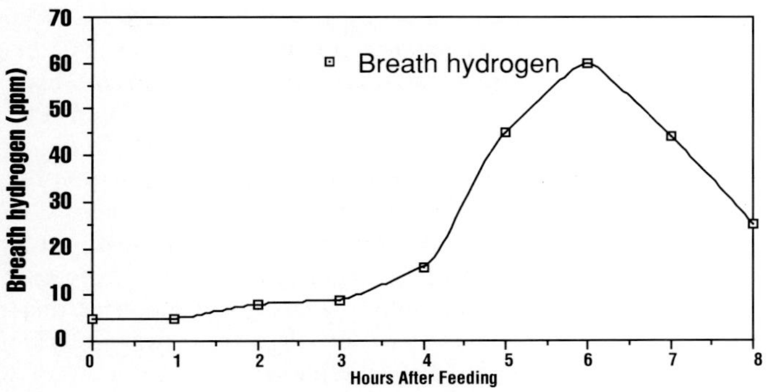

Figure 17-20. Graph showing breath hydrogen results in a dog with lymphangiectasia.

iectasia if the other features of the "stress leukogram", such as eosinopenia and neutrophilia, are absent.

Clinical Findings in Protein-Losing Enteropathy

The clinical findings vary with the cause and severity of the protein loss. Diarrhea is a consistent finding except with lymphangiectasia. Weight loss is usually present and is often marked. When hypoalbuminemia becomes profound, pleural fluid, ascites and dependent edema appear. The dependent edema is usually bilaterally symmetrical but occasionally local venous hypertension created by prolonged recumbency on one or other limb will create a non-symmetrical collection of fluid.

Laboratory Findings & Diagnosis of Protein-Losing Enteropathy[80,82,96]

The diagnosis of protein-losing enteropathy usually begins with a series of diagnostic tests to rule out diseases of the kidney and liver that may result in hypoalbuminemia, and is then continued with procedures aimed at discerning potential causes of protein loss from the bowel. Protein-losing enteropathy can only be definitively confirmed by identifying excess excretion of a radio-labeled protein from the bowel.

In protein-losing enteropathy, hemograms and blood chemistries will usually identify both hypoalbuminemia and hypoglobulinemia. Edema and ascites are consistently present when albumin concentration decreases to 1.0 g/dl, and may occur at higher albumin values if there is concomitant capillary hypertension from such causes as congestive heart disease. Ascitic fluid from congestive heart disease has a relatively high protein content. Ascites can also develop because of lymphatic hypertension, resulting in the accumulation of an ultrafiltrate of lymphatic or interstitial fluid. The intestinal serosa and muscle layers effectively exclude movement of protein molecules from the interstitial space so the ascitic fluid is virtually free of protein. The fluid does contain fats, however; they are solubilized in micelles so the fluid appears clear and colorless, like water. Staining the fluid sediment with Sudan stain reveals the fat. A urinalysis should be performed to rule out glomerular protein loss. Proteinuria can be confirmed by a protein-creatinine ratio. Blood chemistries are used to screen for hepatic disease as the cause of hypoproteinemia, and a liver function test should be considered to rule out hepatic insufficiency. Hypocalcemia is sometimes present. This finding is primarily a reflection of decreased serum albumin but calcium absorption is also reduced because excess unabsorbed free fatty acids bind dietary calcium to form insoluble salts. Vitamin D malabsorption may also play a role in the hypocalcemia, but the intestinal absorption of calcium has been reported to be normal in humans with lymphangiectasia.[97] Hypocholesterolemia is common in dogs with lymphangiectasia, and presumably results from the fat malabsorption.[90]

Multiple fecal examinations are conducted to rule out parasite infestation. If hookworm or whipworm infestation is present, this is assumed to be the cause of protein-losing enteropathy until failure to respond to anthelmintic therapy suggests otherwise. Increased fecal fat content is a consistent feature of lymphangiectasia, since the transport of chylomicrons through lymphatics is impaired, and is also seen in many other protein-losing enteropathies.

Digestion tests are usually normal; pancreatic function testing with BT-PABA is normal. In lymphangiectasia xylose absorption is also often normal. Breath hydrogen testing usually shows carbohydrate malassimilation (Figure 17-20). Gastrointestinal excretion of radio-labeled tracers can be used to identify the gastrointestinal tract as the site of plasma protein loss, but reveal little about cause. Such tests are primarily indicated to confirm concomitant bowel protein loss in hypoalbuminemic patients which have evidence of hepatic or renal disease of apparent insufficient severity to explain the full extent of the hypoalbuminemia. These tests are discussed in Chapter 6.

Radiographic studies usually add little information useful for assessing protein-losing enteropathy, but occasionally gastrointestinal masses or mucosal abnormalities may be tentatively identified. If ascites is present without a marked hypoalbuminemia, radiographic evaluation for cardiovascular disease is indicated.

Endoscopy and endoscopic biopsy are the diagnostic techniques of choice for the differential diagnosis of protein-losing enteropathy. With lymphaniectasia, the mucosa may appear more granular, and on occasion, circular patches of white, lipid-filled dilated villi may be apparent. Blind biopsy of the colon or stomach using suction capsules will sometimes reveal the pathologic process. Biopsy of the small intestine is required to definitively diagnose lymphangiectasia, however. Celiotomy will also provide diagnostic biopsies but the risk of dehiscence of full thickness biopsies in debilitated hypoalbuminemic animals is high. During celiotomy, the major intestinal lymphatics of patients with lymphangiectasia will often appear dilated and prominent.

The histologic changes of lymphangiectasia are characteristic. Dilatation of the lymphatics in the mucosa and submucosa are seen (Figure 17-21 and 17-22). The villi enlarge, and structures of the lamina propria are displaced by the dilated lymphatics. Lipids are not transported from the villi, and the retained chylomicrons are phagocytized by macrophages, giving them a foamy appearance. Granulomas can usually be found with acquired lymphangiectasia. Lymphedema is found only if the mucosa is in the absorptive state.[98] Mild diffuse accumulations of plasma cells and lymphocytes are also often apparent.

Management of Protein-Losing Enteropathy

When possible, the management of protein-losing enter-

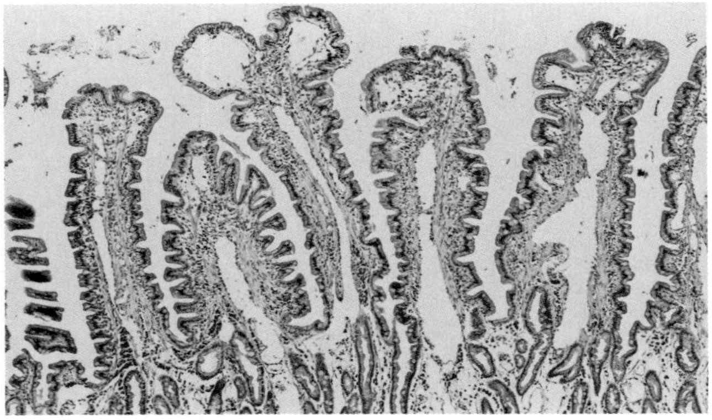

Figure 17-21. Lymphangiectasia. Marked dilation of lymphatics in lamina propria of villi and crypt. From dog with hypoproteinemia and diarrhea.

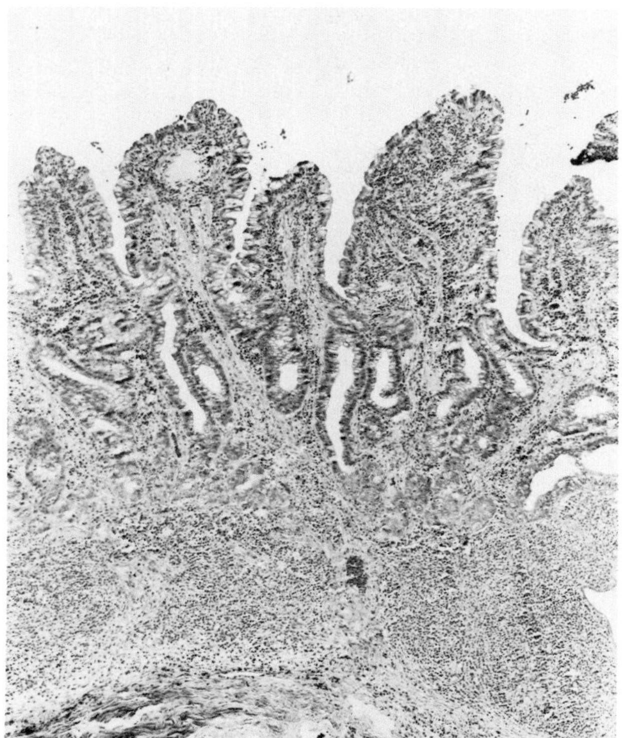

Figure 17-22. Lymphangiectasia with granulomatous lymphangitis. Marked distension of lymph vessels by proteinaceous material was evident grossly. Granulomas found in and around intestinal lymphatics.

opathy is directed at the primary cause of the protein loss. On some occasions, the cause will not be apparent, or will be without specific treatment such as in lymphangiectasia. In all cases of protein-losing enteropathy, intensive nutritional support is of prime importance.

Dietary Management. Protein-losing problems involving the gut are best treated with a high energy-high protein-low fat controlled diet. The controlled diet should initially consist of a single source of carbohydrate and a single source of protein. The carbohydrate source should consist only of starch, excluding glutens. The best sources of carbohydrates are boiled rice and synthetically prepared oligosaccharides. The protein source should be highly digestible, contain minimal fat and, if a food intolerance or allergy is suspected, should be a protein to which the patient has not been exposed. Suitable proteins are boiled beef, poultry, or lamb, low fat cottage cheese, or a protein hydrolysate. Th diet should be supplemented with vitamins and minerals.

High fat diets are avoided in protein-losing enteropathies, whether the disease is due to lymphangiectasia or mucosal inflammatory processes. In the latter disorders, fats are avoided because of the difficulty with which they are assimilated. In lymphangiectasia, triglycerides made up of long-chain fatty acids must be excluded from the diet because the absorption of long-chain triglyceride is a major stimulus for intestinal lymph flow. After digestion and absorption, these lipids are reesterified and incorporated into chylomicrons that must be transported out of the gut through the intestinal lymphatics. Restriction of dietary long-chain triglyceride will reduce lymphatic hypertension and reduce gastrointestinal protein loss and lipid exudation into the perilymphatic tissues.

Lipid sources that contain triglycerides synthesized from medium-to short chain fatty acids do not require all the steps that are necessary for normal assimilation of triglycerides made up of long-chain fatty acids.[99] Medium-chain triglycerides are readily hydrolyzed by pancreatic lipase but a considerable proportion of medium-chain triglyceride is absorbed intact without prior lipolysis. The medium-chain fatty acids are not dependent on micellization for absorption. Once absorbed, they need not be reesterified, and instead rapidly enter the portal circulation, thus bypassing the lymphatics and minimizing lymphatic hypertension. MCT oil (Mead Johnson) is a commercially available source of medium-chain triglycerides that has been used successfully in treating some cases of protein-losing enteropathy in dogs. It has been used in dogs with chylous ascites associated with a profound hypoproteinemia. Its use is not limited to such problems. It can be used to treat steatorrhea of any cause. The usual dose is 1-2 ml/kg. MCT oil does not provide the essential fatty acids. They can be provided at a later time by incorporating a small amount of vegetable oil in the diet. In addition MCT oil is expensive, and palatibility can be a problem. An alternative to MCT oil is a powdered elemental diet mix (Portagen).

Low fat commercial reducing diets such as Hills r/d have been recommended for the management of lymphangiectaisa. In our opinion these diets are not suitable for use in this condition because protein-losing enteropathies are very energetically expensive diseases, and even with high energy supplements such as MCT oil, it becomes difficult to meet the animals energy requirements with diets that are purposefully calorie restricted and often of below average palatibility.

Medical Management. Drugs are used to correct precipitating causes of protein-losing enteropathies such as parasitism and inflammatory bowel disease. Corticosteroids have been the most widely used of these agents. Azathioprine, antiplasmin drugs, and atropine have been shown to reduce the amount of protein lost into the stomach in various experimental models. The value of these drugs in clinical cases has not been explored.

The management of acquired lymphangiectasia can be occasionally assisted by use of immunosuppressive agents such as corticosteroids, azathioprine, and cyclophosphamide, singly or in combination. These drugs may reduce the perilymphatic granulomatous response. Response to these drugs is often poor, however.

Surgical Management. Surgery corrects protein-losing gastroenteropathy when a localized chronic inflammatory, ulcerative, or neoplastic lesion can be successfully removed from the stomach or the intestinal tract.

Prognosis and Complications

The prognosis for protein-losing enteropathies of inflammatory origin is guarded. Many patients with severe inflammatory bowel disease will eventually respond, but the therapy is often protracted and fraught with complications. Lymphangiectasia also carries a guarded prognosis. Response to therapy is unpredictable, and is dependent to a large extent on the severity of the disease process at presentation. Patients that are inappetant and severely malnourished at presentation should receive a poor prognosis.

Complications of these disorders are frequent, and include pleural and abdominal effusions, wound dehiscence, pulmonary thromboembolism, lung lobe torsions, and portal vein thrombosis.

REFERENCES

1. Wilson, F.A. and Dietschy, J.M.: The differential diagnostic approach to clinical problems of malabsorption. Gastroenterology 61:911-931, 1971.
2. Wormsley, K.G. and Goldberg, D.M.: The interrelationships of the pancreatic enzymes. Gut 13:398-412, 1972.
3. Sateri, H.: Investigations on the exocrine pancreatic function in dogs suffering from chronic exocrine pancreatic insufficiency. Acta. Vet. Scand. Suppl. 53:1-86, 1975.
4. Wormsly, K.G.: Pancreatic Function Tests. Clinics in Gastroenterology 1:27-51, 1972.
5. Garvey, M.S. and Zawie, D.A.: Feline pancreatic disease. Vet. Clin. N. Am. 14:1231-1246, 1984.
6. Batt, R.M. and Mann, L.C.: Specificity of the BT-PABA test for the diagnosis of exocrine pancreatic insufficiency in the dog. Vet. Rec. 108:303-307, 1981.
7. Lebenthal, E., Antonowicz, I. and Schwachman, H.: Enterokinase and trypsin activities in pancreatic insufficiency and diseases of the small intestine. Gastroenterology 70:508-512, 1976.
8. Ovesen, L., Bendtsen, F., Tage-Jensen, U., Pedersen, N.T., Gram, B.R., Rune, S.J.: Intraluminal pH in the stomach, duodenum, and proximal jejunum in normal subjects and patients with exocrine pancreatic insufficiency. Gastroenterology 90:958-962, 1986.
9. Williams, D.A., Batt, R.M. and McLean, L.: Bacterial overgrowth in the duodenum of dogs with exocrine pancreatic insufficiency. JAVMA 191:201-206, 1987.
10. Genell, S. and Gustafsson, B.E.: Impaired enteric degradation of pancreatic endopeptidases in antibiotic-treated rats. Scand. J. Gastroenterology 12:801-809, 1977.
11. Liebow, C. and Rothman, S.S.: Enteropancreatic circulation of digestive enzymes. Science 189:472-474, 1975.
12. Pidgeon, G. and Strombeck, D.R.: Evaluation of treatment for pancreatic exocrine insufficiency in dogs with ligated pancreatic ducts. AJVR 43:461-464, 1982.
13. Shimoda, S.S., Saunders, D.R., Schuffler, M.D. and Leinbach, G.L.: Electron microscopy of small intestinal mucosa in pancreatic insufficiency. Gastroenterology 67:19-27, 1974.
14. Meyer, J.H., Stevenson, E.A. and Watts, H.D.: The potential role of protein in the absorption of fat. Gastroenterology 70:232-239, 1976.
15. Saunders, D.R. and Sillery, J.: Another absorptive defect in pancreatic insufficiency: Unhydrolyzed lecithin can depress absorption of free fatty acid. Gastroenterology 70:934, 1976.
16. Binder, H.J.: Fecal fatty acids - mediators of diarrhea. Gastroenterology 65:847-850, 1973.
17. Binder, H.J. and Sandle, G.I.: Electrolyte absorption and secretion in the mammalian colon. In, Physiology of the Gastrointestinal Tract. 2nd edition. Edited by Johnson, L.R. 1389-1418, 1987.
18. Saunders, D.R., Hedges, J.R., Sillery, J., Esther, L., Matsumura, K. and Rubin, C.E.: Morphological and functional effects of bile salts on rat colon. Gastroenterology 68:1236-1245, 1975.
19. Dobbins, J.W. and Binder, J.J.: Effect of bile salts and fatty acids on the colonic absorption of oxalate. Gastroenterology 70:1096-1100, 1976.
20. Washabau, R.J., Strombeck, D.R., Buffington, C.A. and Harrold, D.: Use of pulmonary hydrogen gas excretion to detect carbohydrate malabsorption in dogs. JAVMA 189:674-679, 1986.
21. Mathews, D.M. and Adibi, S.A.: Peptide absorption. Gastroenterology 71:151-161, 1976.
22. Borgstrom, B.: Fat digestion and absorption. In, Biomembranes, Vol. 4B. Edited by D.H. Smyth. Plenum Press, London, 555-620, 1974.
23. DiMagno, E.P., Go, V.L.W., and Summerskill, W.H.J.: Relations between pancreatic enzyme outputs and malabsorption in severe pancreatic insufficiency. N. Eng. J. Med. 288:813-815, 1973.
24. Strombeck, D.R.: New method for evaluation of chymotrypsin deficiency in dogs. JAVMA 173:1319-1323, 1978.
25. Strombeck, D.R. and Harrold, D.: Evaluation of 60-minute blood p-aminobenzoic acid concentration in pancreatic function testing of dogs. JAVMA 180:419-421, 1982.
26. Stradley, R.P., Stern, R.J. and Heinhold, N.B.: A method for the simultaneous evaluation of exocrine pancreatic function and intestinal absorptive function in dogs. AJVR 40:1201-1205, 1979.
27. Williams, D.A. and Batt, R.M.: Sensitivity and specificity of radioimmunoassay of serum trypsin-like immunoreactivity for the diagnosis of canine exocrine pancreatic insufficiency. JAVMA 192:195-201, 1988.
28. Williams, D.A. and Reed, S.D.: Comparison of two methods for evaluation of pancreatic function in cats by assay of fecal proteolytic activity. ACVIM Proceedings, 1047, 1989.
29. Valerio, D., Whyte, E.H.A., Schlamm, H.T. and Blackburn, G.L.: Enzyme replacement therapy in pancreatic insufficiency. Scientific Exhibit, Digestive Diseases Week, Las Vegas, Nevada, May 20-26, 1978.
30. DiMagno, E.P., Go, V.L.W., Malagelada, J.R. and Moertel, C.G.: Fate of orally ingested pancreatic enzymes in severe pancreatic insufficiency. Gastroenterology 70:878, 1976.
31. Pilsworth, R.C. and Lehner, R.P.: Use of cimetidine as an aid to the control of pancreatic insufficiency in a German Shepherd bitch. Vet. Rec. 119:240, 1986.
32. Madrid, J.A., Salido, G.M., Martinez de Victoria, E. and Mataix, F.J.: Cimetidine and postprandial pancreatic exocrine secretion in dogs. Agents and Actions 17:145-149, 1985.
33. Regan, P.T., Malagelada, J.R., DiMagno, E.P., Glanzman, S.L. and Go, V.L.W.: Comparative effects of antacids,

cimetidine and enteric coating on the therapeutic response to oral enzymes in severe pancreatic insufficiency. New Eng. J. Med. 297:854-858, 1977.
34. DiMagno, E.P.: Controversies in the treatment of exocrine pancreatic insufficiency. Dig. Dis. Sci. 27:481-484, 1982.
35. Isaksson, G., Lundquist, I. and Ihse, I.: Effect of dietary fiber on pancreatic enzyme activity in vitro. Gastroenterology 82:918-924, 1982.
36. Stock-Damage, C., Bouchet, P., Dentinger, A., Aprahamian, M. and Grenier, J.F.: Effect of dietary fiber supplementation on the secretory function of the exocrine pancreas in the dog. Am. J. Clin. Nut. 38:843-848, 1983.
37. Hofmann, A.F.: Functions of bile in the alimentary canal. In, Handbook of Physiology, Sect. 6, Alimentary Canal, Edited by C.F. Code, American Physiological Society, Washington, DC, Vol. 5:2507-2533, 1968.
38. Hofmann, A.F.: Consequences of bile acid malabsorption. Mayo Clin. Proc. 48:656-659, 1973.
39. Hadorn, B., Hess, J., Troesch, V., Verhaage, W., Gotze, H. and Bender, S.W.: Role of bile acids in the activation of trypsinogen by enterokinase: Disturbance of trypsinogen activation in patients with intrahepatic biliary atresia. Gastroenterology 66:548-555, 1974.
40. Hill, F.W.G. and Kelly, D.F.: Naturally occurring intestinal malabsorption in the dog. Am. J. Dig. Dis. 19:649-665, 1974.
41. Hoffbrand, A.V. and Broitman, S.A.: Effect of chronic nutritional iron deficiency on the small intestinal disaccharidase activities of growing dogs. Proc. Soc. Exp. Biol. Med. 130:595-598, 1969.
42. Symons, L.E.A. and Fairbarin, D.: Pathology, absorption, transport and activity of digestive enzymes in rat jejunum parasitized by the nematode, *Nippostrongylus brasilie*nsis. Fed. Proc. 21:913-918, 1962.
43. Alpers, D.H. and Seetharam, B.: Pathophysiology of diseases involving intestinal brush border proteins. New Eng. J. Med. 296:1047-1050, 1977.
44. Klipstein, F.A. and Corcino, J.J.: Malabsorption of essential amino acids in tropical sprue. Gastroenterology 68:239-244, 1975.
45. Bond, J.H. and Levitt, M.D.: Quantitative measurement of lactose absorption. Gastroenterology 70:1058-1062, 1976.
46. Popovic, O.S., Kostic, K.M., Milovic, V.B., et al.: Primary bile acid malabsorption. Gastroenterology 92:1851-1858, 1987.
47. Kim, Y.S., Sprtiz, N., Blum, M., Terz, J. and Sherlock, P.: The role of altered bile acid metabolism in the steatorrhea of experimental blind loop. J. Clin. Invest. 45:956-962, 1966.
48. Gangl, A. and Ockner, R.K.: Intestinal metabolism of lipids and lipoproteins. Gastroenterology 68:167-186, 1975.
49. Brindley, D.N.: The intracellular phase of fat absorption. In, Biomembranes. Vol. 43, Edited by D.H. Smyth, Plenum Press, London 621-671, 1974.
50. Freind, S.C.E., Barr, S.C. and Embury, D.: Fucosidosis in an English Springer Spaniel presenting as malabsorption syndrome. Aust. Vet. J. 62:415-420, 1985.
51. Edwards, D.F. and Russell, R.G.: Probable vitamin K deficient bleeding in two cats with malabsorption syndrome secondary to lymphocytic-plasmacytic enteritis. J. Vet. Int. Med. 1:97-101, 1987.
52. Dobbins, J. and Binder, H.J.: The colon: The site of oxalate absorption in patients with hyperoxaluria and steatorrhea. Gastroenterology 70:879, 1976.
53. Earnest, D.L., Gancher, S. and Admirand, W.H.: Treatment of enteric hyperoxaluria with calcium and aluminum. Gastroenterology 70:881, 1976.
54. Clain, J., Malagelada, J.R., Chadwick, V. and Hofmann, A.F.: Bile acid binding properties of antacids: An in vitro study. Gastroenterology 80:871, 1976.
55. Dyer, N.H. and Hawkins, C.: Blind loop syndrome. In, Recent Advances in Gastroenterology, Edited by J. Badenoch and B.N. Brooke, Churchill and Livingston, London, 250-275, 1972.
56. Leib, M.S.: Stagnant loop syndrome in the dog and cat. Sem. Vet. Med. Surg. 2:257-265, 1987.
57. Banwell, J.G., Kistler, L.A., Giannella, R.A., Weber, F.L., Lieber, A. and Powell, D.E.: Small intestinal bacterial overgrowth syndrome. Gastroenterology 80:834-845, 1981.
58. Whitbread, T.J., Batt, R.M. and Garthwaite, G.: A relative deficiency of serum IgA in the German shepherd dog: a breed abnormality. Res. Vet. Sci. 37:350-352, 1984.
59. Batt, R.M. and Hall, E.J.: Chronic enteropathies in the dog. J. Sm. An. Pract. 30:3-12, 1989.
60. Abrams, G.D.: Microbial effects on mucosal structure and function. Am. J. Clin. Nutr. 30:1880-1886, 1977.
61. Toskes, P.O., Giannella, R.A., Jervis, H.R., Route, W.R. and Takeuchi, A.: Small intestinal mucosal injury in the experimental blind loop syndrome. Light- and electron-microscopic and histochemical studies. Gastroenterology 68:1193-1203, 1975.
62. Klipstein, F.A. and Schenk, E.A.: Enterotoxigenic intestinal bacteria in tropic sprue. II. Effect of the bacteria and their enterotoxins on intestinal structure. Gastroenterology 68:642-655, 1975.
63. Goldstein, F.: Bacterial populations of the gut in health and diseases: Clinical aspects. In, Gastroenterology, 3rd edition, Edited by H.L. Bockus, W.B. Saunders, Philadelphia, 152-173, 1976.
64. Batt, R.M.: New approaches to malabsorption in dogs. Comp. Contin. Ed. Pract. Vet. 8:783-794, 1986.
65. Donaldson, R.M.: Role of indigenous enteric bacteria in intestinal function and disease. In, Handbook of Physiology, Sect. 6, Alimentary Canal, Edited by C.F. Code, American Physiological Society, Washington, DC, Vol 5:2807-2837, 1968.
66. Drasar, B.S. and Hill, M.J.: Human intestinal flora. Academic Press, London, 1974.
67. Williams, R.C., Showalter, R. and Kern, F.: In vivo effect of bile salts and cholestyramine on intestinal anaerobic bacteria. Gastroenterology 69:483-491, 1975.
68. Milne, M.D.: Hereditary disorders of intestinal transport. In, Biomembranes, Vol. 4B, Edited by D.H. Smyth, Plenum Press, London 961-1013, 1974.
69. Gracey, M., Papadimitriou, J., Burke, V., Thomas, J. and Bower, G.: Effects on small intestinal function and structure induced by feeding a deconjugated bile salt. Gut 14:519-528, 1973.
70. Gracey, M., Houghton, M. and Thomas, J.: Deoxycholate depresses small intestinal enzyme activity. Gut 16:53-56, 1975.
71. Prizont, R., Whitehead, J.S. and Kim, Y.S.: Short chain fatty acids in rats with jejunal blind loops. I. Analysis of SCFA in small intestine, cecum, feces, and plasma. Gastroenterology 69:1254-1264, 1975.
72. Ammon, H.V. and Phillips, S.F.: Inhibition of ileal water absorption by intraluminal fatty acids. Influence of chain length, hydroxylation, and conjugation of fatty acids. J. Clin. Invest. 53:205-210, 1974.
73. Cline, W.S., Lorenzsonn, V., Benz, L., Bass, P. and Olsen, W.A.: The effects of sodium ricinoleate on small intestinal function and structure. J. Clin. Invest. 58:380-390, 1976.
74. Stewart, J.J. and Bass, P.: Effects of ricinoleic and oleic acids on the digestive contractile activity of the canine small and large bowel. Gastroenterology 70:371-376, 1976.
75. Gaginella, T.S, Stewart, J.J., Gullikson, G.W., Olsen, W.A. and Bass, P.: Inhibition of small intestinal mucosal and smooth muscle cell function by ricinoleic acid and other surfactants. Life Sciences 16:1595-1606, 1975.
76. Lamabadusuriya, S.P., Guiraldes, E. and Harries, J.T.: Influence of mixtures of taurocholate, fatty acids, and monolein on the toxic effects of deoxycholate in rat jejunum in vivo. Gastroenterology 69:463-469, 1975.
77. Fordtran, J.S., Scroggie, W.B. and Potter, D.E.: Colonic absorption of tryptophan metabolites in man. J. Lab. Clin. Med. 64:125-132, 1964.
78. Mayer, P.J. and Beeken, W.L.: The role of urinary indican as a predictor of bacterial colonization in the human jejunum. Am. J. Dig. Dis. 20:1003-1010, 1975.
79. Batt, R.M., Needham, J.R. and Carter, M.W.: Bacterial over-

growth associated with a naturally occurring enteropathy in the German Shepherd dog. Res. Vet. Sci. 35:42-46, 1983.

80. Finco, D.R., Duncan, J.R., Schall, W.D., Hooper, B.E., Chandler, F.W. and Keating, K.A.: Chronic enteric disease and hypoproteinemia in 9 dogs. JAVMA 163:262-271, 1973.

81. Mattheeuws, D., DeRick, A., Thoonen, A. and Van Der Stock, J.: Intestinal lymphagiectasia in a dog. J. Sm. An. Pract. 15:757-761, 1974.

82. Waldmann, T.A.: Protein-losing gastroenteropathies. In, Gastroenterology, 3rd edition. Edited by H.L. Bockus, Vol. 2. W.B. Saunders Co., Philadelphia, 1976.

83. Sherding, R.G.: Canine intestinal lymphangiectasia. Proceedings ACVIM 406-408, 1988.

84. Tidball, C.S.: The nature of the intestinal epithelial barrier. Am. J. Dig. Dis. 16:745-767, 1971.

85. Katz, J., Rosenfeld, S. and Sellers, A.L.: Sites of plasma albumin catabolism in the rat. Am. J. Physiol. 200:1301-1306, 1961.

86. Munor, D.R.: Route of protein losing during a model protein-losing gastropathy in dogs. Gastroenterology 66:960-972, 1974.

87. Kondo, M., Nakanishi, K., Bamba, T., Hosokawa, K. and Masuda, M.: Experimental protein-losing gastroenteropathy. Role of tissue plasminogen activator. Gastroenterology 71:631-634, 1976.

88. Meschter, C.L., Rakich, P.M. and Tyler, D.E.: Intestinal lymphangiectasia with lipogranulomatous lymphangitis in a dog. JAVMA 190:427-430, 1987.

89. Van kruiningen, H.J., Lees, G.E., Hayden, et al. Lipoganulomatous lymphangitis in canine intestinal lymphangiectasia. Vet. Pathol. 21:377, 1984.

90. Burns, M.G.: Intestinal lymphangiectasia in the dog: A case report and review. JAAHA 18:97-105, 1982.

91. Pedersen, N.C.: Personal communication.

92. Fossum, T.W., Sherding, R.G., Zack, P.M., Birchard, S.J. and Smeak, D.D.: Intestinal lymphangiectasia associated with chylothorax in two dogs. JAVMA 190:61-64, 1987.

93. Bank, S., Fisher, G., Marks,I.N. and Groll, A.: The lymphatics of the intestinal mucosa. A clinical and experimental study. Am. J. Dig. Dis. 12:619, 1967.

94. Danese, C.A., Georgulas-Penesis, M. and Kark, A.: Studies of the effects of blockage of intestinal lymphatics. Am. J. Gastroenterology 57:541, 1972.

95. Kaup, F.J., Drommer, W., Kersten, U. and Thissen, H.J.: Ultrastrukturelle untersuchungen bei einem Fall von intestinaler Lymphangiektasie. Kleintierpraxis 33:81-86, 1988.

96. Hill, F.W.G. and Kelly, D.F.: Naturally occurring intestinal malabsorption in the dog. Am. J. Dig. Dis. 19:649-665, 1974.

97. Nicolaidou, K., Ladefoged, K., Hylander, E., Thale, M. and Jarnum, S.: Endogenous faecal calcium in chronic malabsorption syndromes and in intestinal malabsorption. Scand. J. Gastroenterology 15:587-592, 1980.

98. Wilk, P., Karipineni, R., Dreiling, D.A. and Danese, C.: Studies of the effects of blockage of intestinal lymphatics. Am. J. Gastroenterology. 63:400-403, 1975.

99. Kalser, M.H.: Medium chain triglycerides. Adv. Int. Med. 17:301-322, 1971.

100. Batt, R.M., Bush, B.M. and Peters, T.J.: Biochemical changes in the jejunal mucosa of dogs with naturally occurring exocrine pancreatic insufficiency. Gut:709-715, 1979.

Chapter 18

Infectious, Parasitic, and Toxic Gastroenteritis

PATHOGENESIS OF ACUTE GASTROENTERITIS DUE TO MICROORGANISMS[1]

Introduction

Transient exposure of the gastrointestinal tract to microoganisms that are not normal members of the intestinal flora is a frequent occurrence that does not often result in clinical evidence of diarrhea. Transient bacteria become pathogenic only when they colonize the bowel. Colonization is prevented in normal animals by: 1) the luxuriant normal microflora, not readily displaced from the mucosal surface; 2) bacterial interactions favoring growth of only the normal microflora; 3) the production of bactericidal agents by the normal flora; 4) the production of bactericidal or bacteriostatic gastrointestinal secretions such as hydrochloric acid and pancreatic and biliary juice; 5) the normal propulsive activity of the intestine in sweeping the organisms in the aboral direction; 6) the complete assimilation of food ensuring a restricted nutrient supply for bacterial growth; and 7) the antiseptic paint of secretory immunoglobulins that prevents adherence of specific pathogens to the mucosal surface. A change in any one of these seven homeostatic mechanisms can cause sufficient disruption of the normal flora or local immune system to allow colonization by foreign microorganisms and signs of disease. For example, diarrhea produced by any means causes profound changes in the normal microflora, in particular reducing the number of anaerobes in the colon because of more rapid transit (and hence less anaerobic environment). This change in the normal flora interferes with the floral resistance to aerobic colonization. Thus, diarrhea resulting from a sudden change of diet may sufficiently disrupt the normal flora to allow the colonization of the intestinal tract by transient pathogens that result in the perpetuation or worsening of the diarrhea. Malnutrition changes the normal bacterial flora so that pathogens can colonize. Stress changes the flora, and severe stress can change intestinal motility so that bacterial numbers increase. Antibiotics often alter the normal flora, permitting antibiotic-resistant transients to colonize and cause disease. Some bacteria have the ability to secrete an IgA protease that degrades immunoglobulins secreted on the mucosal surface. This property enables the bacteria to colonize.[2] Once colonized, microorganisms multiply and produce diarrhea by one of three means.

Enterotoxigenic Infectious Agents[3]

Some bacteria and protozoa attach to the mucosal surface without penetrating, and produce diarrhea by releasing an enterotoxin. This type of toxin is produced by many organisms normally found in the intestines of small animals. The bacterial enterotoxin that has received the most investigation is that produced by *Vibrio cholera*. This bacteria is not a pathogen in small animals, but its pathomechanisms are similar to many other enterotoxins.

Vibrio cholera enterotoxin is a heat-labile protein made up of 7 subunits forming one molecule with a weight of about 80,000 daltons. The toxin's structure is disorganized at acid pH, so that toxin entering orally is inactivated in the stomach. Part of the toxin molecule binds to a receptor on the epithelial cell. Following its mucosal attachment a subunit of the cholera toxin diffuses through the cell to the basal lateral membrane where, after a latent period of 15 to 60 minutes, the toxin activates adenyl cyclase producing cyclic AMP. The net effect of cyclic AMP on the intestinal epithelial cell is to inhibit linked sodium and chloride absorptive process and increase electrogenic chloride and potassium secretion.[4] The composition of the secretion induced by cyclic AMP is similar to that of normal intestinal secretions. The majority of the cyclic AMP effect on apical membrane permeability is related to phosphorylation of protein kinases, a phosphatase, and several substrate proteins in the apical membrane.[4] Part of the cyclic AMP effect may be mediated by an interaction with calcium-mediated processes. While direct activation of the cyclic AMP system is considered the major way by which cholera toxin initiates diarrhea, an interaction of the toxin with the enteric nervous system has also been proposed.[4] Copious amounts of fluid can be secreted and lost. Secretion of fluid continues for the life of the villus cell, which may be for two to five days or until the secreting cells desquamate and are replaced by newly matured cells that have migrated from the crypt. The secreting mucosa's absorptive functions remain intact, permitting the treatment of cholera-induced fluid losses with oral fluid replacement. The administration of balanced solutions with added glucose takes advantage of the mechanisms that provide for the mutual absorption of sodium and glucose. The transmucosal facilitated transport of glucose and sodium chloride permits more effective absorption of fluid than does the transport of salt solution alone.[5]

The intestinal secretion induced by the enterotoxins produced by *Vibrio cholera, Salmonella, Campylobacter jejuni, Pseudomonas aeruginosa, and Shigella,* and the heat-labile

Escherichia coli enterotoxin are all mediated predominantly through the cyclic AMP mechanism described above. In contrast, the intestinal secretion induced by the enterotoxins produced by *Yersinia enterocolitica*, and *Klebsiella pneumoniae*, and the heat-stable *Escherichia coli* enterotoxin are mediated predominantly through cylic GMP-dependent mechanisms.[4] The enterotoxin secreted by *Clostridium difficile* is thought to result in calcium-dependent intestinal secretion. The effects of the cyclic GMP and calcium second messenger systems on intestinal secretion are not well understood. They are thought to be similar to the effects of cyclic AMP but the magnitude of the chloride secretory response induced by agents acting through cyclic AMP is greater than that caused by agents acting through cyclic GMP and calcium.[4] The second messengers of the enterotoxins produced by *Clostridium perfringens* and *Staphylococcus aureus* are unknown.

More details of the enterotoxins produced by each species of bacteria are provided in the discussion of the diarrheal syndromes pertaining to each species. *Entamoeba histolytica* is a protozoa which excretes an enterotoxin capable of producing secretory diarrhea. Like many of the bacteria, however, this organism also secretes cytotoxic products that allow mucosal invasion.

The importance of enterotoxigenic organisms in producing disease in small animals is unknown.

Enteroadherent Infectious Agents

Certain strains of *E. coli* are able to tightly adhere in an extensive coat to the gastrointestinal mucosa. After occupying this position they efface the microvilli over broad expanses of mucosa and produce a chronic diarrheal process.[6] The incidence of diarrhea due to enteroadherent organisms in cats and dogs is unknown. Enteroadherent *E. coli* have been reported in cats with diarrhea. Heavy infections with *Giardia* may also produce diarrhea by occlusion of the mucosa and damage to the brush border.[7]

Mucosal-Invading Infectious Agents

Some pathogenic microorganisms are able to attach to and penetrate mucosal epithelial cells. *Shigella, Salmonella, Campylobacter, Yersinia* and invasive strains of *E. coli* are enteroinvasive bacteria. *Shigella* invade epithelial cells and produce cytotoxic enterotoxins that destroy the cell. Other enteroinvasive bacteria appear to damage the mucosa in a manner similar to Shigella. Disruption of the mucosal surface leads to the clinical signs of enterocolitis that include watery diarrhea, and as the condition progresses, dysentery. The mechanism of fluid production in invasive diarrhea may be multifactorial. As discussed previously, damage to the epithelial surface, results in an inability to resorb fluid creating a passive intestinal secretion. Furthermore, invasive organisms increase local synthesis of prostaglandins which may mediate the diarrhea. Moreover, villus atrophy as a result of epithelial cell destruction and increased turnover may lead to malabsorption. In addition, many invasive organisms concurrently produce enterotoxins that stimulate surviving enterocytes to secrete fluid. And finally, if the permeability breakdown of the mucosal barrier is sufficient, the exudation of interstitial fluid, protein and blood is unrestricted.

Bacteria are not the only microoganisms capable of producing diarrhea by mucosal invasion. Protozoa such as *Entamoeba histolytica, Balantidium coli,* and Coccidia, also invade the epithelium or lamina propria. Giardia has been demonstrated within intestinal epithelial cells.

All enteropathogenic viruses invade the intestinal epithelium. The site at which they invade markedly affects their pathological potential. Thus coronaviruses, rotaviruses, and reoviruses infect and destroy the mature enterocytes on the tips of the villi. The result is mild villus atrophy, malabsorption, and a passive secretory diarrhea as a result of deficient intestinal fluid absorption. In contrast, canine parvovirus and feline panleukopenia virus infect and destroy the epithelial cells in the small intestinal crypts. The consequence of this cytotropism is denudation and collapse of the villi because of failed enterocyte replication. Diarrhea results from failed absorption of digestive organ secretions and from increased permeability.

Collectively, diarrhea due to one or another of these enteroinvasive organisms is relatively common in cats and dogs.

Submucosal-Invading Infectious Agents

If not kept in check by the immune system, many of the mucosal-invasive infectious agents discussed above may go on to invade the submucosa. After they penetrate the submucosa they stimulate marked inflammation characterized by neutrophil accumulation, and in the latter stages by macrophage infiltration. Septicemia often develops when submucosal invasion occurs and normal defense mechanisms are overwhelmed. Invasive strains of *E. coli* and *Salmonella* are the most important bacteria to cause septicemia from an intestinal infection. Some salmonellae are resistant to the effects of leukocytes and can replicate in macrophages, in which they can be transported to other parts of the body. They may even persist in the presence of antibiotics that retard multiplication. After the antibiotics are discontinued, the salmonellae are then able to multiply rapidly. That is a basis for the carrier state that can develop after an acute attack of *Salmonella* enteritis. There is little information on the incidence or characteristics of the invasive *E. coli* that produce septicemia in small animals. In humans, *Yersinia enterocolitica* infection may also progress from the mucosa into the submucosa to cause septicemia, as can *Balantidium coli*. Fungi such as *Absidia, Mucor, Rhizopus, Aspergillus, Histoplasma,* and *Candida* may also invade the intestinal wall. The portal of entry may be a preexisting defect or could result from the carriage of fungal spores from the lumen into the mucosa by macrophages.

BACTERIAL GASTROENTERITIS

Tyzzer's Disease[8,9]

Tyzzer's disease is caused by *Bacillus piliformis*, a spore-forming, gram-negative, intracellular, pleomorphic bacillus. Tyzzer's disease is an important disorder of laboratory rodents, but only rarely affects the dog and cat. The disease is primarily seen in neonates of weaning age, but will occur in immunosuppressed adult animals. Most feline cases have occurred in laboratory-reared kittens. An outbreak also occurred in kittens with familial hyperlipoproteinemia.[10] Rodents or their feces may be the source of the infection. The organism proliferates in the intestinal epithelial cells producing an enterocolitis, and spreads by way of the portal system to the liver where a periportal multi-focal hepatitis develops. The most consistent clinical signs are a rapid onset of depression, and abdominal discomfort. Death usually occurs within 24-48 hours although recurrent weight loss and recurrent attacks of diarrhea extending over several weeks was reported in one affected cat.[11] Furthermore, 2 kittens have been reported in which the primary manifestation of the infection with *Bacillus piliformis* was a relatively mild colitis that progressed over a 5 day period to central nervous system signs and death.[12] Diarrhea is infrequent, scant and pasty. Diagnosis is most often made at necropsy. Multiple 1-2 mm diameter necrotic foci are apparent in the liver, and the ileal and colonic mucosa appears thickened and congested. Histology reveals intracellular filamentous organisms, provided special stains such as Giemsa are utilized. To date, therapy has been unsuccessful. The disease does not affect people.

Campylobacteriosis

Clinical Synopsis

Diagnostic features

* Young animal; recently kenneled
* Acute onset of mild, mucoid diarrhea; rarely hemorrhagic
* *Campylobacter jejuni* cultured from feces

Standard treatment

* Erythromycin: 10-15 mg/kg q 8 h PO for 5 days
* Quarantine away from children
* Advise owner on hygiene

Follow up

* Reculture feces 1 & 4 weeks following therapy

Etiology and Epizootology. Interest in *Campyobacter jejuni* has burgeoned recently and the reader is referred to several detailed articles for in depth discussion of this pathogen.[8,13,14] *Campylobacter jejuni* is a small, curved, motile, microaerophilic, gram negative rod. It can be isolated from the feces of a high percentage of young animals that have been kenneled, particularly in animal control facilities. Isolations from adult household pets are relatively rare. A number of *Campylobacter jejuni* serotypes have been associated with diarrhea in humans, dogs, cats, and a variety of domestic animals. A related bacterium, *Campylobacter pylori* is a suspected cause of gastritis and peptic ulcerations in humans.

As with many enteric pathogens, *Campylobacter jejuni* can be isolated from the feces of normal dogs. Futhermore, many studies have not found a significant difference between the frequency of isolation between normal and diarrheic dogs and cats. Moreover, experimental infection of dogs and cats with *Campylobacter jejuni* has met with inconsistent results, probably due to strain differences, and variations in the susceptibility of the host populations studied.[15-17] There seems little doubt, however, that in young dogs and cats some strains of *Campylobacter jejuni* can act as a primary enteric pathogen. In older animals it is likely that *Campylobacter* acts more as an opportunist, producing disease only when appropriate predisposing factors lower the host's resistance. Predisposing factors include stress, concurrent infection with other enteric pathogens such as parvovirus, coronavirus, and *Giardia*.

Campylobacter can survive for days in surface water and as long 4 weeks in feces. The duration of excretion in infected dogs and cats can be as long as 4 months. Asymptomatic carriers are frequent.[18] Contamination of food and water sources with *Campylobacter* infected feces is the most likely mode of transmission. The incubation period is 3-7 days.

Pathogenesis. *Campylobacter jejuni* can colonize the jejunum, ileum, cecum, and colon, but histopathologic changes are largely restricted to the large bowel. *Campylobacter jejuni* produces a secretory diarrhea and less frequently invades the epithelium.[17] The organism produces an enterotoxin that has immunologic similarity to both the cholera toxin and the *E. coli* heat-labile toxin. The secretory diarrhea resulting from *Campylobacter jejuni* is mediated by cyclic AMP. *Campylobacter* also elaborate a cytotoxic enterotoxin which is presumably responsible for the epithelial damage. Bacteremia, an extraintestinal colonization, particularly in the early stages of infection, has been reported.[17,19]

Clinical Features. Clinical signs of campylobacteriosis in dogs have ranged from mild transient diarrhea to mucus-laden bloody stools with associated tenesmus and systemic signs of vomiting, anorexia, and depression.[8,16,17,20-22] In cats diarrhea is sometimes profuse and watery but is most often soft and mucoid.[23] In both species fever is usually absent, except in the severe cases. Rare fatal cases have been recorded.[24,25] Clinical signs are usually self-limiting within several days to several weeks. Young animals exposed to a kenneling situation are most likely to be affected, particularly with the more severe signs. At necropsy, the most consistent gross abnormality is mesenteric lymphadenopathy.[17] Histological changes are usually restricted to the large bowel and have included mucosal hyperplasia, a reduction in crypt height, a change to a cuboidal epithelium, and infiltration of the lamina propria with a mild, mixed inflammatory infiltrate. A proliferative enteritis has also been attributed to *Campylobacter*.[26] Some strains produce no histologic abnormalities.

A tentative diagnosis rests on a positive fecal culture in an animal with appropriate clinical signs. The organism is fastidious and fecal samples must be submitted to the laboratory immediately or, if delay is expected, placed in appropriate transport material. As mentioned above, *Campylobacter jejuni* can be cultured from normal animals, and so circumspection is required before a diarrheal process is ascribed to Campylobacteriosis.

Public Health Concerns and Therapy. The zoonotic potential is high. It is estimated that 5-11% of all human diarrhea cases results from *Campylobacter jejuni*.[27] As many as 5% of these cases may have resulted from exposure to campylobacter infected dogs and cats.[28] Humans appear to be considerably more susceptible to *Campylobacter* infection than are dogs and cats, and the diarrheal process is predictably more severe. In view of the high risk to humans, antibiotic therapy of animals with positive *Campylobacter* cultures is warranted. Erythromycin (10-15 mg/kg q 8 h PO) or tylosin (20 mg/kg q 12 h PO) for 5 days appear to eradicate infection from dogs and cats.[8] Aminoglycosides, tetracyclines, chloramphenicol, and fluoroquinolones are also usually successful. Ampicillin and trimethoprim-sulfonamides are less effective. The effectiveness of therapy should be confirmed by fecal cultures performed 1 and 4 weeks following therapy.[8] Occasionally additional supportive therapy such as fluids may be required. Owners should be advised on appropriate hygienic measures. The animal should not be allowed to come in contact with children. Most commonly used disinfectants, including hypochlorite, will kill the organism. Consideration should be given to the possibility that the source of bacteria that infected the dog might also be a potential source for human members of the family.

Clostridium Perfringens-Associated Diarrhea

Clinical Synopsis

Diagnostic features

* Acute onset of watery or hemorrhagic diarrhea
* Hospitalized patients predisposed
* *Clostridium perfringens* enterotoxin isolated from the feces
* Heavy, relatively pure growths of *Clostridium* species on fecal culture

Standard treatment

* Oral or intravenous fluid therapy
* Withhold food for 24-48 hours
* Ampicillin 20 mg/kg q 8 h PO, IV, SC, or IM for 3-5 days if hemorrhagic diarrhea

Etiopathogenesis. *Clostridium perfringens* is a gram positive, anaerobic, bacillus that is a normal resident of the intestinal flora of dogs and cats. The organism produces an enterotoxin that is cytotoxic in addition to altering the absorptive and secretory functions in the cell.[29] The enterotoxin can result in clinical evidence of gastroenteritis if increased quantities of the toxin are ingested on contaminated food or if overgrowth of *Clostridium perfringens* occurs in the intestine. Intestinal overgrowth with *Clostridia* can occur with any disorder that results in intestinal stasis such as intestinal obstruction or adynamic ileus. Heavy and relatively pure growths of *Clostridia* have been consistently recovered from the feces of dogs affected with parvovirus.[30] Furthermore, *Clostridium perfringens* has been associated with severe, peracute hemorrhagic gastroenteritis,[31] and is now emerging as an important cause of outbreaks of nosocomial diarrhea in dogs.[32,33]

Clinical Features. The clinical signs of a series of dogs with nosocomial diarrhea associated with *Clostridium perfringens* of a variety of serotypes included mild depression and soft watery diarrhea with or without frank blood, mucus, and tenesmus.[32] Dogs with diarrhea had significantly higher fecal clostridial counts than did dogs without diarrhea. *Clostridium perfringens* enterotoxin was found in the feces of 41% of diarrheic dogs but in only 7% of dogs without diarrhea.[32] Histopathological examination of the intestine of one dog showed a hemorrhagic necrotizing enteritis with a prominent neutrophilic component and evidence of bacteria resembling *Clostridia* in the tissues. The changes were most pronounced in the ileum. Most dogs recovered within 2-3 days; all recovered within a week with or without treatment. The role of *Clostridium perfringens* in chronic diarrhea is less well established, but dogs with antibiotic-responsive chronic intermittent diarrhea that were excreting excess quantities of Clostridial enterotoxin have been described.[33]

Diagnosis. *Clostridium perfringens*-associated diarrhea should be suspected in dogs with excess quantities of enterotoxin in their feces, or histopathological evidence of a suppurative, necrotizing, or mucofibrinous colitis, that respond promptly to ampicillin or metronidazole. Some dogs with *Clostridium perfringens*-associated diarrhea may shed endospores that can be observed on fecal smears[33] and others have a fecal smear almost exclusively composed of gram positive bacilli.

Therapy and Summary. Acute, mild cases of watery diarrhea are likely to be too self-limiting and require only supportive care such as easily digestible diets and appropriate fluid therapy. Dogs with acute hemorrhagic diarrhea should be promptly treated by withholding food, and, if clostridial overgrowth is confirmed, ampicillin (20 mg/kg q 8 h, PO, IV, SC, or IM) or metronidazole (10-15 mg/kg q 12 h, PO) for 3-5 days is recommended.

It is probable that most enteritis associated with *Clostridium perfringens* is opportunistic, but it is possible that some serotypes may be primary gastrointestinal pathogens. A zoonotic potential has not been proven.

Clostridium Difficile

Clostridium difficile may be transiently isolated from the feces of up to 21% of dogs.[34] The organism responsible for antibiotic-associated, pseudomembranous colitis. This entity is not uncommon in humans treated with antibiotics that suppress the normal colonic flora such as clindamycin, lincomycin, ampicillin, and cephalosporins. Pseudomembranous colitis is very uncommon in dogs or cats, but has been reported in 1 dog treated with clindamycin.[35] Association with *Cl. difficle* was not established in this case.

Clostridium difficile infection has also been incriminated as a cause of chronic diarrhea in 3 dogs.[34] The animals had chronic watery diarrhea. *Cl. difficile* and *Cl. difficile* toxin were recovered from the dogs, and the response to metronidazole was prompt. Metronidazole administration was required on a long term basis in two of the dogs to maintain remission. Unfortunately, no colon biopsies were taken to confirm pseudomembranous colitis, and the authors mention no attempt to rule out other metronidazole-responsive diseases such as chronic idiopathic colitis and giardiasis.

Escherichia Coli Enteritis[4]

Clinical Synopsis

Diagnostic features

* Acute onset of watery or hemorrhagic diarrhea
* Pathogenic *E. coli* subtype cultured from feces

Standard treatment

* Oral or intravenous fluid therapy
* Withhold food for 12-24 hours
* Bismuth subsalicylate 0.25 ml/kg q 4-6 hr for 3-5 days
* Trimethroprim-sulfa 15 mg/kg q 12 h for 5 days (hemorrhagic form)

Etiology and Epizootiology. *Escherichia coli* are a major component of the intestinal flora. There are a very large number of *E. coli* subtypes. Most are harmless, but through refined identification techniques over 100 potentially pathogenic subtypes of *E. coli* have been defined.[4,27] In humans, *E. coli* is now thought to be one of the most common causes of acute diarrhea. Enterotoxigenic *E. coli* are isolated from 40-70% of people with the very common syndrome of "travellers" diarrhea.[27] Invasive *E. coli* are isolated in 0-4% of the same syndrome.

The importance of *E. coli* infections in cats and dogs is unknown.

Pathogenesis. Enterotoxigenic strains of *E. coli* are a cause of secretory diarrhea in many species. Some strains produce a heat-labile toxin that increases adenylate cyclase activity. Several types of heat-labile toxins have been identified in different species. Other strains of *E. coli* produce a heat-stable enterotoxin that induces secretory diarrhea through cyclic GMP-mediated mechanisms. Enterotoxigenic strains of *E. coli* depend on specific fimbrial antigens (colonization factor antigens) for adherence to the mucosa and subsequent colonization. The antigenic structure of the fimbriae determine the species specificity of the enterotoxigenic *E. coli* strains. Thus, *E. coli* bearing K88 antigen are pathogenic for piglets, while those bearing K99 antigen cause diarrhea in calves and lambs. The ability to produce enterotoxins is under genetic control that can be transferred from one strain to another through plasmids. Some strains of *Escherichia coli* produce enterotoxins but do not cause disease since the organism is normally restricted to the colon, which is a site where the toxin does not act.[36] They are pathogenic only when they colonize the small intestine. A strain of E. *coli* (0157:H7) produces an enterotoxin-mediated acute hemorrhagic colitis.[37] This so-called "enterohemorrhagic" *E. coli* produces an enterotoxin that resembles *Shigella* toxin. It is cytotoxic and results in mucosal erosions and ulcerations. The 0157:H7 *E. coli* has been responsible for deaths in a number of humans and the reservoir of infection is thought to be cattle, an observation which reinforces the necessity of responsible antibiotic usage by veterinarians. The importance of 0157:H7 *E. coli* in dogs and cats has not been established.

Other strains of *E. coli* have been shown to diffusely coat the jejunum and ileum. These so-called "enteroadherent" or "effacing" strains of *E. coli* have been reported in rabbits, children, calves, and cats with diarrhea.[6,27] The diarrhea tends to have a chronic course. The mechanism of the diarrhea appears to relate to a diffuse effacing of the microvilli,perhaps by the release of a cytotoxin.[6] Finally, several *E. coli* strains induce diarrhea by mucosal invasion. These strains are termed enteroinvasive *E. coli* .

In all species studied, immunity to most pathogenic *E. coli* and their toxins develops readily. Older dogs are resistant to colonization by enterotoxigenic *E. coli* given orally.[36] Resistance to colonization is as great in 10-to-12-week-old pups as in adult dogs. Dogs are partially resistant to *E. coli* enterotoxin placed directly in the lumen of the small intestine. With a few subsequent challenges, they become completely resistant to the toxin. Since circulating antitoxin levels do not change, the local immune system is thought to be responsible for the resistance. The immunogenicity of the enterotoxins of most enterotoxigenic bacteria argues against an important role for enterotoxigenic bacteria in chronic diarrhea. There is evidence to suggest, however, that the heat-stable enterotoxin produced by some *E. coli* strains is less immunogenic and can be a cause of more persistent diarrhea. Furthermore, the enteroadherent strains of *E. coli* appear to be able to colonize the mucosa for prolonged periods of time.

Clinical Features. Puppies and kittens within the first few weeks of life can succumb to neonatal colibacillosis.[8,38] Clinical signs shown include acute depression, weakness, hypothermia, and cyanosis and CNS signs immediately before death.[8] The diagnosis is confirmed by culture of *E. coli* from tissues such as the spleen and liver.

Transient gastroenteritis associated with pathogenic strains of *E. coli* have occasionally been reported in the cat.[38] Strains of *E. coli* that secrete a shigella-like toxin have been isolated from cats with diarrhea.[39] Strains of *E. coli* that secret a shigella-like toxin have been associated with outbreaks of human neonatal diarrhea.[27] In an outbreak of diarrhea in a cattery, hemolytic *E. coli* with recognized pathogenic O groups were isolated from 93% percentage of affected cats, whereas only 22% of normal cats carried pathogenic strains.[40] Recovered cats carried the pathogenic serotype for greater than 10 months after recovery. The pathogenic serotypes most commonly implicated in feline diarrhea are O6, and to a lesser extent O78, O25, 0141, and K80.[38,41] Diarrhea resulting from enteroadherent effacing *E. coli* has been diagnosed in two cats presented with anorexia and diarrhea.[6] Light microscopy revealed mild neutrophilic infiltration with diffuse atrophy and focal fusion of villi. An extensive layer of bacteria were demonstrated attached to the villi in association with extensive microvilli effacement. Both the colon and small intestine were affected.

A relatively slow-acting heat-labile enterotoxin of *E. coli* origin has been isolated from dogs with diarrhea,[42] and entero-invasive strains are suspected to occur occasionally.

The predominate clinical signs of enterotoxigenic *E. coli* infection is watery diarrhea, and that of enteroinvasive *E. coli* is hemorrhagic "large bowel" type diarrhea. Laboratory changes are non-specific. Diagnosis can not be made by routine culture of the feces. It is dependent on animal inoculation studies, cytotoxicity in vero cell cultures, or serotyping.

Therapy. Therapy of colibacillosis depends on the presenting signs. In neonatal colibacillosis antibiotic therapy may be attempted but is rarely successful unless begun prior to all but the mildest clinical signs. All members of the litter should be treated. The most suitable antibiotics are cephalosporins or ampicillin. In older animals, colibacillosis is usually rapidly self-limiting and therapy is primarily supportive. Treatment may include oral or intravenous fluids in association with bismuth subsalicylate. In humans, antibiotic therapy has minimal influence on the course of the enterotoxigenic diarrhea, but is recommended for therapy of the enteroinvasive *E. coli* infections. It is probable that antibiotic therapy may also be required for the enteroadherent forms of *E. coli* . Antibiotics usually effective against *E. coli* are trimethoprim-sulfa, chloramphenicol, aminoglycosides, tetracycline, doxycycline, ampicillin, and fluoroquinolones.[27,43]

Public Health Aspects. Most enterotoxigenic *E. coli* are species-specific so it is unlikely that they are public health risks. As mentioned above, however, enterohemorrhagic and entero-invasive strains are potentially important public health risks.

Summary. In summary, evidence is accumulating that pathogenic serotypes of *E. coli* are a cause of diarrhea in both neonatal and adult dogs and cats. The incidence of diarrhea due to *E. coli* is unknown. Enteropathogenic and enteroinvasive*E. coli* are most likely to be responsible for acute, self-limiting diarrhea in animals exposed to a kennel or cattery environment. Enteroadherent*E. coli* may be responsible for chronic diarrhea.

Salmonellosis[44-46]

Clinical Synopsis

Diagnostic features

* Young animal; recently kenneled
* Acute onset of watery or hemorrhagic diarrhea
* *Salmonella* species cultured from feces and/or extraintestinal tissue
* Other intestinal pathogens not isolated

Standard treatment

* Oral or intravenous fluid therapy
* Withhold food for 12-24 hours
* Advise owner on hygiene
* Bismuth subsalicylate 0.25 ml/kg q 4-6 hr for 3-5 days
* Norfloxacin 22 mg/kg q 12 h PO for 7 days (hemorrhagic form)
* Trimethroprim-sulfa 15 mg/kg q 12 h for 7 days (hemorrhagic form)

Follow up

* Reculture feces 4 weeks following therapy

Etiology and Epizootiology.[8] *Salmonella* organisms are gram negative, aerobic bacilli with a propensity for intracellular persistence. The *Salmonella* isolated most frequently from dogs and cats are various subtypes of the genus *Salmonella enteritidis*. This species has over 1700 potentially pathogenic serotypes. As many as 53 serotypes have been isolated from dogs.[45] The most frequently isolated serotypes are *S. typhimurium*, and *S. anatum*. *S. krefeld* was isolated from a nosocomial outbreak at the UCD VMTH.[47] *Salmonella* can be cultured from the feces of normal as well as diarrheic animals. The frequency of isolation from normal animals varies considerably. Isolation frequencies as great as 36% have been reported from clinically normal dogs. In cats isolation frequencies as high as 18% have been reported.[48] Cats appear to be more resistant to salmonellosis than dogs. At the UCD, VMTH, *Salmonellae* are rarely cultured from the feces of healthy household pets. Positive cultures are usually found in animals debilitated by other diseases such as parvovirus, suggesting an opportunistic behavior. The frequency of *Salmonella* isolation and *Salmonella*-associated diarrhea is highest in young, stressed, or diseased cats and dogs housed in poorly sanitary, overcrowded conditions. There may be a seasonal prevalence, with peak incidence at the coldest time of the year. Obesity, glucocorticoid therapy, and antecedent or concomitant antibiotic therapy (particularly ampicillin) are additional risk factors.[8,47,49]

Salmonellae are readily transmitted from carriers by fecal contamination of food and water. Wild animals and birds are a reservoir. An outbreak of *Salmonella* in cats has been linked to an epidemic of salmonellosis in a population of song birds.[50] Products of the poultry industry are the largest reservoir of *Salmonellae*. Also sources are other domestic animals raised for consumption. Commercial pet foods that are not cooked during processing are a potential source. Dehydrated dog food has been found to be a source of *Salmonella*. Canned or kibbled products are cooked during processing, so that any *Salmonellae* are destroyed. Other uncooked foods can also contain *Salmonellae* and be a source of infection.

Salmonella can survive for prolonged periods outside the host, particularly in aquatic environments. As with all enteric pathogens that are zoonoses consideration must be given to the possibility that the source of bacteria that infected the dog might also be a potential source for human members of the family.

Pathogenesis. The primary pathogenic mechanism of *Salmonella* is mucosal invasion, that induces inflammation, necrosis, and increased synthesis of prostaglandins. However, cell-free lysates of *Salmonella* intestinal secretion, and it appears that Salmonella enterotoxin is involved in the pathogenesis of salmonellosis by the production of a cyclic AMP-mediated secretory diarrhea.[4] The organism preferentially localizes in the ileum and affects the colon to a lesser extent. The infectivity of *Salmonella* varies with the strain and the size of the inoculum. The incubation period is 3-5 days. Shedding may continue for 3-6 weeks, but can be reactivated at a latter date by any intercurrent stress.

Clinical Features. The clinical signs are highly variable. Most animals infected with *Salmonella* are asymptomatic. Mild to severe acute gastroenteritis may be seen. This may progress to septicemia. The septicemia can be acute and progress rapidly to collapse and death or it may be less fulminating. The more severe cases of gastroenteritis are characterized by fever, vomiting, abdominal pain, and diarrhea. The diarrhea varies from watery to mucoid and fresh blood may be present. Some cats[51] and dogs may present with a chronic febrile illness without specific gastrointestinal signs. Hematologic abnormalities are variable, but in the acute stage a degenerative left shift is not uncommon. A fecal smear often reveals leukocytes. Diagnosis rests on appropriate clinical signs in association with positive fecal or blood culture. As with the other enteric pathogens, a positive fecal culture proves infection, but does not establish that the clinical signs are a result of the *Salmonella*. Culture of the organism from blood or other body fluid is more definitive but does not detect infections limited to the mucosa. A negative culture result does not rule out Salmonellosis because the organism can be difficult to isolate. Histologic changes in the intestinal mucosa vary from mild catarrhal inflammation to extensive mucosal sloughing. Invasion of the lamina propria with neutrophils and to a lesser extent macrophages are also seen. Less than 10% of infected animals die within the acute stages of salmonellosis,[8] although occasional outbreaks have been associated with mortalities as high as 61%,[52] and salmonellosis as a complication of protracted medical problems has a 50% mortality rate.[49] Recovery usually occurs within 1 week but may take 3-4 weeks.

Therapy. Recommendations on antibiotic usage in the therapy of salmonellosis are at present undergoing a reevaluation because of the advent of a new class of antibiotics, the fluoroquinolones. Fluoroquinolones appear to be highly effective against all aerobic bowel pathogens; they minimally disrupt normal flora, and rapid acquisition of resistance does not occur. Therefore, these antibiotics have become the drug of choice in the treatment of human salmonellosis, and early evidence suggests that they may be able to eliminate the carrier state. The latter feature is a tremendous advance in the therapy of salmonellosis, because in the past antibiotics were known to prolong the carrier state. Proposed reasons for the prolonged carrier state included the inability of antibiotics to destroy organisms localized within macrophages, and the development of resistant strains. Amidst this uncertainty the following recommendations can be made.

Salmonella invasion limited to the superficial mucosa produces a self-limiting gastroenteritis. In such uncomplicated cases, treatment with antibiotics are unnecessary, and therapy is best restricted to supportive measures in association with advice on appropriate hygiene and/or quarantine procedures. In contrast, antibiotic therapy is indicated, if the diarrhea is hemorrhagic, the dog depressed or febrile, or laboratory evidence of sepsis such as a degenerative left shift, or a positive blood culture are observed. If blood culture or fecal culture results are available, therapy may be based on sensitivity patterns. Unfortunately, the sensitivity pattern of *Salmonella* organisms can be poorly predictive of in vivo response to antibiotics.[51] If blood culture results are unavailable, the antibiotics of choice are a member of the fluoroquinolones, chloramphenicol, or a trimethoprim-sulfonamide. Fluoroquinolone antibiotics should probably be avoided in young animals.

If the fluoroquinolones live up to their promise, another potential indication for fluoroquinolone therapy will be to shorten the carrier state in pets potentially exposed to very young, elderly, or debilitated people.

Salmonella resist common forms of disinfection. Activated aqueous glutaraldehyde (2%) applied for 30 minutes to an hour is usually effective and is suitable for most surfaces and equipment.[8]

Yersiniosis[52]

Yersinia enterocolitica is a gram negative, facultative coccobacillus. The bacteria induces secretory diarrhea by virtue of a cyclic GMP-mediated enterotoxin. Some subtypes of *Yersinia* are invasive and may also secrete a cytotoxic enterotoxin. It is an important enteric pathogen in people, and an important cause of diarrhea in farm animals. The importance of this bacteria in diarrhea of the dog and cat, however, is unknown. *Y. enterocolitica* can be isolated from the feces of normal dogs and cats, but has been isolated in large numbers from two dogs with 2 week histories of large bowel type diarrhea that responded rapidly to antibiotics.[54] Tetracyclines, and trimethoprim-sulfonamides are usually effective. In humans it is not uncommon for *Yersinia enterocolitica* to invade from the intestine to cause a septicemia. Thus there is a possible serious public health problem.[55,56]

Y. enterocolitica has not yet been reported in the cat. Another species of *Yersinia*, however, *Y. pseudotuberculosis* can result in vomiting, diarrhea and eventually jaundice as part of a septicemic disease in cats.[38] *Y. pseudotuberculosisis* is also a public health risk producing a mesenteric lymphadenitis with associated abdominal pain in people. Tetracycline, chloramphenicol, and trimethoprim-sulphonamides are suitable antibiotics for the therapy of *Y. pseudotuberculosis*. Therapy must be prolonged in advanced cases and the prognosis guarded.

MISCELLANEOUS BACTERIAL ENTERITIS

Shigellosis

Shigella have been infrequently isolated from the bowel movements and mesenteric nodes of dogs.[57] *Shigella* are known to produce enterotoxins with both secretory and cytotoxic properties. The cytotoxic toxin is responsible for the dysenteric appearance of the stools of patients with Shigellosis. *Shigella* toxins are heat-labile and readily degraded by proteolytic enzymes. The virulence of these organisms is dependent on both their invasive properties and the ability to produce the cytotoxin.[58] *Shigella* infection results in rapid production of a toxin-neutralizing antibody of the IgM class that persists for 9 to 18 months. *Shigella* are unlikely to be important in causing disease in animals, but it is possible that dogs and cats contaminated by human Shigella could act as a transient zoonotic reservoir.

Tuberculosis

Tuberculosis is uncommon in the dog and cat. The cat is most commonly affected by *Mycobacterium bovis* whereas the dog is most commonly affected by *M. tuberculosis*. Gastrointestinal infection is more common with *M. bovis* and respiratory infection more common with *M. tuberculosis*. Cats develop intestinal localization more commonly than dogs. In cats the clinical signs include weight loss, anemia, vomiting, diarrhea, and palpable masses in mesenteric lymph nodes, intestine, and other abdominal organs.[8,38] Some cats develop ascites. In dogs, the signs are primarily respiratory but in a series of 5 Basset Hounds infected with *Mycobacterium avium* complex most dogs exhibited gastrointestinal signs in association with granulomatous mesenteric masses and granulomatous enterocolitis.[59] Basset hounds appear to be predisposed to avium tuberculosis and the gastrointestinal route appears to be the portal of entry. Diagnosis of tuberculosis can be made by intradermal skin testing but this test has inconsistencies.[8] The best test site appears to be the pinna. Definitive diagnosis is usually made by demonstration of acid-fast intracellular bacteria in biopsies of lesions. Successful treatment has been reported,[8] but infected animals are a public health risk and in some situations therapy may not be appropriate.

Klebsiella Pneumoniae[60]

Klebsiella produces an enterotoxin that at low doses stimulates secretion of fluid and at high doses produces morphological changes in the mucosa. The intestinal secretion is mediated through a cyclic GMP mechanism. The importance of this bacteria in diarrheal diseases of dogs and cats is unknown.

Staphylococcus Aureus[61]

Overgrowth of the small intestine by *Staphylococcus aureus* can be caused by broad-spectrum antibiotic therapy, resulting in diarrhea of variable severity. This microorganism produces an enterotoxin that inhibits fluid absorption in the jejunum by unknown mechanisms. It also produces a cytotoxic enterotoxin.

VIRAL GASTROENTERITIS

A large number of enteric viral pathogens affect dogs and cats. The relative prevalence of these viruses in the canine and feline population is unknown. The clinical signs range from mild transient gastroenteritis such as characterizes enteric coronavirus infection to life-threatening necrotizing enteritis such as can occur with canine and feline parvovirus infections. The primary pathogenic mechanism of enteric viruses is mucosal invasion followed by varying degrees of villus atrophy and denudation. As discussed above, viruses that affect the rapidly dividing crypt cells have more pathogenic effects than those that invade the crypts. Epithelial denudation is followed by massive secondary bacterial invasion that is responsible for the mortality. The panleukopenia virus produces few signs of disease in germ-free cats.[62] Its ability to produce severe disease in conventional cats illustrates the synergism between a virus and bacteria in producing disease. Understanding of the role of viruses in causing enteritis is hampered by the need for special techniques to identify viruses,[63] and the difficulty of reproducing the disease by viral inoculation.

Clinical signs common to the enteric viruses include acute onset of clinical signs, evidence of rapid contagion, and a predisposition for young animals. Treatment is always symptomatic, with particular attention being paid to fluid therapy and prevention of secondary bacterial invasion. Prevention of enteric viral diseases by appropriate quarantine, hygiene and vaccination practices is of prime importance in limiting the morbidity and mortality from enteric viruses.

Canine Coronavirus Enteritis[8]

Clinical Synopsis

Diagnostic features

* Young animal; recently kenneled
* Acute onset vomiting and soft to watery diarrhea
* Fever and leukopenia rarely seen.
* Coronavirus particles in feces
* Other intestinal pathogens not isolated

Standard treatment

* Oral or intravenous fluid therapy
* Withhold food for 12-24 hours

Etiology and Epizootiology. Cornaviruses are pleomorphic, single-stranded, enveloped RNA viruses. The virus appears to be widespread in the canine population with up to 70% of dogs demonstrating serological titers. Feces are the primary source of infection. Coronaviruses are heat labile but may persist in the environment during cooler times of the year, leading to increased outbreaks in the winter months. The virus appears to affect only dogs.

Following ingestion it localizes in the epithelial cells of the upper two-thirds of the villi. It enters the cell by pinocytosis and replicates in the cell cytoplasm. Replication occurs by budding into cytoplasmic vesicles, and eventually results in cell death, with epithelial desquamation, shortening of the villi, decreased intestinal fluid absorption (passive secretory diarrhea) and malabsorption. Rupture of the infected cell releases the progeny virions to infect other enterocytes. Mucosal immunity plays an important role in the immunity to canine coronavirus. The duration of immunity following infection is unknown but recurrent attacks of coronavirus appear rare in pet animals either as a result of longterm immunity or frequent reexposure.

The incubation period ranges from 1-4 days. Viremia is not seen. Following infection, dogs shed the virus for at least 2 weeks in their feces. The disease is highly contagious and often occurs as outbreaks in susceptible populations.

Clinical signs are most common in dogs less than 1 year. Experimental and clinical evidence suggest that uncomplicated canine coronavirus induces a relatively mild, non-fatal, self-limiting gastroenteritis.[64-66] Fever and leukopenia are usually not seen. The diarrhea is rarely bloody. Clinical signs usually resolve within 1-12 days but the diarrhea may persist on an intermittent basis for 3-4 weeks. Opportunistic enteric pathogens such as *Clostridium perfringens*, *Campylobacter*, and *Salmonella* may increase the severity of the clinical signs, although their role in this regard remains unconfirmed.

Diagnosis is made on the basis of appropriate history and clinical signs in association with isolation of the virus from the feces, or the demonstration of viral particles in the feces by electron microscopy.

Therapy is symptomatic. Effective vaccination is difficult because of the existence of multiple antigenic strains and the importance of local rather than systemic immunity in the protection against the virus. The mild nature of uncomplicated coronaviral gastroenteritis suggest that vaccination should be considered only in dogs likely to suffer from concomitant infection with another pathogen. Thus vaccination may be considered in dogs "stressed" by heavy work schedules, substandard nutrition or hygiene, intercurrent disease, and frequent exposure to other animals. An alternative and more sound approach is to remedy the predisposing causes. Vaccination against coronavirus infection is not recommended in the healthy household pet. During an outbreak strict quarantine, careful hygiene, and thorough disinfection (1:30 dilution of bleach) may help limit the extent of the spread.

Feline Enteric Coronavirus[38]

Feline enteric coronaviruses are pleomorphic, enveloped RNA viruses. Two strains have been characterized to date, one of which has a demonstrated cytopathic effect in tissue cultures. Feline enteric coronaviruses are antigenically and morphologically similar to feline infectious peritonitis virus. A spectrum of feline coronaviruses exist ranging from those that produce purely enteritis and those that produce purely FIP. The major source of the infection appears to be asymptomatic carrier cats. Transfer by fomites appears possible. Kittens become infected at weaning. The virus replicates in the apical epithelial cells of the intestinal villi. Clinical signs are usually not apparent but some kittens develop transient mild gastroenteritis. A fatal hemorrhagic diarrhea associated with feline enteric coronavirus infection has been described but is very uncommon. Histopathological changes are usually mild but villus atrophy and fusion may be seen.

Diagnosis can be made by demonstrating a rising coronavirus titer (tests for FIP can be used) or by detecting virus particles in the stool using electron microscopy. Treatment is symptomatic. Prevention is difficult (because the virus is enzootic) and unnecessary in view of the mild clinical signs.

Feline Infectious Peritonitis[38]

Feline infectious peritonitis is caused by a coronavirus antigenically and morphologically similar to feline enteric coronavirus. In addition to the classical effusive inflammatory serosal form of FIP, a second form of the disease characterized by granulomatous inflammation of parenchymous organs including the mesenteric nodes, bowel wall, liver, and pancreas may be seen. At times, the granulomatous inflammation is largely restricted to the colon producing a granulomatous colitis.[67] Diagnosis may be made by detection of pyogranulomatous inflammation on biopsy in association with a high FIP titer (>1:32,000). Alternatively, fluorescent antibody staining may be used to demonstrate FIP in the tissues. Brief remission of granulomatous FIP may occur in a small percentage of cats treated by immunosuppressive drugs. The disease is invariably fatal.

Canine Parvovirus Enteritis[8]

Clinical Synopsis

Diagnostic features

* Young dogs primarily affected
* Acute onset of hemorrhagic diarrhea
* Fever and leukopenia commonly seen.
* Fecal parvovirus hemagGlutination or ELISA test may be positive
* 4-fold rise in serum IgG titer over a 7-14 day period;
* Detection of serum IgM titer in an unvaccinated dog

Standard treatment

* Intravenous fluid therapy
* Withhold food for 24-72 hours
* Trimethoprim-sulfa 15 mg/kg q 12 h SC PO for 5-10 days (if signs of moderate severity)
* Ampicillin (20 mg/kg q 8 h IV) and gentamicin (2.2 mg/kg q 8 h IV, SC) for maximum 5 days (if signs severe)
* Metoclopramide 2.0 mg/kg/24 h as a continuous IV infusion
* AVOID oral aminoglycosides, flunixin meglumine, glucocorticoids, anticholinergics, opioids

Follow up

* Continue easily digestible diet for minimum of 2 weeks

Etiology and Epizootiology. Canine parvoviral enteritis is caused by an unenveloped DNA virus (canine parvovirus 2) that has an affinity for rapidly dividing cells. The disease first became apparent in 1978 when epizootics of severe gastroenteritis simultaneously afflicted canine populations about the world. The origin of canine parvovirus has not been determined. The virus is antigenically distinct from a non-pathogenic parvovirus of dogs called "minute virus of canines" (canine parvovirus 1), but bears antigenic similarity to feline parvovirus from which it may have mutated. Three syndromes of parvovirus infection have been reported: hemorrhagic gastroenteritis; acute myocarditis; and neonatal mortality. This discussion refers to only hemorrhagic gastroenteritis, the more common of these syndromes.

The virus appears to be widespread in the canine population with most dogs being exposed to the virus at an early age either by vaccination or contact with the street virus. Canine parvovirus can survive for months or years in feces, and contact with feces is the primary mode of infection. Fecal contaminated fomites are important sources of spread. The virus is able to infect most Canidae. Cats are susceptible to a self-limiting inapparent infection. The Rottweiller and perhaps the Doberman Pinscher appear predisposed.[68]

Factors such as crowding, concurrent disease, and other pathogens increase the severity of the clinical signs. Opportunistic enteric pathogens such as, *Campylobacter, Salmonella*, coronavirus, and various parasites may increase the severity of the clinical signs. The normal bacterial flora are important in the pathogenesis of the disease since infection of gnotobiotic dogs with parvovirus produces an inapparent disease. The normal flora increase the rate of epithelial turnover thus exacerbating the disease, and invade the mucosa to produce sepsis.

Pathogenesis. Following ingestion the virus replicates in the lymphoid tissue of the oropharynx from where it spreads to the blood stream in greater or lesser amounts depending on the level of immunity (Figure 18-1). This initial immune response determines the magnitude of the viremia and the severity of the ensuing clinical signs. The viremia deposits virus in rapidly dividing cells throughout the body. Cells affected include the bone marrow, the lymphopoietic tissue and the crypt epithelium of the jejunum and ileum. Viremia is terminated by increased serum neutralizing antibody which first appears 5-6 days post-infection. The replication of the virus in the lymphopoietic system and bone marrow results in lymphopenia and neutropenia, respectively. The replication of the virus in the cryptal epithelial cells results in rapid collapse of the intestinal villi, epithelial necrosis, and hemorrhagic diarrhea. Normal bacterial flora enter the denuded mucosa and, as a result of the deficient neutrophil numbers and depressed immune response, gain rapid access to the blood stream resulting in fulminant sepsis and death.

In animals with a partial immunity to the virus, from either previous exposure or maternally derived immunoglobulin, the initial viremia is less intense, and the immunosuppression and intestinal necrosis less severe. The result is mild or inapparent clinical signs. The resistance to infection, and the severity of the signs correlate better with coproantibody levels than with serum titers. The duration of immunity following infection is prolonged, perhaps measured in years. The immunosuppression resulting from parvovirus infection can predispose dogs to other infectious diseases such as distemper, hemobartonellosis,

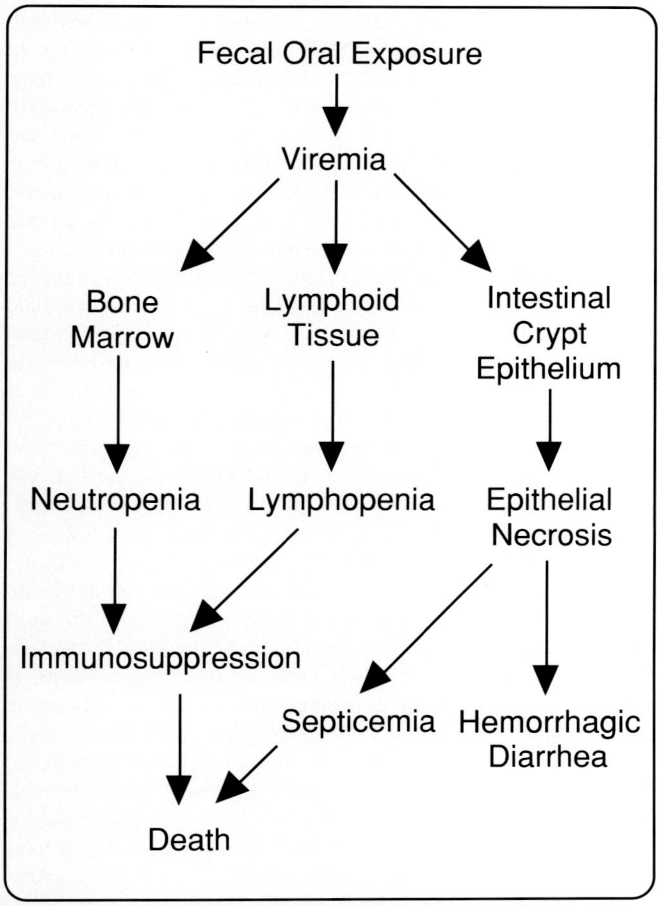

Figure 18-1 Pathogenesis of Canine Parvoviral Enteritis

and distemper vaccine-associated encephalitis.

Clinical Features. The incubation period ranges from 5-10 days. The duration of fecal shedding following parvoviral infection is controversial. Virus is difficult to recover within 2-8 days after the onset of clinical signs, however feces may still contain sufficient, albeit small, quantities of virus to infect susceptible dogs for as long as 3 weeks after the onset of clinical signs. As with coronavirus, the disease is highly contagious and often occurs as outbreaks in susceptible populations.

Clinical signs are most common in dogs less than 1 year,[68,69] with more than 75% of cases occurring within the age bracket from 6-18 weeks of age.[70,71] Not all puppies of a litter need be clinically affected. Depression, anorexia, pyrexia, and vomiting are early clinical signs, followed by diarrhea. The vomitus is usually scant, clear or bile-stained fluid. Large volumes of vomitus are unusual and should raise the suspicion of intussusception. In mild cases the diarrhea is soft or watery. In severe cases the diarrhea is hemorrhagic, and has a fetid smell. The same smell is associated with other causes of hemorrhagic diarrhea and is not specific for parvovirus. A rapid progression to hypothermia, septic shock, and death occur in some dogs.

Leukopenia is present in approximately 80% of dogs at some time during their illness.[68,69] Both lymphopenia and neutropenia are common with the former slightly more common than the latter.[69] Occasionally atypical reactive lymphocytes are seen in the peripheral blood. These changes should raise the index of suspicion for parvovirus but they are not pathognomonic for the disease. Leukopenia is also seen in salmonellosis, for instance. The serum chemistry profile usually shows non-specific changes. Hypoalbuminemia and electrolyte abnormalities such as hyponatremia, hypokalemia, and hypochloremia are seen in 25-33% of dogs.[69] Plasma ALT is elevated in approximately 25% of dogs.[69] Acid-base abnormalities may be seen in severely affected dogs and are usually suggestive of metabolic acidosis (13%).

Diagnosis. Diagnosis is made on the basis of appropriate history and clinical signs in association with any of the following: a 4-fold rise in serum IgG titer over a 7-14 day period; detection of serum IgM antibody against parvovirus in a dog that has not been vaccinated within the last 3-4 weeks; a positive parvovirus fecal hemagglutination or ELISA test; isolation of parvovirus from the feces; detection of parvovirus particles in the stool using immunoelectronmicroscopy; indirect fluorescent antibody tests of tissues at necropsy. The fecal hemagglutination and ELISA tests are simple to perform and reasonably specific but less sensitive than the other tests because of the rapidity with which viral numbers decline in the feces of affected dogs. Necropsy usually reveals fibrin-covered serosal surfaces, a congested, hemorrhagic mucosa often covered with a pseudomembrane, thymic atrophy, and enlarged mesenteric nodes. Histology reveals epithelial necrosis and denudation, collapse of the villi, and inflammatory infiltrates in the lamina propria.

Therapy. Supportive therapy is necessary for the treatment of most cases of parvovirus, and antibiotic administration is required for many. The details of supportive therapy for acute gastroenteritis is found in Chapter 16. Of paramount importance is the selection of an appropriate volume and composition of fluid. In most situations, lactated Ringer's solution with an additional 10-15 mEq of potassium chloride per liter is appropriate. The volume administered is dependent on the patient's body weight, estimated degree of dehydration (5-12%), basal requirements and on-going losses. The rate of administration should be sufficiently rapid to replace the patient's fluid deficit in as short a time as the patient's cardiovascular, respiratory, and renal systems will permit. Administration of plasma or blood is occasionally required in anemic or hypoalbuminemic animals. The role of hyperimmune serum has yet to be defined. Supplemental nutritional support is often required.

Antibiotic usage for the treatment of parvovirus is justified if the dog shows hemorrhagic diarrhea or evidence of sepsis such as fever, depression, degenerative left-shifted leukograms, or positive blood cultures. Our first choice antibiotic for patients with hemorrhagic diarrhea but no evidence of sepsis is trimethoprim-sulphadiazine. This antibiotic is preferred because of a broad spectrum of activity against pathogens invading the mucosa but minimal effects on the normal flora. However, if the patient is severely depressed, shows evidence of sepsis, or has a profound neutropenia (<1000/μL), we institute a combination of parenteral ampicillin and gentamicin with the aim of broadening the spectrum of activity against gram negative and anaerobic pathogens. We do not use ampicillin as our routine first choice antibiotic, as has been recommended by others, because of the disruptive effect this antibiotic has on the normal flora, and its documented ability in our clinic and in human hospitals to predispose patients to overgrowth with particularly lethal aerobic bacteria such as *Salmonella*.[47] Gentamicin should only be used after rehydration of the patient and the duration of administration should be limited to 5 days.

An additional drug of value in the supportive therapy of dogs with parvovirus is metoclopramide. Adynamic ileus is not uncommon in association with parvovirus and predisposes the patient to bacterial overgrowth. Metoclopramide has been shown to be effective in the treatment of experimentally-induced adynamic ileus in the dog and may assist a return to normal intestinal motility in parvoviral enteritis. An additional beneficial aspect of this drug is its antiemetic activity. If vomiting is persistent, therapy with a phenothiazine antiemetic may be required.

Drugs that should be avoided in the therapy of parvovirus are oral aminoglycosides, flunixin meglumine, glucocorticoids, and anticholinergics. Oral aminoglycosides disturb the normal flora, may induce diarrhea as an adverse drug reaction, and have a high risk of toxicity because of increased absorption through the denuded mucosa. Flunixin meglumine is associated with a high incidence of gastrointestinal ulceration and ischemic renal disease. It should only be used in animals with clear clinical evidence of septic or endotoxic shock and then only as a single injection after rehydration. It should not be used in association with corticosteroids as synergistic damage to the intestinal mucosa will result. The effectiveness of corticosteroids in the treatment of septic or hypovolemic shock has still not been clearly demonstrated. In addition to predictable detrimental effects on a wide range of body systems, corticosteroids may adversely affect the outcome in gram positive septic shock.[72] They have no place in the routine treatment of parvoviral enteritis. If used at all, their use should be restricted to single injections of "shock" doses administered early in the therapy of patients suffering from shock. Anticholinergics compound any adynamic ileus that may be present as a result of the disease process, and are contraindicated. Opioids have potential detrimental effects when used during infective diarrheal processes and should be avoided in the treatment of parvoviral enteritis except on rare occasions when fluid therapy cannot keep up with ongoing losses. The fetid material that is defecated by many patients with parvovirus is likely to contain a large quantity of potentially lethal materials such as gram negative endotoxins and clostridial enterotoxins. These materials are best passed from the body rather than kept in prolonged contact with the denuded mucosa by the use of potent agents such as opioids.

Complications. The most important complication of parvovirus infection is septicemia. Sepsis may promote the lethal complications of shock and DIC. Another complication occurring with reasonable frequency is intussusception. Patients hospitalized for parvoviral enteritis should undergo a minimum daily physical examination, including abdominal palpation, to ensure that complications such as intussusceptions are not overlooked. As mentioned above, adynamic ileus is also common as a result of parvovirus enteritis. A complication that can occur following recovery from the acute phase of the disease is intractable diarrhea as a result of irreparable mucosal damage or persistent inflammation, perhaps a result of the deranged mucosal barrier. An association between non-regenerative anemia and parvovirus infection has also been proposed. Miscellaneous complications include pneumonia, and candidiasis.

Prevention. Prevention is based on proper vaccination schedules in association with correct hygiene practices. The most appropriate vaccine is a modified-live preparation of parvovirus of canine origin. These products break through maternal immunity earlier, produce a more rapid immunity in seronegative dogs and result in a more long lasting immunity. They may also induce some degree of local immunity because of replication in the bowel and subsequent transient fecal shedding. The vaccination schedule used in most practices is administration of a modified-live parvovirus vaccine of canine origin every 2-3 weeks from 6-9 weeks of age until the puppy reaches 16-20 weeks of age. Vaccination of pups earlier than 6 weeks of age is rarely necessary unless the pup did not receive colostrum. Modified-live virus vaccinations should not be used in pups less than 6 weeks of age as they may cause vaccine-related morbidity. Animals not receiving colostrum should be given oral plasma (2-4 ml/kg) from a vaccinated donor if presented within the first few days of birth. If presented later, the same dose of serum may be given subcutaneously or intraperitoneally. Rottweillers should receive an additional vaccination at 18-20 weeks of age. If so desired, the adequacy of immunization can be established by post-vaccine titers. Revaccination is usually carried out at yearly intervals.

The most common cause of a vaccine failure is inadequate quarantine or hygiene practices. No matter what the vaccination schedule, there will be a time in a pup's life when its maternal immunity will be sufficient to prevent the development of active immunity from a vaccination, but inadequate at the same time (or in the ensuing 2 weeks until the next vaccination) will be inadequate to protect the pup against serious infection by the more virulent "street" virus. The only way these gaps in immunity can be minimized is to reduce the likelihood of exposure of the pup to large quantities of the virus. This is achieved by careful hygiene and by restricting the pups access to poorly cared for dogs. The immunity "gaps" cannot be filled by more frequent vaccination because intervals of less than 10-14 days result in "vaccine interference".[8]

During an outbreak strict quarantine, careful hygiene, and thorough disinfection (1:30 dilution of bleach) may help limit the extent of the spread. Vaccination of unaffected dogs with modified-live vaccine of canine origin in the face of the outbreak is recommended. Protective immunity may be obtained as early as 3-4 days following a single vaccination in seronegative dogs.

Prognosis. In mild cases the dogs make rapid recoveries over a 2-3 day period. Most dogs that survive the initial 2-3 days of therapy will eventually go on to recover. If severely affected animals survive, recovery from the acute signs may take a week or more and diarrhea can persist for several weeks. The mortality associated with parvovirus infection has been variously reported as 16-35%.[68,69] Mortalities are now considerably less common then in the early stages of the parvovirus epidemic. The reasons for the decline in mortality is unknown but may be a result of more widespread immunity, a shift in the virulence of the organism or perhaps improved therapeutics. Prognostic factors have proved difficult to identify. The presence of, hemorrhagic diarrhea, fever, depression, or leukopenia were not found to correlate to survival.[68,69] In our experience, however, patients with septic or hypovolemic shock at presentation, fibrinous mucosal casts or severe hemorrhagic diarrhea, and pronounced neutropenia (less than 500/μL) should receive a guarded prognosis.

Feline Panleukopenia[8,38]

Feline panleukopenia is caused by a feline parvovirus. Its epidemiology, pathophysiology, clinical signs, hematological findings, and treatment are essentially the same as that for canine parvovirus. A difference between feline and canine parvoviruses is the propensity of the feline parvovirus to produce cerebellar disease in cats infected in utero or during the early neonatal period. As with canine parvovirus, the tissues preferentially affected in the bowel are the jejunum and ileum. Cats with panleukopenia tend to need blood transfusions more frequently than their canine counterparts because of more rapidly progressive anemia. Furthermore, earlier initiation of supplemental nutrition protocols inclusive of vitamin B are recommended. The prognosis is poor. Prevention is by vaccination with a modified live vaccine. Vaccination is usually begun at 8-9 weeks of age and a second vaccination administered at 12 weeks or older. Colostrum-deprived kittens may receive serum as described for the pup. Modified-live vaccines should not be given to kittens less than 4 weeks of age. Inactivated vaccines may be used instead from birth to 4 weeks of age.

Miscellaneous Enteric Viral Infections

Many other types of viruses have been intermittently identified in the feces or vomitus of dogs and cats with acute gastroenteritis. These include rotaviruses, astroviruses, caliciviruses,[73] and reoviruses. At present, the importance of many of these viruses as enteric pathogens remains to be defined.[38,71,74-79,83] Relatively few virus identification surveys of the feces and vomitus of dogs and cats with acute gastrointestinal disease have been conducted and no multidisciplinary surveys of viral, bacterial, and parasitic agents and their interrelationships in producing gastrointestinal disease have been reported, even though a number of mixed viral,[71,76-80] viral-bacterial,[30,81] and viral-parasitic[81] enteric infections have been reported.

Several other viruses have been associated with chronic gastrointestinal disease in the cat. These include feline leukemia (FeLV) and feline immunodeficiency virus (FIV).

Astrovirus. Astroviruses have been isolated from both kittens and pups with diarrhea.[79,84] The epithelium of the tips of the small intestinal villi appears to be the primary target.[85,86] The clinical signs associated with experimental transfer of this virus have included mild self-limiting diarrhea. Clinical cases have had a more prolonged course. Inapparent infections also occur.[80]

Feline Immunodeficiency Virus.[38] Serological studies of cats with FIV have revealed a significant incidence of chronic oral inflammation (50%) and chronic enteritis or enterocolitis (20%).[87] The clinical signs associated with these lesions included anorexia, chronic diarrhea, dehydration, and emaciation. The diarrhea may be persistent and progressive intestinal thickening develops. Leukopenia is common. A high mortality was seen in the cats showing gastrointestinal signs. Histopathology shows a diffuse enterocolitis characterized by enterocyte necrosis in the glandular epithelium, villus atrophy and fusion, multiple foci of subacute ulceration, and transmural pyogranulomatous inflammation. A role for the virus in a panleukopenia-like syndrome of cats has also been proposed. The pathogenesis of these gastrointestinal disorders is unknown, but it is of interest to note that gastrointestinal manifestations of the human immunodeficiency syndrome are common and have a variety of cases including *Cryptosporidium, Giardia, Coccidia, Candida*, certain viruses, and *Salmonella*. In some of the cats Yersinia pseudotuberculosis was isolated from the affected bowel, and the type of lesion suggests that viral invasion, such as the enteric coronavirus may be involved . Lymphosarcoma may be a possible sequelae. At present, diagnosis is made by compatible clinical-pathological signs in association with a positive FIV titer.

Feline Leukemia. FeLV has been associated with a fatal peracute enterocolitis (panleukopenia-like syndrome).[88] It is also thought to be involved in the development of alimentary lymphosarcoma, even though many cats with alimentary lymphosarcoma have negative FeLV tests.[8]

Canine Distemper. Canine distemper produces a transient gastroenteritis characterized by vomiting and diarrhea in the early stages of the disease process. In a small number of dogs, severe enteritis is the principal manifestation. The diarrhea may be bloody and tenesmus has been observed. Leukopenia can also occur. Differentiation of this distemper variant from parvovirus is difficult because of similar clinical signs. If respiratory or neurological signs become apparent distemper should be suspected. Rarely the diseases can be differentiated by finding intracytoplasmic distemper inclusions in red or white blood cells. Distemper immunofluorescent antibody tests on conjunctival epithelium or urinary sediment may reveal distemper antigen.[8]

Rotavirus. Rotavirus has been associated with transient diarrhea in neonatal dogs,[89,90] and cats.[85,86] The prevalence of rotavirus in diarrheic stools in the USA has been reported to be very low[71] but in other countries it is higher.[91] Inapparent rotavirus infection of adult animals may be reasonably common.[71,83,91,92] Canine rotavirus have been reported to produce pathologic changes in the small intestine of dogs that are recognizable at both the light and electron microscopy level. Epithelial necrosis and mild villus atrophy were noted.[93] Recently, a rotavirus-like agent has been implicated as a cause of acute gastroenteritis of adult humans, piglets, calves, lambs, chickens, and rats,[94] and may also infect cats.[95] Diagnosis of rotavirus infections in dogs and cats can be made by a fecal ELISA test.

FUNGAL GASTROENTERITIS[96-98]

Low numbers of fungi are found in the normal intestinal microflora. They are not considered pathogenic. If their numbers increase, however, they can colonize parts of the intestine that they normally do not populate, they can invade the mucosa, and they can disseminate through the blood stream.

Candidiasis

Candida are dimorphic fungi that normally inhabit the gastrointestinal tract. They are opportunist pathogens. *Candida albicans* has been used in animal models to study how the fungi can become pathogenic. Fungemia can be produced by direct instillation of large amounts of yeasts into the duodenum of dogs. Gastrointestinal candidiasis can be produced by administering antibiotics and steroids, and by immunosuppressive therapy. Alteration of the normal bacterial microflora by antibiotics makes overgrowth by fungi possible. The use of corticosteroids with antibiotics potentiates the problem. Gastrointestinal candidiasis is rare in dogs and cats.[99-101] It has been reported in the aftermath of a case of canine parvovirus infection.[100] Candidal stomatitis is occasionally seen in the dog. The lesion appears as a raised white plaque or plaques on the mucosa. The diagnosis is confirmed by impression smears, biopsy, and culture. The treatment of choice for candidiasis restricted to the gastrointestinal tract is nystatin. The recommended human dose is 4.5-20 million units q 6-8 hours PO. Systemic candidiasis is best treated with ketoconazole or itraconazole (2-2.5 mg/kg PO).

Histoplasmosis.[8,38,102,103] Histoplasmosis is caused by a pleomorphic fungus, *Histoplasma capsulatum*. The disease is widely distributed in the world and in the United States is endemic in States about the Mississippi. The fungus grows particularly well in soil enriched by bird or bat feces. The fungus can enter the body through the respiratory or gastrointestinal tract. Localized pulmonary disease or systemic histoplasmosis can result.

Gastrointestinal involvement of the systemic form of the disease is more common in dogs than in cats, but chronic diarrhea as a result of histoplasmosis has been reported in the cat[8,103] as well as the dog. Gastrointestinal histoplasmosis is a chronic debilitating diarrheal disease. The diarrhea is usually profuse, intractable and occasionally bloody when the colon is involved. The bowel wall becomes thickened by a granulomatous inflammation. Malabsorption and protein-losing enteropathy are common. Physical examination or diagnostic evaluations will often reveal involvement of other tissues such as the eyes, lungs, liver, joints, bones, and spleen. A diagnosis is usually made by observation of the organism inside macrophages from colon scrapes, buffy coats, or bone marrow aspirates, or by biopsy of the colon or small intestine. Serum tests such as the agar gel diffusion test are available but can be unreliable. Treatment is with amphotericin B followed by ketoconazole.[8] The prognosis is guarded to poor. The newer imidazoles such as itraconazole may prove more efficacious.

Miscellaneous Fungi.[8,104] Disseminated aspergillosis and Mucormycosis can be responsible for diarrhea in cats.[8,38,103,105] Approximately 40% of cases have intestinal involvement with both small bowel and large bowel being affected. Panleukopenia, or antibiotic and corticosteroid administration appear important predisposing causes. In dogs, aspergillosis is rarely associated with gastrointestinal signs, but a variety of zygomycetes including members of the class *Mucorales* have been responsible for canine intestinal zygomycosis (phycomycosis).[8] The zygomycetes are opportunist fungi that are widespread in nature. In dogs they are thought to gain entrance to the intestinal wall as a result of mucosal trauma. The affected area of bowel becomes greatly thickened and eventually results in partial or complete intestinal obstruction. Clinical signs generally include a chronic history of diarrhea, or a palpable abdominal mass. Vomiting may occur, particularly once a partial obstruction develops. Radiography, ultrasound, or exploratory celiotomy may be required to detect the mass. Diagnosis is made by intestinal biopsy. Granulomatous lesions full of branching nonseptate hyphae are characteristic. In dogs the fungi may spread to the mesenteric nodes, and in cats disseminated disease has been reported. Treatment is surgical resection of the mass with subsequent amphotericin B therapy. The prognosis is poor.

PROTOTHECOSIS[8,106]

Gastrointestinal protothecosis is a rare disease of the dog caused by microorganisms morphologically similar to the green algae. In tissues the organisms are spherical to oval in shape. The organisms are ubiquitous in the environment. They appear to be opportunists. When they infect the bowel they most commonly colonize the colon and produce a severe chronic colitis that is characterized by intermittent, protracted bloody diarrhea. The disease eventually disseminates, often causing blindness. The disseminated disease is invariably fatal. Diagnosis is usually made by biopsy of the colon, vitreous taps, or evaluation of urinary sediment all of which may show the organism. In cats the disease is relatively benign and is usually localized to the skin.

SALMON POISONING[8]

Salmon poisoning isan often fatal disease of dogs caused by the rickettsial organism *Neorickettsia helminthoeca*. A second rickettsia-like organism, "Elokomin fluke fever agent" may also be involved in the disease process. This organism is probably another strain of *Neorickettsia helminthoeca*. Dogs acquire the rickettsial organism by the ingestion of fish (usually a salmon or trout) that harbour in their tissues (in particular the kidneys) metacercaria of the canine intestinal fluke *Nanophyetus salmincola*. The life cycle of the fluke has an obligate requirement for a developmental stage in a particular species of freshwater snail called *Oxytremma silicula*. It is the narrow geographic distribution of this snail that has restricted the occurrence of salmon poisoning to an endemic area in the Northern West Coast of North America.

Clinical signs of salmon poisoning include an acute onset of pyrexia, anorexia, vomiting and diarrhea. If untreated the diarrhea becomes progressively worse and may become grossly hemorrhagic. Peripheral and mesenteric lymphadenopathy are common. Important differentials are parvovirus and distemper. Either leukopenia or leukocytosis can occur. The incubation period following the ingestion of fish is usually 5-7 days although periods as long as 19-33 days have been reported.

The disease should be strongly suspected in dogs in endemic areas that develop acute gastroenteritis after documented or suspected access to salmon fish. Tentative diagnosis may be made by the demonstration of operculated fluke eggs in the feces of the dogs, indirect evidence of *Neorickettsia helminthoeca* infection. Fluke eggs are most reliably demonstrated by sedimentation techniques. More definitive diagnosis can be made by aspiration cytology of enlarged lymph nodes which often reveals reactive inflammation with macrophages containing rickettsial bodies.

The rickettsial infection is best treated with tetracyclines. In profusely vomiting animals parenteral administration is preferred until vomiting is controlled (oxytetracycline 7mg/kg q 12 h IV for 3 days). Oral tetracycline therapy 20 mg/kg PO q 8 h for 7 days is successful in dogs with less profuse vomiting. Treatment of the fluke infection may be accomplished by praziquantel (Droncit) at standard cestode doses. Even though Nanophyetes causes few clinical signs in of itself, eradication of fluke is recommended because it continues to shed eggs for as long as 250 days contributing to the contamination of more waterways. Prevention relies on restricting dogs access to fresh fish. Immunity following infection may be long lasting.

Other rickettsia that affect the dog produce occasional gastrointestinal signs. In ehrlichiosis these signs are generally restricted to hematochezia as a result of the bleeding tendencies that accompany rickettsial infection. Rocky Mountain spotted fever, however, can result in vomiting, diarrhea, abdominal pain and melena.

PARASITIC INFECTIONS[107-112]

Intestinal parasites are often associated with acute diarrhea. It is not always known to what degree they contribute to clinical signs. Protozoa are normally found in the feces of some species of animals, and their numbers usually increase with the onset of diarrhea due to any cause. In this case the protozoa are a consequence and not a cause of the diarrhea. Cestodes are commonly found in dogs and cats but their is little evidence they cause clinical signs other than perhaps perianal irritation. The appearance of these worms causes aesthetic displeasure, however, and some species such as *Echinococcus, Mesocestoides*, and *Dipylidium caninum* are public health risks.

Nematode Parasites

The most important intestinal nematode parasites of the dog and cat are ascarids, hookworms, whipworms, and *Strongyloides*. Ascarids are most commonly associated with ill thrift in pups and kittens. Heavy burdens may result in a pot-bellied appearance, mild diarrhea and intermittent vomiting. Migration of larval stages through the lungs can result in a pneumonitis with associated soft cough. The treatment of choice is piperazine or pyrantel pamoate. Intestinal obstruction due to the death of large quantities of worms following treatment has been recorded. Ascarids are an important public health risk.

Hookworms are of most importance in the young dog although they can also affect the cat. They are primarily a small bowel parasite, but will occasionally infect the large bowel if the parasite burden is sufficiently heavy. Clinical signs primarily pertain to blood loss anemia. The treatment of choice is pyrantel pamoate.

Whipworms are an important cause of chronic enterocolitis in dogs. They are infrequently seen in cats. The clinical signs can vary from blood tinged mucoid feces with associated tenesmus to a profuse watery diarrhea. Diagnosis is usually made by fecal flotation. Several flotations may be required. Occasionally whipworm eggs cannot be detected in the stool and the diagnosis is made by endoscopic examination of the large bowel. Treatments of choice are fenbendazole (Panacur) and butamisole (Styquin). Panacur is administered at 50 mg/kg q 24 h PO for 3 days. The course is repeated after 3 weeks and 3 months. Fecal flotations should be repeated to verify effectiveness of therapy. The parasite egg persists well in many environments including concrete runs and may result in persistent reinfection. Adequately cleaning the environment is difficult but flaming of concrete runs, or scrubbing them with dilute sodium hypochlorite has been recommended. Feces should be collected and disposed of appropriately. it is difficult to eradicate the parasite from grassed areas. In extreme cases, removal of heavily contaminated topsoil has been advocated.

Strongyloides stercoralis infection is seen most frequently in pups from a kennel or pet shop with unsanitary conditions. A diarrhea is consistently associated with this parasite. The animal with *Strongyloides* is a public health problem since humans can be infected with the parasite. The parasite is difficult to eradicate, compounding the problem. Thiabendazole (100-150 mg/kg for 3 days) maybe effective. Prevention aims at eradicated moist areas where the parasite larvae can persist.

Coccidia[8]

Coccidia are an important subclass of parasites that contains many species of veterinary importance including members of *Cryptosporidia, Sarcocystidae, Hammondia, Toxoplasma, Besnoitia*, and *Cystoisospora*. The coccidia of dogs and cats that were formly placed in the genus Isospora have now been placed in the genus *Cystoisospora*. The pathogenicity and life cycles of the coccidia vary considerably. Most species multiply in the epithelium of the distal small intestine. Generally, these organisms are not highly pathogenic and inapparent infections are common. However, clinical signs of diarrhea often with mucus or hematochezia, may be seen in young animals especially if they are debilitated or have been exposed to large numbers of coccidia through poor hygiene. Moreover, there is evidence to suggest that some species of intestinal coccidia and some strains of those species are more pathogenic than others. The usual therapy is sulfonamides (25-30 mg/kg PO q 12) or nitrofurazone (15 mg/kg PO q 24 h) administered for 7-21 days. These agents are coccidiostats and do not necessarily eliminate infection.

Cryptosporidia are extremely small coccidian parasites that have been responsible for chronic and severe diarrhea in immunosuppressed dogs and cats and which have also been held responsible for diarrhea in neonatal puppies and kittens. As with the other coccidia, asymptomatic infections can occur. The organism is very small (4-8 μm) and is difficult to demonstrate in the feces by routine microscopy. Sheather's sugar flotation solution is used to concentrate the organism in fecal samples. Phase contrast microscopy assists identification. Diagnosis is most often made by intestinal biopsy. An unusual feature of the organism compared to other coccidia is that it only penetrates the mucosa to the level of the brush border. There is little if any host specificity and this agent is a health risk for immunosuppressed people. Treatment is difficult in immunosuppressed patients but clindamycin may be tried.

Entamoeba Histolytica[113]

Entamoeba histolytica is a protozoan parasite of the large bowel that has been found in the United States, and is suggested to be more prevalent in dogs than generally believed. It is found most commonly in the tropics. Dogs are most likely to be infected through ingestion of water contaminated by the feces of infected humans. *E. histolytica* can produce hematochezia or a watery secretory diarrhea. Amebae possess multiple degradative enzymes, including hyaluronidase, mucinase, trypsin, pepsin, collagenase, and multiple other proteinases.[4] In addition, they can produce a cytotoxin that inhibits DNA and protein synthesis in target cells. These degradative enzymes and cytotoxins are presumably responsible for the hemorrhagic diarrhea associated with many cases of the disease. The secretory diarrhea of amebiasis is thought to be the result of either a heat-labile enterotoxin, or neurohumoral substances such as serotonin, substance P and neurotensin, released from the amebae. Some of these changes may in part be mediated by increased mucosal prostaglandin secretion. Extraintestinal infection can occur but is rare in dogs. The diagnosis is made by observing the trophozoite in smears of warm feces, or in colon biopsies. The treatment of choice is metronidazole.

Balantidium Coli and Trichomonas

Balantidium coli has been detected in several dogs with acute ulcerative colitis in association with *Trichuris* infection. It is possible that the protozoa is a secondary invader. The parasite is more common in pigs. Diagnosis is made by detecting the trophozoite or cyst in feces or by colonic biopsy. Clinical signs usually resolve following treatment of the trichuris infection. Metronidazole is an effective therapy.

No pathogenic trichomonas species have been found in the United States. The nonpathogenic *Pentatrichomonas hominis* is found in up to 15% of normal dogs.

Giardiasis[8,114]

Giardia species are flagellate protozoa that resides as motile trophozoites in the small intestine and to a lesser extent the large intestine of both dogs and cats. There is confusion over the number of *Giardia* species and the infectivity of different species for various hosts. The life cycle of giardia is direct and fecal-oral transmission occurs. Cysts can survive for weeks or months in cool, moist conditions. Contaminated waterways are a major source of infection. The latency period in dogs from ingestion to cyst excretion ranges from 5-12 days. The prevalence of *Giardia* in dogs and cats is less than 10%. In some areas the incidence of *Giardia* is higher, up to 33% of dogs being infected, many of which have no clinical signs of disease.1[15,116]

After ingestion, *Giardia* attach themselves to the small intestinal surface where they can induce malassimilation, steatorrhea, and chronic enteritis. Infections can also be inapparent. The pathophysiology of the malassimilation is unknown, but a multitude of processes maybe involved. *Giardia* appear to incite a T cell-mediated increase in epithelial turnover rate, which results in cryptal hyperplasia and villus atrophy.[4] They may also damage the brush border or, in large numbers, form a physical blockage to nutrient absorption by coating the mucosa. *Giardia* are able to interfere with lipase activity against triglyceride, and can reduce brush border disaccharidase activity, and glucose and amino acid transport. Most infections are self-limiting and acquired resistance, involving both humoral and cellular mechanisms, is thought to occur.

Clinical findings vary from inapparent infections (most common) to evidence of malassimilation characterized by chronic, continuous or intermittent, soft or watery diarrhea. Mucus is occasionally seen, and steatorrhea is common. On occasion, *Giardia* are associated with an ulcerative colitis, and may perhaps result in signs of large bowel dysfunction including tenesmus.

Diagnosis is made by fecal examinations including fresh smears for trophozoites, and various flotation and staining techniques (see Chapter 6). Zinc sulfate has been recommended as the preferred flotation media. Diagnosis can also be made by intestinal biopsy, aspiration of duodenal fluid by the endoscope, or the peroral string technique, or immunofluoresence for antigen in feces.

The recommended therapy is metronidazole 20-25 mg/ kg q 12 h PO for 5-7 days. In the dog, treatment failures are not uncommon, but in the cat metronidazole appears reasonably reliable.[117] In a study of a kennel infected with endemic giardiasis metronidazole only effected a cure rate of 67%.[118] Treatment failures have been approached by repeating the therapy at a higher dose (50 mg/ kg q 12 h for 5 days) or for more prolonged periods (weeks to months). High dose metronidazole therapy can induce serious neurological dysfunction, however, and should be avoided if at all possible. Another treatment option for cats (and probably dogs) is furazolidone (4 mg/kg q 12 h PO for 5 days).[119] Quinacrine (11 mg/kg daily for 12 days) eliminated the clinical signs but not cyst shedding in a cat.

Quinacrine (6.6 mg/kg PO for 5 days) has been reported to be the drug of choice for the therapy of intractable canine giardiasis.[118] The high incidence of side effects such as anorexia, lethargy, fever, and vomiting, restrict this drug to a second choice pharmaceutical in spite of its apparent efficacy.

In view of the potential public health risk of *Giardi*a, treatment of animals with positive *Giardia* examinations is recommended regardless of whether the infection is causing diarrhea. Without therapy, dogs can remain infected with Giardia for as long as six to 36 months.[110] The recommended disinfectants are the quaternary ammonium products.

TOXIN-INDUCED ACUTE GASTROENTERITIS

A list of toxins commonly resulting in gastrointestinal signs is provided in Table 16-9. Additional information on toxin-induced gastroenteritis including specific antidotes for the various toxins may be found in several recent publications.[120,121] The therapy of gastrointestinal toxicities is largely dependent on cause, but certain guidelines for the symptomatic therapy of toxin-induced gastroenteritis may be given. The first rule of the treatment of any toxic problem is to limit further absorption. In the gastrointestinal tract, this is achieved by the judicious use of emetics, cathartics, and absorbents.

In general, emesis should be induced only if the time from ingestion of the suspected toxin to the time of presentation is less than 4 hours. Most toxic materials will have completed their emptying from the stomach within this period of time. Exceptions to this rule include the ingestion of heavy objects such as metals, and the ingestion of indigestible materials such as plant leaves. These materials may remain in the stomach for prolonged periods of time. Unfortunately, because of their weight or large size, induced-emesis will often be unsuccessful in ridding the stomach of these types of foreign objects. If emesis is unsuccessful, endoscopy or gastrotomy is indicated. The induction of emesis is contraindicated in moribund animals for fear of inhalation pneumonia. It is also contraindicated in animals suspected of ingesting caustic agents or sharp metallic objects. The vomiting of the caustic material may create further damage to the esophagus which may result in esophageal stricturing. Furthermore, the violent abdominal contractions associated with vomiting may result in perforation of the stomach or esophagus. A consistently effective emetic agent is apomorphine (Eli Lilly & Co.). Apomorphine is an opioid dopaminergic agonist that induces emesis by an effect on the chemoreceptor trigger zone of the vomiting center. An appropriate dose in the dog and cat is 0.04 mg/kg IV or 0.08 mg/kg IM or SC. An alternative, route is to place an apomorphine tablet in the conjunctival sac. The tablet is removed as soon as the patient shows evidence of nausea after which vomiting will soon follow. The advantage of this technique is the accurate titration of the apomorphine dose, thus avoiding some of the complications of excessive apomorphine such as protracted vomiting and CNS depression. Syrup of ipecac (1-2 ml/kg, maximum 15 ml)[120] has been used as an emetic agent but it has several drawbacks including an efficaciousness of only 50%, a cardiotoxic effect, and a reduction of the effectiveness of activated charcoal.[120] Xylazine is an effective emetic in the cat but is less reliable in the dog. The dose of xylazine required for emesis (0.2 mg/kg IV) is far below that necessary for tranquilization. At these doses bradycardia is usually not a significant problem but heart rate should be monitored.

Moribund animals suspected of the recent ingestion of toxins should undergo gastric lavage by stomach tube. The procedure is thought to be effective if utilized within 2 hours of ingestion.[120] Its major disadvantage is the requirement for tranquilization or anesthesia in non-moribund patients. Ten to fifteen infusion-and-drainage cycles are performed with 5-10 ml/kg of lavage solution instilled at each infusion. Water or activated charcoal and water are the preferred lavage solutions.

Cathartics or lavage solutions are indicated if the ingestion of the toxic material has been within 8-12 hours of presentation and enemas may be considered within anytime period from several hours to several days after ingestion. Suitable cathartics are any of the osmotic laxatives including sodium sulfate (1 gm/kg), magnesium hydroxide (Milk of Magnesia - 3 ml/kg), and magnesium sulfate (Epsom's salts - 0.5 gm/kg). A suitable lavage solution is CoLyte (Reed and Carnrick) administered at 30 ml/kg by stomach tube. If the toxin is fat soluble, the cathartic may be preceded by a small quantity of mineral oil. Products, such as castor oil, and bisacodyl that increase the permeability of the epithelium should be avoided. Warm water enemas are the preferred enema technique. Soap should not be included as it can irritate the mucosa sufficiently to produce colitis and therefore increase mucosal permeability.

The most widely used and effective absorbent is activated charcoal. This product is usually administered in association with a cathartic. The powdered form is preferred and the recommended dose is 1-5 gm/kg made into a slurry at a concentration of 1 gm of charcoal per 10 ml of water. The slurry is administered by stomach tube and may be repeated several times a day.

REFERENCES

1. Drachman, R.H.: Acute infectious gastroenteritis. Ped. Clin. N. Amer. 21:711-737, 1974.
2. Plautt, A.G.: Microbial IgA proteases. New Eng. J. Med. 298:1459-1463, 1978.
3. Banwell, J.G. and Sherr, H.: Effect of bacterial enterotoxins on the gastrointestinal tract. Gastroenterology 65:467-497, 1973.
4. Donowitz, M. and Welsh, M.J.: Regulation of mammalian small intestinal electrolyte secretion. In, Physiology of the Gastrointestinal Tract. 2nd edition, Edited by L.R. Johnson. Raven Press, New York, 1351-1388, 1987.
5. Klipstein, F.A. and Engert, R.F.: Reversal of jejunal water secretion by glucose in rats exposed to coliform enterotoxins. Gastroenterology 75:255-262, 1978.
6. Pospischil, A., Mainil, J.G., Baljer, G. and Moon, H.W.: Attaching and effacing bacteria in the intestines of calves and cats with diarrhea. Vet. Pathol. 24:330-334, 1987.
7. Owens, R.L.: Parasitic diseases. In, Gastrointestinal Disease. Edited by Sleisenger, M.H., Fordtran, J.S. WB Saunders Co, Philadelphia, 1153-1191, 1989.
8. Greene, C.E.: Clinical Microbiology and Infectious Diseases of the Dog and Cat. WB Saunders Co, Philadelphia, 1984.
9. Qureshi, S.R., Carlton, W.W. and Olander, H.J.: Tyzzer's disease in a dog. JAVMA 168:602-604, 1976.
10. Jones, B.R., et al: Tyzzer's disease in kittens with familial hyperlipoproteinemia. J. Sm. An. Pract. 26:411-419, 1985.
11. Schneck, G.: Tyzzer's disease in an adult cat. VM/SAC 70:155-156, 1975.
12. Wilkie, J.S. and Barker, I.K.: Colitis due to *Bacillus piliformis* in two kittens. Vet. Pathol. 22:649-652, 1985.
13. Dillon, A.R., Boosinger, T.R. and Blevins, W.T.: Campylobacter enteritis in dogs and cats. Comp. Contin. Ed. Pract. Vet. 9:1176-1182, 1987.
14. Shane, S.M. and Montrose, M.S.: The occurrence and significance of *Campylobacter jejuni* in man and animals. Vet. Res. Commun. 9:167-198, 1985.
15. Prescott, J.F. and Karmali, M.A.: Attempts to transmit *Campylobacter enteritis* to dogs and cats. Can. Med. Assoc. J. 119:1001-1002, 1978.
16. Prescott, J.F., Barker, I.K., Manninen, K.I. and Miniats, O.P.: *Campylobacter jejuni* colitis in gnotobiotic dogs. Can. J. Comp. Med. 45:377-383, 1981.
17. MacCartney, L., Al-Mashat, R.R., Taylor, D.J. and McCandlish, I.A.P.: Experimental infection of dogs with *Campylobacter jejuni*. Vet. Rec. 122:245-249, 1988.
18. Newton, C.M., Newell, D.G., Wood, M. and Baskerville, M.: *Campylobacter* infection in a closed dog breeding colony. Vet. Rec. 123:152-154, 1988.
19. Blaser, M.J. and Reller, L.B.: *Campylobacter* enteritis. N. Eng. J. Med. 305:1444-1452, 1981.
20. Fox, J.G., Moore, R. and Ackerman, J.I.: *Campylobacter jejuni*-associated diarrhea in dogs. JAVMA 183:1430-1433, 1983.
21. Fox, J.G., Moore, R. and Ackerman, J.I.: Canine and feline Campylobacteriosis: epizootiology and clinical and public health features. JAVMA 183:1420-1424, 1983.
22. Olson, P. and Sandstedt, K.: *Campylobacter* in the dog: a clinical and experimental study. Vet. Rec. 121:99-101, 1987.
23. Junttila, J., Crispin, S.M. and Ophthal, D.V.: *Campylobacter*-associated epidemic in cats. Compan. An. Pract. 1:16-18, 1987.
24. Murtaugh, R.J. and Lawrence, A.E.: *Campylobacter jejuni*-associated enteritis. Feline Pract. 14:37-42, 1984.
25. Peel, R.N. and McIntosh, A.W.: The dog it was that died. Lancet 2:1212, 1978.
26. Collins, J.E., Libal, M.C. and Brobst, D.: Proliferative enteritis in two pups. JAVMA 183:86-889, 1983.
27. Gorbach, S.L.: Infectious diarrhea. In, Gastrointestinal Disease. Edited by Sleisenger, M.H., Fordtran, J.S. WB Saunders Co, Philadelphia, 1191-1232, 1989.
28. Skirrow, M.B.: *Campylobacter* enteritis in dogs and cats: a new zoonosis. Vet. Res. Commun. 5:13-19, 1981.
29. McDonel, J.L. and Duncan, C.L.: Histopathological effect of *Clostridium perfringens* enterotoxin in the rabbit ileum. Infect. Immun. 12:1214-1218, 1975.
30. Jones, B.D. and Kirby, R.: Acute hemorrhagic diarrhea. Proc 7th ACVIM forum 435-437, 1989.
31. Prescott, J.F., Johnson, J.A. and Patterson, J.M.: Haemorrhagic gastroenteritis in the dog associated with *Clostridium welchii*. Vet. Rec. 103:116-117, 1978.
32. Kruth, S.A., Prescott, J.F., Welch, M.K. and Brodsky, M.H.: Nosocomial diarrhea associated with enterotoxigenic *Clostridium perfringens* infection in dogs. JAVMA 195:331-334, 1989.

33. Twedt, D.C., Jones, R.L., Collins, J.K. and Ogilive, G.: *Clostridium perfringens* enterotoxin associated with diarrhea in dogs. Abstract Proc 7th ACVIM forum 1046, 1989.
34. Berry, A.P. and Levett, P.N.: Chronic diarrhoea in dogs associated with *Clostridium difficile* infection. Vet. Rec. 118:102-103, 1986.
35. Burrows, C.F.: Diseases of the colon, rectum, and anus in the dog and cat. In, Veterinary Gastroenterology. Edited by Anderson, N.V. Lea & Febiger, Philadelphia, 553-592, 1980.
36. Sack, R.B., Johnson, J., Pierce, N.F., Keren, D.F. and Yardley, J.H.: Challenge of dogs with live enterotoxigenic *Escherichia coli* and effects of repeated challenges on fluid secretion in jejunal Thiry-Vella loops. J. Infect. Dis. 134:15-24, 1976.
37. Sack, R.B.: Enterohemorrhagic *Escherichia coli*. New Eng. J. Med. 317:1535-1537, 1987.
38. Pedersen, N.C.: Feline Infectious Diseases. American Veterinary Publications Inc, Goleta, CA, 1988.
39. Abaas, S. and Franklin, A.: Shigella-like toxin production from *Escherichia coli* associated with cat diarrhea. Abstracts World Vet Congress XIII, Montreal, Canada, 167, 1987.
40. Rhoades, H.E., et al: Serological identification of *Escherichia coli* isolated from cats and dogs. Can. J. Comp. Med. 35:218-223, 1971.
41. Wilkinson, G.T.: Diseases of the Cat and Their Management. Blackwell Scientific, Melbourne, 1984.
42. Oslon, P., Hedhammar, A. and Waddstrom, T.: Enterotoxigenic *Escherichia coli* infection in two dogs with acute diarrhea. JAVMA 184:982-983, 1984.
43. Moss, S. and Frost, A.J.: The resistance to chemotherapeutic agents of *Escherichia coli* in dogs and cats. Aust. Vet. J. 61:82-84, 1984.
44. Morse, E.V. and Duncan, M.A.: Salmonellosis - An environmental problem affecting animals and man. Proc. 78th Annual Meeting U.S. Animal Health Assoc. 288-299, 1974.
45. Morse, E.V. and Duncan, M.A.: Canine Salmonellosis: Prevalence, epizootiology, signs, and public health significance. JAVMA 167:817-820, 1975.
46. Morse, E.V., Duncan, M.A., Estep, D.A., Riggs, W.A. and Blackburn, B.O.:Canine Salmonellosis-A review and report of dog to child transmission of Salmonella enteritis. Am. J. Public Health 66:82-84, 1976.
47. Uhaa, I.J., Hird, D.W., Hirsh, D.C. and Jang, S.S.: Case-control study of risk factors associated with nosocomial *Salmonella krefeld* infection in dogs. AJVR 49:1501-1505, 1988.
48. Shimi, A. and Barin, A.: *Salmonella* in cats. J. Comp. Pathol. 87:315-318, 1977.
49. Calvert, C.A. and Leifer, C.E.: Salmonellosis in dogs with lymphosarcoma. JAVMA 180:56-58, 1982.
50. Scott, F.W.: *Salmonella* implicated as a cause of song bird fever. Feline Hlth. Topics 3:5-6, 1988.
51. Dow, S.W., Jones, R.L., Henik, R.A. and Husted, P.W.: Clinical features of salmonellosis in cats: Six cases (1981-1986). JAVMA 194:1464-1466, 1989.
52. Timoney, J.F., Neibert, H.C. and Scott, F.W.: Feline salmonellosis. Cornell Vet. 68:211-219, 1978.
53. Pai, C.H. and Mors, V.: Production of enterotoxin by *Yersinia enteroxolitica*. Infect. Immun. 19:908-911, 1978.
54. Papageorges, M., Higgins, R. and Gosselin, Y.: *Yersinia enterocolitica* enteritis in two dogs. JAVMA 182:618-619, 1983.
55. Vantrappen, G., Agg, H.O., Ponette, E., Geboes, K. and Bertrand, Ph.: *Yersinia* enteritis and enterocolitis: Gastroenterological aspects. Gastroenterology 72:220-227, 1977.
56. Wilson, H.D., McCormick, J.B. and Feeley, J.C.: *Yersinia enterocolitica* infection in a 4 month old infant associated with infection in household dogs. J. Pediatr. 89:767-769, 1976.
57. Varela, G., Perez-Rebelo, R. and Olarte, J.: *Salmonella* and *Shigella* organisms in the intestinal tract of dogs in Mexico City. JAVMA 119:385-386, 1951.
58. Keusch, G.T., Jacewicz, M., Levine, M.M., Hornick, R.B. and Kochwa, S.:Pathogenesis of *Shigella* diarrhea. J. Clin. Invest. 57:194-202, 1976.
59. Carpenter, J.L., Myers, A.M., Conner, M.W., Schelling, S.H., Kennedy, F.A. and Reimann, K.A.: Tuberculosis in five Basset Hounds. JAVMA 192:1563-1568, 1988.
60. Klipstein, F.A., Horowitz, I.R., Engert, R.F. and Schenk, E.A.: Effect of *Klebsiella pneumoniae* enterotoxin on intestinal transport in the rat. J. Clin. Invest. 56:799-807, 1975.
61. Kapral, F.A., O'Brien, A.D., Ruff, P.D. and Drugan, W.J., Jr.: Inhibition of water absorption in the intestine by *Staphylococcus aureus* delta-toxin. Infect. Immun. 13:140-145, 1976.
62. Carlson, J.H., Scott, F.W. and Duncan, J.R.: Feline panleukopenia. I. Pathogenesis in germfree and specific pathogen-free cats. Vet. Path. 14:79-88, 1977.
63. England, J.J., Fry, C.S. and Enright, E.A.: Negative contrast electron microscopic diagnosis of viruses of neonatal calf diarrhea. Cornell Vet. 66:172-182, 1976.
64. Keenan, K.P., Jervis, H.R., Marchwicki, R.H. and Binn, L.N.: Intestinal infection of neonatal dogs with canine coronavirus 1-71: Studies by virologic, histologic, histochemical, and immunofluorescent techniques. AJVR 37:247-256, 1976.
65. News: Infectious canine enteritis caused by a coronaviral type virus. JAVMA 173:247-248, 1978.
66. Takeuchi, A., Binn, L.N., Jervis, H.R., Keenan, K.P., Hildebrandt, P.K., Valas, R.B. and Bland, F.F.: Electron microscope study of experimental enteric infection in neonatal dogs with a canine coronavirus. Lab. invest. 34:539-549, 1976.
67. Van kruiningen: The classification of feline colitis. J. Comp. Path. 93:275-294, 1983.
68. Glickman, L.T., Domanski, L.M., Patronek, G.J. and Visintainer, F.: Bred-related risk factors for canine parvovirus enteritis. JAVMA 187:589-594, 1985.
69. Jacobs, R.M., Weiser, M.G., Hall, R.L. and Kowalski, J.J.: Clinicopathologic features of canine parvoviral enteritis. JAAHA 16:809-814, 1980.
70. Pollock, R.V.H.: The parvoviruses. Part II Comp. Cont. Ed. Pract. Vet. 6:653-?1984.
71. Hammond, M.M. and Timoney, R.J.: An electron microscope study of viruses associated with canine gastroenteritis. Cornell Vet. 73:82-97, 1983.
72. Hinshaw, L., et al: Effect of high-dose glucocorticoid therapy on mortality in patients with clinical signs of systemic sepsis. New Eng. J. Med. 317:659-665, 1987.
73. Evermann, J.F., McKeirnan, A.J., Smith, A.W., Skilling, D.E., Ott, R.L.: Isolation and identification of calicivirues from dogs with enteric infections. AJVR 46:218-220, 1985.
74. Mebus, C.A.: Infectious enteric viruses of neonatal animals. J. Clin. Nutr. 30:1851-1856, 1977.
75. Schreiber, D.S., Trier, J.S. and Blacklow, N.R.: Recent advances in ural gastroenteritis. Gastroenterology 73:174-183, 1977.
76. Hoffmann, R. and von Pock, U.: Zur epidemiologie und symptomatologie der parvovirusinfektion des hundes. Praktische tierarzt 62:16-23, 1981.
77. Roseto, A., Lema, F., Cavalieri, F., Dianoux, L., Sitbon, M., F., Lasneret, J. and Peries, J.: Electron microscopy detection and characterization of viral particles in dog stools. Arch. Virology 66:89-93, 1980.
78. McNulty, M.S., Curran, W.L., McFerran, J.B. and Collins, D.S.: Viruses and diarrhea in dogs. Vet. Rec. 106:350-351, 1980.
79. Williams, F.P.: Astrovirus-like, coronavirus-like, and parvovirus-like particles detected in the diarrheal stools of beagle pups. Arch. Virol. 66:215-226, 1980.
80. Marshall, J.A., Healey, D.S., Studdert, M.J., Scott, P.C., Kennett, M.L., Ward, B.K. and Gust, I.D.: Virus and virus-like particles in the faeces of dogs with and without diarrhoea. Aust. Vet. J. 612:33-37, 1984.
81. Vandenberghe, J., et al: Coronavirus infection in a litter of pups. Vet Quarterly 2:136-141, 1980.
82. Chalifoux, A., Elazhary, Y. and Frechette, J.L.: Canine parvovirus enteritis: possible role of endoparasites. Med. Vet. du Quebec 11:66-70, 1981.

83. McNultey, M.S., Allan, G.M., Thompson, D.J. and O'Boyle, J.D.: Antibody to rotavirus in dogs and cats. Vet. Rec. 102:534-535, 1978.
84. Harbour, D.A., Williams, P.D., Gruffydd-Jones, T.J. and Ashley, C.R.: Natural and experimental astrovirus infection of cats. Vet. Rec. 120:555-557, 1987.
85. Snodgrass, D.R., Angus, K.W. and Gray, E.W.: A rotavirus from kittens. Vet. Rec. 104:222-223, 1979.
86. Snodgrass, D.R., Angus, K.W., Gray, E.W., Menzies, J.D. and Paul, G.: Pathogenesis of diarrhea cause by astrovirus infections Arch. Virol. 60:217-226, 1979.
87. Yamamoto, J.K., Hansen, H., Ho, E.W., Morishita, T.Y., et al.: Epidemiologic and clinical aspects of feline immunodeficiency virus infection in cats from the continental United states and Canada and possible mode of transmission. JAVMA 194:213-220, 1989.
88. Reinacher, M.: Feline leukemia virus-associated enteritis. A condition with features of panleukopenia. Vet. Pathol. 24:1-4, 1987.
89. Johnson, C.A., Snider, T.G., Fulton, R.W. and Cho, D.: Gross and light microscopic lesions in neonatal gnotobiotic dogs inoculated with a canine rotavirus. AJVR 44:1687-1693, 1983.
90. Fulton, R.W., Johnson, C.A., Person, N.J. and Woode, G.N.: Isolation of a rotavirus from a newborn dog with diarrhea. AJVR 42:841-843, 1981.
91. Osterhaus, A.D.M.E., Drost, G.A., Wirahadiredja, R.M.S. and van den Ingh, Th.S.G.A.M.: Canine viral enteritis: prevalence of parvo-, corona-,and rotavirus infections in dogs in the Netherlands. Vet. Quarterly 2:181-190, 1980.
92. Oldenburg, V.U., Danner, K. and Krass, H.: Importance of rotavirus infections in the dog. Zentralbatt fur Veterinarmedizin 31:297-302, 1984.
93. Johnson, C.A., Snider, T.G., Henk, W.G. and Fulton, R.W.: A scanning and transmission electron microscopic study of rotavirus-induced intestinal lesions in neonatal gnotobiotic dogs. Vet. Pathol. 23:443-453, 1986.
94. Voderfecht, S.L., Miskuff, R.L., Eiden, J.J. and Yolken, R.H.: Enzyme immunoassay inhibition assay for the detection of rat rotavirus-like agent in intestinal and fecal specimens obtained from diarrheic rats and humans. J. Clin. Micro. 726-730, 1985.
95. Farrar, P.: Personal communication, 1987.
96. Stone, H.H., Geheber, C.E., Kolb, L.D. and Kitchens, W.R.: Alimentary tract colonization by *Candida albicans*. J. Surg. Res. 14:273-276, 1973.
97. Evas, P., Goldstein, M. and Sherlock, P.: *Candida* infection of the gastrointestinal tract. Medicine 51:367-379, 1972.
98. Buttner, D.W. and Matthieseen, B.: Gelangen lebende Hefezellen beim Gesunden regelmassig aus dem dermlungen in die blutbahn? Mykosen 12:387-390, 1969.
99. Anderson, P.G. and Pidgeon, G.: Candidiasis in a dog with parvoviral enteritis. JAAHA 23:27-30, 1987.
100. McClausland, I.P.: Systemic mycoses of two cats. N. Zeal. Vet. J. 20:10-12, 1972.
101. Ossent, P.: Systemic aspergillosis and mucormycosis in 23 cats. Vet. Rec. 120:330-333, 1987.
102. Clinkenbeard, K.D., Cowell, R.L. and Tyler, R.D.: Disseminated histoplasmosis in cats: 12 cases (1981-1986). JAVMA 190:1445-1448, 1987.
103. Stark, D.R.: Primary gastrointestinal histoplasmosis in a cat. JAAHA 18:154-156, 1982.
104. Ader, P.L.: Phycomycosis in fifteen dogs and two cats. JAVMA 174:1216-1223, 1979
105. Stokes, K.: Intestinal mycosis in a cat. Aust. Vet. J. 49:499-500, 1973.
106. Migaki, G., Font, R.L., Sauer, R.M., Kaplan, W. and Miller, R.L.: Canine protothecosis: Review of the literature and report of an additional case. JAVMA 181:794-797, 1982.
107. Roudebush, P.: An updated guide to the chemotherapy of small animal intestinal parasites. Canine Pract. 12:7-20, 1985.
108. Brightman, A.H. and Slonka, G.F.: A review of five clinical cases of giardiasis in cats. JAAHA 12:492-497, 1976.
109. Erlandsen, S.L.: Scanning electron microscopy of intestinal giardiasis:Lesions of the microvillous border of villus epithelial cells produced by trophozoites of giardia. In, Scaning Electron Microscopy/1973. Edited by O. Johari. IIT Research Institute, Chicago, IL, 775-782, 1973.
110. Levine, H.D.: Protozoan Parasites of Domestic Animals and of Man. Second Edition. Minneapolis, Minnesota, Burgess Publishing, 1973.
111. Petersen, H.: Giardiasis (lambliasis). Scand. J. Gastroent. 7, suppl. 14:1-44, 1972.
112. Roberts-Thomson, I.C., Stevens, D.P., Mahmoud, A.A.F. and Warren, K.S.:Giardiasis in the mouse: An animal model. Gastroenterology 71:57-61, 1976.
113. Wittnich, C: Entamoeba histolytica infection in a German Shepherd dog. Can. Vet. J. 17:259-262, 1976
114. Kirkpatrick, C.E.: Feline giardiasis: A review. J. Sm. An. Pract. 27:69-80, 1986.
115. Baker, D.G., Strombeck, D.R. and Gershwin, L.J.: JAVMA 190:53-56, 1987
116. Hahn, N.E., Glaser, C.A., Hird, D.W. and Hirsch, D.C.: Prevalence of *Giardia* in the feces of pups. JAVMA 192(10):1428-1429, 1988.
117. Zimmer, J.F.: Treatment of feline giardiasis with metronidazole. Cornell Vet. 77:383-388, 1987.
118. Zimmer, J.F. and Burrington, D.B.: Comparison of four protocols for the treatment of canine giardiasis. JAAHA 22:168-172, 1986.
119. Kirkpatrick, C.E. and Farrell, J.P.: Feline giardiasis: observations on natural and experimental transmission. Am. J. Vet. Res. 45:2182-2188, 1984.
120. Bailey, E.M.: Emergency and general treatment of poisonings. In, Current Veterinary Therapy. Edited by R.W. Kirk. W.B. Saunders, Philadelphia, 116-125, 1989.
121. Clark, M.L.: Poisoning. In, Canine Medicine and Therapeutics. Edited by E.A. Chandler, J.B. Sutton, D.J. Thompson. Blackwell Scientific, Oxford, 482-498, 1984.

Chapter 19

Acute Hemorrhagic Enterocolitis and Gastroenteritis

ACUTE HEMORRHAGIC GASTROENTERITIS (HGE)

Clinical Synopsis

Diagnostic features.

* Peracute onset of vomiting and bloody diarrhea
* Often aged between 2-4 years
* Toy and miniature breeds predisposed
* Vaccination history, environment and age help rule out parvovirus and toxic causes
* Usually do not appear dehydrated
* PCV very high; 60-75 in most

Standard treatment

* NPO 2-3 days
* Lactated Ringers solution 45-90 ml/hr within the first hour; thereafter maintenance rates
* Trimethroprim-sulfa 15 mg/kg q 12 h SC and then PO for 3-5 days; or Ampicillin 20 mg/kg q 8 h IV and then PO for 3-5 days

---

Small animals can develop acute hemorrhage enterocolitis or gastroenteritis for which there is no apparent cause. This entity is often merely a more severe manifestation of acute diarrhea. Many cases of acute hemorrhagic enterocolitis, however, have unique features that warrant discussing it as a separate entity. Although animals usually recover from acute hemorrhagic enterocolitis, the problem is important because a significant number do not survive despite prompt and vigorous treatment.

Acute hemorrhagic enterocolitis usually appears in adult dogs two to four years old.[1] Incidence appears to be a greater than expected in Miniature Schnauzers, Dachshunds, and small Poodles, and greatest in Schnauzers. The incidence is much lower in large dogs. Dogs developing acute hemorrhagic enterocolitis have usually been restricted to their home environment and have had not contact with other animals. The problem occurs in dogs receiving the best care, following a daily routine in its eating habits and living in an environment that is remarkable constant from day to day.

ETIOLOGY AND PATHOGENESIS

The cause of acute hemorrhagic enterocolitis is not known. There is no evidence that a transmissible infectious agent is involved. Cultures of diseased tissues do not reveal any pathogens. The problem appears randomly in animals that live in relative isolation, which suggests that acute hemorrhagic enterocolitis is not a contagious disease caused by an infectious agent. The great number of microorganisms in the normal colonic microflora are opportunists and can invade the body when acute inflammation of the colonic mucosa causes it to lose its function as a barrier. Thus, these organisms can be cultured form the tissues of animals dying from acute hemorrhagic enterocolitis, but that is not evidence that they initiate the process. It is possible that bacterial invasion is an important factor in the progression of lesions to their severest form. Pathogenic bacteria, if found in the colon with acute hemorrhagic enterocolitis, could not be attributed to the pathogenesis since the known pathogens cause different pathological changes. Invasive organisms such as *Salmonella, Shigella, E. coli*, and enterotoxigenic bacteria do not cause as striking morphological changes in the mucosa as seen with acute hemorrhagic gastroenteritis. Endotoxins cause some changes but they are more likely secondary effects following endotoxin absorption from the diseased bowel. There are no toxins (other than chemical) that cause the pattern of lesions seen with this disease. Dietary factors are an unlikely cause, since most dogs have been on an unchanging diet.

The clinical and pathological features of acute hemorrhagic enterocolitis suggest that the most likely basis for its pathogenesis is an abnormal immune response. This is based on the exclusion of other causes through lack of evidence. infectious, toxic, or dietary factors cannot be incriminated in naturally occurring acute hemorrhagic enterocolitis, and they are not able to cause the disease in experimental animals. The pathology produced by any of these etiologic agents is different from that of acute hemorrhagic enterocolitis. There are several experimental models of acute enterocolitis that are similar to the naturally occurring hemorrhagic variety.

Hemorrhagic enteritis consistently develops in dogs with experimentally produced hemorrhagic shock. Hemorrhagic lesions do not develop unless blood is reinfused during the irreversible stage. When blood is not reinfused, the intestine remains ischemic, and hemorrhagic enteritis does not develop.[2] One can speculate that other stresses, such as trauma, cold, infection, and endotoxin, could cause vascular changes that produce hemorrhagic enteritis. In this case, the pathogenesis of the lesion would involve an initial ischemia followed by tissue necrosis and hemorrhage. Such changes can be produced by intravenous administration of bacterial endotoxins to cause immediate intestinal ischemia[3] and severe mucosal congestion with hemorrhage within 24 hours.[4] Some situations may result in high concentrations of endotoxin in the intestinal lumen, which could provide the conditions for absorption of significant amounts, resulting in mucosal ischemia, necrosis, and hemorrhage. Accumulation of gut endotoxin is seen in at least one clinical situation. Obstruction of the small intestine causes fluid to accumulate cranial to the obstruction, and this fluid contains lethal amounts of endotoxin.[4] Hemorrhagic enteritis does not develop, suggesting that endotoxins are not readily absorbed from the intestine. Endotoxins are not absorbed until after the bowel becomes ischemic, and only then do they cause all the effects of endotoxic shock. Thus, it is unlikely that endotoxin is absorbed as the primary cause of acute hemorrhagic enterocolitis; instead, its absorption is secondary to the damage to the mucosal barrier. Severe ischemia produces endotoxemia almost immediately, indicating that reduced mesenteric blood flow does not interfere with toxin absorption. Endotoxin is absorbed from the peritoneal cavity after leaving the gut, and it reaches the liver via the systemic circulation.[5]

Shock producing intestinal ischemia could initiate acute hemorrhagic enterocolitis. Shock due to severe trauma, however, seldom results in this type of bowel pathology. In addition, experimental models used to study shock-induced bowel ischemia do not produce the same type of lesion. A necrotizing lesion is produced, not a hemorrhagic lesion. One model uses very young animals to reproduce a type of problem seen in newborn infants,[6] while another involves ligating the arterial supply to the colon and making the animal hypovolemic.[7] In all experimentally induced hemorrhagic enterocolitis, shock is produced first; thus, systemic signs of shock are evident before signs of diarrhea. In naturally occurring hemorrhagic enterocolitis, bloody diarrhea is evident before signs of shock. If the problem were secondary to the shock and subsequent ischemia, signs of shock would precede the diarrhea. The appearance of shock as a secondary event and the pathologic dissimilarity between acute hemorrhage enterocolitis and intestinal ischemia make the latter an unlikely primary event.

Clinical cases of canine hemorrhagic enterocolitis are most likely immune-mediated problems. They most closely resemble

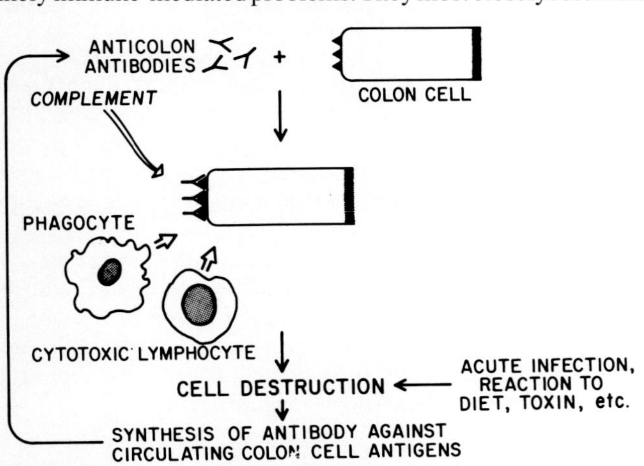

Figure 19-1. Colonic cell destruction by anticolon antibodies. Can be created in experimental animal by injection of anticolon antibodies. Is also initiated by acute diarrhea due to many different causes. Disease process is perpetuated as shown in positive feedback cycle. Minimization of cell destruction necessary to break cycle.

some experimentally induced models of immune-mediated colitis in dogs.[8-10] These are the only immune-mediated experimental models that produce a hemorrhagic enteritis. Different kinds of intestinal lesions are produced when other types of immune responses are stimulated in animals. Hemorrhagic lesions are produced by antibodies against canine colonic antigens produced in rabbits. Injection of antibodies into normal dogs causes diarrhea. Severe mucosal hemorrhage and varying degrees of necrosis are consistently seen in most dogs. Some animals develop watery diarrhea following the initial injection of antibodies, and reinjection some months later produces severe hemorrhagic lesions. In one model, dogs develop hemorrhagic jejunitis and colitis with massive rectal bleeding with a second injection of antibodies is given 24 hours after an initial one that caused no reaction.

Inflammatory reactions begin within two hours of the administration of anticolon antibodies. Microscopic lesions consistent in all models include necrosis, ulceration, marked infiltration by inflammatory cells, congestion, and hemorrhage. In one study, dogs had recurring episodes of watery or bloody diarrhea for as long as a year after the initial injection.[9] The patterns seen resembled those of naturally occurring cases of recurring enterocolitis. Serum anticolon antibody levels were elevated as long as the dogs had recurring episodes. Passive immunity from antibody injections disappears by three weeks. Thus, antibodies found six months or a year later are synthesized by the dog. The severity of the recurring colitis correlated with the serum levels of anticolon antibodies. When dogs were reinjected with a dose of anticolon antibodies similar to that which produced the initial acute hemorrhagic enterocolitis, the pathology was more severe than in the initial episode, causing death within 48 hours, if the dogs were not treated.

Fulfilling Koch's postulates for attribution of an immunogenic etiology requires that this disease must be induced in experimental animals by injection of antibodies. This criterion is fulfilled since anticolon antibodies precipitate acute hemorrhagic enterocolitis. Anticolon antibodies bind colonic cell antigens, and the complexes formed can: 1) fix and activate complement to cause cell lysis; 2) cause phagocytosis of the cell through opsonic (Fc) or immune (C_3) adherence; and 3) cause cytotoxic attack by normal lymphoid cells. Thus, the response initiates a positive feedback that perpetuates the problem, as diagrammed in Figure 19-1. Management of this problem must consider that a vicious cycle can be perpetuated and that an extended period may be required before relapses cease and anticolon antibodies disappear. The antibodies are not specific exclusively for colonic tissue. They cross-react to an equal degree with ileum and jejunal antigens.

It is uncertain how dogs could be come sensitized, allowing acute enterocolitis to develop. A dietary ingredient could initially cause subtle mucosal changes too mild to cause diarrhea but releasing colonic antigens. The colonic bacteria may play an important role. Some bacteria stimulate synthesis of antibodies that can react to colonic antigens, and thereby may sensitize a dog.

The susceptibility of animals to antibody-mediated pathologic changes varies with the species. Acute hemorrhagic enterocolitis cannot be produced experimentally in some laboratory animals, such as the guinea pig. Within the canine species not all breeds show the same incidence of disease. As stated earlier, the Miniature Schnauzer is the most susceptible. This may represent a genetic defect that is retained and harms the animal. Antibody production is controlled by genes that function through the immunocytes, each of which produces only a few different antibodies. The immunocyte that would synthesize anticolon antibodies is abnormal and would cause destruction of the animal. The normal animal tolerates its own antigens and does not produce antibodies against them. If a few such abnormal cells survive and are passed down through the generations the animal is able to produce clones that generate antibodies against its own tissues.

CLINICAL FINDINGS

Clinical findings with acute hemorrhagic enterocolitis are variable, especially the severity and duration of signs. Severe bloody diarrhea can appear and spontaneously go in remission within 24 hours in untreated dogs. More often, bloody diarrhea persists and becomes more severe. The feces often look like dark raspberry jam. In some cases the diarrhea is not noted by the owner; instead, the chief complaints are anorexia and severe depression that began abruptly less than eight hours earlier. The problem is identified in such dogs by finding dark-red blood on the rectal thermometer. Vomiting and any of the secondary signs can be seen. The history usually does not reveal any changes in diet, environment, animal contact or daily routine. Physical findings usually reveal a well-cared-for dog that appears to have been in good health. Some may show signs of shock by rapid weak pulse and poor capillary refill time.

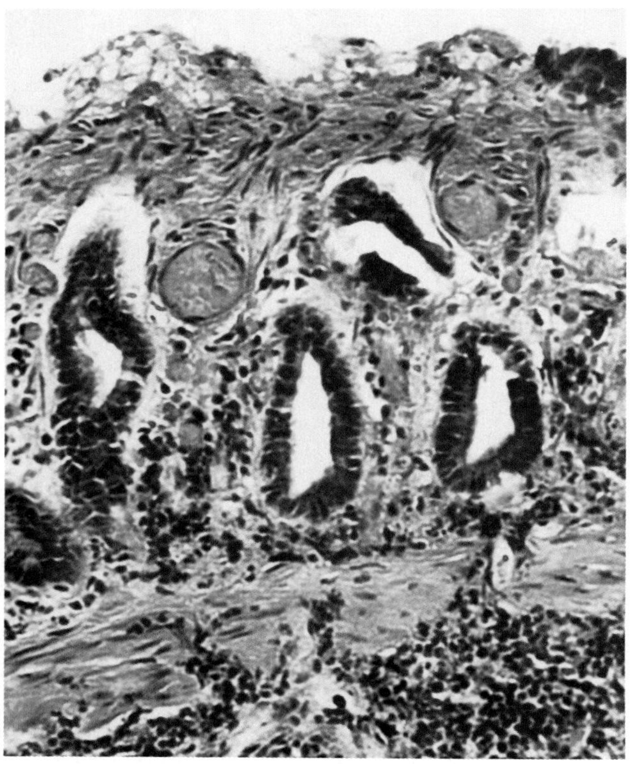

Figure 19-2. Acute necrotizing colitis: Biopsy specimen shows necrosis and desquamation of epithelium and lamina propria, plasma cell infiltration of lamina propria, necrosis in submucosal lymphoid nodules.

Abdominal palpation often reveals the colon to be enlarged, doughy, and sensitive to manipulation. Rectal examination identifies the characteristic dark bloody feces. The physical examination is otherwise usually unremarkable.

LABORATORY FINDINGS

The need for laboratory evaluation of the patient with acute hemorrhage gastrointestinal disease is based on the clinical and physical findings. With bleeding and few indications that the problem is serious, a minimum of further evaluation is needed. Very depressed and shocky dogs should be investigated for complications. A hemogram to evaluate for fluid losses usually shows elevated hematocrit and plasma proteins. The hemogram sometimes shows a degenerative left shift, with toxic leukocytes.

Measurement of serum electrolytes can show changes from the loss of fluid into the intestine and from shock. The fluid lost into the intestine contains higher concentrations of potassium and bicarbonate than plasma, and its loss can produce hypokalemia and acidosis. Acidosis is also produced by shock but causes potassium to leave cells and produce a hyperkalemia. Tissue destruction also causes escape of potassium from damaged cells. The net effect of these two influences on potassium metabolism is to cause depletion of total body potassium. Plasma potassium levels do not reflect the total body deficit of potassium, and they can be high, low, or normal.

Results of blood chemistry reveal secondary changes. Increased serum alanine transaminase activity indicates liver-cell damage that can be caused by toxins absorbed from the gut and by hypoxia developing from shock-induced hepatic ischemia. Increased blood urea nitrogen reflects prerenal uremia caused by reduced renal blood flow. Measurement of urine production often reveals oliguria.

Circulation in the critically ill patient is evaluated by measurement of arterial blood pressure and central venous pressure, both of which are often decreased.

Bleeding patients should be evaluated for coagulopathies since disseminated intravascular coagulation (DIC) can be a cause or a complication. Decreased platelet numbers, reduced fibrinogen content, and prolonged activated clotting time[11] identify DIC as a problem. Radiographic procedures are of little value in providing useful information on bleeding lesions in the small and large intestine. Proctoscopy yields no useful additional information, and there is the possibility that proctoscopy will damage the mucosa further.

Gross pathologic findings include marked congestion of parts of the entire intestinal tract. The mucosa is dark-reddish-black in affected areas. Hemorrhage is found in the lumen. Histology shows marked autolysis, which precludes the provision of useful information. In less severe cases colon biopsy can be used to evaluate the changes (Figure 19-2).

MANAGEMENT

Successful management of acute hemorrhagic enterocolitis depends on minimizing bacterial invasion of the body and managing shock and fluid derangements. Specific treatment includes corticosteroids for shock, and heparin for DIC. Motility modifiers are of little value, and intestinal protectives are of no value. Dietary management is important during recovery.

Antimicrobial Therapy

Antibiotics are always used to treat acute hemorrhagic enterocolitis since the barrier that protects against bacterial invasion is lost. The antibiotics used must be effective against anaerobes, which make up 99.9% of the colonic microflora. Penicillin is the best choice since it is effective against anaerobes in the canine colon, is bactericidal, and does not disrupt the normal microflora so as to allow one species to overgrow and become a pathogen. Penicillin is given parenterally to minimize invasion. Trimethoprim sulfa combinations also have a broad spectrum of activity against anaerobes, and aerobes as well, and they minimally disrupt the intestinal microflora. Ampicillin and amoxicillin are also effective against anaerobes, but they are highly disruptive of the normal microflora. Metronidazole, an antimicrobial with broad activity against intestinal anaerobes, can be used for preventing or treating sepsis.

The aerobes constitute only 0.1% of the total colonic bacteria but include some important types, such as the coliforms. Aerobes produce both endotoxins and enterotoxins. Endotoxins contribute to shock after their absorption from the gut.[11] Unfortunately, aerobes can rapidly develop resistance to antibiotics, making it difficult to generalize on use of a single likely effective antibiotic. Most aerobes are resistant to streptomycin and kanamycin. Other antibiotics effective against aerobes have the disadvantage of being expensive, toxic, or damaging to the normal microflora. Some with nephrotoxic effects, such as gentamicin, should not be given when renal function is reduced by shock. Gentamicin, an effective antibiotic against aerobes, is used when the patient's condition is critical and it is essential to control invasion by aerobes. First generation cephalosporins have limited effectiveness against intestinal aerobes. Fluoroquinolones can be very effective and without an effect to cause the appearance of resistant strains. Clindamycin can also be effective but with the disruption of the normal microflora. These antibiotics are all given by injection. Unabsorbed antibiotics given orally, such as neomycin, are of no value. Many intestinal bacteria are resistant to neomycin, and that antibiotic can damage the mucosa further. The goal of antibiotic therapy is to treat against bacterial invasion, not to sterilize the intestine. In summary, it is unknown how the normal microflora contributes to the pathogenesis and pathology in acute hemorrhagic gastroenteritis. Animals in experimental studies are seldom treated with antibiotics, yet they recover within a matter of days. Some clinical cases die so rapidly that it seems unlikely that a peracute bacteremia or septicemia could contribute to the fatal outcome. There is no doubt, however, that antibiotics should be given, and drugs are selected that are effective against both anaerobes and aerobes in the gut.

Fluid Therapy

Management of fluid and electrolyte derangements is often more important than all other treatments for acute hemorrhagic enterocolitis. When serum electrolytes are measured, the fluids used can be tailored to meet the animal's needs. With no measurements, the fluid used is the one most likely to replace the losses. Fluid lost into the intestine is similar to extracellular fluid and is replaced with a balanced electrolyte solution such as Ringers or lactated Ringers solution. If hyperkalemia exists where electrolytes are not measured, the administration of Ringers containing potassium at a level of 4 mEq/L does not increase serum potassium levels but reduces them. Thus, with suspected hyperkalemia a balanced solution is still indicated since potassium depletion is a problem. With hypokalemia the amount of potassium in a balanced solution may be inadequate to replace the total-body deficits. The renal losses of potassium are accelerated with hypovolemia and may be of such magnitude that large amounts of Ringers solution must be given for replacement. In anorectic animals, the administration of balanced solutions is not adequate to replace the continuous normal losses of potassium. Potassium therapy is usually not necessary with anorexia of a few days. With resumption of feeding, potassium intake resumes and body deficits are repaired. Specific therapy to repair potassium deficits is not usually required early in the disease.

Balanced electrolyte solutions are administered only by the intravenous route. With hypovolemia and shock, fluids are given at rates and in amounts determined by monitoring the character and rate of the pulse and the central venous pressure. Administration of fluids is sometimes different to animals in shock from that to dehydrated animals. If the animal is in shock and there is no question that fluids should be given, they are administered until the central venous pressure increases, regardless of the initial pressure before fluids are given.[12] Even if the pressure is higher than normal, fluids are given until an increment is observed. In general, animals that require fluid therapy are more often undertreated than overtreated. A fear of producing pulmonary edema frequently causes insufficient amounts of fluids to be used. The effectiveness of restoring fluid deficits and returning circulatory function to normal can be assessed also by measuring urine production. Arterial blood pressure is not as sensitive an indicator of the size of the extracellular fluid compartment as the central venous pressure.

Modified balanced solutions are sometimes indicated. Acute shock in animals is treated more effectively with Ringers containing 5% dextrose.[13] The use of dextrose and water or dextrose in a solution that does not contain potassium is contraindicated since the monosaccharide aggravates any existing hypokalemia. Solutions containing glucose and without potassium can be used only when serum electrolytes are measured to identify hyperkalemia.

Bicarbonate is used to correct acidosis. It should be given only to replace deficits calculated from measured plasma bicarbonate concentrations. Bicarbonate is normally not given empirically to treat a hypothetical acidosis in hemorrhagic enterocolitis. There is little reason to give bicarbonate to replace small deficits estimated to be 5 mEq/L.

After several days, potassium replacement therapy may become important. Serum potassium levels are used as an aid in replacing deficits. Extracellular fluid potassium represents less than 2% of all potassium in the body. Concentrations are 30 times lower in the plasma than in cells. Thus, serum potassium levels do not necessarily reflect total-body stores. Deficits develop in anorectic animals from ongoing renal losses and are magnified by losses of intestinal fluid. To replace major deficits, potassium can be added to Ringers solution to a final concentration of 44 mEq/L (by adding a vial of 40 mEq KCl to a liter of Ringers) and the fluid administered at 1 mEq per pound of body weight per hour. The amount to give can be estimated by monitoring electrocardiograms or by serial measurement of plasma electrolyte levels. Deficits of potassium in extracellular fluid can be calculated from plasma levels and estimation that body weight is four times as great. It may require up to five times this calculated extracellular fluid deficit of potassium to restore plasma levels to normal with fluids given slowly over two hours. That is possible because potassium enters the cell rapidly. The movement of potassium into cells is facilitated by glucose and bicarbonate, which are sometimes added to minimize any hazards of giving potassium. In general, the most common error in potassium therapy is under treatment because of an old fear of the toxic effects of the potassium ion.

Corticosteroids

Corticosteroids are frequently used to treat acute hemorrhagic gastroenteritis or enterocolitis. Although corticosteroids have not been shown to affect survival rate in animals with shock, they ameliorate some of the changes that contribute to the shock syndrome. Corticosteroids also depress the natural defense mechanisms and handicap the ability to respond to bacterial invasion from the gut. The use of corticosteroids to treat shock may have an effect on later complications. Steroids used on humans in shock greatly reduce the incidence of gastric ulcer formations.[14] Steroids are given at doses up to one mg per pound body weight, which can be repeated every six hours.

Adjunct Therapy

Motility modifiers and intestinal protectives, often used to treat acute hemorrhagic enterocolitis, are of little benefit. The goal in using intestinal protectives is to protect the severely damaged mucosa from the normal contents of the intestine. Bacteria are invading, and in sections of the intestine where stasis exists they are multiplying and producing many types of toxins. The mucosa is severely damaged by the initial insult, and the presence of bacteria, toxins, and pancreatic proteases[15] contributes to the problem by determining the final severity of the insult and the speed with which the mucosa returns to normal. Experimental studies show that other forms of treatment can be used to protect the intestinal mucosa. Necrosis and inflammation of the mucosa can be produced by acute and complete ischemia lasting for two hours. When the loop of ischemic intestine is perfused with any type of solution there is good protection against the development of pathological changes.[16] The addition of glucose to the perfusate provides substrate for the ischemic tissue to survive, and protection produced by perfusion is augmented further.[17,18] Thus, bathing the mucosal surface reduces the ability of the normal intestinal microflora to damage the mucosa further. Hence, an ideal goal of treatment is to simulate this perfusion. This effect is produced by enemas and by cathartics given orally to clean out the gastrointestinal tract. They were once a part of common treatment for diarrhea. The perfusion can be mimicked by giving a balanced electrolyte solution orally in amounts that exceed the absorptive capacity of the intestine. Saline cathartics such as magnesium sulfate and sodium phosphate can be used for the purpose.

Motility modifiers of any type are better not used. Anticholinergics reduce motility further in the already hypomotile intestine. The loss of motility ranges from stasis in a single segment to paralytic ileus involving the entire intestine. Hypomotility results in bacterial multiplication and the production of toxins. Motility modifiers to stimulate rhythmic segmentation may also be contraindicated in dogs with acute hemorrhagic enterocolitis. These drugs, the opioids, retard the passage of contents, and if the stasis produced is sufficient, undesired effects are produced. Thus, the desired goal is to have the mucosa washed down, but either of the motility modifiers can interfere with that. Persistent fluid loss from the colon is not a devastating problem, since fluids are easily replaced. In humans, the motility modifiers are either ineffective or are contraindicated or both in the management of very acute enterocolitis.[19,20]

Intestinal protectives such as pectin or kaolin are misnomers in that they do not coat the mucosal surface of the intestine and protect it. The only manner by which some of these agents are effective is if they have properties to bind and inactivate bacteria and toxins. Chemicals with these binding properties include some of the antacids. Plant fiber is also capable of binding toxins in addition to absorbing water.[21] A resin, cholestryamine, binding bile acids and preventing their toxic effect on the colonic mucosa has been used to treat diarrhea.[22]

Patients recognized as developed coagulopathies as a complication are treated accordingly. Disseminated intravascular coagulation (DIC) is treated with heparin. If liver failure is a complication that initiates the coagulopathy and if the liver is unable to respond with the synthesis of clotting factors, the latter must be replaced by administering plasma before the animals are treated with heparin. DIC is treated by giving heparin at 100 units per kg body weight, repeated every six to eight hours.

Diet and Recovery of Function

The dietary management of patients with acute hemorrhagic enterocolitis is based on how rapidly the mucosa regains its integrity and functions. Mucosal integrity is important to minimizing the absorption of antigens in the colon. Feeding should not begin before the mucosal functions are renewed. The length of time for recovery of normal function has been studied in the dog following complete ischemia of the colon and small intestine for one to two hours.[16,23,24] Pathologic changes in acute hemorrhagic enterocolitis are comparable. Immediate changes in experimental dogs are severe, including necrosis and desquamation of villus tips, edema, vascular stasis, and hemorrhage in the lamina propria. Dye injected intra-arterially reveals that there is no circulation to the villi. Within 24 hours the mucosa has regained almost complete normal histological appearance, and circulation is almost normal again. The ileum is more sensitive than the colon to the effects of ischemia, but its mucosa returns to a normal appearance more rapidly. Mucosal functions return quite rapidly. Net absorption of fluid and nutrients is apparent in 24 hours, and within three days the regenerated mucosa has fully regained normal function except that function for water and ion absorption requires a week to return.

The normal colon absorbs small amounts of intact proteins at a rate only one-tenth of that in the small intestine.[25] The absorption of antigens in colonic contents increases with colonic inflammation or following trauma to the intestine such as surgery. Dietary proteins are antigenic, as can be shown by the consistent appearance of circulating antibodies synthesized against specific dietary antigens. The antigens escape processing by the local immune mechanisms, overwhelmed during the acute problem, and they reach the systemic circulation. The choice of a diet to feed an animal with acute hemorrhagic enterocolitis and the time that feeding is resumed become important when it is apparent that the animal is in a state where it can be readily "immunized" against nutrients that are antigenic. A usual observation made on the lifelong history of an animal that has had a bout with acute hemorrhagic enterocolitis is that the patient was originally able to eat all varieties of foods, both table and commercial preparations. After the acute bout, however, the animal cannot tolerate many foods previously tolerated. At the time of the acute attack these animals develop sensitivities that are most likely related to the absorption of abnormal amounts of dietary antigens. It is not possible to determine whether the sensitization occurs by antigens in the gut at the time of the acute attack or by antigens introduced too early in the recovery phase. The former possibility is more likely, though the antigens introduced during later stages should be controlled. As the first step, this problem is solved by feeding nutrients that are nonantigenic. Purified carbohydrates fit that requirement and can be fed as a solution of glucose, oligosaccharides, or starches. Proteins are antigenic. The type to choose should be one that is not likely to have constituted a major part of the animal's diet in the past. This reduces the possibilities of feeding foods that the animal developed sensitivity to at an earlier date. Meat protein such as lamb, being seldom fed, meets the requirements. This procedure also reduces the chances that the animal will develop a sensitivity to a major ingredient of a diet likely to be fed in the future. Another means of supplying nitrogen in a form that is minimally antigenic or nonantigenic is to feed a hydrolysate of protein. Products that are enzymatically hydrolyzed contain peptides that may still be antigenic but are absorbed more efficiently and are less expensive than mixtures consisting only of pure amino acids. There is no great urgency about restoring nitrogen intake in an animal with severe intestinal lesions. Protein should be withheld from the diet until four to five days after the acute clinical signs of the bleeding problem subside. Fats are not added to the diet until later.

PROGNOSIS

Clinical cases are like experimental dogs with acute hemorrhagic enterocolitis in that they both have recurring problems that persist for indeterminate periods. Management of this problem is similar to that for chronic colitis. Long term successful management is based on control of the diet rather than medications. All measures are used to prevent or minimize colonic inflammation. Inability to maintain complete remission is associated with indefinite persistence of the problem. As with the experimental cases, the naturally occurring disease may show complete and lasting remission a variable number of months after the acute bout. In some dogs, clinical signs of vomiting, diarrhea, and anorexia will reappear at an interval of days to weeks. Without effective management the interval shortens and instead of the problem cycling, the problem becomes continuous. The basis for the worsening is unknown.

REFERENCES

1. Burrows, C.F.: Canine hemorrhagic gastroenteritis. JAAHA 12:492-497, 1976.
2. Swan, H. and Nelson, A.W.: Experimental lethal canine hemorrhage:Ischemic abdominal viscera; absence of hemorrhagic gut or portal congestion. J. Surg. Res. 11:620-628, 1971.
3. Brungardt, J.M., Reynolds, D.G. and Swan, K.G.: Route of endotoxin delivery: Effects on canine mesenteric hemodynamics. Am. J. Physiol. 223:565-568, 1972.
4. Weipers, W.L., Hagy, L., Pirie, H.M., Sanford, J. and Pillinger, R.: A comparison of the toxic effects of intestinal obstruction fluid with those of certain endotoxins. J. Path. 110:295-304, 1973.
5. Cuevas, P. and Fine, J.: Route of absorption of endotoxin from the intestine in nonseptic shock. J. Reticuloendothelial Soc. 11:535-538, 1972.
6. Barlow, B. and Santulli, T.V.: Importance of multiple episodes of hypoxia or cold stress on the development of enterocolitis in an animal model. Surgery 77:687-690, 1975.
7. Matthews, J.G.W. and Parks, T.G.: Ischaemic colitis in the experimental animal. Gut 17:677-684, 1976.
8. Bicks, R.O. and Walker, R.H.: Immunologic "colitis" in dogs. Am. J. Dig. Dis. 7:574-584, 1962.
9. LeVeen, H.H., Falk, G. and Schatman, B.: Experimental ulcerative colitis produced by anticolon sera. Ann. Surg. 154:275-280, 1961.
10. Shean, F.C., Barker, W.F. and Fonkalsrud, E.W.: Studies on active and passive antibody induced colitis in the dog. Amer. J. Surg. 107:337-339, 1964.
11. Jacob, A.I., Goldberg, P.K., Bloom, N., Degenshein, G.A. and Kozinn, P.J.: Endotoxin and bacteria in portal blood. Gastroenterology 72:1268-1270, 1977.
12. Wilson, R.F. and Sibbald, W.J.: A new look at an old approach to resuscitation: Early aggressive fluid administration. Circulatory Shock. 2:1-3, 1975.
13. Hinshaw, L.B.: The role of glucose in endotoxin shock, Circulatory Shock 3:1-10, 1976.
14. ama, R.H., Perman, M.H. and Matsumoto, T.: Incidence of stress ulcer formation associated with steroid therapy in various shock states. Am. J. Surg. 130:328-331, 1975.
15. Bounous, G., Menard, D. and de Medicis, E.: Role of pancreatic proteases in the pathogenesis of ischemic enteropathy. Gastroenterology 73:102-108, 1977.
16. Robinson, J.W.L. and Mirkovitch, V.: The recovery of function and microcirculation in small intestinal loops following ischaemia. Gut 13:784-789, 1972.
17. McArdle, A.H., Chiu, C.-J. and Gurd, F.N.: Intraluminal glucose, substrate for ischemic intestine. Arch. Surg. 105:441-445, 1972.
18. Mirkovitch, V., Menge, H. and Robinson, J.W.L.: Protection of the intestinal mucosa during ischaemia by intraluminal perfusion. Res. Exp. Med. 166:183-191, 1975.
19. DuPont, H.L. and Hornick, R.B.: Adverse effect of Lomotil therapy in shigellosis. JAMA 226:1525-1528, 1973.
20. Portnoy, B.L., DuPont, H.L., Pruitt, D., Abdo, J.A. and Rodriguez, J.T.: Antidiarrheal agents in the treatment of acute diarrhea in children. JAMA 236:844-846, 1976.
21. Brodribb, A.J.M. and Groves, C.: Effect of bran particle size on stool weight. Gut 19:60-63, 1978.
22. Tamer, M.A., Santora, T.R. and Sandberg, D.H.: Cholestyramine therapy for intractable diarrhea. Pediatr. 53:217, 1974.
23. Robinson, J.W.L., Haroud, M., Winistorfer, B. and Mirkovitch, V.: Recovery of function and structure of dog ileum and colon following two hours acute ischaemia. Eur. J. Clin. Invest. 4:443-452, 1974.
24. Robinson, J.W.L., Menge, H., Sepulveda, F.V., Cobo, F., and Mirkovitch, V.: The functional response of the dog ileum to one hour's ischaemia. Clin. Sci. Mol. Med. 50:115-122, 1976.
25. Warshaw, A.L., Bellini, C.A. and Walker, W.A.: The intestinal mucosal barrier to intact antigenic protein: Difference between colon and small intestine. Soc. for Surg. of the Alimen. tract. abstract, 1976, Abs. 76.

Chapter 20

Adverse Reactions to Food

INTRODUCTION

Adverse reactions to food are frequently observed in dogs and cats. They are comprised of a variety of subclassifications including food allergies, food anaphylaxis, food intolerances, food poisoning, food idiosyncrasy, anaphylactoid reactions to food, pharmacologic reactions to food, metabolic adverse reactions to food, and dietary indiscretions. In general, the pathogenic mechanisms that lead to an adverse reaction to food include ingestion of the inciting agent followed by interaction of the agent with a cellular or noncellular biological amplification system that leads to inflammation and the generation of clinical signs (Figure 20-1).[1] The amplification system varies considerably with the inciting agent but may include the immune system, the arachidonic acid cascade, the complement cascade, chemotaxis of phagocytes, and generation of kinins. At times, sufficient toxic material may be present in the food to produce clinical signs without need for amplification.

TERMINOLOGY[2]

The terminology applied to adverse reactions to food is confused. The following terms and definitions are those recommended by the American Academy of Allergy and Immunology.[2] Minor degrees of overlap occur between some of these definitions.

"Adverse reaction to food" is a general term that can be applied to a clinically abnormal response attributed to an ingested food or food additive. Adverse reactions to food are further categorized according to pathomechanism (Figure 20-2).

"Food allergy" (hypersensitivity) (sensitivity) refers to an adverse reaction to a food or food additive with a proven immunologic basis. The reaction occurs only in certain animals, may occur in response to a small amount of ingested substance, and is unrelated to any physiologic effect of the food or food additive. Food allergy is but one cause of adverse reactions to food. The majority of adverse reactions to food in humans are thought *not* to be triggered by immunological mechanisms.[1] The term "food allergy" has been greatly misused in the veterinary literature. While there seems little reason to doubt that food allergies occur in dogs and cats, adequate documentation of an allergic response to food, has rarely been provided in spite of a wealth of literature on the subject.

"Food anaphylaxis" is an acute food allergy with systemic consequences resulting from an IgE-mediated release of chemical mediators. The anaphylaxis is characterized by respiratory distress, vascular collapse, urticaria, pruritus, and angioedema.

"Food intolerance" is a general term describing an abnormal response to an ingested food or food additive that does not have an immunological basis. It includes, idiosyncratic, meta-

Figure 20-1. Pathogenic mechanisms involved in the generation of an adverse reaction to food.

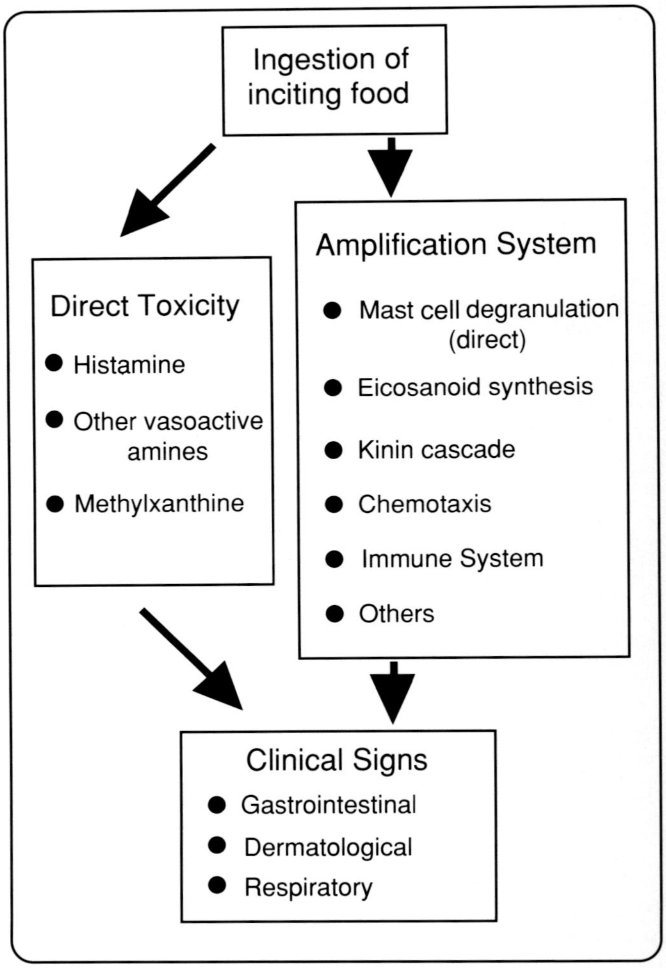

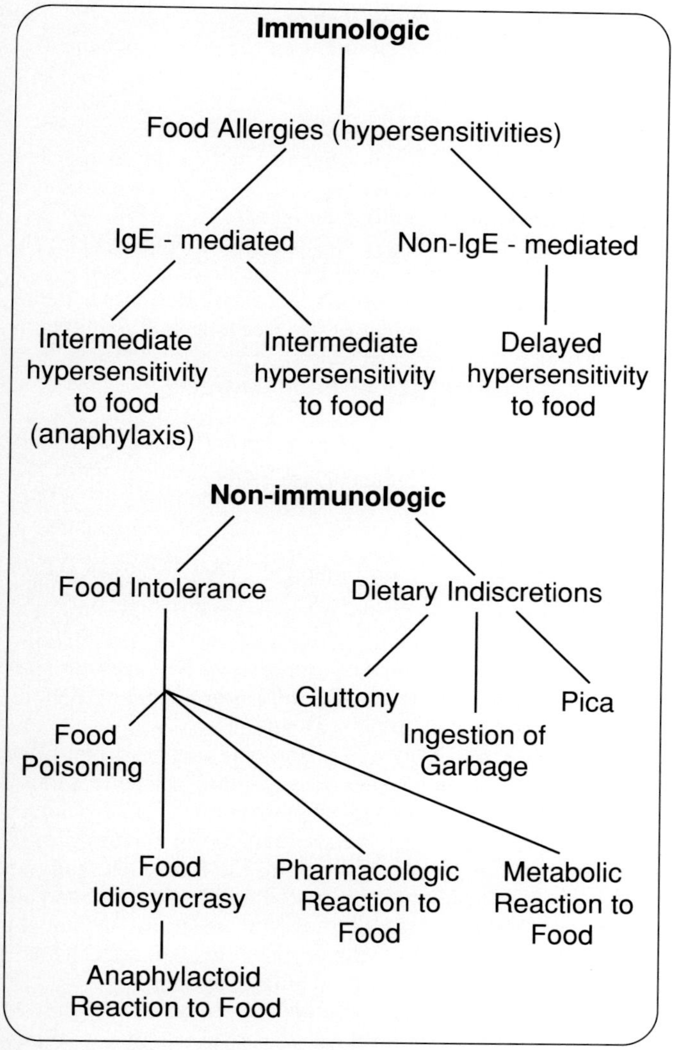

Figure 20-2. Adverse reaction to food.

Figure 20-3 Suggested Protocol for Elimination-Challenge Trials for the Diagnosis of Adverse Reactions to Food

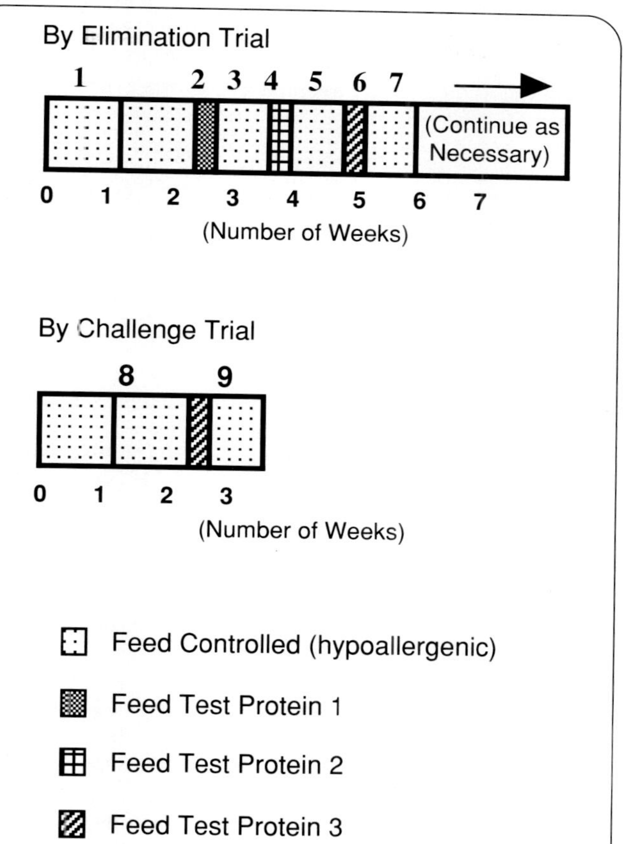

A) Elimination trial

1. Place the patient on a controlled diet of single protein source and a single carbohydrate source until signs resolve. e.g. lamb and boiled white rice, or cottage cheese and rice, or tofu and rice.
2. After 2 symptom-free weeks, add a small quantity (100g) of a protein source to which the patient has been previously exposed, and which may be the cause of the clinical signs, to the controlled diet and feed for 3 days (or less if clinical signs are observed).
3. Observe for clinical signs during the feeding period and for 4 days thereafter.

4-7. If no evidence of clinical abnormality after 4 days, repeat the procedure using another protein or foodstuff every week, until a dietary component is identified that appears to cause clinical signs.

If a prolonged trial becomes necessary supplement the diet with appropriate quantities of vitamins and minerals.

B) Challenge trial

8. After a suspect allergen has been identified, remove the protein from the diet, and observe for evidence of resolution of signs.
9. Wait a minimum of 1-2 weeks from the last ingestion of the suspected allergen and until the patient is symptom free and then, under close observation, challenge the patient again with the suspected allergen to ensure that similar signs are manifest on the second exposure.

bolic, pharmacologic, or toxic responses to foods. Adverse reactions to food with a suspected but not proven immunologic basis, for instance gluten-induced enteropathy, are also sometimes termed food intolerances.

"Food poisoning" results from direct nonimmunologic action on the host of a toxin contained within the food or released by organisms contaminating the food.

"Food idiosyncrasy" is a quantitatively abnormal response to a food substance or additive that resembles a hypersensitivity response but does not involve immune mechanisms. Food idiosyncratic reactions include those which occur in specific groups of individuals who may be genetically predisposed. If the idiosyncratic reaction resembles anaphylaxis (but is nonimmunologic) it is termed an anaphylactoid reaction to food.

"Pharmacologic" reactions to food are adverse reactions as a result of a drug-like or pharmacologic effect in the host. An example of a pharmacologic reaction to food is the adverse reactions of dogs to the methylxanthines in chocolate. "Metabolic" reactions to food are adverse reactions as a result of an effect of the substance upon the metabolism of the host, or as a result of defective metabolism of the nutrient by the host.

"Dietary indiscretion" is a term that overlaps with the term food intolerance. Dietary indiscretions are adverse reactions resulting from such behaviors as gluttony, pica, or ingestion of various indigestible materials or garbage. Gastric dilatation and "garbage can enteritis" are examples of disorders resulting from dietary indiscretions.

CLINICAL SIGNS & DIAGNOSIS OF ADVERSE REACTIONS TO FOOD

Adverse reactions to food are usually suspected when a client or veterinarian establishes an historical association between the ingestion of a certain foodstuff and the appearance of a particular clinical sign or group of signs. The clinical signs are usually dermatological or gastrointestinal but, on occasion, may be respiratory. The diagnosis is confirmed by the resolution of clinical signs after the elimination of a component of the diet followed by recrudescence of the signs when the patient is subsequently challenged with the suspected foodstuff.

A suggested protocol for elimination-challenge trials is listed in Figure 20-3. The constituents of suitable elimination diets are described in the chapter on nutrition. A major disadvantage of challenge trials is that some patients can experience severe reactions to the reexposure. Any patient undergoing a challenge trial must be maintained under close observation and the owner appraised of potential complications.

For complete validity of the trial, the owner and veterinary participants should be blinded as to whether the patient is being challenged with the suspected antigen or a placebo. This involves placing dried, powdered foods in capsules and administering initial doses of between 0.25-50 mg/kg depending on the apparent degree of hypersensitivity. If no reaction occurs within 24 hours, the dose is usually increased to a maximum of 125-250 mg/kg in subsequent tests. Practical constraints have limited the application of such double-blind placebo trials in veterinary medicine, however. This is unfortunate, because the "placebo effect" has been shown to be of great importance in humans participating in food trials,[3] and is also likely to play a role in the reporting by the client or veterinarian of clinical signs expressed by a small animal patient.

To reiterate, such dietary trials confirm or rule out adverse reactions to food. To make a diagnosis of food allergy, the clinician must go on to establish that the adverse reaction to food has an immunologic basis. The latter step is often omitted from the diagnostics because in most patients the management of the case will not be altered whether the clinical signs result from a food allergy or from a food intolerance.

FOOD ALLERGY[4-6]

Clinical Synopsis

Diagnostic features

* Historical association between a particular diet and gastrointestinal, dermatological or multisystemic signs compatible with an adverse reaction to food
* Elimination trial identifies suspect food antigen
* Recrudescence of clinical signs on reexposure
* Documentation of an immunological pathomechanism

Treatment

* Avoidance of the food antigen to which the animal has confirmed hypersensitivity
* Avoidance of related food antigens
* Benadryl (0.5-1.0 mg/kg IV once; 2.0-4.0 mg/kg PO q 8h) for mild to moderate acute to subacute clinical signs
* Epinephrine (0.1-0.5 ml SC, IM, IV of 1:10,000 aqueous solution q 15-20 minutes as required) for food anaphylaxis

Chemistry of Food Antigens

Food allergies are caused by over 6000 antigens.[6] Food allergens are almost exclusively proteins, and in particular glycoproteins with a molecular weight in the range of 18,000-36,000 daltons.[2] Most food allergens are partially resistant to heat and digestion, two properties which help ensure the maintenance of antigenicity. Denaturing of most proteins by heat reduces their antigenicity. Complete enzymatic digestion renders proteins non-antigenic. In contrast, on occasion, incomplete degradation can enhance antigenicity by exposing antigenic determinants. Often only a small component of the total protein component of a food is allergenic.

In humans, a wide variety of antigens have been identified as causing IgE-mediated reactions, including substances found in cow's milk, soybeans, egg white, seafoods, and peanuts. Casein, alpha-lactalbumin, beta-lactoglobulin, bovine gamma globulin, and bovine serum albumin, the five most common proteins in cow's milk are considered highly antigenic and are considered the cause of many allergic reactions in humans including a proctocolitis.[6] Milk protein is also thought by some to be an important cause of food allergy in dogs.[7-9]

Soybean proteins are a potentially important cause of food allergy in dogs because of the widespread use of soy in dog foods and the documented allergenicity of soy proteins in humans and farm animals. In one study of food allergy in dogs, 54% of dogs suspected of food allergy had positive cytotoxic reactions to soy (see below).[7] Soy proteins consist of a globulin and whey fraction. The globulin fraction comprises 85% of the total protein and consists of four subgroups with different sedimentation constants. The 2S globulin subfraction has been found to be the most allergenic.[10] The 2S subfraction is the most heat-stable of the soy globulin fractions. Another allergenic soy protein is a soybean trypsin inhibitor found in the whey fraction. This protein is resistant to acid pH and proteolytic digestion.[2]

Other foods that have been suggested to be prevalent causes of food allergy in dogs include wheat, beef, eggs, horse meat, chicken, corn meal, pork, yeast, and a variety of commercial foods of varying protein base.[7-9,11] In the cat, the foods most often incriminated are similar but also include fish. The validity of these suggestions need to be confirmed. Egg-sensitive humans usually only react to proteins in the egg white.[2] Psyllium is a documented cause of IgE-mediated anaphylaxis in humans.

In some food groups, allergy to one member of the group may result in a variable degree of allergy to other members of the same group. This cross-reactivity is particularly common amongst the seafoods and the legumes, but is less apparent amongst some other foods even when derived from the same species.[2] For example, humans allergic to cows milk can usually tolerate beef. A partial list of foods with an increased likelihood of cross-reactivity are listed in Table 20-1. In humans cross-reactivity between milk and soy hypersensitivity has been reported in spite of the widely different biological origin of these foodstuffs. Other such unexpected cross sensitivities may exist.

Oral Tolerance and Etiopathogenesis of Food Hypersensitivity

The defense against hypersensitivity to dietary antigens is a well developed, multi-tier, system dependent on an effective mucosal barrier in association with oral tolerance generated by the cellular immune system of the gut-associated lymphoid tissue (GALT). The mucosal barrier and oral tolerance are discussed in more detail in Chapters 3, 16, and 21. The following reiterates some of the major points of those discussions pertaining to food allergies.

The first component of the defense against mucosal antigens that may cause food hypersensitivity is an effective mucosal barrier that prevents overwhelming uptake of food antigens. The mucosal barrier is composed of a number of interrelated immunologic and non-immunologic components which include effective digestion (renders proteins non-antigenic); the epithelial cell and its secretions, in particular mucus (mucus glycoproteins act as receptors for the attachment of bacteria and other antigens); IgA; and the mononuclear-phagocyte system (RES) of the liver.[12] Efficient functioning of the mucosal barrier excludes the majority of antigen, thus minimizing the exposure of GALT to reaginic antigens, and minimizing the likelihood that the antigen trapping potential of GALT and the mononuclear-phagocyte systems will be unable to prevent antigen entering the systemic circulation.

Table 20-1 Foods Grouped According to Biological Relationship and Potential Immunologic Cross-Reactivity[2]

BIRDS	**EGGS**	**MILK PRODUCTS**
Chicken	Ovomucoid	Milks
Turkey	Ovovitellin	Milk replacers
Others	White	Creams
BOVIDAE	Yolk	Cheeses
Beef	**FISH**	Cottage cheese
Goat	Salmonidae	Yogurt
Sheep meats	Tuna	Ice cream
Gelatin	Others	Casein and other milk products
Sweatbread	**LEGUMES**	
CEREALS	Peas	**SUIDAE**
Barley	Beans	Bacon
Corn	Lentils	Pork
Oat	Licorice	Ham
Rice	Peanut	Sausage
Rye	Soybean	
Sorghum	Others	
Wheat *		
Others		

*(bran, germ, gliadin, globulin, glutenin, leucosin, proteose)

It is now known that the mucosal barrier is not impervious to macromolecules. Dietary proteins cross the intact small intestinal mucosa of normal animals in small but significant amounts. Up to 2% of fed protein may be absorbed in this way.[13] Some of this protein enters by pinocytosis by the absorptive enterocyte and some passes between cells but it appears, that the majority of absorption occurs by active uptake by the mucosal M cell (see Chapter 3). Much of the antigen absorbed by the enterocyte is degraded intracellularly by lysosomal proteases. A small amount of the antigen may be deposited in the lamina propria where it may stimulate the synthesis of secretory antibodies (IgA) by plasma cells in the lamina propria. The protein absorbed by the M cell is carefully presented as intact antigen to GALT in such a manner that a potent gut-associated, cell-mediated suppressor response to that antigen develops. It is this suppressor response that is the basis of oral tolerance, and may be the primary site of the defect in food allergic animals and people. In addition to the suppressor response, the gut-associated humoral immune system generates IgA antibody which acts to reinforce the mucosal barrier against that antigen, and to eliminate antigen in the lamina propria by forming immune complexes which do not fix complement but which can be taken up by the liver and excreted in the bile. The majority of any antigen that escapes the lamina propria is removed by the mononuclear-phagocytic system of the liver and mesenteric nodes. The prevention of escape of antigens into the systemic circulation is important, because when exposed to gut antigens, the systemic lymphoid tissues do not respond with active immune suppression (tolerance) but rather active immunoreactivity that results in attempted antigen elimination, inflammation, and hypersensitivity.

A food protein, therefore, has the potential to incite an allergic response if it is incompletely digested in the bowel, absorbed across the mucosa intact (or partially intact), and then escapes to the systemic lymphoid tissue. Alternatively, the allergic response may result if the antigen encounters a defective suppressor arm of GALT. In either case, the result is the stimulation of the synthesis of immunoglobulins such as IgE and IgG, and the sensitization of peripheral lymphocytes both of which can go on to generate immunosensitivity to the food antigen rather than tolerance.

In normal animals and people only very small amounts of gut antigens reach the systemic immune system. In normal people, the levels of circulating antibodies to food antigens are low or not measurable. They increase, however, when any of interrelated processes that contribute to exclusion of gut antigens from the systemic circulation and to oral tolerance are compromised. Increased serum antibodies, and in some cases increased food antigen-antibody immune complexes have been clearly demonstrated in human patients with IgA deficiency, portasystemic shunts, and gastrointestinal inflammation. Thus, the feeding of poorly digestible proteins, incomplete digestion, increased mucosal permeability, decreased IgA secretion, deranged cell-mediated responses of GALT, and portasystemic shunts all predispose patients to food allergies.[2]

As discussed previously, any inflammatory process has the potential to increase gastrointestinal permeability. The increased mucosal permeability results in increased absorption of gut antigens at sites other than the intestinal M cell. This results in local inflammation (see discussion of inflammatory bowel

Table 20-2 Proven or Suspected Symptoms or Disorders Associated with Food Allergies in Humans [2]

Anaphylaxis	Anal pruritus
Urticaria	Gastrointestinal bleeding
Angioedema	Protein-losing enteropathy
Pruritus	Gluten-sensitive enteropathy
Dermatitis herpetiformis *	Eosinophilic gastroenteritis
Allergic (eosinophilic) rhinitis	Hemorrhagic proctocolitis
Allergic (eosinophilic) conjunctivitis	Oral and pharyngeal pruritus
	Oropharyngeal fissuring
Bronchitis	Headache
Asthma	Lassitude
Pulmonary infiltrates	Hyperactivity
Vomiting	Vasculitis
Diarrhea	Chronic arthropathies
Constipation	
Abdominal pain	

* Symmetrically distributed, erythematous, pruritic, papulovesicular eruptions

disease) and also increases the likelihood that the suppressor response of the GALT will be bypassed and that intact antigen will enter the systemic circulation, to generate hypersensitivity rather than tolerance to gut antigens such as food proteins. Thus it should not be surprising, that dogs and cats with acute gastrointestinal inflammation frequently do not recover normal intestinal function rapidly and completely. Many must be managed with controlled diets, since transient adverse reactions to foods are often evidenced for some time after the initial insult.

Clinical Features

The history usually reveals an adverse reaction(s) to a food that is both uniform in its clinical manifestation and consistently occurs on subsequent rechallenges. On rare occasions a suspected food may fail to consistently lead to the expected clinical signs. Reasons for such inconsistency in patients with food allergy include variations in dose of the allergen ingested, the presence of simultaneously ingested foods which interfere with the reaction, altered methods of preparation of the food, and antecedent treatment with antiinflammatory agents. The clinical signs are non-seasonal (in contrast to many inhalation allergies) and often occur suddenly after months or years of consuming the diet containing the inciting foodstuff. A wide age range of animals can be affected. No breed or sex predilections have been established.

The clinical signs of food allergy in dogs and cats may vary from local gastrointestinal reactions such as vomiting and diarrhea (with or without blood and protein loss into the bowel) to systemic reactions such as urticaria, angioedema, pruritus, rhinitis, conjunctivitis, bronchoconstriction, and anaphylaxis. Head and neck pruritus is reputed to be a particularly common manifestation of food "allergy" in cats. Dermatologic manifestations in cats may include miliary dermatitis. Whether dermatologic, respiratory, or gastrointestinal manifestations predominate in food allergies (or food intolerances) of dogs and cats has yet to be conclusively determined. Not surprisingly, most dermatologists report that cutaneous manifestations of food allergy are more prevalent than gastrointestinal manifestations. This point is also controversial in humans.[14,15] What does seem clear, is that gastrointestinal signs need not be present to attribute a dermatologic abnormality to a food allergy.

The gastrointestinal lesions in food hypersensitivities can be sufficiently severe to result in protein and blood loss. On most occasions, the gastrointestinal signs relate to gastric and small bowel dysfunction (vomiting and small bowel-type diarrhea) but on some occasions, at least in humans, proctocolitis can occur and result in signs of large bowel dysfunction.[6]

The severity and nature of the immune response is dependent on the type of ingested antigen to which the animal is sensitive, the sensitivity of the patient (in part determined by the number of mast cells that bear IgE antibody), and the amount of allergen ingested. Repeat exposure to the antigen causes an increase in the mast cell population in the lamina propria. The clinical signs associated with food allergies in humans are listed in Table 20-2. Some or all of these signs may occur in animals.

Pathophysiology

Immediate Hypersensitivities to Food. Immediate hypersensitivities to food are well characterized in human medicine but are less well described in dogs and cats. They occur within minutes of ingestion of the offending antigen, and the more severe of these reactions (food anaphylaxis) are easily recognized because of their dramatic clinical signs and life-threatening consequences. Vascular collapse, bronchoconstriction, pruritus, and angioedema are prominent clinical features of food anaphylaxis. Concurrent vomiting, diarrhea, and abdominal pain may also occur. Most canine and feline cases of presumed immediate hypersensitivity to food result in gastrointestinal signs such as an acute onset of transient vomiting, or dermatologic signs such as pruritus rather than systemic, anaphylactic reactions.

Immediate hypersensitivity responses result from type 1 hypersensitivity reactions mediated by IgE. This is thought to be true even for cats, a species in which IgE has not as yet been characterized. In susceptible individuals an IgE immune response develops in response to certain food antigens instead of an IgA response. The basic defect that results in the preferential production of IgE in these individuals is unknown. Genetic factors and age appear to influence the propensity to produce a specific IgE response.[15] In rats, the IgE response appears to be maximal in the young as a result of reduced suppressor activity. Predisposing factors such as a defective mucosal barrier are discussed above. As mentioned in Chapter 3, the source of the IgE in the lamina propria is uncertain but is probably primarily the mesenteric lymph nodes. The IgE binds to gastrointestinal and, on occasion, peripheral mast cells priming them for a response to the inciting antigen if it is represented.

If the sensitized mast cells are restricted to the gastrointestinal tract, the ingestion of antigen will cause a local intestinal type 1 hypersensitivity. If the sensitized mast cells are more widespread, or if basophils are also sensitized, more generalized reactions occur when antigen escapes from the intestine. IgE can be synthesized and fix to the mast cells in the skin or respiratory tract. Antigen contact with those cells following the subsequent absorption from the gut causes hives, urticaria, and similar kinds of inflammatory responses in the airways.

The exposure of the sensitized mast cells to the inciting antigen leads to mast cell degranulation and the release of a variety of mediators, including histamine, kinins, prostaglandins, leukotrienes, and proteases (see Chapter 4). In the bowel, these mediators collectively cause loss of fluid and plasma proteins from the capillaries and into the lumen of the gut, stimulate intestinal chloride secretion, and cause motility derangements all of which culminate in vomiting and diarrhea.[15] If the reaction is severe, the vascular changes can cause extensive loss of plasma proteins and occasionally blood into the gut. Histology can show mucosal edema, separation of the epithelium from the lamina propria, enterocyte shedding, and widespread ultrastructural disruption of the basement membrane and collagenous matrix of the lamina propria.[15] Milder immediate hypersensitivities lead to transient mucosal erythema, and edema which rapidly resolve and need not be apparent on subsequent bowel biopsy. Repeated mast cell degranulation may eventually lead to eosinophil accumulation in the bowel and may be the cause of some cases of eosinophilic gastroenteritis (see Chapter 21).

Recent evidence in humans has demonstrated that patients with food hypersensitivities have increased rates of release of histamine from basophils that appears to be due to the secretion of a cytokine by mononuclear cells stimulated by the food antigen.[16] The cytokine interacts with IgE bound to the basophil causing them to release histamine. Thus the release of histamine from mast cells may occur as a direct result of the interaction of the antigen with IgE bound to mast cells or indirectly in response to allergen-induced cytokine binding. The release of the cytokine only diminishes after prolonged avoidance of the dietary allergen, and it is proposed that this phenomenon explains the cutaneous hyperactivity of to a variety of minor stimuli that are commonly seen in food allergic patients.

Intermediate Hypersensitivities to Food

Intermediate hypersensitivities to food are also common in humans and have been suspected on a number of occasions in cats and dogs. These reactions occur within two hours of antigen ingestion and may result in gastrointestinal signs, urticaria, rhinitis, and mild bronchoconstriction. Intermediate hypersensitivity responses are also mediated by IgE (at least in part) but the clinical signs are probably due primarily to a type 3 hypersensitivity response to immune complexes rather than direct IgE-mediated mast cell degranulation.[16] IgE and IgG complexes accumulate in the gastrointestinal mucosa[17] and other organs leading to an inflammatory response by the fixation of complement and the attraction of phagocytes. Complement fixation leads to non-specific mast cell degranulation by the generation of the anaphylatoxins (C3a & C5a). Immune complexes are another stimulus for eosinophil migration (as well as other phagocytes) and may contribute to the eosinophilic infiltration seen in some cases of food allergy. This contrasts to normal individuals in which IgA complexes predominate in the lamina propria. IgA complexes are non-inflammatory and are rapidly cleared by the liver. Altered complement components have been observed in the sera of some human patients with food allergies.

Delayed Hypersensitivities to Food

Delayed hypersensitivity responses to food are considered by some the most prevalent classification of food allergy in humans.[6] They appear two hours to several days after the ingestion of the antigen and produce nonspecific diverse symptoms such as chronic headaches, recurrent abdominal pain, fatigue, arthropathies, oral ulcers, and chronic cough, all with or without gastrointestinal signs. Little is known about the pathophysiology of delayed hypersensitivities to food but limited evidence suggests that they are mediated by type 3 and delayed hypersensitivity reactions. On rare occasions, delayed reactions may result from the exposure of reaginic antigenic determinants on a food protein by a late phase of the digestion process.[18] In delayed hypersensitivity reactions sensitized lymphocytes release a variety of lymphokines that are responsible for the clinical manifestations. The prevalence of delayed hypersensitivity responses to food in the canine and feline population is unknown, but clinical experience indicates that they do occur and that, as in humans, they may be a relatively prominent classification of food allergy.

Diagnosis of Food Allergy[19]

The diagnosis of food allergy requires that an adverse reaction to an offending antigen is first established by appropriate history, physical examination, elimination and challenge trials. Secondarily, the adverse reaction to the antigen must be proven to have an immune-mediated basis. Demonstration of hypersensitivity to a food antigen is not a simple matter. The enormity of the number of possible dietary antigens that cause food allergy is one stumbling block. Furthermore, whether or not an animal manifests clinical signs following the ingestion of an antigen to which it is sensitive may depend on a number of different factors including synergism with concomitant sensitivities to other allergens, and emotional and various environmental factors that may lower the "allergy threshold".

Tests that have been employed to date include skin testing, radioallergosorbent test, tests of cell-mediated immune reactions and mast cell degranulation, and endoscopic challenge tests. The accuracy of many of these tests is poor in human patients. Their diagnostic utility has not been adequately examined in the dog and cat. A persistent eosinophilia is present in some patients with food allergies.

Skin Tests. Skin tests are performed by inoculation of a small quantity of the suspected antigen into the skin along with a positive control (histamine) and a negative control (saline). A positive reaction appears as an area of swelling and induration sometimes with erythema.

Skin tests are a sensitive technique for the detection of antigen-specific IgE in the skin. Unfortunately, the presence or absence of IgE in the skin need not bear any relation to the presence or absence of IgE in the lamina propria. Thus allergies with signs restricted to the gastrointestinal tract cannot be confirmed by skin tests or, for that matter, measurement of serum IgE levels. Furthermore, non-reaginic (non-IgE) food allergies, such as delayed hypersensitivity reactions will not be diagnosed by this technique. This is a major disadvantage because, as mentioned above, delayed hypersensitivity food allergies are thought to be the most common form of food allergy in humans and may also be common in dogs and cats.

One study in humans demonstrated that only 10% of people allergic to milk proteins had positive skin tests.[20] A second study suggested that skin testing yields a high incidence of false positive results,[21] suggesting that results of skin testing can neither be used to confirm food allergy or to predict which food antigens the patient should avoid. Another draw back is that an extensive range of purified food allergens is not widely available. Skin tests are also thought to be of limited value in the diagnosis of food allergies in dogs and cats.[8]

Oral Challenge Tests

A simple way to evaluate allergens, or food additives suspected of causing reactions in the mouth and adjacent areas is to spread the substance on the oral mucosa. Within 15-20 minutes swelling of the oral mucosa, lips or throat, or rhinitis and conjunctivitis may appear. A positive test identifies the responsible agent but does not always differentiate immunologic from non-immunologic mechanisms as non-immunologic contact urticarial-like reactions to certain substances such as spices can occur.[3]

Measurement of Antibodies

Antibodies (IgG & IgA) specific to food antigens have been demonstrated in the serum of patients with suspected food allergies but also in the serum of normal individuals and in patients with inflammatory bowel disease but no evidence of food allergy.[2] The significance of the majority of these antibodies is unknown. A small percentage may have a pathogenic role but many appear to be epiphenomena.

Fecal antibodies (IgG) against food proteins have also been demonstrated, and again do not have a confirmed pathological role.[22] Increased levels of IgE have been observed in the intestinal juice of humans with food allergies and may provide a means of screening for food allergies.[23]

Total serum IgE levels tend to be elevated in patients with food allergy, but there is considerable overlap with the normal range.[15] The concentration of antigen-specific IgE in the serum can be measured by a radioallergosorbent test (RAST) or ELISA. In humans, RAST is less sensitive and, with the exception of a limited number of proteins, does not correlate well with skin tests[6] or intragastric tests.[24] The greater availability of purified food antigens may, however, improve the accuracy of the RAST.[2] As with skin tests, RAST is committed to the diagnosis of only one form of food allergy, that mediated by IgE released in sufficient quantities to enter the systemic circulation. A canine RAST (A & M Biosciences; Mesa AZ) and ELISA (Bioproducts for Medicine; Tempe AZ) are available, and objective evaluation of the tests for the diagnosis of canine atopy has begun.[25,26]

Assay of Products of Mast Cell Degranulation

Marked increases in the serum concentrations of histamine have been observed following challenge in children with suspected food allergies. Assay difficulties and the rapid metabolism of histamine have prevented routine application of this test.[15] Histamine is also known to increase in concentration in the intestinal fluid following challenge of food sensitive rats. In rats sensitized to egg albumin, oral challenge is associated with the local and systemic release of a protease (rat mast cell protease II) that is a specific product of intestinal mast cells. The systemic release of such a product may prove a useful serum test for food allergies associated with intestinal mast cell degranulation.[15]

Measurements of Cell-Mediated Responses

Techniques to measure cell-mediated responses to food antigens are at present in their infancy. Skin tests with food antigen have not produced characteristic delayed hypersensitivity reactions.[27] Lymphocyte blastogenesis and measurement of migration inhibition factor production in response to food antigens are sometimes abnormal.[28,29]

Miscellaneous Techniques

The basophil or leukocyte histamine release assay is a specific and reproducible diagnostic technique based on the observation that in the presence of antigen peripheral blood leukocytes from allergic individuals release histamine. The phenomenon depends on basophil-fixed IgE.[30] Technical difficulties have limited this assay to the research setting.

A test has been described to evaluate dogs and cats for food allergies that is based on the appearance of cytotoxic changes in neutrophils, and on platelet agglutination when blood from allergic dogs is reacted with food antigens. The test may be useful, but validation in the dog has been inadequate, and the procedure has not found widespread application.[7] The cytotoxic test has been used in humans, but the American Academy of Allergy has stated that the technique is unproven and does not recommend its use.

Endoscopy

Endoscopic examination of patients in the acute phase of a hypersensitivity to food is rarely done because of the transient nature of the clinical signs and increased anesthetic risk. Endoscopic abnormalities that have been noted in food hypersensitive patients include hyperemia, edema, increased nodularity, and excess mucus production.

Endoscopic challenge tests have been used to diagnose food allergies. Antigen solutions, usually a maximum of three per procedure, are sprayed on an area of gastric mucosa and the mucosal response observed. In hypersensitive people, erythema, edema, and petechiation can appear within seconds of application of the test solution.[31] To establish an immune-mediated basis to the inflammation, the tissues can be biopsied and histamine or other mediators measured, or the degree of mast cell degranulation assessed.[31] In vitro tests of mast cell degranulation in intestinal biopsies obtained from food sensitive people have also been reported to be a useful diagnostic technique.[24] These testing methods would appear to have application in veterinary medicine for the definitive confirmation of food allergies mediated by mast cell degranulation. Their disadvantages are expense, the requirement for anesthesia, and the limited number of antigens that can be detected per procedure.

Gastrointestinal Biopsy

Biopsy is rarely helpful in the confirmation of food allergy because many of the acute phase changes such as edema are transient, and gastrointestinal biopsy is always performed during the fasting state. Furthermore, in food allergies, such as celiac sprue that produce morphologic mucosal disease easily recognizable by light microscopy, there are no pathognomonic histologic features that differentiate food hypersensitivity from the other causes of chronic intestinal inflammation such as lymphocytic-plasmacytic enteritis. Eosinophilic infiltration is suggestive of food allergy but, as discussed in Chapter 21, many humans and animals with eosinophilic gastroenteritis do not have evidence of food allergy. IgE containing plasma cells increase in the lamina propria of humans with type 1 hypersensitivity reactions to food.[6,15] This may help differentiate some food allergies from idiopathic inflammatory bowel disease. Caution in interpretation is required, however, because it has also been observed that IgE plasma cells will increase in number as a secondary complication of a variety of chronic gastrointestinal inflammatory disorders.[32]

Treatment of Food Allergy

Treatment is dependent on identification of the responsible allergens by elimination and challenge diets. These antigens and, where possible, any related foodstuff should be omitted from the diet. Care should be taken to ensure that the controlled diet remains balanced, palatable, and practical. Antihistamines (H_1 blockers) administered prior to meals may decrease some of the systemic symptoms of food hypersensitivity but usually do not prevent gastrointestinal symptoms. Corticosteroids are reserved for the induction of a more rapid remission in severe conditions such as allergic chronic gastroenteropathies and for those patients in which avoidance of the offending antigen is impossible. Epinephrine is reserved for food anaphylaxis. Hyposensitization therapy either through oral or parenteral routes has no proven benefit in food hypersensitivity.

FOOD INTOLERANCES

Clinical Synopsis

Diagnostic features

* Historical association between a particular diet and gastrointestinal, dermatological or multisystemic signs compatible with an adverse reaction to food
* Elimination trial identifies suspected inciting food or food additive
* Recrudescence of clinical signs on reexposure
* No documentation of an immunological pathomechanism

Treatment

* Avoidance of the suspected food or food additive

Food Idiosyncrasy[3]

A wide variety of food additives have been noted to produce adverse reactions to food in susceptible people. These reactions can closely mimic food allergies. One distinguishing feature is that they usually do not require prior sensitization, and thus may occur on the first exposure to the inciting agent. By far the majority of reactions to food additives are due to idiosyncratic food intolerances and not immunologic mechanisms. The reactions may be dermatologic, respiratory and, perhaps to a lesser extent, gastrointestinal. The prevalence of adverse reactions to food additives has been estimated to range from 0.3-0.15% of the whole human population.[3] The same reactions are likely to occur in animals but remain to be proven. Diagnosis of food idiosyncracy most often requires the use of elimination-challenge diets. No *in vitro* tests are available. It is difficult to rule out an immunological basis to a food idiosyncracy. RASTs for food additives are not available, and skin testing using chemicals, many of which are known contact irritants, would appear unreliable because a positive test may develop through irritation just as it may develop through immune-mediated mechanisms.

Metabisulfite and sulfur dioxide, used as preservatives, can precipitate asthmatic attacks, hypotension, and flushing in intolerant people. The pathomechanism is unclear but may involve aerosolization and inhalation of the product during mastication. Azo dyes, particularly tartrazine yellow, and benzoate preservatives may trigger asthmatic and urticarial attacks in susceptible individuals. Monosodium L-glutamate ingestion can result in severe headache, and chest pain. Sodium nitrite can cause urticaria, intestinal disorders, or headache. Sorbic acid, canthaxanthine, beta-carotene, annatto, quinoline yellow, butylhydroxytoluene (BHT), butylhydroxyanisole (BHA), and various spices can all cause or aggravate urticaria and angioneurotic edema. Many of these agents also produce a contact urticaria. Penicillin-contaminated milk and other animal products can induce apparent food hypersensitivities in susceptible individuals.

The mechanisms by which these chemical additives produce such clinical symptoms without involvement of the immune system is a matter of continuing investigation. Suggested possibilities include perturbations of eicosanoid pathways, alteration of cell membrane permeability, enzyme inhibition, direct release of histamine, and independent activation of the complement and kinin cascades.

Anaphylactoid Reactions to Food

Anaphylactoid reactions mimic anaphylactic reactions yet laboratory tests fail to establish an immune basis. Immediate anaphylactoid reactions can occur after ingestion of spoiled tuna, mackerel or mahi-mahi, which contain large amounts of histamine. The contamination of the fish with *Proteus morganii* or *Klebsiella* pneumoniae results in microbial decarboxylation of histidine to yield histamine.

Pharmacologic Reactions to Food

A variety of foods contain vasoactive amines and other pharmacologically active substances capable of inducing a wide variety of signs that particularly affect the gastrointestinal tract and nervous system. The vasoactive amines include tyramine, tryptamine, phenylethylamine, dopamine, norepinephrine, serotonin, and histamine. They are usually produced by bacterial decarboxylation of amino acids. Tyramine is common in cheese, histamine in spoiled tuna, and phenylethylamine in chocolate.

Psychoactive agents and stimulants are contained in some foods. The most important example in dogs is chocolate toxicosis resulting from methylxanthines.

Metabolic Adverse Reactions to Food

Metabolic adverse reactions to food usually occur only in a susceptible subpopulation. The diarrhea, bloating, and abdominal discomfort that repeatedly occur on exposure of animals with carbohydrate malabsorption to carbohydrates is a metabolic adverse reaction to food that is relatively common in small animals. Inborn errors of metabolism collectively are important causes of metabolic adverse reactions to food in humans and also occur in animals (for example urea cycle enzyme deficiencies). The site of the defect in the metabolic pathway determines the specificity of the resultant clinical signs for a particular nutrient. For example, inherited defects in the metabolism of most of the amino acids have been reported in humans. Many of these have vomiting, diarrhea, or skin rashes amongst their clinical signs, and many can be controlled by modifications in the type or quantity of amino acids or protein provided in the diet. Occasionally an excessive intake of a food will produce a metabolic derangement. For instance avidin ingestion in raw egg white can induce biotin deficiency.

Food Poisoning

Food poisoning is a not infrequent cause of gastrointestinal disease in small animals. The diagnosis is usually made by historical association of the onset of the clinical signs with ingestion of a particular foodstuff that is suspected to be inadequately prepared, spoiled or contaminated. This is most rewarding when the poisoning is due to a toxin inherent to the food or derived from a microorganism that has secreted an exotoxin on to the food, where upon clinical signs will occur within a few hours of ingestion. More delayed symptoms will occur if the food poisoning results from a microorganism which must colonize the bowel for pathogenicity. In these cases, diagnosis is usually made only by careful epidemiological investigations of outbreaks of poisoning. Obviously, unlike other forms of food intolerance, dietary elimination and challenge trials have no place in the diagnosis of food poisoning.

Ingestion of a variety of toxic plants mistaken as food can cause poisoning. An important example is *Amanita* mushrooms. Ingestion of commonly used foods after inadequate preparation or in excessive quantities can result in food poisoning. For examples green potatoes have high levels of glycoalkaloids; excessive quantities of onions cause Heinz body anemia probably due to N-propyl disulfide; large quantities of inadequately cooked lima beans, sorghum, sprouts, maize or chick peas can lead to cyanide toxicity; excessive quantities of spinach or preserved meats contain nitrates and nitrites that can lead to methemoglobinemia; high levels of oxalates and anthraquinone glycosides contained in rhubarb, spinach, and beet can lead to a corrosive gastroenteritis; large quantities of spices such as peppers can cause abdominal discomfort; excessive ingestion of the fat soluble vitamins A and D can lead to vomiting, diarrhea, and other adverse signs.

Contamination of foods by microbial products can result in food poisoning. Examples include: aflatoxins which cause hepatotoxicity and liver cancer; a wide variety of other mycotoxins that cause vomiting and diarrhea as well as a number of other signs; and bacterial exotoxins such as that produced by *Clostridium botulinum, Cl. perfringens* and *Staphyloccus aureus*.

Dietary Indiscretions

Gluttony by dogs can result in gastric dilatation with or without subsequent volvulus. "Garbage can enteritis" is a frequent problem in unrestrained dogs. The history usually provides the diagnosis. Clinical signs vary with the toxic principles concerned but usually include an acute onset of vomiting and diarrhea sometimes with blood. The condition is usually self-limiting but dogs often require symptomatic therapy to maintain fluid, electrolyte, and acid-base homeostasis. The pathophysiology of the disorder involves a multitude of potential injurious products found in decomposing garbage. They include bacterial and fungal toxins, vasoactive amines such as histamine, and indigestible materials such as bone and tin foil that can physically abrade the mucosa.

GLUTEN-INDUCED ENTEROPATHY[33.34]

Clinical Synopsis

Diagnostic features

* Historical association between gluten-containing diets and malabsorption
* Elimination of gluten-containing grains results in resolution of signs
* Recrudescence of clinical signs on reexposure to one or, preferably, more than one gluten-containing grain
* Intestinal biopsy showing at least some degree of villus atrophy and cellular infiltration

Standard treatment

* Elimination of wheat, barley, rye, buckwheat, and oats from the diet

Introduction

Gluten-induced enteropathy (celiac disease) is an important chronic inflammatory disease of the small intestine of humans. In some populations the prevalence of the disease may reach as high as 1 in 300 people.[34] The prevalence of gluten intolerance in dogs and cats is unknown. Recent work has conclusively demonstrated that an analogous disorder affects the Irish Setter dog[35-37] and clinical experience suggests that other breeds may also be affected. Cytotoxic testing has suggested that 36% of dogs suspected of suffering from food allergies are sensitive to gluten.[37] Idiopathic lymphocytic-plasmacytic enteritis is a very prevalent disorder in the dog and cat. On many occasions the inflammatory infiltrate of this disorder is associated with villus atrophy and the other histologic features found in gluten-induced enteropathy. Therefore, it is possible that some cases of presumed idiopathic lymphocytic-plasmacytic enteritis (improperly diagnosed without use of prior elimination diets) are due to gluten intolerance.

Etiopathogenesis[34,38]

Gluten is a protein found in many cereals. It has two component parts, gliadin and glutenin. The human disease appears to be caused by the gliadin polypeptide of gluten.[39] Gliadin, is a glutamine and proline rich polypeptide with a molecular weight of 15,000 daltons. It is comprised of four major fractions, the most toxic of which appears to be alpha-gliadin. Completely hydrolyzed gliadin is non-toxic. These peptides are normally digested by pancreatic enzymes in the intestinal lumen, and the process is completed by brush border and intracellular enzymes of the mucosa.

How gluten damages the intestinal mucosa remains unknown.[34,40,41] Possible mechanisms include that gluten-induced enteropathy is a metabolic disease in which inadequate digestion of the gluten fraction results in accumulation of a toxic fraction that directly damages the mucosa; or that an abnormal immune reaction to gluten or its breakdown products causes the pathological features of the disease. Of these theories, the evidence that the disease results from an aberrant immune response is most compelling.

The idea that inadequate digestion of gluten is responsible for the disease was based on the observation that humans with gluten-induced enteropathy have reduced enzyme activities in the brush borders and epithelial cells of the mucosa. Subsequently, the brush border enzyme defects have been proven to be a result, not a cause of the disease. Brush border enzyme defects have also been demonstrated in gluten-induced enteropathy of Irish Setters.[36] These brush border defects include a decrease in the activity of aminopeptidase, the most abundant brush border peptidase. As with humans, the level of these enzymes returned to normal on a wheat-free diet, suggesting they are a result and not a cause of the disease. It has also been proposed that the changes in brush-border enzymes may be age-related because dramatic differences in the activities of the enzymes were seen in two groups of dogs from the same litter, one group biopsied at 8 months and the other at 9 months of age.[36] In humans, additional work has shown that the epithelial cell enzymes from patients with the disease in remission are unable to digest gliadin completely, to render it nontoxic. Moreover, when these homogenates containing gliadin are added to lysosomes they are able to disrupt them more readily than normal. This work suggests that patients with gluten-induced enteropathy lack enzymes that completely degrade gliadin, and that one of the effects of the undigested toxic fragment is to disrupt intracellular lysosomes, releasing enzymes that cause cell autolysis.[42,43] This may indeed be one important factor in the pathogenesis of gluten-induced enteropathy, but it is not a popularly held view. In vitro studies have been made of the effects of gliadin on mucosal tissue.[44,45] When mucosal tissue from patients with gluten-induced enteropathy is removed and maintained in vitro, the cells change toward the normal state, and enzyme activity returns. If glutens are added to the culture medium, however, those morphological and enzymatic changes do not occur. Glutens added to a culture medium of mucosal tissue from normal individuals cause no pathological changes - nor do they in mucosal tissue from patients with gluten-induced enteropathy in remission on a gluten-free diet (at least in most studies). Hence, gliadin appears not to be directly toxic to the epithelial cell. In summary, the glutens must activate an endogenous effector mechanism, that is not present in the epithelial cell, to cause the toxicity.

It now appears probable that the endogenous effector mechanism that mediates epithelial cell destruction in the presence of gliadin operates through the immune system. Knowledge of the complete sequence of immunologic events is far from complete, but it appears the immune damage is not mediated by IgE. Instead, evidence suggests that the type III or delayed hypersensitivity response is responsible. Evidence for an immune mechanism in the disease remains indirect and includes the demonstration that: affected patients have an increased incidence of HLA-B8, HLA-DQW2, and HLA-DR3 histocompatibility antigens, certain alloantigens on B cells, and Gm allotype markers on the IgG heavy chain; challenge with gluten stimulates synthesis of IgA and IgM at a rate two to five times normal, and the antibodies produced have antigluten specificity; complement levels fall in the plasma and increase in the mucosa during disease, which makes it possible that complement mediated cytolysis causes the mucosal changes; circulating antibodies to gliadin are present in high titers; functional T-cell suppressor defects specific to gluten have been demonstrated; and normal lymphocytes can be given cytotoxic properties by incubation with serum from patients with gluten-induced enteropathy.[46,47] The pathology of gluten-induced enteropathy indicates that the putative immune process is specifically cytotoxic to epithelial cells of the mucosa.

Recently, sequence homology of a 12 amino acid segment in alpha-gliadin and a human adenovirus protein, along with immunological cross-reactivity, have been observed.[48] This raises the possibility that viral infection may be the initiating event in the development of sensitivity to gliadin. Studies of gluten intolerant Irish Setters have demonstrated that increased mucosal permeability predates the development of the disease.[49] This finding supports the possibility that increased mucosal permeability may be the basis for an acquired sensitivity to gluten. Composite theories including the interaction of one or more of the genetic factors mentioned, inadequate digestion of the peptide, and an aberrant immune response have also been proposed.

Histopathology

The histopathological changes in dogs and humans with gluten-induced enteropathy are similar. As would be expected from the pathophysiology, the lesions of gluten-induced enteropathy are more prominent in the cranial part of the small intestine, where the exposure to gluten is the greatest. In severe cases the entire length of the small intestine is affected. Sparing of the proximal intestine with involvement of the distal intestine does not occur in gluten-induced enteropathy.

Histopathological changes are restricted to the mucosa. The early changes following gluten challenge develop in the connective tissue under the epithelial surface. They include swelling of the basement membranes of the epithelial and capillary endothelial cells. Eosinophils and neutrophils are the first inflammatory cells to appear, and after four days lymphocytes and plasma cells rapidly accumulate.

The later morphological changes are primarily the result of a faster loss of epithelial cells on the villus. The affected villus columnar epithelial cells also show changes. Their height is reduced, and they have irregular nuclei and immature microvilli. The epithelial tight junctions appear focally disrupted. Overall, the mucosa is flattened, with very blunted or no villi, and the crypt layer markedly thickens as a result of reactive hypertrophy. The lamina propria of jejunal tissue from patients with gluten-induced enteropathy is densely infiltrated with plasma cells containing IgA, IgM, and IgG. IgA cells predominate, but the greatest relative increase is in IgM secreting cells. The number of intraepithelial lymphocytes increases per unit length of epithelium, but the total number of intraepithelial cells is not increased, because the absorptive surface is markedly decreased.[34,50] Granulomas can be seen.[51] As with any chronic inflammatory process, a persistent contact with glutens will cause more permanent changes to develop, such as fibrosis. Otherwise, the lesions are to a great degree reversible.

Villus atrophy and infiltration of the lamina propria are nonspecific changes that accompany many other pathological processes in the intestinal tract (Figure 17-4) including the idiopathic inflammatory bowel diseases, marked bacterial overgrowth, parasitism, and neoplasia.

Pathophysiology

The initial clinical signs associated with gluten-induced enteropathy are related to the changes in the small-intestinal mucosa. Villus atrophy and crypt hyperplasia result in a reduced absorptive capacity and increased secretion by the crypt epithelium. Many mucosal-enzymes that contribute to the digestive-absorption process, are decreased. The pathology is most striking in the cranial part of the small intestine, however, and since there is a large reserve capacity for absorption the pathological changes must be advanced and extensive to cause malabsorption by themselves. Another important cause of the malassimilation, at least in humans, is reduced cholecystokinin and secretin release due to the pathological changes in the duodenal mucosa.[34] Enterogastric reflexes may also be impaired. The duodenum bears the greatest insult from the gluten antigens presented to the intestines, and the damage results in a functional inability to respond with a normal secretion of bile and pancreatic enzymes, and perhaps deranged gastric emptying. Chronic malassimilation in humans has resulted in deficiencies of the fat-soluble vitamins, iron, folate, cobalamin, and various electrolytes including calcium, potassium, sodium, chloride, magnesium, and zinc.

Clinical Findings and Diagnosis

The clinical-laboratory findings are those of malassimilation (Chapter 17). In Irish Setters with the disease, the onset of clinical signs occurs between 4-7 months of age. The dogs present with poor weight gain or weight loss, in most cases accompanied by chronic diarrhea.[52] Serum folate concentrations are low in a few dogs whereas cobalamin concentrations are unaltered. Xylose absorption is subnormal in a small number of affected animals.

A promising screening test for the disease in humans is the assay of serum levels of IgG and IgA antigliadin antibodies.[53]

The diagnosis is made on the response to an elimination-challenge trial (see above).[54] The usual test diet contains a single source of carbohydrates and a single source of proteins. They are selected so that they are gluten-free. The most common nutrients used are rice, to meet carbohydrate needs, and cottage cheese, eggs, or meat, to supply protein. With chronic mucosal changes, several weeks are required for morphology and function to begin to return to normal. The controlled diet should be fed for two weeks before evaluations or changes are made. A presumptive diagnosis is made on the response to the test diet, and the diagnosis is confirmed if the diarrhea returns when gluten-containing grains are reintroduced to the diet. A more definitive diagnosis of gluten sensitivity is provided by the observation that the diarrhea may be induced by the use of purified gluten, or by challenge by more than one gluten-containing grains. These precautions rule out or reduce the likelihood (respectively) of the possibility that the diarrhea arises from an allergy to a grain antigen other than gluten. These additional diagnostic challenges are rarely performed, however, because of practical constraints, and because of the high likelihood that an adverse reaction to a gluten-containing grain will prove due to gluten.

A significant number of humans with gluten-induced enteropathy do not respond to a gluten-free diet. They are usually long-standing cases, with mucosal changes that are irreversible. Thus, as long as there are no laboratory procedures that can provide a definitive diagnosis, the possibility of gluten-induced enteropathy should not be excluded if a patient with advanced mucosal changes does not respond well to a gluten-free diet.

Biopsy of the small intestine supports but does not confirm the diagnosis, because the histologic changes seen in gluten enteropathy are nonspecific for a number of pathologic processes.

Management and Prognosis

The treatment for gluten-induced enteropathy is to exclude gluten-containing grains such as wheat, barley, rye, buckwheat, and oats from the diet. If the client chooses to prepare the patient's diet, there are many ingredients to select from. Many foods prepared for human consumption, however, contain cereal byproducts, and such must be excluded from the diet. Thus, most prepared foods cannot be used; instead, the formulation must consist of fresh foods prepared by the client. When an owner refuses to prepare a diet, a commercial food free of glutens or immunosuppressive therapy can be used. Most commercial pet foods contain glutens. The prescription diet d/d is formulated with mutton and rice and contains no glutens. The formula for i/d is also gluten free. Some of the Science diets (Maximum Stress) contain no glutens. The toxic response to glutens is related directly to the amount of glutens in the diet. Since the amount varies with the amount of grain in the diet, it is not unusual to find dogs showing fewer signs on one brand of food than another. The use of cereals in commercial foods is determined by economics. Thus, carbohydrate sources vary, depending on the price of cereal grains. Vitamin and mineral supplementation is an important adjunct to the nutritional therapy.

Two weeks is the earliest to expect improvement from severe mucosal changes complicated by hypoproteinemia, anemia, and mineral imbalances. Studies in humans show that mucosal changes require months for correction, and some may persist indefinitely. Clinical improvement often occurs despite little improvement in mucosal morphology. Any improvement in mucosal pathology is noted first in the caudal small intestine, where the mucosa has been exposed to less glutens than in the cranial part. Malabsorption continues to be a potential problem, supporting the long-term use of low-fat diets. There can be a persistent reduction in brush-border enzymes, which may prevent feeding excessive disaccharides or starches. On most occasions, gluten-free diets must be fed for the remainder of the animal's life. Transient gluten sensitivity has been reported in children but it is not known if dogs can outgrow the problem.

In summary, patients with gluten-induced enteropathy are placed on a high-protein diet not only to correct the malnutrition but because it is the nutrient whose absorption is least affected by mucosal pathology. The carbohydrate content is restricted, so that malabsorption does not develop from the mucosal enzyme deficiency and reduced absorptive area. Particularly avoided are foods containing any disaccharides. The diet should be low in lipids since the mucosal disease reduces the absorptive areas, making lipid malabsorption a real problem. Thus, other aspects of the diet are almost as important as its being gluten-free, at least during the recovery phase.

An alternate or supplemental means of managing gluten-induced enteropathy is with immunosuppressive agents directed against the humoral and cell-mediated hypersensitivity responses to glutens. Corticosteroids cause a remission of clinical signs, and mucosal morphology returns to normal. Both *in vivo* and *in vitro* studies show that when corticosteroids are given and glutens are not removed from the diet, the mucosa returns to morphologically normal and remains normal.[55] Steroids must be used indefinitely since the pathologic changes return when the drug is discontinued. The amount of steroids to use has not been precisely defined. Their use is reserved for patients that have marked histologic changes and do not respond well to the gluten-free diet. Such patients can be given up to one mg of prednisone per pound of body weight for seven days, after which the dose is reduced to one-half. Steroids should be used as adjunct therapy to a gluten-free diet, not as a substitute for gluten exclusion.

The prognosis is generally good. A significant number of humans with gluten-induced enteropathy do not respond to a gluten-free diet, however. They are usually long-standing cases, with mucosal changes that are irreversible. Additionally, the incidence of neoplasia, in particular lymphosarcoma, is increased in human patients with gluten-induced enteropathy.

Prevention

It is likely that current feeding practices can increase the risk for some animals developing gluten-induced enteropathy. Dogs predisposed to the problem have increased intestinal permeability before the disease appears.[47] Feeding gluten-containing cereals sensitizes the intestine and it may be only because the permeability is increased. If the intestine becomes less permeable with age or maturity, it is less likely glutens could induce an enteropathy. Humans are less likely to develop gluten-induced enteropathy when feeding of gluten-containing cereals to young children is delayed.[56] Removal of gluten-containing cereals from infant foods and nursing human infants for a longer period of time reduces the incidence of gluten-induced enteropathy. Young animals may also be less likely to develop dietary intolerances and gluten-induced enteropathy when feeding gluten-containing commercial pet foods is delayed. Young animals often have access to such foods before they have the ability to develop oral tolerance to dietary constitutents. Developing such tolerance may not be possible until after six or more weeks of age.

REFERENCES

1. Kniker, W.T.: Immunologically mediated reactions to food: state of the art. Ann. Allergy 59:60-69, 1987.
2. Adverse Reactions to Foods. Committee on adverse reactions to food. American Acadamy of Allergy and Immunology. National Institute of Allergy and Infectious Diseases. U.S. Depart. Health and Human Services. National Inst. of Health. NIFA Publ. No. 84-2442, July 1984.
3. Hannuksela, M. and Haahtela, T.: Hypersensitivity reactions to food additives. Allergy 42:561-575, 1987.
4. Ferguson, A.: Models of intestinal hypersensitivity. Clinics Gastroenterology 5:271-288, 1976.
5. Roitt, I.M.: Essential Immunology. Blackwell Scientific, Oxford, 1971.
6. Heyman, M.B.: Food sensitivity and eosinophilic gastroenteropathies. In, Gastrointestinal Disease. 4th Edition. Edited by Sleisinger, M.H., Fordtran, J.S. WB Saunders Co, Philadelphia, 1113-1134, 1989.
7. Cheung, G. and Plechner, A.J.: Diagnosis of canine and feline food sensitivities: A new method. New Methods Oct:20, 1982
8. Conroy, J.D.: Immune-mediated diseases of the skin and mucous membranes. In, Textbook of Veterinary Internal Medicine. 2nd edition, Edited by Ettinger, S.J. WB Saunders, Philadelphia, 2140-2158, 1983.
9. August, J.R.: Dietary hypersensitivity in dogs: Cutaneous Manifestations, diagnosis, and management. Comp. Contin. Ed. Pract. Vet. 7:469-477, 1985.
10. Shibasaki, M., Suzuki, S., Tajima, S., Nemoto, H. and Kuroume, T.: Allergenicity of major component proteins of soybean. Int. Arch. Allergy Appl. Immun. 61:441-448, 1980.
11. White, S.D.: Food hypersensitivity in 30 dogs. JAVMA 188:695-698, 1986.
12. Walker, W.A.: Pathophysiology of intestinal uptake and absorption of antigens in food allergy. Ann. Allergy 59:7-20, 1987.
13. Mowat, A.M.: The regulation of immune responses to dietary protein antigens. Immunology Today 8:93-98, 1987.
14. Farah, D.A., Calder, I., Banson, L. and Mackenzie, J.F.: Specific food intolerance: its place as a cause of gastrointestinal symptoms. Gut 26:164-168, 1985.
15. Patrick, M.K. and Gall, D.G.: Protein intolerance and immunocyte and enterocyte interaction. Pediatr Clin N Am 35:17-34, 1988.
16. Sampson, H.A., Broadbent, K.R. and Bernhisel-Broadbent, J.: Spontaneous release of histamine from basophils and histamine-releasing factor in patients with atopic dermatitis and food hypersensitivity. New Eng. J. Med. 321:228-232, 1989.
17. Matthews, T.S. and Soothill, J.F.: Complement activation after milk feeding in children with cow's milk allergy. Lancet 2:893-895, 1970.
18. Haddad, Z.H., Kalara, V. and Verma, S.: IgE antibodies to peptic and peptic-tryptic digests of betalactoglobulin: Significance in food hypersensitivity. Ann. Allergy 42:368-371, 1979.
19. Bjorksten, B.: New diagnostic methods in food allergy. Ann. Allergy 59:150-152, 1987.
20. Bock, S.A.: The natural history of food sensitivity. J. Allergy Clin. Immunol. 69:173, 1982.
21. Sampson, H.A. and Albergo, R.: Comparison of results of skin tests, RAST, and double-blind, placebo-controlled food challenges in children with atopic dermatitis. J. Allergy Clin. Immunol. 74: 26, 1984.
22. Davis, S.D., Bierman, C.W., Pierson, W.E., Maas, C.W. and Iannetta, A.: Clinical nonspecificity of milk coproantibodies in diarrhea stools. New Eng. J. Med. 282:612-613, 1970.
23. Belut, D., Moneret-vautrin, D.A., Nicolas, J.P. and Grilliat, J.P.: IgE levels in intestinal juice. Dig. Dis. Sci. 25:323-332, 1980.
24. Selbekk, B.H.: A comparison between in vitro jejunal mast cell degranulation and intragastric challenge in patients with

suspected food intolerance. Scand. J. Gastroenterology 20:299-303, 1985.
25. Halliwell, R.E.W. and Kunkle, G.A.: The radioallergosorbent test in the diagnosis of canine atopic diseases. J. Allergy Clin. Immunol.62:236, 1978.
26. Griffin, C.: RAST and ELISA testing in canine atopy. In, Current Veterinary Therapy X. Edited by Kirk, R.W. WB Saunders, Philadelphia, 592-595, 1989.
27. May, C.D. and Alberto, R.: In vitro responses of leukocytes to food proteins in allergic and normal children: Lymphocyte stimulation and histamine release. Clin. Allergy 2:335-344, 1972.
28. Minor, J.D., Tolber, S.G. Frick, O.L.: Leukocyte inhibition factor in delayed-onset food allergy. J. Allergy Clin. Immunol. 66:314-321, 1980.
29. Valverde, E., Vich, J.M., Garcia-Calderon, J.V. and Garcia-Calderon, P.A.: In vitro stimulation of lymphocytes in patients with chronic urticaria induced by additives and food. Clin. Allergy 10:691-698, 1980.
30. Lichtenstein, L.M., Ishizaka, K., Norman, P.S., Sobotka, A. and Hill, B.M.: IgE antibody measurements in ragweed hayfever: Relationship to clinical severity and the results of immunotherapy. J. Clin. Invest. 52:472-482, 1973.
31. Reimann, H.J., Ring, J., Ultsch, B. and Wendt, P.: Intragastral provocation under endoscopic control (IPEC) in food allergy: Mast cell and histamine changes in gastric mucosa. Clin. Allergy 15:195-202, 1985.
32. Van Spreeuwel, J.P., Lindeman, J., Van Maanen, J. and Meyer, C.J.L.M.: Increased numbers of IgE containing cells in gastric and duodenal biopsies. An expression of food allergy secondary to chronic inflammation? J. Clin. Pathol. 37:601-606, 1984.
33. Strober, W.: Gluten-sensitive enteropathy. Clinics Gastroenterology 5:429-452, 1976.
34. Trier, J.S.: Celiac Sprue. In, Gastrointestinal Disease, 4th Edition. Edited by Sleisinger, M.H., Fordtran, J.S. WB Saunders Co, Philadelphia, 1134-1152, 1989.
35. Batt, R.M., Carter, M.W. and McLean, L.: Morphological and biochemical studies of a naturally occurring enteropathy in the Irish setter dog: a comparison with coeliac disease in man. Res. Vet. Sci. 37:339-346, 1984.
36. Batt, R.M., Carter, M.W. and McLean, L.: Wheat-sensitive enteropathy in Irish setter dogs: possible age-related brush border abnormalities. Res. Vet. Sci. 39:80-83, 1985
37. Hall, E.J. and Batt, R.M.: Challenge studies demonstrate gluten sensitivity of a naturally occurring enteropathy in Irish setter dogs. Gastroenterology 94:A167, 1988.
38. Strober, W., Falchuk, Z.M., Rogentine, G.N., Nelson, D.L. and Kleaveman, H.L.: The pathogenesis of gluten-sensitive enteropathy, Ann. Intern. Med. 83:242-256, 1975.
39. Kasadra, D.D., Bernardin, J.E. and Nimmo, C.C.: Wheat proteins. In, Advances in Cereal Science and Technology. Edited by Pomeranz, Y., Vol. 1. Amer. Assoc. Cereal Chemists, St. Paul, 158-236, 1976.
40. Peters, T.J. and Bjarnason, I.: Coeliac syndrome: biochemical mechanisms and the missing peptidase hypothesis revisited. Gut 25:913-918, 1984.
41. Davidson, A.G.F. and Bridges, M.A.: Coeliac disease: A critical review of aetiology and pathogenesis. Clin Chim Acta 163:1-40, 1987.
42. Cornell, H.J. and Townley, R.R.W.: Investigation of possible peptidase deficiency in coeliac disease. Clin Chem Acta 43:113-125, 1973.
43. Townley, R.R.W., Cornell, H.J., Bhathal, P.S. and Mitchell, J.D.: Toxicity of wheat gliadin fractions in coeliac disease. Lancet, i:1363-1665, 1973.
44. Falchuk, Z.M., Gebhard, R.L., Sessoms, C. and Strober, W.: An in vitro model of gluten-sensitive enteropathy. J. Clin. Invest. 53:487-500, 1974.
45. Jos, J., Lenoir, G., deRitis, G. and Rey, J.: In vitro pathogenetic studies of coeliac disease. Scand. J. Gastroenterology 10:121-128, 1975.
46. O'Donoghue, D.P., Lancaster-Smith, M., Laviniere, P. and Kumar, P.J.: T cell depletion in untreated adult coeliac disease. Gut 17:328-331, 1976.
47. Corazza, G.R., Sarchielli, P., Londei, M., Frisoni, M. and Gasbarrini, G.: Gluten specific suppressor T cell dysfunction in coeliac disease. Gut 27:392-398, 1986.
48. Kagnoff, M.F., Austin, R.K., Hubert, J.J., Bernardin, J.E. and Kasarda, D.D.: Possible role for a human adenovirus in the pathogenesis of celiac disease. J. Exp. Med. 160:1544, 1984.
49. Hall, E.J. and Batt, R.M.: Abnormal intestinal permeability in a wheat a wheat-sensitive enteropathy of Irish setter dogs. Gastroenterology 92:1422, 1987.
50. Lancaster-Smith, M., Packer, C., Kumar, P.J. and Harries, J.T.: Cellular infiltrate of the jejunum after re-introduction of dietary gluten in children with treated coeliac disease. J. Clin. Path. 29:587-591, 1976.
51. Bjorneklett, A., Fausa, O., Refsum, S.B., Torsvik, H. and Sigstad, H.: Jejunal villous atrophy and granulomatous inflammation responding to a gluten-free diet. Gut 18:814-816, 1977.
52. Batt, R.M. and Hall, E.J.: Chronic enteropathies in the dog. J. Sm. An. Pract. 30:3-12, 1989.
53. Kelly, J., O'Farrelly, C., Rees, J.P.R., Feighery, C. and Weir, D.G.W.: Humoral response to alpha gliadin as serological test for coeliac disease. Arch. Dis. Child. 62:469-473, 1987.
54. Chua, Y.Y., Bremner, K., Lakdawalla, N., Llobet, J.L., Kokubu, H.L., Orange, R.P. and Collins-Williams, C.: In vivo and in vitro correlates of food allergy. J. Allergy Clin. Immunol. 58:299-307, 1976.
55. Katz, A.J., Falchuk, Z.M., Strober, W. and Shwachman, H.: Gluten-sensitive enteropathy. Inhibition by cortisol of the effect of gluten protein in vitro. New Eng. J. Med. 295:131-135, 1976.
56. Logan, R.F.A., Rifkind, E.A., Busuttil, A., Gilmour, H.M. and Ferguson, A.: Prevalence and "incidence" of celiac disease in Edinburgh and the Lothian region of Scotland. Gastroenterology 90:334-342, 1986.

Chapter 21

Idiopathic Inflammatory Bowel Diseases

The idiopathic inflammatory bowel diseases are a group of disorders characterized by persistent clinical signs of gastrointestinal disease associated with histological evidence of inflammation of undetermined cause in the lamina propria of the small or large intestine. The diagnosis of these disorders carries stringent diagnostic obligations, not the least of which is establishing their idiopathic nature. The inflammatory bowel diseases are frequent causes of chronic vomiting and diarrhea in both cats and dogs. They may strike the small intestine, the large intestine, or both. In cats the disease complex most commonly affects the small intestine. In dogs it is more common in the large intestine.

CLASSIFICATION OF IDIOPATHIC INFLAMMATORY BOWEL DISEASES

The idiopathic inflammatory bowel diseases are usually classified according to the type of inflammation present and the area of the gastrointestinal tract in which the inflammation predominates. It is important to realize that this classification is an arbitrary system forced onto disease processes which have overlapping clinical-pathological features. Thus, it should not be of suprise to find inflammatory bowel diseases that do not easily fit into the standard classifications. For the purposes of this discussion, canine and feline idiopathic inflammatory bowel diseases will be classified into lymphocytic-plasmacytic enteritis, chronic (lymphocytic-plasmacytic) colitis, eosinophilic gastroenteritis, eosinophilic colitis, eosinophilic granulomas, the hypereosinophilic syndrome, histiocytic colitis, granulomatous enteritis, granulomatous colitis, transmural granulomatous enterocolitis, suppurative colitis, and the diarrheal syndromes of the Basenji and Ludenhund.

Canine chronic colitis has similarities to ulcerative colitis and "microscopic colitis" of humans. Canine granulomatous enteritis resembles Crohn's disease of humans. Current evidence in humans suggests that ulcerative colitis and Crohn's disease are the two ends of a spectrum of idiopathic inflammatory bowel diseases.[1] These two diseases are commonly grouped together under the term "inflammatory bowel disease." The justification for such a communal grouping is that in 5%-10% of cases they share overlapping clinical-pathological features, that a patient with one disease not infrequently has a relative with the other disease, that the diseases share certain immunologic abnormalities, and finally that they are both idiopathic.[1] While the etiopathogenesis of the idiopathic inflammatory bowel diseases of dogs and cats has been inadequately examined, there is no doubt that the pathophysiology of these diseases has an immune-mediated component, that they have overlapping clinical-pathologic features, that some breeds are predisposed to more than one type of idiopathic inflammatory bowel disease (Boxers, German Shepherds), and that the disorders are idiopathic. Therefore, for purposes of this discussion the diverse group of canine and feline idiopathic inflammatory bowel diseases will be placed in one clinical-pathological category and given the general term "inflammatory bowel disease"(IBD). The pathomechanisms that result in these different morphological expressions of inflammatory bowel disease are as yet poorly defined.

ETIOLOGY

Introduction

The cause or causes of IBD in animals and man remain unknown, in spite of intensive research into the etiopathogenesis of human ulcerative colitis and Crohn's disease. Proposed causes include defective immunoregulation of the gut-associated lymphoid tissue; genetic,[2] ischemic,[3] biochemical,[4,5] and psychosomatic[6] disorders; infectious,[7] and parasitic agents; permeability defects;[8] dietary allergies;[9-11] and adverse drug reactions.[9-10]

Whatever the cause of IBD, there is a general consensus that the pathogenesis of the syndrome involves hypersensitivity responses to antigens in the bowel lumen or mucosa. In the dog, such a conclusion is supported by several experimental studies which have demonstrated that sensitizing dogs to fecal or colonic antigens can produce chronic colitis.[12,13] While there is agreement that hypersensitivity reactions are important in the pathogenesis of IBD, there is as yet no widespread agreement as to the cause of the hypersensitivity responses. Whether the hypersensitivity results from a primary immune disorder or whether the numerous immunologic events associated with the disease are simply secondary to mucosal damage from an undefined primary cause remains to be settled. The nature of the inciting antigens and the reason for the unrestrained immune response against these putative antigens remains unresolved. In addition, which of the immunologic events associated with the disease are pathological and which are epiphenomena have as yet to be determined.

The Immunopathology of IBD

Mucosal Immunopathology. The immunopathology of IBD has been extensively investigated in humans.[1,14] Discrepancies exist in the data, partially as a result of methodology variations (immunohistopathology versus tissue digestion studies), and partially due to variations in the stage and class of IBD investigated. Most investigators are in agreement with the following observations. IBD lesions contain a twofold to fourfold increase in inflammatory cells, with B lymphocytes somewhat more prominent than T lymphocytes. The B lymphocytes are composed of an increased proportion of IgG-secreting lines. IgA secretion at the mucosal level may be depressed in spite of raised serum levels, and there is evidence that a higher percentage of monomeric IgA is secreted than in normal patients.[15] The T lymphocyte population, on the other hand, contains a more or less normal proportion of subpopulations as defined by various monoclonal antibodies. In addition to the increased numbers of lymphocytes, there are increased numbers of macrophages, neutrophils, mast cells, eosinophils, plasma cells, and intraepithelial lymphocytes, the proportion of which varies with the particular class of IBD. Opinion as to the relative numbers of NK cells in the tissues of IBD patients is divided. Their numbers probably change little, but their activity seems to decline.

The mucosal immunopathology of canine and feline IBD remains to be investigated.

Circulating Immunologic Elements in IBD.[1,14,16] Humans with IBD generally manifest normal or mildly increased immunoglobulin levels, particularly of the IgA class. In addition, they demonstrate elevated titers to various bacterial antigens, such as bacterial cell wall constituents of *Enterobacteriaceae* (the common antigen of Kunin) and food antigens such as bovine serum albumin. Antibodies to various colonic epithelial antigens, and mucus glycoproteins are also increased in many patients.

In contrast to the increased serum antibody levels, the percentage and number of circulating B lymphocytes are decreased during active IBD, either as a consequence of sequestration at sites of inflammation or exudation into the bowel lumen. Circulating T lymphocytes are generally normal to decreased. The activity of B lymphocytes, especially those that secrete IgA, as judged by lymphocyte blastogenesis tests is often increased. The reactivity of T lymphocytes to mucosal antigens, such as subcellular fractions of colonic epithelial cells and the common antigen of Kunin, is also often increased, although peripheral blood T cell responsiveness to non-mucosal antigens is often slightly depressed. The increased immunoreactivity of mucosal lymphocytes to mucosal antigens may result from increased exposure of the immune system to these antigens as a result of increased permeability. Alternatively, it may be due to a fundamental mucosal immunoregulatory defect.

Defective Immunoregulation in IBD. Unlike most other lymphoid tissues, GALT cannot rely on elimination of antigen to terminate an immune response. Instead, GALT has evolved a complex system to suppress the interminable immune response to familiar enteric antigens. The details of this oral tolerance are discussed in Chapter 3. Essential components of tolerance are an effective permeability barrier to macromolecules; maintenance of the non-phlogistic, predominantly IgA antibody response of GALT; and effective T suppressor cell activity. Effective T suppressor cell function requires constant surveillance and active suppression by the suppressor limb of the gut-associated lymphoid tissue. A breakdown in the suppressor function of GALT is currently thought by many to be the cause of the hypersensitivity response characteristic of IBD[1,8,9,17] (Figure 21-1). It is hypothesized that a defect in this system results in the escape of a reactive clone of lymphocytes that goes on to incite an immune response against a gut antigen, whether that antigen be a bacterial product, a food antigen, or a self-antigen (autoimmunity). The ensuing immune response would induce gastrointestinal inflammation, which in turn would increase bowel permeability, flooding the lamina propria with additional antigen of a variety of types. Eventually, the suppressor function of the GALT to a variety of antigens is thought to be overwhelmed, resulting in a vicious cycle of further inflammation, further permeability increase, and eventually overt tissue damage.[1]

In support of this hypothesis, defects in the activity of both circulating and mucosal T suppressor cells have been detected in humans with IBD. These defects have not been present in all patients studied or demonstrated in all in vitro assay systems

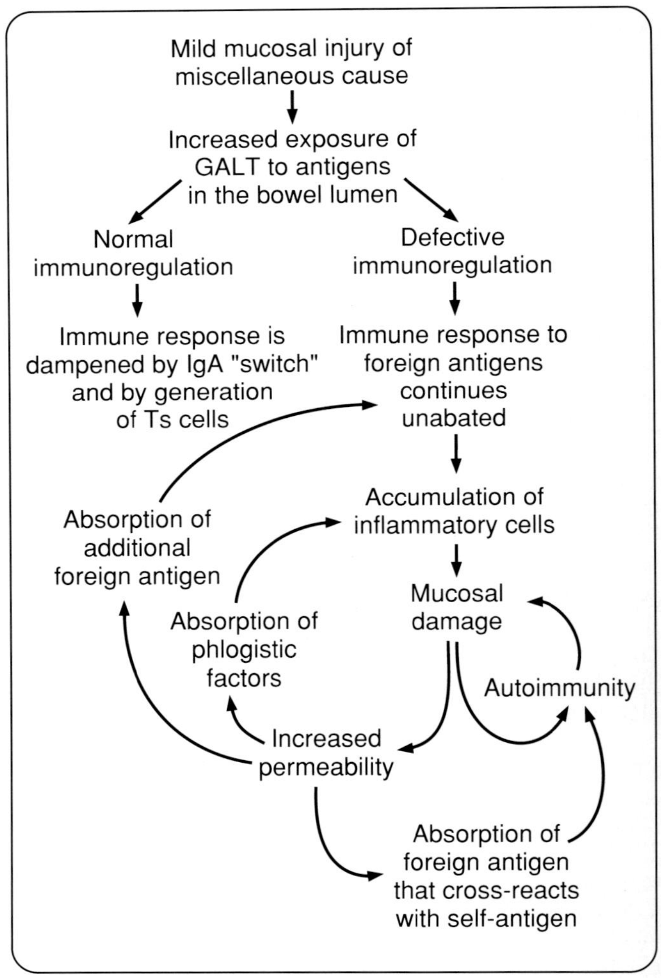

Figure 21-1. A defect in the suppressor function of the gut-associated lymphoid tissue has been proposed as the cause of inflammatory bowel disease.

used, however, and their importance remains to be established.[1,16]

Autoimmunity in IBD. Autoimmune disease of the bowel could result from a number of mechanisms. As discussed above, a T suppressor cell failure may result in the escape of an autoreactive lymphocyte clone. Alternatively, an immune response against a foreign gut antigen that shares antigenic determinants with self tissue could result in an inappropriate attack against self-tissue in addition to the inciting agent. The latter suggestion has received some prominence because of the demonstration that antibodies to the common enterobacterial antigen of Kunin will cross-react with antigenic determinants on colonic epithelial cells.[18]

To establish an autoimmune basis for the disease, researchers must first prove that IBD is associated with disease-specific and tissue-specific autoantibodies or self-reactive lymphocytes, that these antibodies or lymphocytes precede the intestinal damage, and finally that they are capable of causing tissue damage. It has been clearly demonstrated that autoantibodies and cytotoxic cells with specificity for intestinal epithelial cells are present in the sera of humans with IBD and that they can precede overt clinical disease.[1,16] What remains to be convincingly demonstrated is that these autoreactive immune components have an important damaging role and are not simply epiphenomena.

As many as 60%-70% of humans with ulcerative colitis have circulating antibodies to colonic tissue, whereas only 10%-15% of normal people are antibody positive.[1] The importance of these antibodies has been questioned because the titer often bore no correlation to the severity of the disease and because the tissue specificity of the initial autoantibody preparations was poor. More recently, however, the existence of antibodies specific for gastrointestinal tract mucin-associated glycoproteins[19] and basolateral membranes of colon epithelial cells[20] has been confirmed. Furthermore, these antibodies were shown to be present in non-diseased relatives of patients with IBD.[21,22] These observations go against the supposition that all the anti-intestinal antibodies are merely secondary to mucosal injury. In spite of these advances, it remains to be shown how important autoantibodies are to the tissue injury of IBD. It is probable that many of the antibodies produced are not pathogenic, but occur as a consequence of the tissue injury. It has been established, however, that some of these antibodies can prime mucosal leukocytes to cause cytotoxicity of colonic epithelial cells via antibody-dependent cellular cytotoxicity.[23]

Antibody-mediated, complement-dependent cytotoxicity of colon cells does not appear to be important in the pathogenesis of IBD.[24] Autoreactive T cell clones are also present in the intestinal tissues of patients with IBD and are capable of cytotoxicity.[25] As with autoantibodies, however, it remains to be established how important this MHC-restricted T lymphocyte cytotoxicity is in comparison to non-specific tissue destruction resulting from the multitude of cytotoxic mediators released in inflammatory processes.

The importance of autoimmunity in canine and feline IBD requires further investigation. An acute onset of a hemorrhagic diarrhea can be induced in dogs by the injection of antisera prepared against canine colonic mucosa.[26,27] The colonic tissues show edema, neutrophil infiltration, and multifocal hemorrhagic necrosis. A mild, persistent colitis has been induced in two dogs by the repeated injection of a homogenate of the dogs' own colonic mucosa, derived by colectomy.[12] Unfortunately, inadequate attempts to ensure sterility of the antigenic material were made in these studies. Nevertheless, they suggest that immune-mediated mechanisms and perhaps autoimmunity may be involved in the pathogenesis of canine enterocolitis.

Genetic Influences

There is a well recognized familial tendency toward IBD in humans. Multiple occurrences of IBD in the same family are identified in 20%-40% of IBD cases.[16] To date, however, a consistent genetic marker of disease predisposition has not been identified. A genetic influence is also well recognized in dogs. The Boxer and the French Bulldog are the only two dog breeds in which histiocytic colitis has been reported. Furthermore, the Basenji and the Ludenhund have well recognized protein-losing enteropathies with a familial component. It is probable that the genetic makeup of the patient establishes susceptibility to IBD, but that the actual disease is precipitated by other factors.

Environmental Influences

Striking differences in the prevalence of IBD occur in human populations throughout the world. Westernization of populations leads to a higher incidence of the disease. The reasons for these environmental variations are unknown.[11]

Drug Therapy

The prostaglandin synthetase inhibitors, cinchophen and indomethacin, have been shown to induce colitis, in dogs, with a resemblance to early Crohn's disease.[28] Lesions developed as early as one day after the initiation of therapy and were centered over the Peyer's patches. Similarly, a strong association between the use of non-steroidal antiinflammatory drugs (NSAIDs) and small intestinal inflammation has been noted in humans.[29] NSAIDs are known to activate quiescent ulcerative colitis in humans.[30]

The reason for the proinflammatory effect of NSAIDs on the intestine is unknown, but proposed causes have included removal of the protective effect of prostaglandins,[30] interference with mucus secretion, increase in bowel permeability,[31] and interference with T suppressor activity resulting in an unrestrained interaction of lymphoid tissue and intestinal antigen.[28]

Chronic hypermotility of the bowel induced by the repeated administration of cholinergic agents can cause an ulcerative colitis in dogs.[32]

Dietary Influences

It is well established that the clinical signs of some dogs and cats with chronic colitis and, to a lesser extent, eosinophilic gastroenteritis will resolve if the patient is placed on a controlled diet.[33,34] Similarly, in humans, there is convincing data to suggest that "bowel rest" by parenteral nutrition or use of elemental diets can reduce the symptoms of Crohn's disease.[11] These observations, while useful from the therapeutic point of view, do not establish a role for diet in the etiology or pathogenesis of IBD, just as the response of this disorder to prednisone does not establish "prednisone deficiency" as the cause of IBD. The apparent response of some of these patients to dietary management may have a number of explanations (Table 21-1). The diet may contain additives which irritate the mucosa or antigens to which the patient is allergic. The diet directly influences intestinal morphology and physiologic functions such as the rapidity of cell renewal, mucus secretion, fluid and electrolyte absorption, and motility patterns. For instance, in pigs, high protein diets are associated with decreased area for absorption and reduced absorption of fluids and electrolytes.[35] High fiber diets promote mucus synthesis and secretion. Experimental dietary deficiencies of vitamin A, folic acid, and pantothenic acid can cause colitis. Deficiencies of these vitamins are unlikely to be important in the spontaneous disease. The composition of the diet has a profound influence on the composition of the intestinal microbial flora. For instance, dietary variation markedly alters the numbers of *Clostridia* and *Fusobacteria* species in human feces.[36] High-protein diets increase colonic anaerobe numbers, and high-carbohydrate diets increase the numbers of aerobes.[37-39] Alteration of the bacterial flora in turn has wide ranging effects on bowel morphologic, physiologic, and immunologic function. Furthermore, many patients with IBD are malnourished for a variety of reasons (Table 21-2) and their clinical improvement may simply result from improved nutritional status.

It is difficult to determine which of these influences of diet on bowel function is the most important in the responsiveness of IBD to dietary manipulation. The wide variety of diets that have met with apparent success (high protein, low protein, high fiber, low fiber, hypoallergenic, easily digestible, enteral, and parenteral) suggests that the beneficial response may operate through more than one mechanism. It is likely that immune responses against food antigens will prove to be relatively more important in small bowel IBD than large bowel IBD, because digestion and absorption of the majority of food proteins is completed in the small bowel. Diet is more likely to influence the etiopathophysiology of chronic colitis through effects on bowel motility and the composition of the fecal flora, although poorly digestible proteins could conceivably induce a colonic hypersensitivity response. Of the diverse influences of diet on gastrointestinal function, dietary additives and antigenic dietary proteins have received the most attention as possible causes of IBD.

Table 21-1. Possible Influences of Diet on the Etiopathogenesis of IBD

Mucosal disease resulting from dietary deficiencies
Provision of toxic food additives
Provision of antigenic dietary proteins
Provision of protein substrate for ammonia generation
Alteration of cell renewal rate
Alteration of bowel morphology
Alteration of bowel motility
Alteration of absorption
Alteration of mucus secretion
Alteration of the number of bowel microflora
Alteration of the composition of bowel microflora
Reconstitution of depressed immunity resulting from malnutrition

Table 21-2. Causes of Malnutrition in Inflammatory Bowel Disease

Inadequate intake
Anorexia
Maladigestion
"Functional" exocrine pancreatic insufficiency
Malabsorption
Bacterial overgrowth
Brush border enzyme derangements
Villus atrophy
Diffusion barriers
Excessive losses
Protein-losing enteropathy
Gastrointestinal bleeding
Increased cellular desquamation
Increased requirements
Inflammation
Fever

Food Additives. Exposure to certain food additives such as carrageenan, an extract of red seaweeds, and several other closely related sulfated polysaccharides, such as sulfated amylopectin and lignosulfonates, is a well recognized method of producing experimental colitis in laboratory animals.[40,41] Lignosulfonate is a binding agent often used in pelleted animal feeds. Surprisingly, sulfated amylopectins are used to treat and prevent gastroduodenal ulcerations, yet they cause ulceration of the colonic mucosa in certain species. The colon degrades these polysaccharides; their by-products in association with colonic bacteria produce mucosal ulcers.

It is not known whether the incidence of colitis has changed since the feeding of prepared foods became popular. As yet, no binding agents, food colorings or preservatives have been shown to be responsible for human, canine or feline IBD, although the vast array of these products precludes discounting this possibility.

Dietary Antigens. An influence of dietary antigens on the etiopathogenesis of IBD seems likely, but the relative importance of that influence is as yet undetermined. The absorption of intact antigenic macromolecules into the lamina propria of patients with IBD is increased because of increased mucosal permeability. Human patients with IBD have an enhanced immunoresponsiveness to food antigens, but also to other antigens in the gut, particularly bacteria and bacterial products.[11] Antibodies against a variety of dietary antigens are found in the plasma of both normal humans and humans with IBD. There is no correlation between their titers, the severity of the disease process, and the responsiveness of the patient to an elimination diet.[42] Thus, these antibodies appear to be an effect of the disease rather than a cause. An investigation of one dog for the presence of fecal and serum antibodies against a variety of food and parasitic antigens was unrewarding.[43]

In spite of these unsupportive findings, it is a reasonable assumption that humoral or cellular immune responses against dietary antigens contribute to the inflammatory process and help perpetuate the disease. Therefore, a change in dietary antigens may temporarily reduce the immune-mediated mucosal inflammatory response. The longevity of this amelioration is questionable, however, since the so-called "hypoallergenic" diets in common use in veterinary medicine contain intact proteins that are hypoallergenic primarily by virtue of their novelty to the host's immune system. The duration of their novelty to GALT is likely to be very limited if the antigen is fed to an animal with a highly porous mucosal barrier.

The results of elimination diets in humans have been inconsistent. Earlier reports of widespread hypersensitivity to cow milk proteins amongst patients with IBD have not been confirmed,[16] with the exception of patients with eosinophilic gastroenteritis, in which evidence of hypersensitivity to milk is common.[44] Dogs with eosinophilic gastrointestinal inflammation often show a complete clinical response to controlled diets, but no information has been accumulated as to which specific nutrients, if any, the dogs are hypersensitive too.

In summary, the apparent success of dietary therapy in the treatment of IBD most likely relates to direct effects of diet on bowel physiologic functions such as motility and to indirect effects such as altered bowel microflora, rather than to the elimination of toxic food additives or allergenic proteins. The most likely disorder in which hypersensitivity to dietary antigens is involved is eosinophilic IBD.

Pathogenic Microorganisms in IBD

A role for pathogenic microorganisms in IBD has been long suspected but, in spite of intensive efforts over the last 50 years, no pathogenic microorganisms have been conclusively identified as a cause of IBD. Most investigators have been unable to incite intestinal inflammation following the administration to various species of materials obtained from intestinal tissues affected by IBD. An exception to this statement is the work of Van Kruiningen and associates, who were able to isolate an as-yet unclassified *Mycobacterium* from the tissues of humans with Crohn's disease, which when administered to goats incited a granulomatous enteritis similar in nature to human Crohn's disease.[7] Other investigators have also been able to culture *Mycobacteria* from tissues of patients with Crohn's disease.[45] The possibility that the *Mycobacteria* isolated are simply commensals of ulcerated mucosal membranes has been raised.[1] Another group has suggested that cell wall-defective variants of pseudomonas-like bacteria can be consistently isolated from humans with Crohn's disease.[47]

Evidence of a role for pathogenic microorganisms in canine and feline IBD is similarly scanty. Coccoid bodies resembling *Chlamydia* particles have been observed in the macrophages of Boxers with histiocytic colitis,[48] but no evidence could be found for an infectious cause in a comparable study.[49] Feline infectious peritonitis virus can cause a granulomatous colitis in cats, and viruses have inconsistently been isolated from the tissues of humans with IBD.[50]

The inability to consistently isolate a pathogen, the lack of epidemiological data supportive of contagion, and the responsiveness of the condition to immunosuppressive therapy strongly rule against an infectious cause in most cases of human and animal IBD.[1,51] The apparent response of IBD to antibacterial agents such as tylosin, metronidazole, and sulfasalazine has been taken by some to indicate a role for a pathogenic bacteria. This need not be the case, however, because both metronidazole and sulfasalazine have well established immunoregulatory and antiinflammatory effects, respectively. The possibility that tylosin and metronidazole exert their beneficial effects through alteration of the composition of normal flora must also be considered.

Normal Flora in IBD

While it is unlikely that pathogenic microorganisms are an important cause of IBD, there is strong experimental evidence to suggest that the ubiquitous and persistent normal bacterial flora are involved in the pathogenesis of the disease. Most evidence indicates that sensitization to bacterial flora will exacerbate the severity and prolong the duration of transient mild bowel inflammation. In laboratory animals, antigens used were certain strains of *E. coli*[52] and the common enterobacterial antigen of Kunin.[46] Similar results were seen following sensitization of dogs with a bacterial-rich fecal extract.[13] Chronic granulomatous inflammation can be induced in the bowel of rats by injecting cell wall fragments of group A Streptoccus.[53] Antibodies reacting with anaerobic but not aerobic fecal bacteria can be demonstrated in the mucosa of patients with ulcerative colitis.[16] Additional evidence for a role for bacterial flora in IBD is provided by the observation that pretreatment with metronidazole[40] or trimethoprim-sulfamethoxazole[54] will protect guinea pigs against ulcerative colitis induced by the administration of carrageenan. Furthermore, immunization against urease-producing bacteria will reduce the severity of experimental ulcerative colitis resulting from uremia and irradiation.[26]

Which enteric bacterial species are the most likely species to be involved in the pathogenesis of spontaneous IBD has yet to be established. Studies of the bowel microflora in ulcerative colitis in humans are highly variable and as yet indecisive.[16] Aerobic and anaerobic bacterial flora influence numerous anatomic, physiologic, and immunologic parameters of the host. Bacterial flora stimulate peristalsis; induce a heavier, thicker intestinal wall; accelerate the transit time of epithelial cells moving from the crypts to the villous tips; accelerate the process of epithelial renewal; influence the activity of brush border enzymes; increase the number of intraepithelial lymphocytes, plasma cells, and Peyer's patches; and modify bile acids by deconjugation and dehydroxylation.[55]

Recently, evidence has emerged that certain bowel bacteria secrete small phlogistic peptides, the most well-characterized of which is N-formyl-methionyl-leucyl-phenylalanine (FMLP). Leukocytes, in particular neutrophils, have high and low affinity receptors for these peptides. The high affinity receptors respond to low concentrations of mediator and induce chemotaxis, whereas the low affinity receptors stimulate degranulation. It appears that these peptides can cross intact bowel mucosa, raising the possibility that the secretory products of bacterial flora may be directly involved in the initiation of IBD. Neutrophils from patients with ulcerative colitis have increased responsiveness to FMLP. Furthermore, any factor that increases bowel permeability or increases the proportion of enteric bacteria that secrete these agents is likely to predispose to IBD. Infusion of N-formylated peptides into the colon of rats or mice can induce experimental colitis.[56]

Parasites

Gastrointestinal parasitism has been proposed as a cause of eosinophilic gastroenteritis and colitis in humans and animals.

Some cases of eosinophilic gastroenteritis have been thought to be associated with visceral larval migrans.[57] However, ascarids or their migrating larvae are rarely identified in dogs with eosinophilic gastroenteritis. Trichuris vulpis infection is sometimes associated with an extensive inflammatory infiltrate, which may have lymphocytic, plasmacytic, granulomatous, and eosinophilic components. Giardiasis is occasionally associated with lymphocytic-plasmacytic inflammation. While there is no doubt that parasites can cause focal inflammatory reactions in the intestine, there is little evidence to support that occult parasitism is responsible for the generalized inflammation characteristic of many forms of IBD.

Permeability Alterations

Inflammation of many causes is known to increase intestinal permeability in humans and animals.[58,59] The increase is thought to relate to epithelial denudation or, in less severe cases, to the development of a less differentiated epithelium as a result of increased cell turnover.[60] Gamma interferon will increase epithelial tight junction permeability.[61]

Not suprisingly, humans with inflammatory bowel disease have increased bowel permeability, raising suspicion that inflammation-mediated breakdown in mucosal barrier function can contribute to the perpetuation of the disease. Recently, however, it has been demonstrated that relatives of people with IBD also have increased bowel permeability. This raises the likelihood that disordered permeability is the primary lesion in IBD, and that the intestinal inflammation is a result of chronic excessive antigenic exposure (Figure 21-2). As yet no cause of the increased permeability has been defined although the recent discovery that humans with IBD secrete increased monomeric IgA and altered IgA subclasses may partly explain the compromised barrier function.[15]

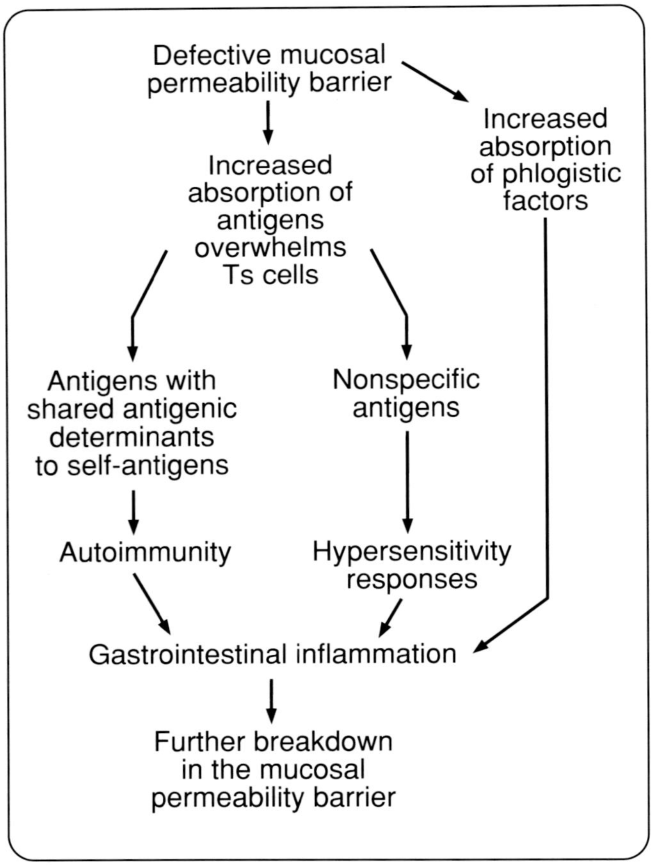

Figure 21-2. A defect in the mucosal permeability barrier has been proposed as the cause of inflammatory bowel disease

Ischemia

Cats and dogs have a low incidence of obstructive vascular disease. Although acute but not slowly developing obstruction of the blood supply to the canine colon results in a hemorrhagic colitis, experimental induction of hypovolemic shock fails to produce colitis in dogs.[3] The possibility has been proposed that intermittent ischemia-reperfusion injury of the colonic mucosa due to intermittent excessive sympathetic activity could result in IBD.[63] Vascular lesions have been identified in histiocytic ulcerative colitis but appear to be a result and not a cause of the ulceration.[62] Thus ischemia would seem to be an unlikely cause of chronic colitis in the dog or cat. The small intestine is more susceptible to ischemic injury than is the colon, but there is no evidence to support a vascular cause for canine or feline small intestinal IBD.

Biochemical Causes

Diminished incorporation of ^{14}C labeled amino acids into colonic mucosal proteins of humans with colitis has been reported, suggesting a defective mucosal regenerative capacity.[16] Rectal biopsies of humans with ulcerative colitis have decreased concentrations of various enzymes, but these are thought to be a consequence rather than a cause of the disease. The metabolism of affected colonic epithelial cells allegedly differs from normal in that butyrate oxidation is impaired and glutamine and glucose oxidation is increased.[16] The significance of these observations is unknown. Alterations in colonic mucin profiles have been reported in human ulcerative colitis.[4,5] The significance of this observation is also unknown, but it is of interest to note that mucin is thought to be a potent scavenger of oxygen-free radicals; furthermore, it affords mucosal protection by way of its lubricant properties and a cooperative role with IgA.

Psychologic Causes

There is as yet no convincing evidence that psychological disturbances can cause IBD, although there is little reason to question that a chronological relationship exists between significant emotional events and the recurrence, or intensification of IBD in both man and animals.[16] The pathomechanism of such exacerbations may involve autonomic and enteric nervous system effects on bowel circulation, motility, secretion or absorption.[6] The observation of increased concentrations of substance P in the IBD lesions of humans provides support for a role of neurogenic inflammation in the pathogenesis of IBD (Chapter 4). Recently it has been proposed that repeated neurogenic-mediated mucosal ischemia resulting from stress may lead to IBD.[63]

PATHOPHYSIOLOGY

Hypersensitivity Responses In IBD[64,65]

Hypersensitivity responses are exuberant inflammatory reactions of immunological origin. It appears that much of the tissue damage of IBD results from hypersensitivity to enteric antigens. As discussed above, it is not clear whether the hypersensitivities result from a primary defect in immunoregulation or whether they are a result of overwhelmed suppressor activity pursuant to a defective mucosal permeability barrier. More than one type of hypersensitivity response is involved in IBD (Figure 21-3).

Type 1, Immediate-Type Hypersensitivity. Eosinophilic gastroenteritis and eosinophilic colitis are probably mediated by an immediate (type 1) hypersensitivity response. Type 1 hypersensitivities are inflammatory reactions mediated by IgE bound to mast cells. Antigens binding to the IgE induce mast cell degranulation. Mast cells release a number of inflammatory mediators, some of which attract eosinophils (Chapter 4). Type 1 hypersensitivity responses also result in acute damage to the enterocytes through unknown mechanisms.[66]

The antigens that induce IgE have no discernable unique features that separate them from the antigens that induce IgG responses.[67] Potent stimulators of this response include pollens, helminth antigens, and some bacteria. In animals and man, there are recognizable genetic predispositions to type 1 hypersensitivities. Evidence that food antigens, such as milk proteins, can induce eosinophilic responses has been presented.[44] Dietary alteration will resolve some cases of canine eosinophilic gastroenteritis or colitis, suggesting but by no means proving that dietary antigens may be involved in the pathogenesis of the inflammation. If eosinophilic gastroenteritis is due to a dietary antigen that incites a type 1 hypersensitivity response, it is likely that the inciting antigen would have to be a regular component of the diet to maintain chronic excitation of what is usually an acute and self-limiting hypersensitivity.

Eosinophils temper some aspects of the inflammatory response but also release toxic products. The pathological consequences of the accumulation of eosinophils is discussed in Chapter 4.

Type II, Cytotoxic-Type Hypersensitivity. Type II hypersensitivity refers to antibody-mediated destruction of cells, either by the activation of complement or through the activities of cytotoxic cells which bind to the antibody-coated cell and induce lysis (antibody-dependent cellular cytotoxicity). This subject is discussed more fully under the section of autoimmunity in IBD. It is possible that antibody-mediated cytotoxicity is important in canine and feline lymphocytic-plasmacytic IBD.

Type III, Antigen-Antibody Complexes. Immune complexes deposited in tissues can fix complement and incite an inflammatory process. Experimental models of colitis induced by immune-complexes have been reported.[68] The majority of human patients with IBD have circulating immune complexes,[1] and in some patients immune complexes can be detected in IBD lesions.[16] However, the pathological role of immune complexes in human IBD is thought to be minor. There is no evidence in humans that immune complex deposition is essential for the development of IBD lesions, and systemic consequences of circulating immune complexes such as vasculitis and glomerulonephritis are not common.[1] The prominent presence of antibody-secreting plasma cells in the IBD lesions of dogs and cats suggests that type III hypersensitivity may be more important in the inflammatory bowel diseases of dogs and cats than it is in humans.

Type IV, Cell-Mediated Hypersensitivity. Cell-mediated or delayed-type hypersensitivity is an immune-mediated response dependent on sensitized T lymphocytes. The primed T lymphocyte releases chemotactic substances that result in inflammation, phagocyte infiltration, and cell death. Expression of this reaction requires several days. Cell-mediated hypersensitivity plays a role in IBD in humans.[25,64] Because of methodology problems in the *in vitro* study of these more delayed processes, there is little definitive information on the importance of T cell-mediated cytotoxicity. Some authors have hypothesized that it is a key mechanism of injury.[1] Certainly, T cell-mediated colitis can be readily induced in laboratory animals by the administration of the contactant dinitrochlorobenzene (DNCB).[69,70] The inflammation produced is non-sustained but

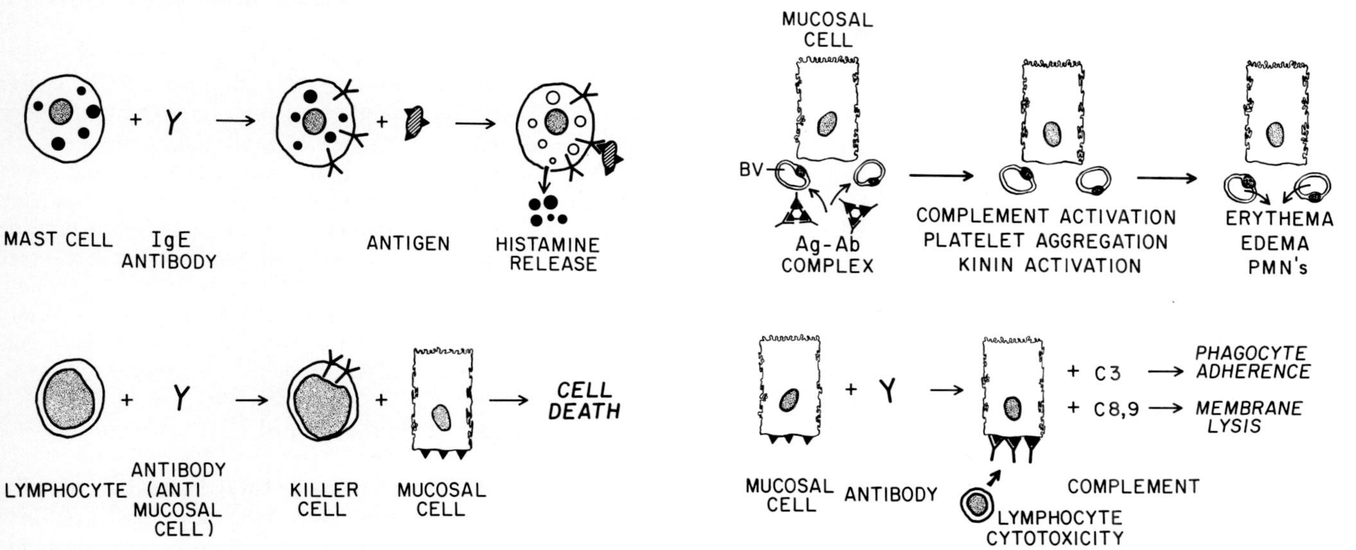

Figure 21-3. The four types of hypersensitivity.

it does demonstrate that T cell-mediated events, no less than B cell-mediated events, can lead to colonic inflammation.

In canine and feline IBD, T cell dependent hypersensitivity is likely to be of prime importance in the few cases of granulomatous enteritis that have been reported. Lymphokines released by activated T cells may also play a role in the induction of the villous atrophy that accompanies many of the inflammatory gastrointestinal disorders.

Gastrointestinal Inflammation in IBD

Gastrointestinal inflammation is the final common pathway to the tissue damage of IBD. The classification, mediators, consequences, and regulation of gastrointestinal inflammation are discussed in Chapter 4. As mentioned above, it is probable that immune-initiated inflammation (hypersensitivity) is an important cause of the persistent inflammation that characterizes IBD, but that other factors such as absorbed bacterial peptides and neurotransmitters are also involved. If inflammation is persistent, fibrosis will result. Leukotriene B_4 and HETEs are found in high concentrations in rectal mucosal samples taken from humans with ulcerative colitis. The severity of the inflammation positively correlates with the concentration of leukotriene B_4. Inhibitors of leukotriene synthesis have resulted in significant decreases in inflammation in various experimental colitis models. It is likely that these eicosanoids are important proinflammatory mediators in inflammatory bowel disease. Other mediators that may be of importance are oxygen-derived free radicals, phagocyte proteases, substance P, lymphokines, platelet derivatives, and prostaglandins.

Pathogenesis of Vomiting in IBD

Vomiting is a frequent sign associated with IBD, whether the disease process is centered in the small or large bowel. The vomiting most often results from either reflexive stimulation of the vomiting center by way of visceral afferent fibers or from stimulation of the chemoreceptor center by way of absorbed toxins. Disrupted gastrointestinal motility and in particular ileus may exacerbate the vomiting.

Pathogenesis of Diarrhea in IBD

The diarrhea associated with IBD has more than one pathogenesis. Inflammatory processes centered in the small bowel result in increased leakage of fluid and electrolytes and, if severe, protein and blood into the bowel lumen. The accumulated inflammatory cells result in a diffusion barrier and release mediators that result in villous atrophy and brush border enzyme damage (Chapter 4). The brush border enzyme defects, villous atrophy, and cellular diffusion barrier result in the malabsorption of nutrients, the consequence of which is osmotic diarrhea. Bacterial overgrowth resulting from intestinal hypomotility, malabsorption, or partial obstruction may contribute to the diarrhea. Concomitant maldigestion as a result of functional pancreatic insufficiency can also occur.

The diarrhea associated with colitis results primarily from disordered colonic motility and reduced water and electrolyte absorption. In an experimental model of feline colitis, a significant overall reduction in both basal and urecholine stimulated colonic motility was observed coincident with the worst colonic ulceration and diarrhea.[71] The pathogenesis of the motility disturbances are not clear but probably result either from a direct effect of the mediators, such as PGE_2 or leukotrienes, on smooth muscle function or from an indirect effect of these mediators on the enteric nervous system (Chapter 4). Inflammatory processes affecting the ascending colon interfere with the reverse peristalsis that characterizes the motility of this segment of the colon in the cat and, to a lesser extent, the dog. This results in more rapid transit of colonic content through the cranial colon, less absorption of water, and a watery diarrhea. In contrast, inflammation of the rectum and distal colon interferes with the reservoir function of the large bowel and can stimulate the defecation reflex. The clinical manifestation is frequent defecation (reservoir fecal incontinence) and tenesmus with small quantities of pasty stool. The inflammation increases bowel permeability and reduces the electrical potential across the colonic epithelial cell, thus interfering with the absorption of fluid and electrolytes. A failure of colonic salvage of fecal carbohydrate may also contribute to the diarrhea.[72] The pathophysiology of diarrhea is discussed in more detail in Chapter 16.

The fresh blood that tinges the feces of dogs and cats with colitis results from vascular engorgement, ulceration, and the development of a friable mucosa and granulation tissue.

Pathogenesis of Abdominal Pain in IBD

Occasionally animals with inflammatory bowel disease will show evidence of abdominal pain. The cause of the abdominal pain is also multifactorial. Gastrointestinal inflammation releases mediators that can directly stimulate visceral pain receptors. The same mediators also reduce the threshold at which muscular stretch is perceived as painful. Thus bowel contractions of normal strength can induce a pain response. In addition, gastrointestinal inflammation is occasionally associated with painful muscular spasms. Furthermore, hypomotility or carbohydrate malabsorption can result in the accumulation or generation of intestinal gas which causes abdominal pain by overdistension of the intestinal tract.

Pathogenesis of Extraintestinal Signs of IBD

A large variety of extraintestinal signs accompany IBD in humans and animals (Table 21-3).[73] Similarly, immunization with intestinal antigens produces striking inflammatory changes in the extraintestinal tissues of laboratory animals.[74] The pathogenesis of these changes remains uncertain. Antibodies to bile ductal cells, liver, kidney, and pancreatic extracts have been observed in the sera of human patients with IBD. The presence of immune complexes does not correlate with the presence of many of the extraintestinal manifestations of IBD,[1] although a correlation has been noted in sclerosing cholangitis. It is possible that the same immunoregulatory defect hypothesized as a cause for IBD results in hypersensitivities in other organs.

Summary of Etiology and Pathophysiology

In summary, the high incidence of IBD, the diversity of the age, breed, and sex of animals affected, and the variations in the site and pathological appearance of the inflammation suggest that there is more than one cause of IBD in dogs and cats (Figure

Table 21-3. Extraintestinal Manifestations of IBD

Weight loss
Growth retardation
Polyarthritis
Ankylosing spondylitis
Nephrolithiasis (oxalate)
Coagulopathies (pulmonary embolism)
Hepatobiliary disease
Skin disease (Pyoderma gangrenosum, erythema nodosum, cutaneous vasculitis)
Autoimmune hemolytic anemia
Hypercoagulability
Uveitis
Pericholangitis and sclerosing cholangitis
Fatty infiltration of the liver
Chronic active hepatitis
Amyloidosis
Chronic obstructive pulmonary disease

21-4). The most likely causes are an as-yet undefined abnormality in the immune response of the suppressor arm of the GALT, or a defect in the mucosal permeability barrier. In some breeds, these defects may have a genetic basis. Either of these abnormalities are capable of inducing a hypersensitivity response to gut antigens, the most important of which are probably normal bacterial flora, but which in some animals may be self-antigens or food antigens. The relative importance of the different hypersensitivity responses to the pathogenesis of IBD has not been determined in the cat or dog, but it is probable that type I hypersensitivity predominates in eosinophilic IBD, and that antibody-mediated hypersensitivities (type II and III) predominate in lymphocytic-plasmacytic IBD. It is likely that inflammation resulting from the absorption of phlogistic factors, as well as neurogenic inflammation, can exacerbate the inflammation resulting from hypersensitivity responses. Neutrophilic infiltrates would be expected to characterize the absorption of phlogistic factors such as FMLP and so might be relatively more important in suppurative IBD. The inflammatory mediators of most importance in IBD appear to be leukotrienes, oxygen-derived free radicals, and leukocyte proteases. The primary clinical signs of IBD directly pertain to gastrointestinal inflammation and its effects on gastrointestinal permeability and motility, nutrient absorption, and the vomiting center. The pathogenesis of the extraintestinal clinical signs remains to be elucidated.

DIAGNOSIS OF INFLAMMATORY BOWEL DISEASE

To make a definitive diagnosis of IBD, the clinician must fulfill certain diagnostic obligations. Not to do so results in the relegation of the term IBD to the status of a "garbage can diagnosis," a front for sloppy medicine. First, the clinician or owner must observe primary or secondary clinical signs of gastrointestinal disease. Secondly, the clinical signs must be determined to be persistent. In general, the duration of such signs should be in terms of weeks rather than days to help

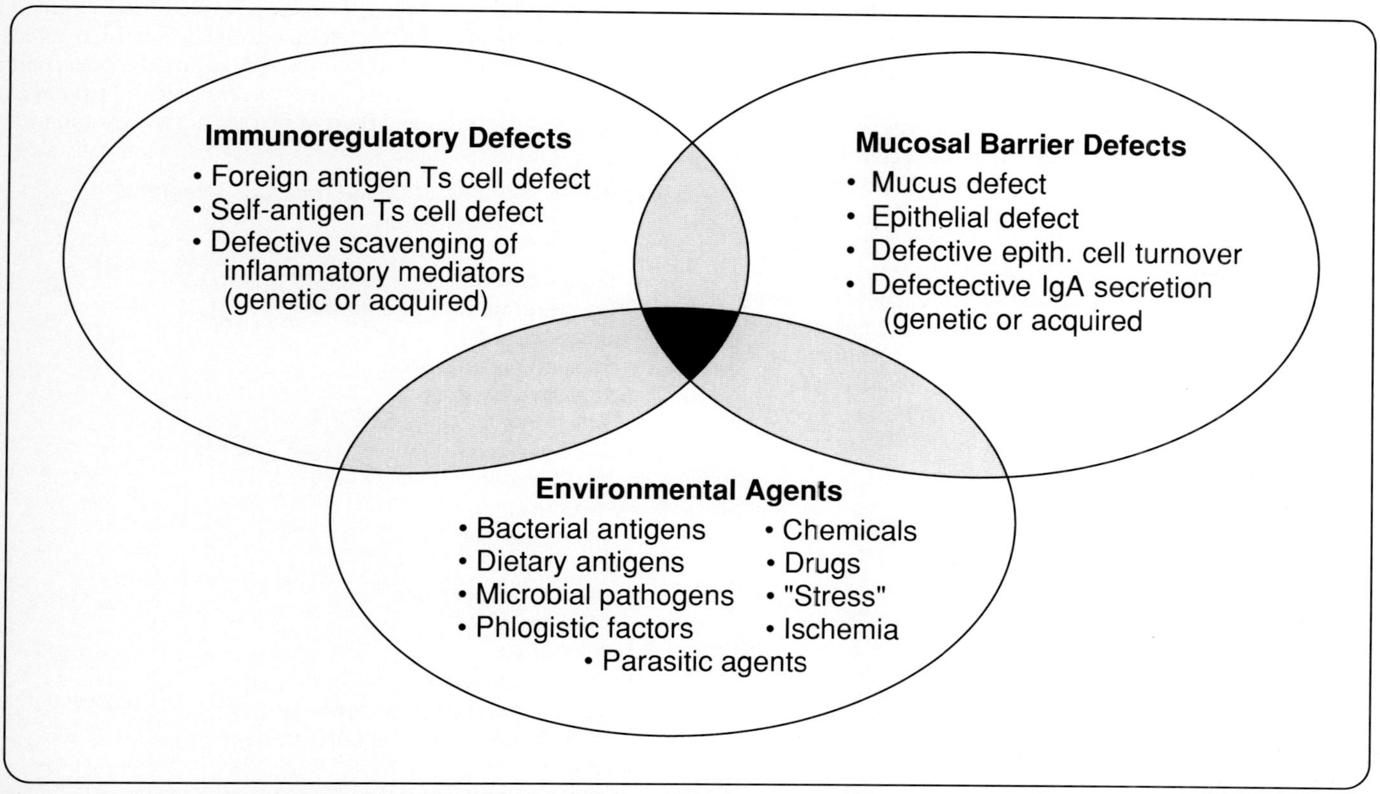

Figure 21-4. The interaction of immunoregulatory defects, increased mucosal permeability, and environmental pathogens in the genesis of inflammatory bowel disease.

differentiate IBD from the inflammatory changes of the acute enteritis. Thirdly, the clinician must go on to demonstrate that the observed clinical signs are associated with chronic inflammation in the lamina propria of the small or large intestine. This is best achieved by thorough endoscopic examination and biopsy of the small and/or large bowel, followed by careful pathologic assessment. Finally, the clinician and pathologist must establish that the gastrointestinal inflammation has no demonstrable cause. This latter step in the diagnostics is commonly overlooked by clinicians, yet it is essential for the diagnosis of IBD.

Clinical Findings

The primary clinical signs compatible with IBD include vomiting, diarrhea, anorexia, weight loss, flatulence, borborygmus, abdominal pain, hematochezia, tenesmus, and mucoid stools. In general, the presence of particular signs in a patient reflects the predominant site of the disease more closely rather than it differentiates the type of infiltrate. There are few if any clinical findings that differentiate the various forms of colitis and enteritis from one another. Signalment provides some help, in that Boxers and French bulldogs are the breeds most likely to be affected by histiocytic colitis, whereas Basenjis and Ludenhunds have their own specific diarrheal syndromes, and Irish Setters are afflicted by wheat-sensitive enteropathy.

Secondary (extraintestinal) signs of IBD seen in humans are listed in Table 21-3. The most frequent of these symptomatic complications is joint disease (26% of patients), closely followed by skin disease (19%).[75] In humans, colitic arthritis is migratory, pauciarticular, and preferentially affects larger joints.[75] In those patients that are affected by joint disease, the severity of the joint disease tends to parallel the severity of the colitis. Common subclinical abnormalities reported in humans include pericholangitis (35%-50%) and fatty livers (40%).

In dogs and cats with IBD, extraintestinal clinical signs are rarely noticed. In a retrospective review of the confirmed cases of canine chronic colitis presented to the VMTH the most common concurrent problems were pruritic skin diseases and otitis externa, but these conditions did not have a greater incidence in dogs with colitis than in our general hospital population. A non-erosive polyarthritis has been recognized in the occasional dog with colitis.[76] Polyarthritis has not been recognized as a complication of IBD in cats, although the sedentary nature of this species may have obscured this clinical sign. Fatty livers are not uncommon in canine and feline IBD, and approximately 20% of dogs with chronic colitis have mild elevations of SAP, ALT, or both.

Diagnostic Tests and Differential Diagnosis

Inflammatory bowel disease is a diagnosis of exclusion. The known causes of intestinal inflammation resembling IBD are many (Tables 21-4, 21-5, 21-6 and 21-7). As a result, the diagnostic testing required to eliminate all known causes of intestinal inflammation is quite laborious and will, by necessity, become more so as our knowledge of the causes of intestinal inflammatory disease increases. Important diagnostic procedures are listed in Table 21-8.

A test of particular importance is a dietary trial for a minimum of two weeks on a controlled diet. Resolution of clinical signs on the controlled diet proves that the patient was suffering an "adverse reaction to food." It does not establish a diagnosis of food allergy or food intolerance, nor does it rule out IBD. It does, however, provide some diagnostic clues. A complete clinical response to food is seen with food allergies, food intolerances, and less commonly with certain forms of IBD such as chronic colitis and canine eosinophilic gastroenteritis. Furthermore, a complete response to controlled diets in most cases obviates further workup. If there is no response to controlled diets, food allergy and food intolerance can be tentatively ruled out, whereas IBD remains a possibility. IBD cannot be diagnosed without a prior dietary trial because the pathological appearance of IBD, food allergies, and food intolerances can be similar.

Table 21-4. Causes of Eosinophilic Intestinal Inflammation

Parasites
- *Trichuris*
- Visceral larval migrans
- Miscellaneous nematode parasites

Immune mediated disorders
- food allergy
- type 1 hypersensitivities
- complement-mediated diseases
- delayed cell-mediated hypersensitivity

Mast cell neoplasia

Miscellaneous causes of mast cell degranulation
- neurogenic?

Idiopathic
- eosinophilic gastroenteritis
- eosinophilic enteritis
- eosinophilic enterocolitis
- eosinophilic colitis
- hypereosinophilic syndrome
- granulomatous enteritis

Table 21-5. Causes of Granulomatous Intestinal Inflammation

Foreign bodies

Non-steroidal antiinflammatory drugs

Tissue trauma
- collagen breakdown

Chronic infections
- *Salmonella*
- *Campylobacter*
- *Mycobacteria*
- Phycomycosis
- Histoplasmosis
- FIP

Parasitic granulomas

Whipworms

Hookworms

Immune-mediated
- miscellaneous delayed hypersensitivity reactions
- miscellaneous complement mediated disease

Idiopathic
- histiocytic colitis of Boxers
- granulomatous enterocolitis

Table 21-6. Causes of Lymphocytic/Plasmacytic Intestinal Inflammation

Bacterial infection
-*Campylobacter*
Bacterial overgrowth (sometimes)
Parasitic disorders
-giardiasis (sometimes)
-cryptosporidiosis
Wheat-sensitive enteropathy
Neoplasia
-lymphosarcoma
-adenocarcinomas
Immune-mediated disease
- miscellaneous chronic antigenic stimulation

Parasitism must be ruled out by several fecal flotations and direct smears, particularly to rule out *Trichuris* infection and the few cases of *Giardia* infection that are associated with a recognizable increase in mucosal lymphocytes and plasma cells. It is possible that overgrowth of some species of bacteria may result in lymphocytic-plasmacytic enteritis. Conversely, malabsorption from any form of IBD can cause bacterial overgrowth. Therefore, tests for bacterial overgrowth should be a routine part of the diagnostic workup of patients with suspected IBD. In those cases of chronic colitis in which there is reason to suspect an infectious cause (see Chapter 5) fecal culture may be required to rule out subacute to chronic bacterial infections such as due to *Campylobacter* and *Salmonella* species. A relationship between feline hyperthyroidism and lymphocytic-plasmacytic infiltrates has been observed.[77] (There may be no relationship but merely that a few animals have several unrelated problems.) It may therefore be prudent to rule out hyperthyroidism with a serum T_4. In cats, FIP can produce a granulomatous colitis. An FIP titer may help rule out this condition, but interpretation of the titer is difficult. FeLV can be associated with inflammatory conditions of the bowel. In both cats and dogs, histoplasmosis can result in a granulomatous enterocolitis that can usually be diagnosed by rectal scrape cytology or intestinal biopsy. Intestinal biopsy is also required to rule out other known causes of intestinal inflammation such as lymphoma, mastocytosis, phycomycosis, prototheca infection, and cryptosporidiosis. Intestinal biopsy provides a more reliable assessment than clinical signs do of whether both small and large bowel are involved in the disease process.

Table 21-7. Causes of Suppurative Intestinal Inflammation

Bacterial infection
-*Yersinia*
-toxigenic *E. coli*
-*Salmonella*
Absorption of bacterial products
- FMLP
Ischemic injury
-shock
Trauma
-bone particles
-indigestible food debris
-fur?
Neoplasia
-necrotizing masses
Immune-mediated disease
- miscellaneous complement-mediated
- miscellaneous immune complex-mediated

Table 21-8. Procedures Commonly Required to Rule Out Known Causes of Intestinal Inflammation

TEST	RULE OUT
Controlled diet	Food allergy, wheat-sensitive enteropathy
Fecal flotation	*Trichuris, Giardia*
Fecal direct smear	*Giardia, Entamoeba*
Quantitative intestinal bacterial count	Bacterial overgrowth
Breath hydrogen	Bacterial overgrowth
Serum cobalamin/folate	Bacterial overgrowth
Fecal culture	*Campylobacter, Salmonella*
Serum T4	Feline hyperthyroidism?
FIP titer?	FIP
FeLV	FeLV
Endoscopic exam and intestinal biopsy	Neoplasia, fungi, algae, Cryptosporidia
Celiotomy & intestinal biopsy	Neoplasia, fungi, algae, Cryptosporidia

Biopsy Interpretation. As described in Chapter 3, the normal intestine has a complement of mucosal leukocytes which varies considerably in number between individual animals and between different bowel locations. For instance, the complement of mucosal leukocytes in the duodenum is usually greater than that of the jejunum.[78] This reemphasizes the issue that consistency in the site of biopsy is essential for proper pathologic interpretation (Chapter 7). Highly discriminant histopathological criteria for the differentiation of IBD from acute inflammatory conditions, or even from normal intestine in the dog and cat, have not been published. A grading system of apparent utility is under development, however.[79,80] Histologic criteria found to be of discriminatory value for the differentiation of ulcerative colitis of humans from non-specific, self-limiting acute colitis include the following: distorted crypt architecture, a villus surface, crypt atrophy, and increased numbers of mixed inflammatory cells in the lamina propria.[81] Of these features, the assessment of cell number had the most inter-observer variability and is felt by many to be an unreliable way to diagnose IBD.[82] Unfortunately, the evaluation of crypt morphology in endoscopic biopsies is very difficult and raises the possibility that, where possible, suction biopsies of the intestine should be obtained to improve diagnostic accuracy. Surgical biopsies provide the best tissue sample but cannot be recommended as a routine procedure. With such biopsies a number of criteria can be used for the differential diagnosis of inflammatory bowel disease (Table 21-9).

Discordance of Biopsy Results and Clinical Signs. Discordant results between clinical signs, endoscopic examination, and biopsy results are sometimes observed. For

Table 21-9. Histopathological Criteria of Possible Use for the Differential Diagnosis of Colitis

Width of mucosa in μm (hyperplasia versus atrophy)
Crypt parallelism
Degree of crypt branching
Proximity of the crypt bases to the muscularis mucosae (crypt shortening)
Mucus content of the goblet cells
Crypt abscesses
Cellular content of the lamina propria with classification of severity and distribution
Cellular content of the remainder of the mucosa
Immunohistochemical staining of plasma cells to differentiate those containing IgA, IgG, IgM and IgE
Granulomas of mucosa or submucosa
Degree of acute inflammation versus chronic inflammation
Presence of a surface exudate
Presence of mucosal necrosis
Degree of fibrosis
Vascular changes: congestion, vasculitis, hemorrhage
Lymphatic changes
Epithelial integrity
Epithelial hyperplasia (hyperchromatism, increased mitoses)
Epithelial regularity
Presence of microorganisms

the clinician, it is most disturbing to receive a normal biopsy report when the clinical signs are suggestive of significant intestinal disease. The reasons for discordance have not been systematically examined. Some suggested causes of discordance are provided in Table 21-10. In our experience the most common discordance is that of essentially normal colon biopsies in spite of concomitant evidence of moderate to severe signs of large bowel function, including tenesmus and hematochezia. It is less common for biopsies of the small intestine to be normal when there is concurrent evidence of moderately severe small bowel disease, but these situations certainly do occur.

Discordance between biopsy results and endoscopic findings is also not uncommon. The concordance between endoscopic examination of the upper gastrointestinal tract and biopsy results in dogs and cats has been the subject of a recent investigation.[80] In about two thirds of cases endoscopic abnormalities were associated with histologic abnormalities. Endoscopically observed mucosal hemorrhage and erythema held the least predictive value for histologic abnormality. Excess mucosal friability was associated with histologic abnormality in 80% of cases. Possible reasons for discordance between endoscopy findings and biopsy are also described in Table 21-10. The most obvious reasons for discordance are inexperienced clinicians, endoscopists, and pathologists. Other explanations are also possible, however, and include the presence of functional rather than morphologic bowel diseases, patchy distribution of mucosal lesions, and failure to place sufficient significance on mild morphologic change. The best example of the latter situation is provided by microscopic colitis of humans, a syndrome in which minimal histologic inflammation of the colon is associated with marked colonic dysfunction.[83]

Post-Treatment Biopsies. Some veterinarians recommend follow-up biopsies of the intestinal mucosa of all patients with moderate to severe IBD after several months of therapy.[77] We have found follow-up biopsies to be helpful in those patients whose clinical signs are not responsive to therapy, as they provide an objective assessment of the intestinal inflammation's response to the therapeutic regimen. Clinically non-responsive patients whose follow-up intestinal biopsies show a reduction in inflammation are maintained on the same therapy, and the client is instructed to allow more time for the disease to resolve. Clinically non-responsive patients whose biopsies show no improvement are changed to a different therapeutic protocol, usually involving another controlled diet and more aggressive immunosuppression.

The question of whether it is justified to rebiopsy patients in clinical remission can not as yet be answered. There is no doubt that many of these patients have evidence of persistent intestinal inflammation in spite of clinical remission. It is not uncommon for patients with subclinical gastrointestinal inflammation to have a rapid recurrence of their clinical signs after the conclusion of the medical therapy. Moreover, it is quite conceivable that in the long term this residual inflammation will lead to intestinal fibrosis and eventually a recurrence of untreatable clinical signs. Whether this theoretical concern justifies the expense of repeated intestinal biopsy can only be determined by carefully controlled prospective studies.

Table 21-10. Reasons for Discordance of Biopsy Results with Clinical and Endoscopic Findings

Incorrect localization of disease process by clinician
Failure to separate large and small bowel diarrheas
Incorrect endoscopic assessment of gastrointestinal mucosa
Inexperience
Inadequate insufflation misread as mucosal thickening, mucosal granularity, or obscured submucosal blood vessels
Scope-induced trauma misread as spontaneous disease
Incorrect biopsy evaluation by pathologist
Inexperience
The unknown significance of mild inflammation
Sample handling error
Non-representative biopsies
Poor biopsy technique
Biopsied incorrect aspect of a lesion (e.g. necrotic center)
Patchy mucosal lesions
Presence of functional rather than morphological disease
Brush-border defects
Motility abnormalities
Secretory diarrheas
Permeability defects

MANAGEMENT OF INFLAMMATORY BOWEL DISEASE

Introduction

The management of IBD varies widely and includes the use of controlled diets, immunosuppressive agents, motility modifiers, antimicrobials, and bulking substances. No controlled studies have been done to evaluate any of these therapies in dogs. They are based on empirical time-honored use in small animals and on controlled studies in humans. Evaluation of therapeutic response is fraught with difficulty because of the often cyclical appearance and disappearance of the signs. The value of any treatment must be based on a well-controlled randomized double-blind study comparing the effects of therapy and placebo. Such a study must use biopsies to establish the diagnosis and evaluate the therapy.

The details of the treatment regimens for each of the different types of IBD are described in the sections pertaining to each disease. It is important to understand that the therapy of IBD must be tailored according to each patient's response. Rapidity of resolution of clinical signs and severity and nature of drug side effects vary tremendously amongst patients. The following discussion consists of general comments on the management of IBD.

Client Education

When IBD is diagnosed, the most important step in achieving successful management is client education. The client is informed that the problem is chronic and in most cases without cure. Regardless of the therapeutic program, relapses are to be expected. Time must be committed to the discussion of the inviolate nature of the controlled diet (see below). Moreover, the client must be made to comprehend that the therapy of IBD must be individualized. So warned, the client will be less likely to lose confidence in the veterinarian.

Fluid and Electrolyte Therapy

The most important component of the symptomatic therapy of IBD is the provision of adequate fluid and electrolyte replacement. In general, fluid and electrolyte derangements are not as frequent in chronic gastrointestinal diseases as in acute gastroenteritis.

Dietary Management

The dietary management of IBD has two basic tenets. The first is that the patient's nutrient requirements must be provided. The IBD patient is often malnourished (Table 21-2), probably has increased energy and protein requirements, and at times must receive intensive nutritional support. The second tenet is that nutrients must be provided in an easily assimilated form. The provision of adequate quantities of easily assimilated nutrients improves the nutritional status of the patient and reduces the quantity of unabsorbed nutrient that can result in osmotic diarrhea, bacterial overgrowth, and antigenic stimulation of the mucosa. Also, dietary antigens may in some cases be the cause of the intestinal inflammation and in other cases be partially responsible for its perpetuation. Since dietary changes alter composition of the bacterial flora, certain diets may significantly change the amount and type of bacterial antigens or bacterial-derived phlogistic factors that are absorbed across the mucosa.

Parenteral Nutrition. Complete bowel rest can be achieved through parenteral nutrition. Results of the treatment of humans with IBD by parenteral nutrition have been mixed.[84-86] There is little doubt that such aggressive nutritional support improves the patient's sense of well-being, primarily by virtue of improving nutritional status. The severity of the diarrhea is also reduced. The greatest success of parenteral nutrition in assisting disease control occurs in patients with newly diagnosed Crohn's disease or in patients with the clinical signs of abdominal pain, anorexia, and weight loss.[87] Ulcerative colitis appears to be more refractory to nutritional therapy than is Crohn's disease.[88] The disappointing response to parenteral nutrition in many patients should not come as a suprise, in view of the well recognized role of bacterial flora in the pathogenesis of the condition. Dietary changes by no means eliminate bowel flora, and so the bowel mucosa is still inundated with potentially highly antigenic products.

Experience with parenteral nutrition in the therapy of canine and feline IBD has been restricted. The primary indication for this type of nutritional supplementation is the support of the anorexic and debilitated patient, particularly if that patient vomits persistently and has small bowel disease that may limit absorption of nutrients. Maintaining nutritional parity is particularly important in those animals destined for full-thickness bowel biopsy.

If carefully performed, parenteral nutrition is practical in dogs and cats for periods of up to a week. The benefits to the animal's attitude and strength are at times remarkable. The severity of the diarrhea also decreases dramatically. There is not enough information available as yet to determine if these short periods of complete bowel rest speed the resolution of the gastrointestinal inflammation.

Elemental Diets. Elemental diets contain nitrogen as protein hydrolysates and carbohydrates as monosaccharides or oligosaccharides. The small size of these products minimizes their antigenicity and reduces the need for digestion, a process which can be impaired in IBD as a result of functional pancreatic insufficiency. Nutrition with elemental diets is only recommended if the animal is anorexic and debilitated. Many studies have shown that enteral diets improve the nutritional status and well being of human patients with IBD.[87] If the small intestine is diffusely involved, the absorption of these highly osmolar solutions is impaired and administration must be very slow to avoid osmotic diarrhea.

Controlled Diets. Controlled diets are the most common dietary manipulation used in veterinary medicine for the therapy of IBD. Controlled diets may be defined as diets in which the clinician has "control" over all or the majority of the dietary ingredients. The weak link in this scheme is the client, and in general the effectiveness of dietary control is directly related to the effectiveness of the client education. The client must be informed that the controlled diet may be less palatable than the animal's standard diet, and that no treats can be fed. The types of IBD most responsive to dietary manipulation are chronic colitis and to a lesser extent eosinophilic gastroenteritis.

The ideal controlled diet has adequate calories and protein provided by a restricted number of easily assimilated nutrients, no dietary additives, and reasonable palatability. A compromise is usually reached between the ideal and what is acceptable to the patient and owner. It is more important to ensure that an overtly malnourished patient is eating a nutritious diet than to be overly concerned about the potential hazards of various foods.

A single source of carbohydrate and protein should be provided initially. Rice is the preferred carbohydrate source since it is more completely assimilated than other carbohydrates.[89] A suitable protein source is low-fat cottage cheese or soy bean protein (tofu). Yogurt should not be used because of its higher lactose content. The controlled diets most commonly utilized in cats at UCD VMTH are baby foods and sliced chicken. The controlled diet most commonly recommended for dogs is one part low-fat cottage cheese or tofu and three parts white rice.

The value of recommending a novel protein such as lamb as the protein source has not been evaluated. Certainly in those rare cases of chronic gastrointestinal inflammation resulting purely from an allergy to a dietary protein source, the feeding of a protein to which the animal has not been previously exposed is likely to meet with success. This is most likely to occur in eosinophilic gastroenteritis. As a general principle, when feeding diets containing intact proteins to animals with an inflamed and porous mucosa, "hypoallergenicity" is most likely to be maintained by the feeding of high digestible proteins rather than novel proteins. Digestion of a protein usually renders it non-antigenic. Feeding of a novel but poorly digestible protein is likely to result in only transient benefit because the intact protein will soon find its way into the mucosa, where it can contribute to the inflammatory response. Oral tolerance is difficult to maintain in the inflammatory milieu, and so the host is likely to become rapidly sensitive to the previously novel antigen. Meat is not assimilated as well as cooked eggs and cottage cheese. Many dogs with inflammatory bowel disease have lost their tolerance for all sources of meat, even novel sources. When remission is achieved on the cottage cheese or tofu and rice diet and the addition of other foods is attempted, most clients will select a meat as the first new food to add. Many dogs relapse and that is difficult for clients to comprehend in dogs that have eaten meat and have never had gastrointestinal problems before.

The amount of protein fed should be just sufficient to satisfy the patient's requirements as dictated by species, growth phase, disease severity, and nutritional status. Most food ingredients have the potential to be antigenic, but the majority of recognized antigens are proteins, and in particular glycoproteins. Furthermore, excess protein's finding its way to the colon can eventually result in the generation of ammonia, which can contribute to colonic injury.[90]

The amount of fat fed should also be kept to a minimum. Fat is the most difficult nutrient to assimilate. Unabsorbed fatty acids can promote colonic secretion. Fecal bile acid excretion also increases when the amount of dietary animal fat is increased. Elevated bile acid concentration in the colon can contribute further to mucosal secretion and degeneration.[91]

Feeding a low-fat diet requires a high-carbohydrate diet for provision of needed calories. Carbohydrates are normally the most abundant nutrient in the diet and with malassimilation the unassimilated carbohydrate is probably the most important nutrient in contributing to the diarrhea. Increases in fecal dry matter with diarrhea are largely due to malassimilated carbohyderate. The increased entry of carbohydrate into the colon increases production of fermentation products that contribute to diarrhea. The increased carbohydrate in the colon also stimulates bacterial growth and colonic bacterial numbers and varieties are factors in the pathogenesis and persistence of colonic disease. Consequently, white rice is fed because it is more completely assimilated than the starch in other cereals.

Consideration should be given to the cessation of all pre-existing medications and dietary supplements until it can be ascertained that they are not contributing to the clinical signs. Oral vitamin and mineral supplements should be avoided in the first few weeks of the controlled diet. They can be carefully reinstituted once remission is attained. In the interim period, parenteral supplementation of vitamins should be considered.

Commercially prepared foods are less ideal as controlled diets because they are less consistent in their formulation and may contain undesirable food additives. The advantages of commercial foods are their convenience and their guaranteed dietary balance.

Some commercial foods are semi-controlled diets in that they contain a limited number of nutrient sources, are highly digestible, and/or contain low fat or so called hypoallergenic proteins. A wide variety of apparently useful diets have been touted. For the dog these include prescription diets d/d and i/d, Science Diets Maximum Stress and Canine Growth (Hill's pet food products); IAMs Chunks and Eukenuba (The Iams Company); ANF (Specialty Pet Products); Gaines Cycle 3, and Gaines Cycle 4 (Gaines Foods). Commercial diets that have been recommended in feline IBD include IAMS Feline, Hill's Science Diet Feline, Prescription Diet c/d, and Tender Vittles (Ralston Purina).

Elimination Diets. With the return of normal bowel movements, new foods such as cooked eggs, lean meats, cereals, vegetables, and vegetable oils can be introduced one at a time. Each one is introduced gradually, and the results are evaluated after they are fed for seven to ten days. Adverse reactions to new additions are not necessarily seen within hours after feeding. Reactions may not be seen for 4 to 5 days in some individuals; the immune response is much delayed, depending on the type of hypersensitivity involved. Adverse reactions to foods can take several days to develop, and adaptive changes in digestive enzyme levels may take seven to ten days. No foods are added that contain more than one ingredient. Unfavorable responses to a food containing several constituents do not help identify nutrients that are not tolerated. Some animals can eventually be successfully weaned back onto commercial diets after months of being sensitive to a number of different foods. Lasting remission results from the patient's regaining oral tolerance. Such tolerance is not regained until the memory for hypersensitivity is lost. When the memory for hypersensitivity is in circulating immunoglobulins, at least a month with no continuing antigenic stimulation is necessary for that memory to disappear. When the memory for hypersensitivity is in cells (lymphocytes), at least three months is required for the memory to be lost. Thus, complete avoidance of antigens stimulating and maintaining the memory for hypersensitivity must be continued for at least three months. Hence, complete compliance is essential to success; an animal being fed a few treats continues to be exposed to antigens maintaining the hypersensitivity and oral tolerance is not regained.

Fiber. Low fiber diets have been recommended for the treatment of IBD on the assumption that fiber results in adverse mechanical trauma to the damaged colonic mucosa. There is no evidence that high fiber diets can exacerbate IBD, however. In contrast, many animals with colitis can be successfully managed by the addition of fiber to their diet. Dietary fiber improves colonic motility, absorbs irritative products such as bile acids, stimulates the production of mucus, and may increase colonic absorption of fluid and electrolytes.

Pharmacological Therapy

Some veterinarians prefer to use pharmacologic therapy only if the patient with IBD fails to respond to dietary management. It is the opinion of one of us (W.G.G.), however, that medical therapy is indicated as an adjunctive therapy to controlled diets in all but the mildest cases of IBD. While it is well established that clinical remission can be obtained in many cases of colitis without medical therapy, it is my (W.G.G.) experience that remission will be more rapid, more complete, and more prolonged if the patient is placed on a short course of antiinflammatory drugs. The rationale for this recommendation is that the more rapidly intestinal inflammation can be controlled, the more rapidly the intestinal permeability barrier will be restored, and the less exposure the patient will have to luminal antigens, including the antigens that are being incorporated in the controlled diet. A large variety of medications have been used on an empirical basis for the treatment of IBD in cats and dogs.

Oral Corticosteroids The value of corticosteroid therapy in canine and feline IBD has not been evaluated by a controlled study, but clinical experience has suggested that corticosteroids are the drugs of choice for the treatment of all inflammatory bowel diseases except chronic (lymphocytic-plasmacytic) colitis. Controlled studies in humans have show that corticosteroids are effective in treating an initial attack or an acute relapse of ulcerative colitis.[92] With prolonged use, however, their effectiveness decreases and the incidence of side effects increases. Similarly, many dogs with acute exacerbations of chronic colitis will respond quickly and completely to corticosteroid therapy. If at all possible sulfasalazine, not corticosteroids, should be used to maintain remission of colitis.

The effectiveness of corticosteroids primarily relates to the potent antiinflammatory and immunosuppressive properties of these drugs. Additional beneficial effects are appetite stimulation and increased small and large intestinal sodium and water absorption. The effect of glucocorticoids on colonic water absorption, at least in the rat, appears to be mediated via specific colonic glucocorticoid receptors that induce an increase in sodium conductance through the apical enterocyte membrane. These effects have been seen with pharmacological doses of methylprednisolone and dexamethasone.[93]

The side effects of corticosteroid therapy are legion. Prolonged usage is associated with predictable iatrogenic hyperadrenocorticism. The onset of this disease is delayed, but not necessarily prevented, by adoption of an alternate day treatment regimen. Side effects of glucocorticoids that are commonly seen include polyuria, polydipsia, steroid hepatopathy, urinary tract infection, and hyperventilation. Behavioral abnormalities are occasionally noted. Rare side effects of great concern are acute pancreatitis, gastric ulceration, and colonic perforation. These adverse drug reactions are most commonly associated with high doses and are rarely apparent during alternate day therapy. The adverse effects of pharmacologic doses of corticosteroids on the gastrointestinal tract include the stimulation of increased gastric acid and pepsin secretion and gastrin cell mass, decreased gastric mucus secretion, and decreased gastric and duodenal epithelial mitotic rate leading to moderate (betamethasone) to mild (prednisolone) epithelial hypoplasia. The latter effect is offset by glucocorticoid-induced increased activity of certain brush border enzymes.[94] In general, cats show fewer adverse clinical signs due to corticosteroids than do dogs, but both species demonstrate marked hypothalamo-pituitary axis depression at the doses utilized for the therapy of IBD. Thus, a tapered withdrawal from the steroid medication is essential. The veterinarian must discuss the ramifications of corticosteroid therapy with the client.

The corticosteroid most frequently used for the therapy of canine and feline IBD is prednisone. Prednisone is suitable because of its availability in a wide range of tablet sizes, its lack of expense, and its short duration of action. Dexamethasone should not be used because it has a longer duration of action than prednisone and therefore is not suitable for alternate day therapy. The prednisone dosages employed in the treatment of canine and feline have been chosen empirically. The initial dose is chosen according to the severity and type of inflammation. Thereafter, it is modified according to clinical response. Consistent beneficial responses are obtained by the short term use of immunosuppressive doses (1-2 mg/kg q 12 hr PO) in association with controlled diets. Higher doses (2-3 mg/kg q 12 hr PO) are required in the cat for the treatment of eosinophilic enteritis, which is considerably less responsive than eosinophilic IBD in dogs.[95] The details of suggested dosage regimens are provided in the discussion of the particular types of IBD.

The eventual aim is to maintain remission by use of a controlled diet. Relapses may require repeated courses of prednisone. As mentioned previously, if at all possible corticosteroids should be avoided for long term maintenance therapy of chronic colitis and also other forms of IBD. In refractory cases, if prednisone must be used for maintenance, then it is best combined with another drug or drugs such as sulfasalazine, metronidazole, or azathioprine to reduce the required prednisone dosage and to allow alternate day prednisone therapy. Treatment of ulcerative colitis in humans with combinations of corticosteroids and sulfasalazine is effective and minimizes side effects of both drugs.[96]

Parenteral Corticosteroids. Parenteral corticosteroid therapy should be considered in non-responsive patients with severe disease. There is some evidence in humans with immune-mediated disease that high dose parenteral therapy will provide a more rapid and predictable remission than oral therapy. In a patient that is vomiting and has diffuse intestinal disease the absorption of oral preparations is likely to be compromised.

Injections of depot preparations of glucocorticoids should be avoided because they produce rapid and profound depression of the hypothalamo-pituitary axis. The only indication for these preparations is in the treatment of intractable cats that cannot be medicated orally. Methylprednisolone acetate (Depo-Medrol — UpJohn) is the most commonly employed product. It is usually used at a dose of 10-20 mg IM and repeated at two week intervals for three injections. Thereafter, injections are administered on an as-needed basis to control the signs. Consistent control of IBD is more difficult to obtain with this drug than with oral corticosteroids.[95]

Corticosteroid Enemas. Patients in the active phase of severe chronic colitis are sometimes treated locally with corticosteroid enemas.[97] In humans these steroids are very effective since very little is absorbed and a high drug concentration is maintained. The value of corticosteroid enemas in the dog and cat remains to be proven. Poor retention of the enema is likely to reduce the effectiveness of this therapy in animals.

Sulfasalazine[98-100](salicylazosulfapyridine). Sulfasalazine (Azulfidine — Pharmacia Laboratories) is a combination of 5-aminosalicylic acid and sulfapyridine, joined through an azo bond. Well-controlled studies have verified that salicylazosulfapyridine is an effective drug for the treatment of ulcerative colitis in humans. No comparable studies have been conducted in small animals, but the drug is in wide usage, and it is the clinical impression of many veterinarians that it is effective for the therapy of chronic colitis in animals. It remains the drug of choice for the pharmacological therapy of chronic colitis in the dog and perhaps the cat.

After administration, a small amount of the intact drug is absorbed in the small intestine (20%-30% in humans), but the majority of the sulfasalazine passes unabsorbed to the colon. The small amount of sulfasalazine absorbed in the small intestine is excreted unchanged in the urine and bile. About 75% of the sulfasalazine reaches the colon, where bacteria break the azo bond and release the component parts of the drug. In humans most of the cleaved sulfapyridine and about 30% of the 5-aminosalicylate is absorbed from the colon. The remainder of the 5-aminosalicylate remains in the colon and is eventually excreted in the feces. After absorption, sulfapyridine is largely metabolized in the liver via acetylation, hydroxylation, and glucuronide formation. The small amount of 5-aminosalicylic acid that is absorbed is metabolized by the liver and excreted in the urine.

The active component of sulfasalazine is 5-aminosalicylate, not sulfapyridine as previously assumed. The 5-aminosalicylate has an antiinflammatory action; it inhibits both cyclooxygenase and lipoxygenase activities. The antiinflammatory action of 5-aminosalicylate results from direct inhibition of lipoxygenase activity and leukotriene synthesis and perhaps from an oxygen-free radical scavenging action. Although both prostaglandins and leukotrienes are produced in chronically inflamed colonic mucosa, only leukotrines are important in the pathogenesis of the lesions. (Drugs such as aspirin and indomethacin which inhibit prostaglandin and not leukotriene formation are ineffective in treating colonic inflammation). The use of 5-aminosalicylate reduces thromboxane and HETE synthesis and interferes with the binding of FMLP to neutrophils. By virtue of the fact that sulfasalazine needs bacterial metabolism to release its active moiety, it is effective only against large bowel inflammation. One reason for treatment failure with this drug is failure by the clinician to recognize concomitant small bowel signs.

Although sulfasalazine is effective for treating ulcerative colitis, it is often ineffective for managing acute exacerbations of colitis. In humans sulfasalazine is the drug of choice for maintaining remission. The drug reduces the frequency of relapses. In one study of canine chronic colitis in which sulfasalazine was used alone and in combination with other drugs, over 80% of the patients improved.[101] Results were poorer with other forms of therapy. There is little doubt that sulfasalazine is the drug of choice for the long-term management of canine chronic colitis. It must be realized that the drug is not a panacea, however, and a significant number of animals do not respond to it, or initially respond to therapy but later relapse.

The possibility of side effects resulting from sulfasalazine therapy should be discussed with the client at the time the drug is prescribed. The most common side effects of sulfasalazine in dogs are anorexia and vomiting. Depression, vomiting, and anemia have been observed in the cat. Keratoconjunctivitis can occur as a result of the sulfasalazine therapy.[102] The keratoconjunctivitis is reversible or partially reversible in only 30% of dogs.[102] The keratoconjunctivitis has been attributed to the sulfapyridine moiety, but this view has recently been challenged by the observation that beagles developed keratoconjunctivitis sicca (KCS) in toxicity trials of 5-aminosalicylate.[103] Dogs maintained on sulfasalazine therapy should have periodic Schirmer's tear testing to identify KCS early.

Azulfidine is supplied as a 500 mg tablet or as a 50 mg/ml liquid formulation, which is particularly useful for the therapy of cats and small dogs. Various dose regimens have been successfully used. The regimen most commonly employed in dogs by these authors is 12.5 mg/kg q 6 hr for two weeks, followed by 12.5 mg/kg q 12 hr for a further four weeks. Others have had success with 20-30 mg/kg q 8 hr administered for three to six weeks. Some intractable cases have been reported to require doses as high as 50 mg/kg q 8 hr.[33] Similarly, in cats a variety of dosages have been reported. We have found 10-20 mg/kg q 24 hr effective, although others have used higher doses without apparent ill effect from salicylate toxicity.

5-aminosalicylate. Preparations of 5-aminosalicylate are now in use in human medicine for the treatment of ulcerative colitis.[104] The drug is administered as an enema or in an enteric coated tablet to ensure the majority of the drug reaches the colon without absorption in the small intestine. These products appear to preserve the effectiveness of sulfasalazine but reduce the incidence of side-effects by dispensing with the sulfonamide moiety. Olsalazine is a drug in which two molecules of 5-aminosalicylic acid are linked by an azo bond, thus serving as their own carriers.[105] The effectiveness of oral 5-aminosalicylate does not appear to be dose dependent above a certain threshold, whereas previous studies had suggested the response to sulfasalazine is dose dependent.[105] This observation implies that perhaps, sulfasalazine does, after all, possess some beneficial activity in addition that of its 5-aminosalicylate. Enemas containing 5-aminosalicylic acid are useful in the treatment of refractory colitis in humans.[106] The value of these products in the treatment of chronic colitis in the dog and cat remains to be established.

Azathioprine. Azathioprine (Imuran - Coopers Animal Health) is a synthetic purine which interferes with DNA formation. Its value in the treatment of human IBD has been questioned.[107] It can be used in cats and dogs as adjunctive therapy in refractory IBD. Azathioprine can also be used if the dosage of prednisone required to maintain remission is unacceptably high. The addition of azathioprine to the treatment regimen usually allows the prednisone dose to be halved. The azathioprine dose most often used in dogs is 50 mg/m^2 or 1-1.5

mg/kg once daily for 2 weeks, followed by alternate day therapy as required. A lower dose has been recommended in cats (0.3 mg/kg q 48 hours).[95] A lag effect of several weeks may occur before the beneficial effects of azathioprine become apparent.

The most important side effect is bone marrow suppression. Mild suppression is common with this drug and of little concern. Severe depression is rare, is most often seen in cats, and is usually reversible on discontinuation of therapy. A complete blood count should be performed within ten days of placing any patient on this drug and should be repeated at monthly to bimonthly intervals thereafter. Other side-effects include anorexia, pancreatitis, and hepatic damage. The drug is supplied only in 50 mg tablets which limits the usefulness of this medication in cats.

Cyclophosphamide and Cyclosporin. Cyclophosphamide (Cytoxan) is a potent immunosuppressive agent that is occasionally of value in the therapy of refractory IBD in dogs and cats. Cyclophosphamide is easier to administer to cats than azathioprine because it requires less frequent dosage and is supplied in a more suitable tablet size (25 mg). The dose is 50 mg/M^2 given four times per week. In most cats this equates to one half to one quarter of a 25 mg tablet at each administration. Side effects include bone marrow suppression and, particularly in dogs, hemorrhagic cystitis. Regular complete blood counts must be performed when using this agent. Cyclosporin is under investigation in humans for the therapy of refractory IBD.

Immunosuppressive Therapy and Oral Tolerance. Most dogs with IBD show some degree of hypersensitivity to many different foods, most of which are ingredients of commercial pet foods. Lasting remission without the need for medication or controlled diets requires the patient to regain oral tolerance for these many foods. The oral tolerance is developed by activity of some suppressor T lymphocytes. Drugs destroying these lymphocytes or drugs inhibiting suppressor activity of these lymphocytes prevent the regaining of oral tolerance. The use of immunosuppressive therapy must be with the recognition that subclinical hypersensitivities will persist while immunosuppressive therapy is continued.

Metronidazole. Metronidazole (Flagyl — Searle Pharmaceuticals) has beneficial effects in the therapy of canine and feline IBD. Metronidazole has a number of different actions. It is an antiprotozoal agent, inhibits cell-mediated immunity,[108,109] and has a broad spectrum of activity against anaerobic bacteria. It is unknown whether the immunosuppressive or antibacterial action of this drug best explains its apparent efficacy in the treatment of IBD. Experimental and clinical studies have shown that it is not possible to suppress the colonic microflora with antibiotics for more than a few days.[110] Metronidazole reduces the number of Bacteroides species in the feces of humans with IBD but has little influence on the fecal flora of healthy individuals. The antibacterial action of metronidazole may be more important in the small bowel, particularly if bacterial overgrowth is present.

Metronidazole is only rarely effective as a single agent in the treatment of IBD and is most often used in combination therapeutic protocols to facilitate control of refractory cases or allow reduction in prednisone dosage. The dosage of metronidazole used in cats and dogs is usually 10-20 mg/kg q 8-12 hr. Metronidazole is supplied as 250 and 500 mg tablets or as a 5 mg/ml oral solution. Side effects are rare, but nausea and vomiting are occasionally seen in the dog and cat. Neurotoxicity has been reported in the dog.[111] The drug is carcinogenic and mutagenic in laboratory animals, and so prolonged high-dose therapy and therapy during pregnancy should be avoided.

Tylosin. Tylosin has been reported to be effective in a variety of IBD-like disorders.[112] The mechanism of action is unknown. Anecdotal reports exist for a response to tylosin in some case of IBD that have been unresponsive to more conventional therapy. Tylosin is supplied as a powder and is licensed for use in pigs. The reported dose range used in small animals is broad 11-200 mg/kg q 12 hr[112] and 20-40 mg/kg q 12 hr.[113] Side effects have yet to be reported.

Miscellaneous Antibiotics. Parenteral antibiotic therapy is required in those animals showing clinical or laboratory signs of sepsis. Sepsis is not a frequent complication of IBD, but it is occasionally observed in those animals with severe mucosal ulceration. Because of the wide variety of possible pathogens, the choice of antibiotic therapy is best based on blood cultures. If expedient therapy is required, trimethoprim-sulfa drugs may be utilized prior to the receipt of blood culture results. These antibiotics combine the advantages of reasonably broad spectrum activity, minimal disturbance of enteric microbial flora, and low toxicity. If life-threatening acute sepsis is suspected, combinations of parenteral aminoglycosides and ampicillin may be utilized.

Oral antibiotics such as tetracycline may be useful in cases in which the IBD is associated with bacterial overgrowth of the small intestine. There is no place for the use of unabsorbable oral antibiotics in the treatment of any form of bowel disease.

Motility Modifiers. Short courses of opiates such as loperamide (Imodium 0.08 mg/kg q 8 hr PO) and diphenoxylate (Lomotil 0.05-0.1 mg/kg q 8 hr PO) are occasionally useful to reduce the severity of watery diarrhea associated with small intestinal and upper colonic IBD. These agents promote segmental contraction of bowel, thus slowing transit time of luminal content and prolonging the period available for water and electrolyte absorption. They should not be used in severe cases of hemorrhagic diarrhea because the retention of necrotizing material and pathogenic microbes may facilitate toxemia and sepsis.

Metoclopramide (Reglan - AH Robins) is an antiemetic and prokinetic. It hastens gastric emptying of solids and liquids and improves upper intestinal motility. It is useful in IBD patients with delayed gastric emptying. The drug has a short duration of action and is best administered four times a day or just prior to meals. A suitable dose is 0.2-0.5 mg/kg PO. Cisapride (Jansen Pharm) is another prokinetic. It appears to be a more reliable agent for the acceleration of gastric emptying of solids in the dog.[114] The effective dose is 5 mg/kg PO administered prior to eating.

Because the bowel is usually hypomotile in chronic colitis, there is no indication for the administration of anticholinergics. Moreover, it is thought that anticholinergics have only minimal influence on colonic motility,[115] and so their benefit in treating colonic spasm is in doubt. Furthermore, it is possible that the intermittent acute abdominal pain demonstrated by some dogs with colitis results from accumulation of gas in the hypomotile colon rather than from colonic spasm.

INFLAMMATORY BOWEL DISEASE-PROGNOSIS AND TREATMENT FAILURES

The prognosis for most patients with IBD is good. Exceptions include those patients with severe mucosal distortion and fibrosis, cats with eosinophilic enteritis or the hypereosinophilic syndrome, and cats or dogs with granulomatous or histiocytic IBD. Treatment failures are usually due to: 1) inadequate client education; 2) noncompliance of owners with the management program; 3) reliance on drugs alone for managing the problem; 4) lack of aggression, persistence, and patience in the tailoring of therapy for individual patients; and 5) misdiagnosis. The most common misdiagnoses are failure to recognize concomitant disease in other parts of the gastrointestinal tract or failure to address the common complications of gastrointestinal inflammation such as delayed gastric emptying, disordered intestinal motility, bacterial overgrowth, and protein-losing enteropathy.

LYMPHOCYTIC-PLASMACYTIC ENTERITIS

Clinical Synopsis

Diagnostic features

* Clinical evidence of "small bowel" signs of greater than several weeks duration
* Biopsy evidence of small intestinal inflammation in which the predominant cells are lymphocytes and plasma cells
* No cause apparent after a thorough work up

Standard treatment

* Controlled diet of cottage cheese and rice (dogs) or sliced chicken (cats)
* Prednisone: 1-2 mg/kg q 12 hr PO for one to two weeks; followed by 0.5-1.0 mg/kg q 24 hr PO for four weeks; followed by 0.5-1.0 mg/kg qod PO for four weeks; followed by a tapered withdrawal over two weeks

Follow up

* Withdraw the pharmacologic therapy and attempt to maintain on controlled diet for several weeks
* Thereafter, attempt elimination diet
* Repeat pharmacological therapy if recurrence occurs

Lymphocytic-plasmacytic enteritis (LPE) is a chronic, idiopathic, inflammatory disease of the small bowel characterized by a mixed inflammatory infiltrate in which lymphocytes and plasma cells predominate.

Incidence and Signalment

The incidence of LPE is unknown, but recent reviews[77,116,117] and our own experience suggest that small intestinal LPE is one of the most frequent causes of chronic vomiting and diarrhea in the cat and dog. LPE is the most common IBD variant affecting the small bowel of the dog and cat. No sex predisposition has been recognized. In both cats and dogs the disease is most common in middle-aged and older animals. However, PLE has been observed in cats as young as five months and dogs as young as eight months.[77,116,117] German Shepherds[118] and Sharpeis, two breeds that have a high incidence of IgA deficiency, may be predisposed. The Basenji and the Ludenhund have their own particular variant of LPE. No breed predisposition has been observed in cats.

Etiopathogenesis

The cause of LPE is unknown.[119] The presence of increased numbers of lymphocytes and plasma cells suggests chronic antigenic challenge of the gut-associated lymphoid tissues. It remains to be established whether this chronic challenge results from a damaged or defective mucosal permeability barrier or a failure of tolerance to self-, dietary-, or bacterial antigens. Moreover, the extent of the role of genetic makeup, psychological factors, enteric pathogens, and mucosal biochemical defects remains to be defined. In all probability there is more than one cause of LPE.

Clinical Findings

Chronic "small bowel" type diarrhea is the most common clinical sign in the dog, whereas chronic intermittent vomiting is the most common sign in the cat. Cats and, less commonly, dogs may manifest vomiting as their only clinical sign. In cats, a presumptive diagnosis of "hair balls" often figures prominently in the history. The clinical signs have a cyclical course, but as the disorder worsens episodes become progressively more frequent and severe. Unless concomitant delayed gastric emptying has developed, patients with LPE will usually vomit only scant volumes of bile-stained or clear fluid. This feature helps differentiate IBD from gastrointestinal neoplasia. Neoplasia also has a progressive course, and if gastrointestinal obstruction occurs the volume of the vomitus tends to be copious. Hematemesis is uncommon and suggests concurrent gastric involvement. Occasionally diarrhea is precipitated by a stressful episode. Additional clinical signs that are often present include weight loss, lethargy, dehydration, and borborygmus. Rarely, abdominal pain, melena, pica, polydipsia, polyuria, and pyrexia may be apparent. Appetite is usually decreased, but in milder cases, particularly in dogs, polyphagia may be apparent. Palpation of the abdomen may reveal abdominal discomfort and thickened loops of intestine.

Laboratory Findings

Hematological findings are usually unremarkable, although leukocytosis as a result of stress or chronic inflammation may be observed. In severely affected animals leukocyte counts can reach 40,000-50,000/mm^3.[77,116] Left-shifted leukograms are rarely observed but can occur, particularly if mucosal ulceration has led to sepsis. Mild normocytic-normochromic-non-regenerative anemia, resulting from chronic inflammation, may be present. Liver enzymes are occasionally mildly elevated. Hypoalbuminemia and hypoglobulinemia as a result of protein-losing enteropathy is common in dogs with moderate to severe disease. In contrast, hypoproteinemia is rare in the cat even with severe disease.[77] Mild hyperglobulinemia is periodically noted in cats. Tests of exocrine pancreatic function are usually normal but laboratory evidence of malabsorption is often noted. Thus, excessive fatty acid droplets in the stool and abnormal absorption tests may occur. Moderate steatorrhea (5-13 gm/day) and excessive fecal nitrogen loss (8.4-11.7 gm per day) have been reported in dogs.[43] Results of xylose, cobalamin, folate, and vitamin A absorption tests are inconsistent. Coagulopathies in association with suspected vitamin K malabsorption due to LPE have been reported in cats[120] but appear to be rare. A partial response to a controlled diet may be observed, but it is uncommon to get complete resolution of signs except on a transient basis.[95] Tests for parasites are usually negative and breath hydrogen tests usually show bacterial overgrowth of the small intestine. In cats, hyperthyroidism can have a similar presentation and so it is important to evaluate a serum T_4. FeLV and FIV titers are usually negative. Fecal cultures do not reveal enteric pathogens.

Radiographic Findings

Survey and contrast radiographs usually reveal few abnormalities. Flocculation and segmentation of barium sulfate suspension is observed in some dogs.[43] Mucosal irregularity and narrowed dye columns have been observed in severely affected cats.

Ultrasound Findings

Ultrasonography will occasionally reveal a diffusely thickened bowel wall or mild mesenteric lymphadenopathy. Marked mesenteric lymphadenopathy is unusual in LPE and should raise suspicion for lymphosarcoma and to a lesser extent hypereosinophilic syndrome. Aspiration of the lymph nodes may provide a diagnosis.

Endoscopy Findings

In mild cases, the endoscopic appearance of the duodenum may be normal. In most cases, however, the duodenal mucosa will appear more granular and friable than normal. Likewise, during celiotomy the bowel may appear normal and this should not discourage biopsy.

Biopsy Findings

Multiple gastric and small intestinal biopsies should be obtained. If concurrent large bowel signs are observed, colon biopsies can also be obtained. It is not unusual for the disease process to involve stomach or colon in addition to the small bowel. The cardinal finding in the intestinal biopsy is an increase in the number of lymphocytes and plasma cells in the lamina propria. The distribution of these cells may widen to extend in heavier numbers into the villi, a position where plasma cells are not commonly found in the normal intestine.[121] The distribution may be patchy with areas of markedly increased cellular infiltrate interdispersed with areas of slightly increased infiltrate. A layer of lymphocytes, plasma cells, eosinophils, and histiocytes may be present along the lamina propria-submucosal junction above the muscularis mucosae. Scattered neutrophils may be seen. In more severe cases there may be villus clubbing, atrophy, and fusion. The surface epithelium may appear normal or low columnar to cuboidal with an indistinct brush border.[121] The crypt architecture may be distorted or hypertrophic. Some crypts may obstruct and dilate with mucus. Occasionally, evidence of rupture of obstructed crypts will be seen, such as mucus in the lamina propria in association with reactive histiocytes and the occasional giant cell.[121] There may be edema of the lamina propria and dilated lacteals, suggestive of concurrent lymphangiectasia. The intestinal biopsy not only helps confirm the diagnosis but also provides information pertinent to prognosis and allows individualization of therapy.

Differential Diagnosis

As discussed previously, the clinician and the pathologist must take great care to differentiate LPE from a variety of known causes of intestinal lymphocytic-plasmacytic infiltrates and from normal intestine which routinely has a small complement of mucosal leukocytes. Important differential diagnoses are provided in Table 21-6. Lymphosarcoma, in particular, can be difficult to differentiate from LPE, and it is not uncommon for patients initially diagnosed as having LPE to later manifest lymphosarcoma. Whether this represents a progression of the disease from LPE to lymphosarcoma or an initial misdiagnosis is as yet uncertain. A similar condition to LPE has been reported in dogs in England and referred to as "tropical sprue-like enteropathy".[122] The information published to date on this enteropathy has not allowed us to clearly differentiate this disorder from LPE.

Treatment

The treatment protocol described in the clinical synopsis is suitable for the therapy of moderate to severe LPE. The higher end of the dosage range recommended is used for the more severe cases. If the inflammatory infiltrates or clinical signs are mild, smaller doses of prednisone may be sufficient to obtain remission. In general, controlled diets used alone are not satisfactory for the induction of remission in patients with LPE.[77,116,117] Controlled diets often ameliorate the signs, but they rarely induce complete remission. Most patients show signs of improvement within a week of therapy. If the clinical signs are non-responsive after two weeks, consider more aggressive immunosuppressive therapy with high dose prednisone in association with metronidazole, azathioprine, or cyclophosphamide. Combination therapy is also useful if unacceptable side-effects from the high-dose prednisone therapy become apparent. Some patients require continued medical therapy throughout their lives, but many can be weaned from medication after three months and maintained in remission on controlled diets. Some patients can eventually be returned to commercial diets. If recurrence of signs occurs, the pharmacological treatment regimen should be reinstituted for the same duration. If recurrence of signs occurs at the end of the second episode of drug therapy, it is probable that indefinite drug administration will be required. Important details concerning the controlled diets and pharmacologic treatment regimens may be found in the section entitled "therapy of inflammatory bowel disease."

Prognosis

The prognosis for LPE is good. The concomitant presence of protein-losing enteropathy, melena, or severe histopathologic changes, however, merits a guarded to poor outlook.[117] In one study, 30% of the dogs were non-responsive to therapy.[118] Forty percent of cats with histologically severe disease are non-responsive.[123]

CHRONIC (LYMPHOCYTIC-PLASMACYTIC) COLITIS

Clinical Synopsis

Diagnostic features

* Clinical evidence of "large bowel" signs of greater than several weeks duration
* Biopsy evidence of colonic inflammation in which the predominant cells are lymphocytes and plasma cells
* No cause apparent after a thorough work up

Standard treatment

* Controlled diet of cottage cheese and rice (dogs) or sliced chicken (cats), with or without metamucil (1-6 tsp/meal)
* Azulfidine (sulfasalazine): Dogs - 12.5 mg/kg q 6 hr PO 14 days followed by 12.5 mg/kg q 12 hr 28 days; Cats - 10-20 mg/kg q 24 hr PO 14 days.

Follow up

* Withdraw the pharmacologic therapy and attempt to maintain on controlled diet for several weeks
* Thereafter, attempt elimination diet
* Repeat pharmacological therapy if recurrence occurs

Chronic colitis is a chronic, idiopathic inflammatory disease of the large bowel characterized by a mixed inflammatory infiltrate in which lymphocytes and plasma cells predominate.

Incidence and Signalment

Chronic colitis is one of the most common causes of chronic diarrhea in dogs presented to the UCD VMTH. Approximately 130 cases of the disease are presented each year, accounting for 5 cases per 1000 canine submissions. Chronic colitis is the most common cause of large bowel disease in the dog. A study of clinically normal dogs in a beagle colony revealed that the incidence of subclinical colonic inflammation is higher, reaching 40 out of every 1,000 dogs.[124] The boxer has an incidence of chronic colitis eight times greater than anticipated. The only other breed with an incidence of colitis greater than expected is the German Shepherd. Its rate of occurrence is 1.7 times the expected. The incidence in purebred dogs is greater than expected, and in mixed-breed dogs is less than expected. This may be a result of genetic predisposition, but the data may be biased by the better medical care afforded purebred than mixed-breed dogs. There is no sex predisposition to chronic colitis.

Chronic colitis appears to be less common in cats than in dogs. Feline colitis accounts for 3.2 cases per 1000 feline submissions. The incidence of colitis may be higher in the feline population than these numbers would suggest, however, because the bowel movements of cats are often not seen or examined by the owner, and because the classical signs of large bowel dysfunction are often less overt in cats. Moreover, diarrhea caused by colitis is less likely to be a nuisance problem in cats than in dogs. Lymphocytic-plasmacytic colitis is recognized in cats, but other variants are also seen, in particular hemorrhagic and suppurative colitis. Some are recognized as having a gangrenous or fibrotic colitis.

Most dogs first present for chronic colitis before six years of age. Thirty percent of dogs first present before one year of age.

Etiopathogenesis

The etiopathogenesis of chronic colitis is presumably similar to that for LPE. A full discussion of the etiopathogenesis of these disorders may be found in the general discussion of IBD.

Clinical Findings

The interview usually reveals a prolonged history of intermittent "large bowel" type diarrhea, characterized by some or all of the following signs: tenesmus, defecation urgency, fecal incontinence, and the frequent passage of diarrhea with fresh blood and mucus. Mucoid stools is usually the earliest sign seen, whereas tenesmus is usually not observed until the disease worsens. Vomiting occurs in as many as 30% of dogs with colitis. The presence of this sign should not mislead the clinician into ruling out a large bowel problem. Anal pruritus is occasionally seen. Borborygmus and excessive flatus are rarely present and suggest concomitant small bowel disease. Occasionally, the only sign is a marked dyschezia. As the severity of the disease increases, other signs develop, including anorexia, weight loss, vomition, fever, and abdominal pain. In multi-pet households only one animal is affected and there should be no evidence of contagion to people. Concurrent involvement of the small intestine is not uncommon. This can lead to animals presented for a mixture of small and large bowel signs.

The physical examination findings are usually unremarkable except for the rectal examination, which often reveals stool with fresh blood or mucus, and occasionally detects a cobblestone mucosal surface or rectal stricture.

Laboratory Findings

Laboratory findings are usually unremarkable. Hemograms can show nonspecific changes in leukocytes that reflect chronic inflammation and stress, such as neutrophilia, monocytosis, lymphopenia, and eosinopenia. Liver enzymes are elevated in about 20% of dogs. Tests for parasites will be negative, and fecal culture (rarely performed) will not reveal pathogens. In cats positive FeLV titer raises the possibility that the colitis is FeLV-associated. In some cats the only manifestation of FIP is persistent colitis, making it important to test for that disease.

Endoscopic Findings

Most cases of chronic colitis in the dog and cat are associated with mucosal abnormalities that can be recognized with a proctoscope. The characteristic findings are generalized erythema and friability, with a patchy or complete loss of the submucosal vascular pattern due to the overlying inflammatory infiltrate and edema in the lamina propria. Additional observations are excessive accumulations of mucus, mucosal granularity, and areas of erosion or spontaneous hemorrhage. The colon is often more difficult to insufflate than the colon of normal dogs, perhaps due to mucosal infiltration by cells or edema or to increased muscular tone. Occasionally circumferential mucosal folds are present that will not yield to the proctoscope (Figure 21-5). Well circumscribed deep ulcers or strictures may be seen but are relatively rare. It is important to emphasize that these features are not specific for chronic (idiopathic) colitis, but rather can be seen in any inflammatory large bowel disease. Furthermore, the colon can appear grossly normal in spite of significant histological abnormalities. Therefore, even normal appearing bowels should be biopsied.

Radiographic Findings

Survey radiographs rarely provide useful information for the diagnosis of chronic colitis. Similarly, barium enemas have poor sensitivity for the diagnosis of this disease and are rarely performed. The few indications for barium enemas are discussed in Chapter 5 and 6 and primarily pertain to the examination of the upper colon if flexible colonoscopy cannot be performed. Changes compatible with chronic colitis that can be recognized by a barium enema include poor colonic distensibility, generalized mucosal thickening and irregularity, and mucosal ulcerations or strictures. The colon can be markedly shortened by disease (Figure 21-6). Endoscopic examination and or "blind" biopsy is necessary subsequent to barium enemas to differentiate the cause of any suspected abnormality.

Biopsy Findings

Colonic biopsy is used to confirm and characterize chronic colitis. Biopsy findings are often useful in suggesting the cause and pathogenesis of the colitis. Moreover, they assist the choice of effective therapy and facilitate the provision of an accurate prognosis. Biopsy of the colon is the single most important diagnostic procedure in evaluation of the clinical signs of colonic disease.

The earliest mucosal change is hyperplasia of crypt cells, reflective of a more rapid epithelial turnover. Additional mild changes include infiltration of the lamina propria with plasma cells, lymphocytes, and eosinophils. The lymphocytes and plasma cells usually predominate. Neutrophils are sometimes present. There is an absence of periodic acid-Schiff (PAS) positive histiocytes. The inflammatory process is confined to the mucosa. In ulcerative colitis of humans, the quantity of eosinophils in the biopsy correlates to disease activity.[125] A mild lesion typical of colitis with plasma cell and lymphocyte infiltration of the lamina propria is shown in Figure 21-7 (normal colonic mucosa is shown for comparison). These mild lesions do not typically alter the endoscopic appearance. It is not uncommon to find profuse diarrhea in association with mild biopsy changes. This syndrome bears a close resemblance to the so named "microscopic colitis" of humans. In microscopic colitis of humans minimal inflammatory infiltrates and mild reactive changes in the epithelium are associated with markedly abnormal colonic absorption of water and electrolytes and clinical signs which include persistent diarrhea with urgency, mild abdominal cramping, but no hematochezia.[83]

In severe cases of chronic colitis, infiltration by leukocytes

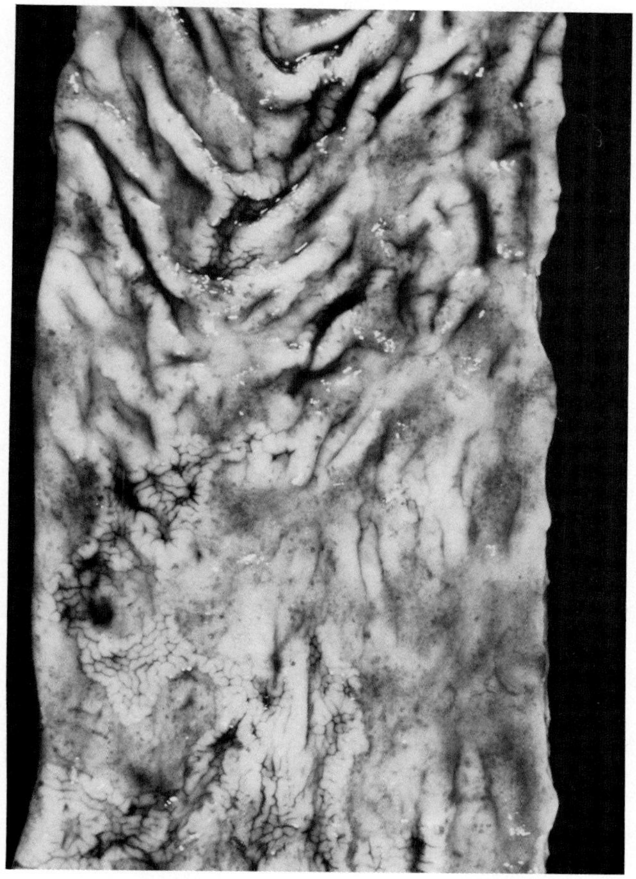

Figure 21-5. Chronic colitis. Inflammation has caused mucosal folds that remain with distention of the colon during endoscopy or barium enema.

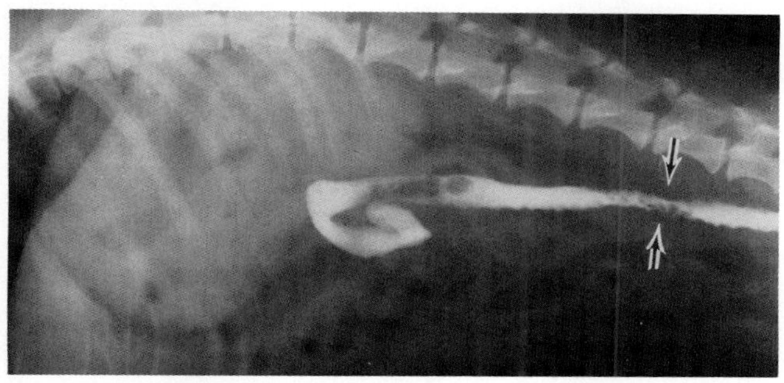

Figure 21-6. Radiograph of one-year-old miniature Dachshund with signs of severe bloody diarrhea. Barium enema reveals the colon to be shortened. The transverse colon is at the level of the first lumbar vertebrae instead of its usual position at the level of the twelfth thoracic vertebrae. The cecum cannot be identified. Stricture of the colon is most evident at the arrows.

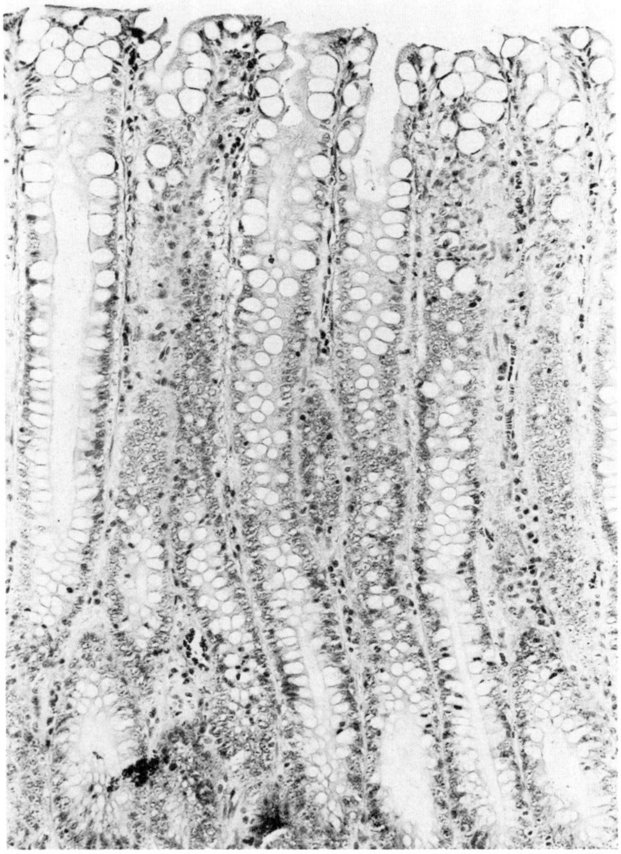

Figure 21-7A. Biopsy of normal canine colon.

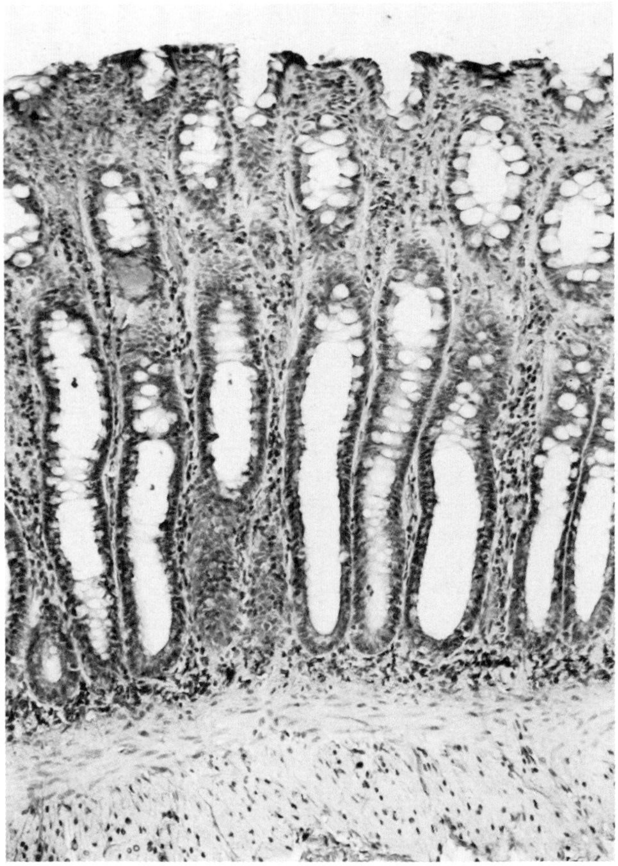

Figure 21-7B. Colitis. Changes include moderate crypt dilation, accelerated regeneration of crypt epithelium (identified by low cuboidal epithelial cells with dark staining nuclei and absence of differentiation to goblet cells) in deepest part of crypt, increased number of inflammatory cells, and degeneration and erosion of surface epithelium.

is more extensive. In some biopsies the lamina propria is so engorged with lymphocytes that the lesions resemble lymphoma. Dilation of the colonic glands and mucus clearance are also observed, and degeneration of the surface epithelial cells is seen. This condition can progress to epithelial desquamation, erosion, and ulceration. In the early stages, degenerating surface mucosal cells are characterized by basophilia, by reductions in height so that they become cuboidal or flattened, and by the appearance of cytoplasmic vacuoles (Figure 21-8). Even with accelerated destruction the surface epithelium can appear normal, but an increase is found in the renewal activity of the crypt epithelium. Thus, the crypt cells in the glands appear hyperplastic and show increased numbers of mitotic figures. With increased severity the goblet cells may virtually disappear from the glandular epithelium, and the protective functions of mucus are lost. Replacement of rapidly desquamating superficial epithelium is a higher priority than maintenance of mucus-secreting cells.

Epithelial cell death is followed by the appearance of acute inflammatory changes characterized by neutrophil accumulation in the lamina propria directly beneath the epithelial surface. Ulceration in chronic colitis results from the failure of crypt-cell proliferation to replace the degenerating surface epithelial cells. Ulceration is usually focal but almost complete loss of the surface epithelium can occur (Figure 21-9). The ulcers may heal with reepithelization of the surface.

Chronic colitis can persist as a mild form that shows nothing more than the early changes of immunocyte infiltration with the addition of fibrosis (Figure 21-7). Fibrosis is usually confined to the lamina propria. Widespread fibrosis at this site eventually results in the loss of colonic glands and a distortion of the normal structure of the lamina propria. Extensive fibrosis causes a loss of the colon's absorptive functions. Inflammation extending into the submucosa stimulates fibrosis and can cause stenosis. Colonic stricture is an unusual sequel to chronic colitis, developing only with improper management or neglect. Advanced lesions can include microabscesses in the lamina propria and submucosa that can rupture and form ulcers. Focal chronic inflammatory changes can result in the formation of granulomas (Figure 21-9), an unusual feature of colitis. Granulomas contribute to stricture formation.

It is important to recall that these changes are not specific for chronic colitis and can be caused by various bacterial and irritative conditions listed in Tables 21-4, 5, 6, and 7.

Treatment

If the inflammatory infiltrates or clinical signs are mild, controlled diets alone are justified. At the UCD VMTH, approximately 50% of dogs with chronic colitis placed on

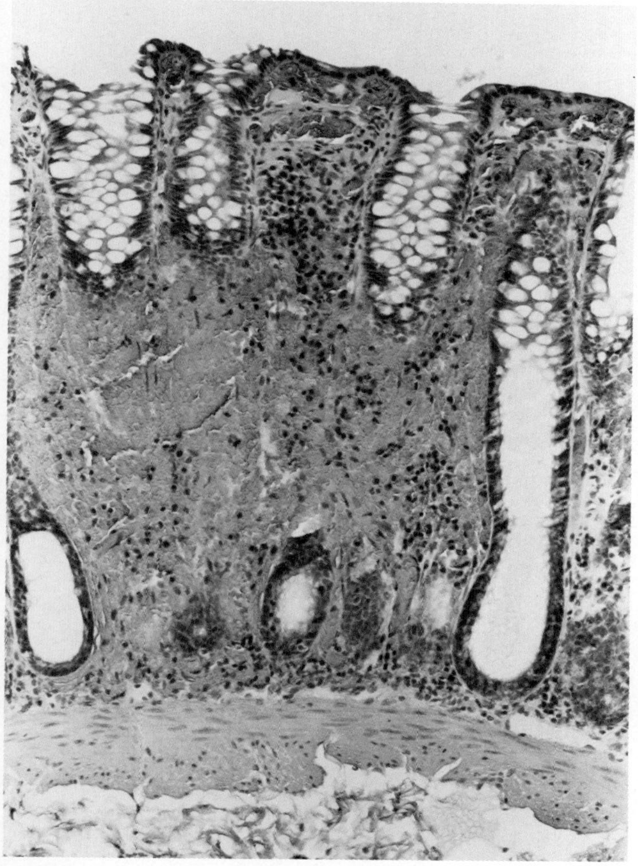

Figure 21-7C. Colitis. Normal mucosal thickness. Surface epithelium is low cuboidal to squamous. Crypts are moderately dilated; lower crypt epithelium is cuboidal with dark nuclei and few goblet cells. Widespread hemorrhage in lamina propria.

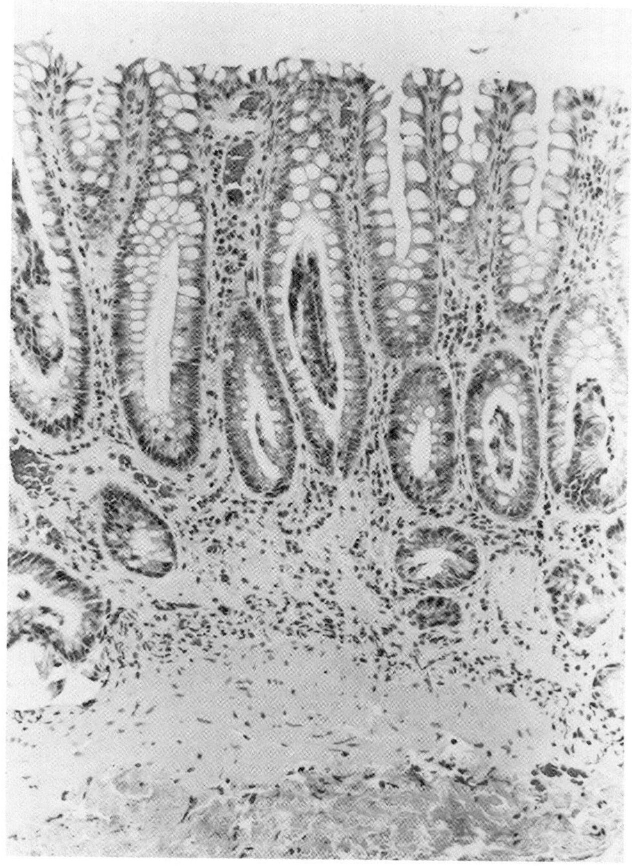

Figure 21-7D. Colitis. Mucosal atrophy caused by inflammatory changes in lower mucosa. Changes characterized by infiltration of inflammatory cells and fibrosis. Surface epithelium is normal.

cottage cheese and rice exclusively had a complete resolution of clinical signs. Approximately 20% showed no improvement, and the remainder of the dogs showed partial remission. In another study, 85% of dogs with chronic colitis showed resolution of their clinical signs within two weeks of the initiation of a cottage cheese and rice diet, and 100% of the dogs were in remission within six weeks.[34] Thirty percent of dogs with chronic colitis have been reported to respond to mutton-based diets such as prescription diet d/d. The addition of fiber such as Metamucil (Searle Laboratories) at one to six teaspoons per meal may be beneficial in some cases.

The treatment protocol described in the clinical synopsis is suitable for the therapy of moderate to severe chronic colitis. If gastrointestinal side effects become apparent from sulfasalazine therapy, the dosage can be lowered and combination therapy with prednisone begun. If more serious side-effects from sulfasalazine such as keratoconjunctivitis occur, the drug must be withdrawn and treatment continued with prednisone. If unacceptable side-effects from high-dose prednisone therapy become apparent, combination therapy with azathioprine or metronidazole in association with a reduced dose of prednisone may be attempted. Disagreement exists over the relative merit of prednisone and sulfasalazine in the treatment of chronic colitis.[95,116,126,127] In our experience and that of others, both drugs are efficacious in the control of acute flareups of the disease, but sulfasalazine is the preferred drug for maintaining remission. Details concerning the formulation of controlled diets and pharmacologic treatment regimens may be found in the section entitled "therapy of inflammatory bowel disease."

Surgical resection of the diseased colon is a last resort option in managing patients with irreversible changes that cannot be treated medically.

Prognosis

Few cases of chronic colitis fail to respond to medical management. Stricture formation and extensive fibrosis of the lamina propria is suggestive of a chronic untreated problem. Such changes are not reversible by medical treatment and adversely affect the prognosis. Failure to recognize concomitant small intestinal involvement is one cause of treatment failure.

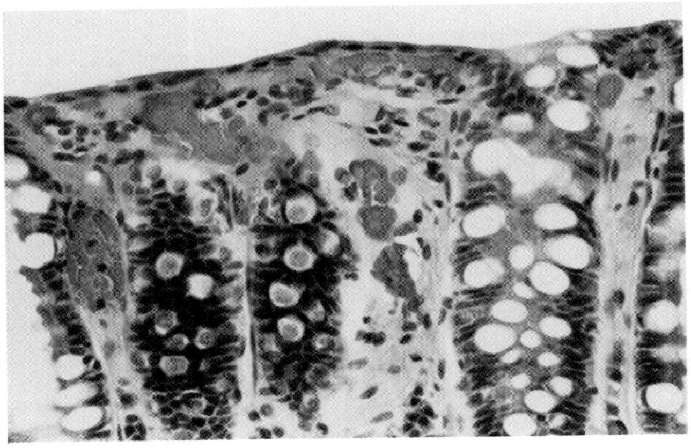

Figure 21-8A. Colitis. Frequent early change with colitis is appearance of squamous or low cuboidal epithelium on absorptive surface. Section also exhibits hemorrhage in lamina propria. High power magnification.

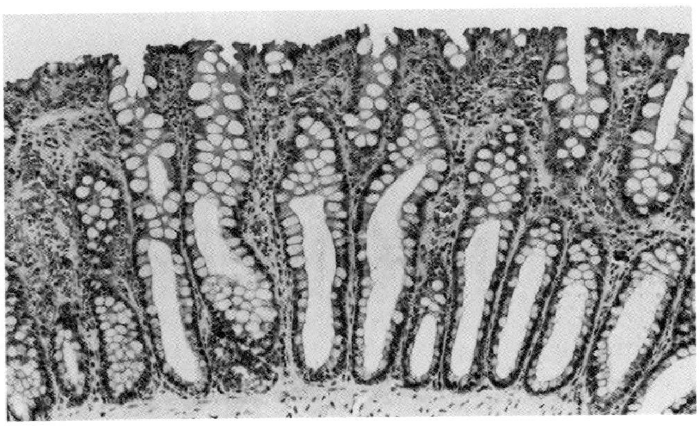

Figure 21-8B. Colitis with atrophy. Reduced mucosal thickness is associated with moderate crypt dilation. Crypt epithelium is normal except in bottom of crypts where many cells are low cuboidal with dark nuclei, suggesting augmented regeneration. Differentiation to goblet cells is normal throughout crypts. Increased inflammatory cells in lamina propria contribute to mild splaying (irregular spacing) of crypts.

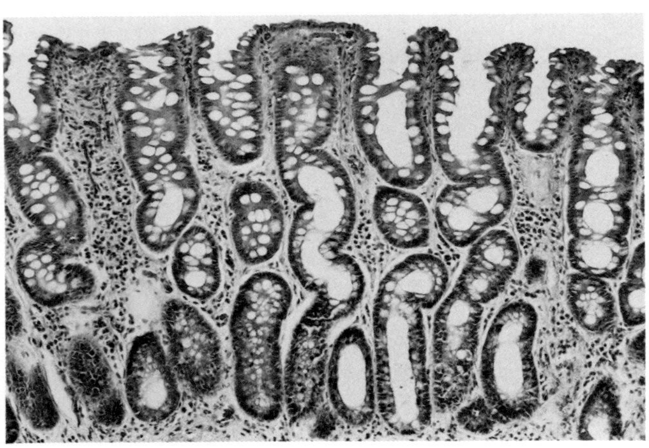

Figure 21-8C. Colitis. Changes are similar to Figure 20-5B except that atrophy is not as severe but mucosal surface epithelium is eroded in places.

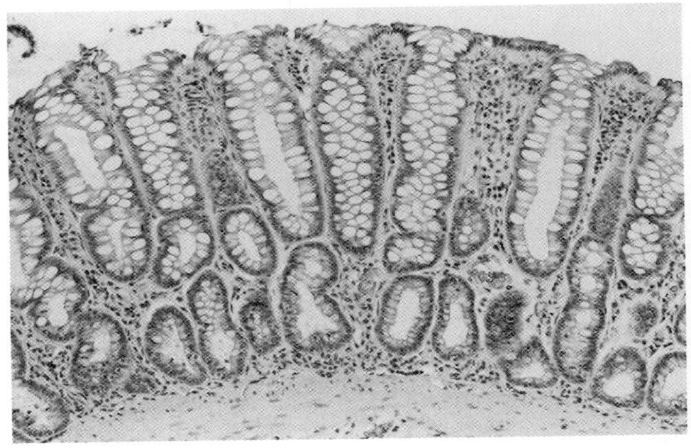

Figure 21-8D. Colitis. Reduced mucosal thickness. Increased number of inflammatory cells in lamina propria. Number of goblet cells on mucosal surface is reduced.

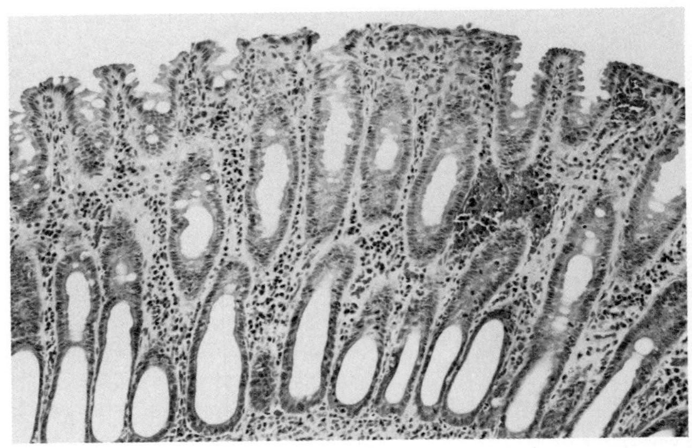

Figure 21-8E. Colitis. Reduced mucosal thickness. Moderate dilation of crypts with epithelium in lower crypts being cuboidal with few goblet cells. Mild to moderate infiltration of inflammatory cells in lamina propria with few areas of hemorrhage.

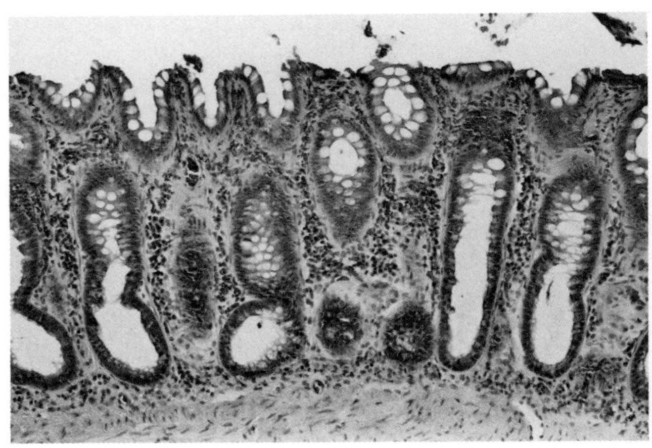

Figure 21-8F. Colitis. Mucosal thickness is 50% to 60% of normal. Moderate crypt dilation and splaying. Epithelial cells in deeper half of crypts are cuboidal with dark nuclei, suggesting increased regeneration. Few goblet cells in crypt depths. Increased number of inflammatory cells in lamina propria. Surface epithelium exhibits thinning and erosions.

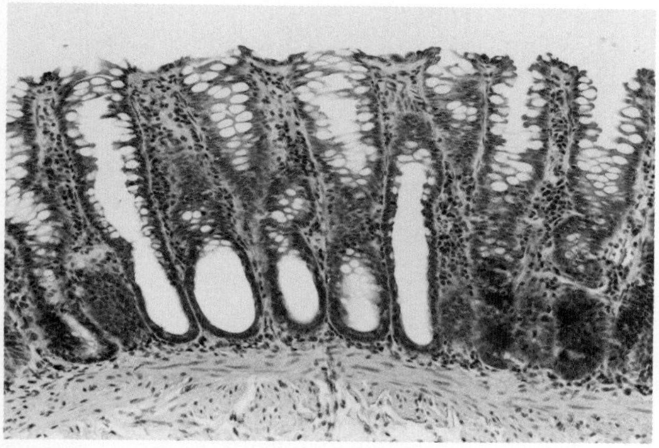

Figure 21-9A. Colitis with mucosal atrophy. Mucosal thickness is about 50% of normal. Moderate crypt dilation with cuboidal epithelium possessing dark nuclei in lower half. Epithelial surface is eroded. Number of inflammatory cells is increased in lamina propria.

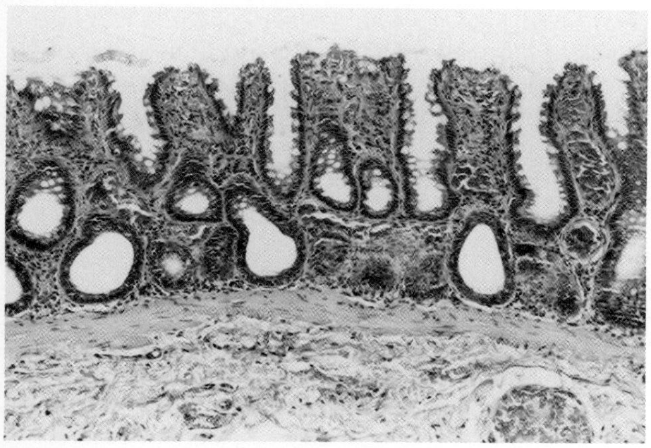

Figure 21-9B. Colitis with atrophy. Changes are similar to Figure 20-6A but are more severe and with hemorrhage.

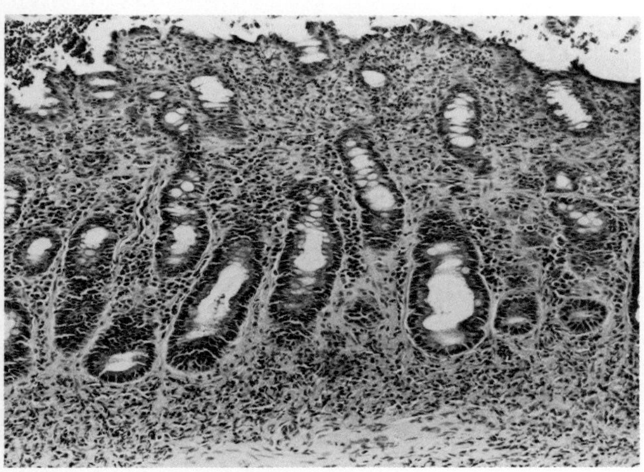

Figure 21-9C. Colitis, Changes include erosion of surface epithelium and ulceration into lamina propria with hemorrhage. Marked infiltration by inflammatory cells. Fibrous tissue is increased. Crypt changes are similar to those with milder forms of colitis.

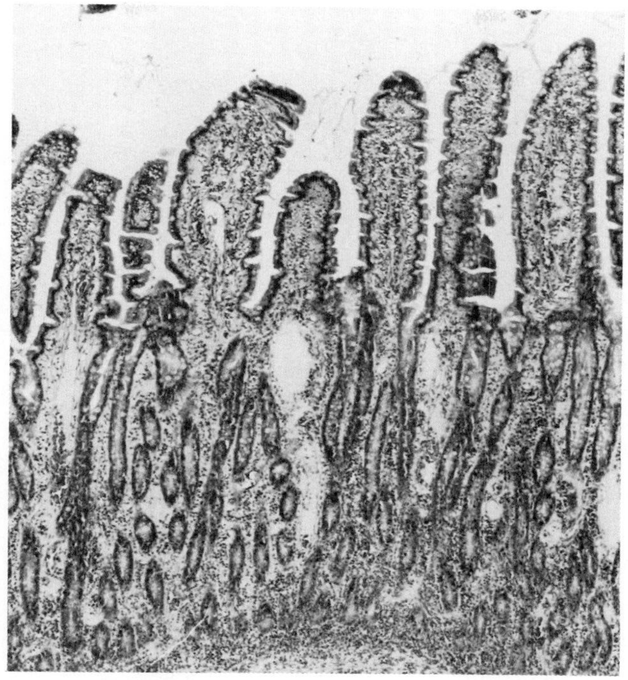

Figure 21-10. Eosinophilic enteritis. Diffuse infiltration of villi and crypts by eosinophils. Dilation of some lymphatics. Changes caused in villus height and crypt depth are minor.

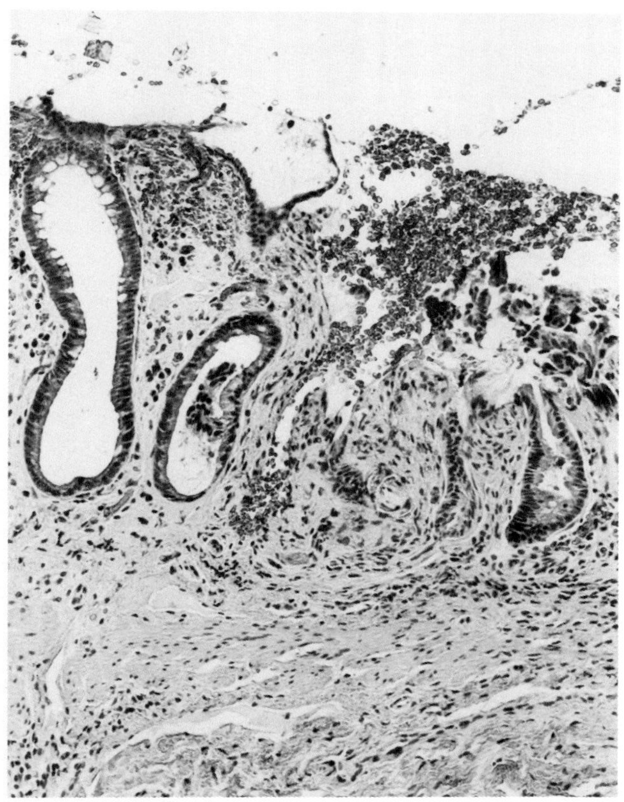

Figure 21-9D. Ulcerative colitis with mucosal atrophy. Changes include ulceration of surface, dilation of crypts, cuboidal crypt epithelium, inflammatory cell infiltration and fibrosis of lamina propria, and hemorrhage.

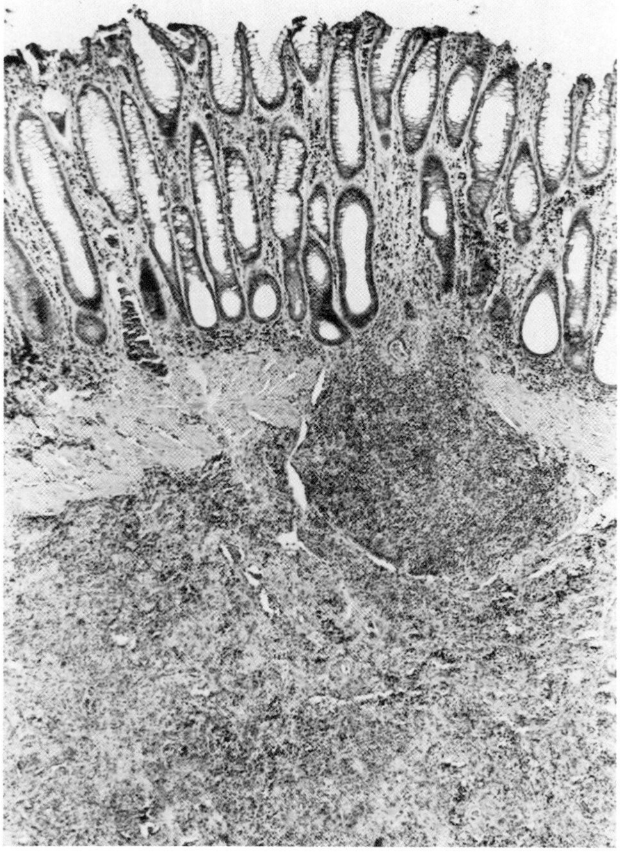

Figure 21-9E. Colitis with severe involvement of submucosa. Marked infiltration by inflammatory cells with granuloma formation. Normal lymphoid follicle is seen in right half at junction of mucosa with submucosa.

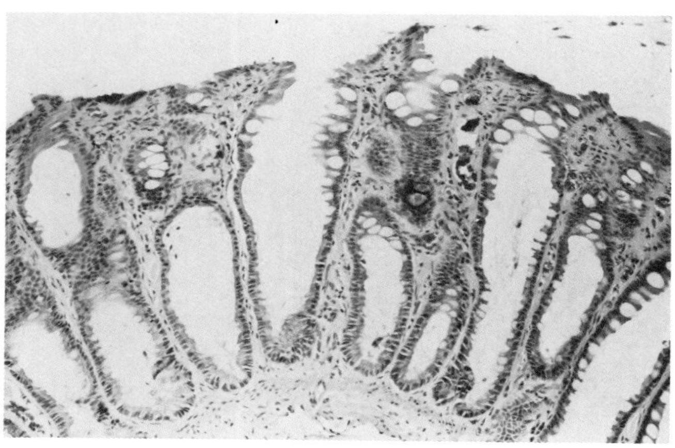

Figure 21-9F. Colitis in cat with feline infectious peritonitis. Biopsy specimen showing changes that include marked crypt dilation. Fip titer was 1 to 1600.

EOSINOPHILIC GASTROENTERITIS, ENTERITIS and ENTEROCOLITIS

Clinical Synopsis

Diagnostic features

* Clinical evidence of small bowel signs, or mixed small and large bowel signs of greater than several weeks' duration
* Peripheral eosinophilia often present
* Biopsy evidence of gastric and/or intestinal inflammation in which the predominant cells are eosinophils
* No cause apparent after a thorough work up

Standard treatment

* Controlled diet of cottage cheese and rice (dogs) or sliced chicken (cats).
* Dogs: Prednisone 0.5-1 mg/kg q 12 hr PO for one to two weeks followed by 0.5 mg/kg q 12 hr PO for four weeks; followed by 0.5 mg/kg qod PO for several weeks.
* Cats: Prednisone 2-3 mg/kg q 12 hr PO for two to four weeks; followed by 1-1.5 mg/kg q 12 hr for two to four weeks; followed by 0.5-1.0 mg q 24 hr for two to four weeks; followed by alternate day therapy for another four months

Follow up

* Withdraw the pharmacologic therapy and attempt to maintain on controlled diet for several weeks
* Thereafter, attempt elimination diet
* Repeat pharmacological therapy if recurrence occurs

Eosinophilic gastroenteritis is a chronic, idiopathic inflammatory disease of the stomach and small intestine that is characterized by a mixed inflammatory infiltrate in which the predominate cell is the eosinophil. If the process involves the small intestine but not the stomach the disease is called eosinophilic enteritis; if it involves both the small and large intestine, it is called eosinophilic enterocolitis. In dogs eosinophilic gastroenteritis is the most common variant of this disease. In cats concomitant involvement of the colon rather than the stomach is more frequently seen.[95,128] In cats eosinophilic involvement of other tissues in addition to the bowel is also common (hypereosinophilic syndrome).[129] Because the cause of eosinophilic IBD has not been proven, it is best classified as a variant of the inflammatory bowel diseases rather than a consequence of food allergy.

Incidence and Signalment

Eosinophilic IBD is less common than LPE. No sex predispositions are apparent. The German Shepherd dog may be predisposed;[130] with the problem more common also in Rottweilers. At the UCD VMTH it is less common in cats than in dogs. In dogs the disorder is most common in animals five years of age or younger.[130] In cats a median age of eight years has been reported with a range of 1.5-11 years.[95,128]

Etiopathogenesis

The most likely cause of eosinophilic gastroenteritis is a type 1 hypersensitivity response to dietary antigens absorbed from the intestine. Eosinophilic gastroenteritis may also result from an immune response to other antigens such as enteric bacteria (Table 21-4). The etiopathogenesis of eosinophilic gastroenteritis is discussed in more detail in the sections in this chapter on type 1 hypersensitivity, IBD differential diagnosis, and the relationship of food and parasitic antigens to IBD.

Clinical Findings

Clinical findings in dogs and cats with eosinophilic IBD are similar to those for other types of chronic gastroenteritis. No pathognomonic findings are seen. Chronic vomiting, "small bowel" type diarrhea, weight loss, and anorexia are the most common clinical signs observed. If the process extends to the colon, signs of large bowel dysfunction may be observed. Occasionally, evidence of chronic blood loss is manifested by anemia and melena. In one report, 50% of cats had evidence of hematochezia and melena.[128] In cats, physical examination often reveals markedly thickened, rigid intestines and may detect peripheral lymphadenopathy, hepatomegaly, or splenomegaly if eosinophilic infiltration of other organs has occurred (hypereosinophilic syndrome).[95]

Diagnostic Findings

Laboratory Findings. A peripheral eosinophilia is invariably present in cats and inconsistently present in dogs. Gastrointestinal parasites, heartworms, hypoadrenocorticism, pulmonary problems, and allergic skin diseases such as flea-allergic dermatitis must be ruled out before the eosinophilia can be attributed to eosinophilic gastroenteritis. Eosinophilia may also occur with mast cell neoplasia and transmural granulomatous enteritis, both of which can mimic many of the clinical signs of eosinophilic gastroenteritis. Resolution of the peripheral eosinophilia after placement of the patient on a controlled diet supports the diagnosis of eosinophilic gastroenteritis. Ninety percent of cats with eosinophilic enteritis have eosinophilic infiltration of their bone marrow.[128] In severe cases, the laboratory work may reveal a panhypoproteinemia suggestive of a protein-losing enteropathy.

Endoscopic, Radiographic, and Ultrasonographic Findings. The endoscopic and radiographic findings are similar to those described for LPE. In severe eosinophilic enteritis the bowel can appear rigid, and insufflation will be difficult. In the dog, there may be increased friability of the gastric mucosa, and erosions or ulcers may be apparent. Rugal folds may appear thickened and edematous. Just as with LPE, the mucosa can look normal to endoscopic examination in spite of the presence of significant disease. Radiography or ultrasonography may reveal organomegaly or mesenteric lymphadenopathy, particularly in cats.

Biopsy Findings. Microscopic changes, found consistently in the small intestine, are a diffuse infiltration of the lamina propria with eosinophils (Figure 21-10). In dogs, cellular infiltration is usually confined to the lamina propria but rarely will involve the submucosa or muscularis.[131] In cats, the infiltration is often transmural.[129] Mucosal atrophy with villus blunting is seen in advanced disease. In dogs, gastric involvement is usually evident; less commonly the eosinophilic infiltrate will also affect the colon. Gastric biopsy often confirms eosinophilic gastroenteritis. When intestinal mucosa is biopsied, multiple samples are obtained since morphological changes of eosinophilic enteritis can be discontinuous.

Treatment

In some, but not many, cases of canine eosinophilic gastroenteritis, remission of clinical signs will occur in response to controlled diet alone.[127] Once signs have resolved, elimination diets should be performed to identify foods that are tolerated and those that are not. In those dogs that do not respond to controlled diets, prednisone therapy should be begun. In cats dietary therapy alone is not sufficient to control the signs, and concurrent prednisone therapy is routinely used. The dosage of prednisone listed in the clinical synopsis controls the disease in most dogs. In cats the refractory nature of the disease demands high prednisone dosages for prolonged periods.[95] Lower prednisone doses (1-2 mg/kg q 24 hr) are associated with temporary remissions but rapid and refractory recurrence of the disease.[128] Additional immunosuppressive drugs such as azathioprine may be useful in some cases. In those animals manifesting a peripheral eosinophilia, the eosinophil count may be used as a guide to the adequacy of therapy. Details concerning the formulation of controlled diets and pharmacologic treatment regimens may be found in the section entitled "therapy of inflammatory bowel disease." Some patients can be treated for short periods with infrequent relapses, whereas others may require medication given continuously.

Disodium cromoglycate is unlikely to be successful in the therapy of gastrointestinal type 1 hypersensitivities because of the minimal influence of this drug on gastrointestinal-type mast cells. Recent experience with this drug in the treatment of humans with IBD has failed to confirm earlier reports of efficacy.

Prognosis

Treatment of eosinophilic gastroenteritis is usually successful in dogs, although controlled diets and glucocorticoids may have to be continued indefinitely. In cats the disease has been traditionally associated with a poor prognosis but recent publications have suggested that very aggressive immunosuppressive therapy can result in resolution.[95] The prognosis in cats is guarded.

HYPEREOSINOPHILIC SYNDROME

The hypereosinophilic syndrome is a common variant of eosinophilic enteritis in the cat, in which the eosinophilic infiltration affects not just the bowel but also other parenchymal organs such as the liver, spleen, mesenteric lymph nodes, kidney, adrenal glands, and heart.[128,129] Involvement of the mesenteric lymph nodes has also been reported in the dog,[131] but more extensive extraintestinal infiltration is rare. The etiopathogenesis is presumably similar to that of eosinophilic enteritis. The reason why some cats (and humans) develop a multisystemic eosinophilic response is poorly understood. Proposed causes are the absorption and widespread dissemination of the inciting antigen or the involvement of the bowel in a multisystemic eosinophilic infiltration due to some defect in eosinophil regulation. The disease is thought to be distinct from eosinophilic leukemia, although the two disorders can be difficult to distinguish.[129] No sex predisposition has been established. The syndrome is most common in cats seven years and older, although cats as young as four years of age have been affected.[129] Clinical findings are similar to the other IBD disorders, with the exception that intestinal thickening is more marked, hepatosplenomegaly may be detected, and bloody diarrhea is frequent.

Peripheral eosinophilia is invariably present and sometimes reaches dramatically high proportions. The diagnosis is usually made by biopsy of a variety of abdominal organs at exploratory celiotomy. The characteristic finding is multiorgan invasion of eosinophils. The only treatment reported to date is aggressive high dose prednisone therapy.[95] Prognosis is guarded to poor.

EOSINOPHILIC COLITIS

Eosinophilic colitis is a chronic, idiopathic inflammatory disease of the large bowel characterized by a mixed inflammatory infiltrate in which eosinophils predominate. It is clinically indistinguishable from chronic (lymphocytic-plasmacytic) colitis.

The etiopathogenesis of eosinophilic colitis is unknown. Pathomechanisms similar to those of eosinophilic gastroenteritis are presumably involved, and it is not uncommon to find eosinophilic infiltration affecting the small intestine in addition to the colon. Dietary antigens are presumably of less importance in the generation of eosinophilic colitis than in eosinophilic gastroenteritis.

Eosinophilic colitis is an uncommon disorder in comparison to chronic colitis. The condition is most frequent in dogs but is occasionally seen in cats. In cats the eosinophilic infiltration is most often a component of eosinophilic enterocolitis or the hypereosinophilic syndrome. It is most common in middle-aged patients. No sex predisposition has been reported.

A peripheral eosinophilia may be present, but otherwise the laboratory work is unremarkable. Particular care must be made to rule out large bowel parasitism by whipworms. Rectal scrapes may reveal large numbers of eosinophils. Endoscopic findings are identical to those with chronic colitis. The predominance of eosinophils in the biopsy distinguishes the disorder from chronic colitis. In dogs, the eosinophilic infiltrate is most commonly confined to the lamina propria, but on occasion it can affect all bowel layers and the mesenteric lymph nodes.[131]

In the dog, the treatment most often used is a controlled diet with the concomitant administration of prednisone (1 mg/kg q 12 hr PO for one to two weeks; followed by 0.5 mg/kg q 12 hr PO for two weeks; followed by 0.5 mg/kg q 24 hr for two weeks; followed by tapering doses of alternate day therapy for two weeks). In cats, higher doses of prednisone are employed because of the likely concomitant hypereosinophilic syndrome. Azulfidine has not found favor in the treatment of eosinophilic colitis. Fiber (Metamucil) is sometimes a useful addition to the standard controlled diet. The response of patients to dietary therapy only is inconsistent. If pharmacologic therapy was used to assist remission, it should be withdrawn after six to eight weeks and the patient maintained on a controlled diet for a further few weeks before elimination diets are begun. Recurrences can occur, but in general the prognosis is favorable.

GASTROINTESTINAL EOSINOPHILIC GRANULOMA

Gastrointestinal eosinophilic granulomas are chronic, idiopathic inflammatory masses of the esophagus, stomach, and small intestine; the predominant cell is the eosinophil. The major importance of this unusual disorder is its mimicry of gastrointestinal neoplasia, a resemblance which may result in inappropriate euthanasia. A related disorder has been reported to occur in the mouth of Siberian Huskies. Eosinophilic granulomas commonly afflict the mouth and lips of cats as a component of the eosinophilic granuloma complex. The following comments apply only to eosinophilic granulomas of the stomach and intestine.

Gastrointestinal eosinophilic granulomas are an uncommon cause of vomiting or diarrhea in the dog.[132] They are most common in middle aged dogs but can occur as early as one year of age.[132] There is some evidence that the Rottweiller dog is predisposed. The most consistent sign of eosinophilic granuloma is vomiting, reflective of either gastric involvement in the granulomatous process or intestinal obstruction. Peripheral eosinophilia may be present. Ultrasonographic evidence of a gastric or small intestinal mass lesion may be noted. Endoscopy may reveal focal thickenings of the gastric mucosa.

Eosinophilic granulomas can look grossly like tumors. They often involve the entire thickness of the bowel wall, as shown in Figure 21-11. Concurrent mesenteric eosinophilic lymphadenopathy may occur.[132] They can be successfully removed surgically, but limited experience has shown that they recur if diet control and glucocorticoid therapy are not continued postsurgically.

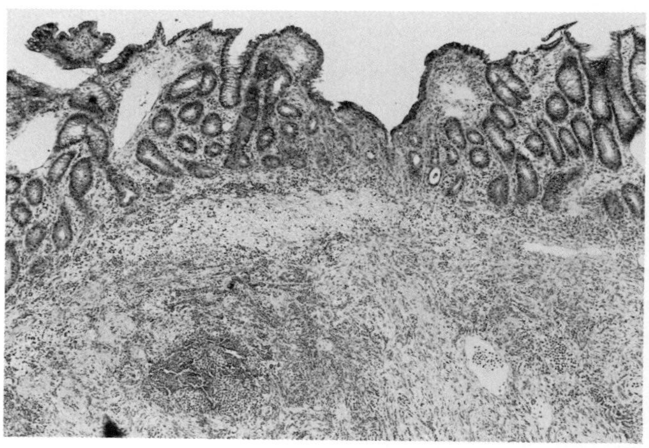

Figure 21-11. Eosinophilic granuloma in intestine. Granuloma in submucosa produced signs of intestinal obstruction. Diffuse infiltration of mucosa by eosinophils. Total villus atrophy at site of granuloma and partial loss of crypt epithelium.

HISTIOCYTIC COLITIS

Clinical Synopsis

Diagnostic features

* Clinical evidence of "large bowel" signs of greater than several weeks duration
* Boxer commonly affected
* Biopsy evidence of colonic inflammation in which the predominant cells are PAS positive histiocytes

Standard treatment

* Controlled diet of cottage cheese and rice with or without fiber added (metamucil (4-6 Tsp per meal)
* Azulfidine: 12.5 mg/kg q 6 hr PO 14 days followed by 12.5 mg/kg q 12 hr 28 days
* Prednisone: 1-2 mg/kg q 12 hr PO for one to two weeks followed by 0.5 mg/kg q 12 hr PO for four weeks, followed by 0.5 mg/kg qod PO for two weeks.

Follow up

* Withdraw the pharmacologic therapy and attempt to maintain on controlled diet for several weeks
* Thereafter, attempt elimination diet
* Repeat pharmacological therapy if recurrence occurs

Histiocytic colitis is a chronic, idiopathic inflammatory disease of the large bowel characterized by a mixed inflammatory infiltrate in which PAS positive histiocytes are a prominent feature. The disease tends to have a more ulcerative nature than chronic (lymphocytic-plasmacytic) colitis and is more refractory to treatment.

Incidence and Signalment

Boxers have a marked predisposition for histiocytic colitis, but the disease has also been reported in the French Bulldog[133] and the cat.[134] It has a relatively high incidence in the Boxer breed as does chronic (lymphocytic-plasmacytic) colitis. It affects primarily young dogs.

Etiopathogenesis

The etiopathogenesis of histiocytic colitis is unknown. Histiocytes, engorged macrophages, accumulate PAS-positive material either because the amount engulfed exceeds the capacity of the macrophage for degradation or because there is a deficiency of lysosomal enzymes for degradation. Early lesions in histiocytic colitis show normal-appearing macrophages near the luminal surface of the lamina propria, while the basilar regions of the mucosa contain distended periodic acid-Schiff (PAS) positive histiocytes, presumably cells transporting engulfed material from the mucosa. Lesions of this severity in other breeds of dogs contain no histiocytes, suggesting that the macrophage in histiocytic colitis is unable to process normal amounts of foreign material absorbed from the colon. When normal animals are fed material that cannot be degraded by lysosomal enzymes, it accumulates and remains in macrophages after being phagocytized.

Ultrastructure studies of engorged macrophages have suggested that they contain an infectious agent that might be the cause of chronic histiocytic ulcerative colitis, making it similar to Whipple's disease in humans. Coccoid bodies have been found, but it is uncertain whether they are nonpathogenic organisms that are phagocytized and not degraded or whether they are indeed pathogens that resist destruction by the inflammatory response in the body.[48] Another ultrastructure study found no evidence for an infectious agent.[49] No studies have shown that histiocytic colitis is a transmissible disease.

Vascular changes as evaluated by microangiography do not appear with early stages of canine histiocytic colitis.[62] Vascular dilation and hypervascularity appear with more extensive inflammatory changes. Ulceration results in complete disruption of the normal mucosal microvascular bed, which is replaced with an unorganized tangle of ectatic vessels. Ulceration of the mucosa results from failure of crypt-cell proliferation to replace the degenerating and desquamating surface epithelial cells. The engorgement of the lamina propria with histiocytes does not cause mechanical rupture.

Clinical and Diagnostic Findings

In general the clinical signs are those of severe large bowel diarrhea and are indistinguishable from chronic colitis. About one-third of the animals with histiocytic colitis show tenesmus, and nearly all pass blood in the feces. Laboratory findings are usually unremarkable. The endoscopy findings are similar to chronic colitis, with the exception of a greater incidence of well-circumscribed ulcers.

Biopsy Findings. Morphological changes characteristic of chronic histiocytic colitis have been well described.[49,135-137] The earliest morphologic change discernible is focal, acute inflammation and epithelial cell degeneration at the luminal surface of the colon. Electron microscopy indicates that epithelial cell injury is the initial morphologic lesion and that acute inflammation appears before necrosis and disruption of the surface epithelium. The inflamed lamina propria contains neutrophils, macrophages, and erythrocytes. Neutrophils appear as a response to nonspecific cell degeneration and do not participate in producing the initial lesion. Histiocytes are normally only present in small numbers in the colonic lamina propria. In histiocytic colitis their numbers increase markedly once the colonic epithelium is disrupted, and they become engorged with PAS-positive polysaccharides (Figure 21-12). Some report that granulomas are a consistent feature of chronic histiocytic ulcerative colitis, whereas others report that this is not the case. The disagreement may be due to differences in chronicity and severity. Epithelioid and giant-cell granulomas, found with advanced disease, can become transmural.

Treatment

The treatment of histiocytic colitis must be more aggressive than that of chronic colitis. A combination of controlled diet, sulfasalazine and prednisone, as described in the clinical synopsis, is a useful starting point. Some dogs will respond to this treatment regimen. Other dogs will require more potent immunosuppression, whereupon combination prednisone and

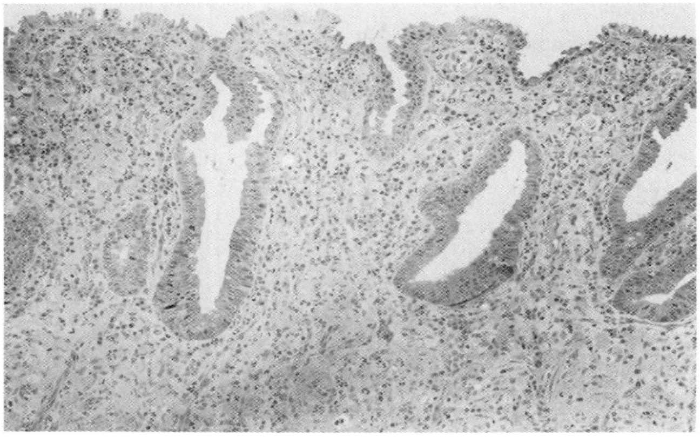

A

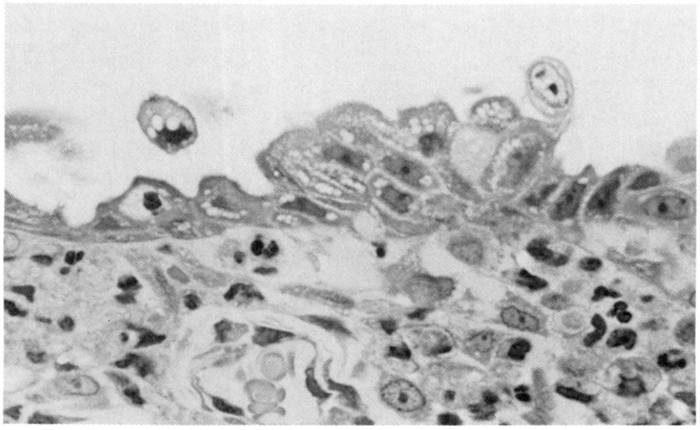

B

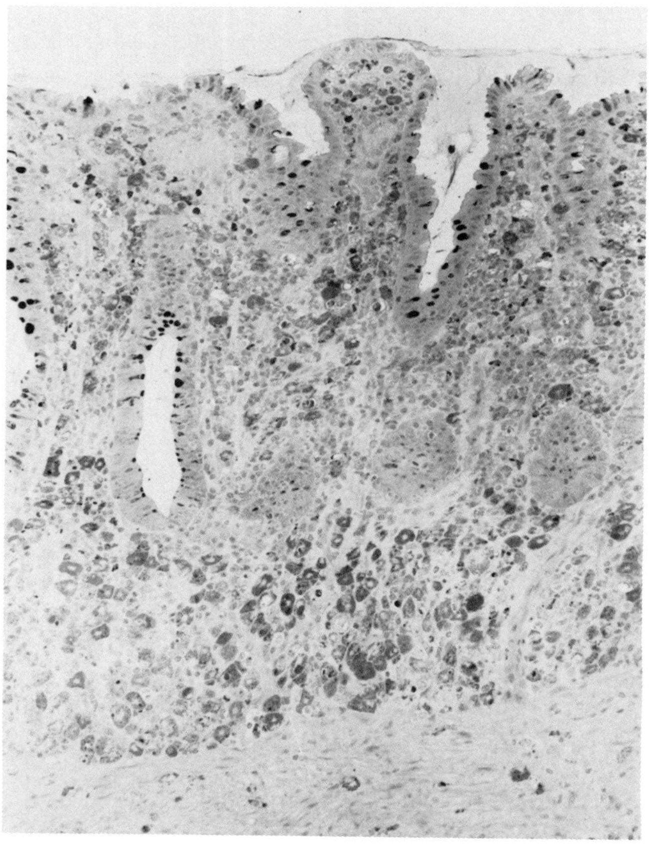

C

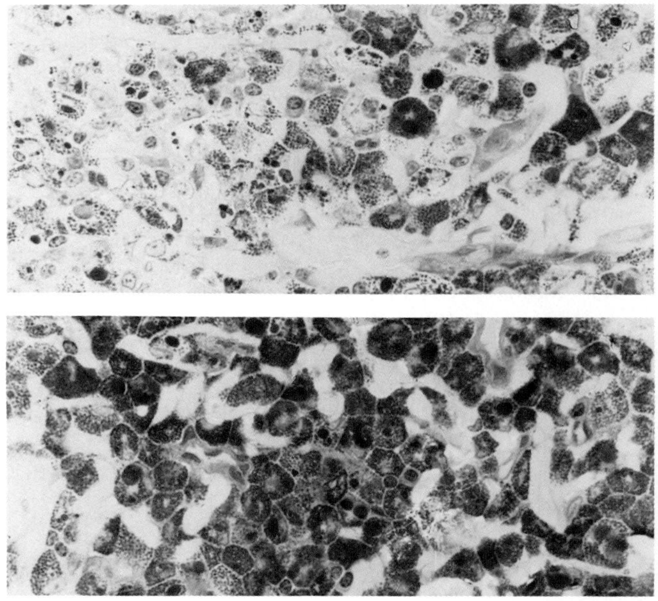

D

Figure 21-12. A) Biopsy of colon from Boxer with chronic histiocytic ulcerative colitis. Marked infiltration of lamina propria with histiocytes. Other forms of inflammatory cells are numerous. Few goblet cells are evident. Cell infiltrate has caused marked splaying of glands. Pathologic changes extended throughout submucosa (not shown). B) Epithelial changes involve all cells lining mucosal surface. C) PAS stained section shows granules in histiocytes with varying amounts of PAS staining material. Goblet cells also stain dark with PAS stain. Relative numbers of goblet cells is low. D) Higher magnification of PAS staining granules in histiocytes showing different degrees of severity.

azathioprine therapy can be utilized. Details concerning the formulation of controlled diets and pharmacologic treatment regimens may be found in the section entitled "therapy of inflammatory bowel disease."

Prognosis

The prognosis is guarded to poor unless treatment is begun very early in the disease course.

GRANULOMATOUS INFLAMMATORY BOWEL DISEASE

Granulomatous Enteritis, Colitis, and Enterocolitis

Granulomatous enteritis, colitis, and enterocolitis are rare, idiopathic inflammatory diseases of the small or large bowel characterized by the presence of aggregates of histiocytes and perhaps giant cells in the lamina propria.[121] PAS positive histiocytes are not a feature. In contrast to transmural granulomatous enterocolitis, this process is more diffuse in distribution. These diseases are seen in both the cat and the dog. Clinical signs and diagnostic procedures are similar to the other inflammatory bowel diseases. Treatment is also similar. Great care must be taken to rule out the infectious causes of granulomatous enteritis such as histiocytic colitis, histoplasmosis, phycomycosis, and tuberculosis (Table 21-5) before a patient is placed on immunosuppressive therapy. The prognosis is guarded.

Transmural Granulomatous Enterocolitis (Regional Enteritis)

Transmural granulomatous enterocolitis is seen rarely in dogs. The majority of affected dogs have been males of less than four years.[138] The disease is usually segmental and discontinuous in distribution and most often affects the lower ileum, cecum, colon, and draining lymph nodes.[121] Clinical signs are similar to chronic colitis with the exception that weight loss is prominent and that violent vomiting, hematemesis, and constipation can occur due to obstruction of the ileum, colon, or rectum by the granulomatous process. Abdominal palpation may reveal an abdominal mass in the ileocecal area. Rectal palpation occasionally will detect strictures or mucosal thickenings. Perianal location of the granulomatous inflammation can lead to perianal fistulation. Mild to moderate peripheral eosinophilia is common, and eosinophils form a significant component of the inflammatory infiltrate.[138,139] Colonoscopy reveals single or multiple discontinuous areas of mucosal proliferation associated with mucosal rigidity, ulceration, and luminal narrowing. Important differential diagnoses are listed in Table 21-5 and include parasitic granulomas from whipworms or hookworms[140] and campylobacter-associated proliferative enteritis.[141] Treatments attempted to date have included surgical resection of affected areas, tylosin, and prednisone therapy. Temporary improvement has been seen following surgery or prednisone therapy, but relapses are common. The prognosis is poor.

CHRONIC SUPPURATIVE COLITIS

Neutrophils are a minor common component of the inflammatory infiltrate of many chronic gastrointestinal inflammatory disorders and a major component of the cellular response in acute gastrointestinal inflammation. The ubiquitous presence of neutrophils is not suprising given the variety of products that causes their chemotaxis (Chapter 4) and the diverse range of pathologic processes that incite the release of these mediators. On rare occasions, the neutrophil will be a prominent or even predominant cell in chronic idiopathic inflammation. This condition is referred to as chronic suppurative colitis. In our experience, and that of others,[142] this entity is most common in cats.

GASTROENTERITIS OF BASENJI DOGS

A spectrum of gastrointestinal pathology including chronic, lymphocytic-plasmacytic inflammation of the stomach and small intestine characterizes Basenji gastroenteritis.[143-146] This syndrome is distinguished from LPE by its high incidence in Basenjis; by a concomitant hypergammaglobulinemia; by its more severe, progressive, and refractory nature; and by the high incidence of a concurrent hypertrophic gastropathy. The disease is thought to bear similarities to immunoproliferative enteropathy of humans. The Basenji disorder has been variously referred to as immunoproliferative enteropathy, immunoproliferative small intestinal disease, and diarrheal syndrome of Basenji dogs. The etiopathogenesis is unknown, although both genetic and environmental factors are involved.

Either sex and a wide age range are affected. Most affected Basenjis develop diarrhea by the time they are three years of age. The incidence in the Basenji breed may approach 3%.[145] The clinical signs include anorexia, progressive weight loss, and intractable diarrhea. Vomiting is occasionally noted. Neurological signs, including incoordination, paresis, circling, and seizures, were seen in some affected Basenjis after vaccination. The gastrointestinal signs are frequently precipitated by a stressful event. Ulcerative dermatitis of the pinnae is occasionally seen.

Hypoproteinemia, hypoalbuminemia, hypergammaglobulinemia, mature leukocytosis, and mild non-regenerative anemia are present in many Basenji dogs.[146] Malabsorption is often present, and concurrent maldigestion is suspected. The maldigestion has been attributed to functional pancreatic insufficiency because the pancreas is histologically normal.[143]

The pathologic findings vary considerably. Gastric rugal hypertrophy, lymphocytic gastritis, and gastric mucosal atrophy occur in 50% of affected Basenjis.[143] Many asymptomatic dogs also have lymphocytic gastritis and a few have rugal hypertrophy. All affected dogs have moderate or severe intestinal lesions dominated by villus clubbing and fusion, increased tortuosity of intestinal crypts, and diffuse infiltration of mononuclear inflammatory cells of which lymphocytes and plasma cells predominate.[143] Mild mononuclear cell infiltrations are also present in the intestine of asymptomatic dogs. The colon is usually not affected by the disease. A mild glomerulonephritis is often present. Progression of the disease to abdominal lymphoma can occur.

Immunosuppressive doses of corticosteroids and therapy with tylosin, metronidazole, or trimethoprim sulfa can ameliorate the signs, but the effect is usually temporary. Affected Basenjis tolerated Iams Diet well (Iams Food Co). The prognosis is guarded to poor. Most dogs die within two years of diagnosis although survival for as long as five years has been reported.

DIARRHEAL SYNDROME IN LUDENHUNDS

A diarrheal syndrome in Ludenhunds characterized by chronic, idiopathic lymphocytic-plasmacytic inflammation of the small intestine has been described.[147] The inflammation is characterized by a mixed infiltrate in which lymphocytes and plasma cells predominate. Intestinal protein loss is common. The disease is distinguished from LPE by its progressive nature and breed predisposition. The prognosis is poor.

REFERENCES

1. Strober, W. and James, S.P.: (a) The immunological basis of inflammatory bowel disease. J. Clin. Immunol. 6:415-432, 1986.

2. McConnell, P.B. and Wyndheim, C.M.: Inflammatory bowel disease. In, The Genetic Basis of Common Disease. Edited by King, R.A., et al. New York, McGraw-Hill (In Press).
3. Matthews, J.G.W.: Experimental ischemic colitis in the dog. In, Animal Models of Colitis. Edited by Pfeiffer, C.J. CRC Press Inc, Boca Raton, Florida, 161-180, 1985.
4. Podolsky, D.K. and Isselbacher, K.J.: Composition of human colonic mucin: selective alteration in inflammatory bowel disease. J. Clin. Invest. 72:142-153, 1983.
5. Podolsky, D.K. and Isselbacher, K.J.: Glycoprotein composition of colonic mucosa. Gastroenterology 87:991-998, 1984.
6. Mayer, E.A., Raybould, H. and Koelbel, C.: Neuropeptides, inflammation, and motility. Dig. Dis. Sci. 33:71S-77S, 1988.
7. Chiodini, R.J., Van Kruiningen, H.J., Thayer, W.R., et al.: Possible role of mycobacteria in inflammatory bowel disease 1. An unclassified Mycobacterium species isolated from patients with Crohn's disease. Dig. Dis. Sci. 29:1073-1079, 1984.
8. Jewell, D.P. and Patel, C.: Immunology of inflammatory bowel disease. Scan. J. Gastroenterology Suppl. 114, 20:120-126, 1985.
9. Strober, S.P., Quinn, T.C. and Danovitch, S.H.: Crohn's disease. New concepts of pathogenesis and current approaches to treatment. Dig. Dis. Sci. 32:1297-1310, 1987.
10. Strober, W. and James, S.P.: The immunopathogenesis of gastrointestinal and hepatobiliary diseases. JAMA 258:2962-2969, 1987.
11. Hodgson, H.J.F.: Inflammatory bowel disease and food intolerance. J. Royal College Physicians, London 20:45-48, 1986.
12. Shean, F.C., barker, W.F. and Fonkalsrud, E.W.: Studies on active and passive antibody induced colitis in the dog. Am. J. Surg. 107:337-339, 1964.
13. Guilford, W.G., Olander, H. and Strombeck, D.R.: Experimental canine colitis. Unpublished observations 1988.
14. Strickland, R.G. and Jewell, D.P.: Immunoregulatory mechanisms in nonspecific inflammatory bowel disease. Ann. Rev. Med, 34:195-204, 1983.
15. MacDermott, R.P., Nash, G.S., Bertovich, M.J.,Mohrman, R. F., Kodner, I.J., Delacroix, D.L. and Vaerman, J-P.: Altered patterns of secretion of monomeric IgA and IgA subclass 1 by intestinal mononuclear cells in inflammatory bowel disease. gastroenterology 91:379-385, 1986.
16. Kirsner, J.B.: Chronic inflammatory bowel disease: Overview of etiology and pathogenesis. In, Bockus Gastroenterology. 4th edition. Edited by Berk, J.E., Haubrich, W.S., Kalser, M.H., et al. W.B. Saunders, Philadelphia. 2093-2126, 1985.
17. Targan, S.R., Kagnoff, M.F., Brogan, M.D., et al.: Immunologic mechanisms in intestinal diseases. UCLA Conference. Ann. Int. Med. 106:853-870, 1987.
18. Lagercrantz, R., Hammarstrom, S., Perlmann, P. and Gustafsson, B.E.: (a) Immunological studies in ulcerative colitis IV. Origin of autoantibodies. J. Exp. Med. 128:1339-1352, 1968.
19. Roche, J.K., Fiocchi, C. and Youngman, K.: Sensitization to epithelial antigens in chronic mucosal inflammatory disease. I. Purification, characterization, and immune reactivity of murine epithelial cell-associated components. J. Immunol. 131:2796-2804, 1983.
20. Vecchi, M., Sakamaki, S., Diamond, B. and Das, K.M.: A human colon specific antigen reactive with ulcerative colitis colon tissue-bound IgG. Gastroenterology 90:1679A, 1986.
21. Lagercrantz, R., Perlmann, P., Hammarstrom, S.: (b) Immunologic studies in ulcerative colitis. V. Family studies. Gastroenterology 60:381-389, 1971.
22. Fiocchi, C., Roch, J.K. and Sapatnekar, W.: Familial immune reactivity to intestinal epithelial cell-associated components in inflammatory bowel disease. Gastroenterology 90:1415, 1986.
23. Shorter, R.G., Huizenga, K.A., ReMine, S.G. and Spencer, R.J.: Effects of preliminary incubation of lymphocytes with serum on their cytotoxicity for colonic epithelial cells. Gastroenterology 58:843-850 1970.
24. Broberger, O. and Perlmann, P.: In vitro studies of ulcerative colitis. I. Reactions of patient's serum with human fetal colon cells in tissue cultures. J. Exp. Med. 117:705-716, 1963.
25. Roche, J.K., Fiocchi, C., and Youngman, K.: Sensitization to epithelial antigens in chronic mucosal inflammatory disease. J. Clin. Invest. 75:522-530, 1985.
26. LeVeen, H.H., Falk, G. and Schatman, B.: Experimental ulcerative colitis produced by anticolon sera. Ann. Surg. 154:275-280, 1961.
27. Bicks, R.O. and Walker, R.H.: Immunologic colitis in dogs. Am. J. Dig. Dis. 7:574-584, 1962.
28. Stewart, T.H.M., Hetenyi, C., et al.: Ulcerative enterocolitis in dogs induced by drugs. J. Pathol. 131:363-378, 1980.
29. Bjarnason, I., Giuseppe, Z., Smith, T., et al.: Nonsteroidal antiinflammatory drug-induced intestinal inflammation in humans. Gastroenterology 93:480-489, 1987.
30. Kaufmann, H.J. and Taubin, H.L.: Non-steroidal antiinflammatory drugs activate quiescent inflammatory bowel disease. Ann. Int. Med. 107:513-516, 1987.
31. Bjarnason, I., Williams, P., Smethurst, P., et al.: Effect of non-steroidal anti-inflammatory drugs and prostaglandins on the permeability of the human small intestine. Gut 27:1292-1297, 1986.
32. Moeller, H.C. and Kirsner, J.B.: The effect of drug-induced hypermotility on the gastrointestinal tract of dogs. 26:303-310, 1954.
33. Leib, M.S., Hay, W.H. and Roth, L.: Plasmacytic-lymphocytic colitis in dogs. In, Current Vet Therapy X. WB Saunders, Philadelphia, 939-944, 1989.
34. Nelson, R.W., Stookey, L.J. and Kazacos, E.: Nutritional management of idiopathic chronic colitis in the dog. J. Vet. Int. Med. 2:133-137, 1988.
35. Dobesh, G.D. and Clemens, T.: Effect of dietary protein on porcine colonic microstructure and function. Am. J. Vet. Res. 48:862-865, 1987.
36. Finegold, S.M., Attebry, H.R. and Sutter, V.L.: Effect of diet on human fecal flora: comparison of Japanese and American diets. Am. J. Clin. Nutr. 27:1456-11469, 1974.
37. Bruns, P., Hood, L.F. and Seeley, H.W.: Effect of modified starch on the microflora of the small intestine and caecum of rats. Nutr. Rep. Intl. 15:131-138, 1977.
38. Dubos, R.: Man Adapting, Yale University Press, New Haven, 1965.
39. Smith, H.W.: Observations on the flora of the alimentary tract of animals and factors affecting its composition. J. Path. Bact. 89:95-122, 1965.
40. Onderdonk, A.B., Hermos, J.A., et al.: Protective effect of metronidazole in experimental ulcerative colitis. Gastroenterology 74:521-526, 1978.
41. Watt, J. and Marcus.: Experimental ulcerative disease of the colon in animals. Gut 14:506-510, 1973.
42. Kraft, S.C. and Kirsner, J.B.: Immunological apparatus of the gut and inflammatory bowel disease. Gastroenterology 60:922-951,1971.
43. Hayden, D.W. and Van Kruiningen, H.J.: Lymphocytic-plasmacytic enteritis in German Shepherd dogs. JAAHA 18:89-96, 1982.
44. Heyman, M.B.: Food sensitivity and eosinophilic gastroenteropathies. In, Gastrointestinal Disease. Pathophysiology, diagnosis, management. 4th edition. Edited by Sleisinger, M.H., Fordtran, J. S. W.B, Saunders, Philadelphia 1113-1134, 1989.
45. Graham, D.Y., Markesich, D.C. and Yoshimura, H.H.: Mycobacteria and inflammatory bowel disease. Results of culture. Gastroenterology 92:436, 1987.
46. Mee, A.S., McLaughlin, J.E., et al.: Chronic immune colitis in rabbits. Gut 20:1-5, 1979
47. Parent, K. and Mitchell, P.: Cell wall-defective variants of pseudomonas-like (Group Va) bacteria in Crohn's disease. Gastroenterology 75:368-372, 1978.
48. Van Kruiningen, H.J.: The ultrastructure of macrophages in granulomatous colitis of Boxer dogs. Vet. Pathol. 12:446-459, 1975.

49. Gomez, J.A. Russell, S.W., Trowbridge, J.W. and Lee, J.: Canine histiocytic ulcerative colitis: An ultrastructural study of the early mucosal lesion. Am. J. Dig. Dis. 22:485-496, 1977.
50. Gitnick, G.L., Rosen, V.J., Arthur, M.H. and Hertweck, S.A.: Evidence for the isolation of a new virus from ulcerative colitis patients. Dig. Dis. Sci. 24:609-619, 1979.
51. Miller, D.S. Keighley, A., Smith, P.G., Hughes, A.O. and Langman, M.J.S.: Acase-control method for seeking evidence of contagion in Crohn's disease. Gastroenterology 71:385-387, 1976.
52. Halpern, B., Zweibaum, R., et al.: Experimental immune ulcerative colitis. In, Immunopathology International Symposium, Basel-Stuttgart, Schwarbe and Co, 161-178, 1967.
53. Sartor, R.B., Schwab, J.H., Powell, et al.: Granulomatous enterocolitis induced by bacterial cell wall fragments. Gastroenterology (Abstr) 80:1271, 1981.
54. van der Waaij, and Cohen, B.J., and Anver, M.R.: Mitigation of experimental inflammatory bowel disease in guinea pigs by selective elimination of the aerobic gram-negative intestinal microflora. Gastroenterology 67:460-472, 1974.
55. Rolfe, R.D.: Interactions among microorganisms of the indigenous intestinal flora and their influence on the host. Rev of Infect Dis 6:S73-S79, 1984.
56. Chester, J.F., Ross, J.S., Malt, R.A., et al.: Acute colitis produced by chemotactic peptides in rats and mice. Am. J. Pathol. 121:284-290, 1985.
57. Hayden, D.W. and van Kruiningen, H.J.: Eosinophilic gastroenteritis in German Shepherd dogs and its relationshiop to visceral larva mirgrans. JAVMA 162:379-384, 1973.
58. Hall, E.J. and Batt, R.M.: Challenge studies deomonstrate gluten sensitivity of a naturally occurring enteropathy in Irish Setter dogs. Gastroenterology 94:A167, 1988.
59. Strober, W.: Animal models of inflammatory bowel disease-an overview. Dig. Dis. Sci. 30:3s-11s, 1985.
60. Ramage, J.K., Hunt, R.H. and Perdue, M.H.: Changes in intestinal permeability and epithelial differentiation during inflammation in the rat. Gut 29:57-61, 1988.
61. Madara, J.L.: Gamma-interferon (Gamma-IFN) enhances intestinal epithelial permeability by altering tight junctions. Gastroenterology 94:A276, 1988.
62. Lawson, T.L., Gomez, J.A., and Margulis, A.R.: Vascular alterations in canine histiocytic ulcerative colitis. Invest. Radiol 10:212-224, 1975.
63. Grisham, M.B. and Granger, D.N.: Neutrophil-mediated mucosal injury. Dig. Dis. Sci. 33:6S-15S, 1988.
64. Thayer, W.R.: Are the inflammatory bowel diseases immune complex diseases? Gastroenterology 70:136-137, 1976.
65. Whorwell, P.J. and Wright, R.: Immunological aspects of inflammatory bowel disease. Clinics in Gastroenterology 5:303-321, 1976.
66. Perdue, M.H., Forstner, J.F., Roomi, N.W. and Gall, D.G.: Epithelial response to intestinal anaphylaxis in rats: goblet cell secretion and enterocyte damage. Am. J. Physiol. 247:G632-G637, 1984.
67. Tizard, I.: Veterinary Immunology. W.B. Saunders, Philadelphia, 1987.
68. Ferguson, A.: Models of intestinal hypersensitivity. Clinics in Gastroenterology 5:271-288, 1976.
69. Rabin, B.S. and Rogers, S.J.: A cell-mediated immune model of inflammatory bowel disease in the rabbit. Gastroenterology 75:29-33, 1978.
70. Glick, M.E. and Falchuk, Z.M.: Dinitrochlorobenzene-induced colitis in guinea pigs. Gut 22:120-125, 1981.
71. MacPherson, B.R., Shearin, N.L. and Pfeiffer, C.J.: Experimental diffuse colitis in cats: observations on motor changes. J. Surg. Res. 25:42-49, 1978.
72. Rao, S.S.C., Read, N.W. and Holdsworth, C.D.: Is the diarrhea in ulcerative colitis related to impaired colonic salvage of carbohydrate? Gut 28:1090-1094, 1987.
73. Danzi, J.T.: Extraintestinal manifestations of idiopathic inflammatory bowel disease. Arch. Int. Med. 148:297-302, 1988.
74. Rabin, B.S. and Rogers, S.J.: Pathologic changes in the liver and kidney produced by immunization with intestinal antigens. Am. J. Pathol. 84:201-210, 1976.
75. Cello, J.P. and Schneiderman, D.J.: Ulcerative colitis. In, Gastrointestinal Disease: Pathophysiology, Diagnosis, Management. 4th edition. Edited by Sleisenger, M.H., Fordtran, J.S. W.B. Saunders, Philadelphia, 1435-1475, 1989.
76. Pedersen, N.C., Weisner, K., Castles, J.J., et al.: Noninfectious canine arthritis: The inflammatory non-erosive arthritides. JAVMA 169:304-310, 1976.
77. Tams, T.R.: Chronic feline inflammatory bowel disorders. Part I. Idiopathic inflammatory bowel disease. Comp. Contin. Ed. Pract. Vet. 8:371-376, 1986.
78. Hart, I.R.: The distribution of immunoglobulin-containing cells in canine small intestine. Res. Vet. Sci. 27:269-274, 1979.
79. Roth, L., Walton, A.M. and Leib, M.S.: Histologic grading of endoscopic biopsies from normal dogs and dogs with colitis. Proc. Am. Col. Vet. Pathol.: Specialty Group Program (Abst), 129, 1988.
80. Leib, M.S.: Gastrointestinal endoscopy: Endoscopic and histologic correlation. Proc 7th ACVIM Forum, 784-786, 1989.
81. Surawicz, C.M. and Belic, L.: Rectal biopsy helps to distinguish acute self-limited colitis from idiopathic inflammatory bowel disease. Gastroenterology 86:104-113, 1984.
82. Goldman, H.: Acute versus chronic colitis: How and when to distinguish by biopsy. Gastroenterology 86:199-201, 1984.
83. Bo-Linn, G.W., Vendrell, D.D., Lee, E. and Fordtran, J.S.: An evaluation of the significance of microscopic colitis in patients with chronic diarrhea. J. Clin. Invest. 75:1559-1569, 1985.
84. Payne-James, J.J. and Silk, D.B.A.: Total parenteral nutrition as primary treatment in Crohn's disease - RIP? Gut 29:1304-1308, 1988.
85. Jones, V.A.: Comparison of total parenteral nutrition and elemental diet in induction of remission of Crohn's disease. Dig. Dis. Sci. 32:100S-107S, 1987.
86. Whittaker, J.S.: Nutritional therapy of hospitalized patients with inflammatory bowel disease. Dig. Dis. Sci. 32:89S-94S, 1987.
87. Fuchs, G.J., Grand, R.J. and Motil, K.J.: Malnutrition and nutritional support in inflammatory bowel disease. Nutritional support services 5:28-33, 1985.
88. Rhodes, J. and Rose, J.: Does food affect acute inflammatory bowel disease? The role of parenteral nutrition, elemental and exclusion diets. Gut 27:471-474, 1986.
89. Washabau, R.J., Strombeck, D.R., Buffington, C.A. and Harrold, D.: Evaluation of intestinal carbohydrate malabsorption in the dog by pulmonary gas excretion. AJVR 47:1402-1406, 1986.
90. LeVeen, E.G., Falk, G., Ip, M., Mazzapica, N. and LeVeen, H.H.: Urease as a contributing factor in ulcerative lesions of the colon. Am. J. Surg. 135:53-56, 1978.
91. Cummings, J.H., Wiggins, H.S., Jenkins, D.J.A., Houston, H., Jivraj, T., Drasar, B.S. and Hill, M.J.: Influence of diets high and low in animal fat on bowel habit, gastrointestinal transit time, fecal microflora, bile acid, and fat excretion. J. Clin. Invest. 61:953-963, 1978.
92. Kaplan, H.P., Portnoy, G., Binder, H.J., Amatruda, T. and Spiro, H.: A controlled evaluation of intravenous adrenocorticotropic hormone and hydrocortisone in the treatment of acute colitis. Gastroenterology 69:91-95, 1975.
93. Binder, H.J. and Sandle, G.I.: Electrolyte absorption and secretion in the mammalian colon. In, Physiology of the Gastrointestinal Tract. 2nd edition. Edited by Johnson, L.R. Raven Press, New York, 1389-1418, 1987.
94. Johnson, L.R.: Regulation of gastrointestinal growth. In, Physiology of the Gastrointestinal Tract. 2nd edition. Edited by Johnson, L.R. Raven Press, New York, 301-333, 1987.
95. Tams, T.R.: Chronic feline inflammatory bowel disorders. Part II. Feline eosinophilic enteritis and lymphosarcoma. Comp. Contin. Ed. Pract. Vet. 8:464-471, 1986.
96. Meyer, J.H.: Ulcerative colitis. In, Gastrointestinal Disease.

Edited by M.H. Sleisinger and J.S. Fordtran, W.B. Saunders, Philadelphia, 1973, 1296-1349.

97. Truelove, S.C.: Treatment of ulcerative colitis with local hydrocortisone hemisuccinate sodium. A report on a controlled therapeutic trial. Brit. Med. J. 2:1072-1077, 1958.

98. Das, K.M. and Sternleib, I.: Salicylazosulfapyridine in inflammatory bowel disease. Am. J. Dig. Dis. 20:971-976, 1975.

99. Goldman, P. and Peppercorn, M.A.: Salicylazosulfapyridine in clinical practice. Gastroenterology 65:166-169, 1773.

100. Schroder, H., Lewkonia, R.M. and Price Evans, D.A.: Metabolism of salicylazosulfapyridine in healthy subjects and in patients with ulcerative colitis. Clin. Pharm. Ther. 14:802-809, 1973.

101. Ewing, G.O. and Gomez, J.A.: Canine ulcerative colitis. JAAHA 9:395-406, 1973.

102. Morgan, R.V. and Bachrach, A.: Keratoconjunctivitis sicca associated with sulfonamide therapy in dogs. JAVMA 180:432-434, 1982.

103. Barnett, KC.: Keratoconjunctivitis sicca and the treatment of canine colitis. Vet. Rec. 119: 363, 1986.

104. Schroeder, K.W., Tremaine, W.J. and Ilstrup, D.M.: Coated oral 5-aminosalicylic acid therapy for mildly to moderately active ulcerative colitis. New Eng. J. Med. 317:1625-1629, 1987.

105. Hawkey, C.J. and Hawthorne, A.B.: Medical treatment of ulcerative colitis: scoring the advances. Gut 29:1298-1303, 1988.

106. McPhee, M.S., Swan, J.T., Biddle, W.L. and Greenberger, N.J.: Proctocolitis unresponsive to conventional therapy. Response to 5-aminosalicylic acid enemas. Dig. Dis. Sci. 32:76S-81S, 1987.

107. Rosenberg, J.L., Wall, A.J., Levin, B., Binder, H.J. and Kirsner, J.B.: A controlled trial of azathioprine in the management of chronic ulcerative colitis. Gastroenterology 69:96-99, 1975.

108. Grove, D.I., et al.: Suppression of cell-mediated immunity by metronidazole. Int. Arch. Allergy Appl. Immunol. 54:422, 1977.

109. Miller, J.J.: The imidazoles as immunosuppressive agents. Transplant Proc. 12:300-303, 1980.

110. Kikuchi, T., Oikawa, T., Inoue, K., Sakai, M., Hara, N., Sunagawa, K. and Ichihashi, Y.: The effect of antibiotics against the intestinal bacterial flora. In, Germ-Free Research, Edited by J.B. Heneghan, Academic Press, New York, 355-359, 1973.

111. Chiapella, A.: Diagnosis and management of chronic colitis in the dog and cat. In, Current Veterinary Therapy IX. Edited by Kirk, R.W. W.B. Saunders, Philadelphia, 896-903, 1986.

112. Van Kruiningen, H.J.: Clinical efficacy of Tylosin in canine inflammatory bowel disease. JAAHA 12:498-501, 1976.

113. De Novo, R.C.: Therapeutics of gastrointestinal diseases. In, Current Veterinary Therapy. Edited by Kirk, R.W. WB Saunders, Philadelphia, 862-872, 1986.

114. Gue, M., Fioramonti, J. and Bueno, L.: A simple double radiolabeled technique to evaluate gastric emptying of canned food meal from dogs. Gastroenterol Clin. Biol. 12:425-430, 1988.

115. Christensen, J.: Motility of the colon In, Physiology of the Gastrointestinal Tract. 2nd edition edited by Johnson, L.R. Raven Press, New York, 665-693, 1987.

116. Tams, T.R.: Canine lymphocytic plasmacytic enteritis. Comp. Cont. Ed. 9:1184-1192, 1987.

117. Magne, M.L.: Canine lymphocytic-plasmacytic enteritis. In, Current Veterinary Therapy X. WB Saunders Co., Philadelphia, 922-926, 1989.

118. Jacobs, G., Lappin, M. and Collins, L.: Lymphocytic-plasmacytic enteritis in 17 dogs. Proc ACVIM 745, 1988.

119. Magne, M.L.: Lymphocytic-plasmacytic enteritis. Pathogenesis. ACVIM proceedings 521-523, 1988.

120. Edwards, D.F. and Russell, R.G.: Probable vitamin K-deficient bleeding in two cats with malabsorption syndrome secondary to lymphocytic-plasmacytic enteritis. J. Vet. Int. Med. 1:97-101, 1987.

121. Barker, I.K., Van Dreumel, A.A.: The Alimentary system. In, Pathology of Domestic Animals. Edited by Jubb, K.V.F., Kennedy, P.C., Palmer, N. Academic Press, Inc., Orlando. 1-202, 1985.

122. Batt, R.M., Bush, B.M. and Peters, T.J.: Subcellular biochemical studies of a naturally occurring enteropathy in the dog resembling chronic tropical sprue in human beings. AJVR 44:1492-1496, 1983.

123. Magne, M.L.: Unpublished observations.

124. Hottendorf, G.H. and Hirth, P.S.: Lesions of spontaneous subclinical disease in Beagle dogs. Vet. Pathol. 11:240-258,1974.

125. Sarin, S.K., Malhotra, V., Sen Gupta, S., et al.: Significance of eosinophil and mast cell counts in rectal mucosa in ulcerative colitis. A prospective controlled study. Dig. Dis. Sci. 32:363-367, 1987.

126. Bush BM. Colitis in the dog. Vet. Annual. 25: 337-347, 1985.

127. Pidgeon, G.L.: Chronic disorders of the exocrine pancreas, small bowel and large bowel. Vet. Clin. N. Am. 13:541-550, 1983.

128. Moore, R.P.: Feline eosinophilic enteritis. In, Current Veterinary Therapy VIII. Edited by Kirk, R.W. WB Saunders, Philadelphia. 791-793, 1983.

129. Hendricks, M.: A spectrum of hypereosinophilic syndromes exemplified by six cats with eosinophilic enteritis. Vet. Pathol. 18:188-200, 1981.

130. Van der Gaag, I., Happe, R.P. and Wolvekamp, W.T.C.: Eosinophilic gastroenteritis complicated by partial ruptures and a perforation of the small intestine in a dog. J. Sm. An. Pract. 24:575-581, 1983.

131. Quigley, P.J. and Henry, K.: Eosinophilic enteritis in the dog: A case report with a brief review of the literature. J. Comp. Path. 91:387-392, 1981.

132. Alliah-Davis, R. and Batdorf, K.: Eosinophilic granuloma complex in a dog. Mod. Vet. Pract. 66:756, 1985.

133. Van der Gaag, I.: Histiocytic ulcerative colitis in a French bull dog. J. Sm. An. Pract. 19:283-290, 1978.

134. Van Kruiningen, H.J. and Dobbins, W.O.: Feline histiocytic colitis. A case report with electron microscopy. Vet. Pathol. 16:215-222, 1979.

135. Russell, S.W., Gomez, J.A. and Trowbridge, J.O.: Canine histiocytic ulcerative colitis. The early lesion and its progression to ulceration. Lab. Invest. 25:509-515, 1971.

136. Kennedy, P.C. and Cello, R.M.: Colitis of Boxer dogs. Gastroenterology 51:926-931, 1966.

137. Van Kruiningen, H.J.: Granulomatous colitis of Boxer dogs: comparative aspects. Gastroenterology 53:114-122, 1967.

138. DiBartola, S.P., Rogers, W.A., Boyce, J.T. and Grimm, J.P.: Regional enteritis in two dogs. JAVMA 181:904-908, 1982.

139. Van der Gaag, I. and van der Linde-Sipman, J.S.: Eosinophilic granulomatous colitis with ulceration in a dog. J. Comp. Path. 97:179-185, 1987.

140. Fletcher, W.D.: Advanced grannlomatons colitis in a Siberian Husky VM/SAC 73:1409, 1978.

141. Collins, J.E., Libal, M.C. and Brost, D.: Proliferative enteritis in two pups. JAVMA 183:886-889, 1983.

142. Leib, M.S., Sponenberg, D.P., Wilcke, J.R., et al.: Suppurative colitis in a cat. JAVMA 188:739-741, 1986.

143. MacLachlan, N.J., Breitschwerdt, E.B., Chambers, J.M., et al.: Gastroenteritis of Basenji Dogs. Vet. Pathol. 25:36-41, 1988.

144. Breitschwerdt, E.B., Halliwell, W.H., Foley, C.W., et al.: A hereditary diarrhetic syndrome in the Basenji characterized by malabsorption, protein losing enteropathy and hypergammaglobulinemia. JAAHA 16:551-560, 1980.

145. Breitschwerdt, E.B., Waltman, C., Hagstad, H.V., et al.: Clinical and epidemiologic characterization of a diarrheal syndrome in Basenji dogs. JAVMA 180:914-920, 1982.

146. Breitschwerdt, E.B., Barta, O., Waltman, C., et al.: Serum proteins in healthy Basenjis and Basenjis with chronic diarrhea. AJVR 44:326-328, 1983.

147. Flesja, K. and Yri, T.: Protein-losing enteropathy in the Lundenhund. J. Sm. An. Pract. 18:11-23, 1977.

Chapter 22

Intestinal Obstruction, Pseudo-Obstruction, and Foreign Bodies

Intestinal obstruction is a familiar presentation to most practitioners. Obstruction can occur in any part of the intestinal tract but most often develops in the small intestine as a result of its narrower luminal diameter. Obstruction can be partial or complete, and in some cases partial obstructions progress to become complete. Intestinal obstruction can be difficult to diagnose, particularly if the obstruction is partial.

CAUSES OF INTESTINAL OBSTRUCTION

Introduction

Intestinal obstruction (ileus) can result from a large number of causes (Table 22-1). Anatomic intestinal obstruction (mechanical ileus) can result from intraluminal foreign objects, intramural masses such as leiomyomas, or extramural compression which can result from abdominal adhesions or entrapment. Functional intestinal obstruction can result from transient hypomotility (paralytic or adynamic ileus) or from persistent intestinal neuromuscular derangements that cause hypomotility (pseudo-obstruction) or spasticity (spastic or hyperdynamic ileus).

Linear Foreign Bodies[1-3]

Most linear foreign bodies, such as pieces of string, cord, or fabrics, pass through the gastrointestinal tract with few clinical signs. They can become fixed at some point, however, and eventually result in intestinal obstruction and perforation. The two most frequent points at which linear foreign bodies will become fixed are the oral cavity and the pylorus. In the oral cavity, the string most commonly loops around the base of the tongue as it is swallowed. The free end is then propelled through the esophagus, stomach and into the small intestine. Linear foreign bodies become fixed at the pylorus if the material bunches up in the stomach. Eventually one free end of the bunched material is propelled through the pylorus. After the linear foreign body reaches its full length in the intestine, peristaltic activity causes the intestine to become pleated by moving proximally around the object. Normally, peristalsis moves intraluminal objects caudally while the intestine remains relatively fixed. Linear foreign bodies are fixed, however, and continual peristalsis causes the gut and luminal contents to move, as normally expected, in opposite directions. Thus, the intestine moves proximally over the fixed string, with the

Table 22-1. Causes of Intestinal Obstruction

ANATOMIC OBSTRUCTION

Intraluminal obstruction
- Linear foreign bodies
- Non-linear foreign bodies

Intramural masses
- Neoplasia (adenocarcinoma, leiomyoma, leiomyosarcoma)
- Inflammatory bowel disease (eosinophilic granuloma, transmural granulomatous enteritis)
- Phycomycosis
- Strictures
- Hematoma[37]

Congenital lesions
- Atresia

Extramural compression
- Adhesions
- Hernias
- Strangulation
- Intussusception
- Volvulus

FUNCTIONAL OBSTRUCTION

Adynamic ileus
- Surgical operations
- Peritonitis
- Unrelieved mechanical obstruction
- Intestinal ischemia
- Gram-negative sepsis
- Electrolyte imbalance (hypokalemia)
- Uremia
- Dysautonomia
- Spinal cord injury
- Anticholinergics
- Lead poisoning

Spastic ileus
- Hirschsprung's disease

Pseudo-obstruction
- Lymphosarcoma
- Idiopathic sclerosing enteropathy
- SLE
- Amanita mushroom poisoning
- Phenothiazines
- Diabetes mellitus
- Others

intestine becoming pleated or bunched up in folds around the string. The string is under tension, seeking to establish a straight line. The intestine is constrained by the mesentery to form circular loops, however, and the extended linear foreign object applies tension on the intestine at regular points in the curved loops. Eventually the pressure of the cord or string perforates the intestine in multiple places and causes peritonitis.

Linear foreign bodies are more common in cats than dogs. Physical examination is more important than radiology in identifying linear foreign bodies. The oral cavity is thoroughly examined for strings fixed around the base of the tongue with the animal under anesthesia if necessary. On palpation of the abdomen accordion-pleated loops of intestine are readily identified.

Non-linear Foreign Bodies

A wide variety of foreign bodies can be ingested by the dog and, to a lesser extent, the cat. Foreign bodies that commonly lodge in the intestine include bones, corn cobs, stones, fruit stones, tampons, fabrics, food wrappings, chew toys, children's toys, bottle caps, plant material, hair, fishhooks, and sewing needles. Foreign bodies can lodge at any point throughout the gastrointestinal tract, but common sites are the esophagus, the pylorus, and the ileocolic junction. The consequences of foreign body ingestion depend on the size of the object, its chemical composition, and whether it has sharp points (Table 22-2). Small foreign bodies with smooth surfaces such as stones will often pass uneventfully. Large foreign bodies may wedge in the bowel lumen, where they mechanically obstruct the gastrointestinal tract and eventually lead to pressure necrosis of the intestinal wall. Many sharp foreign bodies will pass uneventfully, possibly as a result of the mural withdrawal reflex which consists of local intestinal dilation in response to mucosal contact with a sharp object.[4] Not uncommonly, however, sharp foreign bodies may penetrate the intestinal tract, where they can lead to peritonitis and a functional intestinal obstruction through adynamic ileus. Toothpicks are seemingly innocuous foreign bodies that are an important cause of intestinal perforation in humans.

Table 22-2. Consequences of Gastrointestinal Foreign Bodies

Passage without complication	
	Small diameter, smooth, foreign bodies
Mechanical obstruction	
	Linear foreign bodies
	Non-linear foreign bodies
Functional obstruction through peritonitis	
	Penetrating foreign bodies
Peritonitis	
	Penetrating foreign bodies
Mural necrosis	
	Impacted foreign bodies
Laceration of adjacent organs	
	Penetrating foreign bodies
Esophageal stricture	
	Impacted foreign bodies
	Caustic foreign bodies
Toxicity	
	Lead foreign bodies
	Zinc foreign bodies

The chemical composition of the foreign body determines its digestibility and the likelihood of the release of toxic products. Lead objects in the gastrointestinal tract rapidly solubilize under the influence of gastric acid.[5] Absorption of lead is fast, particularly in young animals. The ensuing clinical signs include abdominal pain, vomiting, bizarre behavior, and seizures. The clinical signs of lead toxicity are accompanied by characteristic hematologic changes, including a neutrophilic leukocytosis, moderate anemia, and large numbers of nucleated and basophilic stippled red blood cells. Surgical intervention to remove lead foreign bodies should be undertaken rapidly and must be accompanied by suitable medical therapy such as calcium EDTA (20 mg/kg q 8hr IV or SQ for 4-5 days). Zinc objects in the intestinal tract can result in vomiting, diarrhea, and life-threatening hemolytic crises.[6] The most common sources of zinc are newly minted pennies and hardware such as nuts from zinc cages.

Intussusception

Intussusception is a unique type of obstructive lesion that is produced by the invagination and telescoping of one segment of the intestine into an adjacent loop.[7,8] Single intussusceptions are most common, but occasionally multiple intussusceptions or compounded intussusceptions occur. The latter results when an entire intussusception undergoes a second invagination. Gastroesophageal, pylorogastric, enteroenteric, enterocolic, and colocolic intussusceptions have been reported in small animals.[8] Intussusceptions most commonly occur at the ileocolic junction.[7,9] Eighty percent of intussusceptions arise in animals younger than one year of age.[7] They occur as a sequelae to a number of conditions, including intestinal parasitism, linear foreign bodies, parvovirus, intestinal neoplasia, and prior abdominal surgery.[8] Many intussusceptions in young animals are idiopathic. An association between idiopathic intussusception and recent dietary change has been observed.[9]

The pathophysiologic events that result in intussusception remain to be elucidated, but an important feature would appear to be the failure of coordinated motor activity in the affected segments. This can result from diseases that produce discontinuous segmental intestinal flaccidity or induration.[8] Another proposed cause is mechanical linkage of non-adjacent segments that result in a kink in the bowel. Such mechanical linkage can occur with linear foreign bodies or fibrous adhesions.[8] Peristaltic activity continues the invagination once it has begun. Mesenteric tension limits the length of the invagination. The consequences of the intussusception are intestinal obstruction and ischemia. The lymphatic and venous drainages are obstructed early in the process, resulting in vascular engorgement, intramural edema and hemorrhage, and loss of plasma and blood into the lumen of the gastrointestinal tract. Exudation of fibrin can, within a short time, render the intussusception irreducible. Mural necrosis may eventually result, but perforation is rare because the ensheathing intestinal segments usually retain their viability.[8]

Adynamic Ileus

Adynamic ileus is defined as intestinal obstruction resulting from inhibition of bowel motility. The lack of peristaltic activity results in a functional obstruction because intestinal content pools in the dependent areas of the gastrointestinal tract instead of being propelled in an aborad direction. A further description of ileus is found in the chapter on functional bowel disorders.

Pseudo-Obstruction Syndrome

Pseudo-obstruction is a poorly defined term used to describe patients that develop clinical and radiographic evidence of mechanical intestinal obstruction but that have no evidence of mechanical blockage at subsequent exploratory surgery.[10] The terms pseudo-obstruction and adynamic ileus overlap somewhat, but pseudo-obstruction has a more chronic duration and often a more segmental appearance than does adynamic ileus. Adynamic ileus, not pseudo-obstruction syndrome, is the most common reason for negative exploratory celiotomy results in dogs and cats with suspected intestinal obstructions.

The primary pathophysiologic process in pseudo-obstruction is distention of a loop or loops of bowel because the smooth muscle of the intestinal muscularis is incapable of normal contraction and even incapable of maintaining tone.[10] The intestinal hypomotility can be caused by intrinsic disease of the smooth muscle, infiltration of the muscle by some abnormal material (amyloid, fibrous tissue), or by impaired neurohormonal regulation of intestinal muscle motility (neuropathic, idiopathic).[11] The sites of intestinal motility dysfunction may be single or multiple, and it can occur in the small or large bowel. Pseudo-obstruction in humans can develop secondary to a variety of systemic diseases such as SLE, diabetes mellitus, hypoparathyroidism, pheochromocytoma, familial dysautonomia, amanita mushroom poisoning, and phenothiazine administration.[11]

Intestinal "pseudo-obstruction" is rarely recognized in the dog or cat.[12-14] Idiopathic sclerosing enteropathy is the most commonly reported cause.[13,14] At the UCD VMTH, we have observed the occasional dog with pseudo-obstruction syndrome in which no abnormality could be demonstrated by routine histology at the site of the intestinal obstruction. We have also recognized the syndrome in a cat with intestinal lymphoma. The lymphoma was diffuse and not grossly visible at surgery, but it was presumably associated with disordered intestinal motility. Treatment of pseudo-obstruction is, where possible, directed at the primary cause. Additional therapy includes prokinetic agents such as metoclopramide.

PATHOPHYSIOLOGY OF INTESTINAL OBSTRUCTION

Intestinal obstruction results in life-threatening complications such as dehydration, hypovolemia, electrolyte imbalances, and toxemia (Figure 22-1).

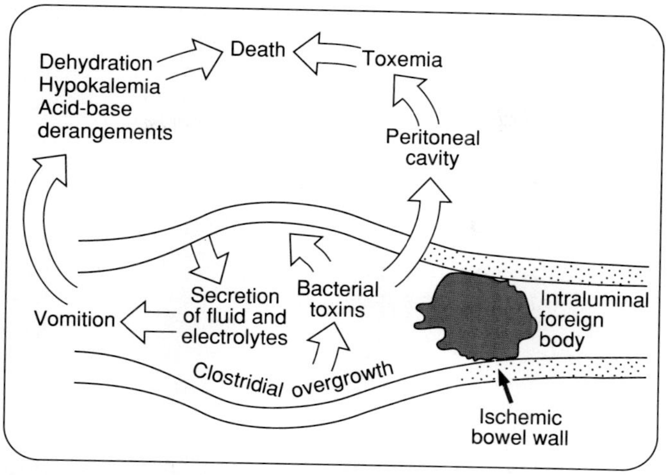

Figure 22-1. The pathophysiology of intestinal obstruction. Bacterial toxins induce intestinal secretion of fluid and electrolytes that is ultimately lost through vomition. Bacterial toxins absorbed through ischemic bowel wall produce toxemia.

Fluid and Electrolyte Homeostasis

Fluid and electrolyte imbalances are caused primarily by losses of fluid through vomiting. Some losses result from the movement of extracellular fluid into the intestine. In the early stages of obstruction, however, vomiting need not be a consistent finding. In an experimental study in which the intestine of dogs was completely obstructed at a cranial site and the dogs then allowed to drink water *ad libitum*, only 10% of dogs vomited over a period of four days, and the amounts of vomitus were small.[15,16] During the first few days after experimental obstruction, fluid does not accumulate in the intestine proximal to the site of obstruction. Thereafter, vomiting becomes more frequent, as fluid is eventually secreted at a rate that causes it to accumulate.

Intestinal mucosa immediately cranial to the obstruction secretes instead of absorbing fluid. The stimulus for the secretion is unknown. The fluid accumulating in obstructed loops may generate enough hydrostatic pressure to cause vascular stasis and mucosal ischemia, with secretion of extracellular fluid following the degenerative changes. However, fluid accumulated with obstruction never generates pressures greater than 5 mm Hg, and there is no morphological evidence of severe mucosal damage. Mucosal changes above the obstruction are limited to blunted thickened villi and shortened crypts. Below the obstruction, villus atrophy is seen. Moreover, it has been demonstrated that the intestinal mucosa above an obstruction maintains its ability to absorb electrolytes, glucose, and amino acids at normal rates.[17] The only change is an increase in the flux of ions and water from the extracellular fluid into the intestine, suggesting the presence of a secretagogue. Compatible with these observations is the proposal that enterotoxins, secreted by the large numbers of bacteria that accumulate in the obstructed loop, activate cyclic AMP-driven intestinal secretion. This suggestion is supported by recent findings, which show that intestinal obstruction in germ-free dogs does not result in secretion of fluid.[18]

The fluid lost contains potassium at higher concentrations than those in the extracellular fluid. Hence, hypokalemia is likely, and depletion of total-body potassium is a consistent feature of intestinal obstruction. Potassium losses contribute to general muscle weakness and to a loss of normal intestinal motility. Since vomition is the most important means of fluid loss, the obstructed animal may also become alkalotic.

If the intestine is strangulated, blood loss can become a

Table 22-3. Clinical Signs of Intestinal Obstruction at Different Sites in the Gastrointestinal Tract

High small bowel	Low small bowel/high large bowel	Low large bowel
Acute onset	Subacute onset	Subacute - chronic
Frequent vomiting	Vomiting less frequent	Vomiting infrequent
Fulminant progression	Insidious	Insidious
Large volume vomitus	Smaller volume of vomitus	May be scant volume
May be feculent odor	Often feculent odor	Rarely feculent
Minimal abd. distension	Often abd. distension	Often abd. distension
No constipation	No constipation	Often constipation
No tenesmus	No tenesmus	Tenesmus
Diarrhea	Diarrhea	Diarrhea

significant problem. Blood is lost into the lumen of the intestine, the wall of the bowel and eventually the peritoneal cavity.[19] The quantity of blood lost will depend on the length of the intestinal segment incarcerated, and whether there is arterial, venous, or combined involvement, with blood loss being greater with only venous obstruction.[19] Strangulation is caused by volvulus of the small or large intestine.[20,21]

Bacterial Flora and Toxins

The numbers of intraluminal bacteria increase in obstructed intestinal segments as a result of mechanical obstruction to flow and/or loss of the migratory myoelectric complex. The migratory myoelectric complex functions to sweep small intestinal contents in the aboral direction, maintaining bacteria at low numbers.[22,23] The number of bacteria in the obstructed loops may approach that usually seen in the large bowel. The composition of the microflora changes toward that found in the feces or mouth.[24,25]

Overgrowth of bacteria and subsequent endotoxic shock is the most important cause of mortality with intestinal obstruction.[26] Experiments in which the small intestine is strangulated in conventional and germ-free animals demonstrate the importance of intestinal bacteria. In conventional animals, strangulation of the intestine with the development of ischemia results in death, usually within 24 hours. Germ-free animals, in contrast, usually survive at least 23 weeks after intestinal strangulation. The survival of germ-free animals is due entirely to the absence of bacteria in the gastrointestinal tract. Instillation of effective antibiotics in loops of strangulated intestine in conventional animals converts a fatal problem to a nonfatal one if fluid and electrolyte balances are maintained.

Clostridia are the most important bacteria contributing to the death of obstructed animals. Compared with other members of its genus, *Clostridium perfringens* is a very lethal organism in strangulated loops of intestine.[27] It is numerically one of the most important microorganisms in the microflora of the dog, and its numbers increase further with bacterial overgrowth. *Clostridium septicum* and *Cl. histolyticum* are also quite deadly, whereas other species are non-pathogenic. Clostridial species produce toxins that, if absorbed, kill the animal. Some of the lethal factors can cross a histologically normal mucosa, but any breaks in the mucosal barrier allow more rapid absorption. The sites of many foreign-body obstructions are ischemic and become necrotic and ulcerated, conditions that allow bacterial toxins to be readily absorbed. Abdominal surgery results in further loss of the barrier to toxin absorption.[28] The toxic products pass from the intestine into the peritoneal cavity from whence absorption into the systemic circulation is very rapid.[19] Fluid collected from an obstructed intestine is rapidly lethal when injected into normal animals. Peritoneal fluid collected during strangulation obstruction of the intestine is also lethal when injected into normal animals.

CLINICAL FINDINGS ASSOCIATED WITH INTESTINAL OBSTRUCTION

The history will reveal the likelihood of the ingestion of a foreign body. Young animals, animals living in an unknown environment, and those with a persistent ravenous appetite are most likely to swallow foreign bodies. One consistent feature of the history is that the clinical signs persist despite medical treatment.

The clinical signs of intestinal obstruction vary with the site of the lesion (Table 22-3), the degree of luminal obstruction, and the severity of the vascular compromise. In general, the higher the obstruction and the more complete the luminal narrowing, the more acute and severe the clinical signs and the more rapid the progression to life-threatening physiologic derangements.

Vomiting is a consistent sign in all but the early phases of intestinal obstruction. Early in the obstructive process the vomiting is thought to be reflexive. As a result it is intermittent, and the volume of the vomitus may be scant. In time the vomiting becomes more regular. With obstruction of the duodenum and proximal jejunum, vomiting is very frequent and occurs soon after eating, whereas with obstruction of the ileum vomiting is less frequent and occurs longer (up to hours) after eating. Proximal intestinal obstruction results in the vomiting of the large volumes of fluid that enter the intestine from the upper gastrointestinal tract. Distal obstructions, in contrast, result in the loss of lesser volumes of fluid because of the greater intestinal area available for absorption of secreted fluid. Complete intestinal obstruction usually produces persistent vomiting of copious volumes of fluid even in anorectic animals. Partial obstruction usually causes intermittent vomiting. Vomiting frequency increases with the progression of obstruction. Some animals continue to eat and pass normal bowel movements with almost no vomiting at a time when obstruction of the intestine is nearly complete. The vomitus from animals with intestinal obstruction may have a fecal odor due to overgrowth of fecal-type bacteria. The vomiting pattern that should most raise the suspicion of intestinal obstruction is the vomiting of copious amounts of feculent fluid by a depressed and anorectic animal. It is important to reemphasize, however, that intestinal obstruction can result in a wide variety of vomiting patterns, none of which are pathognomonic for the disease.

Diarrhea is common in animals with partial obstruction of the large or small bowel. Following obstruction of the large bowel by impaction or stricture, the animal becomes constipated, but liquid feces usually pass around the impaction or though the stricture. The diarrhea develops from a combination of derangements brought on by the obstruction, including morphological and functional mucosal changes. With partial obstruction of the small bowel, diarrhea usually results from bacterial overgrowth. Intussusception often results in bloody diarrhea. Intussusception usually does not cause complete obstruction, and some animals with chronic intussusception will continue to eat and pass regular bowel movements. Complete obstructions are less frequently associated with diarrhea. On occasion intestinal obstruction is associated with a dry and tacky rectal mucosa, presumably as a result of hypovolemia and incipient shock.

Additional consistent clinical signs with intestinal obstruction are partial to complete anorexia, weakness, and depression. These signs often persist when fluid abnormalities are corrected, probably because of persistent absorption of toxins from the obstructed intestinal loops. Abdominal pain may be apparent. In humans, abdominal pain from an intestinal obstruction is said to be initially episodic as a result of distension of the bowel and peristaltic efforts at moving the foreign body.[19] Early acute obstruction results in increased intestinal motility cranial to the obstruction and reduced motility caudal to the obstruction. The changes are due to stimulation of cholinergic nerves and the toxic effects of luminal contents.[29,30] Thereafter, the pain becomes more continuous and dull, a reflection of the onset of adynamic ileus or peritonitis.

Daily patient reevaluation, especially physical examination, is important when signs that are consistent with intestinal obstruction persist. Subsequent examination may reveal an obstruction initially overlooked. Furthermore, intestinal obstructions can develop after the initial examination. For instance, a foreign body may move from the stomach into the intestine where it can be palpated. Particularly in young dogs, intussusception can develop subsequent to enteritis.

Physical examination is the most important procedure in identifying intestinal obstruction. Dehydration is a consistent finding, with the degree paralleling the frequency of vomiting. Diarrhea is usually not severe enough to contribute to dehydration. The oral cavity must be examined for linear foreign bodies. Thorough palpation of the abdomen is possible in most animals with intestinal obstruction. Sometimes, examination of the abdomen is assisted by raising the forequarters of the animal or by placing the patient under tranquilization or anesthesia.

Obstructing mass lesions of the intestine must be differentiated from normal or abnormal intestinal or extraintestinal structures. Particular care must be taken not to confuse kidneys, fecal material, or the ileocecal area with an obstructing lesion. Palpation of obstructing lesions usually causes the animal more discomfort than the palpation of normal structures. Furthermore, concurrent accumulations of excessive intestinal gas and fluid are often palpable. Intestinal intussusceptions palpate as firm, tubular masses.

Auscultation of the abdomen can contribute information on intestinal motility. Excessive noise is sometimes heard early in the obstructive process, possibly as a result of peristaltic rushes. Peristaltic rushes are thought to represent an attempt by the intestine to force content past the point of obstruction. The noise results from frequent peristaltic movements that propel fluid and gas rapidly through flaccid loops of intestine. These types of movement require the disappearance of segmentation motility. A silent abdomen identifies a loss of motility (adynamic ileus) and is suggestive of protracted obstruction or peritonitis.

Rectal examination is mandatory in evaluating all signs of gastrointestinal disease. Rectal impactions or strictures may be palpable.

LABORATORY FINDINGS ASSOCIATED WITH INTESTINAL OBSTRUCTION

Hemograms usually show nonspecific changes such as a stress response. A degenerative left shift is occasionally seen in severely affected animals, particularly following intestinal perforation.

Serum chemistry, electrolyte, and blood gas estimations are an invaluable aid to the selection of the appropriate fluid therapy for the patient. The laboratory findings with intestinal obstruction are variable and primarily reflect the severity of the fluid and electrolyte imbalances. Hypokalemia, acidosis or alkalosis, hyponatremia or hypernatremia may be seen. Pyloroduodenal obstructions often result in alkalosis and at times paradoxical aciduria. The PCV and total protein concentration may be elevated. The serum chemistry panel helps rule out renal, hepatic, and metabolic diseases, all of which are more common causes of the clinical signs that are seen with obstruction. Measurement of plasma electrolytes aids in identifying adrenocortical insufficiency. A normal serum lipase helps rule out acute pancreatitis, a disease with clinical signs that resemble those of intestinal obstruction. Provided it is carefully interpreted, the urinalysis provides valuable information on renal and liver function as well as hydration status. Fecal examinations are required to identify the predisposing cause for obstruction (i.e., intussusception) or the cause for acute signs resembling those of obstruction (i.e., Salmon poisoning).

RADIOGRAPHIC FINDINGS WITH INTESTINAL OBSTRUCTION

Radiographic procedures are an important aid in identifying intestinal obstruction, although radiology is not a substitute for a well conducted examination of the patient's abdomen.[31,32] When radiographs are the only means used to identify intestinal obstruction, some cases will present artifacts that, interpreted as signifying an obstruction, will be used to justify surgical exploration.

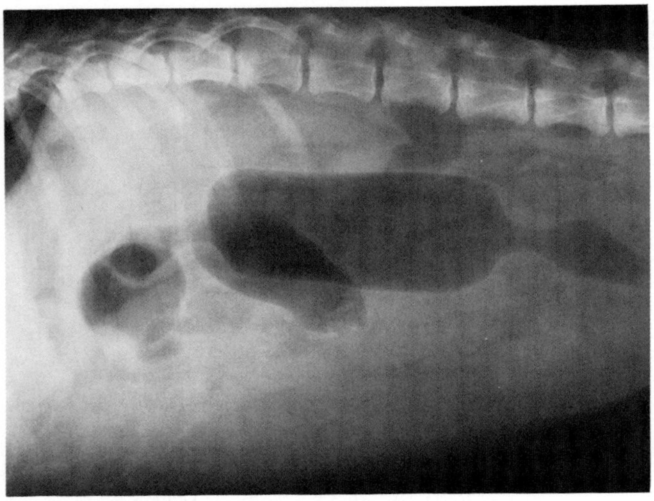

Figure 22-2. Lateral radiograph of abdomen of dog presented with clinical signs of intestinal obstruction. The loops of bowel are distended with fluid and gas. Diagnosis was made of intestinal obstruction, which turned out to be due to an intussusception in the caudal small intestine. Homogenous pattern of abdomen is due to accumulation of abdominal fluid.

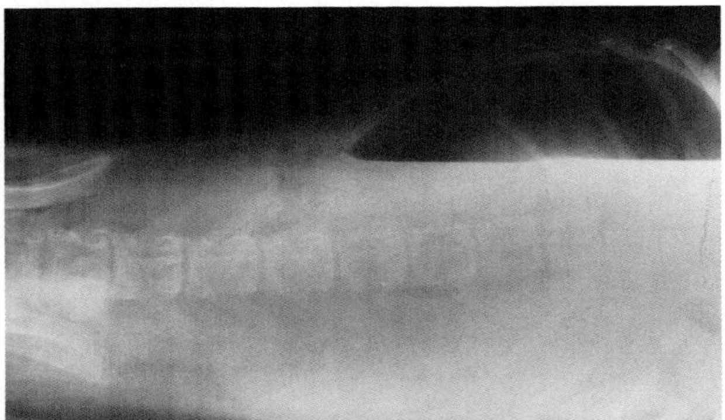

Figure 22-3. Lateral radiograph of same dog as in Figure 2. Radiograph was taken with a horizontal beam and shows gas-capped fluid level. Gas accumulation at only one horizontal plane is evidence for bowel stasis.

Survey Films

Initial radiographic evaluation of intestinal obstruction involves the use of survey radiographs. Obstructed loops of small intestines usually accumulate fluid or gas and consequently appear distended (Figure 22-2). The volume of gas formed usually exceeds the amount that can dissolve in the accumulated fluid, with the excess appearing as free gas. Thus, a large amount of gas trapped in loops of small intestine suggests obstruction. Radiographs taken with a horizontal beam show separation of the fluid and gas (Figure 22-3). Gas-capped fluid, a typical sign of intestinal obstruction, can be seen at different horizontal planes. Fluid at different levels indicates that motility can still move fluid through the intestine (Fig 22-4). With adynamic ileus loss of motility is complete, and gas-

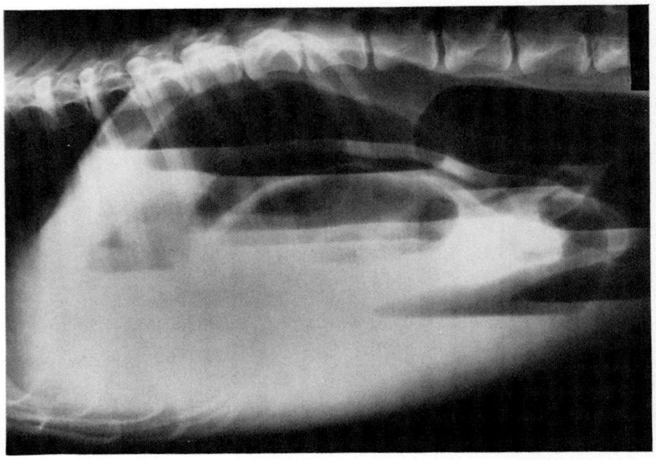

Figure 22-4. Lateral radiograph of a one-year-old German Shepherd with clinical signs of intestinal obstruction. Radiograph was taken with a horizontal beam. Multiple gas-capped fluid levels are seen in different horizontal planes. This suggests that motility is present in the intestine and is able to move the gas and fluid from one segment to another. The homogenous appearance of the abdomen suggests that either peritonitis or peritoneal fluid is present.

capped fluid levels are in the same horizontal plane throughout the obstructed intestine since there is no resistance to the fluid's seeking a common level under the force of gravity. Adynamic ileus must be differentiated from mechanical obstruction, since ileus is managed medically whereas mechanical obstruction requires surgical intervention. The level of the obstruction determines the number of gas-capped loops of intestine. A greater number indicates obstruction in a more caudal part. If the obstruction is complete and has been present longer than several hours, there will be little if any gas in the large intestine. Some obstructing lesions need not cause gas retention in the small bowel (Figure 22-5). The absence of accumulated gas makes the diagnosis of obstruction by survey radiography more difficult, but careful examination of the film may reveal fluid distended loops. If difficulty is experienced in determining whether a large diameter loop of bowel is abnormally dilated small intestine or normal large intestine, an air enema should be performed.

Radiopaque foreign bodies are readily demonstrated with plain films. Deciding whether they are causing obstruction is based on clinical and radiographic findings. Intraluminal air-fluid levels indicate that a foreign body is causing obstruction, as shown in Figure 22-4.

Positive-Contrast Studies

Contrast studies of the upper gastrointestinal tract are often necessary to identify intestinal obstruction. Obstruction of the small intestine delays gastric emptying and the transit of contrast medium through the small intestine. The delay is greatest with a more complete intestinal obstruction. Intestinal obstruction causes fluid accumulation cranial to the lesion, dilating the segment of intestine and diluting the contrast entering the fluid. Both of these changes are apparent on radiographs. Radiolucent

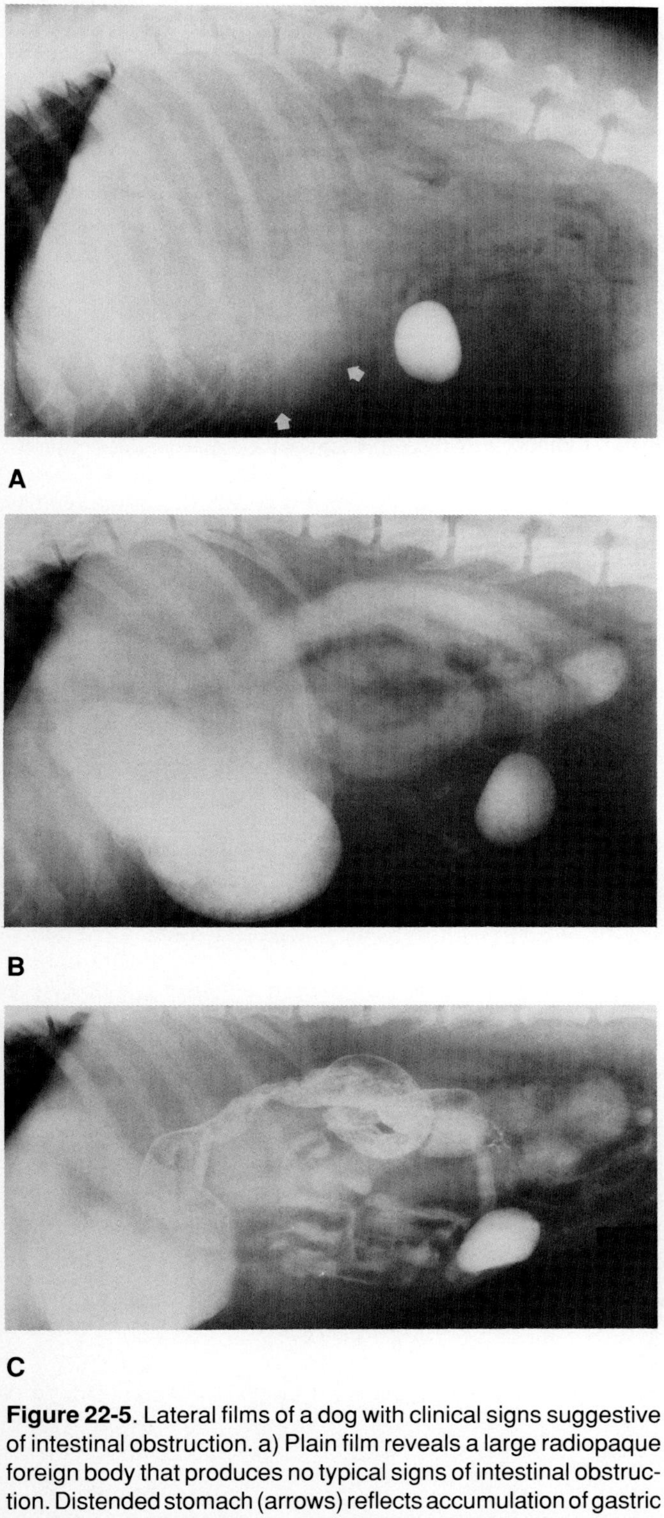

A

B

C

Figure 22-5. Lateral films of a dog with clinical signs suggestive of intestinal obstruction. a) Plain film reveals a large radiopaque foreign body that produces no typical signs of intestinal obstruction. Distended stomach (arrows) reflects accumulation of gastric and refluxed intestinal secretions of fluid. b) Lateral film taken 2 hours after administration of positive contrast medium. Shows dilated loops of jejunum and duodenum proximal to site of obstruction; very little contrast medium has passed this point. c) Lateral film taken at 24 hours shows that obstruction was not complete. The dog had been eating some and passing bowel movements. Obstruction was caused by a stone, which was surgically removed.

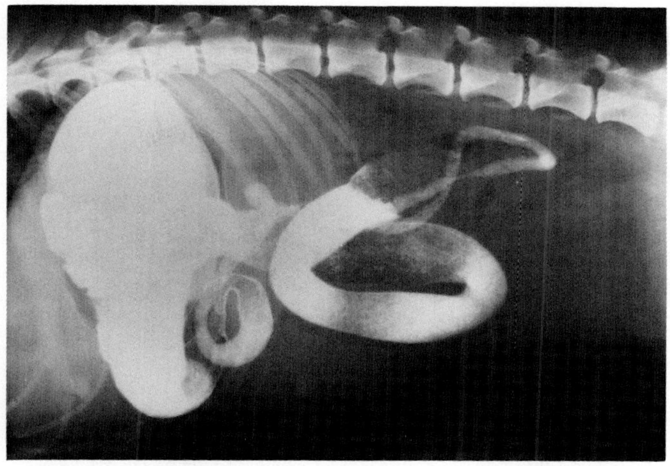

Figure 22-6. Lateral radiograph of 10-year-old Beagle with signs of acute intestinal obstruction. Positive contrast medium was administered. The film shows retention of contrast medium in the stomach, a distended loop of small intestine and an abrupt end to the movement of the contrast through the small intestine. This film suggests the presence of a complete obstruction since the contrast medium is not seen caudal to this point. The obstruction was caused by a corn cob. This study illustrates the use of positive contrast medium to delineate a radiolucent foreign body when there may be no strong radiographic evidence for intestinal obstruction on plain films.

foreign bodies are outlined by contrast medium. Some foreign bodies produce complete stasis, and all that is seen is a column of contrast medium ending with a broad front at the cranial edge of the obstruction (Figure 22-6). Annular lesions, produced by neoplastic or inflammatory disease, cause the column of contrast medium to taper into a relatively thin line (Figure 22-7).[33] The lumen, although narrowed, is consistently seen since annular lesions rarely develop to the point of causing a complete obstruction. When intestinal obstruction is complete, regard-

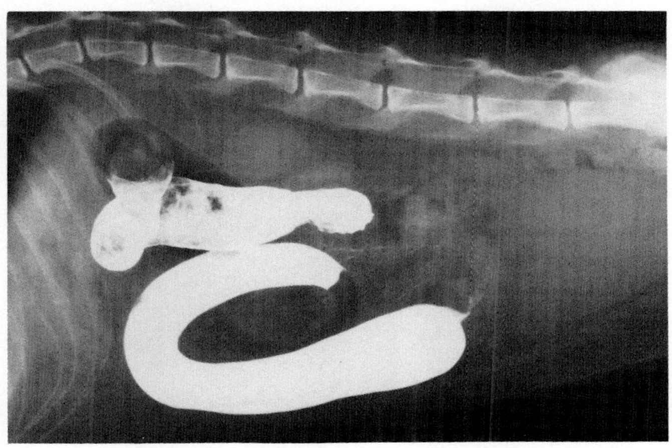

Figure 22-7. Lateral radiograph of an 8-year-old cat with clinical signs of anorexia and intermittent vomiting. Positive contrast medium was administered and the 3-hour film shows an obstruction that is partial since there is considerable contrast in the colon at this time. An adenocarcinoma of the small intestine caused the annular constriction

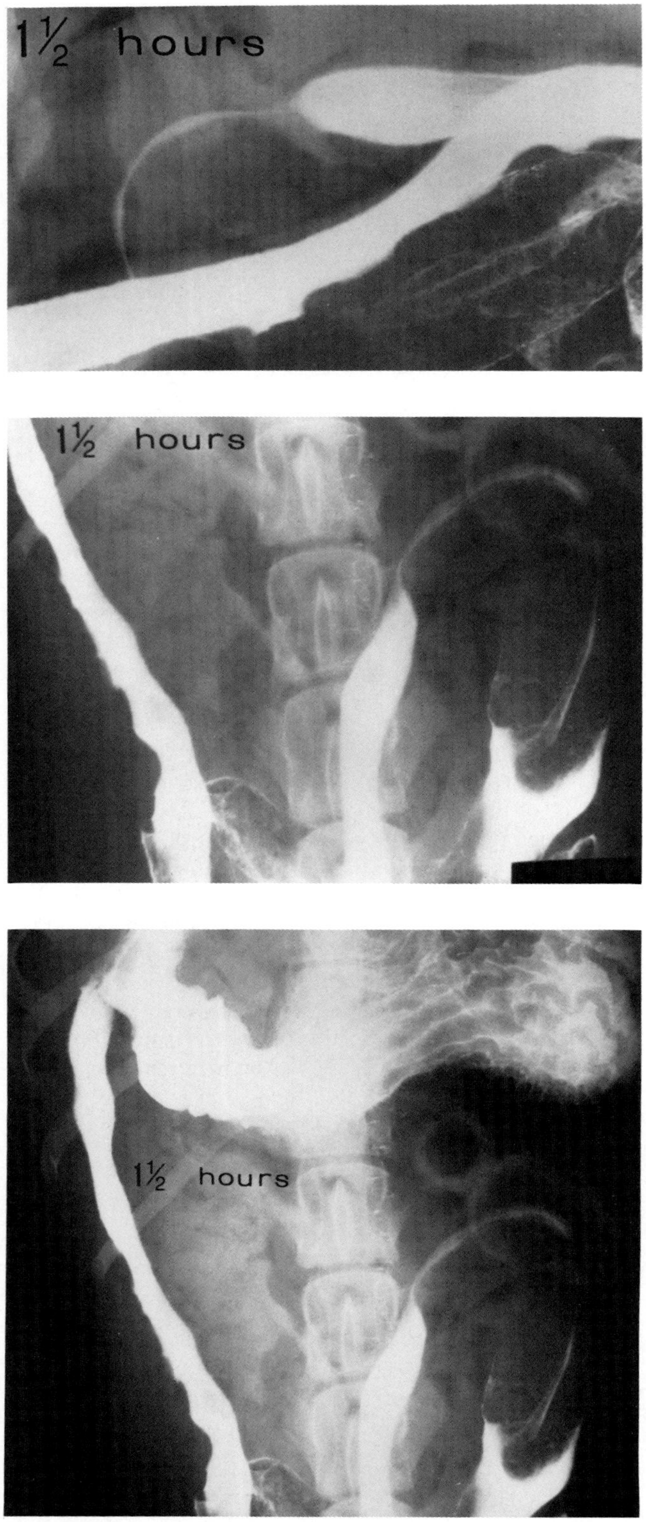

Figure 22-8. Lateral and dorsoventral radiographs of one-year-old Golden Retriever with signs of intestinal obstruction. Positive contrast medium was administered and radiographs 1.5 hours later show intussusception of a loop of jejunum into the adjacent distal part. The size of the lumen is reduced in the intussuscepted part, and some contrast moves retrograde around the intussuscepted part of its distal end.

less of the cause, the leading edge of the contrast column may never reach the point of obstruction. Thus, it is not always possible to define the site of the lesion. As discussed in Chapter 5, enteroclysis is a more sensitive contrast radiographic technique for the diagnosis of partial intestinal obstructions.

Radiographic Appearance of Intussusception

Intussusceptions have a radiographic appearance suggestive of partial obstruction.[7] Gas and fluid accumulation occur cranial to the lesion; horizontal X-ray beams can detect gas-fluid levels. Accumulations of gas are often noted in segments of intestine on the side of the abdomen opposite to the intussusception. Most intussusceptions are ileocolic, in which case the radiographic pattern shows an increase in tissue density caudal to the stomach, with displacement of the small-bowel segments to the right side and caudally. Contrast studies will better identify such obstructive lesions (Figure 22-8). Barium enemas can be used to outline intussusceptions that involve the ileum or the cecum with the colon. The radiographic findings include distention of the segment of colon into which the cecum or ileum is telescoped. The space occupied by the segment of bowel that has telescoped contains no contrast and appears radiolucent. It is outlined only by the small amount of contrast medium that surrounds it. When the cecum invaginates into the colon, it is not outlined by contrast medium although it is normally opacified (Figure 22-9).

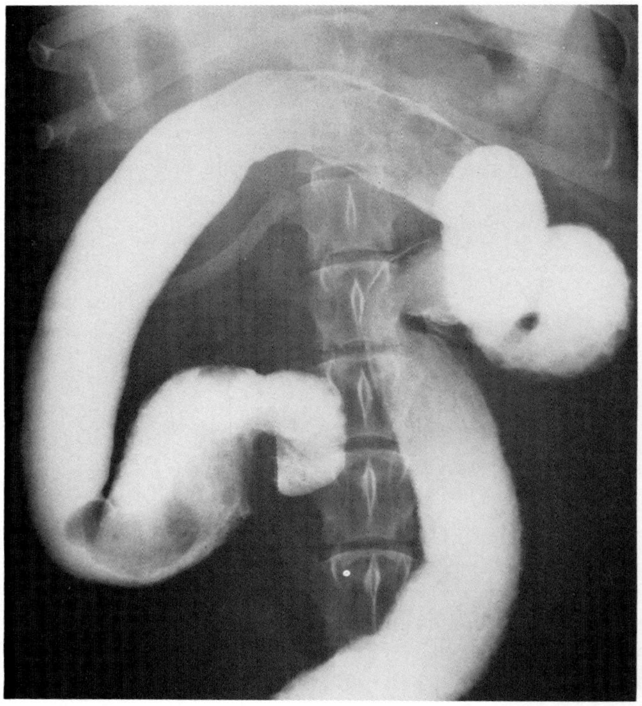

Figure 22-9. Dorsoventral radiograph of a one-year-old Basset Hound that was presented with clinical signs of an enterocolitis. Barium enema shows a filling defect in the cranial end of colon, which is distended. The cecum is not filled with positive contrast medium. Diagnosis is cecal inversion.

Radiographic Appearance of Linear Foreign Bodies

Linear foreign bodies produce characteristic but at times subtle changes that are frequently overlooked.[3] On survey radiographs affected loops of small intestine appear gathered or convoluted and may be bunched up at one site (Figure 22-10). Multiple gas bubbles can appear throughout the affected loop. Contrast studies reveal eccentric pleating, convolution, and foreshortening of the duodenum and jejunum. The duodenum's position often appears fixed in successive films. These are consistent findings. The radiographic appearance of linear foreign bodies must be differentiated from the changes resulting from an increased amount of segmentation activity in the small intestine. Hypersegmentation can produce a pleating appearance to the gut, but the constrictions in the small intestine are symmetrical with centrally located air bubbles, whereas linear foreign bodies create asymmetric convolutions and eccentrically located gas bubbles. The radiographic findings resulting from a linear foreign body can also resemble those from some types of mucosal disease, fixation of loops of intestine by peritoneal adhesions, and occasionally ascarids. A linear foreign body is difficult to distinguish from peritoneal adhesions, but surgical intervention is the treatment for both. Chronic linear foreign body is a cause of peritoneal adhesions.

Ultrasonography

Ultrasonography is an effective tool for the detection of intestinal obstructions. Both radiopaque and some radiolucent foreign bodies may be revealed. Intussusception has a characteristic ultrasonographic appearance, in which the multiple layers of overlapping intestinal wall are readily apparent.

MANAGEMENT OF INTESTINAL OBSTRUCTION

Preoperative Management

Fluids and Electrolytes. Intestinal obstruction should be expediently corrected by surgery, but celiotomy must be preceded by effective management of fluid and electrolyte derangements and toxemia.

The volume of fluid to be administered and the rapidity of administration are best based on clinical assessment of the severity of dehydration and the presence or absence of shock. Central venous pressure monitoring allows an objective assessment of the adequacy of volume replacement therapy. The type of fluid administered is based on the particular fluid, electrolyte, and acid-base derangements present in each individual patient. The wide variation in these derangements makes laboratory assessment of these parameters a necessity for accurate fluid therapy. If laboratory assessments of electrolyte and acid-base abnormalities are unavailable, the most appropriate replacement fluid is a balanced electrolyte solution such as lactated Ringer's solution, supplemented with potassium chloride to approximately 20 mEq/L of fluid. Potassium-free solutions are contraindicated in treating obstruction. Administration of glucose or bicarbonate promotes potassium movement into cells and may aggravate hypokalemia. In animals with ischemic loops of bowel, plasma and blood loss into the bowel may be sufficient to require plasma or whole blood administration.

There is experimental evidence to suggest that colloidal fluids such as plasma or dextrans have considerably different effects than crystaloid fluids do during the resuscitation of dogs with intestinal obstruction.[34] Both colloids and crystaloids will increase systemic arterial pressure and intestinal blood flow, but crystalloid fluids result in a marked decrease in plasma oncotic pressure and enhance transmucosal fluid movement into the bowel. In comparison to crystalloid fluids, colloidal fluids maintain plasma oncotic pressure and result in net fluid movement from the lumen to the blood. Thus colloids will provide better cardiovascular volume support, but in view of the toxic nature of intestinal content it remains to be seen whether colloidal fluid administration will increase or decrease the dogs' survival rate.

Antibiotics. The adverse effects of the bacterial flora in

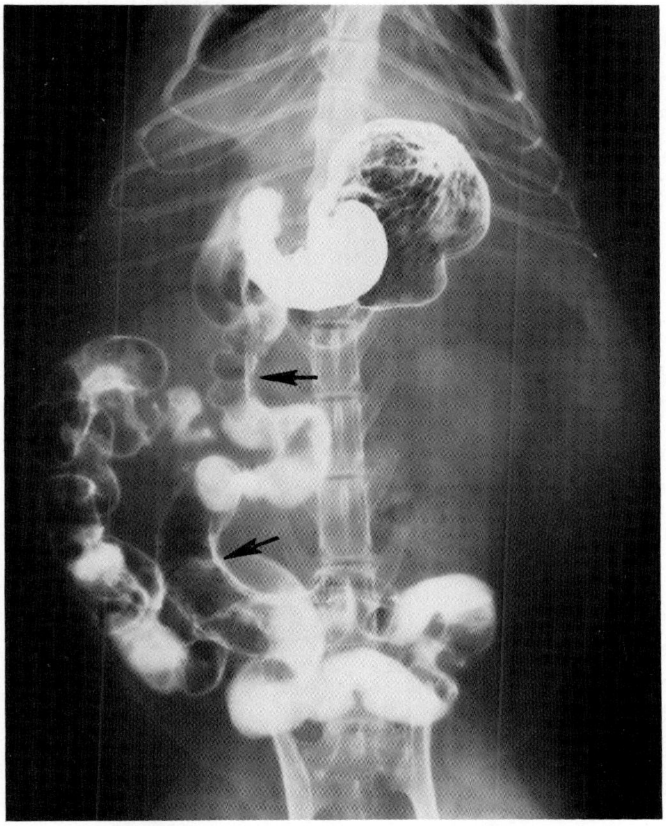

Figure 22-10. Dorsoventral radiograph of 10-year-old cat with clinical signs of vomiting and anorexia. Positive contrast medium was administered. The small intestine is distended and pleated, and the position of the duodenum is altered. A linear foreign body, in this case string, absorbed the contrast medium and can be seen (arrows). The contrast medium in the string and air in the intestine provides double contrast, which assists in evaluation of the abnormality. The string was fixed by forming a clumped mass in the stomach, which retains barium and becomes radiographically visible. Examination of the film should include reading carefully for localized peritonitis.

the intestine of the obstructed patient are more difficult to manage than the fluid and electrolyte derangements. Antibiotics are used to reduce numbers of bacteria in the intestine and to prevent them from invading through the mucosal barrier. Broad spectrum antimicrobials must be used to cover both aerobic and anaerobic spectra. In life-threatening situations, suitable choices include combinations of ampicillin (20 mg/kg IV q 8 hrs) and gentamicin (2 mg/kg IV q 8 hr). Penicillin G (20,000 units/kg q 6 hr) may be used instead of the ampicillin. Amikacin (2 mg/kg IV q 8 hr) is a suitable replacement for the gentamicin. The aminoglycosides should not be administered until fluid therapy has successfully rehydrated the patient. Partial obstructions, in which the clinical signs are not as fulminating, may be treated with tetracyclines (20 mg/kg q 12 hr PO) or metronidazole (15 mg/kg q 12 hr). The effectiveness of antibiotics against aerobes is quite variable since some, such as coliforms, can develop resistance to antibiotics within 24 hours.

Nasogastric Tubes. During the stabilization period, gastrointestinal fluid can be aspirated by a nasogastric tube. The removal of the accumulated fluid minimizes the absorption of bacterial toxins and lessens the chance of leakage of fluid into the abdomen before and during surgery. In humans it has been demonstrated that nasogastric drainage provides decompression comparable to drainage provided by longer intestinal tubes.[10] Data on survival of obstructed germ-free animals indicate that any reduction of intestinal bacterial numbers will benefit the patient.

Celiotomy

Once the animal is adequately stabilized, celiotomy is performed to relieve the obstruction. The surgical management of the obstructed intestine may require enterotomy only or, in cases of intestinal ischemia, may demand bowel resection and end-to-end anastomosis. The surgical management of intussusceptions can also include some form of prophylactic enteropexy or enteroplication. In one study in which no form of preventative enteropexy was performed, 20% of the dogs underwent a surgery for recurrence.[8]

Complications of the surgery include wound dehiscence and peritonitis. Wound dehiscence is not uncommon in debilitated patients with intestinal foreign bodies. These patients benefit greatly from pre-operative and post-operative parenteral nutrition. Consideration should be given at the time of surgery as to whether to place an enteral or gastrostomy feeding tube in an anorectic, debilitated patient. The patient should be allowed to take water orally within 12-24 hours of the surgery and should be offered small amounts of gruel within 24-48 hours. Intravenous fluid therapy should be continued until the animal is maintaining its own fluid and electrolyte homeostasis.

Ileus is a common complication of intestinal obstruction. Intestinal myoelectric activity is depressed, and abnormal activity persists longer in the intestine that is obstructed for a longer time.[35] Abnormal motility persists for at least 48 hours. Restoring intracellular potassium is essential for recovery of normal motility. Treatment with metoclopramide may also be beneficial.

MANAGEMENT OF GASTROINTESTINAL FOREIGN BODIES

Foreign bodies may be managed by conservative, endoscopic, or surgical means. Factors that influence this decision include the type of foreign object and its anatomic location, the clinical appearance of the animal, and the attentiveness with which the owner observes the pet.

Conservative management, consisting of close observation, high fiber diets, and radiographic observation of the aboral progress of the foreign object are recommended for non-traumatic, small-sized foreign bodies (eg pebbles) detected in the stomach or small intestine. Small gastric foreign objects may be given three to four weeks to pass before endoscopic removal, if the owner is capable of appropriately close observation and the animal remains asymptomatic. Conservative management of linear foreign bodies that fix about the tongue of cats is successful in many cases.[2] The conservative management consists of the cutting free of the string from around the tongue, followed by parenteral fluid administration and careful observation of the cat in the hospital. In many cats the string passes in the feces within one to three days. Conservative management should not be attempted or continued if the cat shows evidence of depression, cardiovascular compromise, or peritonitis.

It is questionable whether a high-fiber diet is of any value in hastening transit for a foreign body. Foreign bodies do not pass through the pylorus in the fed state because phasic contractions of the pylorus are maximum at that time.[36] Gastric foreign bodies with a diameter greater than five mm. pass through the pylorus in the unfed state during phase III contractions of the interdigestial motility complex (IDMC). Those contractions occur at about hourly intervals and last for five mm. Phasic pyloric contractions are minimal during the interdigestive periods, thus providing conditions for particulate material to leave the stomach. Drugs cannot be recommended to promote the movement of gastric foreign bodies through the pylorus. Metoclopramide stimulates antral motility and gastric emptying of food, but the drug may increase rather than decrease phasic contractions of the pylorus and thereby inpede any exiting of a foreign body from the stomach.

Surgical removal of a foreign body is indicated if signs of gastrointestinal perforation are observed or if an intestinal foreign body remains stationary for several days. If a hazardous foreign body is out of reach of the endoscope (for example in the periesophageal tissues or intestinal tract), or if a foreign body can be reached but not removed by the endoscope, surgical removal is necessary. If endoscopy reveals significant laceration or pressure necrosis of a viscus, surgical exploration to determine its mural extent is prudent.

All esophageal foreign bodies should be rapidly removed because of the accompanying pain and dysphagia and the possibility of esophageal stricture. Endoscopic removal is particularly desirable in view of the possible complications of esophageal surgery and thoracotomy. Timely endoscopic removal of all non-digestible sharp objects from the stomach is recommended because of the risk of perforation of the stomach or, should the object leave the stomach, perforation of the intestine. To avoid gastrointestinal obstruction, the early endoscopic or surgical removal of foreign bodies judged too large to pass through the gastrointestinal tract is suggested. Foreign bodies suspected of containing lead, zinc, or caustic materials (batteries) must be removed from the gastrointestinal tract immediately.

REFERENCES

1. Felts, J.F., Fox, P.R. and Burk, R.L.: Thread and sewing needles as gastrointestinal foreign bodies in the cat: A review of 64 cases. JAVMA 184:56-59.
2. Basher, A.W.P. and Fowler, J.D.: Conservative versus surgical management of gastrointestinal linear foreign bodies in the cat. Vet. Surg. 16:135-138, 1987.
3. Root, C.R. and Lord, P.F.: Linear radiolucent gastrointestinal foreign bodies in cats and dogs: Their radiographic appearance. J. Am. Vet Radiol. Soc. 12:45-53, 1971.
4. Carp, L.: Foreign bodies in the intestine. Ann. Surg. 85:575, 1927.
5. Kowalczyk, D.F.: Lead poisoning. In, Current Veterinary Therapy IX. Edited by Kirk, R.W. W.B. Saunders, Philadelphia, 145-150, 1986.
6. Torrance, A.G. and Fulton, R.B.: Zinc-induced hemolytic anemia in a dog. JAVMA 191:443-444, 1987.
7. Wilson, G.P. and Burt, J.K.: Intussusception in the dog and cat: a review of 45 cases. JAVMA 164:515-518, 1974.
8. Lewis, D.D. and Ellison, G.W.: Intussusception in dogs and cats. Comp. Contin. Ed. Pract. Vet. 9:523-533, 1987.
9. Weaver, A.D.: Canine intestinal intussusception. Vet. Rec. 100:524-527, 1977.
10. Bynum, T.E.: Intestinal obstruction and peritonitis. In, Internal Medicine. 2nd edition. Edited by Stein, J.H. Little, Brown And Co, Boston. 152-156, 1987.
11. Jones, R.S. and Schirmer, B.D.: Intestinal Obstruction, pseudoobstruction and ileus. In, Gastrointestinal Disease. Edited by M.H. Sleisenger and J.S. Fordtran. W. B. Saunders 369-381, 1989.
12. Arrick, R.H. and Kleine, L.J.: Intestinal pseudoobstruction in a dog. JAVMA 172:1201-1205, 1978.
13. Moore, R. and Carpenter, J.: Intestinal sclerosis with pseudoobstruction in three dogs. JAVMA 184:830, 1984.
14. Swayne, D.E., Tyler, D.E., Farrell, R.L. and Cornelius, L.M.: Sclerosing enteropathy in a dog. Vet. Pathol. 23:641-643, 1986.
15. Mishra, N.K., Appert, H.E. and Howard, J.M.: The effects of distension and obstruction on the accumulation of fluid in the lumen of small bowel of dogs. Ann. Surg. 180:791-795, 1974.
16. Shields, R.: The absorption and secretion of fluid and electrolytes by the obstructed bowel. Brit. J. Surg. 52:774-779, 1965.
17. Mirkovitch, V., Cobo, F., Robinson, J.W.L., Menge, H. and Gomba, S.Z.: Morphology and function of the dog ileum after mechanical occlusion. Clin. Sci. Mol. Med. 50:123-130, 1976.
18. Heneghan, J.B., Robinson, J.W.L., Menge, H. and Winistorfer, B.: Intestinal obstruction in germ-free dogs. Eur. J. Clin. Invest. 11:285-290, 1981.
19. Cohn, I.: Intestinal obstruction. In, Gastroenterology. 4th ed. Edited by Berk, J.E. W.B. Saunders Co., Philadelphia, 2056-2080, 1985.
20. Harvey, H.J. and Rendano, V.T.: Small bowel volvulus in dogs. Vet. Surg. 13:91-94, 1984.
21. Marks, A.: Torsion of the colon in a rough colic. Vet. Rec. 118:400, 1986.
22. Donaldson, R.M.: Small bowel bacterial overgrowth. Adv. Intern. Med. 16:191-212, 1970.
23. Summers, R.W., Helm, J. and Christensen, J.: Intestinal propulsion in the dog. Its relation to food intake and the migratory myoelectric complex. Gastroenterology 70:753-758, 1976.
24. Bishop, R.F. and Allcock, E.A.: Bacterial flora of the small bowel in acute intestinal obstruction. Brit. Med. J. 1:766-770, 1960.
25. Sykes, P.A., Boulter, K.H. and Scofield, P.F.: Alterations in small bowel microflora in acute intestinal obstruction. J. Med. Micro. Biol. 9:13-22, 1976.
26. Yale, C.E. and Balish, E.: The importance of six common bacteria in intestinal strangulation. Arch. Surg. 104:438-442, 1972.
27. Yale, C.E. and Balish, E.: The importance of clostridia in experimental intestinal strangulation. Gastroenterology. 71:793-796, 1976.
28. Rhodes, R.S. and Karnovsky, M.J.: Loss of macromolecular barrier function associated with surgical trauma to the intestine. Lab. Invest. 25:220-229, 1971.
29. Summers, R.W., Yanda, R., Prihoda, M. and Flatt, A.: Acute intestinal obstruction: an electromyographic study in dogs. Gastroenterology 85:1301-1306, 1983.
30. Prihoda, M., Flatt, A. and Summers, R.W.: Mechanisms of motility changes during acute intestinal obstruction in the dog. Am. J. Physiol. 247:G37-G42, 1984.
31. Gomez, J.A.: The gastrointestinal contrast study. Methods and interpretation. Vet. Clinics N. Am. 4:805-842, 1974.
32. O'Brien, T.R.: Radiographic Diagnosis of Adominal Disorders in the Dog and Cat. W.B. Saunders, Philadelphia, 1978.
33. Feeney, D.A., Klausner, J.S. and Johnston, G.R.: Chronic bowel obstruction caused by primary intestinal neoplasia: A report of five cases. JAAHA 18:67-77, 1982.
34. Allen, D., Kvietys, P.R. and Granger, N.: Crystalloids versus colloids: Implications in fluid therapy of dogs with intestinal obstruction. AJVR 47:1751-1755, 1986.
35. Brolin, R.E. and Reddell, M.T.: Gastrointestinal myoelectric activity in mechanical intestinal obstruction. J. Surg. Res. 38:515-523, 1985.
36. Keinke, O. and Ehrlein, H.J.: Effect of oleic acid on canine gastroduodenal motility, pyloric diameter and gastric empting. J. Exp. Physiol. 68: 675-686, 1983.
37. Moore, R. and Carpenter, J.: Intramural hematoma causing obstruction in three dogs. JAVMA 184:186-188, 1984.

Chapter 23

Miscellaneous Disorders of the Bowel, Anorectal Normal Structure and Function, Anorectal Disorders

MISCELLANEOUS DISORDERS OF THE BOWEL

Torsion and Strangulation of the Bowel

Small Intestinal Volvulus. Small intestinal volvulus is a rare and often fatal disorder resulting from a rotation of the intestine about its mesenteric axis. The degree of rotation, the severity of the ensuing gaseous distension of the intestine, and the duration of volvulus determine the severity of the ischemic insult. The duodenum is usually not involved in the volvulus because of its relatively fixed position in the abdominal cavity. Clinical signs are of intestinal obstruction. Vomiting, abdominal distension, abdominal pain, and bloody diarrhea are common, and death is rapid. The treatment is surgical. The small intestine is highly susceptible to reperfusion injury mediated by oxygen-free radicals (see Chapter 14). Premedication of the patient with oxygen-radical inhibitors or scavengers before surgical derotation may eventually prove to reduce morbidity. The prognosis depends on the clinical condition of the patient at presentation and the extent of the bowel requiring resection. If extensive small bowel is resected, malassimilation will result (the short bowel syndrome).[1] The management of short bowel syndrome follows the general principles outlined in the discussion of malassimilation.

Small Intestinal Strangulation. Strangulation of the small intestine by entrappment in mesenteric openings, tears, hernias, or adhesions results in similar signs. The amount of bowel involved is usually less extensive, but the prognosis is still guarded because of potential complications such as peritonitis.

Colon Torsion. Colon torsion is a rare disorder that results from a twist of the colon on its long axis. The cause is unknown. The condition has been reported in dogs.[2,3] The presentation is of acute onset of abdominal pain and distension in association with the rapid onset of shock. Physical examination may reveal a gas distended abdomen or a painful mass in the caudal abdomen. Radiography can show a gas or fluid distension of the colon that ends abruptly at the pelvic inlet. Ischemic necrosis of the colon is rapid, and death usually occurs within 24 hours. Surgical resection of the involved ischemic colon may be attempted. If the period of ischemia is less than 2 hours, the colon may retain its viability and resection may not be necessary. In these cases, reduction of the torsion and colopexy are advised.

Intestinal Recovery from Ischemia. The length of time for recovery of normal intestinal function has been studied in the dog following complete experimental ischemia of the colon and small intestine for one to two hours.[4-6] Immediate changes are severe, including necrosis and desquamation of villus tips, edema, vascular stasis, and hemorrhage in the lamina propria. Within 24 hours the mucosa has regained almost complete normal histological appearance, and circulation is almost normal again. The ileum is more sensitive than the colon to the effects of ischemia, but its mucosa returns to a normal appearance more rapidly. Mucosal functions return quite rapidly. Net absorption of fluid and nutrients is apparent in 24 hours, and within one week the regenerated mucosa has fully regained normal function.

Perforation of the Bowel; Peritonitis

Cause. Perforation of the bowel is an infrequent but extremely serious condition. Perforation may accompany a variety of conditions including ingestion of foreign bodies, neoplasia, adrenocortical adenoma, antiinflammatory drug administration, surgery, intestinal torsion or incarceration, penetrating abdominal wounds, perforating peptic ulcers, and intestinal biopsy. The gastrointestinal tract is the source of peritoneal contamination in approximately 60% of the cases of peritonitis in dogs.[7]

Colonic ulcerations and perforations are most frequently observed in patients treated surgically for neurological disease and concurrently medicated with dexamethasone.[8] Combination corticosteroid and non-steroidal antiinflammatory drug (NSAID) therapy has been associated with colonic perforation in dogs undergoing non-neurological surgical procedures. The colonic perforations are found most commonly on the antimesenteric border of the proximal portion of the descending colon but can appear anywhere in the large bowel including the cecum. Colonic or cecal perforation has also been associated with adrenal adenomas.[9]

Glucocorticoids or NSAIDs can cause upper as well as lower gastrointestinal ulceration and perforation.[10] When NSAIDs and corticosteroids are combined, the development of the lesions is particularly rapid.[11]

Pathogenesis. The pathogenesis of most intestinal perforations is self-explanatory although that of drug-associated and neurosurgery-associated perforation have not been completely resolved. Proposed precipitating factors of colonic perforation in neurosurgical cases include the administration of glucocorticoids, surgical stress, neurological damage, and fecal retention.[8] Localized colonic ischemia as a result of pain-induced increased sympathetic tone is a likely contributor, especially in view of the location of the lesions at the antimesenteric border. Inadequate post-surgical fluid therapy with resultant hypovolemia and release of angiotensin II is likely to compound the intestinal vasoconstriction. Angiotensin II is a potent vasoconstrictor of the canine vascular bed. Once mucosal injury occurs, ischemia may be perpetuated because of the absorption of bacterial endotoxins which are known to increase sympathetic tone and, albeit transiently, portal pressure.

Possible mechanisms, by which corticosteroids could predispose the colon to perforation include the inhibition of the immune response and collagen synthesis, and damage to the mucosal barrier. The pathogenesis of bowel injury resulting from NSAIDs is also thought to be multifactorial and includes inhibition of cytoprotective prostaglandins, compromised bowel permeability, and depressed gut-associated lymphoid tissue suppressor activity.

Diagnosis. The clinical signs are referable to the peritonitis and include depression, anorexia, vomiting, abdominal pain and evidence of sepsis. In some animals, melena may be apparent. An important differential diagnosis is acute pancreatitis. The clinical signs of pancreatitis and intestinal perforation are similar and furthermore, at least in humans, serum amylase can be high in both conditions. The diagnosis of perforation is usually made by observation of free fluid or gas on abdominal radiographs, and a septic exudate containing many different bacterial species on paracentesis. Culture of the abdominal fluid may be necessary to differentiate septic from non-septic peritonitis in some patients. Amylase concentration may be high in the abdominal fluid as a result of leakage from the bowel. On occasion, particularly following colonic perforation, the diagnosis can be elusive because of the antiinflammatory nature of concomitantly administered corticosteroids, peracute onset of clincal signs, and rapid death (within 24 hours) of the patient.[8] Perforations that result in localized areas of peritonitis may require diagnostic peritoneal lavage to detect. Ultrasonography or exploratory surgery may be necessary to locate walled-off abscesses resulting from previous perforation.

Treatment. The treatment for perforation and peritonitis is surgical. The patient is first rapidly stabilized with intravenous fluids in association with intravenous ampicillin (20 mg/kg IV). As soon as any hypovolemia has been corrected, gentamicin therapy (2.2 mg/kg IV) is begun. During surgery the cause of the perforation is determined and corrected, and the abdominal cavity is flushed with copious quantities of warm sterile saline. No antimicrobials need be added to the flush solution. At the conclusion of the surgery, the abdomen is left open and subsequent abdominal drainage and flushing is then continued by the open-abdominal-drainage technique.[12-14] The open-abdominal drainage technique is the prefered technique for the drainage of heavily contaminated abdomens. Hypoproteinemia is a common complication of the procedure.[12-14] Antimicrobial therapy is continued during the post-operative period. A combination protocol is essential to prevent abscess formation by the intestinal anaerobic bacteria, and sepsis from the intestinal (and perhaps nosocomial) gram negative bacteria. A suitable antimicrobial combination is ampicillin (20 mg/kg q 6-8 h IV, PO) to cover the aerobic gram positive spectrum, gentamicin (2.2 mg/kg q 8 h IV, SC) to cover the gram negative aerobic spectrum, and metronidazole (10-15 mg/kg q 12 h PO) to cover the anaerobic population (including *Bacteroides* species). Another suitable combination is clindamycin and gentamicin.[15] The use of gentamicin combined with first generation cephalosporins has been recommended but is not likely to adequately cover the anaerobic spectrum. Once the peritoneal discharge abates, usually 3-5 days after the surgery, the abdominal fluid is cultured both aerobically and anaerobically, the abdominal lavage is repeated, and the abdomen closed. Subsequent antibacterial therapy can be based on these culture results.

Prognosis and Prevention. In spite of properly applied open-drainage techniques, the mortality attributable to generalized peritonitis in dogs and cat ranges from 20-48%.[12,14] The mortality associated with antiinflammatory drug-associated or neurosugery-associated colonic perforation has been close to 100%.

The post-operative patient (particularly following neurosurgery) should be considered at high risk for gastrointestinal perforation.[8] Preventative measures are important to the avoidance of this complication. Maintain adequate hydration status and plasma protein concentration by the use of parenteral fluids or plasma administration to prevent hypovolemia and angiotensin II release. Do not use glucocorticoids in the post-operative period if at all possible. If glucocorticoids are essential, restrict the course of therapy to 2-3 days post-surgery. Correct fecal retention before surgery and prevent constipation by use of bulk promoting agents and laxatives. Avoid the use of NSAIDs and, in particular, do not use combinations of glucocorticoids and NSAIDs.

MISCELLANEOUS DISORDERS OF THE CECUM AND COLON

Diseases of the Cecum

The cecum can be involved in a number of disease processes including ileocolic intussusuception; typhilitis; and cecal abscessation,[16] perforation,[9] dilatation, neoplasia, and inversion. Typhlitis is most commonly due to whipworm infection or occurs along with generalized inflammatory diseases of the large bowel. Ileocolic intussusception is a common cause of intussusception that often involves the cecum. Intussusception is discussed in Chapter 22. Cecal dilatation usually occurs as a component of ileus and of itself has unknown significance. Cecal neoplasia is discussed in Chapter 24. With the exception of typhlitis and cecal dilatation due to ileus, most diseases of the cecum are treated by typhlotomy or typhlectomy.

Cecal Inversion. Cecal inversion is a rare disorder in which the cecum invaginates into the colon. The cause is unknown, but presumably prolapse of the cecum into the colon requires laxity in the ileocecal colic ligament. Whipworm infection is thought to predispose to the condition.[17] The most consistent clinical sign is chronic intermittent diarrhea with hematochezia. Tenesmus is often absent, as would be expected in a lesion that does not involve the distal colon and rectum. The inverted segment will occasionally produce intestinal obstruction resulting in vomiting and rapid deterioration of the patient's condition. Careful abdominal palpation may detect a mid-abdominal mass. Diagnosis is made by barium enemas, air enemas, or colonoscopy. Treatment is surgical resection.

Miscellaneous Causes of Colitis

There are over 25 known causes of colitis in the dog and cat (Table 23-1). The most common cause is idiopathic chronic (lymphocytic-plasmacytic) colitis. This disease along with eosinophilic colitis, suppurative colitis, granulomatous colitis, and histiocytic colitis is classified as an idiopathic inflammatory bowel disease and is discussed in Chapter 21. Colitis can also be caused by a wide variety of infectious agents. These disorders are discussed in Chapter 18. There are a number of other causes of colitis that are less common then the infectious and idiopathic inflammatory colitis conditions.

Table 23-1. Causes of Colitis in the Dog and Cat

Idiopathic inflammatory disorders
- Acute non-specific colitis
- Chronic (lymphocytic-plasmacytic) colitis
- Eosinophilic colitis
- Granulomatous colitis
- Histiocytic colitis
- Suppurative colitis

Bacterial
- *Bacillus piliformis*
- *Campylobacter*
- *Clostridium perfringens*
- *Clostridium difficile?*
- Enterotoxigenic *E. coli*?
- *Salmonella*
- *Yersinia enterocolitica?*

Viruses
- FeLV
- FIP
- FIV

Protozoa
- *Giardia**
- *Balantidium coli*
- *Entamoeba histolytica*

Fungi or algae
- Aspergillosis
- Histoplasmosis
- Mucormycosis
- Protothecosis

Parasites
- Hookworms*
- Whipworms

Miscellaneous
- Antibiotic-associated colitis
- Hemorrhagic gastroenteritis (HGE)
- Pancreatitis
- Traumatic colitis
- Uremic colitis

* Usually small bowel infections

Acute Non-Specific Colitis

Acute onset of large bowel diarrhea is not an uncommon clinical presentation in the dog and cat. The signs are probably a manifestation of a group of poorly defined diseases, and the specific cause is rarely determined. Fecal cultures are indicated to rule out known enteric pathogens. Proposed etiologies have included toxin ingestion (particularly as a component of "garbage can enteritis), abrasion of the colonic mucosa by indigestible material such as bone fragments, unidentiifed bacteria such as enterotoxigenic *E. coli*, and allergic proctocolitis. Coagulation necrosis of the colonic mucosa is a feature of mercury, bismuth, and arsenic poisoning.[18] An important differential diagnosis is ileocolic intussusception. The clinical signs are an acute onset of explosive watery diarrhea, often with blood and tenesmus. Vomiting and depression are not uncommon. The diagnostic work up for large bowel diarrhea is described elsewhere. Treatment is symptomatic and usually includes fluids, bismuth subsalicylate, and antibiotics. Food is withheld for 24-48 hours after which a bland easily digestible diet such as cottage cheese and rice is fed for 5-7 days. The addition of Metamucil (1-6 tsp per meal) may hasten recovery of normal colonic function. The prognosis is good.

Antibiotic-Associated Pseudomembranous Colitis

Antibiotic-associated pseudomembranous colitis has been reported in the dog in association with the administration of clindamycin.[19] The clinical signs included severe mucoid diarrhea beginning 10 days after commencement of the antibiotic. At colonoscopy, the mucosa appeared erythematous and friable and was covered by 1-5 mm raised yellowish-white plaques. The dog recovered when the medication was withdrawn. Fecal culture results were not reported. In humans, the disorder is due to *Clostridium difficile* infection. Antibiotics most often incriminated are clindamycin and lincomycin.

Colitis Associated with Pancreatitis

Acute, severe, necrotizing pancreatitis can be associated with a segmental colitis. The presumed pathogenesis is involvement of the transverse colon (against which the pancreas is anatomically apposed) in the peripancreatic inflammation. The disorder should be suspected in dogs showing concomitant signs of colitis and clinical or laboratory evidence of pancreatitis, or in patients in which colonoscopy determines that colonic inflammation is confined to the transverse colon.

Traumatic Colitis

Trauma to the colon can result from abdominal trauma, or the ingestion of indigestible material such as stones, bones, sticks, aluminum foil, plastic, and wire. Most often such objects are passed with minimal clinical signs except for some fresh blood on the stool. If the mucosal damage is sufficiently widespread, however, acute colitis may result from secondary invasion of bacterial flora. Occasionally, a foreign body may get lodged in the colon or rectum and result in tenesmus and dyschezia. The condition is usually self-limiting and only supportive therapy is required. Lodged foreign bodies may require endoscopic removal.

Uremic Colitis

Colitis can be a complication of advanced renal insufficiency. It is usually but one of a constellation of gastrointestinal signs that are associated with uremia. Other common gastrointestinal signs in the dog and cat include anorexia, nausea, halitosis, oral ulceration, ischemic necrosis of the distal tip of the tongue, vomiting, gastritis, and gastroduodenal ulceration. Additional gastrointestinal disorders have been ascribed to uremia in humans. These include xerostomia, parotitis, esophagitis, duodenitis, bacterial overgrowth, adynamic ileus, intestinal perforation, and colonic intussusception.[20] The pathogenesis of uremic gastrointestinal lesions is probably multifactorial. Factors that are involved include hypergastrinemia, secondary hyperparathyroidism, uremic vasculitis, the microbial breakdown of urea to ammonia, and altered bile salt metabolism.[20]

The treatment is directed at the renal insufficiency.

Non-Inflammatory Large Bowel Diarrheal Disease

As many as 15-20% of dogs presenting for signs of large bowel diarrhea have no evidence of "significant" colonic inflammation on proctoscopy or biopsy.[19] The clinical appearance of these patients is similar to that of dogs with inflammatory colitis. The appearance of the diarrhea can range from small volumes of soft feces with occasional blood to watery diarrhea. The cause of the condition is unknown. Analogies have been drawn to the irritable bowel syndrome in humans based on the favorable response of many affected dogs to supplemental dietary fiber.[21] Some dogs with the syndrome may indeed be suffering from a disorder analogous to irritable bowel syndrome, but in our experience few affected dogs show any of the other clinical signs consistently demonstrated by human patients with the disorder, such as abdominal distension or abdominal pain (see Chapter 25). Furthermore, responsiveness to fiber can occur in a number of secretory large bowel

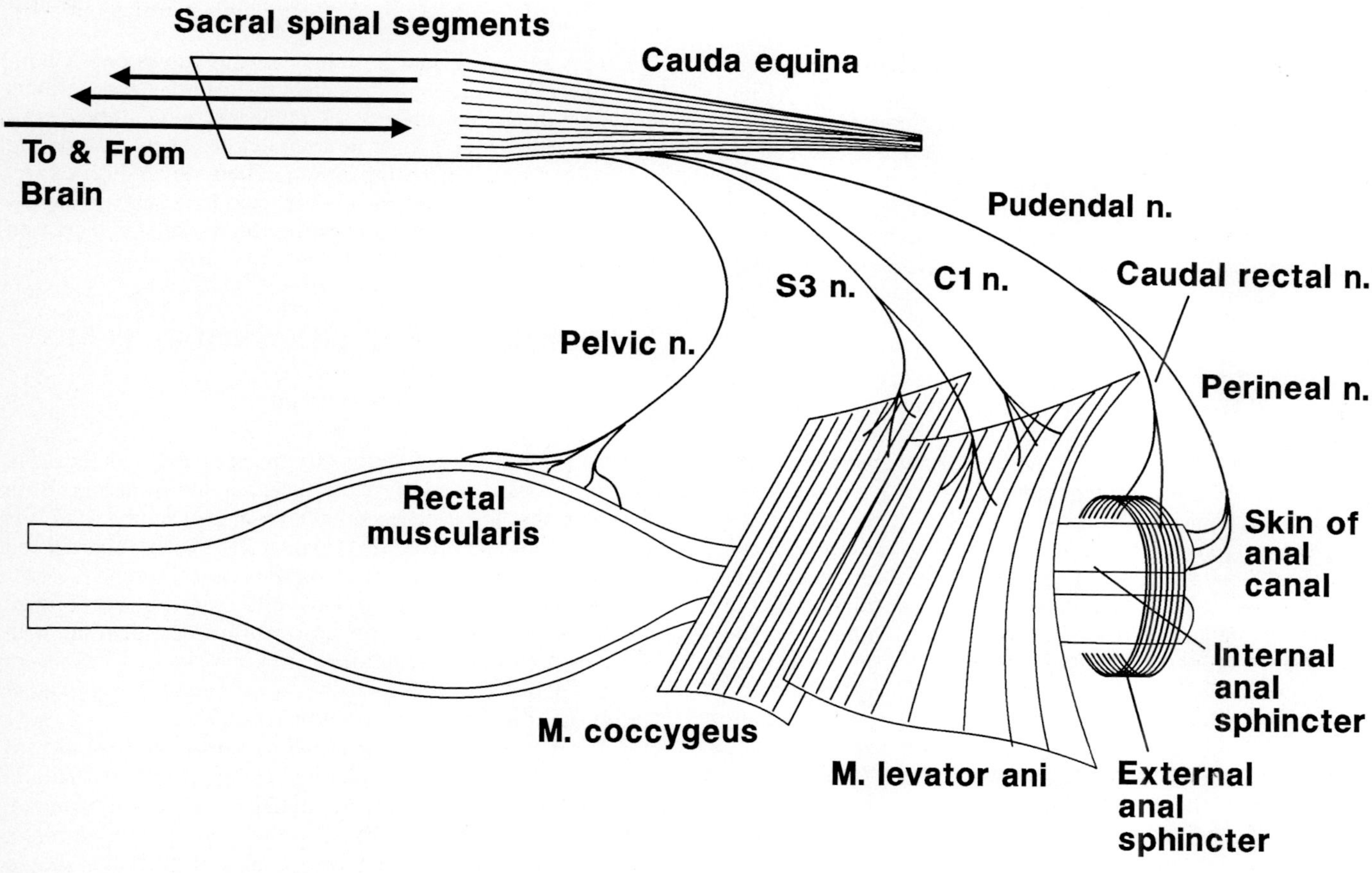

Figure 23-1. Neural control of defecation. Sensory information from wall of rectum and anal canal relayed to sacral synaptic centers. Response carried by parasympathetic fibers is to stimulate contraction of rectal muscles and inhibit motor activity in the internal anal sphincter. Response carried by somatic efferents is to inhibit the external anal sphincter muscle. These events mediate defecation which is reinforced by local reflexes within the rectal wall to stimulate contraction and by voluntary reinforcement of external anal sphincter relaxation and contraction of abdominal perineal muscles. Sympathetic innervation (not shown) is inhibitory to rectal wall and facilitory to internal anal sphincter. The muscles fo the continence reaction in the dog may include coccygens, levator ani, and external anal sphincter muscles. The continence reaction may be initiated by rectal distention, by stretch of pelvic girdle muscles, or by stimulation of anal canal epithelium.

diarrheas including those induced by bile salts and fatty acids. If a comparison is required to a human disease, a closer analogy might be microscopic colitis. In this syndrome minimal inflammatory infiltrates and mild reactive changes in the epithelium are associated with markedly abnormal colonic absorption of water and electrolytes and clinical signs which include persistent diarrhea with urgency, mild abdominal cramping, but no hematochezia.[22] The responsiveness of the diarrhea in this condition to fiber supplementation has not been established, but one publication, linking microscopic colitis and bile-salt malabsorption, described a clinicopathological response to cholestyramine.[23]

The treatment of non-inflammatory large bowel diarrhea is based on fiber administration to which 50% of dogs reportedly respond.[21] If irritable bowel syndrome is suspected, attempts to eliminate stress may be useful. A trial with cholestyramine may be of value and opioids may be effective in some cases.

ANORECTUM - NORMAL STRUCTURE AND FUNCTION[24]

The rectum serves as a reservoir, collecting and holding fecal material. The rectal wall is essentially the same in structure as the colon. The rectal mucosa contains glands of Lieberkuhn with more mucous cells than the colon. At the rectal-anal junction the mucosal surface changes to stratified squamous epithelium. Smooth muscle composes the two rectal muscularis layers, and at the caudal end these muscles form the internal anal sphincter. At the end of the rectum are layers of well defined striated muscle bundles surrounding the inner internal anal sphincter and forming the external anal sphincter.

The rectum contains receptors that are sensitive to changes in intraluminal pressure but not to touch or pain. The anal canal situated between the rectum and the perianal region possesses receptors that respond to pressure, temperature, touch, and pain. The afferent nerve pathway for the rectal receptors is in pelvic nerves, while that for the most caudal receptors is in the pudendal nerve (Figure 23-1). Afferent fibers synapse in the sacral spinal cord, and efferent motor fibers are contained in the pudendal, hypogastric, and pelvic nerves. The rectum and internal anal sphincter are supplied by autonomic nerve fibers. Parasympathetic fibers are motor to the rectum, as in the colon, are inhibitory to the internal anal sphincter, and are carried in the nervi erigentes. Sympathetic fibers are inhibitory to the rectum and motor to the internal anal sphincter, and are carried in the hypogastric nerves coming from the inferior mesenteric ganglia. The external anal sphincter's striated muscle is innervated by somatic nerve fibers in the pudendal nerve.

The receiving, storage, and defecation of rectal contents, controlled by reflex events in the rectum, can be modified by voluntary control exerted via function in the external anal sphincter. As the rectum receives colonic contents, it distends, which stimulates receptors and initiates a reflex act. The reflex consists of sensory reception in the rectum, transmission of information through the afferents in the pelvic nerves, synaptic transmission in the sacral cord, and a motor response to the rectal muscles to cause contraction. Another part of the motor response inhibits tone in the internal anal sphincter, so that, as the rectum contracts, the internal anal sphincter relaxes. Fecal contents distending the more sensitive anal mucosa stimulate receptors to send information to the cord, from where it is relayed to higher cortical centers. Conscious control can be evoked to facilitate or inhibit defecation. For inhibition the external sphincter is voluntarily constricted, closing the anal canal, and stimulation of the receptors ceases. Facilitation is mediated by relaxation of external anal sphincter muscles and contraction of the diaphragm and abdominal muscles, with closing of the glottis to increase intra-abdominal pressure. When defecation is suppressed the rectum adapts to a larger volume by receptive relaxation, and the stimulation of sensory receptors stops.

The anal canal is always normally closed by tonic contraction of the external anal sphincter. Persistent tone is produced by a reflex stimulated by proprioceptive feedback stimuli from muscle spindles in the sphincter. The afferent nerves extend through the dorsal roots of the second sacral nerves. The motor pathway from synaptic centers in the cord is via the pudendal nerves. The cord centers are caudal to the fourth lumbar nerves, since transection of the cord cranial to that point does not abolish the reflex whereas transection caudally causes a loss of sphincteric function. Loss of tone is also caused by transection of the second sacral dorsal roots. Unilateral transection of a pudendal nerve has no effect on maintaining tone in the anal canal.

With an appropriate stimulus the anus shows phasic contractions. This reflex is mediated by afferent nerve fibers traveling through the third sacral dorsal roots. The motor pathway is the same as for tonic contractions. These reflexes are evoked by circumanal stimulation, called the anal reflex; by penetration of the anal canal, the guarding reflex; and by increased intra-abdominal pressure, which results in increased pressure in the rectum.

DISORDERS OF THE ANORECTUM

Constipation[25]

Constipation is defined as infrequent or absent defecation. The term obstipation refers to intractable constipation. Both disorders should be differentiated from megacolon which is defined as colonic dilatation (Chapter 25). Not all constipated animals have megacolon.[25] Constipation is a common presenting complaint. The reason a client believes a pet is constipated should be sought. Many owners confuse constipation with tenesmus. The latter condition has a considerably different range of potential causes than does constipation. The prevalent causes of constipation are listed in Table 23-2.

The evaluation of patients with constipation should include a detailed history of diet and a very careful visual and digital examination of the anorectum. Some painful anorectal lesions such as perianal fistula can be easily missed during a cursory examination. Survey radiographs of the pelvis should be taken to rule out obvious obstructive lesions.

The first considerations in the treatment of constipation are correction of any fluid and electrolyte derangements and attention to the primary cause if one can be identified. In our experience, the initial approach to severely constipated patients should include anesthesia, the administration of a lubricating warm water enema, and manual fragementation and removal of the hardened stool. Precautions include adequate preparation of

Table 23-2. Prevalent Causes of Constipation[25]

Ingestion of indigestible material	
	Bones, wool, cloth, hair
Lack of exercise	
	Hospitalization
Painful defecation	
	Anorectal lesions (perianal fistula, anal sac abscess)
	Pelvic trauma
	Painful hindlimb musculoskeletal diseases
Mechanical obstruction	
	Healed pelvic fractures
	Prostatomegaly
	Intrapelvic masses
	Colonorectal mass
	Perineal hernia
	Congenital anorectal lesions (Imperforate anus, intestinal atresia)
	Pseudocoprostasis
Neurological disease	
	Paraplegia
	Sacral spinal cord deformity (Manx cats)
	Idiopathic megacolon
Miscellaneous	
	Endocrinopathies (hypothyroidism, hyperparathyroidism)
	Hypokalemia
	Debility
	Dehydration
	Opioids
	Cholestyramine

the patient for anesthesia and the use of endotracheal intubation to prevent aspiration of regurgitated gastrointestinal content (which can be induced by the enema procedure). The enema is performed and the fecal mass is carefully but firmly kneaded through the abdominal wall until it softens and can be fragmented into small pieces. These pieces can be subsequently removed by the gloved finger or with the use of whelping forceps. A suitable enema solution is warm water mixed with generous quantities of methylcellulose lubricant. Enema fluid should be run into the rectum under the force of gravity only. Pumping the fluid in can lead to through-and-through rectal to oral lavages. A standard volume used is 5-10 ml/kg. High concentrations of soap should not be used in enema fluids as they can damage the colonic mucosa. Phosphate (Fleet) enemas are contraindicated because of the likelihood of intoxication.[26]

Animals with less severe constipation do not require anesthesia and manual breakdown of the stool. They can be treated by regular warm water, lubricating enemas in association with softening agents such as dioctyl sodium sulfosuccinate (Colace; Surfak; Coloxyl; 50 mg (cats), 50-200 mg (dogs) q 12-24 hr PO) and bulk-forming laxatives such as psyllium (Metamucil; 1-6 tsp mixed with each meal) or bran (1-2 tblsp per 400 gm canned food).

Prevention of subsequent constipation is best achieved by education of the client about suitable diet and exercise for their pet, and the use of bulk-forming laxatives or lubricant laxatives (white petrolatum - Katalax, Laxatone). Lactulose (Chronulac; 1 ml/5kg q 8 hr) may be useful in some cats. Mineral oil should be avoided.

Fecal Incontinence[27]

Definition and Incidence. Fecal incontinence is the inability to retain feces until defecation is appropriate. Failure of fecal continence is a disastrous occurrence for the household pet. Fifty percent of dogs and cats with fecal incontinence are euthanized within several days of presentation. The recorded incidence of fecal incontinence is 43 out of 260,000 admissions to the UMC and UCD VMTHs. This is probably an underestimation of the true incidence of the disease. There is no sex predilection, but the majority of affected animals are 11 years of age or older. Two major subcategories of fecal incontinence are recognized. These are "reservoir incontinence" and "sphincter incontinence".[28] The putative anatomic structures involved in the maintenance of fecal continence are depicted in Figure 23-1.

Reservoir Incontinence. A reservoir mechanism is essential for continence, because the maximum period of sustained voluntary contraction of the striated anal sphincter muscles is brief.[29,30] Reservoir incontinence results from a failure of the large bowel to adapt to, and contain within its length, the colonorectal content. Animals with reservoir incontinence are usually aware of feces in the rectum and are able to sense the imminence of defecation. Reservoir incontinence is most often characterized by frequent, conscious defecation and *not* by inadvertent anal dribbling. The adequacy of large bowel reservoir function is affected by colonorectal irritability, capacity, compliance, and motility, and by the volume of feces.

Sphincter Incontinence. Sphincter incontinence is due to a failure of the sphincteric mechanisms to resist the propulsive forces of the rectum.[29,30] It is characterized by the involuntary passage of feces. Sphincter incontinence is largely dependent on the "continence reaction", a reflexive or conscious contraction of the muscles of the external anal sphincter and the pelvic girdle after sensation of the fecal mass.[31]

Nervous Pathways of the Continence Reaction. Three afferent nervous pathways, each with different sensory triggers, may be involved in the continence reaction (Figure 23-2). Which of these nervous pathways are the more important is somewhat controversial. The majority of evidence in humans favors the afferent nervous pathways triggered by stimulation of the anal epithelium, or stretching of the muscles of the pelvic girdle.[31-33] The issue has not been adequately addressed in the dog or cat. The hypogastric nerves transmit pain resulting from excessive dilatation of the bowel,[34] and probably do not have an important role in the maintenance of fecal continence. The information derived from the three major afferent pathways is integrated in the sacral spinal cord. The reflex arc is completed by efferent nerve fibers to the muscles of the pelvic girdle (via S3 and C1 and to a lesser extent S2 spinal nerves) and to the external anal sphincter (via the caudal rectal nerve, a distal branch of the pudendal nerve).[35,36] Very little specific information exists on the areas of the brain involved in the control of continence and the perception of the urge to defecate, but similar brain stem centers, to those which control micturition are thought to be important.[37]

Muscles of the Continence Reaction. In humans, the

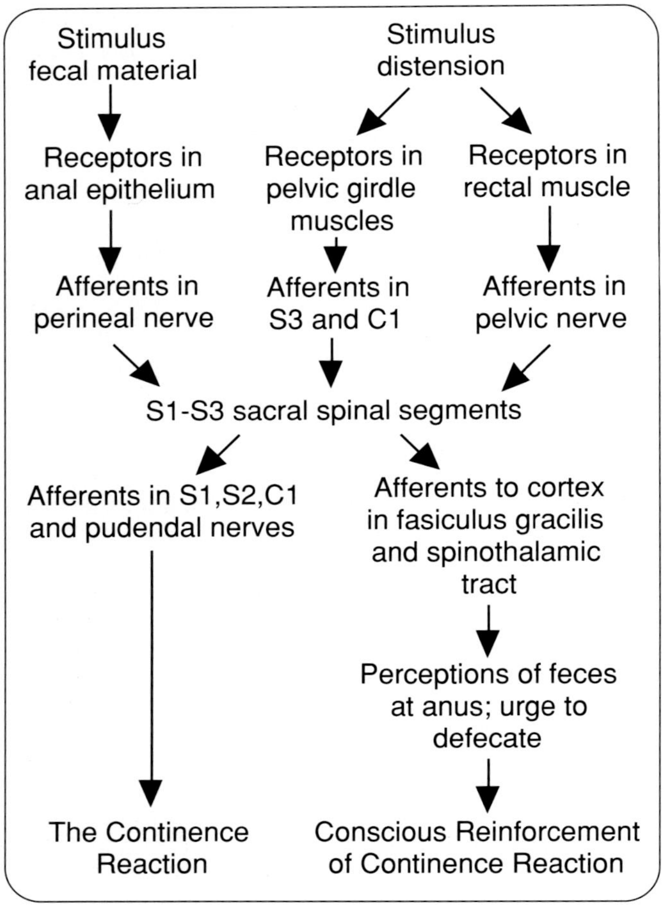

Figure 23-2 Hypothetical reflexes involved in the continence reaction. This figure has been compiled from often conflicting papers and texts that deal with the problem of human and, to a lesser extent, canine incontinence.[4,6,8-10,12,15,25,40,62-65]

muscle that is most important in the resistance of the anal canal to propulsive waves appears to be the puborectalis.[31] Contraction of the external anal sphincter can further raise pressure in the anal canal. It appears that the external anal sphincter and puborectalis muscles are closely related and synergistic in action, acting as consecutive sphincteric muscular loops.[38]

In the dog it is likely that the external anal sphincter plays an important role in the maintenance of continence. The levator ani muscle may also play a role. The levator ani is the most likely canine equivalent of the human puborectalis muscle.[39]

Miscellaneous Factors Contributing to Sphincter Continence. Factors, other than the continence reaction, may also play a contributory role in the maintenance of sphincter continence.[40] Their relative importance is controversial in man[40] and poorly addressed in the dog.[39] The internal anal sphincter, a thickening of the smooth muscle of the rectum,[39,41] appears to be important in maintaining the resting pressure of the anal canal, but in response to a propulsive wave, and even slight distension of the rectum of humans or dogs this muscle relaxes (recto-sphincteric reflex).[31,41-43] Therefore, contraction of the internal sphincter is unlikely to be important in maintaining continence when pressure in the rectum becomes high, but may help guard against incontinence of small amounts of liquid stool.[44] The relaxation of the internal sphincter following rectal distension shortens the functional length of the anal canal allowing rectal pressure and content to contact the highly sensitive anal skin.[33] This may perhaps allow discrimination of the material distending the rectum (eg. gas, fluid or formed stool) and allow

Table 23-3. Possible Causes of Fecal Incontinence

Anorectal Disease
- Lacerations
- Neoplasia
- Anal sac removal
- Perianal fistulas and fistula repair
- Perineal hernia repair
- Rectovaginal fistula

Colonorectal Disease
- Proctitis
- Colitis
- Neoplasia
- Constipation

Myopathies or Neuromuscular Junction Disorders
- Trauma
- Myopathies?
- Myasthenia?

Peripheral Neuropathies
- Trauma
- Drug-induced eg. vincristine
- Polyneuropathies
- Dysautonomia
- Chronic tenesmus?
- Obstetric trauma?
- Diabetes mellitus?
- Pelvic radiation?

Cauda Equina
- Congenital vertebral malformations
- Compressive vertebral malformations
- Traumatic vertebral damage, e.g. sacrococcygeal subluxation
- Lumbosacral instability
- Anomalous lumbosacral vertebral nerve roots
- Infection
- Neoplasia
- Vascular compromise

CNS Disease
- Congenital, e.g. spina bifida
- Traumatic
- Infectious, e.g. distemper
- Degenerative myelopathy
- Vascular compromise
- Neoplasia
- Confusional states

Miscellaneous
- Aging
- Constipation
- Loose fecal consistency
- Increased fecal volume
- Anury

KEY: ?- Causes of fecal incontinence documented in the human literature only conscious reinforcement of the continence reaction.[33]

If low intra-rectal pressures are maintained by effective reservoir function, passive factors are able to preserve some semblance of continence, even in those animals in which the neuromuscular components of the sphincter mechanisms are damaged. These passive mechanisms include a proposed flutter-valve-like action of the anorectum in response to increases in intra-abdominal pressure,[40,45] the inherent resistance to expansion exhibited by any tissue in a collapsed state,[39,40] and the horizontal stance of the dog and cat.

Causes of Fecal Incontinence. The causes of fecal incontinence are varied (Table 23-3). Important causes include anal diseases that interfere with sensory information from the anal epithelium and may disrupt the integrity of the anal canal; colonorectal diseases, such as colitis, and neoplasia which compromise the reservoir function of the large bowel; constipation ("overflow" fecal incontinence); diarrhea; damage to the muscles and nerves of the continence reaction, in particular due to caudal equina syndrome; CNS injury; and aging. Aging is a common "cause" of fecal incontinence in humans[46] and dogs.

Table 23-4. Diagnostics Useful for the Differential Diagnosis of Fecal Incontinence

History
Physical Examination
Neurological Examination
-perception of perineal and anorectal sensation
-perineal reflex
-pudendal-anal reflex
-rectal-inflation reflex
-manual stimulation of erection
Data Base
-CBC
-serum chemistry profile
-urinalysis
-fecal
Radiography
-lumbosacral survey radiographs
-radiographs of stressed lumbosacrum
-myelogram
-epidurogram
-discogram
-intraosseous vertebral venogram
-CAT scan
Electrodiagnostics
-conventional EMG
-single fiber EMG
-anal mapping
-pudendal-anal reflex
-pudendal and perineal nerve motor latencies
-spinal motor latencies
-Hind limb NCV and evoked potentials
CSF Tap
-fluid analysis
-distemper titer
Colonoscopy
Anorectal/Colonorectal Pressure Profiles
Surgical Exploration

The exact site of the defect or defects is unknown. It is likely that multiple factors are involved. Suggested contributory causes include senility, neuropathies, weakness and atrophy of the muscles of fecal continence, diminished rectal compliance and a higher incidence of diarrhea in the older patient.[46-48] Diagnosis is by exclusion.

Diagnosis of Fecal Incontinence. It is important to determine the site and the cause of fecal incontinence because the treatments and prognoses of the different conditions vary considerably. As is evident from the above discussion, in order to determine the cause, the clinician must first obtain a thorough history, perform a thorough physical examination and, if necessary, complete a number of diagnostic tests. Evaluations of value in some cases for the diagnosis of fecal incontinence are listed in Table 23-4.

History. The history may help determine if systemic diseases are involved, may suggest cause (eg poor diet, trauma, difficult whelping, drug or toxin exposure, chronic constipation etc.), and is invaluable in the differentiation of reservoir and sphincter incontinence.

The history should include inquiry as to whether the animal consciously defecates (ie. adopts a posture appropriate to defecation) and, if it does posture to defecate, whether the time and place chosen is appropriate. Failure to make any attempt at conscious defecation suggests a severe anorectal sensory derangement. These animals usually have a history of unconscious anal dribbling, often occurring at times of increased abdominal or rectal pressures such as while coughing or during exertion. In a previously house trained animal, conscious defecation at inappropriate times or places, without the associated distress and urgency of reservoir incontinence, is more suggestive of a behavioral problem or a confusional state. In a young animal, inappropriate defecation may be simply due to a failure of house training.

Inquiry should also be made as to whether the animal has the ability to urinate normally and, in intact males, if the dog can attain an erection and subsequently achieve normal detumescence. Both micturition and erection rely on similar nervous pathways to those of fecal continence,[49] and, therefore, concurrent abnormalities in these functions suggest that the fecal incontinence is of neurogenic origin.

Physical Examination. Close visual inspection of the anal area must be accompanied by careful digital examination of the anorectum to facilitate the detection of anorectal lesions. At this time anal tone may be assessed, but anal tone is poorly correlated with more objective measures of anal sphincter function.[47] This may relate to the fact that a denervated external anal sphincter does not readily atrophy.[28] Abdominal palpation assesses colonorectal content and bladder tone. Bladder tone may be altered by neurological lesions. The skin of the hind limbs should be carefully examined for areas of self trauma, which may be suggestive of paresthesias, and the dorsal lumbosacral skin and musculature should be palpated for evidence of hyperesthesia. Such hindlimb paresthesia and hyperesthesia are both suggestive of cauda equina syndrome.

Neurological Examination. A thorough neurological examination including observation of gait, cranial nerves, myotatic reflexes and postural reactions is an integral part of the work up. Depressed hind limb myotatic reflexes may occur with lumbosacral spinal lesions, cauda equina syndrome, polyneuropathies, neuromuscular junction diseases or myopathies.

Special attention should be paid to the presence or absence of the anal reflex, the rectal-inflation reflex, the pudendal-anal (bulbocavernosus) reflex, and the central recognition of perineal and anorectal sensation. The anal reflex is evaluated by pricking or pinching the perianal skin and looking for contraction of the anal sphincter. The rectal-inflation reflex is induced by inflating with 15-30 ml of air a Foley catheter that has been placed in the caudal extremity of the rectum. This induces anal contraction in both dogs and humans. The pudendal-anal reflex is evaluated by applying digital pressure to the penis while observing for anal contraction. All three reflexes assess sacral spinal segments, motor neurons in the pudendal nerves, and the external anal sphincter. The anal and pudendal-anal reflexes test perineal nerve afferents, whereas it is likely that the "rectal-inflation reflex" tests pelvic or S3 and C1 nerve afferents (Figure 23-2). These reflexes are usually preserved in patients with suprasacral spinal transverse myelopathies, whereas the conscious perception of perineal and anorectal sensation (induced by the inflated Foley catheter) is not.

Diagnostic Evaluations Proctoscopy with biopsy is indicated if reservoir incontinence is suspected. Radiography may reveal diseases of the vertebral column responsible for the incontinence. Myelography, epidurograms, and discography[50] are of value for the diagnosis of deforming lesions affecting the spinal cord and cauda equina. Electrodiagnostic evaluation of the fecal incontinent animal greatly facilitates diagnosis. Electromyographical examination of the continence muscles may reveal denervation or myopathy.[51] The clinical assessment of the pudendal-anal reflex can be made more objective by the electrophysiologic evaluation of the reflex.[52] The CSF examination may include a CSF distemper titer to assist diagnosis of canine distemper.

Treatment of Fecal Incontience. Before treatment of fecal incontinence is instituted, the veterinarian is prudent to discuss with the owner the public health risks of canine and feline feces. Therapy of fecal incontinence is more likely to be successful following identification and treatment, where possible, of the primary cause. For instance, resolution of the incontinence may follow successful treatment of diarrhea.[40,53] Symptomatic surgical therapy by way of implantation of a perianal silastic sling is of demonstrated value for the therapy of fecal incontinence in dogs.[54] Symptomatic medical management aims at reducing fecal water content, decreasing fecal bulk, slowing colonic transit time, and increasing external anal sphincter tone. The use of low residue diets such as cottage cheese and rice reduces fecal volume by up to 85%. They also reduce the frequency of defecation. Bowel transit time may be slowed by the use of opioids such as diphenoxylate or loperamide. These drugs also increase the tone of the anal sphincter in humans.[55] They may be given for prolonged periods with little development of tolerance to their effects.[55] A suggested dosage is: Diphenoxylate at 0.1 mg/kg or Loperamide at 0.08 mg/kg PO q 8h initially and to effect thereafter. It is possible to manage the occasional patient with a dedicated and competent owner by the use of daily warm water enemas administered in a place where defecation is appropriate. Many animals may be induced to defecate by the inflation of a Foley catheter in their rectums. This technique will not produce conscious defecation in animals with anorectal anesthesia but it will often produce involuntary rectal evacuation, a phenomenon also described in humans suffering from traumatic spinal lesions.[42]

In animals with chronic posterior paralysis due to spinal cord damage, a minor stimulus to the hind limbs or perineum, such as a light toe pinch or warm washcloth, may stimulate appropriate elimination (the mass reflex).

Proctitis

Proctitis, inflammation of the rectum, usually occurs in association with acute or chronic inflammatory bowel diseases of the colon. The rectal mucosa, essentially the same in structure as the colon, is subjected to greater numbers of bacteria, larger amounts of toxic substances, and greater abrasion by dehydrated fecal contents. Evaluation and treatment of inflammatory diseases are the same for the rectum as for the colon. Severe inflammatory processes that extend into the submucosa cause strictures to form. Some foreign objects can lacerate the rectal mucosa and lead to strictures. The stenotic areas can be surgically removed.

Rectal Prolapse

Rectal prolapse is occasionally seen in dogs and cats. It is particularly common in young animals and usually results from a secondary complication of diseases causing persistent diarrhea and tenesmus. It is occasionally observed as a complication of the megacolon syndrome in cats. On most occasions just the rectal mucosa prolapses, but occasionally the prolapsed segment involves the entire rectal wall. Prolapsed mucosa usually appears as a small rosette-like area of red and swollen mucosa in the anal canal. When the entire rectal wall is prolapsed, a tubular mass will be observed. The major differential diagnosis in the latter case is intussusception of a more proximal section of bowel through the anus. The two conditions are differentiated by use of a rectal probe. In the case of a proximal intussusception no rectal "cul-de-sac" will be encountered by a probe placed between the anal skin and the rectal prolapse. Small prolapses can usually be replaced manually. Lubrication and use of topical dessicants such as powdered dextrose may facilitate replacement. Once the prolapse is reduced it is usually held in place by way of a temporary purse string suture, and medical treatment is directed at any identifiable cause of tenesmus. Intrarectal administration of topical anesthetic ointments such as 1 per cent dibucaine (Nupercainal Ointment-Ciba) has been recommended in the immediate postoperative period.[56] More extensive prolapse, particularly if the tissue appears to have questionible viability, requires surgical excision of the mucosa or rectum.

Congenital Anorectal and Colon Disorders

Imperforate anus is a congenital disorder with a number of different causes that include persistence of the anal membrane, atresia ani, and rectal agenesis.[56] Imperforate anus results from abnormal embryological development. Atresia ani results from failure of the rectum and embryological cloaca to fuse. One proposed cause of rectal agenesis (atresia) is an *in utero* vascular accident.[57] There is little evidence that intestinal atresia is inherited.[57]

The deformity may be noticed within days of birth, or the owner may not realise there is a problem until the pup or kitten is several weeks old by which time constipation is marked, abdominal distension is apparent, and the neonate has lost its vigor. Radiography helps differentiate these three conditions by deliniating where the rectal gas shadow stops. The view of choice is a horizontal beam radiograph of the neonate suspended by its hind limbs. Treatment of a persistent anal membrane simply consists of perforating the anal membrane with an instrument such as a thermometer followed by trimming of the remaining tissue tags. Treatment of the other conditions involves more extensive surgery. The prognosis is favorable for imperforate anus and atresia ani, but is guarded for rectal agnesis.

Other anorectal deformities also occur in the neonate. Many of these conditions are associated with imperforate anus, such as anovaginal fistula, rectovaginal fistula, and rectourethral fistula.[58-60] Diagnosis of these disorders is usually made by physical examination and contrast radiography.

Other congenital abnormalities of the large bowel of dogs and cats include congenitally short colon,[61] colonic duplication,[62] and enterocyst formation.[63]

Anorectal Strictures

Anorectal strictures are uncommon in the dog and cat. They most commonly result from neoplasia and occasionally from severe inflammatory diseases of the large bowel or anus. They are a recognized complication of perianal fistula. The clinical signs usually pertain initially pertain to the primary disease process, and then are superceded by progressively greater tenesmus, dyschezia, and thinning of the diameter of the stool. Diagnosis may be made by digital palpation in many cases or by contrast radiography or proctoscopy. Treatment is surgical resection. Prognosis is guarded.

Anal Pruritis - Anal Sac Diseases

In dogs, anal pruritus is usually manifested by "scooting" of the perineal region on the ground, or frequent licking of the anal area. In cats, frequent licking of the anal area is seen. The most common cause in dogs is anal gland problems. Cats are rarely presented for anal gland impaction. The cause of impacted or inflammed anal sacs is usually not apparent. Occasionally the disorder is precipitated by a period of diarrhea during which incomplete evacuation of the sac results. It may also be a component of a generalized seborrheic disease.

Other postulated causes of perianal pruritis include tapeworm segments, irritant substances passed in the stool, and frequent perianal soiling by feces. Occasionally, perineal diseases such as perianal fistula, perianal dermatitis, fold pyodermas, vaginitis, and flea bite allergies may be apparent. When no specific cause can be determined, treatment considered should be regular baths or frequent gentle perianal washes (to minimize fecal soiling), a change of diet, and the discontinuation of any non-essential medications. Impacted anal sacs are usually evacuated by digital pressure. Concurrent anal saculitis may be treated by instillation of antibacterial-corticosteroid combinations such as Panalog into the anal sac. If repeated evacuations prove necessary chemical cautery with 1-2 ml of tincture of iodine or a variety of other chemical agents may be performed.[64] Alternatively, surgical resection may be undertaken.

Perianal Fistula

Perianal fistulas are chronic inflammatory lesions of the area around the anus. They are most frequently seen in the middle-aged to older German Shepherd dog and, to a lesser extent, in Irish Setters and Labradors but a wide variety of dog breeds and occasionally cats[65] can be affected. Perianal fistulas cause enough pain that the afflicted dogs usually cannot be examined without sedation. The owner is seldom able to examine the area under the tail. Clinical signs include licking of the anal area, and scooting to relieve the irritation, which may leave a discharge of pus or blood on the floor. More advanced cases show signs of dyschezia and tenesmus.

The cause of perianal fistulas is unknown. One proposed pathomechanism is fecolith impaction in the anal sinuses which is thought to eventually lead to pressure necrosis and fistulation. Another proposed cause is contamination of the hair follicles or anal, tubular, or sebaceous glands with a film of feces that eventually leads to infection and fistulation.[66] Detailed histopathological studies of the early lesions (see below) support this latter proposal as do some perculiarities of the German Shepherd breed. It is entirely possible that both pathomechanisms are operative.

The German Shepherd has a broad tail-base and a low tail carriage which predisposes it to the maintenance of a moist perianal fecal film in which bacteria can proliferate. In a detailed histological analysis of the perianal area of dogs, German Shepherds were noted to have an increase in density of apocrine sweat glands in the zona cutanea and increased evidence of chronic inflammation in the anal glands (modified tubuloalveolar sweat glands that ring the anal canal).[67] German Shepherds are predisposed to deep pyodermas in other parts of the body, and as a breed they are known to have low seum IgA levels, perhaps implying a deficient defence of cutaneous follicular structures. Of 5 consecutive German Shepherds presented to the UCD VMTH for perianal fistula, 3 were observed to have moderately low IgA levels (0.20-0.26 mg/dl).[27] In a more extensive evaluation of immune function in German Shepherds, however, only 2/15 dogs had a low serum IgA.[68] Lymphocytic blastogenesis tests were persistently abnormal in 5/33 dogs.[68] There is also a high incidence of concomitant diarrhea in affected dogs. This diarrhea often persists after surgical correction of the perianal disease. Thus, tenesmus caused by the anal problem is not the sole cause of the diarrhea. Colonic biopsy often identifies chronic colitis. This relationship raises the possibility of an immune-mediated cause for perianal fistulas. Alternatively, the chronic diarrhea may contribute to the condition by encouraging more frequent perianal soiling.

Perianal fistula lesions appear initially as small ulcerations in the perianal area, and when they are probed it is discovered that considerable adjacent subepithelial tissue is involved. In addition to the involvement of the subepithelial space, chronically infected tracts often extend into the loose tissue between the anal sphincters and the wall of the pelvis. Occasionally they can penetrate to depths cranial to both sphincters. The tracts do not usually penetrate the rectal mucosa, submucosa, or the anal sacs. In one study, histopathology of the anal area demonstrated five distinct lesions.[69] Four of these were relatively common and included hidradentitis of the cutaneous zone of the anal canal that was responsible for superficial cutaneous sinuses;

fistulae of the anal sinuses which extended either directly to the skin or into large perianal subcutaneous abscesses that in turn opened to the skin; rupture of the anal sac; and submucosal sinuses of the terminal third of the rectum. A less frequently observed lesion was rectal fistulation. In another study, early lesions were classified as inflammation associated with epidermal appendages; intermediate lesions were considered inflammation of the epidermal appengages in association with cutaneous ulceration and nonaborizing sinus tracts; and late lesions were described as aborizing epithelial-lined sinus tracts extending through the perirectal stroma.[70] Aerobic cultures of deep perianal tissues revealed bacterial growth in 85% of dogs with *E. coli* being the predominant isolate.

Antibiotic therapy of perianal fistulas at best only temporarily ameliorates the disease. The disease is managed surgically, although the best surgical technique remains mired in controversy. The most frequent complication is fecal incontience. In dogs with concomitant diarrhea, a colon biopsy should be obtained at the time of the surgical correction of the fistulas. If concurrent chronic colitis is present it should be managed by standard measures. Recurrence is common. The prognosis is guarded.

Perineal Hernia

Perineal hernias are a relatively common problem in the older male dog. The hernia results from age-related changes in the pelvic girdle, particularly the levator ani muscle. The presence of the hernia results in deviation of the rectum into the hernial sac and/or the development of a rectal diverticulum or sacculation in which fecal material collects. The result is tenesmus, dyschezia, and constipation. Incaceration of the bladder in the hernial sac can result in more severe clinical signs. The diagnosis is usually made by physical examination of the perineal area which reveals a fluctuant swelling lateral to the anus. The process is usually unilateral, but bilateral hernias can occur. The treatment is surgical.

REFERENCES

1. Williams, D.A. and Burrows, C.F.: Short-bowel syndrome - a case report in a dog and discussion of the pathophysiology of bowel resection. J. Sm. An. Pract. 22:263-275, 1981.
2. Marks, A.: Torsion of the colon in a rough collie. Vet. Rec. 118:400, 1986.
3. Endres, W.A., Remondini, D.J. and Graver, E.R.: A case report of torsion of the descending colon in a six-minth-old female collie. VM/SAC 954, 1968.
4. Robinson, J.W.L., Haroud, M., Winistorfer, B. and Mirkovitch, V.: Recovery of function and structure of dog ileum and colon following two hours acute ischaemia. Eur.J. Clin. Invest. 4:443-452, 1974.
5. Robinson, J.W.L., Menge, H., Sepulveda, F.V., Cobo, F., and Mirkovitch, V.: The functional response of the dog ileum to one hour's ischaemia. Clin. Sci. Mol. Med. 50:115-122, 1976.
6. Robinson, J.W.L. and Mirkovitch, V.: The recovery of function and microcirculation in small intestinal loops following ischaemia. Gut 13:784-789, 1972.
7. Hosgood, G. and Salisbury, K.: Generalized peritonitis in dogs: 50 cases (1975-1986). JAVMA 193:1448-1450, 1988.
8. Toombs, J.P., Collins, L.G., Graves, G.M., Crowe, D.T. and Caywood, D.D.: Colonic perforation in corticosteroid-treated dogs. JAVMA 188:145-150, 1986.
9. Moore, M.P. and Robinette, J.D.: Cecal perforation and adrenocortical adenoma in a dog. JAVMA 191:87-88, 1987.
10. Sorjonen, D.C., Dillon, A.R., Powers, R.D. and Spano, J.S.: Effects of dexamethasone and surgical hypotension on the stomach of dogs: clinical, endoscopic, and pathologic evaluations. AJVR 44:1233-1237, 1983.
11. Dow, S.W., Rosychuk, R.A., McChesney, A.E. and Curtis, C.R.: Adverse effects of flunixin meglumine, administered with and without prednisone on the gastrointestinal tract of dogs. Proc. 7th ACVIM forum, 1045, 1989.
12. Greenfield, C.L. and Walshaw, R.: Open peritoneal drainage for treatment of contaminated peritoneal cavity and septic peritonitis in dogs and cats: 24 cases (1980-1986). JAVMA 191:100-105, 1987.
13. Orsher, R.J. and Rosin, E.: Open peritoneal drainage in experimental peritonitis in dogs. Vet. Surg. 222-226, 1984
14. Woolfson, J.M. and Dulisch, M.L.: Open abdominal drainages in the treatment of generalized peritonitis in 25 dogs and cats. Vet. Surg. 15:27-32, 1986.
15. Green, C.E.: Gastrointestinal intra-abdominal, and hepatobiliary infections. In, Clinical Microbiology and Infectious Diseases. WB Saunders, Philadelphia, 247-268, 1984.
16. Levine, S.H.: Ruptured cecum due to abscessation in a dog. A case report. JAAHA 18:337-?, 1982.
17. Miller, W.W., Hathcock, J.T. and Dillon, A.R.: Cecal inversion in eight dogs. JAAHA 20:1009-1013, 1983.
18. Bush, B.M.: Colitis in the dog. Vet. Ann. 25:337-347, 1985.
19. Burrows, C.F.: Diseases of the colon rectum and anus in the dog and cat. In, Veterinary Gastroenterology. Edited by Anderson, N.V. Lea & Febiger, Philadelphia, 553-592, 1980.
20. Sack, T.L. and Sleisenger, M.H.: Effects of systemic and extraintestinal diseases on the gut. In, Gastrointestinal Pathophysiology Diagnosis and Management. 4th edition. W.B. Saunders, Philadelphia 488-528, 1989.
21. Leib, M.S.: Dietary fiber and large bowel diarrhea. 359-360. Proc. of 7th ACVIM Forum, 1989.
22. Bo-Linn, G.W., Vendrell, D.D., Lee, E. and Fordtran, J.S.: An evaluation of the significance of microscopic colitis in patients with chronic diarrhea. J. Clin. Invest. 75:1559-1569, 1985.
23. Rampton, D.S. and Baithun, S.I.: Is microscopic colitis due to bile-salt malabsorption? Dis. Colon Rectum 30:950-952, 1987.
24. Schuster, M.M.: Motor action of rectum and anal sphincters incontinence and defecation. In, Handbook of Physiology. Sec. 6, alimentary canal, Vol 4. Edited by C.F. Code, American Physiological Society, Washington, DC, 1968, 2121-2146.
25. Burrows, C.F.: Constipation. In, Current Veterinary Therapy IX. Edited by Kirk, R.W. WB Saunders, Philadelphia, 905-908, 1986.
26. Atkins, C.E.: Hypertonic sodium phosphate enema intoxication. In, Current Veterinary Therapy IX. Edited by Kirk, R.W. WB Saunders, Philadelphia, 213-216, 1986.
27. Guilford, W.G.: Unpublished observations. 1987.
28. Gaston, E.A.: The physiology of fecal continence. Surg. Gynecol. Obstet. 87:280-290, 1948.
29. Gaston, E.A.: Physiological basis for the preservation of fecal continence after resection of rectum. JAMA 146:1486-1489, 1951.
30. Karlan, M., McPherson, R.C. and Watman, R.N.: An experimental evaluation of fecal continence- sphincter- and reservoir- in the dog. Surg. Gynecol. Obstet. 108:469-475, 1959.
31. Scharli, A.F., Kiesewetter, W.B.: Defecation and continence: Some new concepts. Dis. Colon Rectum 13:81-107, 1970.
32. Parks, A.: Anorectal incontinence. Proc. Royal Soc. Med. 68:681-690, 1975.
33. Duthie, H.L. and Bennett, R.C.: The relationship of sensation in the anal canal to the functional anal sphincter: A possible factor in anal continence. Gut 4:179-182, 1963.
34. De Lahunta, A.: Veterinary Neuroanatomy and Clinical Neurology. 1st edition. Philadelphia, WB Saunders Co, 288-295, 1977.
35. Martin, W.D., Fletcher, T.F. and Bradley, W.E.: Innervation of

feline perineal musculature. Anat. Rec. 180:15-30, 1974.
36. Evans, H.E. and Christensen, G.C.: Miller's Anatomy of the Dog. 2nd edition. Philadelphia, WB Saunders Co, 331-337, 1979.
37. De Lahunta, A.: Veterinary Neuroanatomy and Clinical Neurology. 1st edition. Philadelphia, WB Saunders Co, 110-124, 1977.
38. Shafik, A.: A new concept of the anatomy of the anal sphincter mechanism and the physiology of defecation. Investigative Urology 12:412-419, 1975.
39. Ashdown, R.R.: Symposium on canine recto-anal disorders. 1. Clinical anatomy. J. Sm. An. Pract. 9:315-322, 1968.
40. Duthie, H.L.: Anal continence. Gut 12:844-852, 1971.
41. Wunderlich, M. and Parks, A.G.: Physiology and pathophysiology of the anal sphincters. Int. Surg. 67:291-298, 1982.
42. Frenckner, B.: Function of the anal sphincters in man. Gut 16:638-644, 1975.
43. Strombeck, D.R. and Harrold, D.: Anal sphincter pressure and the rectosphincteric reflex in the dog. AJVR 49:191-192, 1988.
44. Schuster, M.M.: Tests related to the colon, rectum, and anus. In, Gastroenterology. 4th edition. Edited by J.E. Berk. WB Saunders Co, Philadelphia, Chapter 28, 388-401, 1985.
45. Phillips, S.F. and Edwards, D.A.W.: Some aspects of anal continence and defaecation. Gut 6:396-406, 1965.
46. Goldberg, S.M.: Anal incontinence. In. Essentials of Anorectal Surgery. Edited by Goldbery, S.M., Gordon, P.H., Nivatongs, S. Lippincott, 282-290, 1980.
47. Read, N.W., Harford, W.V., Schmulen, C.A., Read, M.G., Santa Ana, C. and Fordtran, J.S.: A clinical study of patients with fecal incontinence and diarrhea. Gastroenterology 76: 747-756, 1979.
48. Schoetz, D.J.: Operative therapy for anal incontinence. Surg. Clin. N. Am. 65:35-46, 1985.
49. De Groat, W.C. and Booth, A.M.: Autonomic systems to the urinary bladder and sexual organs. In, Peripheral Neuropathy. 2nd edition. Edited by Dyck, P.J.,
50. Morgan, J.P.: Vertebral column. In, Radiology in Veterinary Orthopedics. Lea & Febiger, Chapt 4, 1972.
51. Swash, M.: Anorectal incontinence: electrophysiological tests. Br. J. Surg. 72:Suppl s14-s15, 1985.
52. O'Brien, D.P. and Dean, P.W.: Pudendo-anal (bulbocavernosus) reflex electrophysiology in the dog. Abstract ACVIM Proc. 1988.
53. Pemberton, J.H. and Kelly, K.A.: Achieving enteric continence: Principles and applications. Mayo. Clin. Proc. 61:586-599, 1986.
54. Dean, P.W., O'Brien, D.P., Turk, A.M., and Bajrab, J.M.: SilasticR sling for fecal incontinence. Submitted to Vet. Surg., 1988.
55. Jaffe, J.H. and Martin, W.R.: Opioid analgesics and antagonists. In, The Pharmacological Basis of Therapeutics. 7th edition. Edited by Goodman, Gilman A., Goodman, L.S. Macmillan, New York, Pg 503, 1985.
56. Seim, H.B.: Diseases of the anus and rectum. In, Current Veterinary Therapy IX. Edited by Kirk, R.W. W.B. Saunders, Philadelphia, 916-921, 1986.
57. Johnson, R.: Intestinal atresia and stenosis: A review comparing its etiopathogenesis. Vet. Res. Commun. 10:95-105, 1986.
58. Amand, W.B.: Nonneurogenic disorders of the anus and rectum. Vet. Clin. N. Am. 4:535-551, 1974.
59. Osborne, C.A., Engen, M.H. and Yano, B.L.: Congenital urethrorectal fistula in two dogs. JAVMA 166: 999-?, 1975.
60. Rawlings, C.A. and Capps, W.S.: Rectovaginal fistula and imperforate anus in a dog. JAVMA 159:320-326 1971.
61. Fluke, M.H., Hawkins, E.C., Elliot, G.S. and Belvins, W.E.: Short colon in cats and a dog. JAVMA 195:87-90, 1989.
62. Jakowski, R.M.: Duplication of colon in a Labrador Retriever with abnormal spinal column. Vet. Pathol. 14:256-260, 1977.
63. Runyon, C.L., Merkley, D.F. and Hagemoser, W.A.: Intussusception associatedwith a paracolonic enterocyt in a dog. JAVMA 185:443, 1984.
64. Halnan, C.R.E.: Therapy of anal sacculitis in the dog. J. Sm. An. Pract. 17:685-691, 1976.
65. Johnson, M.E.: Perianal fistula-like disease in a cat. Comp. An. Prac. 1:16-19, 1987.
66. Harvey, C.E. Perianal Fistula in the dog. Vet Rec. 91:25-32, 1972.
67. Budsberg, S.C., Spurgeon, T.L. and Liggitt, H.D.: Anatomic predisposition to perianal fistulae formation in the German Shepherd Dog. AJVR 46:1468-1472, 1985.
68. Killingsworth, C.R., Walshaw, R., Reimann, K.A. and Rosser, E.J.: Thyroid and immunologic status of dogs with perianal fistula. AJVR 49:1742-1746, 1988.
69. Johnston, D.E.: Rectum and anus: Surgical diseases In, Textbook of Small Animal Surgery. Edited by Slatter, D.H. W.B. Saunders, Philadelphia, 770-794, 1985.
70. Killingsworth, C.R., Walshaw, R., Dunstan, R.W. and Rosser, E.J.: Bacterial population and histologic changes in dogs with perianal fistula. AJVR 49:1736-1741, 1988.

Chapter 24

Neoplasms of the Gastrointestinal Tract, APUD Tumors, Endocrinopathies and the Gastrointestinal Tract

NEOPLASMS OF THE GASTROINTESTINAL TRACT[1-4]

Incidence of Gastrointestinal Tumors

Neoplasms of the gastrointestinal tract of small animals occur infrequently compared to neoplasms in other body systems. At the VMTH at Davis the incidence of all intestinal and rectal tumors is 9.9 cases per 10,000 in the dog and 8.8 cases per 10,000 in the cat. Tumors of the canine and feline esophagus are very rare, accounting for less than 1 per cent of all neoplasms and less than 5 percent of gastrointestinal tract neoplasms.[4] Similarly, gastric cancer is uncommon in the dog accounting for less than 1 percent of all neoplasms.[4] In the cat, gastric cancer is relatively more common because of the high incidence of lymphosarcoma. In the dog, neoplasms of the small intestine are less frequently recognized than those of the stomach or colonorectum, but in the cat neoplasms occur more frequently in the small intestine.[1] In the intestine of the dog, the most common sites for intestinal cancer are the rectum, colon, and duodenum. Tumors of the large intestine represent 36-60 percent of all canine gastrointestinal tract neoplasms and 10-15 percent of all feline gastrointestinal neoplasms. The incidence of large bowel neoplasms is greatest in the rectum. The respective incidences of tumors of the colon and rectum in the dogs presented to the VMTH are 2.8 and 4.1 per 10,000. These data are similar to findings elsewhere.[5-7]

The majority of intestinal neoplasms are malignant types, such as lymphosarcoma, adenocarcinomas, leiomyosarcomas, and hemangiosarcomas. The most common benign tumors include leiomyomas, adenomas, fibromas, and adenomatous polyps. Less frequent intestinal tumors include plasmacytomas,[8] fibrosarcomas,[2] ganglioneuromas,[9] and neurilemmomas.[10]

About one-fourth of all tumors are found in each of the 4-to-7 year and 7-to-10 year age groups, with the remaining half found in dogs 10 to 15 years old.

Location of Gastrointestinal Tumors

The relative frequency of occurrence of different types of tumor varies according to site in the bowel. In the dog, the most frequent oropharyngeal neoplasm is melanoma followed in incidence by squamous cell carcinoma, fibrosarcoma, and epulides. In the feline oropharynx, the neoplasm with the highest incidence is the squamous cell carcinoma. About 50% of all feline oral neoplasms occur in the tongue.

In the esophagus of dogs, the most common neoplasm in endemic areas is esophageal sarcoma associated with *Spirocerci lupi*. Other reported esophageal neoplasms in the dog and cat include squamous cell carcinoma, undifferentiated carcinoma, leiomyoma, osteosarcoma, and fibrosarcoma.[1] Leiomyomas occurring at the gastroesophageal junction are a relatively common esophageal tumor. The occurrence appears age-related with the incidence reaching 80% in 17-18 year old beagles.[11]

In the stomach of dogs, gastric carcinoma is the most frequent tumor, whereas in the stomach of cats lymphosarcoma is most frequent. In the intestine of dogs intestinal lymphosarcomas are most commonly recognized, with adenocarcinomas and smooth muscle tumors also having a relatively high prevalence. In the small intestine of cats lymphosarcoma is the most common neoplasm, followed by adenocarcinoma (particularly of the ileum). The duodenum of both species is more likely to be invaded by carcinomas from other organs such as the pancreas and liver, than to develop primary neoplasia. In the large bowel of dogs, the most frequent neoplasm is adenocarcinoma. In the cat, lymphosarcoma is the most common neoplasm of the large bowel, followed in frequency by adenocarcinoma.

Etiopathogenesis of Gastrointestinal Tumors[12]

The cause of gastrointestinal neoplasia in rarely evident with the exception of *Spirocerca lupi*-induced esophageal sarcoma. Other postulated causes are listed in Table 24-1.

Clinical Findings and Evaluation of Gastrointestinal Neoplasia

A variety of clinical signs can accompany gastrointestinal neoplasia. The signs may result from the local "mass effect" of the tumor, whereupon the clinical manifestation is primarily dependent on the site of the tumor in the intestinal tract. Thus the most prominent manifestation of esophageal neoplasia is regurgitation, that of gastric neoplasia is vomiting, that of small intestinal neoplasia is small bowel-type diarrhea with or without vomiting, and that of large bowel neoplasia is large bowel-type diarrhea. Alternatively, the clinical signs may result from metastatic lesions. Examples include the compression of adjacent organs by expansive lymph nodes, or infiltration of distant organs such as the liver, spleen, and central nervous system producing dysfunction of these organs and signs such as jaun-

Table 24-1. Postulated Predisposing Causes of Gastrointestinal Neoplasia

Esophageal Sarcoma	**Gastric Carcinoma**
Spirocerca lupi	dietary carcinogens (mycotoxins, nitrosamines)
chronic esophagitis	gastritis
thermal injury	gastric polyps
Colonorectal Adenocarcinoma	achlorhydria
polyposis	nitrosamines
chronic colitis	**Alimentary Lymphosarcoma**
low fiber diets	FeLV
high fat diets	lymphocytic-plasmacytic enteritis
bile salt malabsorption	

dice, abdominal hemorrhage, and seizures. Moreover, clinical signs can result from paraneoplastic syndromes such as the hypercalcemia of apocrine adenocarcinoma, resulting in bowel stasis and renal disease. Diagnosis of gastrointestinal neoplasia follows the principles outlined in the chapter on the approach to gastrointestinal problems. It is important to remember that not all nodular lesions of the gastrointestinal tract need be neoplastic. Differentials include granulomas from inflammatory bowel disease, fungal infections, or foreign body penetration.

Neoplasms of the Small Intestine

Clinical Signs. Prominent clinical signs of small intestinal neoplasia are chronic diarrhea, vomiting, inappetence, and weight loss. The characteristics of the diarrhea and accompanying secondary signs such as borborygmus, and weight loss often support a disease process causing malassimilation. The pathogenesis of the malassimilation is probably multifactorial, but may include defective diffusion of nutrients through the bowel wall because of widespread mucosal tumor infiltration, bacterial overgrowth as a result of deranged intestinal motility and partial obstruction, and maldigestion as a result of bacterial overgrowth and functional pancreatic insufficiency. Occasionally, animals will present with a history of a slowly progressive increase in vomiting frequency. This history is also compatible with inflammatory bowel disease, but if the vomitus becomes odiferous and of large volume, an obstructive neoplasm such as annular adenocarcinoma should be suspected. Not infrequently, melena may be observed, and abdominal masses or thickened intestines palpated. Rarely, the initial presentation is acute abdomen as a result of intestinal perforation.

Diagnosis. Laboratory evidence of blood loss, protein-losing enteropathy, bacterial overgrowth, maldigestion, or malabsorption may be apparent. Contrast radiographic studies, particularly enteroclysis, may reveal mucosal abnormalities or obstructive lesions. Ultrasonography is a major advance in the diagnosis of gastrointestinal neoplasia. The ultrasonographic appearance of gastrointestinal neoplasms in the dog has recently been described.[14] Ultrasonography may reveal bowel thickenings, localized ileus, or enlarged mesenteric nodes. Enlarged mesenteric nodes are highly suggestive of neoplasia but can also occur with other conditions (Table 24-2).

Diagnosis is usually made by ultrasound-guided aspiration of enlarged lymph nodes, percutaneous or ultrasound-guided aspiration of abdominal masses, or intestinal biopsy via endoscopy or celiotomy. Placement of a gastrostomy tube for purposes of nutritional support should be considered at the time of intestinal biopsy in inappetant animals. Occasionally, histological differentiation of lymphosarcoma and lymphocytic-plasmacytic enteritis is difficult.[15]

Treatment and Prognosis. If the process is localized to one segment of the bowel, surgical resection is indicated. If metastasis has occurred, a systemic treatment such as chemotherapy must be selected. Because of the complexities of chemotherapeutic usage and the inherent danger to patient, owner, and veterinary staff, the veterinarian interested in administering chemotherapeutic agents should do so only after consulting with a veterinary oncologist or reading recent in depth reviews on the subject of cancer therapy.[1,4,13] The prognosis for all non-resectable gastrointestinal neoplasia is guarded to poor.

Neoplasms of the Large Intestine[8,16]

Clinical Signs. The clinical signs associated with colonic and rectal neoplasia are essentially the same as with inflammatory and obstructive diseases of those organs. The signs are caused by neoplastic invasion of the bowel wall that causes stricture formation and obstruction (Figure 24-1). Neoplasms cause the mucosa to become friable, subject to bleeding, and easily infected (Figure 24-2). Adenocarcinomas spreading from the colon into adjacent blood vessels and lymphatics sometimes obstruct regional circulation to cause marked edema of the inguinal area and the rear legs. This may develop before signs of intestinal disease appear.

Diagnosis. The clinical and physical findings are evaluated with proctoscopy or colonoscopy of the rectum and colon. Many large bowel neoplasms are detectable by digital examination and most are within view of a proctoscope. In the absence of an endoscope, radiographic studies using positive- and double contrast methods are sometimes useful in gaining more information on colonic lesions (Figure 24-3).

Treatment and Prognosis. The treatment of colonorectal neoplasia is surgical (adenocarcinoma) or medical (lymphoma). The prognosis is guarded. Mean survival time for malignant tumors of the rectal wall irrespective of tumor type was 6.9 months in one study.[16]

Table 24-2. Causes of Mesenteric Lymphadenopathy

Reactive Lymph Node	**Lymphadenitis**
lymphocytic-plasmacytic enteritis (mild lymphadenopathy)	salmon poisoning
	Salmonella sp
	Campylobacter sp
eosinophilic enteritis	*Ehrlichia*
idiopathic	FIP
Neoplasia	*Leishmania*
lymphosarcoma	histoplasmosis
mast cell neoplasia	*Mycobacterium*
metastatic adenocarcinoma	parvovirus
metastatic leiomyosarcoma	protothecosis
other neoplasia	*Yersinia pseudotuberculosis*
	zygomycosis
	other enteric pathogens

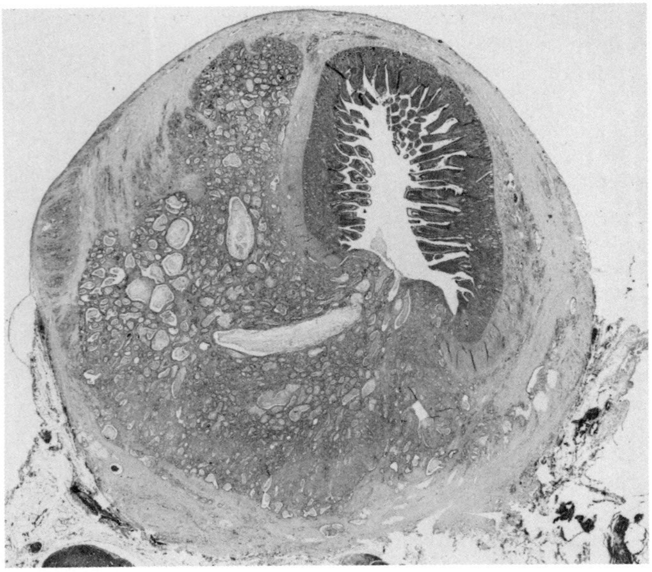

Figure 24-1. Adenocarcinoma of jejunum. (cat) (neoplastic involvement of greater part of circumference produces partial obstruction which usually causes diarrhea.

Alimentary Lymphosarcoma

Several recent reviews provide detailed discussion of gastrointestinal lymphosarcoma.[13,15-18] Lymphopoietic neoplasms are classified as alimentary lymphosarcoma if the involved organs are restricted to the mesenteric nodes, intestine, liver, kidney, and spleen. Alimentary lymphosarcoma constitutes 36 percent of feline lymphosarcoma and 7 percent of canine lymphosarcoma. The intestinal tract can also be affected by multicentric lymphosarcoma which comprises 18 percent of feline lymphosarcoma and 84 percent of canine lymphosarcoma.

Lymphosarcoma can occur at any site along the length of the gastrointestinal tract. The neoplasm may appear as a solitary mass, a generalized diffuse thickening of the wall, and perhaps as "skip" lesions. Lymphosarcoma is the most common cause of small intestinal neoplasia. In cats it is particularly common at the ileocolic junction. Concomitant involvement of other organs resulting in hepatosplenomegaly is frequent, and a variety of paraneoplastic findings and extraintestinal manifestations may be apparent. Occasionally lymphoblasts will be seen in peripheral blood, especially if a buffy coat examination is performed.

Treatment of the localized form is usually by surgical resection followed by adjuvant chemotherapy. The generalized form is treated by combination chemotherapy only. A popular

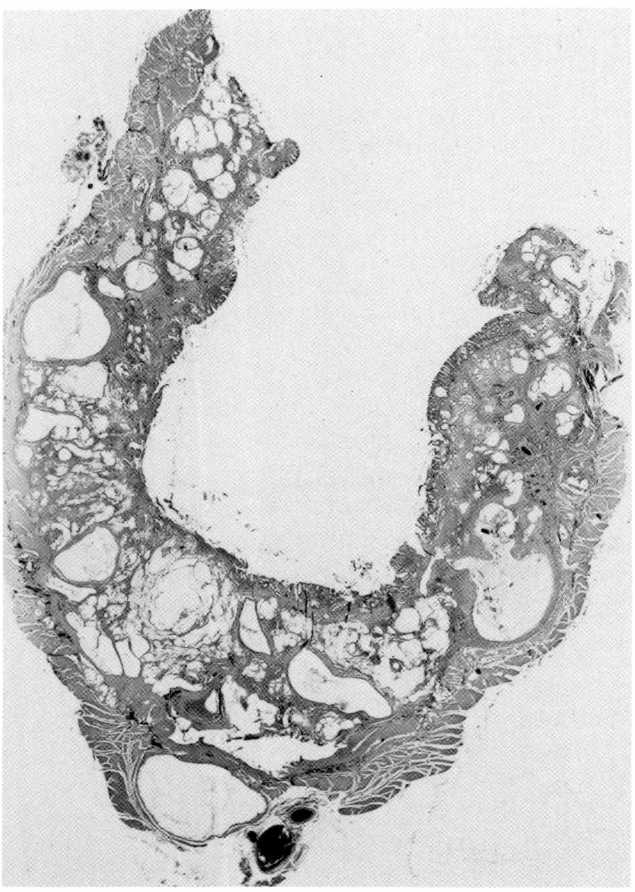

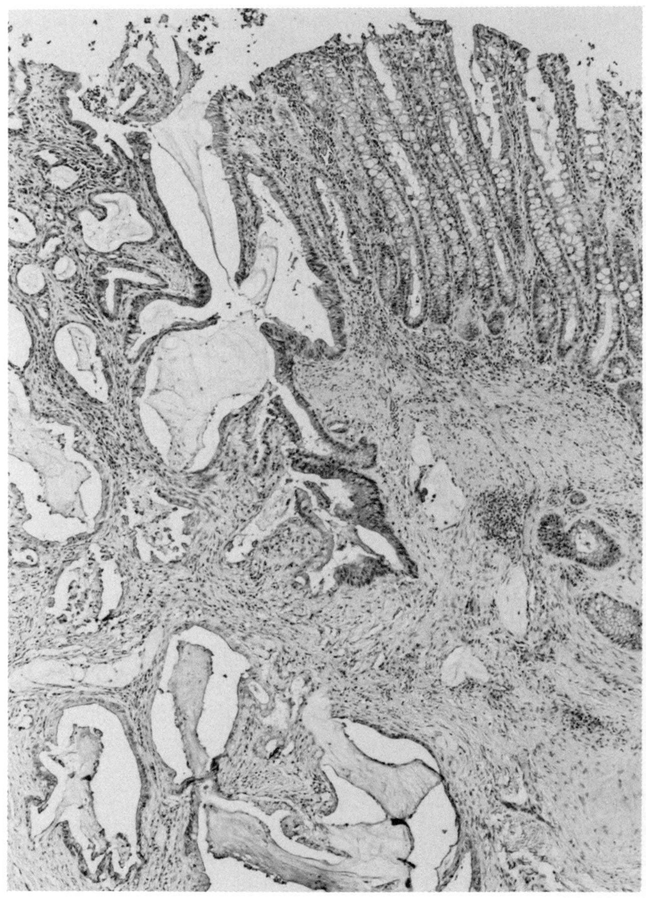

Figure 24-2. Adenocarcinoma of colon (a and b). Neoplastic involvement of wall of colon has resulted in loss of normal mucosa on left side (b).

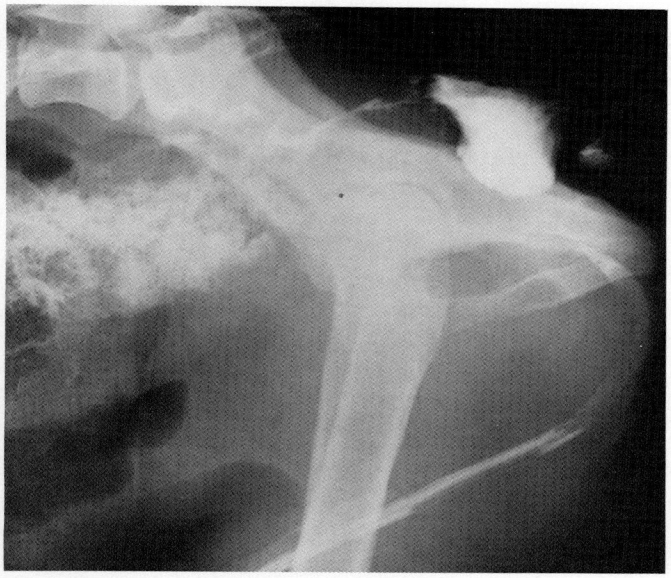

Figure 24-3a. Lateral radiograph of a 9-year-old German Shepherd that presented with signs of tenesmus and chronic diarrhea. Rectal examination revealed a stricture, the length of which could not be determined. Positive contrast medium was introduced into the rectum with a bulb syringe. The mural lesion produced a "ring like" constriction of the rectum. A urethrogram done at this time revealed that the suspected tumor did not involve the urethra. Biopsy identified the cause of the stricture to be an adenocarcinoma.

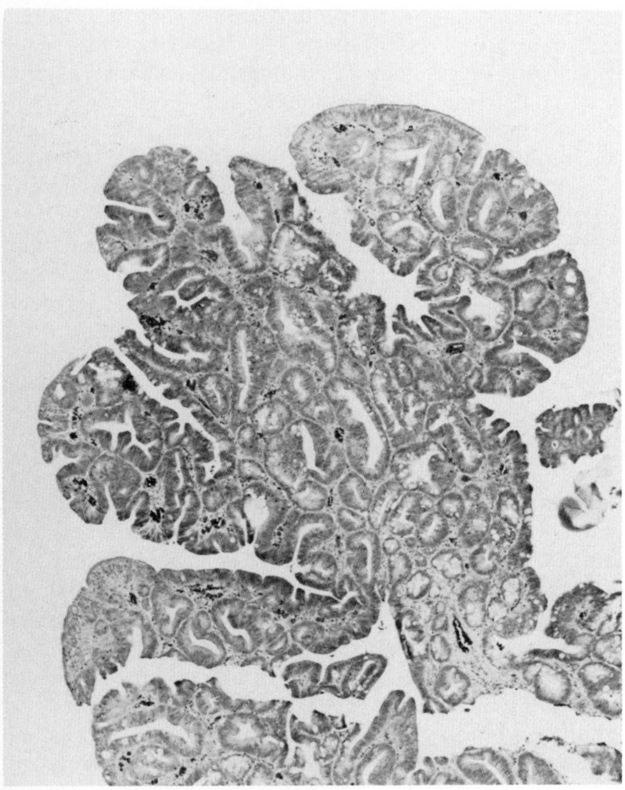

Figure 24-3c. Adenoma of colon. Epithelium is tall columnar, cells are hyperchromatic with large nuclei and several with mitotic figures. There was no evidence for invasion through the basement membrane.

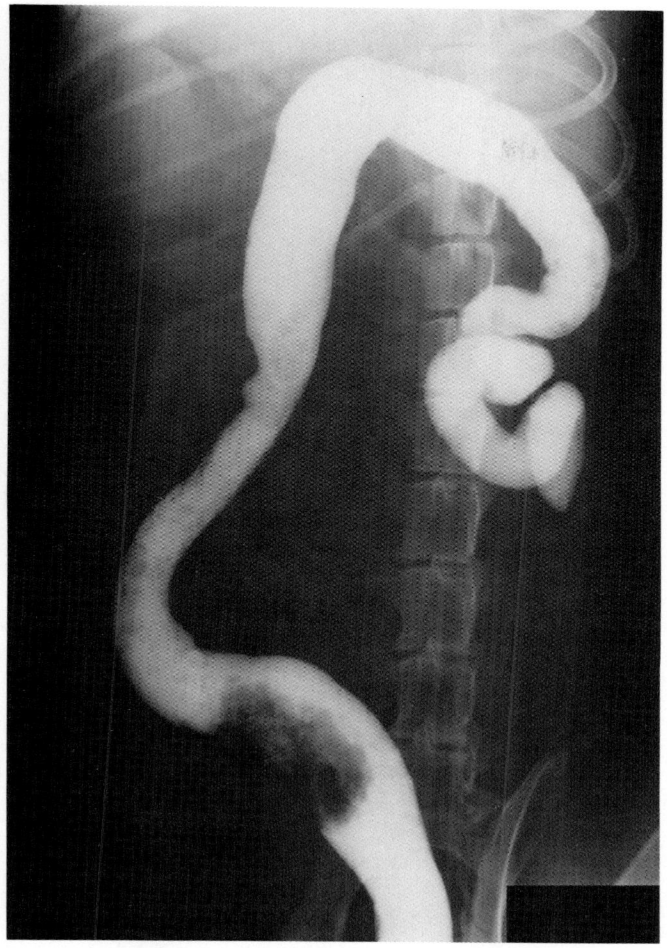

Figure 24-3b. Dorsoventral radiograph of an 8-year-old Airedale Terrier with chronic signs of passing blood in the feces. Proctoscopy was done but with its use the dimensions of the lesion and its involvement could not be ascertained. A barium enema revealed a mural lesion that invades the lumen. The lesion is pedunculated and creates an intraluminal mass. The filling defects proximal to the lesion are due to an inability to completely clean the bowel. The mass was an adenoma which was surgically resected.

drug combination is cyclophosphamide, vincristine, and prednisone.[13,16] Alimentary lymphosarcoma is considered more refractory than multicentric lymphosarcoma. In view of this observation, doxorubicin is sometimes included in the combination protocol.[15] The disease has a guarded prognosis. Response rates of 30-60% can be expected with median remissions of 4-5 months reported.[4,18]

Gastrointestinal Mast Cell Neoplasia[1,19,20]

Visceral mastocytosis is uncommon in the dog but is seen with reasonable frequency in cats. Occasionally the viscera become involved in systemic mastocytosis. Clinical signs most often include vomiting, diarrhea, and weight loss. The diagnosis is made by finding large numbers of mast cells in a peripheral smear or buffy coat, or in a bone marrow, spleen, liver, or mass aspirate. Mast cell tumors appear anywhere throughout the small intestine as segmental thickenings of the gut. Occasionally, they will occur in the colon. They commonly infiltrate the liver and spleen. Prolonged survival times have been reported following splenectomy to remove part of the tumor burden, prednisone therapy (as a chemotherapeutic), and H_2 receptor blockers to limit histamine induced gastric acid secretion. The prognosis remains poor.

Intestinal Adenocarcinoma

Intestinal adenocarcinoma is the most common large bowel neoplasm of the dog and cat.[2] Adenocarcinoma is also a common tumor of the lower small intestine of the cat, particularly the Siamese breed.[21,22] They are most often seen in the older animal, but dogs as young as 2 years have been afflicted with large bowel adenocarcinoma.[23] Adenocarcinoma of the small intestine tends to be annular and produce intestinal obstruction after a sometimes prolonged period (weeks) of vague inappetence and lethargy. Large bowel adenocarcinoma more often manifests as rectal bleeding with or without tenesmus and dyschezia. Gross appearance of adenocarcinomas is variable. They may appear as an expansive, plaque-like, ulcerated masses; they may invade adjacent bowel walls producing an annular or fusiform obstruction; they may cause discrete ulcers; or may diffusely invade the submucosa without causing obstruction. Metastasis to mesenteric lymph nodes is common in cats but need not necessarily warrant a poor prognosis.[21]

Recent reviews of gastrointestinal adenocarcinomas have been published.[21-23] Treatment of localized disease is by surgical excision. Pelvic splitting can usually be avoided by appropriate technique. Single high-dose radiation therapy has been reported to be effective.[50] If sublumbar or mesenteric metastasis is apparent, adjuvant chemotherapy can be attempted but is rarely successful.

Prognosis is guarded. Local recurrence or distant metastasis can occur as late as 1 year after excision.[4] Polypoid forms of adenocarcinoma have a better prognosis than annular lesions.[23] Long term survival is common if patients with slow-growing adenocarcinomas survive the immediate post-operative period.[21]

Smooth Muscle Tumors[2,4,24]

Leiomyomas and leiomyosarcomas can appear at any level of the gastrointestinal tract, but sites of predeliction include the gastroesophageal junction (leiomyomas), and jejunum and cecum (leiomyosarcomas). They usually are single nodules that may eventually produce clinical signs through causing obstruction or perforation. Treatment is by surgical resection. Prognosis is good with leiomyomas and guarded with leiomyosarcomas. Fortunately, leiomyosarcomas are slow to metastasize, and long term survival after resection is not uncommon.[24]

Intestinal Polyps

Hyperplastic polyps can occur in the stomach, duodenum, and rectum of dogs.[2] Rectal polyps are the most common.[8,16,25,26] Most canine rectal polyps are benign although precancerous polyps have been reported.[16,27] Large polyps are particularly likely to be precancerous. They appear as friable, lobulated sessile or pedunculated growths protruding from the rectal mucosa. Sometimes they can be associated with chronic inflammation. Polyps may be single or multiple. They are most often located in the distal rectum and may protrude through the anal canal during defecation. Hematochezia is a common sign. The cause of polypoid growths is usually unknown. The treatment is surgical. Pelvic splitting is usually not necessary. The prognosis is good but local recurrence is common.[16]

Apocrine Adenocarcinomas

Apocrine adenocarcinomas are malignant tumors of the anal sacs. They are most common in older spayed females. They should be differentiated from benign perianal adenomas which are almost exclusively seen in older, uncastrated males. Apocrine adenocarcinomas often produce hypercalcemia due to the secretion of a parathyroid hormone-like substance. The presenting signs most often pertain to the hypercalcemia rather than the perianal mass. Signs include weakness, anorexia, constipation, polyuria, and polydipsia. The prognosis is guarded. Local recurrence can occur and metastasis to the regional lymph nodes occurs in approximately 50% of the dogs.[16]

AMINE PRECURSOR UPTAKE AND DECARBOXYLATION CELLTUMORS[28-31]

Amine precursor uptake and decarboxylation (APUD) cells are a diffuse system of endocrine cells that have in common certain cytochemical, ultrastructural, and metabolic features that allows them to secrete biogenic amines from amino acid precursors. Most APUD cells share a common neuroectodermal source. They often retain the ability to secrete more than one hormone.[32] They are found in many organs of the body including the pituitary gland, intestine, pancreas, adrenal medulla, and thyroid. These features of APUD cells are responsible for the potent secretory function of many APUD tumors and for the occasional development of concomitant neoplasia at apparently disparate sites. The latter syndromes are referred to as the multiple endocrine neoplasm syndromes.

APUD tumors are rare neoplasms in the dog and cat. Those that have been reported include insulinomas, gastrinomas, pheochromocytomas, thyroid medullary carcinoma, a pancreatic polypeptide secreting tumor, and carcinoid tumors of the small intestine.

Gastrinomas (Zollinger-Ellison Syndrome)

Gastrinomas are rare neoplasms in the dog and cat. Detailed description is provided elsewhere.[28,29,33-35] They are most common in older dogs although a dog as young as 3.5 years has been affected. The gastrin-secreting tumor is usually located in the pancreas. The clinical signs include vomiting, weight loss, anorexia, and diarrhea particularly with steatorrhea. Hematemesis, melena, abdominal pain, and polydipsia may be seen. Gastroduodenal ulceration is common. Ulcers of the esophagus and jejunum may also be seen. Diagnosis is usually made by exploratory celiotomy which on most occasion reveals a small pancreatic nodule with metastases to the liver. High gastrin levels support but do not confirm a diagnosis. Provocative testing with calcium or secretin, or the assessment of gastric pH, may enhance the discriminatory value of the serum gastrin (see Chapter 6). Treatment is usually palliative because of early metastasis. Therapy includes surgical removal of visible tumor, and administration of H_2 receptor blockers to decrease gastric acid secretion. Treatment with a somatostatin analogue provided successful palliation in one dog. The prognosis is poor. Expected survival is less than 5 months.

Carcinoid Tumors of the Stomach and Intestine

These tumors have been reported infrequently in the dog and cat.[2,4,36,37] They arise from enterochromaffin cells, which produce a variety of vasoactive amines capable of producing secretory diarrhea. Most carcinoids reported to date in dogs and cats have been clinically silent.[30]

Pancreatic Polypeptide Secreting Pancreatic Tumor

A pancreatic polypeptide secreting adenocarcinoma in a dog has been reported.[38] Associated clinical signs were chronic vomiting, anorexia, and weight loss. The tumor was metastatic and was associated with duodenal ulcers.

ENDOCRINOPATHIES AND THE GASTROINTESTINAL TRACT

Many other endocrinopathies in addition to the APUD tumors can adversely affect the gastrointestinal tract.

Hypoadrenocorticism

Hypoadrenocorticism results in the clinical signs of depression, weakness, vomiting and diarrhea. The vomitus and diarrhea may contain blood, and abdominal pain may be present. Regurgitation can accompany the vomiting as a result of a concomitant megaesophagus. The megaesophagus is reversible, and is thought to result from the generalized muscle weakness that affects these patients.[39] The cause of the vomiting and diarrhea remain uncertain, but it is thought that corticosteroids in physiologic amounts have a trophic action on the gastrointestinal mucosa. Adrenalectomized cats undergo gastric and intestinal atrophy.[40] Gastritis accompanies hypoadrenocorticism in some dogs.[39]

Compatible electrolyte changes include a low serum sodium and a high serum potassium concentration. Gastrointestinal fluid loss from primary gastrointestinal diseases can also produce these electrolyte changes, however, and they should by no means be considered pathognomonic for hypoadrenocorticism.[41] Additional laboratory findings include the presence of an azotemia that responds rapidly to fluids, hypercalcemia, low urine specific gravity, eosinophilia, and lymphocytosis. Diagnosis may be confirmed rapidly by a modified Thorn's test and more definitively with an ACTH test. Therapy is described elsewhere.[28,29]

Hyperadrenocorticism

Aside from the characteristic hepatic vacuolization and cholestasis associated with elevated serum concentrations of glucocorticoids, Cushing's syndrome is generally thought to have minimal effect on the bowel. However, two cases of bowel perforation have been associated with hyperadrenocorticism.

Hypoparathyroidism

Hypoparathyroidism leads to hypocalcemia which depresses gut motility. Constipation and even pseudobstruction can occur in humans. Vomiting and diarrhea are also seen in some patients. Similar signs can occur in dogs, but they are usually overshadowed by other signs of hypocalcemia such as seizures.

Hyperparathyroidism

Constipation, vomiting, anorexia, and peptic ulcers are common in humans with hyperparathyroidism. Pancreatitis is a rare complication.[42] In hyperparathyroid dogs, constipation and vomiting have been observed.[28] The signs appear to be due to the hypercalcemia, but the exact pathogenesis is unknown. High calcium concentrations dampen neuronal transmission and may be responsible for gastric atony. Acute elevations in serum calcium cause increased gastric acid secretion via gastrin release, but this is not a feature of chronic hypercalcemia.[43] The relationship between hypercalcemia and pancreatitis is also obscure. One explanation is that high calcium concentration in pancreatic fluid can activate trypsinogen.[42,44]

Hyperthyroidism

Hyperthyroid cats show a number of gastrointestinal signs. Diarrhea occurs in 45 percent of the cases and vomiting in one third.[28] Additional signs include increased fecal volume, foul smelling stools, increased frequency of defecation, steatorrhea,[28,29] and lymphocytic-plasmacytic enteritis. The causes of these signs in hyperthyroid cats are unknown, but similar signs in humans with thyrotoxicosis have been investigated. Transit time through the small intestine of hyperthyroid people is hastened and correlates well with the presence of diarrhea. Thus, deranged intestinal motility is thought to be of prime importance in the pathogenesis of the diarrhea due to thyrotoxicosis.[45] Additionally, increased thyroid hormone is able to produce a secretory diarrhea via elevating cAMP in the enterocyte. Furthermore, a relative deficiency of pancreatic trypsin secretion is thought to occur[46] and, in the small bowel, hyperthyroidism is associated with mucosal edema and round cell infiltration.[47] The malassimilation is compounded by the polyphagia of the hyperthyroid cat which increases the total amount of nutrient presented to the bowel for digestion and absorption.

Similarly, the pathogenesis of the vomiting in hyperthyroid cats is unknown. In humans hyperthyroidism is associated with a myopathy that can interfere with the striated musculature of the pharynx and upper esophagus resulting in dysphagia. In addition, gastric hypoacidity, hypergastrinemia, and superficial gastritis occur in some people.[42] Gastric emptying time is usually normal. In addition to the possibility that the vomiting exhibited by hyperthyroid cats is due to gastritis or esophageal dysfunction, a direct effect of thyroid hormone on the chemoreceptor trigger zone has been proposed.[28,48]

Hyperthyroid cats commonly also have elevated plasma levels of SAP and ALT liver enzymes. In some cats, a periportal mixed inflammatory reaction and focal areas of fatty degeneration may be seen in the liver. The cause of these lesions is unknown.

Medullary Carcinoma of the Thyroid

Diarrhea has been described in association with medullary carcinoma of the thyroid in dogs.[49] The diarrhea is proposed to result from the secretion of serotonin and/or prostaglandins by the tumor.[28,29]

Hypothyroidism

Hypothyroidism in humans can be associated with reflux esophagitis, gastric hypomotility, constipation, rectal prolapse, and rarely megacolon or diarrhea.[42] The cause of these signs is depressed gastrointestinal motility resulting from myxedema and decreased electrical control activity. In dogs with marked hypothyroidism both diarrhea and, alternatively, constipation have been reported.[28,29,39]

Diabetes Mellitus

Diabetes mellitus has been associated with vomiting due to delayed gastric emptying and gastric hypomotility in dogs.[28] The vomiting responded to metoclopramide therapy. Diabetic gastroparesis is a common complication of human diabetics. The cause appears to be a diabetes-induced degeneration of the parasympathetic innervation of the gastrointestinal tract. Idiopathic chronic diarrhea has also been seen in a diabetic dog, and may have been analogous to idiopathic diabetic diarrhea of humans. The pathogenesis of diabetic diarrhea is multifactorial. In some patients bacterial overgrowth, exocrine pancreatic insufficiency, deranged intestinal motility, and secretory diarrheas have been documented. Management of diabetic diarrhea is usually determined by a trial and error basis. Suggested therapies have included antibiotics for bacterial overgrowth, pancreatic enzyme replacements, opioids, psyllium, cholestyramine, or clonidine.[42] The latter agent has shown considerable promise.

Diabetes mellitus in humans has a wide range of additional deleterious effects on the gastrointestinal tract including esophageal dysfunction, chronic gastritis, idiopathic abdominal pain, constipation, and fatty liver.[42] The cause of these conditions is not completely clear but suggestions have included autonomic degeneration, microcirculatory disease, electrolyte imbalances, and metabolic derangements.

Diabetic ketoacidosis is a well recognized cause of acute vomiting and diarrhea in dogs and cats. Abdominal pain and abdominal distension may also be apparent. Proposed causes for these acute gastrointestinal signs are impaired gastrointestinal motility with resultant gaseous abdominal distension, or a direct effect of the acidosis on the vomiting center.

REFERENCES

1. Theilen, G.H. and Madewell, B.R.: Tumors of the digestive tract. In, Veterinary Cancer Medicine. 499-534, 1987.
2. Head, K.W. and Else, R.W.: Neoplasia and allied conditions of the canine and feline intestine 1980. Vet. Ann. (21st issue) 21:190-208, 1981.
3. Birchard, S.J., Couto, C.G. and Johnson, S.: Nonlymphoid intestinal neoplasia in 32 dogs and 14 cats. JAAHA 22:533-537, 1986.
4. Crow, S.E.: Tumors of the alimentary tract. Vet. Clinics N. Am. 15:577-596, 1985.
5. Brodey, R.S. and Cohen, D.: An epizootiologic and clinicopathologic study of 95 cases of gastrointestinal neoplasms in the dog. Proc. 101st annual meeting AVMA, Chicago 1964, 167-179.
6. Cotchin: Some tumors in dogs and cats of comparative veterinary and human interest. Vet. Rec. 71:1040-1054, 1959.
7. Hayden, D.W., and Nielsen, S.W.: Canine alimentary neoplasia. Zen Tralbl. Veterinaer Med. 20:1-22, 1973.
8. Holt, P.E. and Lucke, V.M.: Rectal neoplasia in the dog. A clinicopathological review of 31 cases. Vet. Rec. 116:400-401, 1985.
9. Patnaik, A.K., Hurvitz, A.I. and Johnson, G.F.: Vet. Pathol. 17:149-163, 1980.
10. Patnaik, A.K. and Hurvitz, A.I.: Neoplasms of the digestive tract in the dog. In, Current Veterinary Therapy VI. Edited by Kirk, R.W. WB Saunders, Philadelphia, 393-394, 1977.
11. Culbertson, R., Branam, J.E. and Rosenblatt, L.S.: Esophageal gastric leiomyoma in the laboratory Beagle. JAVMA 183:1168-? 1983.
12. Haubrich, W.S., and Berk, J.E.: Malignant tumors of the colon and rectum. In, Gastroenterology, 3rd Ed. Edited by H.L. Bockus, W.B. Saunders Co., Philadelphia, 1009-1044, 1976.
13. Cotter, S.M.: Treatment of lymphoma and leukemia with cyclophosphamide, vincristine, and prednisone. II Treatment of cats. JAAHA 19:166-172, 1983.
14. Penninck, D.G., Nyland, T.G., Kerr, L.Y. and Fisher, P.E.: Ultrasonographic evaluation of gastrointestinal diseases in small animals. Vet. Radiol. In press.
15. Couto, C.G., Rutgers, H.C., Sherding, R.G. and Rojko, J.: Gastrointestinal lymphoma in 20 dogs. J. Vet. Int. Med. 3:73-78, 1989.
16. White, R.A.S. and Gorman, N.T.: The clinical diagnosis and management of rectal and pararectal tumors in the dog. J. Sm. An. Pract. 28:87-107, 1987.
17. Couto, C.G.: Canine extranodal lymphomas. In, Current Veterinary Therapy IX. Edited by Kirk, R.W. 473-477, 1986.
18. Tams, T.R.: Chronic feline inflammatory bowel disorders. part II. Feline eosinophilic enteritis and lymphosarcoma. Comp. Contin. Ed. Pract. Vet. 8: 464-471, 1986.
19. Allroy, J., Leav, I., De Ellis, R.A., and Weinstein, R.S.: Mast cell tumors. Lab. Invest. 33:159-167.
20. O'Keefe, D.A., Couto, C.G., Burke-Schwartz, C. and Jacobs, R.M.: Systemic mastocytosis in 16 dogs. J. Vet. Int. Med. 1:75-80, 1987.
21. Kosovsky, J.E., Matthiesen, D.T. and Patnaik, A.K.: Small intestinal adenocarcinoma in cats: 32 cases (1978-1985). JAVMA 192:233-235, 1988.
22. Cribb, A.E.: Feline gastrointestinal adenocarcinoma: A review and retrospective study. Can. Vet. J. 29:709-712, 1988.
23. Church, E.M., Mehlhaff, C.J. and Patnaik, A.K.: Colorectal adenocarcinoma in dogs: 78 cases (1973-1984). JAVMA 191:727-730, 1987.
24. Brueckner, K.A. and Withrow, S.J.: Intestinal leiomyosarcomas in six dogs. JAAHA 24:281-284, 1988
25. Seiler, R.J.: Colorectal polyps of the dog: a clinicopathologic study of 17 cases. JAVMA 174:72, 1979.
26. Seim, H.B.: Diseases of the anus and rectum. In, Current Veterinary Therapy IX. Edited by Kirk, R.W. W.B. Saunders, Philadelphia, 916-921, 1986.
27. Silverberg, S.G.: Carcinomas arising in adenomatous polyps of the rectum of a dog. Dis. Colon Rectum. 14:191, 1971.
28. Feldman, E.C. and Nelson, R.W.: Canine and Feline Endocrinology and Reproduction. WB Saunders, Philadelphia, 1987.
29. Chastain, C.B. and Ganjam, V.K.: Clinical Endocrinology of Companion Animals. Lea & Febiger, Philadelphia, 1986.
30. Morrison, W.B.: The clinical relevance of APUD cells. Comp. Contin. Ed. Pract. Vet. 6:884-890, 1984.
31. Willard, M.D. and Schall, W.D.: APUDOMAS. In, Current Veterinary Therapy VIII. Edited by Kirk, R.W. WB Saunders, Philadelphia, 771-773, 1983.
32. O'Brien, T.D., Hayden, D.W. and O'Leary, T.P.: Canine pancreatic endocrine tumors: Immunohistochemical analysis of

hormone content and amyloid. Vet. Pathol. 24:308-314, 1987.
33. Middleton, D.J. and Watson, A.D.J.: Duodenal ulceration associated with gastrin-secreting pancreatic tumor in a cat. JAVMA 183:461-462, 1983.
34. Shaw, D.H.: Gastrinoma (Zollinger-Ellison syndrome) in the dog and cat. Can. Vet. J. 29:488-452, 1988.
35. Wolfe, M.M. and Jensen, R.T.: Zollinger-Ellison Syndrome. Current concepts in diagnosis and management. New Eng. J. Med. 317:1200-1209, 1987.
36. Brodey, R.S.: Alimentary tract neoplasms in the cat. A clinicopathologic survey of 46 cases Am.J.Vet.Res. 27: 74-80, 1966.
37. Giles, R.C., Hildebrandt, P.K. and Montgomery, C.A.: Carcinoid tumor in the small intestine of a dog. Vet. Pathol. 11:340-349, 1974.
38. Zerbe, C.A., Boosinger, T.R., Grabau, J.H., Pletcher, J.M. and O'Dorisio, T.M.: Pancreatic polypeptide secreting tumor in a dog. Proceedings 6th ACVIM Forum, 1988.
39. Burrows, C.F.: Reversible mega-oesophagus in a dog with hypoadrenocorticism. J. Sm. An. Pract. 28:1073-1078, 1987.
40. Johnson, L.R.: Regulation of gastrointestinal growth. In, Physiology of the Gastrointestinal Tract. Edited by Johnson, L.R. Raven Press, New York. 301-333, 1987.
41. Di Bartola, S.P., Johnson, S.E., Davenport, D.J., Prueter, J.C., Chew, D.J. and Sherding, R.G.: Clinicopathologic findings resembling hypoadrenocorticism in dogs with primary gastrointestinal disease. JAVMA 187:60-63, 1985.
42. Sack, T.L. and Sleisenger, M.H.: Effects of systemic and extraintestinal disease on the gut. In, Gastrointestinal Disease. Pathophysiology, Diagnosis, Management. Edited by Sleisenger, M.H., Fordtran, J.S. WB Saunders, Philadelphia, 488-528, 1989.
43. Wilson, S.D., Singh, R.B., Kalkhoff, R.K. and Go, V.L.W.: Does hyperparathyroidism cause hypergastrinemia? Surgery 80:231-237, 1976.
44. Geokas, M.C., Baltaxe, H.A., Banks, P.A. and Silva, J.: Acute pancreatitis. Ann. Intern. Med. 103:86-100, 1985.
45. Thomas, F.B., Caldwell, J.H. and Greenberger, N.J.: Steatorrhea in thyrotoxicosis. Relation to hypermotility and excessive dietary fat. Ann. Int. Med. 78:669-675, 1973.
46. Wiley, Z.D., Lavigne, M.E., Liu, K.A. and MacGregor, I.L.: The effect of hyperthyroidism on gastric emptying in pancreatic exocrine biliary secretion in man. Dig. Dis. 23:1003-1008, 1978.
47. Hellesen, C., Friis, T., Larsen, E. and Pock-Steen, O.: Small intestinal histology, radiology, and absorption in hyperthyroidism. Scan. J. Gastroenterology 4:169-175, 1969.
48. Rosenthal, F.D., Jones, C. and Lewis, S.I.: Thyrotoxic vomiting. Br. Med. J. 2:209-211, 1976.
49. Rijnberk, A. and Leav, I.: Thyroid tumors. In, Current Veterinary Therapy VI. Edited by Kirk, R.W. WB Saunders, Philadelphia, 1020-1024, 1977.
50. Turrel, J.M. and Theon, A.P.: Single high-dose irradiation for selected canine rectal carcinomas. Vet. Radiol. 27:141-145, 1986.

Chapter 25

Motility Disorders of the Bowel

IRRITABLE BOWEL SYNDROME[1,2]

Clinical Synopsis

Diagnostic features

* Chronic, intermittent, gastrointestinal dysfunction of variable character exacerbated or initiated by stress
* Alternate periods of diarrhea and constipation are common
* Diarrhea usually has a large bowel character
* Clinical signs should preferably include at least two of the following: abdominal distension, abdominal pain or discomfort that is relieved by defecation; more frequent and/or more fluid bowel movements during periods of abdominal discomfort
* Diagnostic evaluations including intestinal biopsy should reveal no evidence of organic disease
* Partial or complete amelioration of clinical signs often accompanies stress reduction and fiber administration

Standard treatment

* Identify and remove stressors
* Administer supplementary dietary fiber (Metamucil 1-6 tsp/meal)

Introduction

Irritable bowel syndrome is a motility disorder of the bowel of humans that is characterized by irregular bowel habits, abdominal pain, and the absence of detectable organic disease.[2] The irritable bowel syndrome has been variously referred to as nervous colon, nervous colitis, unstable colon, spastic colon, spastic colitis, and mucus colitis. The term irritable bowel syndrome is at present favored because the disorder is thought to be a conglomerate of diseases of different causes, because inflammation is not a feature (thus "colitis" is inappropriate), and because areas of the bowel other than the colon are thought to be involved.[2] The syndrome is considered a functional bowel disorder. The term "functional" is used in this contex to denote a disease syndrome with a definable group of symptoms but no organic lesion or at least no lesion that can be consistently demonstrated at our present level of expertise.[3] As time has passed, the syndrome of irritable bowel disease has become more defined. In humans it is now not just a diagnosis of exclusion, but can be confirmed by the presence of certain clinical and motility findings.[2]

Whether a disorder analogous to irritable bowel syndrome afflicts the dog and cat is unknown. There is no doubt that stressful situations can precipitate acute diarrhea in dogs and to a lesser extent cats. Many of these instances, however, are acute responses (apparently physiologic) to extremely stressful situations (such as the waiting room of a veterinary clinic) occuring in animals with no history of preexisting gastrointestinal dysfunction. These acute "nervous diarrheas" are presumably mediated by the autonomic and enteric nervous systems, and are not analogous to irritable bowel syndrome which has a chronic course. Other causes of stress-induced diarrhea are due to recognizable organic diseases of the large bowel which reduce its reservoir and absorptive capacity predisposing the animal to diarrhea from any preciptiating cause. In these patients stress no longer results in diarrhea once the underlying disease (usually chronic colitis) is successfully treated. However, there is a subgroup of animals with stress-related diarrhea (particularly dogs) that have chronic clinical signs of gastrointestinal dysfunction compatible with irritable bowel disease, in which we and others[4,5] have been unable to demonstrate any organic lesion, and which have responded either to fiber or to avoidance of stressful situations. This latter group of patients have been tentatively designated as suffering from the irritable bowel syndrome.

Irritable bowel syndrome is one of the most commonly encountered human gastrointestinal disorders. The veterinarian is perhaps fortunate that this at times vague and frustratingly ellusive disease is not a major cause of gastrointestinal disease in animals.

Etiology, Pathogenesis and Pathophysiology

The cause of irritable bowel syndrome is unknown. The pathogenesis involves a myoelectric abnormality in the bowel and perhaps to a lesser extent generalized autonomic dysfunction. A variety of pathophysiological abnormalities have been observed and are listed in Table 25-1.

During the times when humans have diarrhea with irritable bowel syndrome, pressures within the colon are low, and segmentation motility is reduced.[6] On the other hand, when constipation prevails, pressure within the colon is high, reflecting increased motility. In this state resistance provided by the segmentation type of motility is high, retarding the movement

Table 25-1. Myoelectric and Motility Abnormalities Prominent in Humans with Irritable Bowel Syndrome

High-amplitude pressure waves a prominent feature of basal motility
Spastic response to rectal distension
Delayed but prolonged colonic hypermotility in response to ingestion of food (particularly fats)
Pronounced colonic hypermotility to cholinergic agents
Increased colonic motility and abdominal pain in response to CCK
Increased frequency of basal electrical rhythm
Colonic motor activity is increased by low concentrations of bile acids
Small bowel transit time is faster when diarrhea is predominant
Small bowel transit is slower when constipation is predominant
Lower gastroesophageal sphincter pressure

of colonic contents, with the result that they are maximally dehydrated. Thus, motility responses in the irritable colon are exaggerated in both directions, suggesting that there is a dysfunction in the control mechanisms that normally modulate motility.

The stimuli that initiate the abnormal motor response are not limited to psychological factors. The abnormal response is stimulated also by food; at times before the meal has had a chance to reach the colon. This suggests that the response is mediated by abnormal events in normal physiological reflexes such as the neural reflexes that affect colonic motility when feeding begins. The postprandial response is abolished by vagotomy, anticholinergic drugs, thoracic spinal cord transection and intake or infusion of amino acids. It is possible that some of the gastrointestinal hormones cause the abnormal motor response in the colon. They all have effects on smooth-muscle motility. Both gastrin and cholecystokinin have been suggested as factors in causing functional bowel disorders. CCK infusion in affected patients produces colonic hypermotility and abdomianl pain. This response is thought to be mediated by opiate receptors because it is blocked by naloxone but not atropine. Bile acids can induce increased motor action potentials in the colon. In dogs, only deoxycholic acid has this ability. Humans with irritable bowel syndrome develop abnormal colonic motility responses to bile acid concentrations one third of that required to produce abnormal responses in normal humans. The motility response of the colon of patients with irritable bowel syndrome to stress includes an increase in spike potentials and motor activity but this response has not proved significantly different from normal people. A spastic response of the large bowel to distension is a consistent feature of patients with irritable bowel syndrome although it also seen in some normal individuals.

Clinical Findings and Diagnosis

If the term irritable bowel syndrome is to retain meaning, the onus is on the veterinary profession not to apply it without discretion to any form of diarrhea that defies definition by current methods. Unknown disease entities are better described as "idiopathic" since that term honestly describes a problem as having an unknown cause.

Suggested criteria to be fulfilled before a diagnosis of irritable bowel syndrome is made are provided in the clinical synopsis. They include a history of gastrointestinal signs that are often (but not always) associated with an identifiable stress, and that are chronic, intermittent, and preferably somewhat variable in nature. Affected animals may be timid, behave nervously, or be under performance stress such as police or show animals. The signs most often include a combination of abdominal discomfort, abdominal distension, and diarrhea alternating with constipation. The diarrhea usually has a large bowel character, most often consisting of small volumes of loose stools. Sometimes the diarrhea is explosive consisting of a mixture of gas and fluid. Mucus may be seen but hematochezia is uncommon. Tenesmus may occur and, in humans, is usually attributed to a sensation of incomplete evacuation rather than colonic irritation. Abdominal pain is an important feature of the disease. It has been attributed to bowel spasms or intraluminal distension. It is usually poorly localized and of variable character ranging from sharp to dull, and acute to chronic. It is often precipitated by meals or defecation. Abdominal distension, increased belching and flatulence are common. In most patients the volume of gas generated is not increased but motility disorders and perhaps increased sensitivity to distension account for the symptomology. Intestinal gaseousness is a common complication of motility disorders and is discussed later in this chapter. Nausea and vomiting, and excessive gastroduodenal and esophagogastric reflux can occur. Other signs such as urinary bladder dysfunction, and difficult or painful coitus are not infrequent and have raised the possibility that the disorder results from a generalized autonomic disturbance. The signs appear after or during periods of stress. It is known that emotional stress can trigger hypermotility in normal subjects but the threshold appears lower in irritable bowel syndrome patients.

If analogy is to be drawn to the human disease, the signs in animals with irritable bowel syndrome should include two or more of the following: bloating; abdominal pain or discomfort that is relieved by defecation; and more frequent and/or more fluid bowel movements during periods of abdominal discomfort.[2] It is difficult to evaluate small animal patients for abdominal distress, but they are seldom recognized as having acute pain in the absence of organic disease. An animal presented with the sole complaint of idiopathic, painless, persistent, chronic diarrhea is unlikely to be suffering from a disorder analagous to human irritable bowel syndrome. Before labeling a patient with the diagnosis of irritable bowel syndrome an extensive work up must be preformed to ensure that serious organic disease is not overlooked by hasty attribution of the signs to a functional disorder. Appropriate diagnostic evaluations are dictated by the particular spectrum of clinical signs shown by the patient but as a minimum should include fecal flotations and fecal fat examinations, dietary trials, and endoscopic examination with mucosal (particularly colon) biopsy. In humans barium enemas sometimes show pronounced haustral contractions.

In veterinary medicine, tentative diagnosis of irritable bowel syndrome is thus largely made by exclusion of organic disease in a patient with history and clinical signs compatible with a functional motility disorder. Successful response to treatment trials that include addition of fiber to the diet and stress reduction help confirm the disease. Fiber-responsiveness in of itself should not be considered diagnostic of irritable bowel syndrome. Fiber has a variety of favorable effects on the bowel in addition to its influences on colonic motility (see nutrition chapter), and many diseases of diverse cause will respond or partially respond to supplementation of the diet with fiber. For instance, in people (and perhaps animals) bile salt malabsorption produces signs of large bowel diarrhea (in spite of a morphologic normally colon mucosa) that will respond to fiber supplementation.

In human medicine application of electrodiagnostic and manometric techniques to the diagnosis of gastrointestinal disease has revealed a spectrum of motility abnormalities that allow positive confirmation of the disorder (Table 25-1). Unfortunately, these diagnostic evaluations have not yet been applied to the confirmation of irritable bowel syndrome in animals.

Management

Well designed clinical trials have yet to be conducted in humans with the syndrome.[7] The principal aspects of treatment are identification and elimination of stressors, and the use of high-fiber diets. Psyllium preparations such as Metamucil are helpful for the treatment of both constipation and diarrhea. The condition of a minority of human patients is aggravated by fiber. Low doses of bile acid binding resins such as cholestyramine have been found useful in humans. Low fat diets may help reduce post-prandial pain. Anticholinergics may be useful for temporary relief of intestinal spasms but they are poorly effective in this regard unless prescribed in anticipation of pain (for instance prior to meals). Gas producing foods such as legumes and aerophagia should be avoided. Short courses of opioids may be useful during periods of diarrhea. Tranquilizers are to be avoided.

ADYNAMIC ILEUS

Introduction

Adynamic ileus is defined as a transient and reversible intestinal obstruction resulting from inhibition of bowel motility. It affects both the large and small bowel. The lack of peristaltic activity results in a functional obstruction because intestinal content pools in the dependent areas of the gastrointestinal tract, instead of being propelled in an aborad direction.

Intestinal obstruction (ileus) can result from a large number of causes in addition to adynamic ileus (Table 22-1) including persistent intestinal neuromuscular derangements that cause hypomotility (pseudo-obstruction). The terms pseudo-obstruction and adynamic ileus overlap somewhat, but pseudo-obstruction has a more chronic duration, and often a more segmental appearance than does adynamic ileus. Adynamic ileus, not pseudo-obstruction syndrome, is the most common reason for negative exploratory celiotomy results in dogs and cats with suspected intestinal obstructions. The etiopathogenesis, pathophysiology, and management of intestinal obstruction are described in Chapter 22. What follows is a brief additional discussion of adynamic ileus with particular reference to its etiopathogenesis.

Cause

Adynamic ileus is a relatively common problem of a variety of causes (Table 22-1). It is seen most frequently as a complication of abdominal surgery, electrolyte imbalance, or inflammatory lesions of the bowel, peritoneal cavity, or other abdominal organs. It is a particularly common complication of canine parvovirus enteritis. Acute inflammation of the duodenum secondary to pancreatitis often produces motility changes that can be permanent. Intestinal ischemia transiently increases but then inhibits intestinal motility. Neuropathies affecting the autonomic nervous system can produce intestinal stasis. Anticholinergic drugs inhibit gastrointestinal motility. When disease has reduced normal motility, anticholinergics will compound the situation, leading to ileus and potentially bacterial overgrowth. Phenothiazines can also inhibit gastrointestinal motility, especially in high doses. Intestinal distension, if pronounced, results in inhibition of motility via the intestinointestinal reflex. Frequently, potassium deficits must be corrected before normal motor function returns. Diarrhea causes an accelerated loss of potassium from the body. The potassium depletion is compounded by inadequate intake.

Pathogenesis

Several neural, humoral, and metabolic factors probably interact to cause ileus.[8,9] Electrical slow waves still occur in the longitudinal muscle but do not initiate action potentials and associated contractile activity within the circular muscle layers. This electromechanical dissociation appears to result from a tonic discharge of inhibitory neurons. Increased adrenergic tone may be partly responsible for the tonic inhibitory discharge. The sympathetic nervous system interacts presynaptically with excitatory synaptic connections in the enteric nervous system. Release of norepinephrine appears to inhibit release of excitatory neurotransmittors such as acetylcholine thus allowing tonic discharge of inhibitory neurons to dominate. The result is a decrease in intestinal motor activity and blood flow, and down-regulation of additional gastrointestinal functions.

It is thought that factors additional to sympathetic discharge are responsible for ileus because alpha and beta blockade in either dogs[10] or people does not prevent ileus. It is also noteworthy, that neither morphine or naloxone relieves postoperative ileus.

Humoral factors are known to contribute to the pathogenesis because the motility of transplanted (denervated) intestinal loops is inhibited during experimental peritonitis in dogs.[8] Putative inhibitory humoral factors include circulating catecholamines. Conversely, impaired release of prokinetic hormones such as neurotensin, or motilin may play a role.

Hypokalemia interferes with normal ionic movements on which smooth muscle contraction is dependent. Potassium deficits may contribute more to the loss of motility than disease-induced stimulation of the sympathetic nervous system.[11]

Management

Management of ileus is by correction of any electrolyte abnormalities, maintenance of gastrointestinal decompression (if necessary by use of a nasogastric tube), and the administration of prokinetic agents such as metoclopramide (0.4 mg/kg IV q 6 hr).[12]

DYSAUTONOMIA

Dysfunction of the autonomic nervous system is referred to as dysautonomia and has been reported in man, cats,[13-15] and dogs[16,17] both in Europe and the United States. Characteristic clinical signs of dysautonomia include dilated pupils, dry mucous membranes, regurgitation, vomiting, constipation, a fixed or bradycardic heart rate and dysuria. Megaesophagus and delayed gastric emptying are usually present. In humans, dysautonomia has been related to a number of different causes including diabetes mellitus, paraneoplastic syndromes, genetic defects, CNS lesions, chronic renal failure, drug reactions, and heavy metal toxicoses.[18] In animals, the causes of dysautonomia remain obscure.

The clinical signs result from a widespread degeneration of the autonomic ganglia. Both parasympathetic and sympathetic systems are affected. The gastrointestinal signs primarily pertain to failure of parasympathetic regulation of esophageal, gastric, and colonic motility. Diagnosis is usually made by the characteristic clinical appearance. If the diagnosis is in doubt various diarnostic procedures can be instituted including the 0.1% pilocarpine and 0.25% physostigmine ocular response tests.[15] Plasma and urinary catecholamines can be assayed. In affected cats catecholamine levels are low or absent.[15]

Treatment relies on prolonged nutritional support in association with the use of 0.25% pilocarpine eyedrops, metoclopramide (0.2-0.4 mg/kg PO, SC q 8 h) or bethanechol (2.5-5.0 mg (Cats) or 5-25 mg (dogs) PO q 8h). The prognosis is guarded, particularly if megaesophagus is present.

MEGACOLON SYNDROME

Megacolon is defined simply as colonic dilatation. In humans, the syndrome of megacolon encompasses a variety of diseases that result in colonic dilatation. The syndrome is usually classified into two categories, congenital megacolon (Hirschsprung's disease) and acquired megacolon. Acquired megacolon in turn is subdivided according to the suspected cause of the disorder or is labelled as idiopathic if no cause is apparent. Megacolon has been reported in both dogs and cats.[5] It is uncommon, occuring in about one case per 10,000 in both dogs and cats at the VMTH at Davis, and many of those are referrals. Both congenital and acquired forms are recognized, but it is unclear if the congenital form is analogous to Hirschsprung's disease.[19] The syndrome is most common in the cat, and on most occasions it is idiopathic.

Pathogenesis

Congenital Megacolon.[20-22] Congenital megacolon has been studied in humans and in experimental animals. In most affected individuals, the pathological lesion that causes fecal retention is a congenital absence of myenteric and submucosal intramural plexi (aganglionosis) in the caudal part of the colon. The aganglionosis is thought to occur due to a defect in the caudal migration of cells from the neural crest.[23] The absence of the ganglionic cells releases the gastrointestinal smooth muscle from phasic inhibition by the enteric nervous system which in turn results in tonic smooth muscle contraction and intestinal obstruction. The colon cranial to the contracted segment dilates because of retained fecal material.

There is considerable heterogeneity of congenital megacolon. In most humans with the disorder, only the rectum and sigmoid colon are affected but in others almost the entire extent of the colon is involved. The variability in the length of the large bowel involved results from fetal events. Plexuses containing the ganglia are formed by neuroblasts that lay them down in an order from cranial to caudal. Thus, the terminal colon is the last to be innervated. Aganglionosis results from arrested development, and when arrest is early in gestation most of the colon is involved. When the arrest is late, only the caudal rectum and internal anal sphincter or, in unusual cases, just the anal sphincter are affected. Further confusion has arisen because there is a variety of clinical presentation for what appears to be a similar lesion. Some patients require immediate surgical relief of obstruction in the neonatal period whereas other patients present much later in life with only constipation. Moreover, there is variability in the histopathological lesion. Patchy or zonal loss of ganglia, and abnormal or dysplastic neurons have been reported. Immunohistochemical staining of affected segments has yielded a variety of results ranging from deficits of adrenergic (relaxant) innervation, increased cholinergic (excitatory) innervation, and a deficit or absence of nerves containing enkephalin, gastrin-releasing peptide, VIP, and substance P.[24,25] Another suggestion is that there is a deficit of inhibitory interneurons of the enteric nervous system.[9] It is this heterogeneity of lesion in the complex neurological control of the function of the colon which presumably explains the variability in the clinical picture.

Diagnosis of Hirschsprung's disease in humans is usually made by manometry. Normally the internal anal sphincter relaxes when the rectum is distended. It remains contracted in patients with Hirschsprung's disease.[26] As mentioned above, it is unclear if true Hirschsprung's disease exists in the dog and cat. Differential diagnoses of importance include intestinal atresia and imperforate anus. Most cases of congenital megacolon seen in dogs and cats would be more appropriately termed idiopathic congential megacolon.

Acquired Megacolon. There are a number of known causes for acquired megacolon (Table 25-2). The most frequent are pelvic trauma and constipation. Megacolon can be associated also with active colonic inflammation. Severe colitis is a prerequisite, and the loss of normal motor function is exacerbated by complicating factors, such as potassium depletion. Megacolon is a frequent complaint in older Manx cats. The

Table 25-2. Causes of Megacolon in the Dog and Cat

Extraluminal constriction	
	Pelvic deformity (trauma, congenital, nutritional osteodystrophia fibrosa)
	Prostatomegaly
	Pelvic masses
Intraluminal constriction	
	Constipation*
	Foreign bodies
	Neoplasia
	Non-neoplastic strictures
Metabolic	
	Hypokalemia
	Hypothyroidism
Neuromuscular abnormalities	
	Sacral spinal cord deformities (Manx cats)
	Pseudo-obstruction*
	Ileus*
	Dysautonomia
	Idiopathic
	Aganglionosis?

* These disorders in turn have a variety of rule outs (see Chapters 22, and 23, and the discussion of ileus in this chapter

pathogenesis of the disorder in these cats is not understood but likely relates to interference with the defecation reflex by the sacral spinal cord deformities that plague this breed. Hypothyroidism is an established cause of megacolon in humans and thyroid replacement can be dramatically effective. Constipation has also been noted in hypothyroid dogs. Other clinical and laboratory features of hypothyroidism should be present before constipation and megacolon are attributed to hypothyroidism.

Megacolon is idiopathic in many cats. Idiopathic megacolon can affect cats of a variety of ages. In one report, affected cats ranged from 1-15 years with a mean of 4.9 years.[27] We have also observed kittens of weaning age with the problem. It is unclear whether idiopathic megacolon in these kittens, and for that matter in many adults, is truely an acquired lesion or whether the origin is congenital. The hallmarks of the disorder are a dilated colon with no evidence of physical obstruction, and normal or near normal numbers of ganglion cells observed histologically in affected segments. A similar condition is seen in humans.[22] In humans as in cats, the "sluggish" colonic activity has no defined cause. Proposed etiologies include an ultrashort area of aganglionosis or a functional defect in the intrinsic innervation of the colon. Rectosphincteric manometry is considered the most definitive diagnostic technique for the differentiation of idiopathic megacolon from Hirschprung's disease.

Clinical Findings

Megacolon causes constipation as the principal sign. With neglect, complications can appear, including signs of obstruction such as anorexia and vomiting. The pathogenesis of these systemic signs is uncertain but most likely result from a breakdown of the mucosal barrier and absorption of toxic luminal products such as those produced by *Clostridia*, thought to multiply in the static colonic content. Chronically affected animals take on an unthrifty appearance. Paradoxically, colonic impaction and megacolon can also cause diarrhea. Fecal incontinence is also often associated with the condition. Abdominal palpation and rectal examination are usually sufficient to identify an impacted colon and to rule out prostatomegaly, intestinal atresia and imperforate anus.

Radiographic, Proctoscopy, and Biopsy Findings

Survey radiographs will allow confirmation of megacolon and assessment of pelvic boney structure. After evacuation a barium or air enema will help establish if a narrowed rectal or colonic segment is present. Proctoscopic evaluation followed by surgical resection of the affected segment differentiates fibrous strictures, neoplastic proliferations and aganglionosis. Full thickness (usually excisional) biopsy is required to detect aganglionosis.

Management and Prognosis

Acquired megacolon may occasionally be successfully managed medically, but ultimately most patients undergo colectomy or are euthanized. Even when the cause of the colonic obstruction that resulted in the acquired megacolon is identified and readily corrected, the changes in the dilated colon are often irreversible.

Palliative medical therapies most often utilized are enemas, bulk promoting agents such as psyllium derivatives, and various other laxatives. Animals showing systemic signs such as depression or anorexia related to their obstipation should be immediately treated with fluids and antibiotics such as trimethoprim-sulfonamide combinations or ampicillin. Unexpected deaths from obstipation are not uncommon in patients showing such systemic signs. Once the animals clinical condition has improved, enemas may be administered. Suitable enema procedures are discussed in the section on constipation (Chapter 23). Once the retained feces are removed, laxatives can be utilized with the aim of preventing recurrence. Bulk promoting agents reduce rectal retention time, and limit water absorption from the stool. The stool can also be made softer by laxatives such as dioctyl sodium sulfosuccinate, which, in addition to softening the feces, causes colonic secretion of fluid and alterations in the colonic mucosa.[28] Another useful agent, better tolerated by cats than many other laxatives, is lactulose (Chronulac). An appropriate starting dose is 1 ml/5 kg PO q 8 hours, after which the dosage is individualized depending on response. Mineral oil is not advised for long term use because of the danger of aspiration during administration. Cisapride, a new prokinetic agent, has been used with variable success in humans recovering from acquired megacolon.

The treatment of choice for idiopathic megacolon is subtotal colectomy.[27,29-33] In cats this results in minimal if any adverse clinical or laboratory abnormalities.[34] In dogs reservoir fecal incontinence is a common complication. Removal of the proximal two thirds of the canine colon results in frequent passage of liquid or, at best, semiformed feces.[35]

INTESTINAL GAS[36,37]

Gaseous abdominal distension is a common complication of ileus and may also be partly responsible for the clinical signs of irritable bowel syndrome.

Gas is swallowed and generated within the gastrointestinal tract and normally passes rapidly from one region to another since there is little resistance to its flow, and little peristaltic activity is needed to propel it. When the intestine has lost its normal motility, gas accumulates and distends the bowel. Gaseous distention of the intestines appears as bloat and causes discomfort. Thus, discomfort is likely greater when no gas is passed than when excessive gas is passed. The quantity of gas normally present is very small, and introduction of little additional gas in humans produces signs of bloat that are disproportionate to the amount introduced. The amount of gas accumulated is difficult to assess radiographically. The failure of gas to move normally through the intestine suggests that abdominal gaseousness is due to disordered intestinal motility rather than excessive generation of gas.

The two most common sources of intestinal gas in dogs and cats are probably swallowed air, and bacterial fermentation of nutrients such as carbohydrate and fiber. Additional sources are the chemical release of carbon dioxide from bicarbonates, and diffusion of gas from the blood.

Intestinal gas consists of nitrogen, carbon dioxide, hydrogen, and small amounts of methane and oxygen. Nitrogen makes up 20 to 90% of intestinal gas. The nitrogen is derived primarily from swallowed air and by diffusion from blood. As other gases are produced in the gut, nitrogen diffuses into the lumen, so that its partial pressure remains the same in the lumen as in the blood.

Up to 50% of intestinal gas can be hydrogen, which is produced by colonic bacteria metabolizing unabsorbed nutrients. Malabsorption of carbohydrates provides substrates to the colon for hydrogen production. Thus, pancreatic insufficiency, intramural mucosal disease, and disaccharidase deficiency all cause excessive hydrogen production and abdominal gaseousness. Certain foodstuffs contain nutrients that are fermented in the colon contributing to intestinal gas.

Carbon dioxide is the third-most abundant gas in the intestine. Carbon dioxide is formed as acid contents leaving the stomach are neutralized by the bicarbonate secretions of the pancreas. Most of the gas in the duodenum is carbon dioxide, but most has been absorbed at the level of the caudal intestine, and the amount in the flatus is less than 20%. As much as one to two liters of carbon dioxide can be produced by the hydrochloric acid-bicarbonate reaction in a 25-Kg animal. Carbon dioxide is also produced by colonic bacteria and by secreted colonic bicarbonate reacting with short-chain acids produced by fermentation. An increase in the amount of unabsorbed fermentable substrates entering the colon causes an increase in the amount of carbon dioxide produced. Small amounts of methane are produced by colonic bacteria. In humans, it is recognized that only certain individual have the ability to produce methane. The factors that determine its production are not dietary, but may reflect the population of the normal resident microflora.

Excessive gas production in association with normal motility most often manifests as flatulence (Chapter 5). In contrast, bloating and its associated discomfort are most often caused by a motility problem which does not properly evacuate the intestinal gas allowing it to accumulate. It is possible that a viscious circle can eventually develop because disordered motility results in bacterial overgrowth which in turn results in increased intestinal gas production. Moreover, accumulation of intestinal gas leads to intestinal distension which in turn can exacerbate ileus through the intestinointestinal inhibitory reflex.

REFERENCES

1. Schuster, M.M. and Whitebread, W.E.: Physiologic insights into irritable bowel syndrome. Clin. Gastroenterology 15:839-853, 1986.
2. Schuster, M.M.: Irritable bowel syndrome. 1402-1418, 1989.
3. Haubrich, W.S.: Recognition of functional disorders. In, Bockus Gastroenterology. Edited by Berk, J.E. WB Saunders, Philadelphia, 236-246, 1985.
4. Leib, M.S.: Dietary fiber and large bowel diarrhea. Proceedings 7th ACVIM Forum, 1989.
5. Lorenz, M.D.: Diseases of the large bowel. In, Textbook of Veterinary Internal Medicine. Edited by Ettinger, S.J. WB Saunders, Philadelphia, 1346-1372, 1983.
6. Christensen, J.: Myoelectric control of the colon. Gastroenterology 68:601-609, 1975.
7. Klein, K.B.: Controlled treatment trials in the irritable bowel syndrome; a critique. Gastroenterology 95:232-241, 1988.
8. Jones, R.S. and Schirmer, B.D.: Intestinal obstruction, pseudo-obstruction, and ileus. In, Gastrointestinal Disease. Pathophysiology Diagnosis, and Management. Edited by Sleisenger, M.H., Fordtran, J.S. WB Saunders, Philadelphia, 369-381, 1989.
9. Wood, J.D.: Physiology of the enteric nervous system. In, Physiology of the Gastrointestinal Tract. Edited by Johnson, L.R. Raven Press, New York 67-109, 1987.
10. Smith, J., Kelly, K.A. and Weinshiboum, M.: Pathophysiology of postoperative ileus. Arch. Surg. 112:203-209, 1977.
11. Mishra, N.K., Appert, H.E. and Howard, J.M.: Studies of paralytic ileus. Effects of intraperitoneal injury on motility of the canine small intestine. Amer. J. Surg. 129:559-563, 1975.
12. Graves, G.M., Becht, J.L. and Rawlings, C.A.: Metoclopramide reversal of decreased gastrointestinal myoelectric and contractile activity in a model of canine postoperative ileus. Vet. Surg. 18:27-33, 1989.
13. Rochilitz, I.: feline dysautonomia (the Key-Gaskell or dilated pupilsyndrome): a preliminary review. J. Sm. An. Pract. 25:587-598, 1984.
14. Sharp, N.J.H., Nash, A.S. and Griffiths, I.R.: Feline dysautonomia (the Key-Gaskell syndrome): a clinical and pathological study of forty cases. J. Sm. An. Pract. 25:599-615, 1984.
15. Guilford, W.G., O'Brien, D.P., Allert, A. and Ermeling, H.M.: Diagnosis of dysautonomia in a cat by autonomic nervous system function testing. JAVMA 193:823-828, 1988.
16. Rochilitz, I. and Bennet, A.M.: Key-Gaskell syndrome in a bitch. Vet. Rec. 112:614-615, 1983.
17. Wise, L.A. and Lappin, M.R.: A syndrome resembling feline dysautonomia the Key-Gaskell syndrome) in a dog. 7th ACVIM Forum Proceedings, 1031, 1989.
18. Bannister, R.: Autonomic failure: a textbook of clinical disorders of the autonomic nervous system. Oxford University Press, Oxford, 1983.
19. Burrows, C.F.: Constipation. In, Current Veterinary Therapy IX. Edited by Kirk, R.W. WB Saunders, Philadelphia, 904-908, 1986.
20. Wood, J.D.: Physiological studies on the large intestine of mice with hereditary megacolon and absence of enteric ganglion cells. In. Proceedings Fourth International Symposium on Gastrointestinal Motility. Mitchell Press, Vancouver, 1974, 177-187.

21. Christensen, J.: Motility of the colon. In, Physiology of the Gastrointestinal Tract. Edited by Johnson, L.R. Raven Press, New York 665-693, 1987.
22. Phillips, S.F.: Megacolon: Congenital and Acquired. In, Gastrointestinal Disease. Pathophysiology Diagnosis, and Management. Edited by Sleisenger, M.H., Fordtran, J.S. WB Saunders, Philadelphia, 1389-1402, 1989.
23. Okamoto, E. and Veda, T.: Embryogenesis of intramural ganglia of the gut and its relation to Hirschsprung's disease. J. Pediatric Surg. 2:437-443, 1967.
24. Larsson, L.T., Malmfors, G. and Sundler, F.: Peptidergic innervation in Hirschsprung's disease. Z. Kinderchir. 38:301-304, 1983.
25. Tsuto, T., Okamura, H., Fuukui, K., Obata, H.L., Terubayshi, H., Iwai, N., Majima, S., Yanaihara, N. and Ibata, Y.: An imunohistochemical investigation of vasoactive intestinal polypeptide in the colon of patients with Hirschsprung's diease. Neurosci. Lett. 34:57-62, 1982.
26. Howard, E.R. and Nixon, H.H.: Internal anal sphincter. Arch. Dis. Child. 43:569-578, 1968.
27. Rosin, E., Walshaw, R., Mehlhaff, C., Matthiesen, D., Orsher, R. and Kusba, J. Subtotal colectomy for treatment of chronic constipation associated with idiopathic megacolon in cats: 38 cases (1979-1985). JAVMA 193:850-853, 1988.
28. Saunders, D.R., Sillery, J. and Rachmilewitz, D.: Effect of dioctyl sodium sulfosuccinate on structure and function of rodent and human intestine. Gastroenterology 69:380-386, 1975.
29. Horney, F.D. and Archibald, J.: Colon, rectum and anus. In, Canine Surgery, 2nd Archibald ed. Edited by J. Archibald. American Veterinary Publications, Santa Barbara, 602-628, 1974.
30. Swenson, O.: The pull-though operation for congenital megacolon. Rev. Surg. 24:229-232, 1967.
31. Yoder,J.J., Dragsted, L.R. and Starch, C.J.: Partial colectomy for correction of megacolon in a cat. VM/SAC 63:1049-1052, 1968.
32. Webb, S.M.: Surgical management of acquired megacolon in the cat. J. Sm. An. Pract. 26:399-405, 1985.
33. Bright, R.M., Burrows, C.F., Goring, R., Fox, S. and Tilmant, L.: Subtotal colectomy for treatment of acquired megacolon in the dog and cat. JAVMA 188:1412-1416, 1986.
34. Gregory, C.R., Guilford, W.G., Berry, C.R. and Pedersen, N.C.: Colonic function in cats after subtotal or total colectomy for megacolon syndrome. Vet. Surg. Abstract 18:69, 1989.
35. Peck, D.A. and Hallenbeck, G.A.: Fecal continence in the dog after replacement of rectal mucosa with ileal mucosa. Surg. Gynecol. Obst. 119: 1312-1320, 1964.
36. Lasser, R.B., Levitt, M.D. and Bond, J.H.: Studies of intestinal gas after ingestion of a standard meal. Gastroenterology 70:906, 1976.
37. Levitt, M.D.: Intestinal gas. Postgrad. Med. 57:77-80, 1975.

Chapter 26

The Pancreas

NORMAL STRUCTURE

Gross Anatomy[1,2]

The pancreas is a small pinkish-gray gland, coarsely lobulated, adjacent to the duodenum and stomach (Figure 26-1). It consists of two limbs forming a V, with the apex closely applied to the caudasinistral portion of the pyloric region. The right limb (or lobe) of the pancreas lies in the mesoduodenum near or in contact with the right flank and it follows the duodenum closely. This lobe is about six inches long in a 30 lb. dog. The pancreas lies ventral and adjacent to the right kidney, ureter, caudate process of the liver, ileum, and cecum. The cranial part is adjacent to the ascending colon dorsally and the jejunum ventrally. The left lobe is smaller than the right, and its dorsal surface is related to the transverse colon caudally and to the dorsal wall of the stomach cranially.

A working knowledge of these anatomical landmarks aids in understanding clinical signs and secondary problems associated with pancreatic disease. When acute pancreatitis involves the right lobe, it may be possible to localize the signs to the dorsal right quadrant of the abdomen. If the part of the pancreas involved is adjacent to the liver, clinical and laboratory signs may indicate liver involvement. Because the pancreas is adjacent to sections of the small and large bowel, an ileus sometimes develops as a complication of acute pancreatitis.

Most exocrine pancreatic secretions are delivered to the intestine through the large accessory pancreatic duct, which opens into an indistinct minor papilla about 28 mm from the entrance of the bile duct. This accessory pancreatic duct is the main avenue of transport from the right lobe of the pancreas. The main avenue of transport from the left lobe is a smaller duct, the pancreatic duct, which enters the duodenum near the opening of the bile duct. Unlike in humans, the pancreatic duct of the dog does not empty into the main bile duct. Therefore, reflux of bile into one of the pancreatic ducts is much less likely in dogs than in humans. The cat is different in that the major duodenal papilla, three cm distal to the pylorus, is the common entry point for the bile duct and pancreatic duct into the intestine. The majority of cats have no accessory pancreatic duct.

The pancreatic branches of the cranial and caudal pancreaticoduodenal arteries supply the major blood perfusion to the pancreas. The pancreatic branch of the splenic artery supplies the left extremity of the pancreas. The pancreaticoduodenal vein drains the pancreas by emptying into the cranial mesenteric vein. Additional drainage is supplied by two veins terminating in the splenic vein. Lymphatics drain into duodenal, hepatic, splenic, and mesenteric lymph nodes.

The vagi and the splanchnic nerves supply parasympathetic and sympathetic efferent fibers to the pancreas.[3] The parasympathetic fibers primarily innervate acinar cells and regulate exocrine secretion, while sympathetics innervate blood vessels and control circulation. The vagal branches follow the splenic branch of the celiac artery and the caudal pancreatic branch of the cranial mesenteric artery. The postganglionic

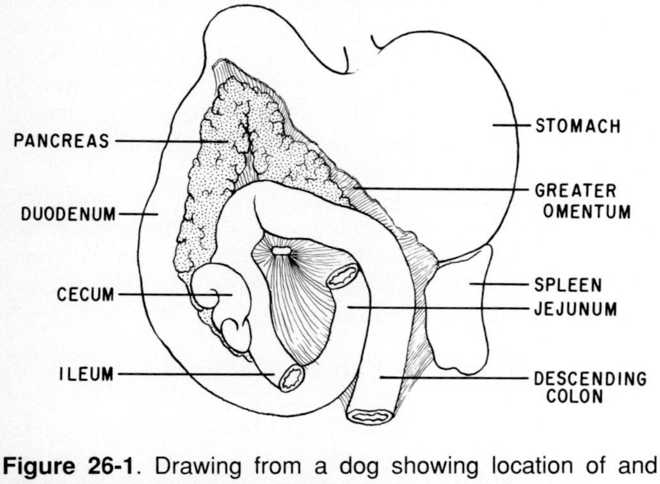

Figure 26-1. Drawing from a dog showing location of and relationships of pancreas to other organs in abdomen.

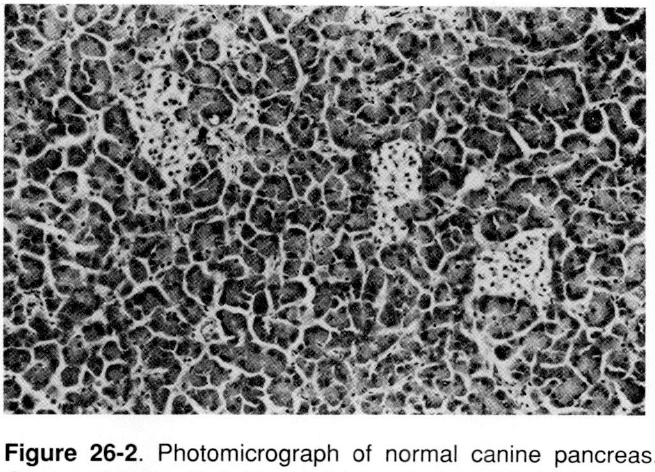

Figure 26-2. Photomicrograph of normal canine pancreas. Groups of cells with lighter staining cytoplasm are islet cells.

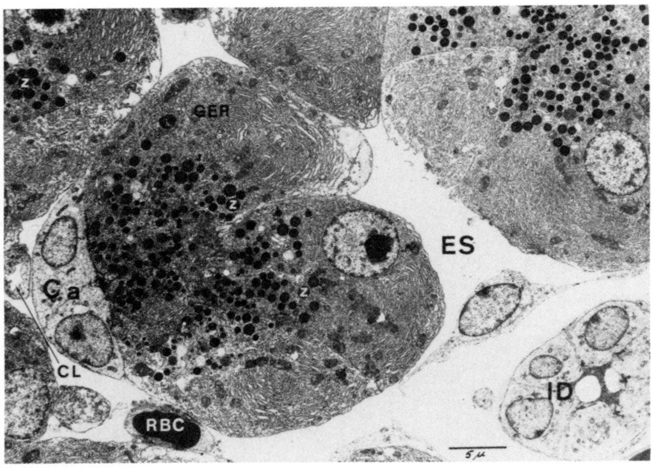

Figure 26-3a. Electron micrograph of normal canine pancreas. X 2100 Z = zymogen granule in an acinar cell; GER = Granular endoplasmic reticulum; Ca = centroacinar cell; ID = intralobular or intercalated duct. Cells lining these ducts appear identical to the centroacinar cells. CL = capillary lumen; ES = extracellular space.

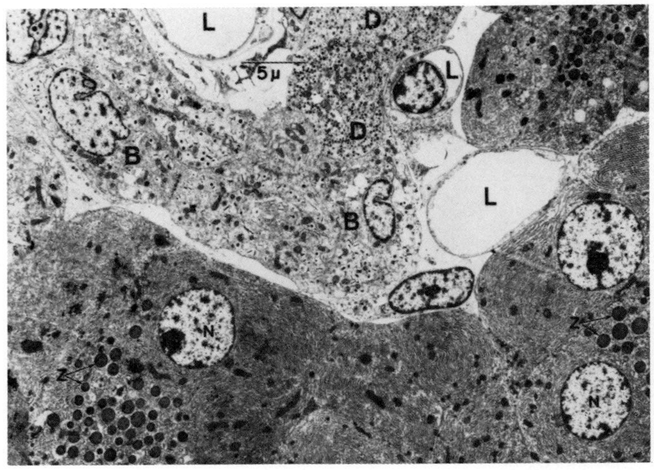

Figure 26-3b. Electron micrograph of normal canine pancreas. X 2400. N = nucleus of acinar cell; B = beta cell; D = delta cell; L = lumen of small blood vessel; Z = zymogen droplet.

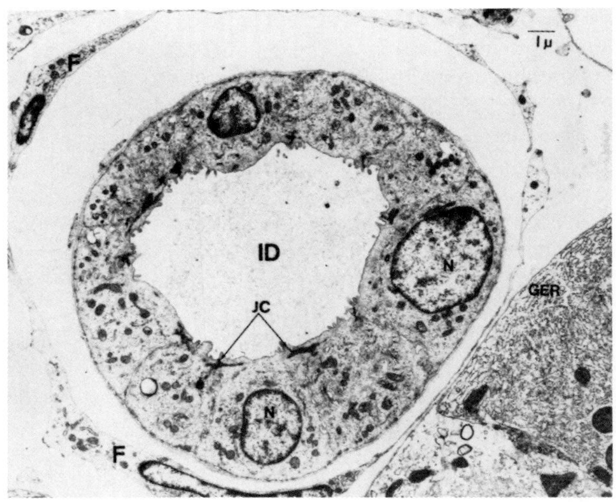

Figure 26-3c. Electron micrograph of normal canine pancreas showing an intralobular duct. X 3540.

sympathetic fibers are derived from the celiac and cranial mesenteric plexuses and follow the pancreatic branches of the caudal pancreaticoduodenal artery.

Histology - Exocrine Pancreas[4]

The pancreas is a compound tubulo-acinar gland that has been described as resembling a bunch of grapes on a stalk (Figure 26-2). The exocrine units of the lobule are called acinar cells. They are arranged side by side in a single row that forms a cul-de-sac. One cluster of acinar cells form small units called acini (Figure 26-3). The bases of the pyramidally shaped acinar cells are adjacent to their basal lamina, and their apices border on the open center of the cul-de-sac. The cul-de-sac is the beginning of the duct system that transports enzymes to the intestine; it is lined by flattened epithelial cells, called centroacinar cells. Nerves, blood vessels, and lymphatics are found at the base of acinar cells and between acini.

Ultrastructure

The pancreas is one of the most metabolically active tissues in the body. This activity is reflected in the subcellular structure of the acinar cell, which contains organelles designed for the synthesis and transport of protein. The acinar cells synthesize and secrete digestive enzymes. Until release, these enzymes are concentrated in secretory granules in the apex of the cell (Figure 26-3). The enzymes are synthesized by endoplasmic reticulum in the more basal part of the cell and packaged in the golgi complex in the center of the cell. Nuclei do not participate directly in the synthesis of enzymes and are therefore located at the basal end of the cell. In addition to synthesizing and secreting enzymes, the pancreatic acinar cells secrete fluid and electrolytes.

The cul-de-sac formed by the acini connects with intralobular ducts lined with low columnar epithelial cells. These ducts empty into interlobular ducts lined with columnar epithelium, a few goblet cells, and an occasional argentaffin cell. The epithelial cells secrete fluid and are similar to cells in other tissues that absorb or secrete fluid and electrolytes. Their similarities include a brush border on their apical surface and large numbers of mitochondria to meet the energy requirements of transport. The interlobular ducts empty into the main pancreatic ducts.

Gastrin and cholecystokinin are trophic for pancreatic acinar cells and promote regeneration after injury and resection.[5] Some normal animals have areas of pancreatic hyperplasia. It is possible that excessive secretion of either of these hormones causes the hyperplasia.

Histology - Endocrine Pancreas

The pancreas is an important site of production and secretion of hormones.[6] Endocrine-producing cells are located in the islets of Langerhans; beta-cells produce insulin, and alpha-cells produce glucagon (Figure 26-3). Cells in the islets of the pancreas also produce other peptide hormones, such as gastrin and somatostatin. All of these cells are of a type found throughout the gastrointestinal tract. Embryologically, they arise from the neural crest and are called foregut endocrine polypeptide-secreting APUD (amine-precursor-uptake and decarboxylation) cells. This designation is based on the cells' properties of: 1) storing fluorescent amines such as catecholamines or 5-hydroxytryptamine; 2) taking up precursors necessary for the synthesis of amines; and 3) decarboxylating amino acids, a necessity for amine synthesis. APUD cells synthesize amines or peptide hormones and release them into the circulation. Half of the types of APUD cells currently recognized are found in the pancreas and gastrointestinal tract; others are located in the pituitary, adrenal, and thyroid glands.

PANCREATITIS

Clinical Synopsis

Diagnostic features

* Acute onset of anorexia, depression, vomiting, diarrhea, abdominal pain
* Dyspnea and weakness are common
* Fever, tachycardia, pulse deficits, dehydration and pain on abdominal palpation are common
* Evidence of coagulapathy occasionally seen
* Serum lipase and amylase increased; ALT and ALp increased; hematocrit increased and plasma protein decreased
* Radiographs may show increased density around pancreas; ultrasound confirms pancreatic inflammation

Standard treatment

* NPO for 5 days
* IV fluid therapy 80-120 ml/kg/day + percent dehydration X body weight (kg) + replacement of losses from vomiting and diarrhea; Plasma may be required
* Antibiotics: procaine pencillin G (20,000 u/kg BID) and an aminoglycoside may be required
* Heparin, dextran, corticosteroid and anticholinergic therapy of no proven value
* Low fat diet is fed after 5 days

Epidemiology of Pancreatitis[7,8]

Acute pancreatitis, a disease of middle-aged obese dogs, has been reported more often in females. The incidence over a six-year period at the VMTH in Davis was 3.2 per 1,000. Equal numbers of males and females were affected. The only breed of dog that showed a greater than expected incidence was the Dachshund (double the anticipated number). The diagnosis of pancreatitis was based on an elevated serum lipase activity and histological evidence of acute pancreatitis detected in animals that did not survive. Figure 26-4 shows the incidence of acute pancreatitis in different age groups. It is interesting that 10% of all the cases seen are in the age group of six months to two years.

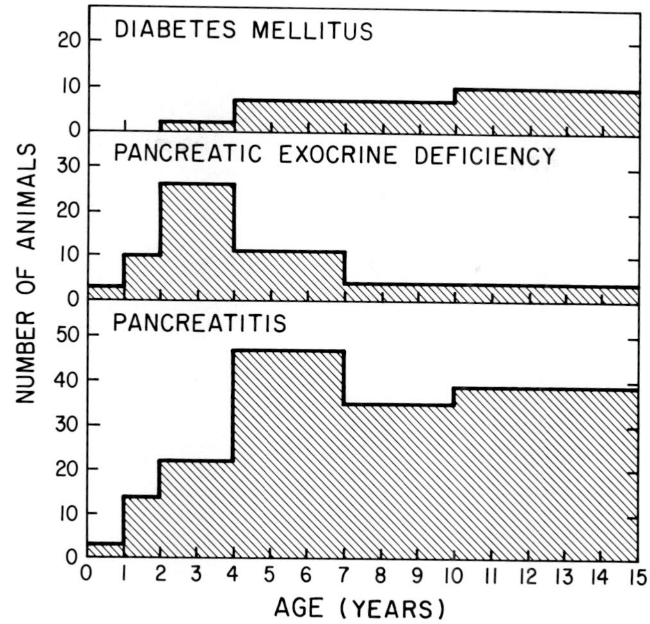

Figure 26-4. Incidence of pancreatitis in different age groups. Comparison is made with the incidences of diabetes mellitus and pancreatic exocrine deficiency which can be complications of pancreatitis. Animals are grouped into ages less than 1 year, 1 to 2 years, 2 to 4 years, 4 to 7 years and 10-15 years.

These animals may represent a group in which the etiology is different, such as viral causes. The true incidence of pancreatitis may be greater than reported here, for histological findings show evidence of pancreatitis in 1% of clinically normal dogs.[8]

The incidence of pancreatic disease in cats at the VMTH over a seven-year period was 1.5 per 1,000 cats seen, with very few of the cases being recognized on the antemortem workup. Few published reports provide information on the incidence of pancreatitis in cats.[9] The true incidence will not be known until a diagnostic procedure is introduced that shows a good correlation between abnormal findings and morphologic evidence of pancreatitis.

Etiology and Pathogenesis[4,10-13]

The etiology of naturally occurring pancreatitis is poorly understood. Nutrition appears to play an important role since pancreatitis in dogs is often found in the obese individual.[14] It

Table 26-1 Pancreatitis - Etiology

	Canine	Feline
Primary	34%	41%
Secondary	66%	59%
Neoplasia	23%	17%
Renal disease	16%	21%
Corticosteriods	12%	
GI disease	12%	16%
Hepatic disease	12%	
Pancreatic tumors	9%	
Infection and DIC	9%	38%
Cardiovascular disease	4%	8%

Table 26-2. Experimental Methods Used to Produce Acute Pancreatitis

Pancreatic intraductal perfusion with:	
	Bile
	Bile and pancreatic juice
	Bile salts and trypsin
	Trypsin
	Activated pancreatic juice
	Long-chain fatty acids
Injection directly into pancreas	
	Trypsin
	Activated trypsin
	Bile salts
Manipulation of pancreatic microcirculation	
	Intra-arterial injection of trypsin
	Obstruction of arterial, venous, or lymphatic flow
	Initiation of local disseminated intravascular coagulation
Toxic and infectious means	
	Endotoxin injection
	Bacterial and viral infection
Closed duodenal loops	

is found less often in dogs that are underfed. The composition of the diet is important, since pancreatitis is often associated with diets rich in fat. Most cases of pancreatitis in dogs and cats are secondary to a nonpancreatic problem (Table 26-1). Drugs can be a cause of pancreatitis, with corticosteroids given at a high level for longer than one week being the most common cause. In some cases pancreatitis develops after acute stress from trauma or surgery. Infectious agents can cause acute pancreatitis in experimental animals and may be an important cause of naturally occurring pancreatitis in cats.[15]

Current concepts on the pathogenesis of pancreatitis are based on information gained from experimental studies. The primary event in the development of pancreatitis involves changes in pancreatic cell membranes. Injury to the membranes of most cells in the body results in rapid cell destruction only if enzymes contained in their lysosomes are released. Lesions in membranes of pancreatic acinar cells can release enzymes prepared for secretion into the intestinal tract. These membranes are more stable than those of other cells, so pancreatic acinar cells are able to withstand ischemic conditions better than cells of the liver, heart, kidney, or brain.[16] Once these membranes are damaged, however, the cells undergo relatively rapid autolytic destruction. Pathogenesis of pancreatitis must explain the initial alterations in membranes. Table 26-2 lists the experimental models used to explain its pathogenesis. Unfortunately, the pancreatic lesions produced in these models vary greatly, and many are quite different from the pathology found in naturally occurring pancreatitis.

Etiologic Factors

Nutritional Factors. Nutrition is considered one of the most important factors in the pathogenesis of pancreatitis in dogs.[14] Extremely imbalanced diets can produce the disease. For example, a means of experimentally creating acute pancreatitis is to feed a dog a diet that is 60% fat.[17] Pancreatitis, while not invariably seen, develops in dogs on the diet for 14 to 38 weeks. Hepatic lipidosis also develops, with hepatic fat content increasing 2.5 to 7 times over normal. Dogs fed a balanced diet with the proper number of calories and proper exercise seldom develop acute pancreatitis, and if the problem does develop it is less severe. A protein deficient diet causes pancreatic atrophy.[18] Alcohol can stimulate caloric imbalances; the dog has the same pancreatic response to alcohol that humans have.[11] When dogs are fed a choline-rich, high-protein diet in addition to alcohol they develop chronic interstitial pancreatitis. Moreover, caloric imbalance created by alcohol can stimulate the development of acute pancreatitis more readily when the diet has been high in proteins and lipids.

Nutritional imbalances cause pancreatic disease either by altering the rate of synthesis, storage, and secretion of pancreatic enzymes or by causing changes in acinar cell membranes. High-fat, high-protein diets in both man and dogs cause increased synthesis and storage of enzymes, an effect also produced by corticosteroids and hypercalcemia, causing acute pancreatitis.

Malnutrition results in a deficiency of pancreatic enzymes,[18] which is the reason that undernourished animals are less susceptible to pancreatitis. The rate of synthesis and secretion of pancreatic enzymes is stimulated by the peptide hormones cholecystokinin (CCK), gastrin, and secretin. Potent releasers of these hormones are factors in producing pancreatitis. Fat and protein are potent stimuli for CCK release, protein for gastrin release, and gastrin-stimulated hydrochloric acid secretion entering the duodenum for secretin release. Thus, a diet rich in protein and fats contains the most potent stimuli for pancreatic secretion; CCK and gastrin are agonists for enzyme secretion, with secretin augmenting the sensitivity of the acinar cell to CCK. High-fat diets are also suggested to reduce the stability of acinar cell membranes, possibly by altering the composition of their lipids. A reduced stability of secretory granule membranes makes the granules more susceptible to lysis by bile and trypsin.

Diets deficient in nutrients required for membrane synthesis can also cause pancreatitis. That is accomplished in experimental animals by interfering with the synthesis of phospholipids, an important component of membranes. Phospholipid synthesis is inhibited by feeding diets deficient in its precursors, such as choline and methionine, or by including ethionine, an analog of methionine that behaves as a counterfeit. Ethionine in the diet can cause acute pancreatitis unless methionine is added. Ethionine added to a choline-deficient diet causes the pancreatitis to be more severe than it would be with a balanced diet.[19] The inhibition of phospholipid synthesis results in inadequate synthesis of membranes for both the storage and secretion of enzymes. Retention of enzymes, followed by progressive degeneration of membranes of the endoplasmic reticulum, characterizes the pathophysiology in the acinar cell . The normal structure of the acinar cell is lost after 24 hours, at which time a release of enzymes causes edema, hemorrhage, and inflammation. Diets deficient in choline and supplemented with ethionine result in a defect in the hormone-stimulated breakdown of phosphoinositides by phospholipase C, an event necessary for secretion of zymogens. The enzymes are retained in large vacoules that fuse with lysosomes. Lysosomal enzymes activate trypsinogen, and the trypsin formed is able to destroy normal pancreatic structures. In summary, nutrition plays a role in the pathogenesis of pancreatitis in that it determines the amounts of enzymes synthesized, stored, and secreted, and the stability of the membranes involved in these processes. It also determines function in secretory processes.

Pancreatitis following consumption of a single high-protein and high-fat meal suggests that maximum stimulation of pancreatic enzyme secretion may be important in the condition's pathogenesis. Pancreatic stimulation by an excessive amount of the cholecystokinin analogue caerulein causes pancreatitis in experimental animals, but not the same as in most clinical cases. The caerulein stimulation causes digestive enzymes to be localized within organelles (vacuoles) containing lysosomal enzymes that are capable of activating trypsinogen. Pancreatitis develops because enzyme secretion is blocked, and the pathogenesis is based on pathology's developing within acinar cells. Obstruction of pancreatic ducts by edema, inflammation, or calculi also blocks enzyme secretion. There is some experimental evidence for the pathology's beginning in ducts, subsequent necrosis of acini following from duct obstruction. Dogs treated with an anticholinesterase insecticide develop a pancreatic lesion similar to that produced by caerulein.[20] Such a chemical would block destruction of acetylcholine and maintain stimulation of pancreatic secretion.

Reflux of Duodenal Contents.[10,11,21] Most theories on the pathogenesis of acute pancreatitis suggest that the initiating factor(s) enter by way of the pancreatic ducts; the most likely factors are refluxed bile or duodenal contents that contain activated enzymes and some lipids that can be toxic. Reflux of bile is an important factor in humans, for biliary-tract disease is found in half of the patients with acute pancreatitis. Infected bile is proposed to reflux from the common bile duct into the pancreatic duct, which is possible in humans since there is a direct communication between the two. It is unlikely for bile to reflux into the pancreatic ducts in dogs since secretions from the biliary tract and pancreas enter the duodenum at separate sites and there is no direct communication between the two. It is possible such a comparison can be made for the pathogenesis in cats and humans since the bile duct and pancreatic duct enter the intestine through a common opening at the major duodenal papilla. The association of biliary infection (cholecystitis) and pancreatitis is difficult in both dogs and cats for another reason: the incidence of cholecystitis is very low in both species. Experimentally induced cholecystitis in dogs can result in acute pancreatitis. In this model, it has been shown that lymphatics from the gall bladder communicate with those in the subacinar spaces of the pancreas. It is postulated that infectious or toxic agents could travel via this route to the pancreas. That may also be an important reason for the association of the two problems in humans.

A widely held theory for the etiology of acute pancreatitis is reflux of duodenal contents into the pancreatic ducts. That has been studied experimentally in the dog[22] and other animals[23] with a closed duodenal loop created by ligation of the intestine cranial and caudal to the entrance of the pancreatic ducts. Acute hemorrhagic pancreatitis develops within 24 hours and is characterized by pancreatic edema, necrosis, and hemorrhage, by intra-abdominal fat necrosis, and by ascites formation. When the pancreatic ducts are also ligated, acute pancreatitis does not usually develop. Duodenal ligation results in gastric distension, which is a stimulus for gastrin release. The possibility that hypergastrinemia is a factor in the development of acute pancreatitis has not been investigated. The suggested cause is the reflux of duodenal contents containing the activated enzymes, bile, and bacteria from the closed loop.

If duodenal contents are to reflux into the pancreatic duct, the pressure of fluids in the duodenum must exceed that in the pancreatic duct. However, pressures increase very little (6 mm Hg) in the intestine, which is an open tube. The only time that intraduodenal pressure exceeds pancreatic duct pressure is during the interval of 20 to 50 minutes after eating.[24] The times that intraduodenal pressure may increase are only 10% of the total in unfed states but increase to 40% after feeding. The maximum total volume refluxing is only 0.1 ml per 15 min in normal medium-size dogs.[21] That is not enough to initiate pancreatitis. On the other hand, fluid secretions can lead to very high pressures in closed loops of small intestine. If reflux were a likely cause in naturally occurring pancreatitis, the intraduodenal fluid pressures required to greatly increase reflux would be greatest in dogs with intestinal obstruction, a problem that is seldom associated with acute pancreatitis.

Experimental production of pancreatitis with closed loops has shown that the loop must contain pancreatic enzymes and bacteria, and ischemia must develop in the intestine and pancreas for lesions to be produced. Pancreatitis is difficult to produce with closed duodenal loops in germfree animals, and the severity of pancreatitis is reduced by ligation of the pancreatic ducts with closed loops in conventional animals. Bacteria proliferate in closed loops of intestine, and pancreatic enzymes secreted into the loop provide the substrate for their growth. Bacterial activity in closed loops produces substances that are toxic if absorbed by the system. Clostridial toxins are the major contributor to death in dogs with obstructed loops of intestine. Toxic macromolecules are absorbed minimally from the intestine of normal animals, and those absorbed are detoxified within the intestine and liver by lysosomal enzymes. High fluid pressure in the closed loop compromises its circulation; pancreatitis can develop, but does not develop if the pressure is kept at a low level. Macromolecules are absorbed faster from an intestine that is ischemic. Since this tissue is then less able to degrade toxins, macromolecules can leave and reach the pancreas via the lymphatics or by direct extension. Evidence from such experimental studies justifies the use of antibiotics and agents to improve circulation, such as heparin, in the management of pancreatitis.

If duodenal reflux could cause pancreatitis in dogs, it is likely that cholecystitis and hepatic necrosis would be problems appearing first. The pressure is greater in dogs' pancreatic ducts than in their bile duct. When the two ducts are connected together they are unable to empty their secretions into the intestine, and death occurs within four days from hemorrhagic necrotic hepatitis and gangrenous cholecystitis. These problems are seldom seen with naturally occurring pancreatitis.

Studies using direct methods have been conducted to determine whether solutions placed in duodenal loops could be shown to reflux. A solution of iron in a duodenal loop at pressures of 100 cm of water administered for an hour does not reflux into the duct. On the other hand, gentian violet placed in closed loops is subsequently found in the pancreas. It is not known, however, whether the dye reaches the organ by reflux through the ducts or by absorption and transport to the pancreas via the circulation.

If duodenal reflux were important in the etiology of acute pancreatitis, surgical widening of the opening of the pancreatic ducts would produce the disease in humans, but, in fact, such treatment of patients who already have the disease results in clinical improvement.

Pancreatic Destruction by Enzymes and Bile. Release and activation of pancreatic enzymes perpetuates the lesion in pancreatitis. It is not known whether the initial event activates the enzymes in the acinar cell or in the pancreatic ducts. The enzymes could also be activated in the intestine and then reflux into the pancreatic ducts, but that is unlikely for reasons already given. Trypsin, chymotrypsin, carboxypeptidase, elastase, and phospholipase are stored in zymogen granules in inactive forms. Trypsinogen is normally activated by enterokinase, an enzyme secreted by the mucosal cells of the duodenum. Trypsin activates the other proteases and phospholipase. Thus, activation of enzymes in pancreatic ducts requires the reflux of enterokinase or trypsin from the lumen of the duodenum. Trypsinogen is also activated within acinar cells as they are destroyed. The activation can be produced by release of acinar cells' lysosomal enzymes or by complement that has been activated. Regardless of whether enzyme activation occurs in the ducts or acinar cells, the initial stages of pancreatic inflammation are most widely believed to occur in the interstitial spaces adjacent to the basal part of acinar cells; the histological changes are caused by trypsin, chymotrypsin, elastase, and phospholipase-A. Infusion of trypsin or chymotrypsin into the canine pancreatic duct results in interlobular edema that can develop into hemorrhagic lesions. Trypsinogen stored in zymogen granules can be activated by trypsin itself, by the lysozomal enzyme cathepsin B, or by the enzymes of the blood-clotting or fibrinolytic systems. Trypsin can initiate the release of histamine from mast cells and endothelial cells and can activate the kinin system. These changes result in the vascular changes leading to edema and hemorrhage. Trypsin, chymotrypsin, and elastase (another proteolytic enzyme) also degrade peptide structures of the pancreas. The activity of elastase is specific in that it digests elastic fibers in blood vessels and is largely responsible for changing pancreatitis from an edematous to a hemorrhagic form. Pancreatic carboxypeptidase, which is nontoxic, is also released.

Phospholipase A can cause pathologic changes by converting membrane lecithin to lysolecithin, resulting in dissolution of the structure. Injection of lysolecithin into the pancreatic duct causes pancreatitis. Pancreatitis in experimental animals and humans is associated with lower levels of lecithin and cephalin in the pancreas, and a higher level of lysolecithin. The phospholipase A activity of plasma and ascitic fluid is sometimes increased. Phospholipase A activity can destroy zymogen granule membranes, thereby perpetuating the destructive process. Active phospholipase A in pancreatic ducts requires the presence of bile before it can cause pancreatitis.

Bile has been used to produce pancreatitis experimentally by injecting it into pancreatic ducts under high pressures. Bile contains lecithin, which must be converted to lysolecithin before it can cause damage. Bacteria or pancreatic phospholipase A makes this conversion, and bile contains bacteria. Bile can activate any trypsinogen released after the pancreatic duct is injected. Phospholipase A released from the acinar cell can also be activated by bile acids in bile.

Activation of pancreatic enzymes and autodigestion of acinar tissue may be an unacceptable explanation for the pathogenesis of pancreatitis. Any trypsin or chymotrypsin activated may not be cytotoxic; these enzymes do not damage cells when they are used to disaggregate them for cell culture. Also, phospholipase A is inactive on phospholipids of intact cellular membranes. An exception may be elastase and its effects on blood vessels. These enzymes without any other insult to the pancreas usually produce no more than a mild edematous pancreatitis that is often self-limiting.

If duodenal contents were able to reflux into the pancreatic ducts, their destructive components would include activated enzymes, lysolecithin, and unconjugated bile acids. Of those, the most potent damaging agent appears to be lysolecithin. The concentrations of lysolecithin in the duodenum of the normal dog are unable to damage its mucosa, which makes it questionable whether the same concentration could cause pancreatitis following reflux into the ducts. Lysolecithin can be produced in high concentrations only where there are high levels of bile lecithin with phospholipase-A activity. That is a likely possibility in humans, whose bile and pancreatic ducts communicate, but not in the dog.

Pancreatic Ischemia.[10,11] Ischemia of the pancreas may be the primary event leading to the development of acute pancreatitis. This may be an important factor in some dogs that develop pancreatitis following extensive trauma or surgery. Surgery intensely stimulating the sympathetic nervous system may produce prolonged ischemia of the pancreas. Pancreatitis is frequent in humans after prolonged periods of extracorporeal circulation, with ischemia the basis for its development. Corticosteroids can also cause acute pancreatitis, and an occlusive vascular problem has been suggested as a contributor to its development. In addition, corticosteroids can cause other changes in the pancreas that may be more important.

The status of circulation in the pancreas is an important determinant of the appearance and severity of the lesions in experimental pancreatitis. In many models, acute severe inflammatory lesions do not develop unless there is stasis in the microcirculation. For example, although ligation of the pancreatic ducts causes no immediate pathological changes, if the gland is stimulated to secrete, edema appears; and if there is the added insult of pancreatic artery occlusion, pancreatic necrosis develops. In another model, intraductal injection of bile produces no changes other than complete microcirculatory stasis, and it is only after 24 hours that pathology appears, a result of the ischemia rather than the bile directly. Intraductal infusion of trypsin produces a mild edematous pancreatitis. This condition can convert to severe necrotizing pancreatitis when ligating a pancreatic vein causes circulatory stasis.

Acute pancreatitis can also be produced by the intra-arterial injection of beads, which compromise pancreatic microcirculation. Stimulated intravascular coagulation in the pancreas produces the same effect. The coagulation must be generalized, however, since the occlusion of isolated vessels by infarcts does not cause pancreatitis.

In other experimental models, an improvement in pancreatic blood flow reduces the severity of pancreatic lesions.

Postganglionic sympathetic denervation increases pancreatic blood flow and in one model results in a mild form of edematous pancreatitis rather than a consistently fatal hemorrhagic form. Agents such as fibrinolysin, heparin, low molecular-weight dextran, glucagon, vasoactive peptide, and vasopressin improve pancreatic circulation that has been reduced 40% to 60% by acute inflammation; this improvement ameliorates the pathologic process and increases survival rates. Prostaglandins are necessary to maintain pancreatic blood flow during pancreatitis since indomethacin causes it to decrease. Drugs should not be used that would inhibit the formation and release of prostaglandins. Some studies suggest that prostaglandins contribute to the pathology developing in acute pancreatitis. Infusion of pharmacologic amounts of some prostaglandins will increase capillary permeability; when that is combined with another chemical capable of producing pancreatitis, a more severe form develops. But that does not support the idea that normal prostaglandin formation should be inhibited in the management of pancreatitis.

Occlusion of lymph drainage in some experimental models causes intensification of mild interstitial inflammation because destructive enzymes and chemicals with vasoactive properties are not removed. This condition occurs in the natural course of development of acute pancreatitis due to the plugging of lymphatics with cells and debris. Improvement of circulation increases lymph flow and minimizes chances of obstruction. Whether the stasis in pancreatic microcirculation found in dogs with spontaneous pancreatitis is the cause or effect of the initial lesion is not known. Circulatory stasis eventually develops when trypsin is released to stimulate intravascular coagulation and thrombosis. The result is areas of ischemia that cannot be replenished with proteinase inhibitors from the circulation and from which tissue-destroying enzymes cannot be washed out.

Obstruction of Pancreatic Ducts. Obstruction of the pancreatic ducts has been suggested as a cause of pancreatitis. Obstruction can be produced by parasites,[25] neoplasms, spasms of the ducts, inflammatory processes around the ducts, and, in rare cases, calculi. Experimental obstruction of the ducts in dogs produces no immediate pathologic changes, however, although serum amylase and lipase concentrations increase. If ligation is accompanied by a stimulus for exocrine secretion, pancreatic edema is the worst that happens. Pancreatic necrosis does not appear unless ligating the pancreatic artery or lymphatics impairs the microcirculation. Drugs such as narcotic analgesics can cause spasms of smooth muscle in the duodenum and pancreatic ducts. A fear exists that such agents would either precipitate acute pancreatitis or intensify an existing problem. Morphine has no effect on serum amylase and lipase levels in normal dogs, however, suggesting that the drug is of no consequence even if it causes partial occlusion of the ducts.[26] Pancreatic enzymes increase in a few humans given morphine, though not to levels diagnostic of pancreatitis.[27] Although occlusion of the pancreatic ducts is not an important factor in the etiology of acute pancreatitis, it may be a factor in causing pancreatic atrophy, which can be produced by ligation of the ducts.

Inhibition of cholinesterase activity does not stop pancreatic secretion but it causes intraductal pressure to increase; pancreatitis can follow.[20] Pancreatitis is not recognized as a problem in dogs poisoned by organophosphates, however. Other studies further illustrate confusion on the role of pancreatic duct occlusion in the pathogenesis of pancreatitis. In one, occlusion of the pancreatic duct appeared to be beneficial to dogs with acute pancreatitis.[28] In another, dilatation of the duodenal papilla and proximal pancreatic duct produced pancreatitis in dogs.[29]

Drugs.[30,31] A number of drugs, including azathioprine, corticosteroids, chlorothiazide, chlorpromazine, estrogens, furosemide, ethacrynic acid, sulfamethazole, and tetracycline have been associated with the development of pancreatitis. Corticosteroids and chlorothiazide can be used to create pancreatitis experimentally. The lesions produced are different from those seen in clinical cases, however. Steroids can produce clinical pancreatitis in dogs, most often when the dose exceeds one milligram per pound of body weight. The pathogenesis of drug-induced pancreatitis is unknown. With steroids it may be due to changes that the drug induces in the physical properties of exocrine secretions, or it may be due to occlusive vascular disease in the pancreas, like the lesions steroids are thought to produce in bone.[32] The steroid effects may reflect the drug's immunosuppressive effects, permitting a bacterial or viral infection to develop. Pancreatitis appearing in steroid-treated animals may be precipitated by other diseases or drugs which are present. Some question whether steroids cause pancreatitis and believe that the other factors are responsible for the disease.[33] Evidence is even cited for steroids being beneficial in the management of pancreatitis. The results of studies in experimental dogs showing steroids to reduce mortality supports that position.[34] Pancreatitis is common in humans given immunosuppressive therapy after renal transplantation.[32] Azathioprine has been implicated as the important reason for pancreatitis in those cases; 5% to 6% of humans receiving that drug develop pancreatitis. Acute pancreatitis has been reported in dogs given azathioprine and prednisone.[35] Azathioprine stimulates pancreatic secretory volume but inhibits trypsin output in experimental dogs.[36]

Chronic Renal Disease. Acute pancreatitis has been associated with uremia[37] and may develop because of pancreatic stimulation by high levels of hormones. Increased serum levels of gastrin accompany chronic renal disease, causing hypersecretion of gastric hydrochloric acid. The subsequent hypersecretion of secretin augments the effect of gastrin, stimulating secretion by the pancreas. The combined effect of these two hormones, plus effects of other substances that may be inadequately cleared during renal disease, could contribute to the pancreatitis. A vascular chronic-fibrosing pancreatitis can be produced experimentally by 5/6-nephrectomy.[38]

Abnormal Lipid Metabolism. Abnormalities in lipid or lipoprotein metabolism are sometimes associated with acute pancreatitis in an unknown way. Fasting lipidemia can appear with clinical pancreatitis and later disappear with recovery.[39] Hypertriglyceridemia and hyperlipemia accompanies experimentally induced acute pancreatitis in dogs in some studies but not in others.[40-42] In the clinical cases, however, it is not known whether the lipidemia precedes and possibly causes the pancreatitis. Familial hyperlipidemia in humans can be associated with recurring pancreatitis. In one instance (Type 1 hyperchylomicronemia), an elevated plasma triglyceride level is associated with a deficiency of lipoprotein lipase activity; in others (Types IV and V), lipoprotein patterns are abnormal. Patients with these problems are subject to recurring bouts of acute pancreatitis unless serum triglyceride levels are controlled.[43] Type V, the most frequent abnormal lipoprotein pattern, changes to Type IV during remission and the absence of a fasting chylomicronemia.[44] The persistence of lipoprotein abnormalities long after an acute attack of pancreatitis suggests a primary defect in lipid metabolism. Similar lipoprotein abnormalities have been reported in dogs.[39] Hypertriglyceridemia can also be caused by estrogen administration or chronic renal disease and can precipitate acute pancreatitis.[45] In all of these cases hypertriglyceridemia is suggested to initiate the acute attacks by an unknown means. One theory is that the high levels of pancreatic lipase activity presumed to be present in the pancreatic capillaries hydrolyze the high circulating levels of triglyceride, releasing large amounts of free fatty acids that initiate the pancreatitis.[46] Other hypotheses suggest that hyperlipidemia causes stasis of the pancreatic microcirculation, and that the ischemia precipitates the acute attack. It is interesting that hyperlipidemia in dogs can cause signs of abdominal distress, as commonly seen with acute pancreatitis, without other evidence of pancreatic disease.[47]

Hypercalcemia.[48,49] Hypercalcemia can precipitate pancreatitis, and the association has been seen with parenteral hyperalimentation, hyperparathyroidism, vitamin-D intoxication, and some malignant neoplasms metastasizing to bones. Parathyroid tumors and some carcinomas of APUD cells found outside the parathyroids cause signs of hyperparathyroidism by secreting hypercalcemia-stimulating substances. A form of pseudohyperparathyroidism is found in some dogs with lymphosarcomas.

Dogs with hypercalcemia uncomplicated by pancreatitis can present with signs of anorexia, vomiting, depression, and muscular weakness. Humans show additional signs also: diarrhea, ileus, and abdominal pain. Thus, hypercalcemia can present signs that are also frequent with acute pancreatitis. Acute pancreatitis can become a problem when the serum level of calcium approaches 15-16 mg/dl. The onset of the problem, however, is determined by the amount of calcium that is ionized (normally 50% of total serum calcium). The ionized fraction is increased by reductions in plasma pH (acidosis) and protein content (hypoproteinemia).

Hypercalcemia produces pancreatitis by an unknown mechanism. One theory suggests that calcium carbonate stones form and obstruct the pancreatic ducts. Although the concentration of calcium in pancreatic secretions increases with hypercalcemia, it does not rise in proportion to elevations in the plasma. Moreover, experimental animals that are made hypercalcemic develop pancreatitis without the formation of calculi, and fewer than half of humans with hypercalcemia and pancreatitis develop calcinosis of the pancreatic parenchyma. A second theory suggests that hypercalcemia-induced increases in calcium levels of pancreatic secretions activate trypsinogen, inducing pancreatitis. Such activation is controlled by calcium. Although the levels of calcium in pancreatic secretions are higher during pancreatitis, they are similar to those in the extracellular fluid; thus, the increase probably represents a diffusion through the damaged membranes of calcium from extracellular fluid. A third hypothesis suggests that acute pancreatitis results from the vasculitis and thromboarteritis caused by hypercalcemia. Lastly, intravenous calcium infusion increases pancreatic secretion of enzymes, fluid and bicarbonate in dogs but only increases enzymes in cats.[50] Whether that is important in the pathogenesis of pancreatitis is unknown.

Prostaglandins. Prostaglandin-E-like activity increases in the pancreatic venous blood of dogs with acute pancreatitis.[51] It has no proven damaging effect and is probably a needed response in order for adequate pancreatic circulation to be sustained.

Infectious Agents. Infectious agents are believed to be a cause of acute pancreatitis in humans.[52] The association of viral hepatitis with acute pancreatitis suggests that the virus attacks cells in both organs. Measurements of antibody titers in humans against many different viruses reveal increased titers against coxsackie B_3 and B_4 viruses.[53] Infectious agents such as feline herpesvirus and feline infectious peritonitis virus are causes of naturally occurring pancreatitis in cats.

There is considerable experimental evidence that viruses can cause acute pancreatic lesions.[54] Picornaviruses, reoviruses, murine hepatitis virus, and the cytomegalovirus, a herpesvirus, have all been shown to cause acute pancreatic lesions in experimental animals. The coxackie-viruses in group-B cause acute necrotic pancreatitis in mice.

Bacteria may play an important role in the pathogenesis of acute pancreatitis. Bacteria can cause pancreatitis by traveling to the pancreas from an infected biliary system through lymphatics or by invading from the lumen of the intestine when the defense barriers are lowered. Certain species of bacteria found in the normal pancreas are suggested as producing some of the complications seen in acute problems. If reflux of duodenal contents into the pancreatic duct is a normal event in dogs, the augmented rate of reflux after feeding could be responsible for bacteria found in the normal pancreas. Bacterial numbers in duodenal contents increase greatly following feeding. The reflux increasing with greater duodenal pressure in dogs with a closed duodenal loop results in numbers of bacteria in the duct that can cause acute pancreatitis. Bacteria can release enzymes that damage cell-membrane phospholipids, toxins that damage parenchymal cells, and chemicals stimulating release of mediators of inflammation from leukocytes. In this sense bacteria may be important in the pathogenesis of some cases of pancreatitis; in others it may be only responsible for infections and abscess formation in the pancreas.

Endotoxemia is a feature of acute pancreatitis. Gram-negative bacterial components may also concentrate in the pancreas and contribute to the pathogenesis of pancreatitis. Local endotoxin accumulation would have its greatest effect disrupting the pancreatic microcirculation.

Immune-Mediated Mechanisms. An immune response may play a role in the pathogenesis of pancreatitis. Studies to support that include the production of pancreatitis by injecting antigens into the pancreatic duct of sensitized animals to initiate an Arthus reaction.[55] Immunization of animals with pancreatic homogenates results in chronic pancreatitis and circulating antibodies.[56] In other studies, injection of heterologous antibodies results in increased serum activity of lipase and amylase and severe edematous pancreatitis.[57]

Immune complexes placed in closed duodenal loops cause more severe acute pancreatitis than saline does when it is placed in the loops.[58] Many such results suggest that circulating antibodies may play a role in the pathogenesis of acute pancreatitis. Immunofluorescent techniques found antibodies to pancreatic tissue in humans a week after onset of acute pancreatitis, but not before.[59] Thus, host antibodies appear to be produced after damaged acinar cells release antigen; they are a sequela of the process rather than its cause. It is possible that antibodies perpetuate the problem and enhance its progress to a chronic state. Other host antibodies against a variety of tissues (including kidney, liver, stomach, and thyroid glands) have been detected in patients with acute pancreatitis. Antinuclear, antismooth muscle, and antireticulin antibodies have also been observed.

Pathogenesis of Pancreatitis

Theories on the pathogenesis of acute pancreatitis must explain the mechanism for creating the initial lesion, which is lysis of cell membranes, a change that must precede the release and activation of destructive enzymes. The initial lesion must be produced by a reaction capable of damaging viable unaltered cell membranes. One system known to be capable of damaging normal cell membranes is the serum complement system, and that may play a role in creating the initial lesion. In most reactions, complement fixed by antibodies directed against antigens on the surface of a cell causes a cytotoxic reaction. Complement does not require antibodies to be activated, since activation can be mediated by the C3 bypass, the serine proteases plasmin and trypsin, and bacterial endotoxins. In experimental animals, complement can be selectively activated in the interstitial fluid around acinar cells by the injection of cobra-venom factor into the pancreatic duct.[60] Acute progressive pancreatitis follows. Activated complement creates the initial lesion since cobra venom does not activate trypsin, phospholipase, or elastase. Acute pancreatitis is produced similarly by intraperitoneal injection of foreign serum, which is suggested to contain components of a complement-dependent cytotoxic heterophile antibody system.[61] The earliest morphological change in these models is swelling of the acinar cell due to movement of extracellular fluid into the cell. Necrosis does not appear until the swelling has progressed and caused a dissolution of zymogen granules and release of pancreatic enzymes. At this point, trypsin, capable of activating complement, perpetuates the progress. Complement can be activated in a number of ways to initiate spontaneous pancreatitis. They include activation by: 1) locally high levels of plasmin in ischemic parts of the pancreas; 2) bacterial endotoxins absorbed from the duodenum and inadequately removed by impaired circulation; 3) movement of toxins or activated enzymes from the pancreatic duct into the interstitial space around acinar cells; and 4) infectious agents that reach the pancreas by the circulation or direct extension from the intestine. Figure 26-5 is a scheme proposing the manner in which the initial lesion of membrane lysis produces the chain of events that leads to acute pancreatitis.

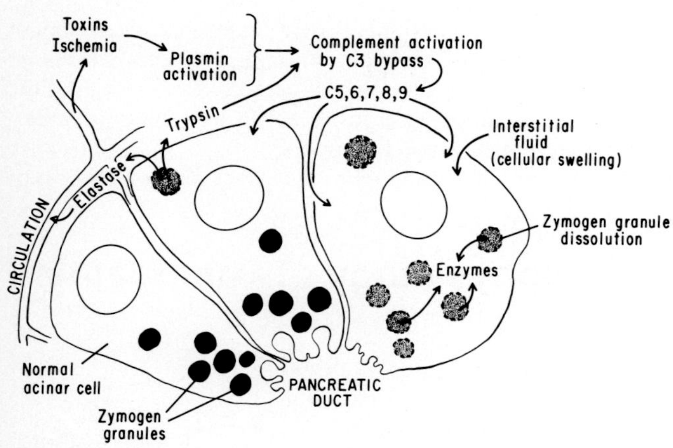

Figures 26-5. Pathogenesis of pancreatitis. Initial change may be activation of complement by toxins or ischemia, causing increased membrane permeability to fluid, followed by cellular swelling and release of zymogens. Activated zymogens trypsin, phospholipase, and elastase destroy cell structures and blood vessels.

Normal cell membranes can also be damaged by oxygen-derived free radicals.[62] These toxic oxygen metabolites are generated during the conversion of hypoxanthine to xanthine by xanthine oxidase. During ischemia and tissue hypoxia the enzyme xanthine dehydrogenase converts to xanthine oxidase. A trypsin inhibitor blocks the conversion, suggesting a protease is released to mediate the effect. During reduced oxygen availability, hypoxanthine forms in excess from breakdown of ATP. When oxygen becomes available in excess, the abundant xanthine oxidase activity converts hypoxanthine to xanthine; producing oxygen-derived free radicals capable of injuring cell membranes by lipid peroxidation. Oxygen-derived free radicals are also capable of producing chemicals that attract neutrophils, macrophages, and platelets. Neutrophils can release lysosomal enzymes that can generate large amounts of oxygen-derived free radicals. The free radicals attack and damage structural lipids of membranes surrounding zymogen granules and lysosomes as well as those of other cell organelles such as mitochondria. The damage releases and can result in activation of any enzymes in the granules or lysosomes. Pancreatitis produced in the canine pancreas by temporary ischemia, perfusion of the pancreas with a fatty acid, or stimulation of pancreatic secretion during partial duct obstruction is prevented by prior treatment with substances preventing damage by oxygen-derived free radicals. That suggests free radical formation is an early essential step in the pathogenesis of pancreatitis. It is evident that the mechanism for free radical formation may be quite different after acute pancreatitis begins, i.e. from the release of neutrophil lysosomal enzymes.

Pancreatic enzymes are probably not essential for the initial events in acute pancreatitis.[63] Phospholipase does not damage intact cell membranes. Trypsinogen is not likely activated to an appreciable degree during acute pancreatitis. Very little active trypsin is found in the affected pancreas. Activation is prevented or eliminated by the low pH in zymogen granules, calcium concentrations that favor trypsinogen degradation rather than activation, and protease inhibitors. Pancreatitis that releases large amounts of trypsinogen results in greatly increased plasma levels of trypsinogen but very little trypsin; little has been activated. Elastase is released, the greatest source possibly being neutrophils. Elastase damages the elastic lamina of small blood vessels, causing hemorrhage and thrombosis.

Neutrophil enzymes act on membrane lipids to release arachidonic acid, which can be metabolized in the cyclooxygenase pathway to prostaglandins that do not promote inflammation and in the lipooxygenase pathway to leukotrienes that amplify the inflammatory process by attracting more leukocytes to the affected tissue.

Natural Defense Mechanisms

Since pancreatic enzymes are easily released by minor trauma or infection,[64] mechanisms must exist to prevent autodigestion. Enzymes released into the interstitial space can be activated by either blood-clotting or kinin-generating enzymes. At the same time, inhibitors are present to prevent the activation of pancreatic enzymes, and of these the protease inhibitors have been characterized the best.[64,65] Endogenous protease inhibitors in tissue fluids are α_1-antitrypsin and α_2-macroglobulins, and pancreatic tissue contains pancreatic trypsin inhibitor. Pancreatic homongenates prepared from an acutely inflamed pancreas usually possess no trypsin activity, and no trypsin activity is found in ascitic fluid from patients with acute pancreatitis. However, immunoelectrophoresis of ascitic fluid reveals a large amount of proteases complexed with inhibitors. Because of their short half-life, these complexes are normally not detected in plasma. The inhibitors are consumed in their inactivating role, and their measurable levels are reduced in the inflamed pancreas. After all the major inhibitors are consumed, proteolytic enzyme activity can be demonstrated in pancreatic tissue, ascitic fluid and thoracic lymph. The activity is associated with arterial hypotension that the generation of kinin by plasma protease activity produces. Inhibitors in extracellular fluid are as important in the defense mechanism as inhibitors in the pancreas. Following consumption they are replenished by the circulation. Microcirculation is severely compromised in the inflamed pancreas, however, and inhibitor levels cannot be restored. In addition, ischemia prevents washout of enzymes released from zymogen granules, and the activity of proteases increases not only for that reason but because of the inability to restore inhibitor levels. One treatment for pancreatitis in humans has been use of the pancreatic trypsin inhibitor aprotinin.[34,66]

Pathophysiology[4,67]

Pancreatitis usually causes altered homeostasis in one or more systems in the body. These secondary events are responsible for pancreatitis' causing death. The secondary pathological changes are due to the activity of released pancreatic enzymes. The enzymes released include: 1) trypsin, which has a broad range of proteolytic activity; 2) kallikrein, which has the specific proteolytic ability to act on plasma kininogens to form kinins; 3) elastase, which may circulate to extra-pancreatic sites and degrade proteins; 4) lipase and phospholipase-A, which can respectively be responsible for fat necrosis (bone marrow and central nervous system in humans) and dissolution of membranes (lung in humans and dogs); 5) amylase, carboxypeptidases, and ribonucleases, which do not contribute to the pathophysiology of pancreatitis; and 6) lysosomal enzymes capable of degrading proteins, lipids, and a variety of polysaccharides. These changes are manifested in clinical signs and in physical findings. Many of the changes cause histologic abnormalities as shown in Table 26-3.

Dehydration and Shock. The most common complication of pancreatitis is fluid and electrolyte imbalance. Dehydration and hypovolemia appear for several reasons (Figure 26-6). Fluids are lost from the extracellular space through vomition and their accumulation in loops of intestine with ileus. The volume of circulating blood can also be reduced by pooling in capillary beds. That is facilitated by kinins that plasma trypsin and kallikrein activity form when protease inhibitor levels are depleted.

Table 26-3 Pancreatitis - Complications

	Canine	Feline
Peritonitis or fat necrosis	21%	52%
Hepatic degeneration necrosis	22%	4%
Renal pathology	12%	
GI pathology	10%	
Pulmonary edema or pleural fluid	6%	11%
Thrombosis or infarction	6%	3%
Myocardial necrosis	5%	11%
Infection	5%	
Diabetes	3%	19%
DIC	3%	
CNS lesions	3%	
Miscellaneous	4%	

Shock can be a sequel to dehydration and hypovolemia. Shock can also be caused by myocardial depressant factor, a toxic peptide produced by enzymes that the ischemic pancreas releases. Toxins produced by bacteria in the intestine can be absorbed and contribute to shock. Ileus, which predisposes to bacterial overgrowth increases toxin production. Impaired intestinal circulation and damage from enzymes released from the adjacent pancreas reduce the preventative barriers to toxin absorption. Hypovolemic shock develops from the reduction of effective circulating blood volume by as much as 30% to 40%. Circulation is compromised throughout the body.[68] Splanchnic circulatory changes are characterized by reduced portal venous flow and increased portal pressure, and increased hepatic arterial flow associated with reduced arterial blood pressure.

Electrolyte imbalances invariably include potassium depletion. Excessive potassium is lost at a rate that exceeds that of fluid volume during vomition. Volume depletion causes an increase in the renal excretion of potassium as the result of the hypovolemia-induced increase in aldosterone secretion. Depletion of body potassium is an important factor contributing to ileus. Moreover, ileus cannot be corrected until tissue stores of

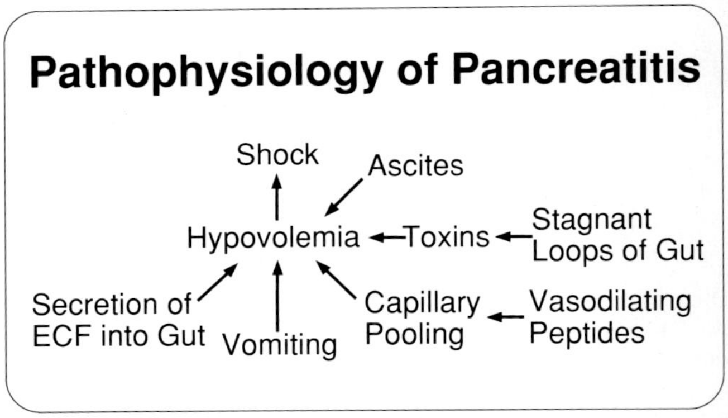

Figure 26-6.

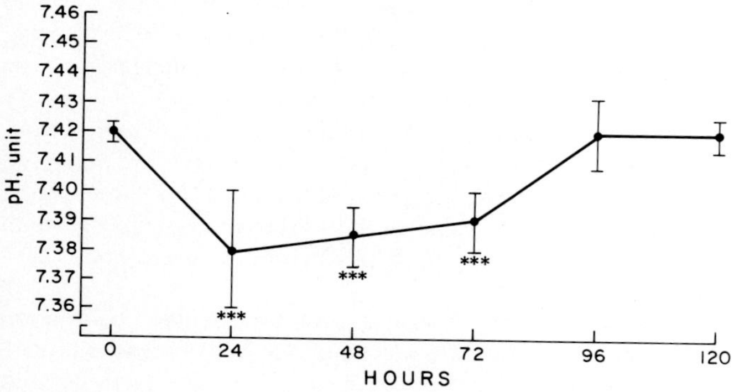

Figure 26-7. Blood pH changes in dogs with acute pancreatitis

potassium are replaced. Acid-base abnormalities usually develop if a significant amount of fluid is lost by vomiting. The loss of hydrochloric acid through vomition produces a net gain of bicarbonate in the extracellular fluid. An accompanying hypovolemia results in maximum retention of all electrolytes, including bicarbonate, and alkalosis should appear. Other changes, most importantly shock, result in acidosis rather than alkalosis, however. Blood pH decreases with experimental pancreatitis despite an early administration of large amounts of fluid to minimize the severity of shock (Figure 26-7).

Altered Gastrointestinal Motility. The pancreas is anatomically related to parts of both the small and large intestine (Figure 10-2). Acute pancreatitis is often accompanied by a local chemical peritonitis that affects function in the adjacent loops of intestine (Figure 26-8). The inflammation causes spasms of smooth muscle at the onset of pancreatitis, and loss of intestinal motility can develop later. Loss of intestinal motility, ileus, results in retention of excessive gas and the appearance of bloat or abdominal distention. Regional ileus can be seen in the duodenum and parts of the ascending and transverse colon from a chemical peritonitis due to pancreatitis. Ileus can sometimes involve most of the intestine. Important to

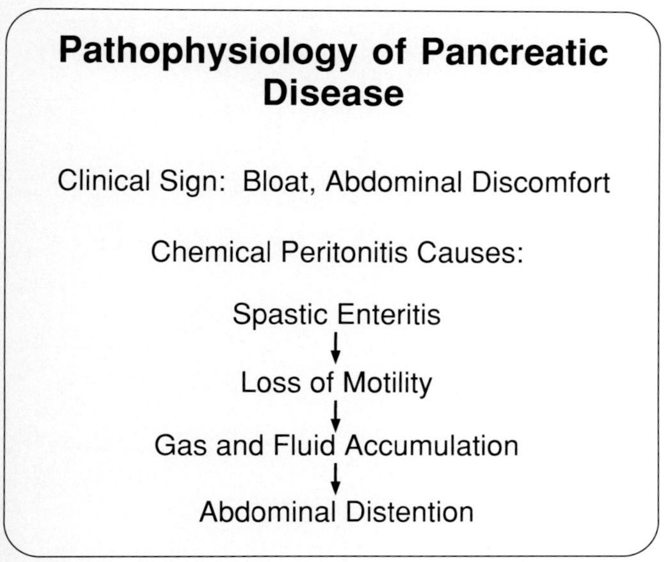

Figure 26-8.

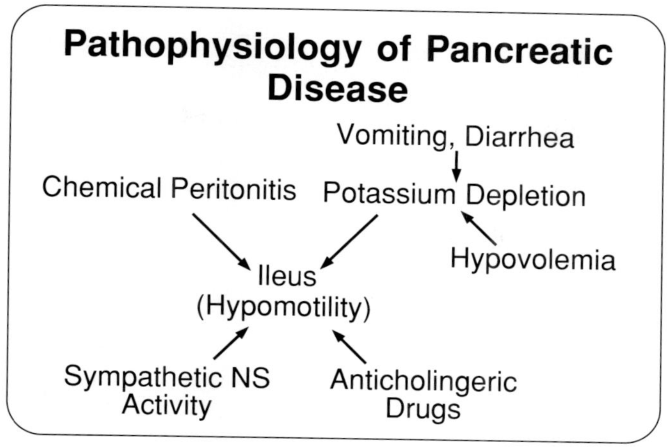

Figure 26-9.

ileus development are stimulation of the sympathetic nervous system by shock and peritonitis, and depletion of body potassium (Figure 26-9). Potassium depletion is the more important factor in dogs since ileus cannot be produced solely by intense stimulation of sympathetics with trauma.[69] Since animals with pancreatitis are potassium-depleted, intestinal hypomotility and ileus are at least impending problems, if not yet realized. The loss of normal motor function is magnified with the use of drugs that reduce smooth muscle contraction. Anticholinergics inhibit intestinal motility, and their use can precipitate ileus that is potential in an animal with pancreatitis. Loss of normal motility is probably the most important reason for diarrhea with pancreatitis.

Peritonitis. Local or generalized peritonitis is a regular feature of acute pancreatitis. Transudation of variable (though usually small) amounts of fluid into the peritoneal cavity can accompany the inflammatory changes. The fluid often resembles an exudate. Without gastrointestinal perforation or pancreatic abscessation, the fluid is sterile. Fluid formation is partly the result of increased vascular permeability produced by substances such as kinins, leukotrienes, and oxygen-derived free radicals.[62,70] High levels of pancreatic lipase, elastase, and trypsin activities found in abdominal fluid can also increase capillary permeability and be associated with high concentrations of plasma proteins.[71] Concentrations of 3.5 to 7.0 g/dl reflect substantial losses of plasma proteins from the vascular compartment. The permeability-enhancing properties of abdominal fluid are significantly inhibited by a trypsin inhibitor.

Renal Complications. Persistent hypovolemia in pancreatitis can be expected to result in prerenal azotemia. Pancreatitis is associated with decreases in gormerular filtration rate and renal blood flow and an increase in renal vascular resistance. Correction of fluid deficits usually improves renal function. The exceptions are patients with a marked and prolonged reduction in renal blood flow, where renal tubular necrosis can result, and patients with compensated renal insufficiency, where damage to a small number of nephrons results in a loss in the compensating ability. The kidneys participate importantly in the disappearance of serum lipase and amylase. With renal insufficiency, their levels will remain higher than expected.

Respiratory Complications. Signs of respiratory distress can be seen with pancreatitis. Seen most commonly is a rapid

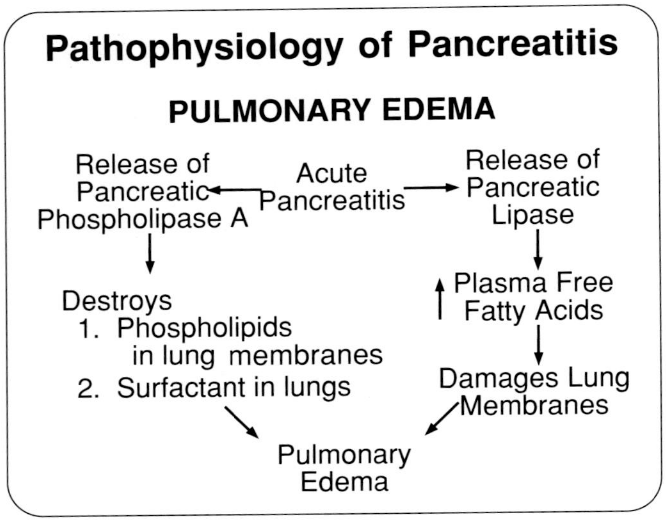

Figure 26-10.

shallow breathing, usually the result of pain-induced splinting of the abdominal wall. Respiratory insufficiency can result from reduced ventilation. Respiratory complications can cause hypoxemia without any clinical or radiographic evidence for respiratory problems. Pancreatitis can also increase the affinity of oxygen for hemoglobin so that less oxygen is available.[72] Respiratory problems can be iatrogenically produced or worsened by the administration of excessive amounts of fluids, resulting in pulmonary edema. Pleural effusion, atelectasis, and pneumonitis can be seen with acute pancreatitis.

Pulmonary edema is associated with acute pancreatitis in the dog as it is in humans under conditions where cardiac function and central venous pressures are normal.[73-75] The pulmonary edema fluid has a high concentration of plasma proteins developing from a disruption of alveolar-capillary membranes, allowing protein-rich plasma to escape into the interstitial space. A suggested cause of the damage is circulating pancreatic enzymes that initiate a cascade of destructive events (Figure 26-10). Plasma-protein-rich pulmonary edema can be produced experimentally in dogs by infusion of phospholipase A to destroy the phospholipid components of the pulmonary membranes, including the surfactants.[76] Thus, high plasma levels of phospholipase A released from the inflamed pancreas may produce the damage. That enzyme is also released by neutrophils attracted to the area. Circulating pancreatic lipase may also be involved. Infusion of large amounts of free fatty acids into normal animals damages alveolar-capillary membranes and results in pulmonary edema.[77] Humans with acute pancreatitis and hyperlipidemia are more likely to develop pulmonary edema than patients with normal serum lipids. Hyperlipidemia could provide the substrate for serum lipase activity to act on, producing large amounts of free fatty acids. Activity of lipoprotein lipase found on pulmonary epithelium increases with pancreatitis and may be a catalyst for triglyceride hydrolysis.

Neutrophils are necessary for increased vascular permeability with some experimental forms of pancreatitis.[75] Complement is activated with pancreatitis and appears to attract neutrophils to pulmonary sites where damage occurs. Neutrophils are responsible for generation of oxygen-derived free radicals that can damage vascular endothelium. Pulmonary edema is also associated with fibrin and platelet microthrombi, reflecting pulmonary intravascular coagulation. These changes increase vascular permeability, and fibrin deposition with pulmonary edema reduces pulmonary compliance, which worsens pulmonary insufficiency.[78] Kinins and histamine levels are increased but appear to play only a minor role in edema formation. Acute pancreatitis should appear in any differential diagnosis in an animal with respiratory problems caused by unexplained pulmonary edema.

Blood-Clotting Disorders. Intravascular coagulation occurs locally in the inflamed pancreas. Widespread intravascular coagulation has been seen in necropsies of dogs with pancreatitis. Proteases released from the pancreas can activate the enzymes involved in the clotting process. They are also capable of splitting and destroying the clotting factors. Contributing to abnormal blood clotting are a combination of excessive clot-promoting substances, deficiencies of clotting factors, and excessive degraded clotting factors. The reduced circulation through an inflamed pancreas is due in part to local thrombosis. Administering fibrinolysin and heparin, agents directed against thrombosis, improves pancreatic circulation and inflammation.

Experimental studies in dogs show acute pancreatitis to reduce platelet numbers and increase times for prothrombin and partial thromboplastin (Figure 26-11).[79,80] In addition, antithrombin III and complement decrease, euglobulin clot lysis time shortens, and fibrin degradation products increase. All these changes are consistent with consumption coagulopathy.

Cardiomyopathy. Acute pancreatitis can cause cardiomyopathies in dogs.[81] They produce arrhythmias that include ventricular premature contractions, atrioventricular dissociation, paroxysmal or persistent supraventricular tachycardia, heart block, and atrial or ventricular flutter or fibrillation.

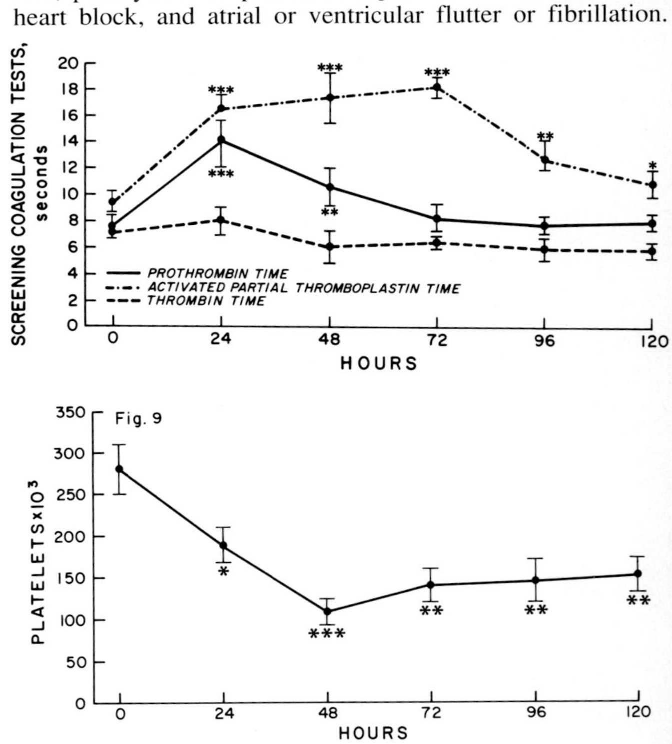

Figure 26-11. Changes in PT, PTT, and platelet numbers in dogs with acute pancreatitis.

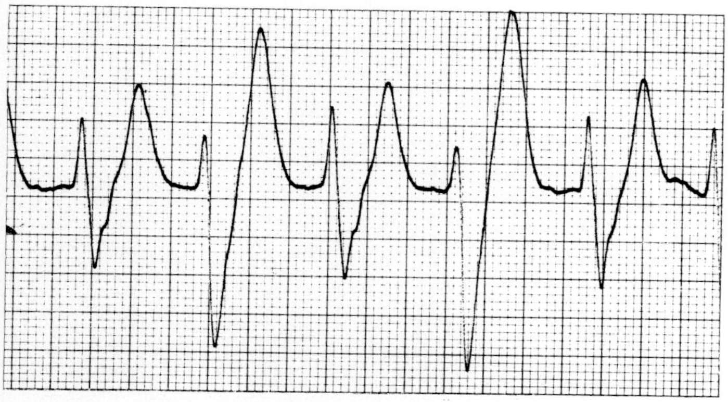

Figure 26-12. Electrocardiogram from dog with acute pancreatitis shows an arrhythmia that can be produced.

Electrocardiograms also show aberrant QRS complexes and changes in the S-T segment (Figure 26-12). The pathogenesis of the cardiomyopathy is not well understood. A possible cause is toxic peptides produced by pancreatic enzyme activity. One such peptide, the myocardial depressant factor, is released from the ischemic pancreas and has a damaging effect on the myocardium. Pancreatic enzymes may also directly damage cardiac muscle, and their promotion of thrombus formation in myocardial vessels may produce myocarditis via an ischemic route. Studies in humans with pancreatitis have correlated changes in electrocardiograms with changes in plasma electrolytes.[82] Pancreatic-induced cardiac arrhythmias seen at the VMTH at Davis have been associated with normal plasma electrolytes.

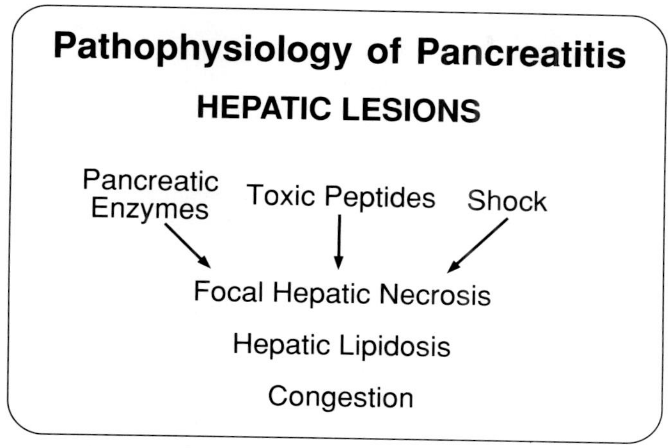

Figure 26-13a.

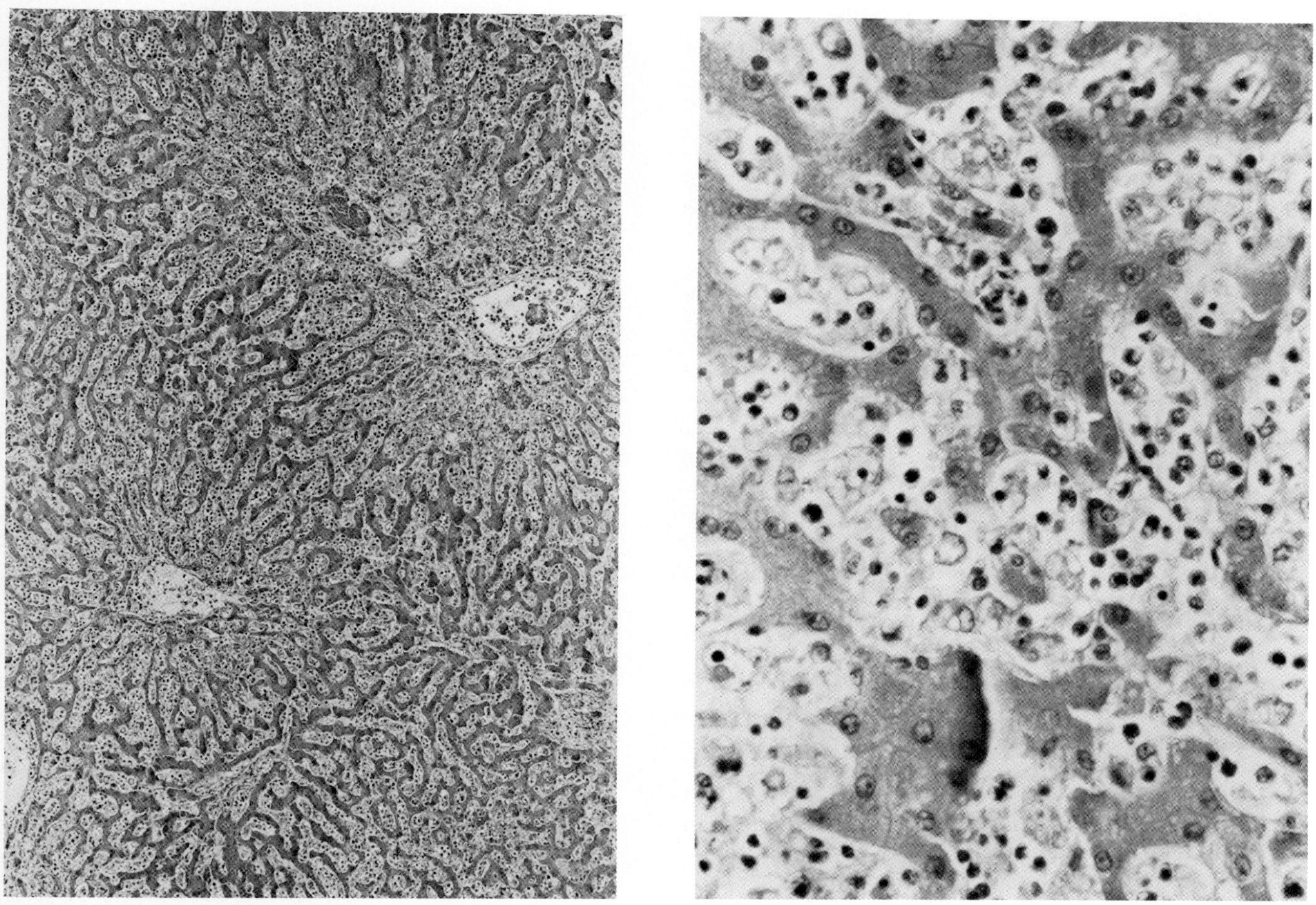

B C

Figure 26-13. b) Hepatic changes with acute pancreatitis. Most striking changes are centrolobular and include thinning of plates of hepatocytes and accumulation of cells in sinusoids. c) Sinusoidal changes include dilation and vacuolation of Kupffer cells and accumulation of many inflammatory cells. Biopsy specimen.

Hepatic Lesions. Acute pancreatitis produces hepatic lesions in dogs and cats with clinical and experimental pancreatitis. Liver changes in experimental hepatitis include necrosis, fatty infiltration, congestion, and loss of normal hepatic architecture. A prominent lesion in some is infiltration by lymphocytes. Chronic pancreatitis causes the same hepatic changes, except that lymphoid infiltration is more frequent, and atrophy and cirrhosis are seen in a few dogs. The pathogenesis of hepatic lesions is thought to involve: 1) changes produced by shock, 2) an etiologic agent that damages both pancreatic and hepatic tissue; and 3) toxic substances released from the pancreas. Hepatic pathology is the most frequently reported lesion in dogs and cats with pancreatitis and the pathology can be severe (Figure 26-13). Early ultrastructural changes in dogs are not different from those produced by ischemia, shock, or endotoxemia.[83]

Hyperglycemia. Hyperglycemia can be associated with acute pancreatitis, developing primarily from excessive amounts of glucagon released from the damaged pancreas. Hyperglycemia can also be due to inadequate release of insulin, especially in animals with an islet-cell population reduced by previous attacks of pancreatitis. The most common cause for diabetes mellitus is pancreatitis.[84] Pancreatitis in experimental dogs causes plasma glucagon to increase and remain elevated for at least four days; increases in plasma insulin are for only two days (Figure 26-14).[85] Catecholamines are probably increased and contribute to hyperglycemia.

Biliary Obstruction and Duodenal Stricture. Pancreatic inflammation can alter function in adjacent structures such as the duodenum and bile duct. Extensive fibrous tissue develops very early with acute pancreatitis. Fibrosis around the bile duct can produce an obstructive type of jaundice.[86] The same process sometimes partially obstructs the duodenum.

Hypocalcemia. Hypocalcemia is sometimes a complication of acute pancreatitis. Its incidence in dogs is unknown. Four theories have been advanced to explain the pathogenesis of this hypocalcemia.

The oldest theory suggests that a significant amount of calcium is removed from the extracellular fluid and sequestered in the abdominal cavity as insoluble salts of fatty acids. Fatty acids are produced when pancreatic enzymes released into the peritoneal tissues hydrolyze lipids. The small amount of calcium bound in this manner is not enough to account for the hypocalcemia, however. Recent studies show the intracellular calcium content of many soft tissues increases during pancreatitis.[87] Circulating enzymes are proposed to alter membrane permeability so calcium enters and plasma concentrations increase.

A second theory suggests that the hypocalcemia develops from increased secretion of thyrocalcitonin. Glucagon stimulates release of this hormone,[88] and hyperglucagonemia is a feature of pancreatitis.[89] Thus, glucagon indirectly produces the hypocalcemia.[90] This effect suggests that glucagon infusion, a treatment for pancreatitis, could precipitate hypocalcemia. In humans with acute pancreatitis, however, glucagon infusion does not reduce the low serum calcium levels further, nor does it stimulate thyrocalcitonin release. Other studies on experimental animals provide evidence that hypocalcemia seen early in acute pancreatitis is not related to a release of calcitonin.[91] Thyroidectomy to remove the source of calcitonin results in a hypocalcemia (24 hours after the onset of acute pancreatitis)

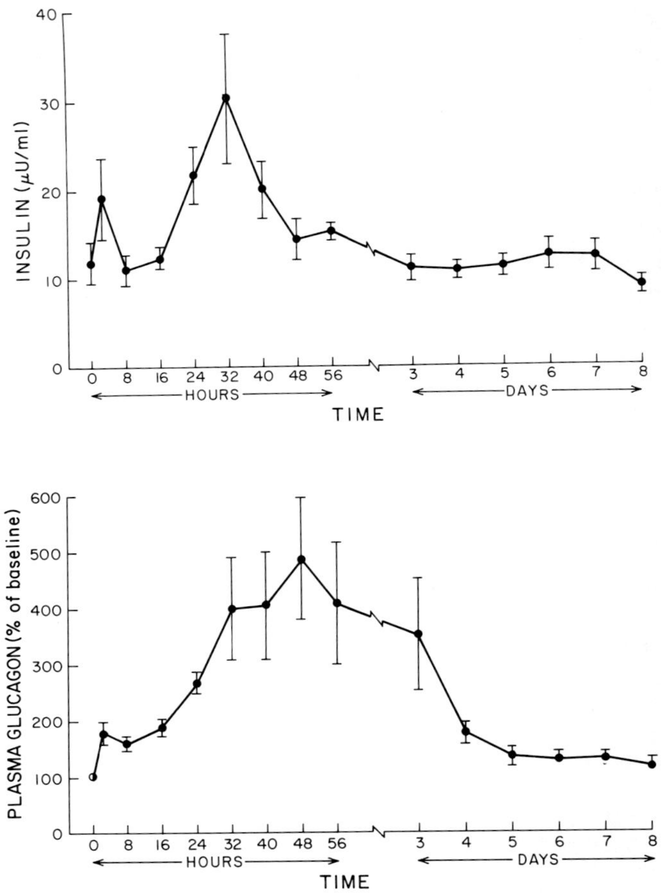

Figure 26-14. Changes in plasma insulin and glucagon levels in dogs with acute pancreatitis.

that is no different from the hypocalcemia in intact animals with pancreatitis.[91] Changes observed at 48 hours, however, suggest that hypocalcemia developing at a later time is related to calcitonin release. Gastrin is also found in the pancreas and is a more potent stimulus of calcitonin release than is glucagon.[90] Its release could contribute to the hypocalcemia.

A third theory suggests that the parathormone-secreting response of the parathyroids to hypocalcemia is abnormal. Supporting this theory is the correction of hypocalcemia by parathormone administration in humans with acute pancreatitis. This hypocalcemia cannot be corrected by calcium infusions.

A fourth theory proposes that the most important factor determining the serum levels of calcium is the concentration of plasma proteins.[92] Severe acute pancreatitis in experimental dogs results in a reduction in plasma ionized calcium but only at 48 hours (Figure 26-15). Plasma total calcium levels decrease only slightly and appear to follow reductions in plasma albumin levels. Infusions of plasma proteins can correct hypocalcemia in experimental animals with pancreatitis. That is in contrast to the failures to correct the hypocalcemia by calcium infusions. Hypocalcemia is not reported to be a problem in dogs and cats with acute pancreatitis; these species are different from others with that problem. Hypoproteinemia with pancreatitis is usually a more important problem to correct, and that will correct an accompanying hypocalcemia.

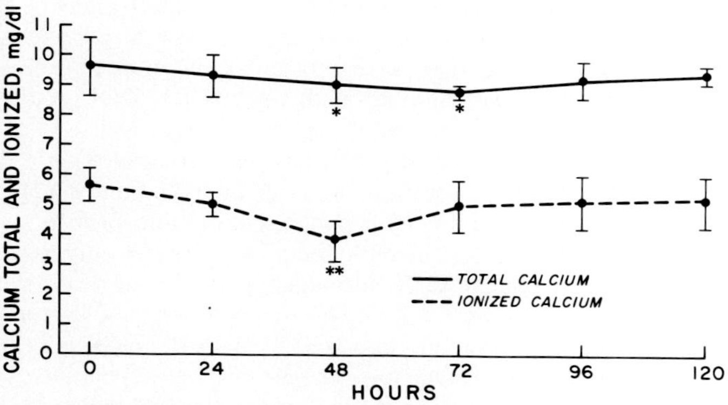

Figure 26-15. Changes in total and ionized calcium in dogs with acute pancreatitis.

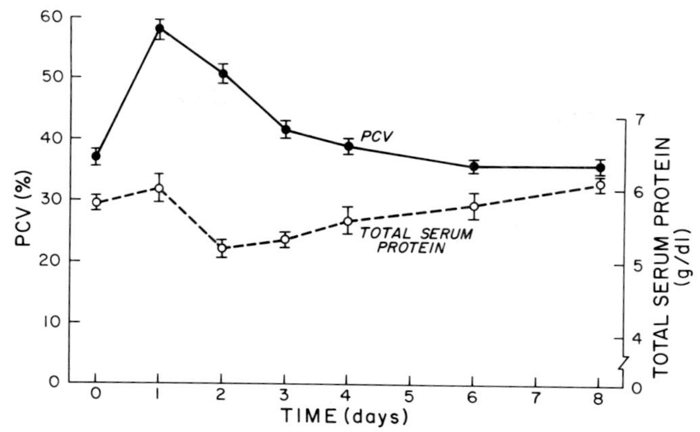

Figure 26-16. Changes in plasma proteins and packed cell volume in dogs with acute pancreatitis.

Acute pancreatitis in experimental dogs causes hemoconcentration and hypoproteinemia by 24 hours (Figure 26-16).[85] The hemoconcentration develops despite early administration of fluids. An increasing hematocrit with falling plasma proteins could be produced by mobilization of erythrocytes from the spleen or a marked loss of plasma proteins from the vascular to the interstitial space. Maintaining plasma protein levels by early plasma infusion does not prevent the hemoconcentration.[93] The hemoconcentration and hypoproteinemia persist for three to four days. Any hemoconcentration would further impair circulation in tissues poorly perfused because of the pancreatitis. These changes may also occur in cats with acute pancreatitis.

Clinical Findings

Pancreatitis presents no pathognomonic signs. The clinical signs are variable and resemble those of a large number of other problems presented with an acute abdomen. A complete history and thorough physical examination of the patient are mandatory in order to raise the level of suspicion so that the possibility of pancreatitis is pursued. Some patients show few if any signs of abdominal pain. Thus, the absence of such pain or any other cardinal feature of pancreatitis is not sufficient evidence to dismiss the possibility of pancreatic disease. In addition, pancreatitis can create so many complications that the secondary problem is sometimes recognized first. Identification of pancreatic disease is a diagnostic challenge.

Vomiting. The predominant clinical signs of acute pancreatitis appear as a result of acute inflammation in and around the pancreas. The stimulation of different types of sensory fibers results in a variety of nonspecific clinical signs, with vomiting being one of the most common. Vomition is stimulated by acute pain, distention or irritation of either the peritoneum or the intestine, and inflammation of the stomach or duodenum. In experimental dogs with acute pancreatitis vomiting is not seen or seen only once or twice in up to 40% of the animals.[85,93] Thus, lack of historical evidence for vomiting does not rule out the possiblity of acute pancreatitis. Cats show similar vomiting responses to pancreatitis.[94]

Pain. Mild to intense abdominal pain, sometimes localized in the cranial dorsal right abdomen, is generally considered to be an invariable sign of pancreatitis. Some dogs with pancreatitis show no signs of abdominal pain. A number of older animals presented with diabetes mellitus or pancreatic exocrine deficiency have no history of any problems suggestive of pancreatitis. Yet pancreatitis is the most common cause of these two problems in older animals. The existence of a group of dogs showing no signs of pain with pancreatitis is similar to a small population of humans who experience no pain with acute or chronic pancreatitis.[95] Experimental dogs with a severe form of acute pancreatitis show variable signs of pain that disappears within three to four days.[85,93] Up to 30% may show little or no evidence of abdominal pain. Thus, acute pancreatitis cannot be ruled out as a problem in patients when no signs of abdominal pain can be recognized.

Anorexia and Depression. Anorexia and depression are frequently associated with pancreatitis. Appetite usually returns before the pancreatitis is in remission as determined by normal plasma amylase and lipase levels. Resumption of feeding with the return of appetite is often followed by relapse. Depression also disappears before recovery is complete.

Fever. Rectal temperatures can increase with pancreatitis. In experimental dogs with acute pancreatitis mean rectal temperature increases from 38.5C to 39.3C at 24 hours and remains over 39C for at least eight days.[85,93] Fever develops as the result of infection, the release of pyrogens from damaged tissue, and the inflammatory process. Fever does not necessarily imply infection, which explains persistent fever despite the use of effective antibiotics.

Diarrhea. Diarrhea can appear with pancreatitis and is seen in 80% of experimental dogs with acute pancreatitis, with the diarrhea lasting at least eight days.[85,93] Up to 40% of these dogs have bloody diarrhea. Parts of the large intestine are normally adjacent to the pancreas. Pancreatic inflammation can extend to the intestine and result in diarrhea. The many other changes with pancreatitis, such as release of polypeptide hormones, can alter intestinal motility or stimulate intestinal secretion to cause diarrhea. Mediators of inflammation have a similar effect. When ileus develops, that by itself is a cause for diarrhea.

Abdominal Distention and Distress. Small animals with pancreatitis are usually uncomfortable, although not necessarily from pain. The discomfort is due in part to distention of the intestines with gas and fluid as a consequence of altered intestinal motility. Intestinal contraction around trapped gas and fluid produces signs of distress that include restlessness, shivering, panting, hiding, assuming a praying position, and seeking cool areas. Abdominal distention is seen in 38% of experimental dogs with pancreatitis.[96]

Dehydration and Shock. Dehydration as judged by skin turgor is evident with loss of excessive fluid through vomiting and diarrhea. Severe depletion of fluid volume sometimes produces few clinical signs of dehydration; that state can be recognized by the weak rapid pulse expected with reduced cardiac output. Shock is identified with heart rate and character of the pulse. Mean pulse rate in experimental dogs with acute pancreatitis increases more than 40% at 24 hours and gradually returns to normal within eight days.[85,93] Similar changes are seen in cats with acute pancreatitis.[94]

Cardiac Arrhythmias. Cardiac arrhythmias normally produce no signs suggestive of cardiac involvement until they become severe. They can appear at any time during the acute phase, making continuous electrocardiographic monitoring advisable in animals with severe pancreatitis. Cardiac complications constitute the most likely cause of sudden unexpected death in dogs with pancreatitis; they have been recognized in 23% of experimental dogs with pancreatitis.[84,93]

Respiratory Distress. Rapid shallow respiration is common in dogs with an acutely painful form of pancreatitis. Physical examination of the thorax is usually unremarkable. Pulmonary edema can also be a reason for respiratory signs and may be suspected from physical findings. Respiratory complications are seen in 8% of experimental dogs with pancreatitis.[96]

Laboratory Findings

A large number of diagnostic tests have been introduced to help the clinician in diagnosis of acute pancreatitis. Nevertheless there is still no one simple reliable test. The diagnosis of acute pancreatitis is based on finding elevated serum activity of amylase and lipase. The major disadvantage in using plasma amylase activity is that hyperamylasemia is not specific for pancreatitis. Plasma lipase activity is currently the most important test, but its specificity is not as great as its sensitivity.

Plasma Amylase. At one time, measurement of plasma levels of amylase was the most important diagnostic tool for pancreatic disease in dogs.[97] Considerable plasma amylase activity is found in normal animals, with levels approaching 1,000 IU/L. Potential sources of this activity are the pancreas, liver, and small intestine.[98] The pancreas does not contribute to the normal levels of activity, for they are unaltered by pancreatectomy. Proposals for the liver as the source are based on observations that plasma amylase activity is reduced one-half in dogs after hepatectomy.[99] The method used to determine amylase activity in this report is unacceptable for diagnosing the dog, however, since it also measures plasma maltase activity, which is considerable in this species. Moreover, hepatectomy rapidly results in hypoglycemia, hyperammonemia, and death within 16 hours, producing a situation where plasma amylase appearance and clearance are studied in a completely unphysiological state. If the large basal levels of amylase did indeed originate from the liver, sizable increases would be expected with acute hepatitis, yet plasma amylase levels do not increase with hepatic disease. It is currently believed that the liver does not contribute significantly to the activity of amylase in plasma.[100] The intestinal mucosa is the most likely source for the normal plasma levels of amylase activity.[101,102] The small intestine contains large amounts of amylase activity, the total amount being comparable to that in the pancreas. Normal plasma amylase activity usually doubles with any inflammatory process involving the gastrointestinal tract.

The half-life of plasma amylase is three to five hours.[103,104] Amylase's site of degradation or route of excretion is not known. The hepatic monocyte phagocytic system probably plays an important role, since blocking its uptake of amylase results in persistence of high plasma activity after infusion.[105] The early changes with a complete hepatectomy include a doubling of the plasma amylase activity, which supports the idea that the liver is responsible for part of its disappearance. The kidney is partly responsible for the disappearance of amylase. Plasma amylase is cleared by the human kidney and appears in the urine. The rate of amylase appearance in the urine is used to differentiate pancreatic disease from biliary obstruction in humans. Quantitation of urine amylase cannot be used to identify pancreatitis in dogs, however, since very little alpha-amylase activity can be detected in the urine of either normal dogs or dogs with acute pancreatitis. Following intravenous infusion of labeled amylase in dogs, only 1% of the label can be recovered in the urine. Little activity appears in the urine following infusion of pancreatic enzymes to produce plasma enzyme activity greater than ten times normal.[104] Hyperamylasemia produced by pancreatic-duct ligation also does not enhance the rate of amylase appearance in the urine. The fact that amylase does not appear in the urine of any dog is remarkable since normal plasma activity of the enzyme is 10 to 30 times greater in the dog than in humans. Since the renal clearance rates for amylase are similar for man and dogs,[106] most of the amylase in the glomerular filtrate is reabsorbed and degraded, probably in the proximal tubular cell. With a molecular weight of 45,000 daltons, pancreatic amylase should have a clearance rate that is 1% to 10% of the glomerular filtration rate. Functional nephrectomy causes the half-life of pancreatic plasma amylase to almost triple,[104] making the kidney an important site for the degradation of that enzyme. The intestinal tract could

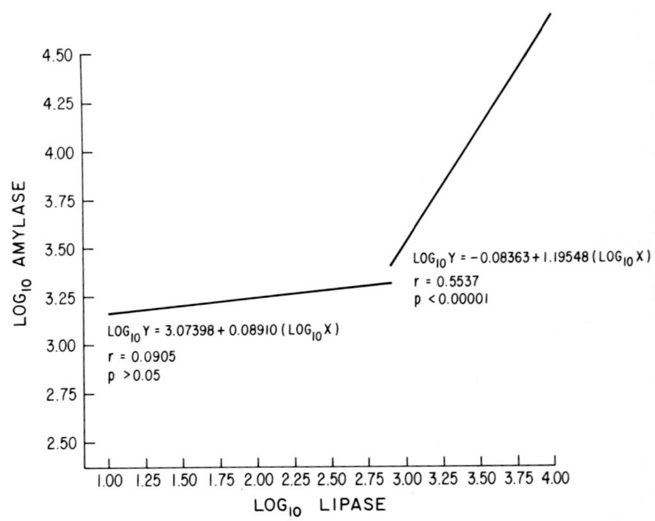

Figure 26-17. Relationships of logarithmic transforms of serum lipase and amylase activities in dogs when (a) lipase activity is < 800 UL and (b) lipase activity is > 800 UL.

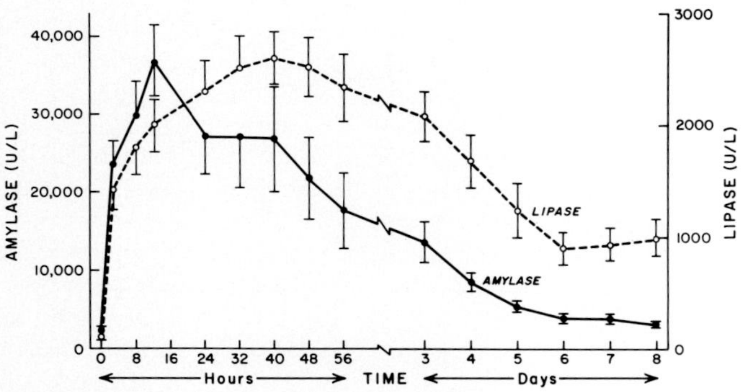

Figure 26-18. Changes in plasma amylase and lipase activities in dogs with acute pancreatitis.

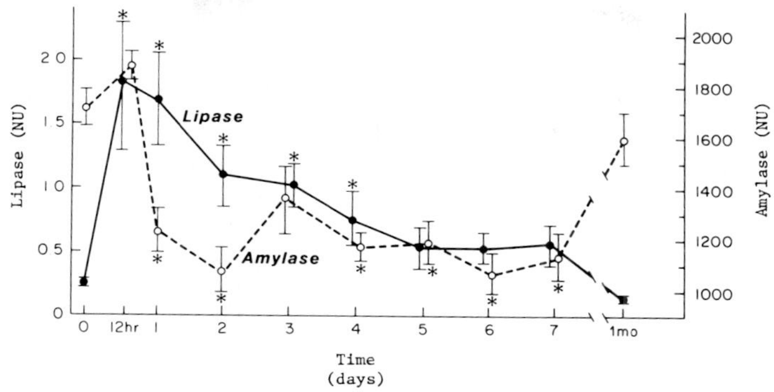

Figure 26-19. Changes in plasma amylase and lipase activities in cats with acute pancreatitis.

play a similar role.

Plasma amylase increases in most dogs with pancreatitis, making its measurement a highly sensitive test. But it also increases often with nonpancreatic diseases, giving it a poor specificity. Plasma amylase increments in pancreatitis do not correlate with lipase activity until lipase values exceed 800 U/L (Figure 26-17).[107] Moreover, the range of plasma amylase activities is the same for dogs with no pancreatitis as for dogs with pancreatitis and lipase values less than 800 U/L. Dogs with plasma amylase increased up to four or five fold over normal are much more likely to have a nonpancreatic problem than acute pancreatitis because there are so many problems that cause plasma amylase to increase compared to the relatively low incidence of acute pancreatitis.

Plasma amylase activity increases to very high levels in experimental dogs with pancreatitis (Figure 26-18).[85,93,108] Within one week its activity returns to levels found with many other diseases. Activities greater than 5000 U/L would seem to be highly suggestive of acute pancreatitis. Finding such a high level is more likely when measurements are made early in the course of the disease.

Plasma amylase activity behaves entirely differently in cats with pancreatitis; its levels decrease (Figure 26-19).[94] Explanations suggested include a decrease in enzyme release, increased amylase catabolism or clearance, or presence of circulating enzyme inhibitory substances. There are no indications for making determinations of plasma amylase activity in cats.

Renal failure is associated with hyperamylasemia, suggesting that plasma amylase activity increases when it is not being cleared by the kidneys. Nevertheless, bilateral nephrectomy does not have a significant effect on plasma amylase activity in normal dogs.[104] Thus, hyperamylasemia with renal failure is not due to a reduction in renal clearance of basal plasma amylase activity, which is most likely intestinal in origin. Being a different enzyme, intestinal amylase may not be cleared by the kidneys. It is possible that pancreatic amylase contributes to the hyperamylasemia with renal failure. This hyperamylasemia may reflect the accompanying increased stimulation of pancreatic secretion, which may be mediated by the high plasma gastrin levels associated with renal failure.[109] In this case, inadequate renal clearance of increased amounts of plasma pancreatic amylase activity could contribute to the hyperamylasemia. The association of pancreatitis with renal failure in humans has led to the suggestion of a cause-and-effect relation, but there is no scientific evidence to support the supposition. Evaluation of the cause of uremia as renal or prerenal has been used to determine the cause of hyperamylasemia. Evaluation of this hyperamylasemia is complicated, however, since amylase can be released at an accelerated rate from the pancreas and intestine and because amylase is not adequately cleared either during the conditions of reduced glomerular filtration in prerenal azotemia or by the kidney in failure.

Plasma amylase activity should be measured with an amyloclastic method, one that measures the disappearance of starch in the assay system.[110] Since maltase activity is high in normal dog plasma, a saccharogenic method (measuring the appearance of glucose in the assay) will indicate a falsely high amylase activity (maltase activity contributes greatly to glucose formed in the assay). Plasma amylase activity represents the sum of up to five isoenzymes. Separation and measurement of activity of one or more of these isoenzymes may be useful for the diagnosis of pancreatitis.[111,112]

Plasma Lipase. The most important means for evaluating a dog for pancreatic disease is determination of plasma lipase activity. Pancreatitis consistently causes the normally low plasma lipase activity to increase many-fold in clinical and experimental dogs (Figure 26-18).[85,107] Measurement of plasma activity and establishing 500 U/L as the cutoff between affected and unaffected gives the test a sensitivity of 98%; thus, few cases of pancreatitis are not identified by lipase determination.[95] The test has a specificity of only 72%, indicating that 28% of dogs with hyperlipasemia have no pancreatic disease. The nonpancreatic problems include hepatic disease, renal disease, and malignancies. The source of the increased plasma lipase is not known for these other problems. The pancreas is the most important source of normal plasma lipase activity, since pancreatectomy causes activity to fall by two-thirds. The gastric mucosa is the only other known source of lipase.

Pancreatic lipase is handled by the kidney in the same manner as amylase. Pancreatic lipase infused into dogs has a half-life of two hours, and nephrectomy increases the half-life to 11 hours.[104] Consequently, chronic renal disease should produce hyperlipasemia, although that has not been seen in humans[113] or reported in dogs. Nephrectomy does not cause

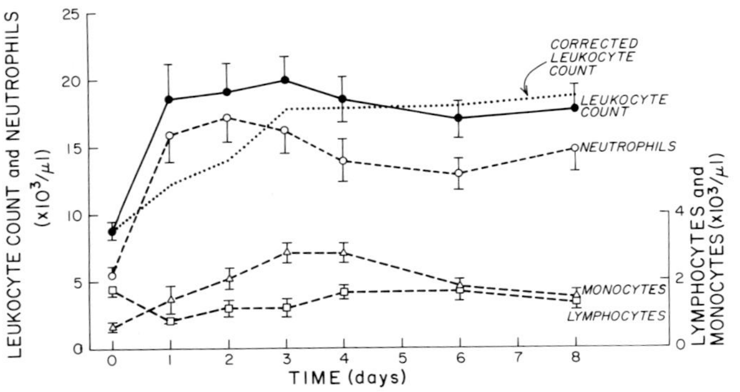

Figure 26-20. Changes in leukocytes in dogs with acute pancreatitis.

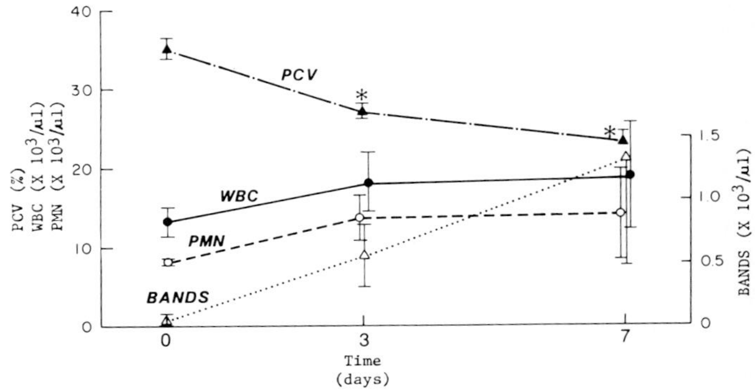

Figure 26-21. Changes in leukocytes in cats with acute pancreatits.

basal plasma lipase activity to increase in the dog.[104]

Plasma lipase activity is technically more difficult to assay than amylase activity. The test is based on hydrolysis of a triglyceride by plasma lipase activity, after which the free fatty acids are titrated with a sodium hydroxide solution to a basic pH. When the customary color pH indicators are used, the end point is difficult and somewhat arbitrary to identify. Use of a pH electrode to identify an endpoint allows precise measurement of serum lipase activity. Methods have been introduced to measure turbidity changes during triglyceride hydrolysis. Lipase determinations are made on serum samples.

Measurement of plasma lipase activity does not identify all cases of pancreatitis in cats.[114,115] Although hyperlipasemia is diagnostic for pancreatitis, normal plasma lipase activity does not rule out the disease.

Plasma lipase in experimental cats with acute pancreatitis increases eight to tenfold and returns rapidly toward normal by four to five days (Figure 26-19).[94] Many cats may have lipase determinations made later in the disease than dogs because the clinical signs are more subtle; measurements made later would show more with normal lipase values.

Plasma Amylase and Lipase Activity Patterns in Pancreatitis. Pancreatitis causes the plasma activities of amylase and lipase to increase simultaneously, but peak amylase activity is over after 24 hours, whereas peak lipase activity remains for at least 48 hours.[85,116] This is consistent with the two enzymes' having similar short half-lives. Plasma lipase activity persists at two times normal for at least seven to eight days, a time when amylase activity has decreased to normal values. On occasion both plasma amylase and lipase activities appear normal in dogs with pancreatitis. That is possible when assays are made after treatment is begun and enzyme levels have returned to normal.

Enzyme Activity in Peritoneal Fluid. Peritoneal fluid can be assayed for amylase and lipase activities; with pancreatitis the activities found will be greater in the fluid than in the plasma.[117]

Plasma Trypsin and Pancreatic Polypeptide. Measurements of plasma trypsin and trypsinogen have been advocated for identifying pancreatitis.[4] The pancreas is the only source of trypsin, and pancreatic disease should result in the release of trypsin to the circulation. Active trypsin is not found in plasma, however; such activity would be incompatible with life. Any trypsin formed is bound and inactivated by α_1-antitrypsin and α_2-macroglobulin. Assays for trypsin are radioimmunoassays for its antigen in trypsinogen and inhibitor-bound trypsin. Both of these forms of trypsin should increase with pancreatitis. Early reports indicate that more information is necessary before their measurement is accepted as a reliable test for pancreatitis. One inadequacy of commercially available tests is that they do not measure all forms of trypsin antigens.

Active trypsin is not found in plasma because of the abundance of circulating antiproteases. Acute pancreatitis reduces antiprotease levels, but only by 20% to 30%.[65]

Plasma levels of pancreatic polypeptide increase in experimental dogs with acute pancreatitis and return to normal within four days.[108] Feeding causes similar increases in unaffected dogs, but no such response is seen in dogs recovering from pancreatitis. If measurement of pancreatic polypeptide is to be used for diagnostic purposes, it is evident that feeding can produce false-positive results, and dogs with chronic recurring pancreatitis may give false-negative results.

Hemogram. In dogs, hemograms show early hemoconcentration and hypoproteinemia, as well as leukocytosis due to neutrophilia and monocytosis that persists for at least eight days (Figure 26-20).[85,93] Similar changes are seen in leukocytes for cats with pancreatitis (Figure 26-21).[94]

Blood Chemistries. Hypocalcemia is a finding that has been more thoroughly documented in humans than in animals with pancreatitis. Hypocalcemia is a feature of severe attacks and appears later in the disease (five to eight days after onset). The physiological effect of calcium in body fluids is due to its ionized fractions, which is the form that should be measured. Plasma calcium levels are evaluated with the knowledge that they parallel the plasma levels of albumin.

Methemalbumin is an abnormal pigment that can be identified in the plasma of animals with hemorrhagic pancreatitis

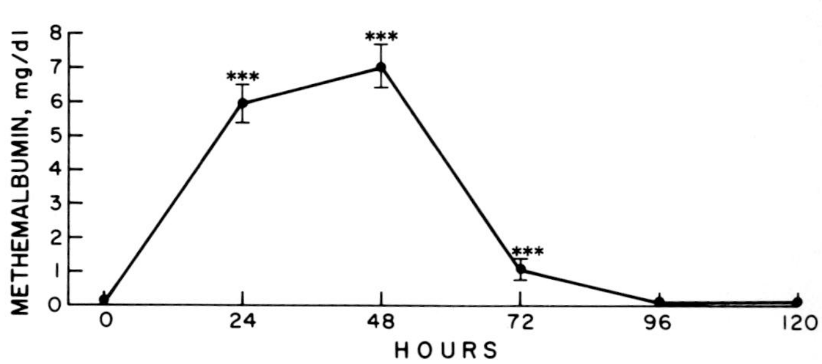

Figure 26-22. Changes in plasma methemalbumin in dogs with acute pancreatitis.

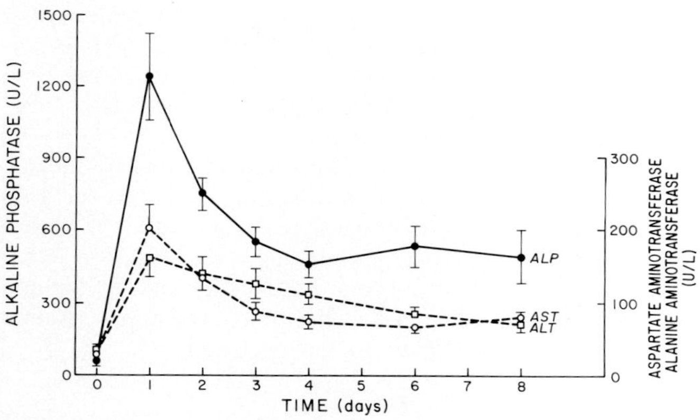

Figure 26-23. Changes in plasma activities of liver enzymes in dogs with acute pancreatitis.

(Figure 26-22).[79] Methemalbumin is produced by the action of pancreatic proteases on hemoglobin to form heme, which subsequently binds to albumin or other plasma proteins. The source of the hemoglobin is hemorrhage from the inflamed pancreas. Methemalbuminemia is not diagnostic for pancreatitis, since it can accompany other acute necrotizing conditions in the abdomen.

Hyperglycemia is often associated with pancreatitis and results from an accompanying hyperglucagonemia. A reduced ability to synthesize and release insulin contributes to hyperglycemia and is a factor in some dogs and cats with a history of pancreatic disease.

Fasting hyperlipidemia is sometimes seen with pancreatitis. Contributing to that are increased plasma triglyceride and cholesterol concentrations, changes not documented for experimental dogs with acute pancreatitis.[85,93] Experimental cats with pancreatitis show a doubling of plasma cholesterol.[94] The hyperlipoproteinemia found in such cases can be the result of pancreatitis, and in some dogs there is evidence that it is the cause. Insulin stimulates postheparin lipoprotein lipase activity and clearance of plasma lipids. A relative deficiency in insulin accompanying pancreatitis could contribute to the hyperlipidemia. Fasting hyperlipoproteinemia is identified and characterized by electrophoresis of the plasma lipoproteins.

Pancreatitis is often associated with hepatic necrosis, causing plasma activities of alanine transaminase and alkaline phosphatase to increase up to ten times normal in dogs (Figure 26-23).[85,93] Hyperbilirubinemia, when seen, usually results from obstruction of the main bile duct. Experimental cats with pancreatitis have only minor changes in plasma ALT and ALP activities, and little change in plasma bilirubin.[94]

Urinalysis can show a proteinuria in some dogs with pancreatitis. Uremia can appear, and is usually prerenal.

Pancreatic function studies on experimental dogs and cats with pancreatitis show a reduction in intestinal chymotrypsin activity.[93,94] One week after pancreatitis begins, the bentiromide test shows a 50% or more reduction in chymotrypsin activity. With more time the results do not improve and often worsen.

Radiographic and Ultrasonic Findings[118,119]

Survey films of the abdomen may provide information supporting a diagnosis of pancreatitis. Findings can include increased density or calcification in the right cranial abdomen (area of the pancreas) and gas in the most cranial part of the duodenum, although those are not diagnostic of pancreatitis. Accumulations of fluid can radiographically create a ground-glass appearance in the entire abdomen. In some cases, gas within an abscess can be demonstrated on survey films. Positive-contrast studies can sometimes provide more evidence for pancreatitis (Figure 26-24). Pancreatic inflammation can extend to the adjacent duodenum, causing spasm and ileus, both radiographically identifiable. Edema and inflammation cause spasm and thickening of the intestinal wall. Inflammation and edema in adjacent tissues "fix" the position of this segment of duodenum. Sequential radiographs taken after rotation of the animal show the affected duodenal loop to remain unchanged in position. A fixed position can persist when ileus develops. With severe damage, the affected duodenal loop may remain hypomotile. Fixation can also persist after remission of pancreatitis. Partial duodenal stricture as a complication is difficult to identify radiographically. Contrast radiography is also used to identify more precisely the locations of abnormal densities seen on survey films. If the history and physical examination indicate pulmonary complications, chest films should also be taken. In summary, rather than being a valuable adjunct in the identification of pancreatitis, radiography is more useful in delineating pathology that accompanies and complicates pancreatitis.

Ultrasonography can be used to visualize the pancreas in experimental dogs with pancreatitis. Gas in the gastrointestinal tract can interfere with the ultrasonographic evaluation so that the pancreas cannot be examined. Gas accumulation is not unusual with pancreatitis because of losses in gastrointestinal motility. The normal pancreas is not seen with ultrasonography. With pancreatitis a uniform but poorly defined density can be seen in the area of the pancreas. That finding in clinical cases helps confirm suspected pancreatitis. There are no reports on the reliability of ultrasonography in identifying or confirming pancreatitis in large numbers of dogs and cats. Some animals with pancreatitis show normal ultrasonographic findings.

Pancreatic Biopsy and Pathologic Findings[120,121]

Biopsy of the pancreas can be done to identify or confirm a pancreatitis. This is useful when clinical signs persist and laboratory test results are not diagnostic. Biopsy is required to identify lesions in a pancreas that grossly appears normal. The pancreas can be biopsied without precipitating a pancreatitis, although many fear such a complication. Needle-aspiration biopsy has been used successfully on the human pancreas[122] and can be a reliable and safe procedure for identifying pancreatitis where diagnosis cannot be confirmed by other means.

The pancreas is grossly normal when edema is the only change. Areas of pancreatic necrosis appear grayish-yellow in the normally grayish-pink pancreas, and they are usually accompanied by varying amounts of hemorrhage. Digestion and liquefaction of normal pancreatic tissue lead to formation of cystic spaces filled with sanguineous fluid and sometimes pus. Parapancreatic fat necrosis appears as chalky areas that can be surrounded by a halo of reddening in the pancreas and adjacent mesentery and omentum. Fat necrosis can be seen in extra-abdominal sites such as the ventral mediastinum; it may be produced by enzymes that lymphatics have transported to the area. Yellow or hemorrhagic adhesions can be found between the pancreas and other organs. The pancreas can be markedly distorted with extensive adhesions to the omentum, stomach, duodenum, jejunum, and spleen. With time large pseudocysts can appear. Chronic pancreatitis can cause pancreatic size to be reduced.

Microscopic changes with acute experimental pancreatitis in dogs can include edema; necrosis involving parenchymal and adipose tissues, blood vessels, nerves, and stroma; thrombosis of vessels; and inflammatory cell infiltration (Figure 26-25).[85,93] Small foci of acinar tissue undergo coagulation necrosis, and inflammatory cells infiltrate and form a yoke between normal and necrotic tissue. Necrosis creates gaps that are filled in by collapse of the adjacent parenchymal tissue. Within eight days histopathologic features are those of an acute exudative pancreatitis with accompanying pancreatic atrophy and fibrosis. When massive, necrosis is outlined by markedly edematous interlobular septa with a profuse fibrin exudate and infiltration of inflammatory cells, mainly neutrophils. As early as one week after onset, extensive granulation tissue can extend into the edematous and necrotic areas, with fibrosis surrounding surviving lobules of acinar cells. The inflammation and fibrosis distorts and obstructs pancreatic ducts. Areas of the pancreas distant from the affected regions show milder reactions: little necrosis, various degrees of edema, dilation of pancreatic ducts, and inter- and intralobular fibrosis.

Chronic interstitial pancreatitis occurs primarily in cats. Grossly the pancreas is smaller, firm, gray, and irregular, with clear retention cysts. Inflammatory cells are mainly mononuclear. Heavy fibrosis develops around the ducts, causing stenosis and an accumulation of catarrhal exudate. Duct epithelium is hyperplastic or metaplastic, becoming squamous. Acinar atrophy develops secondary to duct occlusion.

Diagnosis

Acute Pancreatitis. Finding increased plasma activity and lipase assists a diagnosis of acute pancreatitis. Lipase determinations increase above normal in 98% of dogs with pancreatitis, but of all high lipase values only 72% reflect pancreatic disease. Since the pancreas is the single primary source of plasma lipase

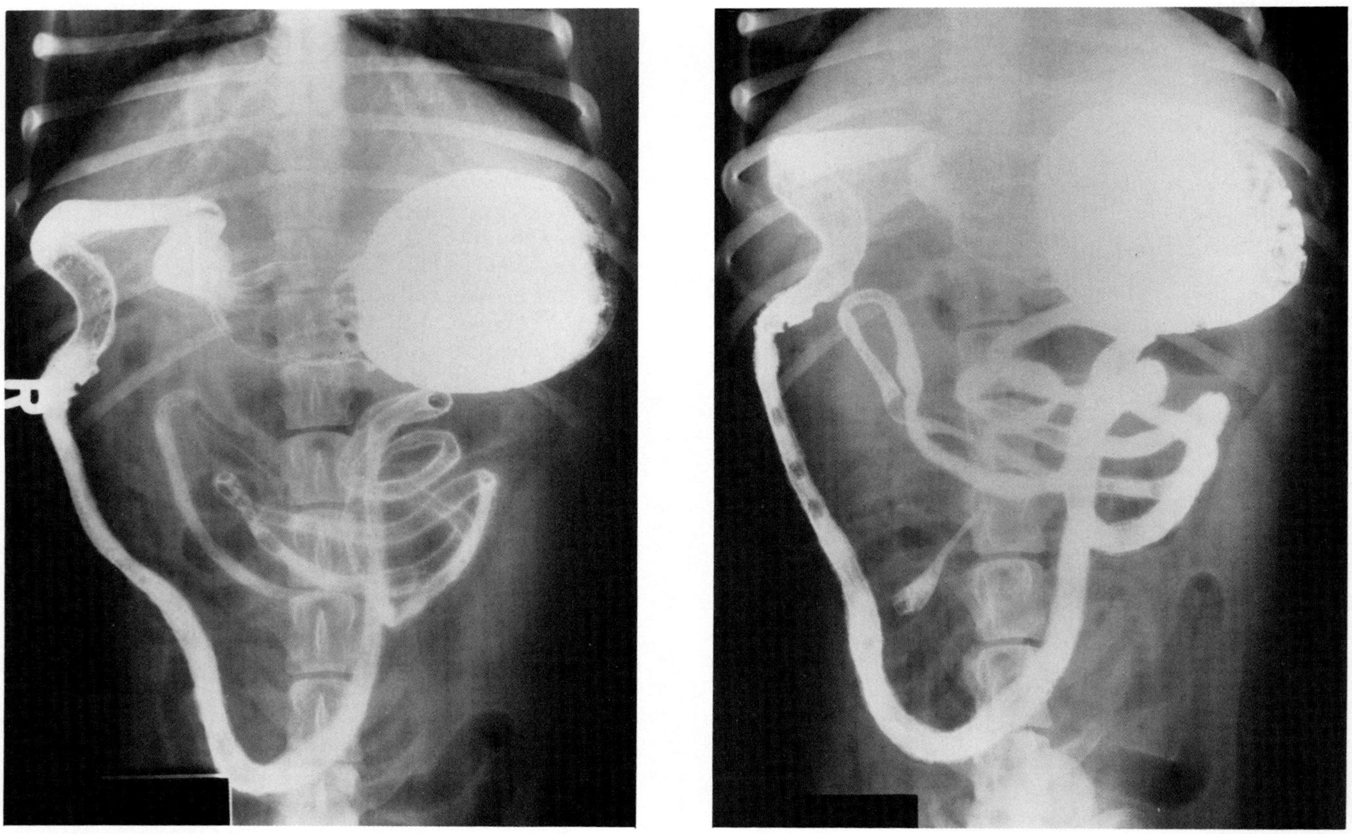

Figure 26-24a. Dorsoventral radiographs taken of a dog with clinical signs of acute abdomen and vomiting. Serum amylase and lipase enzymes were increased to ten times normal to confirm a diagnosis of acute pancreatic inflammation. Positive contrast medium was given and films taken at 10 and 30 minutes show the descending part of the duodenum to be in a fixed position. Films taken at other times showed the same fixed duodenal position. The duodenum shows irregularities along the visceral border. Acute inflammatory lesions in this area often cause the region to appear homogenous, a finding of local peritonitis. The inflammatory changes fix the duodenum's location. Radiographic changes are compatible with a pancreatic problem (tumor or inflammation), abscess or granuloma. Diagnosis was acute pancreatitis.

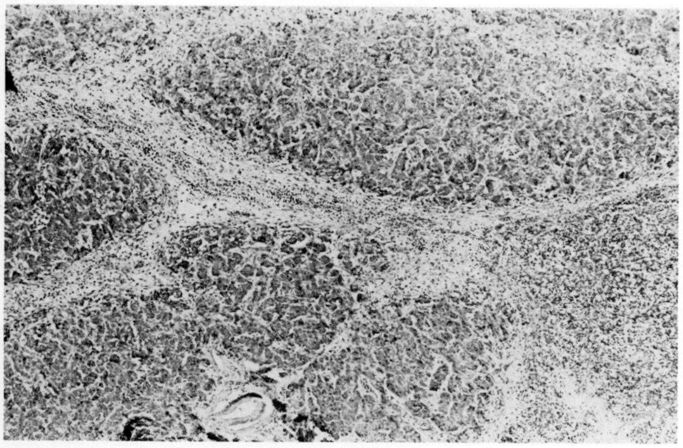

Figure 26-25. Acute pancreatitis. Areas of acute necrosis are identified by the disappearance of parenchymal cells and the presence of inflammatory cells. Edema is evident between some lobules.

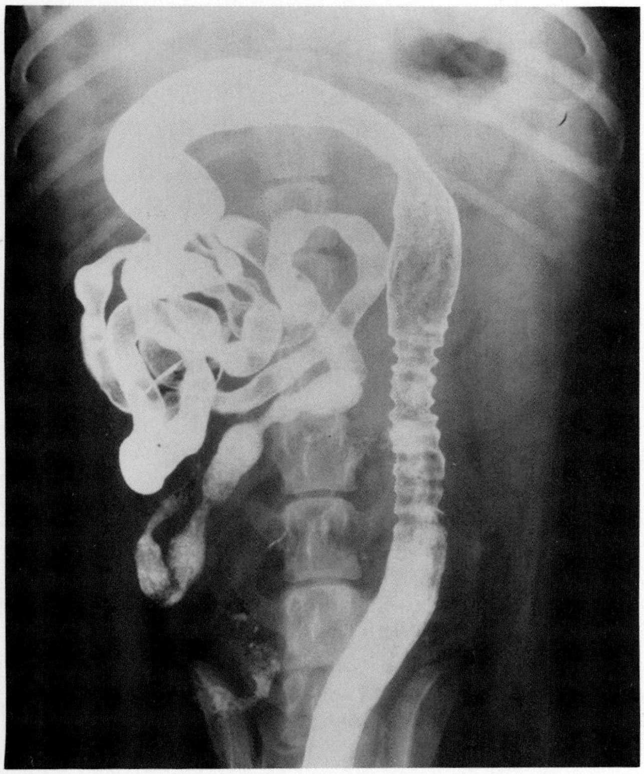

Figure 26-24b. Radiograph taken 7.5 hours after positive contrast medium was given. The descending colon shows shortening and spasms. The homogenous appearance of the abdomen in the adjacent area is suggestive of peritonitis. However, this area is not in close proximity to the pancreas. The colitis evident in this radiograph is consistent with signs of diarrhea that is frequently seen with acute pancreatitis.

activity, it can be assumed to release any significant increment above normal. One must decide whether the release reflects pancreatic disease or possibly some other cause such as hepatic, renal, neoplastic, or cardiovascular disease. Information gained from clinical signs, hemograms, blood chemistries, radiographs, and ultrasound examinations cannot be used to prove or disprove pancreatitis. Acute pancreatitis remains a difficult disease to confirm, and a best judgment on whether it is a problem requires information from all evaluations that can be made. Some cases are not recognized until surgical exploration for an acute abdomen with an unknown cause.

Pancreatitis is difficult to identify in cats primarily because their plasma lipase values correlate poorly with pancreatic inflammation. In addition, there are no pathognomonic clinical signs or biochemical abnormalities for pancreatitis in cats. Pancreatitis can be associated with specific infectious diseases such as panleukopenia, feline leukemia, and feline infectious peritonitis, in which cases the animal is not evaluated for pancreatic involvement. In summary, pancreatitis can be diagnosed with high plasma lipase values, which may be a manifestation of infection with one of the feline viruses, but pancreatitis is not ruled out by normal plasma lipase values.

Chronic Pancreatitis. After recovery from clinical signs of acute pancreatitis, experimental dogs with chronic pancreatitis show virtually no indications of having a serious medical problem.[93] After eight to ten days affected dogs show no clinical signs for at least three months despite having severe pancreatic pathology. They eat normally and maintain their body weight. Within three weeks after acute pancreatitis is produced plasma amylase and lipase activities return to normal and remain so. Determination of pancreatic function with the bentiromide test shows a marked reduction of 50% or more in small intestinal chymotrypsin activity. It is not known whether such experimental dogs show any radiographic or ultrasonographic evidence for pancreatic disease. Histopathology shows the pancreas to have extensive fibrosis with only islands of acinar cells by three weeks; at twelve weeks only remnants of acini may remain (Figure 26-26). Fibrosis' occlusion of ducts causes duct dilation. Later large pseudocysts form with thick fibrous walls. At any time pockets of histiocytes, neutrophils, and debris are scattered throughout the fibrous tissue. Similar changes are found in clinical cases of chronic pancreatitis in dogs. Experimental cats with acute and chronic pancreatitis have histopathologic changes like those in dogs.[94]

Management

Acute pancreatitis is managed by minimizing the synthesis and secretion of pancreatic enzymes. Without a stimulus for secretion, the enzymes are not synthesized and pancreatic inflammation can subside. Dietary management and pharmaceuticals are used to reduce pancreatic exocrine secretion. The value of drugs to reduce secretion is questionable.

Management of Pancreatic Inflammation

Inhibition of Enzyme Secretion. *Diet*. Animals with acute pancreatitis are given nothing by mouth. No food is given because food is the most important stimulus for pancreatic secretion. Amino acids and fatty acids in the small intestine cause the release of cholecystokinin (CCK), the most potent

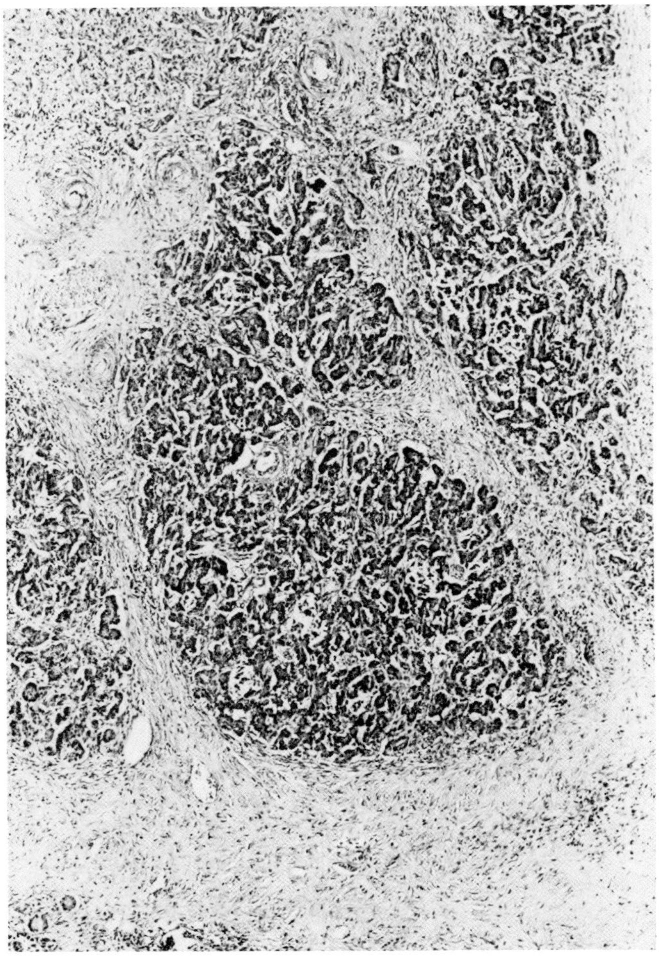

Figure 26-26. Chronic pancreatitis. Chronic inflammation has destroyed acinar cells and caused formation of extensive fibrosis.

stimulus for pancreatic secretion. Other hormones such as gastrin, whose biologic activity resembles that of CCK, stimulate the pancreas. Gastrin is released primarily from the gastric antrum by protein digestion products and by distention. Thus, oral fluids as well as food are withheld since they both cause gastric distention and the release of gastrin.

Oral intake of fluid and nutrients is resumed with remission of clinical signs. Studies in experimental dogs show that feeding can be resumed after five days.[85,93] Used first are nutrients that stimulate enzyme secretion the least. Carbohydrates have that property and are given in a form that requires minimum digestion. Glucose or small polymers of glucose result in minimal pancreatic secretion. With improvement, the carbohydrate source is gradually changed to a source of starch (such as boiled rice), and proteins are introduced. Proteins should be of high biological value, and levels should not exceed minimum requirements. Cottage cheese or lean meat are gradually added to the diet. With improvement, commercial products can be fed. Since protein is more potent than lipids as a stimulator of pancreatic secretion, a high-protein diet should not be fed. Since high levels of dietary fat are an important factor in the development of acute pancreatitis, dietary lipid levels should be as low as possible. Commercial dog foods differ in their fat content. Low-fat prescription diets can be used.

Satisfaction of nutritional requirements may be necessary before oral feeding can be resumed. Those can be met by total parenteral nutrition, which does not affect pancreatic secretion.[123] Elemental diets may be used, but pancreatic secretion of fluid and enzymes is as great with orally administered elemental diets as with conventional diets.[123] Infusion of an elemental diet directly into the duodenum results in the normal response of secreting enzymes but not fluid and bicarbonate. The acid-pH stimulus for secretin release is lacking during this infusion. If, however, an elemental diet with a neutral pH is infused into the jejunum, the pancreas secretes neither enzymes nor fluid and bicarbonate.[124]

Anticholinergics. Drugs have been used to inhibit enzyme synthesis and secretion. Anticholinergic drugs such as atropine and propantheline bromide inhibit the neurogenically stimulated secretion of pancreatic enzymes. Anticholinergic drugs inhibit secretion in the actively secreting pancreas, although it has not been shown that they inhibit the low basal level of secretion in the gland not stimulated to secrete. Since secretion ceases in the acutely inflamed pancreas,[125,126] the use of anticholinergics to reduce enzyme secretion is questionable. Moreover, anticholinergics have other effects that may make their use contraindicated. Inflammation often extends from the pancreas to the adjacent stomach and intestines, causing a loss of normal motility. Anticholinergics reduce motility further and can precipitate an ileus if that is not already a problem.

Anticholinergics reduce normal gastric motility to the extent that gastric retention develops. With resumption of oral feeding, anticholinergic drugs cannot be expected to reduce food-stimulated pancreatic enzyme secretion in order for pancreatic inflammation to subside. In experimental dogs anticholinergics do not show any benefit in recovery from pancreatitis, and they may contribute to complications.[85,127]

Glucagon and Somatostatin. Glucagon has been used to treat acute pancreatitis. Glucagon inhibits pancreatic secretion following stimulation by secretin or CCK.[128] Glucagon, being a member of the secretin family, could competitively inhibit secretin-stimulated secretion. The effect of glucagon on the resting pancreas, however, is to stimulate the basal rate of secretion.[129] Secretin does not stimulate enzyme secretion, and the diseased gland responds poorly to secretin.[126] Glucagon may exert a beneficial effect by stimulating splanchnic blood flow; improvement in pancreatic blood flow reduces the severity of acute pancreatitis. Glucagon has undesired effect of reducing gastrointestinal motility. No benefit has been shown for using glucagon to manage pancreatitis. Somatostatin, a hormone inhibiting pancreatic exocrine secretion, has little to no beneficial effect on acute experimental pancreatitis in dogs.[34]

Improvement of Pancreatic Circulation. Pancreatic blood flow is reduced with pancreatitis.[130] In some experimental models it is not possible to produce pancreatitis without causing pancreatic ischemia. Thus, reduced microcirculation is an important factor in the pathogenesis. Local thrombus formation, vessel destruction, and intrapancreatic shunting of blood contribute to the ischemia. The impaired circulation is also a factor in the persistence and progress of the pathology; any means of improving pancreatic microcirculation improves the chances for resolution of the problem.

Low-molecular-weight dextrans improve the survival rate

of animals with experimental pancreatitis. Given intravenously, the dextrans decrease blood viscosity, prevent thrombosis, and improve peripheral circulation. Dextrans prevent the marked decrease in pancreatic blood flow seen with pancreatitis. Dextran should be used with caution in patients with hemorrhagic pancreatitis since excessive amounts promote bleeding.[131,132]

Vasoactive peptides have been used to increase pancreatic blood flow in experimental dogs with pancreatitis. Vasopressin, which has a general vasoconstrictive effect on peripheral blood flow, has no effect on blood flow in the normal pancreas, but in the acutely inflamed pancreas it restores the reduced blood flow to normal.[133] Vasopressin (five units in oil given before experimental pancreatitis and repeated every six hours) is effective in doubling survival time and reducing the severity of acute pancreatitis in dogs.[134] Vasopressin also has a beneficial effect when given after the onset of inflammation.[135] Glucagon, as mentioned earlier, increases splanchnic blood flow, which may be the basis for a beneficial effect.

Pancreatic circulation can be improved by preventing thrombus formation and promoting clot dissolution.[136] Experimentally induced hemorrhagic pancreatitis (normally fatal), was prevented from developing in a group of dogs by heparin administered at a dose of 1.0 mg/kg, one-half intravenously and one-half subcutaneously, followed by a single subcutaneous dose at 12 hours. Treatment with heparin is important if disseminated intravascular coagulation develops. Fibrinolysin, used to dissolve thrombi in the vessels of the acutely inflamed pancreas, produces a greater improvement than heparin. Thrombi are already a problem in the clinical case before treatment is begun, which suggests that fibrinolysin should be more effective than heparin. Fibrinolysin was given intravenously to experimental dogs every eight hours at a dose of 50,000 units in 25 ml of 5% dextrose.[136] It remains to be determined whether heparin and fibrinolysin are effective in clinical cases. Heparin is also of value in managing the peritonitis accompanying pancreatitis.[137]

Enzyme Inhibitors. Enzyme inhibitors could be used to effectively treat acute pancreatitis if trypsin, elastase, and phospholipase-A are important in the pathogenesis and progress of acute pancreatitis. A trypsin inhibitor, with a wide range of inhibition on many proteases, isolated from bovine salivary glands (aprotinin and distributed commercially as Trasylol) has been evaluated in experimental dogs with pancreatitis.[34] Aprotinin reduces mortality in such dogs, but any clinical use is restricted by its high cost.

Insulin. Insulin is suggested to be of benefit in the treatment of acute pancreatitis; it inhibits a hormone-sensitive lipase that may cause the fat necrosis accompanying acute pancreatitis. Insulin markedly alleviates pain in humans.[138] Its effects on serum enzyme levels and morphological pancreatic changes, however, have not been determined.

Corticosteroids. Corticosteroids are used as part of the standard treatment for all types of shock. Corticosteroids are known to stabilize lysosomal membranes and inhibit release of the destructive lysosomal enzymes that play an important role in the pathogenesis of shock. Corticosteroids' beneficial effect on survival rates, however, has not been well-documented. Experimental dogs with one form of pancreatitis live longer when given steroids, but even then they do not live more than an average of 40 to 45 hours.[67] Other experimental dogs with acute pancreatitis who live more than one week demonstrate no beneficial effect from corticosteroid therapy.[85] Studies on the isolated canine pancreas with pancreatitis also show no beneficial effect from such therapy.[139] Although the results of steroids in experimental studies are difficult to translate into an assessment of their value in clinical problems, steroids have been advocated to reduce pancreatic inflammation. That practice may be contraindicated if steroids can cause pancreatitis, for which there is some evidence. Since their effectiveness in treating pancreatitis has not been established, and since it is believed that they can cause pancreatitis, corticosteroid use should be limited to treating shock and not extended to arresting the inflammatory process in the pancreas.

Management of Complications

Fluid and Electrolyte Abnormalities. Replacement of fluid deficits and management of hypovolemia constitute the most important therapy for pancreatitis. Experimental dogs with acute pancreatitis survive when vigorous fluid therapy is instituted.[85,93,140,141] Fluid must be given at a rate of 6.5 ml/kg/hr to prevent decreases in central venous pressure and to maintain normal pancreatic blood flow. Without such fluid therapy circulatory shock develops and early death rate is high. Fluid therapy is also important for management of the primary problem since pancreatic microcirculation does not improve until any hypovolemia is corrected. Fluid deficits develop, primarily due to losses from vomiting and diarrhea. Hypovolemia develops from fluid losses and from pooling of plasma fluid in capillary beds as a result of changes in the microcirculation.

Decisions on fluid therapy are based on information from the history and physical examination (Table 26-4).[96] Measurements of arterial blood pressure, central venous pressure, blood gases, and plasma electrolytes permit selection of a fluid for meeting specific requirements and for determining amounts to give.

Physical signs of dehydration, tachycardia, and pulse deficits determine the requirements for volume replacement. Deficits should be corrected as rapidly as possible by intravenous administration of fluids. The size of the deficits can be calculated from an estimation of the degree of dehydration. The disadvantages of this method include the possiblity of underestimating volume requirements and of causing or aggravating pulmonary edema. A more accurate means of determining the animal's volume needs is measurement of central venous pressure during fluid administration. This method solves the common problem of underestimating needs. Monitoring central venous pressure helps prevent pulmonary edema during fluid administration unless hypoproteinemia is severe or excess plasma protein is lost into the alveoli. In addition to monitoring arterial and central venous pressures, one can assess the results of fluid therapy by measuring urine output and by monitoring body weight.

Generalized increased capillary permeability, often seen with pancreatitis, results in movement of albumin into the extravascular space. Hypoproteinemia is predictable in experimental dogs. Circulating albumin volume can be reduced to the extent that plasma volume and cardiac output cannot be maintained at normal levels. Hence, if fluids do not restore central venous pressure, plasma or other colloids may be required. Pulmonary edema resulting from a loss of plasma proteins into the alveolar interstitial space can become more severe with the

Table 26-4. Management of Acute Pancreatitis

First 5 days after onset - IV fluids - **Day 1**: 80-120 ml/kg/day + percent dehydration X body weight in kilograms (for existing deficit) + continual losses due to vomiting, diarrhea, and ascites. Flow rates should initially be high (monitor central venous pressure) and then gradually decreased toward basal requirements **Day 2**:Evaluate effectiveness of fluid therapy from Day 1 and modify fluid composition and flow rates accordingly. **Days 3 to 5**:Fluid deficit should be corrected at this point, continual losses should be minimal to nonexistent; maintenance requirements must be satisfied (50/mg/kg/day).

Food and water - Nothing per os

Antibiotics

Procaine penicillin G (20,000 U/kg BID)
aminoglycoside, in some cases

Days 6 and thereafter onset - Stop IV fluids and antibi - otics; give free-choice water. Initially, give small amounts of low-fat, high-carbohydrate diet five to six times per day; by two weeks the dog should be fed once a day; after this time gradually wean from low-fat diet to a normal balanced diet.

administration of plasma. Plasma administration is monitored by measurement of the central venous pressure.

Plasma electrolyte derangements are usually the result of fluid losses through vomiting. Metabolic acidosis develops in experimental dogs with pancreatitis and is usually found when looked for in clinical cases. Bicarbonate can be given to correct that problem. Electrolyte derangements are often seen for potassium and sometimes sodium. Potassium is at high concentration in gastric secretions. Its loss causes a depletion of body potassium and frequently hypokalemia. Thus, potassium must be given. Gastric secretions contain sodium at concentrations less than those of plasma. Hypernatremia develops when water is lost through vomiting at a rate that is greater than the loss of sodium. With access to water, vomiting patients drink to replace volume deficits. Despite repeated vomition, some water is absorbed after drinking, causing hyponatremia from progressive dilution. Continued loss of sodium in the vomitus and through the kidneys intensifies the problem. Ringer's solution is used to correct electrolyte abnormalities when plasma electrolytes and blood gases are not measured. This solution meets volume needs and partly replaces potassium losses. The lactate in Ringer's solution helps to correct metabolic acidosis.

Antibiotics. Antibiotics have been an important part of the treatment of acute pancreatitis despite the lack of controlled studies to support their value in clinical cases. Bacteremia is documented in experimental animals with pancreatitis.[143] Enteric organisms are responsible, which justifies the use of antibiotics effective against bacteria invading from the gastrointestinal tract. The efficacy of antibiotic therapy has been demonstrated in experimental animals with severe pancreatitis. Invasive bacteria can multiply in areas of necrotic or devitalized tissue and cause abscesses. Both aerobic and anaerobic bacteria are normally found in the intestine. Invasion by aerobes is related to increased mortality rates, and invasion by anaerobes is the cause of abscess formation.[143] Treatment is directed against both types of organisms, with penicillins the most effective against anaerobes, and gentamicin effective against aerobes. One controlled clinical study used only ampicillin to treat pancreatitis, and the results were no better than when using no antibiotic.[144] Treatment must be directed against every type of bacteria potentially invading from the intestine.

Vomiting. Vomiting is controlled with thorazine, given at the smallest recommended dose. Like any other tranquilizer, thorazine has hypotensive properties and is used with caution in the hypovolemic patient. Antiemetics acting at the chemoreceptor trigger zone may not control vomiting.

Analgesics. Narcotic analgesics such as meperidine can be used to relieve pain but are used with caution since they depress central nervous system centers controling circulation, and that worsens shock. Narcotic analgesics have other pharmacologic effects, including stimulation of intestinal smooth muscle contraction. Such constriction in addition to that of the pancreatic duct could worsen pancreatitis if duct obstruction was an important factor in its pathogenesis. In humans, narcotic analgesics cause serum amylase to increase, presumably by closing the pancreatic duct or sphincter of Oddi, but serum levels of lipase do not change.[27] The increment of serum amylase is more likely to derive from intestinal mucosa than from the pancreas, since lipase is unchanged. In normal dogs, morphine does not cause serum amylase or lipase to increase.[26] Narcotic analgesics have not been shown to increase damage in the inflamed pancreas. Moreover, they inhibit pancreatic secretion, a desired goal.[145] Meperidine or butorphanol, but not morphine, can be used and repeated as necessary.

Hypocalcemia. Hypocalcemia is treated by correction of the hypoproteinemia that causes its appearance. Plasma proteins are administered, with monitoring of central venous pressure. Calcium infusions cannot correct this hypocalcemia.

Cardiac Arrhythmias. The cardiac arrhythmias are treated with lidocaine, quinidine, and procainamide, and they require continuous electrocardiographic monitoring.

Pulmonary Edema. Pulmonary edema develops because of a loss of plasma proteins into the alveolar interstitial space. Diuretics do not remove this edema, and if the problem causes hypoxia the patient must be ventilated on a respirator using positive end-expiratory pressure.

Adjunct Therapy

Peritoneal Lavage. Peritoneal lavage is beneficial in treating some humans with pancreatitis.[146] From results of an experimental study in dogs,[147] peritoneal lavage may be of value in treating pancreatitis. More dogs survived when lavaged with a balanced electrolyte solution than when managed only with intravenous saline administration. The difference was attributed to the washing of destructive pancreatic enzymes from the abdomen in the lavaged group. The difference in survival, however, could have been due also to the benefits of receiving a balanced electrolyte solution, which the unlavaged group did not receive. Clinical studies have been reported on the use of peritoneal lavage for treatment of pancreatitis in humans with no value found.[34] Similar clinical studies have been reported in dogs.[148]

Peritoneal lavage is indicated in patients with septic peritonitis but remains of doubtful value in the treatment of chemical peritonitis caused by pancreatitis. Moreover, some risk

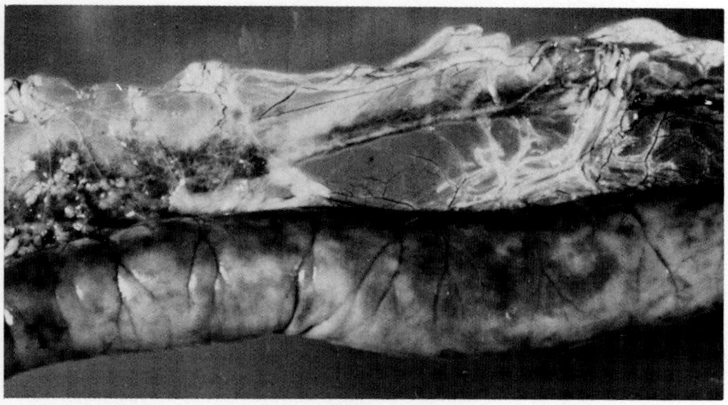

A

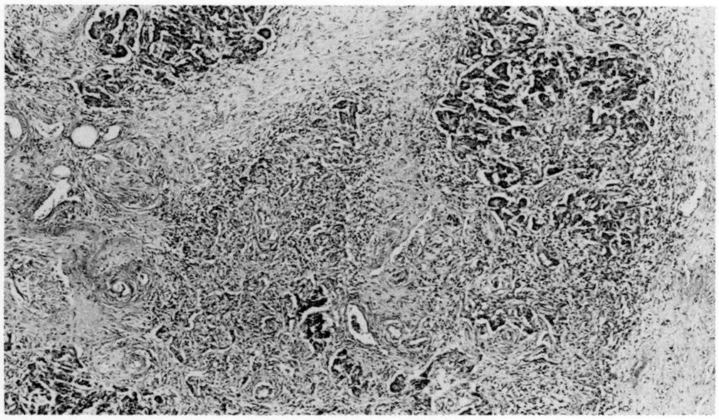

B

Figure 26-27. a) Juvenile pancreatic atrophy. Gross specimen shows only traces of pancreatic tissue in mesentery of duodenum. b) Chronic pancreatitis as cause of pancreatic exocrine deficiency. Most of acinar cells are lost and replaced by fibrous tissue.

accompanies the lavaging procedure, which requires restraint of the patient and minor surgical procedures. Those are important when shock is a complication. Peritoneal lavage or dialysis can be important therapy for the renal failure that can accompany pancreatitis. The techniques and solutions are the same for dialysis as for lavage.

Surgery. Indications for surgical intervention in animals with acute pancreatitis are borrowed from experience in human medicine. At one time, surgery was the popular treatment for acute pancreatitis, but current treatment is primarily by medical management, with some indications for surgery.[149] Species differences between humans and dogs reduce the indications for surgery in dogs. Acute biliary tract disease in man is a surgical problem that is difficult to differentiate from acute pancreatitis, and it can itself cause acute pancreatitis. Since acute biliary tract disease is rare in dogs, there are fewer indications for surgery. Surgical dilation of the common bile duct and sphincteroplasty are used to treat humans with recurring pancreatitis. Because of differences in the anatomy of the bile and pancreatic ducts in humans and dogs, there are no indications to use these procedures in a dog that has recurring pancreatitis.

Exploratory surgery is often performed on animals with signs of an acute abdomen if no diagnosis can be made from the history, physical examination, and laboratory findings. When acute pancreatitis is found, the most important problem becomes management of shock. Surgical intervention in animals with acute pancreatitis and shock is accompanied by mortality rates up to 50%. Partial or complete pancreatectomy may be indicated when acute pancreatitis is unresponsive to treatment. But that is done only with an understanding of a high rate of mortality. Experimental dogs with untreated severe acute pancreatitis, had a mortality rate of 93%.[140] Fluid therapy in such dogs reduced mortality to 25%, but mortality was 54% when fluid therapy and total pancreatectomy were done. Postoperative management following complete pancreatectomy includes replacement of insulin and pancreatic enzymes. Diabetes mellitus is more difficult to regulate if accompanied by pancreatic enzyme deficiency. In summary, acute pancreatitis is managed medically at present, and surgical procedures in animals to resect diseased tissue must be considered experimental. Pancreatectomy has not been shown to improve shock or renal shutdown. In humans, additionally, surgery increases both the length of illness and the mortality rate.[150]

There are three indications for surgery on animals with pancreatitis. One is persistent obstructive jaundice, in which case surgery is performed to decompress the biliary tract. A transient jaundice is due to either inflammation around the bile duct or hepatic damage caused by the pancreatitis. Intestinal obstruction is a second indication for surgery in patients whose clinical signs of anorexia and vomition persist as laboratory findings show improvement. A positive-contrast radiographic study may or may not provide evidence for the obstruction. In either case, exploratory surgery is performed to evaluate and correct the problem. A third indication for surgery is for identification and treatment of a suspected abscess or intestinal perforation causing peritonitis. It is difficult to identify those complications by other means. Culturing and staining abdominal fluid will sometimes identify an infection. Pyrexia and leukocytosis are not diagnostic of septic peritonitis since they can be caused by a sterile inflammatory process in the pancreas and by substances released into the circulation during pancreatitis. The three indications for surgical intervention are found in patients that fail to respond to treatment. They are not seen in the early acute phase unless the animal has had a problem with a recurring pancreatitis.

Partial pancreatectomy is not greatly associated with risk of initiating acute pancreatitis in segments left in the animal. There is no justification for following a partial pancreatectomy with administration of antibiotics, fluids, anticholinergics, and agents to maintain optimum pancreatic circulation.[151] Partially pancreatectomized dogs given no postoperative supportive care do not develop pancreatitis.

Diabetes Mellitus. The complications of diabetes mellitus are treated with insulin and supportive therapy as indicated. The complete loss of islet cell function may be managed in the future by transplantation of pancreatic islets. Autotransplantation of pancreatic islets has been accomplished in experimental dogs.[152,153] Transplants of pancreatic islets into histoincompatible recipients may be successful when the islets are cultured in vitro, a procedure which enhances host tolerance to the transplant.[154] Thus, transplants of pancreatic islets from random dogs would not be rejected by the diabetic patient.

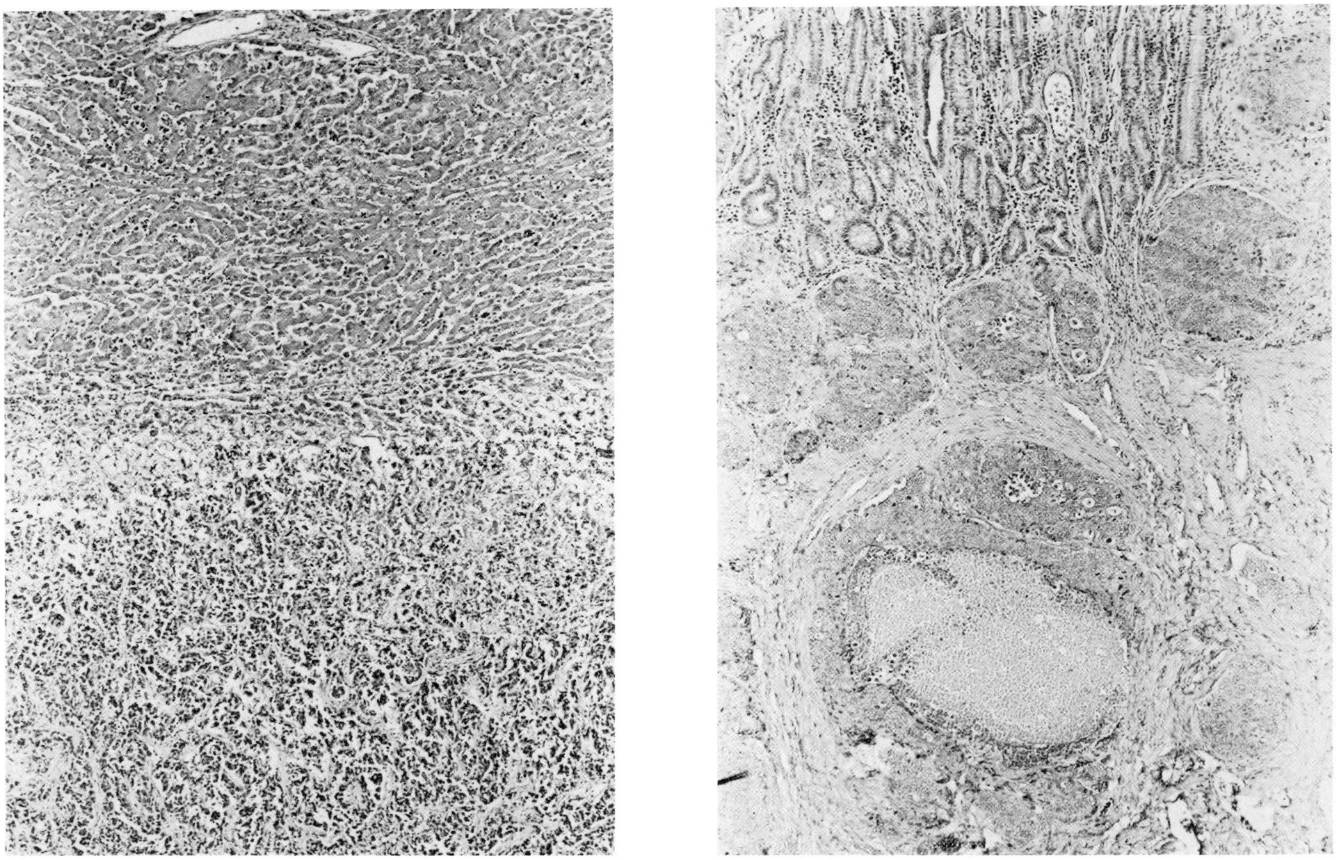

A B

Figure 26-28. a) Adenocarcinoma of pancreatic acinar cells metastasized to liver (normal liver at top). b) Spread is often by direct extension into the duodenal wall and around the bile duct, causing obstructive jaundice.

Evaluation of Management

Few acute inflammatory processes create as many complications that seriously effect normal function in most body systems as pancreatitis does. Hence, function must be evaluated and monitored frequently in many organ systems. Plasma enzyme levels are used to evaluate the status of the inflammatory process in the pancreas. Cardiovascular functions are monitored with electrocardiograms. Fluid and electrolyte homeostasis is evaluated with measurements of arterial blood pressure, central venous pressure, blood gases, and plasma electrolytes. Urine output is quantitated, and renal function is assessed through determination of blood urea nitrogen.

Prognosis

A good prognosis can be expected with pancreatitis. The exception is the severe case that is not managed properly. Sudden unexpected death, sometimes seen, is usually due to cardiovascular collapse. The overall prognosis improves in patients with complications when electrocardiographic and blood pressure monitoring are routinely used to identify cardiac complications and evaluate the response to therapy. Very few patients fail to survive if managed properly. The most important reasons for a poor prognosis are: 1) failure to recognize complications; 2) failure to treat complications adequately; and 3) premature resumption of feeding. Sequelae to pancreatitis include diabetes mellitus (incidence about 15% that of pancreatitis) and pancreatic enzyme deficiency.

PANCREATIC ATROPHY

The pancreas can atrophy following pancreatitis, and atrophy of unknown etiology has been found in younger dogs. Atrophy, defined as a loss of acinar cells, causes diarrhea, steatorrhea, and weight loss when more than 85% of the pancreatic enzymes are lost.

Epidemiology

The incidence of pancreatic atrophy at the VMTH in Davis is 1.4 cases per 1,000. The age distribution is shown in Figure 26-4. German Shepherd dogs represent half of the total cases, with an incidence five times greater than expected.

Etiology and Pathogenesis

Pancreatitis is the most likely cause of pancreatic atrophy in older dogs, where chronic inflammation progresses through the pancreas and eventually destroys enough acinar cells to make the animal deficient in the amount of enzymes secreted.

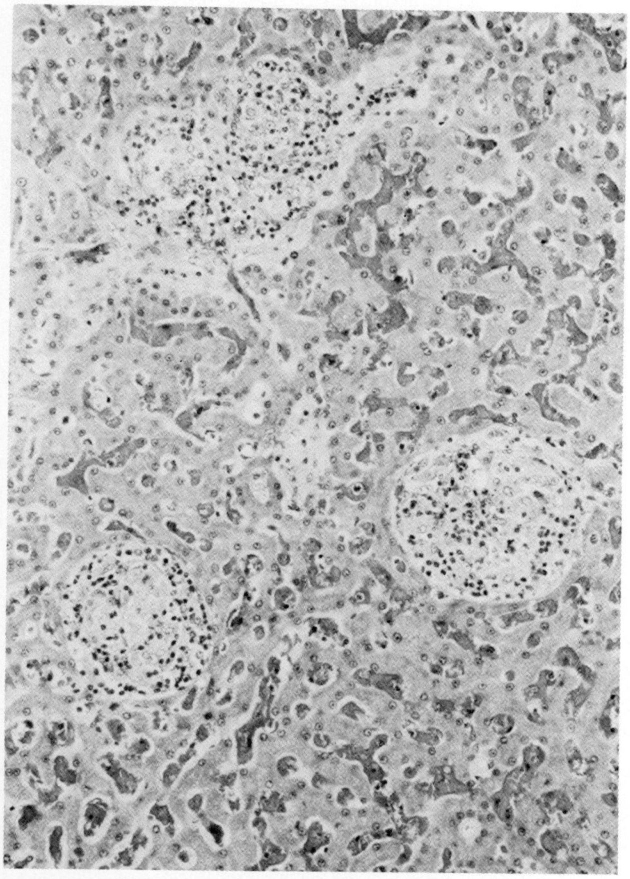

Figure 26-28. c) Islet cell tumor metastases in liver. Clusters of islet cells stand out in sharp contrast to adjacent normal hepatic tissue. Hepatic metastases are usually grossly visible and offer poor prognosis. Tumors confined to the pancreas only can be surgically removed with a good prognosis.

Atrophy can also appear without any evidence of pancreatitis as the cause. It is uncertain whether this is atrophy or hypoplasia, and since it appears early in life it has been called juvenile pancreatic atrophy (Figure 26-27). The cause is unknown. It may be a congenital or genetically transmitted problem, since it predominates in young German Shepherds. Clinical signs frequently do not appear until the animal is six to twelve months old, which suggests than enzyme secretion is adequate in very early life. Other possible causes include viral infections and abnormal immune-mediated responses that are able to destroy pancreatic acinar tissue, so that the nature of the pathogenic process cannot be identified once atrophy is complete. Protein starvation can produce reversible pancreatic atrophy in monkeys, but such circumstances would be rare in dogs. Atrophy is also produced by obstruction of pancreatic ducts, but that has not been found in juvenile pancreatic atrophy.

Canine juvenile pancreatic atrophy has a somewhat similar counterpart in children, described as congenital hypoplasia of the pancreas or the Schwachman syndrome. It is characterized by dwarfism, neutropenia or pancytopenia, metaphyseal dysostosis of the femoral necks, and recurrent infections and replacement of pancreatic tissue by fat (lipomatosis). These problems are dissimilar to pancreatic atrophy in dogs.

Cystic fibrosis, another human disease causing pancreatic exocrine deficiency, has not been recognized in small animals. It is different from juvenile pancreatic atrophy in both clinical manifestations and pathological changes. A defect in mucin secreting tissues throughout the body causes cystic fibrosis. The pancreatic changes are primarily diffuse fibrosis, with secondary atrophy of normal tissue. Chronic interstitial pancreatitis occurs occasionally in the cat, with heavy fibrosis as the main lesion. This is similar to cystic fibrosis in that inflammatory cells are found. No involvement of other systems has been described in cats with chronic interstitial pancreatitis. The causes for the entity in cats and for cystic fibrosis in humans are unknown.

Clinical evaluation and management of pancreatic atrophy are described in Chapter 17.

PANCREATIC NEOPLASMS[120,121,155]

Tumors in the pancreas arise from the acinar and endocrine-secreting cells. Adenomas of acinar cells cause no clinical signs. Adenocarcinomas of acinar cells, found one-tenth as often as pancreatitis, cause clinical signs of pancreatitis and increases in plasma amylase and lipase activity. The tumors are usually not recognized before they have grown quite large and have metastasized. Pancreatic adenocarcinomas can compress and obstruct the bile duct and duodenum, producing additional clinical signs. The most frequent sites of metastasis are regional lymph nodes, stomach, duodenum, and liver. Pancreatic adenocarcinoma can be identified only by biopsy (Figure 26-28).

Tumors can also arise from any of the endocrine-secreting cells of the pancreas. The cell most commonly involved is the insulin-secreting islet cell,[156,157] which produces either adenomas or adenocarcinomas (Figure 26-28). No cellular morphological features allow differentiation of the two. Invasiveness is the criterion to identify an adenocarcinoma. Their differences can be determined by the stage at which they are recognized. Two or three cases per 10,000 are seen in dogs at the VMTH, but the actual incidence is much lower since a number of those are referrals. Such animals manifest seizures and other central-nervous-system signs related to the hypoglycemia produced by release of large amounts of insulin.

Other cells in the pancreas produce hormones such as glucagon and somatostatin. Tumors can arise from those cells and secrete excessive amounts of hormones.[6] Those APUDomas have been described in man, with most of them secreting gastrin or vasoactive intestinal peptide (VIP). The hypersecretion causes gastric or duodenal ulceration when gastrin is the hormone secreted, and diarrhea when VIP is secreted. This description of these entities is oversimplified, for they are increasingly recognized as secreting a number of other substances that participate in causing the clinical signs. Gastrin-secreting tumors have been recognized in the dog.[158-161]

REFERENCES

1. Miller, M.E., Christensen, G.C. and Evans, H.E.: Anatomy of the dog. First edition. W.B. Saunders Co., Philadelphia, 1964.
2. Nickel, R., Schummer, A., Seiferle, E. and Sack, W.O.: The viscera of the domestic animals. Springer-Verlag. New York, 1973.

3. Lenninger, S.: The autonomic innervation of the exocrine pancreas. Med. Clinics. No. Amer. 58:1311-1318, 1974.
4. Go, V.L.W., Gardner, J.D., Brooks, F.P., Lebenthal, E., DiMagno, E.P. and Scheele, G.A.: The exocrine pancreas. Raven Press, New York, 1986.
5. Dreiling, D.A.: Symposium on diagnosis of pancreatic disease. Pancreatic secretory testing in 1974. Gut. 16:653-657, 1975.
6. Welbourn, R.B., Pearse, A.G.E., Polak, J.M., Bloom, S.R. and Joffe, S.N.: The APUD cells of the alimentary tract in health and disease. Med. Clinics No. Am. 58:1359-1374, 1974.
7. Anderson, N.V.: Pancreatitis in dogs. Vet. Clinics No. Am. 2:79-91, 1972.
8. Hottendorf, G.H. and Hirth, R.S.: Lesions of spontaneous subclinical disease in beagle dogs. Vet Path. 11:240-258, 1974.
9. Garvey, M.S. and Zawie, D.A.: Feline pancreatic disease. Vet. Clin. No. Am. 14:1231-1246, 1984.
10. Banks, P.A.: Acute pancreatitis. Gastroenterology 61:382-397, 1971.
11. Schiller, W.R., Suriyapa, C. and Anderson, M.C.: A review of experimental pancreatitis. J. Surg. Res. 16:69-90, 1974.
12. Steer, M.L. and Meldolesi, J.: The cell biology of experimental pancreatitis. New Eng. J. Med. 316:144-150, 1987.
13. Keynes, M.: Heretical thoughts on the pathogenesis of acute pancreatitis. Gut 29:1413-1423, 1988.
14. Anderson, N.V.: The pancreas. JAAHA 9:89-100, 1973.
15. VanPelt, C.S. and Crandell, R.A.: Pancreatitis associated with a feline herpesvirus infection. Compan. An. Pract. 7-10, 1987.
16. Jones, R.T. and Trump, B.F.: Cellular and subcellular effects of ischemia on the pancreatic acinar cell. Virchows Arch. B. Cell Path. 19:325-336, 1975.
17. Lindsay, S., Entenman, C. and Chaikoff, I.L.: Pancreatitis accompanying hepatic disease in dogs fed a high fat, low protein diet. Arch. Pathol. 45:635-638, 1948.
18. Kirsch, R.E., Saunders, S.J. and Brock, J.F.: Animal models and human protein-calorie malnutrition. Amer. J. Clin. Nutr. 212:1225-1228, 1968.
19. Lombardi, B., Estes, L.W. and Longnecker, D.S.: Acute hemorrhagic pancreatitis (massive necrosis) with fat necrosis induced in mice by DL-ethionine fed with a choline-deficient diet. Amer. J. Path. 79:465-480, 1975.
20. Dressel, T.D., Goodale, R.L., Zweber, B. and Borner, J.W.: The effect of atropine and duct decompression on the evolution of Diazinon-induced acute canine pancreatitis. Ann. Surg. 195:424-434, 1982.
21. Hendricks, J.C., DiMagno, E.P., Go, V.L.W. and Dozois, R.R.: Reflux of duodenal contents into the pancreatic duct of dogs. J. Lab Clin. Med. 96:912-921, 1980.
22. Schapiro, H., Britt, L.G., Blackwell, C.F. and Gaines, K.J.: Acute hemorrhagic pancreatitis in the dog. Arch Surg. 107:608-612, 1973.
23. Nevalainen, T.J. and Seppa, A.: Acute pancreatitis caused by closed duodenal loop in the rat. Scand. J. Gastroenterology. 10:521-527, 1975.
24. Owyang, C., Dozois, R.R., DiMagno, E.P. and Go, V.L.W.: Relationshiops between fasting and postprandial pancreaticoduodenal pressures, pancreatic secretion; and duodenal volume flow in the dog. Gastroenterology 73:1046-1049, 1977.
25. Sheldon, W.G.: Pancreatic Flukes (Eurytrema procynis) in domestic cats. JAVMA 148:251-253, 1966.
26. Strombeck, D.R.: Unpublished observations.
27. Bogoch, A., Roth, J.L.A. and Bockus, H.L.: Effects of morphine on serum amylase and lipase. Gastroenterology. 26:697-708, 1954.
28. Estourgie, R.J.A., Yap, S.H., van Haelst, U.J.G. and deBoer, H.H.M.: The clinical and histopathological effects of pancreatic duct occlusion in experimental acute pancreatitis in dogs. J. Surg. Res. 34:164-170, 1983.
29. Blackstone, M.O., Ito, Y., Brown, S. and Moossa, A.R.: Endoscopic traumatic dilatation of the duodenal papilla and proximal pancreatic duct in dogs: a model of acute pancreatitis. 24:191, 1978.
30. Nakashima, Y. and Howard, J.M.: Drug-induced acute pancreatitis. Surg. Gynecol. Obstet. 145:105-109, 1977.
31. Mallory, A. and Kern, F.: Drug-induced pancreatitis: a critical review. Gastroenterology 78:813-820, 1980.
32. Corrodi, P., Knoblauch, M., Binswanger, U., Scholzel, E. and Largiader, F.: Pancreatitis after renal transplantation. Gut. 16:285-289, 1975.
33. Steinberg, W.M. and Lewis, J.H.: Steroid-induced pancreatitis: Does it really exist? Gastroenterology 81:799-808, 1981.
34. Steinberg, W.M. and Schlesselman, S.E.: Treatment of acute pancreatitis. Comparison of animal and human studies. Gastroenterology 93:1420-1427, 1987.
35. Moriello, K.A., Bowne, D. and Meyer, D.J.: Acute pancreatitis in two dogs given azathioprine and prednisone. JAVMA 191:695-696, 1987.
36. Broe, P.J. and Cameron J.L.: Azathioprine and acute pancreatitis: Studies with an isolated perfused canine pancreas. J. Surg. Res. 34:159-163, 1983.
37. Merrill, J.P. and Hampers, C.L.: Uremia, New Eng. J. Med. 282:953-961, 1970.
38. Putzke, H.-P., Jonas, L. and Bienengraber, A.: Vascular chronic fibrosing pancreatitis of the rat after 5/6 nephrectomy. Exp. Path. 14:113-121, 1977.
39. Rogers, W.A., Donovan, E.F. and Kociba, G.J.: Lipids and lipoproteins in normal dogs and in dogs with secondary hyperlipoproteinemia. JAVMA 166:1092-1100, 1975.
40. Stackhouse, K.L, Glass, D.D. and Zimmerman, B.: Relationshiops of lipoprotein lipase and hyperlipemia in pancreatitis. Surg. Forum. 17:343-347, 1966.
41. Whitney, M.S., Boon, G.D., Rebar, A.H. and Ford, R.B.: Effects of acute pancreatitis on circulating lipids in dogs. Am. J. Vet. Res. 48:1492-1497, 1987.
42. Bass, V.D., Hoffman, W.E. and Dorner, J.L.: Normal canine lipid profiles and effects of expermentally induced pancreatitis and hepatic necrosis on lipids. Am. J. Vet. Res. 37:1355-1357, 1976.
43. Fredrickson, D.S., Levy, R.I. and Lees, R.S.: Fat transport in lipoproteins — an integrated approach to mechanisms and disorders. New Eng. J. Med. 276:34-44, 94-103, 148-156, 215-226, 273-281, 1967.
44. Cameron, J.L., Capuzzi, D.M., Zuidema, G.D. and Margolis, S.: Acute pancreatitis with hyperlipemia. Evidence for a persistent defect in lipid metabolism. Amer. J. Med. 56:482-487, 1974.
45. Brunzell, J.D. and Schrott, H.G.: Interaction of familial and secondary causes of hypertriglyceridemia: Role in pancreatitis. Clin. Res. 21:723, 1973.
46. Saharia, P., Margolis, S., Zuidema, G.D. and Cameron, J.L.: Acute pancreatitis with hyperlipidemia: Studies with an isolated perfused canine pancreas. Surgery 82:60-67, 1977.
47. Rogers, W.A., Donovan, E.F. and Kociba, G.J.: Idiopathic hyperlipoproteinemia in dogs. JAVMA 166:1087-1091, 1975.
48. Hochgelerent, E.L. and David, D.S.: Acute pancreatitis secondary to calcium infusion in the dialysis patient. Arch. Surg. 108:218-219, 1974.
49. Manson, R.R.: Acute pancreatitis secondary to iatrogenic hypercalcemia. Arch. Surg. 108:213-215, 1974.
50. Layer, P., Hotz, J., Schmitz-Moorman, H.P. and Goebell, H.: Effects of experimental chronic hypercalcemia on feline exocrine pancreatic secretion. Gastroenterology 82:309-316, 1982.
51. Glazer, G. and Bennett, A.: Prostaglandin release in canine acute hemorrhagic pancreatitis. Gut. 17:22-26, 1976.
52. Ham, J.M. and Fitzpatrick, P.: Acute pancreatitis in patients with acute hepatic failure. Am. J. Dig. Dis. 18:1079-1083, 1973.
53. Capner, P., Lendrum, R., Jeffries, D.J. and Walker, G.: Viral antibody studies in pancreatic disease. Gut. 16:866-870, 1975.
54. Craighead, J.E.: The role of viruses in the pathogenesis of pancreatic disease and diabetes mellitus. Prog. Med. Virol. 19:161-214, 1975.
55. Thal, A.: Studies on pancreatitis. II. Acute pancreatic necrosis produced experimentally by the Arthus sensitization reaction. Surgery 37:911-917, 1955.
56. Murray, M.J. and Thal, A.P.: The clinical significance of circulating pancreatic antibodies. Ann. Intern. Med. 53:548-555, 1960.
57. Fonkalsrud, E.W. and Longmire, W.P.: The occurrence of pancreatic antibodies and the experimental production of pancreatitis with pancreatic antiserum. Surgery. 50:134-142,

1961.
58. Durst, A., Dishon, T., Rosenmann, R. and Boss, J.H.: Factors in the pathogenesis of experimental acute pancreatitis in the rat. Eur. Surg. Res. 5:348-361, 1973.
59. Lendrum, R. and Walker, G.: Serum antibodies in human pancreatic disease. Gut. 16:365-371, 1975.
60. Seelig, R., Ehemann, V., Tschahargane, C. and Seelig, H.P.: The serum complement system - a mediator of acute pancreatitis. Virchows Arch. A Path. Anat. Hist. 365:193-199, 1975.
61. Janigan, D.T., Nevalainen, T.J., MacAulay, M.A. and Vethamany, V.G.: Foreign serum-induced pancreatitis in mice. I. A new model of acute pancreatitis. Lab. Invest. 33:591-607, 1975.
62. Sanfey, H., Bulkley, G.B. and Cameron, J.L.: The role of oxygen-derived free radicals in the pathogenesis of acute pancreatitis. Ann. Surg. 200:405-413, 1984.
63. Rinderknecht, H.: Fatal pancreatitis, a consequence of excessive leukocyte stimulation. Intl. J. Pancreatology 3:105-112, 1988.
64. Ohlsson, K. and Eddeland, A.: Release of proteolytic enzymes in bile-induced pancreatitis in dogs. Gastroenterology. 69:668-675, 1975.
65. Murtaugh, R.J. and Jacobs, R.M.: Serum antiprotease concentrations in dogs with spontaneous and experimentally induced acute pancreatitis. AJVR 46:80-83, 1985.
66. Trapnell, J.E., Rigby, C.C., Talbot, C.H. and Duncan, E.H.L.: A controlled trial of trasylol in the treatment of acute pancreatitis. Brit. J. Surg. 61:177-182, 1974.
67. Studley, J.G.N. and Schenk, W.G.: Pathophysiology of acute pancreatitis. Am. J. Surg. 143:761-764, 1982.
68. Skjennald, A.: Aniography in acute experimental pancreatitis correlated to hemodynamic changes. Scand. J. Gastroenterology 17, Suppl. 73, 1982.
69. Mishra, N.K., Appert, H.E. and Howard, J.M.: Studies of paralytic ileus. Effect of intraperitoneal injury on motility of the canine small intestine. Am. J. Surg. 129:559-563, 1975.
70. Ryan, J.W., Moffat, J.G. and Thompson, A.G.: Role of bradykinin system in acute hemorrhagic pancreatitis. Arch. Surg. 91:14-24, 1965.
71. Takada, Y., Appert, H.E. and Howard, J.M.: Vascular permeability induced by pancreatic exudate formed during acute pancreatitis in dogs. Surg. Gynecol. Obstet. 143:779-783, 1976.
72. Greenburg, A.G., Terlizzi, L. and Peskin, G.W.: Oxyhemoglobin affinity in acute pancreatitis. J. Surg. Res. 22:561-565, 1977.
73. Lees, G.E., Suter, P.F. and Johnson, G.C.: Pulmonary edema in a dog with acute pancreatitis and cardiac disease. JAVMA 172:690-696, 1978.
74. Warshaw, A.L., Lesser, P.B., Rie, M. and Cullen, D.J.: The pathogenesis of pulmonary edema in acute pancreatitis. Ann. Surg. 182:505-510, 1975.
75. Malik, A.B.: Pulmonary edema after pancreatitis: Role of humoral factors. Circ. Shock 10:71-80, 1983.
76. Morgan, A.P., Jenny, M.E. and Haessler, H.: Phospholipids, acute pancreatitis, and the lungs: Effect of lecithinase infusion on pulmonary surface activity in dogs. Ann. Surg. 167:329-335, 1968.
77. Ashbaugh, D.G. and Uza, T.: Respiratory and hemodynamic changes after injection of free fatty acids. J. Surg. Res. 8:417-423, 1968.
78. Berry, A.R. and Taylor, T.V.: Effect of drugs on the pulmonary changes in experimental acute pancreatitis in the rat. Gut 23:481-484, 1982.
79. Feldman, B.F., Attix, E.A., Strombeck, D.R. and O'Neill, S.: Biochemical and coagulation changes in a canine model of acute necrotizing pancreatitis. AJVR 42:805-809, 1981.
80. Satake, K., Uchima, K., Umeyama, K., Appert, H.E. and Howard, J.M.: The effects upon blood coagulation in dogs of experimentally induced pancreatitis and the infusion of pancreatic juice. Surg. Gynec. Obstet 153:341-345, 1981.
81. Ettinger, S.J. and Suter, P.F.: Canine cardiology. W.B. Saunders, Co., Philadelphia, 1970.
82. Tuzhilin, S.A. and Dreiling, D.A.: Cardiovascular lesions in pancreatitis. Am. J. Gastroenterology. 63:381-388, 1975.
83. Andrzejewska, A., Dlugosz, J. and Kurasz, S.: The ultrastructure of the liver in acute experimental pancreatitis. Exp. Path. 28:167-176, 1985.
84. Ling, G.V., Lowenstine, L.J., Pulley, L.T., and Kaneko, J.J.: Diabetes mellitus in dogs: A review of initial evaluation, immediate and long-term management and outcome. JAVMA 170:521-530, 1977.
85. Attix, E., Strombeck, D.R., Wheeldon, E.B. and Stern, J.S.: Effects of an anticholinergic and a corticosteroid on acute pancreatitis in experimental dogs. AJVR 42:1668-1674, 1981.
86. Cribb, A.E., Burgener, D.C. and Reimann, K.A.: Bile duct obstruction secondary to chronic pancreatitis in seven dogs. Can. Vet. J. 29:654-657, 1988.
87. Bhattacharya, S.K., Luther, R.W., Pate, J.W., Crawford, A.J., Moore, O.F., Pitcock, J.A., Palmieri, G.M.A. and Britt, L.G.: Soft tissue calcium and magnesium content in acute pancreatitis in the dog: Calcium accumulation, a mechanism for hypocalcemia in acute pancreatitis. J. Lab. Clin. Med. 105:422-427, 1985.
88. Avioli, L.V., Birge, S.J., Scott, S. and Shieber, W.: Role of the thyroid gland during glucagon induced hypercalcemia in the dog. Am. J. Physiol. 216:939-945, 1969.
89. Donowitz, M., Hendler, R., Spiro, H.M., Binder, H.J. and Felig, P.: Glucagon secretion in acute and chronic pancreatitis. Ann. Intern. Med. 83:778-781, 1975.
90. Canale, D.D. and Donabedian, R.K.: Hypercalcitoninemia in acute pancreatitis. J. Clin. Endocrinol. Metab. 40:738-741, 1975.
91. Peoples, J.B., Webster, M.W. and Carey, L.C.: Mechanisms of hypocalcemia in acute hemorrhagic pancreatitis. Surg. Gynecol. Obstet. 141:724-726, 1975.
92. Peoples, J.B., Eberlein, T. and Webster, M.W.: Prevention of hypocalcemia by administration of homologous plasma during experimental hemorrhage pancreatitis in the pig. Am. J. Surg. 133:42-45, 1977.
93. Strombeck, D.R., Wheeldon, E.B. and Harrold, D.: Model of chronic pancreatitis in the dog. AJVR 45:131-136, 1984.
94. Kitchell, B.E., Strombeck, D.R., Cullen, J. and Harrold, D.: Clinical and pathologic changes in experimentally induced acute pancreatitis in cats. AJVR 47:1170-1173, 1986.
95. Fitzgerald, O.: Painless pancreatitis and other painless pancreatic disorders. Clinics Gastroenterology. 1:195-218, 1972.
96. Mulvany, M.H., Feinberg, C.K. and Tilson, D.L.: Clinical characterization of acute necrotizing pancreatitis. Comp. Contin. Educ. 4:394-405, 1982.
97. Perman, V. and Stevens, J.B.: Clinical evaluation of the acinar pancreas of the dog. JAVMA 155:2052-2058, 1969.
98. Goldberg, D.M. and Spooner, R.J.: Amylase, isoamylase and macroamylase. Digestion. 13:56-75, 1975.
99. Notheman, M.M. and Callow, A.D.: Investigations on the origin of amylase in serum and urine. Gastroenterology. 60:82-89, 1971.
100. Salt, W.B. and Schenker, S.: Amylase - its clinical significance: A review of the literature. Medicine. 55:269-289, 1976.
101. Boyd, T.F., Traad, E.M. and Byrne, J.J.: Serum amylase levels in experimental intestinal obstruction. J. Surg. Res. 1:128-131, 1961.
102. Hiatt, N.: Investigation of the role of the small intestine in the maintenance of the serum amylase level of the dog. Ann. Surg. 154:864-873, 1961.
103. Appert, H.E., Dimbiloglu, M., Pairent, F.W. and Howard, J.M.: The disappearance of intravenously injected pancreatic enzymes. Surg. Gynecol. Obstet. 127:1281-1287, 1968.
104. Hudson, E.B. and Strombeck, D.R.: The role of the kidneys in the disappearance of serum amylase and lipase. JAVR 39:1316-1321, 1978.
105. Hiatt, NH. and Bonorris, G.: Removal of serum amylase in dogs and the influence of reticuloendothelial blockade. Amer. J. Physiol. 210:133-138, 1966.
106. Eto, K., Pairent, F.W., Appert, H.E. and Howard, J.M.: Renal excretion of amylase and lipase by dogs. Arch. Surg. 98:241-244, 1969.
107. Strombeck, D.R., Farver, T. and Kaneko, J.J.: Serum amylase and lipase activities in the diagnosis of pancreatitis in dogs. AmJVR 42:1966-1970, 1981.
108. Martaugh, R.J., Jacobs, R.M., Sherding, R.G. and O'Dorisio, T.M.: Serum pancreatic polypeptide and amylase concentrations

in dogs with experimentally induced acute pancreatitis. AJVR 46:654-656, 1985.
109. Fleischer, K. and Kasper, H.: Exocrine pancreatic function in uraemic rats. Acta Hepato-gastroenterol. 21:398-403, 1974.
110. Rapp, J.P.: Normal values for serum amylase and maltase in dogs and the effect of maltase on the saccharogenic method of determining amylase in serum. AJVR 23:343-350, 1962.
111. Martaugh, R.J. and Jacobs, R.M.: Serum amylase and isoamylases and their origins in healthy dogs and dogs with experimentally induced acute pancreatitis. AJVR 46:742-747, 1985.
112. Onishi, T. and Hoshino, T.: Amylase activity and its isoenzymes in normal canine serum and tissues. J. Jap. V.M.A. 39:498-503, 1986.
113. Sommer, H., Kasper, H., and Fosel, T.: Serum lipase activity in chronic renal failure. Acta Hepato-gastroenterol. 22:248-252, 1975.
114. Duffell, S.J.: Some aspects of pancreatic disease in the cat. J. Small An. Pract. 16:365-374, 1975.
115. VMTH: Davis, CA. unpublished cases.
116. Brobst, D., Ferguson, A.B. and Carter, J.M.: Evaluation of serum amylase and lipase activity in experimentally induced pancreatitis in the dog. JAVMA 157:1697-1702, 1970.
117. Munoz, J.N. and Bose, S.: Pancreatic ascites. Amer. J. Dig. Dis. 20:1178-1183, 1975.
118. O'Brien, T.R.: Radiographic diagnosis of abdominal disorders in the dog and cat. W.B. Saunders, Philadelphia, 1978.
119. Nyland, T.G., Mulvany, M.H. and Strombeck, D.R.: Ultrasonic features of experimentally induced, acute pancreatitis in the dog. Vet. Radiol 24:260-266, 1983.
120. Jubb, K.V.F. and Kennedy, P.C.: pathology of domestic animals. Vol. 2 Academic Press, New York, 1970.
121. Owens, J.M., Drazner, F.H. and Gilbertson, S.R.: Pancreatic disease in the cat. JAAHA 11:83-89, 1975.
122. Kline, T.S., Abramson, J., Golstein, F. and Neal H.S.: Needle aspiration biopsy of the pancreas at laparotomy. Am. J. Gastroenterology. 68:30-33, 1977.
123. Kelly, G.A. and Nahrwold, D.L.: Pancreatic secretion in response to an elemental diet and intravenous hyperalimentation. Surg. Gynecol. Obstet. 143:87-91, 1976.
124. Ragins, H., Levenson, S.M., Signer, R., Stamford, W. and Seifter, E.: Intrajejunal administration of an elemental diet at neutral pH avoids pancreatic stimulation. Am. J. Surg. 126:606-614, 1973.
125. Scratcherd, T.: Symposium on diagnosis of pancreatic disease. Pancreatic function tests: the physiological background. Gut. 16:648-653, 1975.
126. Wormsley, K.G.: Pancreatic function tests. Clinics Gastroenterology. 1:27-51, 1972.
127. Soergel, K.H.: Medical treatment of acute pancreatitis. What is the evidence? Gastroenterology 74:620-628, 1978.
128. Dyck, W.P., Rudick, J., Hoexter, B. and Janowitz, H.D.: Influence of glucagon on pancreatic exocrine secretion. Gastroenterology. 56:531-537, 1969.
129. Iwatsuki, K., Ond, H. and Hashimoto, K.: Effects of glucagon on pancreatic secretion in the dog. Clin. Exp. Pharmacol. Physiol. 3:59-65, 1976.
130. Schiller, W.R. and Anderson, M.C.: Microcirculation of the normal and inflamed canine pancreas. Ann. Surg. 181:466-470, 1975.
131. Carey, L.C.: Low molecular weight dextran in experimental pancreatitis. Am. J. Surg. 119:197-199, 1970.
132. Wright, P.W. and Goodhead, B.: The value of dextrans in the treatment of experimental pancreatitis. Surgery 67:807-815, 1970.
133. Pissiotis, C.A., Condon, R.E. and Nyhus, L.M.: Effect of vasopressin on pancreatic blood flow in acute hemorrhagic pancreatitis. Am. J. Surg. 123:203-208, 1972.
134. Schapiro, H., Britt, L.G., Brooks, J., Campbell, D. and Blackwell, C.F.: Acute hemorrhagic pancreatitis in the dog. II. Effect of vasopressin on survival times. Am. J. Dig. Dis. 18:1075-1078, 1973.
135. Schapiro, H., McDougal, H.D., Morrison, E.J. and Wan, A.T.: Acute hemorrhagic pancreatitis in the dog. IV. Treatment with vasopressin. Am. J. Dig. Dis. 21:286-290, 1976.
136. Wright, P.W. and Goodhead, B.: Prevention of hemorrhagic pancreatitis with fibrinolysin or heparin. Arch. Surg. 100:42-46, 1970.
137. Hau, T. and Simmons, R.L.: Heparin in the treatment of experimental peritonitis. Ann. Surg. 187:294-298, 1978.
138. Svensson, J-O.: Role of intravenously infused insulin in treatment of acute pancreatitis. Scand. J. Gastroenterology. 10:487-490, 1975.
139. Kimura, T., Zuidema, G.D., and Cameron, J.L.: Acute pancreatitis. Experimental evaluation of steroid, albumin and trasylol therapy. Am. J. Surg. 140:403-408, 1980.
140. Henry, L.G. and Condon, R.E.: Ablative surgery for necrotizing pancreatitis. Am. J. Surg. 131:125-128, 1976.
141. Knol, J.A., Inman, M.G., Strodel, W.E. and Eckhauser, F.E.: Pancreatic response to crystalloid resuscitation in experimental pancreatitis. J. Surg. Res. 43:387-392, 1987.
142. Webster, M.W., Pasculle, A.W., Myerowitz, R.L., Rao, K.N. and Lombardi, B.: Postinduction bacteremia in experimental acute pancreatitis. Am. J. Surg. 138:418-420, 1979.
143. Bartlett, J.G., Louie, T.J., Onderdonk, A.B. and Gorbach, S.L.: Experimental intraabdominal sepsis. Gastroenterology 68:861, 1975.
144. Howes, R., Zuidema, G.D. and Cameron, J.L.: Evaluation of prophylactic antibiotics in acute pancreatitis. J. Surg. Res. 18:197-200, 1975.
145. Konturek, S.J., Tasler, J., Cieszkowski, M., Jaworek, J., Coy, D.H. and Schally, A.V.: Inhibition of pancreatic secretion by enkephalin and morphine in dogs. Gastroenterology 84:851-855, 1978.
146. Ranson, J.H.C. and Spencer, F.C.: The role of peritoneal lavage in severe acute pancreatitis. Ann. Surg. 187:565-575, 1978.
147. Rodgers, R.E. and Carey, L.C.: Peritoneal lavage in experimental pancreatitis in dogs. Am. J. Surg. 111:792-794, 1966.
148. Parks, J., Gahring, D. and Greene, R.W.: Peritoneal lavage for peritonitis and pancreatitis in twenty-two dogs. JAAHA 9:442-446, 1973.
149. Smith, R.: Progress in the surgical treatment of pancreatic disease. Am. J. Surg. 125:143-153, 1973.
150. Babb, R.R.: The role of surgery in acute pancreatitis. Am. J. Dig. Dis. 21:672-676 1976.
151. Dingwall, J.S. and McDonell, W.: Partial pancreatectomy in the dog. JAAHA 8:86-92, 1972.
152. Kolb, E., Ruckert, R. and Largiader, F.: Intraportal and intrasplenic autotransplantation of pancreatic islets in the dog. Eur. Surg. Res. 9:419-426, 1977.
153. Kretschmer, G.J., Sutherland, D.E.R., Matas, A.J., Cain, T.L. and Najarian, J.S.: Autotransplantation of pancreatic islets without separation of exocrine and endocrine tissue in totally pancreatectomized dogs. Surgery 82:74-81, 1977.
154. Kedinger, M., Haffen, K., Greiner, J. and Eloy, R.: In vitro culture reduces immunogenicity of pancreatic endocrine islets. Nature 270:736-738, 1977.
155. Kircher, C.H. and Nielsen, S.W.: Tumors of the pancreas. Bull. World Health Organ. 53:195-202, 1976.
156. Njoku, C.O., Strafuss, A.C. and Dennis, S.M.: Canine islet cell neoplasia: A review. JAAHA 8:284-290, 1972.
157. O'Brien, T.D., Hayden, D.W., O'Leary, T.P., Caywood, D.D. and Johnson, K.H.: Canine pancreatic endocrine tumors: Immunohistochemical analysis of hormone content and amyuloid. Vet. Pathol. 24:308-314, 1987.
158. Jones, B.R., Nicholls, M.R. and Badman, R.: Peptic ulceration in a dog associated with an islet cell carcinoma of the pancreas and an elevated plasma gastrin level. J. Small Anim. Pract. 17:593-598, 1976.
159. Straus, E., Johnson, G.F. and Yalow, R.S.: Canine Zollinger-Ellison syndrome. Gastroenterology 72:380-381, 1977.
160. Hoppe, R.D., van der Gaag, I., Lamers, C.B.H.W., van Toorenberg, J., Rehfeld, J.F. and Larsson, L.I.: Zoolinger-Ellison syndrome in three dogs. Vet. Pathol. 17:177-186, 1980.
161. Boosinger, T.R., Zerbe, C.A., Graban, J.H. and Pletcher, J.M.: Multihormonal pancreatic endocrine tumor in a dog with duodenal ulcers and hypertrophic gastropathy. Vet. Pathol. 25:237-239, 1988.

Chapter 27

Liver: Normal Structure

STRUCTURE

The liver is the largest organ of the body. It has a highly vascularized structure, receiving venous blood from the spleen and gastrointestinal organs in addition to its arterial supply. The many functions of the liver enable it to participate in carbohydrate, lipid, and protein metabolism; temperature regulation; regulation of circulation; detoxification and excretion of useless substances; storage of nutrients; and host defense activities.

GROSS STRUCTURE[1,2]

Anatomic Relationships

The liver comprises 3.4 percent of the body weight in adults with the percentage higher for young animals. The normal liver, being recessed cranial to the last rib, cannot be palpated. The convex surface is in contact with the diaphragm primarily, and the visceral concave surface is in contact with the stomach, duodenum, pancreas, and right kidney, all of which produce impressions on the liver. The liver consists of four lobes: right and left hepatic, quadrate, and caudate. The left lobe represents a third to almost a half of the total liver. The right hepatic lobe is smaller than the left. Both the right and left lobes can be divided morphologically into medial and lateral sublobes. The smaller quadrate lobe lies in the median plane between the medial portions of the right and left hepatic lobes. The gallbladder lies in a fossa between the quadrate lobe and the medial part of the right lobe. The caudate lobe is a tongue-shaped portion that lies almost entirely on the visceral aspect of the liver. The papillary process of this lobe lies in the gastric impression on the left side, and the caudate process of the caudate lobe forms the most caudal portion of the liver. The duodenal impression crosses this process, and the renal fossa lies in its most caudal aspect. Figure 27-1 shows the relationship of the liver to other abdominal organs.

The peritoneum, almost completely covering the liver, forms ligaments called the coronary, right triangular, left triangular, falciform, and hepatorenal ligaments.

Blood and Lymph Vessels[1-3]

The hepatic artery and portal vein supply the hepatic blood flow (Figure 27-2). One-fourth to one-third of the cardiac output can perfuse the liver in the resting state. Of the total

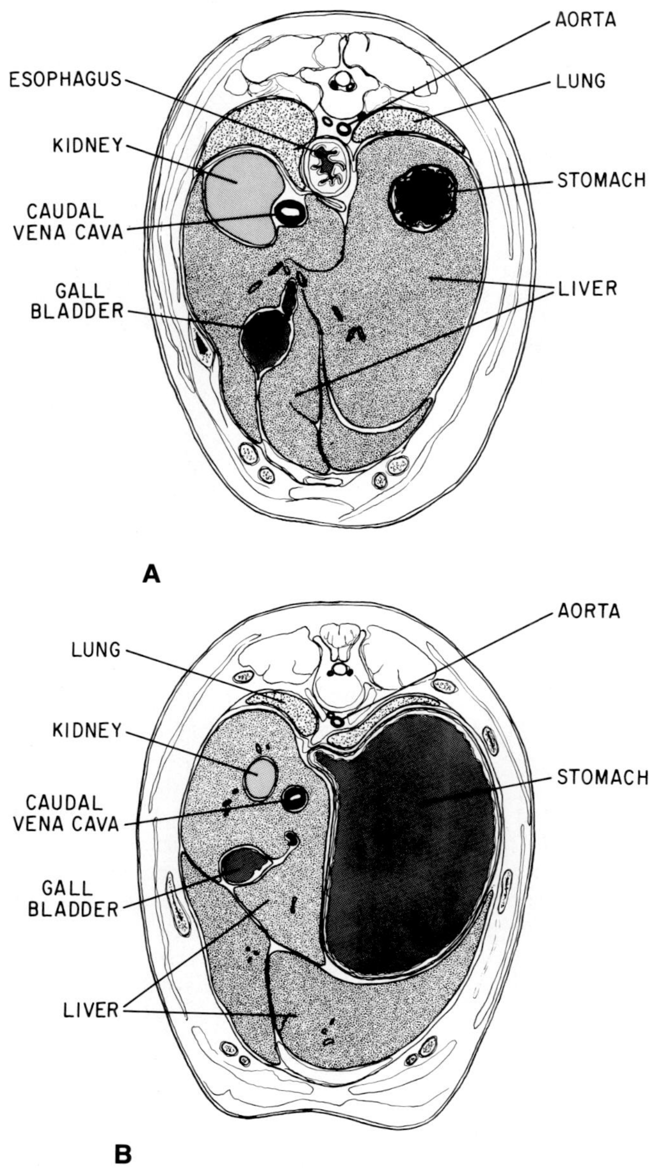

Figure 27-1. Drawings of transverse sections of dog showing relationship of liver to adjacent structures. Drawing a) at level of thoracic vertebrae 12 and b) at level of thoracic vertebrae 13.

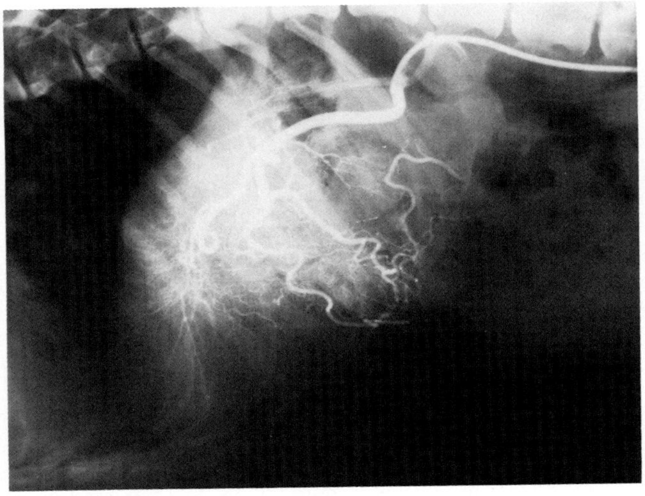

Figure 27-2a. Arteriogram of hepatic artery in a normal dog. Number of branches is variable, being two in this case. (By permission, Sibylle Schmidt)

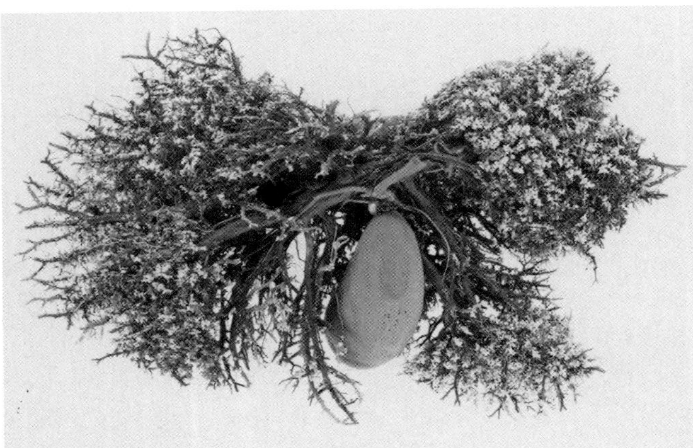

Figure 27-2c. Corrosion cast of hepatic circulatory and biliary systems after injection of the portal, arterial and biliary system with different color plastex. The smaller vessels have been removed from parts of the periphery to show distribution of larger vessels.

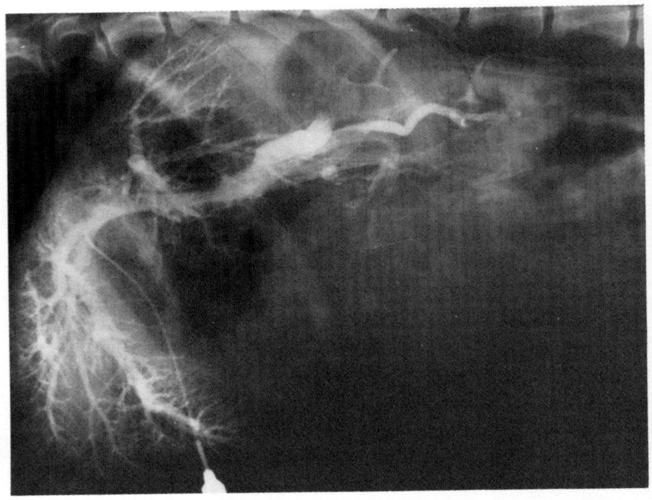

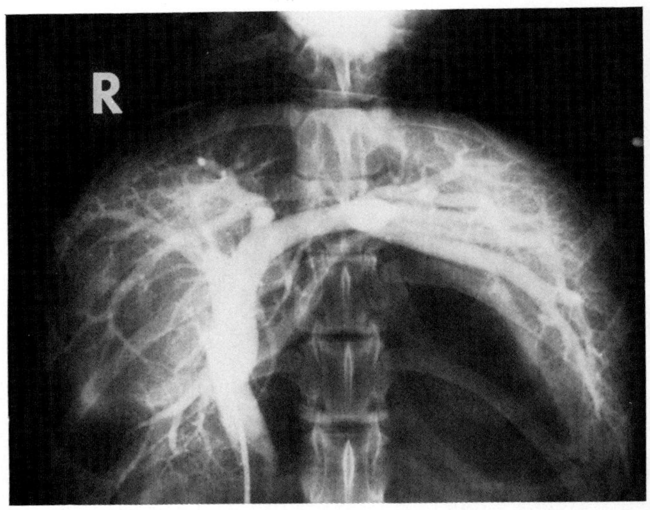

Figure 27-2b. Venograms of portal vein of a normal dog shown in lateral and ventrodorsal views. (By permission, Sibylle Schmidt).

hepatic blood flow, 20% is from the hepatic artery, and the remainder is from the portal vein. The hepatic artery is a branch of the celiac artery. The portal vein carries venous blood from the stomach, intestines, pancreas, and spleen. The hepatic artery and portal vein enter the liver at the isthmus between the two processes of the caudate lobe and at the central point formed by the merging of the other lobes. This is the hilus of the liver, a site where the bile duct emerges from the liver and gallbladder. Lymphatic drainage of the liver moves through vessels to the hepatic lymph nodes (on the sides of the portal vein near the hilus of the liver); to splenic nodes adjacent to the splenic artery; and to the gastric node (in the lesser omentum, near the pyloric end of the stomach).

Neural Innervation[1,2]

The vagus nerves carry afferent nerve fibers from the liver. Hepatic efferent fibers are vagal parasympathetics and splanchnic sympathetics. Sympathetics are from the celiac ganglia and celiac plexuses, with the fibers following the hepatic artery.

Gallbladder Structure[1,2]

The gallbladder is a reservoir that stores and modifies bile secreted by the liver. The gallbladder can be divided regionally into a fundus, body, and a neck that is continuous with the cystic duct. Its capacity is about 1 cc per Kg of body weight. The wall of the gallbladder, from inside out, consists of epithelial cells on a lamina propria; a muscular layer; a perimuscular layer of connective tissue; and a peritoneal covering (Figure 27-3). The epithelium consists of columnar cells containing microvilli on the luminal surface. The muscular layer consists of poorly defined groups of longitudinal, transverse, and oblique fibers.

A number of hepatic biliary ducts carry bile to the common

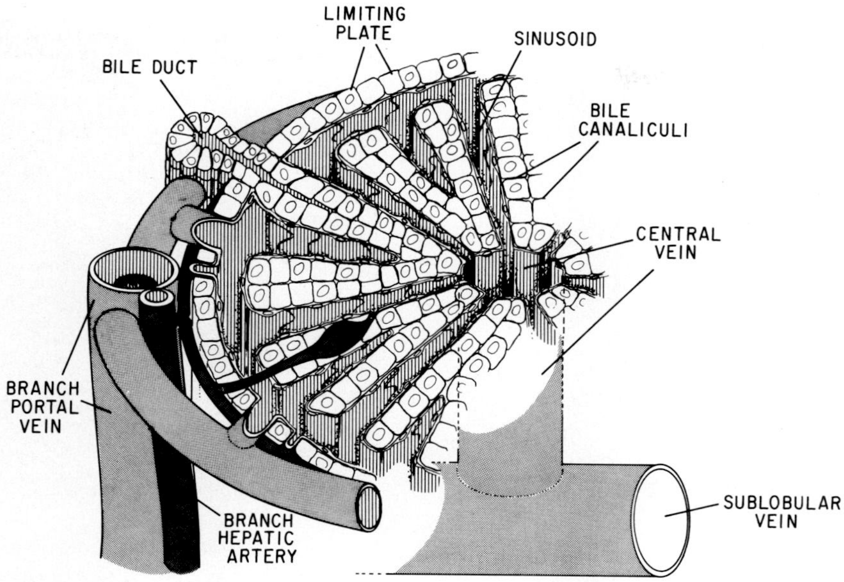

Figure 27-2d. Drawing of hepatic lobule showing circulation entering the liver by the branches of the portal vein and hepatic artery. After circulation through hepatic capillaries (sinusoids), blood leaves the lobule by central and sublobular veins.

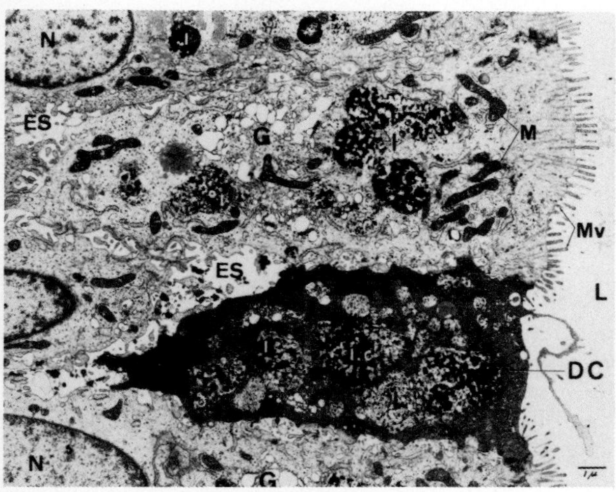

Figure 27-3. Electron micrograph of gall bladder epithelium from a normal dog. L = lumen of gall bladder, Mv = microvilli, M = mitochondrion, I = inclusion, G = golgi apparatus, ES = extracellular space, N = nucleus, DC = degenerating cell.

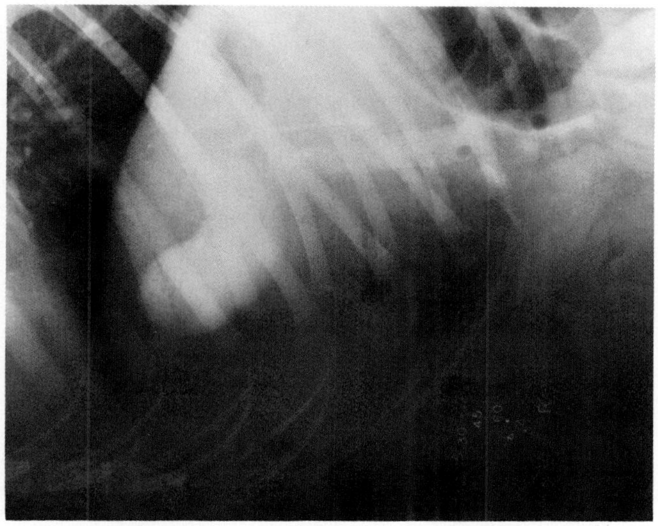

Figure 27-4. Lateral radiograph of dog 60 minutes after receiving iodipamide identifies the position of the normal gallbladder.

bile duct. The segment of the common bile duct from the neck of the gallbladder to the point where the first hepatic duct enters is called the cystic duct, and the remainder of the main duct to the duodenum is the common bile duct, which empties into the duodenum about 2.5 to 6 cm from the pylorus in the dog (Figure 27-4). In the cat the bile duct ends at the intestine, together with the pancreatic duct, about 3 cm distal to the pylorus. Release of bile into the intestine is controlled by the sphincter of Oddi, consisting of two layers of muscle, one being derived from the duodenum.

Microscopic Structure[3-6]

The liver is made up of hepatocytes, the most predominant cell type; bile ducts; blood vessels; and sinusoidal cells that include Kupffer cells, endothetial cells, fat-storing (Ito) cells, and pit cells.

Hepatocytes are large cells richly supplied with mitochondria and endoplasmic reticulum. They possess the abilities to synthesize, store, secrete, and detoxify. Hepatocytes are arranged in one-cell-thick radiating cords, or plates, with blood perfusion on two sides (Figure 27-5). That arrangement overcomes problems associated with the perfusion by blood that contains both oxygen at a low tension and an abundant supply of substances from the intestinal tract that have to be removed.

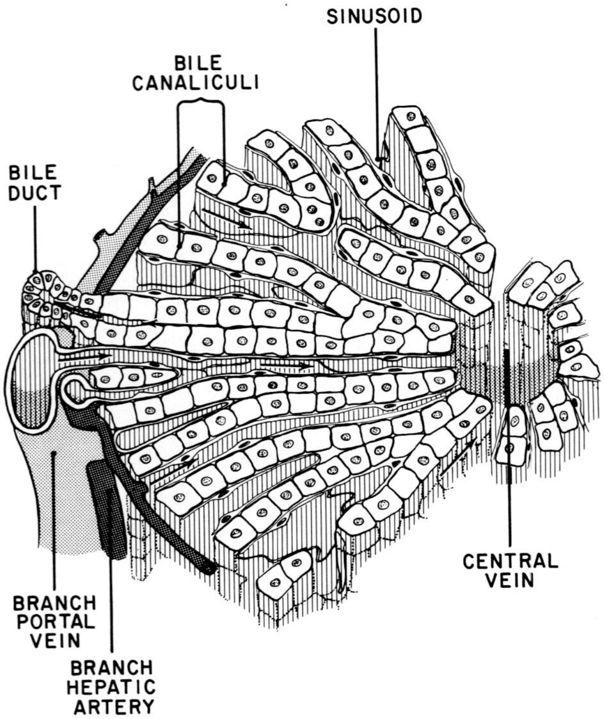

Figure 27-5. Drawing of normal hepatic lobule. Blood normally perfuses two sides of hepatocytes. Bile canaliculi are formed by specialization of hepatocyte membranes. Arrows show the directions of blood and bile flows which are opposite.

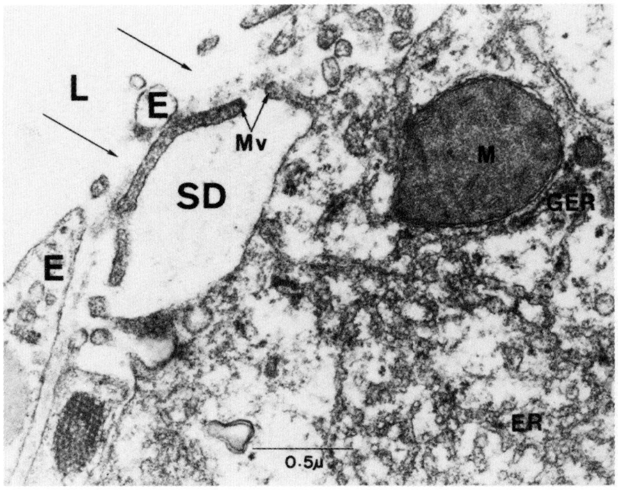

Figure 27-6. Electron micrograph of canine liver showing relationship of hepatocyte, space of Disse, and sinusoid. X 26,930. L = lumen of sinusoid, E = part of endothelial cell, SD = space of Disse, Mv = microvilli of hepatocyte, M = mitochondria, GER = granular (rough) endoplasmic reticulum, ER = a granular endoplasmic reticulum. Arrows from sinusoidal lumen = pores in endothelial lining.

This relationship of a cell to its circulation permits a maximal rate of exchange of substances between the two. The vascular channels that perfuse each side of these cords or sheets are called sinusoids, and they contain no valves. The sinusoids, communicating with each other, form a honeycomb within the liver mass. The cords, or plates, appear to radiate from a central point, or axis, the central vein. The aggregation of radiating plates around one central vein has been called a lobule, with the periphery of each lobule being bounded and outlined by the structures in portal triads. The afferent blood flow supplied by the portal vein and hepatic artery enters the lobule from vessels in the portal triad (Figure 27-5). The normal direction of blood flow is from the portal triads through the sinusoids to the central vein and into the hepatic vein and caudal vena cava. Bile ducts, collecting bile secreted by hepatocytes, leave through the portal triads.

The portal triads resemble diamond-shaped islands of fibrous tissue containing vessels. Branches of the vessels from the triads radiate out to meet the branches from adjacent triads. These structures have more connective tissue than do other parts of the lobule. Branches of the hepatic artery enter the lobules through the portal triads and terminate in arterioles to sinusoids. Sphincters at the end of the arterioles regulate the rate of flow and pressure in sinusoids. The arterioles terminate at all levels of the lobule, that is, near the central vein as well as near the portal triads; however, most arterial blood is supplied by short vessels that terminate close to the portal triads or periphery of the lobule. A red blood cell entering the liver at the portal vein is not committed to follow the shortest route to the central vein. The contractibility of sinusoids enables them to contribute to proper distribution of blood flow so that perfusion is uniform to all hepatocytes. In addition, the redistribution of blood from one area to another is assisted by sphincters in the venules and by branches of distributing vessels from the portal vein supplying the sinusoids. Sphincters around sinusoids entering the central vein also control the distribution of blood flow through a lobule. Central veins circulate blood to sublobular veins, which unite in hepatic veins and subsequently deliver blood to the caudal vena cava. Sphincters where central veins join sublobular veins also regulate hepatic circulation.

The hexagonal shaped lobule around one central vein has been thought of as the functional unit comprising the liver. The functional unit is currently conceived to be the small mass of parenchyma, irregular in shape and size, arranged around a terminal portal vein and its accompanying hepatic arteriole and bile duct. This unit, called an acinus, lies between two or more terminal hepatic venules into which it drains; in the hexagonal description of the liver it occupies only part of two adjacent classic lobules. The acinus as a functional unit provides a concept upon which a clearer understanding of hepatic pathophysiology and pathologic changes is based.

Sinusoids are lined with fenestrated sheets of endothelial cells acting as a barrier that prevents direct contact of blood with hepatocytes. A space, the space of Disse, can be found between endothelial cells and hepatocytes (Figure 27-6). This space contains fine collagen fibers (reticulin) that provide the framework supporting the plates of hepatocytes. Endothelial fenestrations permit substances to move between the circulation and hepatocytes. Microvillous projections on the surface of hepatocytes increase the surface area available for exchange of substances between the hepatocyte and the circulation.

Bile is secreted by hepatocytes into small bile canaliculi found between adjacent hepatic cells (Figure 27-7). The walls

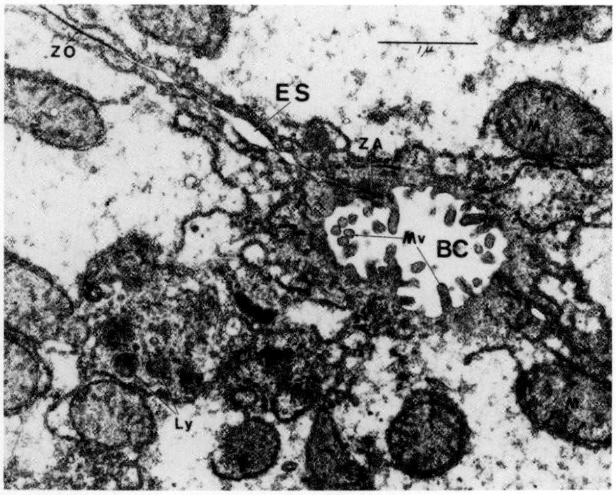

Figure 27-7. Electron micrograph of canine liver showing a bile canaliculus between two hepatocytes. X 12,920. BC = bile canaliculus, Mv = microvilli, ZO = zonula occludens (tight junction), ZA = zonula adherens, M = mitochondrion, Ly = lysosomes, ES = extracellular space dilated by perfusate.

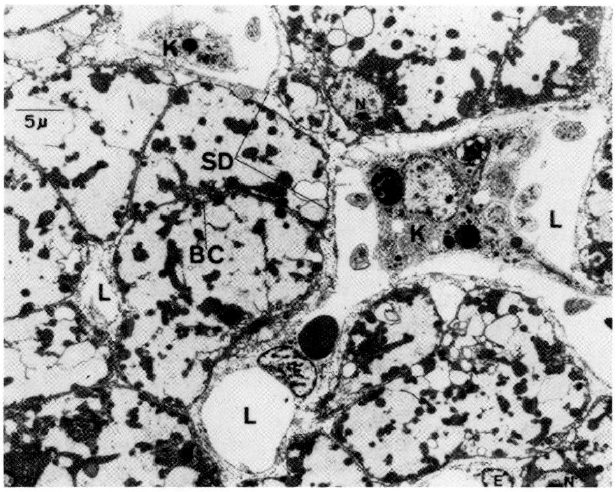

Figure 27-8. Electron micrograph of normal canine liver. X 1260. N = nucleus of hepatocyte, BC = bile canaliculus, L = lumen of sinusoid, K = Kupffer cell, E = nucleus of endothelial cell, SD = space of Disse. Extensive gray areas are rich in glycogen.

of these ducts are formed by cell membranes of hepatocytes and contain numerous microvilli. Bile canaliculi begin near central veins and extend to the periphery of hepatic lobules. Bile flows from the center of the lobule toward the portal triads, opposite to blood flow. Since bile is normally compartmentalized and separated from blood by a barrier at least half a cell thick, little regurgitates into the circulation. Bile canaliculi empty into larger ducts, called cholangioles (canals of Hering), which are formed by four or five modified liver cells arranged in a circular fashion. These modified cells morphologically have a mixture of features of hepatocytes and bile duct cells. They possess fewer organelles and more intracellular fibrils than hepatocytes. Cholangioles deliver bile to bile ducts in portal triads. Bile ducts are lined with cuboidal or columnar epithelial cells, with some mucin-secreting cells.

Hepatocytes are hexagonal-appearing cells that have three different types of surfaces (Figure 27-8).[7] Surfaces facing sinusoids are adapted for exchange of fluid and substances with the blood. The area of this surface is greatly magnified by numerous microvilli projecting into the space of Disse. A major part of a hepatocyte's surface, about 70%, contacts sinusoidal blood flow. On the side of a hepatocyte opposite to the sinusoid, a small percentage of the surface area, about 15%, is specialized to form the walls of the bile canaliculi. The surface is modified to form microvilli for secretion of bile. This surface is further modified to become relatively impermeable to the movement of fluid and solutes by a sealing of the intercellular junctional complexes of the bile canaliculi. Actin microfilaments surround bile canaliculi, and with their contractile properties they are able to promote bile flow. The third type of cell membrane forms the borders between adjacent hepatocytes. These membranes form a relatively impermeable barrier to the movement of fluid and ions between adjacent cells. At the same time they contain pores for the movement of substances from one cell to another, thus forming an intercellular communication system.[8] Hepatocyte cell membranes possess receptors for many hormones, plasma proteins, and glycoproteins.

The microscopic appearance of hepatocytes reflects their many functions (Figure 27-9). Hepatocytes have a relatively large nucleus, which is consistent with cells actively engaged in protein synthesis. The synthesis of large amounts of protein is also reflected in the abundant rough endoplasmic reticulum, the site of its manufacture. Smooth endoplasmic reticulum is prominent and can increase greatly by demand to increase its functions. Its metabolic functions include synthesis of triglycerides from free fatty acids, the production and metabolism of cholesterol and possibly bile acids, the metabolism of drugs such as phenobarbital, and possibly some aspects of glycogen metabolism. The golgi complex is evident in cells designed to store and

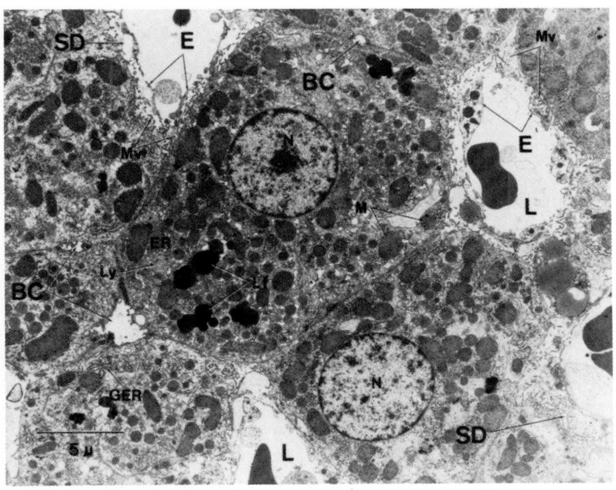

Figure 27-9. Electron micrograph of normal canine liver, X 2310. N = nucleus of hepatocyte, BC = bile canaliculus. L = lumen of sinusoid, E = part of endothelial cell, SD = space of Disse, Mv = microvilli of hepatocyte, M = mitochondrion, Ly = lysosome, Lf = lipofuscin, GER = granular endoplasmic reticulum, ER = agranular endoplasmic reticulum

export some of the materials they produce; the liver actively exports many of its products. Lysosomes provide cells the ability to degrade intracellular constituents for provision of nutrients during nonfed states. That catabolic function is also important during periods of rapid growth and differentiation, both in development and in regeneration. Lysosomes store elements such as copper and iron and products of lipid catabolism such as lipofuscin pigment. Mitochondria are abundant in hepatocytes with more in those around central veins than around the portal areas. They are concerned with fatty acid oxidation, citric acid cycle activity, and oxidative phosphorylation, all of which function to meet the large energy requirements of hepatocytes.

Hepatocytes store substances such as glycogen (which can be seen) and lipid-soluble vitamins (which are not evident). The hepatocyte also accumulates substances that are often of no value. Some partially degraded substances do not leave the hepatocyte but accumulate and appear as pigments, such as lipofuscin. There may be abnormal storage not only of normal pigment, such as iron, but also of foreign substances. They accumulate in lysosomes, forming residual bodies.

Kupffer cells lining sinusoids are part of the monocyte-macrophage system that removes material from the circulation and degrades much of it. Endothelial cells providing the structure of hepatic sinusoids are designed to provide fenestrae of varying sizes. These openings permit the passage of certain size particles and exclude larger ones. The fenestrae are larger in pericentral than in periportal sinusoids. That is important in directing some chylomicron remnants to pericentral hepatocytes and preventing their access to periportal hepatocytes. Endothelial cells also take up some viral agents and produce anti-viral substances in response. Lipid-storing (Ito) cells, found in sinusoids, store fats and vitamin A and can be transformed into cells with fibroblastic activity. Pit cells found in sinusoids have vesicles that were once thought to reflect an endocrine function, but the cells may actually have a natural killer cell function.

REFERENCES

1. Miller, M.E., Christensen, G.C. and Evans, H.E.: Anatomy of the Dog. W.B. Saunders Co., Philadelphia, 1964.
2. Nickel, R., Schummer, A., Seiferele, E. and Sack, W.O.: The viscera of the domestic animals. Springer-Verlag. New York, 1973.
3. Bradley, S.E.: The hepatic circulation. In, Handbook of Physiology, Section 2, Circulation, Vol. 2. Edited by W.F. Hamilton, P. Dow. Amer. Physiolo. Soc., Washington D.C. 1387-1438, 1963.
4. Rappaport, A.M.: Anatomic considerations. In, Diseases of the Liver. 6th edition. Edited by L. Schiff and E.R. Schiff. J.B. Lippincott, Philadelphia, 1-46, 1987.
5. Schaffner, F. and Popper, H.: Electron microscopy of the liver. In, Diseases of the Liver. 6th edition. Edited by L. Schiff. J.B. Lippincott, Philadelphia, 47-76, 1987.
6. Millward-Sadler, G.H. and Jezequel, A.M.: Normal hilstology and ultrastructure. In, Liver and Biliary Disease. 2nd edition. Edited by R. Wright, G.H. Millward-Sadler, K.G.M.M. Alberti and S. Karran. W.B. Saunders, Philadelphia, 13-44, 1985.
7. Heath, T. and Wissig, S.L.: Fine structure of the surface of mouse hepatic cells. Am. J. Anat. 119:97-127, 1966.

Chapter 28

Liver: Normal Function and Pathophysiology

METABOLIC FUNCTION - ANABOLIC

Carbohydrate Metabolism

Physiology.[1-5] The liver is the center of carbohydrate metabolism due to its role in maintaining normal blood glucose levels; complete hepatectomy results in hypoglycemic shock and death within a few hours. Carbohydrate metabolism involves glucose storage and release, glucose production, and the metabolic conversion of some non-glucose hexoses to glucose. Glucagon, insulin, catecholamines, glucocorticoids, thyroid hormone, and growth hormone regulate these function through their effects on metabolic enzyme activity and to some extent on transport of carbohydrates and amino acids across cell membranes.

Glucose is stored as glycogen after entering hepatocytes by a non-insulin-dependent mechanism (Figure 28-1). Glycogen formation is maximum after a meal when portal blood glucose increases and insulin, at levels three to ten times those in the systemic circulation, stimulates glucokinase activity and promotes phosphorylation. In dogs the liver takes up glucose very efficiently until portal blood glucose levels fall below 120 mg/dl of glucose. Low blood glucose stimulates glucose-6-phosphatase activity to degrade glycogen for the release of glucose, a process stimulated during hypoglycemia by such hormones as catecholamines, glucagon, corticosteroids, and growth hormone. The liver normally stores one gram of carbohydrate per kilogram of an animal's total body weight.

Starvation for 24 hours depletes glycogen stores. Since the brain's daily requirement of glucose is greater than the amount stored in the liver, gluconeogenesis is necessary to prevent glucose deficiency during this state of starvation. Gluconeogenesis is also important to and may be continuous in animals fed diets containing little available carbohydrate. Precursors for gluconeogenesis are primarily lactate, pyruvate, glycerol, and alanine.

Following a meal, the liver removes the largest part of the amino acids absorbed, with the exception of the branched-chain amino acids. Under this condition, alanine is by far the most abundant amino acid available for gluco-neogenesis, not only because of its levels in the diet but also because of its formation from the intestine's metabolism of glutamine. During fasting, glucose is primarily produced by the amino acids alanine and glutamine, which together account for over 50% of those released from skeletal muscle. Acting as the donor of precursors for glucose synthesis, skeletal muscle protein undergoes proteolysis and release of amino acids, events controlled by insulin levels. In the catabolic state the skeletal muscle is energy requirements are sustained by the metabolism of branched-chain amino acids released from muscle protein, a glucose conserving process. The nitrogen produced is incorporated into pyruvate to form alanine and glutamate to form glutamine. The pyruvate is derived largely from the carbon remains of other amino acids. The small intestine metabolizes glutamine to alanine, with over one-half of the ammonia in the portal blood from that conversion; the kidneys metabolize glutamine to alanine and serine. Alanine is transaminated in the liver, and eventually the pyruvate formed can be converted to glucose and the nitrogen to urea. With minimal carbohydrate intake and inadequate glycogen stores, gluconeogenesis from amino acids is the most important source for glucose.

Glucose produced in the liver from lactate, pyruvate, and glycerol is greater than that from glycogen after a 12-hour fast. Most of these precursors are derived from glucose metabolism in extrahepatic tissues and from muscle glycogen accumulated from glucose originally released, largely from the liver. Thus, the glucose from these sources represents more of a recycling rather than a *de novo* synthesis.

Glucose produced from the non-glucose hexoses, fructose and galactose, is unimportant in small animals, since these carbohydrates are not an important part of their diet. Before they can be used, these hexoses require metabolism in the liver.

Hepatic metabolism of glucose is regulated by substrate availability and by a number of hormones. After feeding, insulin-stimulating glucokinase activity and the phosphorylation of glucose are essential for hepatic uptake of glucose; increasing portal blood glucose content without a change in portal insulin concentration results in unchanged hepatic glucose uptake. When hepatic glucose concentration is high, phosphorylase activity is inhibited so that glucose is not released from glycogen. Higher insulin concentrations postprandially affect substrate availability indirectly, while having no effect on glucose production. Insulin inhibits gluconeogenesis, resulting in the accumulation of lactate and pyruvate, which are normally converted to glucose.

During fasting, glycogenolysis increases because of lack of its inhibition by both glucose and insulin and because of its stimulation by glucagon and catecholamines. Gluconeogenesis increases because of glucagon's enhancing the hepatic uptake of alanine and because of an increased uptake of other substrates for glucose production. Proteolysis and release of amino acids from skeletal muscle increases with a reduction in

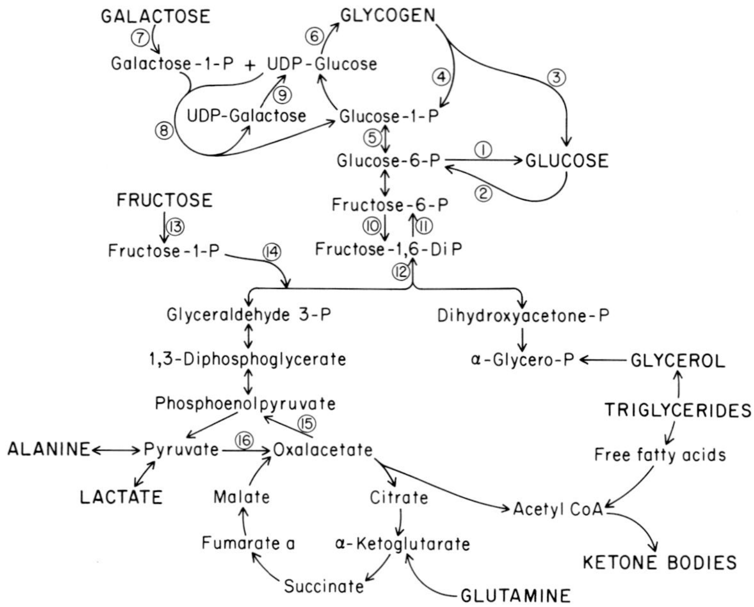

Figure 28-1. Metabolic pathways involved in glycogen synthesis and degradation and gluconeogenesis. Enzymes designated by number, are 1) glucose-6-phosphatase, 2) glucokinase, 3) amylo-1, 6-glucosidase, 4) phosphorylase, 5) phosphoglucomutase, 6) glycogen synthetase, 7) galactokinase, 8) galactose-1-phosphate uridyl transferase, 9) uridine diphosphogalactose-4-epimerase, 10) phosphofructokinase, 11) fructose-1, 6- diphosphatase, 12) fructose-1, 6-diphosphate aldolase, 13) fructokinase, 14) fructose-1-phosphate aldolase, 15) phosphoenolpyruvate carboxykinase, 16) pyruvate carboxylase.

insulin's effects to promote amino acid uptake and protein synthesis and inhibit protein catabolism. Glucagon's ability to stimulate branched-chain amino acid oxidation, to inhibit amino acid incorporation into protein, and to increase the release of animo acids from muscle also promotes this catabolic effect. Glucocorticosteroids, catecholamines, and growth hormone have similar effects. The liver's gluconeogenic function is essential to life; following complete hepatectomy, hypoglycemia and death rapidly develop unless glucose is administered.

Pathophysiology.[1,4,5] (Table 28-1) With extensive hepatic disease, blood glucose levels are not maintained within the normal range of 75 to 100 mg/dl, and hypoglycemia or, less commonly, hyperglycemia follows.

Liver disease can cause fasting hypoglycemia, in which the diseased liver is unable to store sufficient glycogen for maintaining normal blood glucose levels and has inadequate gluconeogenic enzyme activity for converting amino acids to glucose. Liver disease can also cause prolonged hyperglycemia following feeding because the activity of carbohydrate-metabolizing enzymes is deficient. The activity of some enzymes normally increases after a meal and insulin secretion. This response lowers blood sugar and maintains it at normal levels.

Concentrations of hormones regulating carbohydrate metabolism are changed by hepatic disease, however. Plasma levels increase for catecholamines which promote hyperglycemia. Plasma glucocorticoid levels may also be higher than normal, and that would promote gluconeogenesis and contribute to hyperglycemia. Plasma concentrations of both glucagon and insulin increase, with glucagon increasing more. Despite that the overall effect of such changes in dogs with hepatic insufficiency is a relative hypoglycemia during fasting. Relative hepatic and peripheral insensitivities to insulin or glucagon have been used to explain the prolonged hyperglycemia after feeding and the fasting hypoglycemia with liver disease.

Hepatic problems must be included in the differential diagnosis of fasting hypoglycemia.[6] The causes of fasting hypoglycemias are listed in Table 28-2. The liver is the cause of hypoglycemia in diffuse liver disease, deficiency of hepatic carbohydrate-metabolizing enzymes, and non-pancreatic tumors in the liver.

Hepatic Disease. A toxic or infectious agent, such as infectious canine hepatitis virus, can often result in hypoglycemia as an early manifestation of diffuse and severe hepatic disease. The hypoglycemia following complete hepatectomy appears before clinical signs due to loss of any other hepatic functions. Some studies indicate that less than 30% of the liver is sufficient to maintain normal blood glucose, for a 70% hepatectomy does not cause hypoglycemia. Reduction of hepatic mass to 50% of normal by toxins results in hypoglycemia that improves with time. Portasystemic vascular shunts cause a relative hypoglycemia in dogs showing no signs of hepatic insufficiency. With most liver disease, hypoglycemia is seldom recognized; substantial hepatic reserves remain to maintain normal blood glucose levels. Increased fasting blood glucose levels are also found with hepatic disease.

Hepatic Enzyme Deficiencies.[7,8] Congenital hepatic enzyme deficiencies causing glycogen storage diseases result in hypoglycemia. Abnormal glycogen retention develops from a deficiency of glucose-6-phosphatase, which catalyzes the hydrolysis of glucose-6-phosphate to free glucose in the conversion of glycogen to glucose. A deficiency of amylo-1,6-glucosidase, the debrancher enzyme, reduces the liver's ability

Table 28-1. Pathophysiologic Correlations in Liver Disease

I. Loss of metabolic functions
- A. Carbohydrate metabolism
  1. Hypoglycemia
  2. Hyperglycemia
- B. Protein metabolism
  1. Hypoalbuminemia
  2. Deficiencies of blood-clotting factors
  3. Hypolipoproteinemia
  4. Hyperammonemia
  5. Abnormal plasma amino acid ratios
- C. Lipid metabolism
  1. Hyperlipemia
  2. Hypercholesterolemia or hypocholesterolemia
  3. Decreased bile salt formation
- D. Vitamin metabolism
  1. Coenzyme deficiencies

II. Loss of catabolic functions (conjugation, detoxification, and excretion)
- A. Bile-pigment metabolism
  1. Hyperbilirubinemia
     - a. Prehepatic
     - b. Hepatic
     - c. Posthepatic
- B. Bile acid metabolism
  1. Pruritus
  2. Malabsorption
- C. Steroid metabolism
  1. Hyperestrogenism
     - a. Gynecomastia, testicular atrophy, alopecia
  2. Hyperadrenocorticism
     - a. Polydypsia, ascites
- D. Drug metabolism
  1. Impaired catabolism of exogenous steroids
  2. Delayed catabolism of anesthetic agents
     - a. Prolonged recovery times
  3. Impaired catabolism of organic dyes
- E. Detoxification and RES function
  1. Hyperammonemia
     - a. Hepatic disease
     - b. Portal-circulation anomaly
  2. Endotoxemia
- F. Excretory function
  1. Intrahepatic or posthepatic biliary stasis

III. Loss of circulatory function
- A. Increased portal blood pressure (ascites)
  1. Prehepatic (thrombosis, anomalies)
  2. Intrahepatic (hepatic malignancy, cirrhosis)
  3. Posthepatic (heart failure)
- B. Portal bypass of liver
  1. Hyperammonemia

IV. Loss of compartmentalization function
- A. Trauma (infection, inflammation, toxins)
  1. Loss of enzymes
  2. Increased utilization of clotting factors
  3. Loss of antigens, immunologic implications
  4. Loss of hepatocyte functions

Table 28-2. Causes of Fasting Hypoglycemias

Organic hypoglycemia
- Pancreatic islet beta-cell disease
  - Adenomas
  - Adenocarcinomas
- Nonpancreatic tumors
- Anterior pituitary hypofunction
- Adrenocortical hypofunction
- Diffuse liver disease
- Severe congestive heart failure

Deficiency of hepatic carbohydrate-metabolizing enzymes

Functional hypoglycemia
- Glucagon deficiency
- Ketotic hypoglycemia
- Starvation

Iatrogenic - insulin administration

to convert glycogen to glucose-6-phosphate.

Deficiency of lysosomal acid α-glucosidase also results in the accumulation of glycogen. Hypoglycemia is possible with deficiencies of fructose-1,6-diphosphatase or glycogen synthetase because glucose cannot be stored as glucose in the liver. Deficiency of an enzyme such as pyruvate carboxylase will impair gluconeogenesis and result in hypoglycemia. A deficiency of other enzymes can cause galactosemia or fructose intolerance. Some of these deficiencies have been reported in dogs, usually in pups as a congenital defect. Suspicion of an enzyme deficiency is usually based on finding unexplained hypoglycemia in a young animal. The glycogen storage diseases will also cause hepatomegaly, due to abnormal glycogen accumulation. These enzyme deficiencies are not diagnosed on the animal's age, clinical signs, blood glucose levels, response to treatment, or absence of any organic disease. Hypoglycemia due to enzyme deficiencies may or may not respond to glucagon. Confirmation of enzyme deficiency is based on glucagon response testing and on biopsies for histology and enzyme assay.

Ketotic Hypoglycemias.[7] Pups presented with self-limiting hypoglycemia are probably similar to children with ketotic hypoglycemia (formerly called idiopathic hypoglycemia). Ketotic hypoglycemia, representing greater than 70% of all hypoglycemias in children, is characterized by hypoglycemia, ketonuria, ketonemia, normal liver size, a normal hyperglycemic response to glucagon, and low plasma alanine levels. Signs appear during fasting or when a provocative ketogenic diet (high fat, low carbohydrate, and hypocaloric) is fed. Plasma insulin levels are decreased, indicating that this hormone does not precipitate the hypoglycemia. Low plasma alanine levels and the beneficial response to alanine infusions suggest that gluconeogenic mechanisms are normal, converting alanine to glucose, but that conversion of muscle proteins to alanine may be abnormal. Exogenous corticosteroids correct the problem in children by promoting protein catabolism and the release of alanine. One case was seen in which a pup did not respond to steroids.[9] The pup outgrew the problem, as do children. The problem may be self-limiting, because glucose requirements are two to three times as great in young animals as in adults. This pup did not have detectable amounts of plasma ketone bodies. Ketones are an important source of energy during fasting, and the pup's hypoglycemia may have been from an enhanced utilization of glucose because of the liver's inability to produce ketone bodies. The greater glucose requirements in young animals may result from an immaturity of the hepatic mechanism for producing ketones.

Tumor Hypoglycemia.[10,11] Hypoglycemia is sometimes associated with neoplastic disease. The hypoglycemia has been attributed to excessive utilization of glucose by the tumor, reduced hepatic glucose production, and the tumor's release of insulin-like activity.

Extrahepatic Causes of Hypoglycemia. In addition to intrahepatic problems that alter carbohydrate metabolism to produce hypoglycemia, extrahepatic problems can cause deranged carbohydrate metabolism. Endocrine abnormalities, including abnormal release of insulin, pituitary hormones, or adrenal hormones, can cause hypoglycemia. Circulatory problems may also be responsible for hypoglycemia. When anemia or cardiac disease reduces arterial blood oxygen tension, peripheral tissues rely more on glucose for energy, and the liver responds by manufacturing more glucose. Sepsis has a similar effect. It reduces circulation and oxygen delivery; in addition, it interferes with hepatic carbohydrate metabolism and the maintenance of normal blood glucose.

Correlation With Clinical Signs. Signs of hypoglycemia range from weakness, ataxia, and collapse to severe CNS manifestations, such as seizures and coma. Severe signs of hypoglycemia usually respond promptly to intravenous glucose. Weight loss may or may not accompany hypoglycemia. Hyperglycemia causes polydipsia and polyuria, but it is not the only reason for polydipsia and polyuria in hepatic disease.

Lipid Metabolism

Physiology.[12-15] The liver is most important in the integration of lipid metabolism. In liponeogenesis it converts excess carbohydrates and proteins to fatty acids, which are esterified and exported in triglyceride-rich very-low-density lipoproteins (Figure 28-2). Lipids absorbed from the intestinal tract and released from adipose tissue are also metabolized in the liver. Excess fatty acids are either re-esterified or converted to detones via ß-oxidation. In normal animals, the anabolic and catabolic processes are in equilibrium.

Lipids absorbed from the small intestine and formed into chylomicrons reach the systemic circulation via the lymphatics. Triglycerides, re-esterified from fatty acids and monoglycerides in the intestine, combine with small amounts of free and esterified cholesterol, phospholipids, and a protein, called apoprotein, to form chylomicrons. (Also a small amount of triglycerides is combined with larger amounts of these same constituents of chylomicrons to form high-density lipoproteins). This formation of chylomicrons and lipoproteins makes it possible for insoluble lipids to be transported from the intestine in aqueous fluids. During circulation through various tissues, notably adipose tissue, capillary endothelial lipoprotein lipase activity hydrolyses the triglycerides in chylomicrons. This releases fatty acids and glycerol to tissues, where they can be re-esterified and stored or used for energy. Upon loss of a substantial part of their triglycerides, the parts of the chylomicrons remaining are high-density lipoproteins.

An organ's regulation and integration of lipid metabolism is dependent on its ability to synthesize and secrete lipoproteins. The intestine assimilates dietary lipids but does not regulate or integrate lipid metabolism. The liver, being the only organ other than the intestine with lipoprotein metabolism functions, has the primary role in overall lipid metabolism. In general most, if not all, lipoprotein traffic requires circulation through the liver. Lipids accumulate in the liver by a number of ways.

High concentrations of glucose and other metabolizable carbohydrates promote Liponeogenesis and the accumulation of lipids in the liver. Fatty acids, formed from the conversion of glucose, are esterified with glycerol to triglycerides that are exported from the liver in very-low-density lipoproteins. Fatty acid synthesis is determined by the activity of acetyl-CoA carboxylase, the rate-limiting enzyme. The activity of this enzyme is reduced by starvation and high levels of serum fatty acids. Glucagon and catecholamines have the same effect. Feeding, high glucose levels, and insulin stimulate this enzyme's activity.

During fasting, fats in adipose tissue are released as free fatty acids and used for energy. They are mobilized by corticosteroids, glucagon, growth hormone, thyroxine, and catecholamines. Their release is inhibited by insulin and high blood sugar levels. Following release, the hepatocyte binds free fatty acids to albumin and removes them from the circulation. When fatty acids are not catabolized, the liver converts them to triglycerides, which are incorporated into very-low-density lipoproteins for transport to adipose tissue.

The release of fatty acids from adipose tissue is not very well controlled; therefore, the amount released exceeds levels which can be used for energy. During all metabolic conditions, hepatic fatty acid uptake is greater than the amount used for energy. The latter amount generally does not exceed 10% of the uptake even during starvation. The amount converted to ketone bodies varies from 10 to 60% depending on the state of nutrition. By far the greatest amount of fatty acids are esterified to triglycerides; that conversion is important in preventing the accumulation of toxic levels of fatty acids in the serum.

The skeletal muscle, myocardium, and the liver extract and use fatty acids equally. They are an important source of energy to the liver. Fatty acids are metabolized to a two-carbon metabolite, acetyl coenzyme-A, primarily in mitochondria. Entry into a mitochondria requires a carrier process involving carnitine. Acetyl-CoA is a substrate for either energy production or ketogenesis. In the former, acetyl coenzyme-A condenses with oxaloacetate to form citrate, a metabolite oxidized in the citric acid cycle. Oxaloacetate must be replenished by glucose metabolism to sustain this form of fatty acid metabolism. With oxaloacetate deficiency, as in diabetes, excess acetyl-CoA condenses to form acetoacetate, a ketone body. The ketone bodies acetoacetate and 3-hydroxybutyrate released from the liver, where they cannot be used for energy, are sources of energy for muscle during short-term postabsorption and for the brain at any time. Ketone bodies supply up to 60% of energy for the brain during starvation.

The pathways for hepatic fatty acid metabolism are regulated by substrate availability and specific enzyme activities. Reduced factors for transfer of fatty acids into mitochondria for degradation, carnitine and the enzymes involved in fatty acid-

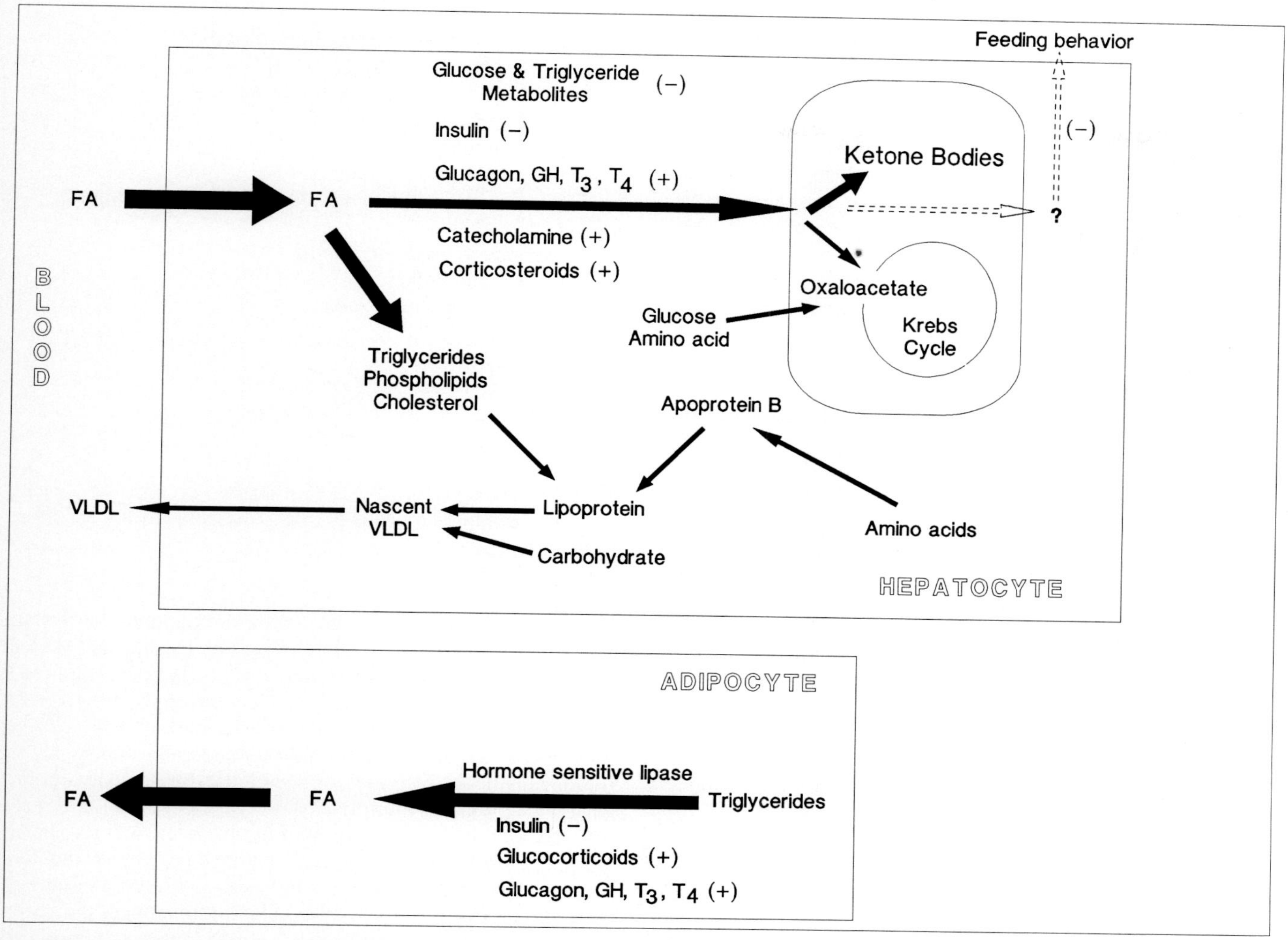

Figure 28-2 Physiology of Lipid Metabolism. Used with permission of Vincent Biourge.

carnitine formation and transport, promote esterification of fatty acids. Esterification also increases with feeding and is inhibited during starvation. Insulin promotes esterification. Fatty acids committed to degradation rather than esterification convert to acetyl-CoA, which can be further metabolized to either citrate or ketone bodies. Citrate formation for the tricarboxylate cycle is promoted by the gluconeogenic substance's increasing the level of oxaloacetate. Decreases in this substance and inhibition of citrate synthesis promote ketogenesis.

The liver has a limited capacity for oxidizing fatty acids to carbon dioxide and water, but it is able to metabolize large amounts of fatty acids to acetyl-Co-A and ketone bodies. This process can be reversed with fatty acids synthesized from acetyl-CoA. An interplay of lipogenic and lipotrophic factors, promoting deposition and mobilization of lipid in the liver, control fatty acid synthesis and degradation. The balance of anabolic and catabolic effects is upset when caloric delivery to the liver is inadequate, excessive, or imbalanced. Such derangements can be produced by consumption of high-lipid or protein deficient diets, overnutrition, starvation, and endocrine imbalances. Most abnormalities are associated with excess secretion of glucagon, corticosteroids, growth hormone, or thyroid hormone; the excess hormone secretion is usually due to low glucose availability. These hormones promote the hydrolysis of adipose lipids and the hepatic uptake and metabolism of fatty acids released. Fatty acids cannot be converted to glucose, and excesses accumulate in the liver as triglycerides.

The liver synthesizes large amounts of cholesterol and accounts for most of the serum cholesterol. Cholesterol synthesis is regulated and is normally related inversely to dietary intake. The liver also metabolizes cholesterol to cholic acid and secretes it in the bile after conjugation with glycine or taurine. Secretion into bile provides a single important pathway for cholesterol excretion from the body.

All plasma triglycerides are of dietary and hepatic origin, since the intestinal mucosa and liver are the only places where triglycerides can be synthesized and prepared for transport. Triglycerides formed in the liver do not leave to enter the circulation until they are coated with an apoprotein, phospholipids, cholesterol, and cholesterol esters, to form very-low density lipoproteins (VLDL). The rates of VLDL synthesis and secretion reflects the rate of triglyceride synthesis; they are increased by insulin and decreased by glucagon. VLDL formation is also determined by the liver's ability to synthesize apoproteins, without which triglyceride formation proceeds unchecked and abnormal amounts of untransportable lipid accumulate in the liver.

Triglycerides in circulating VLDL are hydrolyzed by lipoprotein lipase activity that is found on the extracellular surface of capillary endothelia. The activity of this enzyme in the myocardium promotes hydrolysis when plasma triglyceride levels are low, whereas its activity in adipose tissue promotes uptake at higher levels. Insulin stimulates lipoprotein lipase activity and lipid uptake by tissues; glucagon, adrenocorticotrophic hormone and thyroid stimulating hormone inhibit lipase activity. Circulating VLDL exchange apoproteins with HDL to gain a cofactor for lipoprotein lipase activity. Exchanges of phospholipids and cholesterol are also made. The products of these exchanges are called remnants and low-density lipoproteins (LDL), which form with a further loss of triglycerides from remnants. These remains of VLDL metabolism, after being carried to membrane receptors, are taken up and catabolized, primarily by the liver. Lysosomal enzymes degrade the proteins, and the cholesterol ester is hydrolyzed to free cholesterol, which is re-esterified and stored.

High-density lipoproteins (HDL), small particles poor in triglycerides but rich in protein, cholesterol, and phospholipid, form by triglyceride depletion in chylomicrons and VLDL and by secretion from the liver and intestine. As stated above, HDL exchange constituents with other lipoproteins in the circulation. These lipoproteins have lecithin cholesterol acyltransferase (LCAT) activity for esterifying free cholesterol. LCAT is produced by the liver and may be important in moving cholesterol from peripheral tissue to the liver for catabolism. The liver removes and catabolizes HDL, but it may not be as important in this role as the kidneys and the tissues that synthesize hormones from cholesterol.

Pathophysiology.[12-15] Lipid metabolism is abnormal with endocrine diseases, nutritional derangements and some forms of hepatic disease. The lipid content of the liver, normally 5% of hepatic weight, increases with these abnormalities; essentially, the deposition of triglycerides is evident histologically as lipidosis. With fatty livers 40% to 50% of hepatic weight can be due to triglycerides. In general, abnormal hepatic lipid accumulation can result from: 1) increased hepatic synthesis of triglycerides; 2) decreased hepatic oxidation of fatty acids; 3) increased mobilization of fatty acids from adipose tissue; and 4) impaired transport of lipids from the liver. It reflects imbalances in cellular metabolism. Specific causes include: 1) abnormalities in the level of caloric intake; 2) a deficiency of one or more essential food factors; 3) an imbalance in dietary nutrients; 4) hepatotoxins; and disease such as diabetes mellitus (Table 28-3).

Table 28-3. Causes of Hepatic Lipidosis

Abnormalities in level of caloric intake	
	Overnutrition
	Starvation
Deficiency of essential food factors - lipotropic agents	
Imbalance in dietary nutrients	
	Protein deficiency
	Carbohydrate excess
Hepatotoxins	
	Chemicals
	Drugs
	Bacterial endotoxins
Metabolic diseases	
	Diabetes mellitus

Imbalances in Caloric Intake. Increased hepatic synthesis of lipids is a potential problem when calories are consumed in great excess, resulting in obesity. Hepatic synthesis of lipids increases, with morphological evidence of lipidosis, when excessive glucose is fed either with or without proteins.[16] The rate of synthesis exceeds the rate triglycerides can be transported from the liver. This is a potential problem in obese patients. Only restricting caloric intake can correct these fatty livers; administration of choline and other lipotrophic agents does not do so.

Fatty livers develop when caloric intake is too low or ceases, as with complete anorexia for two weeks. During starvation, blood glucose levels are maintained by the catabolism of body protein. Another source of energy is triglycerides released from adipose tissue. This metabolism is controlled by glucagon, corticosteroids, growth hormone, and catecholamines. Most fatty acids are metabolized by cardiac and skeletal muscle for energy. Approximately one third of the plasma fatty acids released from adipose tissue is removed by the liver and oxidized to ketone bodies or re-esterified to triglycerides. Ketone bodies become an important source of energy for the brain, and the triglycerides are secreted as low-density lipoproteins. The liver has a limited capacity for oxidizing fatty acids to ketone bodies, and the limitation promotes their re-esterification. During starvation, triglycerides remain in the liver because lipoproteins are not synthesized at rates adequate for their transport from hepatocytes. Starvation reduces the availability of amino acids and other nutrients such as choline for synthesis of apolipoproteins and lipoproteins. Choline, being necessary for phospholipid synthesis, reverses hepatic lipidosis when administered to starving animals. During starvation extrahepatic tissue such as muscle and brain adapts to using fatty acids for 95% of their energy requirements. This adaptation conserves glucose and reduces the need for converting amino acids to glucose. The effect is a less-than-expected accumulation of fat in the liver. With less than total starvation, the ingestion of some carbohydrate can interfere with the adaptation to use fatty acids for energy, and more fat can accumulate in the liver than with total starvation.

Fatty changes developing in response to inadequate intake of calories appear initially in the periportal area. This region of the functional unit receives blood before the pericentral area. Initial fatty changes with excessive calorie intake appear in the pericentral area.

Deficiency and Imbalances of Nutrients. Some food factors are essential to prevent fatty livers. Inadequate intake of either choline or choline precursors results in fatty livers. Choline is important for normal fat metabolism since it is an essential part of phospholipids, which are necessary for the synthesis of lipoproteins. These proteins transport lipids from the liver to adipose tissue. Lipotrophic agents promote the transfer. Precursors for lipoprotein synthesis are lipotrophic. Choline is lipotrophic, as are methionine and betaine, used to synthesize choline. Metabolic processes synthesizing and transporting triglycerides from hepatocytes are rapidly occurring, dynamic events. Increased hepatic deposition of lipid can be detected within a few hours of the feeding of a choline-deficient diet. Substances such as vitamin B_{12} and folic acid are choline-sparing, and if they are absent from diets low in choline, fatty livers can develop. Inositol also spares choline. In experimental animals, administration of pantothenic acid, pyridoxine, or riboflavin does not prevent fatty livers. Deficiencies of those or other vitamins do not cause fatty livers.

The amounts of choline in the diet are usually adequate. Choline is readily absorbed from the small intestine unless pancreatic exocrine deficiency is causing maldigestion and malabsorption. Choline requirements depend on the level of food intake. Additional choline is needed to prevent fatty liver when diets are rich in either cholesterol or fats containing long-chain fatty acids. If glucocorticoids, estrogens, or thyroid hormones are administered, less choline is needed to prevent fatty changes in the liver. Ovariectomy or administration of testosterone causes an increase in minimum choline requirements. Less choline is needed by animals in a cold environment.

Dietary protein is important in preventing hepatic lipidosis. Fatty liver develops from protein-deficient diets even if they contain all other essential nutrients, including choline. Protein deficiencies initiate fatty changes primarily in periportal areas, while choline deficiency produces changes in pericentral areas. With a deficiency of both protein and choline, hepatic lipidosis progresses to cirrhosis. That is the only dietary means of producing hepatic cirrhosis.

Fatty liver occasionally develops from dietary imbalances in the relative amounts of carbohydrates and lipids, such as when the primary source of energy is lipids. With a protein-calorie malnutrition, lipid first accumulates in the periportal area. Dietary supplementation with choline, vitamins, and protein minimizes fatty changes due to these imbalances.

Hepatotoxins. Different toxic compounds, such as carbon tetrachloride and endotoxin, cause abnormal fat accumulation in hepatocytes. Toxins cause lipids to accumulate by impairing their transport from the liver. A defective synthesis of very low-density lipoproteins prevents the packaging of triglycerides for transport from the liver. Fatty acids delivered continuously to the liver are synthesized to triglycerides, which are retained.

Hepatocyte injury results from metabolites of carbon tetrachloride produced in the liver. An NADP cytochrome P-450 electron-transfer system in microsomes metabolizes carbon tetrachloride, as well as many other chemicals, to form free radicals, which initiate lipid peroxidation. The activity of all microsomal enzymes is depressed by peroxidation, disrupting the lipid structures of microsomes. Small nonlethal doses of carbon tetrachloride depress microsomal enzyme activity to the extent that normally fatal doses given later are not lethal, since the compound cannot be transformed into toxic metabolites. Lipid peroxidation also damages structures required for lipoprotein synthesis, contributing to hepatic lipidosis. Hepatic microsomal enzymes are important in transforming many drugs to allow for their excretion. Thus, the pharmacologic biological activity of drugs is prolonged when microsomal enzyme activity is reduced by metabolites of carbon tetrachloride.

Antioxidants are normally available to protect hepatocytes against lipid peroxidation. If vitamin E, a naturally occurring antioxidant, is administered before exposure to carbon tetrachloride, it protects the liver from damage. Unfortunately, antioxidants have not been found to be effective when given after exposure to a toxin. Glutathione also protects against peroxides. Hepatocytes contain a glutathione peroxidase system that rapidly converts lipid peroxides to alcohols.

Naturally occurring toxins can produce fatty livers. Intestinal aerobes produce *E. coli* endotoxin and possibly other bacterial toxins, although the amounts absorbed are normally small. When large quantities are absorbed, fatty liver can develop. Mild hepatic lipidosis induced by moderate choline deficiency develops into severe lipidosis with an intraperitoneal injection of endotoxin. The mechanism for this potentiation is unknown. It could result from the endotoxin's effect of compromising hepatic circulation, or possibly from its known effect of altering hepatic carbohydrate metabolism. Intestinal anaerobic bacteria have an effect similar to that of aerobes. Hepatic lipidosis develops with bacterial overgrowth of the small intestine, such as seen with chronic disease or the exclusion of a large section of small intestinal tract from the alimentary flow. The bacterial overgrowth would contribute to endotoxin absorption, but it could also contribute to protein deficiency and protein-calorie malnutrition and to the formation and absorption of toxic metabolites of bile acids. Antibiotic suppression of intestinal bacteria ameliorates some forms of fatty livers. Tetracycline as well as removal of the excluded bowel will prevent hepatic lipidosis in animals with a bypassed section of the small intestine.

Ethionine, phosphorus, and puromycin are like carbon tetrachloride in impairing hepatic protein synthesis. Their action stops apolipoprotein production, whereupon triglycerides cannot be mobilized from the liver. These compounds disrupt protein synthesis by causing detachment of the ribosomes and disaggregation of the polysomes. Additional effects include a mobilization of free fatty acids, which may be mediated by abnormal levels of hormones that regulate carbohydrate and lipid metabolism. These changes reduce hepatic synthesis of all proteins, with those having the shortest half-lives being affected first. The liver loses its normal ability to respond to increased demands for apolipoprotein synthesis. In these cases fatty livers do not develop unless there is an ongoing fatty acid influx into the liver. That can be prevented by glucose infusions or by feeding.

Abnormal Cell Metabolism. Hepatic lipidosis accompanies diabetes mellitus. Hypoinsulinemia causes hyperglycemia and intracellular glucose deficiency in nonhepatic tissues. In response, hormones are released in a pattern similar to that in starvation, and they stimulate the mobilization of adipose triglycerides. The pathogenesis of fatty liver, however, differs somewhat from starvation. Since glucose does not require insulin for transport into hepatocytes, these cells are not glucose-starved. Insulin is necessary, however, for optimum activity of some enzymes in glycolysis and the citric acid cycle. Consequently, the liver is unable to remove glucose from the portal circulation at a normal rate following feeding. It removes about half the normal amount. Insulin is not available to promote glucose entry into nonhepatic cells, so the signal to hepatocytes is to produce more glucose for glucose-starved cells. Gluconeogenesis is stimulated to increase the production of glucose from amino acids and glycerol. When hyperglycemia is attained, however, there is no signal to terminate glucose production. Thus, the abnormality is glucose over-production rather than decreased utilization. Production is sustained by persistent secretion of glucagon. Ketogenesis is also stimulated; the high levels of circulating ketones do not result merely from increased delivery of fatty acids to the liver. Fatty acids not metabolized to ketones are re-esterified to triglycerides. Apolipoprotein synthesis is reduced, however, so lipoprotein formation is not adequate to transport lipids from the liver. Reduced availability of amino acids and disruption of ribosomes bearing endoplasmic reticulum contribute to decreased protein synthesis. The net result is increased deposition of lipids in the liver. There are similarities in the pathogenesis of fatty livers with diabetes, overnutrition, and undernutrition. Found in all three are increased mobilization of fatty acids from peripheral stores, increased intrahepatic synthesis of triglycerides, and impaired transport of lipids from the liver. Hepatic oxidation of fatty acids also increases and is the only regulatory response able to modify the severity of the problem.

Hyperadrenalcorticism, whether due to iatrogenic causes or to naturally occurring Cushing's disease, is frequently associated with morphological changes resembling hepatic lipidosis. Since corticosteroids mobilize triglycerides from adipose tissue and increase plasma levels of free fatty acids, the morphological changes and hepatomegaly associated with Cushing's syndrome are often thought to be due to hepatic accumulation of triglycerides. These changes are not due primarily to lipid accumulation, but represent hepatocyte swelling due to glycogen accumulation and possibly some edema. Corticosteroids cause the swelling by promoting gluconeogenesis, which results in accelerated amino acid catabolism. It is uncertain whether the excess fatty acids, contributing to increased hepatic triglycerides and a potentially reduced capacity for apolipoprotein synthesis, account for a possible abnormal retention of triglycerides, which contribute to the morphological changes.

Hepatic lipidosis results from metabolic derangements. Cellular hypoxia, due to abnormal hepatic circulation and reduced oxygen-carrying capacity of the blood, causes these derangements. Hepatic lipidosis appears around central veins, and when sinusoidal oxygen tension is severely reduced by circulatory problems and anemias, little remains for use by the pericentral hepatocytes, which are the last to be supplied. Congestive heart failure, shock, anesthetic agents, and drugs or toxins with vasoactive properties all reduce circulation. Lipidosis appears because the liver responds by engaging all its resources for maintaining normal blood glucose, thereby reducing energy available to supply the hepatocytes' own needs. The oxygen deficiency reduces the liver's capacity to oxidize free fatty acids, an alternate source of energy. Some forms of hepatic lipidosis can be prevented or reversed by promoting adenosine triphosphate (ATP) formation and thereby supporting the ability to metabolize fatty acids and synthesize apolipoproteins. Administration of glucose, ATP or an ATP precursor such as adenine, furthermore, can prevent or reverse fatty changes caused by ethionine and other toxic agents. Apolipoprotein synthesis, however, may be inadequate to provide sufficient lipoproteins, a response required whenever the mobilization of adipose lipids is increased. Structural changes probably occur with hypoxia and affect the activity of enzymes participating in hepatic fat metabolism. As the hypoxia progresses, fatty changes become more severe and can lead to necrosis. The distribution of fat around pericentral hepatocytes is similar to that seen with obesity, protein-calorie imbalance, choline deficiency, or diabetes mellitus. Most normal functions usually continue in fatty livers; thus, in contrast to liver necrosis, fatty changes can be relatively benign.

Cholesterol.[12-15,17] Cholesterol is synthesized by a number of tissues, the liver being the most important. Its rate of synthesis is related inversely to the dietary intake of cholesterol. Small amounts of cholesterol are used to synthesize all steroid hormones. Sizable amounts are used for the synthesis of bile salts. Cholesterol is also a component of plasma membranes. Cholesterol is always found in plasma, where most is esterified. Following hepatic uptake of chylomicrons or hepatic cholesterol synthesis, dietary and *de novo* cholesterol not metabolized further are secreted as a component of lipoproteins. Free cholesterol on the surface of lipoproteins is esterified by lecithin cholesterol acyl transferase (LCAT). This enzyme catalyzes transfer of fatty acids from the ß-position of lecithin to the 3-ß-OH group of free cholesterol, producing cholesterol ester and lysolecithin. LCAT is synthesized in the liver, and hepatic disease can decrease plasma LCAT activity, which increases plasma levels of free cholesterol and decreases the levels of esterified cholesterol. In humans, obstructive jaundice consistently produces low LCAT activity and reductions in the ratio of esterified to free cholesterol. Dogs with obstructive jaundice and acute hepatitis have an abnormal ratio (less than 0.64).[18] Some cases of hepatic tumors and cirrhosis also have low ratios. Plasma total cholesterol levels are markedly increased with biliary obstruction.[19,20] This is due to an unexplained increase in the rate of hepatic synthesis and to interruption of the release of bile into the intestine. The synthesis of bile acids from cholesterol and their secretion represent the only means of excreting cholesterol from the body. Parenchymal hepatic disease can cause total plasma cholesterol to increase, probably by the same means as obstructive jaundice. Severe and diffuse hepatocyte damage, on the other hand, causes plasma cholesterol levels to fall below normal. Hepatic damage induced by nitrosamines, reducing liver mass by one half, has no effect on total plasma cholesterol levels.[21] Hepatic insufficiency resulting from portasystemic vascular shunts reduces plasma cholesterol in about 50% of clinical cases and is an invariable finding in dogs with experimentally created shunts.[22,23] Thus, either hypercholesterolemia or hypocholesterolemia can be seen with hepatic disease. Plasma cholesterol levels can also be reduced with fat malabsorption and with accelerated loss of bile acids from the body.

Plasma Lipids. The metabolism of triglycerides is regulated by the activities of extrahepatic lipoprotein lipases and hepatic lipases which are bound to capillary endothelia. The extrahepatic lipoprotein lipases promote the hydrolysis of triglycerides in chylomicrons and very low density lipoproteins. Its hydrolytic activity requires a lipoprotein produced by the liver or intestine. Triglyceride hydrolysis results in the formation of chylomicron remnants which are removed by the liver, where hepatic lipase hydrolyzes remaining triglycerides. Plasma levels of lipids increase with some forms of hepatic disease.[24] They consistently increase with biliary obstruction and fatty livers. Hepatic lipase activity is reduced in humans with hepatic cirrhosis, which is suggested to be the basis for the hypertriglyceridemia observed. In dogs with hepatic insufficiency caused either by nitrosamine toxicity or by portasystemic vascular shunts, plasma triglyceride levels are normal.[21,23]

Plasma free fatty acids contribute to signs of hepatic encephalopathy. They directly interfere with ammonia metabolism and act synergistically with ammonia and mercaptans to

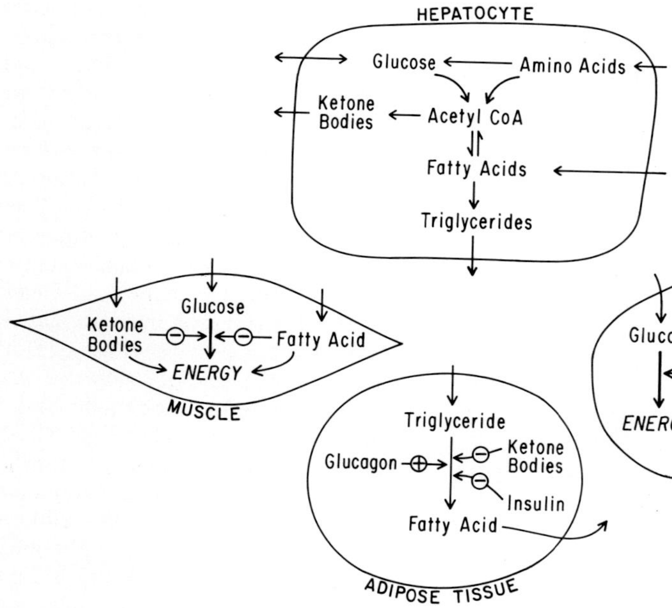

Figure 28-3. Interrelationships of carbohydrate and lipid metabolism in liver, muscle, adipose tissue, and brain. See text for explanation.

alter brain function. Octanoic acid is more effective than longer chain fatty acids in producing signs. Plasma octanoate concentrations increase up to 15 times normal with hepatic disease. This fatty acid is produced by the partial beta-oxidation of long chain fatty acids such as palmitic.[25] Plasma palmitic acid concentrations increase with hepatic disease, partly because of impaired hepatic metabolism of lipids. They also increase during fasting or anorexia, with four-fold increases occuring within 24 to 48 hours.[26] It is apparent that dietary therapy should be directed at maintaining plasma free fatty acids at low concentrations.

Correlation With Clinical Signs. No specific clinical signs are pathognomonic for hepatic lipidosis. Extreme obesity and undernutrition are signs often associated with fatty liver. Hepatomegaly, a usual result from lipid engorgement of hepatocytes, is identified by abdominal palpation or radiography. Some liver disease, including fatty livers, can be accompanied by a marked fasting lipemia that may or may not be associated with clinical signs. Lipemia can be associated with abdominal distress but has not been shown to be the cause. Lipemia is often associated with abdominal pain in dogs with acute pancreatitis. Hepatic lipidosis often accompanies clinical signs of chronic congestive heart disease and anemia. Some endocrine diseases consistently cause fatty livers. Since many nonspecific signs are seen, it is not possible to attribute any one to hepatic lipidosis. Clinical signs cannot be attributed to abnormal concentrations or ratios of plasma cholesterols. Prolonged high plasma cholesterol levels produce atherosclerotic lesions in dogs. These vascular changes can be produced by feeding a high-fat and high-cholesterol diet.

Integration of Carbohydrate and Fat Metabolism[3] (Figure 28-3)

Glucose is the primary source of energy during absorption of a meal. Glucose is less important at other times, when products of lipid metabolism are used for energy. Proteins are used to produce glucose, and if that were important for energy during fasting, body protein depletion would rapidly cause death. The limited ability to replenish glucose during starvation results in decreased glucose utilization by muscles, an effect of low insulin levels. Adipose tissue releases free fatty acids for energy in muscles where fatty acid oxidation increases. Release of free fatty acids is controlled to prevent toxic plasma levels.

Many fatty acids are converted to ketone bodies, which are important sources of energy during fasting. Plasma ketone bodies are unbound, entering cells readily. Levels of ketone bodies in plasma can increase to approach plasma glucose levels during starvation. Ketone bodies are used for energy by brain and muscle tissues. Ketone bodies inhibit further lipolysis of adipose lipids not only directly, but also indirectly when the plasma levels of ketone bodies stimulate insulin release. Ketone bodies spare the use of body proteins for energy. Elevated ketone-body levels are associated with positive nitrogen balance in situations where negative nitrogen balance would otherwise exist. Glucose infusion reduces plasma fatty acid and ketone-body concentrations, with the effect of promoting negative nitrogen balance.

Protein Metabolism

Physiology - Amino Acids, Ammonia.[12,27,28]

Amino Acids.[29-31] The liver is important in the regulation of protein metabolism. The liver maintains a pool of free amino acids, representing 5% of the total body amino acid pool, at a fairly constant level. Increased amino acid levels are toxic, as seen during acute hepatic failure. Reduced amino acid levels result in impaired synthesis of important proteins such as albumin and blood clotting factors. Catabolic and anabolic functions in normal livers respond to alterations in nutritional conditions to maintain a normal-size pool of free amino acids. Following a protein-rich meal, amino acid absorption from the intestine results in a 20-fold increase in portal amino acid content. The liver takes up a large fraction of all of these, except for the branched-chain amino acids, and as a consequence arterial plasma levels vary little. Arterial amino acid levels are also maintained following a protein-poor meal since the hepatic uptake of amino acids is reduced, and in times of need there is even release of amino acids from the liver to the circulation.

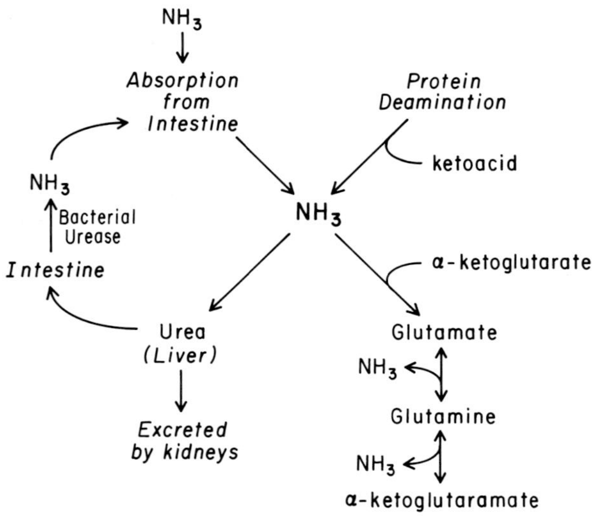

Figure 28-4a,b. a) Overall scheme of ammonia production and disposition. The urea produced from ammonia is an important source of ammonia, produced by intestinal bacterial urease activity. b) Urea cycle in hepatocyte for conversion of ammonia to urea. CPSase = carbamyl phosphate synthetase, OTCase = ornithine transcarbamylase, ASSase = argininosuccinate synthetase. Part of events take place in mitochondria with the remainder being in the cytoplasm.

Hepatic catabolism of amino acids prevails when their levels exceed that necessary to sustain protein synthesis for export or use in the liver. Amino acid degradation provides carbon for gluconeogenesis, ketogenesis, or fatty acid synthesis. Alanine, serine and threonine are primary substrates for gluconeogenesis. Most of the essential amino acids are catabolized primarily in the liver. Some, such as the aromatics, are not degraded outside the liver, so that with hepatic insufficiency their circulating levels increase. During postabsorptive times the primary source of alanine is skeletal muscle, where it is produced to carry nitrogen, derived from primarily branched-chain amino acids, to the liver. The only other postabsorptive source of alanine is the intestine, where it serves as the carrier of nitrogen derived from glutamine, a major source of energy in the intestine. Hepatic deamination of alanine produces substrates for gluconeogenesis or liponeogenesis and nitrogen that is converted to urea or used for the synthesis of other amino acids.

The liver synthesizes amino acids from intermediates of carbohydrate and lipid metabolism by amination and transamination. An amine group can be transferred from one amino acid to many alpha-keto acids to synthesize amino acids in particular demand.[32] Only lysine and threonine cannot be produced by transamination of keto acids.

The liver's ability to take up and release amino acids to the circulation determines hepatic regulation of the pool of free amino acids. The extraction of amino acids is achieved by transport systems on the hepatocyte membranes. Amino acids compete for transport by one or more of four systems. For one important amino acid, alanine, the rate of membrane transport

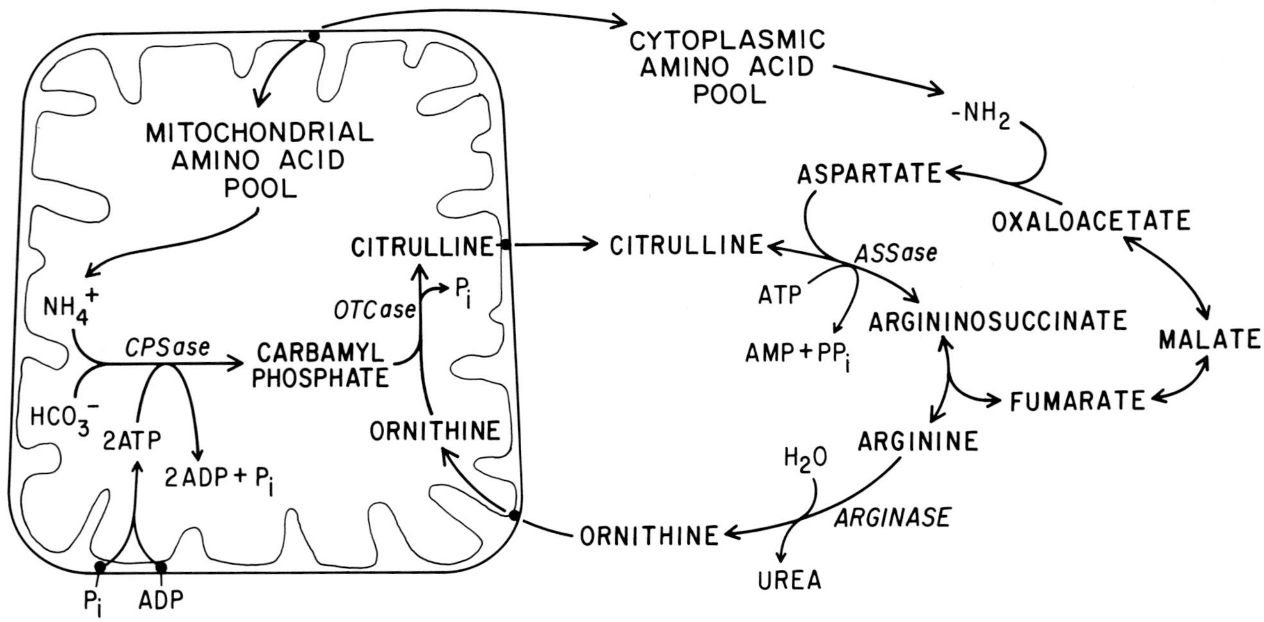

is limited and controls the rate of alanine metabolism. Nutritional states influence transport rates, with alanine uptake increasing during starvation or the feeding of a high-protein diet. Alanine transport is also increased by glucagon, insulin, glucocorticoids, thyroid hormone, and catecholamines. Its transport is reduced by competition from serine, glycine, proline and histidine, as well as by acidosis. Transport of other amino acids such as glutamate and glutamine is rate-limiting for their metabolism, but the regulation of that transport is different; the system is not the same.

Hepatic extraction of amino acids maintains intracellular amino acid pools that maintain their catabolism. The rate-controlling steps in that process for alanine, aspartate, or glutamate are not in their transamination or deamination, but rather in the gluconeogenic or oxidative pathways, which are controlled by hormones such as glucagon, insulin, glucocorticoids, thyroid hormone, and catecholamines. Thus, these hormones direct the activity of both hepatic catabolic enzymes and hepatic transport rates. In addition, they regulate amino acid release by extrahepatic tissue and hepatic protein synthesis and degradation. The rate-controlling steps in the catabolism of other amino acids may be the result of enzyme activity acting directly on the amino acid. The degradation of glutamine, for instance, is controlled by the activity of hepatic glutaminase.

Ammonia.[33-35] Ammonia is an important product of amino acid metabolism (Figure 28-4). Mechanisms operate to maintain ammonia at low levels, without which important signs of toxicity appear. The intestine and kidney are the important sites for ammonia production; the liver is the only organ equipped to convert ammonia to a product that can be excreted from the body.

The intestine is the most important site for ammonia production; it generates one half of its production in the small intestine and the other half in the colon. The small intestine produces ammonia during the metabolism of glutamine which is an important source of energy in the small intestine. The amount produced is directly related to portal glutamine concentrations which determine glutamine extraction and metabolism. Ammonia is produced in the large intestine when bacterial ureases act on urea diffusing into the lumen from the extracellular fluid; this accounts for 40% of the colonic production and represents hydrolysis of 20%-30% of the urea produced by the liver. The small intestine, unlike the large intestine, is highly permeable to diffusion of urea. The bacterial conversion of urea to ammonia occurs primarily in the colon, after the delivery of urea from the small intestine. Intestinal mucosa contains no ureases to reduce urea to ammonia.[36] Some ammonia is also produced by intestinal bacteria acting on proteins entering the colon.

A number of different intestinal bacteria produce ammonia.[37] The most potent producers are the gram-negative aerobic bacilli *E. coli*, *Klebsiella*, *Proteus*, and *Pseudomonas* species. *Proteus mirabilis* produces ammonia from urea, but only when the pH of the medium is greater than 5.3. *E. coli* produces ammonia from peptides when the pH is greater than 4.6. At lower pH's the amounts of ammonia produced are small and not related to numbers of intestinal bacteria. Urease producers also include *Bacteroides*, *Bifidobacteria*, and *Clostridium* species. Little ammonia is produced from urea in the intestine of germfree animals.

Drugs such as sodium sulfate, mannitol, sorbitol, and lactulose cause osmotic diarrhea and reduce colonic bacterial numbers and pH, thereby reducing the production of ammonia. Lactulose is a disaccharide not digested and absorbed in the small intestine. It is fermented by colonic bacteria to produce acid pH and increased numbers of particles, resulting in osmotic diarrhea. The rate of ammonia absorption from the colon is determined by the pH of the medium. Most ammonia is un-ionized (NH_3) at a higher pH, and as the pH of the medium becomes acid, more ammonia is ionized (NH_4^+). The un-ionized form is relatively lipid-soluble and readily crosses lipid cell membranes. Ionized ammonia is less able to diffuse across membranes since it carries a charge and behaves like a water-soluble particle traversing pores in a membrane. Thus, reductions in the pH of colonic contents reduce the amounts of ammonia absorbed. Ammonia also diffuses from the extracellular fluid to the intestine, and when the pH of intestinal contents is low the ammonia ionizes and is trapped in the bowel.

There are other sources of ammonia production in the body. The kidneys extract glutamine from the circulation, and its nitrogen is released as ammonia for regulation of acid-base homeostasis. Free un-ionized ammonia can diffuse into the blood and contribute to the circulating pool of ammonia. Renal ammonia release into the blood is increased by acidosis or hypokalemia.

Skeletal muscle produces and takes up ammonia. At rest, no ammonia is released to increase circulating levels. During exercise, the production and release exceeds the uptake, and blood ammonia levels can increase. The liver produces ammonia, which may represent a considerable amount, during catabolism of primarily glutamate and glutamine. That ammonia is not normally released but is converted to urea; the liver is, therefore, not considered a producer and releaser of ammonia.

Following absorption, ammonia is delivered to the liver by the portal vein, where its concentration is 350 µg/dl in fasting dogs and 700 µg/dl in fasting cats.[38] In contrast, ammonia concentration in the systemic circulation is normally less than 100 µg/dl. This species difference reflects a greater dietary protein requirement for cats as well as greater hepatic capacity to metabolize ammonia to urea. Marked elevation of portal ammonia concentration has little effect on hepatic-vein concentrations in normal dogs. With different amounts of ammonia entering the normal liver, the percentage removed remains at 85 to 90%.[39] The liver has a remarkable capacity to remove ammonia even when the amount it receives doubles. Consequently, hyperammonemia does not appear unless liver damage is extensive and severe, or portal blood flow bypasses the liver.

Ammonia is also taken up and released from peripheral tissues. In general, there is a small uptake during resting; with exercise, large amounts can be released. In clinical cases signs of hepatic encephalopathy improve with cage rest. These changes in uptake or release are a reflection of the metabolic activity of peripheral tissues. Other peripheral changes affect plasma ammonia levels. Loss of potassium from the body results in the movement of potassium from intracellular stores to maintain normal extracellular potassium. Outward movement of potassium requires inward movement of other ions into the cell, which in this case are predominantly hydrogen and sodium ions. That movement results in reduced intracellular and increased extracellular pH. The greater resulting pH gradient favors the movement of ammonia into cells, and greater toxic effects may be seen. Thus it is possible to see falling or relatively low blood ammonia levels with worsening signs of hepatic encephalopathy. It is apparent that changes in muscle mass, such as with wasting, would affect the capacity of peripheral tissues to control blood ammonia levels.

The most important mechanism for detoxifying ammonia is conversion of ammonia to urea, a process that occurs only in the liver in the krebs ornithine or urea cycle (Figure 28-4). Ammonia combines with carbon dioxide and phosphate to form carbamyl phosphate, which combines with ornithine to form citrulline. A second ammonia molecule is added, producing arginine, which is converted to urea and ornithine, completing the cycle. The capacity of this cycle is determined by the activity of all its enzymes, but especially argininosuccinate synthetase and carbamyl phosphate synthetase. Since they are lower in activity than the other enzymes, they represent the rate-limiting steps. The intermediate products must be continuously supplied to maintain activity in the cycle. A large ammonia infusion in dogs causes depletion of one intermediate, arginine, so that its level falls.[40] In cats the availability of dietary arginine for urea cycle activity is critical; an arginine deficient diet results in hyperammonemia and coma within a few hours after eating.[41] Others have proposed that increased arginine availability may prevent ammonia toxicity,[42] presumably by increasing urea-cycle activity. The beneficial effects, if any, are currently regarded as unimportant. Ammonia is also detoxified when used to aminate ketoacids. Some ammonia absorbed into portal blood condenses with ketoglutarate to form glutamate, which can react with more ammonia to form glutamine.

Regulation of animals' urea-synthesizing capacity is not well understood. Metabolism of ammonia to urea increases with the feeding of high-protein diets, fasting, or increased corticosteroid or glucagon release, all of which increase activities of the urea-cycle enzymes. These hormones increase ammonia formation by stimulating gluconeogenesis, resulting in amino acid catabolism. Sustaining urea-cycle activity are aspartate for conversion of citrulline to argininosuccinate and ammonia for carbamylphosphate formation. The normally low activity of carbamylphosphate synthetase is augmented by N-acetylglutamate and by bicarbonate. Bicarbonate reduction by acidosis or inhibition of carbonic anhydrase activity reduces urea-cycle activity and urea formation.

Zinc determines plasma ammonia levels by an unknown means; zinc deficiency results in plasma increases for ammonia and decreases for blood urea nitrogen. The animal with hepatic insufficiency is often assumed to have a zinc deficiency.

There are interrelations in hepatic metabolism between ammonia and other substances. Mercaptans produced in the intestine from methionine interfere with the conversion of ammonia to urea. Small amounts of mercaptans cause blood ammonia levels to increase.[43] Fatty acids have a similar effect, and they inhibit the activities of carbamyl phosphate synthetase and argininosuccinate synthetase enzymes,[44] octanoate being more potent than oleic acid. Hepatic insufficiency causes increased levels of intermediate length fatty acids presumably due to incomplete catabolism by the liver.

Ammonia is also detoxified by its incorporation into glutamate to form glutamine.[45] This process occurs in the liver, skeletal muscle, brain and kidney and must be viewed as a means of temporary storage rather than a means for excretion of ammonia. The detoxification into glutamine proceeds at rates as rapid as urea synthesis, but that proceeds relatively slowly when substrate levels decrease for glutamine formation. Glutamine provides a carrier for ammonia excreted by the kidneys, but renal excretion provides a very limited means for elimination of excess nitrogen from the body.

Pathophysiology - Hepatic Encephalopathy.[46,47]

Clinical Signs. When amino acid and ammonia metabolism are abnormal, clinical signs of hepatic encephalopathy are possible. The earliest sign is reduction in food intake, which can be documented before any changes in an animal's activity.[48] Often early signs are subtle and not recognized by the owner until hepatic disease is advanced. The most frequent signs of hepatic encephalopathy are nonspecific signs such as depression, listlessness, polydipsia, vomiting, diarrhea, and unexplained weight loss. Neurologic and neuromuscular signs such as seizures, ataxia, and behavioral changes occur in less than half the animals. Coma is an infrequent and usually terminal sign of hepatic encephalopathy. Although plasma ammonia and amino acid levels are abnormal with hepatic encephalopathy, there is no proof that they are the cause.

Pathology. Signs of hepatic encephalopathy appear because of changes in metabolic activity in the brain. These changes result from abnormalities in the kinds and amounts of chemicals that enter the brain. To some extent these changes are the result of alterations in the relatively impermeable blood-brain barrier, changes caused by hepatic disease. These functional changes may be accompanied by morphologic changes. Pathologic evaluation can show gross cerebral edema and microscopic evidence of swollen astrocytes, focal necrosis of neurons, or gliosis, but in many cases no abnormalities are found.

Amino Acid Metabolism. Maintenance of normal plasma amino acid concentrations is lost with liver disease. Different patterns of amino acid changes are seen with acute and chronic hepatic disease (Figure 28-5). Similar alterations in plasma amino acids are seen in dogs with portacaval shunts and chronic hepatitis.[23,49-51] Plasma levels of phenylalanine, tryptophan, tyrosine, and glutamic acid increase. Aromatic amino acids are metabolized only in the liver, and with hepatic insufficiency their plasma levels increase. Plasma levels of threonine decrease despite the fact that it is also metabolized in the liver. Plasma levels of methionine consistently increase with chronic hepatic disease. However, levels of methionine and lysine, both metabolized by the liver, are unchanged in experimentally produced portacaval shunts. Branched-chain amino acids, used primarily by muscle to build protein or as a source of calories, are found at reduced levels with portacaval shunts and chronic hepatitis. Alanine is also reduced in the plasma of dogs with chronic hepatic insufficiency. Other hepatic diseases resulting in inflammation and hepatocellular necrosis are associated with similar amino acid changes. Bile duct obstruction in dogs produces moderate to severe histologic changes within one month that correlate with significant plasma changes in the amino acids metabolized in the liver.[52]

The changes in plasma amino acid concentrations are caused both by an inability of the liver to metabolize those requiring normal liver function and by a release of hormones affecting their metabolism. With hepatic disease, the plasma levels of aromatic amino acids increase because they are not removed and metabolized. The metabolism of most other amino acids occurs primarily in nonhepatic tissues, and is

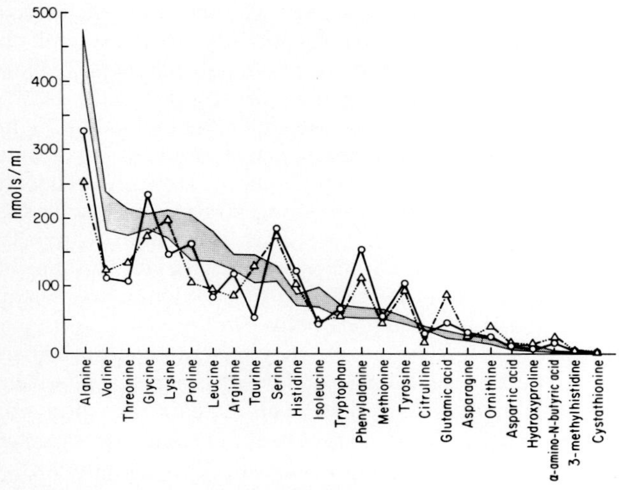

Figure 28-5. Graph showing plasma amino acid concentrations in clinically normal dogs (shaded area representing Mean ± SE), in dogs with chronic active hepatitis (Mean values represented by Δ), and in dogs with portosystemic vascular anastomoses (Mean values represented by O). The amino acid concentrations in normal dogs are plotted from left to right in an order for those with highest to those with lowest concentration. Glutamine, having the highest concentration, is not shown on this graph.

regulated by insulin, glucagon, catecholamines, and possibly other hormones. Plasma levels of these hormones increase partly because they are not adequately removed by the diseased liver,[53,54,55] and also because hyperammonemia stimulates their release directly or indirectly.[40] Normally, 40% to 50% of insulin secreted into portal blood is removed during a single transit through the liver.[56] With hepatic insufficiency both hyperinsulinemia and hyperglucagonemia are found, but the increase for glucagon is greater than that for insulin. The resulting decreased molar ratio of insulin to glucagon is a stimulus for gluconeogenesis at the expense of body proteins.[57] Body protein broken down to sustain gluconeogenesis releases amino acids, a process which increases blood levels of amino acids metabolized only by the liver.

Hyperammonemia does not change plasma amino acid levels in adrenalectomized dogs.[40] In intact dogs catecholamine infusion without any changes in insulin and glucagon plasma levels results in plasma changes for amino acids metabolized outside the liver, and those changes are the same as ones seen with hepatic insufficiency.[58] Since plasma catecholamine levels increase with hepatic disease, that change may be the most important for shifts in amino acid metabolism. A long-term study on chronic hepatic insufficiency in dogs reported that no significant correlations were found to explain plasma amino acid changes by changes in insulin and glucagon levels.[21]

Glucagon decreases plasma alanine concentrations with or without the presence of insulin or catecholamines. The net effect is increased conversion of alanine to glucose. Plasma concentrations of branched-chain and most other amino acids are reduced by increased catecholamines; with normal background levels of insulin and glucagon, taurine and ornithine increase under those conditions. Glutamine's plasma concentrations are reduced by glucagon, but not catecholamines. Normally, the ratio of the sum of three branched-chain amino acids to that of phenylalanine and tyrosine should be 3.0 or 3.5.[59] When the ratio is reduced to 1.0, signs of hepatic encephalopathy appear.

Acute and diffuse hepatic necrosis causes a different pattern of plasma amino acid changes with experimental hepatic necrosis in dogs; plasma levels of all amino acids increase, which is similar to the increase in dogs with fulminant hepatitis (Figure 28-6).[49] Amino acids released from degenerating hepatocytes are not metabolized by the liver. The net effect of high levels of catecholamines, insulin, and glucagon is the catabolism of extrahepatic proteins, the release of amino acids that cannot be metabolized by the liver, and increases for plasma levels of all amino acids. In contrast, arginine levels can decrease with acute hepatic disease. Damage to hepatocytes releases arginase to the circulation, where it can rapidly degrade arginine to ornithine and urea.[60]

Plasma levels of glutamine are normally about 1000 nanomoles per ml, twice that of the next-most abundant amino acid, alanine. Glutamine levels can increase dramatically with hyperammonemia, with glutamine formation representing a temporary means of protection against ammonia toxicity. Its levels return to normal within hours after blood ammonia concentration returns to normal.

Inborn errors of metabolism can cause derangements in plasma amino acid levels. In humans, deficiencies in either the transport mechanisms or the enzymes involved in the metabolism of an amino acid cause the imbalances.[61] Hyperammonemia is frequently an associated problem.

Ammonia and Brain Metabolic Activity.[35] Ammonia is one toxin able to readily cross the normal intact blood-brain barrier. For many years hyperammonemia was considered the most important abnormality causing hepatic encephalopathy. Yet, hyperammonemia does not fully explain the phenomenon of

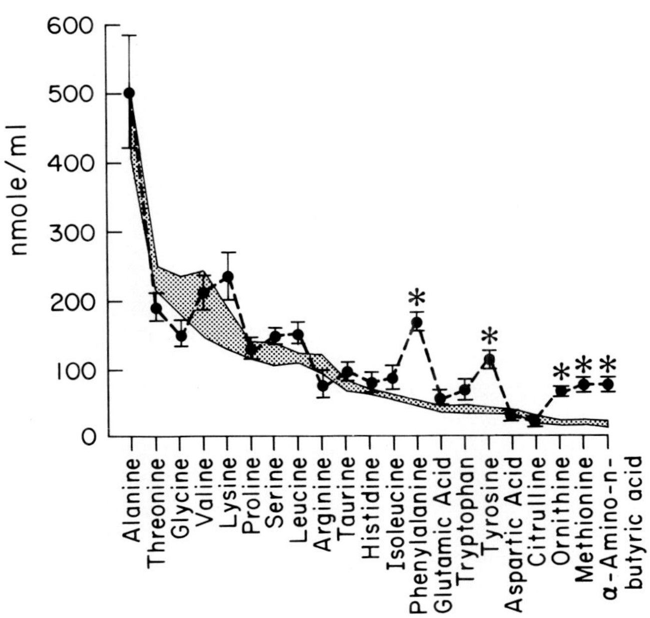

Figure 28-6. Changes in plasma amino acids in dogs two to four weeks after exposure to nitrosamines. Normal range of values for dogs are in shaded area.

hepatic encephalopathy. Signs of encephalopathy appear within minutes of the infusion of ammonia into dogs, and coma is produced within a short time.[40] These signs appear long before plasma amino acids are deranged, suggesting that ammonia plays a very important role in hepatic encephalopathy. In clinical cases, however, blood ammonia levels do not correlate with the severity of encephalopathy. Some dogs with blood ammonia levels of 500 µg/dl show few signs, whereas others have severe clinical signs with blood levels of 200 µg/dl. Transient elevation of blood ammonia does not appear to affect animals with hepatic encephalopathy. The ammonia tolerance test to evaluate liver function consists of administering ammonia orally and measuring blood ammonia before and 30 minutes after administration. Blood ammonia can increase transiently in 30 minutes to over 1000 µg/dl without other or more severe clinical signs.

Ammonia causes toxicity by an unknown means.[35] Signs appear in experimental dogs before neurotransmitter levels change; brain serotonin and acetylcholine levels are unchanged. High levels of ammonia entering the brain react primarily with glutamate, forming glutamine, a reaction requiring energy in the form of ATP. Hyperammonemia is proposed by some to cause hepatic encephalopathy by interfering with brain energy metabolism. Brain ammonia content is normally twice that of plasma, and increases in the brain levels have been associated with reduced overall oxidative metabolism. Less glucose is converted to brain glutamate, aspartate, and gamma-aminobutyric acid (GABA); ammonia may interfere directly with the tricarboxylic acid cycle; more glucose and/or CO_2 carbon could be diverted to glutamine, resulting in a reduction of potentially oxidizable carbon and a drain on ATP reserves; and ammonia may interfere with the formation of glutamate, affecting the metabolic shuttle between malate and aspartate and its affect on ATP formation. The oxidative metabolism of glucose in the brain is important in that 90% is oxidized to CO_2 and only 10% converted to lactate.

Ammonia toxicity may result from the formation of toxic metabolites in the brain. Ammonia entering the brain reacts with glutamate, forming glutamine. With hyperammonemia brain glutamine and glutamate concentrations increase in the dog.[58] The glutamate is not derived from the circulation since it does not easily cross the blood-brain barrier. Aspartate and GABA metabolism are also affected by hyperammonemia. High concentrations of glutamine, glutamate, alpha-ketoglutarate, aspartate, and GABA all have the potential to be neurotoxic.

Hyperammonemia interferes with normal neural physiology. It causes changes in resting membrane potentials and neural excitability so that depression, seizures, behavioral changes, and coma are all possible. These changes can be accompanied by morphologic changes.

Synergistic Neurotoxins. Ammonia can act synergistically with mercaptans and short-chain fatty acids to produce hepatic encephalopathy. Plasma concentrations of each one of these, which when alone are too low to cause signs, will produce hepatic encephalopathy when combined. The intestinal tract is the primary source of the mercaptans and short-chain fatty acids (Figure 28-7). Of these, the mercaptans, deaminated products of sulfur-containing amino acids, are produced by intestinal bacteria. The most important is methyl mercaptan, produced from methionine. Nanomole concentrations of this mercaptan can induce coma, acting synergistically with ammonia and fatty acids.[43] The liver normally removes methyl mercaptan from the portal circulation and converts it to a less toxic derivative, dimethyl sulfide. When hepatic disease interferes with the function of removing and metabolizing mercaptans, blood levels increase. The metabolism of mercaptans is related to that of ammonia and fatty acids. Mercaptan detoxification by the liver is inhibited by hyperammonemia and short-chain fatty acids. Oral administration of methionine causes signs of hepatic encephalopathy to worsen, producing coma in dogs with portacaval shunts.[62] Antibiotics are used in attempts to manage hepatic encephalopathy. Some of their beneficial effects are due to reducing bacterial degradation of methionine to mercaptans.[63] Bacteria fermenting carbohydrates produce short-chain fatty acids in the large bowel. They are readily absorbed and removed by the liver. With hepatic insufficiency that removal is impaired and plasma fatty acid levels increase. The shorter the chain, the more toxic a fatty acid is. If fatty acids are important in hepatic encephalopathy, measures to reduce their production and absorption could be important in hepatic disease.

Abnormal Neurotransmitters.[64] Changes in the composition of plasma supplying the brain alter biochemical events across the blood-brain barrier.[46,65] As a consequence plasma changes can affect metabolism in the brain; they include altered amino acid levels as well as hyperammonemia. Biochemical changes in the brain involve alterations in its concentrations of excitatory and inhibitory neurotransmitters. Levels of the excitatory transmitters norepinephrine and dopamine decrease, and levels of the inhibitory transmitter serotonin increase. Neurons also accumulate octopamine and phenylethanolamine, which are suggested to function as false neurotransmitters and inhibit activity in a manner like serotonin. Relationships between the abnormalities on each side of the blood-brain barrier are not understood well.

Altered plasma amino acid levels cause a marked imbalance in the ratio of amino acids crossing the blood-brain barrier. Amino acids cross by special transport mechanisms, with a single one for phenylalanine, tyrosine, tryptophan, and the branched-chain amino acids. Since these amino acids compete with one another for transport, transport will increase for some when levels of others are low. When plasma levels are low for branched-chain amino acids and high for aromatics, phenylalanine, tyrosine, and tryptophan are transported at an accelerated rate, producing high levels of aromatic amino acids in the brain. In addition, brain glutamine is suggested to be involved in the transport process, efflux of this amino acid from the brain being involved in an exchange process for amino acids entering. Since increased brain ammonia promotes the formation of glutamine, hyperammonemia results in increased synthesis and efflux of glutamine from the brain, thereby facilitating the influx of aromatic amino acids into the brain.

The amounts of aromatic amino acids entering the brain determine the brain levels of excitatory and false neurotransmitters. High intracellular levels of phenylalanine compete with tyrosine for binding to the enzyme tyrosine-3 hydroxylase (Figure 28-8). Phenylalanine is converted to tyrosine, which, not able to be metabolized to dopa, is transformed into tyramine and octopamine. This process results in increased levels of octopamine and low levels of dopamine. Conversion of tyramine to octopamine is catalyzed by the relatively nonspecific enzyme dopamine beta-oxidase. Since little dopamine is formed,

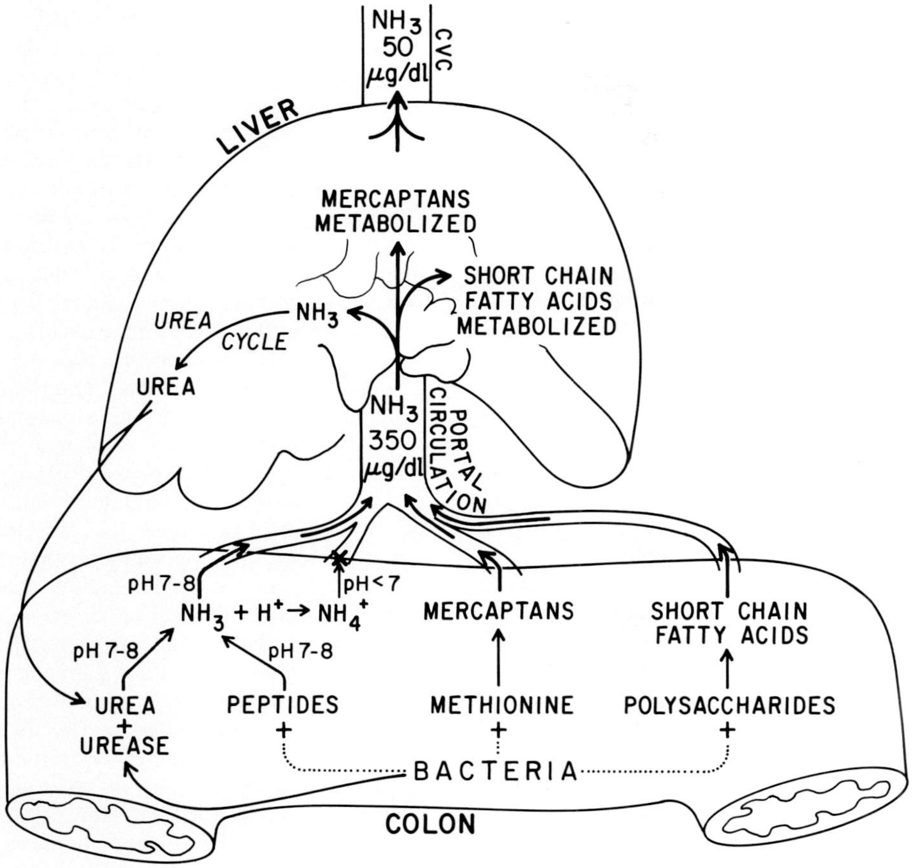

Figure 28-7. Scheme of formation and absorption of ammonia, mercaptans and fatty acids. Their formation is dependent on intestinal bacteria and their removal requires normal hepatic function. Ammonia formation and absorption is pH dependent.

there can be little production of norepinephrine. L-dopa has been suggested as a chemical to ameliorate the signs of hepatic encephalopathy. It is suggested that this compound supplies substrate for synthesis of norepinephrine and enters the pathway beyond the site of the block. Tryptophan is the substrate for synthesis of serotonin, and high tryptophan concentrations in the brain inhibit hydroxylation of tyrosine to dopa. Excess levels of tryptophan should also increase levels of the important inhibitory neurotransmitter serotonin, in addition to inhibiting synthesis of the important excitatory neurotransmitter.

Octopamine and phenylethanolamine, being false transmitters, are believed to be packaged in place of the normal neurotransmitters and stored at high levels in vesicles at the synapses. Like the normal neurotransmitters, they are released during stimulation of the nerve, but their biological activity is only a fraction of that of the normal transmitters, so that neural transmission across the synapse is ineffective. The false neurotransmitter hypothesis, however, is inconsistent with the results of many other studies. Some studies have shown that increasing plasma aromatic amino acid levels by feeding dogs with hepatic insufficiency does not precipitate signs of hepatic encephalopathy.[48] In others studies feeding high levels of branched-chain amino acids to reduce the influx of aromatic amino acids into the brain does not improve hepatic encephalopathy despite correcting the abnormal ratio of the branched-chain to the aromatic amino acids. Also, chemicals such as L-dopa have

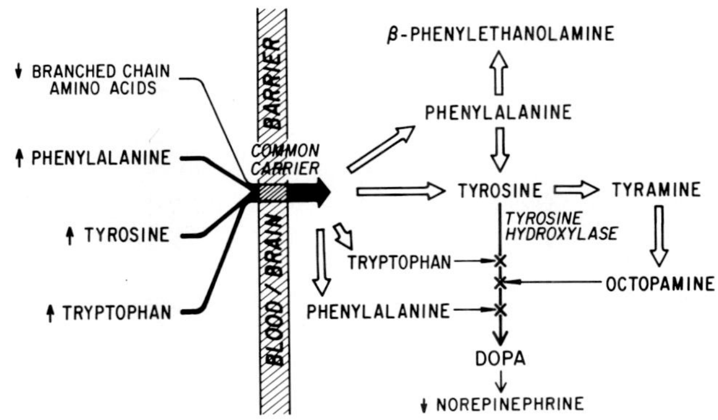

Figure 28-8. Schematic of pathogenesis of abnormal brain neurotransmitter levels. Amino acid precursors enter brain by a common carrier for which they compete. Increased plasma concentrations of aromatic amino acids results in greater amounts in brain with the effect being reduced amounts of the excitatory neurotransmitter norepinephrine and increased amounts of the false transmitters ß-phenylethanolamine and octopamine.

been shown to have no effects on ameliorating hepatic encephalopathy even though they may increase brain norepinephrine levels.

Normal Neurotransmitter Changes. Hepatic encephalopathy could also be due to increased brain levels of the most important inhibitory neurotransmitter, serotonin.[66] Serotonin is synthesized from tryptophan; its rate of production reflects tryptophan plasma levels, brain uptake and brain levels. Tryptophan circulates at relatively low levels, bound to albumin. That binding limits the rate at which tryptophan is taken up by the brain. Plasma tryptophan concentrations do not usually change with hepatic disease, but it is believed that the amount of free plasma tryptophan increases so that more is available to the brain. Experimental studies have shown that infusions of tryptophan, increased to 20 times the normal brain level, have no effect on normal dogs' mental and physical activity despite an increase in serotonin levels.[58] Something other than increased brain serotonin is necessary to explain hepatic encephalopathy.

Amino Acid Neurotransmitter Changes. Chemical neurotransmitters in the brain also include gamma-aminobutyric acid (GABA), glutamate, aspartate, and glycine. These four amino acids, along with glutamine, are the most abundant in the brain. Glutamate and aspartate are excitatory neurotransmitters.[67] GABA, a metabolite of glutamate, and glycine are inhibitory neurotransmitters. With hepatic encephalopathy the density of receptors for GABA and glycine can increase in the brain, and this suggests that there is increased sensitivity of the brain to GABA- and glycine-included neural inhibition due to increased binding of these amino acids.[68] Some forms of hepatic encephalopathy are associated with no increase in reception density or binding.[69] Under the same conditions receptors for glutamate and aspartate are decreased, suggesting reduced binding by these excitatory neurotransmitters. There is an accumulation of GABA in the circulation with hepatic encephalopathy, explained by increased production in the intestine and reduced clearance by the liver, and that is the source for some of the increased brain levels. Receptor density also increases for some sedatives, which may explain why animals with hepatic disease show an increased sensitivity to such drugs.

The importance of the amino acid neurotransmitter in hepatic encephalopathy is questioned. When ammonia produces CNS signs, the brain levels of the inhibitory amino acids GABA and glycine decrease; the levels of glutamate increase greatly, while those for aspartate decrease modestly.[58] Whereas these acute changes are most likely not associated with changes in receptor densities, the basis for hepatic encephalopathy in a chronic state may be entirely different and based more importantly on changes in densities for these receptors. Drugs may someday be found to be effective in blocking the effects of glycine and GABA on the increased receptor population.

Hepatic encephalopathy may be associated with abnormal functioning of the autonomic nervous system. Both serotonin and norepinephrine function in this system. Serotinin is suggested to participate in peristalsis and fluid secretion, and in diseases where increased amounts of serotinin are released, diarrhea is a consistent sign. Levels of the autonomic neurotransmitters could be altered with hepatic encephalopathy and explain the gastrointestinal signs frequently seen.

Management of Pathophysiology.[70,71] One goal in treating hepatic encephalopathy is to correct the hyperammonemia and plasma amino acid abnormalities. The amount of ammonia delivered to the liver is determined by levels of protein in the diet, activity of colonic bacteria, and the amount of nondietary nitrogen entering the colon. Hyperammonemia is managed, though not very successfully, by reducing both protein in the diet and the numbers of colonic bacteria. Dietary protein restriction can worsen already impaired hepatic protein synthetic functions and, for example, cause plasma albumin to decrease further where it is already low. The production of ammonia from glutamine is reduced by restricting protein intake. Its production is also reduced by decreasing colonic bacterial numbers and by reducing the pH of colonic contents. This is accomplished by administering carbohydrates, such as lactalose, which is unabsorbed in the small intestine and fermented in the colon; enemas containing diluted acetic acid or betadine; and/or some laxatives, and unabsorbed antibiotics.

The colonic microflora is not changed by feeding cultures of lactobacillus acidophilus. The pH of the colonic contents can be reduced to 5.5 by lactulose or lactitol and to 6.1 by a combination of neomycin and sorbitol. Absorbed antibiotics such as ampicillin, metronidazole, and sulfonamides can also be used because enough remains unabsorbed to change the colonic microflora. Oral or intravenous glucose lower blood ammonia levels, and that is reflected in the brain by a reduction in glutamine levels.[72] Adding branched-chain amino acids to the glucose offers no additional benefit. Hyperammonemia may also be aided by correction of any zinc deficiency.[73] Nondietary nitrogen increases in the colon with uremia and with bleeding or increased loss of plasma protein and mucosal cell protein in the small intestine. The ensuing hyperammonemia can be treated by management directed at those causes.

Hyperammonemia can improve with correction of hypokalemia and alkalosis, which can accompany hepatic insufficiency. Management with arginine has been advocated with the idea that provision of that substrate will help sustain the urea cycle activity of converting ammonia to urea. The use of glutamate has also been recommended since it can remove ammonia in its conversion to glutamine, but only outside the brain.

Correction of plasma amino acid abnormalities has not proven to be effective treatment for hepatic encephalopathy. Oral or parenteral administration of branched-chain amino acids or their ketoanalogs corrects the abnormal ratio of those amino acids to the aromatics, but while it may provide the benefit of improving a negative nitrogen balance with wasting conditions, it has no beneficial effects on hepatic encephalopathy. Dogs with portosystemic vascular shunts do not survive as long on diets rich in tryptophan and tyrosine as on conventional diets.[74] But the difference may not be due to the abundance of these amino acids metabolized by the liver. Dogs with portosystemic vascular shunts fed a liquid diet, Isocal, did not develop signs of hepatic encephalopathy, whereas those fed standard dry dog food developed signs in a long-term study. The most striking manifestations in the encephalopathic groups were a 40% reduction in food intake, weight loss, and hypoalbuminemia. There were no differences in these diets in the distribution of branched-chain to aromatic amino acids. The dry food had a higher content of glycine, an amino acid that is an important source of ammonia. Most importantly, the liquid diet had a higher ratio of carbohydrate to protein, which would minimize gluconeogensis and promote the conversion of dietary protein to body protein rather than favoring its catabolism with the release of ammonia. Thus, the protein content of the diet and the abundance of amino acid sources of ammonia appear to be the most important determinants of hepatic encephalopathy.[75] The sources of nitrogen in the liquid diet are milk protein and soybean protein. That may be important in that these proteins are not as rich in methionine as meat protein. The liver is the main site of methionine metabolism, which is abnormal with hepatic disease since plasma levels of methionine, cysteine and taurine are increased.[76] Vegetable proteins also have a beneficial effect on hepatic encephalopathy; it is not known whether that is because of their amino acid composition or their high fiber content, which increases fecal nitrogen excretion and reduces the amount of urea available in the colon for ammonia generation.[77] Purified diets with soybean protein as the source of nitrogen maintained dogs with portasystemic vascular shunts in a chemically normal state for as long as one year;[23] such animals die within threeour months when fed commercial dry dog food. A similar purified diet with milk protein (casein) as the protein source was fed to dogs that survived longer than two years with 50% of normal liver mass following acute nitrosamine toxicity.[21] There are probably unknown reasons for these diets having such a beneficial effect on animals with hepatic insufficiency.

Physiology - Proteins. The liver synthesizes many proteins, including plasma albumin and fibrinogen, most alpha-globulins, and half of the beta-globulins.[78,79] Prothrombin and clotting factors V, VII, VIII, IX, and X are produced in the liver, as well as ceruloplasmin, ferritin, and many serum enzymes. Plasma and lymphoid cells synthesize gamma-globulins in lymph nodes, spleen, and bone marrow.

Hepatic protein synthesis and degradation are very active, resulting in a complete turnover of liver proteins each day. Part of this turnover involves structural proteins, and a large part of it represents protein produced for export.

Factors affecting hepatic production of proteins include hepatic amino acid pool size and the levels of some hormones.[27,80] Amino acid levels must be maintained to sustain synthesis of proteins for export, the most important quantitatively being albumin. Reduced protein intake rapidly results in decreased albumin synthesis. Following long-term protein deprivation, albumin synthesis does not return immediately following increased protein intake. This decrease reflects the need for restoration of normal protein synthesizing capability, which is dependent on restoration of hepatic structure. Of all the amino acids, tryptophan may be unique as a requirement for stimulating or maintaining normal protein synthesis. Insulin also stimulates synthesis of proteins for both structure and export and inhibits protein degradation. Thyroid hormone and corticosteroids have similar anabolic effects. Abnormally high levels of corticosteroids increase rates of both synthesis and degradation of albumin.

Gluconeogenesis, necessary to maintain blood glucose, is one of the liver's highest priorities. During fasting the liver becomes the first source of substrates for gluconeogenesis. Hepatic structural proteins are degraded before those of skeletal muscle to provide those substrates. Fasting and glucagon stimulate hepatic autophagy, which continues through the activity of primarily lysosomal proteases. Amino acid levels determine the catabolism of liver proteins. Hepatic proteolysis is inhibited by amino acids, especially by alanine, glutamate, and glutamine, and by ammonia. Synthesis of proteins for export or hepatic structure is reduced with decreased amino acid concentrations and by glucagon and catecholamines, which reduce alanine, glutamate and glutamine levels. These conditions lead to increased proteolysis. A lack of insulin or thyroid hormone also reduces hepatic protein synthesis. It is evident that extremes in degradation of hepatic structure would affect overall hepatic size.

Regulation of hepatic protein synthesis and degradation is coordinated with the needs for such proteins as reflected in their half-lives. The half-lives of some plasma proteins are estimated to be less than 20 days for albumin, approximately two to three days for fibrinogen, eight to ten days for alpha-globulin, and 20 to 35 days for gamma-globulin. Proteins synthesized for structural needs of hepatocytes have half-lives shorter than those of proteins in other tissues.

Albumin.[78,80-83]

Albumin Synthesis. The liver synthesizes albumin, and since it is the most abundant large molecule in plasma, constituting 60% of the plasma protein mass, its level determines the most (80%) of the plasma colloid osmotic pressure. Plasma concentrations of albumin represent the net result of its rates of synthesis and degradation and its volume of distribution.

Albumin represents 25% of all protein synthesized by the liver. Hepatic function and the animal's nutritional status determines the rate of albumin synthesis. Portasystemic vascular shunts, cirrhosis, and severe chronic hepatitis reduce albumin production. Nutritional derangements compound reduced synthesis caused by liver disease. The nutritionally deprived diseased liver does not permanently lose the capacity to produce albumin but often returns to a normal rate of synthesis when adequate nutrition is resumed. Signs of hyperammonemia and hepatic encephalopathy are usually managed with low-protein diets. With pre-existing hypoproteinemia, restriction of dietary protein is likely to decrease albumin levels further. Albumin synthesis does not have a high priority. Reduction in its plasma level is not life-threatening. Albumin synthesis proceeds with adequate nutrition and decreases with inadequate nutrition, hepatocyte damage, or increased colloid osmotic pressure. Following refeeding after a fast, albumin synthesis is rapidly resumed, reflecting a relatively long half-life for the ribosomes and mRNA needed for its production, compared to those for synthesis of other proteins by the liver.

Severe malnutrition reduces albumin synthesis when amino acid deficiencies are produced by protein-deficient diets, malabsorption, and increased utilization of dietary nitrogen by abnormal numbers of bacteria in the small intestine. Animals with portasystemic vascular shunts have abnormal plasma amino acid levels; essential or rate-limiting amino acids are not available in normal ratios for normal albumin synthesis. In addition, plasma concentrations of glucagon and insulin are altered so that protein synthesis is reduced and hyperammonemia inhibits albumin release from hepatocytes.[84] With nutritional deficiency due to any cause the protein content of the liver decreases, resulting in hepatocyte atrophy and reduction in the albumin-synthesizing machinery. Complete restriction of food induces a 50% reduction in albumin synthesis within a few hours. Even though liver disease can be a cause of hypoalbuminemia, measurement of plasma albumin concentration is not a good index of liver function; many other factors contribute to reductions in plasma albumin levels.

Albumin synthesis depends primarily on adequate supplies of amino acids in the liver. The rate of synthesis is augmented or maintained by corticosteroids, growth hormone, sex hormones, thyroid hormone, and insulin. Corticosteroids act directly by stimulating RNA synthesis and indirectly by increasing the hepatic pool of amino acids. Thyroid hormone stimulates hepatic RNA synthesis; hypothyroidism has the opposite effect. Insulin maintains the endoplasmic reticulum. Glucagon depresses hepatic protein synthesis. During hypoalbuminemia the liver cannot compensate to increase the rate of albumin synthesis above normal. Compensatory mechanisms to maintain a normal pool of albumin alter its rate of degradation. Albumin synthesis proceeds at an optimum rate when all nutrients and hormones are available. Control mechanisms exist only to inhibit synthesis so that hyperalbuminemia does not appear. Plasma oncotic pressure regulates albumin synthesis in that synthesis is inhibited when plasma levels reach normal. Whereas infusions of colloids other than albumin inhibit albumin synthesis, the infusion of albumin does not affect its synthesis but increases its rate of degradation and disappearance.

Albumin Distribution. Albumin's volume of distribution determines plasma levels of albumin. One-third of all albumin in the body is in the intravascular space. The remaining two-thirds is in the extravascular space, primarily the interstitial fluid, in which half of the albumin is in the skin. The plasma concentrations of albumin do not necessarily reflect the size of the total pool. The plasma concentration of albumin usually increases with dehydration when the total body pool is normal, and it can be normal in a dehydrated patient with reduced total-body albumin. The size of the total-body pool of albumin cannot be predicted accurately without measuring its volume of distribution. With hypoproteinemia and ascites, the rate of albumin synthesis may be normal; and the total amount of albumin in the body may be normal. Albumin lost directly into the peritoneal cavity may be the reason for the accumulation or persistence of ascitic fluid. Thus, hypoalbuminemia can result from an increase in its space of distribution where rate of albumin synthesis remains normal. Volumes of ascitic fluid are usually in a steady state; that is, bidirectional fluxes of fluid into and out of the abdomen are equal. When ascitic fluid is removed by paracentesis, it usually reforms completely, often within 24 hours. Removal of ascitic fluid represents a means of accelerating the loss of albumin from the body.

Albumin Degradation. The most important variable influencing the amount of albumin in the body is its rate of degradation. The gastrointestinal tract is only a minor pathway for degradation, amounting to 10% of the total. An equivalent amount is degraded in the liver. The major site of albumin catabolism is undetermined. Degradation is variable, regulating the pool size of albumin (synthesized at a constant rate) by maintaining a fractional rate of catabolism directly proportional to the plasma concentration or pool size. Thus, when pool size increases, the degradation of albumin increases to maintain its normal size. Conversely, with reductions in pool size, the albumin degradation decreases so that ongoing synthesis can return the pool to its normal size. Thus, hypoalbuminemia is automatically accompanied by a degradation of less albumin. The absolute rate of degradation depends on rates of albumin synthesis in nutritionally deprived animals, one of the few situations in which synthesis changes.

The half-life of plasma albumin labeled with a radioisotope is subject to wide fluctuation, with values reported for dogs ranging widely. The half-life is determined by the degradation rate (which can fluctuate), the rate of loss through normal channels of excretion from the body, and, indirectly, by the rate of synthesis. Thus for example, in a nutritionally deprived animal with a very low rate of albumin catabolism, albumin has a long half-life.

Albumin loss is accelerated with some forms of intestinal and kidney disease. Increased permeability of the intestinal mucosa and glomerular membranes accounts for most of the losses. Diseased epithelial cells may also be capable of increased albumin catabolism, so that the amount of albumin lost in feces or urine represents only a part of the total loss. Renal and intestinal epithelial cells are capable of degrading albumin, and disease may allow more albumin to enter those cells and be degraded. The rate of albumin degradation in renal disease is greater than can be accounted for by the appearance of protein in the urine. With chronic toxic, infectious, and neoplastic processes, plasma albumin may undergo structural changes, allowing it to be catabolized faster. Stress from surgery or injury can increase albumin degradation so that the albumin pool can decrease by 20% to 75% in the more severe cases. Albumin degradation also increases with inflammatory problems that induce increases in plasma levels of fibrinogen and haptoglobin. These effects of stress on albumin can also be due to reduced synthesis. Plasma proteins can be taken up by neoplastic cells to provide amino acids for their growth. Hypoalbuminemia can be associated with cardiovascular disease, probably because of increased albumin loss into the intestine and, possibly because of increased loss by the kidneys. Impaired lymphatic circulation such as with lymphangiectasia results in a major loss of plasma proteins to the body.

In conclusion, most hypoalbuminemias are due not to decreased albumin synthesis but to increased degradation or loss. The site of the loss, often difficult to identify, can be determined when albuminuria is found. When diarrhea is a major sign, the likely cause of hypoalbuminemia is increased loss into the intestine. Reduced hepatic synthesis is assumed to cause hypoalbuminemia only in select cases. Even with advanced cirrhosis, the hypoalbuminemia accompanying ascites is usually thought to result from losses to ascitic fluid. The fluid loss is caused by portal hypertension secondary to increased resistance to hepatic blood flow. In these cases, intestinal losses also increase, contributing to hypoalbuminemia.

Hypoalbuminemia is seen in dogs with the liver reduced to one-half its size by the toxin nitrosamine.[21] That reduction is believed to be due to reduced albumin synthesis by the liver. Chronic hepatitis also results in hypoalbuminemia due to reduced synthesis; the problem correlates with survival time, which suggests hypoalbuminemia reflects the degree of hepatic insufficiency.[85] Dogs with portasystemic shunts are unable to maintain normal plasma albumin levels despite being clinically normal and consuming adequate proteins and calories to maintain normal levels.[23]

Clinical Correlation. Hypoalbuminemia is usually accompanied by reductions in the other plasma proteins, producing hypoproteinemia; the low levels result from increased degradation or loss. Therefore, the usual clinical signs accompanying hypoproteinemia are those of chronic renal disease, protein-losing enteropathy, and malignancies. Some hypoproteinemias develop from hepatic disease, in which case the associated signs are nonspecific. Hypoalbuminemia is usually associated with renal or hepatic disease, and a reduction in both albumin and globulins usually reflects gastrointestinal disease or blood loss.

Hypoalbuminemia can cause fluid to be lost from the intravascular to extravascular compartments, such as seen with ascites, edema, and thoracic transudate. Plasma albumin represents greater than half of the mass of the plasma proteins. Albumin is small in molecular size compared with other plasma proteins, so that the number of albumin molecules is far greater than the remaining total. Thus, albumin most importantly determines plasma oncotic pressure. Globulins, being larger molecules, contribute less to this pressure. Only when plasma globulins greatly increase do they exert an important osmotic force in maintaining plasma volume size. Peripheral edema and transudation of fluid into the thoracic and abdominal cavities occur when plasma albumin levels approach 1.0 g/dl. When ascites is the only evidence for fluid retention, and hypoalbuminemia is only moderate, an additional problem is usually found. Portal hypertension or obstruction of lymphatic circulation in splanchnic viscera contributes to ascites in these cases.

Albumin contains a large number of the charged amino acids glutamic acid, aspartic acid, lysine, and arginine, which enables it to bind and transport many electrolytes, nutrients, hormones, pigments, and drugs. Other plasma proteins are synthesized for specific transport of certain nutrients or hormones. Albumin levels determine plasma calcium concentrations. Hypocalcemia accompanying acute pancreatitis is corrected only by restoring circulating albumin levels. Fatty acids and tryptophan bind to albumin, an interaction that determines their metabolism. Albumin also binds drugs, so that pharmaceutical activity is determined by the amounts bound and free (Table 28-4). Thus, the blood levels, biological activity, and clearance rates resulting from therapeutic doses differ with hypoalbuminemia.

In summary, albumin in its two major functions maintains the osmotic force within the vascular compartment and binds substances for transport in the blood. Hypoalbuminemia causes clinical signs to appear because of loss of one or both of those functions.

Alpha- and Beta-Globulins.[27,79,86] The plasma alpha- and beta-globulins are synthesized in the liver, and their levels may be altered with hepatic disease. The α_1-globulin fraction contains high-density and very high-density lipoproteins; haptoglobulin, which binds and transports hemoglobin; a glycoprotein component; and a mucoprotein. The α_2-globulin fraction consists of ceruloplasmin, the carrier of copper; plasminogen; prothrombin; another glycoprotein component; and a macroglobulin. The levels of α_2-globulins sometimes increase with extra-hepatic obstruction and metastatic tumors. This fraction can also increase in bacterial and viral infections. The α_2-globulins are lost at a rate similar to that for albumin in protein-losing enteropathies.

The ß-globulins consist of low-density and very low-density lipoproteins and the iron metal-binding protein transferrin. This fraction is more consistently elevated in liver disease. It can be increased with acute and chronic hepatitis, with cirrhosis, and with extrahepatic obstruction. Since lipoproteins are the most important contributor to this fraction,

Table 28-4. Drugs with Strong Binding to Albumin

CNS Active	**Antiinfective**
Diazepam	Sulfaphenazole
Imipramine	Dicloxacillin
Chlorpromazine	Sulfaethidole
Chlordiaezepoxide	Cloxacillin
Desipramine	Oxacillin
Phenytoin	Flucloxacillin
Thoipental	Doxycycline
Antiinflammatory	Nafcillin
Fenoprofen	Cefazolin
Phenylbutazone	Sulfadimethoxine
Indomethacin	Sulfamethoxypyridazine
Oxyphenbutazone	Sulfisoxazole
Salicylic acid	**Miscellaneous**
Cardiovascular-renal	Tolbutamide
Propranolol	Warfarin
Diazoxide	Chlorpropamide
Quinidine	Tolazamide
Hydralazine	Methotrexate
Renal	Clofibrate
Probenecid	
Furosemide	
Chlorothiazide	
Trichlormethiazide	
Ethacrynic acid	

abnormalities in protein, carbohydrate, or lipid metabolism changes plasma ß-globulins and to some extent plasma α-globulins. The ß-globulins contain cholesterol-transporting lipoproteins.

Plasma globulin levels are frequently not reduced with hypoalbuminemia, especially in renal disease where glomerular membrane permeability is increased. Lesions are severe enough to permit increased filtration and loss of albumin to the urine, but not enough to allow the loss of larger globulin molecules. Globulins are lost at a rate equal to albumin losses in protein-losing enteropathy. In the cachectic animal consuming inadequate nitrogen hepatic synthesis of globulins is maintained when albumin production is reduced.

Control of synthesis is more specific for most globulins than for albumin. Proteins must be synthesized at established rates when they are catabolized after completing their function. An example is haptoglobin, which binds hemoglobin, transports the pigment to its destination in the body, and is then degraded. Prothrombin and plasminogen are also consumed on fulfillment of their biological role. Some other plasma proteins, such as transferrin, are not degraded but are reused. Some of the globulins are called "acute phase reactant protein" and are produced for response to tissue injury. With disease the production of these protective proteins increases, at the expense of the transport proteins such as albumin. The protective proteins include alpha-1-antitrypsin, alpha-1-antichymotrypsin, and haptoglobin.

Plasma protein electrophoresis is not completely reliable for evaluating levels of globulins produced by the liver, since gamma-globulins may be found in the α- and ß-globulin fractions.[87] Changes in α- and ß-globulins should be evaluated by quantitation of each of the different globulins. Increases are found with some hepatic diseases that accelerate the release of specific plasma proteins from hepatocytes.[88] Plasma globulin levels decrease with some hepatic problems because synthesis is decreased. A combination of increases and decreases in individual globulins can be seen in some specific hepatic diseases.[89]

Fibrinogen. Fibrinogen is a plasma globulin produced in the liver. Its plasma levels usually do not reflect hepatic function. Plasma fibrinogen levels increase in inflammatory diseases that may or may not involve the liver. Decreased plasma fibrinogen reflects either reduced synthesis or increased consumption, but synthesis decreases only in diffuse fulminant hepatitis. With moderately severe acute hepatic disease, fibrinogen synthesis is usually adequate to meet normal requirements. Synthesis of fibrinogen seldom fails to meet needs in chronic hepatic disease. Death results from other complications before hypofibrinogenemia becomes a problem. The most likely cause of hypofibrinogenemia with hepatic disease is accelerated consumption resulting from disseminated intravascular coagulation.

Normal disappearance of fibrinogen from the circulation follows first-order control. The fractional rate of degradation remains constant, so that the amount catabolized is directly proportional to its level in the plasma. Thus, hyperfibrinogenemia represents an increase in synthesis and release by the hepatocyte. It is seen after extensive surgery[90] as well as with inflammatory processes.[27]

Gamma-Globulins.[91-93] Since gamma-globulins are synthesized by lymphoid cells, their levels do not reflect the capacity of the liver to synthesize proteins. Serum levels of gamma-globulins are often elevated with liver disease.

Gamma-globulins can increase following stimulation by an infectious agent causing hepatic disease. A damaged liver releases antigens that stimulate synthesis of antibodies against nuclear, smooth muscle and mitochondrial cell components. Gamma-globulin synthesis is also stimulated when extraction of antigens in the portal circulation is inadequate, such as occurs with hepatic insufficiency and intrahepatic or extrahepatic vascular shunts. Small shunts develop in cirrhotic livers and produce the same effect as a single large portacaval shunt. Increased gamma-globulin synthesis is not seen in shunted animals when intestinal bacterial numbers are reduced, indicating that the antigens absorbed are products of bacteria.

Immunoglobulins are produced by lymphocytes and plasma cells in nonhepatic tissues. When hepatic immunocyte infiltration is a feature of hepatic disease, the liver synthesizes antibodies. Most immunoglobulin alterations with hepatic disease are polygammopathies. Monoclonal gammopathies are seen in small animals, and although most are not related to hepatic diseases the liver should not be overlooked as the site of the problem.

Some antibodies of the IgG, IgM, and IgA types are precipitated by cold. They produce cryoglobulinemia, which is seen most often with autoimmune diseases, malignant proliferative diseases, and chronic infections. Cryoglobulinemia can be seen with hepatic disease in which hepatic injury is either caused by the deposition of cyroprecipitates in the hepatic vasculature or is the cause for the globulin response to develop.

Blood-Clotting Factors.[94-98] Blood-clotting abnormalities can be associated with liver disease. Bleeding can be the primary clinical sign. Hepatic disease disrupts normal hemostasis by a number of ways. The initial step in hemostasis is aggregation and adherence of platelets to collagen-like proteins exposed at the site of vascular injury. The enzyme thrombin, activated from its precursor prothrombin, splits off peptides from fibrinogen, forming fibrin monomers, which are polymerized by calcium. The polymer is irreversibly stabilized by fibrin-stabilizing factor (Factor XIII). Fibrin polymers are degraded by the enzyme plasmin. This scheme is diagramed in Figure 28-9. Thrombin is activated by the intrinsic pathway, involving a cascade dependent on clotting Factors V, VIII, IX, X, XI, and XII. The extrinsic pathway requires Factors V, VII, and X to activate thrombin. Liver disease can affect any step in the clotting process.

The liver synthesizes all of the plasma-clotting Factors (Figure 28-10). The production of activated prothrombin-complex Factors II, VII, IX, and X is dependent on vitamin K. Fat-soluble vitamin K is seldom deficient; its hepatic concentrations depend on adequate dietary amounts and normal intestinal absorption of fats. Deficiencies can develop with fat malabsorption. Vitamin K is rapidly concentrated in the liver following absorption, but when absorption ceases it disappears within 24 hours. Since another source of vitamin K is synthesis by intestinal bacteria, it may take one to two months for a deficiency to develop when vitamin K is lacking in the diet. Antibiotics reducing the microflora should cause a deficiency to develop sooner. Synthetic vitamin K, menadione, being water-soluble, is absorbed more readily than the natural lipid-soluble form.

The vitamin K-dependent blood coagulation proteins contain carboxylated glutamic acid residues. Vitamin K is necessary for that carboxylation. Without that conversion the glutamic acid prevents the protein from having normal structure and activity. Prothrombin formed without adequate vitamin K is unable to bind calcium and is not converted to thrombin. The factors also fail to gain enzymatic activity because a deficiency of metal-binding sites results in protein structural abnormalities. Compounds structurally similar to vitamin K, such as the coumarin drugs, inhibit activation of the prothrombin complex. They inhibit the carboxylation of glutamic acid by preventing the recycling and reuse of vitamin K. Drugs such as aspirin, sulfonamides, and tetracycline directly antagonize vitamin K.

Fibrinogen is produced almost exclusively by the liver and factor XIII, the fibrin stabilizing factor, is synthesized in both the liver and megakaryocytes. Factor VIII (at least its von Willebrand portion) is produced in a number of sites, but primarily in endothelial cells.

The half-life of clotting factors in the prothrombin complex can be estimated to be about 2.5 days for prothrombin, 0.2 day for VII, 1.2 days for IX, and 1.7 days for X. They are all available in fresh-frozen or stored plasma. The half-life is about four days for Factors I and XIII, 1.5 days for Factor V, and 0.5 day for Factor VIII. All except V, VII, and VIII are available in both fresh-frozen plasma and stored plasma; V, VII, and VIII are available in fresh-frozen plasma only. The rate of disappearance of some factors is more rapid than estimated following total hepatectomy in dogs where there is no evidence of disseminated intravascular coagulation (Table 28-5).

Plasma clotting is also controlled by substances that inhibit the enzyme activities of clotting factors. The activities of these proteases are inhibited by antithrombin III, alpha-2-macroglob-

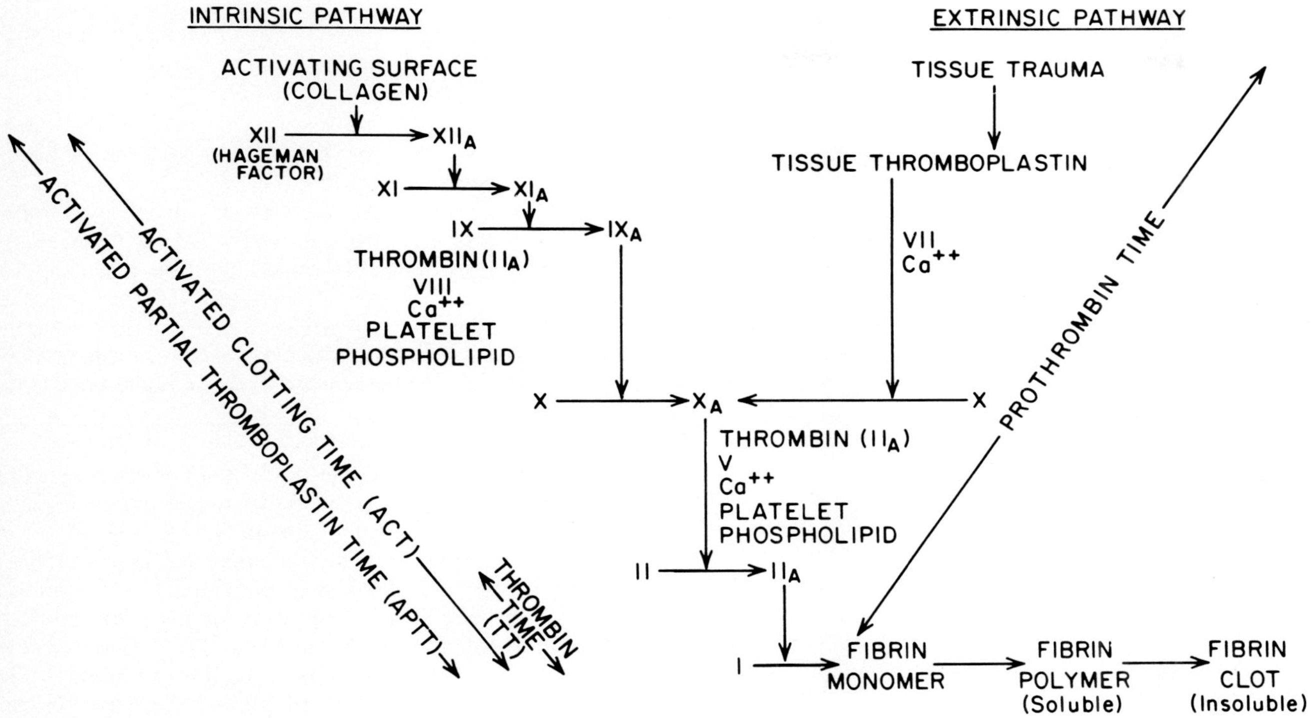

Figure 28-9. Physiology of blood clotting. Used with permission of B.F. Feldman

ulin, alpha-1-antitrypsin, and alpha-2-antiplasmin (the latter two may be the same protein). These inhibitors are believed to be produced in the liver and their levels can fall with hepatic disease. Antithrombin III, believed to be the most important, inhibits activities of thrombin, plasmin, and activated forms of Factors VIII, IX, X, XI, and XII.[99] Heparin combines with antithrombin III to produce a strong inhibitor of the serine proteases and of kallikrein.

The liver removes active clotting factors from the circulation. The Kupffer cells remove thromboplastin (intrinsic prothrombin activator) from plasma, minimizing or preventing intravascular clotting. In addition, activated clotting Factors IX, X, and XI and possibly plasminogen activator, are removed. The Kupffer cells also remove fibrin degradation products, which interfere with normal clot formation if they accumulate. Some factors participating in the removal of blood clots are made in the liver. Plasminogen, precursor of the protease plasmin, which degrades fibrin clots, is synthesized in the liver and granulocytes, especially eosinophils. Plasmin's proteolytic activity is inhibited by antiplasmin, also synthesized by the liver.

Pathophysiology of Clotting Factors in Liver Disease. Coagulopathies related to severe liver disease[95,100] are caused by deficiency of clotting factors and their inhibitors, increased fibrinolysis, circulating anticoagulants, increased levels of circulating thromboplastin, and either reductions or abnormalities in thrombocytes. A combination of abnormalities frequently contributes to increased bleeding tendencies (Table 28-6).

Deficiency of clotting factors is produced in both clinical and experimentally induced hepatic disease.[96,97,101] Reductions are due in part to decreased hepatic synthesis and increased consumption by an accompanying disseminated intravascular coagulation. There is no evidence to identify one as being more important than the other. With severe hepatic disease the clotting factors with the shortest half-lives are most likely to be depleted, such as Factors VII and VIII, with half-lives of 0.2 and 0.5 day. Hepatitis caused by the infectious canine hepatitis virus results in a precipitous fall in Factor VII levels within two

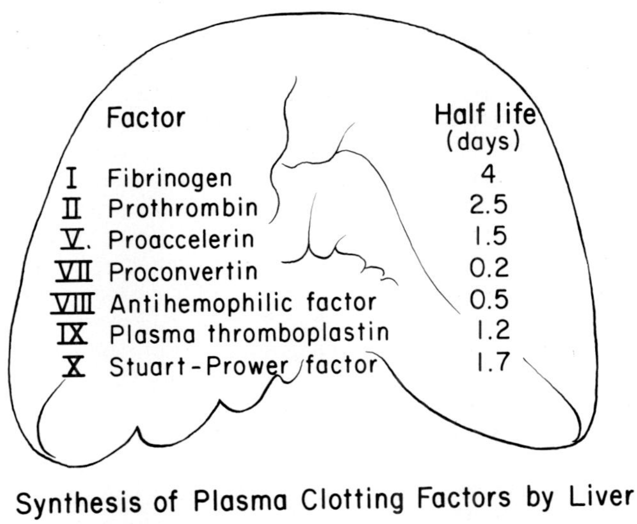

Figure 28-10. Blood clotting factors synthesized by the liver and their half lives.

Table 28-5. Effect of Hepatectomy on Clotting Factors in the Dog.

Clotting Factor	Time after Hepatectomy				
	Pre	0.5 hr	3 hr	6 hr	8 hr
Factor V	100*	90	38	18	5
Factor VII	100	81	35	14	5
Factor VIII	100	73	38	25	10
Factor X	100	91	40	17	10
AT III	100	63	62	38	14
Factor VIII:RA	100	236	298	374	266
Fibrinogen	100	93	38	16	5

*All values are percentages of presurgical factor levels; in addition the times for PT, PTT and thrombin time increased to greater than 10-fold by 6 hours. Fibrin split products were detected at no time. Unpublished observations of B.F. Feldman and D.R. Strombeck.

days.[102] Factor I, also synthesized by the liver but having a longer half-life, shows a more modest decrease. In dogs with partial hepatectomy, Factor VII levels decrease to almost zero within one to two days, while Factor V levels are reduced only 50%.[90] Thus, reduction of the capacity to synthesize protein-clotting factors by either disease or hepatectomy is manifested by decreases that are most acute for the circulating factors having the shortest half-lives. In general, the clotting factors whose synthesis is most likely to be affected by hepatocellular disease are those in the prothrombin complex.

Clotting factors are depleted by disseminated intravascular coagulation, whether the coagulapathy is caused by hepatic disease or by another problem. Clotting-factor consumption increases and production by the liver is unable to restore circulating clotting factor levels to normal. Clotting factors are destroyed by proteolytic enzymes; increased thrombin activity found in disseminated intravascular coagulation can deplete Factors I, II, V, VIII, IX, X, and XII. Clotting factors are usually depleted by a combination of changes, and determining which change is most important in causing the depletion is difficult. The liver removes activated clotting factors. With severe hepatic disease, high circulating levels of activated factors can persist.

Disseminated intravascular coagulation can be precipitated by thromboplastic substances released from the liver during acute hepatic disease. Substances with thromboplastin activity generate thrombin activity, which has many effects besides converting fibrinogen to fibrin monomers. Thromboplastin increases utilization or destruction of Factor VIII, which appears sooner than changes in other clotting factors and can be reversed by heparin infusion.[103] With increased thrombin activity, fibrinogen utilization increases, producing hypofibrinogenemia. That is followed by increased consumption of Factors V and XIII, platelets, plasminogen, and antithrombin. These primary events deplete most clotting factors and activate coagulation factors subsequently removed by the liver. Prolonged intravascular coagulation is also seen with a loss of the liver's ability to synthesize antithrombin III and the other protease inhibitors. Sinusoidal deposition of fibrin contributes to liver damage associated with disseminated intravascular coagulation. Treatment with antithrombin III minimizes that damage as well as contributing to improvement in most other signs of liver function. Disseminated intravascular coagulation is managed with heparin, but that will not be effective without antithrombin III; it may be necessary for use of both in patients found to be unresponsive to heparin therapy.

When hepatic "clearing" functions are impaired, the pathophysiology of disseminated intravascular coagulation becomes more complicated. Inability to remove activated clotting factors perpetuates bleeding disorders. The diseased liver may be unable to clear plasminogen activator, so that high levels accumulate, causing increased plasmin activity. Excessive splitting of fibrinogen and fibrin by plasmin produces more degradation products than the diseased liver can adequately remove. These degradation products interfere with fibrin polymerization and platelet function, so that clots cannot form.

The liver not only sometimes initiates disseminated intra-

Table 28-6. Causes of Coagulopathies Associated with Hepatic Disease

Deficiency of clotting factors
- Increased utilization, disseminated intravascular coagulation (DIC)
- Increased rate of destruction, excessive thromboplastic activity
- Decreased rate of synthesis, hepatic failure

Increased rate of fibrinolysis
- Increased plasminogen activator, hepatic failure

Increased levels of fibrin degradation products and other anticoagulants
- Increased rate of formation, DIC
- Decreased rate of removal, hepatic failure

Increased release of tissue thromboplastin
- Massive hepatic injury

Abnormal platelet function
- Secondary to hepatic disease

Abnormal clotting factors
- Secondary to hepatic disease

vascular coagulation but often is the target of most of the resulting secondary damage, which worsens any pre-existing problems. Deposition of fibrin in the liver and spleen is greatest during hepatic necrosis.[104] This event, which potentiates the necrotic process, can be retarded by heparin infusion (and may also require antithrombin III). Heparin is not proven to be effective in treating coagulopathies associated with liver disease, however. Heparin can cause massive bleeding in coagulopathies due to deficiency of clotting factors, high levels of circulating anticoagulants, or abnormal clotting factors. The many events contributing to coagulopathies in hepatic disease make it difficult to determine which change is the most important cause of bleeding.

Bleeding tendencies can result from abnormal clotting factors. In man, hepatic disease can result in the synthesis of abnormal fibrinogen molecules that lack the glucose residues necessary for fibrin polymerization, resulting in prolonged times for prothrombin and thrombin clotting tests and in abnormal clots.

Thrombocytopenia associated with liver disease can result from increased clearance of thrombocytes by the spleen; from increased consumption, as in disseminated intravascular coagulation; and possibly from secondary reduction of thrombocyte production. Abnormal platelet function is sometimes seen and contributes to increased bleeding tendency.

Hepatic disease can increase clotting-factor concentrations. Levels of Factor VIII frequently increase with obstructive jaundice, hepatic cancer, inflammatory hepatic diseases, and fatty degeneration of the liver. That is not surprising since Factor VIII is produced by vascular endothelium in nonhepatic tissues. In fact, levels of this factor do not decrease but if anything increase following complete hepatectomy in the dog.[101] Fibrinogen also increases with inflammatory diseases.

Bleeding problems in small animals can result from hepatic problems such as infections, toxic and chronic hepatitis, leukemic involvement of the liver, cirrhosis, obstructive jaundice, cholangitis, biliary cirrhosis, hepatic lipidosis, and cancer of the liver.[96,97,105-107] Bleeding can be a worsening problem in patients given large amounts of stored blood to replace acute losses. In such cases the stored blood is deficient in clotting factors and platelets, and replacement of blood does not restore the circulating levels of these clotting requirements.

Correlation With Clinical Signs. Hemorrhage is seldom seen with hepatic disease even when the liver is severely damaged. Clotting abnormalities are more likely to contribute to increased bleeding tendency than to cause spontaneous bleeding. Abnormal bleeding is more likely to be recognized after a venipuncture or biopsy procedure. The prothrombin complex is normally in excess, since prothrombin time remains normal while prothrombin clotting factors are reduced to 25% of normal. The partial thromboplastin test, which evaluates the levels of more clotting factors and is more sensitive than the prothrombin test, can also give normal readings despite substantial reductions in Factors I, II, V, VIII, IX, X, XI, XII.

With hepatic disease bleeding is most likely to begin in the gastrointestinal tract. Liver disease is accompanied by elevated gastrin levels since hepatic removal of gastrin is impaired. Consequently, the secretion of hydrochloric acid increases, contributing to gastric ulcer formation. An association between hepatic disease and gastric ulceration has been reported in dogs.[108] Endotoxin absorbed from the intestine and inadequately removed by the diseased liver contributes both to shock and circulatory collapse and to disseminated intravascular coagulation. Reduction of gastrointestinal blood flow produced by shock and DIC-initiated thrombus formation results in mucosal ulceration. Massive hemorrhage often follows ulceration associated with increased bleeding tendency, and can be seen with near normal prothrombin and partial thromboplastin times associated with only marginal levels of clotting factors. There may be no evidence to predict a potential bleeding problem, and when low levels of clotting factors are reduced further, for example by liver biopsy, the remaining clotting factors may be insufficient to prevent spontaneous and uncontrolled bleeding. That sometimes occurs when blood-clotting tests give normal results. Thus, increased bleeding tendencies are not always identified before the liver is biopsied.

Hepatic failure or insufficiency can be evaluated by directly or indirectly measuring the liver's ability to synthesize protein. That is done by determination of plasma albumin levels and times for prothrombin (PT) and partial thromboplastin (PTT). The PT and PTT times correlate with severity in chronic hepatitis to the extent that their values can be used to aid in predicting survival time.[85] The PT and PTT can be made more sensitive indicators of hepatic disease when their determinations are made on diluted plasma. In one study only 15% of dogs with hepatic disease showed abnormal PT and PTT, but with testing done on diluted plasma this figure increased to 66%.[109] Determination of clotting factor levels provides a direct test that is more reliable that the PT and PTT tests for evaluating liver function. As many as 93% of all dogs with hepatic disease have an abnormality in the level of at least one clotting factor. This makes the clotting factor assay more sensitive than the PT or PTT in identifying hepatic disease. This is not surprising since plasma dilution reducing clotting factor concentration to one-half has very little effect on PT and PTT in the normal animal.

Biopsy of the liver occurs without complications unless an animal is bleeding or is on the verge of bleeding as judged by very abnormal PT and PTT. Most animals with hepatic disease accompanied by abnormal PT and PTT are not at risk to prolonged bleeding from liver biopsy. In fact, in non-bleeding animals there may be no value in PT and PTT determination for predicting bleeding complications from a biopsy. Despite any confirmation of that, these tests will continue to provide a means for evaluating liver function.

Apolipoproteins.[15,17,110,111] To make their transport possible, plasma lipids are almost always combined with proteins, producing soluble aggregates. Lipoproteins, constituting an important group of these aggregates, are a combination of lipids with specific proteins called apolipoproteins (Figure 28-11). The liver synthesizes and degrades both lipoproteins and apolipoproteins. Lipoproteins are separated by plasma electrophoresis and are identified as an alpha band of high-density lipoproteins (HDL), a beta band of low-density lipoproteins (LDL), and a prebeta band of very low-density lipoproteins (VLDL). The extent of their migration during electrophoresis is determined primarily by their apolipoproteins. Lipoprotein density is determined by their flotation rates during centrifugation. HDL are the smallest lipoproteins and have the highest protein content. Lipids in HDL are primarily cholesterol esters and phospholipids. Cholesterol esters are synthesized in HDL by the enzyme lecithin cholesterol acyltransferase (LCAT) in its apolipoprotein. Proteins in HDL also participate in the metabolism of triglycerides transported in VLDL and chylomicrons. VLDL contain mostly triglycerides, with the remainder consisting of phospholipids and cholesterol esters. HDL proteins contain activators and inhibitors of lipoprotein lipase, which splits VLDL triglycerides at the adipocyte. Cholesterol and phospholipids accumulated on VLDL during transport are removed by LCAT in HDL. When free fatty acids are released, the residue of the VLDL becomes LDL. The apolipoprotein that is the major carrier of cholesterol is degraded in the liver.[112]

Pathophysiology in Liver Disease.[15,113,114] Liver disease can change the normal structure and amount of apolipoproteins synthesized. Although many other factors can alter plasma lipoprotein levels, the liver is assumed to be the cause until proven otherwise. Hepatocellular damage and biliary obstruction cause abnormal lipoprotein metabolism. Liver disease can decrease apolipoprotein synthesis, resulting in the reduction of lipoprotein formation. Hepatic disease can also cause synthesis of abnormal apolipoproteins. The apolipoproteins produced may have lost their lipid-binding properties, their regulatory effects on lipoprotein lipase, or their ability to esterify cholesterol. Blood cholesterol levels are thereby increased primarily from an increase in unesterified cholesterol. Thus, the ratio of free cholesterol to cholesterol ester is increased in the plasma. A decrease of a lipoprotein such as HDL can result from impaired lipid-binding capacity of abnormal apoplipoprotein so that little lipid is present to accept stain when identification is attempted. Thus, the concentration of this lipoprotein appears to be reduced. In other cases, abnormal apolipoproteins may bind lipids normally, but changes in their mobility cause them to appear in a different globulin fraction, giving that fraction an apparent increase in quantity.

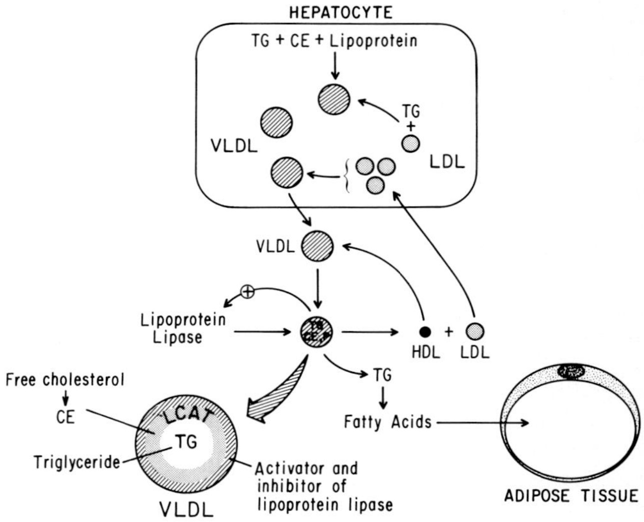

Figure 28-11. Diagram depicting lipoprotein metabolism. Enlargement in lower left corner shows composition of VLDL, containing the enzyme LCAT, cholesterol ester esterified by LCAT activity, triglyceride, and regulators of lipoprotein lipase activity. VLDL under lipoprotein lipase activity releases fatty acids from its triglycerides. Having lost triglycerides VLDL become HDL and LDL which return to the liver to pick up more triglyceride. TG = Triglyceride, CE = Cholesterol Ester, VLDL = Very Low Density Lipoprotein, LDL = Low Density Lipoprotein, HDL = High Density Lipoprotein, LCAT = Lecithin: Cholesterol Acyl Transferase.

Vitamin Metabolism[115,116]

The liver has an important role in vitamin metabolism; it produces bile for absorption of fat-soluble vitamins, stores vitamins, and converts them to metabolically active chemicals.

Vitamin A is stored in both Kupffer cells and hepatocytes. About 95% of total-body vitamin A is stored in the liver, which represents a one- to two-year supply. The liver continues to release vitamin A to maintain normal blood levels despite reductions in its hepatic content. Circulating vitamin A is bound to retinal binding protein, an α-1-globulin produced in the liver and complexed in the plasma with a pre-albumin protein. Malnutrition, liver disease, and intestinal malabsorption reduce liver and plasma vitamin A levels, but signs of deficiency do not appear until abnormalities become severe. Cholestasis of long enough duration to cause bile deficiency and vitamin A malabsorption is not recognized in small animals. The vitamin A content in the liver is also reduced by ACTH and corticosteroids.

Excess vitamin A in the liver is a greater threat than its deficiency; once an excess is stored in the liver there is no effective means for accelerating its removal.[117] Excess hepatic vitamin A would not be unusual in a patient receiving a vitamin supplement or consuming liver regularly over a long period of time. That excess can cause hepatocellular damage and hepatic fibrosis, producing hepatomegaly, portal hypertension, splenomegaly, and ascites. Vitamin A supplementation can act synergistically with hepatotoxins to cause liver damage, whereas either one at low levels would cause no pathology. Thus, supplementation of this vitamin for animals receiving drugs known to be hepatotoxic bears some risk. Vitamin A also accumulates in the liver's fat-storing cells (Ito cells) during hepatic disease where there are defects in retinol-binding protein metabolism and vitamin A is not mobilized from the liver. Renal failure and protein-calorie malnutrition also create a greater risk for vitamin A retention and toxicity.

Vitamin D is stored in the liver as well as other tissues. Vitamin D is hydroxylated in the liver to form 25-hydroxycholecalciferol, which when released to the plasma is bound to a specific transport protein and represents the major form of the vitamin in the circulation. Vitamin D deficiency can result from inadequate absorption or from defective conversion to its metabolically active form, 25-hydroxyvitamin D. Vitamin D malabsorption can be a consequence of intestinal diseases causing fat malabsorption. That can be caused by intralumunal bile salt deficiency resulting from chronic cholestatic disease, a problem seldom important in small animal patients. Chronic hepatic disease can reduce vitamin D 25-hydroxylase activity so that deficiency develops despite adequate intestinal absorption. In such cases, greatly increased amounts of parenterally administered vitamin D are required to reverse signs of deficiency.

Vitamin E is also stored in a variety of tissues, including the liver, with the amounts related to dietary levels. With respect to the liver, this vitamin's most important role may be to offer protection by inhibiting lipid peroxidation. Many chemicals and metals are known to cause liver damage. The effects of some substances are prevented or inhibited by vitamin E.

The liver's vitamin K stores are limited and can be rapidly depleted when dietary sources are inadequate or lipid malabsorption is severe. Depletion occurs within one week when none is absorbed from the intestine. Vitamin K is synthesized by intestinal bacteria, an important source. When the diet contains no vitamin K, the endogenous production is able to meet needs for a month. Vitamin K is essential for synthesis of the prothrombin-complex clotting factors, of a metal-binding amino acid necessary for the function of the coagulation proteins, and of a protease which inactivates several clotting factors and facilitates clot lysis.

When hepatic disease destroys hepatic functions, the last functions lost are those relating to the storage of fat-soluble vitamins. With bleeding due to hepatic disease, the function for synthesis is always lost before the storage of vitamin K is depleted; hence, parenteral administration of vitamin K is consistently ineffective in initiating synthesis of prothrombin-complex factors. There is little indication that fat-soluble vitamins are a necessary adjunct therapy for liver disease. When lipid malabsorption accompanies hepatic disease, additional vitamins are given.

The liver, of all tissues, is the richest source of water-soluble vitamins, present in the form of coenzymes. The liver's vitamin requirements are related directly to its metabolic workload. Water-soluble vitamins, except vitamin B_{12}, are readily absorbed from the small intestine and are used primarily to make coenzymes employed in metabolic processes. Vitamin phosphorylation, occurring primarily in hepatocytes, is required to produce some coenzymes. Thiamine is phosphorylated to thiamine pyrophosphate, primarily in the liver and kidney. Pyridoxine is phosphorylated to its active form in the liver, as is the transformation of pantothenic acid to coenzyme-A. Nicotinic acid is a precursor in pyridine nucleotide synthesis, and an initial step in its conversion is nicotinamide synthesis in the liver. Folic acid is converted to its active form in the liver. Large amounts of all water-soluble vitamins except vitamin C are stored in the liver as coenzymes, which can be released to supply vitamins to peripheral tissues. Vitamin C is produced in the liver; with hepatic insufficiency, usual dietary levels of vitamin C may be inadequate to maintain normal plasma levels.

During anorexia the liver atrophies and releases part of its coenzymes. Most are excreted by the kidneys, but some are used by other tissues. Supplementation of water-soluble vitamins is not required during starvation. When a normal intake of calories resumes, however, water-soluble vitamins are necessary to replenish coenzymes involved in metabolic processes in all tissues, most importantly in the liver. Thus, deficiencies in water-soluble vitamins are unlikely in anorectic animals but can develop when large amounts of calories are fed with small amounts of vitamins. Water-soluble vitamins, combined with small amounts of calories in glucose- or lactate-containing solutions, are of little value. With hepatic disease, the metabolic conversion of vitamins to coenzymes is decreased and contributes to the reduced metabolism of carbohydrates.

Iron Metabolism[118,119]

The liver stores iron, which can be toxic in excessive amounts. The amount of iron in the body is determined by regulation of its absorption in the upper small intestine. Dietary iron is usually in the ferric form, and gastric acidity must change iron to the ferrous form before it is absorbed. Ferrous iron rapidly enters mucosal epithelial cells, possibly by a carrier protein similar to transferrin. Intracellular iron is oxidized to the ferric form, which binds to a protein, apoferritin, to form ferritin.

The most important step in regulating iron metabolism is the controlled-release of iron from the mucosal cell to the circulation. Iron is released at a rate determined by the animal's needs. With large amounts of stored mucosal iron, release is minimal (see Chapter 15). Ferric iron, released to the circulation, binds transferrin, a plasma ß-globulin protein, synthesized in the liver (Figure 28-12). This protein transports iron from the intestinal tract to reticulocytes and tissue stores, and from the latter to bone marrow. The rate of transferrin synthesis is regulated by levels of stored iron. Increased stored iron decreases transferrin synthesis.

Iron is stored intracellularly as ferritin in a number of tissues, with the liver having a large storage capacity. When the capacity is exceeded iron accumulates as hemosiderin, which is thought to be large aggregates of colloidal iron attached to ferritin molecules. No pathway is designed for excretion of iron from the body, and repeated administrations of iron as injections or blood transfusions result in hemosiderin accumulation in hepatocytes and Kupffer cells, ultimately leading to their degeneration. Increased hepatic storage of iron also accompanies hemolytic anemia and excessive and prolonged oral intake of iron. Iron released from hemolyzed erythrocytes binds to apoferritin and is stored.

Iron in hepatic ferritin and hemosiderin can be used to synthesize hemoglobin. The mechanism for releasing this form of iron is not precisely understood. It involves reduction of iron to the ferrous form, which may require xanthine oxidase. This enzyme couples the reaction in which ferric iron is reduced to ferrous iron, and xanthine is oxidized to uric acid.

Copper and Zinc Metabolism[120]

Small amounts of copper normally found in the diet are readily absorbed, enter the circulation and bind to albumin and amino acids, and are readily taken up and deposited in the liver. Hepatic copper levels are the highest of any tissue in the body, stored in a protein-bound cytosolic pool and in lysosomes. Copper leaves the liver by incorporating with liver-produced ceruloplasmin and entering the circulation. Its excretion in bile is the primary means for mobilization of copper from the liver. That copper is bound to a carrier which prevents its absorption in the intestine. This represents the only significant means for copper excretion and hence for maintaining copper balance in the body. Canine hepatic copper metabolism is different from that of other species. Canine hepatic copper levels do not decrease as the neonate matures, a unique feature that may be related to dogs' having different copper binding proteins in the liver.

Zinc is also readily absorbed in the intestine, and its level in the ingesta affects the absorption of copper. Zinc absorption competes with that of copper. Zinc induces synthesis of the metal-binding protein metallothionein, which binds copper in intestinal epithelial cells and blocks its absorption. Binding of zinc to that protein is weaker and does not prevent its absorption. Following absorption, zinc binds to albumin and an α-macroglobulin and is transported to the liver. Zinc is stored in the liver as a complex with a binding protein.

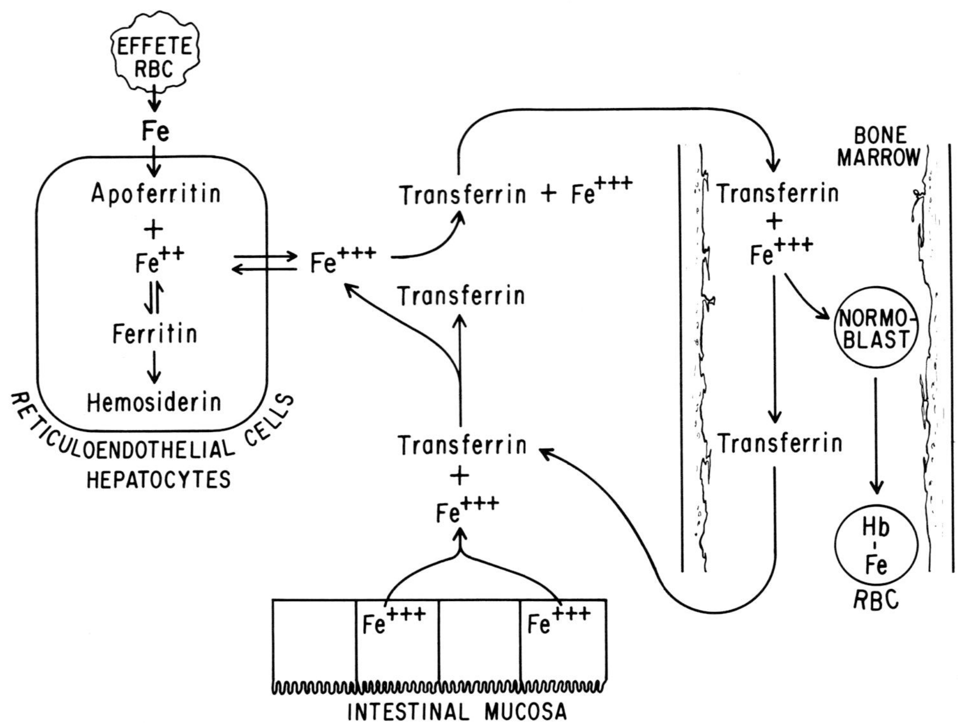

Figure 28-12. Overall scheme of iron transport and storage.

METABOLIC FUNCTION - CATABOLIC (CONJUGATION, DETOXIFICATION, EXCRETION)

Bile Metabolism and Excretion

Bile Formation and Secretion.[121-125] Bile is a slightly alkaline isosmotic solution of bile salts, bile pigments, phospholipids, and cholesterol, secreted by hepatocytes and delivered by the biliary system to the intestine. Bile is formed by an energy-requiring active transport of solutes from hepatocytes into bile canaliculi. Bile acids are the major solute in bile, constituting three-fourths of the total solids. Bile acids are actively transported into bile canaliculi; water and plasma electrolytes follow passively to maintain isosmosity. Hepatocytes actively secrete small amounts of other organic anions. Bile also contains small amounts of lipids, proteins, blood constituents, substances detoxified by the liver, and certain enzymes such as amylase and phosphatase.

During transport of bile through biliary ducts, it is modified by the addition of an electrolyte solution. This secretion is produced by active sodium transport, with water following passively, accompanied by other plasma electrolytes. Bile leaving the liver is more alkaline than plasma, which is produced by an ion-exchange process in bile ducts in which chloride is removed and bicarbonate is added. Bicarbonate concentration approximates 70 mEq per liter, making the pH of bile 8 to 9 as it enters the gallbladder.

Hepatic secretion of bile is regulated, with the total rate determined by rates of secretion by hepatocytes and bile ducts. Choleretic agents stimulate secretion, the most important natural ones being bile acids absorbed from the intestine. Bile released from the gallbladder into the intestine is reabsorbed and delivered by the portal circulation to the liver. With enterohepatic circulation of bile acids back to the liver, hepatocytes are stimulated to take up and resecrete bile acids. Other choleretics augment hepatic bile flow by stimulating the secretion of fluid and electrolytes in bile ducts. They include secretin, gastrin, cholecystokinin, glucagon, prostaglandins, and cyclic AMP, all of which increase both bile flow rate and bicarbonate content. Parasympathetic activity stimulates secretion, and drugs affecting the parasympathetic nervous system affect bile secretion. Exogenous agents with a choleretic effect include sulfobromophthalein (BSP), indocyanine green, rose bengal, salicylates, hydrocortisone, and phenobarbital. Cholestasis (reduced bile secretion) is induced by somatostatin; it is also observed after administration of estrogens and in animals with hepatic insufficiency.

Hepatobiliary excretion of bile acids and other organic compounds requires hepatocellular uptake; intracellular transport, conjugation and storage; and secretion into bile canaliculi. Organic compounds compete for processing through the different stages. High levels of bile acids decrease excretion of dyes such as BSP or indocyanine green. Their excretion is enhanced when choleresis is stimulated by agents not competing with the organic dyes for excretion. Choleretic agents enhance excretion of bile acids and bilirubin. Many drugs are excreted in bile after being metabolized by the liver.

Bile Storage and Modification.[121,126] The gallbladder stores bile and modifies its composition. The capacity of the gallbladder is small compared with the amounts secreted by the liver during fasting. Thus, bile secreted by the liver must be concentrated before it can be stored within the gallbladder. Bile is concentrated by the absorption of water and electrolytes. Sodium is removed by an active transport mechanism similar to that in the small intestine. Water and other ions are absorbed passively, following concentration gradients. Bile's concentration of bicarbonate is reduced so that the pH is less than seven. The acid pH minimizes precipitation of calcium salts since their solubility is inversely related to pH. Calcium salts are poorly absorbed and precipitation is more likely as their concentration increases. Bile acids and cholesterol are not absorbed in the gallbladder. As bile is concentrated, cholesterol remains in solution due to the solubilizing effects of bile salts and lecithin.

Biliary-Tract Evacuation.[127] The active secretion of bile can generate pressures in the biliary tract as high as 35 cm of water. When pressures reach 20 cm of water, bile constituents diffuse back across the walls of biliary ducts into the hepatic parenchyma. During fasting, bile is retained in the biliary system by pressures of five to 10 cm water at the sphincter of Oddi. This diverts bile to the gallbladder, where the total pool of bile acid can be stored after its concentration. Evacuation during a meal occurs when neural and humoral stimuli contract the gallbladder and relax the sphincter of Oddi. Neural stimulation is achieved by the vagal parasympathetics, and humoral stimulation by cholecystokinin. Parasympathomimetic drugs contract the gallbladder, and anticholinergic drugs inhibit contraction. Morphine causes biliary-tract spasm and increases intraductal pressure. Evacuation of the biliary system is also affected by smooth-muscle activity in the duodenum around the sphincter of Oddi.

Bile Acid Metabolism[128,129]

Physiology. The synthesis and secretion of bile acids provides a single important avenue for the excretion of cholesterol and provides a compound necessary for normal digestion and absorption of dietary lipids. Bile acid is the most abundant compound in bile.

Bile acids are synthesized from cholesterol (Figure 28-13), the primary ones being cholate and chenodeoxycholate. Both are hydroxylated at carbon-7 of the steroid nucleus, and cholate is further hydroxylated at carbon-12.

The rate-limiting step in bile-salt synthesis is the hydroxylation of cholesterol at the 7-alpha position of the sterol nucleus by the hepatic microsomal enzyme cholesterol-7α-hydroxylase. In both bile acids, the terminal methyl group at carbon 24 of the side chain is oxidized to an acid group, to which is conjugated an amino acid, either taurine or glycine. Conjugation is required for secretion.

The conjugation of bile acids lowers their pKa. The pKa of glycine-conjugated acids is pH 4, and that of taurine-conjugated is pH 2, in contrast to pKa of pH 6 for the unconjugated acids. The pKa of a bile acid is that pH where half of the bile acid is ionized and half is un-ionized. Bile acids with a low pKa have a strong tendency to remain ionized at low pH. Un-ionized bile salts are lipid-soluble and readily cross lipid cell membranes. Ionized and water-soluble bile acids cross cell membranes slowly. At the pH of the intestinal contents (between six to seven), unconjugated bile acids are rapidly absorbed since they are largely un-ionized and lipid-soluble. Thus, these bile acids are not available to form micelles. With conjugation lowering their pKa, bile acids are ionized and are not readily absorbed.

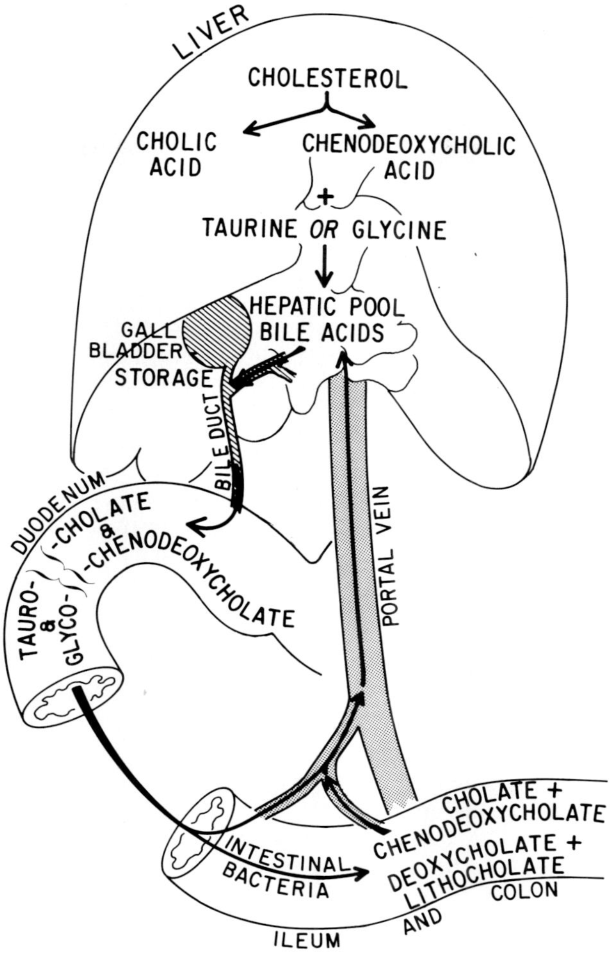

Figure 28-13. Scheme of bile acid synthesis, secretion, release into the intestine, bacterial degradation, absorption from intestine and resecretion by the liver.

After discharge into the intestines, some of the conjugated bile acids are lost in the feces, some are absorbed unaltered, and about 5% are altered by intestinal bacteria. The end product of bacterial activity on chenodeoxycholic acid is lithocholic acid, and that on cholic acid is deoxycholic acid, which are the compounds formed after the amino acid and the hydroxyl groups at carbon-7 are removed. Both unaltered bile acids and most deoxycholic acid are absorbed in the ileum by an active transport process; most lithocholic acid is excreted in the feces. Absorbed bile acids bind to plasma albumin and lipoproteins and are carried by the portal circulation to the liver, where they are very efficiently removed, reconjugated if necessary, and resecreted in the bile. Therefore, bile contains conjugates of lithocholic and deoxycholic acids as well as those of cholic and chenodeoxycholic acids. Some bile acids are sulfated, which enables them to be excreted by the kidneys and minimizes their reabsorption in the intestine. With obstruction of the biliary system, renal excretion can become an important means for the elimination of bile acids.

The rate of bile acid synthesis is determined largely by the amount delivered to the liver for uptake and resecretion. Any factor increasing the loss of bile acids from the body stimulates the rate of bile acid synthesis. When enterohepatic circulation is interrupted so that bile acids are lost in feces, bile acid synthesis can increase tenfold and is able to replace smaller losses but not large losses. The size of the bile acid pool is limited. Thus, the pool must be cycled twice through the enterohepatic circulation during a single meal. A small amount of bile acids is excreted in urine. The fecal loss of bile acids represents the major pathway for cholesterol excretion in the body. The amount not absorbed and lost in the feces is determined by dietary levels of fiber. Cellulose, and possibly bran, are fibers that bind bile acids and increase their rate of fecal excretion. Diets low in fiber minimize fecal losses of bile acids, which reduces the rate of their synthesis from cholesterol.

The hepatic regulation of bile acid metabolism is important for several reasons. The rate of secretion of cholic and chenodeoxycholic acid must be maintained to ensure normal digestion and absorption of lipids. Lithocholic acid is hepatotoxic, and deoxycholic acid can damage the surface of the intestinal mucosa. Those substances should therefore be excreted, if possible. Some lithocholic acid is sulfated in the liver, so that it is only poorly absorbed in the renal tubule and intestine and is lost from the body. Deoxycholic acid is largely absorbed in the small intestine when the diet contains no fiber. Under these circumstances, its half-life in the body increases three to four times, possibly up to a month, and bile acid synthesis decreases since little is bound to fiber and lost in the feces. With cholic acid continuing to be converted to deoxycholic acid, the greater amounts of deoxycholic acid secreted in bile increase the possibility of a toxic effect. Dietary fiber is important for bile acids to have the normal turnover that helps maintain their proper ratios. A bile-acid-binding resin, cholestyramine, is sometimes used to increase losses of bile acids through the intestine.

In general, diet has little influence on the rate of bile acid synthesis unless fecal excretion changes. Cholesterol levels in the diet or plasma do not influence the rate of bile salt synthesis. Unsaturated fatty acids in the diet increase the rate of fecal bile acid excretion, which increases bile acid synthesis and thereby lowers plasma levels of cholesterol.

Hormones affect bile acid synthesis, with thyroid hormone stimulating it. Thyroid hormone also regulates the activity of hydroxylating and conjugating enzymes since it influences the ratio of cholic to chenodeoxycholic acids and the ratio of glycine-conjugated to taurine-conjugated acids. Corticosteroids, estrogens, and androgens also affect bile acid synthesis, with some of the effect via cholesterol metabolism.

Pathophysiology. Liver disease can change both the rate of synthesis and the pool size of bile acids. Abnormal bile salt metabolism results from: 1) reduction of the parenchymal cell mass; 2) impaired hepatocyte function as a result of disease; and 3) disturbance of enterohepatic circulation of bile acids. The abnormal metabolism can increase or decrease plasma concentrations of total bile acids. Changes can occur in the rate of bile acid synthesis, in the ratios of their respective concentrations, or in their rate of uptake and secretion by the liver.

Bile acid synthesis is reduced in cirrhosis primarily for cholate; chenodeoxycholate synthesis is nearly normal. This selective inhibition, reflecting impairment of carbon-12 hydroxylation, results in altered ratios of cholate to chenodeoxycholate plasma concentrations. The total bile acid pool is reduced by one-half in cirrhosis; since plasma levels are usually increased, hepatic uptake and secretion must be affected. Cirrhosis reduces secretion of bile acids and to some degree that also reflects both a reduced synthesis and impaired uptake. The reduced bile acid secretion should contribute to lipid maldigestion and malabsorption. Signs of bile acid deficiencies are recognized infrequently with hepatic disease, however. Acute hepatitis and most other hepatic diseases have the similar effect of reducing synthesis and the size of the total pool, impairing uptake and secretion, and increasing plasma bile and levels. In general, hepatocyte damage releasing its bile acid content has little effect on increasing plasma levels since only 5% of the bile acid pool is in the liver.[130]

Cholestasis, preventing the secretion and discharge of bile into the biliary system, increases plasma bile acid levels.[131-133] High levels of bile acids inhibit synthesis, primarily by affecting carbon-7 hydroxylation. With reduced secretion, much smaller amounts of bile acids enter the intestine and are available for conversion by bacterial activity to deoxycholic acid or lithocholic acid; hence, their plasma levels are low.

Plasma bile acid levels can increase with portasystemic shunts where hepatic clearance is reduced.[134-136] Although shunts reduce liver mass, the total pool of bile acids is unchanged.[137] Bile acid synthesis can increase to maintain normal release of bile acids into the intestine. The plasma pool of bile acids increases, but in this case the increase does not inhibit synthesis. Both intra- and extrahepatic vascular shunts develop with loss of hepatic architecture due to disease. It is not clear whether plasma bile acids increase because of loss of hepatocyte functions, portasystemic shunts, or both.

Intestinal conditions can alter plasma bile acid concentrations.[138-140] Inadequate reabsorption of bile acids in the ileum contribute to reducing plasma bile acids. Only partial emptying of the gall bladder during feeding reduces bile acids available for absorption, and postprandial plasma levels could be less than expected. Such changes could mask an effect of concurrent liver disease to raise plasma bile acid levels. Conversely, intestinal bacterial overgrowth deconjugates bile acids and accelerates their rate of absorption to raise plasma levels. Under such conditions both unconjugated and total plasma bile acids increase, and that finding could mislead one to believe that hepatic disease is a problem. Bacterial deconjugation is due to anaerobes in concentrations greater than 100/ml. Fasting bile acid determinations are made on the premise that there is no release of bile into the intestine. Bile can intermittently be released, making fasting plasma bile and concentrations higher than expected. Plasma bile acid concentrations are normally higher in the very young animal.[141]

Clinical Application. Early use of plasma bile acid measurements to identify hepatic disease was accompanied by the hope that an ideal diagnostic test had been found.[142,143] An understanding of bile acid metabolism with various diseases is much better for human than for small animal patients, and there are far more data on its use in humans. The current status of plasma bile acids as a diagnostic tool for humans probably reflects what it is or will become for small animals.[140,144] The routine use of plasma bile acid determination for the diagnosis of hepatobiliary diseases does not appear to be warranted, however, because the routine biochemical tests are, in the vast majority of cases, sufficiently sensitive (see Chapter 30). Textbooks on liver disease in humans state that bile acid measurements are unlikely to enter routine clinical practice in the future. Determination of ratios of cholate to chenodeoxycholate have also not been found reliable for evaluating suspected hepatic disease. Clearance tests to follow the disappearance of bile acids after oral administration are not proven to be useful. Evaluation of any plasma bile acid level must be based on an understanding of all the hepatic and nonhepatic factors that affect bile acid metabolism.

Bile Pigment Metabolism (Figure 28-12)[145-147]

Bile Pigment Formation. Bilirubin, the major bile pigment, is a product of hemoprotein catabolism. Erythrocyte hemoglobin is the primary source of bilirubin. Hemoglobin constitutes over 90% of all heme in the body, but its turnover rate is low, with the life span of normal erythrocytes being up to 120 days. Myoglobin is another abundant hemoprotein, but its turnover rate is so low that it contributes little to the formation of bilirubin. Many hemoproteins with shorter half-lives contribute significantly to the total daily production of bilirubin, accounting for 25% to 35% of the total. The liver is a major source of these hemoproteins, which include cytochromes, catalase, and peroxidases. Cytochrome P-450, a coenzyme in the liver, has a rapid turnover rate, making it a significant source of bile pigments. In normal dogs, 67% of total bilirubin produced is from erythrocytes, 28% from hepatic hemoproteins, and 5% from ineffective erythropoiesis. Of the bilirubin in plasma 79% is from erythrocytes and 15% from hepatic hemoproteins. The mononuclear phagocytic system (MPS) phagocytizes senescent erythrocytes and free hemoglobin, and the catabolism of hemoglobin that follows is a function of both the Kupffer cell and the hepatocyte (Figure 28-14, 28-15).

Hemoglobin consists of four peptide chains with a heme group bound to each. When released by erythrocyte destruction, hemoglobin combines with haptoglobin and α_2-globulin (a mucoprotein), forming a weak peroxidase that is transported to the MPS, where it is phagocytized. Other plasma carrier proteins have less affinity for heme and are not used to form circulating complexes unless excessive amounts of hemoglobin and heme are formed. The MPS cells are primarily those in

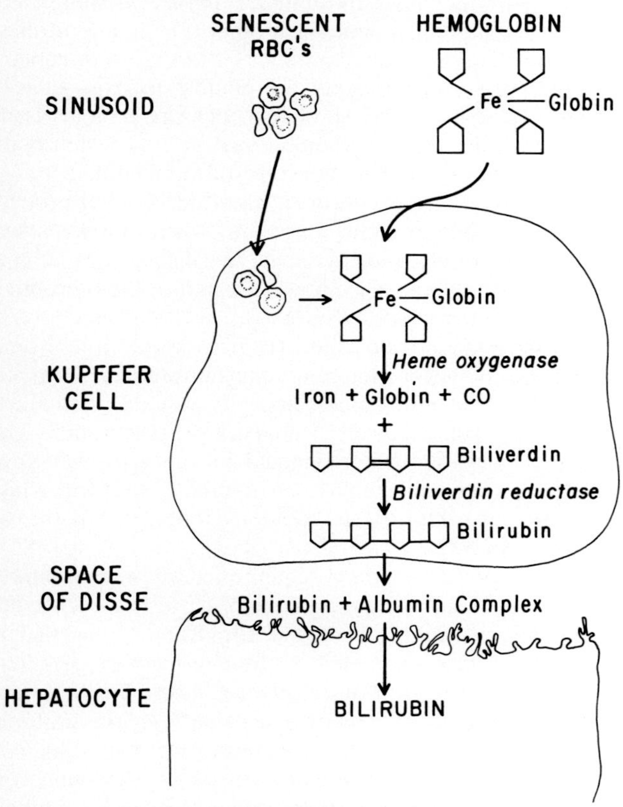

Figure 28-14. Schematic showing catabolism of hemoglobin by Kupffer cell to bilirubin.

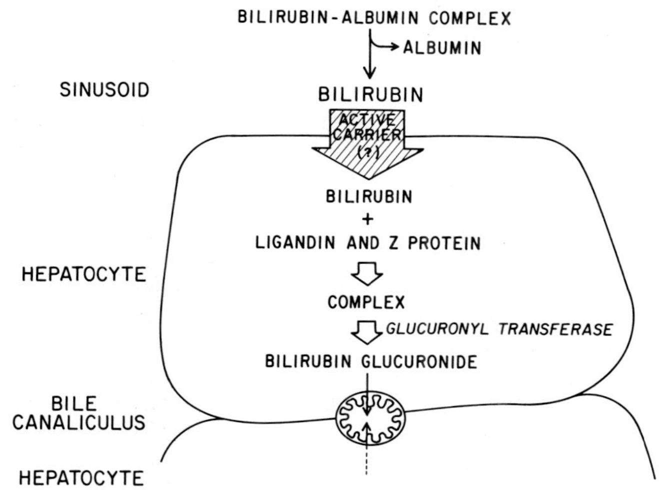

Figure 28-15a. Schematic showing catabolism of bilirubin by hepatocyte and its secretion into bile canaliculi.

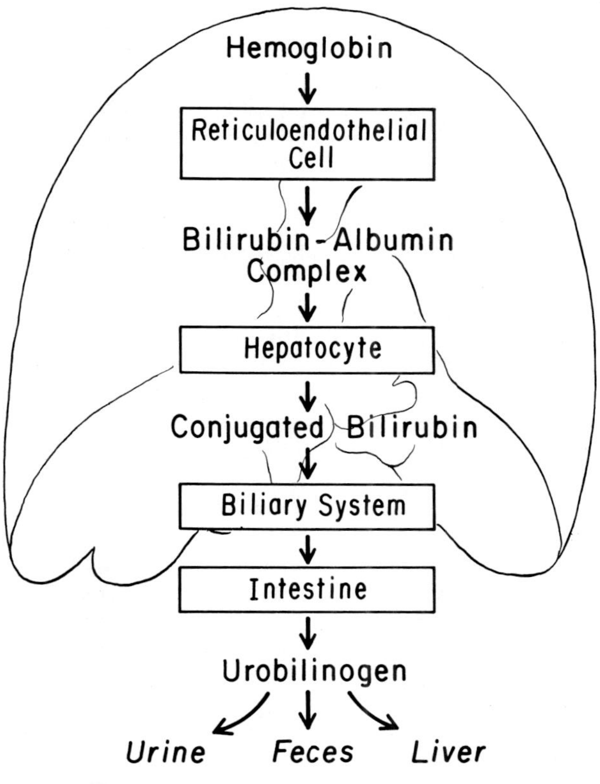

Figure 28-15b. Scheme of bile pigment metabolism from its formation to its conversion to various metabolites in the intestine.

the bone marrow, spleen, and liver, the last being the most important. Both the Kupffer cells of the MPS in the liver and the hepatocyte participate in the catabolism of hemoglobin. Other hemoproteins produced from hemoglobin include oxyhemoglobin, methemoglobin, and methemalbumin. During heme catabolism the carrier protein is also degraded except with methemalbumin, where albumin is the carrier.

Hemoproteins are taken up by Kupffer cells and hepatocytes, where they are catabolized to bilirubin. The proteins are removed and degraded to amino acids. The remaining heme is a complex of iron and a ring structure of four pyrrole rings forming a ferroprotoporphyrin ring. The microsomal enzyme heme oxygenase degrades heme by splitting the ring to produce the four pyrrole rings in a chain, biliverdin, carbon monoxide, and free iron (Figure 28-14). Another microsomal enzyme, biliverdin reductase, converts biliverdin, a green pigment, to bilirubin, an orange pigment. The iron binds to iron-carrying proteins, transferrin and ferritin, for storage and transport to sites for reuse. Kupffer cells degrade hemoglobin from erythrocytes removed by the MPS; hepatocytes degrade hemoproteins circulating in plasma whether in the form of hemoglobin, methemoglobin or methemealbumin. Most heme-oxygenase is found in the liver and spleen with some in bone marrow, renal tubular epithelium, and tissue macrophages. Biliverdin reductase is found in the liver and spleen.

Plasma Bilirubin Transport

About two-thirds of the bilirubin produced is released from hepatocytes and Kupffer cells to the circulation. This bilirubin, not yet conjugated, is relatively insoluble in aqueous solutions at physiological pH; hence, it is transported only when bound to albumin. Although the albumin-binding capacity is great and the relative affinity for unconjugated bilirubin and albumin is high, some bilirubin remains unbound. Since that bilirubin is lipid-soluble, it crosses all membranes readily. Because of the interaction with albumin, little is filtered at the glomerulus, and virtually none appears in urine. At relatively high concentrations, exceeding 30 mg/dl, bilirubin binds to other sites on albumin molecules. The affinity for these sites is less than that for the primary binding sites. Bilirubin bound loosely to these sites is easily displaced by competing agents such as organic anions, sulfonamides, hydrocortisone, digoxin, Valium (diazepam), mercuhydrin, oxacillin, salicylates, thyroxine, and free fatty acids, and conditions such as acidosis. Such substances can increase the rate of deposition of unbound bilirubin in nonhepatic tissue, but plasma bilirubin levels are infrequently seen to exceed the capacity for primary site binding. It is evident that hypoalbuminemia increases the amount of unbound pigment.

Bilirubin circulating with albumin is next transferred to hepatocytes for conversion to a water-soluble pigment that can be excreted from the body (Figure 28-15). Bilirubin uptake is rapid and efficient and is preceded by disassociation of the bilirubin-albumin complex. With any substance bound avidly to a carrier protein, the rate of uptake by the liver is determined by the efficiency of the method rather than hepatic blood flow. Bilirubin competes with sulfobromophthalein and other organic anions for uptake by hepatocytes, possibly by competing for carrier sites in an active transport system. Bile acids do not compete for this uptake. The rate of bilirubin uptake is not affected by high intracellular concentrations of unconjugated or conjugated bilirubin in hemolytic or obstructive jaundice. Unconjugated bilirubin causes hyperbilirubinemia when icterus is due to a failure in uptake. Uptake deficiency is undoubtedly a problem in hepatocellular disease. Humans can have congenital defects in bilirubin transport into hepatocytes. That condition has been reported also in a dog. High plasma levels of unconjugated bilirubin do not necessarily reflect inability of the liver to remove the circulating bilirubin mass since up to 40% of the bilirubin taken up by the liver can reflux unchanged to the plasma. Any study on hepatic uptake of unconjugated bilirubin must take that into consideration.

Bilirubin binds to specific intracellular proteins in hepatocytes.[123] One of the bilirubin-binding proteins is ligandin, which has a nonspecific affinity for anions including corticosteroids; dyes such as sulfobromophthalein, indocyanine green, and rose bengal; fatty acids; antimicrobials such as sulfonamides, penicillin, tetracycline, and nitrofurantoin; and ethacrynic acid. Unconjugated bilirubin has a marked affinity for ligandin, and it is suggested that transport into hepatocytes results from a greater affinity for ligandin than for serum albumin. However, albumin's greater affinity identifies the role of ligandin as a binding rather than transport protein. Hepatocytes also contain Z protein, which binds unconjugated bilirubin but has less affinity than ligandin. Ligandin and Z proteins have similar properties; Z protein's major function is likely involved in the uptake and metabolism of fatty acids. These proteins are essential for clearing organic anions from the circulation. They do not appear in humans and some animals until five to ten days after birth. Until that time there is a marked delay in the removal of organic anions, including bilirubin, from the circulation. Since organic anions compete with each other for binding to these proteins, the binding of these proteins by excessive amounts of bilirubin reduces the capacity for binding to dyes such as sulfobromophthalein. The amount of binding proteins is increased by drugs such as phenobarbital, a drug which is the basis for treating some forms of hyperbilirubinemia.

Bilirubin is transferred from intracellular binding proteins to the smooth endoplasmic reticulum, where a microsomal enzyme, glucuronyl transferase, catalyzes the pigment's conjugation with glucuronic acid. A smaller part of the bilirubin is conjugated with glucose and xylose.

During esterification with glucuronide, the microsomal enzyme bilirubin UDP-glucuronyl transferase transfers glucuronic acid from uridine diphosphate glucuronic acid to bilirubin. Most of the conjugated bilirubin is the diglucuronide. This esterification changes unconjugated bilirubin from a lipid-soluble, water-insoluble molecule to its conjugated form, which is rended water-soluble by the addition of polar groups, the two glucuronic acids.

The rate of this reaction is determined by enzyme activity and the availability of glucuronic acid. There is evidence that enzyme activity is in great excess in normal animals and that the availability of glucuronic acid is the rate-limiting step. That enzymatic conversion of unconjugated bilirubin is the rate-limiting step is supported by evidence that 70% of bilirubin in the liver is unconjugated. Deficiencies of the glucuronic acid donor or of transferase enzyme activity cause inadequate conjugation, with jaundice resulting. Phenobarbitol stimulates glucuronic transferase activity. Two other enzymes conjugate bilirubin with glucose or xylose.

Other factors influence bilirubin conjugation. A regular intake of calories is necessary to prevent fasting unconjugated hyperbilirubinemia. During fasting there is a reduction in the concentrations of the intracellular binding protein and in intrahepatic uptake. Glucuronyl transferase activity also decreases. These changes in two of the steps of bilirubin metabolism readily reverse when caloric intake is resumed. Conjugation of sulfobromophthalein is also reduced during fasting. Another factor influencing bilirubin conjugation is competition for glucuronic acid. Drugs conjugated as glucuronides during detoxification by the liver compete with bilirubin for glucuronic acid. Microsomal glucuronyl transferase activity is not specific for glucuronidation of bilirubin. Activity of this enzyme is also necessary for the metabolism of testosterone, estradiol, chloramphenicol and morphine. It is possible that the metabolism of each of these substances affects that of the others.

Bile Pigment Excretion[148-150]

Conjugated bilirubin is transported into bile canaliculi by a poorly understood process. A special mechanism may be involved since other anions in high concentration compete for transport. Other evidence suggests that transport is merely passive, with bilirubin movement following a concentration gradient. This scheme proposes that conjugated bilirubin diffuses across membranes in a nonmicellar phase, and, after reaching bile canaliculi, reacts with bile to form micelles, in which it is trapped. This maintains an effective concentration of almost zero for bilirubin on the bile duct side of the membrane, consequently maintaining a gradient for diffusion. This mechanism is supported by the fact that stimulation of bile acid secretion enhances the amount of bilirubin transferred from the hepatocytes. The rate-limiting step in bilirubin uptake, conjugation, and secretion has been assumed to be its transport into bile. Recent evidence identifies conjugation as the rate-limiting step, however. In either case, with liver disease changes in uptake should have less influence on the development of hyperbilirubinemia than do changes in conjugation of bilirubin or its secretion into bile. The liver, having a large reserve capacity to secrete bilirubin, can excrete 30 times the normally small amounts of bilirubin produced daily. Thus, liver disease must be extensive for this reserve to be reduced significantly.

Abnormalities involving only bilirubin secretion are difficult to identify. Defects in secretion in humans are called Dubin-Johnson and Rotor's syndromes. A similar congenital defect is described in Corriedale sheep.[151] When hepatocellular disease impairs bilirubin secretion, the pigment usually found is both conjugated and unconjugated. Finding about half of each is generally considered pathognomonic for hepatocellular disease causing icterus, but that view has to change, as described later. With uptake and conjugation unaffected but secretion inhibited, conjugated bilirubin is regurgitated and appears in plasma. In normal dogs, however, all bilirubin in the plasma is unconjugated. Plasma unconjugated bilirubin can be produced from conjugated bilirubin that is deconjugated by lysosomal beta-glucuronidases released from injured hepatocytes or inflammatory cells invading the liver. In recent studies no significant role was found for glucuronidase deconjugation of bilirubin, however.

Conjugated bilirubin released to the circulation binds albumin but with less affinity than unconjugated bilirubin. Although less than 2% of conjugated bilirubin is filtered at the renal glomerulus, the dog's renal threshold for the pigment is very low, with it almost invariably appearing in the urine; with obstruction of the bile duct, renal excretion becomes important for elimination of the pigment. Renal excretion of bilirubin is not efficient compared with excretion by the biliary system. Unconjugated bilirubin does not appear in urine because the complex it forms with serum albumin is too large to be filtered by the glomerulus. An exception is possible since the kidney can degrade hemoglobin and excrete the unconjugated bilirubin formed in urine. That exception is probably seldom identified, however.

Bile pigments secreted in bile, conjugated primarily as glucuronides, are deconjugated and hydrogenated by large intestinal bacteria, producing a colorless pigment, mesobilirubinogen. That product is subsequently reduced by bacteria to urobilinogen (colorless), which is then oxidized to urobilin or stercobilin (brown). The type of bacteria in the intestine determines the final pigment formed. Small amounts of urobilinogen are absorbed from the intestine and are either resecreted by the liver or eliminated by the kidneys. Conjugation minimizes absorption of bilirubin in the small intestine, and this maximizes its fecal excretion. Appearance of colonic-type bacterial flora in the small intestine, such as with bacterial overgrowth, favors bilirubin deconjugation at a site where unconjugated bilirubin can be readily absorbed. Thus, some intestinal problems can contribute to hyperbilirubinemia.

Urobilinogen binds to plasma proteins, but a small fraction is free and can be filtered by the glomerulus. This pigment can also be secreted by the proximal tubule. Some urobilinogen is reabsorbed in the distal tubule by back-diffusion, which is pH-dependent. More urobilinogen is excreted in alkaline urine. With increasing acidification of urine in the distal nephron, more urobilinogen is absorbed.[152]

Pathophysiology of Bilirubin Metabolism[145,147]

Hyperbilirubinemia. Hyperbilirubinemia (icterus or jaundice) is one of the more pathognomonic signs of hepatic disease. The cause can usually be readily determined with a minimum of diagnostic procedures, although the pathophysiology sometimes remains elusive. Normal and abnormal bilirubin metabolism is of interest because plasma levels of unconjugated and conjugated bilirubin reflect hepatic metabolic and excretory functions, not because those pigments are toxic. Hyperbilirubinemia of short duration causes no clinical signs other than imparting a yellow color to the tissues of the body. One exception, icterus, is toxic in human infants,[153] but is not important in small-animal medicine, where few cases have been reported.[154]

Hyperbilirubinemia results from: 1) production of bilirubin exceeding the liver's capacity for metabolism and excretion; 2) an abnormality in uptake, conjugation, or secretion of bilirubin by hepatocytes; and 3) interference with the excretion of bilirubin through intrahepatic or extrahepatic biliary ducts. The last two causes of hyperbilirubinemia often exist together, producing icterus.

The clinical signs of hyperbilirubinemia are easily recognized by scleral pigmentation when blood levels exceed 2 mg/dl. With levels reaching 4 to 5 mg/dl, a yellowing of unpigmented mucous membranes is apparent. The upper limit of normal plasma bilirubin is somewhat arbitrarily established at about 0.4 to 0.6 mg/dl in the dog and 0.2 mg/dl in the cat; the normal icterus index is less than 5 units. Most normal animals have plasma levels less than 0.2 mg/dl. Early changes in plasma bilirubin can be recognized most easily by determining the icterus index. Most, if not all, of the plasma bilirubin in normal animals is unconjugated.

Increased production of bilirubin as a cause of icterus results from an increased destruction of mature erythrocytes. Hemolytic diseases are usually regarded as the primary cause of decreased erythrocyte life-span. Hemolytic forms are readily identified from the results of a hemogram. Erythrocyte survival is also reduced in most dogs with hepatic disease, and that is explained by cell membrane alterations and hypersplenism.[147] From a normal life span of 94 to 102 days, reductions to a range of 44 to 60 days are found with extrahepatic cholestasis, chronic hepatitis, and cirrhosis, and reductions to a range of 20 to 27 days are seen for acute or fulminant hepatitis and hepatic lymphosarcoma. Increased production of bilirubin from hepatic hemoproteins is less likely an important contributor since the percentage of hemoproteins refluxing from the liver is essentially unchanged with hepatic disease.

Hyperbilirubinemia due to increased bilirubin production is usually thought to reflect increases in unconjugated bilirubin. With hemolytic disease approximately 38% of plasma bilirubin is unconjugated, and that is similar to its levels in dogs with different forms of hepatic disease.[147] Thus, determination of whether bilirubin is largely unconjugated or conjugated is of no value in distinguishing hepatic from nonhepatic causes of hyperbilirubinemia.

Unconjugated hyperbilirubinemia can also be caused by reduced uptake and clearance by hepatocytes. Bilirubin clearance is reduced to 30-50% of normal in most cases of hepatobiliary disease and in primary hemolysis.[147] Reduced clearance results from limits on glucuronidation or secretion of conjugated bilirubin. With decreases in conjugating activity the ratio of monoglucuronide to diglucuronide increases, but that is not seen in the bile of dogs with hepatic disease. Glucuronyltransferase activity changes little with hepatic disease. The rate-limiting metabolic step most important and affected by hepatic disease may well be secretion into the biliary system.

Conjugated hyperbilirubinemia appears when conjugated pigment is not secreted by hepatocytes or when the biliary system is obstructed. Considerable amounts of conjugated pigment must be regurgitated in dogs to increase plasma concentrations significantly. The plasma level of conjugated bilirubin in the dog is relatively low compared to humans because of a more efficient clearance by the liver and a low renal threshold. With excessive regurgitation of bilirubin, hyperbilirubinemia appears later in the dog than in other animals, including man. Thus, slight plasma elevations of the conjugated pigment in dogs suggest hepatocellular disease. Dogs with hepatocellular disease may have normal plasma levels of bilirubin, where the only evidence for excessive regurgitation is large amounts of bilirubin in the urine. Measurement of plasma conjugated bilirubin in dogs does not identify mild cases of regurgitation that readily produce icterus in other species.

Obstruction of the biliary system is the most common cause of conjugated hyperbilirubinemia. Obstruction can be in the liver or can be extrahepatic. Intrahepatic biliary obstruction or cholestasis develops with acute hepatitis, where hepatocyte swelling and inflammatory changes occlude small bile ducts and increase membrane permeability to bilirubin. Chronic inflammation in the portal area and involving bile ducts, bile-duct hyperplasia and biliary cirrhosis results in cholestasis. Hepatic architecture is changed by fibrosis to occlude bile channels. Fibrosis is often striking, and it is not difficult to understand why conjugated hyperbilirubinemia develops. Intrahepatic cholestasis sometimes develops without striking morphological changes in the liver. Mild inflammatory changes produced experimentally in periportal areas of the liver cause marked hyperbilirubinemia.[155] The pathology affects bile flow from canaliculi into larger bile ducts. Severe parenchymal damage inflicted away from periportal areas, however, does not cause hyperbilirubinemia. Loss of normal hepatic architecture in regenerative nodules, can preclude normal bile secretion so that icterus develops.

Extrahepatic biliary obstruction is caused by intra- or extraluminal problems that mechanically obstruct the duct. The most common cause of conjugated hyperbilirubinemia due to extrahepatic obstruction is neoplastic disease in and around the gallbladder and cystic duct. Carcinomas of the pancreas can constrict the cystic duct passing through the pancreas. Neoplasms arising from the lymph tissue or gastrointestinal tissues in the region of the biliary tract can mechanically obstruct the excretory ducts. Other problems causing obstruction from without are abscesses, granulomatous masses, and fibrosis, which can be sequelae to acute pancreatitis.

Less-frequent causes of extrahepatic biliary obstruction are problems involving the walls or lumen of the biliary system that obstruct bile flow. Chronic inflammation sometimes obstructs the bile duct. A hematoma has been reported in the wall of the common bile duct of a cat. Neoplasms of the biliary system also cause obstruction.

The biliary system is seldom obstructed in the dog and cat by intraluminal causes. In humans, cholelithiasis commonly causes obstruction and icterus. Calculi seldom develop in gallbladders of small animals, for reasons discussed later. Intestinal parasites occasionally migrate into and occlude the bile duct.

Extrahepatic icterus also occurs where bile flow is not obstructed, such as with traumatic rupture of the biliary tract, so that bile drains into the peritoneal cavity.

Bilirubin can increase to high plasma levels, exceeding 30 mg/dl, in dogs with hepatic disease. They do not increase to such concentrations following complete obstruction of the bile duct. After increasing to about 5 mg/dl, plasma bilirubin levels plateau for 2-3 weeks and then gradually decrease to near normal. The bilirubin is mostly conjugated, 90% of the total, and being in a water soluble form can be excreted by the kidneys. The daily urinary excretion of 2 mg/kg bilirubin is less than daily production; the difference with unchanging plasma levels is that increase in bilirubin stored in a volume-expanded biliary system.[156] Prevention of biliary excretion of bilirubin by a different means, diversion of bile into the vena cava, results in much greater plasma bilirubin levels than with bile duct ligation. Those results may more closely resemble the hyperbilirubinemia found with hepatic disease.

The capacity of the liver to metabolize bilirubin and maintain normal plasma levels is greater than for many of the liver's other functions. Nitrosamine toxicity results in hyperbilirubinemia and a return to normal plasma bilirubin levels within a few months.[21] Normal levels are maintained by a liver less than half its normal size, one that is unable to maintain normal plasma albumin, glucose and urea levels.

Pathophysiology of Urobilinogen Metabolism.[145] Normally, bilirubin conjugated with glucuronic acid is excreted almost entirely through bile ducts into the intestine. The glucuronide conjugate is a larger and more water-soluble molecule than unconjugated bilirubin. Both of these physical properties minimize intestinal absorption of conjugated bilirubin. Intestinal bacteria transforms bilirubin glucuronide to a number of different compounds. Bacterial glucuronidases begin the transformations by deconjugating bilirubin in the terminal ileum and colon. Other bacterial transformations produce pigmented compounds and a colorless one, urobilinogen. The clinical significance of these compounds is related to the color they impart to feces and to the appearance of urobilinogen in urine after its absorption from the intestine.

Since fecal color requires both bilirubin and bacterial activity to change bilirubin to different-colored pigments, a lack of fecal pigmentation can reflect a deficiency of either biliary secretions or bacterial activity in the intestine. Only small amounts of bile pigments are needed to impart normal color to the feces, and complete biliary obstruction is usually required for stools to become acholic, a sign not usually seen until long after clinical signs of icterus appear. Obstruction is seldom so complete that no bile can be released into the small intestine. Fecal color can change with antibiotics, diarrhea and different diets, causing numbers and activity of intestinal bacteria to change, which may alter bilirubin metabolism in the intestine to change fecal color.

Urobilinogen is formed from bilirubin by the action of intestinal anaerobic bacteria (Figure 28-16). Urobilinogen is not produced in germfree rats, and antibiotics suppressing the intestinal microflora can cause its disappearance from the urine in conventional animals. Considerable amounts of bilirubin are reduced to urobilinogen, which is largely lost in the feces, although some is absorbed from the ileum and colon. After absorption, the liver removes urobilinogen from the portal circulation and secretes it into the bile. The liver has a large capacity for taking up urobilinogen, which does not require conjugation for secretion. Plasma urobilinogen not removed by the liver is excreted in the urine. Urobilinogen is freely filtered at the glomerulus and is secreted by the proximal tubule. Some is passively reabsorbed in the distal nephron. The quantity of urobilinogen reabsorbed is greater when urine is acid, a pH at which the pigment is largely un-ionized and, being more lipid-soluble, readily crosses lipid cell membranes and is absorbed.

Semiquantitation of urinary urobilinogen is often used for differential diagnosis of hepatobiliary problems. Urinary levels are determined by factors influencing its rate of formation in the intestine. Large amounts of bilirubin, the precursor of urobilinogen, are formed during hemolysis, which increases the urinary excretion of urobilinogen. With increased numbers of bacteria in the small intestine, bilirubin is reduced to urobilinogen sooner than in the usual sites of ileum and colon. More urobilinogen is absorbed since its absorption is more efficient from the small intestine than from the colon. Both the hepatic uptake of urobilinogen from the circulation and its biliary secretion are decreased with hepatocellular disease, causing renal excretion to increase. Conversely, suppression of intestinal bacterial numbers may result in no pigment appearing in the urine. With fairly complete biliary obstruction, little or no urobilinogen is detected in urine, and with diarrhea little is absorbed from the intestine. Renal function determines the amount of urobilinogen appearing in the urine. Its rate of renal excretion is determined by fluid balance and the degree of urine acidification. Little urobilinogen is detected in very dilute urine. In addition, very little appears when oliguria accompanies renal shutdown or when the glomerular filtration rate is reduced by chronic renal disease. Urine acidified in the distal nephron loses appreciable amounts of urobilinogen by reabsorption. Urobilinogen is rapidly oxidized to urobilin by light at room temperature, and urobilin does not react in the Ehrlich test.

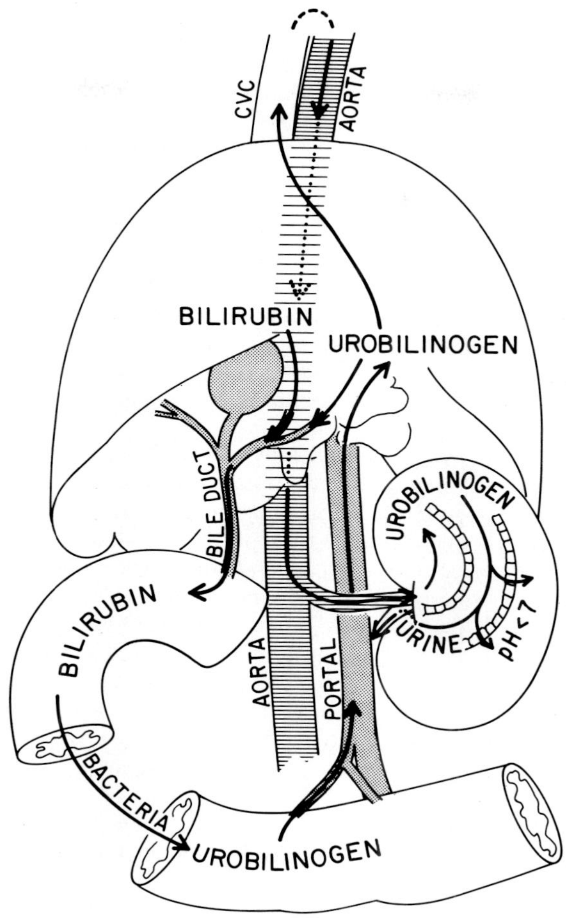

Figure 28-16. Schematic showing metabolism of urobilinogen. Urobilinogen, formed from bilirubin by intestinal bacteria, is absorbed from the intestine and secreted into bile or excreted by the kidneys (a pH determined process).

Urinary Excretion of Bilirubin Conjugates.[145] Unconjugated bilirubin is bound to plasma proteins, and since it is not filtered at the glomerulus it does not appear in urine. Conjugated bilirubin is filtered and represents essentially all of the urinary bilirubin. The amount of bilirubin in the urine generally reflects plasma levels. In dogs, however, urine levels must be interpreted with the knowledge that the renal threshold for conjugated bilirubin is very low; bile is found regularly in normal dog urine, with the low renal threshold maintaining low plasma conjugated bilirubin levels. Increased bilirubin production increases urinary levels before plasma levels increase. Since fasting causes hyperbilirubinemia, bile appears regularly in urine from anorectic patients. Hyperbilirubinuria is also found with fever, hepatic disease, and biliary obstruction. Large amounts of bilirubin in dilute urine are likely to be significant. High concentrations of bile in urine with a high specific gravity is often unremarkable. Conjugated bilirubin is not normally found in the urine of cats.

The renal proximal tubule is able to absorb the hemoglobin sometimes found in the glomerular filtrate. This hemoglobin is converted to bilirubin in renal epithelial cells and subsequently excreted in the urine. Thus, bilirubin in the urine can result from hemoglobin filtered and metabolized by the kidney. This bilirubin is not conjugated.

Clinical Correlations. Early hyperbilirubinemia is identified with the icterus index, while more advanced stages are identified through physical examination or are recognized by the owner. Primary unconjugated bilirubinemia due to a hemolytic disease is identified with a hemogram. When conjugated pigment is more than half of the total, the cause can be either hemolytic or hepatocellular disease. With extrahepatic biliary obstruction, bilirubin is mostly conjugated. These generalities are unreliable, however. The commonly used methods for measuring plasma bilirubin have limitations and provide only estimates of their concentrations. Variations of the diazo reaction used most often provide unreliable measurements that are greatest for that of conjugated bilirubin. Where only unconjugated bilirubin is present, the diazo test can identify 65% of the pigment as being conjugated. Thus, the test cannot be used for differential quantitation of different bilirubins. In addition, the diazo test returns considerably higher values for total bilirubin levels than actually exist. Thus, at best, determination of plasma bilirubin provides an estimation of whether or not hyperbilirubinemia is a problem.

Plasma bilirubin levels also are influenced by renal function and bilirubin urinary excretion, and by intestinal disease with bacterial overgrowth that may be deconjugating bilirubin and allowing its absorption to increase. As described earlier, drugs and other chemicals can affect bilirubin metabolism, and that must be considered when evaluating the patient with hyperbilirubinemia.

Drug, Steroid and Peptide Hormone Metabolism[157-160]

Physiology

Drugs. Many chemicals affect physiologic function in the body, the extent of the effect being related to the chemical's concentration at the site of action. That level is determined by the chemical's rate of release or introduction into the body, extent that it reaches the circulation and distributes to various tissues, binding to extracellular and intracellular proteins, and rate of elimination from the body. All of these may be influenced by hepatic function. The liver is important for the metabolic regulation of endogenous substances, such as steroid and peptide hormones, and waste products, such as phenol, indole, and skatole. It is also important for regulation and elimination of exogenous chemicals, such as most drugs.

Drugs introduced orally are readily absorbed if they are relatively small or are lipid soluble, un-ionized at the pH of intestinal contents. A readily absorbed drug is not one that necessarily reaches optimum blood concentrations after oral administration. The liver may have the ability to extract most of a chemical in the portal flow from the intestine, in which case it may not be practical to produce therapeutic levels from oral administration; in such cases drugs are given by an injectable route. Chemicals distribute in tissues according to their size, with larger molecules restricted to the plasma compartment, and their lipid-solubility, with lipid-soluble chemicals distributing to the intracellular as well as extracellular compartment.

Drug concentrations in the body are determined more importantly by their processes of elimination than those of absorption because absorption is usually relatively more rapid. The liver and kidneys handle elimination for most drugs. The liver primarily metabolizes drugs to water soluble metabolites, and the kidney primarily excretes drugs without biotransformation or after they have been metabolized by the liver. Many drugs administered in a highly polar form are not metabolized in the body.

Lipid-soluble chemicals are generally not eliminated from the body until converted to a water-soluble form. The kidneys are then able to excrete a chemical that would be reabsorbed when the chemical's lipid-soluble form passed through renal tubules from which it is readily reabsorbed. Thus, the lipid solubility that facilitates a chemical's absorption from the intestinal tract prevents its excretion through the kidney. The liver converts lipid-soluble substances to a water-soluble form able to be readily excreted in urine or bile from, which they are not easily reabsorbed.

The transformation of drugs from lipid- to water-solubility requires two metabolic steps. The important site for most metabolic changes is the liver's smooth endoplasmic reticulum, although some drug metabolism occurs in nonhepatic tissues. The initial metabolic changes alter drugs by introducing hydroxyl, carboxyl, amine, or sulfhydryl groups. This metabolism begins by the drug's binding to cytochrome P-450, a hemoprotein component of the endoplasmic reticulum. The drug is metabolized by cytochrome P-450, in conjunction with a cytochrome-c reductase. This metabolic process alters the drug in one of a number of ways. It can change the drug into a different compound with similar or different pharmacological activities. It can activate an inactive compound, or inactivate an active drug. In the second phase, drug metabolites formed in the initial step are conjugated with glucuronides, sulfates, and some amino acids. The side groups created in step one provide the site for conjugation. Methylation and acetylation of drugs are other means of metabolic transformations that occur in this phase.

The hepatic elimination of chemicals is determined by the activity of these enzymes and the availability of substrates for conjugation. Their activity can be induced, augmented, or inhibited by a variety of chemicals (Table 28-7). Induction of microsomal enzyme activity by such chemicals will increase the metabolic transformation of others converted by this enzyme system. That effect persists for two to three weeks after the induction ceases. Such induction also increases hepatic mass by an increase in microsomal smooth endoplasmic reticulum structure; whether that can be appreciated in an apparent increase in overall liver size is debatable.

The hepatic elimination of a chemical is also determined by

Table 28-7. Chemicals Inducing, Augmenting, or Inhibiting Hepatic Microsomal Enzymes.

Inducers	Inhibitors
Chlorcyclizine	Allopurinol
Chlorinated hydrocarbons	Chloramphenicol
Diphenhydramine	Cimetidine
Griseofulvin	Iproniazid
Meprobamate	Methylphenidate
Nikethamide	Morphine
Pentobarbital	Organophosphate insecticides
Phenobarbital	Oxyphenbutazone
Phenylbutazone	Quinidine
Phenytoin	Quinine
Polycyclic hydrocarbons	

hepatic blood flow and the capacity or ability of the liver to extract it from the circulation. Chemicals usually circulate bound to protein; only the free unbound chemical exerts a pharmacologic effect. Hepatic uptake is also only for unbound forms and depends on size and lipid solubility; to some extent it also depends on hepatic metabolic conversion rate. The influence of binding to a plasma protein determines a chemical's availability. The availability is determined by the binding protein's concentration, number of binding sites, and strength of binding to the chemical. Avidly bound chemicals are eliminated more slowly; only the free form is available to be metabolized. Thus, their effect is longer lasting. Different chemicals often compete for binding, so their mutual presence will affect each one's rate of elimination.

When strong binding factors are important determinants of clearance, a chemical is described as having a low-extraction ratio. Hepatic clearance rates depend on the degree of protein binding for chemicals that are highly bound, and only the free form can be extracted by the liver. Reductions in binding protein, i.e. hypoalbuminemia, or competitive displacement of binding by other chemicals results in more rapid clearance of chemicals at greater levels in the unbound form. In such cases, the chemical can also be available to exert a pharmacologic or toxic effect, but for a shorter time because clearance is faster.

Clearance of chemicals readily extracted by the liver is determined more by hepatic blood flow. Reduced blood flow caused by cardiac disease or chronic hepatic disease can result in greatly decreased clearance of such chemicals, and clearance rate increases with increased hepatic blood flow. Chemicals not highly extracted by the liver are relatively insensitive to changes in hepatic blood flow.

Adrenal Steroids.[161,162] Natural and synthetic steroid hormones are metabolized in the liver. Adrenocortical hormones are lipid-soluble and must be converted to biologically inactive water-soluble derivatives before excretion by the kidneys. This transformation is achieved by reduction of the 4,3-ene group of ring A to inactivate the hormone, and by subsequent conjugation with glucuronide or sulfate to render it water-soluble. Drugs may be inert in the form given and changed by the liver to become active. Prednisone is such a drug, converted to biologically active prednisolone by reduction of the 11-oxy group.

Steroids bind to serum albumin and to transcortin, a corticosteroid-binding globulin produced by the liver. A reduction in the amounts of plasma-binding proteins results in elevated levels of unbound steroids in plasma. That increases the likelihood of a steroid overdose since unbound steroids are biologically active, in contrast to the bound, which are not.

Aldosterone, a natural mineralocorticoid, is also inactivated and rendered water-soluble in the liver by reduction of the A-ring and conjugation with a water-soluble compound. This function is reduced by hepatic disease, whereupon blood levels of aldosterone can increase. In contrast, plasma levels of endogenous glucocorticoids usually remain normal with liver disease because high plasma levels of aldosterone do not feed back to inhibit hormone release from the adrenal gland, whereas corticosteroids can. The primary signal for aldosterone release is renin, which is also metabolized in the liver. The state of renal blood perfusion controls the release of renin. Renal blood flow is often completely independent of any influence exerted by blood levels of aldosterone. Thus, if aldosterone synthesis and release is continuous, its rate of hepatic degradation is important in maintaining normal blood levels.

Sex Steroids.[162,163] Reproductive hormones produced in tissues other than the pituitary or placenta are steroid hormones, which are largely metabolized by the liver before excretion.

Androgens are metabolized by the liver before excretion, in urine (primarily) and in bile. Enzymes catalyze the reversible conversion of testosterone to a product containing a ketone group at carbon-17 instead of a hydroxyl group. Reductases catalyze the addition of hydrogens in ring-A. Hydrogenases participate in the reversible interconversion of 3-hydroxy and 3-beta derivatives. Conjugation with glucuronides or sulfates completes the inactivation and solubilization of androgens so they can be excreted. Total plasma testosterone is often decreased in humans with chronic hepatic disease. Testicular secretion of testosterone is markedly reduced; because the concentration of testosterone's plasma binding protein is increased, there is less biologically available testosterone, and tissues are deprived of its influence. Increases in plasma binding delay testosterone metabolic clearance, and so near normal plasma levels are possible with reduced availability for hormonal effects. Testosterone is also converted to estradiol in nonhepatic tissues; an increase in this conversion with hepatic disease may also contribute to decreased plasma testosterone.

Estrogens are metabolized in the liver for inactivation and excretion. Beta-estradiol, the natural ovarian hormone, is interconverted with estrones, estriol, and other estradiols in the liver. Different enzymes catalyze oxidation, reduction, and methylation reactions, producing a number of different metabolites that are subsequently excreted as glucuronide and sulfate conjugates. Liver disease should reduce the capacity for such metabolic transformation, but that has not been demonstrated for humans with hepatic disease. Estrogens are normally produced in males as well as females by the conversion of testosterone to estradiol, and blood levels can increase in males with liver disease, causing changes in secondary sexual characteristics. But plasma estrogen levels are often normal with hepatic disease, which may reflect an increase only in tissue levels of estrogens or possibly an increase in tissue estrogen receptors, something shown to happen in experimental animals with hepatic disease. Metabolites of estrogens which retain some biological activity can be increased in humans with hepatic disease. Bile provides an important means for the excretion of all estrogens. Some estrogen metabolites in bile are absorbed in the small intestine, resulting in an enterohepatic circulation of estrogens. These estrogens are biologically active when given orally. The enterohepatic cycling of estrogens may be important in maintaining high plasma levels of biologically active compounds. Like androgens, estrogens are excreted in urine.

Progesterone is metabolized chiefly in the liver, by reduction of the A-ring and coupling with glucuronic acid, forming pregnanediol, which is excreted in urine. In contrast to some of the androgens and estrogens, neither progesterone nor pregnanediol impairs liver function, as determined by sulfobromophthalein retention, or interferes with bile secretion. Progesterone is the precursor in the biosynthesis of androgens, estrogens, and adrenal steroid hormones. Progesterone has salt-retaining properties resulting from its structural similarity to mineralocorticoids.

Pathophysiology.[164-166] The most important site in the body for the metabolism and detoxification of drugs is the hepatic microsomal enzyme system. Some drugs and their metabolites formed, by hepatic enzymes, produce liver damage which reduces drug catabolism and excretion. Primary hepatic disease also reduces drug metabolism, so that plasma and tissue levels are abnormally high following the administration of therapeutic doses. Thus, drugs cause hepatopathies, and impaired hepatic function reduces drug inactivation and excretion.

Damage by drugs can produce severe hepatic necrosis, chronic hepatitis, or relatively mild lesions that are associated with few if any clinical signs. The changes can include hepatocyte damage, cholestasis, or a mixture of the two. In small animals the importance of drug or chemical-induced hepatopathies has been largely unknown, but more cases have been reported in the last decade; as a result, some drugs have been well-documented as potential hepatotoxins.

Most drugs, like other chemicals foreign to the body, would be toxic if they were not given at a safe dose and if they could not be eliminated from the body. The agent's effects are usually eliminated by biotransformation to a nontoxic compound. In some cases a nontoxic agent can be converted to a potentially toxic product. If metabolism increases for this conversion, the level of toxic products can increase to that necessary for hepatic damage. The metabolic biotransformation of most chemicals involves oxidizing isoenzymes of cytochrome P-450. Activity of these enzymes is increased by other chemicals, such as phenobarbital, which they metabolize. That activity increases twelve- to fourteen-fold after four days of phenobarbital; with longer treatment it can increase ninty-fold and increase susceptibility to the effects of a hepatotoxin given at a nontoxic dose. The biotransformation and elimination of a potentially toxic drug can also be delayed in the presence of another chemical competing with it for metabolism by the cytochrome P-450 enzymes.

Host factors influence the possibility of toxic and drug-induced hepatitis. Reaction to certain drugs is recognized for certain species and breeds of animals; thus there may be a genetic factor determining drug-induced hepatitis. In humans, females appear to be more vulnerable than males to drug-induced disease. Also in humans, age can be a factor, susceptibility to some drugs being greater with advancing age and to others being greater in young individuals. Nutritional status is another factor; feeding a high protein diet stimulates cytochrome P-450 activity and increases the risk for hepatic damage upon administration of a drug metabolized to a toxic compound by that enzyme system. Feeding diets deficient in the antioxidant vitamin E increases the risk for damage by peroxidation when a drug capable of that result is given. Obesity also increases susceptibility to drugs that are converted to hepatotoxins under conditions of relative hypoxia in the liver. A variety of diseases which alter hepatic metabolism by affecting oxygen or glucose availability affect the metabolism of drugs, and that can also lead to drug-induced hepatic damage.

Chemicals that can predictably produce hepatic damage are called intrinsic hepatotoxins. Other chemicals that can damage the liver but not predictably, are called idiosyncratic hepatotoxins. Intrinsic hepatotoxins consistently produce lesions in experimental animals, and the effects are dose dependent. Idiosyncratic hepatoxins do not produce lesions in experimental animals but only in susceptible individuals, and the effect of the chemical is not dose related.

Intrinsic and Idiosyncratic Hepatotoxins. A hepatotoxin can damage a hepatocyte and its organelles by a direct physicochemical effect that is mediated by peroxidation of membrane lipids and by other chemical changes that lead to membrane distortion and destruction. Either the chemical or its metabolic products can cause the damage. Less severe damage is characterized by hepatic lipidosis. Lipid accumulates when lipoprotein and apolipoprotein production are reduced and moreso if adipose lipid is mobilized and transported to the liver. With greater damage, intracellular calcium increases and is associated with cell necrosis. Carbon tetrachloride, a direct hepatotoxin, produces primarily centrolobular lesions because that location is the richest source of enzymes for its metabolism and formation of free radicals. Other such toxins are phosphorus, which produces a periportal lesion, and chloroform. No hepatotoxic drugs in current use exert their effect by a direct means.

Intrinsic hepatotoxins can damage hepatocytes indirectly, by selective interference with a specific metabolic pathway or a component maintaining normal structure. Structural damage develops indirectly and follows the metabolic disruption or interference with a select cellular function. The hepatotoxins interaction with cell molecules leads to diversion, competitive inhibition, or structural distortion of molecules essential for metabolism, or to interference with specific metabolic pathways necessary for maintaining structural integrity. The biochemical lesions of indirect hepatotoxins most commonly cause lipidosis and necrosis (Table 28-8). The pathogenesis of lipidosis is similar to that produced by direct toxins; lipids are not metabolized or able to be mobilized from hepatocytes, and greater amounts of adipose lipids may be mobilized and transported to the liver. Hepatic necrosis is produced by the indirect hepatotoxin's or its metabolite's depleting the cell of UTP, alkalating or arylating cell macromolecules, or attaching to cell membranes (Figure 28-17). Alkylation or arylation of DNA by indirect hepatotoxins can produce hepatic carcinoma.

Intrinsic hepatotoxins can interfere with hepatic bilirubin metabolism and be potentially cholestatic. Prolonged administration of organic arsenicals, chlorpromazine, erythromycin, and anabolic steroids can produce cholestasis. In general, steroids with an alkyl group at carbon 17 have the ability to

Table 28-8. Indirect Toxins Causing Necrosis and Lipidosis

Hepatotoxin	Action
Phalloidin	Binds to membranes
Paracetamol Bromobenzene	Arylation of cell proteins
Nitrosamines	Alkylation of cell molecules
Tetracycline	Blocks tRNA
Ethionine	Depletes ATP
Galactosamine	Depletes UTP
Arsenic	Binds thiol group
Aflatoxin Pyrrolizidine	Binds cell molecules

produce icterus by selectively interfering with the mechanisms that remove substances from the blood and secrete them into the bile. These steroids include anabolic derivatives of testosterone and derivatives of estradiol. Some of the other drugs produce cholestasis by damaging the ductal system. The development of cholestasis with bile casts is dependent on drug dose and can generally be readily produced in experimental animals.

Drugs which are unpredictable in damaging the liver are called idiosyncratic hepatotoxins. Appearing in a small population of patients, the hepatotoxicity is an expression of individual susceptibility. It can be a drug hypersensitivity in which the sensitization develops over a period of weeks. An allergic reaction manifested by fever, skin manifestations, and eosinophilia is possible. Liver involvement may not be apparent unless icterus develops. Drugs shown to cause hepatic disease in humans by an allergic reaction include phenytoin, sulfonamides, chlorpromazine, halothane, and possibly methoxyflurane. Methoxyflurane usually has no harmful effects on hepatic function in dogs.[167] Other drugs injure the liver without causing any clinical manifestation. Some drugs usually causing mild hepatic changes can cause severe hepatic changes with added factors. For example, halothane hepatotoxicity is an unusual clinical problem, but it can be readily produced by pretreatment with phenobarbital or hypoxia. Idiosyncrasy to a drug can also be explained by a metabolic abnormality in which the drug is converted to a hepatotoxic rather than nontoxic metabolite. Halothane is one such example. Hepatic injuries caused by drug idiosyncrasies are characterized by low incidence, prolonged or repeated exposure to the drug, and hepatotoxic morphological changes in the liver.

Mechanisms of Toxicity. The specific mechanisms for drug hepatotoxicity are largely unknown. In many cases the drug is not toxic at therapeutic levels, becoming toxic only at very high doses. For example, the analgesic acetaminophen is detoxified in the liver by conjugating its metabolites with the sulfhydryl tripeptide glutathione. If the latter is not available, the metabolite, being a reactive alkylating or arylating agent, will bind to tissue macromolecules to form chemically stable substances that cause tissue necrosis (Figure 28-17).[168] In this case, pretreatment with barbiturates will increase the activity of microsomal enzymes, so that subsequent administration of the analgesic results in an increased rate of metabolism of the acetaminophen. Administration of pentothal as a sedative just prior to acetaminophen worsens the hepatic necrosis seen without that sedative. As a result, toxic metabolites are formed faster than glutathione can be supplied for conjugation and detoxification. (Acetaminophen can also induce granulomatous hepatic lesions, suggesting hypersensitivity is one means for expression of the hepatotoxicity.) In animals, glutathione appears to be essential for the protection of tissues against a variety of toxic drug metabolites and other alkylating agents. Furosemide is normally conjugated with glucuronide and metabolized to nontoxic derivatives. However, the drug can also be converted to toxic arylating metabolites that are capable of covalently binding to tissue macromolecules. Depletion of the supply of glutathione causes more covalent binding of furosemide metabolites with cell proteins.

Microsomal enzyme activity is essential for the formation of many toxic metabolites. Metabolic activation of halothane is required for hepatotoxicity.[169] Toxic products are produced by the approximately 20% of halothane that is metabolized. Pretreatment with phenobarbital to increase cytochrome P-450 cytochrome oxidase activity augments metabolism of halothane. With reduced oxygen tension halothane is not oxidized but is reduced after binding to the cytochrome, and the product is a hepatotoxin. The metabolite formed binds covalently to cellular macromolecules. At low oxygen tension, halothane also induces lipid peroxidation. Inhibitors of microsomal enzyme activity prevent the toxic effects of some drugs. For example, dibenamine inhibits this activity and reduces the toxicity produced by carbon tetrachloride, since less is converted to free radicals and chloroform.

Effects of Liver Disease on Drugs Disposition. The blood levels of drugs are determined by the dose, rate of absorption,

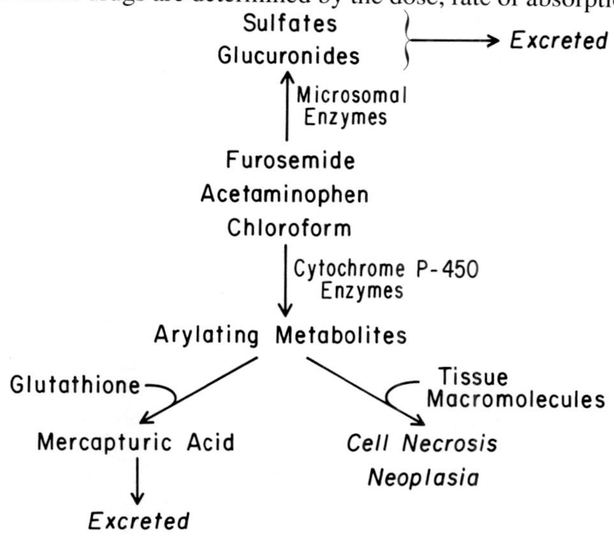

Figure 28-17. Mechanism for drug induced hepatic necrosis and neoplasia. Drugs can be conjugated and excreted or metabolized to metabolites that bind to tissue macromolecules. Ample availability of glutathione prevents toxicity by enabling the metabolites to be catabolized for excretion.

rate of inactivation, and rate of excretion.[170-171] The rates of inactivation and excretion are interrelated in that many drugs cannot be excreted until they are transformed into a water-soluble metabolite. Hepatic disease alters blood and tissue levels of both drugs and endogenous steroids.

Both the half-life and the biological activity of a drug can be affected by hepatic parenchymal disease. Liver disease increases half-lives for antibiotics, narcotics, barbiturates, tranquilizers, and antiinflammatory agents such as phenylbutazone and corticosteroids. With liver disease, factors influencing the elimination of a drug from the body by the liver include plasma protein binding, hepatic blood flow, and intrinsic ability of the liver to take up and excrete a drug.

Hepatic disease frequently causes a reduction in the plasma proteins synthesized by the liver. When hypoproteinemia results, less drug is bound in plasma, which increases its biological activity. Unbound drugs are cleared more rapidly if they do not require hepatic metabolic conversion before excretion. The clearance of drugs from the plasma is a function of blood flow through the liver; hence, either reductions in hepatic blood flow or circulatory bypass of the liver prolongs the half-life of drugs metabolized there. Drug clearance is also a function of the liver's capacity to remove and metabolize a drug. Thus, a pharmaceutical agent not metabolized at a normal rate by a diseased liver is retained for a longer time in the body.

Drug disposal is influenced not only by hepatic disease but by nutrition. When nutritional intake is maintained, a diseased liver metabolizes drugs more completely than during starvation. The duration of therapeutic blood and tissue levels is also influenced by the drug dose and whether another drug is competing for metabolism in the diseased liver. All factors increasing a drug's half-life must be considered in determining proper doses. Patients with hepatic disease are easily overdosed with some drugs.[170]

Normal hepatic metabolism is necessary to convert at least one drug from an inactive to active form.[161] Prednisone is not biologically active until the liver converts it to prednisolone. The liver also conjugates corticosteroids in preparation for excretion. Corticosteroids bind to plasma proteins, and their biological activity should change in patients with hypoproteinemia. Hepatic disease in dogs does not appear to significantly affect prednisone metabolism, either its conversion to prednisolone or clearance from the body; prednisone is effective in managing chronic hepatitis. Data from humans with chronic active hepatitis show no changes in the half-life and clearance of prednisone when compared with healthy controls. Thus there is no evidence that the selection of prednisone or its dose should be modified in the treatment of chronic hepatitis in dogs.

The clearance of highly extracted drugs is affected more and in a more predictable way than of poorly extracted drugs. The former is determined more by hepatic blood flow than hepatic function or plasma protein binding. Hepatic disease reduces effective blood flow to the liver by reductions in total flow and by intrahepatic or extrahepatic shunts that result in part of the flow bypassing the liver. Chronic liver disease in humans increases half-lives for highly extracted drugs to the extent that recommendations are made to reduce the dose by at least 50 percent. The amount of drug needed to achieve a desired plasma concentration does not change, but the rate of administration is reduced to compensate for the reduced clearance and to maintain the desired level.

The clearance of a poorly extracted drug is affected more by changes in its plasma protein binding and in the intrinsic ability of the liver for its elimination. Hepatic disease affects that clearance less predictably. Unchanged, decreased, or even increased drug clearance is reported for humans with hepatic disease. Changes in plasma binding may alter clearance of a drug but not its pharmacologic effect. That can happen when binding changes result in plasma clearance changes that alter total plasma drug but not unbound-drug concentrations. With no change in unbound-drug levels, no changes are needed in drug dosage. When clearance of unbound drugs decreases, the dosage must be reduced.

The sex steroid hormones are an important group of lipids metabolized by the liver.[172] If they are not converted to an excretable form, their levels can increase. Prolonged or exaggerated effects are possible from sex hormones administered to a patient with reduced liver function. Another type of response is seen in male dogs with a liver that cannot metabolize the normal physiological amounts of hormones produced each day. In this case, the liver is unable to conjugate and excrete the small amounts of estrogens normally produced in the adrenal gland and testes. Estrogen blood levels may increase, causing gynecomastia, hair loss, and testicular atrophy. Furthermore, androgens, also produced in the adrenals and testes, can be converted to estrogens and add to the problem. Transformation of androgens to estrogens is increased with hepatic disease,[173] and biliary excretion of estrogens is decreased, as is their conjugation with sulfate or glucuronic acid. As with other steroid hormones, the biological effect of estrogen is presumably determined by the amounts free in the plasma, thus being related to plasma protein levels.

Peptide Hormones. The gastrointestinal tract is a rich source of peptide hormones that regulate and integrate gastrointestinal functions. For many peptide hormones, the liver is an important site of metabolic degradation. The liver thereby determines their half-lives and consequently their blood levels. Most gastrointestinal peptide hormones are produced for a local physiologic effect. Some are degraded before they leave the intestine. Those released from the intestine must pass through the liver, where most are removed. The liver removes approximately 50% of the insulin and 80% of glucagon activity on their first pass through the liver. Peptide hormones escaping hepatic removal are usually catabolized in the kidneys and gastrointestinal tract. Hepatic insufficiency causes their plasma levels to increase by increasing their half-lives, and that may result in clinical signs from pathology in the gastrointestinal tract before those from liver disease. Plasma gastrin levels increase with hepatic disease; that helps to explain the gastric ulcers that sometimes develop. Carbohydrate metabolism is abnormal in animals with portasystemic shunts, and hypoglycemia can become a problem. Part of the loss of homeostasis in that metabolism is due to abnormal insulin and glucagon levels because of altered hepatic hormone clearance. For hormones avidly taken up by the liver a change in hepatic blood flow is more important than hepatic insufficiency in influencing blood levels. Shunting of portal circulation away from the liver greatly increases the blood levels of such hormones. In summary, it is evident that normal liver function and circulation are mandatory for the homeostasis maintained by humoral agents, the levels of which are partly controlled by the liver.

Clinical Correlations. With intrinsic or idiosyncratic drug reactions, clinical signs of acute hepatitis appear. Nonspecific signs such as vomiting, polydipsia, and abdominal pain can be accompanied by icterus. Drugs with cholestatic effects may result in icterus as the only sign. Prolonged cholestasis can be associated with signs of chronic hepatitis and loss of normal liver function.

The increase of the half-life of drugs or hormones from hepatic disease is often important in producing clinical signs. The signs often appear in patients given an anesthetic agent or sedative, where its effects are prolonged. Thus, a surgery case that requires 24 to 48 hours to recover from anesthesia may have a markedly reduced hepatic capacity to metabolize anesthetic agents. Another example suggesting hepatic dysfunction is sedation that persists for several days after a tranquilizer is administered. A drug such as phenylbutazone can cause serious anemia, which is a greater threat when there is a reduced hepatic capacity to metabolize the drug to an excretable form for maintenance of therapeutic blood levels.

Hyperadrenocorticism can be produced iatrogenically by normal doses of glucocorticoids given patients with hepatic disease. Thus, clinical signs of Cushing's syndrome can result from liver disease. Polydipsia, polyuria, hair loss, and redistribution of body fat appear. Cushing's syndrome is likely only in animals with a diseased liver than cannot metabolize a normal dose of an active steroid.

Gynecomastia, testicular atrophy, and hair loss are clinical signs associated with the hyperestrogenism that may accompany liver disease. Normal plasma levels of androgens do not aid in restoring the normal male appearance, and they can contribute to the signs if androgens are converted to estrogens in significant amounts. Clinical signs can appear from elevated blood levels of hormones secreted by organs of the gastrointestinal tract. These hormones primarily affect secretion and motility.

Mononuclear Phagocytic System and Catabolic Function[174]

The mononuclear phagocytic (reticuloendothelial) system in the liver is important for the removal of many endogenous and foreign substances from the circulation that may be either harmful or are no longer needed.

They include inert metabolizable foreign material, effete autologous tissue debris, antigens, cholesterol, hemoglobin, denatured proteins, drugs, steroids, microaggregates of fibrin, and endotoxins or exotoxins. The mononuclear phagocytic system (MPS) also metabolizes some of these substances. Only a small part of the capacity of the MPS is normally used, leaving a large reserve available to remove a heavy load of substances from the circulation.

The MPS is situated as a barrier across the main avenues that foreign substances follow after gaining entrance into the body. The sites most accessible to their entry are the intestine and lungs. Phagocytic function to clear blood of the many substances is found in spleen and lymph nodes. The hepatic MPS in its Kupffer cells contributes more than the total of all others to the vascular clearance capacity. With depression of hepatic MPS activity, the other sites can compensate by increasing their activity.

A number of individual factors contribute to overall MPS activity. Total Kupffer cell activity is proportional to hepatic blood flow; an increase in hepatic portal perfusion increases that activity. Liver and spleen mass relative to total body mass determines MPS activity. Animals with a relatively large liver and spleen have greater activity. Metabolic activity of hepatic cells determines clearance of blood. Phagocytosis by Kupffer cells is an active process dependent on the availability of oxygen, glucose, and other sources of energy.

Clearance by the MPS is also determined by opsonins, specific serum antibodies, and the properties of the particles to be phagocytized. Opsonins, called recognition factors, are like natural antibodies; fibronectin is the major "nonspecific opsonin."[175] They are plasma proteins that coat unwanted substances so they can be phagocytized. Opsonins increase phagocytic rates and may be important in partly mediating recognition in nonimmune animals. Specific antibodies also interact with antigens to form complexes that increase vascular clearance of antigens by the MPS.

A number of factors affect function within individual Kupffer cells. For example, estrogens, endotoxin, and BCG (*Bacillus Calmette-Guerin*) potently stimulate MPS function, whereas cortisone potently depresses it. Phagocytosis is determined also by: 1) the size of the phagocytized particle, with a larger particle being cleared faster than a smaller one; 2) the amount of the particles to be cleared, since the MPS can be saturated; and 3) the particle properties, such as surface charge and configuration. The amount of particle phagocytized is important in that large amounts of material engulfed by the MPS prevent the uptake of additional material, resulting in blockade. Opsonins are largely consumed during overload with foreign materials.

Function can be activated or depressed by numerous endogenous and exogenous factors that become very important in a number of pathologic processes. Clearance by the MPS is altered during hemorrhagic shock, traumatic shock, endotoxic shock, tumor growth, bacterial infection, viral infection, atherosclerosis, radiation injury, autoimmune disease, immunologic depression, starvation and any condition reducing hepatic circulation. An increase in MPS function is the normal host-defense response to bacterial infections, neoplastic disease, and autoimmune diseases, which suggests that MPS function is regulated. On the other hand, MPS activity is depressed by circulatory failure (as seen with shock), which contributes to the pathogenesis of shock.

Substances reaching the MPS after absorption from the intestine include microorganisms and their endotoxins, enterotoxins, and exotoxins; undegraded nutrients; and chemicals ingested. The MPS participates in the metabolism and occasional storage of these substances. The MPS also removes and metabolizes hormones and chylomicrons from the gastrointestinal tract. The MPS is important for maintaining a normal immunologic state. It removes antigenic substances, primarily proteins, and processes them for the development of oral tolerance. Blocking MPS uptake of these substances prevents the development of oral tolerance, and hypersensitivity to such antigens can develop. The phagocytozing and storage capacity of the MPS is limited; saturation of the MPS allows foreign substances to escape to the circulation. Escape is also seen when hepatic disease or diversion of portal flow to bypass the liver reduces MPS capacity.

Whereas the hepatic MPS renders antigenic material from

the intestine nonimmunogenic, activity in lymph nodes and often MPS promotes the development of immune responses to antigenic substances. The predominance of antigens exposed to one or another determines whether oral tolerance or hypersensitivity develops. Diversion of antigens from MPS activity of the liver to that of lymph nodes and spleen increases hypersensitivity to the diverted substances. Such diversion is caused by portasystemic shunting of portal flow away from the liver, hepatic disease that reduces clearance capacity of the hepatic MPS, and any of the problems and drugs described earlier that reduce hepatic MPS activity. That complication is illustrated by an endotoxemia that can complicate hepatic disease. Bacterial endotoxin, normally absorbed in small quantities from the intestine, is removed from the portal circulation by the liver. Hepatic disease can allow some endotoxin to escape phagocytosis by hepatic Kuppfer cells and cause an endotoxemia. Another manifestation of antigens escaping from hepatic MPS activity is a hypergammaglobulinemia often found with hepatic disease.

IMMUNOLOGIC FUNCTIONS[176-178]

The liver can be viewed as an innocent bystander suffering injury from problems in other organs, the damage often being from an immune attack. But the liver is also an active component of the host's immune defenses. The normal liver has activated macrophages, T and B lymphocytes, and natural killer cells as well as mechanisms to contribute to the maintenance of humoral immunity at the intestinal surface.

Normal macrophage function is required for oral tolerance to develop, without which an animal readily develops hypersensitivity responses to antigens absorbed from the intestine. Some of the macrophages and lymphocytes may function in the normal turnover of hepatocytes. Some of the lymphocytes may be of a depressor variety to prevent damage by some immune responses. Hepatocytes also produce proteins that are specific in suppressing immunologic responses specific to the liver. In addition to regulating immune responses, the liver participates in macrophage function by producing and releasing fibronectin. Plasma fibronectin binds particulate matter so that it can be phagocytized and removed by the mononuclear phagocytic system. Low plasma fibronectin is associated with severe hepatic necrosis due to various insults where pretreatment with fibronectin protects against the damaging effects.[175] Fibronectin with a half-life of one to three days will be reduced with chronic hepatic disease, and that results in a loss of the normal protective mechanism to ameliorate further damage.

The liver secretes immunoglobulin A into bile, which upon reaching the intestine coats and contributes to a protective layer of immunoglobulins. Most of that coating is provided by IgA that is synthesized in the intestine and transported directly to the mucosal surface. All of that IgA is polymeric, whereas most serum IgA is a monomer (90%) produced in bone marrow and peripheral lymphoid tissue. The liver can take up the small amount of dimeric IgA in plasma for secretion into bile. But bile IgA can also be synthesized in the liver by plasma cells that have migrated from the intestine to periportal areas of the liver. Normally such cells must migrate back to the intestine in their maturation from B lymphocytes to IgA secreting cells. Cells sensitized to eventually produce IgA against a specific antigen, i.e. a pathogen, would produce antibody for quicker delivery to the intestine if the cells migrated to the liver for IgA secretion than if they had to return to the intestine. Thereby, an earlier immune response can be made against an intestinal pathogen; it may represent an early first line of defense. Liver produced IgA represents about one-half of the total found in bile. The amount of plasma dimeric IgA secreted into bile is relatively small in dogs, with no more than 1% of that in plasma being transported in eight hours. The total hepatic daily contribution is only 1.5 mg IgA per Kg; obstruction of the bile duct in dogs results in only minor and late increases in plasma dimeric IgA levels. Mechanisms other than biliary excretion are responsible for the disappearance of dimeric IgA, which has a half-life of three to four days in dogs.

In addition to secreting IgA into bile, IgA immune complexes can be transported from plasma into bile. That may be an important mechanism for eliminating potentially harmful antigens from the circulation, antigens crossing the intestinal mucosa that subsequently react with IgA to form immune complexes. Elimination through bile entering the intestine minimizes the possibility of such immune complexes activating a cascade of immune-mediated inflammatory reactions.

Secretion of dimeric IgA by salivary glands appears to be more important than the secretion of IgA in bile, with five to ten times more appearing each day in salivary secretions.

CIRCULATORY FUNCTION[179-181]

Physiology

One-fourth of the cardiac output circulates through the liver, by way of the hepatic artery and the portal venous system; at any time 30% of hepatic volume is blood. The liver is a unique organ, receiving blood from both an arterial and a venous source. The liver regulates hepatic arterial flow. Portal venous flow is not regulated, but portal pressure is regulated. Interaction of these two regulations maintains hepatic circulation within a defined range. That is essential to the maintenance of normal circulation throughout the entire splanchnic bed, as well as the rest of the body. Changes of cardiac output from the 25% flowing through the liver will affect blood flow in the rest of the body. For example, hepatic blood flow increases secondary to splanchnic blood flow during digestion and absorption of a meal. Hepatic blood flow can also be reduced when a part of the 25% is needed to support more important metabolic events in other organs. Hence, the normal hepatic blood flow during the unfed state represents a reserve. Examples of higher-priority needs include maintaining oxygenation of the brain and heart tissue during shock and diversion of energy to skeletal muscles during exercise.

Perfusion through the hepatic arterial system is similar to arterial perfusion in other organs. Pressure is high in the hepatic artery, as in the aorta, and the pressure of arterial blood flowing into sinusoidal vessels is regulated by resistance in the network's arterioles. The resistance vessels are sensitive to vasoactive agents and show autoregulation; they make appropriate responses to changes in arterial pressure in order to maintain normal sinusoidal blood pressure. Perfusion through the portal system is at low pressures, 6 to 10 mmHg, and its vessels are much less sensitive to vasoactive substances. Autoregulation is not seen in the portal system, which behaves as a conduit that passively responds to changes in perfusion pressure. Vasoactive drugs reducing splanchnic blood flow by arteriolar vasoconstriction in mesenteric arteries reduce hepatic blood flow, but this response is secondary to the reduction in intestinal venous outflow.

Hepatic arterial blood flow interrelates with flow in the portal vein so that normal sinusoidal circulation is maintained. The only control of blood flow within the liver is via the hepatic artery. Reducing portal blood flow decreases hepatic arterial resistance, leading to an increase in arterial flow. Complete diversion of portal circulation to systemic veins results in a 50% to 100% increase in hepatic arterial flow. Vasoactive chemicals released locally mediate the augmented flow. Unlike the arterial flow, portal blood flow is not autoregulated. The portal system is a passive circulatory bed; its blood flow remains unchanged by complete occlusion of the hepatic artery. Portal resistance and pressure reductions are relatively small following hepatic artery occlusion. With arterial blood pressure in the normal range, from 80 to 120 mmHg, total hepatic blood flow remains normal. The hepatic artery contributes 30% of the flow when blood pressure is at the high end of this normal range (120 mmHg). Hepatic arterial flow increases to 70% of the total when arterial pressure is 80 mmHg. At this low normal pressure, less blood flows through the intestines, and as a result less blood enters the portal circulation. With selective reduction of pressure in the hepatic artery, total hepatic circulation also remains unchanged because hepatic arterial flow increases to compensate for reduced portal blood flow.[182]

Reduction in portal blood flow can result in a drop in intrahepatic sinusoidal blood pressure. Constriction of hepatic venous sphincters maintains sinusoidal blood volume and uniform distribution of flow when increased arterial flow is inadequate to prevent a fall in sinusoidal pressure. These sphincters regulate that pressure by regulating outflow of blood from the liver. In the normal state the hepatic venous sphincters are responsible for virtually all of the resistance to portal blood flow through the liver. There is essentially no resistance to flow through presinusoidal portal or sinusoidal vessels in the normal state. A presinusoidal site for resistance can be demonstrated during infusion of vasoconstricting agents such as norepinephrine, angiotensin (cats and dogs), or histamine (dogs) to cause an increase in portal pressure that is greater than that in sinusoids.

Regulation.[183,184] Portal blood flow varies greatly depending primarily on whether the animal is in the fed or unfed state. Because the liver is not capable of controlling portal blood flow, the liver must regulate its arterial flow in order to prevent great variations in total hepatic blood flow. Arterial flow could be determined by the liver's metabolic requirements for oxygen, but reduced oxygen tension or increased oxygen needs does not increase hepatic arterial flow. Neither portal venous pressure nor hepatic arterial pressure via a myogenic response mechanism is responsible for regulation of hepatic arterial flow. Continuous release of the vasodilating chemical, adenosine and may be the most important regulator. Reduced portal blood flow does not wash away adenosine, and so it accumulates and dilates resistance vessels controlling arterial flow. Increased portal flow washes it away, resulting in vasoconstriction of the arterial resistance vessels and reduction of arterial blood flow. In the fed state arterial flow is not reduced, despite increased portal flow. The chemicals and conditions mediating a persisting vasodilator effect include bile salts, gastrin, secretin, glucagon, and hypertonicity. Total hepatic blood flow increases after feeding, representing an increase for both portal flow and hepatic arterial flow.

Hepatic portal pressure, not blood flow, is regulated by hepatic venous sphincters, located in the third-order branches of the hepatic vein in cats and in the terminal 1 to 2 cm of the lobar vein in dogs. The sphincters constrict to maintain intrahepatic blood pressure; that constriction can protect against increases in central venous pressure. With greater increases in central venous pressure the sphincters are distended and their resistance or competence is diminished. Hepatic venous sphincters constrict in response to norepinephrine, angiotensin, and hepatic nerve stimulation, and to histamine in dogs.

The overall regulation of hepatic blood flow necessitates a complex interaction of flow through the hepatic artery and portal circulation. Hepatic nerve activity and a number of chemicals also have a role. Their relative importance is largely unknown in animals during normal physiological conditions. Regulated hepatic blood flow is essential for regulated clearance of hormones and nutrients. Hepatic blood flow determines the uptake and clearance of some hormones (aldosterone and corticosteroids). Reductions in total sinusoidal flow reduce their clearance, and homeostasis is disrupted for the endocrine systems involved.

The portal circulation is estimated to supply half of the liver's oxygen requirements, with the hepatic artery supplying the remainder. Oxygen tension in portal blood is low, as in venous circulation in other systems. Despite that low oxygen concentration, the liver survives reduction of oxygen delivery in dogs following complete ligation of hepatic arterial flow. With a reduction in oxygen delivery of up to 50%, the liver continues to meet its needs by extracting oxygen from blood with very low oxygen content. The liver is not an organ verging on hypoxia in the normal state. The liver is now thought to receive more oxygen than it requires, and any changes in liver metabolism result in changes in the amount of oxygen extracted from blood. Hyperthyroidism increases metabolic rates, and it is suggested that hepatic oxygen uptake can double to meet the needs of the liver with that problem. Hepatic cells counter reduction in hepatic blood flow and oxygen delivery from shock or anesthetic agents by extracting more oxygen from what blood is provided. Oxygen deprivation, as caused by hepatic artery ligation, reduces Kupffer cell function, resulting in inadequate removal of bacteria and toxins from portal blood.[185] In this case the liver requires a normal supply of oxygen to prevent septicemia. Septicemia is a cause of death in dogs with ligated hepatic arteries; survival is usual when they are pretreated with antibiotics.[186]

Clostridia are reported to inhabit the normal canine liver, and it is suggested that penicillin suppresses them following artery ligation. It is questionable whether any microorganism survives in normal canine livers. Older experiments to identify microorganisms growing in normal liver were fraught with problems, a major one being contamination of culture samples. Later microbiological studies cast doubt on the results of older procedures used to identify bacteria in the liver.[187] Moreover, if clostridia were a normal inhabitant of the liver, these bacteria would often produce intrahepatic abscess or bacteremia. The incidence of such complications would be high with severe trauma, following shock, with acute hepatic necrosis and regional vessel thrombosis, and with reduced oxygen tension caused by general cardiovascular disease. Nevertheless, intrahepatic abscesses or hepatitis due to infection is seldom encountered. Bacterial endocarditis occurs more frequently in humans with cirrhosis, presumably due to intestinal bacteria bypassing hepatic Kupffer cells through arteriovenous shunts.

The hepatic lymphatic system transports extracellular fluid and large molecules, such as plasma proteins, tissue debris, and foreign substances, from the liver. The plasma protein content of hepatic lymph is similar to that of plasma because hepatic sinusoids are very permeable to the movement of large molecules. The rate of lymph flow is related to hepatic blood flow and intrahepatic sinusoidal pressure; that serves to remove excess fluid from hepatic tissue.

The liver is an important reservoir for blood that can be mobilized for essential needs elsewhere. Approximately 50% of the hepatic total blood volume can be expelled within 90 seconds by sympathetic nerve activity. Catecholamines and angiotensin agonists have a similar effect. During hemorrhage such a response does not impair hepatic function; hepatic blood flow, intrahepatic blood pressure, cardiac output, and venous return to the heart are all protected. Such protection is possible because the blood expelled from the liver is a part that is not contributing to effective circulation of blood through the liver; it may be thought of as pooled blood.

Pathophysiology

Regulation of hepatic circulation is achieved by humoral and neural control and by autoregulation of resistance vessels in the splanchnic microcirculation. Two types of abnormalities can disrupt the capacity of regulatory mechanisms to maintain normal hepatic circulation. In one case, hepatic circulation is impaired and portal pressure increases due to increased resistance to blood flow. In the other, hepatic circulation is reduced because part of the portal flow bypasses the liver. Bypassing blood may open an avenue of lesser resistance around the liver as a consequence of increased portal blood pressure, or the blood flow may be following an abnormal pathway present since birth, in which case portal pressure is not elevated.

Portal Hypertension.[188,189] In medium-size and large dogs, blood pressure in the portal vein is normally 6 to 10 mmHg (8 to 13 cm H_2O), and blood flow is 600 to 650 ml/minute.[183] Pressure is reduced following a gradient through the portal system into the hepatic veins and vena cava (Table 28-9). Pressures in central veins and sinusoids are essentially the same as portal pressure. Free hepatic vein pressure is the same as that in the caudal vena cava.

Portal hypertension can be caused by increased total portal blood volume, increased resistance to portal or intrahepatic blood flow, hypertension in the vena cava, or a combination of blood volume, pressure, and resistance changes.

Total blood volume correlates well with portal blood pressure in humans with cirrhosis, suggesting that increases in portal blood volume contribute to portal hypertension. Mesenteric blood flow dramatically increases two to three times in normal dogs infused with pharmacologic doses of glucagon, but that does not raise portal pressure significantly. On the other hand, portal blood flow increases to the same degree following creation of a shunt between the aorta and portal vein, in which case portal pressure increases to 15 mmHg. In portal hypertensive dogs with portal fibrosis, total hepatic blood flow increases 60% over normal.[190] That is largely due to an increase in portal venous flow, which doubles despite a marked increase in portal vascular resistance. The increased flow circulated entirely through the liver since portasystemic shunting of blood is not evident. Portal venous flow correlates directly with portal pressure up to pressures of 20 mmHg; the flow increases as pressure increases. Thus, the pathogenesis of portal hypertension must be explained partly by a substantial increase in portal blood flow or blood volume, as well as by an increased resistance to flow. In clinical cases arteriovenous fistulae increase hepatic blood flow and produce portal hypertension.[191,192]

Table 28-9. Hepatic Blood Flow and Pressures in Normal Dogs

Hepatic arterial pressure	109 mmHg
Hepatic arterial flow	77 ml/min/100 gm
Portal blood pressure	5.8 mmHg
Hepatic venous pressure	1.7 mmHg
Portal blood flow	88 ml/min/100 gm
Data are from reference 183	
Splenic pulp pressure	12.5-13.5 cm H_2O
Hepatic vein, wedge	12-13 cm H_2O
Hepatic vein, free	5-7.5 cm H_2O
Porta cava, abdomen	3-3.5 cm H_2O
Porta cava, thorax	0.5-1.0 cm H_2O
Right atrium	0-0.5 cm H_2O

All values corrected to level of right atrium.
Reproduced with permission of P.F. Suter.

Based on studies in the dog with induced portal fibrosis, clinical cases with portal hypertension due to hepatic fibrosis may actually experience an increase in hepatic blood flow rather than a decrease, predicted on suspicion of increased resistance to portal blood flow. Blood flow may be augmented because the portal vascular bed can expand passively to accommodate great increases in blood flow without changing portal pressure. Vasodilators (one suggestion is glucagon) that escape degradation by the liver may play a role in the hepatic portal vascular changes. They may also contribute to a general hyperdynamic circulation involving all of the splanchnic viscera where blood flow can double; consistent with these changes is an increase in cardiac output. An oral antibiotic normalizes the hyperdynamic features of portal hypertension produced by partial portal vein ligation, suggesting that the features are caused by products of intestinal bacterial metabolism (but not ammonia).[193]

Resistance to portal blood flow can increase due to changes within or outside the liver and are described as prehepatic, intrahepatic, and posthepatic (Figure 28-18). These increases in resistance combine with increases in hepatic blood flow to produce portal hypertension. The most common causes are intrahepatic and posthepatic.

Prehepatic portal hypertension develops from lesions obstructing portal blood flow before it enters the liver. Tumors

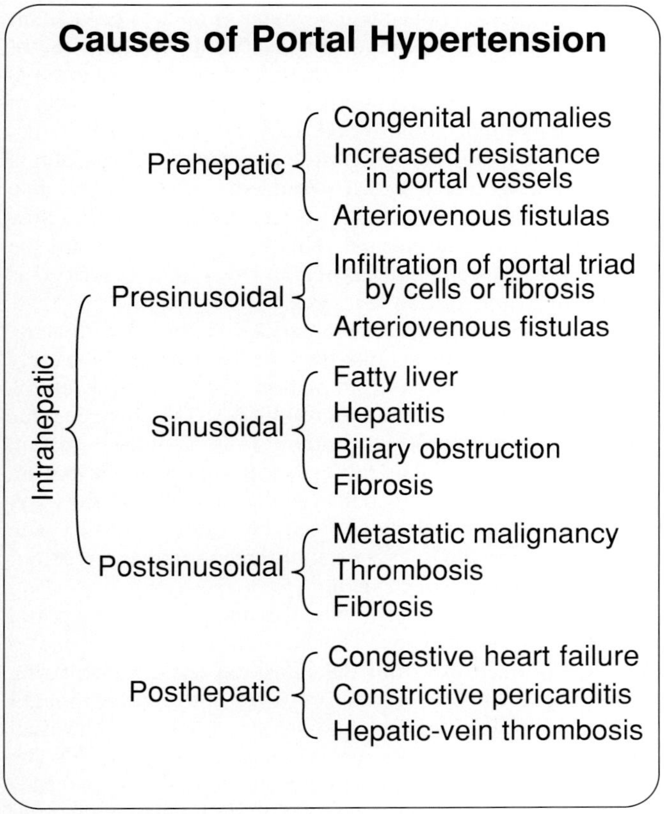

Figure 28-18

can compress the portal vein to produce hypertension. Inflammatory diseases such as pancreatitis can result in lesions constricting the portal vein. Thrombosis of the portal vein can also be a cause. Prehepatic portal hypertension also develops from increased hepatic arterial blood flow resulting from trauma- or tumor-induced arteriovenous fistulae. Portal venous pressure increases but intrahepatic portal pressure remains normal. Mechanisms for escape from the hypertension include splenomegaly and the development of portasystemic shunts; ascites usually does not develop.

Intrahepatic lesions cause portal hypertension by increasing resistance at a site that is presinusoidal, sinusoidal, or postsinusoidal. Presinusoidal resistance increases from lesions involving the periportal area of the hepatic acinus or lobule. Involvement of the portal triad due to inflammation, fibrosis, or neoplastic cells characterizes much of this type of hypertension. Nodular regeneration disrupting normal hepatic architecture can cause presinusoidal portal hypertension. Copper toxicosis and hypervitaminosis A are also described as causing this form of portal hypertension. Manifestations of presinusoidal hypertension include normal sinusoidal blood pressure, splenomegaly, development of portasystemic shunts, and seldom the development of ascites.

Sinusoidal portal hypertension develops from increased resistance to blood flow with or without increased blood flow in sinusoids. Hepatocyte enlargement or increased deposition of collagen around sinusoids increases resistance to blood flow. Hepatocyte enlargement can be caused by acute hepatitis and storage diseases where the cell retains abnormal amounts of nutrients or waste products. Hepatic cirrhosis and chronic hepatitis are usually manifested by fibrosis around sinusoids with the result being hypertension. Chronic bile duct ligation in dogs leads to these kinds of changes within a few months. Sinusoidal hypertension can be a problem with nodular regeneration of the liver. Splenomegaly and the development of portasystemic shunts are manifestations, as they are with presinusoidal portal hypertension. In contrast to presinusoidal hypertension, ascites formation is commonly seen with sinusoidal hypertension.

Postsinusoidal portal hypertension develops from increased resistance to blood flow through any part of the venous system draining the sinusoids. Venoocclusion is a part of cirrhosis and chronic hepatitis. Any disease producing fibrosis of terminal central veins, such as chronic bile duct obstruction in the dog, is a cause as is. Venous thrombosis caused by a coagulopathy or by sclerotic or fibrotic changes produced by chemicals such as nitrosamines and senecio alkaloids. Inflammatory and neoplastic diseases involving the terminal hepatic veins are occasional causes. Lesions confined to the terminal hepatic veins may be associated with few other morphological hepatic abnormalities. Postsinusoidal portal hypertension is manifested by splenomegaly, portasystemic vascular shunts, and ascites. Postsinusoidal portal hypertension also causes hepatomegaly when pooling of blood is not restricted by cirrhosis or fibrosis.

Any disease that increases pressure in the vena cava causes posthepatic portal hypertension, and the increase is transmitted backwards so portal hypertension appears both in the liver and in the portal circulation to the liver. Causes include any heart disease resulting in congestive failure and any lesion in the heart or caudal vena cava, such as a tumor, restricting vena caval blood flow to the heart. These diseases result in splenomegaly, hepatomegaly, and ascites. Portasystemic shunts do not develop because hypertension in the systemic venous system results in no significant pressure gradient between it and the portal circulation. Whereas portal and total hepatic blood flow increase despite sinusoidal resistance increases with presinusoidal portal hypertension, hepatic blood flow decreases with postsinusoidal and posthepatic causes of portal hypertension. Similarly, in dogs with chronic bile duct ligation and morphologic evidence for increases in sinusoidal and postsinusoidal resistance, total hepatic blood flow decreases to half of normal flow, which is due primarily to a reduction in portal rather than arterial flow. Increases in caudal vena cava pressure, as seen with congestive heart failure, are associated with and follow linearly reductions in flow in the hepatic artery and portal vein.[194]

In clinical cases portal hypertension is caused by a combination of increased portal blood flow or volume and increased resistance to flow. Neither alone readily sustains portal hypertension; both are interrelated. Where portal hypertension due to cirrhosis is associated with consistently increased portal blood volume, portal pressure is directly proportional to the total blood volume in the body.[195] Portal hypertension may be transient and seen only at times of increased blood flow. Intestinal blood flow increases during feeding, and so portal hypertension may develop or is potentiated at that time. Successful treatment directed at reducing blood volume is difficult with portal hypertension. The blood volume increases to sustain normal cardiac output and normal function in nonhepatic organs. Treatment to reduce blood volume to alleviate portal hypertension decreases circulation in these other organs.

Increased resistance to portal flow, as already discussed, can increase portal blood pressure. In experimental dogs acute constriction of the portal vein promptly increases portal pressure, reduces mesenteric arterial flow, and decreases blood oxygen saturation of portal blood. On the other hand, chronic obstruction of portal venous flow does not result in portal hypertension and ascites formation. Compensatory mechanisms intervene to maintain homeostasis in hepatic circulation.

Maintenance of Homeostasis in Portal Circulation. Compensatory mechanisms maintain homeostasis in the portal circulation. They effectively maintain normal blood pressure but are not always as effective in maintaining hepatic circulation. When portal blood flow and resistance increase to cause portal hypertension, compensatory responses to minimize those changes are an increase in the size of venous capacitance beds and the opening of alternate routes of blood flow.

Portal hypertension reflexly reduces the volume of blood entering the mesenteric microcirculation. Increased venous pressure reflexly constricts arterioles, by autoregulation, so that less blood enters intestinal capillary beds. Another response to portal hypertension is vasodilation of venous capacitance vessels so that they can contain more blood, resulting in its intestinal pooling. Portal hypertension in the liver and spleen causes a similar response for restoration of normal pressures. Pooling of blood is primarily passive in those organs. Arterial inflow is reduced by a response similar to that seen in the intestine. Liver and spleen sizes increase with increased portal and mesenteric venous pressure. Hepatomegaly is characterized by dilated sinusoids, which appear to have the greatest capacity to enlarge and contain more blood. Thus, the initial major compensatory mechanisms responding to portal hypertension are a reduction of arterial inflow and a dilation of capacitance vessels to pool blood.

Lymphatic drainage increases during portal hypertension as a means of compensation. When gastrointestinal and hepatic blood flow increase, lymphatic circulation increases to maintain homeostasis.

The splanchnic circulation contains a number of vessels or remnants of fetal blood vessels that are virtually closed in normal animals. Other small vessels communicate between different circulatory beds and normally carry very little blood in normal adults. In the fetus, some of those vessels enable blood to bypass the liver since gastrointestinal function is minimal and no gastrointestinal microflora is yet present. These vessels close at birth and remain closed unless portal pressure increases. Microscopic shunt vessels normally found in the entire splanchnic circulation carry blood directly from the arterial inflow to the venous outflow, thereby bypassing the capillary bed. They divert blood flow from one capillary bed to another. With portal hypertension, these vessels divert blood flow away from congested capillary beds. A major fraction of an organ's blood flow can bypass the capillary circulation by collaterals of this type.

Collateral circulation developing during portal hypertension has been studied in dogs with obstruction of the portal circulation.[196] Diverting blood from the portal system to the vena cava compensates for the portal hypertension. Collaterals appear between the left gastric and left phrenicoabdominal veins; between the pancreaticoduodenal vein and the phrenicoabdominal, left renal, or left gonadal vein; between the splenic vein and left gonadal or left renal vein; between the left colic vein and the left gonadal, renal capsular, or deep circumflex iliac vein; and from the hemorrhoidal veins to the internal iliac veins. This collateral circulation reverses the direction of blood flow, so that portal blood does not reach the liver but passes directly into the systemic circulation, by hepatofugal (away from the liver) flow. In contrast, collaterals can also develop around a site of portal obstruction, allowing portal flow to the liver to remain normal. This hepatopedal (toward the liver) collateral circulation has not, however, been described as a means of compensation for portal hypertension.

Hepatic blood flow can dramatically increase with acute liver inflammation, by an unknown means that may be merely a nonspecific response to inflammation. The blood flow returns to normal when the inflammation subsides. The change is due primarily to increased hepatic arterial flow. In order to sustain a high flow this extra blood must pass through channels that are the equivalent of arteriovenous fistulas. This blood flow bypasses functional hepatocytes since the arteriovenous oxygen difference across the liver is smaller than normal as a result of decreased extraction of oxygen.

Hepatic blood flow also increases and persists with portal inflammation and fibrosis. The increase is primarily due to increased portal flow from the intestinal tract. Vasodilating agents produced by bacterial activity in the intestine are thought to be responsible, since oral antibiotics reducing the intestinal microflora return the hyperdynamic state to normal.[193] The increased blood flow accompanies portal hypertension, and it is not until weeks later that collateral circulation develops.

Collateral circulation develops when the initial responses are inadequate to resolve portal hypertension. With resolution of an underlying hepatic disease portal hypertension may never be a problem long enough for collateral circulation to develop. It is evident that in both normal animals and those with hepatic disease portal pressure fluctuates. Blood flow determines absolute pressures, and that changes with normal events like feeding as well as with disease. Portal pressure measurement must be made in the unfed state and in animals under anesthesia. Since these two conditions reduce portal flow and hence pressure, normal pressures can be recorded in dogs with portal hypertension when fed and unsedated. Greater flow rates and pressures anticipated in the fed and awake state may be of a great enough magnitude to cause collaterals to open and persist, given enough time for the primary problem to persist.

Ascites.[47] Ascites, the accumulation of fluid in the abdominal cavity, can develop when the limits of an animal's compensatory mechanisms are exceeded (Figure 28-19). Portal hypertension remains at this point despite changed resistance of arterial and capacitance vessels, increased hepatic lymph flow, and the opening of shunt vessels. In addition, an imbalance develops in the Starling forces that normally maintain a steady state in fluxes of fluid in and out of the capillaries. At the arterial end of capillaries, hydrostatic pressure is relatively high and promotes the movement of fluid from vessels into the extravascular space. At the venous end of capillaries, the hydrostatic pressure has fallen and the colloid osmotic pressure has increased due to increases in albumin concentration from the loss of plasma water. These changes, in addition to increased tissue hydrostatic pressure and decreased tissue colloid osmotic pressure, favor the movement of fluid from the extravascular space into capillaries. A hypoalbuminemia causing reduced colloid

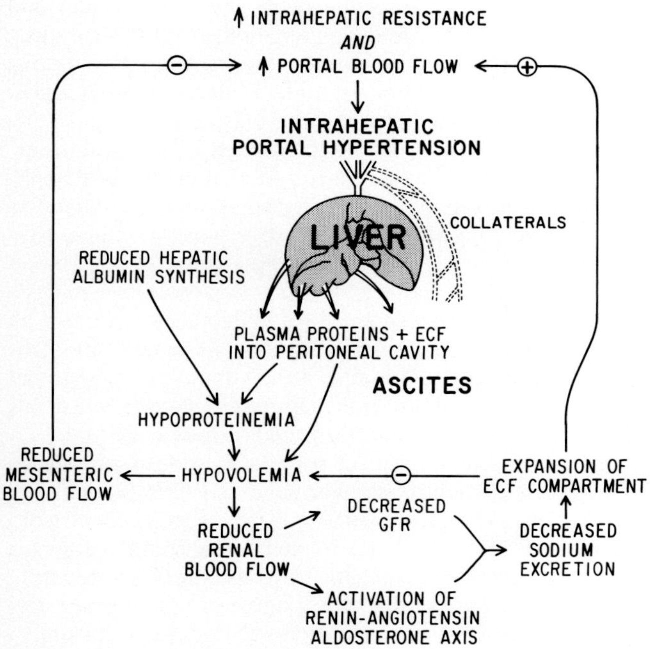

Figure 28-19. Pathogenesis of ascites due to hepatic disease. See text for description.

osmotic pressure would reduce the force promoting return of extracellular fluid to the capillary. The imbalance which develops after compensation is caused primarily by increased capillary hydrostatic pressure resulting from the portal hypertension. Hypoalbuminemia usually accompanies ascites and frequently contributes to the formation of ascitic fluid but is seldom the primary cause. With normal portal blood pressure, plasma albumin concentration must approach 1.0 g/dl before ascites appears. Hypoalbuminemia that severe also causes peripheral edema, which is usually more obvious and recognized sooner than ascites. Hypoalbuminemia is sometimes accompanied by transudation of fluid into pleural spaces.

Altered albumin metabolism is the result of portal hypertension and ascites formation, not the cause. After hypoalbuminemia appears, however, there is no doubt that it contributes to the progressive development and persistence of ascites. Reduced hepatic synthesis of albumin is unimportant in most cases of hypoproteinemia with ascites. A more frequent cause of hypoalbuminemia is the expansion of plasma volume in an attempt to maintain normal cardiac output, in which case the expansion dilutes plasma protein. An expansion in plasma volume is secondary to a pooling of blood in the splanchnic circulation and a reduction in effective circulating blood volume.

When ascitic fluid contains plasma proteins, the normal albumin space is further expanded to include the ascitic fluid. That fluid dilutes albumin in the total body pool, which worsens hypoalbuminemia. The concentration of protein in ascitic fluid is determined by the location of increased resistance causing portal hypertension. Ascites' source is interstitial fluid; it should have similar composition. Interstitial fluid in splanchnic viscera has a relatively high albumin concentration. Interstitial or lymph-like fluid moves under the influence of increased capillary and tissue hydrostatic pressure from the tissue spaces into the lymphatic circulation. When lymph flow reaches its maximum, a continuing increased tissue pressure causes fluid to move into the abdomen and ascites forms. The interstitial fluid is modified in its movement across tissues, and the fluid entering the abdomen has a different albumin content depending on the tissue which is its source. Intestinal lymphatic hypertension caused by lymphatic obstruction produces an abdominal transudate very low in protein, less than 0.5 g/dl. Thus, the high concentrations of plasma proteins in the intestinal interstitial space do not escape into the abdominal cavity with the movement of fluid producing ascites. On the other hand, when portal hypertension develops within the liver, plasma proteins readily escape in the fluid entering the abdominal cavity. Sinusoidal capillaries are more permeable to large molecules, and once they enter the interstitial space of Disse, only the thin hepatic capsule prevents their escape. Thus, increased sinusoidal hydrostatic pressure promotes the movement of interstitial fluid from the space of Disse out into the abdominal cavity, and large amounts of plasma proteins follow.

Sinusoidal capillaries are semipermeable to proteins to the extent that the albumin space is about 64% of the sodium space in the normal liver. These capillaries become more permeable as sinusoidal pressure is increased, so that the protein concentration of interstitial fluid exuding from the liver surface is 90% that of plasma. It is evident that gaps between hepatic cells can increase, so that there is little resistance to the movement of albumin into the abdomen. During portal hypertension the intestine does not lose its ability to sieve and retain albumin since fluid lost from that organ into the intestine is virtually protein-free. Thus, the liver lacks the mechanisms for protecting against fluid loss, such as are found in the intestine and other tissues. Ascitic fluid albumin concentration is high under conditions of high sinusoidal blood pressure, the basis being posthepatic and sinusoidal or postsinusoidal hepatic causes. Prehepatic and presinusoidal hepatic causes result in formation of ascites fluid with relatively low albumin content.

Portal hypertension, as the most important factor determining the development of ascites, results in loss of fluid from nonhepatic splanchnic viscera as well as the liver. The plasma-ascites filtration rate is nearly maximum in stable human cirrhotics. Expansion of the extracellular fluid compartment with saline solution does not increase that filtration rate but increases it for nonhepatic splanchnic tissues. Thus, further increases in portal pressure affect filtration of fluid from the latter with minimal effect on filtration across the liver. Recent studies suggest that diuretics are useful in managing ascites because they reduce the liver's plasma-ascites filtration rate, an effect that is not dependent on any reductions in plasma volume or portal pressure.[197]

Ascitic fluid is in a dynamic equilibrium with fluid elsewhere in the body. With portal hypertension, water or protein cannot be returned from the ascitic fluid to the portal circulation. The fluid is removed from the abdomen by lymphatics in the peritoneal cavity. The compensation that develops takes the form of a ten- to twelve-fold increase in lymph flow in some lymphatics. That causes lymphatic vessels to enlarge and increases lymphatic hydrostatic pressure. Hence, increased lymphatic size and pressure does not necessary indicate obstruction to flow but can indicate merely an increased rate of flow.

Ascites is associated with reduced effective circulating plasma volume. With normal return of blood to the heart and normal cardiac function, the effective plasma volume and cardiac output are normal. When blood-return to the heart is reduced, both of those parameters are reduced. Homeostatic mechanisms attempt to return the effective plasma volume to normal so that cardiac output will be normal. Effective plasma can be reduced with normal or increased cardiac output, however. In fact, cardiac output increases in the hyperdynamic circulatory state that can develop with chronic hepatitis. Generalized arterial vasodilation can be associated with increased cardiac output and hepatic disease. That vasodilation is responsible for the reduced effective blood volume and provides the signal for release of chemicals promoting sodium and water retention. The vasodilation may be recognized by a subtle decrease in arterial blood pressure. Sodium retention is a very early response in hepatic disease; ascites is a secondary manifestation. The peripheral vasodilation, despite an increased cardiac output, thereby causes sodium retention. The resulting volume expansion, when associated with portal hypertension, promotes the formation of ascites. The response to reduced effective plasma volume results in increased total plasma volume. Total plasma volume increases do not necessarily restore normal effective plasma volume, however. Normally 80% of the blood volume is in the low-pressure part of the vascular compartment, with 20% in the high-pressure side. Reductions in effective plasma volume involve the high-pressure side, and the compensations increase the size of the low-pressure compartment without necessarily returning the high-pressure side to normal. Consequently total blood volume can be increased without rectifying the reduced effective blood volume and cardiac output.

With ascites and reduced effective plasma volume, the decreased cardiac output is used to maintain normal circulation in tissues vital for survival, and as a result the splanchnic blood flow is reduced. Normally, the 25% of the cardiac output perfusing the kidneys represents a reserve for use by other tissues when the need arises. During stress or exercise, part of the renal blood flow is diverted away by the same homeostatic mechanisms, shunting blood flow from the kidneys during reduced cardiac output and decreased effective plasma volume. However, these mechanisms are unable to correct the imbalances associated with ascites, and others are invoked to correct the reduced effective plasma volume.

The reduced effective plasma volume is corrected by increasing the total plasma volume, which involves mechanisms regulating fluid and electrolyte metabolism.[198] All mechanisms invoked are aimed at reducing the daily loss of body fluids through the kidneys. Renal conservation of fluid and electrolytes is mediated by changes in renal blood flow and glomerular filtration rate; the physiological action of aldosterone; the effects of antidiuretic hormone (ADH); the effect of natriuretic hormone; and the effects of other hormones such as catecholamines and ones with vasoactive properties.

The reduction in renal blood flow by diversion to other tissues contributes to the conservation of body fluids by reducing glomerular filtration rate (GFR). Renal blood flow and GFR are directly related, and blood flow determines the amount of salt and water excreted from the body. In general, when less sodium is filtered with reduced GFR, less is excreted and more is retained in the extracellular fluid. Since the amount of sodium in this fluid determines the fluid's content of water, the consequence of sodium retention is water retention. Therefore, the kidney filters less sodium as one means of retaining water, and that is accomplished by reducing renal blood flow. The reduction in blood flow is mediated by the sympathetic nervous system and by catecholamines, both of which constrict arterioles in the glomerular circulation.

Sodium is also retained by the adrenal hormone aldosterone, which stimulates a mechanism located in the distal nephron to reabsorb sodium and secrete potassium. The signal to release aldosterone is reduced effective plasma volume (hypovolemia). That is detected in the kidney, where reduced blood perfusion initiates the events leading to aldosterone release. Low renal perfusion pressure results in the release of renin, an enzyme catalyzing conversion of the plasma protein angiotensinogen to angiotensin. Angiotensin acts directly on the adrenal gland to stimulate aldosterone secretion. It also constricts glomerular vessels to reduce GFR and sodium excretion.

A less important means of stimulating aldosterone secretion is adrenocorticotrophic hormone (ACTH), which acts directly on the adrenal, similarly to its effect on glucocorticoid secretion. ACTH is released by stress via neural pathways through the hypothalamus. In this case, the stress is a reduction in effective blood volume. Another signal stimulating aldosterone secretion is a low plasma ratio of sodium to potassium.

Aldosterone, like the other steroid hormones, must be metabolized by the liver before it can be excreted. When hepatic disease accompanies ascites, the transformation of aldosterone to an excretable form is reduced, and blood levels usually remain elevated.

Unlike other endocrine systems, the renin-angiotensin-aldosterone system is not regulated by a precise negative feedback system. Normal effective blood volume is the signal to reduce aldosterone secretion. With ascites caused by portal hypertension, high levels of aldosterone do not necessarily return effective blood volume to normal. Therefore, aldosterone secretion continues despite an increase in total body sodium, the ion that the hormone functions to retain. Thus, aldosterone levels can be increased with ascites due to portal hypertension, with or without liver disease.

Low GFR and high aldosterone levels are not the only reasons for renal retention of fluids. The expanded volume of extracellular fluid that accompanies the ascites should be a stimulus for increased urine output. In normal animals, expansion of the extracellular fluid volume causes diuresis. A normal animal given excessive doses of both aldosterone and antidiuretic hormone will diurese when infused with fluids, whereas the animal with ascites does not respond to the same conditions. Normal animals will respond to the expanded extracellular fluid, despite the presence of large amounts of aldosterone and ADH, by release of atrial natriuretic factor, a peptide hormone. That hormone inhibits sodium reabsorption in the proximal renal tubule. With ascites, failure of an appropriate renal response to atrial natriuretic factor is more important to the retention of fluid than is either reduced GFR or increased aldosterone secretion performed in experimental dogs to produce a model for studying sodium retention and ascites formation due to enhanced tubular sodium absorption.

Hepatic insufficiency and ascites is associated with abnormalities in the renal regulation of water balance as well as that for sodium balance.[199] Hyponatremia can be seen, indicating a defect in the ability of the kidneys to excrete water and produce dilute urine. Humoral agents other than antidiuretic hormone appear to contribute to the derangement.

A sequence of events has been described to explain ascites formation. The sequence began with portal hypertension that progressed to ascites formation and eventually to hypovolemia and secondary renal sodium and water retention. Some recent studies suggest that the renal sodium and water retention is the initial event that progress to the others. That retention is suggested to follow an initial peripheral vasodilation that reduces effective arterial blood volume.[200] A fall in arterial blood pressure is evident with the onset of sodium and water retention. It is evident that the concepts for ascites formation are changing.

Hepatorenal Syndrome.[201] The changes in renal function to retain sodium may progress to the development of hepatorenal syndrome. This term describes an oliguric renal failure, functional renal failure, spontaneous renal failure, or hemodynamic failure of the kidney. The syndrome represents a functional failure of the kidneys to maintain fluid and electrolyte homeostasis; examination of the kidneys reveals no morphologic changes. Hepatorenal syndrome appears with hepatic disease and may be precipitated by changes that reduce effective blood volume and renal blood flow. Paracentesis to remove ascites fluid, forced diuresis, and gastrointestinal hemorrhage are potential causes. The important renal manifestation is a reduction in glomerular filtration rate due to potent vasoconstriction in the outer renal cortex, with relative preservation of blood flow to the remainder of the kidney. A number of chemicals released by reduced effective blood volume to mediate this effect include renin, angiotension, catecholamines, and vasopressin. In the normal state, at least three hormones are released to maintain normal renal circulation and mitigate against the effects of the vasoconstrictors. Atrial natriuretic factor or hormone increases glomerular filtration rate (and hence renal blood flow) as well as stimulating natriuresis and diuresis. Atrial distension stimulates its release, and that can be reduced when chronic hepatic disease reduces the volume of blood returning to the heart. A deficient release of atrial natriuretic factor may contribute to hepatorenal syndrome. Plasma levels of that hormone are often normal or increased with hepatic disease, however. There is evidence now for the renal tubule being unresponsive to its effects. Eicosanoids may also be important for the syndrome to develop.[202] The kidneys appear to synthesize and release prostaglandins to promote vasodilation, glomerular filtration, natriuresis, and diuresis. Nonsteroidal antiinflammatory drugs markedly reduce glomerular filtration rate in cirrhotic patients, and deficiencies of prostaglandin's release and effects may contribute to hepatorenal syndrome. Another eicosanoid, a thromboxane, is a vasoconstrictor and its increased renal level with hepatic disease probably contributes to the reduced glomerular filtration and oliguria. A third type of hormone, glomerulopressin, regulates renal blood flow and glomerular filtration by increasing both. Glucagon, reaching the liver in the portal circulation, releases glomerulopressin from the liver. Plasma glucagon levels increase with hepatic disease, but the liver loses its ability to release glomerulopressin and less is available to sustain renal blood flow and maintain normal fluid and electrolyte balance.

Electrolyte abnormalities are predictable with chronic hepatic disease. Potassium depletion is common and results from anorexia, vomiting, diarrhea and greater than usual renal losses of potassium. Potassium deficits contribute to the functional renal failure by impairing renal tubular concentrating ability. Alkalosis becomes a problem because of the potassium depletion and because of the loss of excess hydrochloric acid from vomiting. Hyponatremia may be encountered when water is retained because of increased antidiuretic activity or when anorexia, diuretics, or diarrhea results in sodium depletion.

Ascites can be managed if normal renal function is regained by normalizing GFR and aldosterone levels and by obtaining a normal diuretic response to volume expansion. That can be achieved with diuretics — not by increasing GFR but by inhibiting the reabsorption of sodium. Animals with ascites have a reduced effective circulating volume, however, which diuretics reduces further. Thus, when blood flow is essentially normal in the brain, heart, and splanchnic bed only because compensatory mechanisms are operating at their maximum limit, diuretics reduce the effective blood volume, with circulatory failure sometimes resulting. Just as the administration of fluids aggravates portal hypertension, the loss of body fluids following diuretics reduces portal pressure. Although there is a direct and almost linear relation between portal pressure and blood volume, normal animals can lose 15% of their blood volume before there are significant changes in other cardiovascular parameters such as cardiac dynamics or hepatic venous pressure. Thus, the substantial reserve in cardiac output of normal animals allows plasma volume to be reduced moderately without danger. With ascites, however, the reserve is used, so small reductions in plasma volume can have great effects on cardiac output and effective plasma volume. Reducing plasma volume with diuretics further reduces renal and hepatic functions, while small increases in plasma volume increase portal pressure and contribute further to ascites. Diuretics may not alter the rate of ascites fluid absorption as is generally thought, and many can accelerate potassium loss already produced by hyperaldosteronism. Complete removal of ascites fluid is not advisable since intraabdominal pressure determines fluid formation. Rapid removal of a large ascitic volume without replacement of plasma colloids can worsen the vascular underfilling already present, and with that there is an augmented release of vasoconstricting chemicals.

Portasystemic Shunting.[204] Normal hepatic circulation is lost with portacaval or portasystemic vascular shunts. These vascular abnormalities are either acquired or congenital. The acquired shunts result from compensation of portal hypertension. Shunting can occur when many small arteriovenous shunt vessels open within an organ, or when larger mesenteric vessels open.

Congenital shunting of blood from the portal circulation directly into the systemic venous circulation occurs through portal-vein anomalies. The most common type of shunt is persistence of the ductus venosus, a fetal vessel that carries blood from the umbilical and portal veins through the liver. Blood bypasses the liver and is delivered to the hepatic vein and vena cava. When the ductus venosus fails to close after birth, a portacaval shunt allows blood to continue bypassing the liver. In most cases of persistent ductus venosus, hepatic portal branches are poorly outlined with angiography, appearing to be hypoplastic.

The second most common type of portal-vein anomaly is the large central portapostcaval anastomosis, in which the portal vein empties into the caudal vena cava before (caudal to) the liver. This type of shunting can also occur through a number of smaller collateral vessels instead of through one large one, a situation that can be either congenital or acquired. Acquired collaterals develop secondary to portal hypertension. Measurement of portal pressure could aid in identifying the hypertension, but after collaterals open, portal pressure approaches normal. When portal blood shunts into systemic veins, the liver atrophies, reducing the capacitance of the hepatic vascular bed. Then, when the congenital portasystemic shunts are completely closed by surgery, the atrophied hepatic portal circulation is unable to accommodate the normal flow of blood received from the gastrointestinal tract. Large central portapostcaval anastomoses are thought to be present from birth. Multiple peripheral portasystemic anastomoses, similar to those developing in experimental dogs with portal obstruction, are thought to be acquired secondary to portal hypertension. Another type of congenital shunt involves anastomosis of the portal vein with the azygos.

The cause of persistent portal-vein anomalies is not known. Some undoubtedly result from abnormal fetal development of blood vessels, such as the portal azygos anastomoses, but that is less likely to be the cause of the failure of the ductus venosus to close. The ductus venosus normally closes 60 to 65 hours after birth in the dog.[205] The failure of this shunt to close may involve a deficiency of the humoral agents that promote its closure. It is possible that infection gaining entrance through the umbilical vein at birth prevents the shunt from closing.

COMPARTMENTATION FUNCTIONS OF LIVER

The compartmentation functions of hepatocytes depend on maintenance of normal architecture and circulation. Metabolic functions are not the same for all hepatocytes, and the cells are organized in a way to provide the optimum overall function. Intracellular organization is also necessary to keep functionally related enzyme systems in close proximity. Disruption of internal structures causes enzymes to be scattered throughout the cell, so that the overall function of metabolic systems is lost.

Zonal Distribution of Metabolic Functions[206,207]

The liver consists of hepatocytes which appear morphologically homogenous regardless of their location in a lobule or functional unit but which are in reality heterogenous in their functions. A knowledge of the distribution of functions can be useful in understanding the relationships between clinical pathologic and pathologic manifestations of liver disease.

Heterogenous zonation for carbohydrate metabolism is expressed by a predominately periportal concentration of metabolic activity for releasing glucose, glycogenolysis and gluconeogenesis to the circulation; activity for glucose uptake, glycogen synthesis and glycolysis concentrates in the perivenous area. Thus, as blood circulates through a lobule, it first contacts glucose-forming hepatocytes and later passes glucose-using hepatocytes. This heterogeneity is also expressed in appropriate differences in receptor numbers for hormones regulating carbohydrate metabolism. The heterogeneity develops in the young animal and is later able to adapt to different nutritional states. During starvation the periportal glucogenic zone enlarges and the perivenous glycolytic zone decreases in size. In cirrhotic nodules the normal heterogeneity of carbohydrate metabolism persists; the centers of such nodules correspond functionally to the periportal zone.

Zonal differences for lipid metabolism include liponeogenic metabolic activity predominating in perivenous hepatocytes; fatty acid synthesis is active in the glycolytic region of the liver, an area where carbohydrate metabolism can support it. After feeding the perivenous area appears to use excess glucose for energy and during fasting to produce ketone bodies for energy. This fatty acid catabolism by ß-oxidation is also active in periportal hepatocytes, where its product of acetyl-CoA is the principle source of energy. Cholesterol and bile acids appear to be synthesized mainly in periportal hepatocytes. The heterogeneity of metabolic activity for lipid metabolism also varies with the nutritional state. Carbohydrate-rich diets stimulate liponeogenesis and the activity of its enzymes in the perivenous zone. That activity becomes very low during starvation.

Amino acid metabolism closely integrates with carbohydrate metabolism. Thus, the zone for gluconeogesis in the periportal area should be the center for metabolic conversion of amino acids to glucose. That zone is predominant for deamination and transamination of the important amino acid precursors, especially alanine, for glucose formation. The periportal hepatocytes are predominant in urea cycle enzyme activity and urea formation. This ability to fix ammonia in the periportal area is complemented by the fixation of ammonia to form glutamine in the perivenous area. One might expect that diffuse, largely periportal hepatic lesions are the most likely to reduce overall urea synthesis and result in low blood urea nitrogen. Changes in zonal patterns for amino acid metabolism follow those for carbohydrate metabolism. The gluconeogenic zone increases with starvation, when enzyme activity increases for the conversion of alanine to glucose.

The synthesis of urea involves the consumption of stoichiometric amounts of bicarbonate and ammonia. The amount of bicarbonate formed from metabolism of a normal size protein meal is greater than can be disposed of by the kidney to prevent an alkalosis. Conversion of bicarbonate to urea is an important means for maintaining acid-base balance following a protein meal. Loss of periportal hepatocyte function can result in a loss of this capacity to buffer a base excess and can contribute to alkalosis. Normally, urea synthesis increases in response to alkalosis, something not possible with liver disease. Conversely, with acidosis urea synthesis decreases, and glutamine synthesis, primarily in the perivenular hepatocytes, increases. The glutamine formed can be used to augment renal excretion of hydrogen ions as a part of the normal compensatory response to acidosis. Thus, perivenular lesions can contribute to and interfere with the normal response to acidosis.

In summary, the interactions between periportal and perivenular zones of the liver allow for fine adjustment of ammonia, urea, and glutamine in terminal hepatic venules. They also assist in responding appropriately to changes in acid base homeostasis.

For many substances, location makes no evident difference in hepatocytes' ability to remove substances for the circulation. Hepatocytes with differences in concentrations of binding proteins, however, will remove certain substances more avidly than others. The capacity to secrete some substances into the bile also varies with location of hepatocytes. For example, the periportal hepatocytes have a greater ability than do perivenular hepatocytes to secrete bile acids.

Hepatic Oxygen Supply

The major blood supply to the liver travels via the portal vein; the hepatic artery contributes much less. The mixture of these two sources of blood provides oxygen to periportal hepatocytes at a concentration approximating 60% of arterial blood. The hepatic venous oxygen concentration is approximately 33% that of portal venous blood, which represents a sizeable oxygen gradient between periportal and perivenous oxygen concentrations. This gradient indicates that the liver is able to extract a greater percentage of oxygen from the circulation than other tissues can. Thus, a heterogeneity exists for sinusoidal oxygen concentrations, but with efficient extraction the liver is not deprived of its oxygen requirements.

Loss of Compartmentation

The loss of intracellular relationships is not identifiable by light microscopy. Electron microscopy has been used to study the early changes caused by agents such as viruses. This is at a time when the hepatocyte has lost important functions, yet light-microscope changes are not apparent.

Causes of a loss of compartmentation include viruses, bacteria, parasites, toxins, trauma, neoplasia, nutritional derangements, and immune-mediated mechanisms; viral and toxic agents cause the greatest losses.

Loss of compartmentation disrupts the normal heterogeneity of hepatocyte functions that simultaneously perform complementary processes. Sometimes it may be possible to correlate histologic findings of changes in hepatic architecture with abnormal clinical pathologic findings reflecting functional changes. More likely, changes are seen in plasma levels of activity for certain enzymes.

Loss of Enzymes. Loss of enzymes from either hepatocytes or biliary epithelial cells increases their plasma activities. Plasma enzymes lost from hepatocytes include alanine aminotransferase, aspartate aminotransferase, arginase, ornithine carbamyl transferase, and lactic dehydrogenase. Plasma enzymes increasing with biliary obstruction are alkaline phosphatase, gamma-glutamyl transpeptidase, and 5'-nucleotidase. These enzymes are used for diagnostic purposes to evaluate for hepatocellular damage or biliary-tract obstruction. Increased alkaline phosphatase activity reflects increased synthesis by epithelial cells of the biliary system rather than a loss of compartmentation function.

Increased plasma activity of most enzymes is significant only for diagnostic or prognostic purposes. With one exception, enzymes with proteolytic activity are the only ones to cause the appearance of clinical signs or losses of normal function. The exception is arginase, which does not have proteolytic properties but can contribute to clinical signs. High plasma arginase activity following hepatic damage can cause plasma arginine levels to decrease to essentially zero. Plasma arginase causes this by converting plasma arginine to ornithine and urea. The deficiency of plasma arginine has an effect on protein synthesis and on the availability of arginine required for ammonia detoxification in the urea cycle. The clinical correlations are signs of hepatic encephalopathy.

The release of proteolytic enzymes from damaged hepatocytes is much more serious than the loss of other enzymes. The liver is a rich source of thromboplastic activity, and when a large amount is released, disseminated intravascular coagulation is initiated. Coagulopathies, a problem with some forms of liver disease, can also be consistently produced by some hepatotoxins and by viruses attacking the liver. Other proteases released from hepatocytes include lysosomal enzymes, which are able to degrade plasma peptides and blood-clotting factors, contributing further to bleeding problems.

Loss of Liver-Cell Antigens. Antigenic components of liver cells are released from damaged hepatocytes and can stimulate the synthesis of antibodies that theoretically can damage normal cells. Plasma immunoglobulin levels increase with hepatic disease but primarily because antigens in portal blood are not taken up by the damaged monocyte phagocytic system. Autoantibodies to hepatic antigens represent a measurable increment in specific autoantibodies, but their sum does not contribute significantly to the hypergammaglobulinemia. The self-directed antibodies are produced in lymph nodes by immunocytes. Some are also produced in the liver by plasma cells that have infiltrated following injury.

Any insult to the liver, whether by trauma, infection, or drugs, releases hepatic antigens to the circulation, against which the synthesis of antibodies is directed. Antiorganelle antibodies are produced but are neither organ-specific nor species-specific. They include antinuclear antibody and the accompanying LE cell phenomenon, antimitochondrial antibody, antismooth-muscle antibody, and antimicrosomal antibody. Of these, only the antimitochondrial antibody is found consistently with virus- or drug-induced hepatitis in humans. This antibody is produced in experimentally-induced toxic hepatitis in animals. It remains to be seen whether any of these antibodies are produced in clinical cases of hepatitis in animals. Other nonspecific autoantibodies are not found consistently with hepatic disease. Their presence does not identify anything other than tissue damage, and can accompany injury to many different tissues.

Chronic hepatitis frequently follows damage by a chemical or infectious agent where pathology persists after the cause is removed. The initial insult probably initiates an immune-mediated process that causes the hepatitis to persist. Cell antigens are released or uncovered to stimulate the immune response. Immunization of animals with liver-specific proteins causes chronic hepatitis. The process is characterized by hepatic necrosis with infiltration of lymphocytes and antibody-producing plasma cells. That is sufficient to cause antibody-dependent cytotoxicity, resulting in pathology that is persistent and self-perpetuating. Thus, loss of compartmentation is important in the pathogenesis of chronic hepatitis initiated by a variety of etiological agents.

REFERENCES

1. Altszuler, N. and Finegold, M.J.: Glucose metabolism. In, The Liver: Normal and Abnormal Functions, Part A. The Biochemistry of Disease. Edited by F.F. Becker. Marcel Dekker, New York 463-529, 1974.
2. Felig, P. and Sherwin, R.: Carbohydrate homeostasis, liver and diabetes. In, Progress in Liver Diseases, Vol. 5. Edited by H. Popper and F. Schaffner. Grune and Stratton, New York, 149-171, 1976.
3. Newsholme, E.A.: Role of the liver in integration of fat and carbohydrate metabolism and clinical implications in pa-

tients with liver disease. In, Progress in Liver Diseases. Vol. 5. Edited by H. Popper and F. Schaffner. Grune and Stratton, New York, 125-135, 1976.

4. Alberti, K.G.M.M., Johnston, D.G. and Taylor, R.: Carbohydrate metabolism in liver disease. In, Liver and Biliary Disease. Edited by R. Wright, G.H. Millward-Sadler, K.G.M.M. Alberti and S. Karran. WB Saunders, Philadelphia, 45-64 1985.
5. Jungerman, K. and Katz, N.: Metabolism of carbohydrates. In, Regulation of Hepatic Metabolism. Edited by R.C. Thuman, F.C. Kauffman, and K. Jungermann. Plenum Press, New York, 211-235, 1986.
6. Fajans, S.S. and Floyd, J.C.: Fasting hypoglycemia in adults. New Eng. J. Med. 294:766-772, 1976.
7. Pagliara, A.S., Karl, I.E., Haymond, M. and Kipnis, D.M.: Hypoglycemia in infancy and childhood. J. Pediatr. 82:365-379, 558-577, 1973.
8. Walvoort, H.C.: Glycogen storage disease type II in the Lapland dog. Vet. Quart. 7:187-190, 1985.
9. Strombeck, D.R., Rogers, Q., Freedland, R. and McEwan, L.C.: Fasting hypoglycemia in a pup. JAVMA 173:299-300, 1978.
10. Leifer, C.E., Peterson, M.E., Matus, R.E. and Patnaik, A.K.: Hypoglycemia associated with nonislet cell tumor in 13 dogs. JAVMA 186:53-55, 1985.
11. Strombeck, D.R., Krum, S., Meyer, D. and Kappesser, R.M.: Hypoglycemia and hypoinsulinemia associated with hepatoma in a dog. JAVMA 169:811-812, 1976.
12. Cooper, A.D.: Role of the liver in the degradation of lipoproteins. Gastroenterology 88:192-205, 1985.
13. Hoyumpa, A.M., Greene, H.L., Dunn, G.D. and Schenker, S.: Fatty liver: Biochemical and clinical considerations. Am. J. Dig. Dis. 12:1141-1170, 1975.
14. Alpers, D.H. and Sabesin, S.M.: Fatty liver: Biochemical and clinical aspects. In, Diseases of the Liver. Edited by L. Schiff and E.R. Schiff. J.B. Lippincott, Philadelphia, 949-978, 1987.
15. Harry, D.S., Owen, J.S. and McIntyre, N.: Plasma lipoproteins and the liver. In, Liver and Biliary Disease. Edited by R. Wright, G.H. Millward-Sadler, K.G.M.M. Alberti and S. Karran. W.B. Saunders, Philadephia, 65-85, 1985.
16. Challenger, F. and Walshe, J.M.: Feator hepaticus. Lancet i:1239-1241, 1955.
17. McIntyre, N., Harry, D.S. and Pearson, A.J.G.: The hypercholesterolaemia of obstructive jaundice. Gut 16:379-391, 1975.
18. Opitz, M. and Lettow, E.: Der cholesterinesterquotient im serum leberkranker hunde. Berl. Munch. Tierarztl. Wschr. 89:32-35, 1976.
19. Van Vleet, J.F. and Alberts, J.O.: Evaluation of liver function tests and liver biopsy in experimental carbon tetrachloride intoxication and extrahepatic bile duct obstruction in the dog. AJVR 29:2119-2131, 1968.
20. Center, S.A., Baldwin, B.H., King, J.M. and Tennant, B.C.: Hematologic and biochemical abnormalities associated with induced extrahepatic bile duct obstruction in the cat. AJVR 44:1822-1829, 1983.
21. Strombeck, D.R., Harrold, D., Roberts, Q., Wheeldon, E., Stern, J. and Schaeffer, M.: Plasma amino acid, glucagon and insulin concentrations in dogs with nitrosamine-induced hepatic disease. AJVR 44:2028-2036, 1983.
22. Whiting, P.: Unpublished Observations.
23. Schaeffer, M.C., Rogers, Q.R., Buffington, C.A., Wolfe, B.M., and Strombeck, D.R.: Long-term biochemical and physiologic effects of surgically placed portacaval shunts in dogs. AJVR 47:346-355, 1986.
24. Muller, P., Fellin, R., Lambrecht, J., Agostinin, B., Wieland, H., Rost, W. and Seidel, D.: Hypertriglyceridaemia secondary to liver disease. Eur. J. Clin. Invest. 4:419-428, 1974.
25. Rabinowitz, J.L., Staeffen, J., Blanquet, P., Vincent, J.D., Terme, R., Series, C. and Myerson, R.M.: Sources of serum (14C) - octanoate in cirrhosis of the liver and hepatic encephalopathy. J. Lab. Clin. Med. 91:223-227, 1978.
26. Brady, L.J., Armstrong, M.K., Muiruri, K.L., Romsos, D.R., Bergen, W.G. and Leveille, G.A.: Influence of prolonged fasting in the dog on glucose turnover and blood metabolites. J. Nutr. 107:1053-1060, 1977.
27. Tavill, A.S.: Protein metabolism and the liver. In, Liver and Biliary Disease. Edited by R. Wright, G.H. Millward-Sadler, K.G.M.M. Alberti and S. Karran. W.B. Saunders, Philadelphia, 87-117, 1985.
28. LeBonton, A.V.: Protein synthesis and secretion. In, Regulation of Hepatic Metabolism. Edited by R.G. Thurman, F.C. Kauffman, and K. Jungerman. Plenum Press, New York, 383-410, 1986.
29. Felig, P.: Amino acid metabolism in man. Ann. Rev. Biochem. 44:933-955, 1975.
30. Haussinger, D. and Gerok, W.: Metabolism of amino acids and ammonia. In, Regulation of Hepatic Metabolism. Edited by R.G. Thurman, F.C. Kauffman, and K. Jungerman. Plenum Press, New York, 253-291, 1986.
31. Christensen, H.N.: Interorgan amino acid nutrition. Physiol Rev. 62:1193-1233, 1982.
32. Walser, M.: Nutritional effects of nitrogen-free analogues of essential amino acids. Life Sciences 17:1011-1020, 1975.
33. Tannen, R.L.: Ammonia metabolism. Am. J. Physiol. 235:F265-F277, 1978.
34. Flannery, D.B., Hsia, Y.E. and Wold, B.: Current status of hyperammonemic syndromes. Hepatology 2:495-506, 1982.
35. Cooper, A.J.L. and Plum, F.: Biochemistry and physiology of brain ammonia. Physiol. Rev. 67:440-519, 1987.
36. Nance, F.C., Kaufman, H.J. and Kline, D.G.: Role of urea in the hyperammonemia of germ-free Eck fistula dogs. Gastroenterology 66:108-112, 1974.
37. Vince, A., Dawson, A.M., Park, N. and O'Grady, F.: Ammonia production by intestinal bacteria. Gut 14:171-177, 1973.
38. Windmueller, H.G. and Spaeth, A.: Uptake and metabolism of plasma glutamine by the small intestine. J. Biol. Chem. 249:5070-5079, 1974.
39. Aldrete, J.S.: Quantification of the capacity of the liver to remove ammonia from the circulation of dogs with portacaval transposition. Surg. Gynecol. Obstet. 141:399-404, 1975.
40. Strombeck, D.R., Rogers, Q.R. and Stern, J.S.: Effects of ammonia infusion on plasma glucagon, insulin, and amino acids in intact, pancreatectomized, and adrenalectomized dogs. AJVR 42:810-818, 1981.
41. Morris, J.G. and Rogers, Q.R.: Ammonia intoxication in the near-adult cat as a result of a dietary deficiency of arginine. Science 199:431-432, 1978.
42. Greenstein, J.P., Winitz, M., Gullino, P., Birnbaum, S.M. and Otey, M.C.: Studies on the metabolism of amino acids and related compounds in vivo, III. Prevention of ammonia toxicity by arginine and related compounds. Arch. Biochem. Biophys. 64:342-354, 1956.
43. Zieve, L., Doizaki, W.M. and Zieve, F.J.: Synergism between mercaptans and ammonia or fatty acids in the production of coma: a possible role for mercaptans in the pathogenesis of hepatic coma. J. Lab. Clin. Med. 83:16-28, 1974.
44. Derr, R.F. and Zieve, L.: Effects of fatty acids on the disposition of ammonia. J. Pharmacol. Exper. Ther. 197:675-680, 1976.
45. Buttrose, M., McKellar, D. and Welbourne, T.C.: Gut-liver interaction in glutamine homeostasis: portal ammonia role in uptake and metabolism. Am. J. Physiol. 252:E746-E750, 1987.
46. Fraser, C.L. and Arieff, A.I.: Hepatic encephalopathy. New. Eng. J. Med. 313:865-873, 1985.
47. Conn, H.O. and Atterbury, C.E.: Cirrhosis. In, Diseases of the Liver. Edited by L. Schiff and E.R. Schiff. J.B. Lippincott, Philadelphia, 725-864, 1978.
48. Rogers, Q.: Unpublished Observations.
49. Aguirre, A., Yoshimura, N., Westman, T. and Fischer, J.E.: Plasma amino acids in dogs with two experimental forms of liver damage. J. Surg. Res. 16:339-345, 1974.
50. Rosen, H.M., Yoshimura, N., Hodgman, J.M. and Fischer, J.E.: Plasma amino acid patterns in hepatic encephalopathy of differing etiology. Gastroenterology 72:483-487, 1977.

51. Strombeck, D.R. and Rogers, Q.: Plasma amino acid concentrations in dogs with hepatic disease. JAVMA 173:93-96, 1978.
52. Rutgers, C., Stradley, R.P. and Rogers, W.A.: Plasma amino acid analysis in dogs with experimentally induced hepatocellular and obstructive jaundice. AJVR 48:696-702, 1987.
53. Holdsworth, C.D., Nye, L. and Kin, E.: The effect of portacaval anastomosis on oral carbohydrate tolerance and on plasma insulin levels. Gut 13:58-63, 1972.
54. Lickley, H.L.A., Chisholm, D.J., Rabinovitch, A., Wexler, M. and Dupre, J.: Effects of portacaval anastomosis on glucose tolerance in the dog: evidence of an interaction between the gut and the liver in oral glucose disposal. Metabolism 24:1157-1168, 1975.
55. Waddell, W.R. and Sussman, K.E.: Plasma insulin after diversion of portal and pancreatic venous blood to vena cava. J. Appl. Physiol. 22:808-812, 1967.
56. Kaden, M., Harding, P. and Field, J.B.: Effect of intraduodenal glucose administration on hepatic extraction of insulin in the anesthetized dog. J. Clin. Invest. 52:2016-2028, 1973.
57. Felig, P. and Sherwin, R.: Carbohydrate homeostasis, liver and diabetes. In, Progress in Liver Diseases. Vol. 5. Edited by H. Popper and F. Schaffner. Grune and Stratton, New York, 149-171, 1976.
58. Strombeck, D.R., Harrold, D. and Rogers, Q.R.: Effects of catecholamines and ammonia on plasma and brain amino acids in dogs. Am. J. Physiol. 247:E276-283, 1984.
59. Fischer, J.E., Rosen, H.M., Ebeid, A.M., James, J.H., Keane, J.M. and Soeters, P.B.: The effect of normalization of plasma amino acids on hepatic encephalopathy in man. Surgery 80:77-91, 1976.
60. Cacciatore, L., Antoniello, S., Valentino, B. and DeRitis, F.: Arginase activity, arginine, and ornithine of plasma in experimental liver damage. Enzyme 17:269-275, 1974.
61. Hsia, Y.E.: Inherited hyperammonemic syndromes. Gastroenterology 67:347-374, 1974.
62. Merino, G.E., Ketzer, T., Doizaki, W.M.D. and Najarian, J.S.: Methionine-induced hepatic coma in dogs. Am. J. Surg. 130:41-46, 1975.
63. Phear, E.A., Ruebner, B., Sherlock, S. and Summerskill, W.H.J.: Methionine toxicity in liver disease and its prevention by chlortetracycline. Clin. Sci. 15:93-117, 1956.
64. Payne, J.A.: False neurotransmitters and portal systemic encephalopathy. Clin. Neuropharm. 5:267-275, 1982.
65. Goldstein, G.W.: The role of brain capillaries in the pathogenesis of hepatic encephalopathy. Hepatology 4:565-567, 1984.
66. Trulson, M.E.: Dietary tryptophan does not alter the function of brain serotonin neurons. Life Sciences 37:1067-1072, 1985.
67. Fonnum, F.: Glutamate: A neurotransmitter in mammalian brain. J. Neurochem. 42:1-11, 1984.
68. Schafer, D.F.: Hepatic Coma: Studies on the target organ. Gastroenterology 93:1131-1134, 1987.
69. Ferenci, P., Zieve, L., Ebner, J., Zimmerman, Ch. and Rzepczynski, D.: Postsynaptic q-aminobutyric acid receptors in hepatic coma following portacaval shunt and hepatic artery ligation in the rat. Metab. Brain Dis. 2:195-200, 1987.
70. Zieve, L.: Hepatic encephalopathy. In, Diseases of the Liver. Edited by L. Schiff and E.R. Schiff. J.B. Lippincott, Philadelphia, 925-248, 1987.
71. Weber, F.L.: Therapy of portal-systemic encephalopathy: The practical and the promising. Gastroenterology 81:174-181, 1981.
72. Mans, A.M., Biebuyck, J.F., Davis, D.W. and Hawkins, R.A.: Portacaval anastomosis: Brain and plasma metabolite abnormalities and the effect of nutritional therapy. J. Neurochem. 43:697-705, 1984.
73. Cossack, Z.T. and Prasad, A.S.: Hyperammonemia in zinc deficiency: Activities of urea cycle related enzymes. Nutr. Res. 7:1161-1167, 1987.
74. Condon, R.E.: Effect of dietary protein on symptoms and survival in dogs with an Eck fistula. Am. J. Surg. 121:107-114, 1971.
75. Zieve, L. and Zieve, F.J.: The dietary prevention of hepatic coma in ECK fistula dogs: Ammonia and the carbohydrate to protein ratio. (Comment) Hepatology 7:196-198, 1987.
76. Benjamine, L.E. and Steele, R.D.: Methionine metabolism after portacaval shunt in the rat. Am. J. Physiol. 249:G321-G327, 1985.
77. Weber, F.L., Minco, D., Fresard, K.M. and Banwell, J.G.: Effects of vegetable diets on nitrogen metabolism in cirrhotic subjects. Gastroenterology 89:538-544, 1985.
78. Rothschild, M.A., Oratz, M. and Schreiber, S.S.: Albumin metabolism. Gastroenterology 64:324-337, 1973.
79. Tavill, A.S.: The synthesis and degradation of liver-produced proteins. Gut 13:225-241, 1972.
80. Maier, K.P.: Protein metabolism and urea synthesis. In, Metabolism and Nutrition in Liver Disease. Edited by E. Holm and H. Kasper. MTP Press Ltd, Boston, 31-41, 1984.
81. Rothschild, M.A., Oratz, M. and Schreiber, S.S.: Albumin metabolism. In, Progress in Liver Diseases. Vol. 4. Edited by H. Popper and F. Schaffner. Grune and Stratton, New York, 19-29, 1972.
82. Sidransky, H.: Regulatory effect of amino acids on polyribosomes and protein synthesis of liver. In, Progress in Liver Diseases. Vol. 4. Edited by H. Popper and F. Schaffner. Grune and Stratton, New York, 31-43, 1972.
83. Rothschild, M.A., Oratz, M. and Schreiber, S.S.: Serum albumin. Hepatology 8:385-401, 1988.
84. Seglen, P.O. and Reith, A.: Ammonia inhibits protein secretion in isolated rat hepatocytes. Biochem. Biophys. Acta 496:29-35, 1977.
85. Strombeck, D.R., Miller, L.M. and Harrold, D.: Effects of corticosteroid treatment on survival time in dogs with chronic hepatitis: 151 cases (1977-1985). JAVMA 193:1109-1113, 1988.
86. Kukral, J.C., Sporn, J., Louch, J. and Winzler, R.J.: Synthesis of alpha-and beta-globulins in normal and liverless dog. Am. J. Physiol. 204:262-264, 1963.
87. Knapp, K.K. and Hunter, R.L.: Serum proteins of the beagle dog: A two-dimensional electrophoretic study. Am. J. Vet. Res. 36:193-195, 1975.
88. Sherry, S., Fletcher, A.P. and Alkjaersing, N.: Fibrinolysis and fibrinolytic activity in man. Physiol. Rev. 39:343-382, 1959.
89. Hiramatsu, S., Kojima, J., Okada, T.T., Inai, S. and Ohmori, K.: The serum protein profile in chronic hepatitis, cirrhosis and liver cancer. Acta Hepato-Gastroenterol. 23:177-182, 1976.
90. Furnival, C.M., Mackenzie, R.J., MacDonald, G.A. and Blumgart, L.H.: The mechanism of impaired coagulation after partial hepatectomy in the dog. Surg. Gynecol. Obstet. 143:81-86, 1976.
91. Thomas, H.C.: Immunologic aspects of liver disease. In, Diseases of the Liver. Edited by L. Schiff and E.R. Schiff. 163-185, 1987.
92. Kleinmaan, R.E. and Walker, W.A.: The liver and intestinal immunoglobulin A: up from the "minors"? Gastroenterology 93:650-651, 1987.
93. Allen, P.M.: Antigen presentation and autoimmunity. Hepatology 8:677-679, 1988.
94. Aledort, L.M.: Blood clotting mechanisms in liver disease. In, Progress in Liver Diseases, Vol. 5. Edited by H. Popper and F. Schaffner, Grune and Stratton, New York. 350-362, 1965.
95. Roberts, H.R. and Cederbaum, A.I.: The liver and blood coagulation: physiology and pathology. Gastroenterology 63:297-320, 1972.
96. Badylak, S.F.: Coagulopathies associated with hepatic disease. Calif. Vet. 14-17, 1982.
97. Badylak, S.F., Dodds, W.J., van Vleet, J.F.: Plasma coagulation factor abnormalities in dogs with naturally occurring hepatic disease. AJVR 44:2336-2340, 1983.
98. Dodds, W.J.: Hemostasis and coagulation. In, Clinical Biochemistry of Domestic Animals. Edited by J.J. Kaneko. Academic Press, New York, 671-718, 1980.
99. Hellebrekers, L.J., Slappendel, R.J. and van den Brom, W.E.:

Effect of sodium heparin and antithrombin III concentration on activated partial thromboplastin time in the dog. AJVR 46:1460-1462, 1985.

100. Verstraete, M., Vermylen, J. and Collen, D.: Intravascular coagulation in liver disease. Ann. Rev. Med. 25:447-455, 1974.

101. Feldman, B.F. and Strombeck, D.R.: Unpublished Data.

102. Wigton, D.H., Kociba, G.J. and Hoover, E.A.: Infectious canine hepatitis: animal model for viral-induced disseminated intravascular coagulation. blood 47:287-296, 1976.

103. Owen, C.A. and Walter Bowie, E.J.: Effect of heparin on chronically induced intravascular coagulation in dogs. Am. J. Physiol. 229:449-454, 1975.

104. Rake, M.O., Flute, P.T., Pannell, G., Shilkin, K.B. and Williams, R.: Experimental hepatic necrosis: studies on coagulation abnormalities, plasma clearance, and organ distribution of 1251-labelled fibrinogen. Gut 14:574-580, 1973.

105. Schaewen, H. von: Sweifalle von Verbrauchskoagulopathie bei akuter hepatitis des hundes. Kleintier-Praxis 18:111-114, 1973.

106. Slappendel, R.J. and Dijk, J.E. van: Diffuse intravasale stolling (DIS). II. Spontane DIS bij de hond. Tijdschr Diergeneeskd 98:615-631, 1973.

107. Strombeck, D.R., Krum, S. and Rogers, Q.: Coagulopathy and encephalopathy in a dog with acute hepatic necrosis. JAVMA 169:813-816, 1976.

108. Murray, M., Robinson, P.B., McKeating, F.J. and Lauder, I.M.: Peptic ulceration in the dog: a clincio-pathological study. Vet. Rec. 91:441-447, 1972.

109. Badylak, S.F. and VanVleet, J.F.: Alterations of prothrombin time and activated partial thromboplastin time in dogs with hepatic disease. AJVR 42:2053-2056, 1981.

110. Margolis, S. and Capuzzi, D.: Serum lipoprotein synthesis and metabolism. In, Blood Lipids and Lipoproteins: Quantitation, Composition and Metabolism. Edited by G.J. Nelson. Wiley-Interscience, New York, 825-880, 1973.

111. Solyom, A., Bradford, R.H. and Furman, R.H.: Apolipoprotein and lipid distribution in canine serum lipoproteins. Biochem. Biophys. Acta. 229:471-483, 1971.

112. Nakai, T. and Whayne, T.F.: Catabolism of canine apolipoprotein A-I: purification, catabolic rate, organs of catabolism, and the liver subcellular catabolic site. J. Lab. Clin. Med. 88:63-80, 1976.

113. Dainelsson, B., Eckman, R., Johansson, B.G. and Peterson, B.G.: Abnormal low density plasma lipoproteins occurring in dogs with obstructive jaundice. FEBS Letters 63:33-36, 1976.

114. Magnani, H.N. and Alaupovic, P.: Utilization of the quantitative assay of lipoprotein X in the differential diagnosis of extrahepatic obstructive jaundice and intrahepatic diseases. Gastroenterology 71:87-93, 1976.

115. Marks, J.: The vitamins in health and disease. Little, Brown and Co., Boston, 1968.

116. White, A., Handler, P. and Smith, E.L.: Principles of Biochemistry, 3rd edition. McGraw Hill, New York, 1964.

117. Leo, M.A. and Lieber, C.S.: Hypervitaminosis A: a liver lover's lament. Hepatology 8:412-417, 1988.

118. Barry, M.: Iron and the liver. Gut. 15:324-334, 1974.

119. Macdonald, R.A.: Hemochromatosis and Wilson's Disease in the Liver. Monographs in Pathology. Edited by E.A. Gall and F.K. Mostofi. Williams and Wilkins Co., Baltimore 466-479, 1973.

120. Cousins, R.J.: Absorption, transport, and hepatic metabolism of copper and zinc: Special reference to metallothionein and ceruloplasmin. Physiol. Rev. 65:238-309, 1985.

121. Erlinger, S. and Dhumeaux, D.: Mechanisms and control of secretion of bile water and electrolytes. Gastroenterology 66:281-304, 1974.

122. Javitt, N.B.: Hepatic Bile Formation. New Eng. J. Med. 295:1464 and 1511, 1976.

123. Schanker, L.S.: Secretion of organic compounds in bile. In, Handbook of physiology. Section 6. Alimentary Canal, Vol. 5. Edited by C.F. Code. Amer. Physiol. Soc., Washington DC, 2433-2449, 1968.

124. Wheeler, H.O.: Water and electrolytes in bile. In, Handbook of Physiology, Section 6, Alimentary Canal, Vol. 5. Edited by C.F. Code. Amer. Physiol. Soc., Washington, DC, 2409-2431, 1968.

125. Erlinger, S.: Secretion of bile. In: Diseases of the Liver. Edited by L. Schiff and E.R. Schiff. J.B. Lippincott, Philadelphia, 77-101, 1987.

126. Diamond, J.M.: Transport mechanisms in the gallbladder. In, Handbook of Physiology, Section 6, Alimentary Canal, Vol. 5, Edited by C.F. Code. Amer. Physiol. Soc., Washington DC 2451-2482, 1968.

127. Banfield, W.J.: Physiology of the gallbladder. Gastroenterology 69:770-777, 1975.

128. Bjorkhem, I. and Danielsson, H.: Biosynthesis and metabolism of bile acids in man. In, Progress in Liver Diseases, Vol. 5. Edited by H. Popper and F. Schaffner. Grune and Stratton, New York, 215-231, 1976.

129. Heaton, K.W.: Bile salts. In: Liver and Biliary Disease. Edited by R. Wright, G.H. Millward-Sadler, K.G.M.M. Alberti and S. Karran. 277-300. W.B. Saunders, Philadelphia, 1985.

130. Ramakrishnan, V.R, Beher, W.T., Lin, G.J., Stradnieks, S., Samhouri, F., Toledo-Pereyra, L.H. and Block, M.A.: Effects of sphincter of Oddi bypass on bile acid metabolism in fed and fasted intact and cholecystectomized dogs. Digestion 21:143-150, 1981.

131. DeNovo, R.C. and Prasse, K.W.: Comparison of serum biochemical and hepatic functional alterations in dogs treated with corticosteroids and hepatic duct ligation. Am. J. Vet. Res. 44:1703-1709, 1983.

132. Center, S.A., Baldwin, B.H., King, J.M. and Tennant, B.C.: Hematologic and biochemical abnormalities associated with induced extrahepatic bile duct obstruction in the cat. Am. J. Vet. Res. 44:1822-1829, 1983.

133. Rutgers, H.C., Stradley, R.P. and Johnson, S.E.: Serum bile acid analysis in dogs with experimentally induced cholestatic jaundice. AJVR 49:317-320, 1988.

134. Horak, W., Gangl, A., Funovics, J. and Grabner, G.: Effect of portacaval shunt and arterialization of the liver on bile acid metabolism. Gastroenterology 69:338-341, 1975.

135. Center, S.A., Baldwin, B.H., Lahynta, A., Dietze, A.E. and Tennant, B.C.: Evaluation of serum bile acid concentrations for the diagnosis of portosystemic venous anomalies in the dog and cat. JAVMA 186:1090-1094, 1985.

136. Meyer, D.J.: Liver function tests in dogs with portosystemic shunts: measurement of serum bile acid concentration. JAVMA 188:168-169, 1986.

137. Herz, R., Paumgartner, G. and Preisig, R.: Bile salt metabolism and bile formation in the rate with a portacaval shunt. Eur. J. Clin. Invest. 4:223-228, 1974.

138. Pare, P., Hoefs, J.C. and Ashcavai, M.: Determinants of serum bile acids in chronic liver disease. Gastroenterology 81:959-964, 1981.

139. Washizu, T., Koizumi, I. and Kaneko, J.J.: Postprandial changes in serum bile acids concentration and fractionation of individual bile acid by high performance liquid chromatography in normal dogs. Jpn. J. Vet. Sci. 49:593-600, 1987.

140. Fromm, H. and Albert, M.B.: Selected Summaries. Gastroenterology 92:829-830, 1987.

141. Kitagawa, H., Ishihara, K. and Yokoyama, S.: Serum total bile acid level in normal dogs. Jpn. J. Vet. Sci. 43:257-260, 1981.

142. Center, S.A., Baldwin, B.H., Erb, H.N. and Tennant, B.C.: Bile acid concentrations in the diagnosis of hepatobiliary disease in the dog. JAVMA 187:935-940, 1985.

143. Johnson, S.E., Rogers, W.A., Bonagura, J.D. and Caldwell, J.H.: Determination of serum bile acids in fasting dogs with hepatobiliary disease. AJVR 46:2048-2053, 1985.

144. Cravetto, C., Molino, G., Biondi, A.M., Cavanna, A., Avagina, P. and Frediani, S.: Evaluation of the diagnostic value of serum bile acid in the detection and functional assessment of liver diseases. Ann. Clin, Biochem. 22:596-605, 1985.

145. Kaneko, J.J.: Porphyrins, heme, and erythrocyte metabolism: The porphyrias. In, Clinical Biochemistry of Domestic Animals. Edited by J.J. Kaneko. Academic Press, New

York, 119-174, 1980.
146. Gollan, J. and Schmid, R.: Bilirubin metabolism and hyperbilirubinaemic disorders. In, Liver and Biliary Disease. Edited by R. Wright, G.H. Millward-Sadler, K.G.M.M. Alberti, and S. Karran. 301-357. W.B. Saunders, Philadelphia, 1985.
147. Rothuizen, J.: Hyperbilirubinemia in canine hepatobiliary disease. Thesis. Sept. 1985.
148. Arias, I.M.: Formation of bile pigment. In, Handbook of Physiology, Section 6, Alimentary Canal, Vol. 5. Edited by C.F. Code. Am. Physiol. Soc., Washington DC, 2347-2374, 1968.
149. Cornelius, C.E.: Liver function. In, Clinical Biochemistry of Domestic Animals, second edition. Vol. 1 Edited by J.J. Kaneko and C.E. Cornelius. Academic Press, New York, 1970.
150. Gray, C.H., Nicholson, D.C. and Quincy, R.V.: Fate of bile in the bowel. In, Handbook of Physiology, Section 6, Alimentary Canal, Vol. 5. Edited by C.F. Code. Am. Physiol. Soc., Washington DC 2483-2505, 1968.
151. Cornelius, C.E.: Hepatic disease in animals. In, Progress in Liver Diseases. Vol. 3. Edited by H. Popper and F. Schaffner. Grune and Stratton, New York, 419-431, 1970.
152. Levy, M., Lester, R. and Levinsky, N.G.: Renal excretion of urobilinogen in the dog. J. Clin. Invest. 47:2117-2124, 1968.
153. Mathis, R.K., Andres, J.M. and Walker, W.A.: Liver Disease in infants. Part II: Hepatic disease states. J. Pediatr. 90:864-880, 1977.
154. Tryphonas, L. and Rozdilsky, B.: Nuclear jaundice (Kernicterus) in a newborn kitten. JAVMA 157:1084-1087, 1970.
155. Gopinath, C. and Ford, E.J.H.: Location of liver injury and extent of bilirubinaemia in experimental liver lesions. Vet. Path. 9:99-108, 1972.
156. Mor, L., Bomzon, A., Mordechovich, D., Blendis, L.M. and Better, O.S.: Renal bilirubin excretion in canine models of jaundice. Biochem. Med. Metabl. Biol. 36:252-259, 1986.
157. Gillette, J.R. and Jollow, D.J.: Drug metabolism in liver. In, The Liver: Normal and abnormal functions. Part A, Vol. 5. Edited by F.F. Becker. The biochemistry of disease. Marcel Dekker, New York, 165-201, 1974.
158. George, C.F. and George, R.H.: The liver and response to drugs. In: Liver and Biliary Disease. Edited by R. Wright, G.H. Millward-Sadler, K.G.M.M. Alberti and S. Karran. W.B. Saunders, Philadelphia, 415-452, 1985.
159. VanThiel, D.H., Stone, B.G. and Schade, R.R.: The liver and its effect on endocrine function in health and diseases. In, Diseases of the Liver. Edited by L. Schiff and E.R. Schiff. J.B. Lippincott, Philadelphia, 129-162, 1987.
160. Thurman, R.G., Kauffman, F.C. and Baron, J.: Biotransformation and zonal toxicity. In, Regulation of Hepatic Metabolism. Edited by R.G. Thurman, F.C. Kauffman, and K. Jungerman. Plenum Press, New York, 321-382, 1986.
161. Powell, L.W. and Axelsen, E.: Corticosteroids in liver disease: Studies on the biological conversion of prednisone to prednisolone and plasma protein binding. Gut 13:690-696, 1972.
162. McKerns, K.W.: Steroid Hormones and Metabolism. Appleton-Century-Crofts, New York, 1969.
163. Wilson, J.D.: Metabolism of testicular androgens. In. Handbook of physiology, Sec 7. Endocrinology, Vol. 5. Edited by R.O. Greep and E.B. Astwood. Am. Physiol. Soc., Washington DC, 491-508, 1975.
164. Sherlock, S.: The spectrum of hepatotoxicity due to drugs. Lancet 2:440-444, 1986.
165. Zimmerman, H.J. and Maddrey, W.C.: Toxic and drug-induced hepatitis. In,Diseases of the Liver. Edited by L. Schiff and E.R. Schiff. J.B. Lippincott, Philadelphia, 591-667, 1987.
166. Read, A.E.: The liver and drugs. In, Liver and Biliary Disease. Edited by R. Wright, G.H. Millward-Sadler, K.G.M.M. Alberti and S. Karran. W.B. Saunders, Philadelphia, 1003-1031, 1985.
167. Pedersoli, W.M.: Serum fluoride concentrations, renal, and hepatic function tests results in dogs with methoxyflurane anesthesia. Am. J. Vet. Res. 38:949-953, 1977.
168. Ortega, L., Garcia, J.I.: Acetaminophen-induced fulminant hepatic failure in dogs. Hepatology 5:673-676, 1985.
169. deGroot, H. and Noll, T.: Halothane toxicity: relation between metabolic activation; hypoxia, covalent binding, lipid peroxidation and liver cell damage. Hepatology 3:601-606, 1983.
170. Williams, R.L.: Drug administration in hepatic disease. New Eng. J. Med. 309:1616-1622, 1983.
171. Wilkinson, G.R. and Shand, D.G.: A physiological approach to hepatic drug clearance. Clin. Pharmacol. There. 18:377-390, 1975.
172. McKerns, K.W.: Steroid Hormones and Metabolism. Appleton-Century-Crofts, New York, 1969.
173. Gordon, G.G., Olivo, J., Rafii, F. and Southren, A.L.: Conversions of androgens to estrogens in cirrhosis of the liver. J. Clin. Endocrinol. Metab. 40:1018-1026, 1975.
174. Saba, T.M.: Physiology and pathophysiology of the reticuloendothelial system. Arch. Int. Med. 126:1031-1052, 1970.
175. Mosher, D.F.: Fibronectin and liver disease. Hepatology 6:1419-1421, 1986.
176. Kleinman, R.E., Harmatz, P.R. and Walker, W.A.: The liver: An integral part of the enteric mucosal immune system. Hepatology 2:379-384, 1982.
177. Delacroix, D.L., Furtado-Barreira, G., deHemptinne, B., Gondswaard, J., Dive, C., and Vaerman, J.-P.: The liver in the IgA secretory immune system, but not rats and rabbits, are suitable models for human studies. Hepatology 3:980-988, 1983.
178. Edgington, T.S.: Immune responses and liver disease, perhaps. But what about target organ defenses. Hepatology 3:767-768, 1983.
179. Bradley, S.E.: The hepatic circulation. In, Handbook of Physiology Sec. 2, Circulation, Vol. 2. Edited by W.F. Hamilton and P. Dow. American Physiological Society, Washington, DC, 1387-1438, 1963.
180. Witte, C.L. and Witte, M.H.: Hepatic circulation. In, The Liver; Normal and Abnormal Functions. Part A. Vol. 5. Edited by F.F. Becker. The Biochemistry of Disease. Marcel dekker, New York, 11-54, 1974.
181. Lautt, W.W. and Greenway, C.V.: Conceptual review of the hepatic vascular bed. Hepatology 7:952-963, 1987.
182. Groszmann, R.J., Blei, A.T. Kniaz, J.L., Storer, E.H. and Conn, H.O.: Portal pressure reduction induced by partial mechanical obstruction of the superior mesenteric artery in the anesthetized dog. Gastroenterology 75:187-192, 1978.
183. Richardson, P.O.I. and Withrington, P.G.: Liver blood flow I. Gastroenterology 81:159-173, 1981.
184. Richardson, P.O.I. and Withrington, P.G.: Liver blood flow II. Gastroenterology 81:356-375, 1981.
185. Schatten, W.E.: The role of intestinal bacteria in liver necrosis following experimental excision of the hepatic arterial supply. Surgery 36:256-269, 1954.
186. Markowitz, J., Rappaport, A. and Scott, A.C.: The function of the hepatic artery in the dog. Am. J. Dig. Dis. 16:344-348, 1949.
187. Lykkegaard Nielsen, M., Justesen, T. and Asnaes, S.: Anaerobic bacteriological study of the human liver - with a critical review of the literature. Scand. J. Gastroenterology 9:671-677, 1974.
188. Crossley, I.R., Westaby, D. and Williams, R.: Portal hypertension. In, Liver and Biliary Disease. Edited by R. Wright, G.H. Millward-Sadler, K.G.M.M. Alberti and S. Karran. W.B. Saunders, Philadelphia, 1283-1316, 1985.
189. Reynolds, T.B.: Portal hypertension. In, Diseases of the Liver. Edited by L. Schiff and E.R. Schiff. J.B. Lippincott, Philadelphia, 875-901, 1987.
190. Sugita, S., Ohnishi, K., Saito, M. and Okuda, K.: Splanchnic hemodynamics in portal hypertensive dogs with portal fibrosis. Am. J. Physiol. 252:G748-G754, 1987.
191. Easley, J.C. and Carpenter, J.L.: Hepatic arteriovenous fistula in two Saint Bernard pups. JAVMA 166:167-171, 1975.
192. Legendre, A.M., Krahwinkel, D.J., Carrig, C.B. and Michel, R.L.: Ascites associated with intrahepatic arteriovenous

fistula in a cat. JAVMA 168:589-591, 1976.
193. Blei, A.T., Gottsten, J. and Ganger, D.: Oral neomycin normalizes hyperdynamic features of awake portal hypertensive rats. Hepatology 8:1253, 1988.
194. Sugar, I., Jakab, F. and Szabo, G.: The effect of increased inferior vena cava pressure on hepatic circulation in the dog. Res. Exp. Med. 171:263-270, 1977.
195. Zimon, D.S. and Kessler, R.E.: The portal pressure-blood volume relationship in cirrhosis. Gut 15:99-101, 1974.
196. Vitums, A.: Portosystemic communications in the dog. Acta Anat. 39:271-299, 1959.
197. Rector, W.G.: Ascites kinetics in cirrhosis: Effects of rapid volume expansion and duiretic administration. J. Lab. Clin. Med. 111:166-172, 1988.
198. Laragh, J.H.: Atrial natriuretic hormone, the renin-aldosterone axis, and blood pressure-electrolyte homeostasis. New Eng. J. Med. 313:1330-1340, 1985.
199. Epstein, M.: Derangements in renal water handling in liver disease. Gastroenterology 89:1415-1425, 1985.
200. Schrier, R.W., Arroyo, V., Bernardi, M., Epstein, M., Henriksen, J.H. and Rodes, J.: Peripheral arterial vasodilation hypothesis: A proposal for the initiation of renal sodium and water retention in cirrhosis. Hepatology 8:1151-1157, 1988.
201. Davidson, E.W. and Dunn, M.J.: Pathogenesis of the hepatorenal syndrome. Ann. Rev. Med. 38:361-372, 1987.
202. Epstein, M. and Lifschitz, M.: Renal eicosanoids as determinants of renal function in liver disease. Hepatology 7:1359-1367, 1987.
203. Zink, J. and Greenway, C.V.: Control of ascites absorption in anesthetized cats: effects of intraperitoneal pressure, protein, and furosemide diuresis. Gastroenterology 73:1119-1124, 1977.
204. Suter, P.F.: Portal vein anomalies in the dog: their angiographic diagnosis. J. Am. Vet. Radiol. 16:84-97, 1975.
205. Lohse, C.L. and Suter, P.F.: Functional closure of the ductus venosus during early postnatal life in the dog. AJVR June, 1977.
206. Traber, P.G., Chianale, J. and Gumucio, J.J.: Physiologic signficance and regulation of hepatocellular heterogeneity. Gastroenterology 95:1130-1143, 1988.
207. Jungerman, K.: Zonal signal heterogeneity and induction of hepatocyte heterogeneity. In, Regulation of Hepatic Metabolism. Edited by R.G. Thurman, F.C. Kauffman and K. Jungerman. Plenum Press, New York, 445-469, 1986.

Chapter 29

Pathogenesis and Incidence of Hepatic Disease

PATHOGENESIS OF HEPATOCYTE INJURY AND DEATH

Numerous experimental studies demonstrate that a wide variety of insults to hepatocytes result in injury and death. Conventional concepts hold that hepatocellular injury and death represent a stepwise and continuous process, where the insult initiates a chain of events which can be compared to a disease process caused by an excess or deficiency of one enzyme or hormone. The pathogenesis of hepatocellular damage is not that straightforward, however. Many interacting factors determine the appearance of hepatocellular damage; a very well-documented insult can cause pathology under certain conditions and no pathology under different circumstances. This diversity has led to the conclusion "that most forms of liver cell injury represent a derangement or malfunctioning of an interlinking network of key factors in which feedback activation may produce not only unfavorable, vicious cycles but also favorable adaptive compensation."[1] With an understanding of that network it is possible to develop methods for modulating the factors involved in order to alter a process moving to cell death. Such a goal would be instituted rather than attempting to inhibit or replace a single factor, an attempt comparable to using an antibody to interact with and neutralize an antigen, or an antibiotic to counteract a microbiological agent.

Hepatocyte injury and death is associated with two intracellular factors: the rate of generation and concentration of toxic forms of oxygen and the concentration of free calcium.[1-5] The abundance of factors inactivating their effects determines the degree of damage by the oxygen species. Hepatocyte injury is also produced by extracellular factors which promote changes in the concentrations of toxic forms of oxygen and of calcium; factors from the outside can also directly damage cell membranes when enzymatic activity degrades structural lipids, carbohydrates, or proteins (see Chapter 4).

The extracellular concentration of calcium is 10^{-3}M; the intracellular concentration is much lower at 10^{-7}M.[4] Since optimum calcium levels are essential for the regulation of many important biological processes, free calcium levels in cytosol are highly regulated. Uncontrolled increases in cytosolic-free calcium are thought to be important for the initiation of toxic cell injury.[1,2,4] Such increases are possible due to an exaggerated release of calcium from endoplasmic reticulum and mitochondria, the calcium-sequestering cellular organelles, and to increases in cell membrane permeability, which permits calcium to move readily from its high extracellular concentrations to the region of normally low intracellular levels. Increasing cytosolic-free calcium results in disruption of the structure of the hepatocyte's cytoskeleton and plasma membrane, both early changes in cell injury. Calcium also activates phospholipases and proteases, which can lead to cell death.

Cytosolic-free calcium is maintained at low levels by active uptake of calcium into the intracellular compartments and by active extrusion of the ion through the plasma membrane. Calcium uptake by endoplasmic reticulum and mitochondria is an energy-dependent process. Competition for the energy used in that process, as from drugs being metabolized by microsomal enzymes, results in an increase of cytosolic-free calcium. As expected, oxygen deficiency reduces calcium uptake by both mitochondria and endoplasmic reticulum, and cytosolic-free calcium increases. Cytosolic factors protecting against the drug- or hypoxia-induced calcium changes include the availability of the reduced nucleotide NADPH as a substrate for energy and glutathione. Glutathione and other thiol-reducing agents protect the microsomal pump for sequestering calcium, probably by preventing the oxidation of protein sulfhydryl groups critical for calcium transport activity. Depletion of glutathione is an early important event preceding changes in protein sulfhydryl groups and cytosolic-free calcium homeostasis. A cytosolic protein, calmodulin, also interacts with glutathione. This protein does not bind calcium at the normally low intracellular levels, but it sequesters calcium as those levels increase.

Increased transport of calcium across plasma membranes is one of the earliest changes evident following injury induced by drugs such as acetaminophen and carbon tetrachloride or by reperfusion after ischemia. Cell membrane injury increases permeability to the movement of calcium from high extracellular concentrations to low intracellular concentrations. But it also damages the plasma membrane calcium translocase system so that the cell loses its ability to extrude calcium from the cell. A calcium ATPase is involved in that transport; its activity is reduced by injury but can be restored by glutathione or other sulfhydryl chemicals. The plasma membrane's restrictions to the inward flux of calcium are partly due to its heparin sulfate and other sulfated glycosaminoglycans, which are lost with injury. Since heparin binds circulating lipases, it is possible that the released heparin may be reflected in the increased plasma lipase activity sometimes seen with liver disease. The increase in cytosolic-free calcium is believed to be more important than either covalent binding or lipid peroxidation in hepatocellular injury.

In biological systems oxygen is ultimately reduced to water. In the process, oxygen gains single electrons to form potentially toxic and highly reactive free radicals, which include superoxide anion-free radical, hydrogen peroxide, and the hydroxyl radical.[1,3,5] These intermediates are formed under physiological conditions as products of normal cell metabolism. They do not accumulate and damage cell structures because of normal defense mechanisms that convert the free radicals to less toxic products. The defense mechanisms include cytosolic and mitochondrial superoxide dismutases and glutathione peroxidases as well as peroxisomal catalase. The critical defense mechanism is the ability of the cell to maintain a pool of reduced glutathione.

Oxygen-derived free radicals are produced by macrophages and neutrophils and represent the principle mechanism for the bactericidal properties of these cells. Increased activity of these cells, releases an abundance of free radicals; if the amount overwhelms the defense mechanisms, hepatocyte damage can follow. Oxygen radicals are also responsible for parenchymal cell injury following reperfusion of ischemic tissues. During ischemia the enzyme xanthine dehydrogenase is converted to xanthine oxidase, which has the ability to produce oxygen radicals. Also during ischemia ATP is used up and catabolized to hypoxanthine. Upon reperfusion and restoration of oxygen delivery, the oxygen reacts with hypoxanthine, catalyzed by xanthine oxidase, to produce the highly toxic oxygen free radicals. Oxygen radical formation has other potential sources in the liver; they can be produced by enzymatic activities of aldehyde oxidase, tryptophan dioxygenase, prostaglandin synthetase, and D-amino acid oxidases. Oxygen radicals are also produced by autoxidation of flavins, catecholamines, ferredoxins, quinols, and hemeproteins. Iron overload results in lipid peroxidation produced by oxygen radicals. Lipid peroxides react with metal ions or with metalloproteins to produce alkoxy radicals and initiate free radical reactions. Breakdown of the products of lipid peroxidation results in the formation of metabolites such as aldehydes, which are cytotoxic, inhibit enzymes and damage DNA.

Oxygen-free radicals have a well-understood effect on membrane lipids, causing their peroxidation and the formation of aldehyde and carboxyl groups in their molecules. These changes were once thought to be most important for cell injury. Lipid peroxidation's most important consequence, however, is its consumption of the cell's defense mechanisms. The peroxides formed in the membranes' unsaturated fatty acids react with and consume glutathione. The oxidized glutathione produced must be converted to reduced glutathione by NADPH in order to replenish the defense capacity. Lipid peroxidation reduces the availability of reduced glutathione for other detoxification processes. Oxygen-free radicals cause more important damage to macromolecules other than lipids, such as proteins, nucleic acids, and carbohydrates. Oxidation of sulfhydryl groups inactivates many intracellular enzymes, any one of which could be critical for cell survival.

Oxygen-derived free radicals are converted from their toxic to less- or nontoxic forms by naturally occurring free-radical scavengers and antioxidant pathways. The most important inactivator is glutathione; others are vitamins A, C, and E. An enzyme in mitochondria and the cytosol superoxide dismutase accelerate the dismutation of the superoxide anion to hydrogen peroxide and molecular oxygen. Another enzyme in peroxisomes, catalase, promotes the conversion of hydrogen peroxide to water and oxygen. Glutathione peroxidase acts to convert organic hydroperoxides to corresponding alcohols, at the expense of oxidation of glutathione to glutathione disulfide. The latter is regenerated to glutathione by glutathione reductase activity using NADPH. The level of reduced or protective forms of glutathione is reduced by ischemia, by an increasing rate of generation of oxygen-free radicals, and by fasting. Greater glutathione levels in the fed state or following glutathione administration help protect the liver against ischemic and other types of insults.

Lysosomal enzymes and mediators of inflammation released by neutrophils and mononuclear phagocytes can damage hepatocytes. The lysosomal enzymes act to degrade protein, lipid, and carbohydrate components of cell membranes. Leukotrienes are probably the key mediators of inflammation in liver disease; they are produced by eosinophils and mast cells as well as neutrophils and mononuclear phagocytes.[6] Many substances can activate macrophages to release their mediators of injury; lipopolysaccharide of endotoxin is the best understood activator.

A number of different conditions can accentuate or attenuate pathogic processes leading to cell injury.[1,3] Such effects have been demonstrated for endotoxin, metals such as iron, high vitamin A levels, drugs such as halothane and acetaminophen, bile acids, toxic metabolites produced in the colon, fibronectin, fasting or feeding, and oxygen availability. Under some conditions a drug produces no injury, whereas under different conditions it can be very damaging.

Small amounts of endotoxin can be absorbed from the colon.[7] The liver is resistant to the endotoxin lipopolysaccharide (LPS) because its Kupffer cells are able to remove and degrade LPS. Very large doses of LPS are required to cause death, but the lethal dose is 600-fold less when combined with small and rather inconsequential doses of another insult, carbon tetrachloride.[8] Thus, liver injury greatly enhances the ability of normally harmless doses of LPS to damage hepatocytes. The toxic effects of LPS are mostly indirect on liver cells. Macrophages (Kupffer cells) mediate the effects by releasing a number of chemicals (Figure 29-1). Hepatocytes have receptors for LPS, and interaction of the two results in an increased lysosomal fragility.[8] The synergistic effects of LPS on liver injury can be minimized by maneuvers to reduce LPS absorption from the

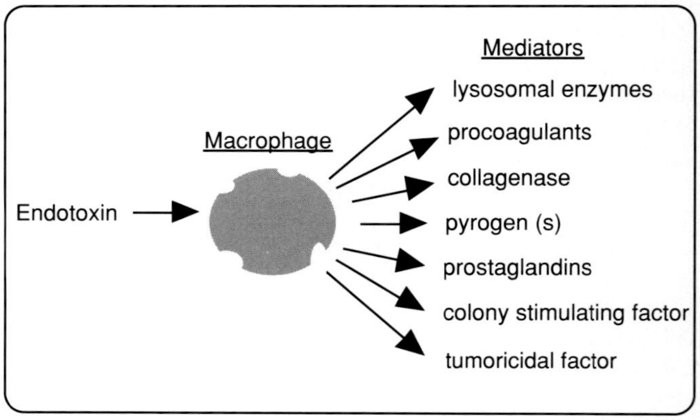

Figure 29-1. Effects of endotoxin lipopolysaccharide on macrophage to release chemical mediators of tissue injury.

colon and to induce tolerance for LPS. Diets or antibiotics that reduce the numbers of enteric bacteria also reduce LPS absorption. For example, neomycin given to animals developing cirrhosis from being fed a choline-deficient diet protects against the pathology; the lesions are known to be caused by LPS's interacting with the diet-induced changes. Another antibiotic, polymyxin B, is protective because of its unique ability to disrupt the cell walls of gram-negative bacteria, rendering LPS nontoxic. Absorption of LPS increases with increased permeability of the intestinal mucosa. That occurs with most intestinal diseases and also with insults that both injure the liver and promote mast cell degranulation to release histamine. Surgery to remove the colon reduces LPS absorption so that hepatic viruses normally able to cause massive hepatic necrosis have no effect on parenchymal cells, even though they are still able to cause massive sinusoidal destruction. Endotoxin absorbed from the intestine can also cause fever due to the pyrogens released from Kupffer cells. Hepatic lipidosis, associated with bacterial overgrowth of the small intestine, may also develop because of increased LPS absorption. The phagocytic function of Kupffer cells may be depressed by hepatic lipidosis, and that may lead to higher circulating LPS levels.

Increased tolerance for LPS can reduce endotoxin toxicity. That tolerance could be gained in the form of an immune response that prevents LPS absorption or minimizes its effects.[8] Tolerance could also be induced by drugs such as corticosteroids, which protect against endotoxin damage by stabilizing lysosomes. Endotoxin absorption can be reduced by drugs such as cimetidine, which block the effects of histamine at H_2 receptors. That drug protects against carbon tetrachloride damage.

Excess iron in the liver can initiate oxygen-free radical generation.[3] The lipid peroxidation that follows is not associated with a depletion of the glutathione stores; the defense mechanisms are not compromised. With the addition of another usually harmless insult, it is possible for the defenses to become exhausted and for hepatocyte damage to ensue. Excess iron stores could put hepatocytes at greater risk for injury by endotoxin, drugs, or hypoxia. Vitamin A has a similar effect; its combination with another insult can result in hepatocyte injury, although at the same low levels either one alone causes no pathology.[9]

Drugs such as halothane and acetaminophen are normally metabolized with no injury to hepatocytes.[10,11] The metabolism of halothane changes with reduced oxygen availability, so that oxygen-free radicals and lipid peroxidation become important enough to injure hepatocytes. Toxicity due to acetaminophen is associated with glutathione depletion and lipid peroxidation. Other factors such as drug metabolism, endotoxin, hypoxia or fasting could consume enough of the defenses that normally harmless doses of acetaminophen could precipitate total depletion. Bacterial metabolism on the many non-nutrient constituents of commercial animal foods undoubtedly produces a host of unknown compounds. There is some evidence that such metabolites can have an adverse effect on the liver. Metabolites of bile acids produced by bacteria and absorbed form the intestine may have similar effects. Problems that reduce fibronectin levels deplete the defenses that the liver has against some toxic insults.

Reduced oxygen availability handicaps hepatocytes' ability to metabolize many substances. Thus any factor reducing circulation and its delivery of oxygen can act synergistically with other potential insults to produce hepatocyte injury. Many metabolic processes consume glutathione, and oxidative metabolism is necessary for its replenishment. Otherwise glutathione is depleted, and with it goes the most important defense mechanism against the oxygen-free radicals that are always being produced. Fasting has a similar effect of reducing glutathione levels and thus affecting the cells' protective mechanisms. Hepatocytes in zone 2, the midzonal region, appear to be the most susceptible to injury after oxygen deprivation.12 That suggests that hypoxia in zone 2 cells is more injurious than more complete anoxia in adjacent zone 3 cells. Zone 1 hepatocytes appear to be less vulnerable because antioxidants are preferentially located in periportal hepatocytes.

Biologically active metabolites of arachidonic acid metabolism may be important in contributing to and ameliorating liver injury caused by different factors. Leukotrienes produced in the lipoxygenase pathway of arachidonic acid metabolism may be one of the most important mediators of injury in liver inflammation.[6] Leukotrienes may be more cytotoxic to hepatocytes with reduced oxygen availability. Leukotrienes are eliminated following metabolism by microsomal cytochromes and dipeptidases on plasma membranes. They are also excreted in bile and by the kidneys. Endotoxin and cholestasis inhibit biliary excretion. Cholestasis results in increased activities for alkaline phosphatase and glutamyltransferase. Alkaline phosphatase activity may stimulate plasma lipocortin activation, an effect also produced by corticosteroids, which results in inhibition of phospholipase activity; less arachidonic acid is released, and the production of leukotrienes falls.[6] Cholestasis thereby provides a means for feedback inhibition of leukotriene formation when its biliary excretion is impaired.

Prostaglandins produced by the cyclooxygenase pathway in arachidonic acid metabolism have a cytoprotective effect throughout the gastrointestinal tract. They provide cytoprotection in the liver that is sensitized to the effects of lipopolysaccharide and in the liver exposed to injury by carbon tetrachloride. Cytoprotection is not seen for hepatocytes exposed to acetaminophen.[13,14]

Because of the many factors interacting to determine whether hepatocytes develop injury, it becomes difficult to establish a simple effective protocol for protecting against or managing parenchymal damage.[1] Of great importance would be approaches to maintain high glutathione levels, the most important of the defense mechanisms. That is done by administering the glutathione precursors cystine, glutamic acid, and glycine. Glutathione levels would probably be reduced in the unfed state. Other antioxidants such as ascorbic acid and vitamin E may be helpful. The movement of calcium into injured cells may be inhibited by calcium channel blockers, but no such effects have been shown for hepatocytes. Phenothiazine derivatives, such as chlorpromazine, may beneficially inhibit phospholipase activity, act as calcium channel blockers, or ameliorate the effects of oxygen deficiency. Flavonoids have similar effects. Corticosteroids can improve hepatocyte injury by suppressing immunologic reactions and by inhibiting phospholipase activity. Antibiotics can be given to reduce the endotoxin that can be absorbed from the intestine. The antibiotic selected must have activity against gram-negative enteric organisms.

PATHOGENESIS OF HEPATIC DISEASE

The specific cause of a particular case of acute or chronic hepatic degeneration or inflammation cannot usually be identified. The causes of hepatitis and hepatopathies are many, including infection by bacterial and viral agents, drug toxicities, endotoxemia, exogenous by many known and unknown agents and immunologic derangements. Chronic hepatitis is thought to require persistent infection or exposure to a toxin, with active hepatic inflammation continuing only as long as the insult remains. That is not so, however; a single insult is often the only stimulus required to initiate chronic active hepatitis. The sequence of events that leads from the initial insult to chronic lesion is often due to immunologic mechanisms.

The canine hepatitis virus is fatal in dogs with no immunity but has no effect on dogs with high antibody titers.[15] Dogs with low levels of antibody survive infection by the virus but develop chronic active hepatitis. A month after exposure the virus can no longer be isolated from the dog's tissues, and no hepatic intranuclear inclusion bodies can be found. Thus, chronic hepatitis develops after the virus has disappeared. An abnormal immune response most likely mediates the pathologic events. It is not unexpected that the liver may be an active component of the animal's immune defenses. Activated macrophages, T cells, B cells, and natural killer cells are present in the liver of normal individuals.

The hepatic cellular infiltrate with chronic active hepatitis consists of immunocytes, plasma cells, and lymphocytes. The appearance of these cells has been associated with the synthesis of antibodies locally within the liver. This evidence for an immunologic basis is supported by clinical evidence that chronic active hepatitis improves upon treatment with corticosteroids.

Immunologic Function in the Normal Liver[16]

The liver contains Kupffer cells, which are fixed macrophages forming the reticuloendothelial or monocyte phagocytic system.[17] Kupffer cells constitute the most important part of the immune surveillance system in the body. The liver's reticuloendothelial system is interposed between the part of the outside environment that is represented by gastrointestinal contents, and the remainder of the body. This portion of the outer environment is a vastly greater potential danger than the outer environment that communicates through the lungs, because the intestines contain high concentrations of microorganisms, dietary antigens, food additives, and toxic metabolites produced by interaction of the flora with its contents.

Macrophages phagocytize foreign and useless substances, and subsequently degrade or store the material to prevent large amounts of immunogenic matter from entering the systemic circulation. Macrophages also participate in immune responses by processing and transferring antigens to antibody-synthesizing cells and by contributing to interactions between T and B lymphocytes. Macrophages can also be cytotoxic for other cells. Kupffer cells are able to phagocytize and degrade circulating intact cells as well as cellular material.

Most antigens in the intestine are degraded before they are absorbed into the portal circulation. The liver removes the small amounts of intact antigens absorbed.[18] Small amounts that escape hepatic removal enter the systemic circulation, where they stimulate the synthesis of antibodies. An antigen's physical properties determine its removal by the reticuloendothelial system.[19] Aggregated substances are readily removed; when they escape phagocytosis, they stimulate antibody synthesis more potently than soluble proteins. The antigens escaping phagocytosis are native proteins in their soluble form. If, however, these proteins form complexes with antibodies produced against them, they become aggregates that are avidly phagocytized. When large amounts of antigens are absorbed from the intestine, the immune system responds with more efficient phagocytosis. That is accomplished by forming antigen-antibody complexes with a greater percentage of the antigen. Thus, antibody synthesis is stimulated, which in this case is T lymphocyte-dependent. Previously sensitized T lymphocytes interact with B lymphocytes to stimulate an immune response. The result of the response is removal of most of the antigen by the liver, and, since antibody is consumed, lower levels are found in the systemic circulation. The animal is described as becoming tolerant to the antigen, since the immune response cannot be characterized by circulating antibodies. Moreover, such animals acquire an impaired delayed hypersensitivity response to injections of antigens after developing the immune response to the orally administered antigen. The liver avidly removes the antigen, preventing the delayed hypersensitivity immune responses. Liver disease or blockage of reticuloendothelial function permits antigens to escape phagocytosis and enter the systemic lymphoid tissue, stimulating antibody formation and other facets of an immune response. Creation of a portacaval shunt allows antigens to escape removal.

It is important that the liver remove many antigens in preventing immune responses. Antigens on colonic epithelial cells are similar to those in the intrahepatic biliary system and in the renal tubules.[20] The colonic antigens are released and absorbed during acute colitis. If the liver's reticuloendothelial system removes and degrades them, no further problems are expected. If they escape phagocytosis and are released into the systemic circulation, however, antibodies can be synthesized against them. These antibodies can damage the biliary epithelia, causing biliary cirrhosis; a similar destructive effect is possible in renal tubules. The lesion initiating this pathology may be reticuloendothelial blockage, so that the immunogenic material is scattered throughout the body. Antigens failing to be phagocytized also include bacterial lipopolysaccharides. This component of bacterial structure can stimulate immune mechanisms to respond to antigens that are normally tolerated.[21] Bacterial endotoxins are B lymphocyte mitogens. Polysaccharides that escape phagocytosis may play a role in the synthesis of self-destructive antibodies. Antigens in bacteria such as E. coli are similar to antigens in the intestine and kidney. Failure to remove these antigens can result in synthesis of antibodies that cross-react and destroy normal intestinal and renal cells. These reticuloendothelial functions prevent initiation of immune responses in lymphoid tissue outside the splanchnic viscera. This immunosuppressive role may be aided by other means. The normal liver is thought to produce a lymphocyte-inhibiting factor that causes the unresponsiveness of T lymphocytes to some antigens not removed by the liver.[22]

The liver's role in removing antigen-antibody complexes is important in preventing complications of hepatic disease. Patients with chronic active hepatitis can develop chronic bowel disease, arthritis, glomerulonephritis, and signs of systemic lupus erythematosus. These are immune-mediated dis-

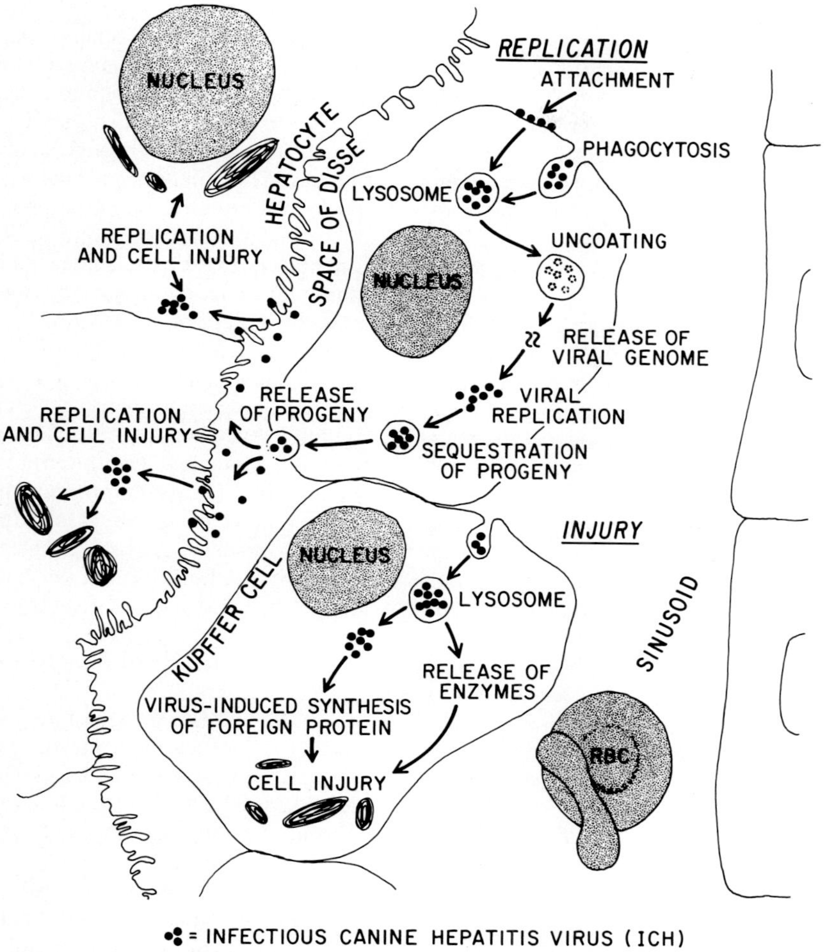

Figure 29-2. Pathogenesis of hepatitis caused by infectious canine hepatitis virus.

eases caused by the deposition of circulating antigen-antibody complexes in extrahepatic tissues.

In summary, although the normal liver is not usually thought of as an immunologic organ, hepatic function does have an effect on an animal's immune response, primarily the function to remove antigens and antigen-antibody complexes from the circulation. The macrophage phagocyte system (MPS) processing antigens for transfer to immunocytes does not produce antibodies. There is some evidence that the normal liver has immunosuppressive properties distinct from its phagocytizing functions.

Immunologic Events Associated with Liver Damage[16,19,23]

Pathogenesis of Viral Hepatitis.[24] Viruses can be an important cause of acute and chronic hepatitis. The infectious canine hepatitis virus produces acute fatal hepatitis in dogs with no immunity, and it can produce chronic hepatitis in partially immune dogs.

Viremia develops soon after exposure to the infectious canine hepatitis virus. Circulating viruses are phagocytized by the hepatic MPS system (Figure 29-2). That provides an avenue for viral entry into the organ involved most importantly. The virus replicates within Kupffer cells. Following phagocytosis by reticuloendothelial cells, virons are found in phagosomes, which are vacuoles containing enzymes to digest engulfed material. Proteolytic digestion aids viral replication by removing the protein coating of the viruses, exposing the viral genome. Kupffer cell proteolytic enzymes are in the cytosol or lysosomes. They are more likely cytosol enzymes, since lysosomes also contain enzymes that destroy viruses; if any lysosomal enzymes were released to digest the viral coating, all other enzymes would be released. The lysosomal viral-degrading enzymes are ribonucleases, degrading DNA and RNA. The release of lysosomal enzymes is reduced to a minimum when their membranes are stabilized with corticosteroids. This reduces the release of ribonucleases, so that viruses replicate more rapidly.

Following viral damage, Kupffer cells release replicated viruses. The virus may alter lysosomal membrane permeability so that enzymes escape and damage Kupffer cells. However, the release of lysosomal enzymes is thought most likely to be a result of damage to the cell. The cell damage is not a mechanical rupture from excessive viral replication; the virus damages the cell without replicating. Damage is caused by synthesis and accumulation of new and foreign proteins induced by the viral genome. This finding is supported by observations that inhibitors of protein synthesis prevent virus-induced morphologic injury.

Replicating viruses are released from damaged Kupffer cells, and, having breached the first line of defense in Kupffer cells, viruses easily enter hepatocytes, where they replicate and destroy the cell. Virons have multiplied many times when released from Kupffer cells, and, when hepatocytes release their virons, massive viremia follows. Uninjured Kupffer cells phagocytize the circulating virions, and all Kupffer cells are eventually involved and become damaged. Kupffer cells may be necessary for access of virons into hepatocytes, and the ability of a specific virus to cause infection may be due to its ability to replicate within the Kupffer cells. Some viruses are able to multiply, whereas others cannot.

Liver Injury by Hepatotoxins[25-28]

Many hepatotoxins cause acute degeneration of hepatocytes. Some drugs consistently cause degeneration, whereas others only infrequently cause unexplained idiosyncratic reactions. Chronic hepatic disease can develop from prolonged exposure to many toxins.

Hepatotoxins damage normal liver cells by interfering with energy production, causing hepatic necrosis, as is seen with bacterial endotoxins.[25] They can also act together with other hepatic insults to hasten the development of hepatic lesions, such as when endotoxin is combined with a potential producer of fat infiltration to precipitate hepatic lipidosis. Ethionine feeding reduces energy availability, causing fatty livers. Ethionine traps adenosine by forming S-adenoxylethionine, thereby depleting ATP. This depletion of energy reduces protein synthesis, and, without apolipoprotein synthesis, triglycerides are retained in hepatocytes.

Hepatotoxins can also damage hepatocytes directly. Drugs can form metabolites that bind intracellular proteins, altering both structure and function. Some chemicals can be metabolized to form free radicals that cause many changes, including peroxidation of lipids in membranes. Peroxidation causes dissolution of ribosomal membranes, whereupon protein synthesis ceases. Thus, these toxins produce multiple damage by multiple effects.

Some hepatotoxins cause part of their damage by reducing hepatic blood flow. Vasoactive compounds reducing hepatic circulation cause fatty changes similar to those seen with cardiovascular disease, while acute reduction in blood flow can cause hepatic necrosis. Toxic compounds can also reduce blood flow by damaging blood vessels or by stimulating thrombosis in the hepatic microcirculation.

Endogenous bacterial toxins contribute to the pathogenesis of hepatic disease. Bacterial endotoxin continuously produced and absorbed from the intestine intensifies the severity of hepatic lesions produced by other insults. For example, choline deficiency causes hepatic cirrhosis, but, when intestinal bacterial numbers are reduced, the lesions develop slowly. They develop rapidly, however, when endotoxin is added to the diet.

Endotoxin causes nonspecific changes in hepatocytes. Extreme hepatocyte vesiculation is seen, with vacuolation and swelling of the endoplasmic reticulum and mitochondria. Hepatic lipidosis is produced and can be associated with hyperlipidemia and abnormal sulfobromophthalein retention. The Kupffer cells have greater numbers of lysosomes and vacuoles, and bile ducts are dilated.

Increased delivery of endotoxin to the liver from increased production or absorption contributes to manifestations of hepatotoxicity. Overgrowth of the intestinal microflora can increase the amount of endotoxin absorbed. Alteration of intestinal microcirculation by shock increases the absorption of bacterial endotoxins, as does inflammatory bowel disease. Failure of the reticuloendothelial system to remove the toxin allows expression of its toxicity, which may be important in many cases of hepatic disease.[26] Decreased hepatic blood flow reduces reticuloendothelial function, a change that can be caused by endotoxin. Reticuloendothelial phagocytic activity is depressed in livers injured by choline deficiency or severe nutritional imbalance. Liver damage caused by depression of reticuloendothelial phagocytic activity can be identified by increased alanine aminotransferase (ALT) activity. Endotoxin is also cleared by activation of the complement system, a deficiency of which causes endotoxemia to persist.

Bacterial endotoxins are toxic to hepatocytes due to an unknown means. They cause changes in membranes of the cell and its organelles and interfere with normal carbohydrate metabolism. One of the consequences of endotoxemia is hypoglycemia, which results, at least in part, from the liver's inability to synthesize glucose.[27] The use of glucose in balanced-electrolyte solutions improves hepatocyte function, as well as functions in other tissues, during endotoxic shock.

Response to Injury[16,23,38]

Liver tissue can regenerate when the insult is removed. Even so, some mechanisms may perpetuate the pathology even though the etiological agent is no longer in evidence. Part of the initial damage during the acute phase and the development of chronic lesions may be due to stimulation or interference of immune responses.

With viral infections involving the liver, necrosis of hepatic parenchymal cells is not caused directly by the virus. In general, hepatic viruses are not cytopathic for hepatocytes, although they may destroy sinusoidal cells. Animals can have serum antibodies to hepadna viruses, including ones infecting humans,[29] which suggests that although some immunoglobulins are produced the body tolerates viruses to the extent that a major immune response is not initiated. Humans are similar in that by middle age over 40% have acquired immunity to some hepatitis viruses; the vast majority having never shown clinical manifestations.

Before hepatocyte damage is evident, antiviral antibodies are produced with an early IgM and later IgG response. That can result in the formation of antigen (virus)-antibody complexes and their deposition in many different tissues. These complexes fix and activate complement, causing inflammation where they are deposited. There is no evidence, however, that this activity contributes to hepatic changes in human viral hepatitis, even though serum immunoglobulins increase, immune complexes are found, and levels of complement are low. The humoral immune reaction leading to immune complexes is most likely responsible for extrahepatic manifestations of arthritis and nephritis, but not for the hepatitis. Although the humoral immune reaction is unable to eliminate the virus infection completely, it is effective in neutralizing extracellular virus. Resolution of infection in hepatocytes is produced by cell-mediated responses.

Cell-mediated responses to resolve viral infection can be inhibited by IgM's and IgG's possessing lymphocytotoxicity. Responses can also be inhibited by factors that interfere with specific helper T cells' production of antiviral antibodies; the factors do not prevent damage but may ameliorate a continuing problem. A decreased number of T lymphocytes characterizes lymphopenia, an initial change during viral infections. Cytotoxicity by T lymphocytes may be the normal response to destroy the etiological agent and terminate the infection. The depression of T lymphocyte numbers seen with human hepatitis infections returns to normal with recovery. With marked reduction in cell-mediated responses, an animal can be persistently viremic, but that can be associated with no damage to the liver. With less reduction in the cell-mediated responses, the body's attempt to eliminate the virus infection can result in liver damage. In one case, the host appears tolerant to the infection and in another there is a reaction, a response that can damage the liver. Hepatocytes are also protected by other immunosuppressive factors produced in the liver, such as alpha-fetoprotein and alpha-globulins. But those factors are not found to be elevated in plasma until after hepatic injury, and so they do not prevent damage but rather ameliorate a continuing problem.

Cell-mediated immune responses injure hepatocytes by reacting to viral antigens, virus-modified antigens produced from normal cell components, virus-induced antigens produced by hepatocytes, or normal cell components. In order for a cell-mediated response to be possible against hepatocytes, antigen in a membrane and an adjacent major histocompatibility complex (MHC) of the cell must both be exposed to the immune system. The antigen and the MHC are recognized by receptors on sensitized lymphocytes, which then respond by damaging the cell. When the antigen is a hepatitis virus, the virus is the target of the immune response and the cell represents an innocent bystander. The antigen can also be a viral component synthesized by hepatocytes from viral DNA left in the cell and integrated with host DNA, so that some of the viral genes are transcribed and translated as though they were hepatocyte DNA. That endogenously synthesized antigen is then transported to the cell surface where it binds with the MHC, allowing it to react with receptors on cytotoxic T cells. All cells have the class I molecules of the MHC. If a cell is able to process a virus and present one of its antigens for binding with the class I MHC, the cell becomes a target for cytotoxic T cells. Cells do not have that ability for most viruses, but the virus may be able to react with class II molecules of the MHC found on the surface of immunocompetent cells and stimulate immunoglobulin production. Many animals have circulating antibodies against the human hepatitis B virus without any evidence of injury to hepatocytes. But autologous liver cells or hepatocytes from individuals carrying the hepatitis surface antigen are destroyed by sensitized T lymphocytes from humans with chronic active hepatitis. Cells laden with surface antigen retain normal structure and function until damaged by lymphocytes. There can be a continued synthesis of viral antigens that do not damage the cell. It is evident that if interaction between lymphocytes and hepatocytes requires exposure of cell's major histocompatibility complex (MHC) as well as an antigen with which to react on the cell membrane, the pathogenesis of hepatitis requires that the MHC must be revealed, if that is not already done.

Chronic active hepatitis in dogs may follow a similar pathogenesis following exposure to infectious canine hepatitis virus.[15] Very little immunity is required to prevent death in dogs challenged with the virus, though they can develop chronic active hepatitis. Within a month of challenge the virus can no longer be isolated, and inclusion bodies typical of hepatitis virus infection can no longer be found. The disease is characterized by a chronic course that persists for months. The progress of the disease may be due to intracellular synthesis of antigens directed by viral genomes left in the cell. Sensitized T lymphocytes are then able to attack and destroy the antigen-laden hepatocytes. The hepatocyte may be the site of foreign-antigen synthesis in animals with mild infection. This suggestion is supported by the finding that hyperimmune serum given to dogs with mild signs of infectious canine hepatitis infection causes a severe and prolonged form of hepatitis to develop.[30] This finding suggests that antibodies are reacting with antigens that are not the virions but are foreign antigens produced under direction of the viral genome and possibly retained in or around the hepatocyte. The pathogenesis of that lesion may also involve natural killer·lymphocytes, which can lyse Ig-coated target cells in the absence of complement. Activity of that lymphocyte increases during acute hepatitis.

Damage to hepatocytes releases or exposes a number of the cells' antigens to the immune system. Production of antibodies and their contact with normal hepatocytes could result in their destruction. The initiation of such an autoimmune disease has been suggested to be involved in the pathogenesis of chronic hepatitis. Both experimental work and clinical findings suggest that this process may play a role after different kinds of hepatic insults.[31,32]

Animals immunized with a protein, believed to be liver-specific, develop either chronic active hepatitis or cirrhosis.[33,34] The severity of the lesion is dose-dependent. It is suggested that antibody-mediated cellular toxicity causes the lesions. No changes are seen in serum immunoglobulin levels during the development of lesions, although immunoglobulin can be demonstrated, bound to hepatocytes. Cellular immunity is evidenced in skin tests. Thus, antibody-mediated lymphocyte toxicity destroys the cells, and cytotoxic lymphocytes can perpetuate a problem that begins with nonspecific injury to hepatocytes. The liver becomes a complete immunologic organ where antibodies are synthesized by the lymphocytes and plasma cells that infiltrate and characterize chronic hepatitis. The antibodies remain within the tissue, form complexes with antigens on normal hepatocytes, and serve as a target for cytotoxic lymphocytes. Evidence for cell-mediated immune responses against antigens in normal liver tissue also includes lymphocyte reactivity to liver extracts. Homogenates of liver tissue excite lymphocyte transformation and inhibit leukocyte migration in cells from humans with chronic liver disease. Thus, these *in vitro* correlates of enhanced cell-immune response agree with the findings of lymphocyte cytotoxicity for homologous liver cells. In the latter case, however, the immune response is not likely to be directed against autoantigens.

Other problems appear in many patients with chronic hepatitis, often producing entities that resemble systemic lupus erythematosus. A number of features of general autoimmune disease are found. Autoantibodies are found, although not to liver-specific antigens, and LE cells are frequently found. The LE phenomenon does not reflect any specific type of etiology or pathogenesis. It does reflect the severity of the disease activity. LE cells and high ALT activity are correlated with morphological confirmation of widespread hepatic necrosis, under which conditions extrahepatic manifestations are more likely to be found. Antinuclear antibodies are demonstrated with positive LE preparations. It is more reliable to measure the antibodies directly. Positive LE preparations do not always reflect the presence of antinuclear antibodies, and the test for LE cells becomes negative on remission or after treatment. The direct test involves measurement of antibodies against native (double-stranded) and denatured (single-stranded) DNA, double-stranded RNA, and histone.

Smooth muscle antibodies commonly appear with many forms of chronic hepatitis, and their production is quite specific for hepatic disease in humans. This antibody does not appear with lupus. The antigenic stimulus for synthesis of antismooth-muscle antibody is not known. The antibody reacts with actin and myosin, which is found in membranes of bile canaliculi and hepatocytes, myocytes found in developing fibrosis, and smooth muscle of blood vessels.

Antimitochondrial antibody is produced in a low percentage of humans with chronic active hepatitis. This antibody is a regular finding in biliary cirrhosis but is not found with extrahepatic biliary obstruction. Thus, antimitochondrial antibody is used to differentiate cases of jaundice to be treated medically from cases to be treated surgically.

A number of other autoantibodies are produced with chronic active hepatitis, although less significance is placed on their appearance. These antibodies are not tissue-specific and not even species-specific. There is no question that they reflect the activity of hepatic disease. Little more is known about them and whether they participate in the persistence of hepatic pathology. Other types of antibodies produced in excess include antibodies directed against antigens absorbed from the intestine. Normally removed by the reticuloendothelial system, these antigens are not removed by the diseased liver, and increased amounts of immunogenic material reach lymphoid tissue. Excess circulating antigen-antibody complexes can deposit in different organs, producing signs of lupus. Some antigens in the intestine are similar to those in normal hepatic and renal tissues. Synthesis of antibodies against excessive antigens escaping from the intestine can result in the antigen-antibody complexes that fix complement and result in the destruction of normal hepatic and renal cells.

Drugs are sometimes believed to be responsible for hepatitis. It is invariably difficult to establish a causal relationship between a drug and any form of liver disease, however. Immunologic mechanisms may mediate hepatotoxic effects whereby the reaction to self-antigens is no longer suppressed or hepatocyte antigens are altered so they are no longer recognized as self-components.[32] Drugs may initiate an immune response by binding to plasma membranes and act as a hapten, or they may denature and alter a membrane antigen so it is no longer recognized as self. Drugs can damage hepatocytes so that antibody is produced against the altered cells. Antibodies can also be produced against the drug so that immune complexes are formed. With drug-associated hepatic disease, antibodies are found against cell organelles such as smooth muscle, nuclear material, and mitochondria. These changes should all be secondary to the hepatocyte damage, with little effect on the pathogenesis of the disease.

INCIDENCE OF HEPATIC DISEASE

In the past decade hepatic disease in small animals has been reported with greater frequency. This is not surprising, because normal animals can have a relatively high incidence of hepatic lesions. In a study on clinically normal Beagle dogs ranging in age from 8 to 20 months, focal hepatic necrosis and inflammation was found in 65%, focal phlebitis in 63%, portal inflammation in 8%, granuloma in 4%, and focal bile duct hyperplasia in less than 1%.[35] Some of these changes were attributed to migrating parasitic larvae.

Table 29-1. Incidence of Hepatic Disease or Lesions, Number of Cases per 1000 Animals Seen at VMTH

	Dog	Cat
Necropsy	18.7	14.1
Biopsy	8.7	—
Case Summaries	12.1	10.7

The incidence of hepatic disease can be based on clinical, biopsy, or necropsy findings and is related directly to the completeness of investigation. When referrals make up a significant part of a practice, the incidence is biased in favor of numbers greater than those for the general population. Only 10% of all cases seen at the Veterinary Medical Teaching Hospital (VMTH) in Davis are referrals, too small a percentage to bias the incidence of hepatic disease. The incidence of significant hepatic lesions in dogs necropsied at the VMTH is 23%. That is an incidence of 18.7 cases of hepatic disease in every 1,000 dogs seen for all types of medical and surgical service (Table 29-1). The incidence of liver disease based on biopsy results is 8.7 cases per 1,000. The incidence of hepatic disease based on data from all case summaries is 12.1 cases per 1,000. These data indicate that hepatic disease is common in dogs, with about one of every 100 cases having some form of hepatic problem. The incidence of hepatic lesions in cats is 14.1% in those necropsied. This represents 17.1 cases of hepatic lesions in every 1,000 cases. Too few biopsies have been obtained from cats at the VMTH to cite any incidence of hepatic disease from biopsy evaluations. The incidence of feline hepatic disease based on information obtained from case summaries is 10.7 cases per 1,000.

Descriptions of hepatic disease in the past have contributed little to the understanding of pathogenesis, treatment, and prognosis, primarily because of the manner of morphological diagnoses. Hepatic disease can be described merely by the lesions that appear (i.e., necrosis), or the pattern of lesions can be used to categorize the pathology (i.e., chronic active hepatitis). For example, the most prominent lesion may be fibrosis, and that may be how the diagnosis is reported. The changes may also include cellular infiltration and necrosis, both of which can be described to characterize the process more completely. Thus, inflammation accompanies fibrosis, and together they may form a typical pattern for chronic active hepatitis, about which incidence, treatment, and prognosis can be predicted. Enlightened understanding of some hepatic lesions has changed the incidence of some forms of hepatic disease, such as hepatic lipidosis. Lipidosis has accounted for as many as half of all the hepatic lesions seen in necropsy cases. One study on biopsies of the liver found that 3.4% showed lipidosis; 33% showed centrilobular vacuolar degeneration, which is not lipidosis but is

Canine	
Hepatitis	18.0
Tumors, metastatic	13.9
Hepatopathy - steroid	11.8
Passive congestion	9.1
Necrosis	8.1
Hepatopathy	7.2
Portasystemic shunts	5.7
Hepatopathy vacuolar	5.6
Fibrosis	4.1
Lipidosis	3.9
Tumors, primary	3.8
Cirrhosis	2.3
Hepatopathy-pigment	1.2
Miscellaneous	5.3

Table 29-2. Distribution by Percentage of Hepatic Disease or Lesions in Dogs. Diagnoses Confirmed by Histology or Radiology (Shunts).

Feline	
Hepatitis	22.9
Hepatopathy	13.5
Tumors metastatic	12.8
Lipidosis	11.0
Passive Congestion	10.7
Necrosis	9.9
Degeneration - atrophy	3.8
Portasystemic shunts	2.5
Myeloproliferative Dis.	2.1
Hyperplasia - nodul-regen	1.9
FIP	1.7
Miscellaneous	7.2

Table 29-3. Distribution by Percentage of Hepatic Disease or Lesions in Cats. Diagnoses Confirmed by Histology or Radiology (Shunts).

due to excessive adrenal corticosteroids.[36] The steroid-induced lesions were once diagnosed as lipidosis because of the similarity in morphologic appearances. Current computer coding procedures still use nonspecific designations to categorize hepatic disease. They include such descriptions as degeneration, proliferation and fibrosis; hepatomegaly; liver disease, cause undetermined; hepatitis due to infection; necrosis; passive congestion; and cirrhosis. It is apparent that statistics on these entities are of little value in understanding the pathogenesis, treatment, and prognosis of hepatic disease.

Many hepatic lesions develop because of pathology in nonhepatic tissues. In such cases the lesions reflect some toxic insult or altered circulation compromising the delivery of oxygen and nutrients to the liver. Often such changes are predictable, as with the hepatic lipidosis accompanying diabetes mellitus or starvation and the centrolobular degenerative changes seen with anemia or circulatory diseases. Table 29-2 and Table 29-3 lists the kinds of lesions found in cats and dogs at the VMTH in Davis. It is important to appreciate that most lesions are not due to primary liver disease. With many clinical pathology procedures to screen for liver pathology, more animals with liver lesions will be identified. With the understanding that primary liver disease is far less common than secondary liver pathology, clinicians will not necessarily focus most of their attention on the liver when a clinical pathologic finding indicates some liver pathology. Having that awareness, better judgments will be made on selecting cases for liver biopsy, and more useful information will be gained from such biopsies. Biopsies are important because patterns of clinical pathologic abnormalities do not reliably for differentiate one form of liver pathology from another.

Most hepatic disease is treatable; the most important diseases — steroid-induced hepatopathies, chronic hepatitis, and hepatic degenerative diseases — can all be treated. A diagnosis is essential for initiating specific management; in the past, nonspecific therapy was frequently used for any non- neoplastic liver disease.

REFERENCES

1. Popper, L. Bianchi and W. Reutter. Falk Symposium 38. MTP Press LTD. Boston, 389-397, 1984.
2. Lanterburg, B.H.: Early disturbance of calcium translocation across the plasma membrane in toxic liver injury. Hepatology 7:1179-1183, 1987.
3. Tribble, D.L., Yee Aw, T., Jones, D.P.: The pathophysiological significance of lipid peroxidation in oxidative cell injury. Hepatology 7:377-387, 1987.
4. Bellomo, G. and Orrenius, S.: Altered thiol and calcium homeostasis in oxidative hepatocellular injury. Hepatology 5:876-882, 1985.
5. Parks, D.A. and Granger, D.N.: Ischemia-reperfusion injury: a radical view. Hepatology 8:680-682, 1988.
6. Keppler, D., Hagmann, W., Rapp, S., Denzlinger, C. and Koch, H.K.: The relation of leukotrienes to liver injury. Hepatology 5:883-891, 1985.
7. van Deventer, S.J.H., ten Cate, J.W. and Tytgat, G.N.J.: Intestinal endotoxemia. Gastroenterology 94:825-831, 1988.
8. Nolan, J.P.: Endotoxin, reticuloendothelial function, and liver injury. Hepatology 1:458-465, 1981.
9. Leo, M.A. and Lieber, C.S.: Hypervitaminosis A: A liver lover's lament. Hepatology 8:412-417, 1988.
10. de Groot, H. and Noll, T.: Halothane hepatotoxicity: Relation between metabolic activation, hypoxia, covalent binding, lipid peroxidation and liver cell damage. Hepatology 3:601-606, 1983.
11. Ortega, L., Garcia, J.I.L., Garcia, A.T., Silecchia, G., Arenas, J., Suarezz, A., Azcoita, M.M., Esponera, J.S., Gonzalez, E.M. and Cantero, J.L.B.: Acetaminophen-induced fulminant hepatic failure in dogs. Hepatology 5:673-676, 1985.
12. Marotto, M.E., Thurman, R.G. and Lemasters, J.J.: Early midzonal cell death during low-flow hypoxia in the isolated, perfused rat liver: Protection by allopurinol. Hepatology 8:585-590, 1988.
13. Burk, R.F.: Hepatocytoprotective substances. Gastroenterology 81:397-398, 1981.
14. Mizoguchi, Y., Tsutsui, H., Miyajima, K., Sakagami, Y., Seki,

S., Kobayashi, K., Yamamoto, S. and Morisawa, S.: The protective effects of prostaglandin E, in an experimental massive hepatic cell necrosis model. Hepatology 7:1184-1188, 1987.

15. Gocke, D.J., Morris, T.Q. and Bradley, S.E.: Chronic hepatitis in the dog: the role of immune factors. JAVMA 156:1700-1705, 1970.

16. Thomas, H.C.: Immunologic aspects of liver disease. In, Diseases of the liver. Edited by L. Schiff and E.R. Schiff. J.B. Lippincott, Philadelphia, 163-185, 1987.

17. Saba, T.M.: Physiology and pathophysiology of the reticuloendothial system. Arch. Int. Med. 126:1031-1052, 1970.

18. Walker, W.A. and Isselbacher, K.J.: Uptake and transport of macromolecules by the intestine. Possible role in clinical disorders. Gastroenterology 67:531-550, 1974.

19. Wright, R. and Rassam, S.: The immunology of acute and chronic hepatitis. Clinics Gastroenterology 5:387-417, 1976.

20. Rabin, B.S. and Rogers, S.: Pathologic changes in the liver and kidney produced by immunization with intestinal antigens. Am. J. Path. 84:201-210, 1976.

21. Whorwell, P.J. and Wright, R.: Immunological aspects of inflammatory bowel disease. Clinics Gastroenterology 5:503-521, 1976.

22. Williams, R.: Hepatic failure and development of artificial liver support system. In, Progress in Liver Diseases, Vol. 5. Edited by H. Popper and F. Schaffner. Grune and Stratton, New York, 418-435, 1976.

23. Glynn, L.E.: Immunopathology of liver disease. In, Progress in Liver Diseases, Vol. 5. Edited by H. Popper and F. Schaffner. Grune and Stratton, New York. 311-325, 1976.

24. Sabesin, S.M. and Koff, R.S.: Pathogenesis of experimental viral hepatitis. New Eng. J. Med. 290:944-950 and 996-1002, 1974.

25. Nolan, J.P.: The role of endotoxin in liver injury. Gastroenterology 69:1346-1356, 1975.

26. Liehr, H., Grun, M. and Brunswig, D.: Endotoxaemia in acute hepatic failure. Acta Hepato-Gastroenterol. 23:235-240, 1976.

27. Zimmerman, H.J. and Maddrey, W.C.: Toxic and drug-induced hepatitis. In, Diseases of the Liver. Edited by L. Schiff and E.R. Schiff. J.B. Lippincott, Philadelphia, 591-667, 1987.

28. Raisfeld, I.H.: Models of liver injury: The effects of toxin on the liver. In, The Liver: Normal and Abnormal Functions. Part A. Edited by F.F. Becker. Vol. 5. The Biochemistry of Disease. Marcel Dekker, New York, 203-223, 1974.

29. Robinson, W.S.: Why do animals have antibodies to hepatitis B surface antigen? Gastroenterology 84:1614-1615, 1983.

30. Preisig, R., Gocke, D., Morris, T. and Bradley, S.E.: Chronic hepatic injury following experimental viral hepatitis in the dog. Experientia 22:701-702, 1966.

31. Allen, P.M.: Antigen presentation and autoimmunity. Hepatology 8:677-679, 1988.

32. Mackay, I.R.: Induction by drugs of hepatitis and autoantibodies to cell organelles: Significance and interpretation. Hepatology 5:904-906, 1985.

33. Hopf, U. and Meyer zum Buschenfelde, K.H.: Studies on the pathogenesis of experimental chronic active hepatitis in rabbits. II. Demonstration of immunoglobulin on isolated hepatocytes. Brit. J. Exp. Path. 55:509-551, 1974.

34. Meyer zum Buschenfelds, K.H. and Hopf, U.: Studies on the pathogenesis of experimental chronic active hepatitis in rabbits. I. Induction of the disease and protective effect of allogeneic liver specific proteins. Brit. J. Exp. Path. 55:498-508, 1974.

35. Hottendorf, G.H. and Hirth, R.S.: Lesions of spontaneous subclinical disease in Beagle dogs. Vet. Path. 11:240-258, 1974.

36. Edwards, D.F.: Blind percutaneous liver biopsy: a safe diagnostic procedure. Calif. Vet. 31:9-17, 1977.

37. Filkins, J.P. and Cornell, R.P.: Depression of hepatic gluconeogenesis and the hypoglycemia of endotoxic shock. Am. J. Physiol. 227:778-781, 1974.

38. Tizard, I.: Veterinary Immunology. W.B. Saunders, Philadelphia, 1987.

Chapter 30

Laboratory Evaluation for Hepatic Disease

CLINICAL SIGNS OF LIVER DISEASE

Historical Findings

Many patients' history contains some information suggesting hepatic disease as a possibility. None of the clinical signs of liver disease (listed in Table 30-1) are diagnostic for hepatic problems. Even more specific signs (e.g., icterus and ascites) are not pathognomonic for hepatic disease. Icterus is often caused by hemolytic disease; ascites is more frequently a complication of cardiac disease. Ascites and icterus usually do not appear until hepatic disease is advanced and severe, and then are not seen consistently. If icterus or ascites were required for hepatic disease to be considered in the differential diagnosis, many hepatic problems would never be detected. The other nonspecific signs offer few clues for suspecting liver disease. Hepatic disease must be included in the differential diagnosis for any of these nonspecific signs.

Physical Findings

Few physical signs are found consistently with hepatic disease. The only specific problems indicating the possibility of hepatic disease are ascites, icterus, and abnormalities in liver size.

Icterus. Clinical manifestations of icterus do not always correlate with either the icteric index or plasma bilirubin levels. Unconjugated bilirubin is practically insoluble at the pH of body fluids and is transported bound tightly to albumin. Albumin-bound pigment distributes only to the vascular compartment and interstitial space. Conjugated bilirubin is water soluble at physiological pH and distributes to most body water. Thus, mucous membranes and skin appear yellow at lower blood levels of conjugated than unconjugated bilirubin, and icterus is detected earlier when most of the retained pigment is conjugated. Determination of the icteric index is a rapid means of identifying icterus in questionable cases. Icterus caused by unconjugated hyperbilirubinemia may not be recognized until plasma levels are quite high. Hyperbilirubinemia that approaches 1.5 mg/dl and is due primarily to conjugated bilirubin is usually recognized as icterus on physical examination.

Hepatomegaly.[1] Abnormal liver size can sometimes be identified on physical examination. Livers of small and normal size cannot be palpated. The borders of enlarged livers can be palpated, and such physical examination then often yields as much information as radiographs. Small livers are seen with portal vascular anomalies and some forms of chronic hepatitis. The liver enlarges as a result of many different problems, and the enlargement can be diffuse or defined (Table 30-2). The liver can expand or contract rapidly. Hepatic size depends on its circulation, with 15% of hepatic size being attributed to sinusoidal and vascular spaces that can expand rapidly and to considerable degrees. This type of hepatomegaly occurs most commonly with cardiac failure causing hypertension in the caudal vena cava. Postsinusoidal blocks such as in the Budd Chiari syndrome, creating obstruction in the hepatic vein, cause hepatic enlargement.

Hepatomegaly can develop from an increase in the size of Kupffer cells and have phagocytized excessive amounts of foreign or endogenous substances. Excessive accumulation enlarges Kupffer cells, which normally represent 10% of all hepatic cells. Kupffer cell hypertrophy and hyperplasia can be seen with septicemias, hepatitis, malignancies, and hypervitaminosis A.

The liver enlarges from growth of nonhepatic and abnormal hepatic cells. Anemic adult animals often develop centers of hematopoiesis in the liver, which is normal in the fetal but not the adult liver. Tumors arising from hepatocytes or biliary duct cells cause enlargement. Enlargement due to hepatocellular carcinomas can be nodular or diffuse. Metastatic tumors, lymphosarcomas, and lymphohistiocytic inflammation are other diseases with cellular infiltration of the liver, but they inconsistently cause hepatomegaly that can be recognized on physical examination.

Excess hepatic storage of normal substances causes hepatomegaly. Lipid accumulation causes hepatic enlargement and is associated with diabetes mellitus, tetracycline toxicity,

Table 30-1. Clinical Signs Associated with Liver Disease

Depression	Weakness
Anorexia	Vomiting
Diarrhea	Weight loss
Fever	Polydipsia
Abdominal pain	Ascites
CNS signs	Coma
Icterus	Change in liver size
Change in spleen size	Dark or light color stools
Dark brown urine	Hemorrhage
Polyuria	Pruritus

Table 30-2. Causes of Hepatomegaly

Congestion
Kupffer cell hyperplasia
Cellular infiltration
Abnormal storage
Inflammation
Fatty infiltration
Intrinsic tumors
Cellular edema-steroids
Amyloidosis
Hemorrhage
Work hypertrophy

chronic endotoxin toxicity, and extreme imbalances in nutrition. Some rare common forms of congenital storage diseases cause hepatomegaly by glycogen retention. Steroids cause a hepatopathy that appears to be due to lipid accumulation but represents an accumulation of glycogen and that results in hepatomegaly.

Inflammation causes hepatocytes to swell, producing hepatomegaly such as seen with infectious hepatitis, parasites, toxins, drugs and biliary tract obstruction.

Sometimes no cause for hepatomegaly is found with no histopathologic changes evident on light microscopy. In such cases discovering the basis for hepatomegaly may require electron microscopy, histochemical techniques, and enzyme assays. With those procedures, the scheme in Figure 30-1 can be used to classify liver enlargement where cardiac disease is not a problem. One occult cause of hepatomegaly is work hypertrophy and the increase in size is due to hypertrophy of hepatocytes following administration of a drug such as phenobarbital. That drug, like some others, stimulates microsomal enzyme activity which is reflected in marked increases in smooth endoplasmic reticulum. Phenobarbital can double liver weight in experimental animals. Since the upper and lower limits of normal liver size have been estimated arbitrarily, a finding of abnormal size must be used in conjunction with all the other information to make a diagnosis. Although a small or large liver may not be indicative of an abnormality, a possible cause of such a finding should be investigated.

LABORATORY EVALUATION

Laboratory procedures must be conducted to provide information essential for the identification, management, and prognosis of hepatic problems. Most patients with hepatic disease are presented with clinical signs that are not specific for any particular problem. In some cases, the signs are not even suggestive of hepatic disease, and only when the organ systems are surveyed with laboratory procedures is a hepatic problem identified. Laboratory procedures help define the type of pathological process involved, the type of management to follow, and the prognosis to expect.

Workup of a suspected hepatic problem includes biochemical tests and morphological evaluation of the liver. Biochemical tests include liver-function tests and measurement of the activities of plasma enzymes originating in the liver. When the liver is screened for disease, the evaluation must often include at least one function test in addition to the measurement of enzymes. Presently, the function test used most commonly is the measurement of plasma bile acids in unfed and fed states. Other function studies include the sulfobromophthalein (BSP) retention test and measurement of blood ammonia concentration. These tests measure hepatocyte function and hepatic circulation, allowing one to assess a completely different aspect of the liver from that gained by measuring the plasma activities of hepatic enzymes. The most important plasma enzyme measured is alanine aminotransferase (ALT), which reflects the integrity of the compartmentalization function of hepatocytes. With hepatocyte damage, plasma ALT activity increases. In some types of problems where plasma ALT levels are normal, plasma bile acids are increased or the BSP retention time is abnormal, notably in animals with a portasystemic vascular shunt. In other forms of hepatic disease the BSP retention time can be normal and the plasma ALT levels increased, such as with hepatic necrosis. If only a single laboratory procedure is conducted, many cases of hepatic disease are never identified. A great number of additional biochemical tests can be conducted, although most indicators are either nonspecific for hepatic disease or are not consistently abnormal in patients with hepatic disease. An example of a non-specific biochemical finding is elevation of plasma alkaline phosphatase (ALP) activity. Blood ammonia levels are also found to be abnormal only inconsistently. The general purpose of biochemically evaluating a liver problem is to document that it indeed exists

Figure 30-1. Occult Causes of Hepatomegaly

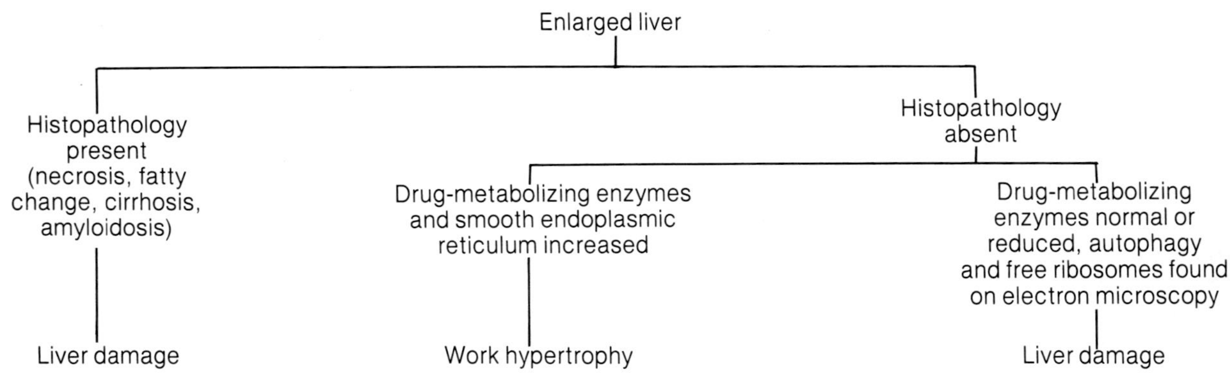

and that identification should be pursued. None of these tests provide information useful for identification of specific problems, proper management of the patient, or accurate prediction of the outcome. Conducting a battery of all available biochemical tests to assess hepatic disease does not provide any better information for answering those questions. At best, the information only complements what is already known.

Morphological evaluation of the liver is required to identify specific pathological processes, to determine proper management, and to predict the results of treatment. Gross morphologic evaluation is less important than microscopic assessment. Microhepatica and hepatomegaly suggest hepatic disease, but many patients with hepatic disease have normal-sized livers. Assessment of liver size is subjective and difficult when changes in the size are not striking, especially when hepatic size is determined from radiographs. The normal-sized liver can be palpated only when changes in the cranial abdominal cavity have moved the liver caudally and ventrally. The enlarged liver can usually be palpated, and radiographic procedures can be used to seek evidence for a liver of abnormal size. Normal liver size cannot be assumed as evidence of either a normal function test or a normal plasma enzyme activity. Thus, radiographic procedures do not substitute for other important parts of the investigation; as in many biochemical tests, the information that radiographs provide complements information already gained from the essential parts of the workup. Once a patient is identified as having liver pathology, the only means of answering the most important questions is liver biopsy. That provides a definitive diagnosis with which to initiate appropriate management and predict the outcome. Liver biopsy is not used to diagnose some problems, such as portasystemic vascular shunts. Even with that problem, however, the pathologist can identify histologic changes highly suggestive of a vascular anomaly.

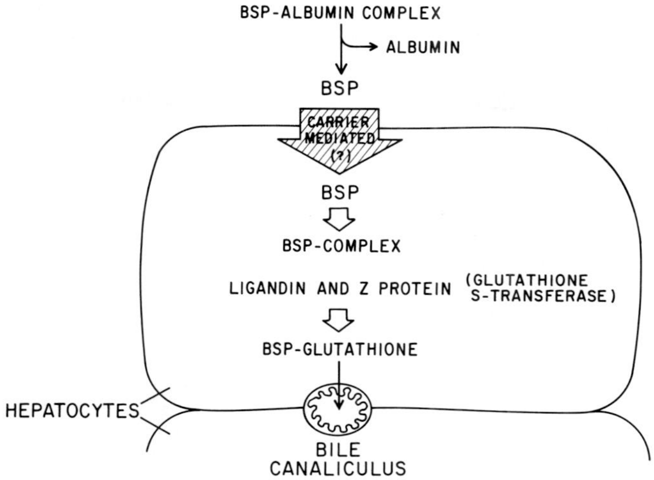

Figure 30-2. Diagram of sulfobromophthalein metabolism in the liver.

FUNCTION TESTS

Sulfobromophthalein Excretion[2]

Sulfobromophthalein (BSP) is an organic dye that, injected into the circulation, is removed by the liver at a rate that reflects the liver's ability to extract and metabolize a number of similar organic dyes. When disease reduces overall hepatic function, the circulation retains the dye for an abnormal time. BSP is cleared in three important steps (Figure 30-2). The dye is transferred from the plasma to the liver. Once inside hepatocytes, BSP binds to intracellular proteins Y and Z and is conjugated with glutathione. The conjugated product is secreted in bile and excreted into the intestine.

Circulatory Effects. The rate of disappearance of BSP is determined by a number of factors (Table 30-3). Since the rate depends on hepatic circulation, reduced hepatic blood flow delivers less dye for uptake, causing prolonged BSP retention. Such reduced hepatic circulation may reflect extrahepatic vascular shunting (such as portasystemic vascular anastomosis), intrahepatic shunting (such as cirrhosis), or cardiac failure. Hepatic or posthepatic causes of ascites predictably prolong BSP retention. Any process that expands plasma volume has a dilution effect on BSP, which causes less to appear to be retained at 30 minutes.

Plasma Protein Binding. BSP disappearance rates are dependent on plasma protein concentrations. The dye rapidly binds to serum albumin and alpha-lipoproteins. BSP retention time is markedly reduced in animals with hypoproteinemia,[3] where the amount of unbound dye is greater than it is when amounts of plasma proteins are normal, so that the liver removes it more avidly. Hepatic diseases may cause abnormal BSP retention time; when associated with hypoproteinemia, however, reduced plasma proteins result in more rapid BSP uptake, so that the prolonged retention may decrease to become normal or only slightly increased. Hypoproteinemia due to

Table 30-3. Causes of Abnormal BSP Excretion

Circulatory
Decreased hepatic blood flow
Cardiac failure
Hypovolemia and shock
Extrahepatic and intrahepatic vascular shunts
Hypoproteinemia
Abnormal hepatic uptake
Abnormal carrier
Congenital - mutant Southdown sheep
Acquired - hepatic disease, drugs and toxins
Competition for uptake - bilirubin, bile salts, drugs
Deficiency of intracellular binding proteins
Storage and conjugation
Deficiency of intracellular binding proteins
Competition for glutathione
Biliary excretion
Abnormal carrier
Congenital - mutant Corriedale sheep
Acquired - hepatic disease, drugs, toxins
Competition for secretion - bilirubin, bile acids, drugs
Biliary obstruction

hepatic disease is most often associated with portasystemic shunts and chronic hepatitis. The evaluation of BSP retention times must consider plasma protein concentrations. Those are more important in younger animals, which have lower plasma protein levels than adults. A dissocation constant determines the binding of BSP to plasma proteins. A substance that competes with BSP for binding and has a stronger affinity for plasma proteins displaces the BSP.

BSP Uptake and Conjugation. The rate of BSP disappearance is determined in part by its rate of uptake by hepatocytes. Uptake is acheived by an unknown mechanism that may involve carrier mediation or merely passive diffusion. The cytoplasmic protein glutathione S-transferase-B binds BSP and catalyzes its conjugation with glutathione. This protein also binds other substances, such as bilirubin and indocyanine green.[4] About 75% of the BSP is conjugated and secreted; the remainder is secreted as unconjugated BSP. Excessive amounts of BSP can enter hepatocytes, and secretion continues until the maximum secretory rate is attained. Then BSP is stored, primarily in the unconjugated form. Small amounts of both conjugated and free BSP normally return to the plasma. When excessive amounts are injected, the amount returning to the plasma increases, a case where hepatic uptake of BSP exceeds the maximum secretory rate. The storage capacity for BSP is great enough that it is never exceeded in normal animals.

BSP Secretion. The disappearance of BSP is determined most importantly by its rate of secretion into the biliary system, making that the rate-limiting step. The nature of the mechanism for its transfer into the bile is not known. Salts of bile acids stimulate BSP excretion to a rate two to three times normal.[5] Bile acids are choleretic agents, stimulating bile flow; they may act by reducing the concentration gradient of BSP across the bile canaliculi membranes that facilitate the back-diffusion of BSP from the ducts into the hepatocytes. Consequently, BSP retention is determined on animals in the fasting state. During feeding, large amounts of bile acids are secreted and cycle through the enterohepatic circulation several times during a single meal.

BSP Retention with Hepatic Disease. Measurement of BSP retention is useful in evaluating a number of hepatic problems. Since its rate of disappearance is a function of hepatic circulation, blood flow altered by portasystemic shunts, cirrhosis, or cardiac failure increases BSP retention time. The uptake, storage, conjugation, and secretion of BSP are all affected by hepatic and biliary disease.

Hyperbilirubinemia. Measurement of BSP retention does not yield additional useful information in animals with hyperbilirubinemia. True, the test can be conducted in icteric animals, since BSP levels can be calorimetrically determined on yellow serum or plasma and since there is no competition between bilirubin and BSP in the disappearance of BSP.[6] The reason BSP retention time cannot be determined in this case is that the abnormal retention of bilirubin reflects a lowered capacity to take up, conjugate, and secrete both bilirubin and BSP. Dogs lose a major part of this function before icterus appears. Only a mild hyperbilirubinemia is evident in most cases of hepatic disease in dogs since they readily take up and conjugate the small amounts of unconjugated bilirubin produced each day. When the rate-limiting step of secretion is affected, conjugated bilirubin is regurgitated and readily excreted in the urine. Abnormal BSP retention with hyperbilirubinemia merely confirms a hepatic or prehepatic cause for the icterus.

Hepatic Insufficiency. BSP retention time becomes markedly abnormal when two-thirds of the liver is removed.[7] When liver weight is reduced by more than half, the amount of BSP excreted into the bile is reduced to 60% of normal. The disappearance rate of BSP from plasma in this case is reduced even further, which reflects the fact that the liver is extracting and storing less BSP besides secreting less. A 70% hepatectomy also reduces the dog's ability to extract indocyanine green, an organic anion similar to BSP.[8] Hepatic regeneration correlates quite well with a return of the normal ability to extract dye, with regeneration proceeding for up to six weeks following hepatectomy. Abnormal BSP retention can persist following hepatic regeneration, which most likely reflects a failure to regain normal hepatic circulation.

Abnormal BSP retention in animals with hepatic necrosis, chronic hepatitis, or lipidosis is partly due to loss of the capacity to extract BSP — a consequence of both abnormal hepatic circulation and abnormal hepatocytes. Retention of BSP is the earliest significant biochemical abnormality in dogs with acute hepatic necrosis due to nitrosamine toxicity (Figure 30-3). Such a change, even before increases in plasma activities of ALT reflecting hepatic necrosis, indicate that BSP retention measurement is in some cases a sensitive indicator of hepatic insufficiency. Retention of BSP can also be one of the few abnormalities persisting after complete clinical remission in dogs with acute or chronic hepatic disease. With only 50% of normal liver mass the BSP retention remains abnormal; plasma enzyme activities and bile acids, blood ammonia, and values for most other hepatic tests return to normal.

Biliary Obstruction. BSP is secreted into the biliary system after uptake by hepatocytes. Thus, secretion of bile and evacuation of the biliary system affect the disappearance of BSP from the plasma. Complete obstruction of the bile duct markedly reduces the rate of BSP disappearance from the circulation.[9] BSP retention is even greater following two-thirds hepatectomy and during acute massive hepatic necrosis from carbon tetrachloride.[9] The reduced BSP disappearance rate during obstruction results from a loss of BSP uptake and storage as well as an inability to excrete the dye.[10] In dogs with a normal BSP retention of 2% at 30 minutes, complete obstruction of the bile duct causes BSP retention to increase to 11% to 12% within two days.[9] It remains elevated at 14% to 18% for another week, after

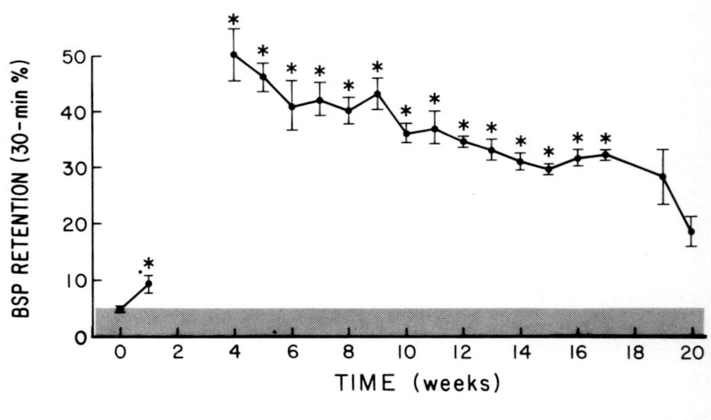

Figure 30-3. Changes in BSP retention percentage before and after exposure of dogs to nitrosamines. *Change is significant.

which it decreases to 7.4%. Biliary obstruction has the same effects on the disappearance of indocyanine green.[9]

Abnormal BSP Metabolism. The BSP retention time can be abnormal in the absence of any other biochemical or morphological evidence for hepatic disease. The abnormal retention can result from a defect in one or more steps in the liver's metabolism of BSP: uptake, storage, conjugation, or secretion into the bile. In humans and some species of animals, laboratory evaluation for liver disease reveals no abnormalities other than hyperbilirubinemia and increased BSP retention time. The problems in humans are characterized by a mild icterus, few clinical signs, and abnormalities in the manner that the liver handles organic anions.[11] Mild hyperbilirubinemia is possible in humans who have only minor defects in bilirubin metabolism. A comparable defect in dogs results in normal plasma bilirubin levels; the renal threshold for conjugated bilirubin is so low that dogs readily excrete moderate increments of conjugated bilirubin entering the circulation.[12] Thus, normal bilirubin levels with abnormal BSP retention are common in dogs. Abnormal BSP metabolism due to a defect in organic-dye metabolism has been reported in a dog.[13] Similar problems have been documented in humans and some other species of animals.[11,14]

Measurement of the rate of BSP disappearance is a valuable function test that can be performed on small-animal patients. Evaluation for suspected liver disease is not complete without a liver function test. In dogs, abnormal excretion of BSP appears before hyperbilirubinemia, which is found inconsistently. When an abnormal BSP retention time is found consistently, the problem is pursued until a cause is found. Abnormal BSP retention is caused almost invariably by hepatic disease that can be characterized morphologically and by circulatory problems.

BSP retention times are only used to identify hepatic disease. It is not possible to make judgments as to the degree of hepatic damage, since a circulatory component as well as a hepatocyte component contributes to the extraction of BSP. In all forms of liver disease, BSP retention time is poorly correlated with the degree of clinical signs of hepatic dysfunction; an animal with one-half of its liver, for instance, can be clinically normal.

BSP Retention Test. BSP retention time is determined by measuring the plasma concentration of BSP 30 minutes after its intravenous injection. The amount of dye given is 5 mg/Kg body weight, with the body weight adjusted in some cases, as follows. Since BSP does not distribute to ascitic fluid over the short period that the dye is in the circulation, the estimated weight of the ascitic fluid is subtracted. BSP distributes to the plasma compartment only, which is about 5% of total body weight, or 50 ml/Kg. Thus, if BSP distributed instantly to the total plasma compartment, the initial concentration would be 10 mg/100ml, which is 100% retention at zero time. The concentration at the end of 30 minutes is 0.5 mg/100 ml, or less. Thus, normal BSP retention is 5% or less at 30 minutes. Of course, any factor that changes the plasma volume from its estimated 5% changes the results of the test. For example, plasma volume does not increase in proportion to body weight in obese animals. Hence, plasma volume in this case is less than 50 ml/Kg, and when BSP is injected in an amount based strictly on body weight, the concentration at zero time will be greater than 10 mg/100 ml. Consequently, BSP retention at 30 minutes can be greater than 5% in obese animals with normal hepatic function. Similar errors can be made following BSP injection into an expanded plasma volume. Since BSP is bound to plasma albumin, Hypoalbuminemia accelerates dye excretion. A BSP retention of 5% or less at 30 minutes cannot be considered normal in a hypoalbuminemic animal. The BSP retention test is not conducted in an icteric animal since the results provide no information that is not already known. Animals are fasted and on no medication when the test is conducted. Values for BSP retention at 30 minutes in normal (not hospitalized) dogs is 1.9 ± 1.1 (mean ± SD) percent and in normal cats 0.6 ± 0.8. In these nonhospital animals the upper limit of normal is 4.2% and 3.0% for dogs and cats, respectively.

Indocyanine Green Excretion[15-18]

The organic anion indocyanine green (ICG) has been used to evaluate hepatic function in a manner similar to that used with BSP. Indocyanine green has become popular for use in humans because of severe reactions that are occasionally seen with BSP injections. That has not been a problem in small animals, so BSP is still the most popular dye for studies of hepatic function.

The metabolism of ICG is not entirely like that of BSP. Both dyes are transported in the circulation bound to serum albumin, and after hepatocyte uptake both are bound to the intracellular binding protein ligandin. Unlike BSP, however, ICG is not conjugated and is excreted unaltered from the hepatocyte into the biliary system. The ICG dye also differs from BSP in that it is not absorbed from the intestine and therefore does not enter an enterohepatic cycle. Although there appear to be advantages in the use of ICG over BSP, there are several reasons that its use has not become widespread. There is little information on its use in clinical cases of hepatic disease in small animals, so guidelines for interpretation are lacking. The BSP retention test is a more sensitive indicator of hepatic disease when it is compared with ICG retention in experimental animals.[9] Although carbon tetrachloride toxicity and bile duct obstruction cause BSP retention times to increase to six- to tenfold within several days, they alter ICG retention to a lesser degree. Moreover, abnormalities in liver function can be detected for a longer period with BSP than with ICG. Hepatic congestion, hepatic artery ligation, or 40% hepatectomy have no significant effect on ICG clearance in dogs.[19,20] Obstruction of a hepatic duct to produce regional cholestasis or 60% hepatectomy have only minor effects. The fact that ICG does not have to be metabolized is the most likely explanation for its more efficient disposal by the diseased liver. There are other differences in metabolism between ICG and BSP. Some humans with normal BSP clearance have abnormal ICG clearance, which suggests that a part of the pathway is different.[21] ICG has been used in small animals primarily to gain insight into the hepatic mechanisms for metabolizing organic anions. It is unlikely that it will ever become popular as a diagnostic test. Such a use would be expensive, require multiple blood samples, and require special spectrophotometers, in addition to being an insensitive test for identifying liver disease.

Blood Ammonia

Blood ammonia concentrations provide an indication of hepatic function. Most ammonia in the blood is produced in the intestines and absorbed into the portal circulation. The liver efficiently removes the ammonia, so that levels in the portal circulation ranging from 350 (dog) to 800 (cat) μg/dl are reduced to 50 μg/dl in blood leaving the liver.[22] Increased blood ammonia concentrations in the systemic circulation always indicate impaired hepatic function. Blood analysis several hours after feeding increases the chances of detecting hyperammonemia.

An ammonia tolerance test is used to semiquantitate hepatic function for converting ammonia to urea.[23] The test is also used to identify hepatic dysfunction that cannot be identified by other means. The test involves administering 100 mg NH_4Cl per Kg of body weight, to a maximum of 3 grams. The NH_4Cl is dissolved in water and placed in the stomach by stomach tube. Blood ammonia levels are measured before NH_4Cl is given and 30 minutes after. Since the normal animal can completely extract the ammonia given, little if any increment is seen in 30 minutes. This test has been most useful in identifying dogs with neurological signs, but no abnormal tests for hepatic disease. It has identified hepatic disease in dogs in which random blood ammonias were normal. Surprisingly, the NH_4Cl does not cause dogs to show any clinical signs other than occasional vomiting, which does not alter the results of the test. Acute ammonia toxicity initially causes hypersalivation and vomition, which is probably the reason for the occasional vomiting with the ammonia tolerance test. A rectal ammonia tolerance test is described where 5% ammonium chloride at a dose of 2 ml/kg body weight is injected into the rectum; blood samples are collected before infusion and at 20 and 40 minutes later for ammonia determinations.[24] Apparently absorption of ammonia is slower and less predictable than when ammonia chloride is given orally; hence, more samples are taken and over a longer period of time. The increases are reported to identify dogs with shunts, but the increments over preammonia infusion are not as great as those following oral administration of ammonia. The great variability in blood ammonia levels after rectal administration makes it more likely that hyperammonemia might not be identified in some dogs. Administering rectal ammonia does not result in hyperammonia in dogs with hepatic disease not associated with portasystemic shunts. Thus, the test is not sensitive enough to identify those patients, whereas they are identified by oral ammonia tolerance testing. Rectal ammonia tolerance testing is not likely to be established as a clinical test for all of these reasons, and also because an enema is required for preparing the patient.

Blood samples for ammonia determination are cooled on ice immediately after collection. Plasma is removed by centrifugation as soon as possible, after which blood ammonia is determined. The plasma can be frozen at -20°C and held for up to 48 hours before analysis. With proper handling, storage for that time does not change plasma ammonia levels. Whole blood cannot be stored and analyzed, since blood ammonia concentrations increase with time.[25] In fact, stored blood can contain enough ammonia to produce signs of hyperammonemia during blood transfusion.

Blood ammonia levels are determined by one of several different methods. The most reliable method involves the use of a binding resin.[26] Plasma is added to a strongly acidic cation-exchange resin, and ammonia is selectively absorbed. The ammonia-resin complex is washed, and the ammonia is subsequently eluted from the resin. Phenol and hypochlorite are added in the presence of sodium nitroferricyanide, and ammonia forms a dark-blue indophenol complex. The test is very accurate for blood levels of ammonia ranging from 0 to 450 μg/dl. Normal blood ammonia concentrations in dogs, determined by this method, are 16 to 48 μg/dl (mean 35).[27] Reagents to conduct this test are available commercially (Hyland Blood Ammonia Test, Travenol Lab.). With this method, as with any other, it is important to prevent contamination of samples by ammonia. Thus, care is taken that ammonia-free water be used at every step in the procedure, including washing the glassware used in the test. Some chemicals can also cause the values for ammonia to increase or decrease.[28] Ammonia-free heparin tubes are used for blood collection; coagulants such as sodium citrate, potassium oxalite, or sodium fluoride can cause ammonia values to increase. Ammonia-based skin disinfectants are not used to prepare sites for venapuncture.

A second method of assay for ammonia is based on an enzymatic reaction.[29] Plasma ammonia is reacted with alpha-ketoglutarate to form glutamate, and in the reaction $NADH_2$ is oxidized to NAD. The enzyme glutamic dehydrogenase catalyzes this reaction. The amount of products formed, glutamate and NAD, is proportional to the amount of ammonia in the sample. The quantitative change of $NADH_2$ to NAD is determined with a spectrophotometer, and the results are used to compute the amount of ammonia converted to glutamate. This method is as accurate as the method using a resin to bind and extract ammonia. Precautions must be taken to ensure that the glassware and water are free of ammonia. The reagents used for this test are available commercially (Sigma Diagnostics). Normal blood ammonia for dogs by this method is 0 to 100 μg/dl.

Miscellaneous Function Tests

A number of hepatic function tests have been used to evaluate the integrity of a single biochemical function of the liver. One such test is based on the liver's ability to metabolize the monosaccharide galactose. The liver is the only site in the body where significant conversion of galactose to glucose occurs. Since hepatic disease reduces this function, galactose injected intravenously disappears from the plasma more slowly than in normal animals. This test is of no value in evaluating for hepatic disease since it only identifies extensive pathology. One of the last liver functions lost with hepatic disease is maintenance of carbohydrate metabolism. Hypoglycemia or hyperglycemia is an infrequent complication.

PLASMA ENZYMES

Hepatocytes contain many enzymes in mitochondria, bound to cell membranes, and in the cytosol. Small amounts of some of these enzymes normally escape to the plasma, where their activities can be measured. Increased plasma enzyme activities for some are associated with hepatic pathology. Increased activity most commonly follows hepatocyte damage. That damage can result from traumatic, hypoxic, toxic, infectious, nutritional, genetic or metabolic problems. The extent, rapidity, and severity of tissue damage, as well as the enzyme's concentration, rate of synthesis, subcellular location, size, and ease of diffusion from the cell, determine the magnitude of the plasma increase. Plasma activities increase greatly with widespread, rapidly developing, and severe cell damage; they also increase when an enzyme is small, rapidly synthesized, and not bound to membranes or organelles, has a high intracellular concentration, and can rapidly diffuse from the cell. Plasma enzyme activity increases because enzyme synthesis is stimulated. Inducement of enzyme synthesis is a normal response to growth, regeneration, drug effects, and biliary obstruction. Plasma enzyme activities can increase because of delayed enzyme clearance; that might be seen with renal failure. The ease with which enzyme proteins can enter the circulation also determines the potential for increases in plasma enzyme activity. The liver is designed with blood bathing two sides of the hepatocytes, which are not separated from the circulation by very restrictive membranes. Thus, enzymes escaping from hepatocytes can readily enter sinusoids. Enzymes lost from cells in other tissues may not reach the circulation until they are transported through the lymphatics.

Most plasma enzymes are found not only in one but in many different tissues of the body, so that many sources contribute to their plasma activities. Changes in any of these tissues can release the enzymes and increase their plasma activity. Increased plasma activity of any one of these enzymes is pathognomonic for hepatocyte pathology when the enzyme's activity is much greater in hepatocytes than any other cells. Two such enzymes are far more abundant in hepatocytes than in any other tissues.

Alanine Aminotransferase

Alanine aminotransferase (ALT) is the most liver-specific enzyme that is measured in the plasma. It is a cytosolic enzyme with concentrations in the liver four times that in the next-most abundant site (the heart) and ten times that in the kidney. The concentration of ALT in hepatocytes is 10,000 times greater than that in plasma. The most common cause for an increase in plasma ALT is hepatic necrosis. Slight to moderate elevations can be seen with myocarditis. Plasma aspartate aminotransferase (AST) activity increases following its release from damaged hepatocytes, but since this transaminase is as abundant in other tissues, or more so, an increment in the plasma is not diagnostic for liver disease. Plasma ALT has a half-life of 2.5 hours, whereas that for plasma AST is greater than 4 hours.[30]

Plasma ALT activity increases markedly with many forms of hepatic degeneration and necrosis. Experimental work has provided an understanding of the relationship of plasma ALT increments to hepatocyte changes.[9] Following hepatocyte necrosis caused by a single episode of carbon tetrachloride poisoning, ALT activity increases dramatically, peaking in three to four days and then gradually decreasing to normal in about two weeks. Some hepatotoxins do not produce such a persisting necrosis. Paracetamol-induced hepatic necrosis markedly increases ALT and AST activities within 24 hours, at which time they correlate well with the degree of hepatic necrosis.[31] The plasma enzyme activities subsequently decrease, so that by 72 hours the elevations are only slight to moderate. The necrosis, however, remains morphologically moderate to severe, and so there is no longer any significant correlation between enzyme levels and the degree of necrosis. Hepatocellular necrosis induced by nitrosamines increases plasma ALT activity, but not significantly, until after one week (Figure 30-4).[32] The increases persist for weeks until the necrosis is resolved. Some drugs cause hepatic pathology and increases in plasma ALT activity. Experimental studies in dogs have demonstrated those results for corticosteroids and some anticonvulsants.[33,34] Hepatocyte pathology is also a feature of portasystemic shunts in experimental dogs, as illustrated by increased plasma ALT activity (Figure 30-5),[35] although histologic changes are not usually evident for hepatocytes. In that case there is a poor correlation between biochemical abnormalities and hepatocyte pathology. Bile duct obstruction in experimental dogs causes plasma ALT increases that peak by five to six days at levels 15 to 20 times normal and thereafter gradually decline.[9] That may not be consistent with early hepatocyte changes (focal necrosis accompanied by inflammation), which can be relatively unremarkable, but the later appearance of marked biliary fibrosis indicates that significant pathologic changes begin after the obstruction. The pathology may be produced by high concentrations of retained bile acids, which damage hepatocytes and biliary epithelium. Hepatic trauma increases plasma transaminase activity, which may not begin returning to normal for a week after the injury.

In clinical cases, plasma ALT activity increases markedly and consistently with acute hepatic necrosis; the degree to

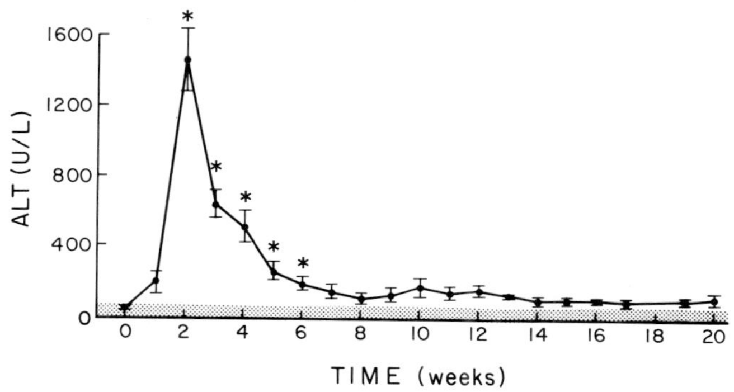

Figure 30-4. Changes in plasma ALT activity before and after exposure of dogs to nitrosamines. *Change is significant.

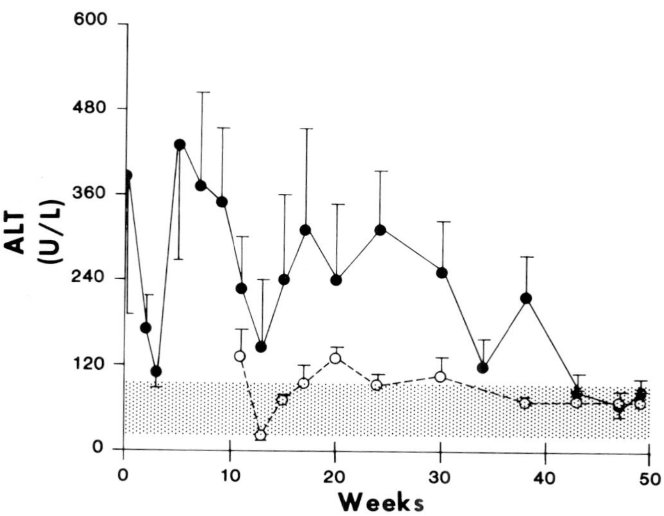

Figure 30-5. Changes in plasma ALT in dogs with portasystemic shunts. Normal range in shaded area.

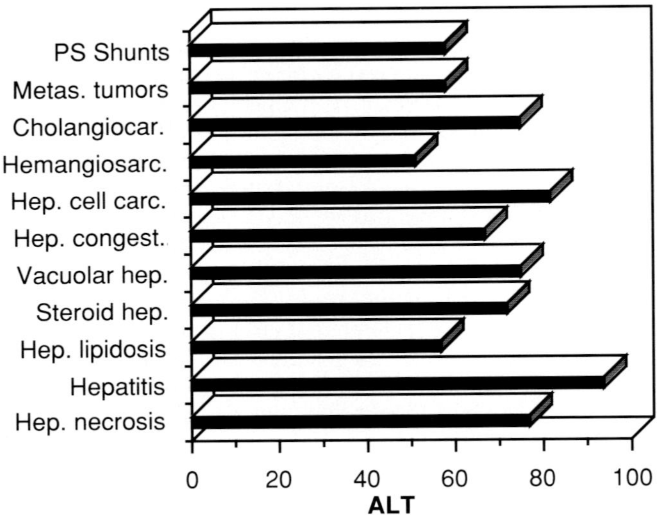

Figure 30-6. Comparison of sensitivities for plasma ALT activity in dogs with different hepatic problems.

which it increases parallels the severity and extent of hepatocyte degeneration. Persisting increments are found consistently with a number of clinical problems (Figure 30-6). Acute hepatic necrosis caused by infectious canine hepatitis increases plasma ALT activity to 30 times normal; activity peaks within four days.[36] Toxic hepatitis causes plasma ALT activity to increase, peak, and return to normal sooner than does virus hepatitis. The magnitude of increases with toxic hepatitis is proportionate to the amount of toxin, and plasma ALT activity can increase to the levels found with virus hepatitis, although they are usually considerably less. Chronic hepatitis, a persistent necrotic process associated with varying degrees of fibrosis, is characterized by mean plasma ALT activity 10 to 12 times the upper limit of normal. The fluctuations in ALT activity reflect activity of the necrotic process at any given time. This fluctuation is in contrast to the animal with hepatic necrosis, where ALT levels decline as the problem resolves.

The peak levels of plasma ALT activity do not show as great an increase in most clinical cases of biliary obstruction as they do during experimental obstruction. Plasma ALT levels in clinical cases may be as high early, but if evaluations are made later, the ALT activity will be lower. Also, plasma ALT may be lower because obstructions are partial and caused by a slowly progressing lesion in clinical cases. An exception occurs with acute inflammatory processes in tissues around the bile duct, such as with acute pancreatitis.

Activities of plasma ALT consistently increase with hepatocellular carcinomas, hepatocellular adenomas, and nodular hyperplasia. Mean increments five to six times over normal are consistent with moderate hepatocellular degeneration. Plasma ALT elevations with these problems are often incidental findings that cannot be related to clinical signs. In contrast, plasma ALT activity increases less frequently and only two to three times over normal in dogs with metastatic neoplastic disease of the liver.

Increased plasma ALT activity is seen more inconsistently with other hepatic problems. In dogs with steroid-induced hepatopathy, ALT activity increases three times over normal. Hepatic lipidosis and vacuolar hepatopathy cause slight plasma ALT increases. Similar changes are seen for chronic passive congestion and portasystemic vascular shunts. Increases in plasma ALT activity are not unusual for a variety of systemic disease processes. Enzyme levels can be expected to increase with septicemias and systemic immune-mediated diseases.

Sorbitol Dehydrogenase

Sorbitol dehydrogenase (SDH) is a cytosolic enzyme released during hepatic degeneration. The concentration of SDH is greater in the liver than in all other tissues.[30] The kidney is the only other organ with significant SDH activity (half that of the liver). The total renal mass as a potential source for SDH is small compared with the liver's, indicating that plasma SDH activity could be more useful in identifying hepatic disease than current usage indicates. The half-life of SDH is about four hours. Measuring plasma SDH activity offers no advantage over measuring plasma ALT activity for identifying hepatic degeneration and necrosis in small animals, and there is some question on its stability in vitro.

Plasma Arginase[12]

Arginase is a urea cycle enzyme found in mitochondria that can be released with hepatic necrosis. Normal plasma arginase activity is 0 to 14 IU/L in normal dogs and cats. Plasma arginase activity increases in dogs following the administration of carbon tetrachloride to peak at 1400 IU/L in 24 hours; it then rapidly decreases to basal levels after two days. Plasma ALT levels also peaks at 24 hours but do not return to normal until two weeks later. Greatly increased plasma arginase activity has been found in clinical cases of hepatic necrosis. In general, if arginase activity is increased with hepatic disease of more than three days duration, the insult causing necrosis is persisting and the prognosis is poor. On the other hand, if plasma arginase activity is low and plasma levels of ALT are still high, the patient is likely to be in the recovery phase at some point more than two days after the insult. Plasma arginase activity can split arginine to urea and ornithine and reduce the plasma levels of arginine to approach zero. Arginine is necessary to maintain urea-cycle activity, and a marked depletion of plasma arginine causes blood ammonia concentrations to increase since conversion of ammonia to urea is reduced.

Plasma Alkaline Phosphatase[37-40]

The alkaline phosphatases are a group of enzymes that catalyze the hydrolysis of a number of organic phosphate compounds to yield phosphate and an organic molecule. The enzymes operate best at an alkaline pH. Alkaline phosphatase (ALP) activity is found primarily in the liver, skeleton, intestine, kidney, and placenta. The activity of the isozymes from any of those tissues can increase in the plasma. However, the increased activity seen in clinical cases is due entirely to the isoenzymes from the liver or bone. Each of those isoenzymes has a long half-life — about three days for the hepatic plasma alkaline phosphatases, in contrast to the half-life of three to six minutes for the placental, intestinal, and renal isoenzymes after their injection into dogs.[41] Thus, disease in one of these organs is not likely to increase ALP activity significantly. It is not known whether these tissues contribute to normal ALP activity. Bone ALP activity increases with osteoblastic activity, as is evident in normal growing animals. Plasma ALP levels can increase with some bone disorders such as osteomalacia, osteogenic sarcoma, and secondary hyperparathyroidism.[12]

Plasma ALP activity increases most often with hepatic diseases associated with biliary obstruction.[42] Plasma ALP activity increases because hepatic enzyme production is stimulated. Alkaline phosphatase is membrane-bound and produced primarily by epithelial cells forming bile canaliculi. These cells proliferate following biliary obstruction, increasing the amounts of enzyme activity that escape to the circulation.[43]. Enzymes can be transported in a retrograde direction from the biliary epithelium or lumen to the sinusoidal border of hepatocytes and from there enter the circulation. Plasma ALP activity also increases with steroid-induced hepatopathy, the liver being the source of the elevated enzyme activity. The increased activity is due primarily to the liver isoenzyme of ALP and to a lesser extent to the corticosteroid-induced isoenzyme of ALP. There is a ten-fold difference in their contributions after a month-long treatment with prednisone.

The function of ALP is unknown.[44] Suggestions have been made that it is involved with the absorption of lipids in the intestine because plasma ALP activity of the intestinal isoenzyme increases in response to a high-fat meal.[45] It may have a similar role in biliary epithelia or may be involved with the transport of calcium, phosphate, or water.

A number of experimental studies show what kind of changes increase ALP activity. Following complete obstruction of the bile duct, ALP activity gradually increases six- to seven fold over a period of five to six days.[9] After this, the activity is 18 to 20 times normal during the period seven to ten days after obstruction. Other studies report similar findings in cats and dogs. The earliest morphological evidence for bile duct proliferation begins within three days of complete obstruction.[46] The marked increases in plasma ALP activity within seven days undoubtedly reflects the proliferative responses manifesting to a maximum degree.

Plasma ALP activity also increases with hepatic necrosis or degeneration in cats and dogs treated with carbon tetrachloride.[9] It increases four- to six fold, peaking at four to six days and then gradually decreasing. These increments parallel those found with biliary obstruction for the first four days. After this, plasma ALP increases due to biliary obstruction far outdistance those for hepatic necrosis. The hepatic necrosis caused by infectious canine hepatitis does not damage the liver as early as carbon tetrachloride toxicity does, and increases in ALP activity are not significant until after three days.[35] Plasma ALP activity increases in the regenerating liver. Following 70% partial hepatectomy, plasma ALP activity peaks at a week and then gradually returns to normal during six weeks.[8] Drugs such as barbiturates and some anticonvulsants also stimulate the activity of hepatic alkaline phosphatase in experimental animals.[40]

Plasma ALP activity increases with many types of clinical hepatic disease.[40,47] The greatest increases are found with cholestasis and steroid-induced hepatopathy. Markedly elevated ALP activities with obstructive jaundice are proportional to the degree of biliary obstruction, reaching 20 to 30 times normal with complete obstruction. Increases with steroid-induced hepatopathy are more variable. Some patients with Cushing's disease have ALP levels 20 to 30 times normal, but in most cases the levels are less than 10 times normal. The activity of ALP does not consistently increase in animals given corticosteroids, but ALP is increased in almost all animals with morphological evidence of steroid-induced hepatopathy.[48] Plasma ALP activity also increases with hepatic necrosis and chronic hepatitis, although not consistently; the elevations found are usually three to six times the upper normal limits. Enzyme activity is increased because of intrahepatic cholestasis caused by bile canaliculi damage and hepatocyte swelling.

Increased plasma ALP activity is usually seen with hepatocellular carcinomas. While the majority of the enzyme levels are four to seven times normal, some have increased to 50 times the upper limit of normal. Only one-fourth of these patients have hyperbilirubinemia, so that intrahepatic cholestasis may not be the only explanation for the high plasma ALP levels. The levels of plasma ALP activity are normal to moderately elevated in patients with metastatic neoplastic disease of the liver. Dogs with portasystemic vascular shunts usually do not have markedly increased ALP activity. In summary, the hepatic diseases that cause plasma ALP to exceed five times the upper limit of normal include most cases of cholestasis and steroid-induced hepatopathy and usually acute hepatitis, chronic hepatitis, and primary hepatocellular carcinoma.

Measurement of ALP activity has not been considered an effective test to evaluate for hepatic disease in cats, since their plasma ALP levels do not increase greatly.[49] Later studies show ALP activity to increase ninefold with bile duct obstruction and sixfold with carbon tetrachloride toxicity in experimental cats.[50] Plasma ALP activity may not be consistently increased because its hepatic concentration is less than the dog's and its half life is only six hours, one-twelfth that for dog's hepatic ALP.[51] Like the dog, ALP activity is normally higher in growing kittens than in adult cats. In comparison, canine lipidosis causes a sixfold increase in plasma ALP, and feline lipidosis causes a fourfold increase over normal. Canine vacuolar hepatopathy results in a fourfold ALP increase, compared to a twofold increase for feline vacuolar hepatopathy. Comparison of other similar hepatic problems shows similar differences. Thus, any two- or threefold increase in plasma ALP activity is much more important as a sign of liver disease in the cat than it would be in the dog, where such an increase may not be sufficient evidence to pursue the possibility of liver disease.

Increased plasma ALP activity is not diagnostic for hepatic disease in dogs and cats. It is found with diabetes mellitus, enteritis, pyometritis, nephritis, cystic calculi, and bone diseases such as malignancies, fractures, and arthritis.[12,37,47] In addition, higher levels of plasma ALP activity are normal in young animals. In general, the increases found with these problems are not as great as those found with hepatic disease. Measurement of plasma ALP activity is used as a screening test to identify possible hepatic problems. When ALP activity is increased, the possibility of hepatic disease can be pursued, although only with the understanding that other problems may be the cause.

Gamma-Glutamyl Transferase

The enzyme gamma-glutamyl transferase (GGT) is synthesized in the liver, and measurement of its plasma activity is used to identify hepatic disease.[52-54] The enzyme, bound to membranes, exists at high concentrations not only in the liver but in the renal tubular epithelium, pancreas, and small intestinal epithelium. The highest concentration is found in the kidney, but plasma GGT levels are seldom elevated with chronic nephritis. Minor increases have been reported for a variety of renal problems, pancreatic diseases, diabetes mellitus, some intestinal problems, and cardiac disease. Marked elevations are found only with hepatic disease, however, which makes GGT a liver-specific enzyme. Plasma GGT levels in normal cats and dogs are 0 to 10 IU/L.

Gamma-glutamyl transferase catalyzes the transfer of the glutamyl part of peptides to gamma-amino acids or other peptides, the most common substrate being glutathione. The hepatic enzyme is concentrated in Kupffer cells, endothelium of periportal vessels, bile-duct epithelium, and hepatocytes. The enzyme is postulated to play a key role in the gamma-glutamyl cycle, which is responsible for the transport of amino acids into the cell. Hepatic levels of GGT increase shortly after birth and gradually decline in the adult to levels that are one-sixth to one-fourth as high. Thus, high levels of the enzyme are associated with the growth phase, which would be consistent with the growing animal's greater need for a system to transport amino acids into the liver. Hepatic levels of the enzyme can increase in adults.

Plasma GGT increases when portasystemic vascular shunts and some forms of steatosis alter the metabolism.[55] Plasma GGT activity increases consistently in experimental animals with primary hepatic neoplastic disease or biliary obstruction. Increased hepatic GGT activity in animals with vascular shunts appears to be an appropriate response to accompanying biochemical defects. Dogs with shunts lose the ability to metabolize aromatic amino acids and a few others, all of which are metabolized in the liver only. Plasma concentrations of aromatic amino acids increase, and increased hepatic GGT activity may reflect an attempt to increase hepatic metabolism by transporting additional amounts of amino acids into hepatocytes. Ethanol and drugs such as phenobarbitol increase plasma and hepatic enzyme activity by increasing hepatic synthesis of the enzyme.[56] Barbiturates stimulate microsomal enzyme activity, and since GGT is an enzyme found in the endoplasmic reticulum, the activity increase may be a nonspecific induction of all microsomal enzymes. The levels of plasma GGT activity increase with biliary stasis. This response is similar to changes in plasma alkaline phosphatase increments during biliary obstruction. The increases in plasma GGT are due to increased hepatic synthesis of the enzyme and possibly due to impaired excretion of enzyme in bile because of biliary obstruction. The enzyme is probably excreted or degraded by the kidneys, since, with anuria, the increments in plasma activity after biliary obstruction are much greater.[57]

Measurement of plasma GGT activity should be useful in evaluating hepatic disease in small animals. In humans, it has been valuable in identifying biliary obstruction, both intrahepatic and extrahepatic, alcoholic hepatic disease, and some neoplastic diseases of the liver. Its potential promise for use in small-animal patients is more accurate identification of patients with all forms of biliary-tract disease and hepatic neoplasms. At present, measurement of plasma alkaline phosphatase activity is the most commonly used means of confirming hepatobiliary disease. Plasma ALP elevations, however, can be due to other problems, making it a nonspecific test.

In dogs, plasma ALP increases can be due to hepatic disease, bone problems, or drugs such as glucocorticosteroids. Plasma GGT increases with two of these problems, however, hepatic disease and corticosteroid excess, giving GGT measurement little advantage over plasma ALP determination in identifying a problem as hepatic.[58] The plasma GGT increase is the same for corticosteroid treatment after 12 days as it is for hepatic duct ligation of the same duration. The plasma ALP increase for corticosteroid is less than that for hepatic duct ligation of the same duration. It is seldom necessary to differentiate between liver disease and a bone problem as the cause for increased plasma ALP activity. Thus, from these experimental studies there appears to be no advantage in determining plasma GGT or plasma ALP levels for evaluation of any hepatic problem, including differentiating intrahepatic from extrahepatic cholestasis.

Plasma GGT activity in clinical cases of hepatic disease increases in 56% of dogs, whereas plasma ALP activity increases in 81%.[59] About one-half of dogs with normal plasma GGT show increases for plasma ALT and ALP activities. Of these three plasma enzymes, the activity of GGT returns to normal sooner than the others. In summary, plasma GGT levels prove less sensitive than plasma ALP for identifying hepatic problems in dogs.

Plasma GGT increases very little and plasma ALP increases threefold five days after carbon tetrachloride is given to cats.[60] Following bile duct ligation in cats, plasma GGT gradually increases to peak at a level four times higher than that of controls; the increase for plasma ALP activity is, in contrast, 18-20 times greater than the controls'. No information is available from studies on clinical cases, but it would appear that, as in the dog, plasma GGT measurement is less sensitive than plasma ALP measurement for determining hepatic disease in the cat. Thus, there would be no advantage to measuring plasma GGT rather than plasma ALP.

PLASMA PROTEINS

Since the liver produces almost all plasma proteins, measurement of their plasma concentrations is used to evaluate hepatic function.[12] The most important of these are albumin, fibrinogen, the prothrombin-complex clotting factors, and both alpha- and beta-globulins. The gamma-globulins, not produced by the liver, can be altered secondarily by hepatic disease. Plasma protein concentrations are evaluated after separation by electrophoresis by measuring total proteins, albumin, and globulin fractions.

Albumin

Plasma albumin increases are attributed to dehydration. Albumin levels decrease because of reduced hepatic synthesis or because of increased loss by degradation or escape into the intestines or urine. The most common causes of increased loss are renal glomerular diseases, protein-losing enteropathies, and some malignancies. Extreme malnutrition and hepatic disease can reduce albumin synthesis. Hepatic albumin synthesis is not severely reduced until hepatic insufficiency becomes marked. Hypoalbuminemia with hepatic disease can be due in part to albumin's expanding volume of distribution, such as with

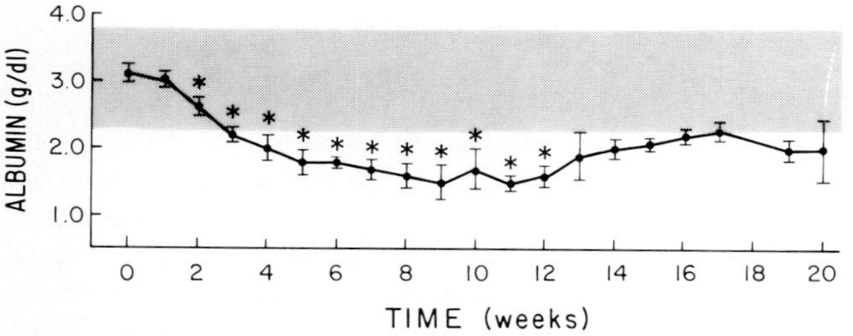

Figure 30-7. Changes in plasma albumin before and after exposure of dogs to nitrosamines. *Change is significant.

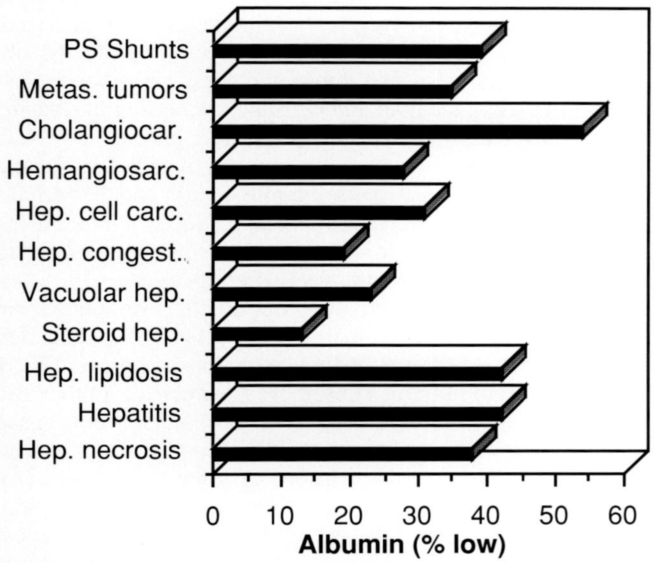

Figure 30-8. Comparison of sensitivities for plasma albumin levels in dogs with different hepatic problems.

ascites, where albumin distributes to ascitic fluid. With total-body albumin remaining constant, a dilutional effect causes hypoalbuminemia. Feeding a low-protein diet to manage hepatic disease and hepatic encephalopathy can produce marginal protein malnutrition, which, when combined with the hepatic disease, results in hypoalbuminemia. Experimental dogs with carbon tetrachloride toxicity have no significant changes in plasma protein concentrations,[9] but those with nitrosamine toxicity do show changes (Figure 30-7).[32] In clinical cases the plasma levels of albumin do not usually decrease unless hepatic disease is marked (Figure 30-8). With severe hepatic disease hypoalbuminemia is of little diagnostic value; that hepatic disease is a problem should be readily recognized from abnormal plasma enzyme determinations and function tests. Measurement of plasma albumin levels is important, however, for recognizing complications of hepatic disease. Its measurement is also useful for predicting the outcome for some problems such as chronic hepatitis.[61]

Globulins

Plasma globulin concentrations can increase or decrease with hepatic disease. Fractionation of serum proteins is used to quantitate changes in any one fraction. This separation allows identification of one or more fractions of alpha-, beta-, and gamma-globulins. Interpretations of electrophoretic patterns must recognize that some immunoglobulins are found in the alpha- and beta- fractions as well as the gamma-fraction.[62] The gamma-globulins can increase with acute and chronic hepatic problems, as a result of a failure of the hepatic mononuclear phagocytic system to remove foreign antigens in the portal circulation. Hypergammaglobulinemia due to this cause can be produced in experimental dogs with portasystemic vascular shunts.[63] Similar changes are seen in dogs with hepatic insufficiency due to nitrosamine toxicity (Figure 30-9). Fractionation of plasma proteins reveals few consistently abnormal patterns with clinical cases of hepatic disease. Changes in globulin levels may be seen with primary hepatocellular carcinomas, where most increases are for gamma-globulins. Gamma globulin increases are seldom documented for other clinical problems; when seen they do not exceed 2 to 2.5 times normal.

Blood-Clotting Factors

Most animals with evidence of liver disease are evaluated indirectly for plasma levels of liver-produced blood-clotting factors. Hemograms provide data on fibrinogen levels, a protein produced in the liver. Hepatic disease does not reduce plasma concentrations of this protein unless nearly all of the organ's functional ability is lost. Low fibrinogen levels usually reflect an increase in fibrinogen utilization, such as with disseminated intravascular coagulation. Measurements of prothrombin time and partial thromboplastin time provide information on prothrombin-complex clotting factors synthesized by the liver. Concentrations of these clotting factors are infrequently low enough to prolong prothrombin and partial thromboplastin times in animals with hepatic disease (Figure 30-10). Blood-clotting ability is usually evaluated before the liver is biopsied. Prolonged prothrombin (PT) and partial thromboplastin (PTT) times are not commonly encountered. Abnormal times are consistently found with hepatic failure due to massive necrosis, a problem usually associated with clinical evidence for increased bleeding tendency. The PT and PTT tests are made more sensitive indicators of hepatic disease when their determinations are made on diluted plasma. In one study, only 15% of dogs with hepatic disease showed abnormal PT and PTT, but

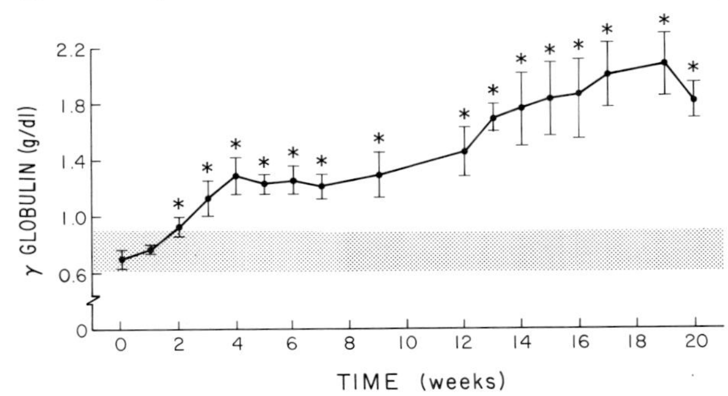

Figure 30-9. Changes in plasma globulins before and after exposure of dogs to nitrosamines. *Change is significant.

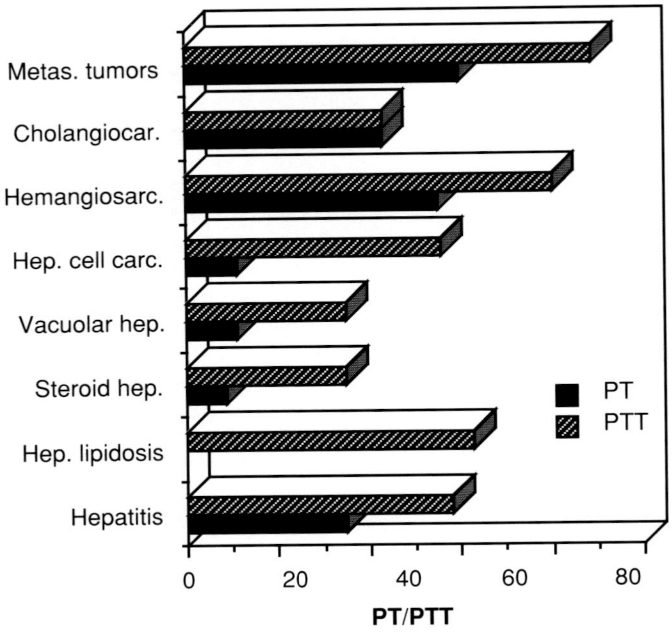

Figure 30-10. Comparison of sensitivities for PT and PTT in dogs with different hepatic problems.

with testing done on diluted plasma, this figure increased to 66%.[64] Determination of clotting factor levels provides a direct test that is more reliable than the PT and PTT tests for evaluating liver function. As many as 93% of all dogs with hepatic disease have an abnormality in the level of at least one clotting factor.[65] This makes the clotting factor assay more sensitive than the PT or PTT in identifying hepatic disease. But blood-clotting factors are not measured to identify hepatic disease; they are used primarily to evaluate the patient's clotting ability before liver biopsy, to characterize clinical evidence for a coagulopathy, and in some cases to help in predicting the outcome. Activated clotting time is also used for indirect evaluation of the adequacy of blood-clotting factors.[66]

Biliary stasis caused by biliary cirrhosis or bile duct obstruction can increase plasma protein concentrations of ceruloplasmin, plasminogen, blood-clotting factors, and immunoglobulins.[67]

PLASMA LIPIDS

Plasma concentrations of a number of lipids can change with hepatic disease. The plasma lipids measured most commonly are free cholesterol and cholesterol esters, which are reported as total cholesterol. Plasma levels of triglycerides and fatty acids are seldom measured, and so there is little information on their value in clinical cases of hepatic disease.

Experimental bile-duct obstruction increases total plasma cholesterol concentrations. In one week-long study on dogs, plasma cholesterol increased within three to four days and peaked at 315 mg/dl by five to six days, from preobstruction levels of 170 mg/dl.[9] In other dogs, total plasma cholesterol concentrations increased gradually from a norm of 184 mg/dl to 322 mg/dl over a 14-day period following bile-duct obstruction.[68] Plasma phospholipid concentrations double eight days after obstruction and then gradually return to levels 50% higher than normal. Triglyceride levels increase transiently and then return to normal. The fractionation of total cholesterol shows that plasma concentrations of cholesterol esters do not change, whereas those of free cholesterol increase four- to five-fold. The percentage of cholesterol ester in total cholesterol decreases from 80% in normal dogs to 50% within eight days of obstruction and remains there. The composition of low-density lipoproteins changes so that levels of free cholesterol increase and levels of cholesterol esters decrease. Measurement of plasma lipoproteins does not differentiate intrahepatic from extrahepatic biliary stasis as is often suggested.[69] The protein content of low-density lipoproteins is reduced to one-third of normal. The increment in plasma free cholesterol is due in small part to a reflux of cholesterol from the obstructed biliary system. The major part of the increase, however, is increased cholesterol synthesis. This is partly due to stimulation of cholesterol production by the increased reflux of lecithin from the obstructed biliary system. Lecithin is a potent stimulus for cholesterol synthesis by the liver and intestine. Increasing the plasma concentration of bile acids in dogs with chronic bile-duct obstruction decreases the plasma levels of free cholesterol and phospholipids. Obstruction of the bile duct in cats has effects similar to those in dogs.[70] Plasma total cholesterol increases to peak at 400 to 500 mg/dl at three weeks and then declines to normal levels by the seventh week after obstruction.

Carbon tetrachloride toxicity has no effect on total serum cholesterol concentrations in dogs.[9] It causes a 35% reduction in cholesterol esters within five to six days, followed by a gradual return to normal. Thus, there is a decrease in the ratio of esterified cholesterol to total cholesterol, but it is not caused by an increase in the free cholesterol content as it is with obstruction of the bile duct. In this case the total cholesterol levels do not change as the cholesterol esters decrease and reduce the ratio of esters to total cholesterol. The pathological changes in cholesterol esters result from the abnormally low plasma activity of lecithin: cholesterol acyl transferase. The liver produces this enzyme, which catalyzes the esterification of cholesterol in plasma; hepatic disease reduces its plasma activity.

Plasma lipid levels are infrequently reported for small animals with hepatic disease. Plasma total cholesterol, routinely measured in most chemistry panels, provides little useful information for identifying hepatic disease. Total cholesterol increases with endocrine diseases such as hypothyroidism, Cushing's syndrome, and diabetes mellitus, and with some renal glomerular diseases. Mild cholesterol increases are difficult to interpret, one reason being the variability in ranges for normal values. One study reports that plasma cholesterol concentrations in healthy dogs range from 125 to 335 mg/dl;[71] another reports the upper limit of normal to be 250 mg/dl.[72] Plasma cholesterol in normal cats is reported to be 116-126 mg/dl by one source[73] and 89-258 mg/dl by another using the same method.[74] If the increment in experimental dogs with biliary obstruction causes total cholesterol levels to increase to the high normal values (320 mg/dl), plasma cholesterol values cannot be used to identify biliary obstruction. On the other hand, the ratio of esterified to total cholesterol can be used to evaluate hepatic disease. The normal ratios of esterified to total cholesterol range from 0.64 to 0.88 (control experimental dogs mean ratio =

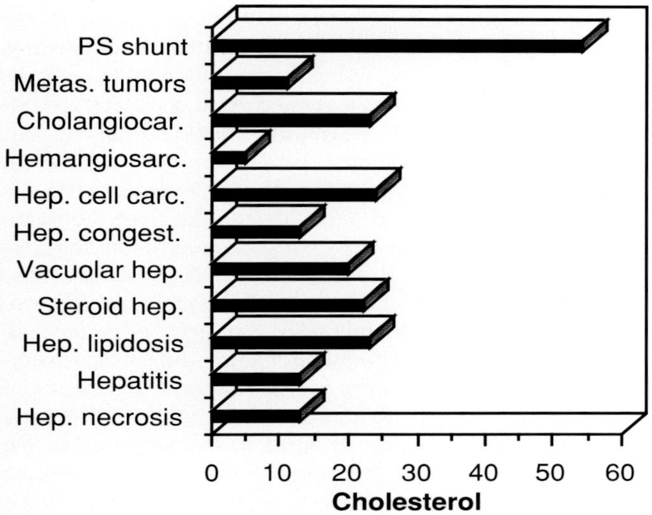

Figure 30-11. Comparison of sensitivities for plasma cholesterol levels in dogs with different hepatic problems. Sensitivity for PS shunt is for low cholesterol; all others are for high cholesterol.

0.80).[71] In dogs with morphologically determined hepatic disease, 90% have ratios that are less than 0.64, and half of those have ratios of less than 0.52. About 20% of those have ratios of less than 0.40. Dogs with acute hepatitis have the highest percentage of abnormal ratios. In descending order, this is followed by obstructive jaundice, liver cirrhosis, and liver tumors. The abnormal cholesterol ester ratio was usually associated with hyperbilirubinemia. The degree of alteration in the ratio could not be correlated with the degree of severity of the hepatic disease. In summary, the ratio of serum cholesterol ester to total cholesterol fairly consistently identifies suspected hepatic disease. Total plasma cholesterol concentrations are of little value in identifying hepatic disease, for they are not usually increased (Figure 30-11).

Some hepatic problems are associated with abnormally low plasma levels of lipids. Plasma total cholesterol and triglyceride concentrations are reduced in animals with portacaval shunts.[75] These changes may result from increased biliary excretion of cholesterol and increased conversion of cholesterol to bile acids. Lower-than-normal cholesterol levels are not pathognomonic for portacaval shunts. Low plasma cholesterol levels are seen also in malnutrition and with small intestinal problems such as lymphangiectasia. Surgical creation of a portacaval shunt has been one means suggested for treating a patient with hyperlipidemia.

PLASMA BILE ACIDS

Measurement of plasma total bile acid levels is used for the identification of hepatic disease in dogs and cats. The liver normally removes bile acids from the portal circulation and secretes them into the biliary system. Increases in plasma bile acid levels identify hepatic insufficiency. Bile acids in portal blood represent only a small part of the pool of total bile acids. In normal nonfed dogs bile acids are distributed in the enterohepatic circulation with 46% in the small intestine, 47% in the gallbladder, 6% in the liver and bile ducts, and less than 1% (.03%) in the circulation.[76] The concentration in portal blood is about six times greater than that in venous blood leaving the liver. It is apparent that bile acid measurements are made on a very small pool that can be affected by a number of different factors.

Total plasma bile acids can be affected by change in their rate of synthesis by the liver. Chronic hepatic insufficiency can reduce synthesis (see Chapter 28). Impairment in synthesis is usually accompanied by a similar abnormality for hepatic secretion of bile acids into the biliary system. Plasma bile acid levels can be affected by pathology that interferes with delivery of bile from the gallbladder to the intestine. Extrahepatic bile duct obstruction can be a cause, but that problem is not common in small animals. Chronic duodenal disease can also be a cause where mucosal pathology is severe enough to impair the synthesis and release of cholecystokinin, the most important stimulator of gall bladder contraction. In such cases, a meal entering the small intestine does not stimulate release of bile into the intestine, and the enterohepatic circulation of bile is interrupted. The rates for intestinal bile acid absorption and for bile acid fecal loss also affect plasma bile acid concentrations. Bile acids are normally absorbed primarily in the ileum; disease of that region can reduce absorption and increase fecal loss. Bacterial deconjugation of bile acids, something important only with bacterial overgrowth of the small intestine, makes them more lipid soluble and therefore readily absorbed in the jejunum. In one case, ileal disease can reduce plasma bile acid levels; in the other, bacterial overgrowth can increase its plasma levels. Fecal losses also increase with increased amounts of bile-acid-binding substances, such as some fibers in the diet. Whether the total flow of portal blood is delivered to the liver or whether some is shunted to the systemic circulation also determines plasma bile acid levels. The effect of shunts can be marked since as little as 5% of portal blood shunting around the liver can increase the fraction of bile acids escaping first-pass extraction by 100%.[77]

Results of experimental studies on dogs and cats indicate the usefulness of plasma bile acid determinations. In an early study, dogs were given carbon tetrachloride; bile acid increases were highly variable and at most increased from a norm of 0.021 to less than 0.06 µmoles/ml.[78] Later studies in dogs treated with nitrosamine showed highly variable plasma bile acid levels with values that were often within the normal range.[32,79] These studies suggest that plasma bile acid determinations are not very sensitive in identifying hepatic necrosis in dogs. Experimental dogs with complete obstruction of the common bile duct have dramatic increases in plasma bile acids that peak at two weeks, a change reflecting complete interruption of the enterohepatic circulation of bile acids.[79] Similar results are reported for cats with bile duct obstruction.[70] Histologic changes with obstruction in dogs correlate the best with both plasma ALP activity and plasma bile acid levels. Thus, determination of plasma bile acids should be as sensitive as that for plasma ALP in identifying extrahepatic obstruction. Plasma ALP increases are likely to be more consistent than bile acid increases in dogs with intrahepatic cholestasis unless the entire liver is affected. Dogs with ligation of a hepatic duct have marked plasma ALP increases but only modest increases for plasma bile acids.[80] Experimental dogs with portasystemic shunts have persistent but variable increases in plasma bile acid levels, which remain around 50 µmol/L for months in dogs with no clinical signs.[35] Experimental dogs given dexamethasone also show plasma bile acid increases that are 20 times normal but with great variability.[80] It is not known whether other drugs may have a similar effect.

Plasma bile acid measurements are believed to be of most value for identifying dogs and cats with portasystemic shunts.[81-83] Abnormal values do not confirm shunts as the cause; that requires other procedures. In 41 dogs reported with shunts that were evaluated with plasma bile acid determinations, increased, abnormal concentrations were found in 80% of the cases. Bile acid measurements reported in a small number of cats with shunts show a similar sensitivity.

Plasma bile acid concentrations increase in dogs with other hepatic problems such as hepatitis, cholestasis (due to either an intrahepatic or extrahepatic cause), hepatic neoplasia, hepatic necrosis, cirrhosis, and glucocorticoid-induced hepatopathy.[84-86] The plasma bile acid levels are highly variable within any one of these groups of hepatic problems. Normal plasma bile acid levels in unfed dogs are 0 to 5 µmol/L. In one large group of dogs with confirmed hepatic disease greater than 13% had bile acids within the normal range.[85] That translates to a sensitivity of 87%. In that same study 25% of dogs with no hepatic disease had plasma bile acid levels exceeding 5 µmol/L, giving a specificity of 75%. In another large group of dogs a range of 0 to 15.5 µmol/L was established as normal.[84] Of 118 dogs with confirmed hepatic disease 25% had values below 15.5 µmol/L, giving the test a 75% sensitivity for identifying hepatic disease. A number of dogs with no hepatic disease had plasma bile acid levels greater than 15.5 µmol/L since at that cutoff the test's specificity is only 72%. The value must be questioned for any diagnostic test with a sensitivity of 75% and a specificity of 72%. That represents a sizeable number of false-negatives and false-positives for hepatic disease. Changing the cutoff for normals from 15.5 to 5 µmol/L increases the sensitivity but worsens the specificity.

Plasma bile acids usually increase in cats with hepatic disease.[87,88] Most consistently they increase with extrahepatic bile duct obstruction and lipidosis. Less consistently they increase with cholestasis due to intrahepatic problems, hepatitis, hepatic necrosis, hepatic neoplasia, and portasystemic vascular shunts. The plasma increases are also greatest for extrahepatic bile duct obstruction and lipidosis. Plasma bile acid concentrations in unfed normal cats are less than 5 µmol/L; in fed cats that value doubles. When 5 µmol/L is used as the cutoff between normal and abnormal, bile acid determinations have a sensitivity of 83% and a specificity of 94%; with a cutoff of 10 µmol/L those values are 80% and 94%, respectively. Consequently, the use of plasma bile acid measurement for screening cats for hepatic problems will not identify about 20% of the cases and will falsely identify about 5% of cats with nonhepatic problems as having hepatic disease. In addition, many abnormal values are near the normal range[87] so that up to 40% of the bile acid measurements when seen as a single test value will be difficult to interpret. As shown later, a comparison of plasma bile acid determinations in the cat with plasma bilirubin indicates that the sensitivity or reliability of bile acid testing is no better, except for cats with portasystemic shunts.

The less than perfect sensitivity for plasma bile acid determination in cats and dogs can be partly explained by a knowledge of the acid's enterohepatic circulation.[89] The major pool of bile acids is stored in the gall bladder, and even during unfed periods contractions promoted by the migrating myoelectric complex release small amounts into the duodenum. When any gastrointestinal disease or drugs disrupt that activity, bile acid flow into the intestine is interrupted, intestinal absorption of bile acids decreases, and plasma bile acid concentrations are decreased. Thus, an animal may have hepatic disease but retain enough function to remove the smaller amounts of bile acids from the portal blood so that the plasma levels are found to be normal. A second reason for less-than-optimum sensitivity is that intestinal bile acid absorption may be reduced because of either ileal disease or binding in excessive amounts to dietary fiber. Both increase fecal bile acid excretion and reduce the amount appearing in the portal circulation. Intestinal absorption and release of bile acids into the intestine are the major determinants of plasma bile acid concentrations in both hepatic disease and normal states.[90] Suggestions have been made that plasma bile acid measurements in the fed state may be more reliable than in the unfed state, but alterations in gall bladder or intestinal motility cause marked variability in plasma bile acids after feeding. Other factors are probably responsible for no better sensitivity in bile acid testing after feeding. In humans, samples from nonfed individuals are more sensitive and discriminant than samples collected after a meal.[90]

The specificity of bile acid testing varies from 94% to values approaching 70%. False positives can appear for a number of reasons. Gastrointestinal problems resulting in bacterial overgrowth of the small intestine deconjugate bile acids to produce a compound that is readily absorbed in the jejunum.[91] That increases portal blood concentrations and can increase levels in the systemic circulation. Bacterial overgrowth is a predictable complication of maldigestion and malabsorption. In a small number of such cases up to 60% of dogs had elevated plasma bile acid concentrations.[92] Plasma bile acids may also increase with significant mucosal disease of the duodenum and beginning of the jejunum. That kind of problem results in the impaired gall bladder's emptying during feeding; the result is increased bile acid synthesis, which increases the total bile acid pool. Consequently, plasma bile acid levels increase. Anticholinergics reduce gall bladder emptying, and that also stimulates bile acid synthesis, which can lead to a 50% increase in its total pool[93]. Other known causes of increased plasma bile acid concentrations include heartworm disease in dogs; that increase may be due to the effects the cardiac disease has in reducing hepatic circulation.[86] Also, young dogs have higher levels of plasma bile acids than those over a year of age.[94] Thus, the young normal animal at greater risk for portasystemic shunts will have higher plasma levels that can complicate an evaluation of mildly increased plasma bile acids.

New clinical diagnostic tests are usually believed to be better than existing tests; after experience in their use on clinical cases many prove that to be true. Plasma bile acid measurements have been used much less frequently for identifying and evaluating hepatic disease in cats and dogs than they have in human medicine. The greater experience has led to the conviction that plasma bile acid determination shows no diagnostic advantage with respect to other routine liver tests; routine biochemical tests are sufficiently sensitive in the vast majority of cases for the identification of hepatobiliary disease.[95,96] Our experiences with the use of plasma bile acid measurements seems to be consistent with these conclusions.

PLASMA BILIRUBIN[12]

Plasma bilirubin concentrations reflect the rates of erythrocyte destruction, of hepatic uptake and metabolism of bilirubin, and of conjugated bilirubin secretion into the biliary system (Table 30-4). There is normally little difficulty in recognizing hemolytic events as the cause of increased bilirubin production. The pathophysiology of bilirubin metabolism is more important to understand in patients with hepatocellular disease and biliary obstruction. However, determining plasma concentrations of conjugated and unconjugated bilirubin is not a reliable discriminator of different causes of hyperbilirubinemia. Plasma bilirubin concentrations in dogs increase only with moderate to severe hepatic disease. Thus, measuring plasma bilirubin to screen patients for hepatic disease fails to identify most cases. Even though jaundice is traditionally associated with hepatic disease, suspicions for hepatic disease should not be based on finding an increased icterus index before the patient is evaluated for hepatic disease.

Hyperbilirubinemia appears with different forms of experimental hepatic problems. Complete obstruction of the bile duct in dogs causes plasma bilirubin levels to increase from normal values of 0.25 mg/dl to almost 5 mg/dl within five to six days, after which they decrease to 2.3 mg/dl at nine to ten days.[9] The plasma concentrations remain two to three times normal for four to six weeks after obstruction.[97] More recent studies show similar results. Biliary obstruction causes a regurgitation of conjugated bilirubin into the plasma. This pigment does not accumulate to extremely high levels since it is water-soluble

Table 30-4. Factors Determining Plasma Bilirubin Level

Increased production	
	Hemolysis
	Shortened RBC lifespan
	Ineffective erythropoiesis
	Hepatic hemoprotein overproduction (cytochrome P-450)
Reduced hepatic uptake	
	Haptoglobin binding
	Albumin binding
	Altered hepatic circulation
	Hepatic binding proteins reduced
	Competition with other molecules
Reduced hepatic conjugation	
	Reduced substrate for conjugation
	Reduced conjugating enzyme activity
	Competition for conjugating activity
Reduced hepatic secretion into bile	
	Reduction in secretory capacity
	Competition for secretion
Reduced excretion of bile	
	Biliary stasis
	Biliary obstruction
	Leak of bile into abdomen
Increased intestinal absorption	
	Bacterial overgrowth
Reduced renal excretion of bile pigment	

and excreted by the kidney. The renal threshold for conjugated bilirubin is very low in the dog, preventing plasma levels from increasing excessively. In contrast to the significant yet only moderate hyperbilirubinemia associated with obstruction of the bile duct, there is virtually no increase observed in dogs poisoned with carbon tetrachloride. The mean normal levels of 0.25 mg/dl increase to only 0.50 mg/dl. Hepatic necrosis must be extensive before hyperbilirubinemia appears. That is demonstrated in dogs with moderate to severe hepatic necrosis produced by nitrosamines. The bilirubin levels return to normal relatively quickly, however, despite the fact that the dogs are living with less than half their liver mass. With that finding there can be little expectation of plasma bilirubin's being a sensitive indicator of hepatic insufficiency. In another type of experimental model, 70% partial hepatectomy in dogs, plasma total bilirubin increases from 0.2 mg/dl to 0.56 mg/dl and returns to low levels within a week. An important determinant of hyperbilirubinemia is the location of lesions within the hepatic lobules.[98] Although severe hepatic necrosis involving the central or midzone of the lobule causes little or no increase in plasma bilirubin, mild lesions in the periportal area consistently produce hyperbilirubinemia.

Obstruction of the common bile duct in cats results in plasma total bilirubin increases peaking at nearly 25 mg/dl at two weeks. At seven weeks plasma bilirubin has decreased to about 5 mg/dl.[70]

Clinical cases of biliary obstruction and hepatocellular disease in dogs cause hyperbilirubinemias that are usually less than 5 mg/dl. Normal plasma bilirubin is less than 0.4 to 0.6 mg/dl.[72] With hepatocellular disease the hyperbilirubinemia is usually half conjugated bilirubin and half unconjugated bilirubin. Theoretically, the liver partially loses its capacities to take up, metabolize, and excrete bilirubin, so that elimination of the pigment is interfered with at every step. Increased bilirubin production may be the most important determinant, however, at least in dogs.[99] The life span of erythrocytes is much shorter in dogs with hepatobiliary disease. Disease reduces the capacity of the liver for bilirubin clearance and, combined with increased production, results in hyperbilirubinemia. With obstruction of the bile duct the bilirubin regurgitating into the plasma is conjugated, so that the hyperbilirubinemia is primarily due to conjugated bilirubin. Determination of the ratio of conjugated to unconjugated bilirubin is often used to support a diagnosis of either biliary obstruction or hepatocellular disease. That ratio is unreliable in distinguishing extrahepatic from intrahepatic causes for hyperbilirubinemia, however. Furthermore, secondary events can change the ratios of conjugated to unconjugated bilirubin so that the predicted ratio is not seen.

Total plasma bilirubin concentrations exceeding 5 mg/dl in dogs are likely to be associated with extensive hepatic disease causing both biliary obstruction and hepatocellular damage (Figure 30-12). Biliary obstruction can be intrahepatic as well as extrahepatic; hepatic problems involving periportal areas cause the greatest increments in serum bilirubin. Cholangiohepatitis and chronic hepatitis are examples of the intrahepatic type of biliary obstruction causing hyperbilirubinemia. The plasma bilirubin is largely conjugated, but some is unconjugated because inflammatory cells release lysosomal enzymes, which in turn deconjugate the conjugated pigment. This type of obstructive jaundice, not correctable by any surgical procedures, is diagnosed by liver biopsy. This condition

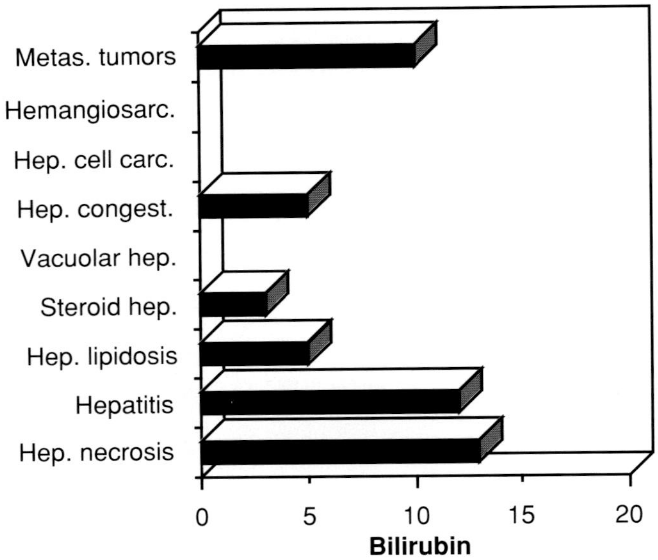

Figure 30-12. Comparison of sensitivities for serum total bilirubin (>5.0) in dogs with different hepatic problems.

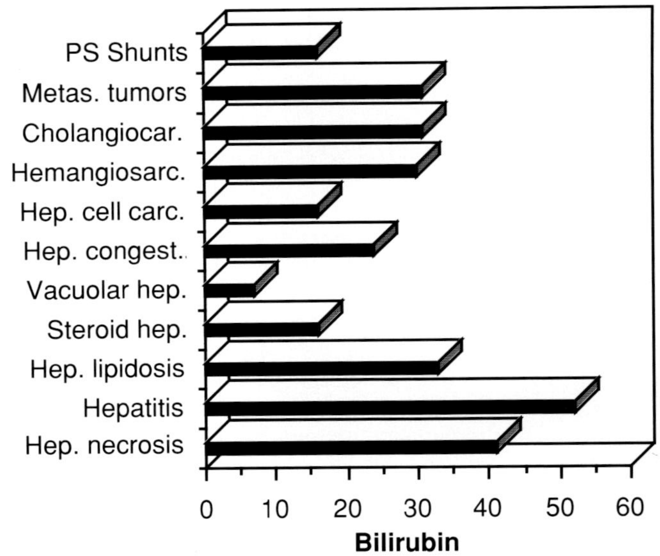

Figure 30-13. Comparison of sensitivities for serum total bilirubin (>0.4) in dogs with different hepatic problems.

illustrates that the relative amounts of conjugated and unconjugated pigments do not provide a definitive diagnosis that allows a decision on whether to perform surgery to correct an obstructive cause of jaundice. Plasma total bilirubin levels are markedly elevated in advanced cases of chronic hepatitis and in those that have progressed to cirrhosis. In such cases, reduced numbers of hepatocytes remain to metabolize bilirubin, and a continuous inflammatory process in periportal areas obstructs bile canaliculi leaving the hepatic lobule to enter bile ductules in portal areas. When liver biopsy reveals that the cause of obstructive hyperbilirubinemia is not intrahepatic, an exploratory celiotomy is performed to determine the cause.

Plasma bilirubin measurements are determined routinely but with the knowledge that levels are not consistently elevated in dogs with primary hepatic disease. Dogs with portasystemic shunts or steroid-induced hepatopathy, among others, rarely have hyperbilirubinemia (Figure 30-13). Thus, bilirubin measurement is a very insensitive test for hepatic disease in dogs. Normal plasma bilirubin levels do not rule out hepatic disease. Diseases causing hemolysis are the most common nonhepatic cause for hyperbilirubinemia in dogs. They are usually suspected from decreased hematocrits; when that is normal, the specificity for bilirubin determination is high. Other nonhepatic problems seldom cause hyperbilirubinemia.

Plasma bilirubin measurement is a sensitive test for identifying hepatic disease in cats for all problems except portasystemic shunts (Figure 30-14). Bilirubin measurement is more reliable than bile acid measurement for all problems except shunts. That greater sensitivity makes it the most useful function test since bilirubin determination is invariably a part of biochemistry screening panels. Many other problems cause hyperbilirubinemia in cats, however, making plasma bilirubin determination a test with poor specificity. A nonhepatic cause for hyperbilirubinemia is more likely when plasma bilirubin is less than 3.0 mg/dl (Table 30-5).[100] Primary hepatic disease is more likely with plasma total bilirubins greater than 3.0 mg/dl. The majority of some forms of feline hepatic disease, such as hepatitis and hepatic necrosis (see Chapters 32 and 33), is secondary to other problems such as infections, renal disease, and gastrointestinal problems. Theoretically, infection can reduce erythrocyte survival time; renal disease can reduce clearance; and small intestinal disease causing bacterial overgrowth can result in bacterial glucuronidases deconjugating the conjugated bilirubin so that bilirubin can be readily absorbed and return to the circulation. In addition, the primary nonhepatic problems causing hyperbilirubinemia are likely to be responsible for a secondary hepatic problem such as hepatic necrosis, hepatitis, or hepatopathies.

Bilirubin does not normally appear in the urine of cats, with only 4% of normal cats exhibiting bilirubinuria. Bilirubin appears in the cat's urine with hyperbilirubinemia before clinical signs of jaundice are apparent. Most cats with hyperbilirubinuria (72%) have liver disease. Most of these cases are likely to be hepatic problems secondary to diseases in another system of the body. Measurement of urine bilirubin is a useful screening test for hepatic problems in cats; whether it is more convenient than using tests on a chemistry panel or evaluating icterus index on a hemogram is questionable.

URINE BILIRUBIN AND UROBILINOGEN[12,101]

Bilirubin is usually found in the urine of dogs. The renal threshold is so low that the pigment appears in the urine even when plasma bilirubin concentrations are normal. Analysis of urine bilirubin is semiquantitative, and the amount found is interpreted with consideration of the urine's specific gravity. A large amount of bilirubin in urine with a high specific gravity cannot be interpreted as being unusual. The same amount in a dilute sample, however, may be an indication of increased production of conjugated bilirubin. That can reflect a hemolytic process, hepatic disease, or biliary tract disease. Finding no bilirubin in the urine does not rule out hepatic disease, and large

Table 30-5. Serum Total Bilirubin Levels in cats. Distribution of Primary Causes

Serum Total Bilirubin			
1.0 to 3.0 mg/dl		**Greater than 3.0 mg/dl**	
Renal disease	21%	Hepatic disease	68%
Infectious panleukopenia	13%	Lipidosis	(24%)
Gastrointestinal disease	12%	Hepatitis	(18%)
Hepatic disease	10%	Hepatopathy	(16%)
Lymphosarcoma	10%	Biliary obstruction	(5%)
Trauma	10%	Hepatic neoplasia	(5%)
FIP	7%	FIP	14%
Pyometra	7%	Hemolytic anemia	7%
Others	7%	Lymphosarcoma	4%
		Others	7%

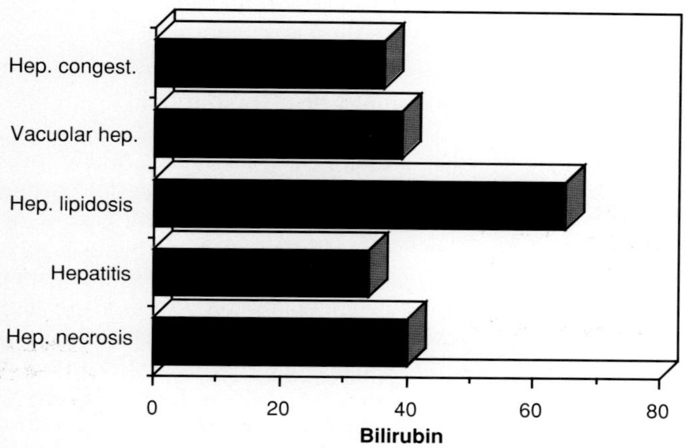

Figure 30-14. Comparison of sensitivities for serum total bilirubin (>0.2) in cats with different hepatic problems.

amounts do not indicate that a hepatic problem exists. Measurement of urine bilirubin concentrations is not a useful screening test for hepatic disease in the dog.

Urine urobilinogen is semiquantitated to identify patients with obstructive jaundice. Bacterial transformation of bilirubin in the intestine forms urobilinogen. It is subsequently absorbed, with part excreted in the urine and part resecreted into the bile. The appearance of urobilinogen in urine is dependent on bile's being secreted and released into the intestine. The absence of any urobilinogen in the urine is suggestive of biliary obstruction, and the presence of large amounts of urobilinogen is indicative of the formation and excretion of large amounts of bilirubin, such as with a hemolytic event. Interpretation of urine urobilinogen levels must be based on a number of variables that can influence its appearance.

Increased amounts of urobilinogen are excreted in urine during constipation, when more urobilinogen is formed and absorbed; after hemolysis, when increased amounts of bilirubin are secreted into the intestine; and with chronic hepatic disease, when absorbed urobilinogen is not resecreted properly by the liver. The amount of urobilinogen excreted in urine is reduced with biliary obstruction, reduction of normal colonic bacteria numbers, rapid intestinal transit such as with diarrhea, and renal insufficiency. Urobilinogen excretion is variable in each individual in that there is a diurnal cycle, with the greatest amount excreted in the early P.M. Renal function and the pH of the urine influence urinary excretion of urobilinogen; Urobilinogen is found in the urine since it is filtered at the glomerulus and secreted by the proximal tubule. Urobilinogen is a weak organic acid existing largely in an un-ionized lipid-soluble form at an acid pH. Thus, as urine is acidified in the distal tubule, urobilinogen, being largely lipid-soluble, is able to diffuse across tubular membranes and return to the circulation. When alkaline urine is produced, urobilinogen is largely ionized and water soluble so that very little back-diffusion occurs. Thus, little or no urobilinogen in an acid urine is difficult to interpret since the pigment that entered the distal nephron could have been completely reabsorbed. Urobilinogen is also unstable in acid urine and in light. Thus, tests for urobilinogen must be conducted soon after the urine samples are collected. The amount of urobilinogen measured is also a function of the specific gravity of the urine. The amount is frequently unmeasurable in very dilute urine.

ASSESSMENT OF HEPATIC DISEASE WITH LABORATORY PROCEDURES

Hepatic disease can cause almost any unexplained clinical signs suggestive of an internal medicine problem in cats and dogs. The initial approach of any evaluation is to rule in or out the possibility of a hepatic problem. That can be done with a biochemical panel that provides information on plasma activities of ALT and ALP. A comparison of the sensitivity of these measurements for a number of hepatic diseases can be helpful in judging their reliability in the evaluation of any single case. Increases in activities of these enzymes call for a judgment on whether they are great enough to pursue further evidence of a hepatic problem or whether the increases can be attributed to another problem that has been verified. Such other problems include a history of drug usage, such as corticosteroids or anticonvulsants; clinical evidence for congestive heart failure or anemia; or confirmation of neoplastic disease, such as

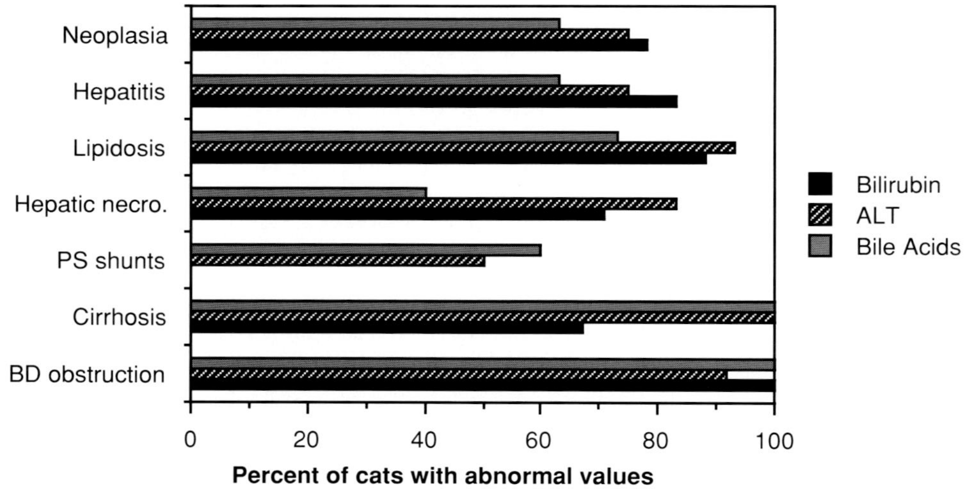

Figure 30-15. Comparison of sensitivities for bilirubin, ALT, and bile acids in cats with different hepatic problems. Data are compiled from many sources.

malignant lymphoma. Often any hepatic involvement is predicted and not confirmed because the relationship of the primary disease and subsequent hepatic involvement is understood. When increases in plasma enzyme activities cannot be explained by a problem in another organ or system, one must decide whether to continue testing to confirm suspicions for a primary hepatic problem or whether to biopsy the liver in order to characterize the problem. It is very important to determine whether the clinical signs can be explained by a liver problem. Often that determination cannot be made solely on the basis of increased plasma enzyme activities. Thus, the conclusions one can draw upon finding increased plasma enzyme activities are that (1) they can be explained by another confirmed problem; (2) they should be pursued with a liver biopsy, with the understanding that primary liver disease may not be found; (3) they should be pursued with further testing to establish a hepatic basis for the clinical signs; or (4) they can be ignored or reevaluated within a few weeks. Finding normal plasma enzyme activities, on the other hand, can suggest that hepatic disease is not a problem, but when clinical signs are still not explained, further testing must be done to rule in or rule out hepatic disease.

Evaluation for hepatic disease is continued, where indicated, by conducting function tests. Measurement of plasma bilirubin is a usual determination on biochemical panels. As already described that test is reliable in identifying hepatic disease in cats although its specificity is poor. Plasma bilirubin's sensitivity is as good or better than other function tests for identifying all hepatic problems except portasystemic shunts in cats (Figure 30-15). It is usually not difficult to determine if increased plasma bilirubin in cats is due to a nonhepatic cause. Even when it is believed that hyperbilirubinemia is due to a hepatic problem, it is understood that many hepatic diseases in cats are secondary to nonhepatic diseases. Plasma bilirubin determination in dogs has poor sensitivity when compared to other function tests for identifying hepatic disease (Figure 30-16). Its specificity is reduced by the many problems causing hemolysis, but that type of problem is usually easy to identify.

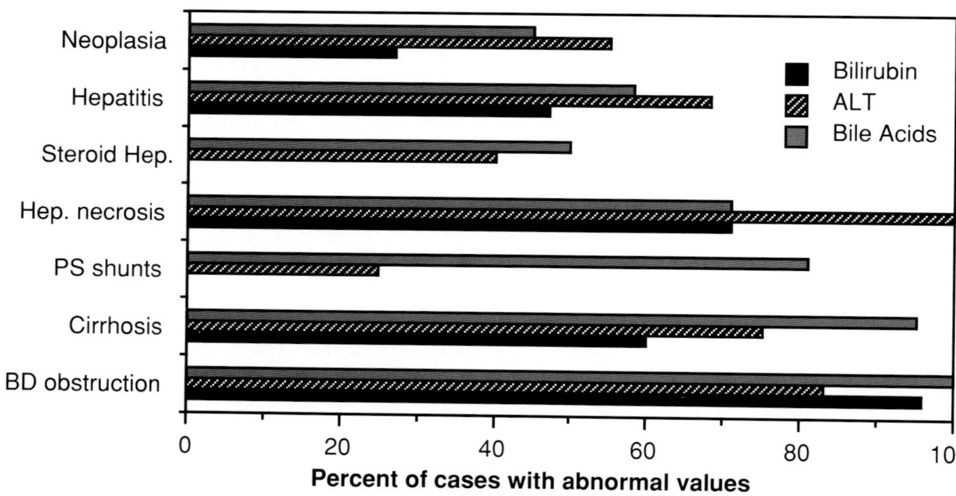

Figure 30-16. Comparison of sensitivities for bilirubin, ALT, and bile acids in dogs with different hepatic problems. Data are compiled from many sources.

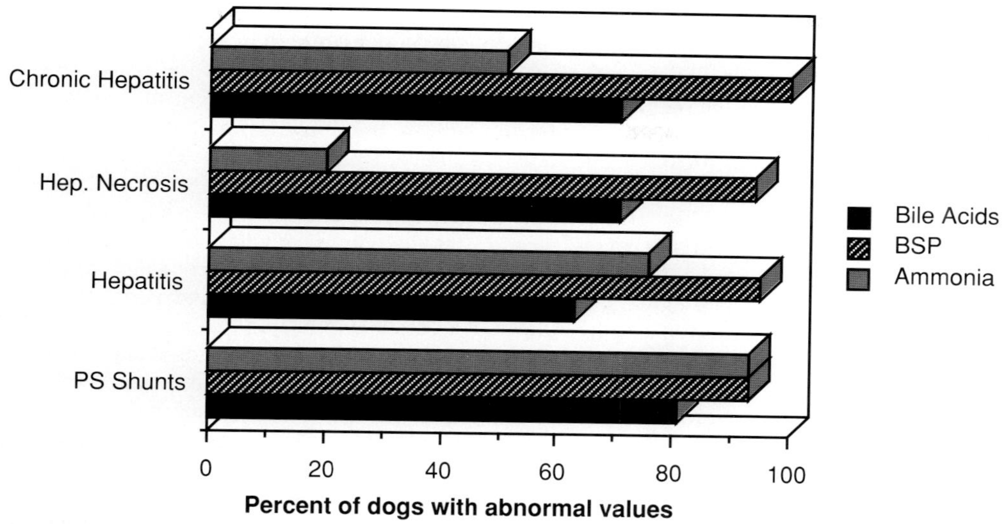

Figure 30-17. Comparison of sensitivities for BSP, ammonia, and bile acids in dogs with different hepatic problems. Data are compiled from many sources.

Dogs with normal plasma bilirubin must be evaluated with another function test in order to rule out hepatic disease. Hyperbilirubinemia in dogs that is believed to be caused by hepatic disease is pursued with biopsy of the liver. That is done less often in cats because the condition can usually be explained without a biopsy.

When clinical signs are still unexplained after a chemistry panel or if further confirmation of hepatic disease is needed, other function tests are conducted. Plasma bile acid, blood ammonia, or sulfobromophthalein tests are indicated in cats only when portasystemic shunts, an uncommon disease, is suspected. For all other hepatic diseases either these tests are no better than plasma bilirubin or little is known about their value in cats. These tests can be conducted in dogs with hepatic problems, and a comparison of their sensitivity shows that some are more effective than others (Figure 30-17), but when convenience and ease of testing is also considered there is no one test that stands out as ideal. In unusual circumstances plasma amino acids can be determined to confirm or deny the attribution of certain clinical signs to hepatic disease.

Evaluation of cats and dogs for hepatic disease often includes other biochemical tests and screening radiographic procedures. Other biochemical tests have a low sensitivity and a low specificity, which make them unreliable when used alone in deciding whether hepatic disease is a problem. Radiographs of the abdomen provide an unreliable estimation of liver size. Moreover, liver disease can be verified in animals with normal-size livers, and liver disease is not a problem in many animals with either small or large livers.

The diagnosis of hepatic disease in small animals is based on liver biopsy findings. It is possible to analyze clinical signs and laboratory findings and use a combination of tests to yield a presumptive diagnosis of hepatic disease, but that is not done with the goal of identifying specific hepatic diseases in small-animal patients. Discriminant analysis of laboratory results has been used to differentiate hepatic problems in humans.[102] In order to achieve this, biochemical tests were used to collect information on five serum enzymes, eleven plasma proteins, and three plasma lipids. Also included were four immunological tests, measurement of plasma iron and bilirubin, and a blood-clotting test. Accurate identification of the pathological process in the liver requires at least fifteen of these tests, and then combinations of some of the tests are used to distinguish between different hepatic diseases. The discriminant analysis for hepatic disease is accomplished with computer programs. A number of other such evaluations have been described. Clusters of laboratory results have not been used to identify and characterize hepatic disease in small animals, however, primarily because so little information is available to perform such analyses. Several reports correlate results of laboratory tests with histological findings in animals with hepatic disease.[42,103,104] Liver biopsy is essential for diagnosis management and prognosis of hepatic disease. The only exception is the animal with a portasystemic shunt, which is diagnosed by radiographic or nuclear medicine procedures. All laboratory testing described in this chapter is intended to aid in the decision of whether biopsy should be done. Some of the testing will also provide information of use for management and prognosis.

HEPATIC IMAGING

Radiography[105-107]

Evaluation of a patient for hepatic disease often includes survey radiographs of the abdomen. Radiography for that purpose is of questionable value, however. Hepatic disease can change liver size, shape, opacity, position and margination, and can cause displacement of adjacent organs such as the stomach, intestines, and spleen. Liver size is difficult to evaluate on plain radiographic films. The precise outline of the organ is seldom clearly demarcated, especially the ventral and caudoventral borders. Even when well-demarcated, evaluation of size is difficult because of the great variability in hepatic mass in normal dogs and cats. Smaller than normal liver size is not abnormal in some animals, where no evidence of any hepatic insufficiency can be demonstrated. The radiographic appearance, leading to an assessment that the liver is small, is influenced by conformation of the thorax. For example, in deep-chested dogs the ventral lobes of the liver appear small and upright and lie within the costal arch. In such dogs measurement of liver size may be possible in up to one-half of radiographs taken in right lateral recumbency. The liver shadow is better delineated with positioning in left lateral recumbency; less mergining of liver and spleen silhouettes is seen. In normal dogs, furthermore, the position of caudal tip of the liver varies and can be up to two times the length of the vertebra beyond the last rib during inspiration. When measured at expiration, total length of the ventral border from the diaphragmatic to the caudal borders varies from five to eight times the length of the eleventh thoracic vertebra. With such great variability in dogs with similar body conformity, it is not surprising that evaluation of hepatic size would be of little use in breeds with great variation in body conformity.

Abdominal radiographs can also indicate intraperitoneal pathology, which produces loss of serosal margin visualization caused by fluid accumulation. Hepatic enlargement, either diffuse or confined to single lobes, can displace the stomach and intestines from the locations in which they are normally found on radiographs. Hepatic enlargement can also round the edges of the liver, something identified with lateral views. Some enlargements displace kidneys or the splenic head, as seen on dorsoventral or ventrodorsal views.

Radiographic evaluations of the liver supplement other information; they are seldom able to confirm that hepatic disease is repsonsible for clinical signs, and they cannot differentiate one hepatic problem from another. Abdominal radiographs usually do no more than confirm what is already known about gross hepatic anatomy from the physical examination.

Ultrasonography[108]

Hepatic structure can be evaluated in a different way by ultrasonography, which is a noninvasive, nonionizing imaging technique using high frequency, low intensity sound. Sound is reflected differently by air, fluid, and tissues with different densities. Reflections are used to produce images that mirror those differences. Ultrasonography is unreliable for predicting liver size, and so evaluation remains a problem, since radiography is also unreliable for sizing the liver.[109] Ultrasonography is valuable for identifying disease of the hepatic parenchyma that change the liver's normal tissue density.[110]

Ultrasonography is used to identify hepatic architecture as abnormal. Changes in architecture may be diffuse, as caused by cirrhosis or widespread nodular hyperplasia. They can be focal, due to neoplasms, abscesses, or cysts. The ultrasonographic hepatic appearance also changes with infiltrative diseases, such as lymphoma or myeloproliferative problems,and metabolic diseases resulting in deposition of unusual amounts of substances such as fat in the liver. The purpose of ultrasonography is to identify changes in hepatic architecture and parenchymal density. Conclusions cannot be made on the basis of such changes; biopsy is required for that. Ultrasonography offers the added advantage of assisting in directing biopsy of focal lesions.

Ultrasonography provides some information on hepatic circulation.[111] Portasystemic shunts are one of the more common circulatory abnormalities seen in small animals. Ultrasonography usually identifies the hepatic hypovascularity found with that problem. Only 40% of the shunts are identified with ultrasonography, however. Further examinations of affected dogs subjected to positive-pressure ventilation under anesthesia results in confirmation of a few more cases. Therefore, ultrasonography is unreliable for identifying animals with shunts. Despite that, with ultrasonography the portal vein and its branches within the liver can usually be seen, and a hypovascularity involving these vessels can be identified. Hepatic veins and their enlargement due ot any cause of increased vena cava pressure can also be seen, and findings may be useful in deciding whether as ascites is due to a posthepatic rather than a hepatic or prehepatic cause. Branches of the hepatic artery are not normally visible on ultrasonography.

The gallbladder and biliary system are well-visualized most easily with ultrasonogrpahy. The gallbladder appears as a fluid-occupying area with its wall not seen unless its thickness is increased because of edema or inflammation. Gallbladder size varies in normal animals, with a greater size during the nonfed state. Biliary sediment described as sludge can be seen during anorexia and is not considered an abnormal finding. Dilatation of the gallbladder, common bile duct, and intrahepatic ducts can be seen and often results from obstruction of one or more ducts. Sometimes that enlargement reflects a functional obstruciton due to disease affecting motility in the biliary system. Calculi, either radiolucent or radiopaque can be visualized when they are of sufficient size. Ultrasonography is also useful in identifying neoplasms and cystic hyperplasia of the gallbladder, both uncommon problems.

Ultrasonography is most useful for assistance in liver biopsy.[112] During imaging the biopsy needle is directed into focal lesions or the hepatic parenchyma most likely to provide tissue representative of a diffuse pathology. Ultrasonography also provides the information to avoid puncturing the gallbladder, major bile ducts, and large intrahepatic blood vessels and thereby minimize complications of bile peritonitis and hemorrhage. Following biopsy the site can be observed for bleeding, which is another advantage for biopsy assisted by ultrasonography. Trucut needles (Travenol Lab) or the equivalent are used to biopsy the liver. Ultrasound scanners are available which automatically display the projected biopsy needle path.

Contrast Radiography and Scintigraphy

Contrast radiography and scintigraphy are useful for identifying portasystemic shunts and arteriovenons fistulas in dogs and cats. These techniques can be used also to image the biliary system.

LIVER BIOPSY

Biopsy of the liver is the single most important procedure in accurate definition of hepatic disease. With biopsy information the proper management can be instituted and the outcome accurately predicted. With only clinical pathologic and radiographic information, definition, management, and prognosis remain a guess. The purpose of the laboratory and radiographic procedures is to determine whether liver biopsy should be performed. The liver is biopsied when the findings are expected to yield useful information.

Table 30-6 - Indications for Performing a Liver Biopsy

Explain abnormal liver tests
elevated serum enzymes
abnormal liver-function tests
Differential diagnosis of icterus
Abnormal liver size
Identify cause of ascites
Identify metastatic neoplastic disease
Evaluate results of management

Indications for Liver Biopsy[113-116]

The objective of histologic examination of the liver is to identify the hepatic disease process, and to provide information for recommending proper management and predicting the outcome. There are a number of indications that justify a liver biopsy (Table 30-6).

Liver biopsy is performed to explain abnormal plasma activity of liver enzymes and abnormal liver function tests. In some cases, liver biopsy is performed with the knowledge that diagnosis of primary hepatic disease may not be forthcoming; biopsy is the easiest means of determining whether primary hepatic disease or disease in another system is causing hepatic lesions responsible for the abnormal biochemical tests.

Liver biopsy is often essential in the differential diagnosis of icterus. Prehepatic (or hemolytic) causes of icterus are usually readily identified from the results of a hemogram. The most challenging differentiation is between cases of intrahepatic and extrahepatic obstructive jaundice. The causes of the former include chronic hepatitis and biliary cirrhosis, while the causes of the latter include neoplastic and inflammatory diseases' obstructing the bile duct. Diagnosis of extrahepatic causes is made by exploratory surgery, while intrahepatic causes are identified with liver biopsy. It is obvious that liver biopsy is an easier procedure that celiotomy, and the biopsy findings will show whether surgery is indicated.

Abnormal liver size is an important indication for liver biopsy. In many cases the cause is apparent, as in patients with congestive heart failure. In less apparent cases the pathologist recognizes changes consistent with circulatory failure. In some cases circulatory problems cannot be identified by the conventional means used for investigating this type of problem. When liver biopsy indicates a circulatory problem, special procedures are subsequently indicated for the problem's identification. Infiltration by unusual cells and storage of abnormally high amounts of substances may enlarge the liver. Hepatocyte swelling frequently causes hepatomegaly, such as with steroid-induced hepatopathy. In some patients, the pathognomonic biopsy lesions for steroid-induced hepatopathy provide the only clue for hyperadrenalcorticism. This finding sometimes diagnoses steroid-induced hepatopathy, whereas an ACTH-response test is not diagnostic. In this case, biopsy findings can be confirmed with dexamethasone suppression tests and ACTH measurement. A liver smaller than normal, microhepatica, is found in some liver diseases, and liver biopsy frequently reveals the cause. For example, the liver eventually atrophies in dogs with portasystemic vascular shunts. That condition is recognized on liver biopsy by morphologic changes that are sometimes diagnostic. Biopsy can also identify microhepatica as a sequel to postnecrotic collapse of hepatic lobules.

Liver biopsy is an important means of identifying the cause of ascites. When the cause of ascites is prehepatic, the liver should be morphologically normal. These findings, with those from analysis of ascites fluid, indicate that other procedures are needed for identifying the cause. Diagnostic morphological changes are found with hepatic and posthepatic causes of ascites. Thus, useful information is returned with all three types of ascites, even when the liver biopsy is normal. Intrahepatic arteriovenous fistula is the only cause in which liver biopsy can appear normal despite a hepatic problem.

In some patients with metastatic neoplastic diseases or granulomatous diseases liver biopsy is the easiest means of confirming a diagnosis. For example, an animal may have pulmonary lesions due to a chronic infectious process or neoplastic disease. The only means of determining whether the problem is treatable is by biopsy of the lesions. Lung biopsies are difficult to obtain, but if the laboratory findings suggest possible hepatic involvement the liver can be biopsied, often providing a definitive diagnosis. Some dogs with lymphosarcoma are most easily identified as having the problem by liver biopsy.

Liver biopsy is usually the most important means of assessing responses to management. Reevaluation with an ammonia tolerance test is more useful than biopsy to assess the results of surgery to correct a portasystemic vascular shunt.

Liver biopsy is suggested to be indicated where hepatic lesions may develop because of systemic inflammatory and metabolic problems. Laboratory findings reveal potential hepatic lesions, but morphological changes found on subsequent liver biopsy seldom generate new information important for evaluating the primary problem. This is generally true in most feline systemic diseases such as feline leukemia or feline infectious peritonitis, which almost invariably include liver lesions. Fever of undetermined origin is suggested to be an indication for liver biopsy, but the biopsy is seldom of diagnostic value. Liver biopsy is of little value in patients with bacterial endocarditis or abscesses in extrahepatic tissues causing secondary hepatic changes. Metabolic diseases frequently cause morphological changes in the liver, such as persistent lipidosis with diabetes mellitus. These hepatic lesions are predictable, and abnormal liver tests do not justify a liver biopsy unless the tests remain normal after the metabolic disease is controlled. Liver-biopsy findings do not change the management of diabetes mellitus. Liver biopsies are not obtained solely for the purpose of examining the liver's morphological appearance. Biopsies can be treated with special stains to identify abnormal pigments and large accumulations of substances that are normally stored only in small quantities. Hepatic concentrations of trace metals can be determined, and the activity of different hepatic enzymes can be evaluated.

In summary, liver biopsy is used to verify hepatic disease as a problem, to define primary hepatic pathological processes, to diagnose metastatic malignant processes not easily determined by other means, and to clarify the cause of abnormal liver function tests and unusual liver size.

Table 30-7. Contraindications for Performing a Liver Biopsy

Absolute contraindications
- High probability for hemorrhage
  - coagulopathies
  - enlarged intrahepatic vessels
- Suspicions of a hepatic abscess or cyst

Relative contraindications
- Inexperience
  - inability to obtain liver tissue
  - retrieval of extrahepatic tissue
- Extrahepatic biliary obstruction
- Ascites
- Possession of a definitive diagnosis

Contraindications[113,114,117,118]

Contraindications for liver biopsy can be categorized into those where an undesirable complication is very likely to occur and where there is a small probability of an undesirable sequel (Table 30-7). Serious complications appearing at a high incidence are classified as absolute contraindications, and less severe complications that are seldom seen are described as relative contraindications.

Absolute contraindications are where needle biopsy could precipitate a life-threatening complication. In some cases the possibility of a particular complication is always suspected, and one or more laboratory tests are conducted to ensure that the complication does not develop. The incidence of coagulopathies is very low, but hemorrhage following liver biopsy is such a serious complication that blood clotting is evaluated before every biopsy. Significant hepatic hemorrhage is possible (though seldom detected) following liver biopsy in dogs with even normal clotting tests. Serial determination of the hematocrit and plasma proteins can be used to identify dogs that are hemorrhaging without clinical signs after liver biopsy. Intrahepatic bleeding can be readily identified with ultrasonography. Biopsy of the liver is risky if performed without correcting any bleeding tendencies. When liver biopsy is performed with the assistance of ultrasonography, postbiopsy bleeding can be seen, which is an important advantage of using that method. Anemia is considered an absolute contraindication, primarily because an additional acute loss of blood could produce a life-threatening situation. Acute blood loss is a likely possibility when needle biopsy is performed in patients with highly vascularized tumors or enlarged intrahepatic blood vessels, as would be seen with arteriovenous fistula or hamartoma. Hepatomegaly is the most consistent sign associated with these problems, and liver biopsy is seldom rejected because of a fear of vascular problems that are seldom encountered. Detection of abdominal bruits and the character of ascites fluid often provides a clue for suspecting one of these vascular problems. Biopsy assisted with ultrasonography helps avoid complications with these problems.

A second absolute contraindication for liver biopsy is suspicion or evidence of an intrahepatic abscess or cyst that may be ruptured by the biopsy needle. Cyst or abscess fluid can contain microorganisms and bacterial toxins, which can be disseminated throughout the abdominal or thoracic cavity following liver biopsy. The release of such toxins can precipitate shock following liver biopsy. Since abscesses and cysts are rarely suspected in patients prepared for liver biopsy, this contraindication is usually academic. Since abscesses and cysts are invariably focal lesions, they are usually identified only by ultrasonography or possibly during laparoscopy or celiotomy. Infections in the pleural or abdominal cavities are also contraindications, since infection can be transferred into the liver by the biopsy procedure.

Relative contraindications are suspected complications that occur at a low incidence and are less threatening to patient survival. Inexperience in performing a liver biopsy has been cited as an important contraindication. The most frequent unwanted sequel of liver biopsy facing the inexperienced operator is obtaining a sample of tissue other than liver. Inexperience results in a higher rate of failure in retrieving hepatic tissue.

Extrahepatic biliary obstruction has been a contraindication for liver biopsy in humans. This is based on a low but unacceptable number of patients who develop biliary peritonitis, which can be fatal. However, complications are unusual following liver biopsy in humans with large-bile-duct obstruction.[119] The same findings have been reported in dogs following liver biopsy.[116] A primary reason for liver biopsy is to determine whether the cause of obstructive icterus is intrahepatic or extrahepatic. That is accomplished most easily by liver biopsy. The causes of extrahepatic biliary obstruction are stricture of the bile duct due to pancreatic disease, bile duct tumors, carcinoma of the pancreas, chronic inflammatory disease of the extrahepatic biliary system, neoplastic disease in the area of bile ducts, and cholelithiasis. These problems can be identified with laparoscopy and exploratory celiotomy, which are more complicated than liver biopsy and not without disadvantages. Ultrasonographic evidence for bile duct obstruction from seeing dilated bile ducts and gall bladder is often unreliable; many are not obstructed. Since complications are rare following biopsy of a liver with large-bile-duct obstruction, suspicion of this problem is not a good reason for not performing liver biopsy. The most frequent cause of bile peritonitis in dogs after liver biopsy has been gallbladder perforation, not associated with large-bile-duct obstruction. This complication correlates better with inexperience in obtaining the biopsy.

Ascites has been considered a complication when percutaneous needle biopsy of the liver is obtained by a transabdominal

Table 30-8 - Complications of Liver Biopsy

- Hemorrhage
- Perforation of gall bladder
- Biopsy of organ other than liver
- Pneumothorax
- Bile pleuritis
- Hemothorax
- Hemobilia
- Bacteremia
- Bacterial peritonitis
- Development of arteriovenous fistulas

approach. Likewise, the presence of pleural fluid has been considered a contraindication for liver biopsy when the transthoracic approach is used. Obtaining a biopsy specimen of the liver is more difficult with ascites, and the fluid should be removed before the biopsy is performed. Under these conditions, ascites does not interfere with liver biopsy.

Relative contraindications also include uncooperative patients, congestive heart failure, neoplastic disease of the liver, amyloidosis, and even icterus and elevated serum alkaline phosphatase levels.[117] These are reported as contraindications because, at one time or another, liver biopsy in patients with these problems has resulted in complications. Uncooperative patients are not a contraindication in small animals because liver biopsy can be obtained with patients under sedation or anesthesia. Patient movement during biopsy can lacerate the liver. During biopsy with the Menghini method, however, the needle is in the liver for 0.1 second, thus permitting little chance of laceration. Neoplastic liver disease is suggested as a contraindication, since the biopsy needle can transfer the tumor to extrahepatic sites. That possibility is remote, however, and if this contraindication were considered important the liver would seldom be biopsied. Furthermore, hepatic neoplastic disease cannot be identified without a biopsy of the liver.

All information on a case is evaluated before the liver is biopsied. Of course, no biopsy is done if little additional useful information would be gained thereby.

Complications[113,114,118,120]

The most important complication of liver biopsy is hemorrhage (Table 30-8). That can occur despite precautions taken to evaluate the animal's blood-clotting ability. An animal with normal clotting tests, platelet numbers, and plasma fibrinogen levels can develop a coagulopathy after liver biopsy. Normal clotting tests do not indicate that levels of blood-clotting factors are normal, but only whether they are adequate to initiate clotting. Blood-clotting tests can be normal when concentrations of blood-clotting factors are low. Biopsy procedures can stimulate the consumption of blood-clotting factors, so that the depletion precipitates a coagulopathy. Some intrahepatic bleeding occurs after all liver biopsies; if excessive, it can be monitored by measurement of hematocrits and plasma proteins and by ultrasonography. Significant bleeding to cause intrahepatic hematomas has been documented in 7% of a small group of humans following percutaneous Menghini needle biopsy.[121] Any vague signs appearing after liver biopsy should be evaluated with a hematocrit.

Biopsy of an organ other than the liver is not an unusual complication. Perforation of the bile duct or gallbladder is possible in animals when the large bile duct is obstructed or the gallbladder is not emptied before liver biopsy. Gallbladder perforation, rarely a complication with experienced operators, frequently results from failure to adhere to proper biopsy technique. When the gallbladder is perforated, the operator is immediately aware of the complication. When there is no obstruction of the bile duct, the perforation usually seals after bile is released into the peritoneal cavity. Bile peritonitis develops when the perforation fails to remain sealed and continues to leak. Perforation of the biliary system in animals with obstruction of the bile duct results in a continuous leakage of bile. Gallbladder perforation with continued leakage and bile peritonitis can be fatal. Vomiting and abdominal tenseness appear within an hour of gallbladder perforation, although they do not persist if the perforation seals spontaneously. If leakage continues, surgical exploration is indicated, and cholecystectomy with decompression of any biliary obstruction is performed. A fatal outcome is predictable if a persistently leaking gallbladder is not surgically corrected. Other organs that have been perforated during biopsy include the pancreas, small intestine, stomach, diaphragm, kidney, and large intestine. The incidence of perforation of extrahepatic organs is probably greater than reported. In most cases, any obviously unsuccessful attempt at biopsy is recognized either by a failure to yield a sample of tissue or by tissue that does not resemble hepatic tissue. Subsequent attempts yield hepatic tissue, and it is usually not known whether the failed attempts have perforated organs other than the liver. Perforation of organs other than the gallbladder rarely causes complications that require management. Perforation without signs of complications is recognized only when biopsy findings indicate that tissue other than liver was submitted for evaluation.

Real or potential complications also include pneumothorax, bile pleuritis, hemobilia, hemothorax, pleural effusion from ascites, development of arteriovenous fistulas, bacteremia, bacterial peritonitis, and dissemination of neoplastic disease. Pneumothorax and pleural effusion from ascites are more likely with the transthoracic approach than the transabdominal approach. The other complications are very remote and have not been observed in small animal patients.

Preparation for Biopsy Procedures[113,114,116]

Preparation of the patient for liver biopsy includes fasting for 12 hours to reduce the likelihood of perforation of a distended stomach or loop of intestine. Blood-clotting ability is evaluated by a hemogram that reports platelet numbers and fibrinogen levels and by a clotting test, such as measurement of activated clotting time or prothrombin time and partial thromboplastin time. Whole-blood-clotting time can also be used in place of the other clotting tests. Normal whole-blood-clotting time and platelet numbers are sufficient for liver biopsy to proceed. Liver biopsy is not performed when one of these parameters is abnormal. One hour before biopsy, a small amount of liquid fat is given orally to stimulate release of cholecystokinin and cause contraction of the gallbladder, thereby reducing the chances of inadvertent perforation. Vegetable oil is given most commonly, at a dose of 5 to 30 ml, depending on body size. Radiographs to determine liver size sometimes aid in performing the biopsy.

The skin is surgically prepared at the site of liver biopsy. Chemical restraint is seldom required for percutaneous blind liver needle biopsies. Where required for dogs, a tranquilizer or narcotic can be given intravenously, and for cats, Ketamine HCl can be given intravenously at a dose of 2 to 4 mg/lb body weight. Premedication with subcutaneous atropine at 0.02 mg/lb may be necessary. Sedation is required with more invasive procedures, such as liver biopsy through a keyhole approach. Directed liver biopsy with laparoscopy requires sedation or general anesthesia; in some cases biopsy is obtained during laparotomy.

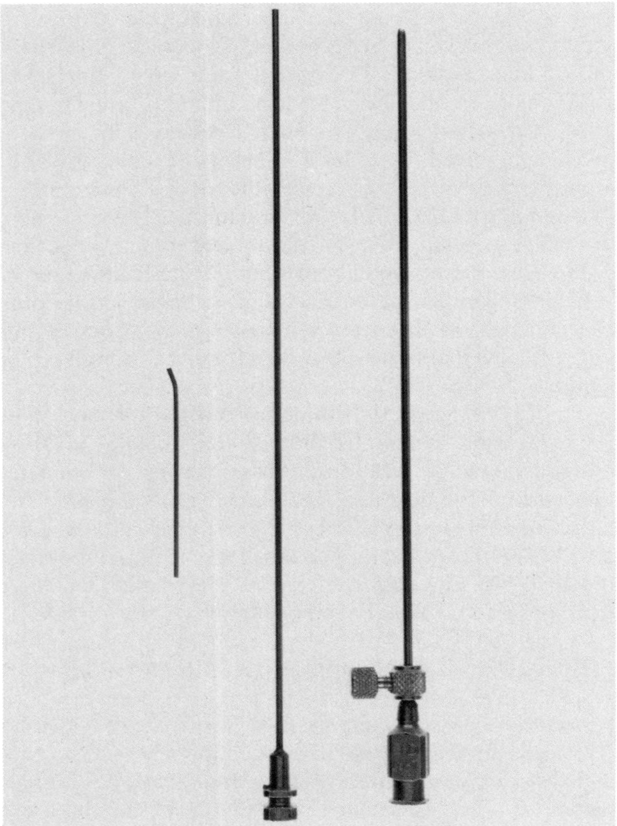

Figure 30-18. Menghini needle for blind percutaneous hepatic biopsy or for directed biopsy with a keyhole. Needle is shown with stylus that is removed after directing needle through abdominal wall and with pin that is placed in needle before biopsy is obtained.

Biopsy Procedures[114-116]

One of three basic types of biopsy procedures can be selected. For most hepatic problems, samples of liver tissue are obtained with a Menghini type of needle. The sizes to use in small animals are 15-, 16-, and 18-gauge thin-wall needles that are 2 3/4 and 4 3/4 inches long. The Menghini biopsy instrument consists of a needle, a needle guard, a blocking pin that inserts into the needle, and a blunt-ended stylet (Figure 30-18). When it is not possible to retrieve a sample of hepatic tissue with the Menghini needle, an alternate method is selected. Since livers with cirrhosis or advanced fibrosis are not biopsied successfully with the Menghini needle, a needle that cuts and removes is used (such as the Trucut and Sherwood). The latter is used also when hepatic disease has caused the tissue to be very friable. Both the Menghini needle and Trucut needle cut liver tissue during biopsy. The basic difference between the two types is that the Menghini relies on suction to remove the biopsy from the liver, whereas the Trucut isolates a core of tissue and

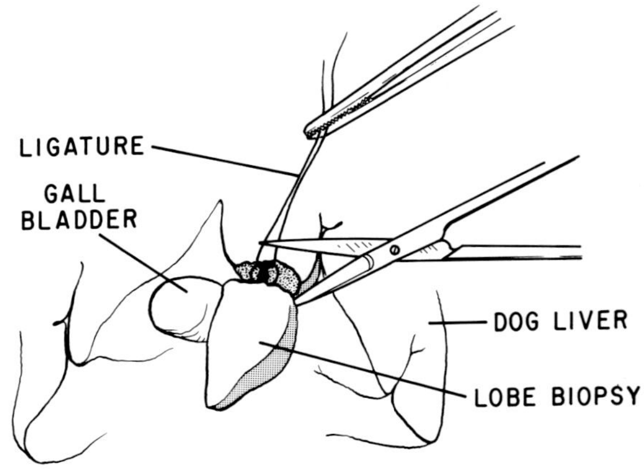

Figure 30-19. Drawing showing how wedge biopsy can be obtained from liver by cutting tissue with a ligature and completing removal with a scissors.

removes it without suction. Cores of biopsy tissues cannot be removed from cirrhotic livers by suction but can be removed by the Trucut needle. Trucut needles guided into the liver during imaging with ultrasound offers a safe and reliable method for obtaining liver biopsies. The third means of sampling the liver is by wedge biopsy during laparotomy (Figure 30-19).[122] Liver sections can be removed by excision and submitted for histology, enzyme assay, and quantitation of stored substances. These three basic biopsy methods have a number of variations for obtaining samples of liver tissue. Some modifications of these needles are purported to have or not have advantages over the originals. In general, proper biopsy technique must be maintained and modification to improve needles does not permit deviation from essential principles and techniques. Laparoscopy equipment is supplied with biopsy instruments that vary in the amount of tissue they can retrieve.

Biopsy Approaches[114,116]

Liver biopsy by a percutaneous procedure can employ a transabdominal or a transthoracic approach. Use of the transthoracic approach has been reported in dogs, with successful retrieval of hepatic tissue in 95% of the cases and no fatalities. Complications included perforation of the gallbladder or bile duct in two dogs, and collection of pulmonary as well as hepatic tissue in three dogs. Pneumothorax was not found to be a complication. The transthoracic approach is the preferred method in humans, on which the method in dogs is based. Transthoracic liver biopsy is performed on the right side. The precise location is determined after evaluation of two radiographic views of the thorax and abdomen. The biopsy needle is passed through the 5th, 6th, or 7th intercostal space at a point slightly dorsal to the costochondral junction. After surgical preparation of the area the biopsy site is infiltrated with a local anesthetic. A small skin incision is made with a number 11 surgical blade. The Menghini needle is introduced into the subcutaneous intercostal structures at a right angle and with the stylet not completely within the needle hub. This allows the cutting edge of the biopsy needle to facilitate passing the needle into the pleural space, after which the stylet is pushed completely into the needle hub. The needle and stylet are then directed caudally and advanced to the diaphragm. After making contact with the diaphragm the needle guard is adjusted and fixed at a point that is 1/2 inch (13mm) from the skin. This limits the depth to which the needle will enter the liver when the biopsy is obtained. The stylet is removed, and a 12-ml syringe containing up to 5 ml sterile saline is attached. This procedure is done rapidly and with the tip of the needle against the diaphragm, both practices that help minimize chances of a pneumothorax. The syringe is used to produce a negative pressure of about 3 ml, and at the end of expiration the needle is rapidly thrust caudally into the liver up to the needle guard and in a continuing motion rapidly removed from the body. The biopsy sample is drawn into the saline-filled syringe, from which it is transferred to a fixative solution of buffered formalin. The patient is placed on its right side for five minutes to cause the weight of body viscera to compress the biopsy site and facilitate hemostasis.

The transabdominal procedure is conducted on animals that are also in left lateral recumbency.[113,116] The liver falls away from the uppermost part of the abdominal wall in this position, so that a needle passed through this part at a right angle may not reach the liver. The approach is through the ventral abdominal wall at a site between the left lateral border of the xiphoid process and the left costal arch. This region is surgically prepared and infiltrated with a local anesthetic. A small skin incision is made with a number 11 blade. The Menghini needle, with stylet and guard, is passed through the abdominal wall. At this point the stylet is removed and the blocking pin is inserted through the hub into the needle. A 12-ml syringe containing 5 to 6 ml saline is attached, and a small amount of saline is flushed through the needle to wash out any blood or tissue collected during the initial part of the procedure. The needle is advanced in a craniodorsal direction until the surface of the liver is reached. The needle guard is adjusted to regulate the depth of penetration during the biopsy. A vacuum of 3 ml is produced with the syringe, and in one continuous motion the needle is rapidly thrust into the liver and removed from the body. The sample of liver tissue is transferred to buffered formalin by flushing saline from the syringe through the needle containing the sample. The post-biopsy complications in a group of patients that were almost all biopsied with the transabdominal approach included one death and major complications in four of 107 patients.[113]

An important difference between the two methods is that the blocking pin is used in the transabdominal approach and not in the transthoracic approach. The pin prevents the sample of tissue from being drawn into the syringe and minimizes the chances of its becoming fragmented. Another difference is the ability to flush the needle with the transabdominal approach and the omission of this step in the transthoracic approach. Flushing the needle reduces the chances of retrieving a sample of blood clot or nonhepatic tissue. The transthoracic approach also requires that the needle pass through the diaphragm without a stylet.

Other approaches must be followed if the liver cannot be identified by blind percutaneous procedures or if the operator lacks skills required to obtain a biopsy. More control over the biopsy procedure can be gained with the keyhole technique.[116] That involves a surgical incision just caudal to the xiphoid through which the index finger is inserted to facilitate the liver biopsy, allowing the operator to identify and avoid puncturing the gallbladder, major vessels, cysts, and abscesses. It also enables immobilization of a lobe of the liver against the abdominal wall or other lobes so that it can be biopsied and not pushed aside as the needle is thrust into the lobe. This procedure allows the operator to identify any unusual contour of the hepatic surface from which retrieval of a biopsy sample can be directed. Abnormalities in other abdominal organs can be identified at this time. The needle biopsy technique is the same as with the blind approach. The needle is introduced through an incision different from the keyhole opening used to immobilize the liver. The keyhole technique is recommended for operators who are relatively inexperienced in biopsying the liver.

A visual examination of the liver or a directed biopsy is sometimes desired. Single large focal lesions in one or two liver lobes or isolated in all the lobes are unlikely to be biopsied by blind percutaneous biopsy procedures. These lesions are not recognized with the keyhole procedure unless they are in liver lobes at the keyhole site. Focal lesions are usually identified with laparoscopy or laparotomy. Laparoscopy is performed through a small abdominal incision, during which the peritoneal cavity is inflated with a gas: air, carbon dioxide, or nitrous oxide. The advantage of the procedure is that the liver biopsy is always directed and that isolated lesions can be biopsied. The ability to direct biopsy instruments visually reduces the number of complications seen with blind percutaneous liver biopsy. An obvious advantage is that the liver's gross appearance can be evaluated. The liver is always biopsied during laparoscopy, regardless of its gross appearance, which is often misleading when compared with its histology. Laparoscopy is the method of choice when both liver biopsy and visual examination of the liver are desired. The primary disadvantage of laparoscopy is the initial expense of the equipment. Other disadvantages are that laparoscopy requires greater sedation, is more invasive, requires pneumoperitoneum, and is more time-consuming than blind percutaneous liver biopsy. Laparoscopy is one of two methods of choice in selected cases where there is a high index of suspicion that some major complication could develop from blind percutaneous liver biopsy. The other method of choice is hepatic biopsy directed by ultrasound imaging.

Complications are prevented by carefully following a standard protocol and are managed as they develop. No postbiopsy treatment is required to prevent complications. Antibiotics are not necessary. There have been no reports of complications caused by infection following liver biopsy.

REFERENCES

1. Walker, W.A. and Mathis, R.K.: Hepatomegaly. An approach to differential diagnosis. Ped. Clin. No. Am. 22:929-942, 1975.
2. Javitt, N.B.: Clinical and experimental aspects of sulphobromophthalein and related compounds. In, Progress in Liver Diseases. Vol. 3. Edited by H. Popper and F. Schaffner. Grune and Stratton, New York. 110-117, 1970.
3. Grausz, H. and Schmid, R.: Reciprocal relation between plasma albumin level and hepatic sulfobromophthalein removal. New Eng. J. Med. 284:1402-1406, 1971.
4. Fleischner, G.M. and Arias, I.M.: Structure and function of ligandin (Y-protein, GSH transferase B) and Z protein in the liver: A progress report. In, Progress in Liver Diseases. Vol. 5. Edited by H. Popper and F. Schaffner. Grune and Stratton, New York. 172-182, 1976.

5. Barnhart, J.L. and Combes, B.: Biliary excretion of dye in dogs infused with BSP or its glutathione conjugate. Amer. J. Physiol. 231:399-407, 1976.
6. Yeary, R.A. and Wise, K.J.: Plasma disappearance of sulfobromophthalein or indocyanine green in unconjugated hyperbilirubinemia. Res. Commun. Chem. Path. Parmacol. 12:125-136, 1975.
7. Klaassen, C.D.: Comparison of the effects of two-thirds hepatectomy and bile duct ligation on hepatic excretory function. J. Pharmacol. Exp. Ther. 191:25-31, 1974.
8. Rikkers, L.F. and Moody, F.G.: Estimation of functional reserve of normal and regenerating dog livers. Surgery 75:421-429, 1974.
9. Van Fleet, J.F. and Alberts, J.O.: Evaluation of liver function tests and liver biopsy in experimental carbon tetrachloride intoxication and extrahepatic bile duct obstruction in the dog. AJVR 29:2119-2131, 1968.
10. Himes, J.A. and Cornelius, C.E.: Hepatic excretion and storage of sulfobromophthalein sodium in experimental hepatic necrosis in the dog. Cornell Vet. 63:424-431, 1973.
11. Berk, P.D., Wolkoff, A.W. and Berlin N.I.: Inborn errors of bilirubin metabolism. Med. Clinics No. Am. 59:803-821, 1975.
12. Cornelius, C.E.: Liver function. In, Clinical Chemistry of Domestic Animals. 2nd Ed. Vol. I. Edited by J.J. Kaneko and C.E. Cornelius. Academic Press, New York. 161-230, 1970.
13. Strombeck, D.R. and Qualls, C.: Hepatic sulfobromophthalein uptake and storage defect in a dog. JAVMA 172:1423-1426, 1978.
14. Cornelius, C.E.: Hepatic disease in animals. In, Progress in Liver Diseases. Vol. 3. Edited by H. Popper and F. Schaffner. Grune and Stratton, New York. 419-431, 1970.
15. Caesar, J., Shaldon, S., Chiandussi, L., Guevara, L. and Sherlock, S.: The use of indocyanine green in the measurement of hepatic blood flow and as a test of hepatic function. Clin. Sci. 21:43-57, 1961.
16. Cherrick, G.R., Stein, S.W., Leevy, C.M. and Davidson, C.S.: Indocyanine green:observations on its physical properties, plasma decay, and hepatic extraction. J. Clin. Invest. 39:592-600, 1960.
17. Center, S.A., Bunch, S.E., Baldwin, B.H., Hornbuckle, W.E. and Tennant, B.C.: Comparison of sulfobromophthalein and indocyanine green clearances in the dog. AJVR 44:722-726, 1983.
18. Center, S.A., Bunch, S.E., Baldwin, B.H., Hornbuckle, W.E. and Tennant, B.C.: Comparison of sulfobromophthalein and indocyanine green clearances in the cat. AJVR 44:727-730, 1983.
19. Prasse, K.W., Bjorling, D.E., Holmes, R.A. and Cornelius, L.M.: Indocyanine green clearance and ammonia tolerance in partially hepatectomized and hepatic devascularized, anesthetized dogs. AJVR 44:2320-2323, 1983.
20. Rakich, P.M., Prasse, K.W. and Bjorling, D.E.: Clearance of indocyanine green in dogs with partial hepatectomy, hepatic duct ligation, and passive hepatic congestion. AJVR 48:1353-1357, 1987.
21. Okuda, K., Ohkubo, H., Musha, H., Kotoda, K., Abe, H. and Tanikawa, K.: Marked delay in indocyanine green plasma clearance with a near-normal bromosulphophthalein retention test: a constitutional abnormality? Gut 17:588-594, 1976.
22. Windmueller, H.G. and Spaeth, A.E.: Uptake and metabolism of plasma glutamine by the small intestine. J. Biol. Chem. 249:5070-5079, 1974.
23. Meyer, D.J., Strombeck, D.R., Stone, E.A., Zenoble, R.D. and Buss, D.D.: Ammonia tolerance test in clinically normal dogs and in dogs with portosystemic shunts. JAVMA 173:377-379, 1978.
24. Rothuizen, J. and van den Ingh, T.S.G.A.M.: Rectal ammonia tolerance test in the evaluation of portal circulation in dogs with liver disease. Res. Vet. Sci. 33:22-25, 1982.
25. Schenker, S., Breen, K.J. and Hoyumpa, A.M.: Hepatic encephalopathy: current status. Gastroenterology 66:121-151, 1974.
26. Miller, G.E. and Rice, J.D.: Determination of the concentration of ammonia nitrogen in plasma by means of a simple ion exchange method. Am. J. Clin. Path. 39:97-103, 1963.
27. Strombeck, D.R.: Unpublished observations.
28. Young, D.S., Thomas, D.W. and Friedman, R.B.: Effects of drugs on clinical laboratory tests. Clin. Chem. 18:1041-1303, 1972.
29. Mondzac, A., Ehrlich, G.E. and Seegmiller, J.E.: An enzymatic determination of ammonia in biological fluids. J. Lab. Clin. Med. 66:526-531, 1965.
30. Zinkl, J.G., Bush, R.M., Cornelius, C.E. and Freedland, R.A.: Comparative studies on plasma and tissue sorbitol, glutamic, lactic, and hydroxybutyric dehydrogenase and transaminase activities in the dog. Res. Vet. Sci. 12:211-214, 1971.
31. Dixon, M.F., Fulker, M.J., Walker, B.E., Kelleher, J. and Losowsky, M.S.: Serum transaminase levels after experimental paracetamol-induced hepatic necrosis. Gut 16:800-807, 1975.
32. Strombeck, D.R., Harrold, D., Rogers, Q., Wheeldon, E., Stern, J. and Schaeffer, M.: Plasma amino acid glucagon, and insulin concentrations in dogs with nitrosamine-induced hepatic disease. AJVR 44:2028-2036, 1983.
33. Badylak, S.F. and Van Vleet, J.F.: Sequential morphologic and clinicopathologic alterations in dogs with experimentally induced glucocorticoid hepatopathy. AJVR 42:1310-1318, 1981.
34. Bunch, S.E., Castleman, W.L., Baldwin, B.H., Hornbuckle, W.E. and Tennant, .C.: Effects of long-term primidone and phenytoin administration on canine hepatic function and morphology. AJVR 46:105-115, 1985.
35. Schaeffer, M.C., Rogers, Q.R., Buffington, C.A., Wolfe, B.M. and Strombeck, D.R.: Long-term biochemical and physiologic effects of surgically placed portacaval shunts in dogs. AJVR 47:346-355, 1986.
36. Wigton, D.H., Kociba, G.J. and Hoover, E.A.: Infectious canine hepatitis: animal model for viral-induced disseminated intravascular coagulation. Blood 47:287-296, 1976.
37. Moore, W.E. and Feldman, B.F.: The use of isoenzymes in small animal medicine. JAAHA 10:420-429, 1974.
38. Milne, E.M. and Doxey, D.L.: Alkaline phosphatase and its isoenzymes in the tissues and sera of normal dogs. Vet. Res. Commun. 10:229-236, 1986.
39. Boyd, J.W.: The mechanisms relating to increases in plasma enzymes and isoenzymes in diseases of animals. Vet. Clin. Pathol. 12(2):9-24, 1983.
40. Hoffman, W.E.: Diagnostic value of canine serum alkaline phosphatase and alkaline phosphatase isoenzymes, JAAHA 13:237-241, 1977.
41. Hoffman, W.E., and Dorner, J.L.: Disappearance rates of intravenously injected canine alkaline phosphatase isoenzymes. AJVR 38:1553-1556, 1977.
42. Brobst, D.F. and Schall, W.D.: Needle biopsy of the canine liver and correlation of laboratory data with histopathologic observations. JAVMA 161:382-388, 1972.
43. Pekarthy, J.M., Short, J., Lansing, A.I. and Lieberman, I.: Function and control of liver alkaline phosphatase, J. Biol. Chem. 247:1767-1774, 1972.
44. Kaplan, M.M.: Serum alkaline phosphatase - another piece is added to the puzzle. Hepatology 6:526-528, 1986.
45. Young, G.P., Friedman, S., Yedlin, S.T. and Alpers, D.H.: Effect of fat feeding on intestinal alkaline phosphatase activity in tissue and serum. Am. J. Physiol. 241:G461-468, 1981.
46. Brooks, S.E.H., Reynolds, P., Audretsch, J.J. and Haggis, G.: Scanning electron microscopy of proliferating bile ductules. Lab. Invest. 33:311-315, 1975.
47. Rogers, W.A.: Source of serum alkaline phosphatase in clinically normal and diseased dogs: a clinical study. JAVMA 168:934-937, 1976.
48. Rogers, W.A. and Ruebner, B.H.: A retrospective study of probable glucocorticoid-induced hepatopathy in dogs. JAVMA 170:603-606, 1977.
49. Kramer, J.W. and Sleight, S.D.: The isoenzymes of serum

alkaline phosphatase in cats. Am. J. Vet. Clin. Path. 2:87-91, 1968.
50. Everett, R.M., Duncan, J.R. and Prasse, K.W.: Alkaline phosphatase, leucine aminopeptidase, and alanine aminotransferase activities with obstructive and toxic hepatic disease in cats. AJVR 38:963-966, 1977.
51. Hoffman, W.E., Renegar, W.E. and Dorner, J.L.: Serum half-life of intravenously injected intestinal and hepatic alkaline phosphatase isoenzymes in the cat. AJVR 38:1637-1639, 1977.
52. Dragosics, B., Ferenci, P., Pesendorfer, F. and Wewalka, F.G.: Gamma-glutamyltranspeptidase (GGTP): Its relationship to other enzymes for diagnosis of liver disease. In, Progress in Liver Diseases. Vol. 5. Edited by H. Popper and F. Schaffner. Grune and Stratton, New York. 436-499, 1976.
53. Goldberg, D.M. and Martin, J.V.: Role of q-glutamyl transpeptidase activity in the diagnosis of hepatobiliary disease. Digestion 12:232-246, 1975.
54. Whitfield, J.B., Pounder, R.E., Neale, G. and Moss, D.W.: Serum q-glutamyl transpeptidase activity in liver disease. Gut 13:702-708, 1972.
55. Colombo, J.P., Peheim, E., Bachmann, C., Muller, E. and Bircher, J.: q-glutamyltranspeptidase in the rat liver after portacaval shunt. Pediat. Res. 10:18-24, 1976.
56. Ivanov, E., Krustev, L., Adjarov, D., Chernev, K., Apostolov, I., Dimitrov, P., Drensak, E., Stefanova, M. and Pramatarova, V.: Studies on the mechanism of the changes in serum and liver q-glutamyl transpeptidase activity. Enzyme 21:8-20, 1976.
57. Adjarov, D., Popov, S. and Ivanov, E.: Studies on the mechanism of changes in serum and liver q-glutamyl transpeptidase activity. Enzyme 21:1-7, 1976.
58. Shull, R.M. and Hornbuckle, W.: Diagnostic use of serum q-glutamyltransferase in canine liver disease. AJVR 40:1321-1324, 1979.
59. Arnold, V.U.: Die wertigkeit der serum-gamma-glutamyltransferase-aktivitat fur die diagnose der hepatopathien des hundes. Kleintierpraxis 32:49-55, 1987.
60. Serum q-glutamyl transpeptidase activity in healthy cats and cats with induced hepatic disease. AJVR 44:2049-2053, 1983.
61. Strombeck, D.R., Miller, L.M. and Harrold, D.: Effects of corticosteroid treatment on survival time in dogs with chronic hepatitis: 151 cases (1977-1985). JAVMA 193:1109-1113, 1988.
62. Knapp, K.K. and Hunter, R.L.: Serum proteins of the Beagle dog: a two-dimensional electrophoretic study. AJVR 36:193-195, 1975.
63. Keraan, M., Meyers, O.L., Engelbrecht, G.H.C., Hickman, R., Saunders, S.J. and Terblanche, J.: Increased serum immunoglobulin levels following portacaval shunt in the normal rat. Gut 15:468-472, 1974.
64. Badylak, S.F. and Van Vleet, J.F.: Alterations of prothrombin time and activated partial thromboplastin time in dogs with hepatic disease. AJVR 42:2053-2056, 1981.
65. Badylak, S.F., Dodds, W.J. and Van Vleet, J.F.: Plasma coagulation factor abnormalities in dogs with naturally occurring hepatic disease. AJVR 44:2336-2340, 1983.
66. Byars, T.D., Ling, G.V., Ferris, N.A. and Keeton, K.S.: Activated coagulation time (ACT) of whole blood in normal dogs. AJVR 37:1359-1361, 1976.
67. Cederblad, G., Korsan-Bengtsen, K. and Olsson, R.: Observations of increased levels of blood coagulation factors and other plasma proteins in cholestatic liver disease. Scand. J. Gastroenterology 11:391-396, 1976.
68. Quarfordt, S.H., Oelschlaeger, H., Krigbaum, W.R., Jakoi, L. and Davis, R.: Effect of biliary obstruction on canine plasma and biliary lipids. Lipids 8:522-530, 1973.
69. Simon, J.B. and Poon, R.W.M.: Lipoprotein-x levels in extrahepatic versus intrahepatic cholestasis. Gastroenterology 75:177-180, 1978.
70. Center, S.A., Baldwin, B.H., King, J.M. and Tennant, B.C.: Hematologic and biochemical abnormalities associated with induced extrahepatic bile duct obstruction in the cat. AJVR 44:1822-1829, 1983.
71. Opitz, M. and Lettow, E.: Der cholesterinesterquotient im serujm leberkranker hunde. Berl. Munch. Tierarztl. Wschr. 89:28-32, 1976.
72. Kaneko, J.J.: Normal values for blood chemistry used at VMTH in Davis, CA.
73. Kirk, R.W.: Current Veterinary Therapy IX. Small Animal Practice. W.B. Saunders, Philadelphia, 1986.
74. VMTH, UCD, Davis, CA - normal values.
75. Coyle, J.J., Schwartz, M.Z., Marubbio, A.T., Varco, R.L. and Buchwald, H.: The effect of portacaval shunt on plasma lipids and tissue cholesterol synthesis in the dog. Surgery 80:54-60, 1976.
76. Ramakrishnan, V.R., Beher, W.T., Lin, G.J., Stradnieks, S., Samhouri, F., Toledo-Pereyra, L.H. and Block, M.A.: Effects of sphincter of Oddi bypass on bile acid metabolism in fed and fasted intact and cholecystectomized dogs. Digestion 21:143-150, 1981.
77. Gilmore, I.T. and Hofmann, A.F.: Altered drug metabolism and elevated serum bile acids in liver disease: an unified pharmacokinetic explanation. Gastroenterology 78:177-178, 1980.
78. Anwer, M.S., Engelking, L.R., Gronwall, R. and Klentz, R.D.: Plasma bile acid elevation following CCl4 induced liver damage in dogs, sheep, calves and ponies. Res. Vet. Sci. 20:127-130, 1976.
79. Rutgers, H.C., Stradley, R.P. and Johnson, S.E.: Serum bile acid analysis in dogs with experimentally induced cholestatic jaundice. AJVR 49:317-320, 1988.
80. DeNovo, R.C. and Prasse, K.W.: Comparison of serum biochemical and hepatic functional alterations in dogs treated with corticosteroids and hepatic duct ligation. AJVR 44:1703-1709, 1983.
81. Meyer, D.J.: Liver function tests in dogs with portasystemic shunts: measurements of serum bile acid concentration. JAVMA 188:168-199, 1986.
82. Center, S.A., Baldwin, B.H., de Lahunta, A., Dietze, A.E. and Tennant, B.C.: Evaluation of serum bile acid concentrations for the diagnosis of portosystemic venous anomalies in the dog and cat. JAVMA 186:1090-1094, 1985.
83. Johnson, C.A., Armstrong, P.J. and Hauptman, J.G.: Congenital portosystemic shunts in dogs: 46 cases (1979-1986). JAVMA 191:1478-1483, 1987.
84. Center, S.A., Baldwin, B.H., Erb., H.N. and Tennant, B.C.: Bile acid concentrations in the diagnosis of hepatobiliary disease in the dog. JAVMA 187:935-940, 1985.
85. Johnson, S.E., Rogers, W.A., Bonagura, J.D. and Caldwell, J.H.: Determination of serum bile acids in fasting dogs with hepatobiliary disease. AJVR 46:2048-2053, 1985.
86. Kitagawa, H., Ishihara, K., Yokoyama, S. and Sasaki, Y.: Serum total bile acid levels in canine dirofilariasis. Jpn. J. Vet. Sci. 44:917-923, 1982.
87. Center, S.A.: Feline liver disorders and their management. Compend. Contin. Educ. Pract. Vet. 8:889-901, 1986.
88. Center, S.A., Baldwin, B.H., Erb, H. and Tennant, B.C.: Bile acid concentrations in the diagnosis of hepatobiliary disease in the cat. JAVMA 189:891-896, 1986.
89. Pare, P., Hoefs, J.C. and Ashcavai, M.: Determinants of serum bile acids in chronic liver disease. Gastroenterology 81:959-964, 1981.
90. Festi, D., Labate, A.M.M., Roda, A., Bazzoli, F., Frabboni, R., Rucci, P., Taroni, F., Aldini, R., Roda, E. and Barbara, L.: Diagnostic effectiveness of serum bile acids in liver diseases as evaluated by multivariate statistical methods. Hepatology 3:707-713, 1983.
91. Carey, M.C.: Bile acids and bile salts: ionization and solubility properties. Hepatology 4:665-715, 1984.
92. Strombeck, D.R.: Unpublished data.
93. Duane, W.C. and Bond, J.H.: Prolongation of intestinal transit and expansion of bile acid pools by propantheline bromide. Gastroenterology 78:226-230, 1980.
94. Kitagawa, H., Ishihara, K. and Yokoyama, S.: Serum total bile acid level in normal dogs. Jpn. J. Vet. Sci. 43:257-260, 1981.
95. Cravetto, C., Molino, G., Biondi, A.M., Cavanna, A., Avagnina, P. and Frediani, S.: Evaluation of the diagnostic

value of serum bile acid in the detection and functional assessment of liver diseases. Ann. Clin. Biochem. 22:596-605, 1985.

96. Fromm, H., and Albert, M.B.: Serum bile acid assays for liver disease: when and how to use them. Gastroenterology 92:829-830, 1987.

97. Shasha, S.M., Better, O.S., Chaimovitz, C., Doman, J. and Kishon, Y.: Haemodynamic studies in dogs with chronic bile-duct ligation. Clin. Sci. Mol. Med. 50:533-537, 1976.

98. Gopinath, C. and Ford, E.J.H.: Location of liver injury and extent of bilirubinemia in experimental liver lesions. Vet. Path. 9:99-108, 1972.

99. Rothuizen, J. and van den Brom, W.E.: Bilirubin metabolism in canine hepatobiliary and haemolytic disease. Vet. Quarterly 9:235-240, 1987.

100. Zawie, D.A. and Garvey, M.S.: Feline hepatic disease. Vet. Clin. No. Am. Sm. Anim. Pract. 14:1201-1230, 1984.

101. Bourke, E., Milne, M.D. and Stokes, G.S.: Mechanisms of renal excretion of urobilinogen. Brit. Med. J. 2:1510-1514, 1965.

102. Solberg, H.E., Skrede, S. and Blomhoff, J.P.: Diagnosis of liver diseases by laboratory results and discriminant analysis. Scand. J. Clin. Lab. Invest. 35:713-721, 1975.

103. Feldman, E.C. and Ettinger, S.J.: Percutaneous transthoracic liver biopsy in the dog: a review of 75 cases. JAAHA 13:17-22, 1977.

104. Hoe, C.M. and O'Shea, J.D.: The correlation of biochemistry and histopathology in liver disease in the dog. Vet. Rec. 77:6614-1171, 1965.

105. Suter, P.F.: Radiographic diagnosis of liver disease in dogs and cats. Vet. Clin. No. Am. Sm. Anim. Pract. 12:153-173, 1982.

106. VanBree, H. and Sacky, A.: Evaluation of radiographic liver size in twenty-seven normal deep-chested dogs. J. Sm. Anim. Pract. 28:693-703, 1987.

107. Evans, S.M.: The radiographic appearance of primary liver neoplasia in dogs. Vet. Radiol. 28:192-196, 1987.

108. Nyland, T.G. and Hager, D.A.: Sonography of the liver, gallbladder and spleen. Vet. Clin. No. Am. Sm. Anim. Pract. 15:1123-1148, 1985.

109. Godshalk, C.P., Badertscher, R.R., Rippy, M.K. and Ghent, A.W.: Quantitative ultrasonic assessment of liver size in the dog. Vet. Radiol. 29:162-167, 1988.

110. Feeney, D.A., Johnston, G.R. and Hardy, R.M.: Two-dimensional, gray-scale ultrasonography for assessment of hepatic splenic neoplasia in the dog and cat. JAVMA 184:68-81, 1984.

111. Wrigley, R.H., Konde, L.J., Park, R.D. and Lebel, J.L.: Ultrasonographic diagnosis of portacaval shunts in young dogs. JAVMA 191:421-424, 1987.

112. Hager, D.A., Nyland, T.G. and Fisher, P.: Ultrasound-guided biopsy of the canine liver, kidney, and prostate. Vet. Radiol. 26:82-88, 1985.

113. Edwards, D.F.: Blind percutaneous liver biopsy: a safe diagnostic procedure. Calif. Vet. 9-17, April 1977.

114. Feldman, E.C. and Ettinger, S.J.: Percutaneous transthoracic liver biopsy in the dog. JAVMA 169:805-810, 1976.

115. Knecht, C.D. and Reynolds, H.A.: Needle punch biopsy procedures for obtaining specimens of the liver, kidney, and lymph nodes of dogs. JAAHA 3:163-170, 1967.

116. Osborne, C.A., Hardy, R.M., Stevens, J.B. and Perman, V.: Liver biopsy. Vet. Clin. N. Amer. 4:333-350, 1974.

117. Conn, H.O.: Liver biopsy in extrahepatic biliary obstruction and in other "contraindicated" disorders. Gastroenterology 68:817-821, 1975.

118. Edmondson, H.A. and Schiff, L.: Needle biopsy of the liver. In: Diseases of the Liver. 4th Ed. Edited by L. Schiff. J.B. Lippincott, Philadelphia. 247-271, 1975.

119. Morris, J.S., Gallo, G.A., Scheuer, P.J. and Sherlock, S.: Percutaneous liver biopsy in patients with large bile duct obstruction. Gastroenterology 68:750-754, 1975.

120. Menghini, G.: One-second biopsy of the liver. Problems of its clinical application. N. Eng. J. Med. 283:582-585, 1970.

121. Raines, D.R., Van Heertum, R.L. and Johnson, L.F.: Intrahepatic hematoma: A complication of percutaneous liver biopsy. Gastroenterology 67:284-289, 1974.

122. Putnam, C.W. and Starzyl, T.E.: Simplified biopsy of the liver in dogs. Surg. Gynecol. Obstet. 144:759, 1977.

Chapter 31

General Pathology of Hepatic Disease

Biochemical and morphological changes are used to identify hepatic disease. The evaluation of biochemical changes is most important in assessing the possibility of a hepatic problem. Morphological changes provide a means of classifying hepatic disease, a prerequisite to proper treatment and accurate prognosis.

Hepatic disease can be caused by infectious agents, toxins, hypoxia, trauma, neoplasms, immune responses, hormone imbalances, nutritional derangements, drugs, and anomalies. Their initial effect on hepatocytes is usually degeneration or necrosis. Normal function and morphology usually return when the cause is removed. The liver readily regenerates and maintains its normal functions despite losing a large amount of its mass. Following resection of 70 to 90% of the liver, regeneration is complete within two weeks.

PATHOLOGIC PATTERNS[1-3]

Pathologic hepatic changes are usually described and interpreted by a scheme based on their location in the hexagonal lobule. The hexagonal lobule, sometimes thought of as the functional unit, is defined as the group of cells and vessels in the hexagon outlined by the portal veins, hepatic arteries, and bile ducts, with the central vein at its center (Figure 31-1). It is unlikely that this morphological unit is a functional one that can be likened to the nephron, the functional unit of the kidney. Rappaport suggests that the functional unit is not the hexagonal lobule, but rather consists of cells and vessels served by the circulation of blood and bile in one branch of a portal triad (Figure 31-2). That unit is triangular-shaped, with the vessels of one branch of a portal triad for its base and the central vein for its apex. In this unit, functional and cellular integrity depend on the unit's blood supply and bile drainage. The portal triad provides an entry for the movement of toxic and infectious agents into the liver through its blood vessels or biliary system. If the functional unit is the hexagonal lobule, any pathology should appear uniformly throughout. Each of the three portal triads forming the unit would contribute to the pathology. In fact, hepatic lesions are not uniform throughout the hexagonal lobule. The pattern of lesions found support the Rappaport scheme of a functional unit (acinus).

The location of liver cells, in zone 1, 2, or 3, usually determines the pattern of pathologic changes. Their location in the acinus reflects how circulation affects liver cells cells in zone 1 receive blood that is richer in oxygen, nutrients, and toxic products than those in zone 3. Their acinar location also reflects the cellular heterogeneity of the unit with cells in zone 1 adapted for gluconeogenesis, urea synthesis, and amino acid catabolism, functions the zone 3 cells are ill-equipped to perform.4 The heterogeneity results in predictable pathologic patterns with a number of metabolic, circulatory, and toxic problems.

Morphologic changes are described by their location and pattern in the functional unit. Lesions in zone 1 are described as periportal in that they are around the portal tracts. Lesions in zone 3 are around or adjacent to central veins and are described as perivenular, pericentral, centrizonal, or centrilobular. These lesions involve the cells most distant from the entry of the blood supply into the functional unit. They are often produced when the amounts of oxygen and nutrients remaining in sinusoidal blood are inadequate after the needs of the periportal part of the lobule are met. Hepatocytes are highly differentiated functional units that possess many biochemical functions and operate with a blood supply at an oxygen tension lower than that of any other organ. Circulatory changes can potentiate this relative tissue hypoxia and precipitate pathological changes. Lesions in zone 2 are described as midzonal or merely as acinar zone 2. Using the terminology reflecting the acinus rather than the lobule as the function unit, more extensive lesions can be described as multiacinar and panacinar.

HEPATOCELLULAR DEGENERATION[1-3]

Hepatocellular degeneration varies with the degree of insult to the hepatocyte. Hepatocyte changes are described morphologically, with the description reflecting the severity of degeneration. There are three ways an insult can trigger degenerative changes that can lead to hepatocyte necrosis. Cell damage can result in hepatocyte swelling or ballooning due to water uptake. Cell damage can also lead to an excessive loss of water, resulting in acidophilic degeneration. Furthermore, cells can disappear through apoptosis, which operates to maintain normal liver size and may be stimulated by specific pathologic stimuli. Apoptosis, as a physiological mechanism for cell deletion, appears as a shrinkage and fragmentation of hepatocytes to form apoptotic bodies. The process is rapid, taking only a few minutes, and the half-life of apoptotic bodies is only several hours.

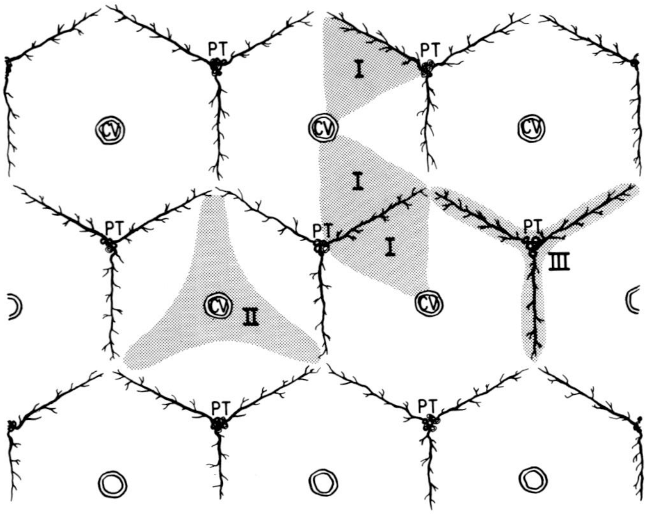

Figure 31-1. Schematic of hepatic lobules formed as hexagons by six terminal branches of the portal vein, two branches from each portal triad (PT). At the center of each lobule is a central vein (CV). In this scheme the hexagonal lobule is considered the functional unit of the liver. Gray zone 1 represents the pattern of pathology seen with paracentral and periportal lesions. Pattern II represents pericentral lesions and Pattern III represents periportal lesions less extensive than those represented by the pattern in I.

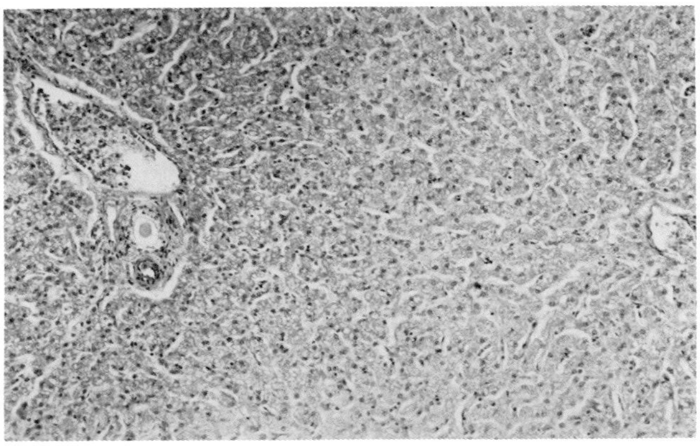

A

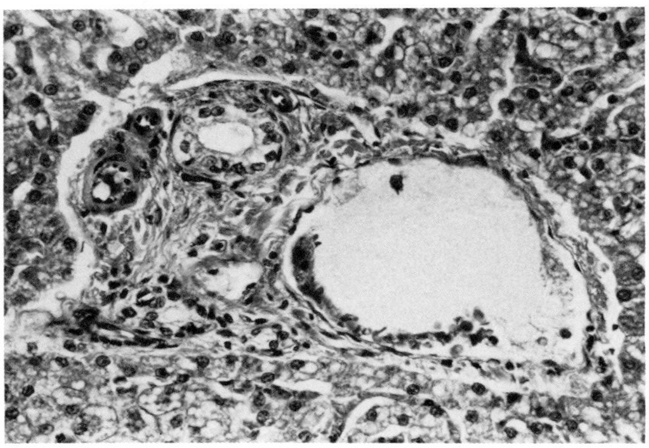

B

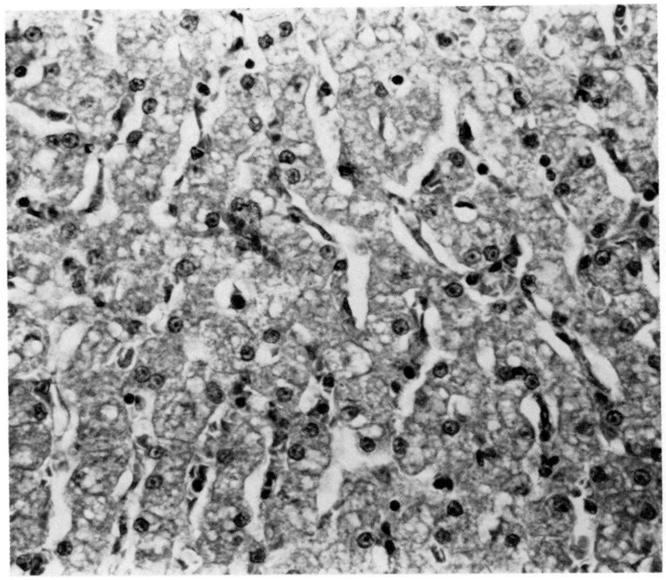

C

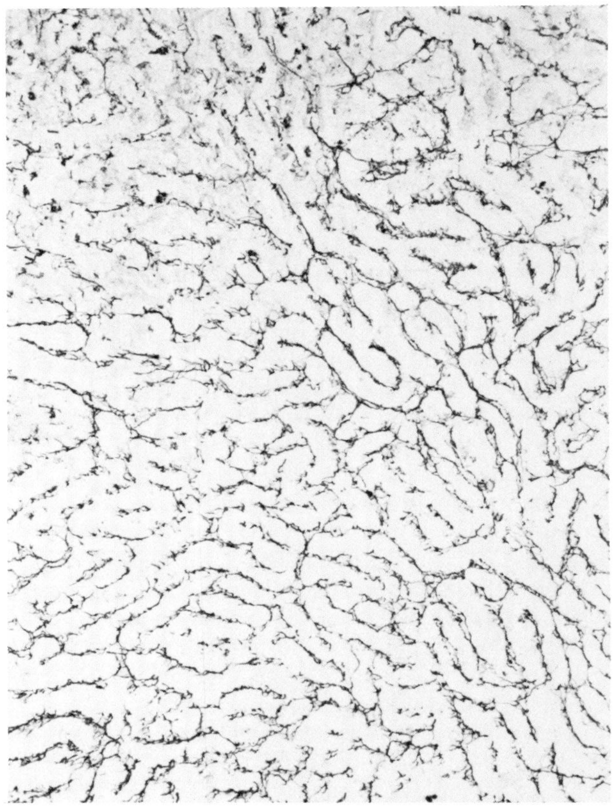

D

Figure 31-2. a) Part of a normal hepatic lobule with portal area on left containing: a large thin-wall portal vein, a bile duct of smaller diameter than the vein and lined with epithelium, and a thick-wall artery with a small lumen, and a central vein in the right. b) and c) Higher magnification of portal area and hepatic cords, respectively. d) Reticulin stain of normal liver.

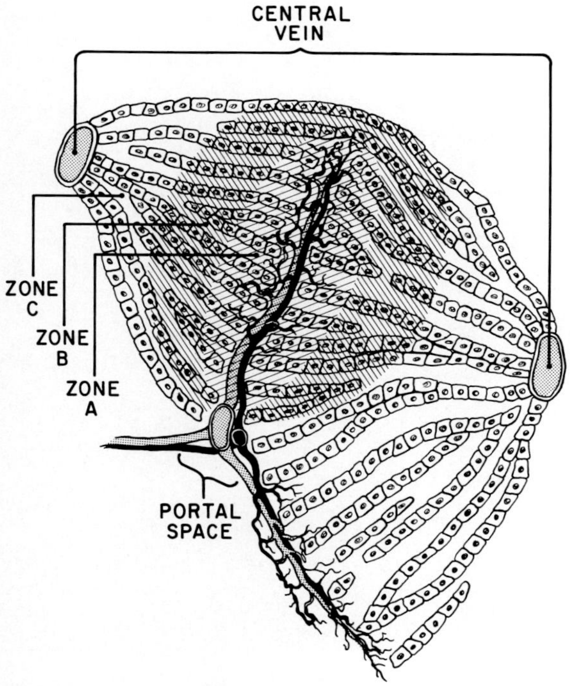

Figure 31-2e. Schematic diagram of the liver lobule illustrating the functional unit of Rappaport (acinus), which consists of the hepatocytes supplied by the terminal branches of one hepatic artery and portal vein. Zones A, B, and C represent the areas that receive the greatest to the least oxygen, respectively.

Hepatocyte Ballooning

Early degeneration can cause hepatocytes to swell up to several times their normal size. Slight ballooning corresponds to cloudy swelling where cytoplasmic granule formation is evident. On electron microscopy, the mitochondria are swollen and rounded. Cloudy swelling is associated with severe infections or toxemias; it may also be found in liver biopsies where its diagnostic significance is unknown. Hydropic degeneration is a more severe form of hepatocyte ballooning. Vacuoles appear in the cytoplasm, reflecting cellular edema. Cell edema appears with a reduction in the availability of cell energy. Energy is required to maintain normal cell volume. Cell size is stabilized by maintaining a constant number of osmotically active particles within the cell, accomplished by actively transporting sodium ions from the cell. Sodium transport is not possible without oxygen or other sources of energy. Sodium leaks continuously into cells from extracellular fluid, accompanied by water, which causes cell edema if not pumped out.

An alternate explanation is suggested for maintaining normal cell volume. By this hypothesis, energy is required to maintain the highly ordered normal tertiary structure of intracellular proteins resulting in maximum structuring of intracellular water. The rigid order effectively excludes larger ions, such as sodium. With reduced energy available to the cell, the structure is lost and the composition of intracellular fluid and electrolytes approaches that of extracellular fluid. Cell-volume changes in ballooning degeneration are reversible. Progression of this form of degeneration leads to lytic necrosis of hepatocytes.

Acidophilic Degeneration

An early morphological change in response to cell injury is eosinophilic, acidophilic, or hyaline degeneration. Hepatocytes lose their basophilia and appear glassy, with an eosinophilic tint. The cause is a loss of cytoplasmic nucleoprotein, and electron microscopy shows a loss of ribosomes and hypertrophy of smooth endoplasmic reticulum. Nuclear changes appear later and may be followed by granular degeneration of the cytoplasm, appearing as bilobular refractile acidophilic bodies. Bodies of clumped cytoplasm are eventually discharged from cells and may be seen in tissue spaces. Acidophilic bodies or remnants can represent apoptotic bodies.

Apoptosis

The rapid time-course for apoptosis minimizes direct evidence for its having occurred. At most, it may represent acidophilic bodies. Indirect evidence includes the disappearance or drop-out of small to large clusters of hepatocytes, leaving no evidence of cell destruction and no inflammatory or fibrotic response. Apoptosis may be assisted by lymphocyte-mediated immune mechanisms. Foci of hepatocytes undergoing apoptosis and appearing as intact shrunken cells may represent what is described as coagulation necrosis.

Feathery Degeneration

Feathery degeneration is associated with cholestasis. Hepatocytes are swollen and appear vacuolated and reticulated. Cellular striations are pigmented brown by retained bile pigments and are usually seen in isolated hepatocytes.

Fat Accumulation

Fatty changes in hepatocytes result from the accumulation of lipids, primarily triglycerides (Figure 31-3). Abnormal lipid deposition results from an imbalance in cellular metabolism that follows a deficiency of one or more essential nutrients, alteration in the level of energy intake, imbalance in the ratio of nutrients, or exposure to a hepatotoxin. The fatty changes can be confined to a region of the lobule or can be diffuse. Fatty changes caused by hepatotoxins are usually diffuse throughout the lobule. Hepatic fatty infiltration frequently accompanies circulatory failure or anemia. The lesions are primarily pericentral in zone 3, since these cells are the last to receive sources of energy brought in by the circulation. Nutrients and oxygen are extracted, and blood reaching the central veins is normally partially depleted. With impaired circulation or reduced oxygen-carrying capacity of the blood, the sources of energy are extracted by periportal cells lining sinusoids, leaving little for the pericentral hepatocytes.

NECROSIS AND INFLAMMATION[1-3]

Hepatic necrosis is an irreversible event, with causes including chemical, parasitic, viral, or bacterial agents, anoxia, nutritional deficiencies, and immune-mediated responses (Figure 31-4). Hepatic necrosis, having different patterns of distribution, is described as focal, pericentral or centrolobular (in zone

A 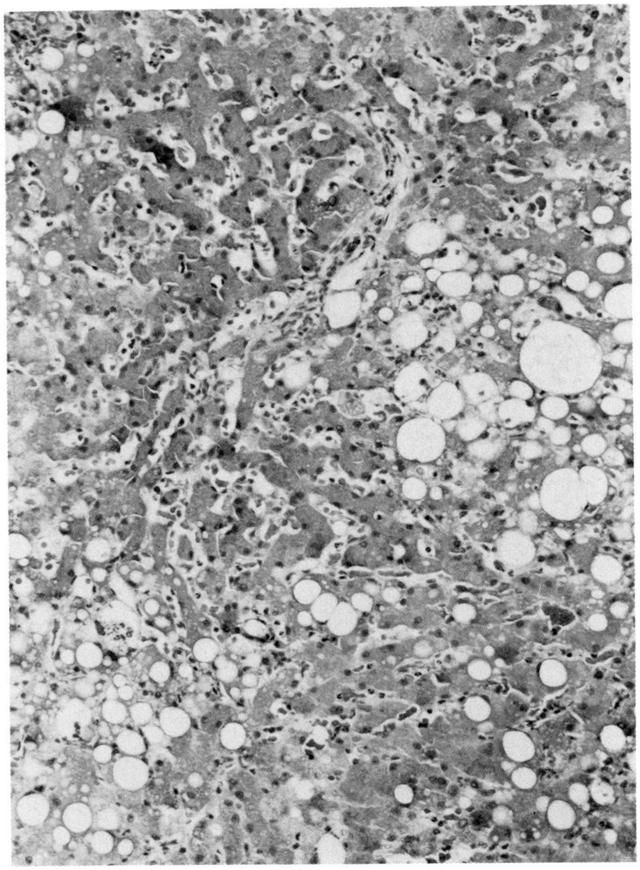 B 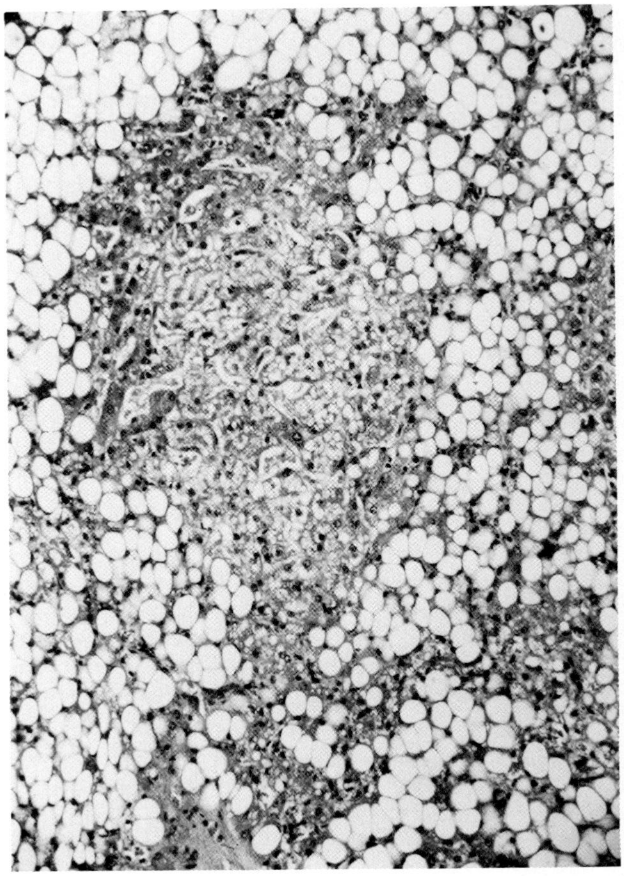

Figure 31-3. a) Mild lipidosis in biopsy specimen from a dog. b) Severe lipidosis surrounding a group of vacuolated hepatocytes.

3), midzonal (in zone 2), periportal (in zone 1), or massive (Figure 31-1). Necrosis can also bridge adjacent central and/or portal areas of the acini. The pattern of necrosis determines its outcome. Inflammatory responses usually accompany necrosis and vary both in degree and cell type.

With most hepatocellular degeneration and necrosis, Kupffer cells and the hepatic stroma remain intact. Necrosis of Kupffer cells and breakdown of stroma occur with interruption of hepatic circulation.

Focal necrosis describes necrosis of single or small groups of hepatocytes scattered randomly throughout the liver. Focal necrosis is usually recognized by the accompanying inflammatory cell infiltration and Kupffer-cell hypertrophy and proliferation. The foci of necrosis are infiltrated with histiocytes, lymphocytes, and plasma cells; sometimes neutrophils predominate. Such focal necrosis occurs with infections, drug reactions, parasitic migration, biliary obstruction, and bacteremia and septicemia. Hepatic function is not lost with focal necrosis, and with recovery only small areas of scarring may be found. Thus, focal necrosis does not cause hepatic failure.

Perivenular, or centrilobular necrosis in zone 3 around central veins is a pattern often caused by circulatory failure. This necrosis is found more frequently at postmortem than in a biopsy from the same animal before death, suggesting that the necrosis is due to agonal events. Cellular hypoxia causes zone 3 necrosis, which can be seen with acute and profound anemia, inadequate circulation secondary to congestive heart failure, and any event that reduces splanchnic circulation sufficiently to cause shock. Zone 3 necrosis can also result from hypoxia due to pulmonary disease. Anoxia can cause a necrosis that appears uniformly eosinophilic with nuclei of connective-tissue cells losing their affinity for stain. Impaired hepatic circulation resulting from swollen and injured hepatocytes can cause local hypoxia and necrosis, as seen in infectious canine hepatitis. Idiosyncratic drug reactions, drug overdoses, and hepatotoxins often cause zone 3 necrosis. With extensive zone 3 necrosis, the pathologic changes can bridge adjacent central veins, giving an appearance of a pseudolobulation (Figure 31-1). With progression of necrosis to zone 2 and into zone 1, bridging necrosis can also be found between central veins and portal areas. Bridging necrosis is sometimes called confluent necrosis. Mild inflammation accompanies zone 3 necrosis, with the inflammation primarily characterized by histiocytes. Lymphocytes, plasma cells, and neutrophils can be found with more pronounced inflammation.

Periportal necrosis is a specific pattern of degeneration seen with inflammatory and infiltrating lesions around vessels in the portal triad. Hepatotoxins and infectious agents entering the liver through its circulation or bile ducts can produce these changes. Proliferation of bile ducts and cholangioles frequently accompany the signs of inflammation.

Midzonal necrosis describes pathology in zone 2 and is an uncommon finding. It is usually associated with degenerative changes in the other two zones. Midzonal necrosis may be a

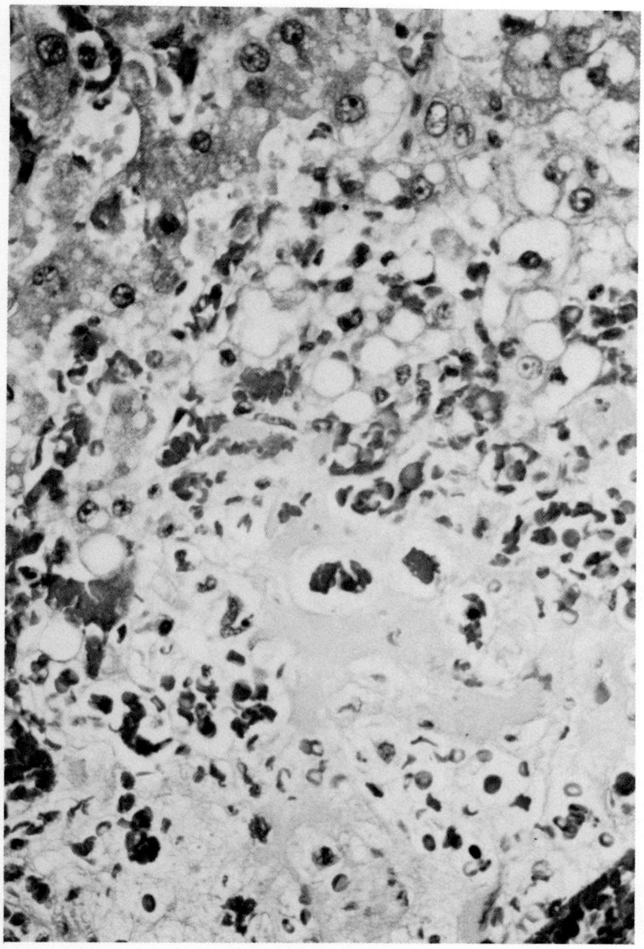

Figure 31-4a. Hepatic necrosis. Hepatocytes in lower half have lost nuclei and cytoplasmic structure and appear hyalinized.

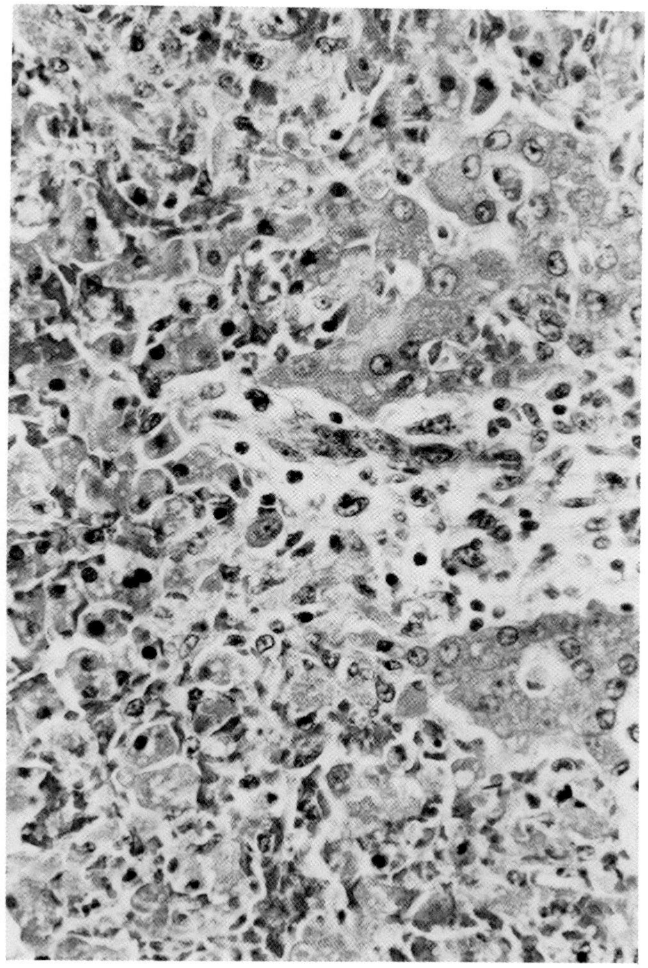

Figure 31-4b. Submassive necrosis. Degenerating hepatocytes throughout but especially in lower third. Disappearance of hepatocytes and collapse of parenchyma is suggested by defect in middle of field. Some hepatocytes surrounding this defect appear like regenerating cells.

pattern of injury following hypotension and shock.[5] Perivenular, periportal, and midzonal necrosis are sometimes described as submassive necrosis because an entire zonal area of an acinus is involved.

Massive or paracentral necrosis describes changes in the triangular-shaped section of the lobule supplied by one branch of a portal triad vessel. It is in reality necrosis of all the cells in a single complete acinus. Massive hepatic necrosis can occur randomly, leaving large parts of the liver unaffected. Massive necrosis tends to develop initially in the left lobes. In the dog, hepatic circulation is streamlined so that the left lobes receive nutrient-poor blood from the spleen and colon, and the right lobes receive mostly nutrient-rich blood from the small intestine. When necrosis involves all cells in an acinus, the supporting framework collapses and regeneration does not occur. Blood may pool in the void created by hepatocyte losses. Acinar collapse can also cause approximation of portal areas to hepatic venular areas. Viable parenchymal cells that survive the insult regenerate in acini with the supporting structure still intact. Collapse of the supporting architecture results in condensation of the hepatic reticulin and fibrous framework to give an appearance of scarification (postnecrotic scarring). Inflammation is mild in areas of massive necrosis.

Massive hepatic necrosis can be caused by virus infections, drugs, toxins, or ischemia. In some cases the pathology may be initially in one or two zones; with progression of the severity all zones become involved. With ischemia due to obstruction of circulation to an acinus, the hepatocytes in zone 1 are usually spared, and only with worsening of the lesion does the pathology progress to involve all three zones. Pathology in zones 2 and 3 may be severe enough to reduce sinusoidal blood flow in zone 1 so that the ischemia may result in necrosis throughout the acinus.

Piecemeal necrosis describes destruction of hepatocytes at their junction with connective tissue of the portal triads or septa that have formed. Periportal (zone 1) piecemeal necrosis is found with chronic active hepatitis, primary biliary cirrhosis, and hepatic cirrhosis. Substantial infiltration of inflammatory cells can accompany piecemeal necrosis.

Necrosis of sinusoidal lining cells can be seen with necrosis of adjacent hepatocytes. Necrosis of bile duct epithelium is usually associated with inflammation of the portal areas.

Necrosis of hepatocytes results in an inflammatory-cell reaction. Necrosis causes nuclear changes (pyknosis, karyor-

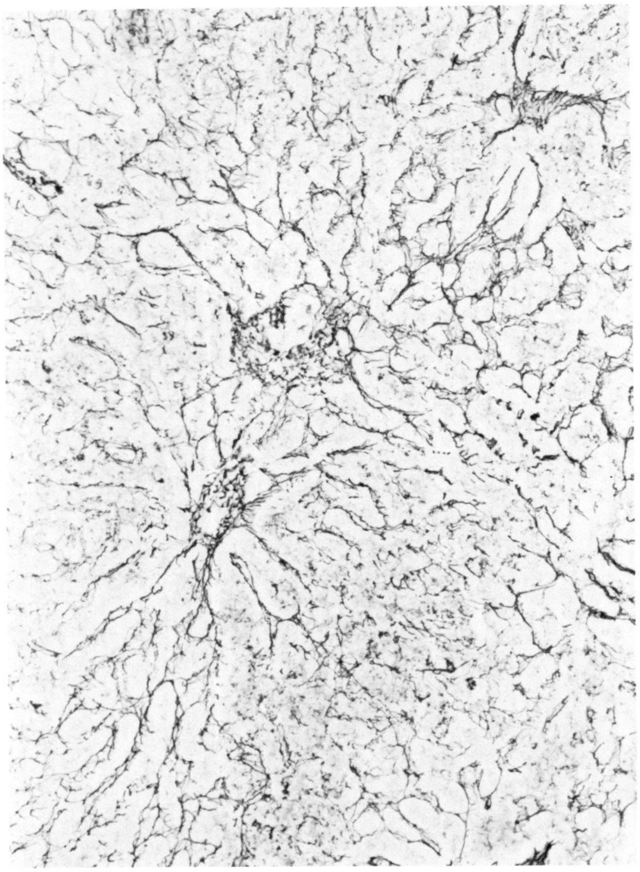

Figure 31-4c. Reticulin stain shows collapse of structural framework of lobules that can accompany hepatic necrosis.

rhexis, and karyolysis) and fragmentation of cytoplasm. Mononuclear cells derived from Kupffer cells phagocytize the cellular remains. Inflammatory cells, polymorphonuclear leukocytes, lymphocytes, and plasma cells infiltrate the area. Foci of neutrophils are commonly found in surgical biopsies and are thought to represent the effects of hypotension and its many ramifications. They may also be a finding in percutaneous biopsies believed to reflect a normal liver.[6] Increased numbers of neutrophils in sinusoids are found with a circulating neutrophilia and may not reflect hepatic disease or damage. Increased eosinophils in sinusoids may be related to either eosinophilia or an immune response to antigenic substances reaching the liver. Neutrophils appear in the portal triads and parenchyma with infection, but also with problems such as drug toxicity and bile duct obstruction. Because of this it is not possible to diagnose hepatitis as due to bacterial infection from neutrophil infiltrations found on biopsy.

CHOLESTASIS

Bile pigments are usually recognized in livers with cholestasis and jaundice. Recognition is easiest when plugs or thrombi of bile are found in bile canaliculi (Figure 31-5) which is a rather consistent finding with biliary obstruction. Bile pigments can also accumulate in hepatocytes and Kupffer cells, although special stains are needed to readily differentiate them from other pigments, such as lipofuscin (Figure 31-5). Accumulated bile pigments in hepatocytes without bile thrombi may be seen with periportal cholestasis caused by primary biliary cirrhosis. Accumulation of bile is seen initially in zone 3 hepatocytes, bile

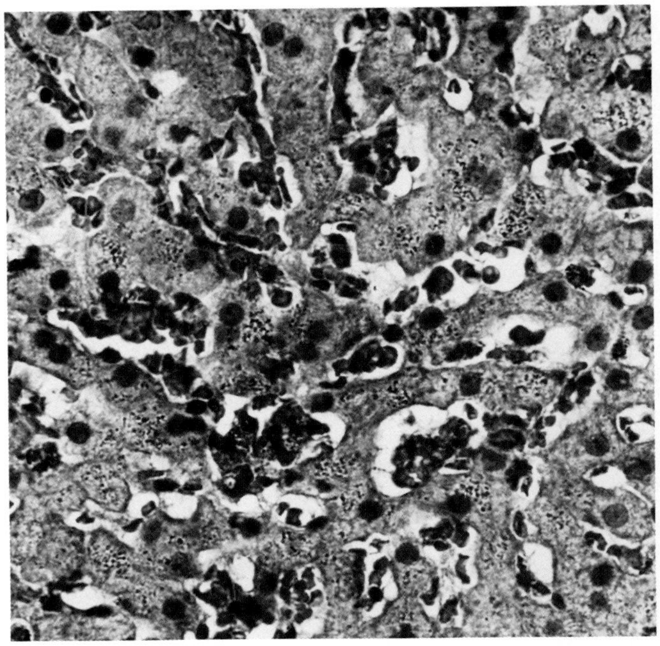

A

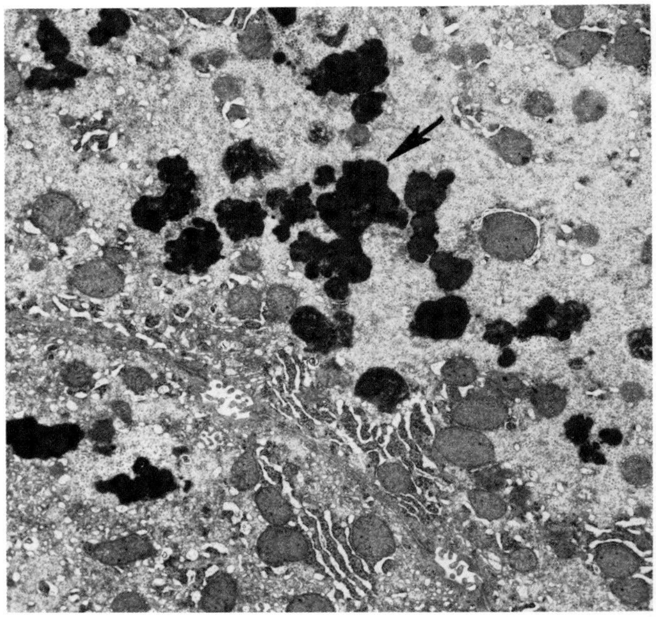

B

Figure 31-5. a) Photomicrograph of liver biopsy showing marked accumulation of a granular pigment within hepatocytes. Pigment could be hemosiderin, bile or lipofuscin. b) Electron micrograph shows granules magnified X5900. This information with results of special staining revealed granules to contain lipofuscin.

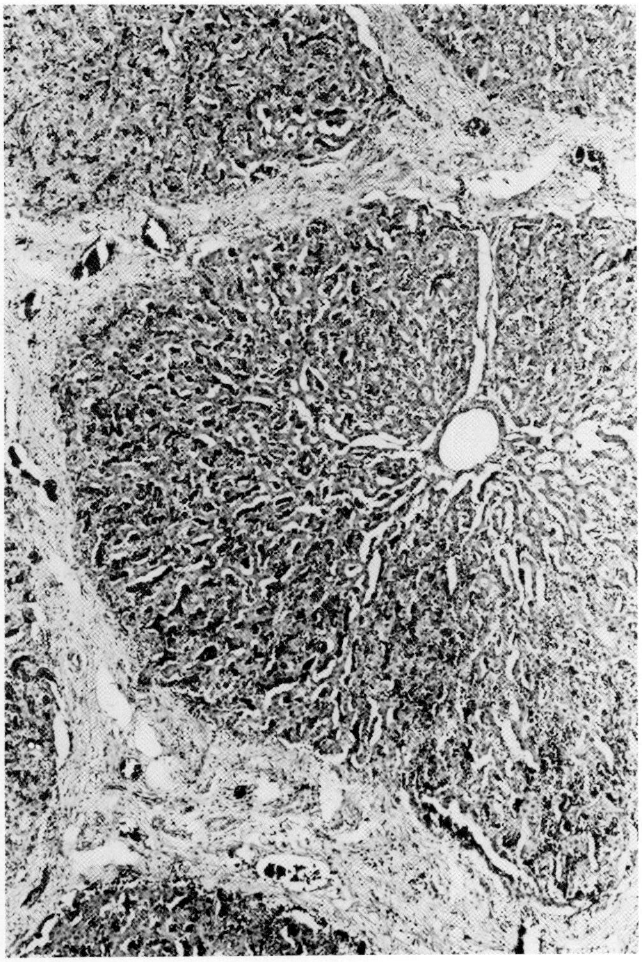

c

Figure 31-5. c) Necropsy specimen from dog with biliary cirrhosis showing bile plugs in both larger bile ducts and biliary canaliculi.

canaliculi, and Kupffer cells regardless of the cause. Intrahepatic zone 3 cholestasis is a minimal histological change seen with icterus. Bile pigments may tend to accumulate there initially because the zone 3 cells function at lower oxygen tension than the other zones; changes in oxygen availability might affect the bile acid independent flow of bile that is most important for bile secretion in zone 3. That zone is the important site for the metabolism of many drugs and toxins that may compete with bile secretion for energy. Active ongoing bile secretion by the bile acid-dependent process most important in zone 1 assures adequate secretion and flow of bile with its pigments; cholestasis doesn't develop until the pathology worsens.

Periportal or zone 1 cholestasis, an accumulation of pigment around portal tracts, is seen with chronic bile-duct obstruction, hepatic fibrosis, and primary biliary cirrhosis. Perivenular or zone 3 cholestasis, an accumulation of bile pigments around central veins, is seen primarily with acute diseases, such as acute hepatitis, systemic infections, acute obstruction of the main bile duct, hepatic lipidosis, and drug-induced cholestasis. With chronicity and progression of pathology, periportal or zone 1 cells show evidence of cholestasis. Periportal hepatocytes show ballooning, and their cytoplasm becomes granular and on special stains show increased copper. These changes are thought to result from the detergent effect of bile acids accumulating in those cells with the highest rate of bile acid transport. Bile canaliculi dilate with a diminution and disappearance of their microvilli, another change that can be attributed solely to bile acids. With cholestasis of greater duration, pigment-laden macrophages and mononuclear cells are found in acini with cholestasis. With persistence of cholestasis, terminal branches of the intrahepatic biliary system proliferate with bile salts as the suspected cause. Newly formed bile ductules may form no communications for draining bile and become another factor resulting in biliary obstruction. Bile leaks from obstructed ducts into the periportal area, causing edema and infiltration by neutrophils. Finding these cells does not necessarily denote a bacterial cholangitis. The ductular proliferation and inflammatory response stimulate fibroplasia that can lead to periportal fibrosis or cirrhosis.

Cholangitis, inflammation of bile ducts, is usually associated with involvement of parenchymal cells to result in cholangio-hepatitis. Cholangitis and cholangio-hepatitis can be caused by bacterial agents, usually enteric organisms. Infection is possible with cessation of bile flow due to obstruction or disease of the biliary system. Bacteria carried to the liver by the blood are cleared in the biliary secretions; bile flow stasis can lead to infection. Infection is also possible by organisms ascending from the intestine through the bile duct. That is possible when pre-existing disease causes stasis of bile flow. Complete stasis of bile flow by bile duct obstruction in experimental animals results in bacteria populating the liver, which provides a rationale for antibiotic therapy in patients with that kind of problem. Periportal inflammation fibrosis can be produced by intraportal injections of killed nonpathogenic enteric bacteria. Some of the pathology in the portal areas may begin from such an insult, especially in animals with chronic intestinal disease where increased amounts of macromolecules are being absorbed.

Many diseases cause pathology in bile ducts as an event that follows damage or disruption of function in hepatocytes. The cholestasis that follows causes further damage. An extrahepatic problem causing complete obstruction of the bile duct produces cholestasis found with tumors and inflammatory processes in the pancreas and around the bile duct. Such an obstruction will eventually produce severe pathology in the liver. Early after obstruction, zone 3 cholestasis appears, followed by bile duct dilation and edema with inflammatory cell infiltration of portal areas. Neutrophil infiltration accompanies proliferation of bile ducts in the margins of portal areas. Within two to three months most dogs with bile duct obstruction have distortion of normal liver architecture. Fibrosis develops in portal and perivenular areas. Broadening of portal fibrosis leads to bridging of portal areas and nodule formation. Central veins also show dilation, congestion, necrosis and distortion with histiocyte infiltration; zone 3 hepatocytes have acute inflammatory changes. These changes develop from a combination of increased hydrostatic pressure in the biliary system and the toxic effects of high bile salt concentrations. These changes represent a model for cirrhosis that is used to study portal hypertension and ascites formation seen with cirrhosis due to other causes.

HEPATIC STORAGE ABNORMALITIES

Liver cells can accumulate excessive amounts of pigments, metals, nutrients, and debris from cell destruction. Lipofuscin, a brown pigment containing some fatty material, is normally found in small amounts in primarily perivenular hepatocytes. The pigment is a breakdown product of lysosomal material, reflecting cell activity, and becomes more abundant with time. Lipofuscin can increase with prolonged administration of some drugs and chronic passive congestion. With increased production, lipofuscin also accumulates in Kupffer cells.

Hemosiderin, an iron bearing pigment, accumulates in hepatocytes and Kupffer cells in iron overload problems such as excessive dietary intake, parenteral injections of iron, or blood transfusions in attempts to manage persistent anemias where there is no blood loss.

Copper storage is excessive in primary copper toxicosis and in any chronic cholestatic disease. Copper granules can resemble lipofuscin, but they have different patterns of appearance in acini. Copper is stored in lysosomes as in lipofuscin, but copper accumulates first and concentrates in periportal cells, whereas lipofuscin accumulates in perivenular hepatocytes. With hepatocyte necrosis, copper is taken up and stored by Kupffer cells.

Excess lipid storage is seen on light microscopy as small and large vesicles. Macrovesicules appear when one or several vacuoles occupy most of a hepatocyte, displacing the nucleus to the cell's periphery. Microvesicules are many small fat droplets that do not displace the nucleus. Macrovesicular lipidosis is seen with obesity, starvation, diabetes mellitus, and some drugs that do not affect any particular zone. Microvesicular lipidosis is associated with drug administration, toxic injury, and the effects of hypoxia. The distribution is uniform throughout the acinus except with tetracycline and circulatory problems causing hypoxia, where the lesion is perivenular. One specific lipid, vitamin A, is stored in perisinusoidal lipocytes (Ito cells); excess vitamin A intake can result in their hypertrophy.

Excessive levels of corticosteroids produce excess glycogen storage, which is usually severe enough to cause hepatomegaly. Excess glycogen is also found with storage diseases, problems rarely seen.

Increased protein content of hepatocytes has not been described as being due to storage diseases in small animals. Cell protein does increase with conditions that cause hypertrophy of the endoplasmic reticulum. Drugs such as phenobarbital induce such a hypertrophy that begins in zone 3 hepatocytes and can spread to other zones. Such cells are swollen and have a ground-glass or faintly vesiculated cytoplasm. Livers in such cases can be markedly enlarged.

Amyloid, a precipitate of protein and polysaccharide, can be deposited and accumulate in the extracellular spaces of the liver (Figure 31-6). The protein consists of abnormal globulins,and the sugar is a mucopolysaccharide. It is amorphous, eosinophilic, glassy, and hyaline-appearing.

Amyloid, by reactions similar to those of starch, is brown when stained with Lugol's solution and blue when subsequently treated with sulfuric acid. Renal is more common than hepatic amyloidosis in dogs,and most cases of hepatic amyloidosis have extensive renal deposits of amyloid. Amyloidosis is not severe enough to cause significant loss of hepatic function, and clinical signs usually develop from pathology in other organs.

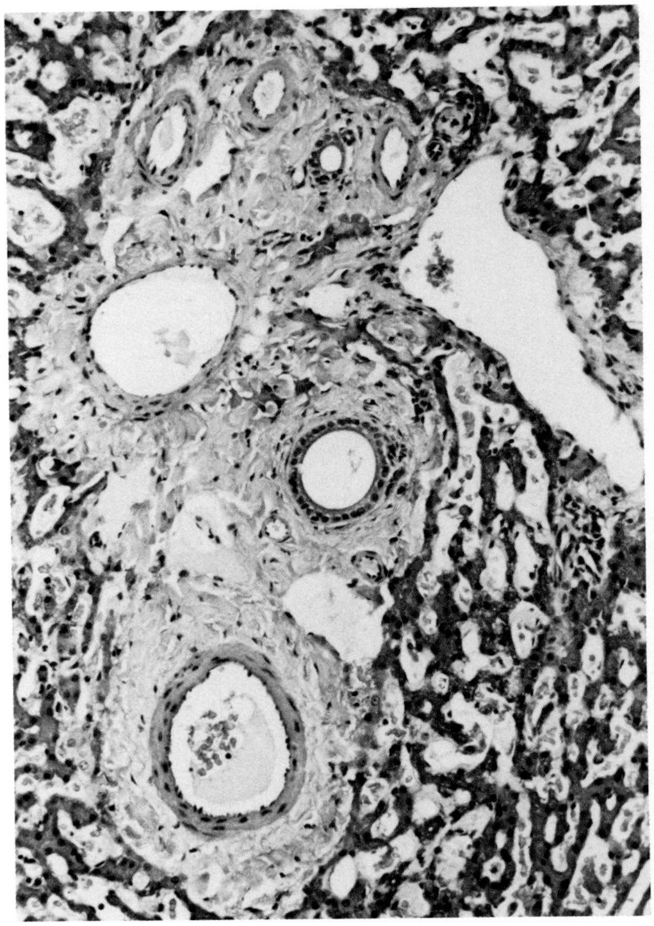

Figure 31-6. Hepatic amyloidosis. Deposition of amyloid has caused marked thickening of vessel walls with some deposition in portal stroma.

SEQUELAE OF HEPATOCELLULAR DAMAGE[1-3]

The liver has a remarkable ability to regenerate its mass after sizable losses by surgery or necrosis. Intracellular pathology can also be reversed, i.e. fatty infiltration of the liver is reversible on removal or correction of the cause. The liver responds to insults at best by regeneration of hepatocytes, with complete recovery, and at worst by diffuse fibrosis. The liver can also respond to insults by bile-duct hyperplasia.

Regeneration (Figure 31-7)[7]

With a loss of 10% or more of the liver, the deficit is corrected by cellular proliferation and hypertrophy. New hepatocytes arise from existing ones in which mitotic activity is normally minimal. Regeneration after resection of a liver lobe is not by regrowth of the lobe but by enlargement of the remaining lobes rather than regeneration that is a process of compensatory growth. Cellular proliferation occurs for biliary epithelial and Ito cells as well as for hepatocytes.

Hepatic regeneration after necrosis is relative, and, to be

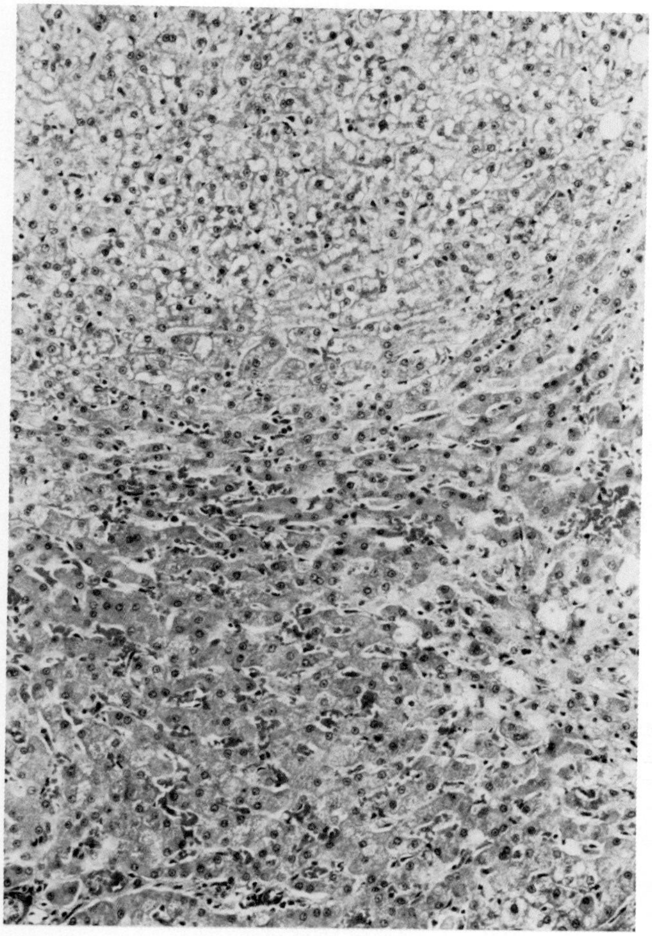

Figure 31-7a. Nodular hyperplasia. Boundary between nodule (upper half) and normal parenchyma (lower half) is marked by compressed hepatocytes in center.

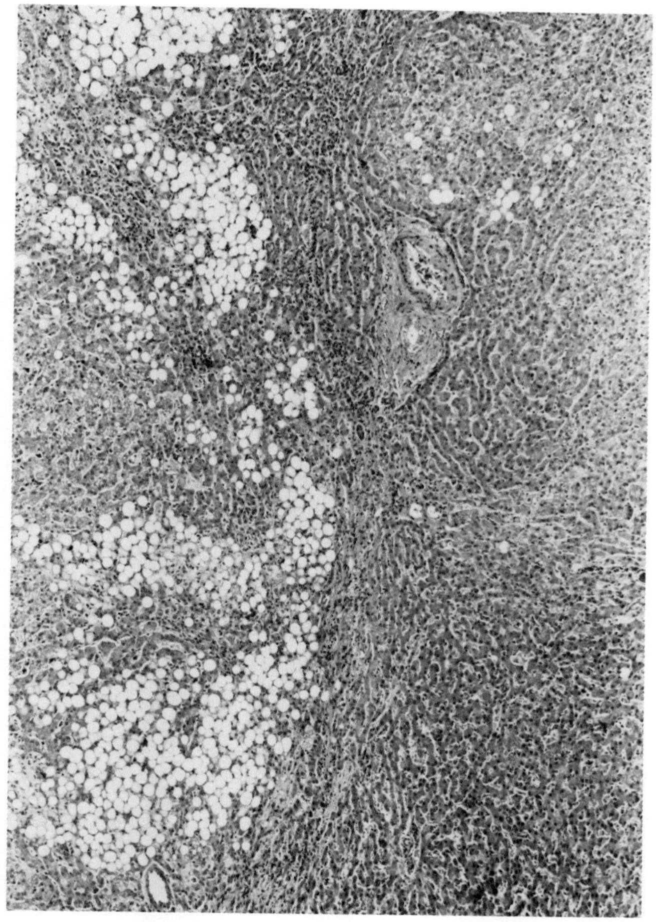

Figure 31-7b. Nodular hyperplasia. Nodules in left half show fatty changes.

complete, circulation must be adequate to each part of the lobule, free drainage of bile must exist, the lobule must be architecturally normal, and regenerating cells must have an intact fibrous and reticulin framework. Regeneration usually does not have the opportunity to progress under ideal circumstances, and newly formed plates of regenerated cells are often two cells thick instead of the normal single-cell thickness. Chronically diseased livers also respond by regeneration, but the constraints on normal regeneration may be so great that normal function remains lost.

Hepatic regeneration begins with a hypertrophy of hepatocytes lasting for 24 hours. Hyperplasia of hepatocytes follows, and shortly thereafter the proliferation involves non-parenchymal cells. Regeneration begins in zone 1 of the hepatic acinus, which may represent an area of germinal cells that eventually migrate to zone 3, where they would represent an older population of hepatocytes. On the other hand, regeneration can be focal anywhere in the liver or in zones 2 or 3 following loss of parenchymal cells. More evidence suggests that proximity to the efferent arterial blood supply is more important in stimulating regeneration. If that supply nourishes zone 3 hepatocytes before those of zone 1, regeneration begins in zone 3.

Hepatic regeneration beginning within 24 hours of cell loss is identified by increased synthesis of RNA and DNA in remaining normal hepatocytes.[8] The stimulus for regeneration is suggested to be humoral agents transmitted to remaining hepatocytes by the circulation or intercellular transport mechanisms. Regeneration of cells is also dependent on maintenance of circulation.

Humoral agents suggested to be responsible for regeneration include substances produced outside and carried by the portal circulation to the liver such as insulin, glucagon, and nutrients such as amino acids.[9] Epidermal growth factor, an albumin-bilirubin complex, glucocorticoids, and thyroxine also act directly to promote regeneration; catecholamines, calcitonin, parathormone, and other peptide hormones act indirectly on regeneration. Intrahepatic sources for promoters of regeneration include a peptide hepatocyte growth factor and unusual purine nucleotides.[10]

Adequate blood flow to remaining parenchymal tissues sustains hepatic regeneration, just as normal flow is essential for maintaining normal size.

Reducing total hepatic blood flow causes hepatic atrophy. A reduced portal blood flow in dogs with portasystemic shunts is associated with hepatic atrophy. The degree of atrophy is proportional to the reduction in hepatic portal blood flow.

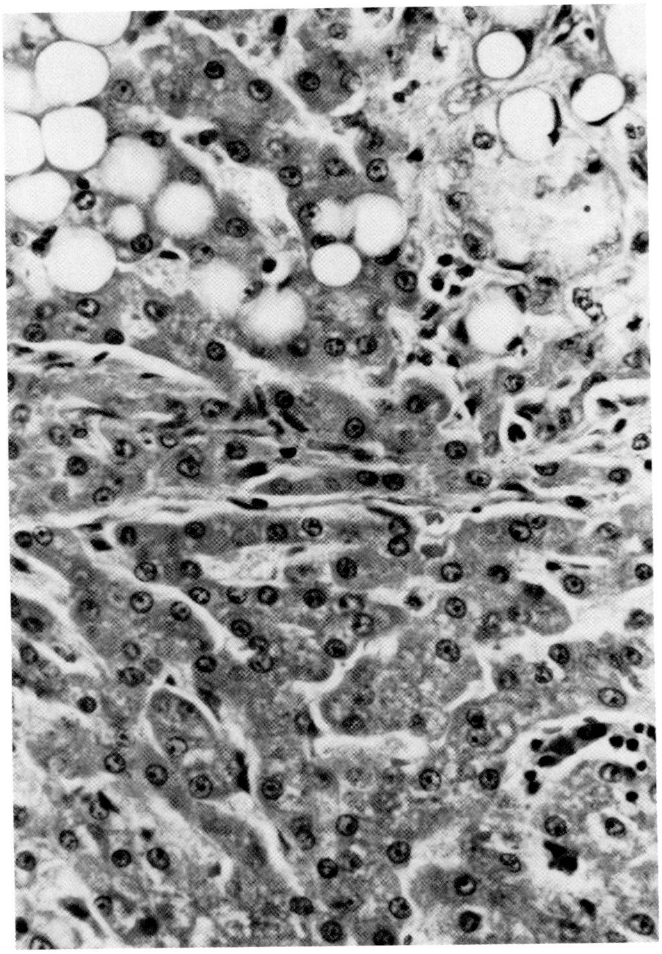

Figure 31-7c. Nodular hyperplasia. Hepatocytes in center of field are compressed between nodule in upper half and normal hepatic parenchyma below.

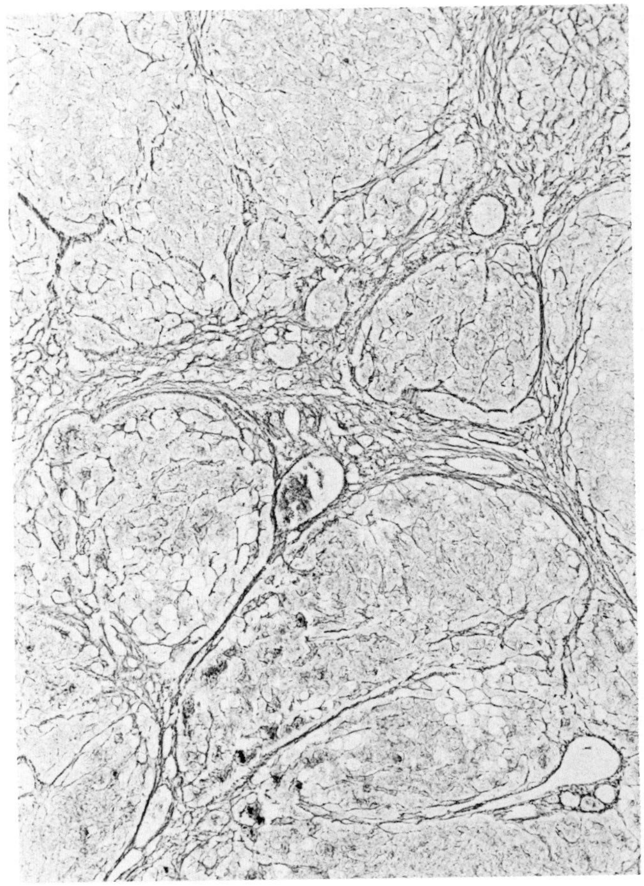

Figure 31-7d. Cirrhosis. Reticulin stain is sometimes used to differentiate nodular hyperplasia (no fibrotic changes) from cirrhosis shown here.

Maintenance of normal liver size is determined by the volume of blood delivered to the liver and by nutrients and hormones delivered from the alimentary tract. Experiments show the relative importance of each. Portacaval shunts cause a loss of 30% of hepatic size, and the size is largely regained when portacaval transposition is added.[11] In this case, normal hepatic volume flow of blood is returned via flow in the caudal vena cava, which contains no hormones or nutrients from the alimentary tract.

Hepatic atrophy in animals with portacaval shunts is prevented by infusing the hepatic portal circulation with arterial blood, whereupon hepatic size remains normal.[12,13] In these experimental models the liver receives only part of the humoral factors delivered in the portal circulation. Pancreatic hormones, insulin and glucagon, are important hepatotrophic factors, although more than likely they play a permissive role. If insulin were a single important factor, hepatic atrophy would be a consistent feature of diabetes mellitus. When insulin is infused into the hepatic portal circulation of dogs with portacaval shunts, the atrophic changes that normally develop are only half as great.[14] Nutrients absorbed from the intestine are also important in maintaining liver size, which decreases during starvation. In summary, normal liver size is maintained and regeneration is sustained by delivery of a normal volume of blood to the liver, by hormones, and by a normal supply of nutrients.

Regenerative changes in the liver sometimes take the form of nodular regenerative hyperplasia, which is characterized by nodules of regenerative hepatocytes diffusely distributed through the liver; the nodules compress and cause atrophy of adjacent hepatic parenchyma; fibrosis is not a feature in or between nodules, which distinguishes it from cirrhosis. The nodules consist of hepatocytes arranged in plates more than one cell thick, and a periportal accentuation may be seen. Hepatomegaly may be evident. The cause and pathogenesis is unknown. It has been associated with drugs, toxins, autoimmune diseases, congestive heart failure, primary vascular diseases, hematological diseases, and chronic inflammatory bowel disease. The nodules may represent a hyperplastic response to an insult of different varieties combined with an alteration in hepatic circulation of blood. Lesions obliterating the portal vein and portacaval shunting of blood combined with partial hepatectomy can result in the development of nodular regenerative hyperplasia. Animals with diffuse nodular regenerative hyperplasia can present signs of severe hepatic insufficiency such as icterus, ascites, and hepatic encephalopathy. In such cases, although the pathology does not appear very striking because hepatocytes seem normal, acinar function is compromised primarily because circulation is not normal in the nodules; that may be evident in manifestations of portal hypertension.

Regenerative nodules are found more frequently focally rather than diffusely distributed in the liver. They appear in dogs after about 6 years of age as focal, usually multiple, lesions that are macroscopically visible and on initial examination appear to be tumors. Nodule incidence is reported to be 15% to 60% of all older dogs, the frequency increasing with age.[15] Focal nodules may be a frequent lesion found with congestive heart failure, and in some cases may be related to long-term drug administration. Histological features are similar to diffuse nodular regenerative hyperplasia with thickened hepatocyte plates, a single prominent portal tract and compression of hepatocytes surrounding the nodule. In addition the population of Ito cells or lipocytes, containing lipid with a high vitamin A content, increases more than tenfold. They also hypertrophy, the two changes result in increased numbers of Ito cells protruding into the sinusoidal lumen and obstructing blood flow. Hypertrophy is due to increased deposition of lipids. The nodules also contain lipogranulomata with accumulations of ceroid pigment, which is an oxidation product of unsaturated lipid. Disturbances in portal or sinusoidal blood flow may be most important in the pathogenesis of focal regenerative nodules.[16] Focal nodules have arterial branches that are larger than normally found in the portal area. That suggests nodules are supplied with a greater flow of arterial blood, something that could be the stimulus for growth of acini benefiting from that circulation. Chronic reduction of portal flow to the acini would be a stimulus for increased arterial flow, and a total flow for that region compared to an adjacent region may be a reason for hyperplasia in one area and not in another.

Biliary Hyperplasia[1]

Hyperplasia of bile ducts is another way in which the liver can respond to injury (Figure 31-8). These changes in small interlobular bile ducts and the intralobular cholangioles can develop independently of events in the hepatocytes. Bile-duct hyperplasia may occur with only a minimal fibrosis necessary to provide structure for new ducts. Thus, changes can occur without affecting other structures in portal triads. When the cause of hyperplasia is removed, excess bile ducts can disappear. Cholangiolar proliferation without other changes in portal triads or parenchymal cells occurs in biliary obstruction and some toxicities. The proliferation of bile ducts can be stimulated by deoxycholate and lithocholate, normal constituents of bile.[17] Increased hydrostatic pressure in obstructed ducts is also important for hyperplasia. Biliary hyperplasia can accompany

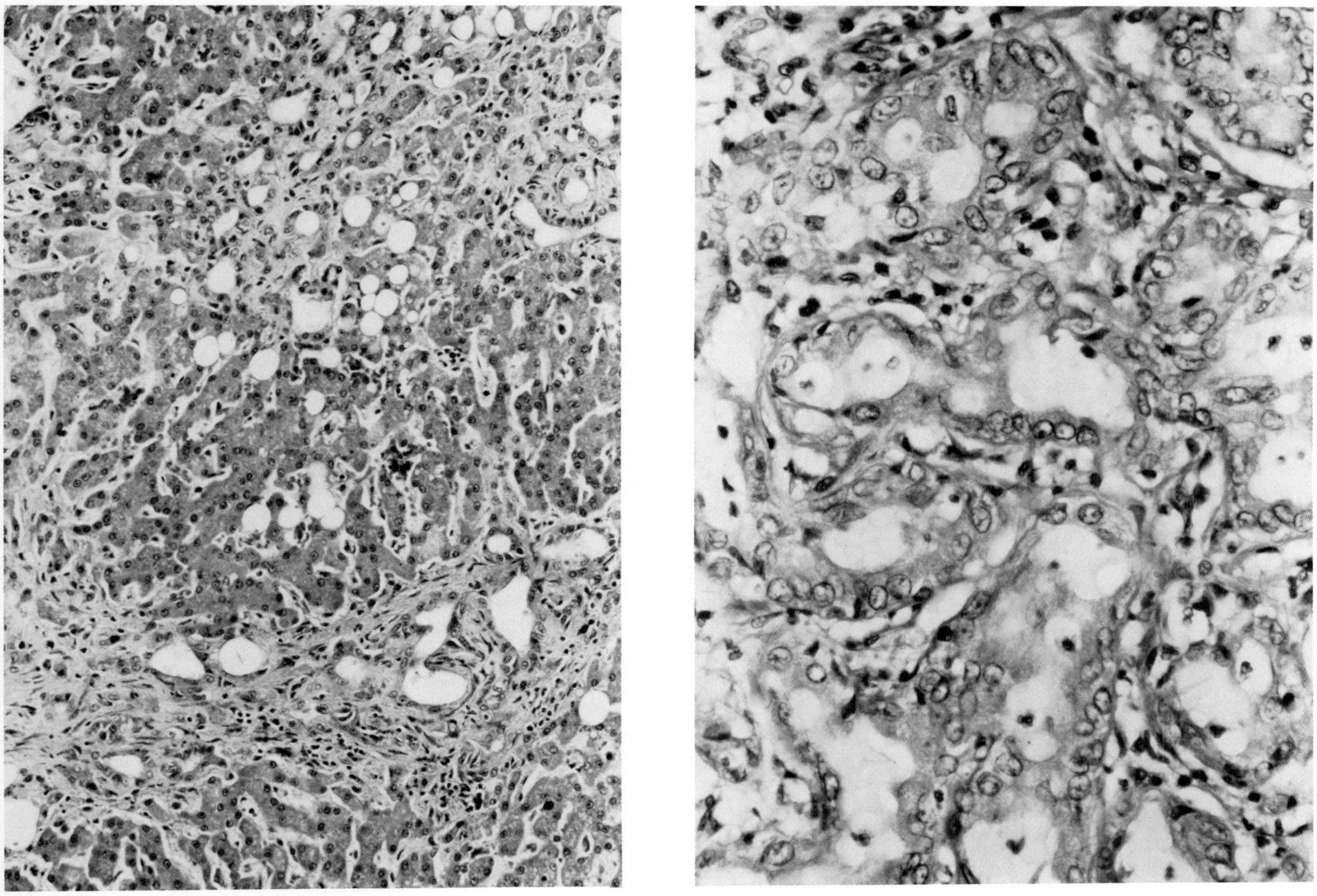

A B

Figure 31-8. a) Bile duct hyperplasia accompanies fibrosis as a response to hepatic injury. Slight lipidosis is evident. b) Marked bile duct hyperplasia.

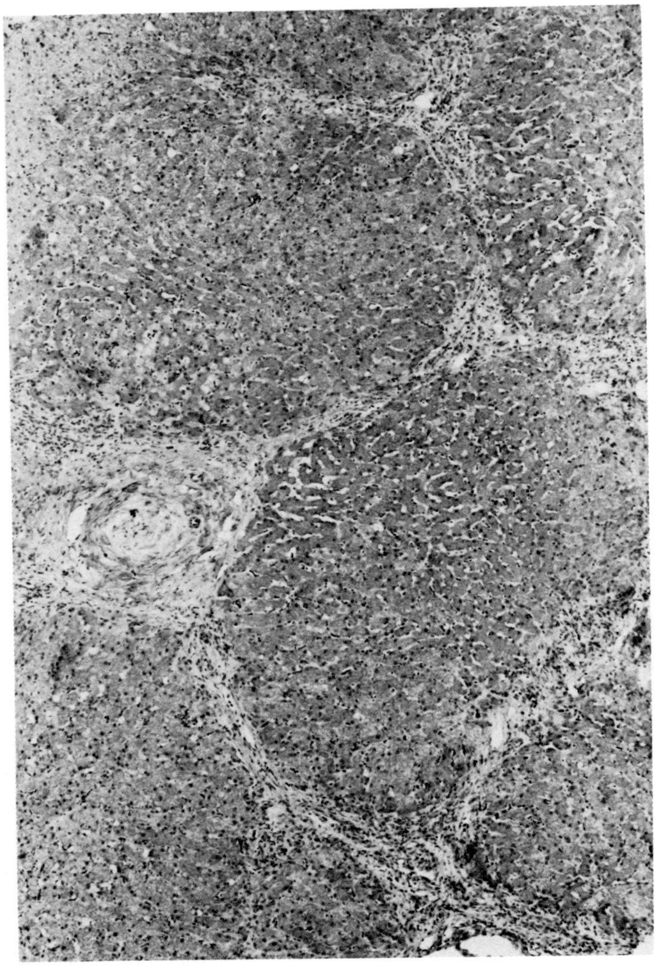

Figure 31-9a. Biliary cirrhosis. Cholangitis in cat progressing to biliary cirrhosis. Moderate amount of inflammation. Lesions caused moderate icterus which improved with corticosteroid therapy.

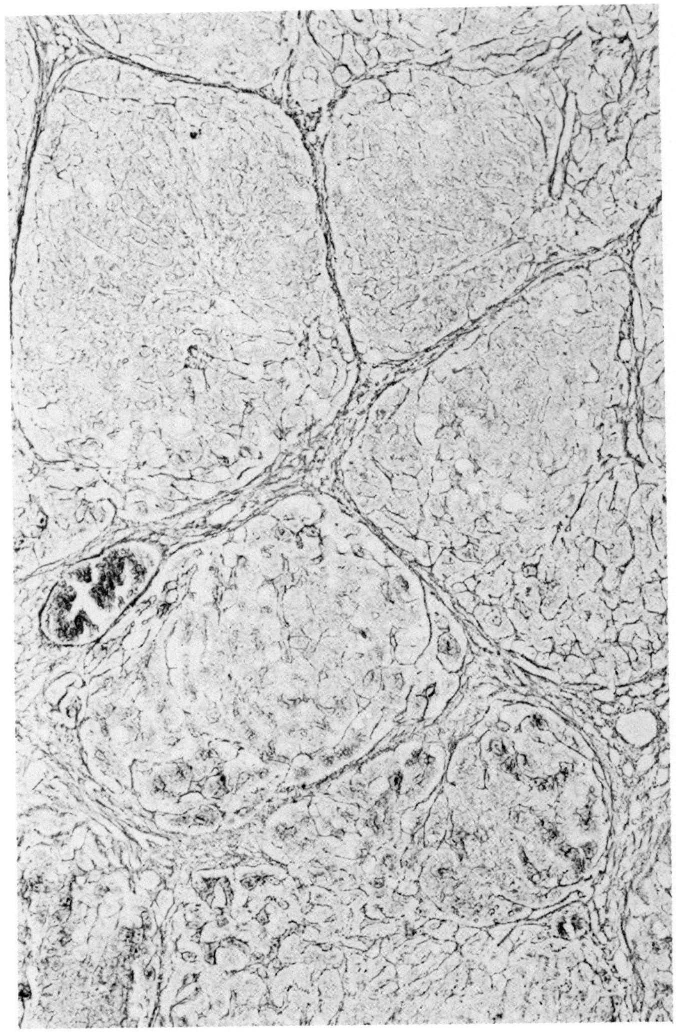

Figure 31-9b. Reticulin stain showing fibrosis developing with biliary cirrhosis in a dog.

fibrosis. Biliary hyperplasia may be an attempt to replace parenchymal cells that cannot be regenerated.

Fibrosis and Cirrhosis[1,3,18-21]

Fibrosis can be another sequel to hepatic parenchymal damage and inflammation (Figure 31-9). Fibrosis is the increased accumulation of collagen and other elements of extracellular connective tissue. Fibrosis may be capsular or subcapsular involving the liver capsule. It may be focal, developing following the healing of abscesses or granulomas. Fibrosis can be diffuse with or without destroying the normal hepatic architecture. Diffuse fibrosis can be seen in zone 3 around central veins with chronic congestive heart failure.

Fibrosis develops around central veins when pericentral or perivenular necrosis is not followed by regeneration, following prolonged passive congestion. With increased severity, bands of fibrosis radiate from zone 3 perivenular areas, bisecting parenchymal tissue out to the periphery. When these septa reach portal triads, anastomotic blood vessels develop between portal and hepatic veins. These vessels bypassing parenchymal cells form internal Eck-type fistulas.

Fibrosis can also develop in zone 1 at the periphery of acini from chronic bile-duct obstruction with bile stasis and low-grade cholangitis or cholangiolitis. It is also stimulated by killed nonpathogenic enteric bacteria in the portal circulation. Hepatic connective tissue is most abundant in portal triads, and proliferates in response to inflammation, resulting in septa that separate portal vessels from parenchymal cells.

These septa can extend into acini, and, radiating from the periphery, they bisect acini down to central veins. Vascular shunts can also develop in these septa between portal and hepatic veins. Periportal fibrosis encroaches on adjacent parenchymal cells, and, by the pressure it exerts, hepatocyte degeneration is continued, further stimulating fibrosis. Inflammation is usually directly responsible for fibrosis following hepatocyte degeneration. Hepatocyte degeneration may also cause differences in tissue pressure throughout acini, creating planes of stress within acini and subsequent fissure formation. Connective tissue is suggested to be laid down in the fissures, eventually forming septa randomly within acini.

With extensive septa formation, hepatocytes attempt to

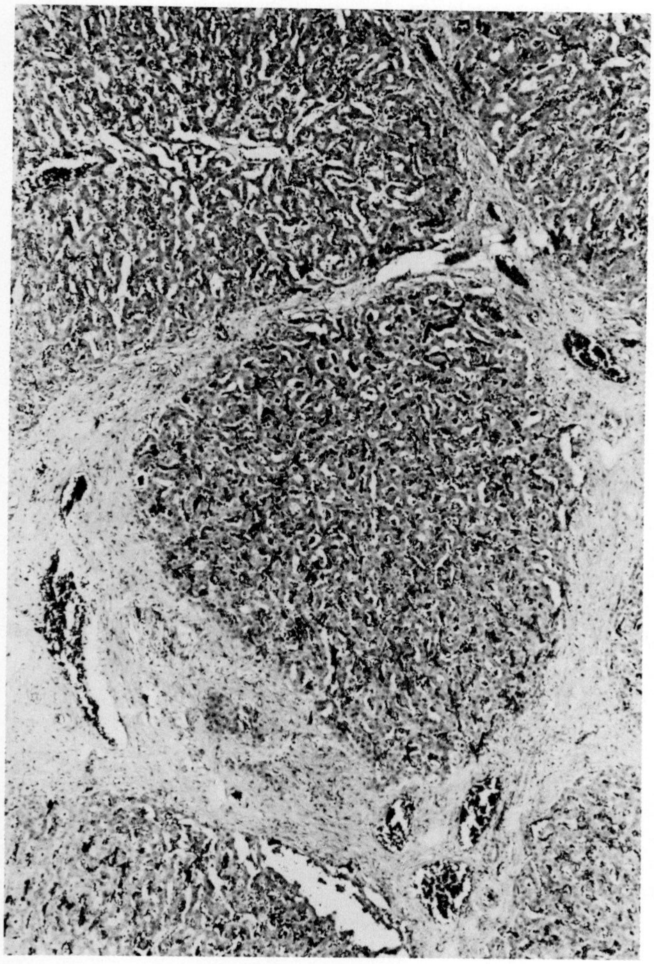

Figure 31-9c. Advanced biliary cirrhosis in a dog causing icterus. Was associated with a chronic colitis.

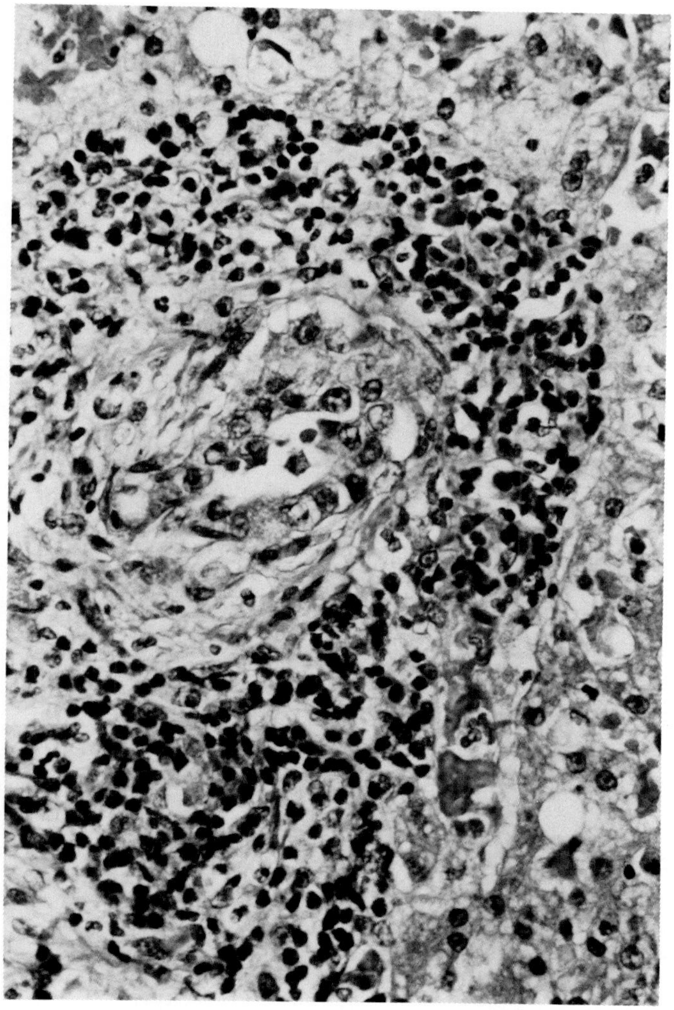

Figure 31-9d. Early changes in biliary cirrhosis include cholangiolitis where inflammation damages bile ducts. Inflammation causes bile ducts to disappear and fibrosis to appear.

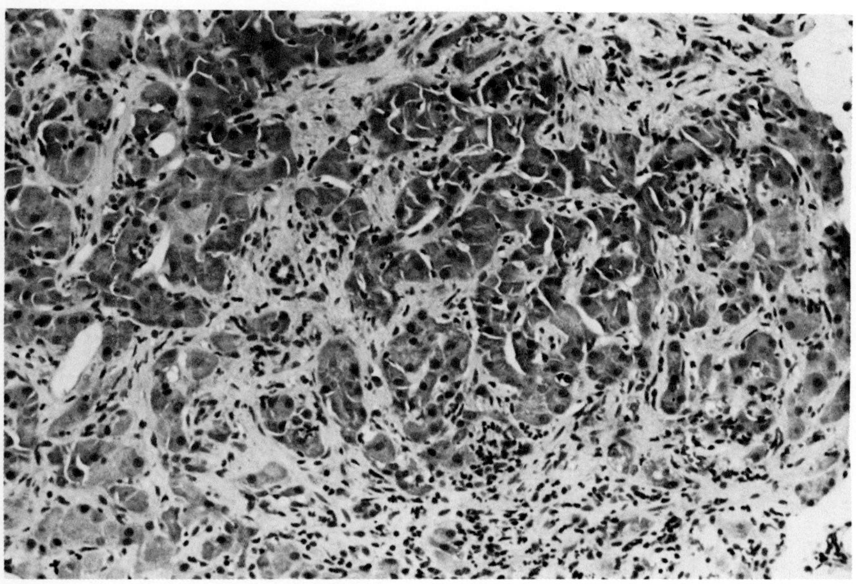

Figure 31-9e. Hepatic cirrhosis as a sequel to chronic active hepatitis. Inflammation is still evident.

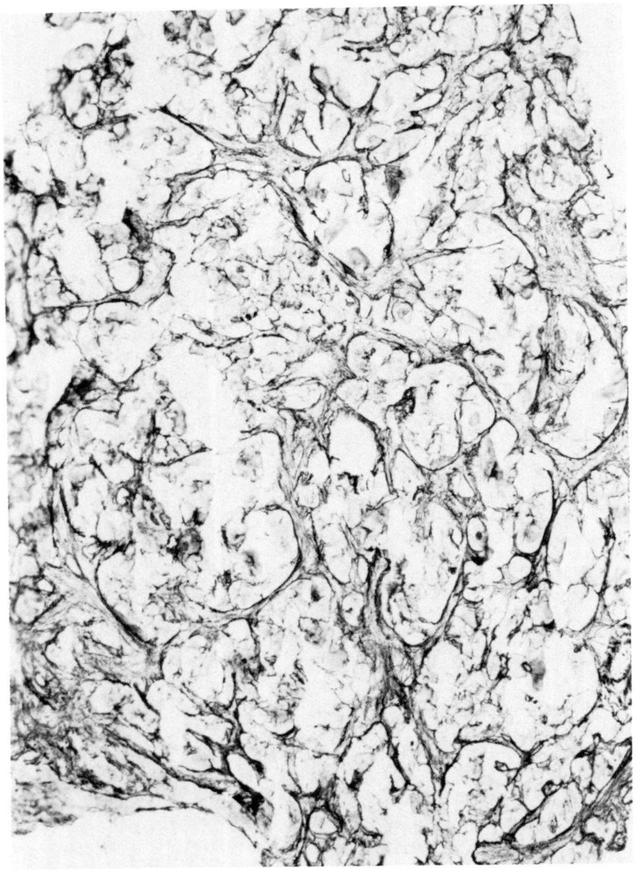

Figure 31-9f. Reticulin stain on same biopsy specimen shows extent of architecture-destroying fibrosis.

regenerate. Regenerating parenchymal cells enclosed in connective-tissue capsules cause the liver to appear nodular. Plates of hepatocytes formed in regenerative nodules are two cells thick. Regeneration of hepatocytes within fibrous capsules increases pressure in the nodules, thereby stimulating further fibrosis in the septa. Thus, regenerative nodule formation is characterized by ongoing division of hepatocytes and continued fibrosis of their encapsulating septa.

Regenerating nodules grow and displace adjacent normal hepatocytes, the degeneration of which further stimulates fibrosis of the encapsulating septa. Connections are not maintained in blood vessels and bile ducts between the nodules and the vessels of the original portal triads. The circulation can bypass many hepatocytes by portal to hepatic vein fistulas. Biliary drainage is also affected in regenerative nodules, and obstructive-type icterus can be seen. Diffuse fibrosis with distortion of normal architecture is cirrhosis. Cirrhosis is characterized by nodules of regenerative hepatocytes that have lost their normal relationship to the hepatic blood supply. Large nodules have impaired perfusion, and areas of intervening connective tissue can be richly perfused with blood by vascular shunts. The imbalance in circulation is more important than the amount of fibrosis. The hepatic insufficiency that develops may be associated with very little fibrosis. The compromised circulation to cirrhotic nodules makes their hepatocytes at greater risk to additional insults by drugs, toxins, ischemia, infections, and biliary obstruction.

Fibrosis can also follow parenchymal damage where all hepatocytes in acini are destroyed and the supporting framework collapses. Postnecrotic fibrosis is produced by fibroplasia in the preexisting and collapsed stroma. This fibrosis appears as broad, irregular bands of scar tissue between lobules of surviving hepatic tissue. Some of that fibrosis represents collapsed and condensed stroma.

Fibrosis develops from increased production of fibronectin,

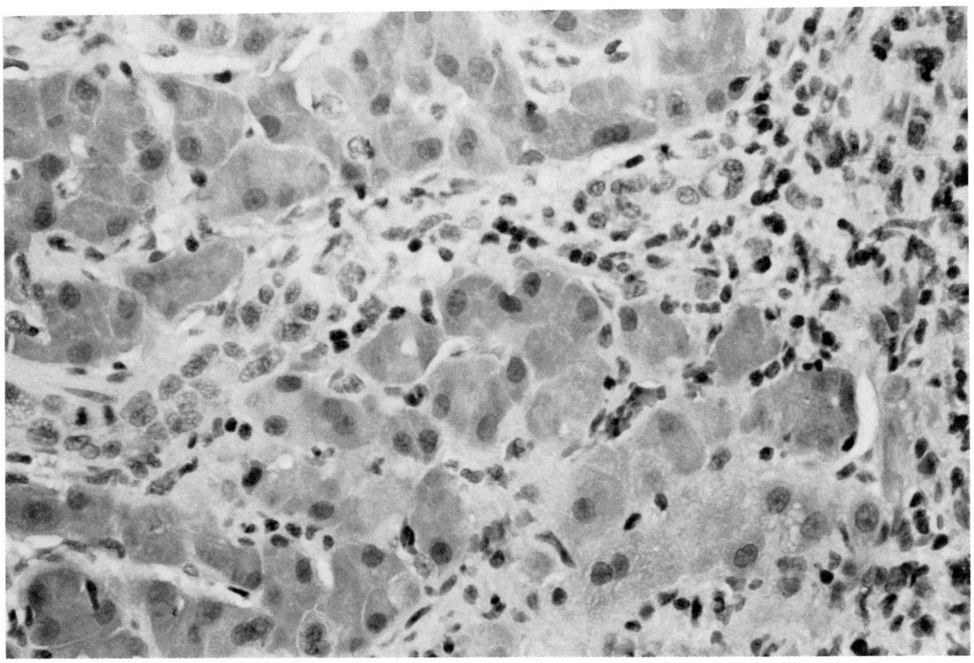

Figure 31-9g. Hepatic cirrhosis. Inflammation and fibrosis beginning in portal area separates vessels from parenchymal cells. This biopsy shows the process extending from the portal area through the lobule to the central vein. Vessels in these dissecting septa can shunt blood from the portal area to central veins thereby bypassing parenchymal cells.

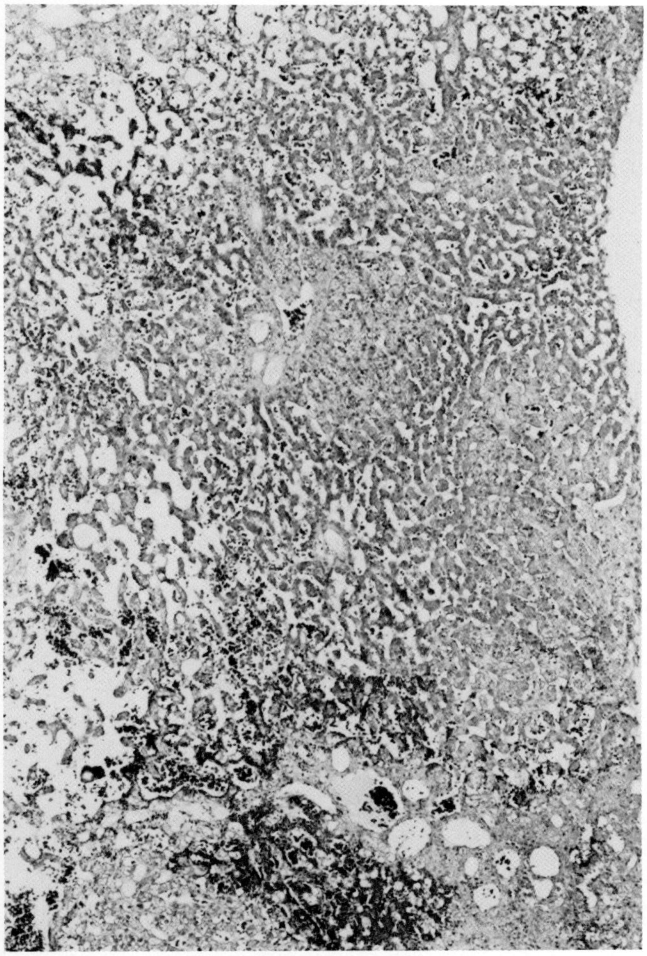

Figure 31-10a. Biopsy of liver from a dog with ascites due to obstruction of blood flow in hepatic vein (Budd Chiari syndrome). The major change is severe congestion resulting in extreme dilation of sinusoids.

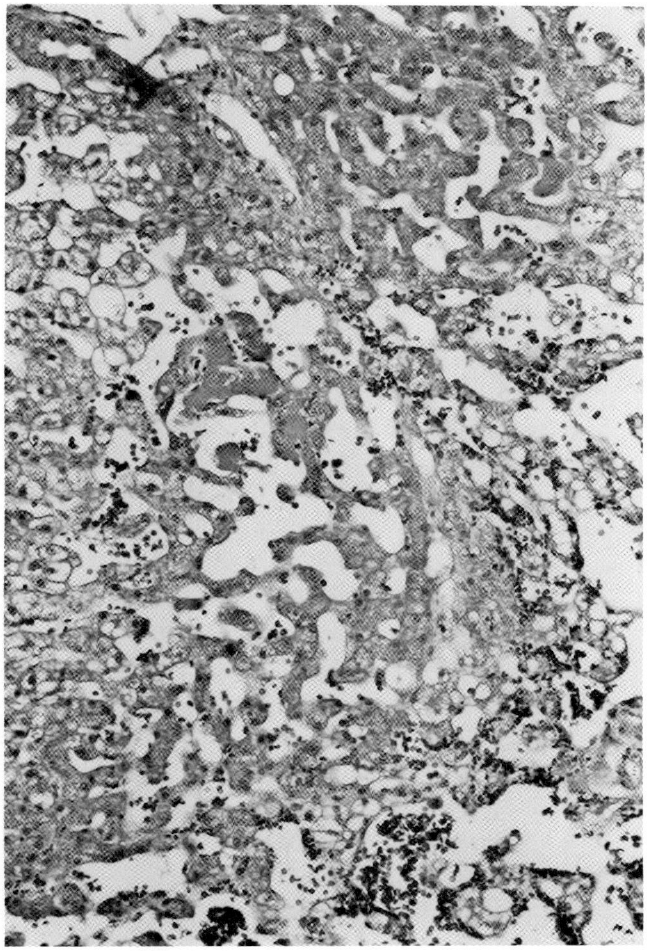

Figure 31-10b. Higher magnification of representative changes found in (a).

laminin, proteoglycans, and five types of collagen by fibroblasts. Fibroblasts are seldom seen in normal livers or under conditions of normal regeneration. The fibroblasts seen during fibrosis are the result of transformation from the lipocytes (Ito cells) that normally store lipids and vitamin A. These cells may also be the origin of myofibroblasts seen with liver injury and fibrosis. Some of the proteins essential to fibrosis are also produced by hepatocytes. Fibroblast activity is stimulated by peptides and biogenic amines produced by inflammatory or Kupffer cells; the products include fibronectin, interleukin-1, histamine, and serotonin. Transforming growth factor ß, a product of hematopoietic cells, and platelet-derived growth factor also promote fibroblast activity and collagen formation. The liver has the ability to degrade collagen as well as to form it. Degradation is due to collagenases, which can show decreased activity with some forms of experimental cirrhosis.

Management of hepatic fibrosis is directed at inhibiting its formation. Collagen polymerization is inhibited by d-penicillamine due to its binding copper, an element essential for the action of lysyl oxidase, the polymerizing enzyme. Collagen release from fibroblasts is inhibited by colchicine, but the drug's effect is short-lasting. Corticosteroids inhibit collagen formation by reducing the inflammatory process that promotes fibrosis. Collagen production is also reduced by chemicals that increase intracellular cAMP levels; B-adrenergic agonists and prostaglandins have that ability. The control of collagenase activity and collagen degradation is not well understood; no therapeutic agents are available for stimulating collagenase activity.

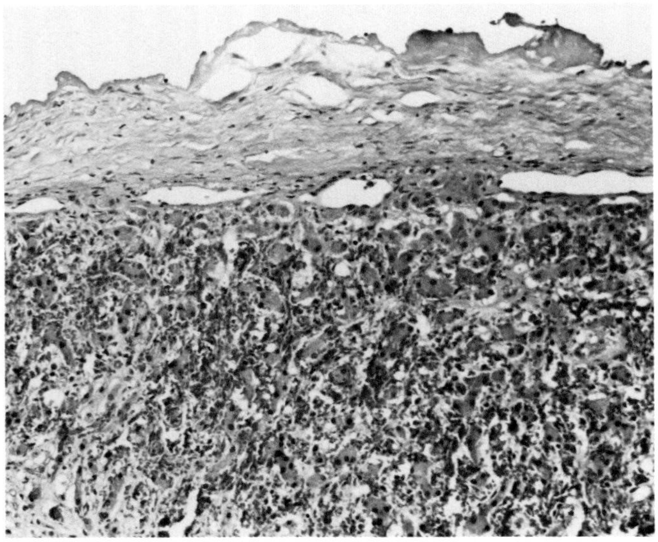

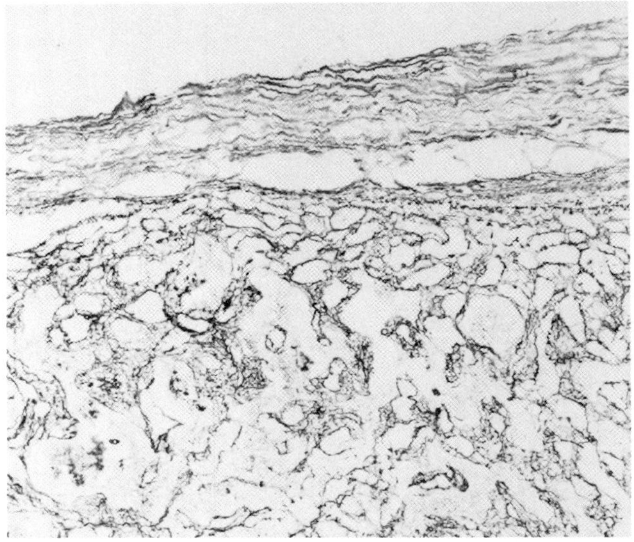

Figure 31-10c. Hepatic changes due to impaired hepatic circulation caused by chronic cardiac disease are shown in biopsy specimen from dog with ascites. The changes shown here include varying degrees of congestion, thickening of hepatic capsule, dilation of lymphatics and fibrosis. Other changes such as centrolobular lipidosis and degeneration were found elsewhere in the biopsy. Lymph flow increases to return extracellular fluid that cannot return at normal rates through the hepatic vein. Reticulin stained preparation shows increased fibrous tissue.

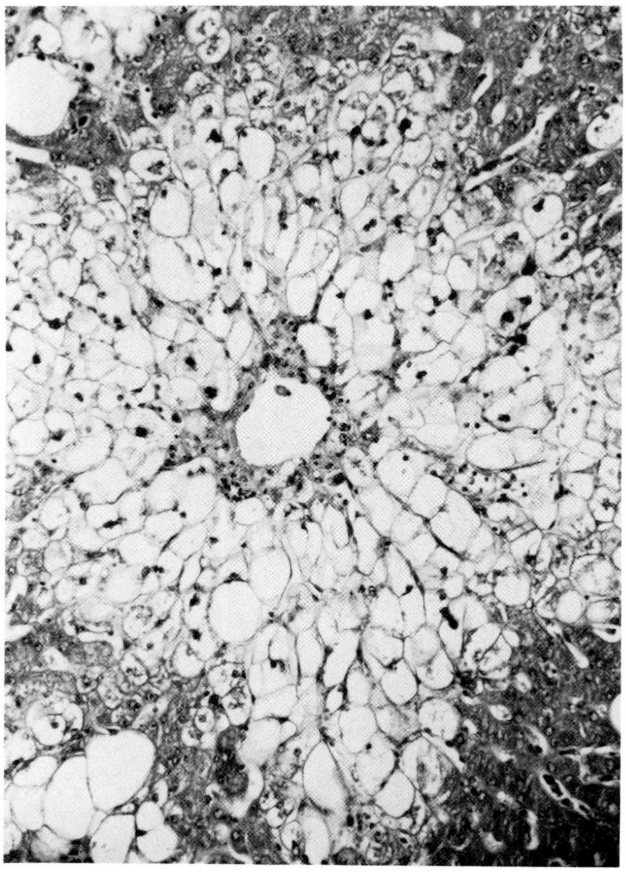

Figure 31-10d. Circulatory failure in a dog caused centrolobular degeneration of hepatocytes that includes necrosis adjacent to central vein and widespread fatty and steroid changes.

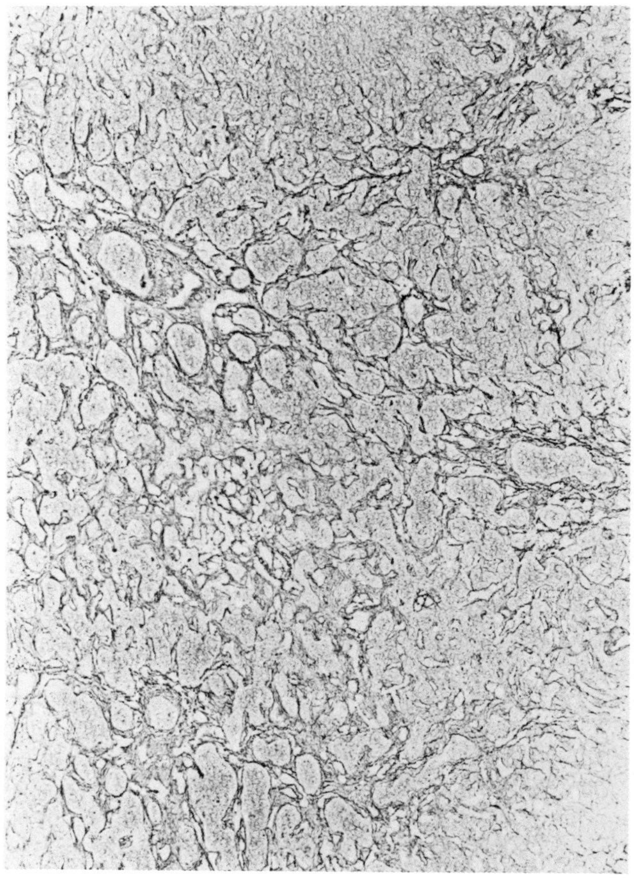

Figure 31-10e. Reticulin stained biopsy specimen from dog with chronic cardiac failure shows increased fibrous tissue (cardiac cirrhosis).

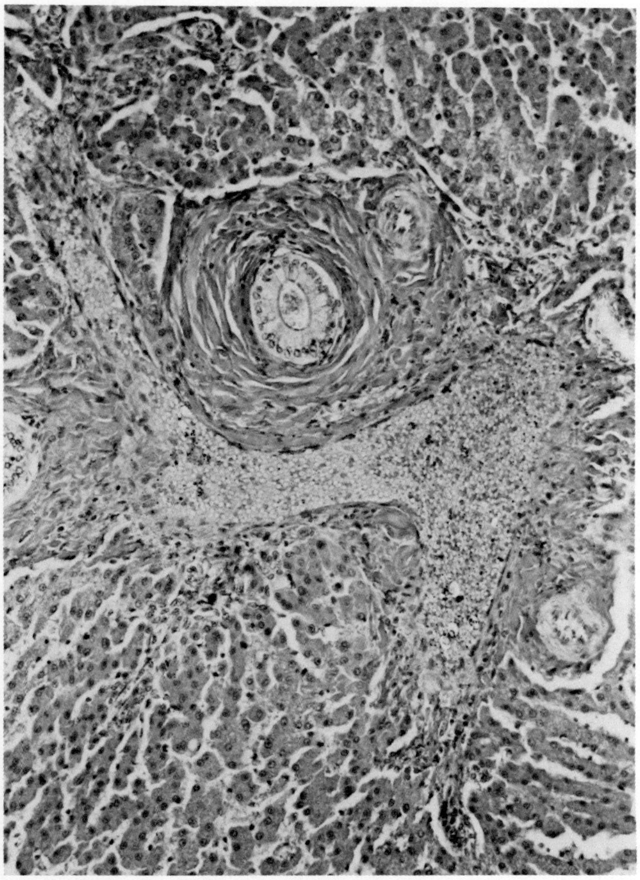

Figure 31-10f. Hepatoportal sclerosis. Portal area from a dog with unexplained chronic ascites associated with portal hypertension. Changes include portal fibrosis and fibrous thickening of dilated portal veins. In other portal areas smaller branches of portal veins were difficult to identify because of thickening and obliteration of the lumen. Organized and recanalized thrombi were found in some larger veins (not shown). Diagnostic lesions were found on wedge biopsy but not on needle biopsy. Cause of lesions is unknown. There is no known treatment.

REFERENCES

1. Jubb, K.V.F. and Kennedy, P.C.: Pathology of domestic animals. Academic Press, New York, 1985.
2. Rappaport, A.M.: Anatomic considerations. In, Diseases of the Liver. Edited by L. Schiff. J.B. Lippincott, Philadelphia, 1-46, 1987.
3. MacSween, R.N.M, Anthony, P.P. and Scheuer, P.J.: Pathology of the Liver. Churchill Livingstone, New York, 1987.
4. Traber, P.G., Chianale, J. and Gumucio, J.J.: Physiologic significance and regulation of hepatocellular heterogeneity. Gastroenterology 95:1130-1143, 1988.
5. de la Monte, S.M., Arcidi, J.M., Moore, G.W. and Hutchins, G.M.: Midzonal necrosis as a pattern of hepatocellular injury after shock. Gastroenterology 86:627-631, 1984.
6. McDonald, G.S.A. and Courtney, M.G.: Operation-associated neutrophils in a percutaneous liver biopsy: effect of prior transjugular procedure. Histopathology 10:217-222, 1986.
7. Becker, F.F.: Regeneration. In, The Liver: Normal and Abnormal Functions. Part A. Edited by F.F. Becker. Marcel Dekker, New York. 69-83, 1974.
8. Fausto, N.: New perspectives on liver regeneration. Hepatology 6:326-327, 1986.
9. Leffert, H.L., Koch, K.S., Moran, T. and Rubalcava, B.: Hormonal control of rat liver regeneration. Gastroenterology 76:1470-1482, 1979.
10. Bissell, D.M.: Peculiar purine nucleotides and liver regeneration. Gastroenterology 89:914-916, 1985.
11. Benjamin, I.S., Ryan, C.J., McLay, A.L.C., Horne, C.H.W. and Blumgart, L.H.: The effects of portacaval shunting and portacaval transposition on serum IgG levels in the rat. Gastroenterology 70:661-664, 1976.
12. Adamsons, R.J., Arif, S., Babich, A., Butt, K., Lam, A. and Minkowitz, S.: Arterialization of the liver in combination with a portacaval shunt in the dog. Surg. Gynecol. Obstet. 140:594-600, 1975.
13. Pector, J.C., Verbeustel, S. and Lambilliotte, J.P.: Effect of portal arterialization on hepatic cytochrome P-450 in rats with portacaval shunt. Digestion 12:144-151, 1975.
14. Starzl, T.E., Porter, K.A. and Putnam, C.W.: Intraportal insulin protects from the liver injury of portacaval shunt in dogs. Lancet 2:1241-1242, 1975.
15. Fabry, A., Benjamin, S.A. and Angleton, G.M.: Nodular hyperplasia of the liver in the Beagle dog. Vet. Pathol. 19:109-119, 1982.
16. Wanless, I.R., Mawdsley, C. and Adams, R.: On the pathogenesis of focal nodular hyperplasia of the liver. Hepatology 5:1194-1200, 1985.
17. Bagheri, S.A., Bolt, M.G., Boyer, J.L. and Palmer, R.H.: Stimulation of thymidine incorporation in mouse liver and biliary tract epithelium by lithocholate and deoxycholate. Gastroenterology 74:188-192, 1978.
18. Schinella, R.A. and Becker, F.F.: Cirrhosis. In, The Liver: Normal and Abnormal Functions. Part B., Vol. 5. Edited by F.F. Becker. The Biochemistry of Disease. Marcel Dekker, New York. 711-723, 1975.
19. Rojkind, M. and Dunn, M.A.: Hepatic fibrosis. Gastroenterology 76:849-863, 1979.
20. Arenson, D.M. and Bissell, D.M.: Glycosaminoglycan, proteoglycan, and hepatic fibrosis. Gastroenterology 92:536-540, 1987.
21. Chojkier, M. and Brenner, D.A.: Therapeutic strategies for hepatic fibrosis. Hepatology 8:176-182, 1988.

Chapter 32

Hepatic Necrosis and Acute Hepatic Failure

ACUTE HEPATIC NECROSIS

Clinical Synopsis

Diagnostic features

* Acute onset of depression and vomiting
* Polydipsia and jaundice may be present
* Abdominal palpation may detect hepatomegaly and pain
* Evidence of a coagulopathy occasionally seen
* ALT and SAP increased (ALT usually greater percentage increase than SAP)
* Bilirubin may be elevated and glucose decreased
* Albumin is usually normal
* Biopsy reveals necrosis

Standard management

* Address primary cause if identified
* NPO for 2-5 days; subsequently cottage cheese and rice based diet or TPN
* IV fluid therapy, with 5% dextrose in Ringer's solution, lactated Ringer's, or 0.45% NaCl depending on fluid and electrolyte status
* Control of hepatic encephalopathy (see Chapter 33)

Additional therapy sometimes indicated (see text) include IV methionine, vitamin E, cimetidine, plasma, heparin, corticosteroids and antibiotics.

The hepatocyte is susceptible to degeneration caused by many etiological agents. Degenerative changes vary in severity and manifestation, from regional lipid infiltration to widespread necrosis. Hepatic necrosis accompanies inflammatory processes such as chronic active and suppurative hepatitis, and some necrosis is usually associated with hepatic tumors, whether primary or metastatic. Necrosis is frequently reported as the primary lesion when no other morphological changes are found. Focal, zonal, or massive necrosis accounts for 8% to 10% of all primary diagnoses of hepatic pathology in biopsy and necropsy cases. Focal hepatic necrosis is likely a common lesion in aged animals. A report that 65% of young dogs in a closed colony had focal hepatic necrosis suggests, furthermore, that its incidence in dogs can be high at any age.[1] Focal necrosis is often an incidental finding in dogs without signs of hepatic disease when a biopsy is performed to evaluate abnormal plasma enzyme activity. It is not known whether focal necrosis consistently causes elevated plasma alanine aminotransferase (ALT) activity or even if it is able to produce clinical signs. Widespread necrosis, however, consistently produces signs of severe hepatic disease. The incidence of all types of necrosis as the primary hepatic lesion in necropsied animals is similar in cats and dogs.

ETIOLOGY AND PATHOGENESIS OF HEPATIC NECROSIS (Table 32-1)

In many cases the etiology of acute hepatic necrosis is unknown. In the majority of cases, however, acute hepatic necrosis is associated with and believed to be caused by another disease or problem. In dogs, nonhepatic problems cause nearly 80% of hepatic necrosis; in cats that percentage is even higher at 90% (Table 32-1). Hepatic necrosis described as primary, where the clinical problems appear to be caused by a disease confined to the liver, has an unknown etiology; when drugs are believed to be the cause, hepatic necrosis is listed under the drug etiology category. Primary hepatic necrosis may be said to have an unknown etiology when a strong association with drugs or chemicals can not be made, or when the clinician bases the diagnosis on biopsy of the liver only and is ignorant of pathology in other organs that may be the cause of the hepatic necrosis. Primary hepatic necrosis is more frequent in dogs than cats, which may reflect cats' tendency to be more discriminating in eating food or substances containing toxins.

In a small percentage of the cases studied, hepatic necrosis was a component of a specific primary liver problem such as chronic active hepatitis, hepatic lipidosis or nodular regeneration. Most lesions of hepatic necrosis were moderate or severe. In both dogs and cats the more severe pathology is found in primary hepatic necrosis and necrosis caused by coagulopathies, thromboembolic problems, and other problems causing hepatic hypoxia and ischemia. Mild hepatic necrosis is infrequently reported, even though it may be a frequent finding on normal liver biopsies. Of nonhepatic diseases with mild hepatic necrosis, steroid-induced hepatopathy is most frequently reported.

The most frequent cause of moderate or more commonly

Table 32-1 Hepatic Necrosis

Etiology	Canine (N = 113)		Feline (N = 49)	
	%		%	
Primary	22	(M,S)	10	(S)
Manifestation of other liver disease	16		12	
DIC, Thromboembolic disease	14	(S)	8	(M,S)
Hypoxia, ischemia, congestion, anemia	10	(S)	26	(M,S)
Generalized or local infection	11	(M)	8	(M)
Neoplastic disease (nonhepatic)	9	(M,S)	12	(M)
Steroid-induced hepatopathy	9	(Mild)	0	
Pancreatitis	6	(M)	2	(S)
Drugs	2	(S)	0	
Hyperthyroidism	0		6	(M)
Enteritis	2	(S)	4	(M,S)
Renal Disease	< 1	(M)	6	
Other	< 1		6	

(M) = moderate (S) = severe

severe hepatic necrosis is a problem that results in reduced delivery of oxygen and nutrients to the liver. That cause accounts for 24% of hepatic necrosis in dogs and 34% in cats. Hepatic necrosis follows from the effects of DIC, thromboembolic disease, hypoxia, ischemia, acute congestion, or anemia due to reduced delivery of oxygen and nutrients to hepatocytes. This effect is most pronounced in zone 3, the group of hepatocytes surrounding central veins, which are the last to receive their metabolic requirements from the circulation.

Circulatory failure due to any form of right-sided heart failure results in a venous hypertension and congestion that is transmitted back through the hepatic vein and into the central veins. With a cardiac failure resulting in peripheral circulatory failure, the congestion does not also involve hepatic sinusoids, but without peripheral failure the sinusoids are congested. Hepatocytes in zone 3 suffer damage from both the venous hypertension and reduced oxygen and nutrient delivery. In one case, zone 3 hepatocytes become necrotic without congestion; in another case, zone 3 necrosis occured with congestion. Congestion associated with venous hypertension can cause hepatocytes to atrophy. Acute circulatory failure or shock, producing a similar type of zone 3 necrosis, can be caused by severe trauma, hemorrhage, septic shock, surgery, pulmonary thrombosis or embolism, and heat stroke. Coagulopathies can regionally or focally restrict circulatory failure to the liver, resulting in thrombosis of hepatic sinusoidal and venous vessels. They are an important cause of severe hepatic necrosis in the dog and cat. A reduction in oxygen supplied to the liver causes the zone 3 necrosis of anemia. Any other cause of local hepatic hypoxia could produce that lesion. Focal hepatic necrosis is a frequent finding in liver biopsies obtained during surgery.[2] The lesion is thought to result from hypotension and local hypoxia, caused by the effects of anesthesia and the stress of surgery. The area of hepatic necrosis may not always be restricted to zone 3 with circulatory failure; zone 2 or midzonal necrosis is sometimes seen.[3]

Hepatic necrosis due to septicemia or bacterial infection in a nonhepatic tissue is diffusely multifocal twice as often as it is restricted to zone 3 (centrolobular). It is possible that shock due to a septicemia is responsible for the central distribution of some of these lesions.

Viral agents may be an important cause of acute hepatic necrosis. Infectious canine hepatitis caused by the adenovirus of Rubarth is thought to be rare because most dogs are vaccinated at an early age. Serological studies performed in some countries indicate that a high percentage of dogs have been infected with the virus without showing any clinical signs.[4] Thus, the presence of the virus may be more common than believed. In contrast to the asymptomatic infections, infected dogs given immunosuppressive therapy develop acute severe hepatic necrosis. Some of the drug-related or primary hepatic necrosis may include such a cause and pathogenesis. Other viruses causing hepatitis in dogs include one identified as a canine acidophil cell hepatitis virus.[5] That virus is responsible for chronic hepatitis, and it is likely that hepatic necrosis predominates as the early lesion. Viral agents have been identified in other morphological studies of canine hepatic disease. Some human hepatitis viral agents appear to survive long enough in animals to cause a serological response. Viruses cause hepatitis in felines, but the primary lesion is not hepatic necrosis. The pyogranulomatous lesion in feline infectious peritonitis is the result of the host's immune response to the virus rather than to the virus' directly damaging the liver. Parasitic diseases involving the liver cause inflammatory lesions rather than primarily hepatic necrosis.

Hepatic metastases of nonhepatic neoplastic disease often show little effect on the necrosis of hepatocytes. When hepatic necrosis is reported as a lesion, there are usually multiple causes of injury to hepatocytes. The metastases can encroach on hepatocytes and cause damage directly, or they can interfere with circulation in the liver and cause hepatic necrosis indirectly.

Hepatic necrosis of steroid-induced hepatopathy is mostly mild and multifocal. Since that lesion is not unusual in normal dogs, it may be insignificant in the steroid-induced hepatic changes.

Acute pancreatitis causes centrolobular degeneration and necrosis, disseminated hemorrhagic focal necrosis, and dilation of sinusoids. In some cases, infiltration of inflammatory cells is seen in periportal areas. These changes are associated with increased plasma ALT and plasma alkaline phosphatase activities. With severe pancreatitis, hyperbilirubinemia can result, although that is more likely due to obstruction of the bile duct by pancreatic inflammation. Acute hepatic lesions develop because shock-producing substances released from the diseased pancreas impair hepatic circulation. These substances, passing through the liver to reach the systemic circulation, damage the hepatic microcirculation, resulting in sinusoidal dilation. With the onset of systemic shock, hepatic circulation is reduced, which causes the centrolobular lesions. The tissue-destroying pancreatic enzymes released from an inflamed pancreas are more concentrated in the portal blood than in the systemic circulation. They remain in the liver longer than usual because of reduced hepatic circulation and are thereby able to initiate necrosis. Trypsin is likely the enzyme that is most damaging to the liver. Pancreatic phospholipase-A and lysolecithin released to the circulation contribute to necrosis. Necrosis persists until circulation improves and pancreatic enzymes are not longer released.

Acute hepatic necrosis can be associated with inflammatory disease of the gastrointestinal tract. It is more likely that hepatic necrosis results from, rather than contributes to, signs of the gastrointestinal problem. It is not unusual to find plasma activity increased for liver-specific enzymes in animals with a gastrointestinal problem. It can be assumed that such increases reflect some degree of hepatic degeneration or necrosis. That is often proven with liver biopsy, but more often the abnormality is monitored during management and resolution of the gastrointestinal problem. Many such cases require dietary management as essential for lasting remission; with such remission the plasma enzyme activities return to normal and liver biopsy, if done, shows no pathology. Evidence for hepatic necrosis is predictable with bacterial overgrowth of the small intestine. That intestinal problem may be more common than realized.

Hepatic necrosis is caused by substances absorbed from the intestinal tract. Such absorption can increase because the substances' intestinal concentrations increase or intestinal permeability increases. Endotoxin, one such substance, increases with bacterial overgrowth, and more is absorbed with acute or chronic gastrointestinal problems. Endotoxin alone can damage the liver; operating synergistically with other factors, smaller amounts of endotoxin cause hepatic necrosis.[6] Other toxins may have similar effects. Chemicals such as carbon tetrachloride are used to produce hepatic necrosis in experimental animals. When such treatment is combined with the oral administration of resins that bind and prevent absorption of both bacteria and toxins by the intestine, such pathology is mild or not seen.[7] Similarly, antibiotics given to suppress the normal intestinal microflora have a protective effect on the livers of animals given hepatotoxic chemicals.[6] It is nonetheless evident that bacteria escaping from the intestine may also contribute directly to hepatic necrosis.

With the increased mucosal permeability predictable during gastrointestinal problems, the absorption of bacterial, dietary, and epithelial cell antigens increases. Their reaction with immunoglobulins to form immune complexes may exceed the capacity of the hepatic Kupffer cells to remove and degrade them. With incomplete removal, immune complexes may deposit in the liver and, by fixing and activating complement, they can cause hepatic necrosis.[8] Some colonic epithelial cell antigens are similar to those found in epithelial cells of the hepatic biliary system and renal tubules. These antigens are also similar to those found in *E. coli*. Antibodies produced against the colonic or bacterial antigens can react with antigens in any of the three types of epithelial cells.[9] Permeability changes, allowing absorption of excess antigen from the intestine, can increase the production of antibodies that can damage both the liver and kidney by an immune-mediated mechanism. This is recognized in animals with chronic bowel disease, where the incidence of hepatic and renal lesions is greater than anticipated. Patients with acute enterocolitis all potentially have hepatic lesions. The restoration of normal plasma liver-specific enzyme activity and the return of normal liver morphology following a controlled diet to manage a persisting problem are most likely due to a reduced absorption of toxins and antigens from the intestine.

Hepatic injury can be caused by toxins, drugs, and other chemicals. Although few cases of hepatic necrosis are documented as having such causes, there are undoubtedly many that are either suspected but unproven or not even suspected. Many drugs can cause hepatic injury, and with evidence of that from increased plasma liver-specific enzyme activity, the drug is often discontinued without a liver biopsy to characterize the injury. Hepatic injury can range from milder forms of degeneration and lipidosis to hepatic necrosis. Some forms of chemical injury manifest themselves as cholestasis, which can be associated with portal inflammation.

Most of the information on hepatic toxicity of drugs and toxins is obtained from their effects on humans and experimental animals.[10-12] They can be classified as drugs and toxins producing necrosis; necrosis and lipidosis; lipidosis; granulomas; or cholestasis (Table 32-2). Many, if not most, cause a specific histologic pattern of lesions. The list includes agents a small animal patient is likely to encounter as well as some no longer posing an important risk. Also included are drugs that are currently used in human medicine and that are being more widely used in veterinary medicine. Long-term exposure to many agents can lead to fibrosis, cirrhosis, and chronic hepatitis. Some agents, such as pyrrolizidine alkaloids, can cause veno-occlusive disease and hepatic vein thrombosis.

Documentation of hepatotoxicity is best for drugs administered over a long time. Anticonvulsants, an important medication given chronically to many animals, may be the most important kind of drug injuring the liver. Primidone given at therapeutic doses can cause hepatic necrosis in dogs.[13] Higher doses, or use in combination with other anticonvulsants such as phenytoin, cause pathology to be more severe. Often seizures are difficult to control and the dose of primidone is increased or the drug is combined with phenytoin in attempts for better control. Such management puts an animal at great risk for developing hepatic necrosis. Phenytoin alone also causes hepatic degeneration and necrosis, but it has not been responsible for frequent hepatic problems in dogs as it has in humans. That

Table 32-2. Drugs with Potential Hepatoxicity

ANESTHETICS
- Chloroform
- Halothane
- Methoxyflurane

ANTICONVULSANTS
- Carbamazepine
- Phenytoin
- Phenothiazines
- Primidone
- Valproic acid

ANTIMICROBIAL
- Amoxicillin
- Ampicillin
- Arsenicals
- Amphotericin
- Carbenicillin
- Cephalosporins
- Chloramphenicol
- Clindamycin
- Erythromycin estolate
- 5-Fluorocytosine
- Griseofulvin
- Isoniazid
- Ketoconazole
- Metronidazole
- Nitrofurantoin
- Oxacillin
- Penicillin G
- Quinacrine
- Sulfonamides
- Tetracyclines
- Thiabendazole
- Trimethoprim-sulfa

ANALGESICS AND NSAIDS
- Acetaminophen
- Allopurinol
- Benoxaprofen
- Colchicine
- Ibuprofen
- Indomethacin
- Naproxen
- Penicillamine
- Phenylbutazone
- Salicylates

CARDIOVASCULAR
- Captopril
- Dihydralazine
- Furosemide
- Hydralazine
- Methyldopa
- Procainamide
- Quinidine
- Thiazides
- Warfarin

ANTINEOPLASTICS
- Busulfan
- Cyclophosphamide
- L-Asparginase
- 6-Mercaptopurine
- Methotrexate
- Mithramycin
- Urethane

ENDOCRINE AGENTS
- Anabolic steroids (C-17 alkylated)
- Corticosteroids
- Methimazole
- Propylthiouracil

TRANQUILIZERS
- Diazepam
- Haloperidol
- Phenothiazines

OTHER DRUGS
- BAL
- Cimetidine
- Danthron
- Dapsone
- Iodochlorhydroxyquin
- Iodine
- Stibophen
- Tannic acid
- Vitamin A

Table 32-2. Toxins with Potential Hepatoxicity

NECROSIS	NECROSIS AND STEATOSIS
Albitocin (PP)	Aflatoxins (PV, PP)
Alloxan (PP)	L-Amanitin (PV)
Allyl compounds (PP)	Arsenic compounds (inorganic)(PV, M)
Aniline (M)	Bromobenzene (PV)
Berylium (MZ)	Carbon tetrachloride (PV)
Chlorinated benzenes (M)	Chlorinated diphenyls (M)
Dioxane (M)	Chlorinated naphthalene (M)
Ferrous sulphate (PP)	Chloroform (PV)
Manganese compounds (PP)	Chloroprene (PV)
Ngaione (MZ)	2-Chloropropane (PV)
Paracetamol (PV)	Dichloropropane (PV)
Paraquat (PV, MZ)	Dimethylnitrosamine
Phalloidin (PV)	Dinitrobenzone (PV, M)
P. vulgaris endotoxin (PP)	Dinitrophenol (M)
Rubratoxin (PV)	Dinitrotoluene (PV, M)
Selenium (M)	Ethylene dibromide (PV)
Sporidesmin (PP)	Ethylene dichloride (PV)
Thioacetamide (PV)	Iodoform (PV)
Urethane (PV)	Islandicum (PV)
	Luteoskyrin (PV)
	Methylchloroform
	Naphthalene (PV)
	Pyrrolizidine alkaloids (PV)
	Synthalin (PP)
	Tannic acid (PV)
	Tetrachloroethane (M)

Key: (PP) = Periportal, (M) = Massive, (MZ) = Midzonal, (PV) = Perivenular

can be explained by the drug's short half-life in dogs, which also explains why phenytoin is not very effective as an anticonvulsant in dogs.

Phenobarbital is a superior anticonvulsant drug and has not been reported to cause hepatic disease in small animals. Phenobarbital stimulates proliferation of the smooth endoplasmic reticulum to the extent that it can cause hepatomegaly with no histologic evidence of hepatocyte degeneration. The hyperplastic smooth endoplasmic reticulum represents an increased capacity for metabolizing a wide variety of chemicals acted on by the cytochrome P-450 enzymes. With that capability an animal is at greater risk when exposed to chemicals that are metabolized to toxic metabolites by that system. Despite all that, phenobarbital is a safe drug and remains the treatment of choice for managing seizures. With the use of any anticonvulsant drug it is likely that plasma activity of liver enzymes will increase, but that activity is not usually associated with morphologic changes in the liver. Dogs with drug-induced morphologic changes have abnormalities in hepatic function in addition to plasma enzyme increases; plasma bilirubin, bile acids, and BSP rate of disappearance are all abnormal.[13]

Antibiotics metabolized by the liver have been shown to cause hepatic degeneration and necrosis. For such lesions to develop, other factors such as preexisting hepatic insufficiency may be necessary. Tetracycline given to normal dogs causes at worst a mild to moderate lipidosis in a few animals. The same therapeutic dose given to dogs with portasystemic shunts precipitates hepatic and renal failure that proves to be fatal.[14] The half-life of tetracycline increases almost three times in shunted dogs, which may be important. Increased toxic agents from the intestine which are not cleared adequately by the liver may also be important. Other drugs metabolized by the liver, and potential causes of hepatic injury, include chloromycetin and erythromycin, as well as a host of newer ones. Sulfonamides are important in considering drug-induced causes of hepatic degeneration and necrosis because use of these drugs is so common. Many animals are on long-term sulfonamide therapy for chronic urinary tract infections and chronic colitis, as well as chronic infections in other organs. That use can also lead to keratitis sicca, maybe a more important complication than the hepatic lesions. The penicillins are included on the list of drugs with the potential for hepatotoxicity. It is difficult to assess the hepatic potential of most of the antibiotics because they are used to treat infection, and infection or septicemia is by itself capable of producing hepatic necrosis. It seems prudent to consider both the metabolism of an antibiotic and the effects of hepatic or renal insufficiency on its half-life when choosing one as part of the management of a patient with hepatic insufficiency.

Non-steroid anti-inflammatory agents are commonly used to manage a wide spectrum of chronic problems. They too have the potential to cause hepatic injury. Their use might be less common in small animals because of steroids' ability to produce gastrointestinal erosions and hence more obvious clinical signs than those of hepatic pathology.

Chemicals used for treatment of parasitic problems can cause hepatic pathology. Arsenicals used for treatment of heartworms are an important cause of hepatic necrosis, sometimes a fatal form. Mebendazole, an anthelmintic drug, was reported to cause moderate to severe hepatic disease in a small group of dogs.[15] Subsequent studies using the drug at several times the therapeutic dose failed to cause any adverse affects in normal dogs.[16] There is probably some risk in using that drug, however, and it may involve some interaction with other factors to synergistically produce hepatic injury. Without further understanding, mebendazole toxicity is regarded as an idiosyncratic and not a predictable, intrinsic hepatotoxicity.

Tranquilizing agents and inhalation anesthetics can also cause hepatic pathology. Halothane hepatotoxicity is precipitated by hypoxic conditions in the liver and can be reproduced in experimental animals. Methoxyflurane on occasion causes hepatic injury; that has been more frequent than injuries from halothane, but the increasing use of halothane may reverse that trend. New agents similar to these drugs may also possess a potential for hepatotoxicity.

Cushing's disease is treated with a drug (o,p,-DDD) metabolized by the liver, a liver with steroid-induced changes that compromise its functions. The difficulty often encountered in treating Cushing's disease is probably in part due to the variability in the drug's metabolism by livers with different degrees of incapacity to metabolize drugs.

Anabolic or any steroid with a C-17 alkylated structure can cause cholestasis. Their long-term use may produce significant hepatic-lesions.

Hepatic necrosis is well-documented following exposure to toxins such as aflatoxin, copper salts, iron salts, pyrrolizidine alkaloids, tannic acid, Amanita phalloides toxin, dimethylnitrosamine, and a host of others. It is unknown how often such toxins are responsible for clinical cases of hepatic disease.

The list of drugs and toxic agents in Table 32-2 may include many of no importance to small animal clinicians. They are included because many more "human drugs" are being used to treat small animal problems. For example, propylthiouracil is used to manage hyperthyroidism in cats. This drug has the potential for hepatotoxicity, although nothing is known of its toxic effect on cats. Many animals are evaluated with biochemical screening panels when they are on drugs. The list allows one to judge whether some drug might explain clinical pathologic abnormalities when biopsy of the liver would be inappropriate and provide no useful information. In a case like this, administration of all drugs is discontinued, and after an interval of 10 to 14 days, the biochemical screening can be repeated to see if the drug may have been the cause of suspected hepatic injury.

PATHOPHYSIOLOGY

Hepatic necrosis causes a loss of hepatocyte structure and function. Loss of structure results in a loss of hepatocytes' soluble intracellular contents. Glutamic pyruvic transaminase or alanine aminotransferase (SGPT or ALT) is lost and its plasma activity increases. The plasma ALT levels increase from a normal level of 50 IU/L to over 1600 IU/L in dogs four days after infection with infectious canine hepatitis virus.[17] This finding applies to dogs that survive only 4 to 7 days and show major clinical signs within the first 36 hours after inoculation. Activity of plasma ALT does not necessarily parallel the degree of hepatic necrosis. In animals given a hepatotoxin, the degree of necrosis correlates well with immediate increases in plasma ALT activity, which are up to 20 to 50 times normal in the first 24 hours.[18] There is considerable individual variation, however, so that an animal may have extensive necrosis without a matching increase in plasma ALT. Three days after the toxic insult the histological appearance of necrosis remains unchanged yet plasma ALT levels are normal or elevated to only four to five times normal. Thus, measurement of plasma ALT activity 3 days after the insult suggests hepatic necrosis in only 50% of the cases. After their release, hepatic transaminases are rapidly degraded and inactivated, so hepatic necrosis is continuing if plasma ALT activity remains elevated. Plasma ALT activity is measured both for diagnosis and to monitor remission of hepatic necrosis. Elevated plasma ALT activity can be seen in animals with no clinical signs of disease. In a closed colony of dogs on the UC campus at Davis, California, a biochemical survey of the entire population revealed that 10% had plasma ALT levels ten to fifteen times normal values without any signs of disease.[19] No biopsies were performed to correlate hepatic morphology with transaminase activity.

Alkaline phosphatase, an enzyme produced in a number of tissues, including the liver, is released at an increased rate during hepatic necrosis, resulting in increased plasma activity. Increased plasma alkaline phosphatase (ALP) activity is not pathognomonic for hepatic disease; it is found whenever the rate of ALP synthesis increases. Intrahepatic and extrahepatic biliary obstruction, and hepatic regeneration following necrosis or with hepatic tumors, are associated with proliferation of biliary epithelium, the site of alkaline phosphatase activity, and with increased plasma ALP activity.[20] Hepatic necrosis caused by infectious canine hepatitis results in increased plasma ALP activity, although not until 3.5 days after inoculation with the virus.[17] Plasma activity increases until death, reflecting an increased synthesis of alkaline phosphatase by proliferating biliary epithelia. A continued increase in plasma ALP activity while plasma ALT returns to normal can signify an unresolved biliary stasis or a regenerating liver.

Hyperbilirubinemia can be produced by hepatic necrosis, especially by necrosis diffusely involving periportal areas. Swelling of degenerated cells and disruption of canaliculi by

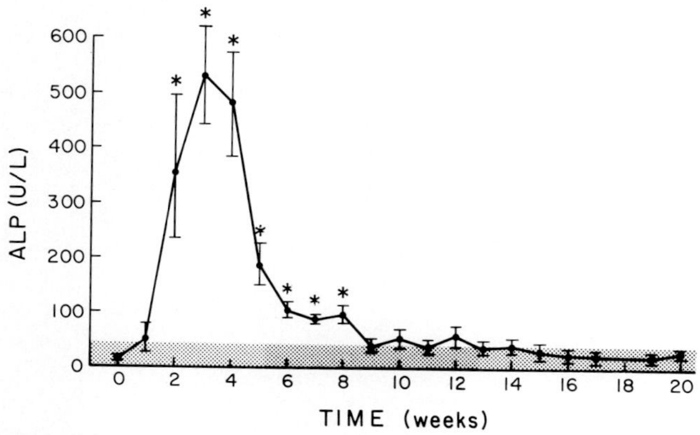

Figure 32-1. Changes in plasma ALP before and after exposure of dogs to nitrosamine.

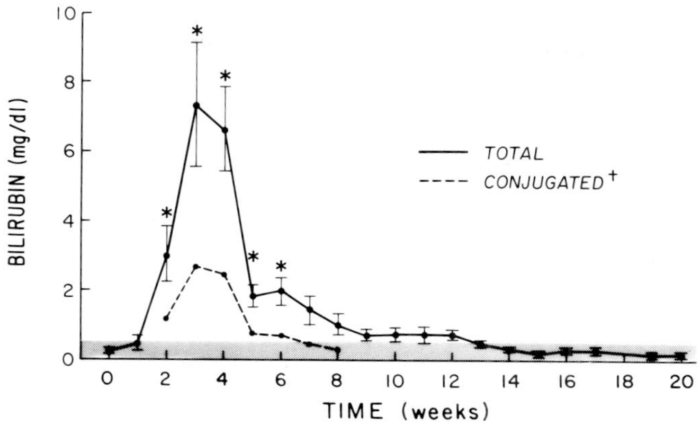

Figure 32-2. Changes in plasma bilirubin before and after exposure of dogs to nitrosamine.

hepatocyte necrosis obstruct biliary flow, producing cholestasis. Only a small percentage of the total liver capacity is required to catabolize the normally small amounts of heme produced each day. With normal periportal hepatocytes and an intact biliary system, hyperbilirubinemia does not develop with hepatic disease.[21] Hyperbilirubinemia is a late and inconsistent finding in dogs with massive hepatic necrosis produced by infectious canine hepatitis.[17]

Massive hepatic necrosis caused by drugs and toxins produces changes in plasma enzyme activities and impairment of hepatic function, as illustrated by the hepatotoxic effects of nitrosamines in dogs.[22] Activity of plasma ALT increases when the toxin is given but begins a rapid return to normal on its discontinuation (Figure 30-4). That is a usual response for many toxic chemicals. The activity of plasma ALP also increases but follows that of plasma ALT and persists for two weeks or longer than the peak plasma ALT activity (32-1). The plasma ALP increase reflects intrahepatic cholestasis and hepatic regeneration. In clinical cases falling plasma ALT activities with increasing or persisting high levels of plasma ALP activity can be viewed as a favorable indication of a healing, i.e. regenerating, liver.

Hepatic function is lost to varying degrees with massive hepatic necrosis. The ability to maintain normal plasma bilirubin levels is lost for a time comparable to the time that plasma activities of ALT and ALP are abnormal (Figure 32-2). At the time of peak ALT activity, blood ammonia levels are still normal and when they do increase they are not a reliable indicator of hepatic pathology. Bile acids are predictably abnormal during the acute phase but not during the recovery or chronic phase. The impairment of the liver to metabolize the dye sulfobromophthalein (BSP) is the earliest significant biochemical abnormality, occurring before significant increases in plasma enzyme activities.[22] The liver's major functions in carbohydrate and nitrogen metabolism are impaired at the time of peak enzyme activities or shortly thereafter. Many of these functions continue to be abnormal after recovery, when dogs appear clinically normal. A relative hypoglycemia and a reduction in the ascorbic acid produced by the liver reflect carbohydrate abnormalities (Figure 32-3). Persisting low plasma levels of blood urea nitrogen, albumin, some globulins, and iron (caused by decreased carrier protein) reflect an impairment in nitrogen metabolism. Plasma amino acid concentrations also change.

Coagulopathies sometimes complicate hepatic necrosis.[23] Massive necrosis produced with hepatitis viruses[17] and with hepatotoxins[24] in experimental animals creates models to study hepatic bleeding disorders. The first event contributing to a coagulopathy is the release of thromboplastic substances from abundant stores in injured hepatocytes. Thromboplastic activity initiates clotting, producing disseminated intravascular coagulation (DIC). With ongoing hepatic necrosis caused by a hepatitis virus, thromboplastic activity release is continuous, making DIC a problem requiring management over a period of days. When DIC is caused by a single insult from a drug or toxin, thromboplastic substance release is more likely to last only for a single day.

After the initial hepatic damage that releases thromboplastic activity, another important result of the coagulopathy is the liver's failure to synthesize clotting factors and to remove activated clotting factors, plasminogen activator, and fibrino-

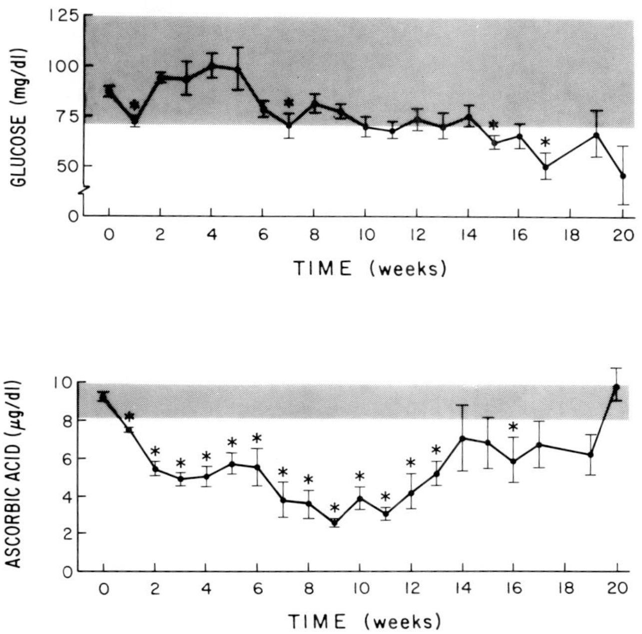

Figure 32-3. Changes in plasma glucose and ascorbic acid before and after exposure of dogs to nitrosamine.

Table 32-3. Blood Clotting in Dogs after Nitrosamine Exposure

	Normal Values	Month 1	2	3	4
PT (sec)	< 8.2	10.7	11.7	10.4	9.2
PTT (sec)	< 12.0	17.4	24.2	27.4	16.7
TT (sec)	5 to 10	10.7	12.9	12.4	15.2
Fibrinogen	>200 mg/dl	76	61	66	73
Factor V	100 %	32	53	41	54
Factor VII	100 %	23	19	19	28
Plasminogen	100 %	50	75	81	89

gen degradation products. The blood-clotting factors that disappear the most rapidly are those with the shortest half-lives, Factors VII and VIII. They have half-lives of 0.5 days or less, and infectious canine hepatitis causes the level of VIII to fall to 5% of normal within two days, whereas the factors with longer half-lives do not decrease for an additional two days, and the decrease is not as great.[17] The same results are seen with Factor VII in partially hepatectomized dogs.[25] Thus, treatment for coagulopathies includes replacement of blood-clotting factors. Complete hepatectomy may be similar to acute massive hepatic necrosis in its production of coagulopathy. Complete hepatectomy, however, causes clotting factors to disappear more rapidly than expected from their half-lives (Table 28-5).[26] Thus, it may not be possible to predict the half-lives of clotting factors with massive hepatic necrosis.

Hepatotoxicity by nitrosamines results in a coagulapathy that involves deficiency of clotting factor synthesis (Table 32-3).[26] The prothrombin time increasing from 8.2 seconds to 10.5 seconds is not as dramatic as the increase in partial thromboplastin time from 12 seconds to 18.9 seconds. Fibrinogen levels decrease from a normal range of 200-400 to 70 mg/dl because of both decreased synthesis and increased consumption. Factor VII, with the shortest half-life, is 22% of normal compared to factor V at 46% of normal. Antithrombin III, the major physiological inhibitor of coagulation, is 55% of normal. Heparin modifies antithrombin III so that it binds and inactivates thrombin. Markedly reduced levels of antithrombin III preclude the possibility of heparin in effectively improving disseminated intravascular coagulation. Plasminogen, produced by the liver, is not greatly reduced at 74% of normal. During recovery, synthesis of clotting factors returns to normal slowly. In this dog model, bleeding may not be seen until clotting factor levels approach 30% of normal.

Massive necrosis incapacitates the liver's function of removing circulating substances that contribute to the coagulopathy.[27] The persistence of activated clotting factors continues to promote hypercoagulability. DIC is promoted by bacterial endotoxins from the endotoxemia that appears with massive hepatic necrosis when plasma fibronectin levels decrease and reticuloendothelial functions fail.[28] The reticuloendothelial system also removes enzymes responsible for splitting fibrinogen and its products. Increased activity of these enzymes results in high levels of fibrinogen degradation products, which interfere with the normal formation of blood clots. High plasma activities of these enzymes, having proteolytic functions, also accelerate the degradation of blood-clotting factors. Thus, the pathology in a continuing coagulopathy primarily involves a reduced availability of blood-clotting factors and the appearance of products that interfere with normal clotting.

Platelet numbers and function are also compromised by massive hepatic failure.[29] Platelet numbers decrease, and their smaller size indicates they are older and that new platelets are not being released properly. The platelets show abnormal morphology and have intrinsic functional defects, resulting in abnormal aggregation and adhesion. Platelets normally interact with a plasma glycoprotein, the von Willebrand factor, in adhering to the surface of exposed connective tissue.

Animals with extensive hepatic necrosis have deranged nitrogen metabolism, causing hyperammonemia and signs of hepatic encephalopathy.[30] Neurological signs are not usually a feature in dogs with focal or moderate hepatic necrosis. Hyperammonemia does not appear until hepatic necrosis becomes

Table 32-4. Plasma Amino Acids in Dogs with Massive Hepatic Failure

Amino Acid	Percent of Normal
Taurine	436
Aspartic Acid	345
Glutamic Acid	403
Proline	323
Glycine	301
Alanine	538
Citrulline	72
Valine	172
Isoleucine	123
Leucine	165
Tyrosine	594
Phenylalanine	392
Ornithine	1070
Lysine	301
Arginine	0

widespread, and then it is accompanied by an abnormal pattern of plasma amino acid concentrations. The levels of almost all plasma amino acids increase markedly with massive hepatic necrosis (Table 32-4). The exceptions are the branched chain amino acids, which increase much less, and arginine, which can fall markedly. The reason suggested for the decrease in branched chain amino acids is that they are used at an accelerated rate by peripheral tissues for energy, a process stimulated by high plasma levels of catecholamines, glucagon, and insulin, hormones not adequately removed by the diseased liver. Low arginine levels may be due to a release of the enzyme arginase from damaged hepatocytes. Plasma arginase activity can increase during hepatic necrosis, and the enzyme can split plasma arginine to form urea and ornithine.[31] Arginine is important in maintaining the urea-cycle activity of converting ammonia to urea. Arginine administered during hyperammonemia due to hepatic failure causes blood ammonia levels to decrease. Reduced plasma citrulline concentrations are consistent with reduced urea-cycle activity. The increase in plasma amino acids is similar in clinical cases to that found in experimental dogs when necrosis is produced with nitrosamines.[30]

None of the increases in plasma amino acids have been fully explained. Amino acids are released from damaged hepatocytes, and their release from muscle is likely promoted by high levels of corticosteroids, catecholamines and glucagon. For reasons unknown, branched-chain amino acids are not used as avidly for calories by peripheral tissues in dogs with hepatic necrosis as it is in dogs with chronic active hepatitis and portasystemic shunts. Plasma levels of amino acids metabolized only by the liver increase with massive hepatic necrosis. Increases are greater than threefold for all except the branched chain amino acids (valine, isoleucine, leucine), citrulline, and arginine. Signs of hepatic encephalopathy with massive hepatic necrosis are not easily explained by abnormalities in the ratio of branched-chain to aromatic amino acids. The pathogenesis of hepatic encephalopathy is not very well understood. The abnormalities in plasma amino acids are a consequence of hepatic injury and probably contribute little to clinical signs.

Acute liver failure often results in the animal's lapsing into an irreversible coma that is considered to be the severest manifestation of hepatic encephalopathy.[32,33] The coma associated with massive hepatic necrosis is often caused by cerebral edema, a situation less often found in animals comatose with chronic hepatic insufficiency. Edema results from increased permeability of the blood-brain barrier and is due to an increase in either extracellular or intracellular fluid. Permeability of the barrier is increased by such toxins as ammonia, mercaptans, octonoate, and phenolic acids, which are not removed adequately by the diseased liver. The increased permeability permits the entry into the brain of some toxins with the ability to disrupt normal neurotransmission. The increased permeability is also associated with the inhibition of some ATPase activity that operates to maintain normal intracellular concentrations of sodium and potassium. Cerebral edema is associated with a loss of autoregulation of cerebral blood flow, resulting primarily from generalized hypotension and hypercapnia. Without autoregulation, cerebral blood flow increases up to threefold with cerebral edema, and that increase is another factor contributing to further edema. The cerebral blood flow could be reduced by hypotensive drugs, but that could reduce cerebral perfusion to a critical level. The increased flow due to hypercapnia can be decreased by hyperventilation to reduce blood carbon dioxide content. Cerebral blood flow is also directly related to brain metabolic activity. Fever, such as seen with hepatic failure, increases that metabolic activity and cerebral blood flow; both can be improved by barbiturates or hypothermia to reduce brain metabolism.

Massive hepatic necrosis leading to hepatic failure is associated with a severe circulatory problem, characterized by a low systemic vascular resistance with a compensatory increase in cardiac output. With generalized hypotension, mesenteric blood flow falls, so that both hepatic arterial and portal flows are reduced. The maintenance of hepatic circulation is further compromised by hepatocyte inflammation and the deposition of fibrin in the microcirculation which further reduces sinusoidal blood flow. Fibrin deposition and thrombi formation are the result of disseminated intravascular coagulation. Compensating for the hypotension, cardiac output increases, and circulation through the hepatic artery can increase selectively to compensate for reduced portal flow.

The critical consequence of circulatory failure is tissue hypoxia. Tissue hypoxia is compounded by pulmonary dysfunction that develops because of low pressure pulmonary edema. Such edema is believed to develop because of increased permeability of pulmonary capillaries, changes similar to that for the blood-brain barrier. Hyperventilation, stimulated by toxins acting centrally, and hypoxia attempt to restore normal oxygen delivery to tissues. It may fail, but the change in ventilation results in a respiratory alkalosis from the carbon dioxide lost.

Tissue hypoxia results in increased anaerobic metabolism, and plasma levels of lactate and pyruvate increase. Excesses of these metabolites are produced because of poor circulation or shunting of blood away from the liver or because of the liver's inadequate metabolic functioning. High lactate levels are not sufficient to cause lactic acidosis unless circulatory failure develops and acidosis produced by shock intervenes. The plasma levels of free fatty acids are high, and the relative amounts of ketone bodies are low. Since ketone bodies are produced from fatty acids in the liver, the abnormally high ratio of free fatty acids to ketone bodies indicates that the hepatic uptake and metabolism of free fatty acids is impaired. Free fatty acids interfere with the synthesis of urea from ammonia, contributing indirectly to the hepatic encephalopathy.

Alkalosis develops that is partly respiratory and partly metabolic.[34] Acute hepatic failure is associated with hyperventilation, and pCO_2 of arterial blood decreases as a result of the greater losses of carbon dioxide. The brain respiratory center is possibly stimulated by toxins accumulating because of hepatic disease. The metabolic alkalosis is also caused by potassium losses. As this ion is lost, intracellular potassium moves into the extracellular fluid, in exchange for hydrogen ions that move into the cell. Thus, hydrogen ions moving intracellularly contribute to the alkalosis. The amount of bicarbonate remaining is in excess and cannot be excreted by the kidneys in oliguric animals, so the alkalosis persists.

Renal dysfunction accompanying massive hepatic necrosis is characterized by oliguria or anuria and is difficult to manage. The renal failure is partly due to the reduction in effective circulating blood flow, but it is also understood to be an example of the hepatorenal syndrome.[35] The many factors contributing to that syndrome include changes in catecholamines, angiotensin, and prostaglandin levels; the syndrome is discussed in Chapter 28.

Massive hepatic necrosis need not represent a hopeless situation. Recovery is possible following injury from a drug or toxin that destroys more than 50% of the liver. Dogs recovering from nitrosamine with a liver mass of 42 to 49% of normal are clinically normal for at least 18 months, although some biochemical abnormalities may continue.[22] Often, radiographic evidence for microhepatica is believed to indicate clinical signs and be responsible for hepatic insufficiency. The studies with nitrosamine show that such a conclusion cannot be made; frequently further evaluation of a small liver reveals no evidence for hepatic disease or insufficiency.

Morphological sequelae to massive hepatic necrosis are largely unknown and speculative. Fibrosis, regenerative nodules, cirrhosis, and possibly chronic hepatitis are suggested to be the outcome. Few long-term studies have been conducted to follow animals recovering from a massive insult to the liver. Following nitrosamine-induced hepatic necrosis, dogs can develop cirrhosis (characterized by sclerosis and regenerating nodules) or hepatitis, or they can recover. In some studies the chronic lesions usually developed, but they followed hepatic biochemical abnormalities that were relatively only modest.[36] In another study, dogs recovering from acute necrosis characterized by severe biochemical abnormalities had normal liver biopsies a number of months later.[22] The difference between these two extremes in pathologic outcome may be due to differences in their management. Dogs fed commercial dog food developed chronic liver pathology. Dogs fed defined diets with casein or soybeans providing the source of protein recovered with nearly normal hepatic histology. Such diets have similar effects on dogs with portasystemic shunts.[37] Rather than the diet having an effect on the animal's nutrition, it may exercise its beneficial effect on minimizing the production and absorption of harmful antigens and toxins from the intestine. Many antigens absorbed from the intestine escape removal and degradation by a liver with compromised function; in dogs recovered from nitrosamine injury, gamma globulins increase by several fold. That increase may also represent an increase in the intestinal absorption of macromolecules, some being substances which can cause hepatic pathology to continue. Bacterial endotoxin absorbed from the intestine acts synergistically to cause hepatic pathology. Anything to reduce its absorption would benefit recovery from any damage to the liver; the nature of the diet may influence that. The absorption of endotoxin and other toxins is reduced by binding resins given orally, and such resins can prevent the hepatotoxic effects of other toxic agents. Some bacterial antigens, such as in *E. coli*, when injected into the portal system of animals, cause portal fibrosis.[38] Increased intestinal permeability allowing increased E. coli absorption may contribute to the progression of hepatic pathology in the animals that do not recover. The nature of the diet may determine the extent of intestinal permeability, toxin production and absorption; it may also determine whether liver pathology worsens or improves. There is good evidence that following recovery from an acute case of a toxic insult the liver is not committed to inevitable fibrosis, cirrhosis, and nodular regeneration.

CLINICAL FINDINGS

Acute and massive hepatic necrosis produces consistent clinical signs, which are usually severe and reflect the degree of hepatic damage. Focal or moderate hepatic necrosis usually causes few if any clinical signs. Signs of acute hepatic failure are nonspecific and consistently include anorexia, depression, vomiting, polydipsia, and dehydration. Icterus is seen invariably when there are significant periportal lesions but does not necessarily develop when massive necrosis involves other parts of the lobule.[21] Fever is seen with infectious hepatitis, with the release of pyrogens from damaged tissue, and when microorganisms and toxins are not removed from the portal circulation. Petechial hemorrhages in the skin and oral mucosa are infrequent. Other manifestations of a coagulopathy causing gastrointestinal bleeding include hematemesis, melena, and rectal bleeding.

LABORATORY FINDINGS

The most consistent finding with hepatic necrosis is increased plasma ALT activity, but that abnormality is found commonly with most other hepatic diseases as well(Table 32-5). The increments correlate with morphologic changes immediately following the initial insult, but plasma ALT activity rapidly returns to normal while the morphological changes are still present. Thus, slight to marked increases in plasma ALT activity suggest hepatic necrosis, and, when necessary, the test is repeated to determine whether necrosis might be a continuing problem. Serum alkaline phosphatase activity can be normal to moderately elevated, with increases reflecting biliary obstruction and regeneration. Other laboratory tests reveal abnormalities less often. Hypoglycemia sometimes accompanies massive hepatic necrosis. Coagulopathies can be associated with hepatic necrosis, and blood clotting is evaluated before liver biopsy by determining bleeding, activated clotting, prothrombin, and partial thromboplastin times. Those tests give normal results in most cases of hepatic necrosis. Hyperbilirubinemia, a variable finding, may not exceed 2.0 to 3.0 mg/dl in dogs with

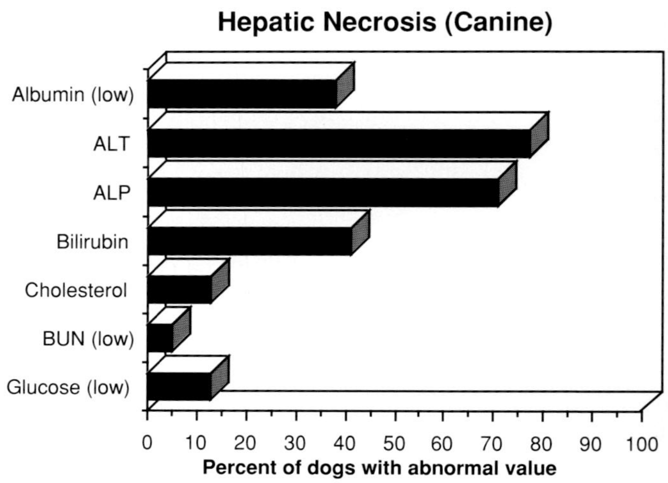

Table 32-5a. Comparison of sensitivities for different tests in dogs with hepatic necrosis.

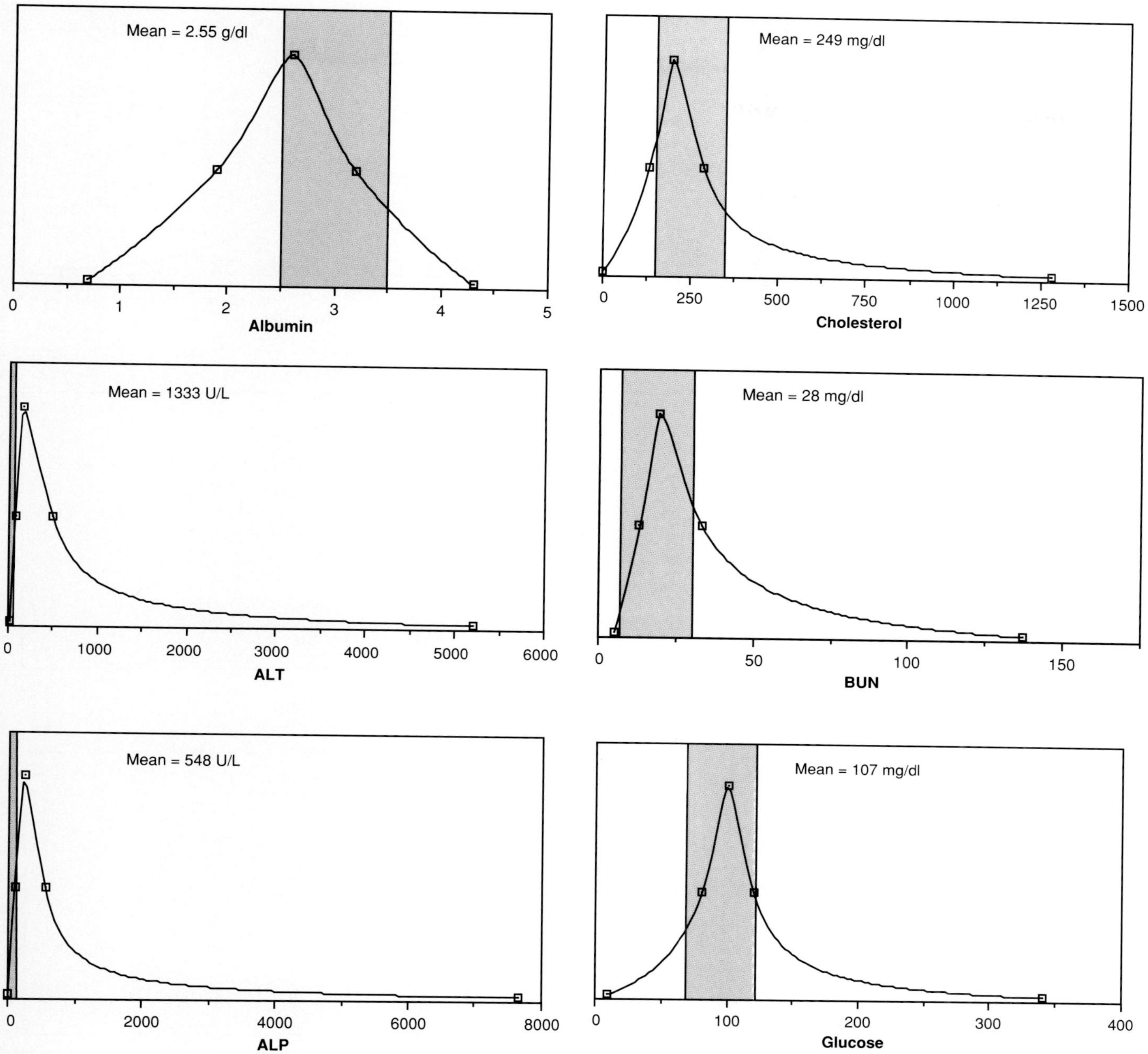

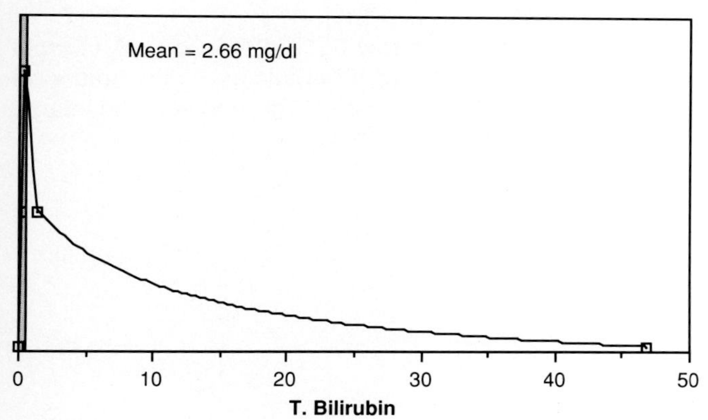

Table 32-5a. Graphs showing distribution of clinical pathology values in dogs with hepatic necrosis. Points on graphs represent 0%, 25%, 50%, 75%, and 100% medians. Normal range is in shaded areas.

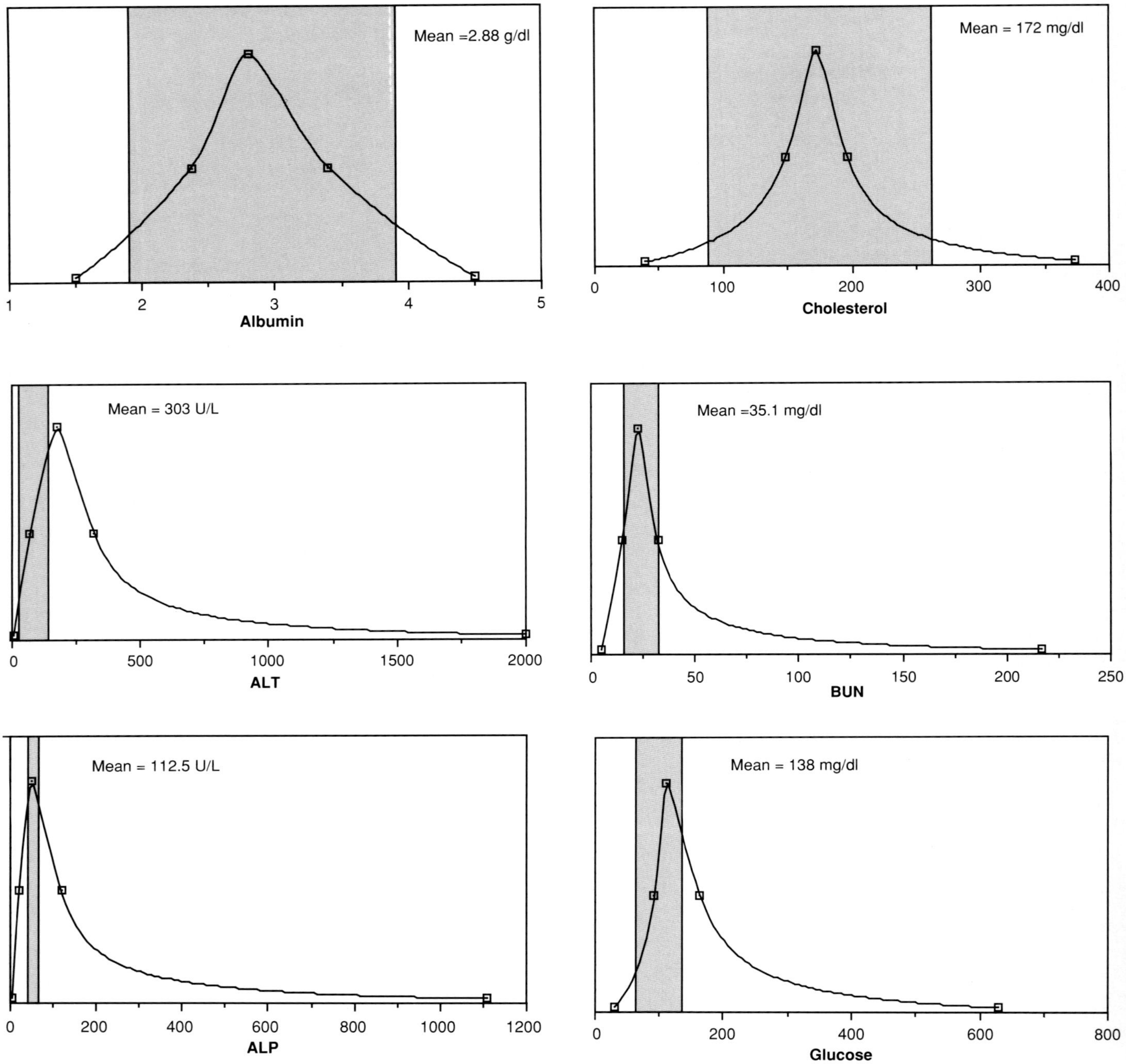

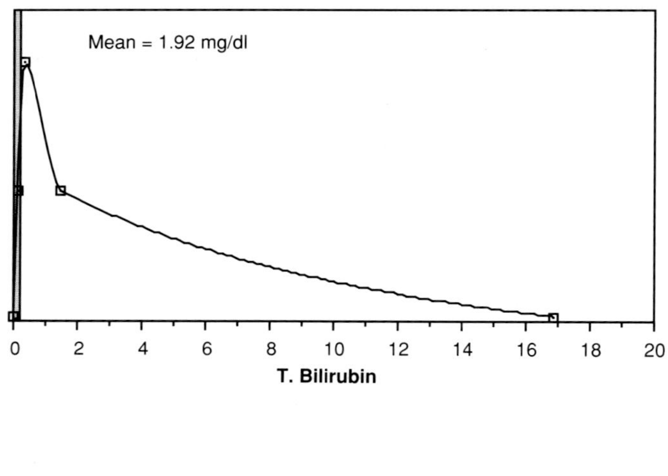

Table 32-5b. Graphs showing distribution of clinical pathology values in cats with hepatic necrosis. Points on graphs represent 0%, 25%, 50%, 75%, and 100% medians. Normal range is in shaded area.

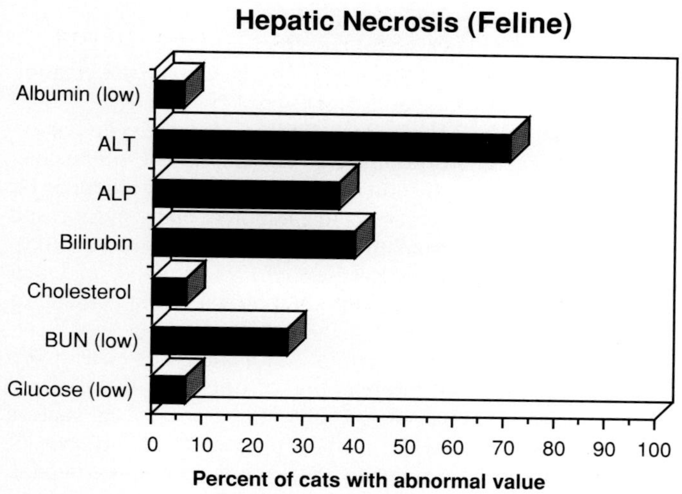

Table 32-5b. Comparison of sensitivities for different tests in cats with hepatic necrosis.

widespread hepatic necrosis. Hyperbilirubinemia usually does not develop unless necrosis involves the periportal hepatocytes. Findings may be normal in function tests, such as sulfobromophthalein retention at 30 minutes and the ammonia tolerance test. They are consistently abnormal, however, with massive hepatic necrosis and hyperbilirubinemia so they need not be determined in those cases. Random blood ammonia determinations are also normal unless hepatic necrosis is severe and diffuse. Plasma amylase and lipase activities are determined to rule out acute pancreatitis as the cause. Most animals with clinical pathologic evidence for hepatic necrosis will have a nonhepatic problem as the cause (Table 32-1). In such cases, confirmation of the necrosis by biopsy is unnecessary.

BIOPSY AND PATHOLOGY FINDINGS

Hepatic necrosis is a morphologic diagnosis made only by histologic examination of the liver. Examples of hepatic necrosis are shown in Figure 32-4.

DIAGNOSIS

Hepatic necrosis cannot be diagnosed from biochemical tests. Moderately to markedly increased plasma ALT activity does not differentiate hepatic necrosis from acute hepatitis, hepatocellular carcinoma, or a variety of other hepatic problems. Slightly increased plasma ALT activity can also be seen with different forms of chronic hepatitis, steroid-induced hepatopathy, and portosystemic vascular shunts. Thus, increased plasma ALT activity is by no means pathognomonic for hepatic necrosis. Additionally, since plasma ALT activity is normal in a few cases, a normal reading does not rule out hepatic necrosis. Diagnosis of hepatic necrosis is made only by liver biopsy.

MANAGEMENT

Focal Necrosis

Since focal necrosis produces few clinical signs, it is seldom identified. When identified, its management should attempt to remove the cause. Management is begun for acute pancreatitis when it is the cause of focal necrosis. Most factors causing focal necrosis are absorbed from the intestinal tract. They include drugs, exogenous toxins, endogenous toxins produced by intestinal bacteria, intestinal microorganisms, dietary antigens, and other antigens able to form immune complexes. An initial goal in managing focal necrosis is to minimize the absorption of such substances. Thus, the patient is evaluated for intestinal disease, which, when found, is managed accordingly. The patient is fed controlled diets free of food additives and preservatives. Some of such chemicals can be hepatotoxic. For example, nitrites used in meat products are converted to hepatotoxic nitrosamines in the intestine. An effectively controlled diet consists of a natural and relatively pure source of carbohydrate and a single protein, such as boiled white rice and cottage cheese. This diet is free also of many antigens that could be potential primary factors causing an intestinal problem that contributes to hepatic necrosis. The diet also affects total numbers and kinds of bacteria in the intestines, and the beneficial effects of a controlled diet may be to reduce the amounts of bacterial toxins produced. Endotoxins contribute to the necrosis of hepatocytes. The net effect of controlled diets is to regulate the entry into the gastrointestinal tract of substances that can affect the formation of absorbable toxins. The diet should contain as much protein as possible without precipitating or aggravating hepatic encephalopathy, since recovery from hepatic necrosis is more rapid on a high-protein than a low-protein diet.

Unless essential to life, drugs are discontinued during the management of focal necrosis. Many drugs are potentially hepatotoxic when used indiscriminately or for extended periods. Focal hepatic necrosis is frequently an incidental finding easily dismissed or ignored as being unimportant. It is unknown what pathological processes result from persistent necrosis, but they could include chronic hepatitis or hepatocellular carcinomas. Chronic hepatic disease often yields no clinical signs until it reaches an advanced stage. Thus, a focal hepatic necrotic process should not be ignored merely because no clinical signs are seen.

Confluent and Massive Necrosis

The management of extensive hepatic necrosis is often unrewarding despite heroic measures. Massive liver necrosis caused by toxins, drugs, and viruses continues when the etiology persists; the liver regenerates when the cause is removed or disappears. The goals of treatment are to remove the cause, prevent signs of hepatic encephalopathy, prevent coagulopathies, prevent massive invasion by intestinal bacteria, maintain normal blood glucose levels, maintain normal hepatic blood flow, and prevent shock and its secondary effects on renal and cardiac function.

The cause of massive necrosis is usually not known. A few cases can be identified as caused by infectious canine hepatitis by finding intranuclear inclusion bodies. The virus replicates in nonimmune dogs and is able to persist for the few days that the animal survives. Nothing can be done to remove this cause of hepatic necrosis. Toxic agents causing massive hepatic necrosis may also remain in the body after the initial insult. Most drugs are toxic because the impaired liver is unable to metabolize them to a water-soluble compound excreted renally or to a form excreted by the biliary system.

An initial approach in the management of massive hepatic necrosis is to assist hepatocytes in rendering toxic substances nontoxic and in maintaining their normal mechanisms for minimizing the effects of toxic substances. Glutathione (glutamyl-cysteinyl-glycine) participates in both of these processes. It binds and inactivates toxic metabolites of many chemicals, and not until hepatic stores of glutathione are reduced to less than 70% do those metabolites bind and damage liver cell macromolecules. The toxic forms of chemicals promote peroxidative damage to lipids and proteins by oxygen-free radicals. The membrane hydroperoxides and hydrogen peroxide formed can be metabolized by the enzyme glutathione peroxidase, and normal structure can return. Reduced glutathione is the substrate for that reaction, being the donor of hydrogen ions.

Intracellular hepatic glutathione synthesis can be promoted by methionine or N-acetylcysteine, each of which acts as a source of cysteine. Glutathione cannot be given because it does not cross cell membranes to enter cells. Of the two, methionine is less effective; it should be given intravenously because given orally it can be converted to mercaptans, which will worsen hepatic encephalopathy. Methionine is given at a dose of 35 mg/kg every 4 hours. Acetylcysteine is available in a form given orally and is currently used specifically for treating acetaminophen toxicity at an oral dose of 140 mg/kg followed by 70 mg/kg every 4 hours.

Vitamin E is a natural antioxidant that protects the liver from injury by oxygen-free radicals. With vitamin E deficiency it is more likely that lipid peroxidation develops as a problem with chemical injury. Vitamin E can be given to minimize or help prevent further peroxidation injury. Administration of vitamin E also protects against the lipid peroxidation produced by excess copper in the liver. Other fat soluble vitamins are not needed. Vitamin A is contraindicated because it acts synergistically with other agents to promote hepatocyte injury.

Some chemicals or toxins are nontoxic until metabolized by the liver. At low rates of metabolic conversion some remain relatively nontoxic; it is only when their conversion is accelerated that toxicity is manifested. There may be some benefit from inhibiting the enzymes involved in the production of toxic metabolites. The cytochrome P-450 enzymes metabolize chemicals such as halothane and acetaminophen to toxic metabolites. Cimetidine is a potent inhibitor of that enzyme system and may be useful in protecting the liver against an ongoing production of toxic metabolites. Cimetidine also helps protect against gastric bleeding, which is a likely problem precipitated by the coagulapathy of massive hepatic necrosis.

Hepatocyte damage may be slowed by protecting the cell against increased influx by calcium.[39] Increased calcium influx is believed by some to be the most important initial event in hepatocyte injury. In the future that may be the basis for the use of calcium channel blockers in treating massive hepatic necrosis. Phenothiazine derivatives, such as chlorpromazine, and flavonoids may protect against calcium influx. Chlorpromazine may also help by inhibiting phospholipase and reducing the production of leukotrienes, which damage hepatic tissue. Glucocorticosteroids have a similar effect. Some prostaglandins appear to be cytoprotective for the liver. There is no information on their use in clinical cases, however.

Hepatic necrosis can induce ornithine decarboxylase activity, which converts ornithine into the polyamine putrescine. That amine inhibits plasmin activity, which is also induced by hepatic necrosis and proceeds to catabolize many plasma and cellular proteins. Administration of putrescine (0.3 mmol/kg) ameliorates the necrosis produced by hepatoxins, and that suggests it may become important in the management of clinical cases.[40]

Whereas drugs are nontoxic until metabolized to toxic products by the liver, the retention of drugs not metabolized during massive necrosis results in a source of toxic substances that destroy hepatocytes as they regenerate. A number of systems have been designed to remove the causes of hepatic necrosis. They are based on dialysis of blood, absorption of toxins from blood by resins, and cross-transfusion, in which normal hepatic function in another animal is used to perform functions lost by the patient.[41-45]

The removal of drugs and toxic substances requires that both renal and hepatic functions be normal. Fluid therapy aids the renal excretion of drugs and substances such as urea, which contributes to hyperammonemia after diffusing into the bacteria-rich environment of the intestine. Renal function is often reduced by massive hepatic necrosis, especially when associated with secondary shock and disseminated intravascular coagulation. In these cases fluid therapy is more important in preventing renal failure than in attempting to wash out toxins.

Theoretically, patients with massive hepatic necrosis should be managed with dialysis therapy, like patients with renal failure.[43] A number of toxic products that cause clinical signs of uremia are removed by dialysis. Dialysis removes the relatively nontoxic urea and other small molecules having molecular weights of less than 300 daltons. Hemodialysis used in dogs with hyperammonemia induced by portacaval shunts removes large amounts of ammonia,[41] and it is of value in humans with hyperammonemia due to chronic hepatitis. Hemodialysis is of no value, however, in treating humans with massive necrosis associated with oliguria and shock. Some important toxins produced with massive necrosis may be large molecules that do not pass through the pores in the membranes normally used in hemodialysis. Membranes with pores able to clear substances of up to 5,000 daltons may prove more useful.[45] Massive hepatic necrosis in humans has been treated with dialysis combined with cross-circulation procedures that use animals for removing the toxins. Dogs have not been used in cross-circulation therapy of hepatic necrosis in canine patients, however. The prognosis is so grave in patients with massive necrosis that if major attempts are made to save an animal's life, they should include the use of normal dogs to remove toxic products via cross-circulation procedures, and that can be combined with hemodialysis.[44] These methods are not designed to sustain life for more than a few days. They are used with the idea that hepatic regeneration is possible, a process that can be rapid.

Circulating toxins associated with massive necrosis can be removed by adsorbents through which the patient's blood is perfused. Activated charcoal is a nonspecific adsorbent given orally to bind toxins in the gastrointestinal tract. It has been used also to treat dogs with experimental acute hepatic necrosis.[42]

Perfusion of the patient's blood through charcoal increased survival times from 9 to 17 hours. Charcoal removes many water-soluble substances such as creatinine, uric acid, and guanidine, and maintains blood ammonia at normal levels. Drugs, biogenic amines, and some of the excess amino acids are removed. Charcoal also removes particles larger than can be removed by hemodialysis. There are some problems with charcoal's removing platelets and leukocytes. When ion exchange and uncharged resins were used in the same manner as charcoal to treat dogs with massive hepatic necrosis, however, the results were not significantly better than in untreated dogs.

Newer approaches have used albumin or enzymes and cells immobilized on charcoal or artificial surfaces for removal of drugs and toxins in the blood. Perfusion of the patient's blood through such an extracorporeal system allows albumin to remove substances such as drugs, hormones, and bilirubin, which have a high affinity for albumin. Enzymes or cells can be immobilized with the capability to remove and metabolize such potentially toxic substances as the aromatic amino acids, ammonia, and phenols.[46]

Blood of patients with massive hepatic necrosis contains cytotoxic factors that inhibit hepatic regeneration.[47] The cytotoxic effect is still found in human patients surviving 10 to 14 days with acute hepatic failure. Attempts to treat such patients fail unless the cytotoxic factors are removed. These factors are heat-labile and removable by charcoal perfusion.

An important part of therapy is to prevent the absorption of toxins from the intestine. It is more important to prevent toxin absorption in massive hepatic necrosis than with any other form of hepatic disease. Patients with massive hepatic necrosis are anorectic, so that dietary considerations are initially unimportant. During fasting, ammonia and other toxins continue to be produced from urea and from nitrogen in desquamated cells and plasma proteins entering the colon. With gastrointestinal hemorrhage, the production of toxin increases greatly, often precipitating a critical condition.[48] Management to minimize toxin production and absorption involves cleansing and irrigating the colon and instilling nonabsorbed antibiotics effective against fecal anaerobic and aerobic bacteria. Cleansing can be with magnesium sulfate or citrate enemas. Neomycin in a 1% solution with the pH adjusted to 4 is introduced as a retention enema. Treatment is continued with the oral administration of lactulose. Flushing and irrigation with antibiotic solutions helps protect the colonic mucosa whose integrity is jeopardized by the shock accompanying hepatic necrosis. That management also ameliorates the signs of hepatic encephalopathy produced by ammonia, mercaptans, and volatile short-chain fatty acids and prevents the absorption of bacterial endotoxins that contribute to hepatic necrosis. The reticuloendothelial system is damaged by acute and massive hepatic necrosis, which allows endotoxin to escape phagocytosis and cause necrosis.[49] Colon cleansing and irrigation also minimizes bacteremia resulting from the failure of the damaged reticuloendothelial system to remove colonic bacteria that are always being absorbed. Parenteral antibiotic therapy is indicated and is discussed in Chapters 16 and 33.

Hepatic circulation is compromised by massive hepatic necrosis. It is corrected by therapy directed against both circulatory deficits and the effects of the ischemia produced. During shock the total hepatic blood flow can decrease 60%. Saline is ineffective in returning the flow to normal. Plasma transfusion or low-molecular weight dextran returns hepatic blood flow to normal and can be used for this purpose unless a coagulopathy has caused an increased bleeding tendency,[50] in which case dextran may worsen the bleeding. Whole blood is not given to treat shock, since that worsens the microcirculation in vascular beds most affected by shock. Vasoactive drugs preventing hepatic ischemia protect against degeneration produced by

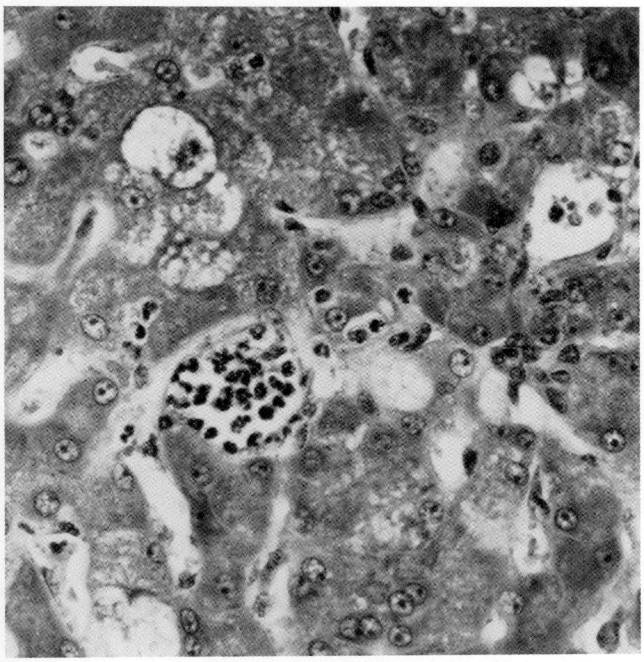

Figure 32-4a. Focal hepatic necrosis. Disappearance of small group of hepatocytes is marked by an accumulation of neutrophils in center of field. Kupffer cell activity is increased.

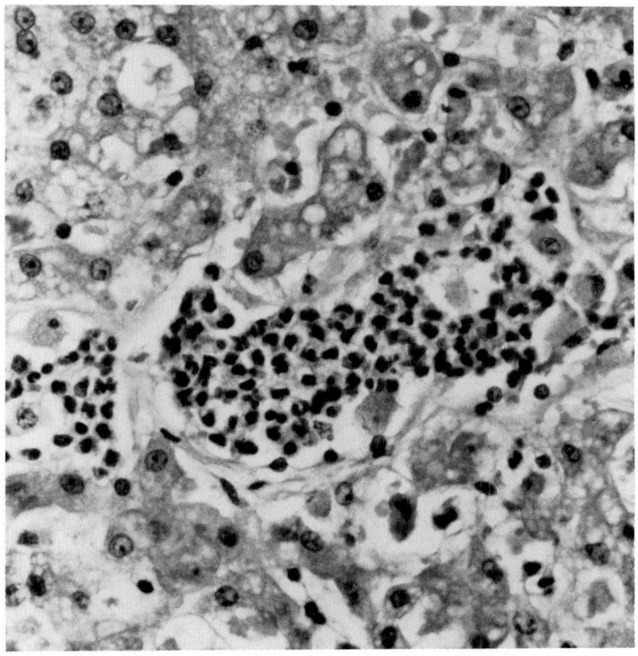

Figure 32-4b. Focal hepatitis secondary to acute pancreatitis. Phlebitis is suggested by engorgement of small vein (portal?) by neutrophils. Kupffer cell activity is increased.

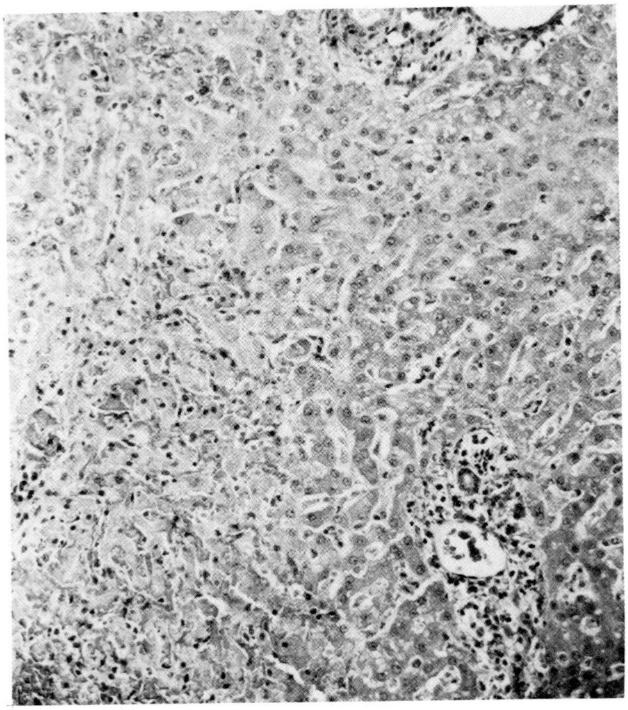

Figure 32-4c. Focal patchy necrosis. Hepatocytes in lower left quarter of field are degenerating. Increased inflammatory cells in portal area on lower right.

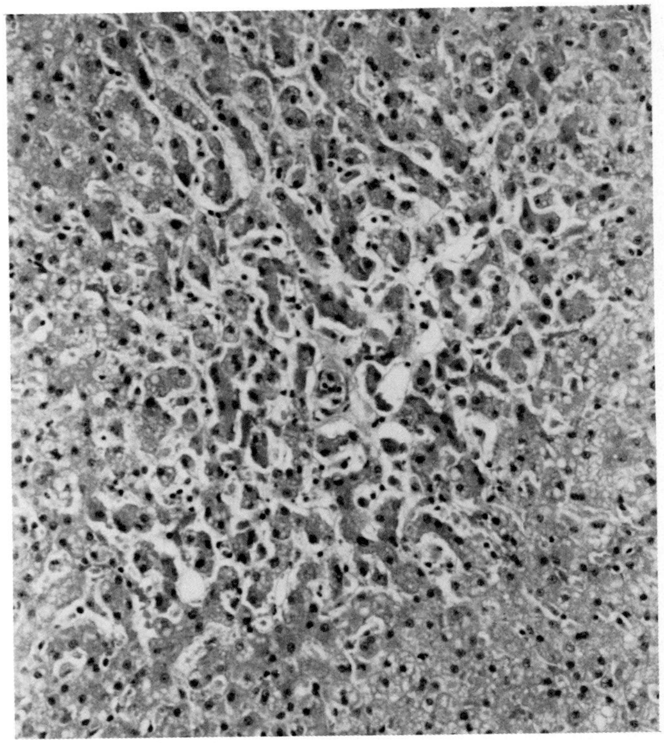

Figure 32-4d. Hepatic necrosis associated with acute pancreatitis. Degeneration of hepatocytes in center of field.

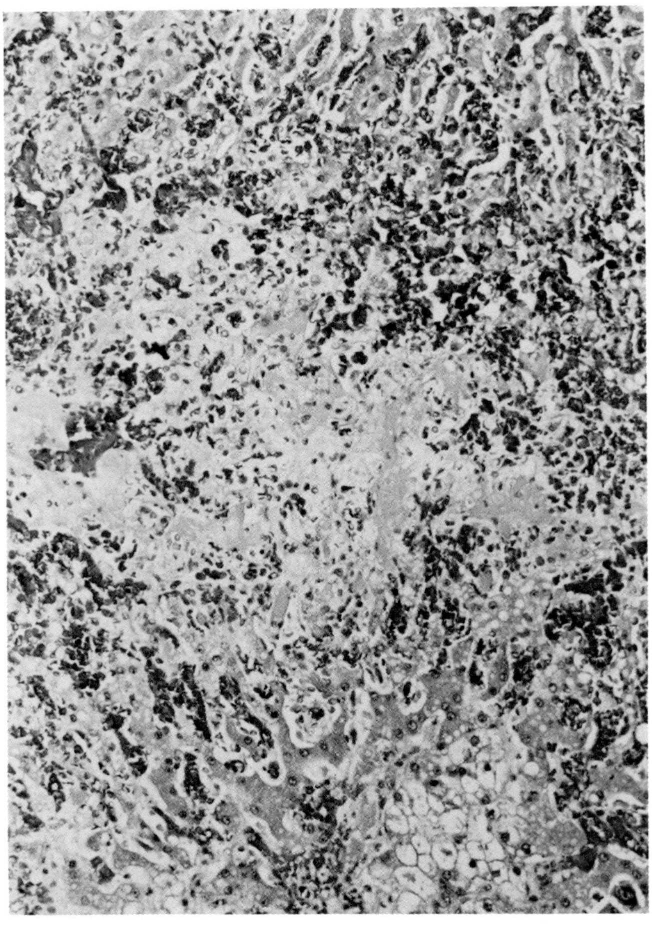

Figure 32-4e. Hepatic necrosis, zonal, centrolobular. In center of field around central vein all hepatocytes have undergone necrosis appearing as a hyaline mass with little visible of nuclear remains. Area around the necrosis is congested. Normal appearing hepatocytes are seen in the top while many of those at the bottom are vacuolated.

agents such as carbon tetrachloride. Vasodilators such as adrenergic-blocking drugs may improve the hepatic problem but are not used with shock since they aggravate hypotension. The anoxic effects of hepatic ischemia are prevented by corticosteroids.[51] Complete 30-minute hepatic ischemia causes a 90% mortality rate, whereas pretreatment with steroids reduces mortality to zero, and steroids given after ischemia appears result in a mortality rate of 54%. Steroids increase the mortality rate in a virus infection.[52] Thus, they must be used with caution with hepatic necrosis from unknown causes. Hepatic circulation is also improved with balanced-electrolyte solutions such as Ringers and lactated Ringers. The lactate may not be metabolized in more severe cases, however. The solutions are given in amounts determined by monitoring central venous pressure, rate of urine formation, and changes in the animal's body weight. For shock therapy, 5% glucose is added to the electrolyte solution. This is beneficial in treating shock and helps maintain normal glucose levels.[53] Low sodium containing fluids may be required if ascites develops.

Management of fulminant hepatic necrosis can include the use of hepatotrophic factors that have been identified as being important in maintaining normal liver size.[54,55] Pancreatic

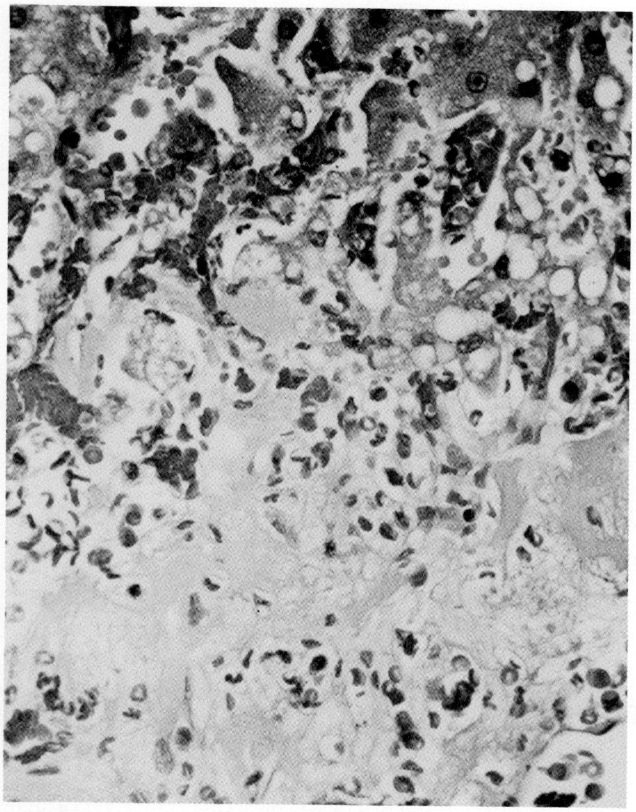

Figure 32-4f. Hepatic necrosis, centrolobular. Necrosis of hepatocytes in middle and lower fields. Some of the hepatocytes in upper field show vacuolation.

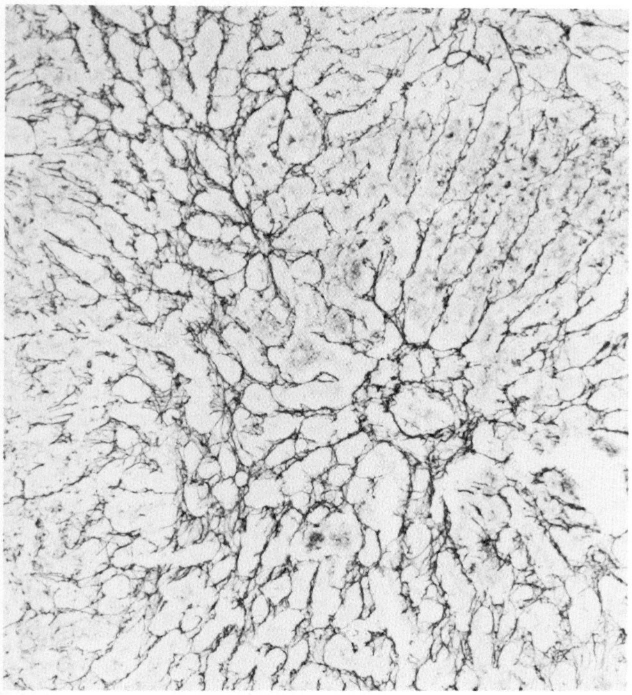

Figure 32-4h. Hepatic necrosis, zonal, centrolobular. Reticulin stain shows collapse of reticulin fibers with loss of hepatocytes due to necrosis. Altered reticulin pattern extends to upper left, reflecting necrosis bridging to an adjacent lobule.

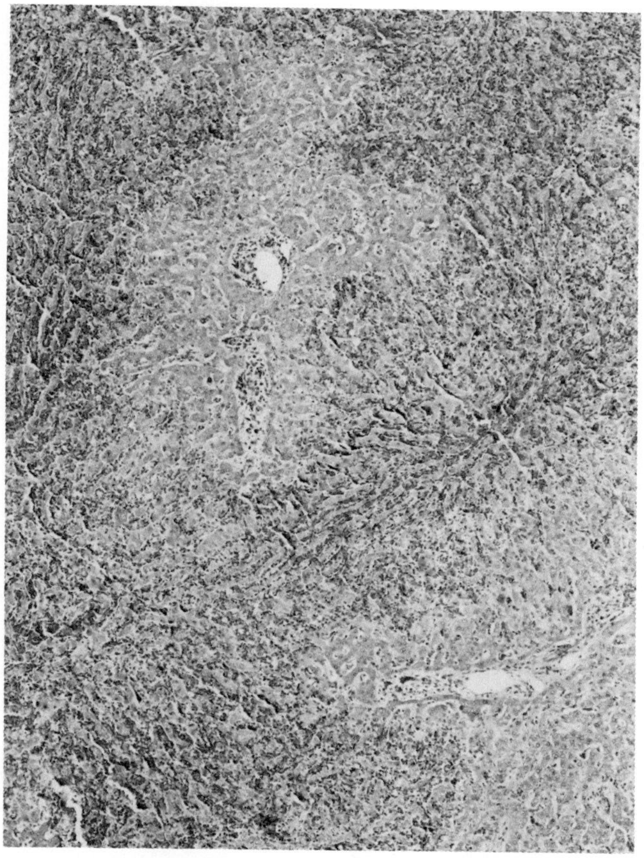

Figure 32-4g. Hepatic necrosis, zonal, centrolobular. Necrosis bridges across lobules from one centrolobular area to adjacent ones. Periportal hepatocytes appear normal in this field.

hormones are important agents, acting in conjunction with the maintenance of normal hepatic blood flow to sustain the normal hepatic mass. There is disagreement, however, on which pancreatic hormone is the most important hepatotrophic agent. Hepatotrophic factors can be used to ameliorate experimental viral hepatitis where mortality is 100% within six days. When glucagon and insulin are infused at the time of challenge with the virus, mortality is only 40%.[55] When animals are treated 24 hours after viral infection, a timing more like that in clinical cases, mortality is 85%. In a model of drug-induced massive hepatic necrosis, glucagon and insulin infusions had no beneficial effects, however.[56] These hormones are normally removed and degraded by the liver, and their blood concentrations increase in chronic hepatic insufficiency. Their plasma levels likely increase with massive hepatic necrosis. Administration of additional hormone may worsen plasma amino acid abnormalities as well as not being of any benefit.

Management of Complications

Coagulopathies are a consistent feature of massive hepatic necrosis. The release of large amounts of thromboplastic substances from damaged hepatocytes causes disseminated intravascular coagulation (DIC). When canine infectious hepatitis is the cause, a generalized vasculitis participates in causing DIC. Thus, therapy is directed against DIC when it is confirmed

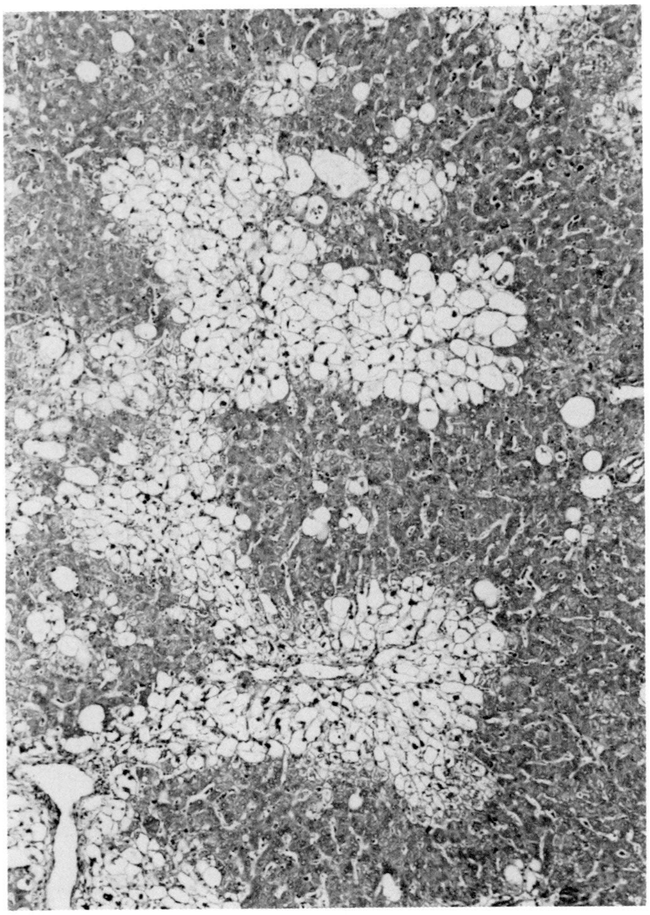

Figure 32-4i. Confluent hepatic degeneration and necrosis, centrolobular. Changes are characterized by lipidosis, steroid changes and necrosis. Dog was completely anorectic and was treated for systemic lupus erythematosus with corticosteroids. A major problem was circulatory failure due to myocarditis and endocarditis. Changes are due to a combination of nutritional deficiency, steroid therapy and reduced hepatic blood perfusion secondary to cardiac failure

Table 32-5. Diet for Management of Hepatic Disease

Ingredient	gm/100 gm Dry Diet
Casein	9.0
Animal fat	20.0
Sucrose	32.35
Corn starch	32.35
Vitamin mix	1.0
Mineral mix	5.0
Choline chloride	0.3

by a thrombocytopenia, hypofibrinogenemia, and prolonged activated clotting time. Heparin is given intravenously three times a day at 100 units/Kg body weight. Hepatic necrosis can reduce levels of clotting factors, especially those with the shortest half-lives. Marked reductions are corrected with fresh blood or plasma. Using only heparin to treat a coagulopathy can cause fatal hemorrhage in patients with a deficiency in blood-clotting factors.[23] Thus, the treatment for coagulopathies caused by hepatic necrosis is heparin combined with fresh blood or plasma. Treatment for DIC minimizes thrombosis in vital organs. Thrombosis of the gastric mucosa produces ischemia, and liver failure results in hypergastrinemia, causing increased secretion of gastric acid. The combination of ischemia and gastric-acid hypersecretion creates ideal conditions for ulceration of the gastric mucosa. Thus, the stomach has the greatest potential for hemorrhage, and other areas in the intestine are also vulnerable. The incidence of gastric ulceration is reduced by administering cimetidine or by giving antacids frequently, at hourly intervals if possible, in order to maintain gastric pH near neutral. Since alkalosis is the most likely acid-base imbalance with massive hepatic necrosis, nonabsorbed antacids are used. DIC is also caused by endotoxins absorbed from the gut;[57] treatment to cleanse the colon is therefore beneficial.

As described earlier, the nature of the diet, once eating resumes, determines whether the liver recovers its normal morphology. That recovery is possible when a defined diet is fed; recovery is less likely with the feeding of commercial animal food. The protein source should be soy beans (tofu) or milk (cottage cheese). That can be combined with a carbohydrate such as rice and an animal fat. When supplemented with minerals and vitamins, a complete and balanced diet is fed (Table 32-5). Commercially prepared enteral diets can also be fed. Such diets sustain dogs with hepatic insufficiency in a relatively normal state compared with the progressive deterioration noted when similar animals are fed a commercial animal food. Those enteral diets have milk and soybeans as the source of their proteins.

REFERENCES

1. Hottendorf, G.H. and Hirth, R.S.: Lesions of spontaneous subclinical disease in Beagle dogs. Vet. Path. 11:240-258, 1974.
2. McDonald, G.S.H. and Courtney, M.G.: Operation-associated neutrophils in a percutaneous liver biopsy: effect of prior transjuglar procedure. Histopathology 10:217-222, 1986.
3. de la Monte, S.M., Arcidi, J.M., Moore, G.W. and Hutchins, G.M.: Midzonal necrosis as a pattern of hepatocellular injury after shock. Gastroenterology 86:627-631, 1984.
4. Kapp, P. and Lapis, K.: Reaction of dogs treated with immunosuppressive agents to infection with the virus of Rubarth disease. Acta Vet. Acad. Sci. Hung. 28:145-157, 1980.
5. Jarrett, W.F.H. and O'Neil, B.W.: A new transmissible agent causing acute hepatitis, chronic hepatitis and cirrhosis in dogs. Vet. Rec. 116:629-635, 1985.
6. Nolan, J.P.: Endotoxin, reticuloendothelial function, and liver injury. 5:458-465, 1981.
7. deHeer, K., Sauer H-D, Werner, B. and Kloeppel, G.: Protective effects of cholestyramine on liver cirrhosis induced by carbon tetrachloride in the rat. Gut 21:860-865, 1980.
8. Thomas, H.C.: Immunologic aspects of liver disease. In, Diseases of the Liver. Edited by L. Schiff and E.R. Schiff. J.B. Lippincott, Philadelphia. 163-185, 1987.
9. Rabin, B.S. and Rogers, S.: Pathologic changes in the liver and kidney produced by immunization with intestinal antigens. Am. J. Path. 84:201-210, 1976.
10. MacSween, R.N.M., Anthony, P.P. and Scheuer, P.J.: Pathology of the Liver. Churchill Livingston, New York, 1987.
11. Zimmerman, H.J. and Maddrey, W.C.: Toxic and drug-induced hepatitis. In, Diseases of the Liver. Edited by L. Schiff and E.R. Schiff. J.B. Lippincott, Philadelphia. 591-667, 1987.
12. Papich, M.G. and Davis, L.E.: Drugs and the liver. Vet. Clin. N. Am. 15:77-95, 1985.
13. Bunch, S.E., Castleman, W.L., Baldwin, B.H., Hornbuckle, W.E. and Tennant, B.C.: Effects of long-term primidone and phenytoin administration on canine hepatic function and morphology. Am. J. Vet. Res. 46:105-115, 1985.
14. Faraj, B.A., Ali, F.M., Fulenwider, J.T., Malveaux, E.J. and Stacciarini, W.M.: Hepatorenal failure induced by tetracycline in dogs with portacaval shunt. J. Pharm. Exp. Ther. 221:558-563, 1982.
15. Polzin, D.J., Stowe, C.M., O'Leary, T.P., Stevens, J.B. and Hardy, R.M.: Acute hepatic necrosis associated with the administration of mebendazole to dogs. JAVMA 179:1013-1016, 1981.
16. Van Cauteren, H., Marsboom, R., Vandenberg, J. and Will, J.A.: Safety studies evaluating the effect of mebendazole on liver function in dogs. JAVMA 183:93-98, 1983.
17. Wigton, D.H., Kociba, G.J., and Hoover, E.A.: Infectious canine hepatitis: animal model for viral-induced disseminated intravascular coagulation. Blood 47:287-296, 1976.
18. Dixon, M.F., Fulker, M.J., Walker, B.E., Kelleher, J. and Losowsky, M.S.: Serum transaminase levels after experimental-induced hepatic necrosis. Gut 16:800-807, 1975.
19. Chrisp, C.E.: Personal communication on data from Radiobiology Laboratories Beagle Colony.
20. Desmet, V.J.: Morphologic and histochemical aspects of cholestasis. In, Progress in Liver Diseases, Vol. 4. Edited by H. Popper and F. Schaffner. Grune and Stratton, New York. 97-132, 1972.
21. Gopinath, C. and Ford, E.J.H.: Location of liver injury and extent of bilirubinaemia in experimental liver lesions. Vet. Path. 9:99-108, 1972.
22. Strombeck, D.R., Harrold, D., Rogers, Q., Wheeldon, E., Stem, J., Schaeffer, M.: Plasma amino acid, glucagon, and insulin concentrations in dogs with nitrosamine-induced hepatic disease. AJVR 44(11):2028-2036.
23. Hillenbrand, P., Parbhoo, S.P., Jedrychowkis, A. and Sherlock, S.: Significance of intravascular coagulation and fibrinolysis in acute hepatic failure. Gut 15:83-88, 1974.
24. Verstraete, M., Vermylen, J. and Collen, D.: Intravascular coagulation in liver disease. Ann. Rev. Med. 25:447-455, 1974.
25. Furnival, C.M., Mackenzie, R.J., MacDonald, G.A. and Blumgart, L.H.: The mechanism of impaired coagulation after partial hepatectomy in the dog. Surg. Gynecol. Obstet. 143:81-86, 1976.
26. Strombeck, D.R., and Feldman, B.F.: Unpublished observations.
27. Roberts, H.R. and Cederbaum, A.I.: The liver and blood coagulation: physiology and pathology. Gastroenterology 62:297-320, 1972.
28. Feldman, B.F.: Disseminated intravascular coagulation. Comp. Cont. Ed. 3:46-57, 1981.
29. Badylak, S.F.: Coagulopathies associated with hepatic disease. Calif. Vet. 14-17, February 1982.
30. Aguirre, A., Yoshimura, N., Westman, T. and Fischer, H.E.: Plasma amino acids in dogs with two experimental forms of liver damage. J. Surg. Res. 16:339-345, 1974.
31. Cacciatore, L., Antoniello, S., Vallentino, B. and DeRitis, F.: Arginase activity, arginine and ornithine of plasma in experimental liver damage. Enzyme 17:269-275, 1974.
32. Zieve, L.: Hepatic encephalopathy. In, Diseases of the Liver. Edited by L. Schiff and E.R. Schiff. J.B. Lippincott, Philadelphia. 925-948, 1987.
33. Wright, R., Alberti, K.G.M.M., Karran, S. and Millward-Sadler, G.H.: Liver and Biliary Disease. W.B. Saunders, Philadelphia, 1985.
34. Record, C.O., Isles, R.A., Cohen, R.D. and Williams, R.: Acid-base and metabolic disturbances in fulminant hepatic failure. Gut 16:144-149, 1975.
35. Davidson, E.W. and Dunn, M.J.: Pathogenesis of the Hepatorenal Syndrome. Ann. Rev. Med. 38:361-372, 1987.
36. Madden, J.W., Gertman, P.M. and Peacock, E.E.: Dimethylnitrosamine-induced hepatic cirrhosis: A new canine model of an ancient human disease. Surgery 68:260-268, 1970.
37. Schaeffer, M.C., Rogers, Q.R., Buffington, C.A., Wolfe, B.M.and Strombeck, D.R.: Long-term biochemical and physiologic effects of surgically placed portacaval shunts in dogs. AJVR 47(2):346-355, 1986.
38. Kono, K., Ohnishi, K., Omata, M., Saito, M., Nakayama, T., Hatano, H., Nakajima, Y., Sugita, S. and Okuda, K.: Experimental portal fibrosis produced by intraportal injection of billed nonpathogenic Escherichia coli in rabbits. Gastroenterology 94:797-796, 1988.
39. Popper, H.: Summary. In: Mechanisms of hepatocyte injury and death. D. Keppler, H. Popper, L. Bianchi and W. Reutter, eds. Falk Symposium 38. MTP Press LTD. Boston, 389-397, 1984.
40. Putnam, C.W., Buckley, A.R., Warneke, J.A., Karrer, F.M., Rhenman, B. and Steinbronn, K.: The mechanism of hepatoprotection by epsilon aminocaproic acid and putrescine. Surgery 96:214-222, 1984.
41. Wallin, V.M., Turcotte, J., Sloan, C.H., Nosanchuk, J.D., Ameriks, J. and Child, C.G.: Conventional and cross dialysis in hepatic failure. Curr. Top. Surg. Res. 2:75-86, 1970.
42. Weston, M.J., Gazzard, B.G., Buxton, B.H., Winch, J., Machado, A.L., Flax, H. and Williams, R.: Effects of haemoperfusion through charcoal or XAD-2 resin on an animal model of fulminant liver failure. Gut 15:482-486, 1974.
43. Berk, P.D., Martin, J.F., Scharschmidt, B.F. and Plotz, P.H.: Current status of artificial hepatic support systems. In, Progress in Liver Diseases, Vol. 5. Edited by H. Popper and F. Schaffner. Grune and Stratton, New York. 398-417, 1976.
44. Burnell, J.M., Dennis, M.B., Clayson, K.J., Smuckler, E.A. and Clift, R.A.: Evaluation in dogs of cross-circulation in the treatment of acute hepatic necrosis induced by yellow phosphorus. Gastroenterology 71:827-831, 1976.

45. Denis, J., Opolon, P., Nusinovici, V., Granger, A. and Darnis, F.: Treatment of encephalopathy during fulminant hepatic failure by hemodialysis with high permeability membrane. Gut 19:787-793, 1978.
46. Demetroiu, A.A., Whiting, J.F., Feldman, D.: Replacement of liver function in rats by transplantation of microcarrier-attached hepatocytes. Science 233:1190-1192, 1986.
47. Williams, R.: Hepatic failure and development of artificial liver support system. In, Progress in Liver Diseases. Vol. 5. Edited by H. Popper and F. Schaffner. Grune and Stratton, New York. 418-435, 1976.
48. Gans, H., Mori, K., Lindsey, E., Kaster, B., Richter, D., Quinlan, R., Dineen, P.A. and Tan, B.H.: Septicemia as a manifestation of acute liver failure. Surg. Gynecol. Obstet. 132:783-790, 1971.
49. Liehr, H., Grun, M., Thile, H., Branswig, D. and Rasenack, U.: Endotoxin-induced liver necrosis and intravascular coagulation in rats enhanced by portacaval collateral circulation. Gut 16:429-436, 1975.
50. Darle, N. and Lim, R.C.: Effect of low molecular dextran on total liver blood flow in hemorrhagic shock. Eur. Surg. Res. 8:132-139, 1976.
51. Figueroa, I., Santiago-Delphin, E.A.: Steroid protection of the liver during experimental ischemia. Surg. Gynecol. Obstet. 140:368-370, 1975.
52. Sabesin, S.M. and Koff, R.S.: Pathogenesis of experimental viral hepatitis. New Eng. J. Med. 290:944-950 and 966-1002, 1974.
53. Wilson, R.F. and Sibbald, W.J.: Editorial: A new look at an old approach to resuscitation: early aggressive fluid administration. Circulatory Shock 2:1-3, 1975.
54. Bucher, N.L.R.: Insulin, glucagon and the liver. Adv. Enz. Reg. 15:221-230, 1977.
55. Farivar, M., Wands, J.R., Isselbacher, K.J. and Bucher, N.L.R.: Effect of insulin and glucagon on fulminant murine hepatitis. New Eng. J. Med. 295:1517-1519, 1976.
56. Minuk, G.Y., Sherman, T.A., Shaffer, E.A. and Kelly, S.K.: A comparative study of the effects of insulin/glucagon infusions, parenteral amino acids and high dose corticosteroids on survival in a rabbit model of acute fulminant hepatitis. Hepatology 6:73-78, 1986.
57. Wilkinson, S.P., Arroyo, V., Gazzard, B.G., Moddie, H. and Williams, R.: Relation of renal failure and haemorrhagic diathesis to endotoxaemia in fulminant hepatic failure. Lancet 1:521-524, 1974.

Chapter 33

Chronic Hepatitis, Chronic Copper Toxicity, Suppurative Hepatitis, Granulomatous Hepatitis

Chronic Hepatitis

Clinical Synopsis - Dogs

Diagnostic features

* Female Doberman Pinschers, predisposed
* Depression, anorexia, vomiting common
* Rarely ascites, icterus, CNS signs
* ALT and SAP usually elevated
* Bilirubin often elevated; hypoalbuminemia frequent
* Liver function tests usually abnormal
* Hepatic biopsy reveals inflammation and provides pathological classification of hepatitis

Standard Management

* Remove any suspected cause
* Restricted protein, low residue, balanced diet fed in small amounts frequently
* Use milk or soy protein not meat
* Prednisilone (or prednisone) 2.2 mg/kg/day 7-20 days, followed by 1.1 mg/kg/day for 7-10 days; followed by 0.6 mg/kg/day until disease judged in remission
* Management of hepatic encephalopathy. Neomycin 20 mg/kg q 6 hr PO for 2-3 days; lactulose 1-2 ml/kg q 6 hr PO as required; saline enema 10-20 ml/kg q 12 hr
* Management of infection. Trimethoprim-sulfa 15 mg/kg q 12 hr 10-14 days or cephalosporins and penicillins
* Management of ascites. Sodium restriction; judicious use of spironolactone 1-2 mg/kg q 12 hr PO; paracentesis (judicious)

Cholangitis - Cholangiohepatitis

Clinical Synopsis- Cats

Diagnostic features

* Adult cats
* Anorexia, depression intermittent vomiting, sometimes icterus
* Increased ALT, ALP, bilirubin common
* Liver biopsy shows suppurative or lymphocytic-plasmacytic inflammation centered about portal triads

Standard treatment

* Prednisone+ 2-3 mg/kg q 12 hr PO for 1-2 weeks; followed by 1 mg/kg q 24 hr for 2 weeks; weaned off over the ensuing 2-4 weeks
* Cephalexin 30 mg/kg q 12 hr PO for 4 weeks
* Dehydrocholic acid (Decholin) 10-15 mg/kg PO 7-10 days (provided no extrahepatic obstruction)

+ There is controversy as to whether prednisone should be used in the suppurative form.

Acute and chronic hepatitis are characterized morphologically by inflammation and biochemically by changes in plasma enzymes and liver function tests. The definition of chronic hepatitis in humans stipulates that the process continues without improvement for 6 months.[1-3] More recently the definition of chronic hepatitis has been restricted to a chronic necro-inflammatory, primarily hepatocytic lesion with or without cirrhosis, in which the lymphocyte dominates the inflammation and in which viral, 'auto-immune,' drug or unknown causes are involved; intra- or extrahepatic bile ducts are not the primary or main targets. Thus, with this classification chronic hepatitis is described according to causes rather than morphologic appearance. Chronic hepatitis in dogs has been described as many different entities based on morphologic criteria (Table 33-1), which has confused our understanding more than it has enlightened our wisdom on hepatic disease. A group of dogs described with chronic active hepatitis in 1978 was studied after visiting professor Sheila Sherlock diagnosed the first one as having chronic active hepatitis.[4] The use of the term continued and along with it the idea that the disease must be like the disease in humans. The adjective active is redundant since hepatitis itself is defined as active to some degree; therefore, the term chronic hepatitis best describes the problem, and any further appropriate description should be limited to a cause, known or unknown. The evolution of current terminology for human hepatitis has developed in a similar way with different groups identifying what appeared to be different diseases. These discrepancies occured despite the fact that hepatologists had a far greater understanding of the etiology and pathogenesis of hepatitis in humans than they had in veterinary cases. This chapter describes chronic hepatitis and, where possible, discusses its cause and pathogenesis.

Table 33-1 Terminology applied to hepatitis

Acute hepatitis
Nonspecific reactive hepatitis
Chronic persistent hepatitis
Chronic aggressive hepatitis
Chronic hepatitis
Chronic cholangiohepatitis
Chronic lobular hepatitis
Lobular dissecting hepatitis
Cholangitis
Drug-induced hepatitis
Toxic hepatitis
Hepatopathy
Primary biliary cirrhosis
Micronodular cirrhosis
Macronodular cirrhosis

Because most cases of chronic hepatitis are not recognized until the pathology has reached an advanced stage, the disease has not been widely understood. A major reason is that clinical signs associated with hepatitis are nonspecific. Jaundice is a relatively consistent feature of chronic hepatitis in most species. In dogs, however, it does not appear as early as in other species, since the renal threshold for conjugated bilirubin in the dog is relatively low, and at low plasma levels the pigment is readily excreted in the urine. Thus, the lack of this almost pathognomic sign in dogs makes it difficult to determine the duration of chronic hepatitis.

Acute and chronic hepatitis can be responsive to treatment when recognized early, but for chronic hepatitis there is often little hope for successful treatment otherwise. Thus, screening with chemistry panels and liver function tests is important whenever patients have nonspecific signs due to an unknown cause. Hepatitis is diagnosed only through liver biopsy. The goal of evaluating clinical findings is to justify collecting enough laboratory information to decide whether hepatic disease is not a problem or whether the laboratory findings merit liver biopsy.

ETIOLOGY

Hepatitis can be primary where the liver is the most important target of the injurious agent. With the primary target in a nonhepatic tissue or system, any resulting hepatitis can be considered secondary or as a consequence of pathology in the primary site. Primary hepatitis is caused by viral agents, drugs, and some immune responses, but in most cases the cause is unknown. Secondary hepatitis represents lesions associated with infections, septicemia, neoplastic disease, and primary disease in the gastrointestinal system, pancreas, and urogenital system. In dogs primary disease represents twice as many cases as secondary hepatitis; in cats only 27% of cases represent primary hepatitis (Table 33-2). That difference is biased by more complete pathology information on cats than on dogs. The diagnosis of hepatitis in cats is from complete necropsy 75% of the time and from biopsy 25% of the time. In contrast, the diagnosis of hepatitis in dogs is from complete necropsy only 33% of the time and is limited to biopsy findings 67% of the time. With more necropsies more dogs may be found to have secondary hepatitis.

Viruses are a well-documented cause of hepatitis in both animals and humans.[5] Chapter 29 describes the pathogenesis of acute and chronic hepatitis caused by the infectious canine hepatitis virus. This virus can initiate an immune response that perpetuates the pathologic process and causes chronic changes.[6] A number of other viruses can cause hepatic lesions in animals. For instance, a viral agent is the probable cause of a newly recognized disease in Great Britain.[7] The agent causes acute hepatitis, chronic hepatitis, and cirrhosis in dogs. The disease is found in an area where the incidence of hepatocellular carcinoma is much greater than expected. It was suggested the disease be called canine acidophil cell hepatitis based on consistent morphologic findings of a strongly acidophilic cytoplasm in hepatocytes. The disease can be readily reproduced by inoculation of normal dogs with serum or liver cell homogenates from infected dogs. That other viruses may cause hepatitis in dogs is supported by occasional reports of viral-appearing agents in electron micrographs of livers with hepatitis. There is also evidence that animals may react to hepatitis viruses from other species. Dogs as well as other animals can have serum antibodies to a human hepatitis virus.[8] For that to happen it is likely that such viruses would replicate even though they do not cause any recognizable pathology. In felines, the feline infectious peritonitis virus is a well-documented cause of hepatitis. With that virus, hepatocytes or cells in other tissues are injured by the immune response directed against eliminating the virus.

Chronic hepatitis has been produced in experimental dogs by infection with leptospires.[9] It is unknown whether leptospires are responsible for clinical cases of chronic hepatitis.

Drugs and chemicals can also cause chronic hepatitis.[1,2,10] Many different drugs and metals can cause acute liver damage as described in Chapter 32, and long-term use of any drug is capable of producing chronic hepatitis. The continuous administration of drugs is sometimes associated with biochemical evidence for hepatic inflammation that disappears with discontinuation of the drug. Few such occurrences are verified by liver biopsy.

Immune mechanisms are important in the development of chronic hepatitis (Chapter 29). There is little evidence that immune responses initiate the pathology, or that antibodies synthesized against smooth muscle, nuclear material, or mitochondria perpetuate injury to hepatocytes. These antibodies appear as a nonspecific response to cellular injury and are not specific for any one organ or species of animal. Chronic liver disease can also be associated with immune-mediated diseases such as autoimmune hemolytic anemia and systemic lupus erythematosus, suggesting that some abnormal immune responses are generalized and include damage to hepatocytes. Studies on the relationship of these immune-mediated diseases to chronic hepatitis do not provide additional evidence that an autoimmune process causes chronic hepatitis. The only evidence for an autoimmune pathogenesis is from animals immunized with liver-specific proteins, where antibodies against these proteins bind to hepatocytes and are associated with cell destruction.[11] A case report describes a dog with chronic hepatitis following immunotherapy; remission was seen upon discontinuation of the treatment.[12]

Chronic hepatitis can develop secondary to problems in

Figure 33-2a.

Causes of Hepatitis - Canine

Pathology *Biopsies 67%* *Necropsies 33%*	Etiology						
	Primary	Infection	Neoplastic Disease	Renal Disease	GI Disease	Steroid Hepatopathy	Misc
Granulomatous	9	7	2	2	---	---	---
Periportal, mild to moderate	27	1	2	6	4	5	---
Periportal, severe	32	3	---	2	1	1	2
Chronic	21	9	---	1	3	---	1
Chronic active	32	---	1	---	3	---	---
Mild	12	4	2	6	2	1	2
Multifocal	9	2	2	2	1	---	2
Multifocal, acute to subacute	18	9	2	---	6	1	---
Cholangiohepatitis	12	---	---	---	4	---	---
	170 (64%)	97 (36%)					

Figure 33-2b.

Causes of Hepatitis - Feline

Pathology *Biopsies 25%* *Necropsies 75%*	Etiology						
	Primary	**Infection**	**Neoplastic Disease**	**Renal Disease**	**GI Disease**	**FIP**	**Misc**
Granulomatous	5		---	1	1	3	---
Periportal, mild to moderate	14	5	5	8	7	---	1
Periportal, severe	4	1	2	2	2	---	---
Chronic	2	---	1	---	1	---	---
Diffuse - mild to moderate	---	3	1	2	1	1	---
Multifocal, acute to subacute, moderate	1	5	5	4	1	3	1
Multifocal, acute, severe	---	5	---	---	2	---	---
Cholangiohepatitis	7	---	3	9	7	---	---
	33 (26%)	93 (74%)					

another system as well as appearing as a single disease entity. Hepatitis sometimes appears with gastrointestinal disease, and biochemical evidence for hepatic disease disappears when the intestinal problem is corrected. The causes of chronic hepatitis with chronic bowel disease are multifactorial and can include bacterial and dietary toxins from the intestine, colonic and dietary antigens initiating destructive immune responses, and invading colonic microorganisms. With immune-mediated diseases the etiology may be found to be viruses affecting a number of different organs.

INCIDENCE

The incidence of acute and chronic hepatitis in the VMTH at Davis is 12.5 cases per 1,000 dogs and 19.0 per 1,000 cats. The incidence of cirrhosis is low at 1 case per 1,000 in dogs. All forms of hepatitis account for 18% of hepatic disease diagnosed by histopathology in dogs and 22.9% in cats. The mean age at which chronic hepatitis is recognized in dogs is between 7 and 8 years. There is no difference in the distribution of males and females in dogs with chronic hepatitis. Doberman Pinschers may be an exception. In some studies there was a strong predisposition for females to have the disease.[13-15] Doberman Pinschers are believed to be more predisposed than other breeds to hepatitis due to an unknown cause.[13-16] The incidence in one study was 4 times greater than the expected incidence according to general hospital population for Dobermans.[16] A high percentage of hepatitis in dogs is primary, with only one third being secondary to some other problem; the opposite is true for cats (Table 33-2).

PATHOGENESIS AND PATHOLOGY

Chapter 29 discusses the pathogenesis of injury included by viruses, drugs, toxins, and immune mechanisms. Following hepatocyte damage regeneration begins, and morphology and function can return to normal if the insult is no longer present. When injury results in inflammation, the sequel is an acute, subacute, or chronic hepatitis. These consequences are likely to persist when the injurious agent continues its effects. With no further injury by a virus, drug, or toxin it is possible for a return of normal hepatic morphology. Some animals with drug-induced chronic hepatitis recover when the drug is discontinued. In other cases the pathology progresses in severity despite removal of the cause. The basis for continuing and worsening pathology in primary chronic hepatitis is unknown but can be surmised from the nature of pathologic changes.

By definition the predominant inflammatory cell type found to establish a diagnosis of primary chronic hepatitis is the lymphocyte. With plasma cells, lymphocytes are suggested to participate in an immune-mediated role perpetuating the problem, regardless of its initial cause (Figure 33-1). These immunocytes can produce cells that are directly cytotoxic for hepatocytes, mount an antibody-mediated cytotoxic response, and produce antibodies enabling complement-fixing antigen-antibody complexes to be formed, which can damage tissue without requiring cytotoxic cells (Chapter 29). Experimental studies show that immunocytes infiltrating the liver can synthesize antibodies directed against liver-specific antigens.[17] The

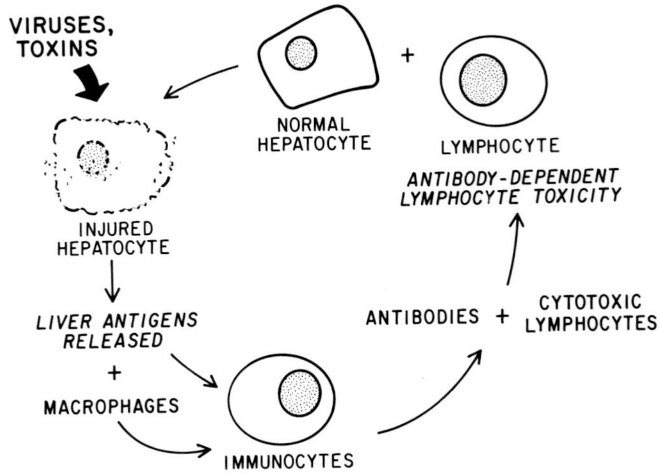

Figure 33-1. Pathogenesis of chronic hepatitis by immune-mediated mechanisms following initial insult by viruses or toxins.

large numbers of lymphocytes and plasma cells found with chronic hepatitis could be synthesizing antibodies against liver-specific proteins.[18,19]

Inflammatory cells are responsible for the necrosis and fibrosis found in chronic hepatitis.[20] Inflammatory cells that cause hepatocyte destruction are found initially in portal areas. Damage to viable liver structure opens up avenues for inflammatory cells to migrate from portal areas and cause widespread fibrosis. Destruction of hepatocytes by massive or bridging necrosis permits the movement of inflammatory cells into the void created (Figure 33-2). With the absence of inflammatory cells, normal lobules collapse into the space created by lost hepatocytes. When hepatic architecture is not destroyed, regeneration is possible. Regeneration following necrosis can be attempted by proliferation of bile ductules; when they extend from portal areas into the parenchyma, they offer another means for inflammatory cells to enter normal areas of the lobule. Bridging necrosis is an extension of inflammation from one portal triad to adjacent ones and from portal areas through the lobule to the central vein. Inflammatory cells are found at all points of bridging necrosis, again suggesting that these cells, finding an avenue out of portal areas, initiate widespread necrosis. Inflammation also causes necrosis of the hepatocytes forming a plate adjacent to portal triads (Figure 33-3). This necrosis of limiting plates is an important feature of chronic active hepatitis, signifying that portal inflammation is destroying hepatocytes. Necrosis of the limiting plate, usually in an irregular fashion, is often called piecemeal necrosis. Another hepatic disease in humans is characterized by portal inflammation, although without necrosis of the limiting plate of hepatocytes even though plasma ALT activity is increased.[1] This entity, benign persistent hepatitis, may have a counterpart in small animals. Chronic persistent hepatitis has a hallmark of predominantly lymphocytic inflammation restricted to widened portal tracts, leaving the parenchymal limiting plate preserved. There is no necrosis of periportal hepatocytes and there may be only slight fibrosis. A morphologically similar entity, periportal hepatitis (of varying severity) accounts for 50% of

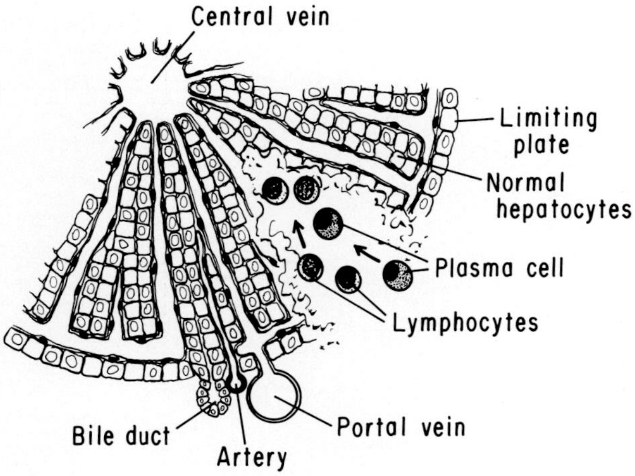

CHRONIC ACTIVE HEPATITIS

PATHOLOGY

INITIAL INSULT

↓

INFLAMMATORY CELL INFILTRATION
PORTAL AREA

↓

PLASMA CELLS AND LYMPHOCYTES
CAUSE NECROSIS OF LIMITING PLATE

↓

INFLAMMATORY PROCESS EXTENDS INTO PARENCHYMA

Figure 33-2. Pathology of chronic hepatitis produced by plasma cells and lymphocytes which destroy the limiting plate of hepatocytes and enter the interior of hepatic lobules.

dogs and 44% of cats with hepatitis. None of these are described as chronic persistent hepatitis, a term usually reserved for the human diseases. The term periportal hepatitis is probably more accurate than chronic persistent hepatitis for describing and understanding these problems in dogs and cats. Periportal hepatitis is more often primary in dogs (with no known cause) and is more often secondary to another problem in cats. There is no information on whether periportal hepatitis is progressive and leads to a more destructive form of hepatitis in small animals. A form of chronic persistent hepatitis is sometimes described as lobular because of its pathologic appearance. Lobular hepatitis in dogs is reported to be progressive and proves to be fatal.[21] Most cases of lobular hepatitis in humans subside without progressing to cirrhosis. Keeping the limiting plate intact in any form of periportal hepatitis prevents the process from developing into the pathology seen in chronic active (or aggressive) hepatitis.

Pathologic assessments vary greatly and result in numerous pathologic descriptions (Table 33-1). Most differences are in evaluation of chronic hepatitis in small animals. Differing evaluations are not unique to veterinary pathologists. A comparison of pathologists' evaluations of human liver biopsies showed difficulty in gaining a consensus on whether a process represented chronic hepatitis or some other form of liver disease.[22] So it is not surprising that there are great differences in the descriptions and assessments of liver biopsies in small animals.

Humans with chronic persistent hepatitis require no therapy, and the process is self-limiting.[1] The disease is characterized by only minor symptoms, which indicates that parenchymal changes are required to produce clinical signs of hepatitis. In humans the causes of chronic persistent hepatitis and chronic active hepatitis are the same; the main difference in pathogenesis between the two is whether the limiting plate of hepatocytes becomes damaged. The different appearances may represent different facets of a similar pathologic process; in one there is a resistance to necrosis of the hepatocytes, and in the other the hepatocytes are susceptible to the effects of immunocytes.

Multifocal hepatitis is documented as secondary to some other problem, most often sepsis outside the liver and/or some gastrointestinal diseases, in nearly 50% of the dogs and in all but one cat with multifocal hepatitis. The 50% of dogs with primary multifocal hepatitis probably represents many cases where pathologic information on the animal was limited to a liver biopsy. With such a biopsy finding, a search should be complete for problems in other organs. Multifocal hepatitis probably represents what is described as nonspecific reactive hepatitis where the liver is injured by disease outside the liver.

Cholangiohepatitis is mostly primary in dogs with one fourth of the cases presumed to be secondary to gastrointestinal disease. Two-thirds of the cases in cats are associated with primary renal or gastrointestinal disease. A relationship can be understood for gastrointestinal disease; it is more difficult for renal disease. A lesion resembling cholangiohepatitis develops in dogs and cats within four to six weeks after obstruction of the bile duct.[23,24] Such obstruction also leads to infection in the biliary system.[25,26] Such infection could be occur when organisms from the intestine invade through the diseased duct or when organisms normally removed by the liver from portal blood and cleared into the biliary system are not cleared and multiply. The obstruction also results in damage from retained bile acids and increased pressure in the biliary system. Both bile stasis and infection can contribute to the pathogenesis, something possible with gastrointestinal disease. With extensive duodenal disease, appropriate release of cholecystokinin is impaired, the most important signal for gall bladder evacuation. Cats in particular have important renal disease as the primary problem in nearly one-half the cases of cholangiohepatitis. An infectious or immune-mediated basis for the relationship can only be speculated.

The liver responds to necrosis by regeneration of hepatocytes and bile-duct epithelial cells. The liver has a greater capacity for regeneration than other tissues. The regeneration can consist of merely replacing isolated cells that are lost. Regeneration that replaces cells lost during destruction of the limiting plate forms a plate that is two cells thick instead of the usual arrangement of a single cord of cells with blood perfusing both sides. Regeneration also occurs in lobules, where hepatocytes are encircled by septa created from chronic inflammation. This results in nodule formation (Figure 33-4). Specialized hepatocytes form bile ductules at the periphery or periportal zone 1 of lobules. The hepatic lobule is sometimes regenerated by a proliferation of these cells, so that bile ductules extend into the lobule's center. Inflammatory cells frequently found around these ductules suggest that the ductules provide a means for inflammatory cells to invade the lobule.

Fibrosis is a regular sequel to inflammation and hepatocyte necrosis.[20,27] Collagen tissue is deposited adjacent to hepatocytes along portal borders of the lobule and in septa of inflam-

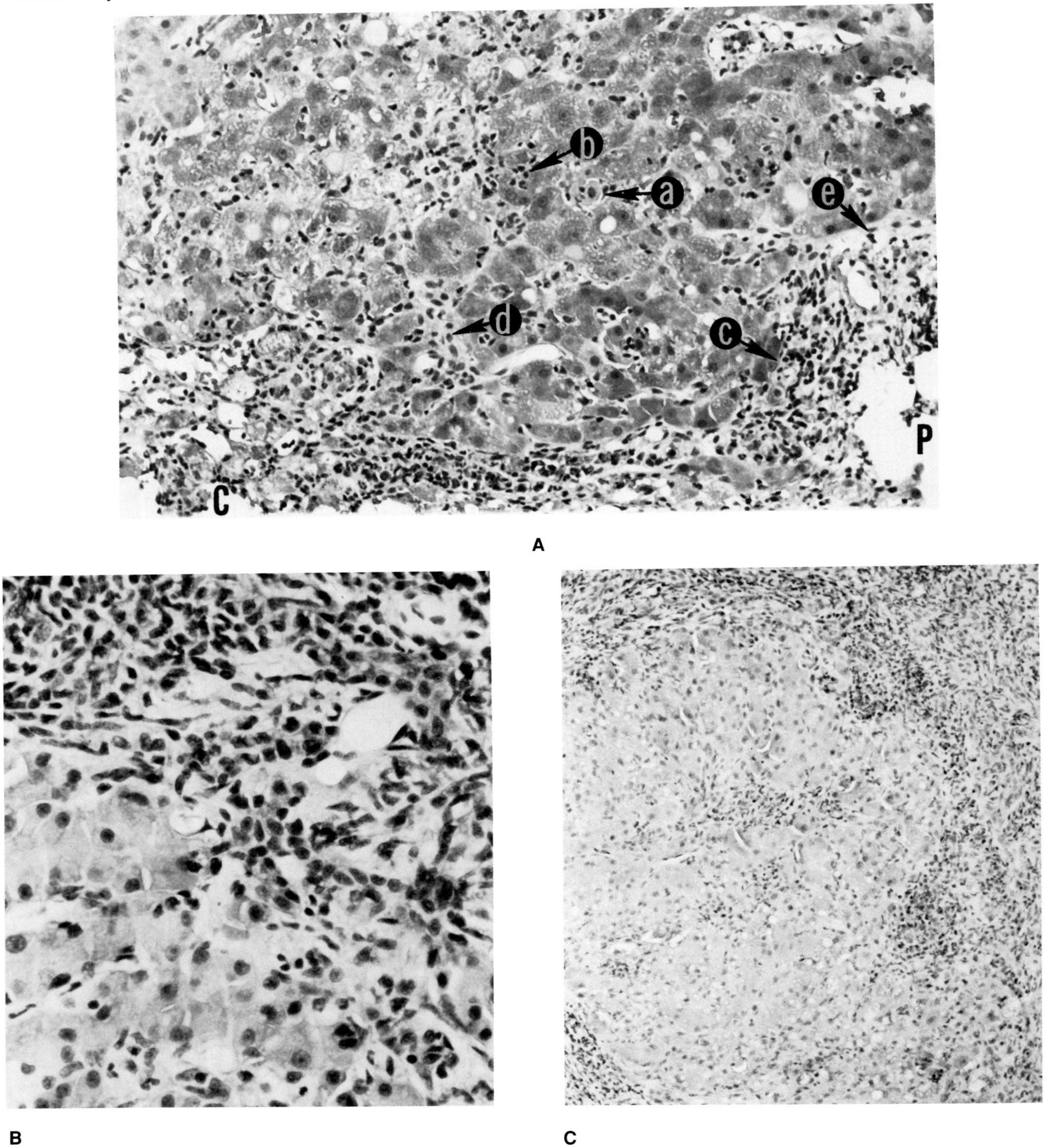

Figure 33-3. (a) Photomicrograph of biopsy specimen from the liver of a dog with chronic hepatitis. Changes include necrosis of hepatocytes (a), foci of inflammation within lobule (b) and at periphery (c), and fibrosis within lobule (d) and at periphery (e). P = portal area; C = central vein area, (b) and (c) Biopsy specimen from dog where most of the inflammatory changes are still confined to the periphery of the lobule, causing piecemeal necrosis of hepatocytes. (d) inflammation and fibrosis that are diffuse throughout liver so that normal architecture is lost.

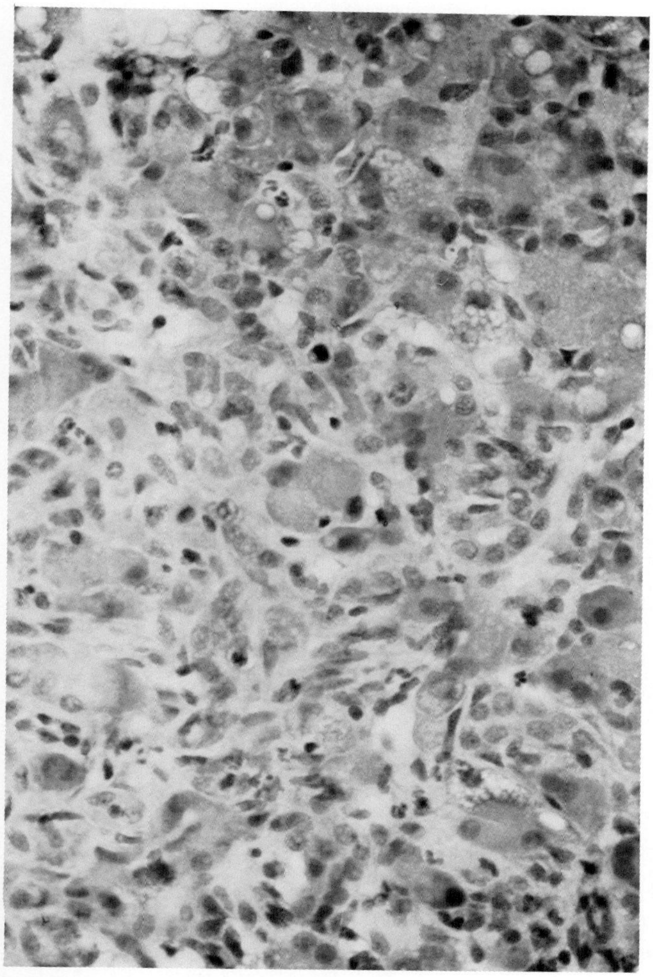

Figure 33-3d.

mation radiating from portal areas to central veins. An abnormal deposition of collagen in the liver without a loss of normal architecture is designated as fibrosis, whereas cirrhosis describes a more diffuse and advanced process that distorts the normal hepatic architecture. As fibrosis develops, the synthesis of collagen is very active, in contrast to the very small synthesis in the normal liver. Livers with active collagen deposition contain fibroblasts transformed from fat-storing cells, which are the source of the collagen. The amino acids glycine and proline are found in high amounts in collagen and cirrhotic livers. The concentrations of these amino acids able to enter collagen-synthesizing cells may determine the rate of collagen synthesis. The amounts of transfer RNAs for glycine and proline are also increased, as well as the activity of collagen propyl hydroxylase, an important enzyme necessary for collagen synthesis. Collagen is secreted as procollagen, which undergoes cross-linking and maturation to produce collagen. Several other enzymes participate in maturation. Fibrosis was once thought to be an irreversible event, but fibrosis produced in experimental animals disappears after the cause is removed. This reversibility is probably due to a collagenase, found in Kupffer cells, which shows increased activity with hepatic fibrosis. Hepatic fibrosis can be reversed with colchicine in both experimental animals and humans with hepatic cirrhosis.

Analogs of proline have been used to prevent fibrosis in experimental animals treated with drugs that consistently cause fibrosis. The analog, acting as a counterfeit proline molecule, inhibits collagen synthesis and deposition in the liver. Plasma proline concentrations decrease in some types of chronic hepatitis in humans. The serum proline level in dogs with chronic active hepatitis is 61% of that in normal dogs. The significance of this reduction is not known at present.

Hepatic fibrosis has major effects on hepatic function. Dogs with chronic hepatitis show major changes in 2 liver-function tests: BSP retention is markedly increased, and ammonia tolerance is consistently reduced.[16] These abnormalities reflect changes in both hepatocyte function and hepatic circulation. The deposition of collagen separates hepatocytes from their circulation, reducing the overall capacity of the liver to remove substances from the portal blood. The formation of a double-cell-thick plate of hepatocytes separated by fibrous septa reduces the exchange of blood-borne substances with hepatocytes. Fibrosis also changes hepatic hemodynamics when fibrous septa develop blood vessels that act as shunts between the inflow and outflow. Thus, blood bypasses the sinusoidal capillary bed and cannot exchange constituents with hepatocytes. The high mean BSP retention in dogs with chronic hepatitis indicates that exchange is poor.

Cirrhosis is advanced fibrosis in which the normal hepatic architecture is lost (Figure 33-5).[1,2] Hepatic cirrhosis is an infrequent problem that often develops insidiously. Cell death, fibrosis, and regeneration combine to produce cirrhosis. Cell death has to be consistent and persistent over a long period of time. Fibrosis can develop without cell death, such as when bacterial products absorbed from the intestine produce portal fibrosis.[28] Cell death can be initiated by any of the agents causing hepatic necrosis. They include drugs, toxins, viruses, metals such as copper and iron, hepatic ischemia or hypoxia, biliary obstruction, and some nutritional abnormalities (see Chapter 29). Death of hepatocytes results from direct damage by the agent, by a metabolite of the agent, or by stimulation of an immune response. Cell death is identified by hepatocyte necrosis or disappearance and can be suggested by infiltrations of lymphocytes and/or macrophages. That cell death must be consistent and persistent is reinforced from the pathologic outcome to massive cell death that is neither consistent nor persistent. Reduction of hepatic mass to less than 50% by the

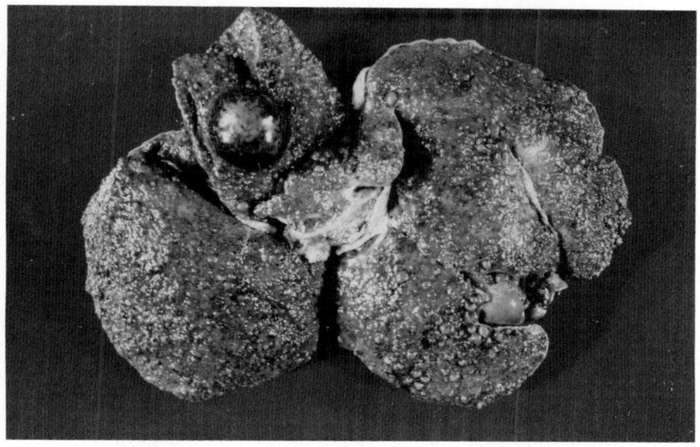

Figure 33-4. (a)Liver with small nodules produced by chronic hepatitis and cirrhosis.

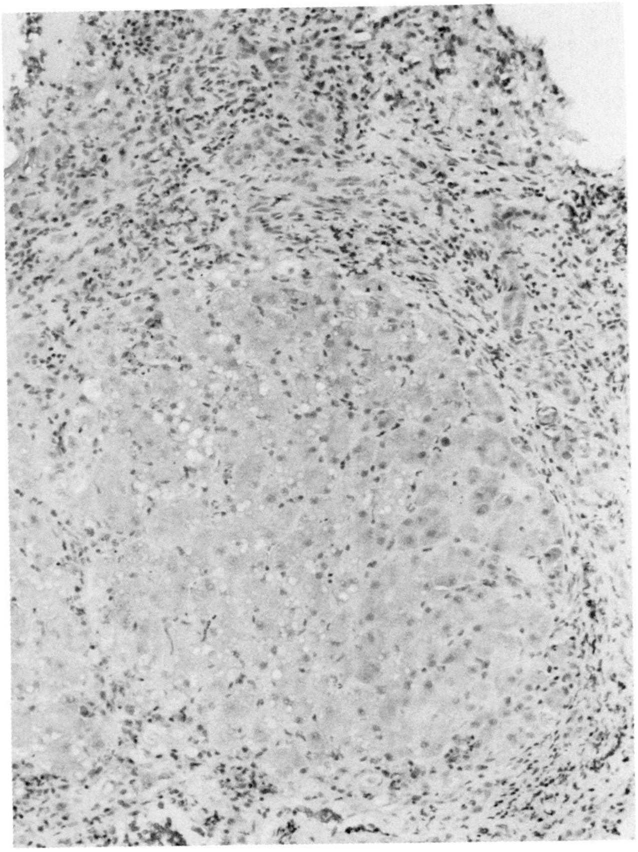

Figure 33-4. (b) Biopsy specimen showing nodule of hepatocytes surrounded by inflammatory cells and fibrosis.

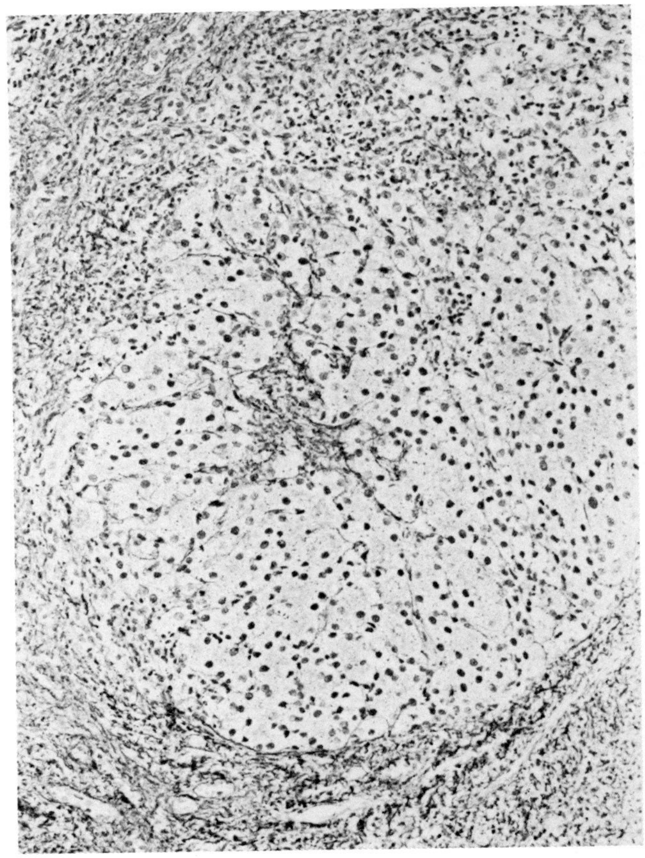

Figure 33-4. (c) Reticulin stain of biopsy specimen in (b) shows constraints placed by encircling fibrous tissue on hepatocyte regeneration.

hepatotoxin nitrosamine given over two to three weeks does not result in the development of cirrhosis when management is instituted to reduce the absorption of toxins from the intestine.[29] Without such management the toxins could be responsible for the development of a consistent and persistent cell necrosis because of a relative hepatic insufficiency produced by the nitrosamines. Any postnecrotic cirrhosis follows long-term hepatocyte injury; it is not seen after an insult inflicted over a short time. With continuous cell necrosis the liver attempts to maintain its normal capacity by regeneration.

Cell death, fibrosis, and regeneration leads to one form of pathology called micronodular cirrhosis and another called macronodular cirrhosis.[12] Sometimes both forms are found. In humans micronodular cirrhosis is caused most often by drugs, chronic obstruction to or impairment of hepatic venous outflow, and chronic biliary disease. Macronodular cirrhosis is most often associated with chronic viral hepatitis and autoimmune forms of hepatitis. Micronodules form when fibrous septa transect zones 1, 2 and 3 of acini. The fibrosis may be greater in one zone than the others. Newly-formed blood vessels develop in the septa and the circulation they carry bypasses the sinusoids. In contrast to septa dividing individual acini into micronodules, fibrous septa dividing the liver and surrounding clusters of acini are called macronodular cirrhosis. Macronodules can be identified by finding more than one portal tract within each nodule. Blood vessels in the septa surrounding nodules also shunt blood away from sinusoids. Regeneration of hepatocytes expands the nodules and compresses adjacent cell plates, further distorting the normal circulation. These events contribute to continuous and persistent cell death within nodules, and that provides a basis for micronodules to develop within macronodules. Now new factors have developed which commit the pathology to worsen, even though the original insult to the liver is gone.

Fibrosis with continuing inflammation leading to the development of cirrhosis can be restricted to the bile ducts and surrounding tissue, characterizing an entity in portal areas called biliary cirrhosis (Figure 31-6). Its cause is unknown but is probably initiated by chronic cholangiohepatitis or bile duct obstruction.[1,2] Biliary cirrhosis may be initiated by portal and periportal hepatitis. Infection, drugs, toxins, parasites, and immune-mediated injury are proposed as specific causes. With cholangiohepatitis accounting for 6% of all hepatitis in dogs and 21% in cats it is expected that some instances would progress to the occasional case of biliary cirrhosis encountered in small animals. Advanced biliary cirrhosis may be difficult to distinguish from chronic hepatitis, especially when inflammation has extended into the interior of lobules.

PATHOPHYSIOLOGY

The primary signs of acute and chronic hepatitis (jaundice, depression, and anorexia) can be explained on the basis of

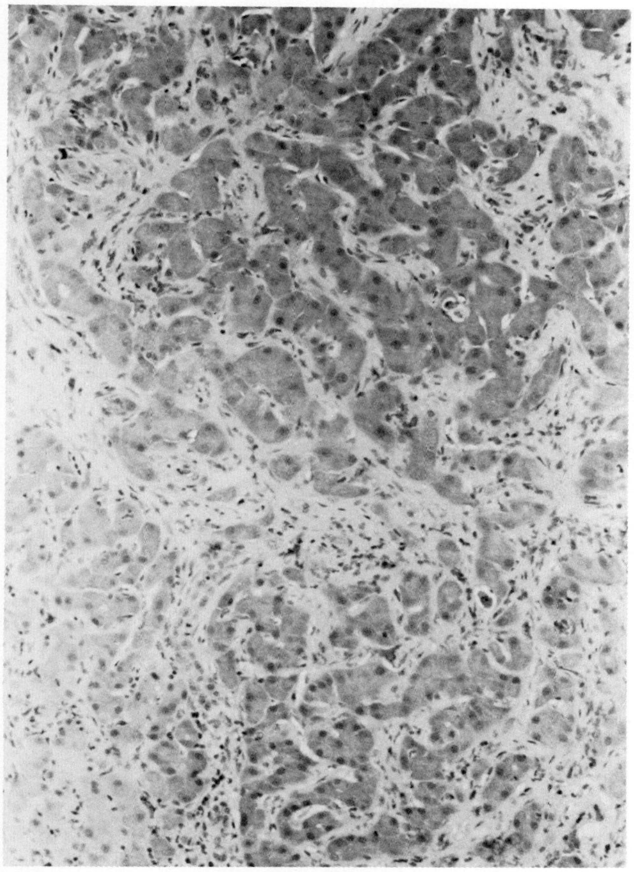

A

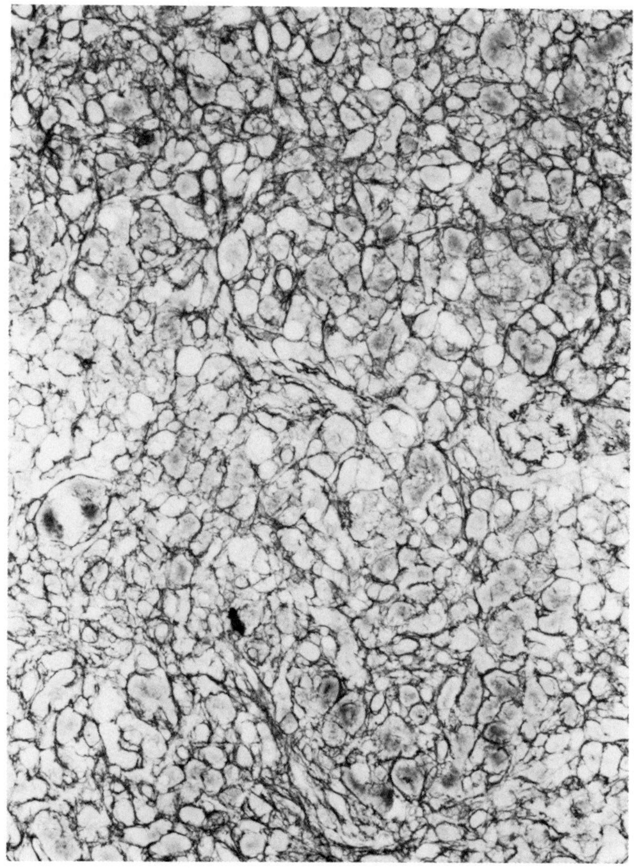

B

Figure 33-5. (a) Biopsy specimen from dog shows marked fibrosis that is widespread and causes loss of hepatic architecture. Changes are easily identified on H and E stained preparation. (b) Reticulin stain on biopsy specimen where diffuse fibrosis was not striking on H and E stained preparation. (c) and (d) Reticulin stained preparations are useful in identifying the extent of fibrosis and hence the prognosis in biopsies where the amount of fibrosis is questionable.

biochemical and morphologic changes. Both acute and chronic hepatitis are insidious in that primary clinical signs are often not readily apparent until a diffuse and well-established pathologic process has developed. In general, the biochemical and morphologic changes are often more striking than the severity of clinical signs.

Bilirubin Metabolism

Jaundice is expected in animals with chronic hepatitis since the lesion develops most often within the portal area. Necrosis of the limiting plate need not be severe to produce jaundice. Experimentally, dogs with limited necrotic lesions confined to the periportal hepatocytes readily become icteric.[30] In contrast, necrosis in other parts of the lobule must be massive before jaundice appears. Periportal inflammation causes cholestasis by obstructing bile flow in the bile ductules entering the portal area. Although the hyperbilirubinemia should be due primarily to conjugated bilirubin, in most cases it is also due to unconjugated bilirubin. The ratio of conjugated to unconjugated bilirubin cannot be used to make a diagnosis of hepatic disease.

Glucose Metabolism

Plasma glucose levels can be abnormal in animals with acute or chronic hepatitis. In dogs hypoglycemia is seen in 8% and fasting hyperglycemia in 10%.[31] The hypoglycemia is not unexpected when the liver loses its ability to produce glucose. Hyperglycemia develops when the liver's capacity is impaired for taking up glucose and because there may be high levels of hormones such as glucagon and catecholamines that promote hyperglycemia. Hypoglycemia is expected to contribute to signs of hepatic encephalopathy, and in some cases the low blood glucose is solely responsible for seizures.

Lipids Metabolism

Plasma cholesterol levels can change with hepatitis but are usually normal. With chronic hepatitis 17% of dogs have hypocholesterolemia and 22% have hypercholesterolemia.[31] The ratio of free to esterified cholesterol also sometimes increases with chronic hepatitis,[32] but the incidence of this abnormality is unknown. Altered ratios of free to esterified cholesterol are a consistent feature of cholestasis, reflecting the

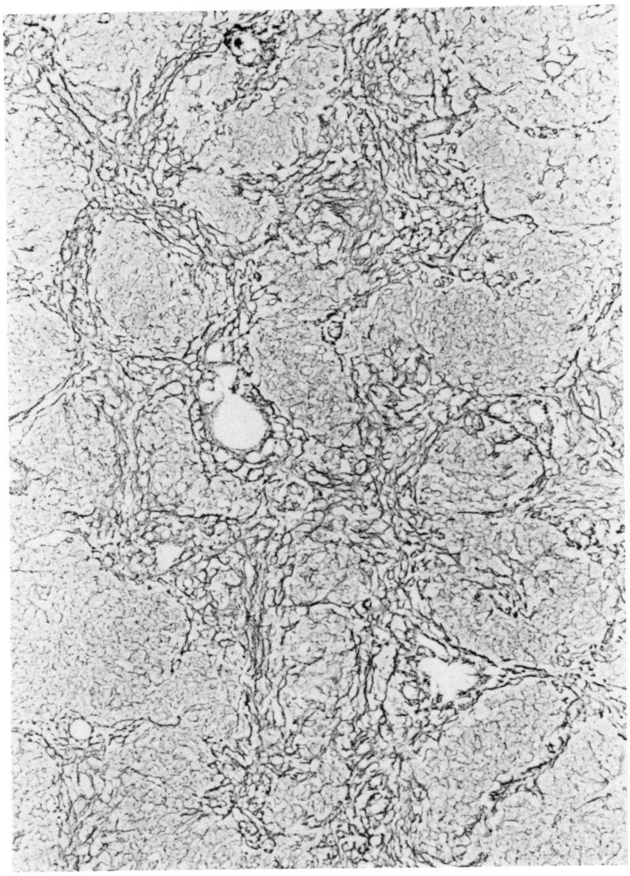

Figure 33-5c. See legend page 601

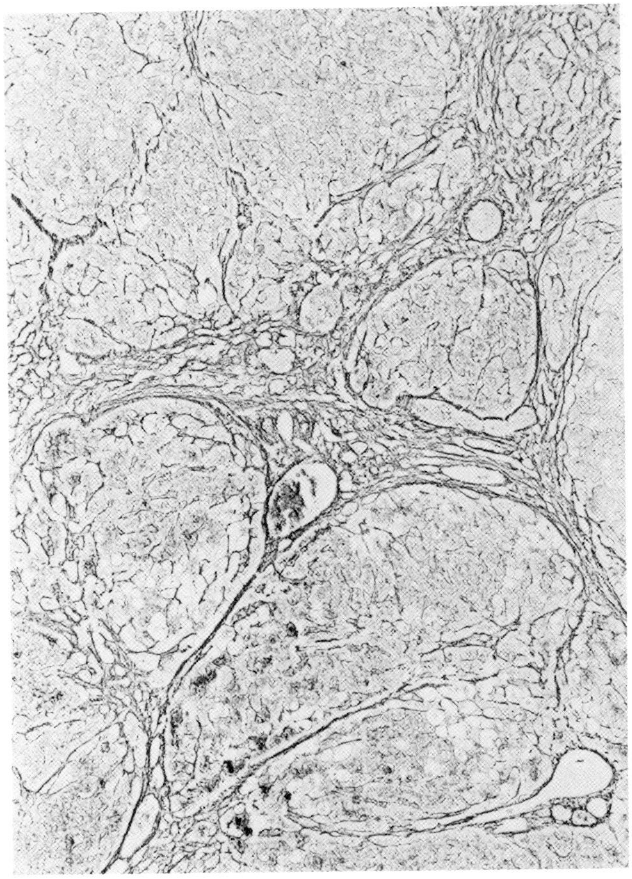

Figure 33-5d. See legend page 601

synthesis of abnormal lipoproteins.[33] Plasma bile acids are also usually abnormal with chronic hepatitis. Cholestasis interrupts the enterohepatic circulation of bile acids, causing plasma levels to increase. Bile acid secretion is reduced, so that less is delivered to the intestine. That reduction appears to be of little consequence for assimilation of a meal since clinical signs of malabsorption and acholic bowel movements have not been described in small animals with chronic hepatitis.

Protein Metabolism and Hepatic Encephalopathy

Hyperammonemia. Depression and anorexia are consistent signs of mild hepatic encephalopathy, with coma sometimes seen in severe forms. Hepatic encephalopathy is a reflection of abnormal nitrogen metabolism resulting in hyperammonemia. The severity of hepatic encephalopathy does not correlate with the degree of hyperammonemia in either random blood samples or in the ammonia tolerance test. Random blood samples show hyperammonemia in 54% of dogs with chronic hepatitis; the ammonia tolerance test is abnormal in 95% of the cases.[31] Neither test correlates well with the overall histologic severity of hepatic changes.[16] Thus, it is not surprising that some animals with moderate to severe hepatic encephalopathy may have few if any clinical signs. Since conversion of ammonia to urea is more important in zone 1 periportal hepatocytes, pathology in that region is more likely to cause hyperammonemia and hepatic encephalopathy than pathology restricted to the zone 3 perivenular area, where the storage of ammonia nitrogen by conversion to glutamine is more important. Urea-cycle activity in zone 3 must adapt to increased needs during hyperammonemia, which is accomplished by increasing substrates required for cycle activity. Citric-acid-cycle intermediates are important substrates that can be supplied by alanine after its conversion to aspartate. Acute ammonia toxicity causes plasma alanine levels to decrease, similar to findings in dogs with chronic hepatitis.[34] Plasma levels of arginine, an amino acid essential for maintaining urea-cycle activity, are also depleted during acute ammonia toxicity, though they are not reduced in dogs with chronic hepatitis. Hepatic capacity for converting ammonia to urea is reflected in blood urea nitrogen levels which are reduced in 25% of dogs with chronic hepatitis.[31]

Amino Acid Abnormalities. Hepatic encephalopathy is also associated with alterations in the levels of some amino acids necessary for the synthesis of neurotransmitters in the brain. The normal ratio of the sum of branched-chain amino acids in the plasma to the sum of the aromatics is 3.0 to 4.1. In dogs with chronic hepatitis the ratio is 1.3, and in experimental animals with portacaval vascular shunts it can approach 1.0.[35] Increased plasma concentrations of aromatic amino acids in relation to branched-chain amino acids result in greater amounts of aromatics crossing the blood-brain barrier, since those two groups of amino acids compete for a single transport system for entry into the brain.[36] Increasing amounts of aromatic amino acids in the brain reduces concentrations of excitatory neuro-

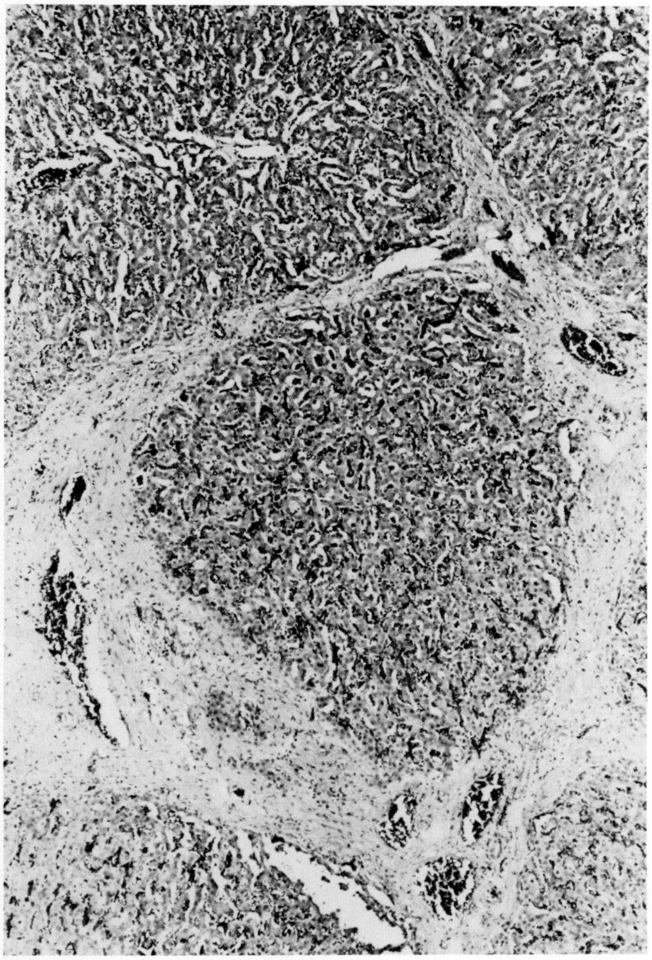

Figure 33-6. Advanced biliary cirrhosis

transmitters and increases concentrations of inhibitory neurotransmitters. The importance of the amino acid abnormality relative to hyperammonemia is unknown. Abnormal plasma amino acids without hyperammonemia do not cause hepatic encephalopathy. Altered amino acid metabolism is caused by hyperammonemia and results in hepatic encephalopathy, but the contribution of each is poorly understood. Other amino acids which change and have been implicated as the cause of hepatic encephalopathy include gamma-aminobutyric acid; its role is discussed in Chapter 28.

Fatty Acids and Mercaptans. Signs of hepatic encephalopathy may also be due in part to increased plasma concentrations of short-chain fatty acids and mercaptans.[36] These products of carbohydrate fermentation, partial lipid oxidation, and methionine degradation in the intestine act synergistically with ammonia to cause clinical signs accompanying hepatic disease.[37] Experimentally, plasma concentrations of these substrates are elevated in dogs with hepatic disease. It is likely that their concentrations are increased in clinical cases. It is possible for dogs with chronic hepatitis to develop hepatic encephalopathy following administration of a therapeutic dose of methionine,[38] a compound used to treat lipidosis.

Plasma Albumin and Clotting Factors. Abnormal nitrogen metabolism with chronic hepatitis is also reflected in plasma albumin levels. Dogs with hypoalbuminemia account for 27% of dogs with chronic hepatitis.[31] That finding is one of the few laboratory findings that correlates with the animal's ability to recover from the disease.[16] The ability to synthesize proteins is also reflected in the capacity for producing and maintaining normal levels of most clotting factors. Increased time for prothrombin and partial thromboplastin found with chronic hepatitis may be largely due to reduced clotting factor synthesis. Increased times for prothrombin are found in 36% and for partial thromboplastin in 60% of dogs with chronic hepatitis.[31]

Abnormal Steroid Hormones

Frequent signs of chronic hepatitis are polydipsia and polyuria. Factors that participate in the appearance of these signs include increased concentrations of hormones such as adrenal corticosteroids that are not adequately metabolized and prepared for excretion by the diseased liver. In normal animals the amount of cortisol released is directed primarily by ACTH, the release of which is controlled by cortisol levels. Severe stress causes cortisol secretion to be maintained despite elevated blood levels. Liver biopsies of chronic hepatitis often show vacuolization, suggestive of excess steroids. The basis for the polydipsia with hyperadrenoalcorticism is not known. It may be due to increased excretion of urinary solutes caused by excess steroids. The polydipsia may be caused by the derangements in neurotransmitters in the brain or by some of the toxins that are inadequately removed by the liver.

Prolonged anestrus as reported in one dog is a regular feature of one-third of human patients with chronic hepatitis.[1] This reflects the impairment in metabolism of all the steroid hormones. In humans, alterations in the levels of these hormones also result in feminization in males and some steroid-induced skin problems.

Renal Insufficiency

The incidence of renal pathology with chronic hepatitis is twice as great in dogs as in the overall population. An unusual number of cats with hepatitis are also found with renal pathology. Some of these animals have glomerulonephritis with the glomerular lesions possibly caused by the deposition of immunoglobulins.[39] Such animals have cholangiohepatitis or periportal hepatitis as the primary lesion; because that may interfere with the secretion of IgA into the biliary system, it may explain why increased IgA and circulating immune complexes are found with some forms of hepatic disease. Thus, renal disease should be suspected as an associated problem until proven otherwise. In addition, these patients sometimes develop imbalances in fluid and electrolyte homeostasis that cannot be explained by morphological changes in the kidneys. Consistent signs in the early stages are polydipsia and polyuria, which can change in advanced stages to oliguria and uremia. The loss of the kidney's ability to maintain fluid and electrolyte homeostasis in association with advanced chronic hepatitis has been termed the hepatorenal syndrome in some cases where the kidneys are morphologically normal.[40]

Oliguria signifies a fluid imbalance characterized by reduced effective plasma volume and a retention of fluid that most likely appears as ascites. Ascites develops as a secondary sign due to intrahepatic portal hypertension and hypoproteinemia, both of which result directly from hepatitis. Ascites formation usually reflects reduced venous return to the heart and reduced cardiac output. The renal response is reduced renal blood flow, a mechanism for oliguria appearing. When severe, renal ischemia can cause acute tubular necrosis. Thus, renal lesions may not be present initially but may develop when patients are not managed properly.

Compensation to increase the effective plasma volume is achieved by diverting circulation away from splanchnic organs and by retaining more sodium. Compensated patients treated with diuretics for ascites can easily decompensate, as characterized by hypovolemia and reduced cardiac output. With preexisting renal disease the ability to compensate is reduced and smaller imbalances in fluids and electrolytes produce oliguria and renal failure. Assessment of patients with chronic hepatitis, oliguria, and uremia includes determination of whether renal complications are due to reduced renal blood flow, acute tubular necrosis, or concurrent chronic nephritis. Oliguria due to reduced renal blood flow is identified by finding urine with a high specific gravity. In the other two cases, urine specific gravity is low and often relatively fixed.

Three factors that determine renal excretion of water and salts and the size of the extracellular fluid compartment are the glomerular filtration rate (GFR), which is a function of renal blood flow; aldosterone secreted when effective circulating blood volume is reduced; and atrial natriuretic factor, operating to promote excretion of salt when the extracellular fluid compartment is expanded. Patients with renal failure usually have reduced GFR and increased aldosterone secretion, contributing to oliguria. However, both GFR and aldosterone secretion may be normal with oliguria. This is due to failure of natriuretic factor to initiate diuresis in animals with ascites, which is an important cause of the hepatorenal syndrome.[40] Natriuretic factor is thought to be mediated by changes in the renal microcirculation. However, the changes are not possible in the kidneys of animals with chronic hepatitis. Disappearance of natriuretic factor is secondary to the overall circulatory disturbances. Effective circulating blood volume is lost by experimentally constricting the vena cava cranial to the liver; the experimental dogs developed ascites and oliguria due to the failure of natriuretic factor to operate. This model is essentially the same in clinical patients with the hepatorenal syndrome. Oliguria persists when chronic hepatic disease maintains significant resistance to hepatic blood flow. Electrolyte alterations contribute to the problem in that, with potassium depletion, expanding extracellular fluid volume does not produce diuresis. The basis for this finding is unknown, but it can be a factor with chronic hepatitis. During compensation, aldosterone secretion increases the renal excretion of potassium, and the loss of fluids in vomiting contributes further to the potassium depletion. Renal failure is now also known to be partly due to failure of prostaglandin production and release in the kidneys. Such release is necessary for sustaining renal blood flow, glomerular filtration rate, natriuresis and diuresis. Non-steroidal anti-inflammatory drugs would have an adverse affect on prostaglandins' participation in normal renal function.

Electrolyte and Acid Base Abnormalities

A slight to moderate total-body deficit of potassium accompanies ascites, regardless of plasma potassium levels. Reduced dietary potassium intake, vomiting, diarrhea, and hyperaldosteronism all contribute to reducing the potassium pool. Potassium deficiency is associated with high intracellular levels of hydrogen ions, which increase renal glutaminase activity, indirectly increasing blood ammonia levels. Ammonia secreted into the renal tubule is normally trapped in the urine by its conversion to ammonium ions. In patients with ascites, the kidney is often unable to acidify the urine and trap ammonia, thereby allowing urine ammonia to diffuse into the circulation and contribute to hepatic encephalopathy.

Alkalosis is another complication of hypokalemia and reduced effective plasma volume. Plasma bicarbonate concentrations increase from vomiting, but, more important, they increase as a result of the body's almost total conservation of sodium when the effective plasma volume is contracted. Almost complete reabsorption of bicarbonate follows that of sodium. In addition, as intracellular potassium is lost during depletion of body stores, hydrogen ions enter cells in an exchange process, creating another means of increasing bicarbonate levels in extracellular fluid. The increased concentration of intracellular hydrogen ions in the renal tubular cells stimulates the hydrogen ion-sodium exchange mechanism in addition to the production of ammonia from glutamine already mentioned. Alkalosis without a hypokalemia is treated with balanced-electrolyte solutions to restore the extracellular and plasma fluid volumes, and the diuresis that follows is accompanied by excretion of excess plasma bicarbonate. Alkalosis is not completely corrected until any potassium deficit is corrected.

Potassium depletion in patients with hepatic disease can cause hypokalemic nephropathy, which is a functional renal defect resulting in a loss of concentrating ability. The renal abnormality is in sodium reabsorption in either the loop of Henle or distal tubule. Without the normal concentrating ability, specific gravity being fixed at 1.010, urea excretion is reduced, with urea being the most abundant solute in urine. Thus, uremia is a consequence of a loss of concentrating ability. Urine is not concentrated in response to ADH, not because the tubule is unresponsive but because the loss of function in the loop of Henle results in a loss of the osmolar gradient in the medullary interstitial space.

Ascites

The pathophysiology of ascites is discussed in Chapter 28.

Gastrointestinal Lesions

Ulceration of the upper gastrointestinal tract is a complication of chronic hepatitis.[41] The pathogenesis of the lesions is not completely understood. Gastric ulceration is produced by a combination of factors. The most important of these is gastric secretion of acid, without which no ulcer can develop. Reduced mucosal blood flow, a loss of the mucous barrier, and the regurgitation of duodenal contents containing bile all contribute to ulcer formation. Part of the gastrin and histamine released is normally removed by the liver from the portal circulation, but that function is impaired by chronic hepatitis. Increased levels of gastrin cause hypersecretion of gastric hydrochloric acid. Impaired mucosal circulation is an important factor when the animal has either disseminated intravascular coagulation or reduced effective circulating plasma volume as an additional problem. Abnormal gastric microcirculation accompanies chronic hepatic insufficiency. Intestinal circulation is also abnormal with portal hypertension, ascites and portasystemic shunting; intestinal absorption is impaired with such problems. Secondary gastrointestinal pathology contributes to the vomiting and diarrhea frequently seen with hepatitis.

Coagulopathies

Increased bleeding tendencies are a serious complication in some patients with hepatic disease. They are a consistent feature of acute hepatitis caused by the infectious canine hepatitis virus.[42] Acute hepatitis severe enough to cause a coagulopathy is infrequent in small animals. Chronic hepatitis also causes coagulopathies, but not very frequently. The general hepatic causes of coagulopathies include decreased synthesis of clotting factors and antithrombin III by the liver, primary fibrinolysis, disseminated intravascular coagulation (DIC), and circulating anticoagulants. In experimental animals with hepatitis, blood levels of clotting factors fall, especially for factors with the shortest half-lives.[42] It can be assumed that reduced synthesis of clotting factors in the prothrombin complex contributes to the coagulopathy in clinical cases of hepatitis. As stated earlier the times for prothrombin and partial thromboplastin increase in dogs with chronic hepatitis. Animals with chronic hepatitis can hemorrhage if treated for DIC with heparin unless blood-clotting factors are also given.

The liver contains large amounts of thromboplastic substances. Hepatocyte damage results in their release and stimulation of the intravascular coagulation of blood. DIC is also initiated when the liver is unable to remove activated clotting factors from the circulation. Both of these factors contribute to the severe coagulopathy seen in some cases of hepatitis. The problem of DIC is identified by finding a thrombocytopenia, hypofibrinogenemia, prolonged prothrombin time and partial thromboplastin time, and increased plasma levels of fibrinogen degradation products. DIC can be consistently produced with acute hepatitis due to infectious canine hepatitis virus. During extensive hepatocyte damage due to chronic active hepatitis, DIC can develop. The pathogenesis is different from the viral-induced DIC, where a generalized vasculitis is suggested to be the basis for thromboplastin release. Multiple factors participate in the chronic active hepatitis-induced DIC. In addition to the release of thromboplastin activity from hepatocytes, there can be decreased removal of activated clotting factors.

The treatment of DIC is with heparin. The dog becomes resistant to the effects of heparin after a few days, however, if it is experimentally infused with thromboplastin.[43] The effectiveness of prolonged therapy is unknown in clinical cases with DIC. The response to heparin therapy can be evaluated with platelet counts, plasma fibrinogen levels, and activated clotting times. Although much less sensitive, activated clotting time provides the same type of information as the prothrombin and partial thromboplastin times. Identification and treatment of DIC is important to prevent a cascade of secondary changes in vital organs that are caused by thrombosis-induced ischemia. Thrombosis of hepatic and renal circulation causes the pathologic changes to worsen in these organs. Ischemic changes in the gastrointestinal tract cause erosions and ulcerations. Hemorrhage into the gut follows, presenting one of the most serious complications. Blood is one of the most potent toxin-producing substrates when bacteria are present for its digestion. Dogs in classical experiments to produce portacaval shunts developed signs of hepatic coma most readily when fed blood, with the severity of coma being greater than when fed any other diet.[44]

Fibrinolysis can be a major problem associated with chronic hepatitis.[45] The persistence of high proteolytic enzyme activity results in the production of large amounts of fibrinogen degradation products that interfere with clotting and thus act as anticoagulants. The liver removes these products, formed in small amounts in the normal animal. Fibrinogen-degradation products are formed at an increased rate with DIC, and with chronic hepatitis the levels remain high since they are not cleared by the liver. High proteolytic enzyme activity is due to decreased hepatic clearance of plasminogen activator, so that the proteolytic enzyme plasmin is continuously activated. Its effects are generally nonspecific in that it can degrade clotting factors. This enzyme is inhibited by proteins normally synthesized in the liver; hepatic disease reduces the amounts synthesized and available to inhibit plasmin activity. The normal process of fibrinolysis is necessary for resolution of thrombi. In the animal with fibrinolysis this process is accelerated, and there is an increased rate of destruction of other plasma proteins, notably clotting factors, and an increased rate of formation of substances with anticoagulant properties. The patient can be easily evaluated for the existence of circulating anticoagulants that are contributing significantly to a coagulopathy. Activated clotting times are determined on a patient's blood with and without addition of a small amount of fresh blood drawn from a normal animal at the same time. If the patient has a problem with DIC or a deficiency of blood-clotting factors, the addition of a small amount of normal blood returns the prolonged activated clotting time to normal. If the patient has high levels of circulating anticoagulants, however, the activated clotting time remains abnormal when the normal blood is added. Fibrinolysis is characterized by poor clot formation, and the clots formed belatedly undergo lysis upon further incubation in the test tube. That is another characteristic used to identify the problem.

CLINICAL FINDINGS

The most frequent clinical signs in dogs with chronic hepatitis are depression, vomiting, and anorexia (Table 33-3). Consistent with this a reduction in food intake is the earliest sign seen in experimental animals with hepatic insufficiency.[46] Signs often thought to be pathognomonic for hepatic disease such as ascites, icterus, and CNS signs are seen infrequently in dogs with chronic hepatitis. Thus, these animals are presented with nonspecific signs as the chief complaint. A small number of dogs with chronic hepatitis show no clinical signs. That is often true in cats, where as a cholangiohepatitis develops, hyperbilirubinemia appears but with no other clinical signs of disease. Comprehensive information on clinical signs has not been reported on cats with hepatitis. Because data on clinical signs is often unreliable, and animals can have marked pathologic changes in the liver with few, if any, clinical signs, it is not

Table 33-3 Frequency of Clinical Signs in Dogs with Chronic Hepatitis

Depression	60%	Seizures	15%
Vomiting	49%	Polydipsia	13%
Anorexia	43%	Fever	11%
Weight loss	31%	Bleeding	11%
Collapse weakness	25%	Coma, ataxia	8%
		Abdom. pain	5%
Diarrhea	24%	Head down	5%
Ascites	21%	Other CNS	5%
Icterus	21%	No signs	6%

possible to classify hepatitis on the basis of clinical findings. Physical signs are usually unremarkable. Ascites or hepatomegaly is reported in few patients. If chronic hepatitis is not recognized early, the number of patients with ascites increases. The liver may be smaller than normal in some animals. Normal size or small livers can not be palpated, however.

LABORATORY FINDINGS[16]

A number of tests for evaluating hepatic function and identifying hepatic necrosis give abnormal results in patients with hepatitis. In dogs with chronic hepatitis plasma alanine transaminase (ALT) or glutamic pyruvic transaminase (SGPT) and plasma alkaline phosphatase (ALP) activities are almost always elevated, although the increases are not always marked (Table 33-4). Mean ALT levels are increased from five to eighteen times the upper limit of normal; ALT is abnormal in 92% of all dogs. Mean plasma alkaline phosphatase activities are increased from two to five times the upper limit of normal; ALP is abnormal in 89% of all dogs. Total bilirubin are at or increased above the upper limit of normal (0.6 mg/dl) in 39% of the cases. Although ALT, ALP, and bilirubin are determined for all patients, function tests are usually conducted only for those not icteric. Mean sulfobromophthalein (BSP) retention percentage is increased two to six times (normal $\leq 5\%$ at 30 min), with 95% of all dogs having abnormal values. This test is not conducted if total bilirubin is greater than 1.0 mg/dl, since the results provide no useful information. Blood ammonia levels were increased in 54% of unfed dogs, and ammonia tolerance tests were abnormal in 95% of the cases. Hypoalbuminemia is seen in 27% of all dogs, and hypergammaglobulinemia is noted in 25%. Other clinical pathologic abnormalities in dogs with chronic hepatitis include increased times for prothrombin (36%) and partial thromboplastin (60%), increased plasma bile acids (63%), hypercholesterolema (22%), hypocholesterolemia (17%), hypoglycemia (8%), and hyperglycemia (10%).

Hepatitis and cirrhosis in cats causes similar biochemical changes. Plasma ALT is increased in most cases, and hypoalbuminemia is usually found. Plasma ALP activity, an insensitive marker for hepatic disease in the cat, is usually normal. Plasma total bilirubin is invariably increased, indicating that it is a very sensitive test for liver disease in cats. Plasma bile acids can be normal in approximately one-half the animals, making it a relatively insensitive indicator of hepatitis and cirrhosis in the cat.

Chronic Hepatitis (Canine)

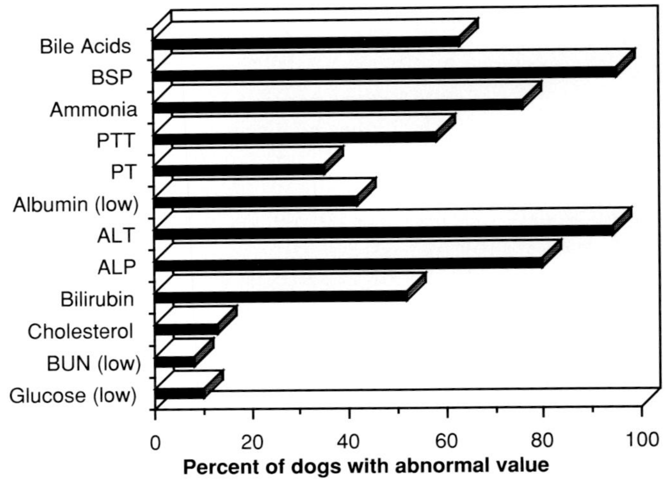

Table 33-4a. Comparison of sensitivities for different tests in dogs with chronic hepatitis. Below: graphs showing distribution of clinical pathology values in dogs with chronic hepatitis. Points on graphs represent 0%, 10%, 25%, 50%, 75%, 90%and 100% medians. Normal range is in shaded area.

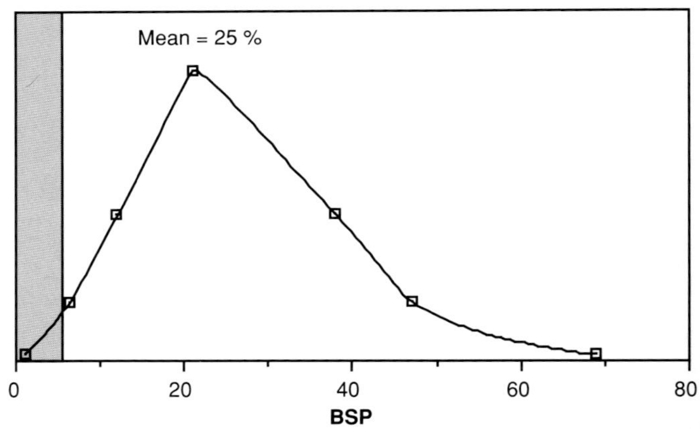

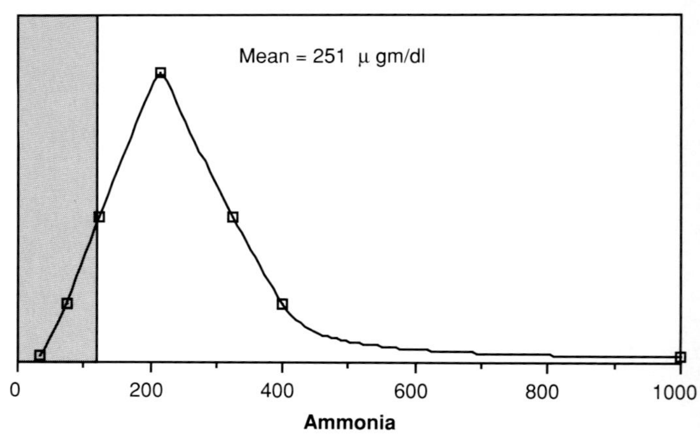

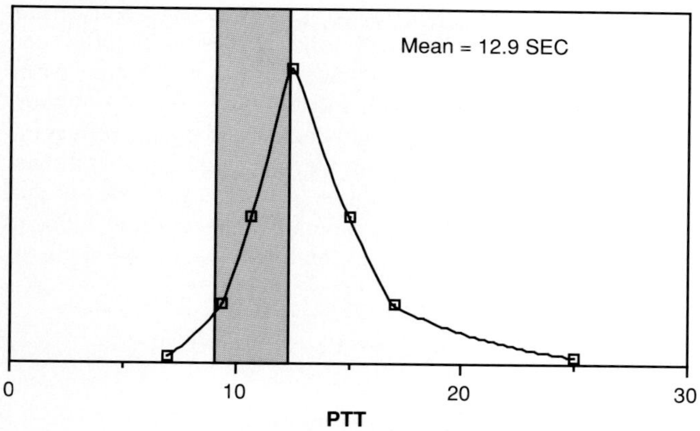
Mean = 12.9 SEC
0
10
20
30
PTT

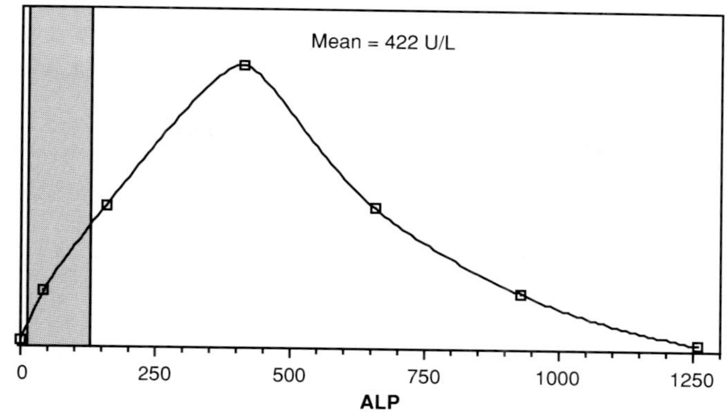
Mean = 422 U/L
0
250
500
750
1000
1250
ALP

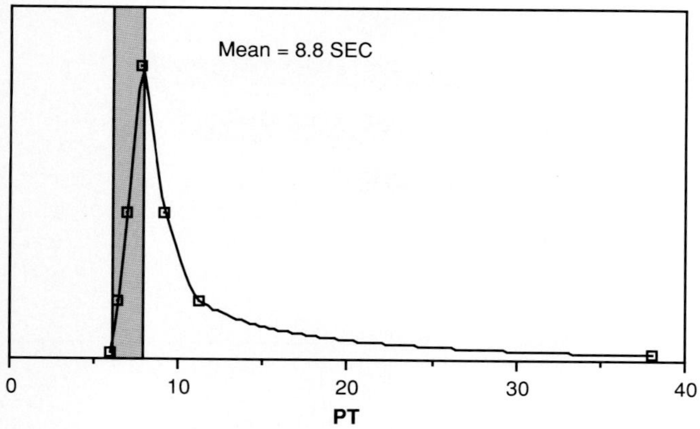
Mean = 8.8 SEC
0
10
20
30
40
PT

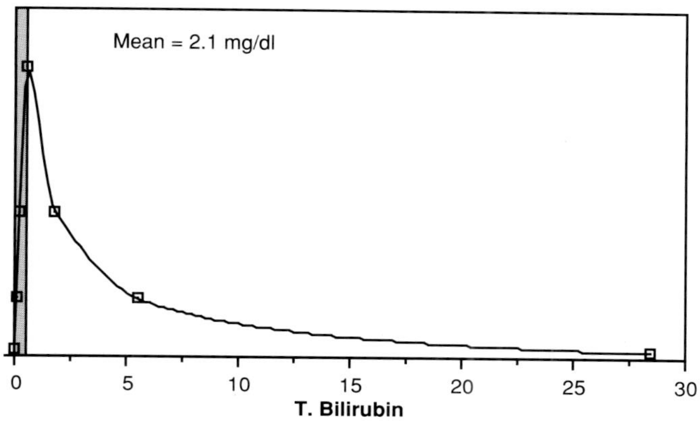
Mean = 2.1 mg/dl
0
5
10
15
20
25
30
T. Bilirubin

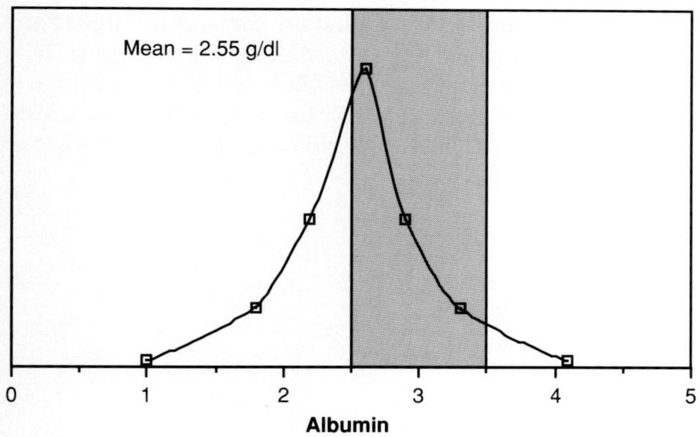
Mean = 2.55 g/dl
0
1
2
3
4
5
Albumin

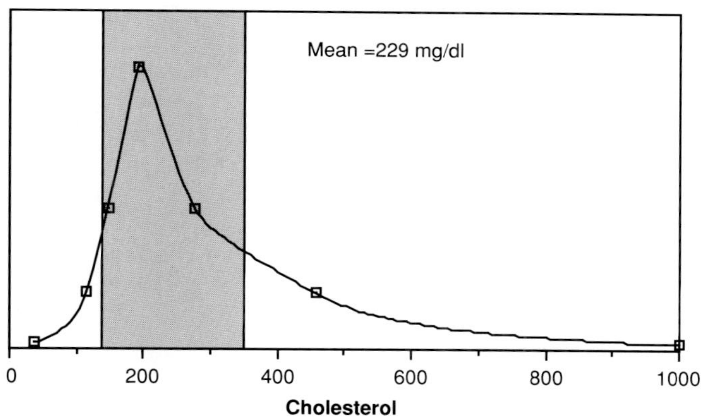
Mean =229 mg/dl
0
200
400
600
800
1000
Cholesterol

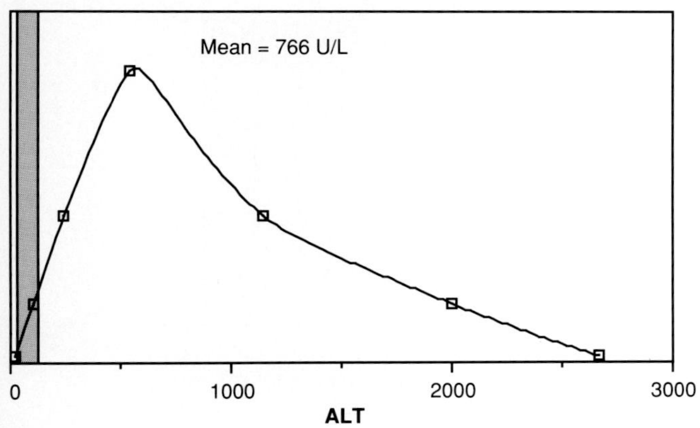
Mean = 766 U/L
0
1000
2000
3000
ALT

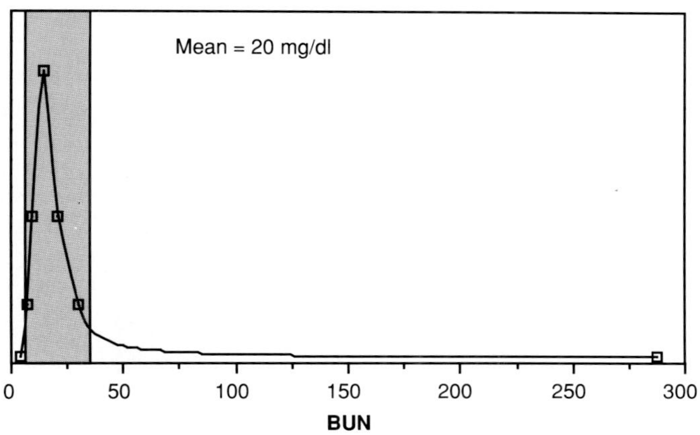
Mean = 20 mg/dl
0
50
100
150
200
250
300
BUN

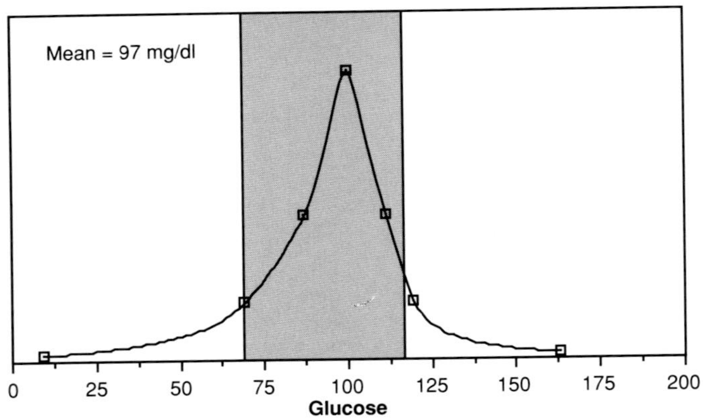

The biochemical studies of patients with chronic hepatitis have included determination of plasma amino acid levels.[47] The significant findings include a decrease in the sum of the branched-chain amino acids valine, isoleucine, and leucine, and an increase in the sum of the neutral aromatic amino acids tyrosine and phenylalanine. The ratio of these branched-chain to aromatics should be 3.0 or greater in normal dogs. The ratio decreases to about 1.0 in dogs with experimentally created portacaval shunts; they do not survive for more than a few months.[35] The ratio of the sums in dogs with chronic hepatitis is 1.3. Plasma glutamine is not elevated, plasma alanine is reduced, and ammonia is increased. The reciprocal changes in ornithine and citrulline reflect the hyperammonemia. The changes in plasma amino acids are marked and associated with a severe functional deterioration of the liver.

Partial biochemical evaluation of animals for chronic hepatitis does not accurately reflect the extent of liver pathology, but, more important, it does not identify all patients with hepatic disease. The ALT and ALP determinations alone, without additional tests, identify up to 92% of the cases. Furthermore, small elevations in plasma enzyme activity can frequently be explained by other problems, and so they may be disregarded and never reevaluated without other evidence for a major hepatic problem. Total bilirubin is elevated inconsistently in dogs with chronic hepatitis, making it a very insensitive indicator. Because of this, function tests must often be used to identify hepatic disease.

BIOPSY AND PATHOLOGY FINDINGS

Hepatitis is diagnosed only on the basis of liver histology (Figure 33-7). The diagnostic features of chronic hepatitis are increased fibroblasts, increased mononuclear cells, and in some cases, biliary proliferation. Histologic evaluation for classification as chronic hepatitis includes assessment of the following characteristics: inflammation (location being periportal, multifocal, or central; cell type being neutrophils, mononuclear cells, or mixed; and severity being mild, moderate or severe); hepatocyte morphology (necrosis location being periportal, multifocal, central, piecemeal or diffuse; necrosis severity being mild, moderate or severe); degeneration (location being periportal, multifocal, central or diffuse; degeneration severity being mild, moderate or severe; and vacuolation of hepatocytes), presence and abundance of sinusoidal leukocytes; fibrosis (location being periportal, central, bridging or focal; severity being mild, moderate or severe); presence and degree of Kupffer cell hyperplasia; number of macrophage clusters; and degree of bile duct proliferation being mild, moderate or severe. Polymorphonuclear leukocytes are usually not abundant and reflect the extent of necrosis. Macrophages are also seen in small numbers and in proportion to the amount of necrosis. Cirrhosis and nodular regeneration are seen often. Lesions of steroid-induced hepatopathy are expected when treatment has included glucocorticosteroids.

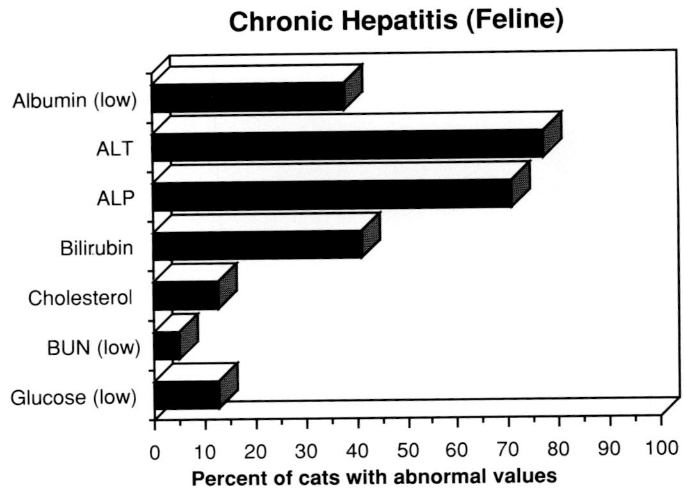

Table 33-4b. Comparison of sensitivities for different tests in cats with chronic hepatitis. Below and on page 609: graphs showing distribution of clinical pathology values in cats with chronic hepatitis. Points represent 0%, 25%, 50%, 75% and 100% medians. Normal range is in shaded area.

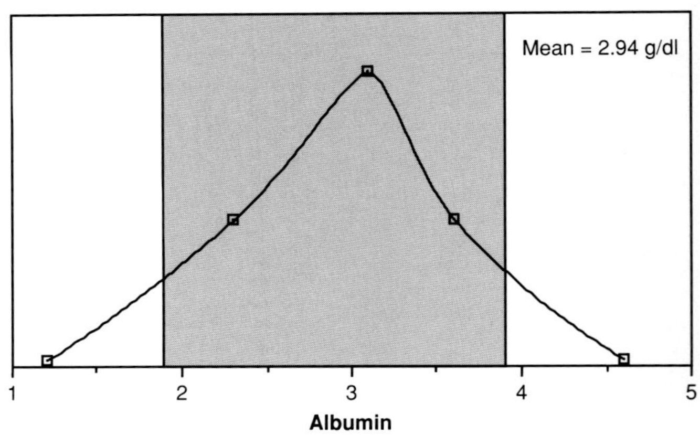

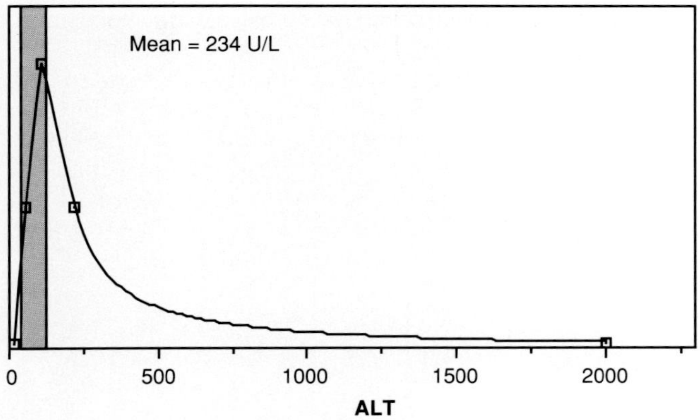
Mean = 234 U/L
0
500
1000
1500
2000
ALT

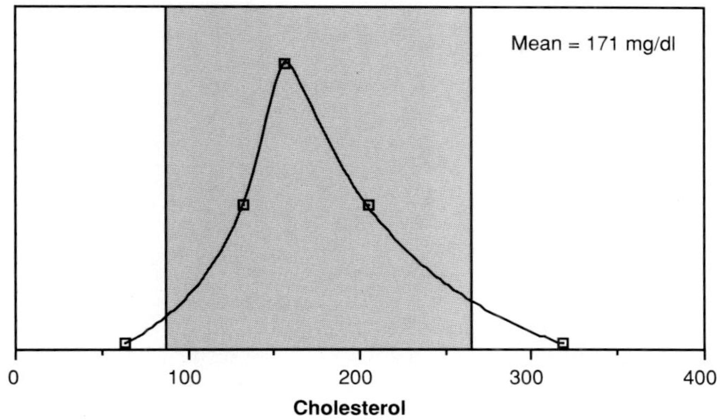
Mean = 171 mg/dl
0
100
200
300
400
Cholesterol

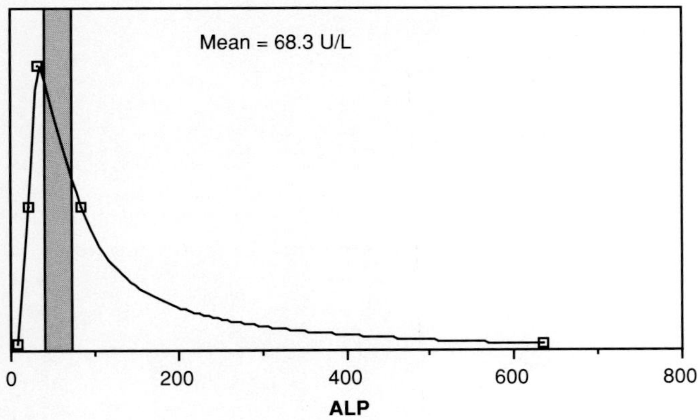
Mean = 68.3 U/L
0
200
400
600
800
ALP

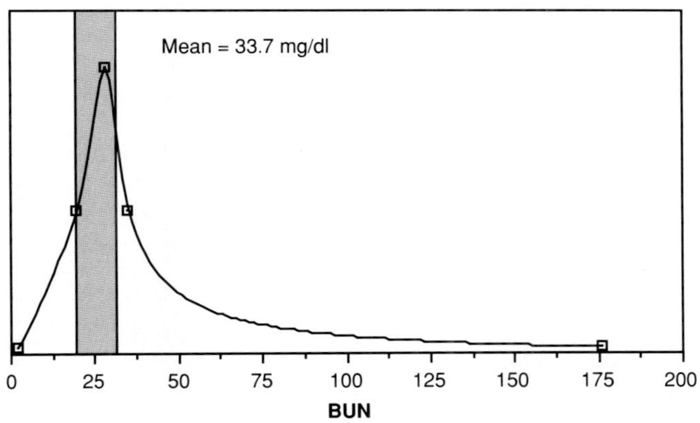
Mean = 33.7 mg/dl
0
25
50
75
100
125
150
175
200
BUN

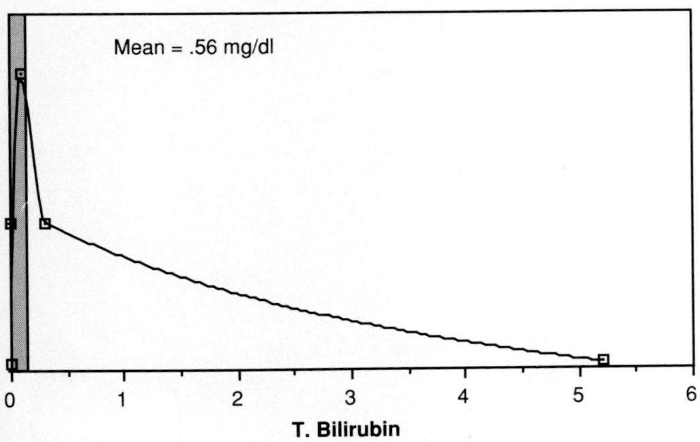
Mean = .56 mg/dl
0
1
2
3
4
5
6
T. Bilirubin

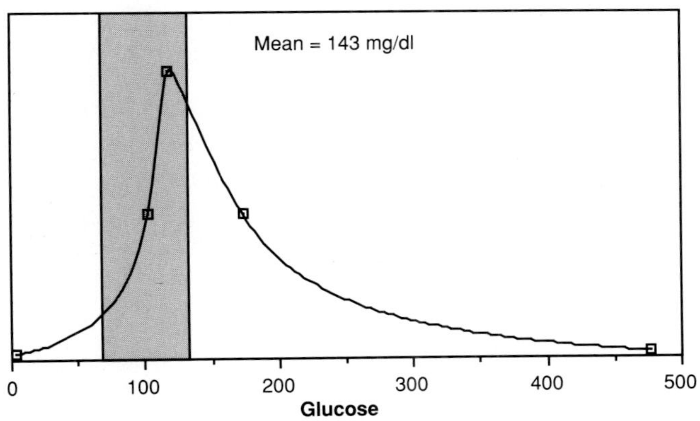
Mean = 143 mg/dl
0
100
200
300
400
500
Glucose

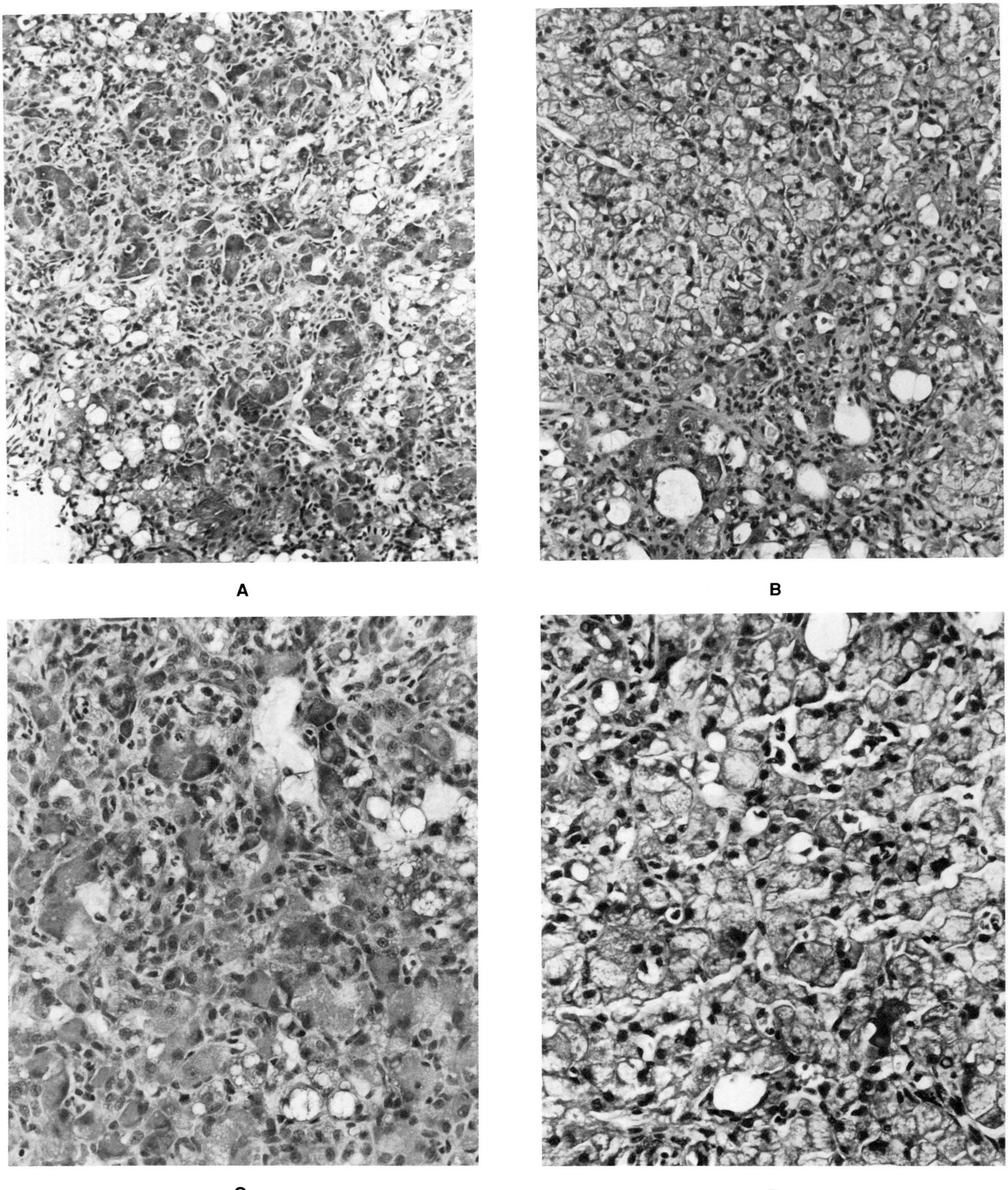

Figure 33-7. (a) Biopsy from liver of a dog with chronic active hepatitis before treatment and (b) rebiopsy after 16 weeks of treatment with corticosteroids. Improvement includes reduction in both inflammation and fibrosis. The vacuolar change in hepatocytes is associated with the use of corticosteroids. (c) and (d) Biopsies before and after treatment in another dog with chronic active hepatitis.

DIAGNOSIS

Diagnosis requires positive biopsy findings.

MANAGEMENT

Treatment of primary chronic hepatitis is directed at arresting inflammation, correcting nutritional derangements, and resolving fibrosis. Management of secondary hepatitis is directed at the primary problem with the expectation the hepatitis will resolve with no additional treatment. No therapy for chronic hepatitis has been evaluated for effectiveness in a controlled study. There are few reports on the results of treating dogs with chronic hepatitis. The earliest studies on dogs report on groups of animals in which most died before any trial of management was possible.[13,14] A few dogs in each report were treated with some form of immunosuppressive therapy but without much success. A recent study on 150 dogs reports a relatively large percentage (37%) died within one week, but that was much better than the 50% death rate for the same institution a few years earlier.[16] That improvement may result from increased awareness of chronic hepatitis and, as a consequence, earlier recognition. A number of reports have described the evaluation and management of cats with chronic hepatitis, but very few cases are included in each report.

Animals with acute hepatitis are seldom biopsied and are usually recognized as having an acute liver problem for which they are managed with nonspecific therapy such as antibiotics and fluids. Acute hepatitis progressing to a chronic form is often recognized, and because that is usually done by biopsy, more is known about the results of management for, in this case, a confirmed diagnosis. The most important specific therapy involves the use of immunosuppressive or anti-inflammatory drugs and diets designed to correct abnormal nitrogen metabolism.

Corticosteroids

The anti-inflammatory drugs used most widely for treating chronic hepatitis are the corticosteroids.[16] Of the types to use, prednisolone may be preferred since it is already biologically active. Since its precursor, prednisone, must be metabolized by the liver to produce the active form, achieving desired blood levels is less predictable with that form.[48,49] For practical purposes prednisone appears to be effective in most animals with chronic hepatitis, so there must be adequate hepatic function for conversion of prednisone to prednisolone.[16] It is probably more important to give prednisone more often than to be concerned about which form to use. Signs of hypercorticism can appear with chronic hepatic disease because steroids are not adequately metabolized and prepared for renal excretion, and continued stress stimulates secretion of excess adrenal corticosteroids. When a steroid is used for treatment, its peak blood levels are predictably higher than normal, making signs of excess possible. To minimize that problem, the daily dose used is divided and given more often than once a day. In dogs prednisone is given at a dose of 2.2 mg/kg/day for seven to twenty days, followed by 1.1 mg/kg/day for another seven to ten days, followed by 0.6 mg/kg/day until the disease is judged to be in remission. That dose is increased by twofold or more in cats because such steroids are metabolized more rapidly in the cat than the dog. Such therapeutic doses of prednisone given to cats produce no biochemical or pathologic signs of iatrogenic Cushings as seen in the dog; the only exception is an inhibited ACTH stimulation of cortisol secretion. In dogs, and probably in cats, reductions in medication by administration of prednisone on alternate days results in treatment failure.

Corticosteroids should not be used in acute hepatitis with an etiology that is unknown but suspected of being viral. Mortality and morbidity rates increase when corticosteroids are used in animals with viral hepatitis or in humans with some forms of acute hepatitis.[50] Viruses may be able to replicate more rapidly when steroids are used in clinical cases, as happens in experimental animals.[5] Corticosteroids have the important catabolic effect of simulating a breakdown of body proteins at a time when protein synthesis must be promoted in order to restore many hepatic functions. Corticosteroids increase urea-cycle activity by stimulating hepatic enzyme synthesis. The diseased liver is handicapped in its ability to synthesize protein, however, and the increase in ammonia produced by corticosteroid-directed protein catabolism can cause clinical signs to worsen.

Other immunosuppressive therapy used to manage chronic hepatitis includes azathioprine and penicillamine. Azathioprine is used in humans in order to avoid the side-effects of corticosteroids. There is no information on any benefits for azathioprine on chronic hepatitis in small animals. If that drug is used, it is essential to monitor the patient for leukopenia and thrombocytopenia that the drug can cause. If steroid therapy results in unacceptable side effects, its dose can be reduced by one half and azathioprine can be added at a dose of 1 mg/kg initially followed by a reduction in the dose for both when improvement can be shown. D-penicillamine at a dose of 10 to 15 mg/kg twice daily is effective when copper toxicosis causes chronic hepatitis. That drug has no effect in managing chronic hepatitis due to other causes, however, other than in its effect of reducing hepatic copper levels. D-penicillamine is also ineffective in managing humans with chronic hepatitis.

Animals are treated with corticosteroids until there is evidence for complete remission; in some cases this may never be found. That evidence is most reliable when gained from a rebiopsy of the liver. Clinical signs are an insensitive indicator of the degree of improvement in liver pathology. That is not surprising because liver pathology is advanced in many cases before any signs appear. Thus, corticosteroid therapy is not discontinued merely because an animal becomes clinically normal. Evaluation of the patient by clinical pathology is not used to determine improvement because corticosteroid therapy causes biochemical abnormalities that would suggest little or no improvement in hepatic pathology. Thus, ideally the liver should be rebiopsied before any recommendations are made to reduce or discontinue immunosuppressive or anti-inflammatory therapy.

Treatment with corticosteroids is effective in improving long-term survival time in dogs with chronic hepatitis that survive at least a week after they are presented for evaluation of their problems.[16] Treated dogs live three times longer than untreated dogs in groups of animals still alive or eventually dying of liver disease (Table 33-5) (Figure 33-8). That is in spite of the treated dogs having significantly worse liver pathology. Other studies report corticosteroid therapy ineffective.[13,14] Some

Table 33-5 Effects of Corticosteroid Treatment on Survival Time of Dogs with Chronic Hepatitis

	Corticosteroid-treated Group			Untreated Group		
Status	Survival time (mo)*	Age (yr)	No. of dogs	Survival Time (mo)	Age (yr)	No. of dogs
Alive	33.1 ± 5.5	6.28 ± 0.81	14	19.3 ± 3.9	6.90 ± 1.06	10
Alive and lost to follow-up	22.1 ± 4.7	6.25 ± 0.77	8	4.3 ± 1.8	7.33 ± 2.60	3
Died of hepatic disease	18.2 ± 3.2	7.61 ± 0.77	23	5.5 ± 1.4	7.24 ± 0.88	23
Died of nonhepatic disease	22.5 ± 9.3	9.38 ± 0.85	13	20.3 ± 9.8	8.67 ± 2.03	3

* P<0.005 significantly different from untreated groups. Data are expressed as mean ± SE

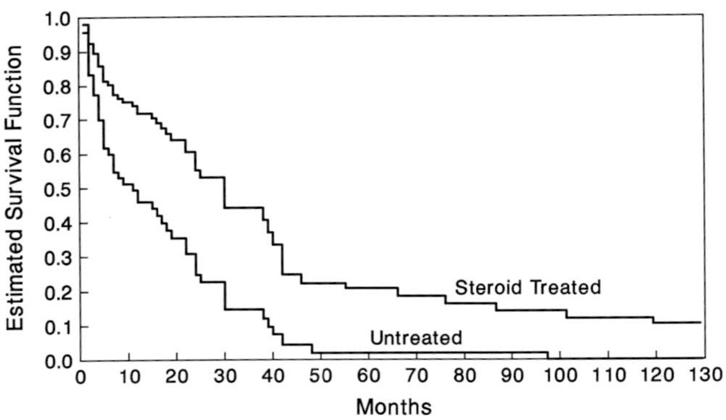

Figure 33-8. Graph showing survival in months of dogs with hepatitis that were treated and untreated.

animals were treated with smaller doses of corticosteroids, and some were managed with alternate day therapy, either of which treatments may explain the poorer results. In another study, treated dogs lived for several years, which may have seemed a poor outcome but could very well represent a long time compared to their survival rate without steroid therapy.[15]

Diet

Dietary management is required to minimize the abnormalities in nitrogen metabolism, which are reflected in hyperammonemia and hypoalbuminemia and alterations in plasma levels of amino acids. Hyperammonemia can be partly managed by feeding a low-protein diet, an acceptable procedure as long as synthesis of body proteins is not severely reduced. Overall protein synthetic functions are evaluated by measurement of plasma albumin, which can be low in dogs with chronic hepatitis, causing such patients to suffer major nitrogen deficiencies if they are fed a low-protein diet. With hypoalbuminemia as a major problem, restriction of dietary protein leads to more profound hypoalbuminemia. (Measurement of total plasma protein is not reliable in identifying hypoalbuminemia because plasma globulin levels often increase with chronic hepatic insufficiency, and when that is associated with low albumin levels the total plasma protein concentration can be normal.) In general, the patient should be fed as much protein as can be tolerated; insufficient amounts result in hypoalbuminemia, and excessive amounts produce signs of hepatic encephalopathy. The restoration of hepatic function requires synthesis of both hepatocyte structure and enzymes; reduction of dietary protein prevents that. Even with feeding more than normal requirements of protein, dogs with hepatic insufficiency may be unable to maintain normal plasma albumin levels; moreover, the levels may progressively decrease despite what is done (Figure 30-7).

The minimum amount of protein to feed daily is 1.0 g/20 calories. If greater amounts can be tolerated, they are of benefit. If early clinical signs (depression, anorexia) of hepatic encephalopathy appear, the amount should be reduced. Caloric requirements must be met with carbohydrate and fats; otherwise, energy needs will be met with the proteins in the diet, with more ammonia produced as a by-product. In addition, adequate carbohydrate diminishes the catabolism of body protein for energy. Frequent feeding is recommended to ensure optimum assimilation of the meal so that little dietary protein enters the colon, where bacterial fermentation produces ammonia amounting to one half of that produced in the small intestinal tract. Feeding a single meal is more likely to let excessive protein enter the colon. The other half of ammonia is produced from metabolism of glutamine by the intestinal mucosa, something that cannot be reduced by dietary modification.

The diet can indirectly reduce intestinal ammonia production and absorption. Ammonia is produced from plasma proteins escaping into the intestine and from desquamated villous epithelial cells. Any event accelerating this protein loss increases the amounts entering the colon, such as intestinal inflammation and intestinal circulatory problems. When diets improve any existing protein-losing enteropathy, ammonia production is reduced. In general, complete restriction of food intake reduces the turnover rate of intestinal epithelial cells. Low-residue diets have a similar effect and reduce the amounts of protein entering the colon.

The source of protein in the diet is important in managing any form of acute or chronic hepatic insufficiency and in reducing the worsening of hepatic pathology.[29,51,52] Certain specific or defined diets allow animals with hepatic insufficiency to survive where animals with the same pathology do not survive when fed commercial dog food. Essential for survival is feeding proteins from milk or soybeans; feeding meat protein has an adverse affect on survival. A number of reasons have been suggested to explain these differences.

Feeding milk protein or vegetable proteins may be beneficial because they improve abnormalities in amino acid metabolism. Experimentally in some early studies, the correction of plasma amino acid imbalances in dogs allowed them to survive with hepatic insufficiency whereas they normally would not. The return toward normal concentrations of plasma amino acids can be accomplished by feeding a protein of amino acid composition that is high in branched-chain amino acids and low in aromatic amino acids. The benefits of feeding milk proteins has been suggested to be due to the favorable composition of the protein's amino acids.[36] The ratio between the branched-chain and aromatic amino acids, however, is essentially the same for proteins in cottage cheese, meat, and fish. The benefits of cottage cheese must therefore be due to properties other than amino acid composition. It might be noted that recent studies show no beneficial effect of using mixtures of branched-chain amino acids to correct the plasma amino acid abnormalities.[53] Although such products are commercially available, there are no justifications for their use in managing chronic hepatitis. The role of aromatic amino acids in contributing to clinical signs is also questioned. Their feeding to dogs with hepatic insufficiency does not cause clinical signs to appear in asymptomatic animals or to worsen in any dogs with signs.[46] A recent study suggests that high levels of amino acids responsible for generating large amounts of ammonia are more important; glycine is one such amino acid.[52]

The benefits of feeding milk or soybean protein may be due to a reduced production and absorption of toxins in the intestinal tract compared to when meat protein is fed. The production of ammonia, one such toxin, may be less. Cottage cheese is optimal in digestibility and biological value, being completely utilized without forming large amounts of ammonia. Protein requirements are much less when the source is used completely than when it is not.[54] Soy bean protein could be beneficial for similar reasons. The defined diets based on milk and soy bean protein may be beneficial because they reduce the production and absorption of bacteria, bacterial antigens, endotoxin, bacterially transformed chemicals, or unaltered chemicals in the diet. Bacterial products are normally found in portal blood. Products of *E. coli* produce inflammation resembling periportal hepatitis and eventually periportal fibrosis.[28] Endotoxin acts synergistically with other agents with a hepatotoxic potential to cause chronic hepatic pathology.[55] Experimental studies show that manipulations to increase endotoxin absorption hastens the pathologic process and that reduction of endotoxin formation and absorption can prevent pathology caused by a proven hepatotoxin. Endotoxin and possibly other toxin effects are reduced by antibiotics that reduce the intestinal bacterial flora and by binding agents such as cholestyramine that reduce toxin absorption. Diets formulated with milk and soy bean proteins may be beneficial in a similar fashion by reducing the formation and absorption of toxins and antigens in the colon. This diet affects the numbers of colonic bacteria because it is free of residue and is completely digested and absorbed. With fewer bacteria, less toxins are produced. Diet composition also influences the type of bacteria flourishing in the intestine, which may be a factor in causing chronic hepatitis to improve. Control of diet composition allows additives to be eliminated. Commercial pet foods contain additives that can be metabolized by intestinal bacteria to produce potent hepatotoxins.

Although the amount and quality of protein in the diet are important, the manner in which they are used is determined by other constituents in the diet. The carbohydrate used should be readily digested and absorbed, leaving little available for fermentation in the colon. Fermentable carbohydrate sustains the colonic bacterial population and thereby influences the production and absorption of toxins. Carbohydrates are fermented to short-chain or volatile free fatty acids, which act synergistically with ammonia and mercaptans to produce signs of hepatic encephalopathy. Chronic hepatitis is also associated with carbohydrate intolerance (identified by fasting hyperglycemia), which may be due to a relative insulin resistance since hyperinsulinemia normally prevails. Such an intolerance may be an indication for limiting carbohydrate in the diet. There are some suggestions, however, that a beneficial criterion of milk- and soy bean-protein diets is a high ratio of carbohydrate to amino acid nitrogen, which has the potential for minimal ammonia production.[56] If that is true it is important to seek a balance with respect to protein and carbohydrate levels.

Lipids should supply most of the calories for a patient with chronic hepatitis even though there are some reasons for limiting dietary lipids.[57] Diets prolonging survival in experimental dogs with chronic hepatic insufficiency contain 25% to 35% fat. That level is necessary to improve acceptance of a meatless diet that is relatively unpalatable. Animal fat adds more flavor than vegetable fat. A higher level of fat also reduces problems with carbohydrate intolerance from feeding a high carbohydrate diet. Some of the plasma amino acid abnormalities are caused by hyperinsulinemia, a problem that is worsened with high carbohydrate diets.

Any reasons for limiting dietary lipids do not appear to be compelling. Free fatty acid levels increase after a meal, especially for shorter-chain fatty acids that can be absorbed without esterification into triglycerides. Fatty acids interfere with the conversion of ammonia to urea and could potentiate a hyperammonemia seen after feeding. Shorter chain fatty acids interfere more effectively with that metabolism. One such fatty acid, octanoic acid is produced by the diseased liver because the long chain fatty acid, palmitic acid, is only partially oxidized. Plasma fatty acid levels also increase during fasting; multiple daily feeding minimizes the release of fatty acids from adipose tissue.

Diets fed to animals with chronic hepatitis are balanced as necessary with vitamin and mineral supplementation. The requirements for B vitamins are determined by the level of caloric intake. With complete anorexia there is no requirement; with resumption of food intake after a period of none there is a greater than maintenance need for these vitamins. Vitamin C supplementation may be necessary even when feeding a diet containing standard amounts of ascorbic acid. An important part of a dog's ascorbic acid is produced in the liver. With hepatic insufficiency plasma ascorbic acid can be lower than normal even when the patient is given recommended additions of a standard vitamin-mineral supplement.[29] Ascorbic acid can be given at levels up to 25 mg/kg per day. Ascorbic acid can cause stored copper to be released in the liver and that can worsen hepatic pathology. Vitamin E can be given at levels of 500 mg/day to dogs and 100 mg/day to cats. Vitamin E is an antioxidant that protects against lipid peroxidation injury and has especially been shown to protect against such injury produced by copper. Vitamin A is not given because it is able to interact synergistically with chemicals and toxins such as endotoxin to injure the liver. That happens with levels of vitamin A that are normally not hepatotoxic. Mineral supplementation can include zinc (3 mg of zinc gluconate/kg/day or 2 mg zinc sulfate/kg/day, each divided into three doses), based on studies that zinc inhibits the intestinal absorption of copper and its deposition in the liver.[58] In some dogs with chronic hepatitis, copper accumulates in the liver, and high copper concentrations in the liver are toxic.

A great amount is known about nutrition in normal cats, but very little is known about feeding cats with hepatic disease. Since most hepatic pathology is secondary to primary disease in some other tissue, dietary management is supportive or directed at the primary problem. In either case cats are fed 80 to 100 Kcal/kg body weight per day, and 12% to 20% of their caloric needs must be provided by protein. The diet must also contain adequate amounts of arginine and taurine. Nothing is known about any benefits when the protein source is milk or soy beans rather than meat, but it can be assumed that with one exception cats are similar to dogs and humans in their response to the type of protein fed. These proteins must be supplemented with taurine. Acceptance of a meat-free diet will be poor. In more severe cases, cats should be managed by feeding an enteral type of diet via a nasogastric or gastrostomy tube. A liquid enteral diet can be slowly dripped into the alimentary tract over an extended period each day. Slow infusion minimizes the possibility of vomiting or diarrhea often seen with the feeding of such diets. Tube feeding eliminates a need to use benzodiazepine compounds or anabolic steroids to stimulate the appetite. These drugs, like many, have side effects that are especially unwanted in a patient with hepatic disease. The enteral diets are ideal because they are meat-free, being formulated from milk and soy bean proteins. Most of these diets have a high fat content, approximating 30% or more. There may be theoretical reasons for a high fat diet contributing to hepatic encephalopathy, but that is not seen. If a high proportion of the calories are provided by carbohydrates, large volumes of such a liquid diet would need to be fed. Enteral diets based on milk and soy bean proteins require supplementation with taurine; 150 mg is added to 8 oz of diet. There is no evidence for any benefit from the addition of branched-chain amino acids to the diet. Diets can also be prepared by the owner for feeding cats with hepatic disease. Such diets are similar to ones prepared for dogs with liver disease, but they must contain more protein and be supplemented with taurine. There are no commercially prepared diets for cats with liver disease. The prescription diet K/D is recommended for that use because of its protein quality and content. There are no studies showing any benefits for that diet in cats with liver disease. In general, many species of animals with hepatic insufficiency do poorer and pathology worsens when they are fed commercially prepared animal foods. Feeding such a diet is probably unimportant in most cats with hepatic pathology, but any commercial diet is likely to be less effective than an enteral diet in cats with serious hepatic disease.

The diet for cats should be supplemented with B vitamins, especially with thiamine because cats can become deficient quite soon during anorexia. Recommendations for supplementation with fat-soluble vitamins is the same as for dogs. No recommendations can be given for supplementation with ascorbic acid and zinc because nothing is known of their need by cats with hepatic disease.

Resolution of Fibrosis[20,59]

Treatment can be directed against advanced fibrosis and cirrhosis. A moderate amount of fibrosis disappears with corticosteroid therapy and dietary management, so that no specific drug therapy directed against fibrosis is necessary. Fibrosis that remains despite this management can be treated by other means. Experimentally, fibrosis in dogs can be treated successfully with colchicine. Controlled studies have shown the drug to resolve cirrhosis in humans. Long-term colchicine treatment dramatically improves hyperbilirubinemia, ascites, acute bouts of hepatic encephalopathy, and survival rate. Colchicine disrupts microtubule formation, interrupting intracellular transport and increasing collagenase activity. By inhibiting microtubule assembly, colchicine interferes with transcellular movement of collagen, so that it is not deposited. Stimulation of collagenase activity removes collagen already deposited. Colchicine is more effective in resolving fibrosis than are proline analogs, which have only a single mechanism to interfere with collagen synthesis. The side effects of colchicine include vomiting, diarrhea, depression, and anorexia, caused by interference of function in gastrointestinal epithelial cells. Less common complications of the drug include fever, loss of hair, hypocalcemia, blood dyscrasias, and possibly liver damage. Little is known on any benefits for using colchicine to resolve fibrosis or cirrhosis in small animals. One report describes improvement following a short course of therapy and relapse on discontinuation of colchicine.[60] Subsequent treatment resulted in no improvement. Two other dogs treated for up to a year with colchicine showed worsening pathology on repeat biopsies and therapy was changed.[31] Thus, there is no evidence that colchicine is effective in managing dogs with chronic hepatitis. Its use on clinical cases must be considered experimental.

The pathogenesis of fibrosis and cirrhosis in animals with biliary cirrhosis may be different from that of chronic hepatitis. It is probably not appropriate to compare biliary cirrhosis in animals with that in humans. In animals, biliary cirrhosis may be simply a sequel to chronic cholangiohepatitis. When the inflammatory process is recognized and managed early, there is little likelihood of biliary cirrhosis developing. Management should include corticosteroid therapy, with prednisone given at doses described for chronic hepatitis. Corticosteroids have the effect of resolving other forms of fibrosis in the liver. D-penicillamine has potential antifibrotic properties in that it interferes with collagen by inhibiting its cross-linking and maturation. D-penicillamine is not effective in managing humans with chronic hepatitis or biliary cirrhosis, however. The drug shows no efficacy for any hepatic problems in small animals except for managing Bedlington Terriers with copper toxicosis.

Management of Hepatic Encephalopathy[61,62]

Severe hepatic encephalopathy is a major complication

possible if protein intake is restricted insufficiently or if there is massive loss of blood or plasma proteins into the alimentary tract. The signs of hepatic encephalopathy are precipitated by absorption of ammonia, mercaptans, and volatile short-chain fatty acids from the intestine. This complication is managed by colonic irrigation to remove all contents. Enemas and cathartics to clean out colonic contents and reduce bacterial numbers reduce both the substrates and agents for ammonia production. Ammonia absorption is reduced by using saline cathartics and mildly acidic enemas to decrease the pH of colonic contents. At lower pH's, ammonia is primarily ionized and, being a charged ion, is largely not absorbed. A cathartic and pH-reducing effect is also produced by a disaccharide, lactulose, or one of its analogues, lactitol. These sugars are not digested in the small intestine. On reaching the colon they are fermented, forming metabolites that produce an acidic environment and cause an osmotic diarrhea (Figure 33-9). Lactulose reduces urea formation from ammonia absorbed from the colon by diverting colonic ammonia into colonic bacteria which are subsequently excreted. It also inhibits urease activity, thereby reducing the production of ammonia from urea in the colon. Lactulose is given at a dose of 1-2 ml/kg every 6 hr PO as required, and when effective, diarrhea develops. Larger doses may be necessary in some individuals. Long-term therapy is usually unacceptable because of diarrhea and complications such as hypovolemia, hypernatremia, hypokalemia and alkalosis are possible. More consistent effects may be seen with lactitol, which may also have fewer side effects in small animals. These compounds are expensive, and the same benefits may be achieved by oral administration of large amounts of lactose (1 gm/kg/day) with the understanding that most small animals do not have the high intestinal lactase activity developed from regular consumption of milk. Lactose in a 20% solution can also be given in an enema.

Lactulose probably reduces ammonia production from other nitrogenous compounds; it has the ability to reduce the incorporation of ammonia into urea by 25%. Although lactulose has properties to cause catharsis and acidify colonic contents, it reduces ammonia production by another means, the alteration of nitrogen metabolism by colonic bacteria. Lactulose also reduces the ammonia produced during glutamine metabolism by the small intestine; that production represents one half of all the ammonia produced in the intestinal tract.

Dietary fiber such as pectin also significantly reduces ammonia and hence urea production. Urea production decreases because urea degradation decreases; fecal nitrogen increases. Increasing dietary fiber increases fecal nitrogen excretion, mostly in fecal bacteria. Management of chronic hyperammonemia can include incorporating fiber in the diet.

Ammonia is produced by colonic urease-producing bacteria, in amounts proportional to blood urea nitrogen levels. Reducing blood urea nitrogen levels is important in treating hyperammonemia. Ammonia production is also decreased by reducing the numbers of colonic bacteria. That reduction is difficult to maintain for more than a few days even when effective antibiotics are used. Bacteria, especially aerobes, rapidly develop a resistance to drugs, terminating their effectiveness.

Neomycin, an aminoglycoside similar to gentamicin and kanamycin, given orally is effective in reducing gram-negative bacterial numbers in the colon. Neomycin at 200 mg/kg (a dose

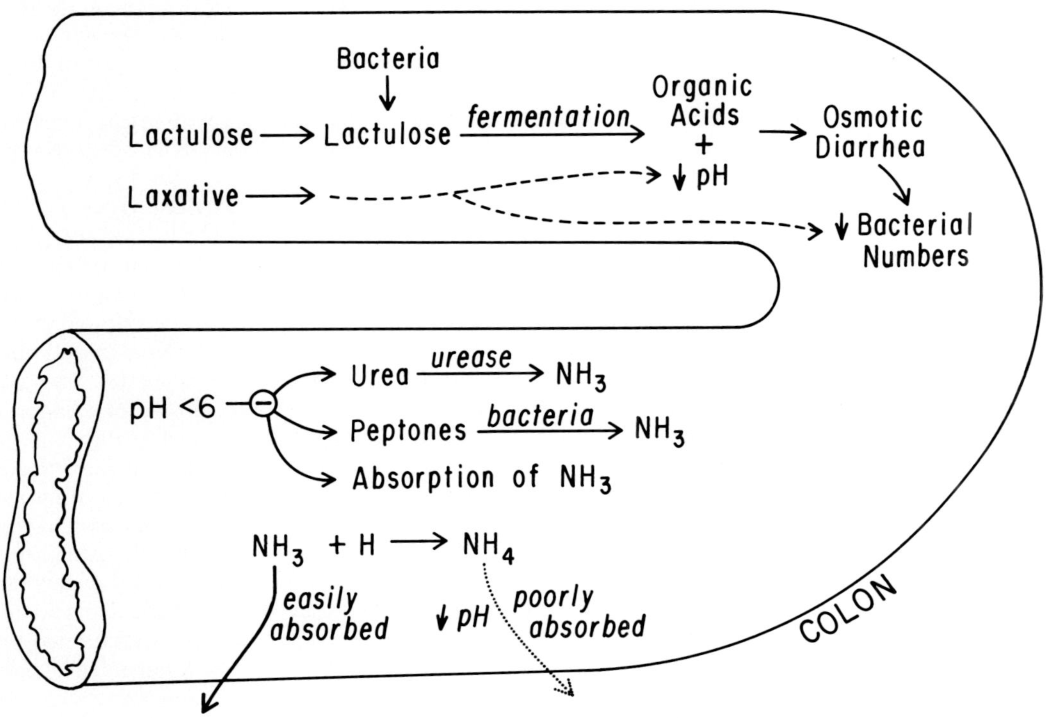

Figure 33-9. Schematic showing factors influencing ammonia production and absorption. Lactulose and conventional laxatives modify the pH and consistency of colonic contents to inhibit ammonia formation and absorption.

that is too high to be recommended - see clinical synopsis) combined with polymyxin B at 20 mg/kg, divided and given in two doses orally, is very effective in reducing fecal numbers of gram-negative bacteria to almost zero within nine days in dogs.[63] Neomycin may be effective for reasons other than reducing bacterial populations. Neomycin reduces the production of ammonia from intestinal glutamine metabolism, similar to that effect shown for lactulose. Neomycin is often combined with lactulose, and the reduction in ammonia production is greater than for either one alone. Neomycin, in reducing colonic bacterial numbers, would be expected to cause incomplete fermentation of lactulose, resulting in a loss of its benefits. Nonappearance of this result may be due to large numbers of anaerobes unaffected by the antibiotic and able to ferment the disaccharide. Other poorly absorbed sugars or their derivatives such as sorbitol and lactitol may have similar beneficial effects when combined with neomycin. Following oral administration, the largely unabsorbed neomycin can reach concentrations in the colon that may importantly reduce numbers of anaerobes.

Many other antibiotics can reduce the numbers of anaerobes, the most numerous bacteria in the colon. These antibiotics reach significant levels in gastrointestinal contents whether given orally or by injection. None have antibacterial activity against all colonic organisms. Most have no activity against bacteroides species. Penicillin is effective against colonic anaerobes, has little effect in reducing total numbers, and does not disrupt the normal microflora. Ampicillin and similar forms of penicillin with an enterohepatic circulation also have little effect in reducing total numbers but they disrupt the normal microflora. Chloromycetin has a similar effect, whereas tetracycline is hepatotoxic and therefore not used. Metronidazole has potent properties to suppress the anaerobic microflora and is sometimes used for that purpose. Erythromycin also has a potent range of activity against anaerobic bacteria. Trimethoprim-sulfa has no effect on the anaerobic microflora although it is effective against gram negative bacteria.

Attempts have been made to alter colonic bacterial activity by introducing nonurease-producing bacteria with the idea that they will displace those producing urease. Lactobacillus cultures have been advocated with the idea that they can repopulate the colonic microflora. Clinical trials show that therapy to be ineffective in humans.[36] Both animal and human studies show that it is difficult to alter bacterial populations in the colon. Bacteria given orally do not remain and multiply in the intestine, but pass out in the feces (Chapter 2). Transients entering through the oral cavity are able to populate only when the bacterial flora is disrupted. An alternate approach of management is to inhibit bacterial urease activity. Some immunity can be produced following immunization of animals with urease or urease-producing bacteria, resulting in some reduction of colonic urease activity.[64]

Hyperammonemia has been treated with substances to augment the fixation of ammonia into nontoxic products. Ammonia is converted most importantly to urea, and any substance supporting urea-cycle activity increases the conversion. Kreb's cycle intermediates providing aspartate are required to maintain urea-cycle activity. Thus, blood glucose levels are maintained, which is obviously important when hepatic disease produces hypoglycemia. Acute hyperammonemia during fasting reduces plasma alanine concentrations, which reflects its deamination and conversion to glucose. Increased urea-cycle activity requires arginine, and acute ammonia toxicity reduces plasma arginine levels.[34] Arginine in-fusions have been used to treat hyperammonemia in animals and humans, although with uncertain effectiveness. Arginine infusion decreases high blood ammonia levels, but that is not accompanied by improved clinical signs. Ammonia is also fixed and detoxified by forming glutamine from glutamic acid and by using alpha-keto acids for amination to form amino acids.[65]

The effects of hyperammonemia in inducing hepatic encephalopathy are reduced by decreasing ammonia diffusion into the brain. Ammonia enters the brain more rapidly during alkalosis, when larger amounts of ammonia are un-ionized, lipid-soluble, and more readily diffusible. Thus, any existing alkalosis is corrected. (In most cases the alkalosis is a metabolic type due to loss of gastrointestinal secretions from vomiting). Alkalosis is treated by replacing fluid deficits and continuing fluid therapy to initiate a diuresis. Since animals become potassium-depleted from vomiting, the potassium must be replaced in managing hyperammonemia and alkalosis. Electrolyte solutions containing glucose will worsen hypokalemia by promoting potassium movement into the cells. Potassium deficiency in itself can cause hyperammonemia.

The major effects of hepatic encephalopathy have been suggested to be due to an unknown toxic effect of ammonia and an alteration of the levels of neural transmitters.[36] Gama-aminobutyric acid, a normal inhibitory neurotransmitter, increases with hepatic encephalopathy.[62] Bacterial activity in the intestine produces that amino acid, and following absorption its blood levels are increased with hepatic insufficiency. That would suggest that administering antibiotics to reduce intestinal bacteria would be helpful in managing hepatic encephalopathy. Gamma-aminobutyric acid does not cross the blood-brain barrier, however, and its brain levels are readily increased by hyperammonemia alone. The increased levels of inhibitory transmitters and reduced levels of excitatory transmitters have been treated by increasing brain levels of the neurotransmitter dopamine using its precursor L-dopa. This treatment gives variable results in humans with severe hepatic encephalopathy, although a general effect is to cause arousal from coma.

Antibiotics

Antibiotics are used with signs of acute hepatitis, though not with the goal of sterilizing the gut. Antibiotics are directed primarily against bacteria absorbed from the intestine and not removed by the liver. Hepatic Kupffer cell function is reduced with hepatitis, so that bacteria are not removed from the portal circulation.[66] Also septicemia severely aggravates hyperammonemia and hepatic encephalopathy, and antibiotics minimize this complication.[26] Antibiotics are directed against intestinal anaerobes and aerobes, with penicillins the choice against the former and kanamycin or gentamicin against the latter. Antibiotics such as tetracycline and chloromycetin are usually not recommended because they are metabolized by the liver (Table 33-6). Tetracycline in particular is not used because it is toxic to dogs and possibly other species with hepatic insufficiency; the drug can be fatal when given to ones with portasystemic shunts.[67] Whether the other drugs can be hepatotoxic is not proven.

Antibiotics can benefit animals with chronic hepatitis. Parenteral antibiotics are indicated in dogs and cats with

Table 33-6 Antibiotics for Managing Hepatic Disease

Use at recommended dosage	Avoid or use at reduced dosage	Avoid
Penicillin (M)	Chloramphenicol (P)	Tetracyclines (G)
Ampicillin (M)	Erythromycin (G)	Aminoglycosides (P)
Other penicillins (M)	Clindamycin (M)	Rifampicin (G)
Cephalosporins (M)	Lincomycin (M)	
Metronidazole (M)	Sulfonamides	
Trimethoprim (M)		

G,M,P = good, moderate and poor antibacterial activity in bile

cholangitis, cholangiohepatitis, or bile duct obstruction. If bacteria are not a cause of cholangitis and cholangiohepatitis, they are a predictable complication. With bile duct obstruction, organisms normally removed by the liver from the portal blood and cleared into biliary secretions are not cleared and multiply in the liver and biliary system. Antibiotics used to treat these infections most effectively include some of the penicillins, trimethoprim, and the newer cephalosporins, all of which are effective in bile and have higher concentrations in bile than in plasma. Metronidazole can be used against anaerobic infections. Erythromycin and chloromycetin are less active in bile than in other media. Aminoglycosides at relatively high concentrations do not reduce bacterial numbers in bile. Aminoglycosides should not be used in animals with any evidence for primary or secondary renal insufficiency because of the drug's renal toxicity when reduced renal blood flow causes delayed clearance.

Untreated chronic hepatitis is a progressive disease that may develop irreversible pathology only after months. Bacterial cell products and toxins act synergistically with other insults to permit or hasten the progression of that pathology.[55] Reducing bacterial numbers and activity by antibiotics reduces the ability for bacteria to contribute to the process. That effect is similar to the goal desired in modifying the intestinal bacterial microflora by diets. Since some of the injury is from interactions, involving endotoxin or *E. coli,* that induce portal inflammation and fibrosis, the most important modification of the colonic bacterial population is reduction of coliform and other gram-negative bacterial numbers.

Bacterial infection is a common problem associated with chronic hepatitis (Table 33-2). A predisposition to bacteremia is well-documented for humans with chronic hepatic disease. Some of that may be due to a reduction of the phagocytic activity of Kupffer cells; circulating bacteria from any source are not removed. Reduced phagocytosis is due to reduced levels of complement and fibronectin or opsonification.[26] Animals with hepatitis should be considered at high risk for infection. Portal blood with bacteria from the intestines, bypassing the liver in portasystemic shunt vessels that develop during portal hypertension, also increases the predisposition to bacteremia. Humans with cirrhosis have increased incidence for bacteremia, urinary tract infections, and a variety of other infections. There is even greater risk for infection following endoscopic procedures and in patients with gastrointestinal problems, such as chronic colitis, where enteric bacteria are more numerous in portal blood. Bacteria can also enter the general circulation through the intestinal lymphatic circulation. Changes in the environment of the duodenum of dogs, such as by instillation of an alkaline solution, can cause enteric organisms to appear in the thoracic duct. Many other factors can change that environment. A fecal type of flora, characterized by coliforms, develops with many forms of acute enteritis, maldigestion, and malabsorption. With that there is increased risk for bacteremia, and when it is associated with hepatitis animals should be considered at high risk for infection.

Ascites and Fluid and Electrolyte Imbalances

Ascites is most often managed with salt restriction and diuretics when its cause, portal hypertension and hypoproteinemia, persists despite any other treatment. Ascites can also be managed by paracentesis and restoration of effective circulating blood volume. Management of a long-term problem is difficult, especially since a number of complications can be associated with any form of management.

Sodium restriction can be the initial approach to management of ascites. A liter of water and two pounds of body weight is lost with the loss of each 140 mEq of sodium. Commercial dog foods contain great excesses of sodium with contents of 0.5% (dry food), 0.7% (semimoist food), and 1.0% (canned food). The diet is gradually modified to reduce its sodium content to 0.1% to 0.3%. That can be accomplished by feeding one of a variety of canine and feline prescription diets or one that the clinician formulates for the owner to prepare (see Chapter 38).[57] An animal with reduced effective circulating blood volume may worsen with restriction of sodium intake exceeding its minimum requirements. That results in reduced renal function, leading to oliguria and enhanced retention of excess body fluid. If in such cases animals increase water intake in attempts to improve the circulating blood volume, a dilutional hyponatremia can develop. During any salt restriction the animal should be monitored for complications of uremia and hyponatremia.

Diuretic therapy employing the most physiological approach is based on the use of spironolactone.[68,69] Since an important factor promoting fluid retention and ascites is increased aldosterone secretion, it follows that a drug blocking aldosterone synthesis and its renal effects, like spironolactone, would be effective in promoting excretion of that fluid. Although spironolactone is relatively free of side-effects, the drug is not commonly used. Diuresis requires three to four days of therapy before an effect is evident. The drug may have to be given in amounts that make treatment costly. The drug promotes the retention of potassium, which could result in hyperkalemia. Spironolactone interferes with aldosterone action in renal tubules and, by reducing aldosterone synthesis, decreases levels of the hormone that are necessary for renal excretion of potassium. Animals with hepatic disease and ascites are usually potassium depleted, however, from vomiting, diarrhea, anorexia, and increased renal excretion of potassium from excess aldosterone. Total body potassium can be reduced by 10% to 30%, and administration of large potassium supplements combined with spironolactone in humans does not easily restore normal potassium content. Spironolactone (Aldactone) given at a dose of 1 to 2 mg/kg repeated every 12 hours is safe and effective; it is a superior diuretic to furosemide or hydrochlorothiazide for the treatment of ascites. Potassium supplements can be used with this potassium-sparing diuretic, but that should be monitored with plasma electrolyte determinations.

Other diuretics, in order of increasing potency, are the thiazides, ethacrynic acid and furosemide. They interfere with sodium reabsorption in the distal loop of Henle and the distal tubule; hence, they are referred to as loop diuretics. Once major effect of these drugs is marked excretion of potassium and chloride, which aggravates any preexisting potassium depletion and alkalosis. When these complications accompany uremia induced by diuretics, hyperammonemia and signs of hepatic encephalopathy worsen. Because of these complications, loop diuretics are not used alone or as the primary therapeutic agent for ascites. Their use is combined with that of spironolactone if a faster diuretic response is desired. Two other diuretics, triamterene and amiloride, have potassium-retaining properties although they do not inhibit aldosterone. Conserving potassium by an effect in the distal tubule, they are sometimes used in combination with the potassium-wasting diuretics for managing potassium-depleted patients. One newer diuretic, ibopamine, improves renal function. The agent is a dopamine agonist and improves renal blood flow and glomerular filtration rate. Another effect is to reduce plasma vasopressin levels, thereby increasing water excretion.

A goal of diuretic therapy with or without sodium restriction is to lose ascitic fluid at a rate that does not exceed 1.5% of body weight per day. When therapy is effective (in many cases it is not), care is exercised to identify the point where diuretics are no longer required. Ultrasound or abdominal radiographs may be necessary to identify that time.

Another means of stimulating diuresis and natriuresis is expansion of the plasma compartment to increase the effective plasma volume. Volume expansion promotes release of atrial natriuretic factor to stimulate sodium excretion. Plasma volume can be expanded with albumin, ascitic fluid, or dextran, but those agents should not be used if central venous pressure is abnormally high and contributing to the portal hypertension. Measurement of central venous pressure aids in determining the amount of fluid to give.

Ascites is commonly treated by removal of ascitic fluid by paracentesis. The removal of ascitic fluid usually results in its reformation, often within hours. The fluid removed usually contains plasma proteins, which are thus lost from the body. Therefore, the removal of ascitic fluid from hypoproteinemic patients further decreases plasma proteins as ascites fluid reforms. Plasma albumin synthesis is usually too slow to replace losses from repeated paracentesis. One advantage to removing ascitic fluid is that its removal from some patients results in increased cardiac output and plasma volume.[70] In addition, paracentesis improves renal function and promotes diuresis in an oliguric animal. These effects may result from reducing intra-abdominal pressure and relieving compression on the caudal vena cava, portal vein, and renal veins. Paracentesis limited to removal of small volumes of fluid two or three times a day has been recommended in the past. Recent studies report that paracentesis to remove large volumes of ascitic fluid in humans is without complication when performed slowly over 30 to 60 minutes. The large volumes removed represented approximately 5% of body weight and were more effective, faster, cheaper, and as safe as conventional diuretic therapy.[71,72] It may be that removal of large amounts of fluid is not associated with the undesirable effects as once thought. Large-volume removal is certainly indicated in some animals in great discomfort and in others as a preparation for further physical or radiographic examinations.

Paracentesis can be combined with plasma volume expansion, so that fluid removed from the abdominal cavity is infused intravenously. Central venous pressure is monitored to determine the rate of infusion. Vigorous treatment with diuretics can be combined with the infusion to maximize the benefits of albumin reinfusion. This procedure speeds the return to normal plasma protein levels. Another means for chronically reinfusing ascitic fluid into the vascular compartment involves permanent placement of a silastic tubing (containing a valve) between the peritoneal cavity and the central venous system.[73] When attempted in small animals, however, that has usually failed.

An effective means of reducing portal hypertension and effecting a reasonable cure for ascites is to create a portasystemic shunt.[74] That can be effective only if the cause of the hypertension is either prehepatic or hepatic, not if the cause is in the heart or vena cava. There are many examples of the naturally occurring model of portasystemic shunts in dogs to illustrate the problems that can occur. From those observations, a portasystemic shunt to treat ascites is a choice of treatment that is likely to create more problems than the original one.

Some animals have hydrothorax complicating ascites with hepatic disease. This has been managed with tetracycline-induced pleural symphysis.[75]

Alkalosis, often accompanying chronic hepatitis, is corrected by fluids (see Chapter 39). Potassium deficits may require oral supplementation or balanced electrolyte solutions fortified with additional potassium. Correction of a total-body potassium deficit may take weeks. Magnesium is usually depleted along with potassium during hepatic disease. Occasionally the potassium deficit cannot be repaired unless magnesium is given first. Magnesium is not a constituent of Ringer's solution.

Renal Insufficiency

Successful management of complicating renal failure is determined by how early it is recognized. Early recognition of oliguria is followed by measures to improve renal circulation and to initiate diuresis. Therapy is directed at improving effective circulating plasma volume. Fluids, fortified with potassium as necessary, are administered to replace deficits and restore renal circulation. Fluid replacement is monitored by measuring central venous pressure. Replacement of fluid to correct the renal insufficiency can increase amounts of ascitic fluid. Albumin or dextran can be used to expand plasma volume and improve renal circulation to initiate diuresis. Diuretics such as furosemide are not used, because they can worsen the conditions responsible for renal insufficiency. Drugs to improve renal circulation, such as dopamine may be of benefit. Since hepatic circulation is also reduced along with the effective circulating plasma volume, treatment of the problems contributing to renal insufficiency also improves splanchnic circulation. Unfortunately, treatment to restore normal renal function is often unsuccessful in patients with chronic hepatitis. The prognosis is poor when oliguria, uremia, and ascites develop. The ensuing uremia increases the amount of substrate, allowing bacterial ureases to produce ammonia, causing signs of hepatic encephalopathy to worsen.

Coagulopathies

The treatment of coagulopathy with chronic active hepatitis is based on the premise that DIC and deficiencies of clotting-factor and antithrombin III coexist. Fibrinolysis is a likely problem, and treatment for DIC and clotting-factor deficiencies can improve fibrinolysis. Heparin given to treat DIC results in decreased plasmin activity and blocks the clotting mechanism. Heparin effectively complexes with and activates antithrombin III, which inactivates serine proteases, especially activated Factor X and thrombin. The liver produces antithrombin III, which can be deficient because of hepatic disease; in that case heparin will be without any effect. The deficiencies of both clotting factors and antithrombin III are replaced by transfusions of fresh blood or plasma, to which heparin is added. (100 units of heparin/kg body weight is added to and given with the blood). That can be followed by subcutaneous injections of 100 units/kg, and that dose should be gradually tapered before discontinuing (to prevent excessive thrombosis). Since using heparin without replacing clotting factors can cause uncontrolled hemorrhage, heparin should not be given alone. Whole blood also provides antiplasmin activity, which inhibits fibrinolysis. Results from experimental dogs indicate that resistance to heparin therapy develops after four to five days, and the prognosis is poor when a coagulopathy does not respond within 24 to 48 hours.

There can be little hope for successful treatment of an animal with hepatic disease that is hemorrhaging into the intestine. Gastrointestinal hemorrhage is difficult enough to manage in patients without associated hepatic disease.

PROGNOSIS[16]

A relatively high percentage (37%) of dogs with chronic hepatitis die within one week despite any management. Few clinical or laboratory findings are reliable in predicting which dogs will not survive beyond one week. The only biochemical changes that correlate with early death are low blood glucose, abnormal ammonia tolerance, and increased times for prothrombin and partial thromboplastin. The best predictors are low blood glucose and prolonged prothrombin time. Biopsy changes correlating with early death are limited to severity of necrosis and severity of fibrosis. In dogs living more than one week the length of survival correlates with only one biochemical test, abnormally low plasma albumin, and with only one biopsy finding, the degree of severity of bridging fibrosis. The prognosis can be good for dogs surviving more than one week, with that being determined by early recognition and appropriate management. Prolongation of life by two to three years or longer can be viewed as a success even though some animals are not cured. There is insufficient information on hepatitis in cats to aid in predicting the outcome with or without management.

CHRONIC COPPER TOXICITY

Chronic hepatitis can be associated with abnormal accumulation of copper in the liver. That accumulation can begin early in life and precede any pathological changes, in which case the excess copper produces a toxicosis that causes the subsequent pathological changes. Copper accumulation can also be caused by liver disease where cholestasis is a problem and copper excretion in bile is impaired. The copper toxicosis that precedes hepatic pathology has been identified and described in Bedlington Terriers.[76-79] The abnormality is inherited, with the inheritance following an autosomal recessive pattern. An inherited defect in copper metabolism has not been proven for any other breed of dog.

Pathogenesis[80-82]

Dietary copper is absorbed from the stomach and small intestine. Most commercial dog foods contain a great excess of copper, so deficiencies are not seen. Other constituents of the diet influence the absorption of copper.[83] Absorption of copper is reduced by zinc, ascorbic acid, bile, and fiber. Its absorption is enhanced by amino acids and high dietary protein. Zinc stimulates synthesis of intestinal metallothionein, a protein that binds both copper and zinc in epithelial cells. That may regulate absorption of these two elements if the binding is strong enough to reduce the amount of copper and zinc that can be released to the circulation. The zinc-induced synthesis of the binding protein results in less copper being absorbed. The portal circulation transports copper, loosely bound to albumin, to the liver. Not being tightly bound to its carrier, copper can be readily removed by the liver. Plasma albumin in the dog does not bind copper, which could be the reason for the liver's more efficient uptake of copper and may be partly responsible for dogs having higher hepatic copper concentrations than other mammals. Following hepatic uptake, copper can be excreted into the biliary system, released into the circulation, or stored in the liver. Copper is excreted into bile tightly bound to a ceruloplasmin-like metallothionein. The avid binding of the copper prevents its absorption when it reenters the intestinal tract. Normal biliary excretion of copper requires synthesis of the binding protein by the liver and normal biliary structure and function. Zinc and glucocorticosteroids, as well as copper, induce synthesis of copper-binding proteins. Thus such steroids may have a beneficial effect on hepatic handling of copper in conditions of excess hepatic copper. The synthesis of metallothionein in such a case would provide a means for detoxification by binding of the protein to metals that are potentially cytotoxic. Copper is released to the circulation tightly bound to ceruloplasmin, a protein made by the liver. That represents 90% or more of total plasma copper and is the form used for synthesis of enzymes and other copper-containing proteins.

Ceruloplasmin levels are increased by zinc, copper, and glucocorticosteroids. Ceruloplasmin levels do not change with copper toxicosis of Bedlington Terriers. Excess hepatic copper can be stored in lysosomes. Lysosomal copper binds to a metallothionein protein that may be resistant to degradation by lysosomal enzymes. Accumulation in lysosomes is also dependent on excessive entry and reduced efflux of copper from hepatocytes. The kidneys also excrete copper when it is free and not bound to ceruloplasm. Tissue damage or wasting releases copper from degradation of copper proteins, and the free copper can be excreted renally.

A combination of factors could contribute to copper's accumulation in the liver. The amount in the diet could be in excess; that is the case for commercial dog foods. A mechanism controlling intestinal absorption may not be operating normally. Zinc deficiency resulting in reduced intestinal metallothionein levels would allow greater absorption of copper. The liver could accumulate copper at a normal rate but have defective means for delivery from the cell. That may result from increased binding to intracellular metallothioneins, which may not be degraded in a normal fashion with such complexes accumulating in lysosomes. The liver may not excrete copper at a normal rate because ceruloplasmin is not synthesized for its transfer to the circulation or for its secretion into bile. Reduced biliary excretion of copper is described in Bedlington Terriers. That reduction could result from inadequate synthesis of the metallothionein required for that excretion or from a defect in the process transporting the copper complex into bile. Animals with cirrhosis have lost their ability for normal protein synthesis. A reduction in ceruloplasmin synthesis may be responsible for copper accumulation in those patients. Animals with cholestasis may have severe enough obstruction of bile canaliculi or damage to biliary transporting structures for copper to accumulate. In one situation the accumulation is primary; in the latter it is secondary. The canine liver is well-adapted for storing copper in that the amount it contains is ten times greater than it is in other species.[84] The hepatic content for copper is greater in neonates than in adults. In dogs the high levels early in life do not change with age, so that normal levels can approach 600 μg/g dry weight. Reported hepatic copper concentrations in dogs have increased in increments to values that are 30 times greater than those reported 50 years earlier. That may reflect changes in feeding practices.

The normal liver has the highest copper content of any organ. Yet copper does not injure the liver until these normally high levels increase seven fold or greater, and even then pathology may not be apparent. Copper induced hepatocyte injury involves changes in plasma membranes, cytosolic proteins rich in sulfhydryl groups, glutathionine, lysosomal membranes, and various other organelles. Lysosomal membrane injury is suggested by increased lysosomal enzyme activity in the cytosol of affected Bedlington Terriers. Eventually the pathology can progress to a hepatitis.

Incidence[76-79]

At one time up to two-thirds of Bedlington Terriers were believed to be affected with copper toxicosis. More recently, hepatic copper determinations on asymptomatic Bedlington Terriers in the United Kingdom showed evidence of abnormality in one-third. There is no sex predisposition for copper toxicosis in the Bedlington Terrier. It is evident that this breed is at high risk for developing a primary copper toxicosis, where abnormal accumulation of copper in the liver results in damage that can progress to chronic hepatitis. Other breeds of dogs reported to be at risk for hepatic disease and copper accumulation include Doberman Pinschers and West Highland White Terriers.[13,14,85] Comprehensive studies to identify the role of copper in the pathogenesis of hepatic disease have not been done in these breeds or in any breed other than Bedlington Terriers, however. The copper accumulations are not a consistent feature of hepatic disease in the other breeds, and copper is seldom increased before pathology develops. The hepatic copper accumulation in the non-Bedlington Terrier breeds may be secondary to various forms of cholestasis. One difficulty in assigning an incidence to primary or secondary copper toxicosis develops because of different ranges for normal hepatic copper concentration.

Clinical Features[76,77,79]

Copper toxicosis in Bedlington Terriers is usually accompanied by few or no clinical signs until the pathology is so severe that management is often unsuccessful. In one study only 28% of affected dogs showed any clinical signs. In another group of asymptomatic dogs 34% had abnormally high levels of copper in the liver. In other reports, when dogs presented clinical signs the liver pathology was usually severe. Acute episodes characterized by anorexia, vomiting, depression and weakness may be more likely in younger animals (less than six years old), and they usually recover with only supportive therapy despite an ongoing hepatitis. Older dogs have signs of chronic hepatitis, including anorexia, weight loss, intermittent vomiting, diarrhea and debilitation, which precede the appearance of jaundice, ascites, and hepatic encephalopathy. Some dogs develop hemolytic anemia and jaundice acutely. Copper toxicosis in Bedlington Terriers does not cause copper deposition in the cornea that produces the Kayser-Fleischer rings seen in Wilson's disease in humans.

Bedlington Terriers with clinical signs invariably have increased plasma alanine aminotransferase (ALT) activity, but in only 45% of the asymptomatic affected dogs was that activity increased. Values for ALT activity correlate with histologic findings. Affected dogs showing only pigment granules have normal ALT activity. With focal hepatitis 50% have increased ALT activity; with chronic hepatitis the incidence increases to 89%. Other clinical pathology findings remain normal until disease becomes advanced; then alkaline phosphatase activity, plasma bilirubin, plasma albumin, and blood clotting become abnormal.

Plasma copper levels of 40 to 70 μg/dl are found in affected or unaffected Bedlington Terriers, which is the same as in normal mixed breed dogs. The plasma levels of ceruloplasmin also do not change with copper toxicosis.

Pathology and Diagnosis[76-79,86,87]

The diagnosis of copper toxicosis of Bedlington Terriers is based on hepatic copper quantitation and biopsy findings.

Normal dogs usually have hepatic copper concentrations of 200 to 400 µg/g dry tissue; some normal dogs have higher values. Normal dogs have copper concentrations that are higher at six months than later in life. A criterion for diagnosis is hepatic copper concentration greater than 850 µg/g dry tissue. For confidence in any assessment of whether or not a Bedlington Terrier is affected, copper should be quantitated on a liver biopsy sample.

Biopsies of the liver are evaluated for histologic changes and for lysosomal granules characteristic of copper accumulation (Figure 33-10). Few if any degenerative or inflammatory changes are seen in most dogs younger than six years of age. The earliest change is the appearance of prominent dark granules resembling lipofuscin diffusely distributed in the cytoplasm of hepatocytes. These changes appear first in zone 3 (perivenular); with increasing accumulation of copper cells, zones 2 and 1 (periportal) contain the granules. Other than the granules, the hepatocytes appear normal. With increasing copper accumulation and time, the granules are more numerous and focal hepatic necrosis appears. With progressive worsening the lesion becomes characteristic of chronic active hepatitis, and that can progress to either or both micro- and macronodular cirrhosis. Identification of the earliest histologic granular changes on hematoxylin and eosin stained biopsies, combined with hepatic copper levels greater than 850 µg/g dry tissue, is diagnostic for copper toxicosis in Bedlington Terriers.

Estimation of hepatic copper content can be made on biopsies prepared with several special stains. Such staining is necessary to differentiate copper granules from those formed from excess iron, lipofuscin or bile pigments. Staining with rhodanine is believed to be more sensitive and specific for evaluating liver biopsies for copper. Rhodanine reacts with copper to form a red precipitate but does not react with iron or zinc. Copper at levels as low as 60 µg/g dry weight is stained with rhodanine. Hepatic copper can also be stained with rubeanic acid, but there is no correlation between staining intensity and hepatic copper concentrations. Orcein-stained preparations are unreliable in identifying excess copper in the liver. Staining for copper is regarded as a screening procedure that is reliable in distinguishing between normal and frankly abnormal copper levels. It does not substitute for spectroscopic quantitation of hepatic copper. Estimation of copper levels on rhodanine-

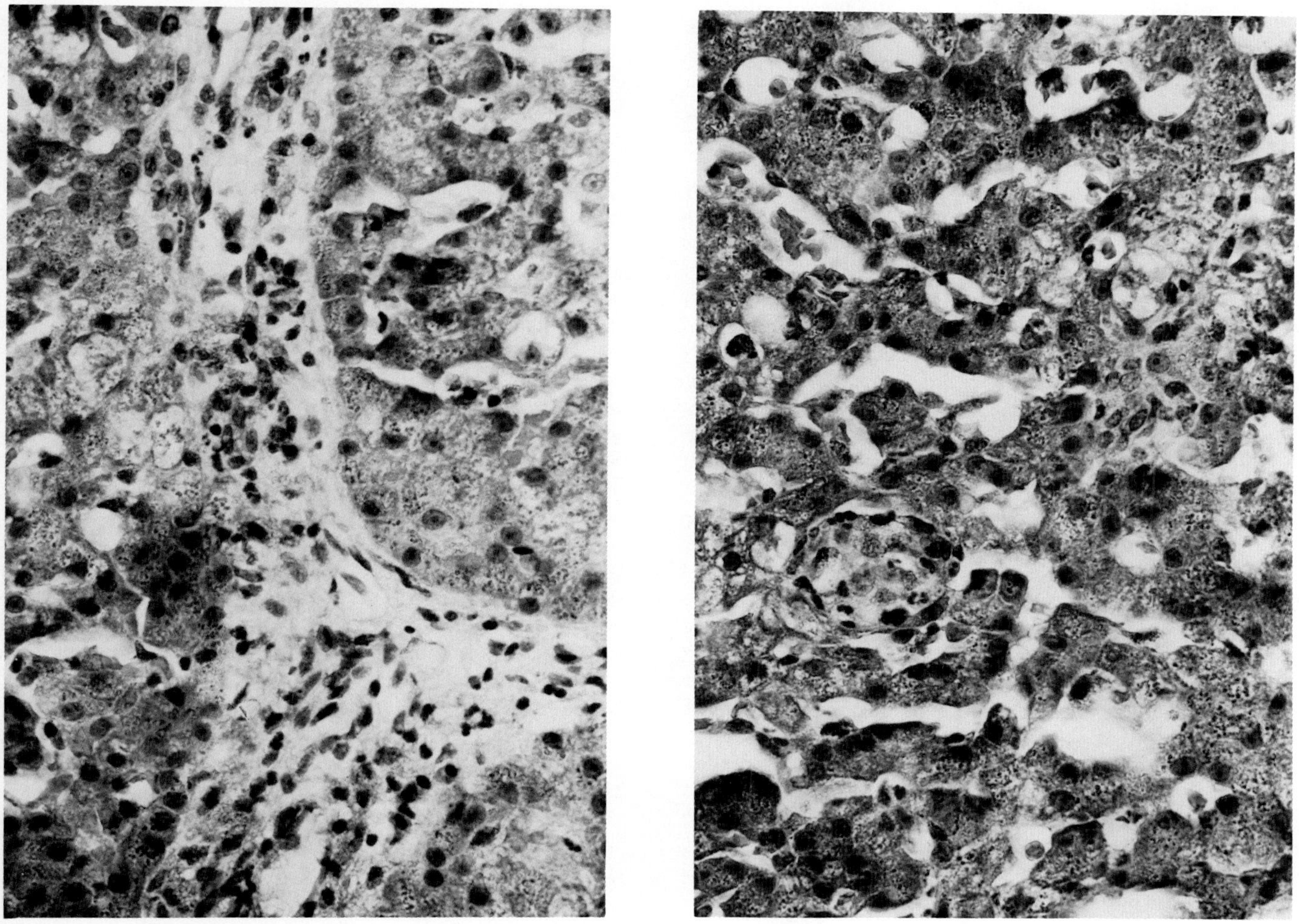

Figure 33-10. Copper toxicity and storage disease. Hepatic biopsy from Bedlington Terrier with no clinical evidence of disease, ALT activity was increased to 10 times normal. Copper content of the liver was 1723 micrograms per gram wet weight (Normal = 40). Plasma copper (91 µg/dl) and ceruloplasmin (27 mg/dl) concentrations were normal. Histology shows infiltration of portal areas with inflammatory cells, focal necrosis with macrophages and hepatocyte changes that include granules and lipidosis. Granules are most likely lipofuscin (PAS positive int his case) which with fat vacuoles are common finding in humans with Wilsons disease.

stained preparations must be done only by a pathologist experienced in evaluating such preparations. Some copper is invariably found in liver biopsies; any estimation on content from a stained preparation is very subjective.

Subjective grading of rhodanine-stained liver tissue provides a range of copper concentrations that have been arbitrarily assigned to one of five groups. Grades 1 and 2 represent unaffected dogs with hepatic copper levels of less than 850 µg/g dry tissue. Grades 3, 4, and 5 represent increasing staining intensity found in affected dogs whose hepatic copper levels range from 850 to over 10,000 µg/g dry tissue.

Hepatic concentrations of iron increase with copper toxicosis of Bedlington Terriers. Quantitation by atomic absorption spectrophotometry shows a fourfold increase in iron. Copper toxicosis infrequently causes hemolytic anemia but that may be subclinical in many cases, and with increased fragility and decreased life-span for erythrocytes there may be more iron released and stored in the liver.

Diagnosis of copper toxicosis in Bedlington Terriers is confirmed by finding hepatic copper levels greater than 850 µg/g dry tissue and histology compatible with the disease. Finding high hepatic copper levels in biopsies from other breeds with hepatic disease can be expected if cholestasis or cirrhosis are part of the pathology. There is no evidence that these problems are the same as the Bedlington Terrier problem.

Management[77,88]

Management is directed at reducing copper stores in the body. That can be approached by using drugs to chelate copper and reduce its intestinal absorption, but also to mobilize copper sequestered in the body so that it can be excreted. Copper binds to chemicals with sulfhydryl groups. Once such chemical, D-penicillamine, a dimethyl derivative of cysteine found in the urine during penicillin therapy, is indicated for reducing abnormal copper accumulations in Bedlington Terriers. The drug increases the urinary excretion of copper. D-penicillamine is given at a dose of 125 mg twice a day or 250 mg once a day 30 minutes before a meal. Vomiting is the only side effect reported; after discontinuation for a few days a resumption of treatment using lower doses slowly increased to the therapeutic dose may avoid further complications. Dogs treated for as long as three years do not develop some of the side effects reported with long-term therapy in humans. Some dogs are reported to have sufficient persistent gastrointestinal side effects to preclude any extended use of the drug. D-penicillamine must be given for an animal's lifetime; copper levels may be reduced, and no cures are realized. There is some question whether D-penicillamine therapy is effective in Bedlington Terriers.[79] Only a few reports, describing only one or two dogs in each, document the results of such therapy. In some animals, reductions in hepatic copper content are modest and achieved only after months of therapy. In others, no reductions in copper content are reported.

Cuprid (2,2,2 tetramine tetrahydrochloride) is another anticopper agent used in humans. Cuprid is four to nine fold less effective than a similar compound 2,3,2 tetramine tetrahydrochloride in dogs.[89] The more effective compound decoppers the liver more rapidly than penicillamine and is not associated with any side effects. Six months of therapy reduce copper levels by one-half. At the present time, however, it is not available commercially. The more effective compound appears to be beneficial in episodes of acute hepatic necrosis in affected Bedlington Terriers where damaged hepatocytes release large amounts of copper and cause acute hemolytic crises. In contrast, D-penicillamine is generally ineffective during such acute episodes.

Zinc given orally is currently being evaluated for its decoppering effects in humans with Wilson's disease.[90] No studies have been done to demonstrate an effectiveness in affected Bedlington Terriers. Zinc reduces the intestinal absorption of copper by stimulating synthesis of copper binding metallothinein, which prevents copper from leaving mucosal cells and entering the circulation. As described earlier, zinc also stimulates the synthesis of similar binding proteins in the liver that detoxify copper and enable it to be transported to and through the circulation. All these effects assist in protecting the animal against copper accumulation and toxicity. Zinc given orally as its sulfate causes gastric irritation and vomiting in humans. That could be a problem in small animals, in which case zinc acetate or zinc gluconate could be given. Such forms are as readily available as any vitamin, mineral, or trace element supplement. Zinc gluconate is given at a daily dose of 3 mg/kg, which is divided into three doses and given 30 minutes before feeding. Currently, zinc supplementation is recommended for management of dogs with chronic hepatitis.[16] Such dogs are often zinc deficient and have accumulations of abnormal amounts of copper. Treatment with zinc may therefore be beneficial, although it is often questionable whether enough copper has accumulated to contribute to the hepatic pathology. Excessive zinc administration can cause a chronic copper deficiency that is manifested in animals by hypochromic-microcytic anemia and neutropenia.

Reduction of copper intake by feeding a low copper diet is mentioned but not emphasized as an important means to manage dogs with abnormal copper accumulation. The difference in daily copper intake may be one reason the canine liver contains ten times more copper than the human liver. Whereas humans consume 1 to 2 mg of copper daily in the average diet, dogs consume 5 to 10 mg copper/kg of commercial dog foods. They all contain that level to meet recommendations of the National Research Council. Studies show 50% of dietary copper to be absorbed, and most of that is deposited in the liver. In humans, 1.5 mg of copper is excreted in bile each day. Thus, most is excreted by the liver. In dogs the small fraction excreted in the urine amounts to about 0.2 mg/day in Bedlington Terriers with copper accumulation. That excretion can be increased to 2.0 - 5.5 mg/day by 2,3,2 tetramine tetrahydrochloride. If a dog consumes food containing 5 mg copper/day and absorbs 50%, excretion must approximate 2.5 mg/day for copper balance to be maintained. Reducing copper intake should be as important in management as any drug therapy. Continuing to feed a copper-fortified commercial dog food may be a reason for reported failures of penicillamine therapy. Feeding a low copper diet and therapy by zinc supplementation may be more effective in reducing hepatic copper content than any other drug therapy. The copper content of different foods is shown in Table 33-7.

Additional therapy can be vitamin E supplementation since that vitamin is protective against lipid peroxidation, which copper induces in hepatocytes. Ascorbic acid can also be given because it reduces the absorption of copper and promotes its renal excretion. The management of the chronic hepatitis associated with the Bedlington Terrier problem may require treatment with an anti-inflammatory agent such as prednisone.

Table 33-7 Food Copper Content

	mg copper/100g food
Beef liver	12.0
Shellfish	.17-7.5
Whole wheat cracker	.87
Beef heart	.73
Lamb	.71
Chicken liver	.54
Pork	.30
Spinach	.25
Beef steak	.18
Fish	.10-.18
Potatoes	.05-.18
Vegetables	.05-.15
Squash	.14
Chicken	.05-.13
Eggs	.08
Cottage cheese	0-.01
Cheeses	0
Rice, white	0
All cereals	0
Tofu	0

Prevention[78,79,91]

Copper-associated hepatitis of Bedlington Terriers is prevented by breeding only dogs that do not carry the gene causing the disease. Many dogs are unaffected heterozygous individuals, carrying one normal and one abnormal controller gene for regulating copper metabolism. The homozygous dogs carrying two abnormal genes are affected. A mating between two unaffected heterozygotes results in 50% heterozygous carriers and 25% homozygous affected dogs. There is little difficulty in identifying the homozygous affected dogs, but there is great difficulty in identifying the heterozygous or carrier dogs. Recommendations have been made to quantitate hepatic copper at five to seven months of age and compare levels at that time with levels found on repeat biopsies at 14 to 15 months of age. Normal dogs have values less than 375 µg/g; heterozygotes have high levels early and normal values on repeat biopsies; and affected dogs have high values on early biopsies and even higher values on later biopsies.

SUPPURATIVE HEPATITIS

Hepatic abscesses are found infrequently in small animals, with only one to three cases reported annually on necropsy in both dogs and cats in the VMTH at Davis. Half of those are in neonates or in animals a few months old. The incidence is likely greater than reported, however, since far fewer neonates than adults are necropsied. Most hepatic abscesses are associated with infections involving other organs and systems.

Etiology and Pathogenesis[26,69]

Suppurative hepatitis is caused by bacterial colonization of the liver. Hepatic abscesses are usually the consequence of the escape from the gastrointestinal tract of large numbers of bacteria. Bacterial contamination of the peritoneal cavity follows gastrointestinal perforations, where bacteria invade the liver by direct extension from the peritoneal contamination and by the portal circulation removing them from the abdomen. The hepatic mononuclear phagocytic (reticuloendothelial) system removes the small numbers of bacteria that normally leave the intestine and enter the portal circulation. The reticuloendothelial system is unable to remove microorganisms in the portal circulation if its normal function is inhibited by the shock of trauma, infection, or surgery. Then intestinal microorganisms escape phagocytosis, allowing hepatic abscessation and septicemia to follow. Suppurative hepatitis results from bacterial contamination of the abdomen during celiotomy or gastrointestinal surgery. Acute pancreatitis can cause abscesses in the pancreas, whereupon liver abscessation can develop by direct extension. In the neonate, suppurative hepatitis develops from bacterial invasion through the umbilical vein at birth. The most common cause for suppurative hepatitis in animals is bacterial invasion of the liver through the umbilical or portal veins.

Abscesses can develop also following hepatic invasion by bacteria brought in by the hepatic artery, which is the means of invasion with primary septicemia or bacteremia. These hepatic abscesses can be associated with bacterial endocarditis.

The biliary system is an avenue whereby bacteria can gain entrance to the liver to cause abscess formation. This is common in species of animals with a high incidence of extrahepatic biliary obstruction where cholangitis is a primary or secondary feature. However, cholangitis is seen infrequently in small animals, and when suppurative hepatitis is found it is seldom associated with cholangitis. Thus, the bile duct does not appear to be an important avenue for bacterial invasion to cause hepatic abscesses. Abscessation of the liver and biliary tract infection can be produced experimentally by intravenous inoculation with the anaerobe *Bacteroides fragilis*, although only when a biliary obstruction has been created.[92] Injection of *E. coli* causes no changes, but when it is combined with *B. fragilis* in smaller doses there is a fivefold increase in the incidence of hepatic abscesses, which contain only *B. fragilis*. It is not known whether a similar pathogenic process contributes to hepatic abscesses in clinical cases.

Suppurative hepatitis develops following regional destruction of hepatocytes by problems such as trauma or neoplastic disease. The devitalized tissue is unable to remove microorganisms the liver normally destroys, and the result is abscess formation. Preventing this complication is partially the basis for using antibiotics following abdominal trauma. The response of some animals with hepatic malignancy to the nonspecific use of antibiotics is explained by the drug's effect against a secondary suppurative hepatitis.

Since bacteriological studies are seldom conducted, the organisms causing hepatic abscesses are seldom identified. Blood cultures performed on animals with septicemia often reveal the organisms that are also causing a suppurative hepatitis. The anaerobic members of the intestinal microflora are the most likely to cause hepatic abscessation.[93] Culture techniques used in the past were not able to isolate and identify the intestinal anaerobes causing hepatic abscesses.[94] Thus, some results have indicated that the abscesses were sterile or contained contaminating organisms that were not the primary cause. Experimental studies on animals show that the abscesses formed following contamination of the peritoneal cavity with intestinal bacteria result from anaerobes, but that the high rate of mortality is caused by the aerobes.[95] Thus, when the organisms causing abscesses are known to have originated from the gastrointestinal tract, the primary treatment for abscesses is directed against intestinal anaerobic bacteria.[25]

Clinical and Laboratory Findings, Diagnosis

Hepatic abscesses cause persistent fever that is frequently unresponsive to antibiotics. Nonspecific signs of depression and anorexia are seen consistently. Hepatomegaly is a usual finding, and peritonitis, pain, and abdominal fluid may be present. Manifestations of systemic infection include lymphadenopathy, orchitis, subcutaneous abscessation, and respiratory involvement with signs of cough and dyspnea. Clinical pathological evaluation reveals changes in the hemogram as expected with chronic infection. Leukocytosis prevails with acute inflammatory changes, and monocytosis appears when the process becomes chronic. Hypergammaglobulinemia can be found in the chronic stage. Blood chemistries reveal increased levels of ALT activity, with the increments reflecting the degree of hepatocyte degeneration. Clinical and routine laboratory findings are not suggestive of hepatic disease; instead, they are changes anticipated with septicemia, making it easy to overlook the possibility of hepatic disease. Examination of peritoneal exudates in the few cases where they can be collected identifies a peritonitis from which hepatic abscessation can be suspected.

Bacterial endocarditis is frequently the diagnosis. Sometimes abscesses are suspected, though they are assumed to be at some unknown site other than the liver. When infectious peritonitis is identified, it is safe to assume that suppurative hepatitis is also a problem. When an infection cannot be found in the abdominal cavity, the diagnosis of hepatic abscessation is difficult. A definitive diagnosis cannot be made on evaluation of standard laboratory and radiographic findings. Biopsy of the liver may be helpful (Figure 33-11), although a blind percutaneous biopsy may miss the lesion. Examination of the liver by laparoscopy or celiotomy is helpful in identifying lesions that are at or near the surface of the liver. Abscesses that are few in number and deep within the interior of the liver, however, are not grossly apparent. They are best identified by ultrasonic examination or by hepatic scans with a gamma counter following injection of a gamma-emitting radioactive isotope preferentially taken up by the liver. Ultrasound examination shows abscesses of density different from the surrounding liver. Abscesses produce filling defects where areas void of normal hepatocytes do not take up and concentrate the radioactive isotope during hepatic scans. Unfortunately, most hepatic abscesses are not suspected, or when they are considered, many are difficult to identify.

Treatment of Suppurative Hepatitis[96]

Suppurative hepatitis is seldom treated successfully. Consequently, a knowledge of the predisposing factors is important so that proper measures are instituted to prevent abscess formation. Thus, the abdomen contaminated with intestinal bacteria is treated vigorously not only to prevent a fatality but to prevent the chronic peritonitis and abscessation that invariably follow.

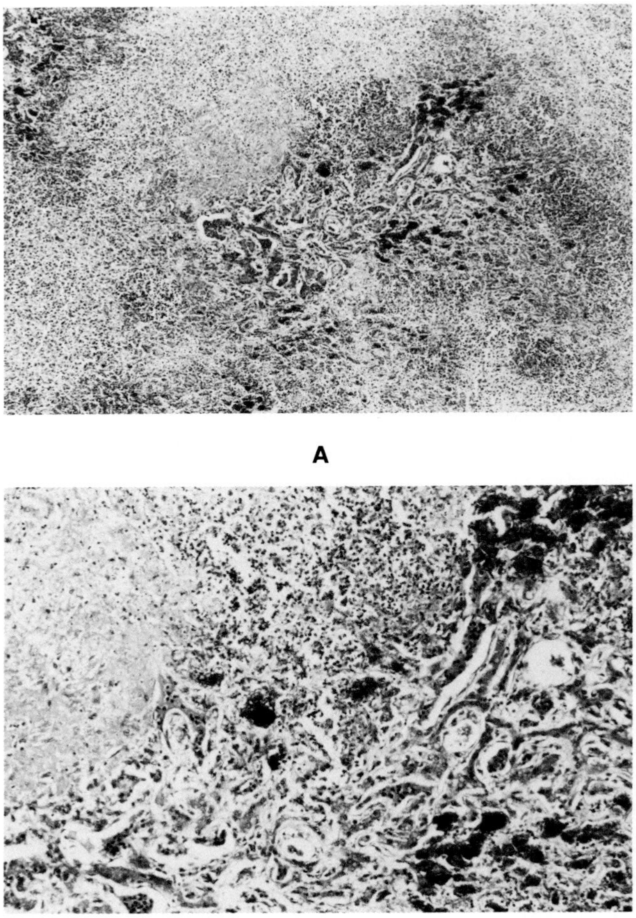

A

B

Figure 33-11. (a) Suppurative Hepatitis. Widespread pericentral necrosis and infiltration of inflammatory cells. Necrosis bridges between lobules. Hepatocytes in a portal area can still be recognized. (b) Higher magnification of (a).

The contaminated peritoneal cavity is thoroughly lavaged to remove microorganisms and foreign debris. The antibiotics used include those directed against both aerobic and anaerobic bacteria. The aerobes are consistently sensitive to gentamicin, and a high percentage are sensitive to kanamycin. The anaerobes are usually sensitive to one of the penicillin's unless *Bacteroides fragilis* is found and could contribute to potential infection. This organism is sensitive to clindamycin, a drug that is recommended only when *Bacteroides fragilis* is identified as a pathogen. It is also sensitive to metronidazole. Chloromycetin is a second, less effective choice against anaerobes.

Treatment of the abscess employs the same antibiotics used for the contaminated abdomen. Treatment is not likely to be successful unless the abscesses can be drained. That is possible only with celiotomy, and care must be taken that surgical drainage does not contaminate the peritoneal cavity and cause additional abscesses. Multiple abscesses cannot be treated by drainage. The prognosis for all types of hepatic abscessation is poor.

GRANULOMATOUS HEPATITIS

Granulomatous hepatitis is usually a biopsy or postmortem finding that is part of a systemic disease process. The usual clinical signs of the overall process are persistent fever, depression, weight loss, anorexia, and leukocytosis. These are nonspecific signs that will not necessarily draw attention to the liver in a workup of the problem. Additional signs reflecting the generalized nature of the disease are lymphadenopathy, lameness, and ulcerative dermatitis and gingivitis. When the clinical signs do not respond to treatment with antibiotics and the patient is euthanatized or dies, the granulomas are recognized on postmortem. Many animals may have an extensive granulomatous hepatitis that is never identified but responds when treated nonspecifically with antibiotics. A number of small animals develop granulomas from parasitic larvae migrating through the liver, though these do not normally cause clinical signs.

The cause of granulomatous hepatitis is unknown in most cases. The potential etiological agents are listed in Table 33-8. The inciting agent initiates a sequence of events that results in a granuloma characterized by giant-cell formation.[97] Microorganisms, sensitizing agents (both endogenous and exogenous), and immune complexes can all cause lymphocytes to become sensitized, after which they cause monocytes and macrophages to be transformed into epithelioid cells. These subsequently develop into multinucleated giant-cells. The histologic appearance of granulomas reveals the presence of lymphocytes and plasma cells surrounding nests of monocytes and macrophages or histiocytes, with giant-cells scattered throughout. The granuloma develops as an immunologic response or as an inflammatory response to a foreign substance. Hence, a wide range of different substances can stimulate granuloma formation. The liver, a primary site, has an active monocytic phagocytic (reticuloendothelial) system that removes all foreign substances from the portal circulation. When that involves an infectious agent or antigen that it cannot destroy, granuloma formation is a possible outcome. The spleen is frequently similarly involved.

Granuloma formation is seen with neoplasms, which may represent the best example of an endogenous antigen as stimulus. Thus, in a sense, some granuloma formation is an autoimmune phenomenon. Granuloma formation accompanying fe-

Table 33-8

Causes of Hepatic Granulomas: Infectious

- Bacterial infections
  - Mycobacterial diseases
  - Brucellosis
  - Nocardiosis
  - Actinomycosis
  - Tularemia
  - Yersiniosis
- Fungal infections
  - Histoplasmosis
  - Cryptococcosis
  - Coccidiodomycosis
  - Candidiasis
  - Aspergillosis
  - Blastomycosis
- Parasitic infections
  - Helminthic diseases
  - Visceral larva migrans
  - Fascioliasis
  - Capillariosis
  - Strongyloidiasis
  - Ascariasis
  - Ancylostomiasis
- Protozoal diseases
  - Amebiasis
  - Toxoplasmosis
  - Viral infections

Causes of Hepatic Granulomas: Noninfectious

- Sarcoidosis
- Primary liver disease
  - Primary biliary cirrhosis
  - Postnecrotic cirrhosis
  - Nutritional cirrhosis
  - Biliary obstruction
  - Acute and chronic pericholangitis
  - Fatty infiltraton
  - Toxic or drug-induced hepatitis
  - Chronic hepatitis
- Collagen vascular diseases
- Immune deficiency diseases
- Malignancies
  - Lymphomas
  - Others
- Other diseases
  - IBD
  - Ulcerative colitis
  - Gluten enteropathy
  - Foreign bodies
- Idiopathic granulomas
- Hypersensitivity reactions: drugs
  - Allopurinol
  - Aspirin
  - Carbamazepine
  - Diazepam
  - Feprazone
  - Halothane
  - Hydralazine
  - Isoniazid
  - Metahydrine
  - Methyldopa
  - Metolazone
  - Nitrofurantoin
  - Oxyphenbutazone
  - Penicillin
  - Phenylbutazone
  - Procarbazine
  - Quinidine
  - Seatone
  - Sulphonamides
  - Sulphonylurea derivatives

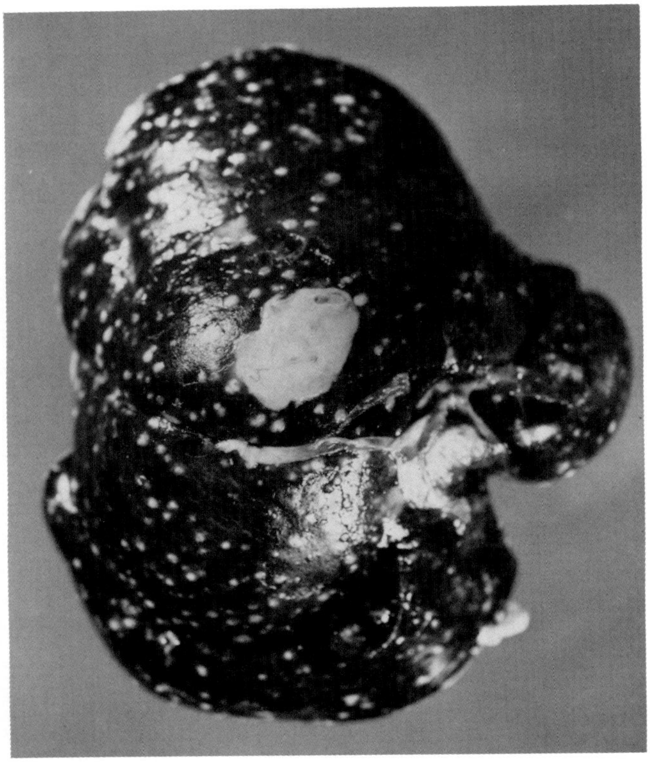

Figure 33-12. Granulomatous hepatitis. Multifocal granulomas are grossly evident in liver from a dog.

line infectious peritonitis virus infection causes many of the clinical signs. This response by the immune system damages tissues more than does the presence of the virus. Cats with only a viremia may show few clinical signs until morphological changes are induced by the response of the immune system to the virus. A high incidence of granulomas was found in a colony of normal Beagle dogs, where it was suggested to be due to migrating parasitic larvae.[98] Coccidioidomycosis and histoplasmosis cause granulomatous hepatitis in dogs living in endemic areas. The cause of granulomas is not identified in most other cases where it is recognized. That may represent granuloma formation stimulated by drugs or manifested by a noninfectious disease elsewhere in the body.

Granulomatous hepatitis is identified through biopsies of the liver. There is no other means of making a diagnosis. Biochemical evaluation of liver disease gives variable results that can be made confusing by persistent fever and treatment with antibiotics or steroids (Figure 33-12). Granulomas do not form a diffuse process throughout the liver. They can be scattered to such an extent that blind percutaneous biopsy of the liver does not retrieve a diagnostic piece of tissue a significant number of times. The biopsy sampling error can be reduced by obtaining more than one biopsy and by examining more than one section at different levels within the same biopsy sample. Biopsy samples can be further evaluated by culturing and special staining for microorganisms.

Treatment of granulomatous hepatitis involves specific measures when a specific treatable etiologic agent is identified. In some cases, improvement may be seen with antibiotics. Nonspecific therapy involves the use of corticosteroids. These agents interfere with the suggested immune response, which begins with the sensitization of lymphocytes and plasma cells. They also interfere with the immune-complex formation, which can be an etiologic agent. Corticosteroids have been shown to be of value in treating the problem in humans.[97] That has not been documented in dogs. A number of animals, however, have a systemic problem that includes granulomatous hepatitis, which does not respond to antibiotics but does respond to corticosteroids. In cases where the etiologic agent persists, long-term corticosteroid therapy is employed. The results are good unless an advanced form of the disease is found. The prognosis is poor in all cats with feline infectious peritonitis. It is not known why granuloma formation does not respond to therapy for this disease.

REFERENCES

1. Boyer, J.L. and Miller, D.J.: Chronic hepatitis. In, Diseases of the Liver. Edited by L. Schiff and E.R. Schiff. J.B. Lippincott Co., Philadelphia, PA 687-723, 1987.
2. MacSween, R.N.M., Anthony, P.O. and Scheuer, P.J.: Pathology of the Liver. Churchill Livingstone, New York, 1987.
3. Wright, R., Alberti, K.G.M.M., Karran, S. and Millward-Sadler, G.H.: W.B. Saunders, Philadelphia, PA. 1985.
4. Strombeck, D.R. and Gribble, D.: Chronic active hepatitis in the dog. JAVMA 173:380-386, 1978.
5. Sabesin, S.M. and Koff, R.S.: Pathogenesis of experimental viral hepatitis. New Eng. J. Med. 290:944-950 and 996-1002, 1974.
6. Gocke, D.J., Morris, T.Q. and Bradley, S.E.: Chronic hepatitis in the dog: the role of immune factors. JAVMA 156:1700-1705, 1970.
7. Jarrett, W.F.H. and O'Neil, B.W.: A new transmissible agent causing acute hepatitis, chronic hepatitis and cirrhosis in dogs. Vet. Rec. 116:629-635, 1985.
8. Robinson, W.S.: Why do animals have antibodies to hepatitis B surface antigen? Gastroenterology 84:1614-1615, 1983.
9. Bishop, L., Strandberg, J.D., Adams, R.J., Brownstein, D.G. and Patterson, R.: Chronic active hepatitis in dogs associated with leptospires. AJVR 40:839-844, 1979.
10. Testas, P., Benichou, J., Perrin, N., Vieillefond, A. and Benhamou, M.: Comparative study of two models for experimental cirrhosis in the dog. Eur. Surg. Res. 10:146-152, 1978.
11. Meyer zum Buschenfelde, K.H. and Hopf, U.: Studies on the pathogenesis of experimental chronic active hepatitis in rabbits. I. Induction of the disease and protective effect of allogeneic liver specific proteins. Brit. J. Exp. Path. 55:498-508, 1974.
12. Leifer, C.E., Page, R.L., Matus, R.E., Patnaik, A.K. and MacEwen, E.G.: Proliferative glomerulonephritis and chronic active hepatitis with cirrhosis associated with Corynebacterium parvum immunotherapy in a dog. JAVMA 190:78-80, 1987.
13. Johnson, G.F., Zawie, D.A., Gilbertson, S.R. and Sternlieb, I.: Chronic active hepatitis in Doberman Pinschers. JAVMA 180:1438-1442, 1982.
14. Crawford, M.A., Schall, W.D., Jensen, R.K. and Tasker, J.B.: Chronic active hepatitis in 26 Doberman Pinschers. JAVMA 187:1343-1350, 1985.
15. Van den Ingh, T.S.G.A.M., Rothuizen, J. and Cupery, R.: Chronic active hepatitis with cirrhosis in the Doberman Pinscher. Vet. Quarterly 10:84-89, 1988.
16. Strombeck, D.R., Miller, L.M., Harrold, D.: Effects of corticosteroid treatment on survival time in dogs with chronic hepatitis: 151 cases (1977-1985) JAVMA 193:1109-1113, 1988.

17. Hopf, U. and Meyer zum Buschenfelde, K.H.: Studies on the pathogenesis of experimental chronic active hepatitis in rabbits. II. Demonstration of immunoglobulin on isolated hepatocytes. Brit. J. Exp. Path. 55:509-513, 1974.
18. Hopf, U. and Meyer zum Buschenfelde, K.H.: Diagnosis of autoimmune chronic active hepatitis a simplified method for the detection of liver membrane autoantibodies (LMA). Zeit Gastroenterologie 16:261-264, 1978.
19. Kawanishi, H.: In vitro morphological studies on antibody-dependent nonimmune lymphocyte-mediated cytotoxicity in chronic active liver disease. Am. J. Dig. Dis. 23:97-109, 1978.
20. Rojkind, M. and Kershenobich, D.: Hepatic fibrosis. In, Progress in Liver Diseases. Vol. 5. Edited by H. Popper and F. Schaffner. Grune and Stratton, New York. 294-310, 1976.
21. Bennett, A.M., Davies, J.D., Gaskell, C.J. and Lucke, V.M.: Lobular Dissecting Hepatitis in the Dog. Vet. Pathol. 20:179-188, 1983.
22. Theodossi, A., Skene, A.M., Portmann, B., Knill-Jones, R.P., Patrick, R.S., Tate, R.A., Kealey, W., Jarvis, K.J., O'Brian, D.J. and Williams, R.: Observer variation in assessment of liver biopsies including analysis by kappa statistics. Gastroenterology 79:232-241, 1980.
23. Bosch, J., Enriquez, R., Grossmann, R.J. and Storer, E.H.: Chronic bile duct ligation in the dog: Hemodynamic characterization of a portal hypertensive model. Hepatology 3:1002-1007, 1983.
24. Center, S.A., Castleman, W., Rother, L., Baldwin, B.H. and Tennant, B.C.: Light microscopic and electron microscopic changes in the livers of cats with extrahepatic bile duct obstruction. AJVR 47: 1278-1282, 1986.
25. Dooley, J.S., Hamilton-Miller, J.M.T., Brumfitt, W. and Sherlock, S.: Antibiotics in the treatment of biliary infection. Gut 25:988-998, 1984.
26. Wyke, R.J.: Problems of bacterial infection in patients with liver disease. Gut 28:623-641, 1987.
27. Chojkier, M. and Brenner, D.A.: Therapeutic strategies for hepatic fibrosis. Hepatology 8:176-182, 1988.
28. Kono, K., Ohnishi, K., Omata, M., Saito, M., Nakayama, T., Hatano, H., Nakajima, Y., Sugita, S. and Okuda, K.: Experimental portal fibrosis produced by intraportal injection of killed nonpathogenic Escherichia coli in rabbits. Gastroenterology 94:787-796, 1988.
29. Strombeck, D.R., Harrold, D., Rogers, Q., Wheeldon, E., Stern, J. and Schaeffer, M.: Plasma amino acid, glucagon, and insulin concentrations in dogs with nitrosamine-induced hepatic disease. AJVR 44:2028-2036, 1983.
30. Gopinath, C. and Ford, E.J.H.: Location of liver injury and extent of bilirubinaemia in experimental liver lesions. Vet. Path. 9:99-108, 1972.
31. Strombeck, D.R.: Unpublished Data
32. Opitz, M. and Lettwo, E.: Der cholesterinesterquotient im serum leberkranker hunde. Berl. Munch. Tierarztl, Wschr. 89:32-35, 1976.
33. McIntyre, N., Harry, D.S. and Pearson, A.J.G.: The hypercholesterolaemia of obstructive jaundice. Gut 16:379-391, 1975.
34. Strombeck, D.R., Rogers, Q. and Stem, J.: Effects of ammonia infusion on plasma glucagon, insulin and amino acids in intact, pancreatectomized, and adrenalectomized dogs. AJVR 42:810-818, 1981.
35. Aguirre, A., Yoshimura, N., Westman, T. and Fischer, J.E.: Plasma amino acids in dogs with two experimental forms of liver damage. J. Surg. Res. 16:339-345, 1974.
36. Fischer, J.E. and Baldessarini, R.J.: Pathogenesis and therapy of hepatic coma. In, Progress in Liver Diseases. Vol. 5. Edited by H. Popper and F. Schaffner. Grune and Stratton, New York. 363-397, 1976.
37. Zieve, L., Doizaki, W.M. and Zieve, F.J.: Synergism between mercaptans and ammonia or fatty acids in the production of coma: a possible role for mercaptans in the pathogenesis of hepatic coma. J. Lab. Clin. Med. 83:16-28, 1974.
38. Merino, G.E., Jetzer, T., Doizaki, W.M.D. and Najarian, J.S.: Mehionine-induced hepatic coma in dogs. Am. J. Surg. 130:41-46, 1975.
39. Gormly, A.A., Smith, P.S., Seymour, A.E., Clarkson, A.R. and Woodroffe, A.J.: IgA glomerular deposits in experimental cirrhosis. Am. J. Pathol. 104:50-54, 1981.
40. Conn, H.O.: A rational approach to the hepatorenal syndrome. Gastroenterology 65:321-340, 1973.
41. Murray, M., Robinson, P.B., McKeating, F.J. and Lauder, I.M.: Peptic ulceration in the dog: a clinico-pathological study. Vet. Rec. 91:441-447, 1972.
42. Wigton, D.H., Kociba, G.J. and Hoover, E.A.: Infectious canine hepatitis: Animal model for viral-induced disseminated intravascular coagulation. Blood 47:287-296, 1976.
43. Owen, C.A. and Bowie, E.J.W.: Effect of heparin on chronically induced intravascular coagulation in dogs. Am. J. Physiol. 229:449-454, 1975.
44. Bollman, J.L.: The animal with an Eck fistula. Physiol. Rev. 41:607-621, 1961.
45. Roberts, H.R. and Cederbaum, A.I.: The liver and blood coagulation: physiology and pathology. Gastroenterology 63:297-320, 1972.
46. Rogers, Q.: Personal Communication.
47. Strombeck, D.R. and Rogers, Q.: Plasma amino acid concentrations in dogs with hepatic disease. JAVMA 173:93-96, 1978.
48. Powell, L.W. and Axelsen, E.: Corticosteroids in liver disease: Studies on the biological conversion of prednisone to prednisilone and plasma protein binding. Gut 13:690-696, 1972.
49. Schalm. S.W., Summerskill, W.H.J. and Go, V.L.W.: Prednisone for chronic active liver disease: pharmokinetics, including conversion to prednisolone. Gastroenterology 72:910-913, 1977.
50. Gregory, P.B., Knauer, C.M., Kempson, R.L. and Miller, R.: Steroid therapy in severe viral hepatitis. New Eng. J. Med. 294:687-690, 1976.
51. Schaeffer, M.C., Rogers, Q.R., Buffington, C.A., Wolfe, B.M. and Strombeck, D.R.: Long-term biochemical and physiologic ewffects of surgically placed portacaval shunts in dogs. AJVR 47:346-355, 1986.
52. Thompson, J.S., Schafer, D.F., Haun, J. and Schafer, G.J.: Adequate diet prevents hepatic coma in dogs with Eck fistuals. Surg. Gynecol. Obstet. 162:126-130, 1986.
53. Ericksson, L.S. and Conn, H.O.: Branched-chain amino acids in the management of hepatic encephalopathy: An analysis of variants. Hepatology 10:228-246, 1989.
54. Fenton, J.C.B., Knight, E.J. and Humpherson, P.L.: Milk and cheese diet in portal-systemic encephalopathy. Lancet 1:164-166, 1966.
55. Nolan, J.P.: Endotoxin, reticuloendothelial function, and liver injury 5:458-465, 1981.
56. Zieve, L. and Zieve, F.J.: The dietary prevention of hepatic coma in Eck fistula dogs: Ammonia and the carbohydrate to protein ratio. Hepatology 7:196-198, 1987.
57. Strombeck, D.R.: Management of canine chronic active hepatitis. In, Current Veterinary Therapy. Edited by R.W. Kirk. Philadelphia, 885-891, 1980.
58. Fisher, P.W.F., Giroux, A. and L-Abbe, M.R.: Effects of zinc on mucosal copper binding and on kinetics of copper absorption. J. Nutr. 113:462-469, 1983.
59. Rojkind, M. and Dunn, M.A.: Hepatic fibrosis. Gastroenterology 76:849-863, 1979.
60. Boer, H.H., Nelson, R.W. and Long, G.G.: Colehicine therapy for hepatic fibrosis in a dog. JAVMA 185:303-305, 1984.
61. Zieve, L.: Hepatic encephalopathy. In, Diseases of the Liver. Edited by L. Schiff and E.R. Schiff. 925-948.
62. Fraser, C.L. and Arieff, A.I.: Hepatic encephalopathy. New Eng. J. Med. 313:865-873, 1985.
63. Hirsch, D.W.: Infectious complications of cancer. In, Current Veterinary Therapy. Edited by R.W. Kirk. Philadelphia, 464-466, 1986.
64. Moreau, M.C., Ducluzeau, R. and Raibaud, P.: Hydrolysis of urea in the gastrointestinal tract of "monoxenic" rats: effect of immunization with strains of ureolytic bacteria. Infect. Immun. 13:9-15, 1976.
65. Maddrey, W.C., Weber, F.L., Coulter, A.W., Chura, C.M., Chapanis, N.P. and Walser, M.: Effects of keto analogues of

essential amino acids in portal-systemic encephalopathy. Gastroenterology 71:190-195, 1976.
66. Rimola, A., Soto, R., Bory, F., Arroyo, V., Piera, C. and Rodes, J.: Reticuloendothelial system phagocytic activity in cirrhosis and its relation to bacterial infections and prognosis. Hepatology 4:53-58, 1984.
67. Faraj, B.A., Ali, F.M., Fulenwider, J.T., Walveaux, E.J., and Stacciarini, W.M.: Hepatorenal failure induced by tetracycline in dogs with portacaval shunt. J. Pharm. Exp. Ther. 221:558-563, 1982.
68. Boyer, T.D. and Warnock, D.G.: Use of diuretics in the treatment of cirrhotic ascites. Gastroenterology 84:1051-1055, 1983.
69. Conn, H.O. and Atterbury, C.E.: Cirrhosis. In, Diseases of the Liver 725-864, 1987.
70. Knauer, C.M. and Lowe, H.M.: Hemodynamics in the cirrhotic patient during paracentesis. New Eng. J. Med. 276:491-496, 1967.
71. Schiff, E.R.: Paracentesis: a safe and effective form of therapy. Hepatology 7:591-592, 1987.
72. Reynolds, T.B.: Therapeutic Paracentesis. Gastroenterology. 93:386-388, 1987.
73. Leveen, H.H., Christondias, G., Ip, M., Luft, R., Falk, G. and Grosberg, S.: Peritoneo-venous shunting for ascites. Ann. Surg. 180:580-591, 1974.
74. Furneaux, R.W. and Mero, K.N.: End-to-side portocaval anastomosis for the correction of ascites in a terrier dog. JAAHA 9:562-566, 1973.
75. Falchuk, K.R., Jacoby, I., Colucci, W.S. and Rybak, M.E.: Tetracycline-induced pleural symphysis for recurrent hydrothorax complicating cirrhosis. A new approach to treatment. Gastroenterology 72:319-321, 1977.
76. Hardy, R.M., Stevens, J.B. and Stowe, C.M.: Chronic progressive hepatitis in Bedlington Terriers associated with elevated liver copper concentrations. Minn. Vet. 15:13-20, 1975.
77. Twedt, D.C., Sternlieb, I. and Gilbertson, S.R.: Clinical, morphologic, and chemical studies on copper toxicosis of Bedlington Terriers. JAVMA 175:269-275, 1979.
78. Johnson, G.F, Sterlieb, I., Twedt, D.C., Grushoff, P.S. and Scheinberg, I.H.: Inheritance of copper toxicosis in Bedlington Terriers. AJVR 41:1865-1866, 1980.
79. Herrtage, M.E., Seymour, C.A., White, R.A.S., Small, G.M. and Wight, D.G.D.: Inherited copper toxicosis in the Bedlington Terrier: the prevalence in asymptomatic dogs. J. Sm. An. Pract. 28:1141-1151, 1987.
80. Johnson, G.F., Morell, A.G., Stockert, R.J. and Sternlieb, I.: Hepatic lysosomal copper protein in dogs with an inherited copper toxicosis. Hepatology 3:243-248, 1981.
81 Su, L.-C., Ravanshad, S., Owen, C.A., McCall, J.T., Zollman, P.E. and Hardy, R.M.: A comparison of copper-loading disease in Bedlington Terriers and Wilson's disease in humans. Am. J. Physiol. 243:G226-G230, 1982.
82. Su, L.-C., Owen, C.A., Zollman, P.E. and Hardy, R.M.: A defect of biliary excretion of copper in copper-laden Bedlington Terriers. Am. J. Physiol. 243:G231-G236, 1982.
83. Cousins, R.J.: Absorption, transport and hepatic metabolism of copper and zinc: Special reference to metallothionein and ceruloplasm. Physiol. Rev. 65:238-309, 1985.
84. Keen, C.L., Lonnerdal, B., Fisher, G.L.: Age-related variations in hepatic iron, copper, zinc, and selenium concentrations in Beagles. AJVR 42:1884-1887, 1981.
85. Thornburg, L.P., Shaw, D., Dolan, M., Raisbeck, M., Crawford, S., Dennis, G.L. and Olwin, D.B.: Hereditary copper toxicosis in West Highland White Terriers. Vet. Pathol. 23:148-154, 1986.
86. Ludwig, J., Owen, C.A., Barham, S.S., McCall, J.T. and Hardy, R.M.: The liver in the inherited copper disease of Bedlington Terriers. Lab. Invest. 43:82-87, 1980.
87. Johnson, G.F., Gilbertson, S.R., Goldfischer, S., Grushoff, P.S. and Sternlieb, I.: Cytochemical detection of inherited copper toxicosis of Bedlington Terriers. Vet. Pathol. 21:57-60, 1984.
88. Strombeck, D.R.: Management of canine chronic active hepatitis. In, Current Vet. Therapy. Edited by R.W. Kirk, Philadelphia, 1980.
89. Twedt, D.C., Hunsaker, H.A. and Allen, K.G.D.: Use of 2, 3, 2-tetramine as a hepatic copper chelating agent for treatment of copper hepatotoxicosis in Bedlington terriers. JAVMA 192:52-56, 1988.
90. Lipsky, M.A. and Gollan, J.L.: Treatment of Wilson's Disease: In D-penicillamine we trust - what about zinc? Hepatology 7:593-595, 1987.
91. Owen, C.A. and McCall, J.T.: Identification of the carrier of the Bedlington Terrier copper disease. AJVR 44:694-696, 1983.
92. Lykkegaard Nielsen, M., Asnaes, S. and Justesen, T.: Susceptibility of the liver and biliary tract to anaerobic infection in extrahepatic biliary tract obstruction. III. Possible synergistic effect between anaerobic and aerobic bacteria. Scand. J. Gastroenterology 11:263-272, 1976.
93. Finegold, S.M.: Intraabdominal, genito-urinary, skin and soft tissue infections due to non-sporeforming anaerobic bacteria. In, Infection with Non-sporing Anaerobic Bacteria. Edited by I. Philips and M. Sussman, Churchill Livingston, London. 160-188, 1974.
94. Lykkegaard Nielsen, M., Justesen, T. and Asnaes, S.: Anaerobic bacteriological study of human liver — with a critical review of the literature. Scand. J. Gastroenterology 9:671-677, 1974.
95. Bartlett, J.G., Louie, T.J., Onderdonk, A.B. and Gorbach, S.L.: Experimental intraabdominal sepsis. Gastroenterology 68:861, 1975.
96. Ranson, J.H.C., Madayag, M.A., Localio, S.A. and Spencer, F.C.: New diagnostic and therapeutic techniques in the management of pyogenic liver abscesses. Ann. Surg. 181:508-518, 1975.
97. Fauci, A.S. and Wolff, S.M.: Granulomatous hepatitis. In, Progress in Liver Diseases. Vol. 5. Edited by H. Popper and F. Schaffner. Grune and Stratton, New York, 609-621, 1976.
98. Hottendorf, G.H. and Hirth, R.S.: Lesions of spontaneous subclinical disease in beagle dogs. Vet. Path. 11:240-258, 1974.

Chapter 34

Hepatic Lipidosis, Vacuolar Hepatopathy, Steroid-Induced Hepatopathy, Hemochromatosis, and Amyloidosis

HEPATIC LIPIDOSIS AND VACUOLAR HEPATOPATHY

Feline Idiopathic Hepatic Lipidosis

Clinical Synopsis

Diagnostic features

* Obese cat with depression and persistent anorexia
* Late signs: vomiting, diarrhea, icterus, hypersalivation, weight loss
* Characteristic elevation of ALP
* Hepatomegaly
* Hepatic lipidosis detected by needle aspiration or hepatic biopsy

Standard management

* Nasogastric or gastrostomy tube placement
* Ensure to meet all caloric and protein requirements
* Restricted protein, low residue, balanced diet
* High fat diets not contraindicated (see text)
* Manage hepatic encephalopathy (see Chapter 33)

Hepatic Lipidosis. Hepatic lipidosis had been one of the most frequently reported of all hepatic problems in small animals; diagnosed on necropsy, it accounts for half of all types of hepatic disease in both dogs and cats. In the past, steroid-induced hepatopathy was often identified incorrectly as lipidosis. The morphological changes in hepatocytes following administration of steroids are due not to fatty infiltration but to changes in the cells' glycogen content. Recent evaluation of pathology material at the VMTH in Davis reveals that the incidence of lipidosis is much lower, with lipidosis representing 11% of the total in cats and 3.9% in dogs. In another survey hepatic lipidosis was diagnosed in 3.4% of feline day-case histology submissions and the prevalence was increasing.[1]

Etiology and Pathogenesis

The causes of hepatic lipidosis in small animals are undernutrition (starvation), overnutrition (obesity), protein-calorie malnutrition, diabetes mellitus, drugs, and toxins.[2,3] The most important type in cats is idiopathic hepatic lipidosis, which probably has starvation or anorexia as one important factor in its pathogenesis (Table 34-1).[1,4-7] The most important cause of hepatic lipidosis in dogs is diabetes mellitus. Hepatic lipidosis in either species develops because of nutritional derangements, caused by starvation or anorexia or precipitated by a metabolic abnormality.

Idiopathic hepatic lipidosis is a serious problem that is difficult to manage successfully in the cat. The history of cats with this problem invariably includes complete anorexia for a week or longer. Dogs or cats not eating for one to two weeks will develop fatty changes in the liver, but they usually do not develop severe illness as a consequence. Other factors are probably necessary for cats to become severely ill with idiopathic hepatic lipidosis. One such factor may be preexisting obesity, which is reported in the history of many cats with this problem. About 5% of the normal liver is lipid; that percentage increases with obesity. The hepatic accumulation results from increased synthesis of fatty acids from the excess calories consumed; presumably hepatic secretion of lipids does not increase enough to prevent hepatic accumulation. Obesity also results in increased plasma fatty acid levels since with increased adipose stores the release of fatty acids increases. Increased plasma free fatty acids promote hyperglycemia and insulin release in response to reduced glucose utilization. Insulin has the effect of inhibiting release of fatty acids from adipose tissue,

Table 34-1 Hepatic Lipidosis

	Canine	Feline
	%	%
Idiopathic anorexia	19	45
Diabetes mellitus	30	9
Gastrointestinal disease	19	17
Pancreatitis	12	9
Neoplastic disease	10	4
Passive congestion or anemia	--	10
Miscellaneous	10	6

but the increased mass of lipid stores is too great and prevents insulin from maintaining plasma free fatty acids at normal levels. Affected cats appear to have a resistance to insulin or possibly an insulin deficiency, and that can explain why fatty acids continue to be released from adipose tissue. Evidence for insulin deficiency is no change in plasma insulin levels during hyperglycemia. Evidence for insulin resistance includes normal or increased plasma insulin levels, prolonged hyperglycemia during an intravenous glucose tolerance test and increased plasma levels of branched-chain amino acids. These amino acids are metabolized in peripheral tissues, and insulin is required for their catabolism. The combination of increased hepatic lipid content, increased plasma free fatty acids, and relative insulin resistance or deficiency may be a means to increase the risk for idiopathic hepatic lipidosis in obese animals. It is evident that insulin therapy should be ineffective in managing a problem caused partly by insulin resistance.

Hepatic lipidosis is predictable in normal, non-obese cats that have eaten nothing for 10 to 14 days. Plasma free fatty acid levels increase, and body protein is degraded for amino acids as a source of energy. In such cats the plasma concentrations of most amino acids are one-half of normal values.[8] The plasma levels of branched-chain amino acids are normal, however, a finding that suggests an insulin resistance in cats not previously obese. The plasma levels of tyrosine and phenylalanine, aromatic amino acids metabolized in the liver, are also normal, which suggest that the hepatic lipidosis reduces the liver's capacity for metabolizing aromatic amino acids. The degree of lipid accumulation may depend on the completeness of starvation. During complete starvation tissues adapt so they can metabolize fatty acids as their primary source of energy. That adaptation is incomplete if small amounts of carbohydrate are fed. With incomplete adaptation it is likely that more lipids will not be metabolized and will accumulate in the liver.[3]

Hepatic lipidosis develops when the diet is deficient in protein or is high in carbohydrate without appropriate amounts of protein so that a protein-calorie malnutrition develops. Protein deficiency should not develop in cats or dogs fed commercial pet food since it contains more than the minimum requirement of protein. Cats fed dog food receive inadequate amounts of protein. Either cats or dogs fed commercial pet food that is supplemented by primarily carbohydrate-rich foods can develop hepatic lipid changes. High-carbohydrate diets produce fatty livers in experimental animals; similar parenteral-nutrition diets have the same effect.[9] Feeding a high-lipid diet does not have that effect. Cats with primary hepatic lipidosis have been successfully managed by feeding them diets containing lipids in amounts providing 30% to 40% of the total calories.[6]

Idiopathic hepatic lipidosis may have developed along with the development of diets intended to change the cat from a carnivore to an omnivore. Despite our knowledge of cats' nutritional requirements, feeding diets relatively high in carbohydrate and lower in fat and protein than is typical for a carnivore's diet may involve a greater risk for developing hepatic lipidosis during times when nothing is eaten.

The severity of idiopathic hepatic lipidosis together with its poor response to treatment and poor prognosis suggests that the entity may be quite different from other forms of hepatic lipidosis. One aspect of that difference may be its cause. The disease may be one manifestation of an infectious or toxic disease. Other animals and humans can develop a severe form of hepatic lipidosis following a viral infection. For example, coronavirus intestinal infection results in a hepatic lipidosis resembling Reyes syndrome in two-thirds of infected mice. Toxins suggested to be a cause include aflatoxin, a metabolite of the fungus *Aspergillus flavus*; the toxin can contaminate commercial pet foods. A number of other chemical toxins can cause hepatic degeneration and lipidosis, but they would be less likely causes in the cat than the dog because of greater discrimination by the cat in what it eats. Of these two types of causes there may be more merit for some kind of viral infection because of the problem's increasing frequency. One pathology service reports an increasing prevalence for feline fatty liver syndrome over the past five years.[1]

Gastrointestinal disease is frequently associated with hepatic lipidosis, both in cats and dogs. Lipidosis may be the most common pathologic change in animals with gastrointestinal problems. The changes are partly attributed to endotoxins and possibly other toxins absorbed from the diseased intestine.[2] The production of such toxins increases with intestinal bacterial overgrowth, an expected complication of maldigestion and malabsorption. The absorption of toxins increases with increased intestinal permeability, a change expected with many gastrointestinal problems. Antibiotics are shown to prevent lipidosis caused by bacterial overgrowth in experimental dogs. Many cats are presented with a history that includes some gastrointestinal signs. It is possible that these events in the gastrointestinal tract may be a factor in the initiation or progression of idiopathic hepatic lipidosis in cats. The management of hepatic lipidosis usually includes antibiotics, which should be selected and used to reduce the contribution of gastrointestinal problems to the lipidosis. Gastrointestinal problems also contribute to hepatic lipidosis by any malnutrition they create.

Diabetes mellitus is a frequent cause of hepatic lipidosis in the dog but not in the cat. Inflammatory disease of the exocrine pancreas is also associated with hepatic lipidosis in both species. It has been recognized for over 50 years that normal pancreatic function is necessary to prevent hepatic lipidosis.[10,11] Pancreatectomy in dogs results in a hepatic lipidosis that persists when insulin is administered but disappears when pancreatic extracts or choline is fed. The pathogenesis of the fatty changes can result from increased transport of fat to the liver, increased lipid synthesis in the liver, a reduction in the oxidation of lipids in the liver, or a reduction in the mobilization of fat from the liver. Most of those factors play a role in the dog and probably in other species of small animals as well. During insulin deficiency there is an increased lipolysis of peripheral lipid stores; the liver removes the resulting increased plasma levels of free fatty acids. In the dog, an increased production of triglycerides follows insulin deficiency.[12] The diabetic does not lose the ability to synthesize lipoproteins for mobilization of fats from the liver. Mobilization is impaired only when protein deficiency or a lack of precursors for phospholipid synthesis becomes a problem. Phospholipid synthesis is not normally reduced in diabetics. Hepatic lipidosis can progress to cirrhosis in dogs that are diabetic for 2.5 to 5 years, and the pathogenesis appears to be the same as in the choline-deficient animal.[13] Hepatic lipidosis is an important problem that should be considered in the management and prognosis for every animal with diabetes mellitus.

Hepatic lipidosis is also seen in hyperthyroid cats. In-

Table 34-2. Drugs and Toxins Causing Hepatic Lipidosis

Alcohol	Flectol H
Antimony	Hydrazine
L-Asparaginase	Hypoglycin
Azacytidine	Methotrexate
Azaserine	Methyl bromide
Azauridine	Methyl chloride
BAL	Methychlorobromide
Barium salts	Methyl dichloride
Bleomycin	Orotic acid
Borates	Phosphorus
Carbon disulphide	Puromycin
Chromates	Rare earth
Dichloreoethylene	Satrole
Dimethylhydrazine	Tetracycline
Ethionine	Thallium compounds
Ethylbromide	Uranium compounds
Ethyl chloride	Warfarin

creased thyroxine levels promote the release of fatty acids from adipose tissue, and excess amounts accumulate in the liver.

Drugs are well-established causes of hepatic lipidosis. They are infrequently reported as the cause in both dogs and cats. Table 34-2 lists drugs and toxins capable of producing hepatic lipidosis. Some of the drugs are used often in small animal medicine; some are rarely or never used.

Vacuolar Hepatopathy. Vacuolar hepatopathy represents 5.6% of total pathologic diagnoses of hepatic disease in dogs and 13.5% of those in cats. Vacuolar hepatopathy can be caused by the same insults that cause hepatic degeneration, hepatic necrosis, and hepatic lipidosis. In dogs, vacuolar hepatopathy is most often associated with another liver problem; in the cat many cases have an unknown cause (Table 34-3).

Clinical and Laboratory Findings, Diagnosis[4-7]

Hepatic lipidosis is the pathologic change developing from a metabolic disorder. That disorder may have no identifiable cause other than a primary sign of complete anorexia, or it may be caused by a disease in another system. The early clinical signs may be merely those of depression and anorexia; later signs such as vomiting, diarrhea, and icterus may appear. It is not possible to determine whether the early signs reflect problems other than hepatic lipidosis and whether the later signs appear only after hepatic lipidosis develops. Also, diseases in other systems can cause different clinical signs, and they may represent the major complaints in animals that prove to have hepatic lipidosis.

Table 34-3 Vacuolar Hepatopathy

Etiology	Canine	Feline
	%	%
Primary or unknown	20	32
Other liver problems	25	18
Nonhepatic neoplastic disease	18	18
GI or pancreatic disease	8	9
Renal disease	6	7
Septicemia or infection	8	4
Circulatory disease	6	7
Miscellaneous	9	5

Cats with idiopathic hepatic lipidosis are invariably reported to show anorexia as the most common sign. Some report vomiting and diarrhea as common signs. Others do not mention these but list other signs as severe weight loss, severe depression, excessive salivation, and signs of hepatic encephalopathy. Many of the cats have a history of obesity, and in some there is a history of trauma, stress, or an illness that preceded the presenting signs. Common physical findings include icterus, hepatomegaly, and dehydration.

Cats with hepatic lipidosis have a nonregenerative, normocytic, normochromic anemia and stress leukocytosis. Consistent increases are reported for plasma activities of alkaline phosphatase (ALP) and alanine aminotransferase (ALT), and for plasma concentrations of total bilirubin (Table 34-4). Many nondiabetic cats have hyperglycemia. Compromise of hepatic function is also reflected in some cats by low albumin, prolonged prothrombin and partial thromboplastin times, and hyperammonemia. Of these changes the biochemical abnormality most unique for feline hepatic diseases is the increased ALP activity. That activity is seldom so greatly or consistently elevated with other feline liver diseases.

Similar biochemical changes are seen in dogs with hepatic lipidosis (Table 34-5). Plasma ALT increases only slightly if at all in dogs with hepatic lipidosis secondary to diabetes mellitus.[14] The mean value of ALT activity in one report was 50% above the upper limit of normal, while another study reported an ALT activity of four times the mean normal value.[14,15] Excessive amounts of this enzyme are released with hepatocyte degeneration and necrosis. Diabetes mellitus can appear concurrently with acute pancreatitis, causing extensive focal hepatic necrosis and increased ALT levels. A high percentage of animals with diabetes mellitus show a microscopic change of acute pancreatitis on necropsy. This association is also supported by the finding that one-third of diabetes mellitus patients have elevated serum levels of amylase and lipase, changes consistent with acute pancreatitis. With biochemical evaluations to screen for liver disease, plasma ALT levels cannot be expected to identify the possibility of hepatic lipidosis. A function test can be used to evaluate such patients, with the expectation that half of those with hepatic lipidosis will show abnormal function. The sulfobromophthalein retention test is abnormal in half of dogs with diabetes mellitus.

Measurement of plasma ALP activity is useful in identifying possible hepatic disease. Increased ALP activity is not diagnostic for liver problems, however, which limits its usefulness in evaluating hepatic lipidosis. Plasma ALP increases in diabetes mellitus to five to six times normal. This increment is most likely due to the secretion of excessive amounts of steroids. Adrenalcortical hyperplasia, found in up to a third of dogs necropsied, suggests that measurement of plasma cortisol levels would identify hypersecretion of adrenal corticosteroids accompanying diabetes mellitus. That is supported by the finding that most animals show a stress response in their

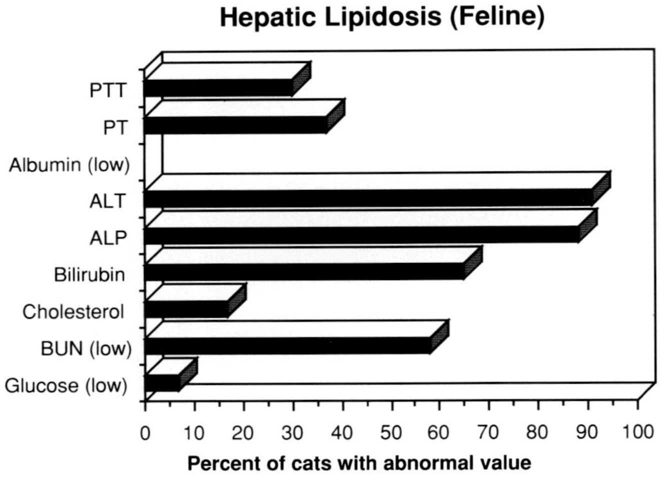

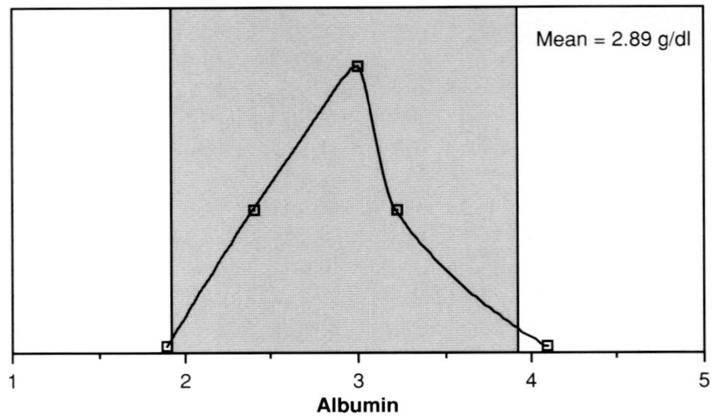

Table 34-4. Comparison of sensitivities for different tests in cats with hepatic lipidosis. Below: graphs showing distribution of clinical pathology values in cats with hepatic lipidosis. Points on graphs represent 0%, 25%, 50%, 75%and 100% medians. Normal range is in shaded area.

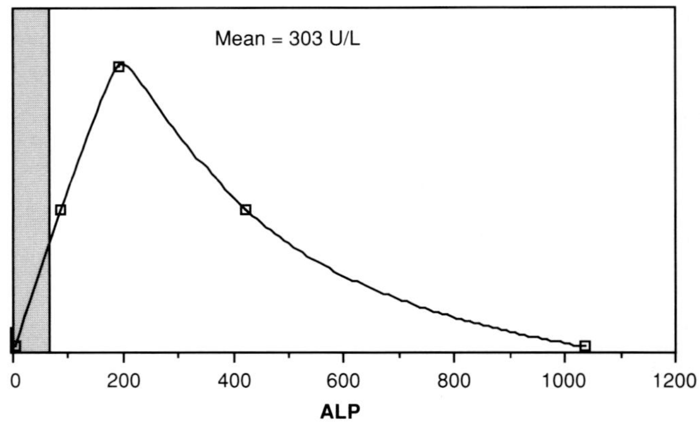

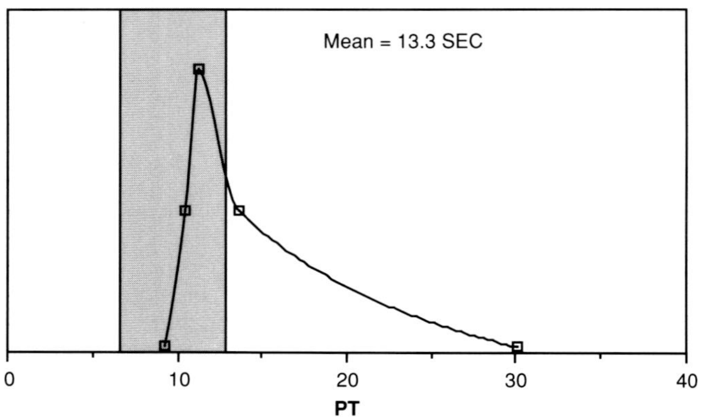

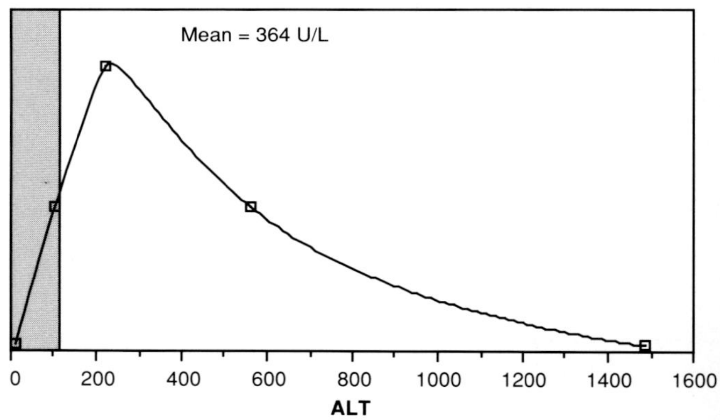

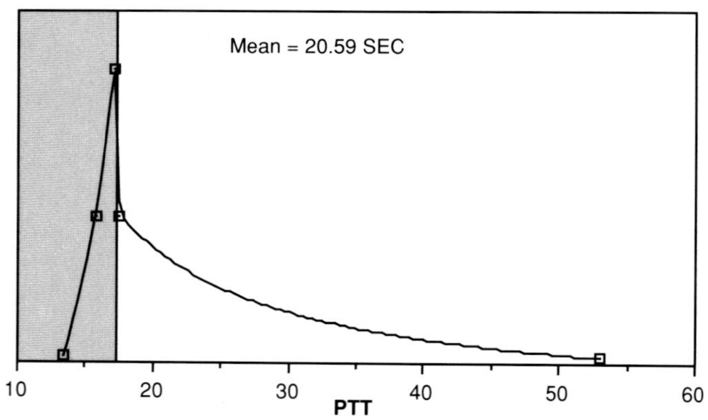

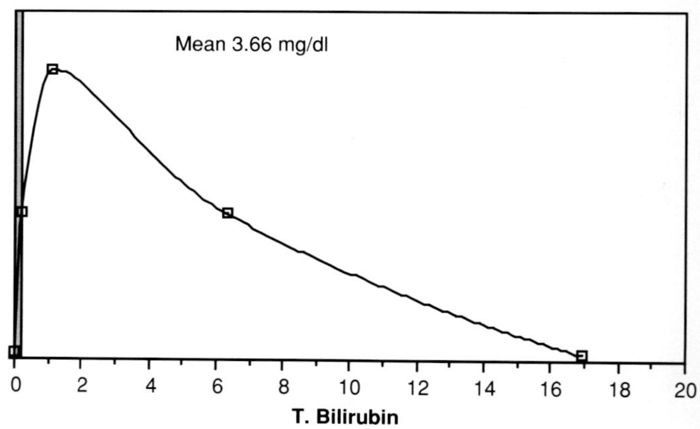

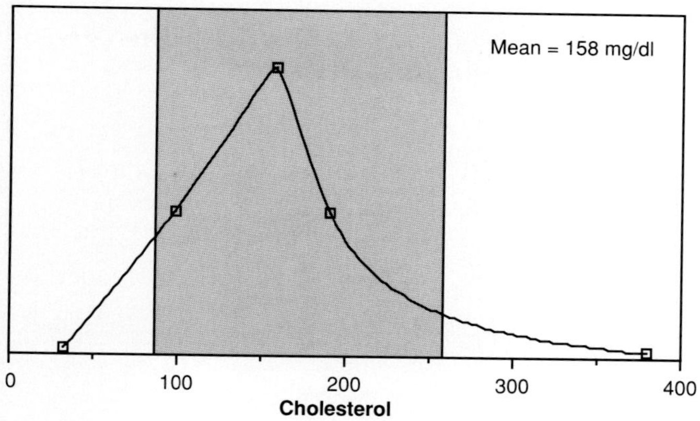

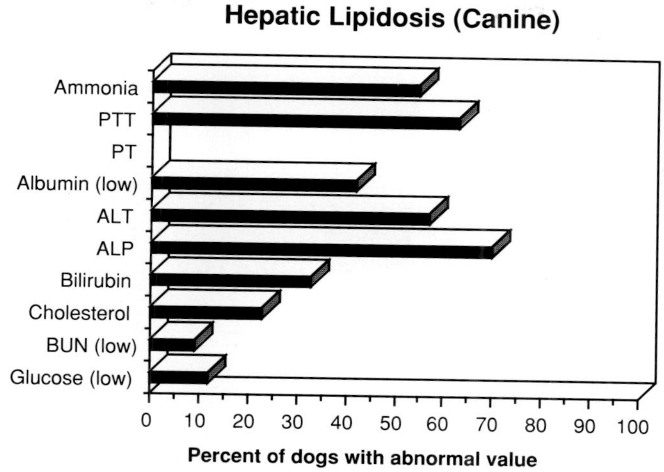

Table 34-5. Comparison of sensitivities for different tests in dogs with hepatic lipidosis. Below: graphs show distribution of clinical pathology values in dogs with hepatic lipidosis. Points on graphs represent 0%, 25%, 50%, 75% and 100%. Normal range is in shaded areas.

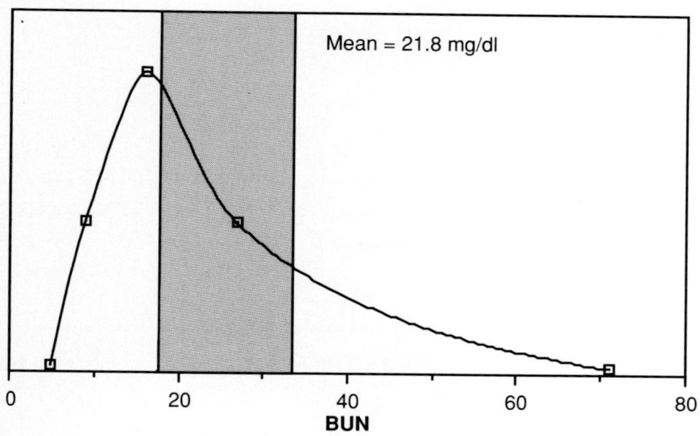

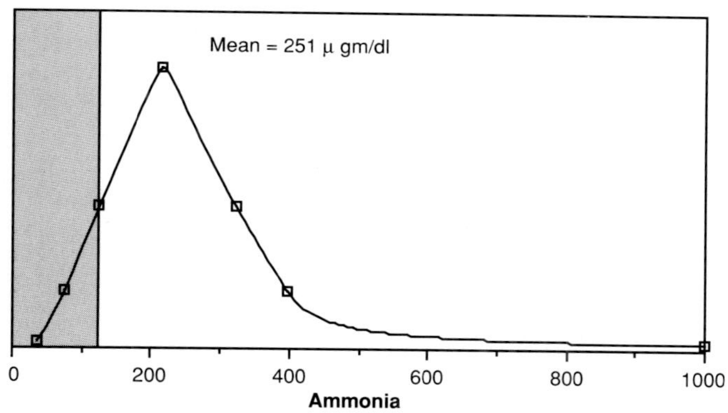

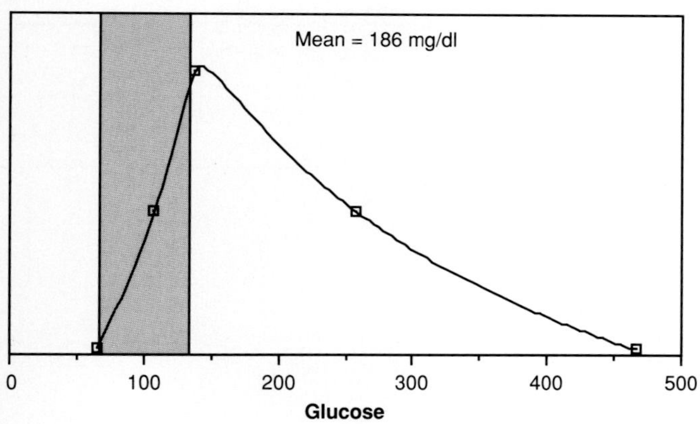

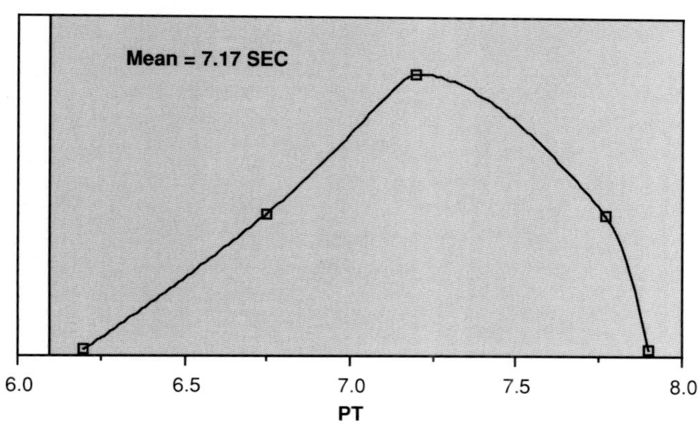

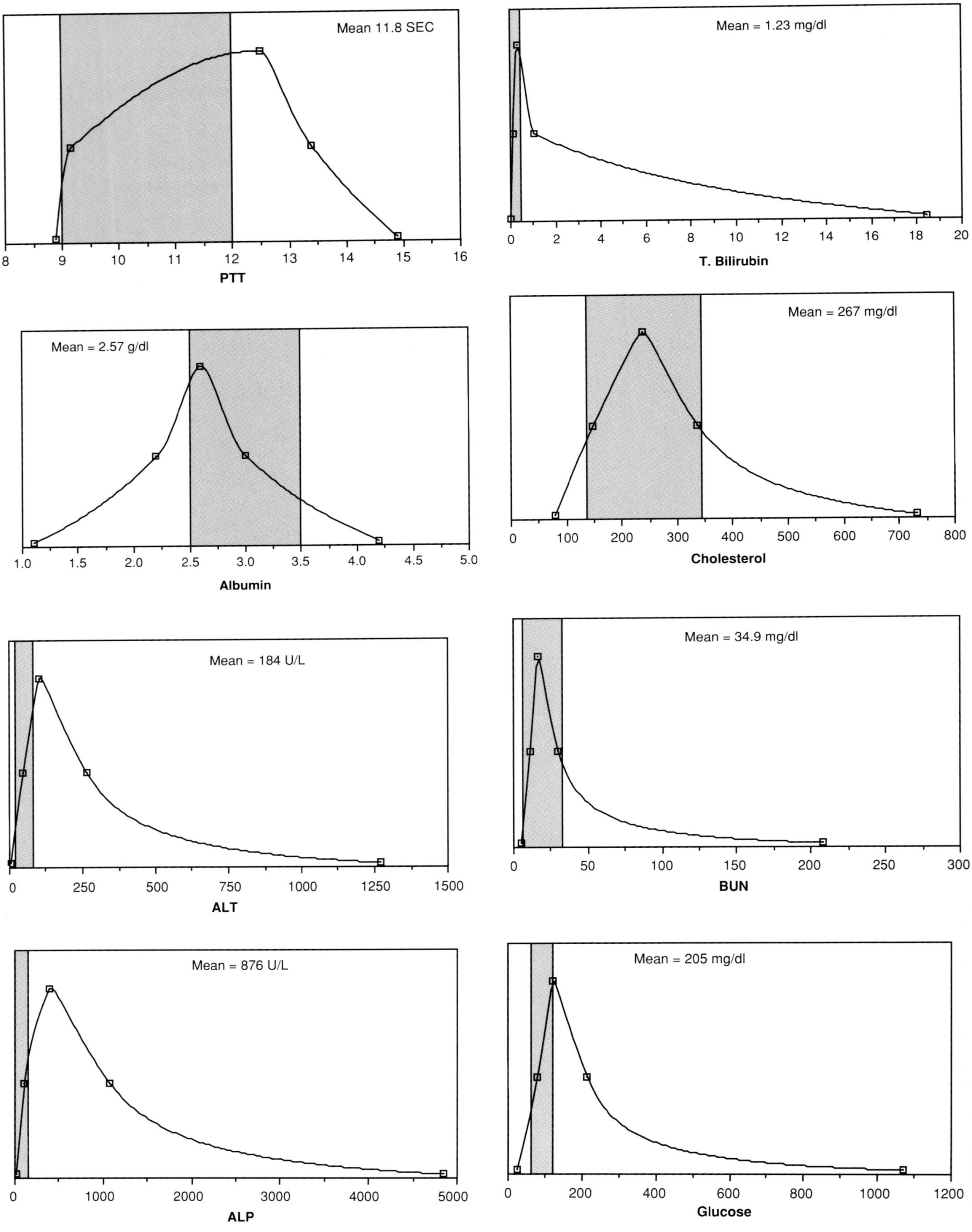
Mean 11.8 SEC
8 9 10 11 12 13 14 15 16
PTT
Mean = 1.23 mg/dl
0 2 4 6 8 10 12 14 16 18 20
T. Bilirubin
Mean = 2.57 g/dl
1.0 1.5 2.0 2.5 3.0 3.5 4.0 4.5 5.0
Albumin
Mean = 267 mg/dl
0 100 200 300 400 500 600 700 800
Cholesterol
Mean = 184 U/L
0 250 500 750 1000 1250 1500
ALT
Mean = 34.9 mg/dl
0 50 100 150 200 250 300
BUN
Mean = 876 U/L
0 1000 2000 3000 4000 5000
ALP
Mean = 205 mg/dl
0 200 400 600 800 1000 1200
Glucose

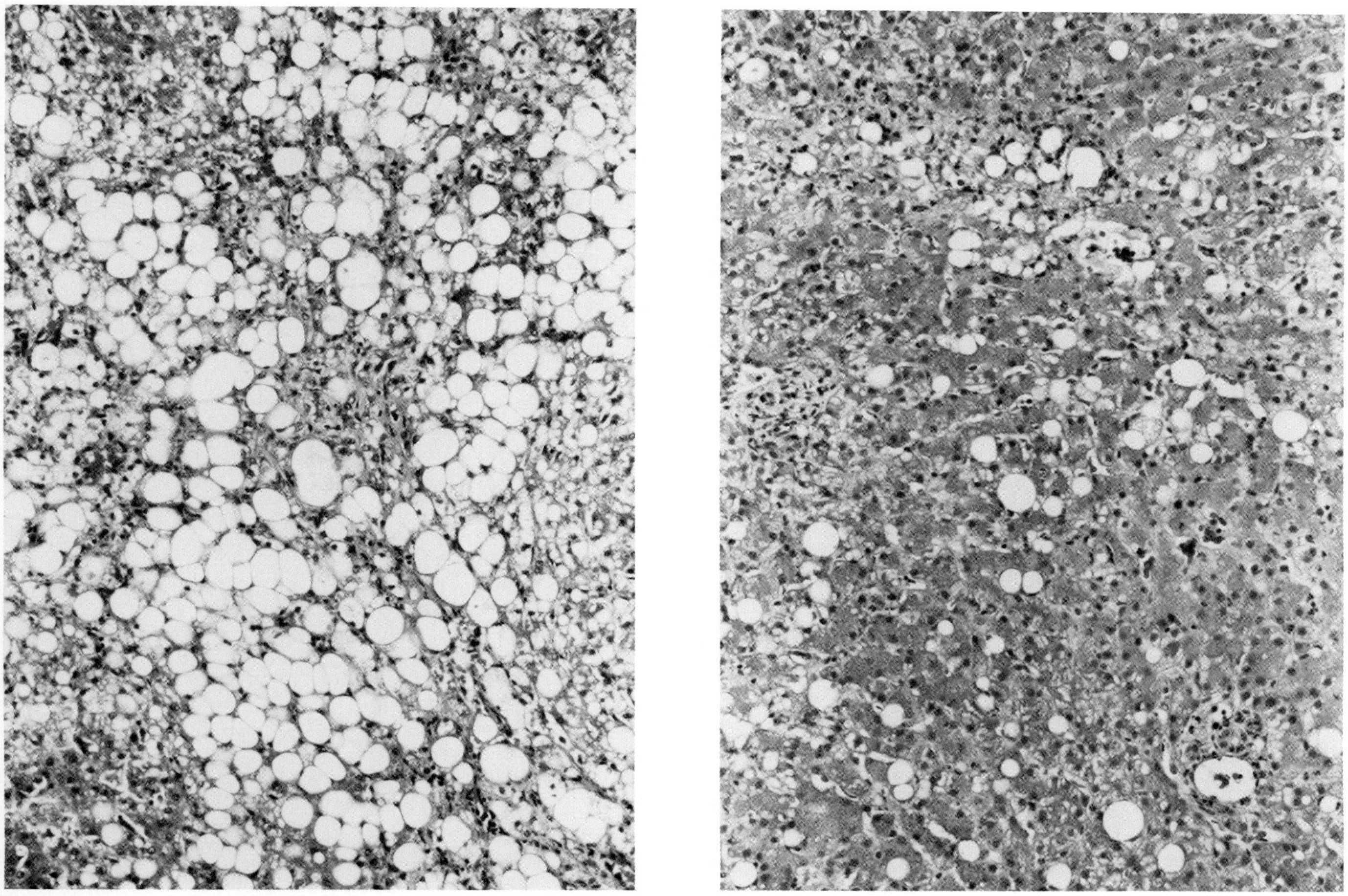

A B

Figure 34-1. Hepatic lipidosis. (a) Diffuse fatty infiltration involves many hepatocytes that contain clear vacuoles and inconspicuous nuclei. (b) Mild lipidosis.

hemogram: a neutrophilia, lymphopenia, and eosinopenia. In summary, there is little evidence in the way of clinical signs or abnormal laboratory data that suggests hepatic disease when lipidosis is a major problem.

Severe hepatic lipidosis causes the entire liver to be yellow, greasy, friable, and enlarged. No gross changes may be apparent with mild to moderate degrees of lipidosis. The histologic distribution of lipid throughout the liver can be diffuse, whereas in other cases of lipidosis it can be located primarily in zone 1 (periportal) or zone 3 (centrilobular). Other changes such as inflammation or necrosis are not usually found.

Microscopically, lipid accumulates in the liver in a microvesicular and macrovesicular form.[3] In the microvesicular form hepatocytes are filled with small fat droplets that give the hepatocyte a foamy appearance and do not displace the nucleus. Macrovesicular lipidosis is characterized by large fat droplets that displace the nucleus to the periphery of the hepatocyte. The form of fat distribution as either large or small droplets is specific for some types of hepatocyte injury. For example, tetracycline and aflatoxins cause microvesicular lipidosis, whereas starvation and malnutrition cause macrovesicular lipidosis. Both forms of lipidosis are described for cats with idiopathic hepatic lipidosis, which indicates that the pathology seen does not provide much insight into its pathogenesis.

Accumulation of fat in the liver appears histologically as a void that takes no stain because fat is lost in the processing of tissues (Figure 34-1). Glycogen is also lost during tissue processing and causes a similar void to appear in stained preparations. Intracellular edema results in a similar appearance. Consequently, vacuoles, whether as macrovesicles or microvesicles, cannot be readily attributed to accumulation of lipid, glycogen or water in hepatocytes. Special staining of tissue not subjected to leaching and loss of lipids and glycogen is sometimes used to verify lipids or glycogen as the cause of vesicles. When the clinical and pathologic findings do not convince the pathologist that the vesicles contain lipid (for hepatic lipidosis diagnosis) or glycogen (for steroid-induced hepatopathy diagnosis) the diagnosis will be vacuolar hepatopathy with no suggestion that it is due to either lipid or glycogen.

In most cases of vacuolar hepatopathy the clinical signs are nonspecific; biochemical abnormalities found on screening tests suggest hepatic disease, and the liver is biopsied. Biochemical findings on cats with vacuolar hepatopathy show abnormalities similar to those for hepatic lipidosis and steroid-

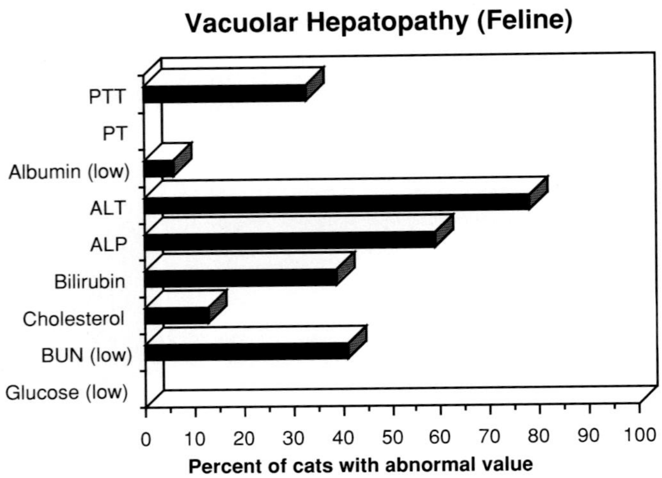

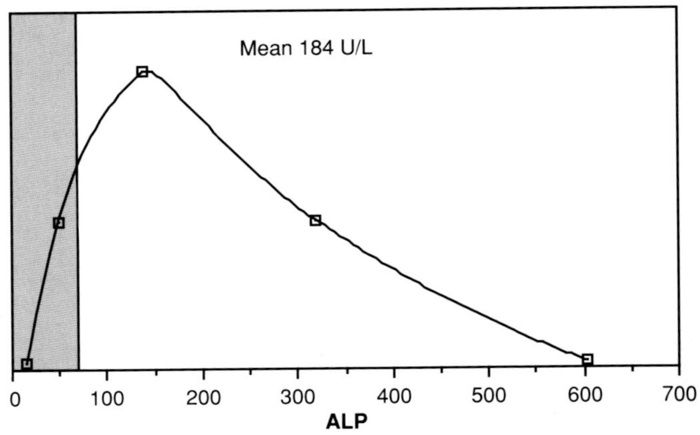

Table 34-6. Comparison of sensitivities for different tests in cats with vacuolar hepatopathy. Below: graphs showing distribution of clinical pathology values in cats with vacuolar hepatopathy. Points represent 0%, 25%, 50%, 75% and 100%% medians. Normal range is in shaded area.

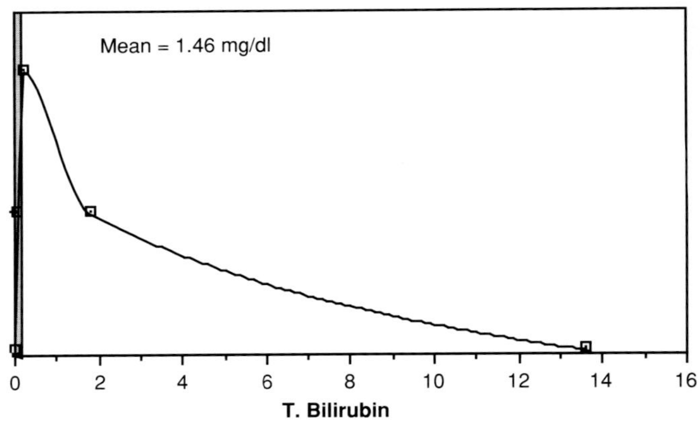

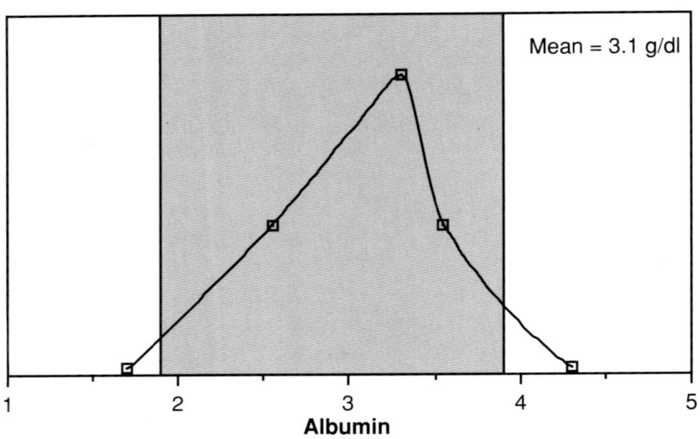

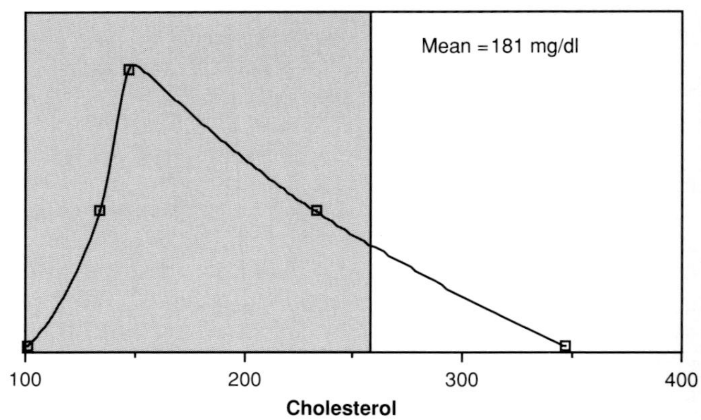

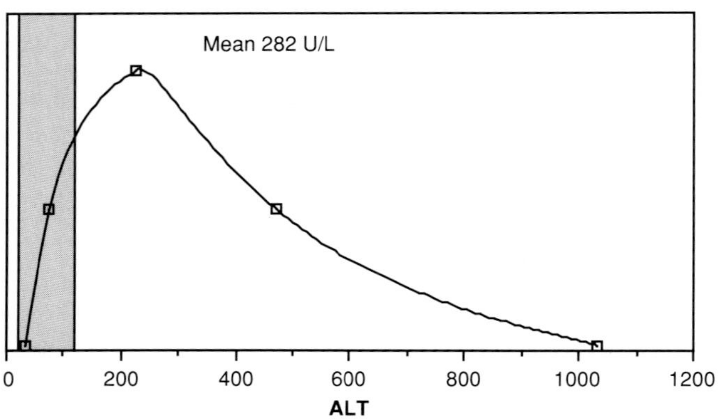

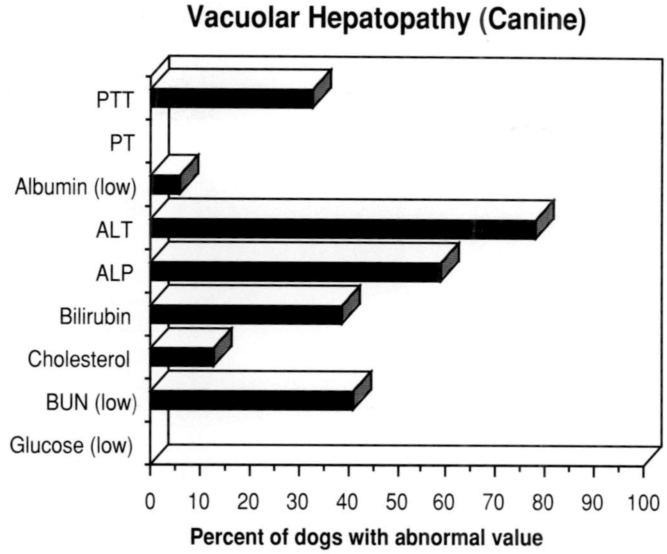

Table 34-7. Comparison of sensitivities for different tests in dogs with vacuolar hepatopathy. Below: graphs showing distribution of clinical pathology values in dogs with vacuolar hepatopathy. Points on graphs represent 0%, 25%, 50%, 75% and 100% medians. Normal range is in shaded area.

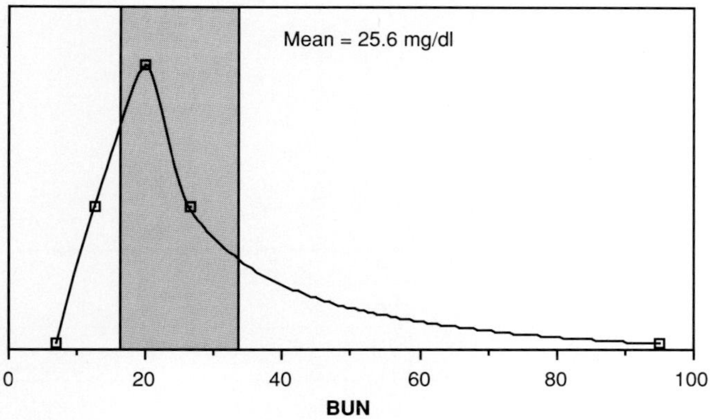

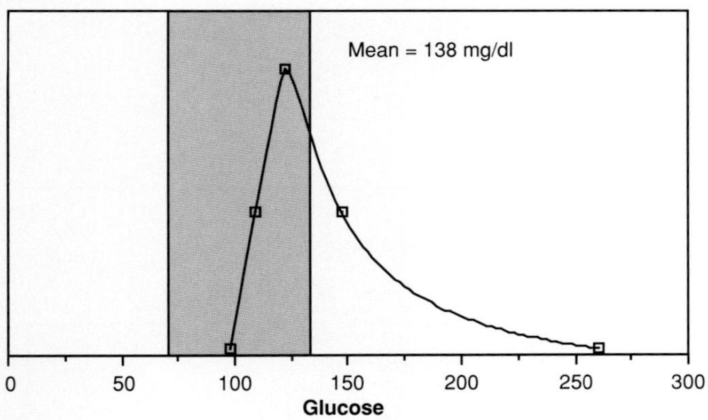

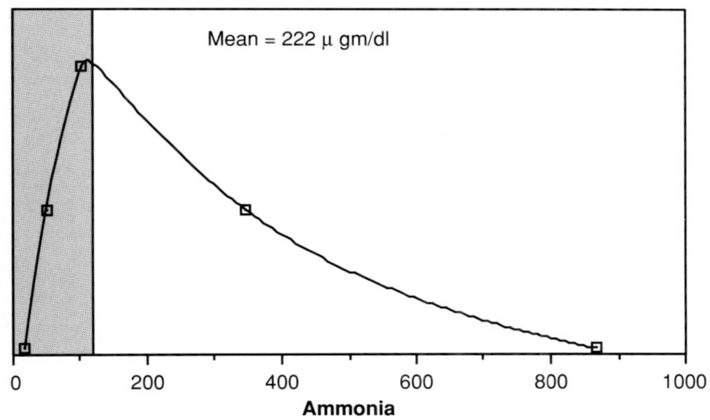

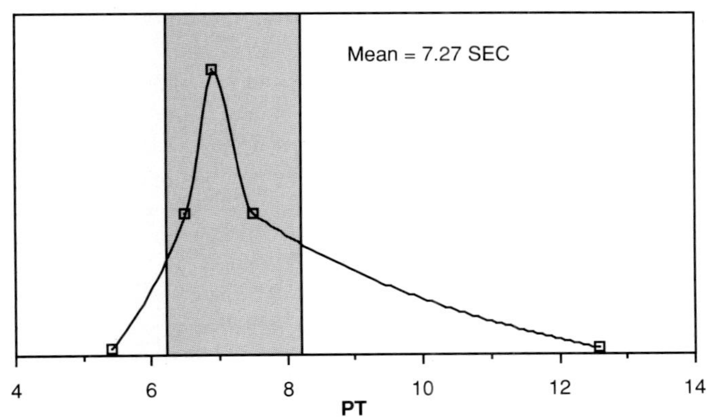

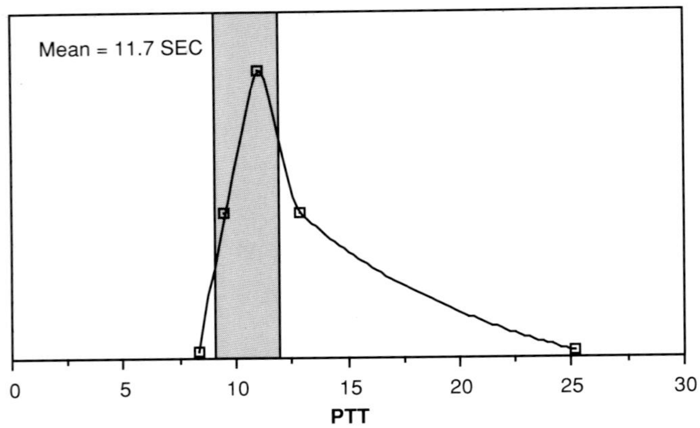
Mean = 11.7 SEC
0
5
10
15
20
25
30
PTT

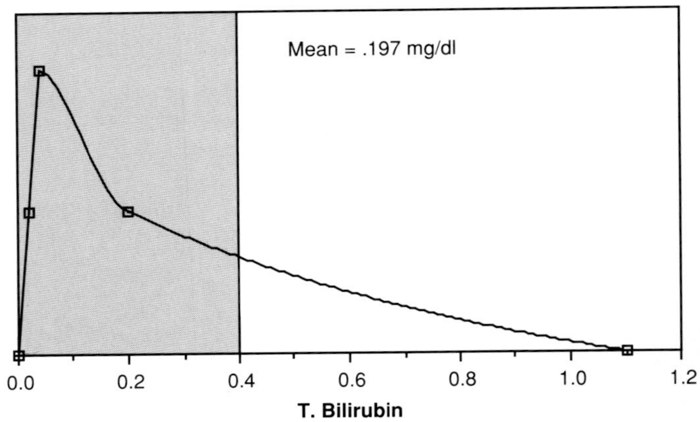
Mean = .197 mg/dl
0.0
0.2
0.4
0.6
0.8
1.0
1.2
T. Bilirubin

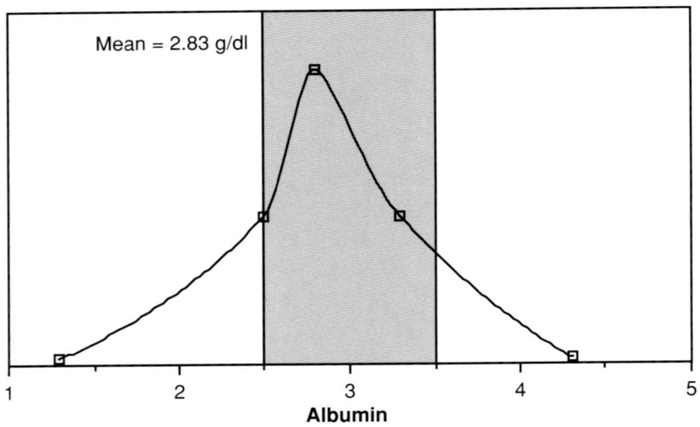
Mean = 2.83 g/dl
1
2
3
4
5
Albumin

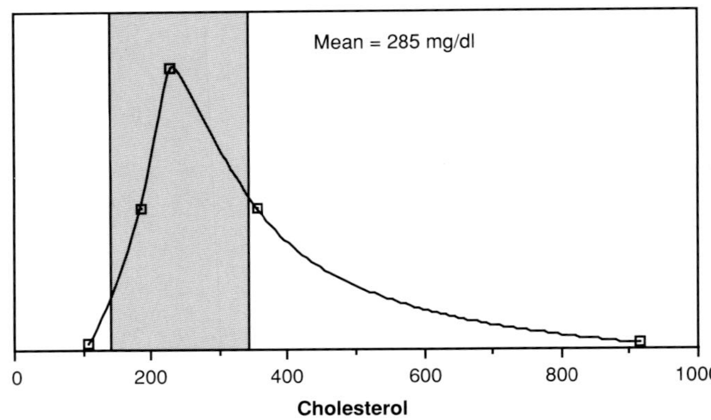
Mean = 285 mg/dl
0
200
400
600
800
1000
Cholesterol

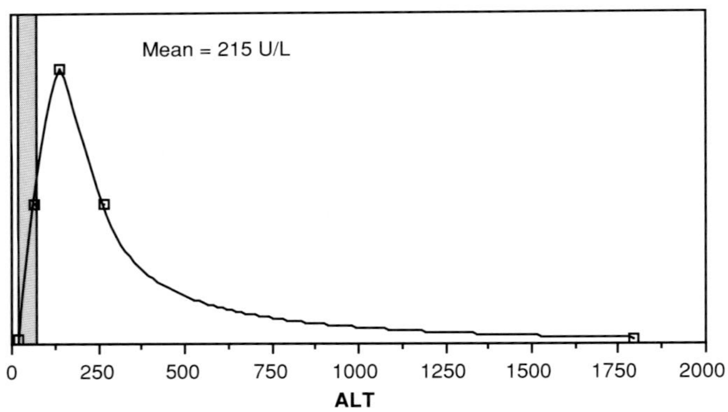
Mean = 215 U/L
0
250
500
750
1000
1250
1500
1750
2000
ALT

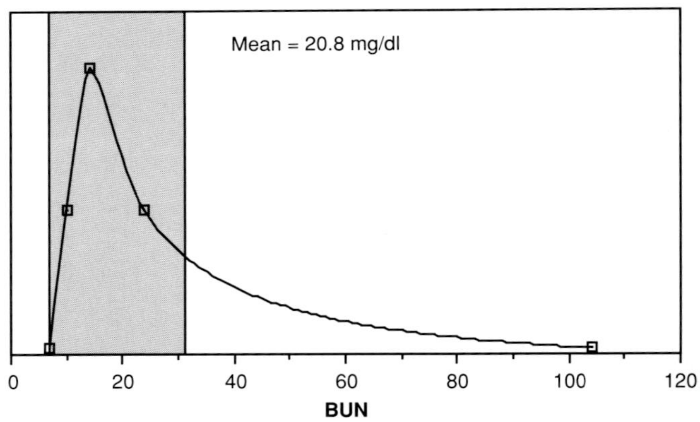
Mean = 20.8 mg/dl
0
20
40
60
80
100
120
BUN

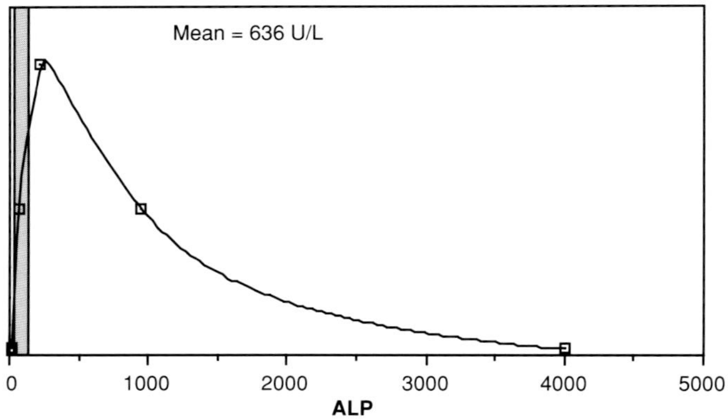
Mean = 636 U/L
0
1000
2000
3000
4000
5000
ALP

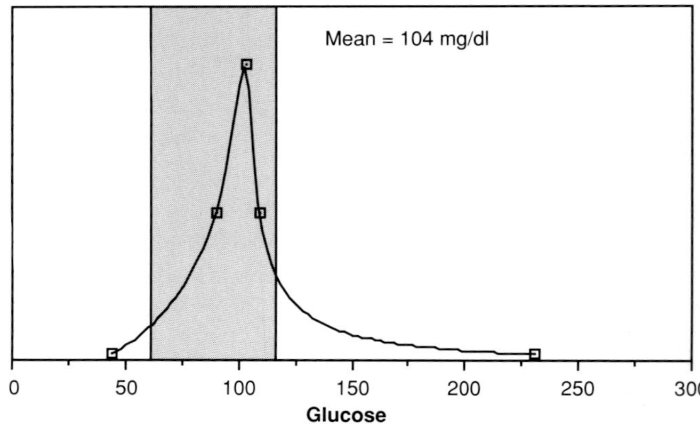
Mean = 104 mg/dl
0
50
100
150
200
250
300
Glucose

induced hepatopathy (Table 34-6). Similar findings are seen in dogs (Table 34-7).

Management

Feline idiopathic hepatic lipidosis is difficult to treat successfully. The experience of many is that only 10% to 20% of affected cats are cured. Most die or are euthanized because the prognosis is so poor. Initial management is directed toward correcting complications such as dehydration, electrolyte abnormalities, hepatic encephalopathy, and infection. The single essential treatment is to restore nutritional intake. As an initial approach, force-feeding of canned cat food can be attempted. If that fails, the patient can be fed a liquid diet through a nasogastric, pharyngostomy, or gastrostomy tube. Selection of the diet takes into consideration the cat's requirement for a high-protein diet and its need for essential amino acids unique to the cat. A diet that does not cause vomiting or diarrhea is also a basis of selection.

A liquid diet is selected to provide 60 to 80 Kcal of metabolizable energy per Kg of body weight. Lipids provide most of the calories. High carbohydrate intake may be more likely to promote an ongoing synthesis and accumulation of hepatic lipids. Diets containing 35% fats are effective in managing cats with idiopathic hepatic lipidosis.[6] As noted earlier these cats have a glucose intolerance, and the effects of that would be worsened by feeding a high carbohydrate diet. The digestion of starch produces an abundance of osmotically active particles that may produce hyperosmotic conditions in the intestinal lumen if there is any delay in absorption. The hyperosmolality can cause vomiting and diarrhea as well as promoting the movement of extracellular fluid into the intestine.

Hepatic lipidosis is a reflection of protein deficiency in the anorectic animal. The problem is not corrected unless the diet contains more than adequate amounts of protein. The diet can contain up to 2g protein per 20 Kcal of total energy. Liquid diets available for feeding cats are enteral diets with a high protein content; examples are Traumacal and Pulmocare. Milk and soy beans are the source of proteins in enteral diets. For cats these proteins are deficient in taurine, and so that amino acid is added to provide a minimum of 80 mg for 1000 Kcal of total energy. The diets should also be supplemented with additional protein, such as more casein in the form of powdered milk. Supplementation with lipotrophic substances such as choline and methionine is not necessary. The diet contains adequate amounts.

A diet can be formulated to meet all of the cat's nutritional requirements (see Chapter 38). With initiation of tube feeding the diet is diluted to reduce osmolality to 200-300 mOsm/Liter, reducing the risk of vomiting or diarrhea. The concentration of the diet is increased over a week to undiluted levels. Tube feeding may have to continue for weeks. Failures and belief in a poor prognosis may occur partly because dietary management is indeed a test of one's patience.

Based on the relative insulin resistance and insulin deficiency, insulin therapy has been used in some cats with hepatic lipidosis. Insulin at a dose of 1/4 to 1 unit, NPH insulin is given daily. It is combined with a slow intravenous glucose infusion (5% - 10%) to avoid hypoglycemia in anorectic cats. Some believe that such low-dose insulin therapy can be dangerous and is indicated only if the cat has diabetes mellitus.

Other treatment is based on theoretical considerations. If hepatic lipidosis predisposes a cat to infection, antibiotics are indicated. Penicillin is safe and relatively effective. Anabolic steroids are sometimes used but with no evidence that they may be effective. Hepatic encephalopathy can be managed with lactulose and other agents to cleanse the colon and reduce the amount of ammonia absorbed. Cats with hepatic encephalopathy caused by lipidosis are usually dying, however, and such treatment is usually futile. It is surprising how severe liver pathology must be before encephalopathy appears. That may be one reason that the problem is not recognized earlier. With early recognition and recommended management, the disease may prove to have a better prognosis.

Treatment of canine hepatic lipidosis through eliminating the cause is usually successful if the cause is overnutrition, undernutrition, a nutritional imbalance, or a toxicity. If the cause is diabetes mellitus, however, management is unsuccessful in many if not most animals. It is not known how frequently lipidosis persists in animals with successfully managed diabetes mellitus. If fatty livers persist as often in dogs with diabetes as in human diabetics, management for lipidosis is unlikely to be successful. Hepatic lipidosis in humans with diabetes is not successfully treated with drugs.[16] The lipotropic agents choline and methionine are of no value in humans with well-regulated diabetes. It is not known how well diabetes is regulated in small-animal patients. Persistence of hepatic lipidosis is more likely when diabetes is not well-regulated.

Management of hepatic lipidosis in the diabetic must correct the overnutrition found in more than half the cases. Continued intake of excessive amounts of calories supports the persistence of hepatic lipidosis,[17] and lipotropic substances do not correct the problem. The problems consist of an increased delivery of fatty acids to the liver and an augmented synthesis of triglycerides. The liver does not reduce the transport of lipids, but it is unable to mobilize the excessive lipids produced. Lipotropic agents do not stimulate increased phospholipid and lipoprotein synthesis when an adequate diet is being fed. Management of hepatic lipidosis includes reducing caloric intake and providing high levels of proteins to maintain adequate lipoprotein synthesis for transporting lipids from the liver. In this case the dietary components provide all the elements that are necessary to produce lipoproteins.

The only type of therapeutic agent that is known to mobilize lipids from the liver is some anabolic steroids.[18] They stimulate the synthesis of proteins, including beta-lipoproteins. These chemicals also increase serum lipid levels, though they may result from increased hydrolysis of either hepatic or adipose lipids. Anabolic steroids have side effects that sometimes result in cholestasis and focal hepatic necrosis. Lipotropic agents and anabolic steroids cannot be used to replace careful regulation of the abnormalities in carbohydrate and lipid metabolism. These drugs may in fact be incapable of correcting hepatic lipidosis that persists in animals with well-regulated diabetes.

The normal animal regulates carbohydrate, lipid, and protein metabolism by appropriate release of hormones, maintaining blood glucose, lipid, and amino acid levels within a relatively narrow normal range. The diabetic animals, unable to show a normal response to many of these stimuli, is treated with insulin, but that cannot restore the normal state. Consequently, there are times when insulin requirements exceed the supply, and there are other times when insulin availability is inadequate. Although the patient may be relatively well-regulated, it is not sufficient to correct hepatic lipidosis.

Hepatic lipidosis is frequently caused or augmented by factors that affect hepatocyte metabolism. These factors include endotoxins absorbed from the intestine, exogenous toxins, and some drugs. Hepatic lipidosis associated with intestinal problems may respond to antibiotics that reduce intestinal bacterial numbers, which may have greatly increased. Endotoxin absorption is reduced by antibiotics given to animals with an intestinal bypass, and this prevents the fatty livers that otherwise consistently develop. Thus, the intestinal microflora can be altered as part of the treatment for hepatic lipidosis. In addition to achieving this with antibiotics, it can be accomplished by providing a readily digested source of nutrients. Intestinal microflora overgrows when nutrients are not digested and absorbed. Hepatic lipidosis that can accompany malabsorption is due in part to absorption of excessive amounts of bacterial products, i.e., endotoxins. This occurs in animals with pancreatic enzyme deficiency, in which the main cause of hepatic fatty changes is undernutrition.

Resolution of hepatic lipidosis associated with pancreatitis, circulatory diseases, infections, nonpancreatic endocrine diseases, and miscellaneous causes is dependent on the success in treating the primary problem.

Vacuolar hepatopathy can be viewed as a pathologic response to a drug, toxin or disease process outside of the liver. The considerations in its management are essentially the same as those for lipidosis, especially since many cases of vacuolar hepatopathy may be merely early or atypical manifestations of hepatic lipidosis.

GLUCOCORTICOSTEROID-INDUCED HEPATOPATHY

Vacuolar hepatopathy is produced in dogs and cats by high plasma concentrations of adrenal glucocorticosteroids, whether given as a part of therapy or appearing because of spontaneous adrenal or pituitary disease. Corticosteroids are widely used to treat many immune-mediated diseases and as a part of nonspecific therapy for inflammatory diseases. For some diseases that cannot be cured, steroid therapy must be continued indefinitely; steroid-induced hepatopathy invariably develops. Liver pathology in dogs at the VMTH at Davis shows 11.8% of all hepatic lesions to be of steroid-induced hepatopathy.

Pathogenesis

Dogs given glucocorticoids (prednisone) daily in large doses, 4 mg/Kg of body weight, develop hepatic lesions within two to three days.[19] In clinical cases, lesions can appear following a relatively small single dose of corticosteroids as well as following prolonged administration of large doses.[20] The vacuolar hepatopathy consistently produced by glucocorticosteroids in dogs is also seen in cats following treatment with prednisilone or megestrol acetate.[21] Severe histologic lesions can develop within one week, or possibly earlier. Glucocorticosteroids given dogs by injection cause the earliest and most severe morphologic hepatic changes. The lesions may appear slower and with less consistent severity when steroids are given orally. Hepatic changes are even possible following application of steroids topically, especially to the cornea and conjunctiva.[22] Evidence for such hepatic changes is the exaggerated glucagon tolerance test responses seen in dogs treated in that way. The exaggerated response reflects accumulation of excess glycogen in the liver.

Hepatic morphologic changes appear within a few days and before any biochemical abnormalities are detected.[19] Vacuolar changes consist of hepatocyte swelling with the cytoplasm containing a fine reticulum that encloses multiple vacuole-like areas. Ballooned hepatocytes can be found among the uniformly enlarged hepatocytes. With increasing severity the ballooned hepatocytes can be two to ten times the size of normal hepatocytes. The nucleus location becomes eccentric; eventually it is displaced with mitochondria, endoplasmic reticulum, and other organelles to the periphery of the cell by large vacuoles. The severity of morphologic changes is dependent on the amount of steroids given. Hepatocyte swelling compresses and reduces the size of sinusoids. The cellular changes result in hepatomegaly.

The vacuolar changes have been attributed to accumulation of lipid, glycogen, and water. Glucocorticosteroids cause no accumulation of lipids, and the water content does not change in affected livers.[23] Hepatic glycogen accumulation is a consistent effect of steroids and is responsible for all the vacuolar changes. With uninterrupted steroid administration the glycogen content gradually increases to reach a maximum after two weeks. After that the glycogen content gradually decreases. Vacuolation and glycogen are distributed diffusely through hepatic lobules early, and later either the midzonal area (zone 2) or the centrolobular area (zone 3) is more severely affected. A study with dexamethasone reports a mainly periportal (zone 1) distribution of vacuolation after one week.[24] These differences in results from experimental studies are consistent with the great variation in patterns of vacuolation in clinical cases.

Glucocorticosteroid-induced hepatopathy causes biochemical abnormalities that are most striking after five days of steroids in experimental dogs.[19,23-26] Although there is great variability, plasma ALP activity continues to increase and reaches a peak of 700-800 U/L at three weeks in dogs given high doses of prednisone daily for two weeks. A similar pattern is seen for plasma ALT activity with mean peak levels at 200 karmen U/ml. Mean plasma γ-glutamyl transpeptidase (GGT) activity increases to peak at 30-40 Sigma U/ml at 30 days. None of these activities return to normal by 40 days after steroids are discontinued. The greatest increase above normal is seen for ALP activity (Figure 34-2). Prednisone treatment greatly stimulates GGT activity in the pancreas and only slightly in the liver. The pancreas may be the source of the increased plasma GGT activity. Similar changes in plasma enzyme activities are not seen in the cat.[21]

Glucocorticosteroids can alter some hepatic functions. Daily dexamethasone treatment causes mean plasma bile acid concentrations to increase from a normal of 1.0 µg/dl to 19.2 µg/dl within 12 days in dogs.[26] The same treatment causes sulfobromophthalein (BSP) retention at 30 minutes to double. Treatment of dogs with prednisone causes no increase in BSP retention, however. Prednisone treatment has no effect on ammonia metabolism; ammonia tolerance tests remain normal.[26] Glucagon tolerance tests have been conducted on dogs treated with relatively small amounts of prednisolone.[22] The

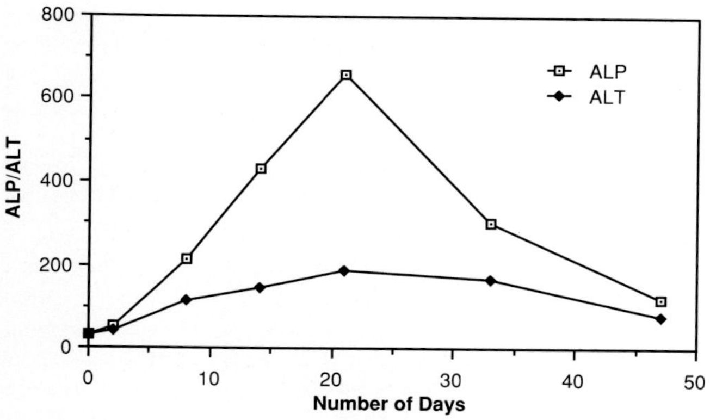

Figure 34-2. Changes in plasma ALP and ALT activities in dogs before, during and after daily treatment with prednisome (4 mg/kg/day). Redrawn from data in reference 19.

results indicate that the test can be a sensitive indicator of hepatic glycogen accumulation in dogs since glucagon injections cause a response of 350 mg glucose/dl rather than a normal hyperglycemic response of 250 mg glucose/dl at 30 minutes.

Clinical and Laboratory Findings

Clinical signs of steroid-induced hepatopathy are nonspecific symptoms of corticosteroid excess, including polydipsia, polyuria, polyphagia, skin changes such as alopecia and pigmentation, and changes in physical activity. Hepatomegaly is frequently found on physical examination. Laboratory findings include increased plasma activities of ALP, ALT, and GGT, and abnormal retention of BSP at 30 minutes (Table 34-8). The clinical signs, abnormal blood chemistry and unexplained hepatomegaly, are often pursued by tests to confirm spontaneous or iatrogenic Cushing's disease. On the other hand, the abnormal findings may lead one to biopsy the liver.

Biopsy and Pathology Findings

Histology reveals morphologic changes that resemble those for hepatic lipidosis and vacuolar hepatopathy. Marked vacuolization and ballooning of hepatocytes predominate in more severe forms (Figure 34-3). The more severe pathology shows lesions with a centrilobular (zone 3) or midzonal (zone 2) distribution. Glycogen accumulation can be identified with PAS stains before and after digestion. Focal necrosis is a frequent feature, marked by aggregation of polymorphonuclear cells. On recognition of the lesions as consistent with steroid-induced hepatopathy, it may be necessary to determine whether they are caused by spontaneous or iatrogenic Cushing's disease. Spontaneous Cushing's disease is confirmed with an ACTH response test and dexamethasone suppression tests. Quantitation of 24-hour urinary excretion of ketogenic steroids and fasting plasma insulin determination are uncommonly done. Iatrogenic Cushing's disease shows low cortisol levels and no response to ACTH. Often the history is all that is needed to know that glucocorticosteroids have been given.

Diagnosis

Glucocorticosteroid-induced hepatopathy can be suspected from a history of steroid therapy; abnormal results from laboratory tests support the diagnosis. The provisional diagnosis is supported by discontinuation of steroid therapy and a subsequent laboratory reevaluation that shows improvement. With no suggestions of corticosteroid excess, diagnosis is assisted by liver biopsy and can be confirmed by ACTH response tests. Steroid-induced hepatopathy cannot be differentiated from any other form of hepatic disease by abnormal plasma activities of ALP, ALT, and GGT and abnormal BSP retention at 30 minutes. Glucocorticosteroids do not cause these tests to be abnormal in cats, but they do cause ACTH response to be minimal or absent.

Management and Prognosis

The pathologic changes caused by steroid therapy are reversible. The only management required is discontinuation of steroid drugs or removal of the cause of excess steroid secretion. Prolonged administration of large amounts of steroids cause most cases. Instead of daily administration, steroids can be given on alternate days, which is likely to reduce the severity of the hepatopathy. Drugs other than glucocorticoids can be used to treat immune-mediated diseases. Management to remove excess glucocorticosteroids results in complete remission. Biochemical abnormalities and hepatic pathology revert to normal, but more than two months is required.[19]

Hemochromatosis[27,28]

The liver is the major organ for storing iron in both the normal state and in animals with excess total body iron. One-third of storage iron is located in the liver, from which it is mobilized in times of need. Most of the nonheme iron is in the form of ferritin and is found in hepatocytes. That iron derives primarily from iron circulating bound to transferrin. Heme iron that accumulates from destruction of erythrocytes, for example, tends to be stored in Kupffer cells as hemosiderin. Ferritin is a diffusely soluble form of iron; hemosiderin is an insoluble aggregate form of iron. Ferritin laden with iron is metabolized within a few days, making iron continuously available from that pool. Hemosiderin is a degraded form of iron.

Plasma contains two iron-binding proteins, transferrin and ferritin. Transferrin carries iron absorbed by intestinal epithelial cells to the liver. Plasma ferritin differs from liver ferritin in that it is virtually free of iron. Although it contains little iron, low plasma ferritin levels with low levels of transferrin reflect a low level of iron stored in the body. Ferritin increases with inflammatory and neoplastic diseases as well as with liver disease. Hepatocytes take up transferrin-bound and non-transferrin-bound iron by endocytosis.

In normal dogs the mean hepatic level of iron is about 1000 μg/g dry weight (range 311-1579).[29] In Bedlington Terriers with abnormal copper accumulation the mean level of iron increases fourfold to about 4000 μg/g dry weight (range 2197-6792). In normal humans hepatic iron levels are similar to those in dogs, and hepatic injury is not evident until they increase ten times, such as seen with hemochromatosis. As the hepatic iron content increases, the proportion incorporated in hemosiderin increases. The excess iron is stored in lysosomes, probably as hemosid-

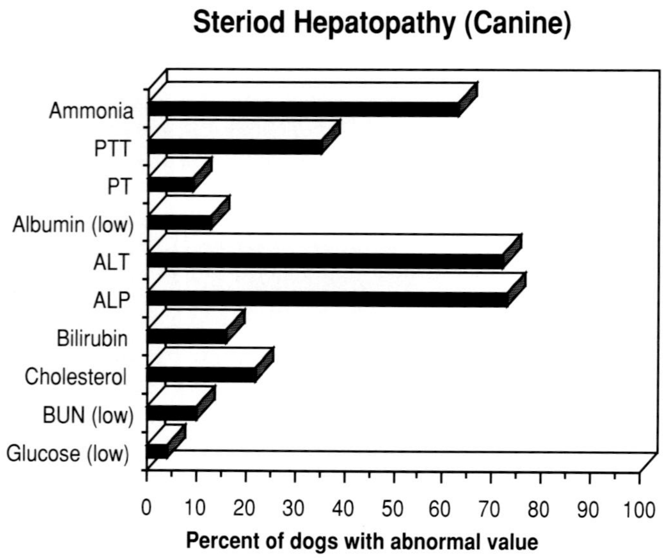

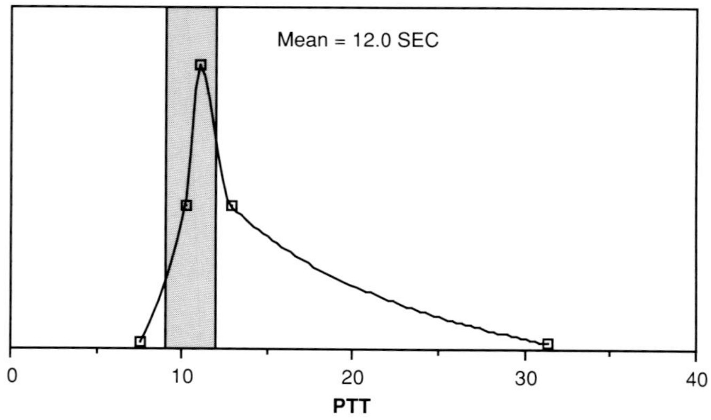

Table 34-8. Comparison of sensitivities for different tests in dogs with steroid hepatopathy. Below: graphs showing distribution of clinical pathology values in dogs with steroid hepatopathy. Points on graphs represent 0%, 25%, 50%, 75% and 100% medians. Normal range is in shaded area.

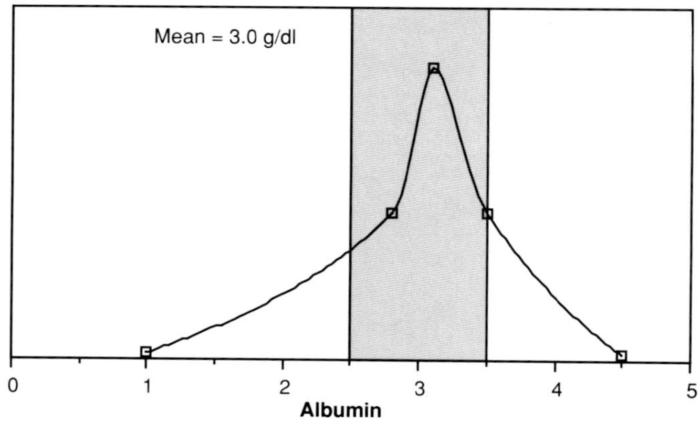

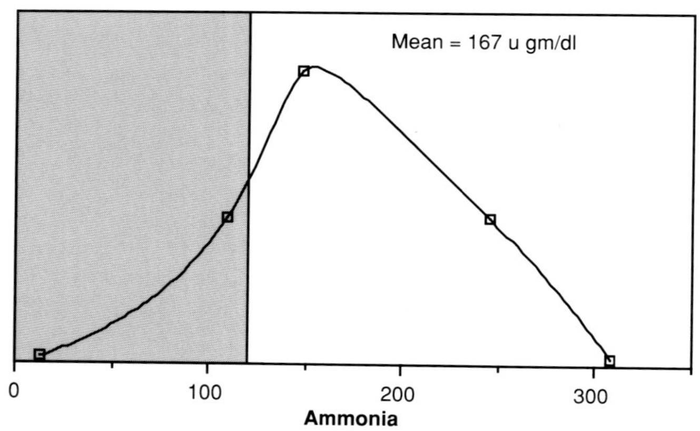

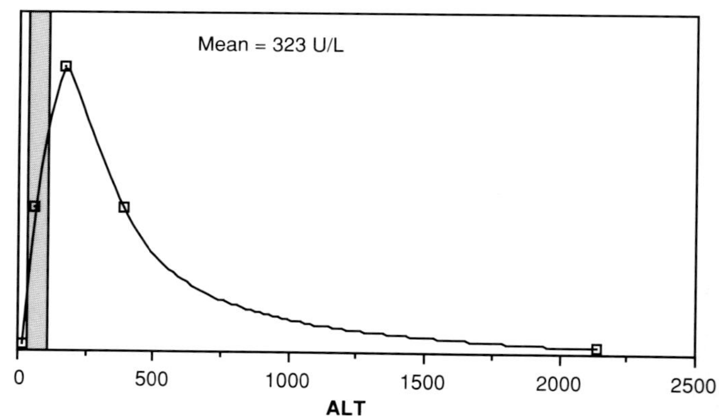

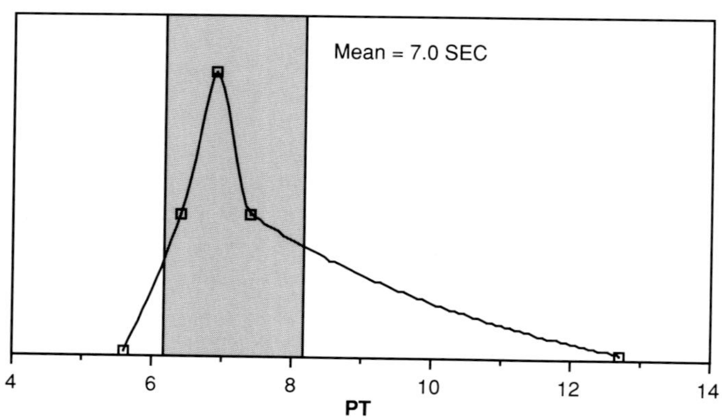

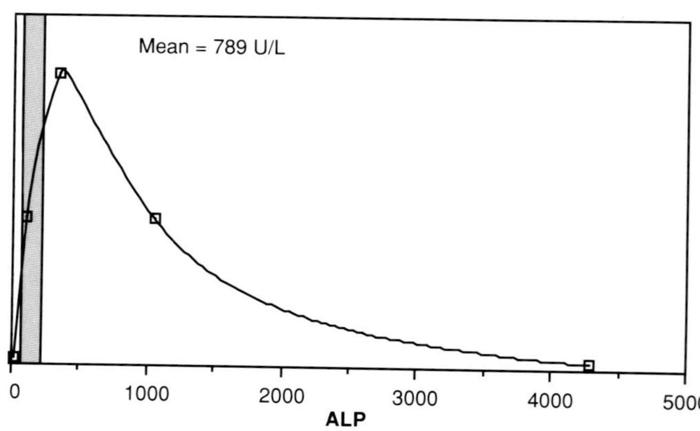

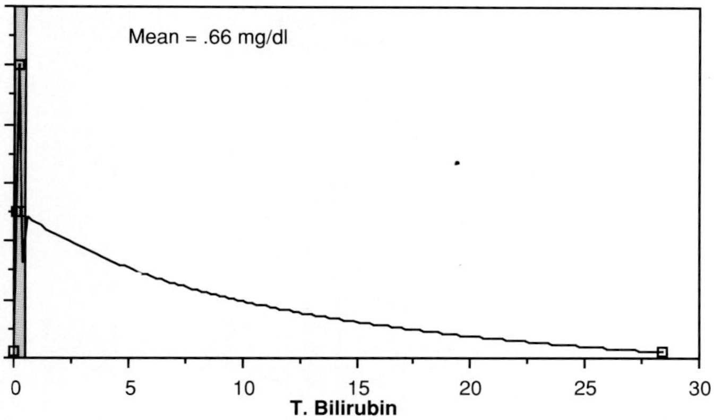

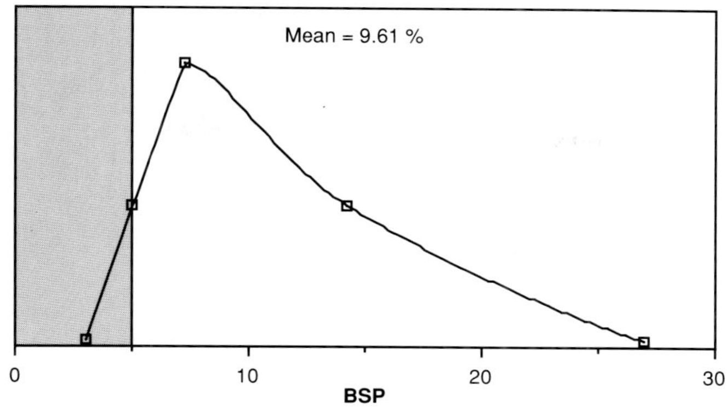

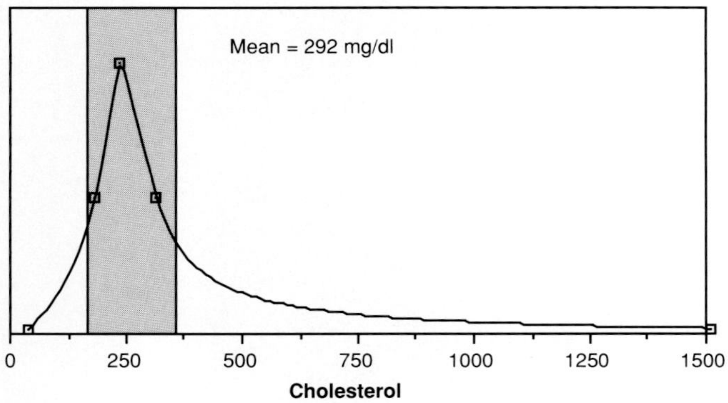

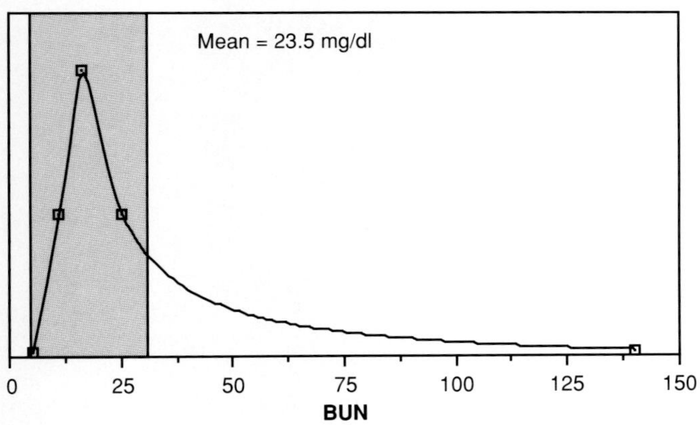

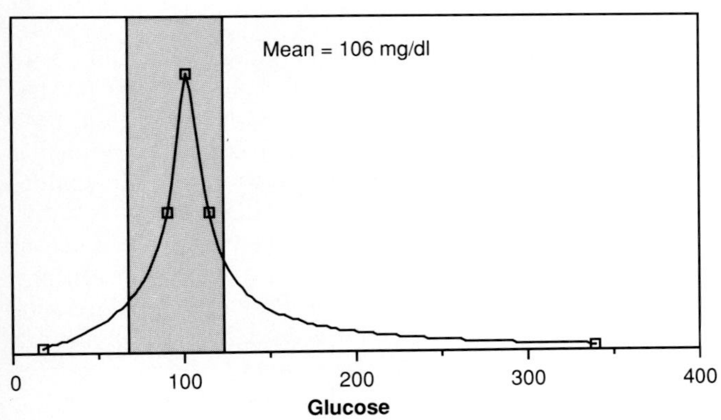

erin. Excess iron accumulating because of transfusions accumulates predominately in Kupffer cells but some of that is redistributed to hepatocytes, which can be overloaded secondarily. Excess iron from increased intestinal absorption or parenteral administration accumulates in hepatocytes, where damage is evident at much lower levels.

Experimental studies show that massive doses of iron given parenterally as iron dextran damage hepatocytes and produce fibrosis.[30] Lower levels of iron combined with other potential hepatotoxins or dietary deficiencies are effective in damaging the liver. It may be that the hepatic iron levels that increase four times in Bedlington Terriers may act synergistically with copper and possibly endotoxin from the intestine to injure the liver. Stored iron is not toxic. Iron released from hemosiderin in lysosomes is damaging and is believed to destabilize lysosomal membranes, releasing lysosomal enzymes that damage cells further. Release of iron in its ferrous form presents an active catalyst for generating free radicals that damage cell structures by lipid peroxidation. Release of iron from hemosiderin is promoted by ascorbic acid and inhibited by its deficiency.[31] Its release is augmented by ascorbic acid supplementation, and that could increase the risk for hepatocyte damage. On the other hand, ascorbic acid deficiency can accompany hepatic insufficiency, and that may promote hemosiderin accumulation in the liver. Ascorbic acid also stimulates intestinal absorption of iron.

The accumulation of abnormal quantities of iron in hepatic parenchymal cells, leading to degenerative changes and eventually fibrosis, is accompanied by a loss of liver functions. Large amounts of iron administered to dogs result in hepatic cirrhosis,[32] with the severity of fibrosis proportional to the concentration of iron in the liver. Hemochromatosis in small animals is most commonly an iatrogenic phenomenon, caused by administering excessive iron to manage an anemia. Repeated blood transfusions to patients with hemolytic or aplastic anemia result in the deposition of excessive iron. Iron released from senescent erythrocytes is stored in the liver, and this iron in the normal animal is used for synthesis of hemoglobin during erythrogenesis. Thus, the pool turns over and excessive amounts do not accumulate. When erythrogenesis is unable to produce new cells fast enough to maintain normal erythrocyte numbers, this store of iron is not used, so that transfused blood adds to the unused pool of iron accumulating in the body. Similar accumulations occur with hemolytic anemia when iron is administered

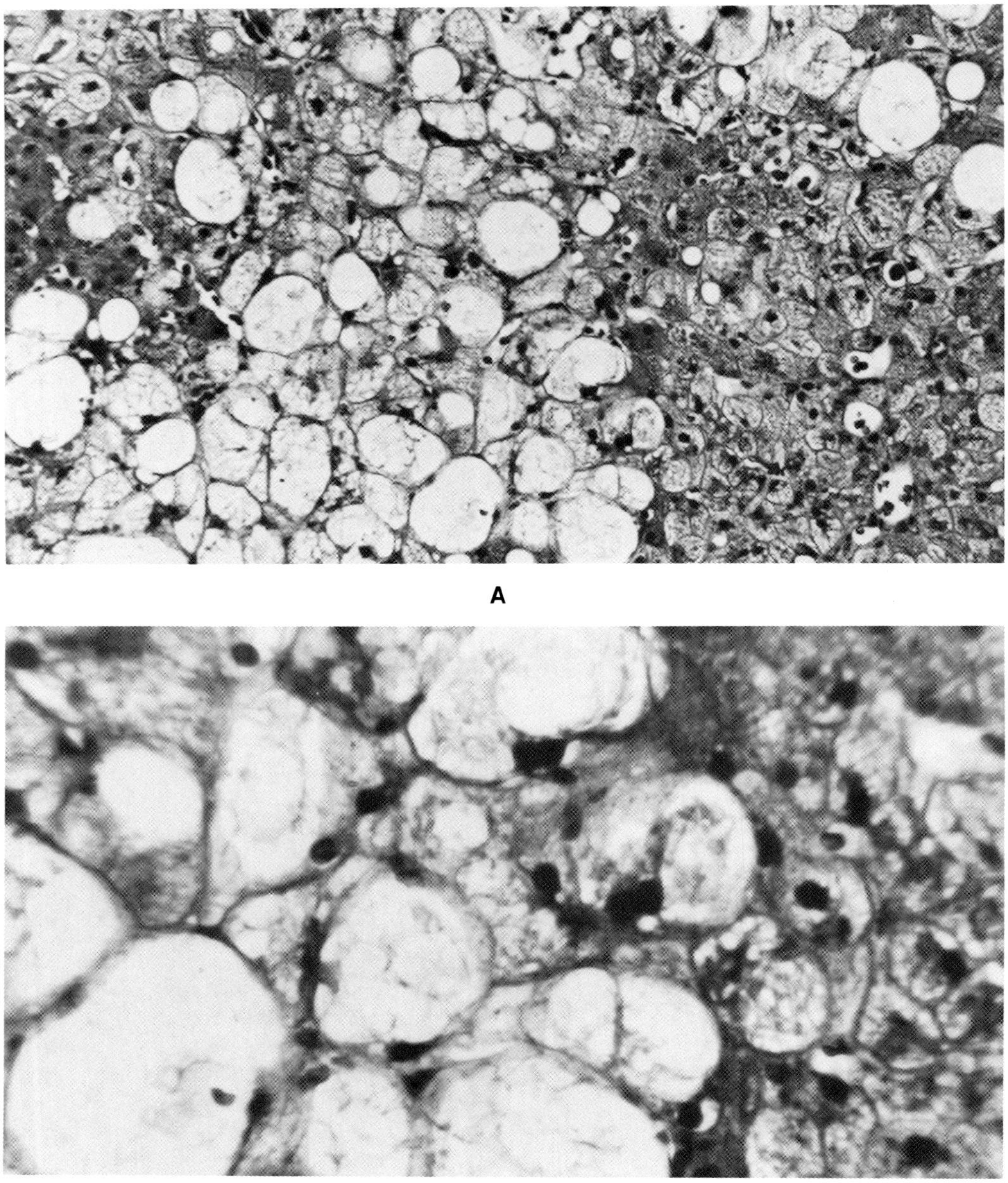

A

B

Figure 34-3. Glucocorticosteroid induced hepatopathy. (a) and (b) Vacuolar changes vary from mild to severe in biopsy specimen from dog with Cushing's disease. Reticulation within hepatocytes is evident in contrast to its absence in lipidosis. (c) and (d) distribution of changes can be diffuse or random with many hepatocytes unaffected.

as part of therapy. Erythrogenesis continues in these patients, but the iron given far exceeds that required to sustain normal erythrocyte production. Some patients are treated with other types of parenteral preparations containing iron that with continued use can cause abnormal accumulations of iron in the liver.

Hemochromatosis can follow increased intestinal absorption of iron. Gastric, pancreatic, and intestinal secretions determine normal iron absorption. Gastric juices maintain iron in a soluble and ferrous form to facilitate absorption. Pancreatic secretions bind part of the dietary iron and thus play a role in determining the amount absorbed. With pancreatic insufficiency, iron absorption can increase. Intracellular apoferritin concentrations regulate the absorption of iron by special mechanisms in epithelial cells. With increased need for iron, little apoferritin is synthesized and the iron absorbed into epithelial cells remains unbound, passing readily into the circulation. When iron reserves are adequate, apoferritin synthesis is stimulated so that this iron-binding protein accumulates in mucosal cells. Iron transported into the cell binds to apoferritin, forming ferritin, which prevents its absorption. Primary hemochromatosis can develop in humans with a deficiency in apoferritin synthesis when the intestinal absorption of iron is excessive. The absorption of iron must be well-regulated because there are

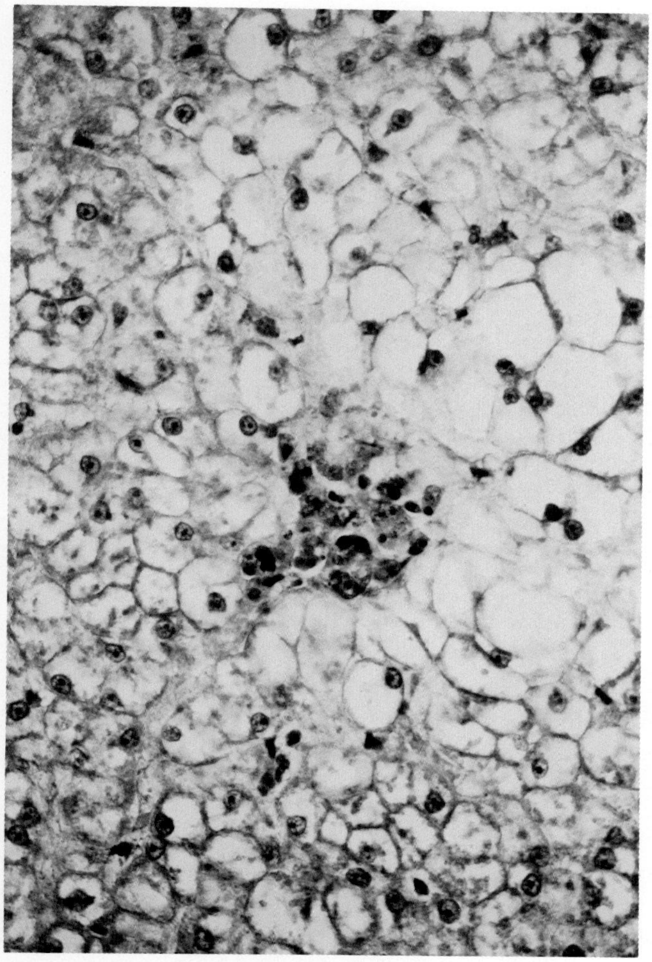

Figure 34-3. c) See legend with A and B

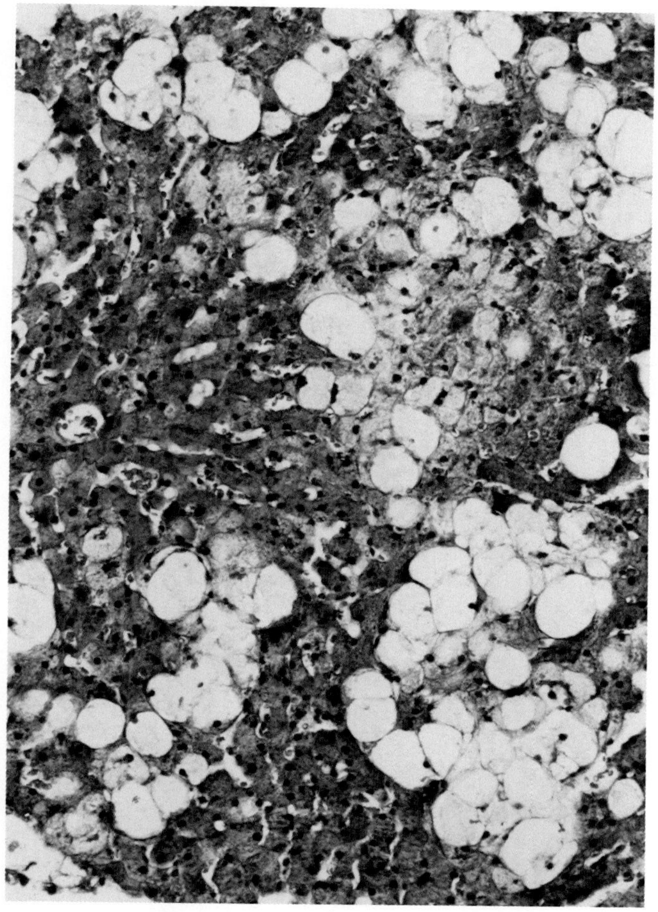

Figure 34-3. d) See legend with A and B

no special mechanisms designed for the excretion of iron from the body. Excess iron introduced or absorbed must accumulate because it cannot be excreted.

The pathogenesis of hepatic fibrosis with an iron excess is probably more complicated than if it were due entirely to the iron. Iron is a factor in the development of fibrosis, and the lesions that accompany iron excess appear earlier when nutritional factors are lacking.[27] For example, fibrosis develops more readily when choline or folate deficiency accompanies the iron excess. Also as mentioned, excess iron potentiates the action of weak hepatotoxins to produce fibrosis.

Biopsy and Pathology Findings

Deposition of visible amounts of iron pigments is described as hemosiderin. That is not unusual in animals, especially those with a history of previous anemia. With excessive retention of iron, deposits are heaviest in the liver and pancreas; concentrations can reach 10 to 20 times normal. Hemosiderin deposition can be primary or secondary, resulting from excessive iron or hepatic pathology. Hepatic fibrosis can cause hemosiderin formation. Thus, hemochromatosis must be distinguished from cirrhosis with accompanying hemosiderin deposits. Hemochromatosis is diagnosed when hepatic iron concentration exceeds 1.0% of the dry weight. Iron deposits are found in lysosomes in periportal hepatocytes. Fibrosis begins in the portal area, histologically resembling chronic biliary disease, and can dissect through the lobule to cause nodule formation. Hemochromatosis is a storage disease in which the accumulation of iron and its damaging effects result in hepatomegaly.

Clinical Findings

Hemochromatosis is associated with the nonspecific clinical signs of chronic hepatic disease. In addition to hepatomegaly, the skin becomes pigmented by increased deposition of melanin and hemosiderin. In humans, excess iron accumulation in the pancreas destroys islet cells, and diabetes mellitus may follow. Testicular atrophy caused by decreased gonadotrophic hormones develops secondary to the destruction of pituitary cells by the deposition of excessive iron. With hemochromatosis, hepatocellular carcinoma is higher in incidence than expected, which reflects the hepatotoxicity caused by long-term iron excess. The diagnosis of hemochromatosis is based on elevated plasma iron levels, histologic evidence for excessive deposition of iron in hepatocytes, increased iron concentration in liver biopsy samples, and clinical signs.

Management of Hemochromatosis

Since hemochromatosis is most often a secondary iatrogenic problem, it can be prevented. Prevention is based on the realization that excessive iron administered to animals is not excreted but is retained in the body. Repeated blood transfusions cause excessive deposition of iron, primarily in the liver and pancreas. With no alternative to using whole blood, hemochromatosis is a predictable consequence. Injectable products containing iron cannot be used indiscriminately. Only small amounts of iron are required for normal erythrogenesis. When injectable iron does not correct what appears to be an iron deficiency anemia, the basis for the defect should be sought rather than continuing a potentially hepatotoxic treatment. Hemochromatosis can be treated successfully only by bleeding to remove iron from the body. Other factors contribute to the pathogenesis of cirrhosis with iron excess. Since these factors are nutritional, any deficiencies are corrected, and a high quality protein diet is fed with vitamin supplementation. Proteins and vitamins are the most important nutrients to prevent cirrhosis and support hepatic regeneration. If possible, dietary levels of iron are reduced to a minimum.

Hepatic Amyloidosis[33]

Hepatic amyloidosis is uncommon in small animals. Amyloid is an amorphous, eosinophilic, glassy, hyaline, extracellular substance that stains a blue-purple color with iodine and diluted sulfuric acid. Amyloid can be deposited in many organs; in the liver it appears between the sinusoids and the cords of hepatocytes in the space of Disse. It can also be found in small arteries and veins. Amyloid is a fibrous protein that consists partly of immunoglobulin light chains in primary and multiple myeloma-associated amyloid, and of other proteins in secondary amyloid. One such other protein is termed AA and has an acute-phase reactant counterpart in the serum. It is unknown why these proteins are deposited in the liver and other tissues. Causes suggested include hyperglobulinemia, abnormal protein metabolism, abnormal Kupffer cell function, immune complex disease, and abnormal delayed hypersensitivity.

Small animals with hepatic amyloidosis are usually presented with persistent gastrointestinal signs. Hepatomegaly and splenomegaly are consistent findings, and the liver appears homogenous on ultrasonic examination. Plasma activities of ALT and ALP are increased. Diagnosis is made on biopsy of the liver; suspicions of amyloid can be confirmed on finding green birefringence after polarization in Congo-red-stained sections. There is no successful treatment for primary amyloidosis. When amyloidosis is secondary to a chronic inflammatory or infectious disease, it may be possible to arrest the progression of amyloid deposition by successful management of the primary problem.

REFERENCES

1. Hazlett, M.J. and Maxie, G.: Feline fatty liver syndrome. Can. Vet. J. 28:207, 1987.
2. Hoyumpa, A.M., Greene, H.L., Dunn, G.D. and Schenker, S.: Fatty liver: biochemical and clinical considerations. Am. J. Dig. Dis. 20:1142-1170, 1975.
3. Alpers, D.H. and Sabesin, S.M.: Fatty liver: Biochemical and clinical aspects. In, Diseases of the Liver. Edited by L. Schiff and E.R. Schiff. J.B. Lippincott, Philadelphia. 949-978, 1987.
4. Burrows, C.F., Chiapella, A.M. and Jezyk, P.: Idiopathic feline hepatic lipidosis: The syndrome and speculations on its pathogenesis. Florida Vet. J. 18-20, Winter 1981.
5. Center, S.A.: Feline liver disorders and their management. Comp. Contin. Educ. 8:889-901, 1986.
6. Biourge, V., MacDonald, M.J. and King, L.: Feline hepatic lipidosis: Pathogenesis and nutritional management of three recoveries. Submitted.
7. Zawie, D.A. and Garvey, M.S.: Feline hepatic disease. Vet. Clin. N. Am. 14:1201-1230, 1984.
8. Buffington, C. and Rogers, Q.: Unpublished observations.
9. Schaffner, F. and Thaler, H.: Nonalcoholic fatty liver disease. In, Progress in Liver Diseases. 283-295, 1986.
10. Allan, F.N., Bowie, D.J., Macleod, J.J.R. and Robinson, W.L.: Behavior of depancreatized dogs kept alive with insulin. Brit. J. Exp. Path. 5:75-83, 1924.
11. Best, C.H., Ferguson, C.C. and Hershey, J.M.: Choline and liver fat in diabetic dogs. J. Physiol. (London) 79:94-102, 1933.
12. Shamoian, C.A., Masoro, E.J., Derrow, A. and Canzanelli, A.: Fatty acid synthesis by surviving hepatic tissue of "acute" and "chronic" diabetic dogs. Endocrinology 74:21-27, 1964.
13. Chaikoff, I.L., Conner, C.L. and Biskind, G.R.: Fatty infiltration and cirrhosis of the liver in depancreatized dogs maintained with insulin. Am. J. Pathol. 13:101-110, 1938.
14. Ling, G.V., Lowenstine, L.J., Pulley, L.T. and Kaneko, J.J.: Diabetes mellitus in dogs: a review of initial evaluation, immediate and long-term management and outcome. JAVMA 170:521-530, 1977.
15. Cotton, R.B., Cornelius, L.M. and Theran, P.: Diabetes mellitus in the dog: A clinicopathologic study. JAVMA 159:863-870, 1971.
16. Creutzfeldt, W., Frerichs, H. and Sickinger, K.: Liver disease and diabetes mellitus. In, Progress in Liver Diseases. Vol. 3. Edited by H. Popper and F. Schaffner. Grune and Stratton, New York. 371-407, 1970.
17. Chang, S. and Silvis, S.E.: Fatty liver produced by hyperalimentation of rats. Am. J. Gastroenterology 62:410-418, 1974.
18. Mendenhall, C.L.: Augmented release of hepatic triglycerides with anabolic steroids in patients with fatty liver. Am. J. Dig. Dis. 19:122-126, 1974.
19. Badylak, S.F. and Van Vleet, J.F.: Sequential morphologic and clinicopathologic alterations in dogs with experimentally induced glucocorticoid hepatopathy. AJVR 42:1310-1318, 1981.
20. Rogers, W.A. and Ruebner, B.H.: A retrospective study of probably glucocorticoid-induced hepatopathy in dogs. JAVMA 170:603-606, 1977.
21. Middleton, D.J., Watson, A.D.J., Howe, C.J. and Caterson, I.D.: Suppression of cortisol responses to exogenous adrenocorticotrophic hormone, and the occurrence of side effects attributable to glucocorticoid excess, in cats during therapy with megestrol acetate and prednisolone. Can. J. Vet. Res. 51:60-65, 1987.
22. Roberts, S.M., Lavach, J.D., Macy, D.W. and Severin, G.A.: Effect of ophthalmic prednisolone acetate on the canine adrenal gland and hepatic function. AJVR 45:1711-1714, 1984.
23. Fittschen, C. and Bellamy, J.E.C.: Prednisone-induced morphologic and chemical changes in the liver of dogs. Vet. Pathol. 21:399-406, 1984.
24. Dillon, A.R., Sorjonen, D.C., Powers, R.D. and Spano, S.: Effects of dexamethasone and surgical hypotension on hepatic morphologic features and enzymes in dogs. AJVR 44:1996-1999, 1983.
25. Badylak, S.F. and Van Vleet, J.F.: Tissue γ-glutamyl transpeptidase activity and hepatic ultrastructural alterations in dogs with experimentally induced glucocorticoid hepatopathy.

AJVR 43:649-655, 1982.

26. DeNovo, R.C. and Prasse, K.W.: Comparison of serum biochemical and hepatic functional alterations in dogs treated with corticosteroids and hepatic duct ligation. AJVR 44:1703-1709, 1983.
27. Powell, L.W., Bassett, M.L. and Halliday, J.W.: Hemochromatosis: 1980 update. Gastroenterology 78:374-381, 1980.
28. Bothwell, T.H. and Charlton, R.W.: Hemochromatosis in the liver. In, Diseases of the Liver. Edited by L. Schiff and E.R. Schiff. J.B. Lippincott Co., Philadelphia, PA 101-1035, 1987.
29. Ludwig, J., Owen, C.A., Barham, S.S., McCall, J.T. and Hardy, R.M.: The liver in the inherited copper disease of Bedlington Terriers. Lab. Invest. 43:82-87, 1980.
30. Tavill, A.S. and Bacon, B.R.: Hemochromatosis: How much iron is too much? Hepatology 6:142-145, 1986.
31. Gollan, J.L.: Diagnosis of hemochromatosis. Gastroenterology 84:418-421, 1983.
32. Lisboa, P.E.: Experimental hepatic cirrhosis in dogs caused by chronic massive iron overload. Gut 12:363-368, 1971.
33. Cohen, A.S. and Skinner, M.: Amyloidosis of the liver. In, Diseases of the liver. Edited by L. Schiff and E.R. Schiff. J.B. Lippincott Co., Philadelphia, PA, 1093-1108, 1987.

Chapter 35

Hepatic Vascular Diseases

PORTASYSTEMIC VASCULAR ANASTOMOSES

Portasystemic Shunts

Clinical Synopsis

Diagnostic features

* Young dogs of specific breeds (see text) predisposed
* Depression or behavioral abnormalities common
* Vomiting and weight loss common
* Hypersalivation common in cats
* Low serum albumin, low BUN, low cholesterol common
* ALT and ALP usually normal or only mildly elevated
* Liver function tests abnormal
* Microhepatica
* Urate crystals may be seen in the urine
* Radiographic or scintigraphic demonstration of a portasystemic vascular anastomosis

Standard management

* Restricted protein, low residue, balanced diet fed in small amounts frequently
* Use milk or soy as protein source
* Surgical ligation or partial ligation of shunt
* Management of hepatic encephalopathy (see Chapter 33)

Circulation leaving the stomach, intestine, spleen, and pancreas enters the portal vein and flows through the liver before returning to the systemic circulation. Blood leaving the gastrointestinal tract is unique in containing nutrients absorbed from the intestine, hormones released by the stomach, intestines and pancreas, toxins produced in the intestine, and bacteria escaping from the intestine. The liver normally removes these substances, so when some escape to the systemic circulation, clinical signs of hepatic disease appear. The liver is designed to process materials from the gastrointestinal tract, and maintenance of hepatic circulation and the workload presented to the liver preserves normal hepatic size. The importance of the relationship of portal blood flow to normal hepatic function and overall homeostasis was recognized a century ago, by Eck, in dogs with experimentally created shunts between the portal vein and vena cava.[1] This partial diversion of blood from the liver produced hepatic encephalopathy. Information from many similar experimental studies has been used to understand the problems associated with congenital and acquired portasystemic shunts in dogs and humans. Most shunts recognized in dogs are congenital, involving a fetal vessel that remains patent after birth. Shunts can also develop secondary to chronic hepatic disease, shunting blood through macroscopic prehepatic vessels or through microscopic vessels within the liver.

The first report of a portal vascular anomaly was made by Hickman in 1949.[2] A dog had a normal arterial supply to the liver, but the portal vein was absent and blood from the intestines entered the azygous vein. No clinical signs of disease were recognized in the dog. The clinical entity caused by portal-vein anomalies was not recognized in clinical small-animal medicine until a report by Ewing et al in 1974.[3] Since then reports have described the entity in both cats and dogs. The incidence of portal vascular anomalies in dogs varies from 0.02% to 0.6% in dogs and from 0.02% to 0.1% in cats.

Portasystemic shunts are reported most often in the Yorkshire Terrier, Miniature Schnauzer, Doberman Pinscher, Golden Retriever, German Shepherd, Poodle, Labrador Retriever, and Cocker Spaniel.[4] The breeds considered to be at higher risk, with shunts occurring at twice or more the expected incidence, include the Miniature Schnauzer, Yorkshire Terrier, Maltese Terrier, Pug, Irish Wolfhound, Cairn Terrier, and Scottish Terrier. The smaller breed dogs usually have single extrahepatic shunts (90%). Intrahepatic shunts are more commonly seen in large breed dogs (65%), especially in the Golden Retriever, Labrador Retriever, and Irish Wolfhound. These two forms of shunts are usually believed to be congenital problems. Multiple shunts account for approximately one-fourth of all shunts and are believed to be acquired secondary to preexisting liver disease. They are reported most often in the Doberman Pinscher, German Shepherd, and Cocker Spaniel. The Doberman Pinscher is recognized as being at high risk for chronic hepatitis. Multiple portasystemic shunt development would be expected as that pathology progresses to cirrhosis.

There is no sex predilection for dogs developing portasystemic shunts.[4] Most dogs with single shunts are diagnosed early, 60% when less than a year of age and 75% when less than two years of age. Dogs with multiple shunts are recognized at an older age, 29% being less than one year and 56% less than two years of age. Although portasystemic shunts are considered to be far more important in the differential diagnosis of problems

Table 35-1 Types and frequency of portasystemic shunts in dogs.

Ductus venosus	26.7%
Single extrahepatic	44.7%
(porta caval)	(37.9%)
porta-azygous	(6.8%)
Multiple	26.3%
No portal vein	2.3%

in young animals, dogs have lived with shunts for as long as ten years before they were recognized.

Portasystemic shunts were first reported in cats in 1980, and since then there have been descriptions of many more.[5-8] The numbers are too few, however, to make any comments on breed or sex distribution. Most of the cats involved had extrahepatic shunts.

Half of the single portasystemic vascular anastomoses in dogs are due to persistent ductus venosus (Table 35-1, Figure 35-1).[4] About one-fourth are due to shunts communicating between the portal vein and the vena cava caudal to the liver. This may be a variation of persistent ductus venosus, in which the fetal vessel enters the vena cava more caudally than usual. The shunts may connect the portal vein and vena cava via the gastroduodenal vein or gastrosplenic vein. Some shunts are communications between the portal circulation and the azygous vein, some of which are found in animals without a prerenal caudal vena cava. Most portasystemic shunts in cats connect vessels to the caudal vena cava from the cranial mesenteric vein, splenic (gastrosplenic) vein, gastric vein, or pancreaticoduodenal vein. A few are communications between the mesenteric or portal circulation to the azygous vein and a few are due to patent ductus venosus. The pathogenesis is probably not the same for the patent ductus venosus and the other shunts.

ETIOLOGY AND PATHOGENESIS

The ductus venosus is a fetal vessel providing a shunt for blood from the gastrointestinal tract and in the umbilical vein to bypass the liver before birth.[9] The ductus venosus closes about 60 hours after birth in the dog,[10] causing the entire portal blood flow to perfuse the liver. Failure of that shunt to close in some animals is suggested to result from several abnormalities. Infection entering through the umbilical vein at parturition and causing phlebitis is suggested to prevent ductus venosus closure. Fetal vessels performing such a shunting function are no longer necessary after birth and close in response to physical and humoral events. Shunts close in response to vasoactive substances, such as prostaglandins, or after changes in blood oxygen tension or pressure. The ductus venosus carries blood with a high oxygen tension in the fetus, and this changes to a vessel carrying blood with a low oxygen tension after birth. The ductus venosus carries a greater flow of blood in the fetus than in the neonate after circulation through the umbilical vein ceases. Thus, changes in oxygen tension, flow, and pressure can contribute to closure of the fetal vessel.

Other portasystemic shunts likely are anomalies due to imperfect embryonic development. The hepatic-portal venous circulation, including that of the hepatic portion of the caudal vena cava, develops from the anastomoses and transformation of the embryo's vitelline veins. A similar development of the embryo's caudal cardinal venous system results in formation of the remainder of the caudal vena cava and the azygous vein. At one time in embryonic development there can be more communication between the two venous systems than is found in the normal animal. Such communications become nonfunctional remnant vessels. In the fetus persistence of one such vessel or its unusual development may explain the various shunts connecting the mesenteric or portal circulation to the vena cava or azygous vein. After birth the nonfunctional remnant vessels can become functional with portal hypertension, and that results in the appearance of many blood vessels described as multiple shunts. Why a normally remnant vessel develops to produce portasystemic shunting is unknown.

Portasystemic shunt vessels appear in animals with portal hypertension.[11] Opening of these vessels serves to buffer the hypertension; relatively high portal pressures do not develop in animals until this form of compensation has been exhausted. The pattern of multiple shunts found in clinical cases resembles that seen in dogs developing collateral circulation that follows portal hypertension produced by constriction of the portal vein. In some clinical cases of multiple shunts there may be a question

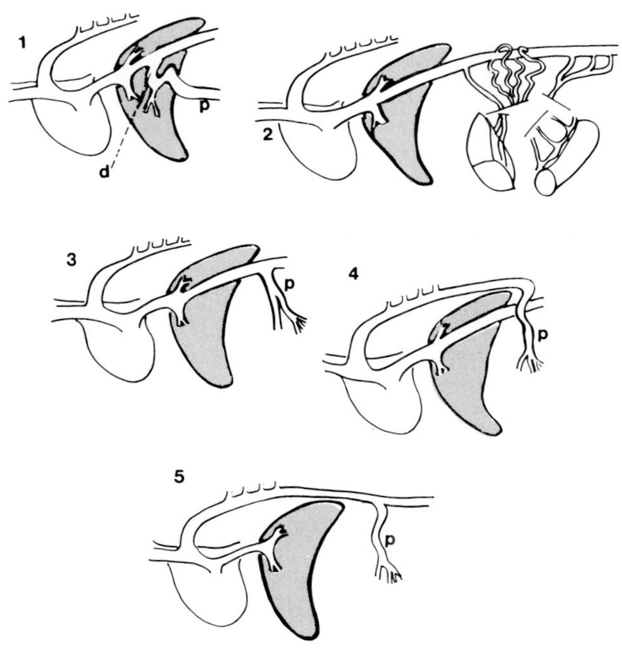

Figure 35-1. Anomalous development of the portal system can produce several different portacaval shunting disorders. Five portacaval shunting patterns visualized radiographically are illustrated. These include: (1) persistent ductus venosus, (d) with or without hypoplasia of the portal system of the liver; (2) peripheral portosystemic collaterals (splenorenal or mesenteric); (3) large central portacaval anastomosis (p); (4) portal azygos anastomosis; and (5) portal azygos anastomosis with discontinuation of the prerenal PVC. (By permission Dr. P.F. Suter, JAVRS.)

of whether they are acquired or congenital. Although increased resistance to portal blood flow is suspected with this type of shunt, it is difficult to determine whether increased resistance is a primary or secondary event. Portasystemic shunting of blood reduces hepatic circulation, causing hepatic atrophy and possibly a secondary increase in resistance to blood flow. That is evident from the portal hypertension that develops when shunts are closed. Most cases of multiple shunts are secondary to hepatic disease that increases the resistance to hepatic venous flow. Some cases of multiple shunts may represent a primary and congenital problem. A lack of hepatic pathologic changes supportive of portal hypertension is often invoked as an argument for the shunt being congenital.

PATHOPHYSIOLOGY

Portasystemic shunts have important effects on carbohydrate metabolism (Table 35-2). In dogs with portasystemic shunts, fasting blood levels of glucose are slightly lower than normal, and plasma levels of insulin are slightly higher than normal.[12] Following intestinal absorption of glucose, insulin is released, with blood levels reaching twice normal in 90 minutes, at which time the blood levels of glucose are 50 mg/dl greater than in dogs without portasystemic shunts. Both the hyperinsulinemic and the hyperglycemic response persist longer than in normal control dogs. A similar, though less marked, response is seen in animals given glucose intravenously. Thus, these animals show impaired glucose tolerance and hyperinsulinemia. Similar experiments on dogs with portacaval transposition show normal glucose tolerance and normal blood insulin levels.[13] Thus, normal carbohydrate metabolism does not require that portal blood be delivered directly to the liver or

Table 35-2. Effects of portasystemic shunts on liver functions

Carbohydrate metabolism

- **Fasting – hypoglycemia (relative)**
  hyperinsulinemia
- **Prandial – hyperglycemia**
  double insulin response

Lipid metabolism

- **Hypocholesterolemia**
- **Hypotriglyceridemia**
- **High serum bile acid levels**
- **Elevated volatile fatty acid levels**

Nitrogen metabolism

- **Low plasma branched-chain amino acid levels**
- **High plasma aromatic amino acid levels**

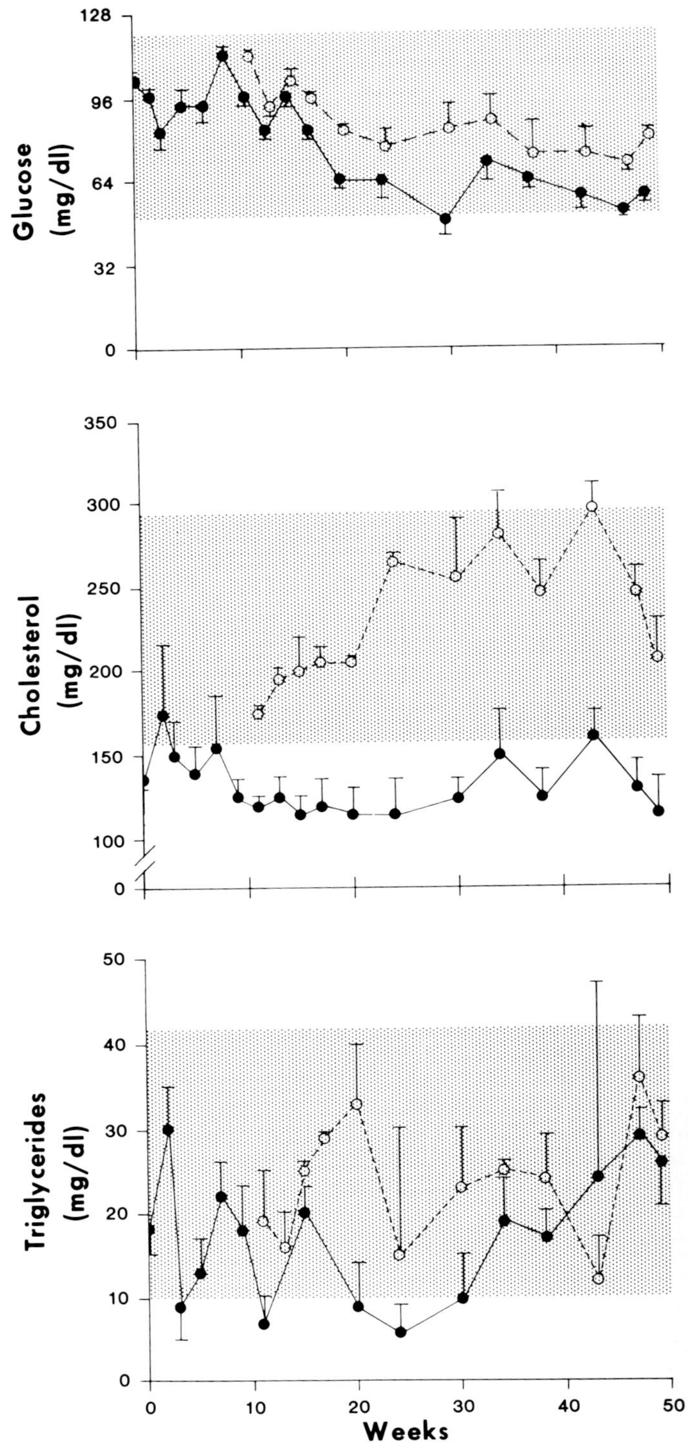

Figure 35-2. Serum cholesterol, triglyceride, and glucose concentration changes with time after portacaval shunting. Mean values for normal dogs (open circles) and dogs with shunts (closed circles) are shown over a period of one year. Shaded areas represent range for normal values. From reference 15. Used with permission.

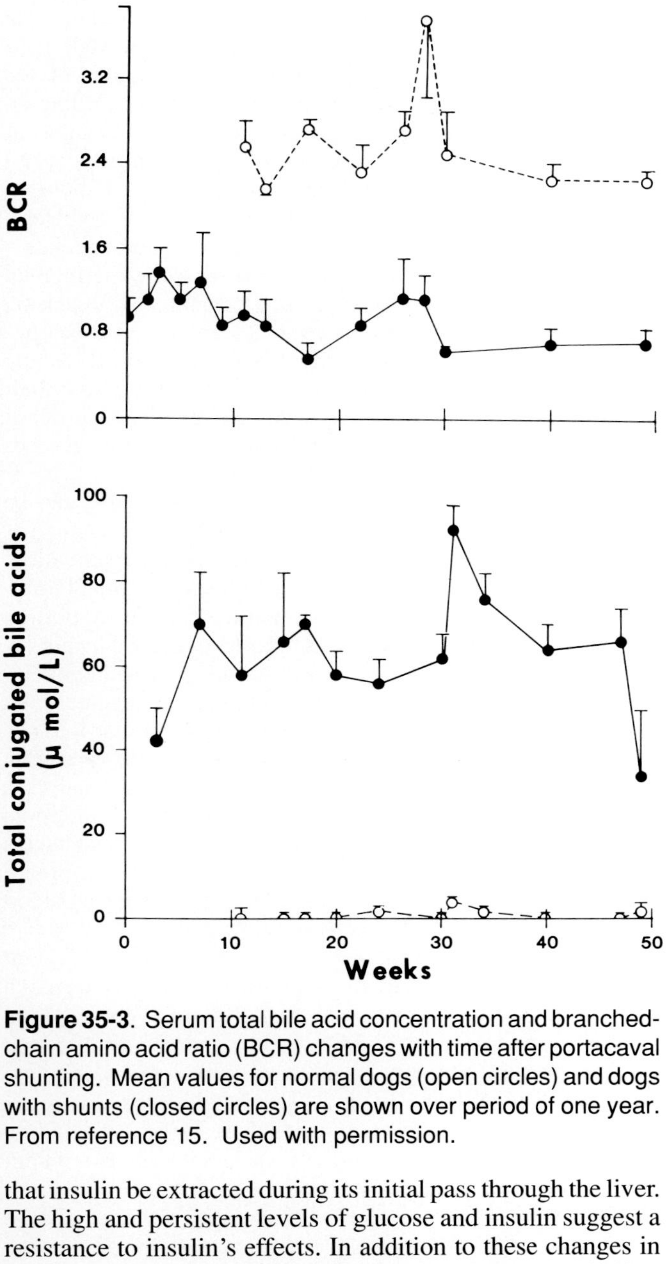

Figure 35-3. Serum total bile acid concentration and branched-chain amino acid ratio (BCR) changes with time after portacaval shunting. Mean values for normal dogs (open circles) and dogs with shunts (closed circles) are shown over period of one year. From reference 15. Used with permission.

that insulin be extracted during its initial pass through the liver. The high and persistent levels of glucose and insulin suggest a resistance to insulin's effects. In addition to these changes in insulin's effects, the abnormalities in carbohydrate metabolism are also explained by changes in glucagon and growth hormone both of which contribute to hyperglycemia. Amino acids as well as ammonia stimulate glucagon release, and portasystemic shunting exaggerates that release.[14] Reduced hepatic mass also contributes to a persisting postprandial hyperglycemia because of a reduction in the liver's capacity to take up glucose. In addition to glucagon and growth hormone, plasma catecholamine levels are increased and contribute to a persisting hyperglycemia.[14] In contrast to these postprandial changes, dogs with shunts have a relative fasting hypoglycemia. Despite persisting elevations of the three hormones promoting hyperglycemia, the capacity of the liver for glucose production is reduced and is unable to maintain normal blood glucose.[15] The relative hypoglycemia of dogs with shunts is illustrated in Figure 35-2.

Derangements in lipid metabolism, not often reported in clinical cases, are documented in dogs with experimental shunts (Figures 35-2). Plasma cholesterol and triglyceride concentrations decrease to 60% of normal in dogs with shunts.[15-17] The reductions are associated with no changes in the distribution of cholesterol in serum lipoprotein fractions and hepatic cholesterol. The content of cholesterol in the atrophied liver remains the same as in control dogs. Serum cholesterol levels most likely decrease because of an increased rate of synthesis that is less than an increased rate of catabolism. Normal hepatic portal circulation is essential to maintain normal plasma cholesterol levels. Hypocholesterolemia still occurs with portacaval transposition or arterialization of the portal circulation, both of which maintain normal values of blood flowing to the liver, although its supply is not entirely portal. The basis for decreased plasma triglyceride concentration found in dogs with shunts is not entirely understood.

Cholesterol synthesis to bile acids decreases in dogs with portacaval shunts, reflecting the marked reduction in hepatic size.[18] The total pool size of bile acids decreases to 30% of normal and the rate of bile acid loss increases. Despite that, serum bile acid concentrations can increase to 80 times normal (Figure 35-3).[15] Thus, bile acids are not removed from the plasma at a normal rate. The reduced pool size and impaired hepatic uptake suggest that decreased amounts of bile acids are delivered to the intestine.

The liver's role in lipid metabolism also includes removing and metabolizing short-chain fatty acids absorbed from the intestine. Hepatectomy in dogs causes blood volatile fatty acid levels to nearly double within 30 hours. Volatile fatty acids are fermentation products of the intestinal anaerobic bacteria. The amount of volatile fatty acids absorbed is determined by the numbers and locations of anaerobes in the intestine and by the composition of the diet. When these lipids accumulate, they contribute to the signs of hepatic encephalopathy by interfering with the activity of carbamyl phosphate synthetase and argininosuccinate synthetase, inhibiting the conversion of ammonia to urea.[19] Plasma volatile fatty acid levels may be elevated in animals with shunts, but any contribution to the signs of hepatic encephalopathy is probably minor.

The pathogenesis of abnormal nitrogen metabolism is described in Chapter 28. Experimental dogs with portasystemic shunts develop abnormalities in synthesis of proteins for export and in nitrogen metabolism, reflected by changes in plasma amino acids, ammonia, urea nitrogen, uric acid, and creatinine. Albumin synthesis decreases in dogs with shunts despite feeding more than adequate amounts of protein. Plasma albumin levels progressively decrease and contribute to a relatively low plasma total protein (Figure 35-4).[15] Total plasma globulins usually do not decrease and in some cases can increase because increased amounts of antigens, absorbed from the intestine and escaping removal by the liver, increase gamma globulin synthesis.

Plasma amino acid changes in dogs with shunts are similar to those seen with chronic hepatitis.[15] In general, the levels of branched-chain amino acids decrease because peripheral tissues catabolize them faster than normal, a change promoted by high plasma concentrations of catecholamines, glucagon, and insulin. Plasma levels of aromatic neutral amino acids increase because the liver must metabolized them, and the capacity for

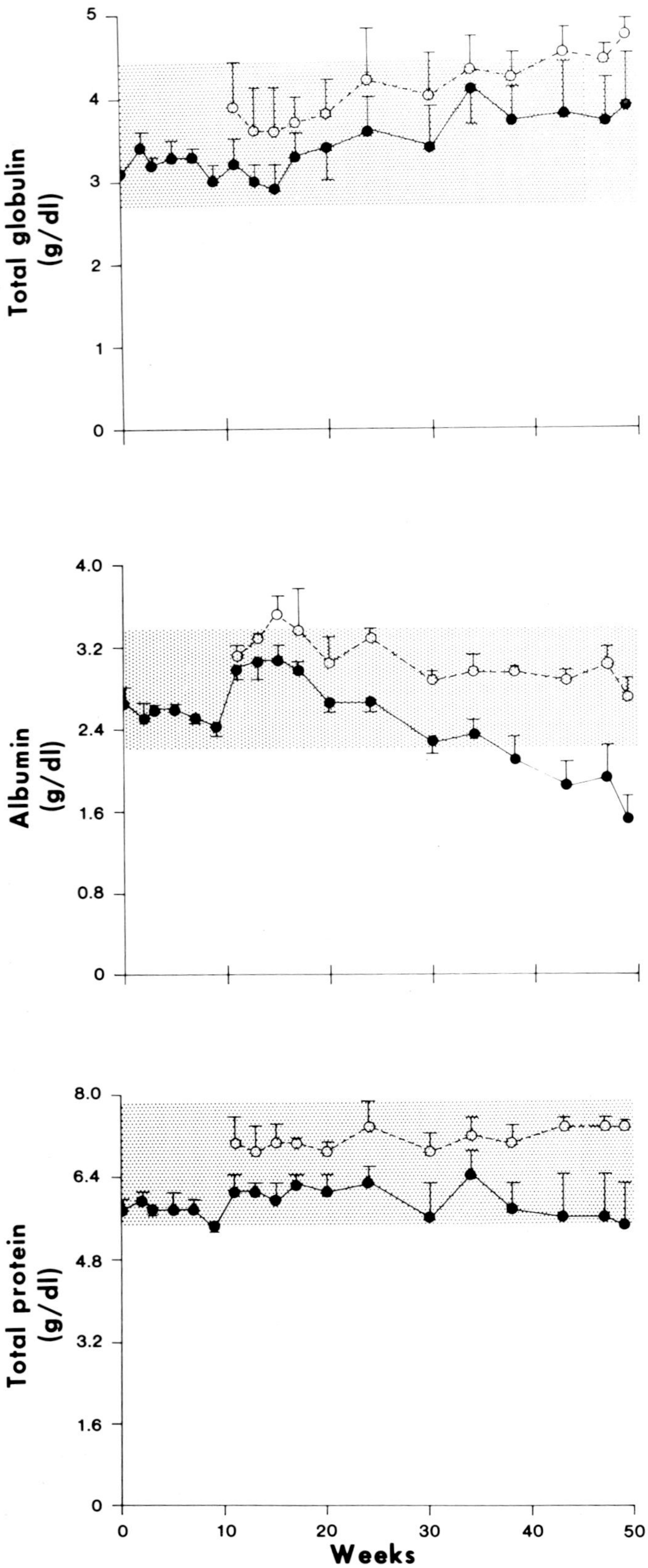

Figure 35-4. Serum albumin and globulin concentration changes with time after portacaval shunting. Mean values for normal dogs (open circles) and dogs with shunts (closed circles) are shown over period of one year. Shaded areas represent range for normal values. From reference 15. Used with permission.

that conversion is reduced in an atrophic liver with partial diversion of its portal circulation. The branched-chain amino acids involved are valine, leucine, and isoleucine, while the important aromatics are phenylalanine and tyrosine. The ratio of the sum of the molar concentrations of the branched-chain amino acids to the sum of the molar concentrations of the aromatics is 3 or greater in normal dogs and 1 in experimental dogs with shunts but not necessarily with clinical signs of hepatic encephalopathy (Figure 35-3).[15] Dogs can survive and be free of clinical signs when the ratio remains at 1, but that depends on how they are managed. Correction of the branched-chain amino acid deficiency does not improve clinical signs; feeding excess aromatic amino acids to dogs with experimental shunts but no clinical signs results in great increases in plasma aromatic amino acid levels, but clinical signs do not develop.[20] In either case blood ammonia levels are unchanged. At the present time there is no good evidence that amino acid imbalances are important in producing clinical signs. The pattern of changes in amino acid metabolism is the same in clinical cases as in dogs with experimentally-produced shunts.

Signs of acute hepatic encephalopathy and coma can be produced in dogs by infusing ammonia salts intravenously.[14] Clinical signs seen within five minutes include hypersalivation, vomiting, and hyperexcitability; coma appears within 30 minutes. These changes appear before marked changes in plasma amino acids, indicating that the signs are not caused by abnormal ratios of plasma amino acids. Within several hours of infusion, plasma levels of arginine, alanine, and branched chain amino acids decrease. These later changes are similar to those seen in dogs with chronic active hepatitis and shunts. Ammonia is toxic, and although fasting hyperammonemia cannot always be demonstrated for dogs with shunts, abnormal ammonia tolerance is an invariable finding, indicating these dogs have a reduced capacity for converting ammonia to urea. Although ammonia is toxic, there is not a good correlation between blood ammonia levels and the severity of clinical signs.

Conversion of ammonia to urea is impaired in dogs with shunts (Figure 35-5). Metabolism of uric acid is also altered, so that plasma levels increase. An effect of these two changes is increased urinary excretion of ammonia and uric acid, which combine to form ammonium urate or biurate and precipitate into crystals with increasing pH. Their solubility is also determined by the concentration of other solutes in the urine. Dilute urine with a low specific gravity is less likely to contain ammonium urate or biurate crystals.

Plasma creatinine decreases in dogs with shunts (Figure 35-5). That may be in part due to reduced creatinine production because of reduced muscle mass from the muscle wasting commonly seen. Plasma creatinine levels are more importantly a reflection of renal glomerular filtration rate. That rate increases in dogs with shunts, and plasma creatinine clearance increases.

The liver also loses its ability to remove and detoxify substances from the portal circulation. The hepatic monocyte phagocytic system is bypassed and its capacity is reduced in experimental animals with portasystemic shunts. That results in persistent endotoxemia[21] and hypergammaglobulinemia caused by the many intestinal antigens' escaping removal.[22] Another toxin is produced from the amino acid methionine in the intestine. Methionine given orally can be converted by intestinal bacteria to methyl mercaptan, which, when absorbed into

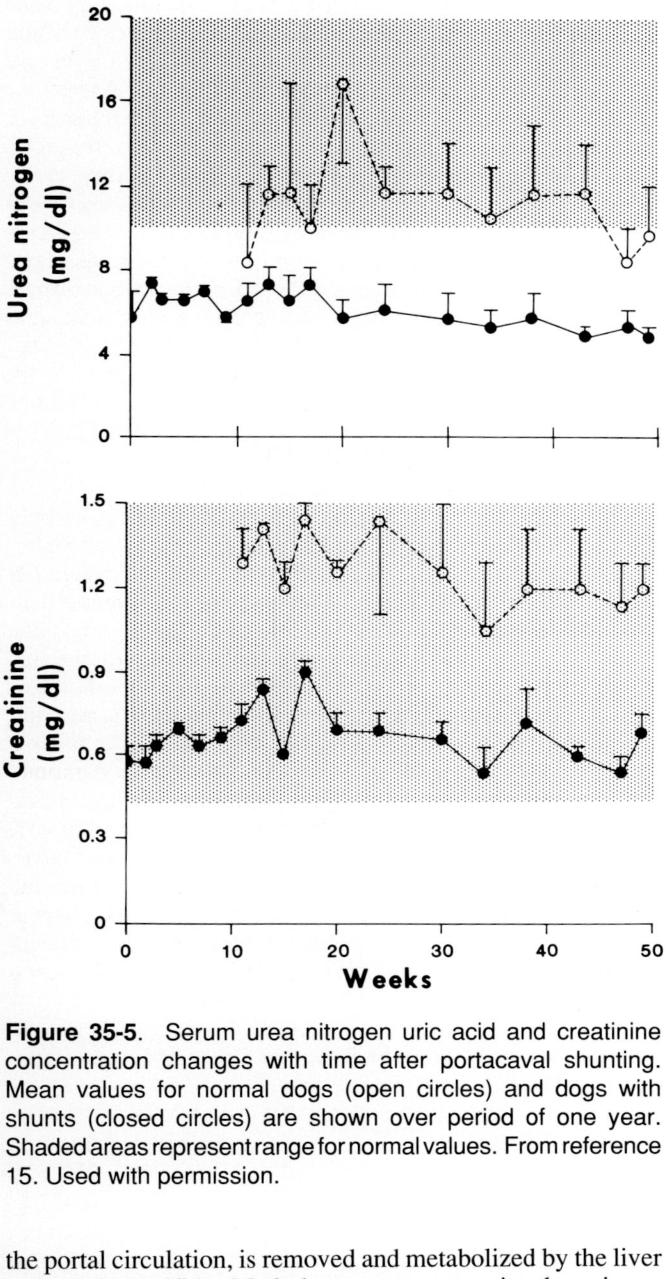

Figure 35-5. Serum urea nitrogen uric acid and creatinine concentration changes with time after portacaval shunting. Mean values for normal dogs (open circles) and dogs with shunts (closed circles) are shown over period of one year. Shaded areas represent range for normal values. From reference 15. Used with permission.

the portal circulation, is removed and metabolized by the liver to dimethyl-sulfide. Methyl mercaptan escaping hepatic removal is toxic in nanomole plasma concentrations. Methyl mercaptan is not adequately removed from the circulation in dogs with shunts. Thus, methionine given orally to dogs with hyperammonemia due to a portacaval shunt can produce hepatic coma.[23]

Portasystemic shunts reduce the ability of the liver to remove and secrete into the biliary system many substances found in bile. In addition to the reduced capacity for uptake (and in some cases metabolic transformation), there is a reduction in biliary secretion. The reduction in bile secretion is greater than the reduction in hepatic size; portasystemic shunts causing a 50% reduction in hepatic size can reduce biliary transport capacity by 70%. Bile acids are one such group of substances cleared by the liver and secreted into bile. Dogs with experimentally-produced shunts have markedly increased plasma bile acid concentrations (Figure 35-3).[15] Another substance, sulfobromophthalein (BSP), is cleared in a similar way but must be metabolized in the liver before secretion is possible. Retention of BSP is invariably abnormal in experimental dogs with shunts. The clearance of the pigment bilirubin may be reduced in dogs with shunts, but it is not severe enough to cause plasma bilirubin to increase.

Gross and microscopic hepatic changes are predictable in dogs with shunts. The liver atrophies up to 50% of normal when portasystemic anastomoses partially divert portal blood from the liver.[24] This is due to a reduction in both number and size of hepatocytes. Hepatocyte loss can approach 50% with the remainder of the liver consisting of atrophied hepatocytes and an increased sinusoidal space. Reductions in smooth endoplasmic reticulum with its cytochrome P-450 enzyme systems are greatest in zone 3.[25] Other microscopic changes consistent with metabolic alterations include reduced glycogen and increased lipid. The liver compensates with hyperplasia (accompanied by an increase in mitotic figures) in zone 1, the periportal area, whereas the centrolobular zone 3 area remains atrophic. Thereby, the functions in zone 1 are preserved better than the functions in zone 3.

Hepatic atrophy results from reduced portal circulation to the liver and a loss of hepatotrophic factors in portal blood. (see Chapter 31, hepatic regeneration). The volume of blood flow to the liver is important for maintaining normal liver size. Reduced total hepatic blood flow in dogs with portacaval shunts can be restored with arterialization of the portal system by anastomosing a small artery to the portal vein.[26] Although the loss of hepatotrophic factors in the portal blood continues, these livers maintain normal size. Portacaval transposition produces similar results when the vena cava is connected to the portal vein entering the liver and the portal vein is anastomosed to the caudal end of the transected vena cava.[27] Normal homeostatic mechanisms attempt to improve hepatic circulation in dogs with portasystemic shunts. Hepatic arterial flow doubles in animals with shunts and hepatic atrophy up to 50% of normal size; this increased flow is magnified, so that blood content per gram of tissue is four times normal.[21,28] The increase is associated with dilation of the arteries and proliferation of arterioles. Total-body blood volume increases by 20%, and cardiac output can increase by 50% to maintain normal hepatic perfusion. Arterial blood pressure decreases from 110 to 81 mm Hg, and pressure in the portal vein decreases from 8.6 to 6.0 mm Hg. Despite these circulatory changes, total hepatic blood flow remains below normal, and the liver stabilizes at the size commensurate with its blood supply.

The portal circulation is a rich source of nutrients and humoral agents important for maintaining normal liver size. Dietary nutrients are important since hepatic size decreases during starvation. Part of the structure of hepatocytes and the protein metabolic machinery turns over at a given rate; when nutrients are not available, the structure that is lost is not replaced until food intake resumes. Hepatic size is also maintained by hepatotrophic factors contained in the portal circulation,[29-31] including insulin, glucagon, and other gut hormones. The importance of insulin as a factor has been studied in animals with portacaval shunts where it has been infused in blood vessels to the liver. Where shunts cause a 50% reduction in the size of hepatocytes, insulin is able to restore half of the loss.[31] Other studies indicate that the important hepatotrophic factor is a hormone(s) other than insulin.[29,30]

Renal function has not been studied in dogs with portasystemic shunts. A number of observations have been made on increased kidney size in patients with naturally occurring shunts, however.[32,33] Increased cardiac output is a consistent change with shunts, as are increases for renal blood flow and glomerular filtration rate. Increased renal blood flow may explain the development of the renal hypertrophy.

Portacaval shunts cause thrombocytopenia and coagulation impairment in experimental animals.[34] This is not associated with abnormal partial thromboplastin time. Similar coagulopathies have not been described in dogs with spontaneous shunts.

Hepatic portal blood flow determines structure and function in the small intestine.[35-37] With normal portal flow through the liver a degree of minimum resistance maintains portal pressure above a certain minimum. Shunting of portal flow around the liver can reduce portal pressure below that minimum. Such a reduction results in simplification of intestinal villi which in essence is the same as villus atrophy, and that can result in intestinal malabsorption. If increased hepatic arterial flow and atrophic changes cause that minimum portal pressure to return, the villus anatomy returns to normal.

CLINICAL FINDINGS

Portasystemic vascular anomalies in dogs cause similiar clinical signs to those seen with other forms of hepatic disease (Table 35-3).[4] Seen most consistently are mild signs of hepatic encephalopathy, manifested as depression. One or more of the neurologic signs were seen more consistently (93%) than gastrointestinal signs (75%) or any of the other abnormalities. Fewer numbers show more severe signs of CNS involvement, such as seizures, blindness, ataxia, head pressing, disorientation, and coma. The milder signs are always evident, though they may be overlooked if they have been present for the entire life of the dog and are considered to reflect its normal personality. Since more severe signs appear in less than a third of the cases, portal vascular anomalies must be suspected with any unexplained nonspecific and mild signs of hepatic disease.

Portasystemic vascular anastomoses in cats are reported to be invariably associated with neurologic signs. Most frequent, when described, are depression or stupor and ataxia. Other frequent signs include behavioral changes, dilated pupils, and excessive salivation. Some cats show disorientation, head pressing, aggressiveness or agitation, blindness, weakness, and seizures. Other signs seen less consistently include anorexia, dysphagia, vomiting, diarrhea, polydipsia, polyphagia, and delayed recovery from anesthesia. Many affected cats are small for their age and may be thin.

LABORATORY FINDINGS

Partial diversion of the portal circulation from the liver causes clinical pathologic changes recognized by routine laboratory tests. Hemograms are often unremarkable except for anemia and hypoproteinemia. Anemia is found in about one-third of dogs with shunts. Many more dogs, up to two-thirds, can have microcytosis with normal packed cell volume and normal corpuscular hemoglobin concentration. Some have normocytic, normochromic, nonregenerative anemia and others have a hypochromic, microcytic nonregenerative anemia consistent with iron deficiency. Erythrocytic microcytosis and hypochromasia may be explained by impaired absorption and metabolism of iron, but the microcytosis commonly seen with no hypochromasia requires other explanations.

Hepatic albumin synthesis is reduced because of hepatic atrophy and disruption of nitrogen metabolism. Reducing protein intake to manage signs of hepatic encephalopathy contributes to defective albumin synthesis. Ascites, by increasing

Table 35-3. Clinical Signs in Dogs Associated with Portasystemic Vascular Anastomoses Listed in Order of Frequency of Occurrence

Clinical Sign	Frequency Seen	Clinical Sign	Frequency Seen
Depression	68%	Related to meals	24%
Vomiting	48%	Seizures	23%
Vague CNS signs	48%	Head pressing	22%
Weight loss, retarded growth	43%	Ascites	20%
Stupor	38%	Hyperactive	17%
Polydipsia	35%	Prolonged anesthesia recovery	15%
Pacing, circling	35%	Head down	14%
Ataxia, staggering	33%	Abdominal pain	14%
Diarrhea	32%	Fever	14%
Blindness	32%	Polyphagia	12%
Anorexia	31%	Head tremors	7%
Hypersalivation	30%	Deafness	4%
Personality change	30%	Coma	4%
Collapse, weakness	29%	Bleeding	2%
		Jaundice	1%

Table 35-4. Clinical Pathology: Incidence of Abnormalities

Abnormality	% abnormal	Abnormality	% abnormal
Post NH_3 tolerance	100	Low cholesterol	54
BSP	90	Urine NH_3 biurate crystals	51
Resting NH_3	88	Leukocytosis	30
Partial thromboplastin time	83	Anemia	30
Serum alkaline phosphatase	71	Prothrombin time	28
Low BUN	70	Hypoglycemia	16
Low plasma protein (albumin)	68	Hyperbilirubinemia	16
Serum ALT	58		

albumin's volume of distribution, worsens hypoproteinemia. Albumin degradation may also be increased by accelerated losses through the intestinal tract.

Some blood chemistries are consistently abnormal in dogs when portal circulation is partially diverted from the liver (Table 35-4 and 35-5). Random fasting blood ammonia concentrations are usually increased above the normal mean value of 50 to 60 µg/dl (range of normals being 20 to 120 µg/dl). Patients with portal-vein anomalies show signs of hepatic encephalopathy, with blood ammonia ranging from 150 to over 1,000 µg/dl. The degree of hyperammonemia does not correlate with the severity of clinical signs. Repeated seizures can be associated with blood ammonia of 200 µg/dl, whereas other dogs with ammonia of 500 µg/dl will show few severe clinical signs. Since the clinical signs of hepatic encephalopathy are produced by alterations not only in ammonia but in plasma amino acid ratios, short-chain fatty acids, and mercaptans, the severity of clinical signs can be independent of blood ammonia concentrations. Normal fasting blood ammonia does not rule out the possibility of a portal shunt. When blood ammonia concentration is normal an ammonia tolerance test must be used to identify the inability to metabolize ammonia properly (Chapter 30). Ammonium chloride is given orally and blood ammonia determinations are made before and 30 minutes after.[38] In normal animals 30-minute samples contain amounts of ammonia similar to those of preammonia samples. With portasystemic shunts, blood ammonia concentration can rise from a normal value below 120 µg/dl to over 1,000 µg/dl.

In dogs with shunts hepatic function evaluated with the sulfobromophthalein (BSP) retention test is abnormal, with retention of more than 5% of the dye at the end of 30 minutes. Hepatic function and blood flow determines dye disappearance. In young dogs, abnormal dye excretion is due primarily to altered circulation, so that retention may not be striking. Following secondary hepatic atrophy, BSP retention reflects reduced hepatic function as well as altered blood flow. With hypoproteinemia the BSP retention time is falsely decreased.

Abnormal nitrogen metabolism as a reflection of reduced hepatic function may be evident in reduced production of clotting factors (abnormal partial thromboplastin and prothrombin times), plasma albumin, and urea. Urine ammonium biurate crystals reflect hyperammonemia and increased renal excretion of uric acid. Other functions of the liver are reduced, as evident in the hypocholesterolemia, hypoglycemia, and occasionally hyperbilirubinemia.

Activities of plasma enzymes are usually increased but only modestly. Mean activity of alanine transaminase (ALT) increases consistently and remains elevated in experimental dogs with shunts (Figure 35-6).[15] But it is evident that there is great variability, and normal activities are often found. The magnitude and unpredictability of ALT activities is the same in clinical cases, where abnormal values seldom exceed 400 U/L; only about one-half of dogs have increased activity. Increased ALT activity reflects hepatocyte degeneration, which can be due to a combination of nutritional derangements and the endotoxemia known to accompany shunts. Plasma alkaline phosphatase (ALP) activity increases modestly in dogs with experimental shunts (Figure 35-6). Most clinical cases have increased ALP activity, but the mean abnormal values approximate only a 50% increase, which is not striking compared to ALP increases seen for most other hepatic diseases. Because increased ALP activity is less specific for hepatic disease than increased ALT activity, there are probably multiple factors for its elevation. Young animals normally have ALP activity that can be twice as great as adults. That difference is due to higher osteoblastic activity in the young. Shunts are recognized in many dogs at a young age. Plasma activity of gamma-glutamyltranspeptidase (GGT) increases in animals with experimental shunts. Activity of that enzyme parallels ALP activity and provides no additional useful information.

Blood glucose concentrations are frequently low normal. Since blood glucose levels are determined by many factors operating to maintain homeostasis, interpretation of blood glucose levels within the normal range is difficult without conducting other tests. In experimental animals, where variable factors such as diet can be controlled, hypoglycemia is a feature of portasystemic shunts, resulting from reduced hepatic capacity to maintain normal carbohydrate metabolism and from increased blood insulin levels. Hypocholesterolemia is a more common finding, as would be anticipated because cholesterol catabolism increases.

Plasma bile acid levels are invariably increased in dogs with experimental shunts and are usually increased in clinical cases. From values on bile acids reported on dogs with shunts, approximately 80% have increased fasting bile acid values; although there is little information on bile acid values after feeding, it appears that they may be consistently elevated.

Urinalysis sometimes provides clues for hepatic disease. Hepatic disease and hyperammonemia frequently cause ammonium biurate, amorphous urate, or bilirubin crystals to appear in the urine. Since these crystals are soluble in dilute urine, they are usually found only in concentrated urine. Plasma uric acid

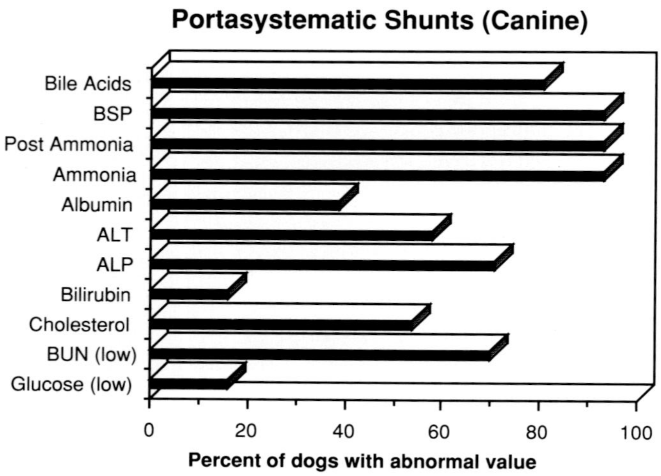

Table 35-5. Comparison of sensitivities for different tests in dogs with portasystemic shunts. Below: graphs showing distribution of clinical pathology values in dogs with portasystemic shunts. Points on graphs represent 0%, 25%, 50%, 75% and 100% medians. Normal range is in shaded area.

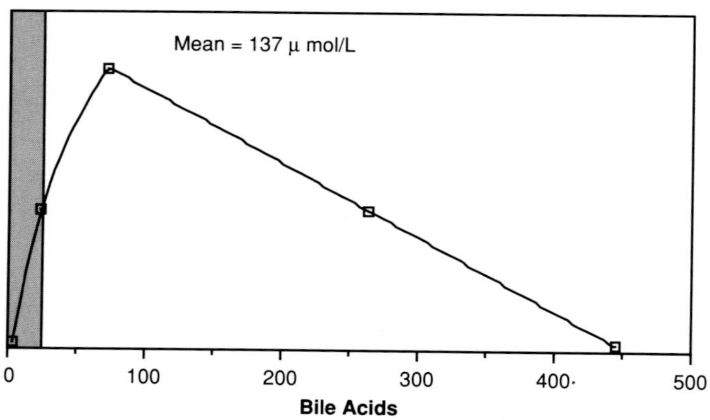

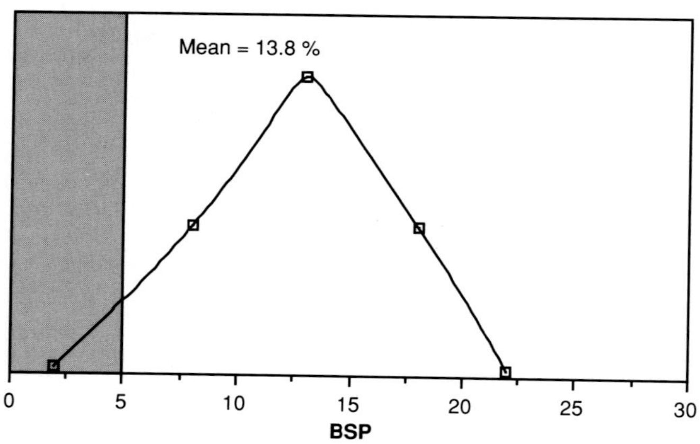

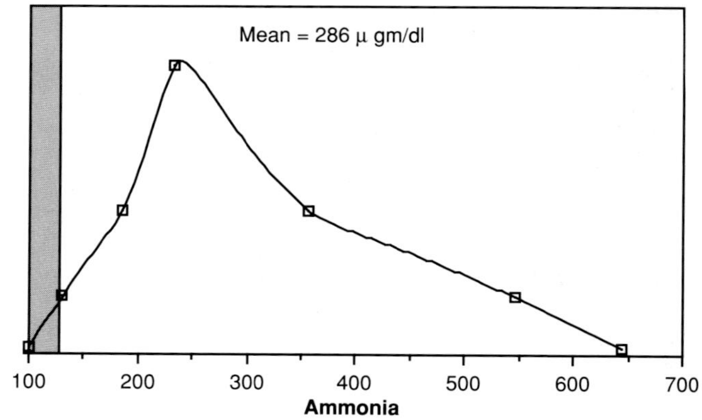

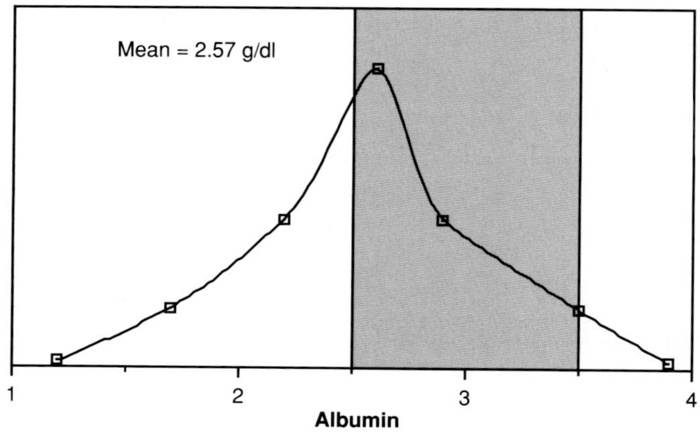

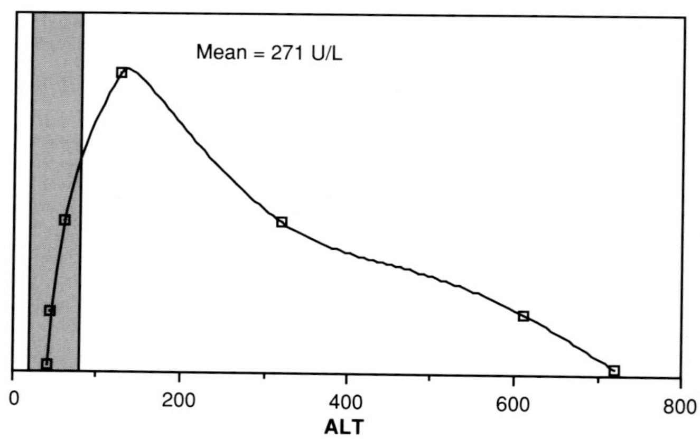

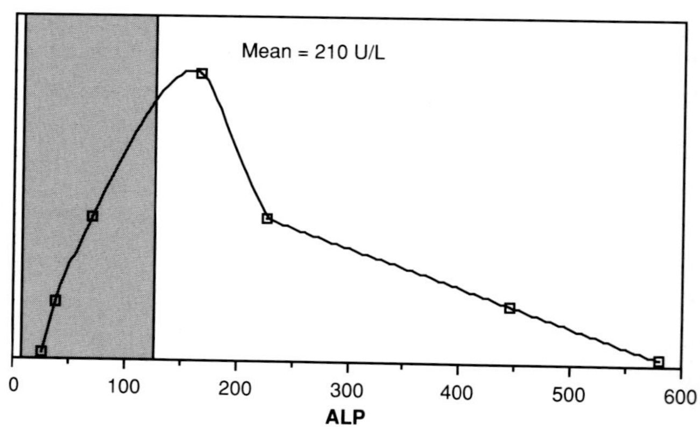

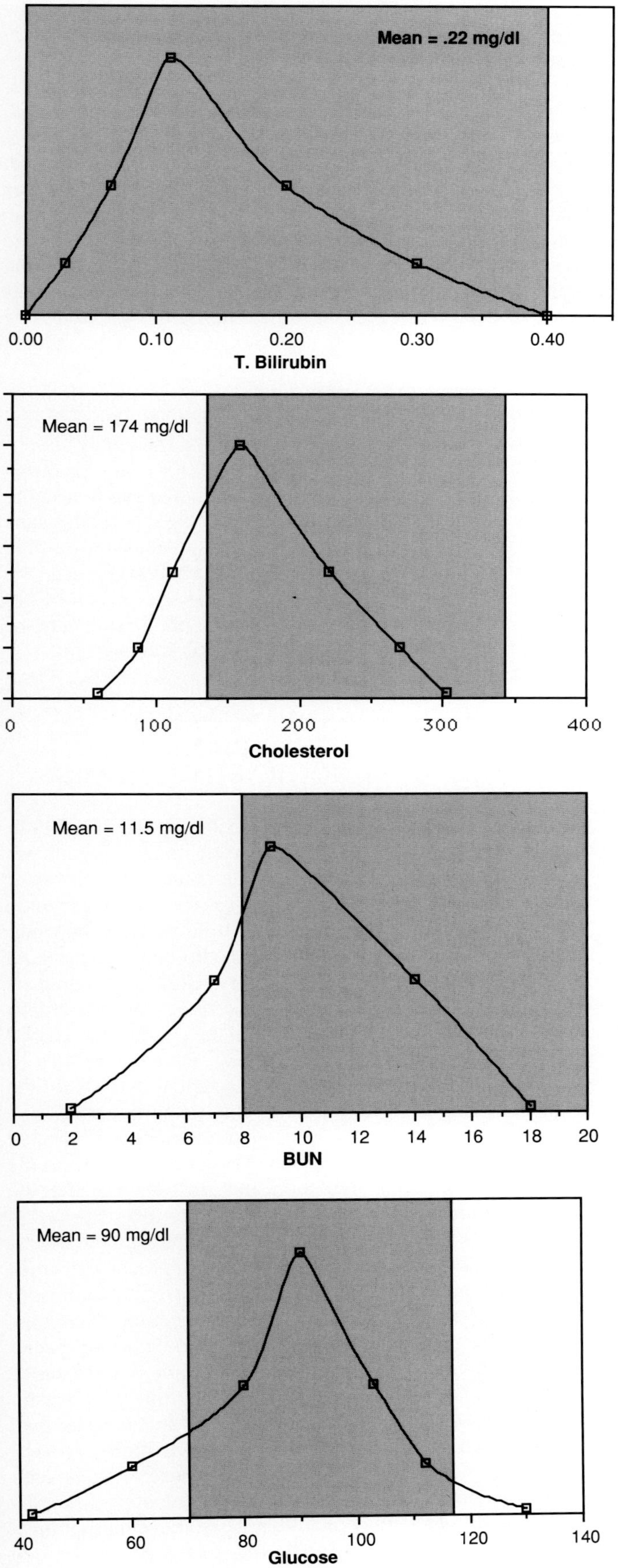

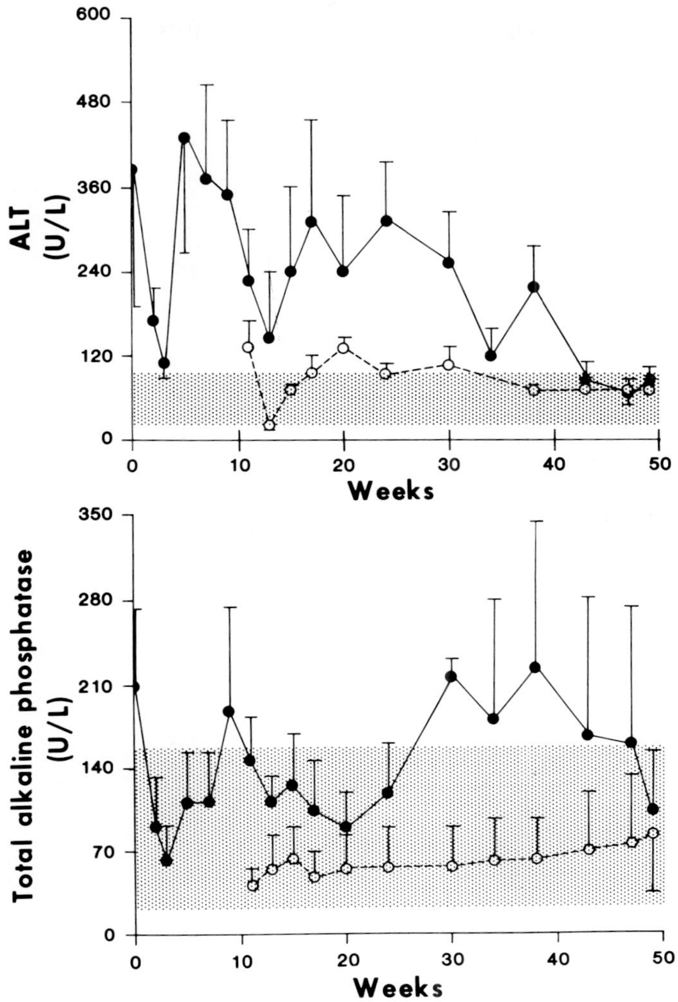

Figure 35-6. Serum alanine transaminase (ALT) and alkaline phosphatase concentration changes with time after portacaval shunting. Mean values for normal dogs (open circles) and dogs with shunts (closed circles) are shown over period of one year. Shaded areas represent range for normal values. From reference 15. Used with permission.

levels are not increased in clinical cases although there is a relative increase in experimental dogs with shunts. An absence of ammonium biurate crystals in concentrated urine does not rule out the possibility of a shunt. Ammonium biurate crystals are not pathognomonic for a shunt; they can be found in nonhepatic as well as hepatic problems. Dogs with portacaval shunts are also at high risk for developing urinary calculi composed of uric acid or urate salts.[39]

There is little information on clinical pathologic findings from cats with shunts. Tests reflecting hepatic function include fasting blood ammonia determination, which in two studies was reported to be consistently abnormal[8] but in another two was often normal.[6,7] Ammonia tolerance testing has not been reported often enough to make any conclusions on its results in

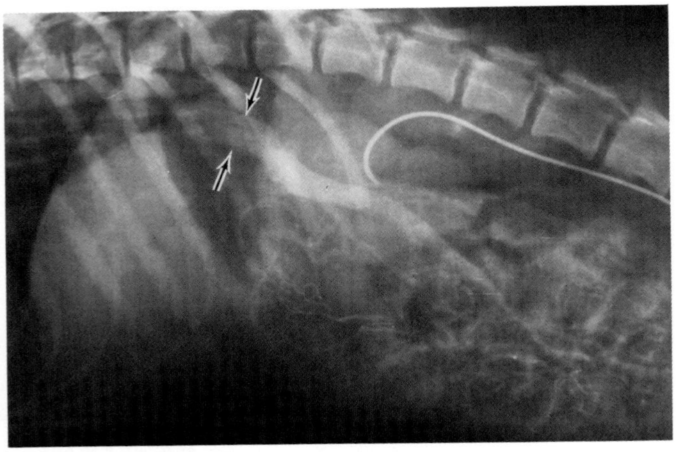

Figure 35-7a. Angiographic study in a dog with a large portasystemic anastomosis between the portal and azygous veins (arrows). Shunt was partially closed achieve remission of clinical signs.

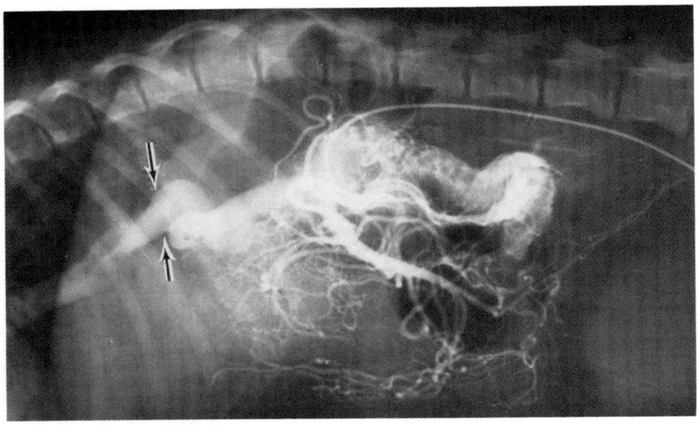

Figure 35-7b. Angiographic study in a dog with a patent ductus venosus (arrows). In this study most of the dye entered the portal vein directly from the mesenteric arterial system (without passing through mesenteric capillary beds, presumably by a shunt) thereby outlining the portal vein and shunt better than in studies where dye is diluted on passing through the mesenteric circulation.

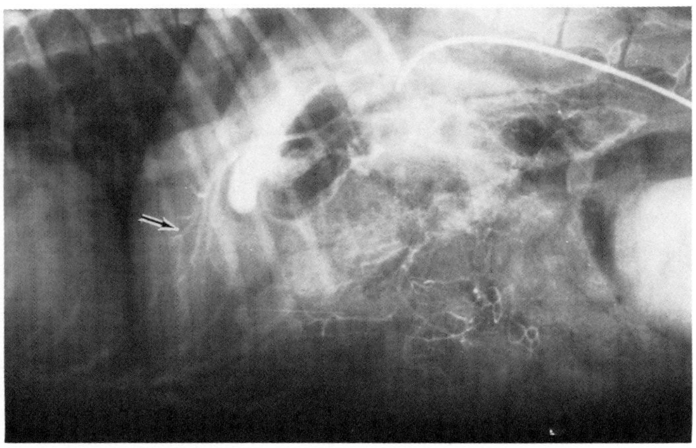

Figure 35-7c. Sometimes the atrophied hepatic portal system is outlined (arrows).

cats with shunts. Up to one-half of cats with shunts have low blood urea nitrogen, and a few have hypoalbuminemia. When done, BSP testing showed fewer than one-half of the cats to have abnormal retention of the dye at 30 minutes. In a small group of cats 75% had increased plasma bile acid concentrations.[7] Low normal glucose has also been reported. Activities of ALT and ALP are increased in no more than 50% of cats with shunts; the increases for each rarely exceed twice the upper limit of normal. Activity of GGT and plasma total bilirubin concentration are invariably normal. Urinalysis findings are unremarkable except for ammonium biurate crystals, found in nearly 40% of the cases reported. Hematologic abnormalities have not been mentioned in most reports. In one, excessive erythrocyte shape variation (poikilocytosis) was a frequent finding.[7]

A suspicion for portasystemic shunt is most reliably strengthened by results from ammonia tolerance, nonfed blood ammonia, BSP, and bile acid test results. Of these only ammonia tolerance has a sensitivity close to 100%. Only abnormal ammonia tolerance or nonfed blood ammonia can be used to attribute CNS signs to hepatic disease. Finding abnormal plasma amino acid levels can lead to the same conclusion, but that testing is seldom done. Abnormal BSP or bile acid results are unreliable in confirming hepatic disease as the cause for CNS signs. With sufficient cause a radiographic or nuclear medicine procedure is performed to confirm a portasystemic shunt.

RADIOGRAPY, NUCLEAR SCINTIGRAPHY, AND ULTRASONOGRAPHY FINDINGS

Portasystemic vascular anastomoses are identified radiographically by arteriography and venography (Figure 35-7).[33,40] Most procedures require catheterization of an artery or vein. One of the least invasive techniques is cranial mesenteric arterial portography, where a catheter introduced into the femoral artery is passed under fluoroscopic control through the aorta and into the cranial mesenteric artery. Contrast medium is injected automatically, and a rapid succession of radiographs are taken. Shunts are not outlined until the contrast has passed through the arterial and capillary phase, which takes 4 to 10 seconds. The venous phase showing the shunt extends for the next 6 to 14 seconds. A second, minimally invasive procedure involves splenoportography, where contrast medium is injected into the parenchyma of the spleen. Venous drainage from the spleen enters the portal circulation, and 2 to 4 seconds after the injection radiographs are taken during a 4 to 6 second period to outline shunts. This procedure is one that small animal practitioners can conduct with radiographic equipment that most use.[41] The most invasive procedure requires celiotomy to catheterize a small mesenteric vein for injection of contrast medium. The advantage of using this procedure is that special rapid cassette-changing equipment is not required, since one or two radiographs taken 5 to 10 seconds after injection usually identify shunts. This technique also outlines shunts better than any other procedure. Contrast medium injected into a mesenteric vein arrives at the shunt in a more compact bolus than with arterial injection, where the dye, diluted by traveling through a large capillary bed, may not identify some abnormalities. Operative mesenteric portography is suggested as the technique

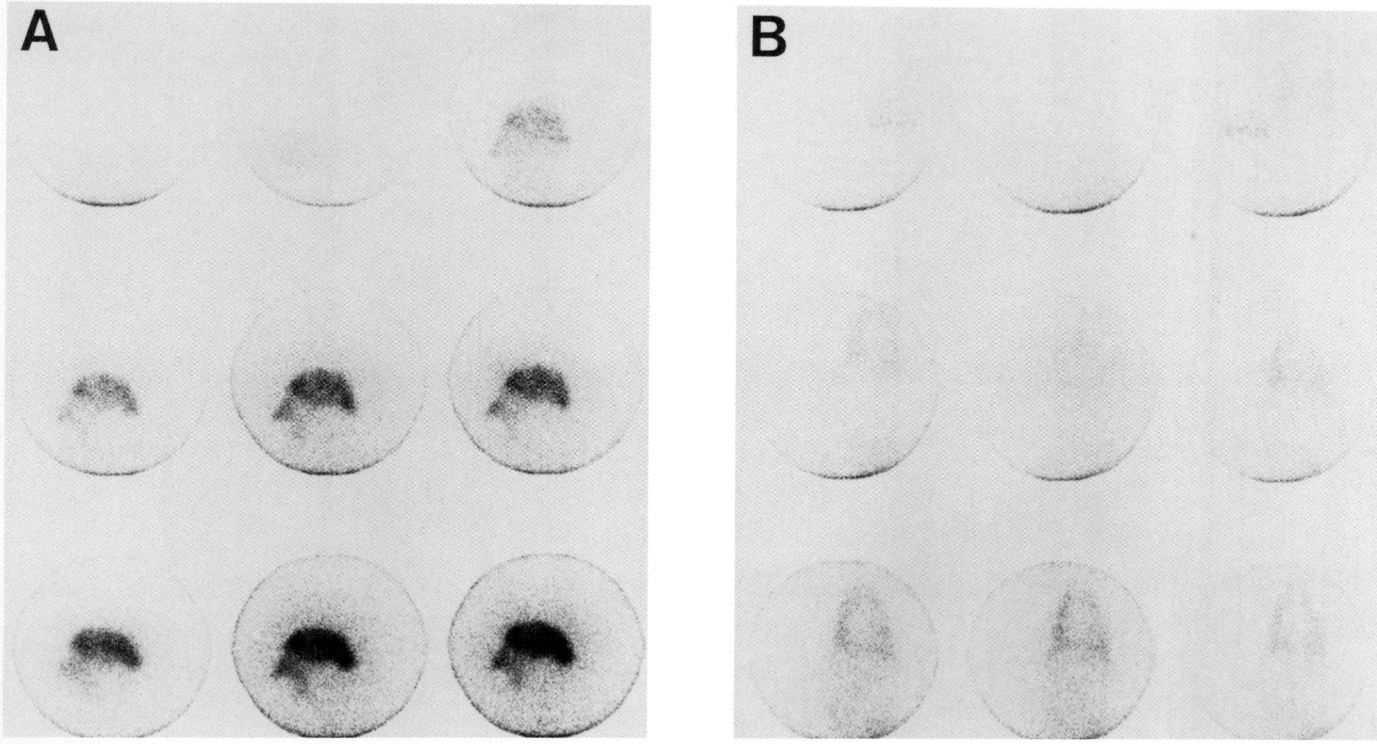

Figure 35-8a. Transcolonic ^{123}I-iodoamphetamine studies performed on a normal dog (A) and a dog with a portasystemic shunt (B). The sequential series of 1 minute ventral microdot images demonstrate exclusive uptake of the tracer by the liver in the normal dog, whereas the dog with the shunt has obvious pulmonary uptake. A ratio of lung counts to lung counts plus liver counts provides an estimate of the relative shunt flow. (from reference 44, used with permission).

for the practitioner to use. It is the least likely to result in complications and the most likely to give results. Celiac arteriography has been used to identify vascular abnormalities of the liver although only the arterial and capillary phases are usually outlined well. Percutaneous transhepatic portography has been described to outline shunts in experimental dogs and may find clinical use.[42]

Although most reported cases of shunts in dogs and cats have been identified with angiographic studies, there are few descriptions on radiographic hepatic size. When size has been reported, 50% or more of the cases are described as having normal-sized livers. Because animals with a shunt or any other form of hepatic insufficiency can have a small liver, it can be misleading to put much importance on small-liver size in any individual case.

Portasystemic shunts are also identified with nuclear scintigraphy, which is less invasive than angiography and does not require anesthesia.[43] A colloid with a radioactive isotope label, after being given intravenously, is removed from the circulation by the monocyte phagocytic system, located primarily in the liver and spleen but also in the lung. Labelled sulfur colloid is used in dogs because the liver is the primary organ for its uptake. The liver is not as well visualized in cats with sulfur colloid since the lung is their primary organ for uptake. The rate of uptake of radioactive technetium is imaged with a gamma camera, which outlines the organs involved (Figure 35-8). The rate of uptake can be graphed and is used to identify a dog with portasystemic shunting of blood. Normal dogs show normal size liver and most of the radioactive label in the liver with little in the spleen and lungs. Time-activity curves reflect the liver's being the primary organ for uptake. Dogs with shunts show a small liver and large uptake by the lungs and spleen; and that is reflected in their time-activity curves. Analysis of the information on the first pass, as derived from a time-activity curve, can be made to identify changes in hepatic perfusion. An arterial venous (A-V) ratio can be calculated that reflects the relative proportion of arterial and venous blood flow. Normal dogs have an A-V ratio of 0.9 to 1.7; dogs with shunts have a ratio of 2.0 or greater. Although it would appear that this nuclear scintigraphy should be a very sensitive test for identifying portasystemic shunting in dogs, the hepatic perfusion ratio has not been completely reliable in over 200 tested dogs both with and without shunts. Difficulties are encountered more often in small dogs, in dogs with small livers, and in dogs with impaired liver function but no shunts.

Nuclear scintigraphy, in which radioisotope is instilled in the colon, can be done on dogs.[44] Following its absorption into the portal circulation, all of the label transported through the liver only is on its first pass. In normal dogs the liver removes nearly all the radioisotope and little is found in the lungs. With portasystemic shunting of blood around the liver the amount of isotope in the lungs increases. Labelled preparations used in these studies include amphetamine labelled with radioactive iodine. The substance is expensive, and its slow absorption precludes outline of the hepatic circulation as provided by angiography. Another preparation is sodium pertechnetate

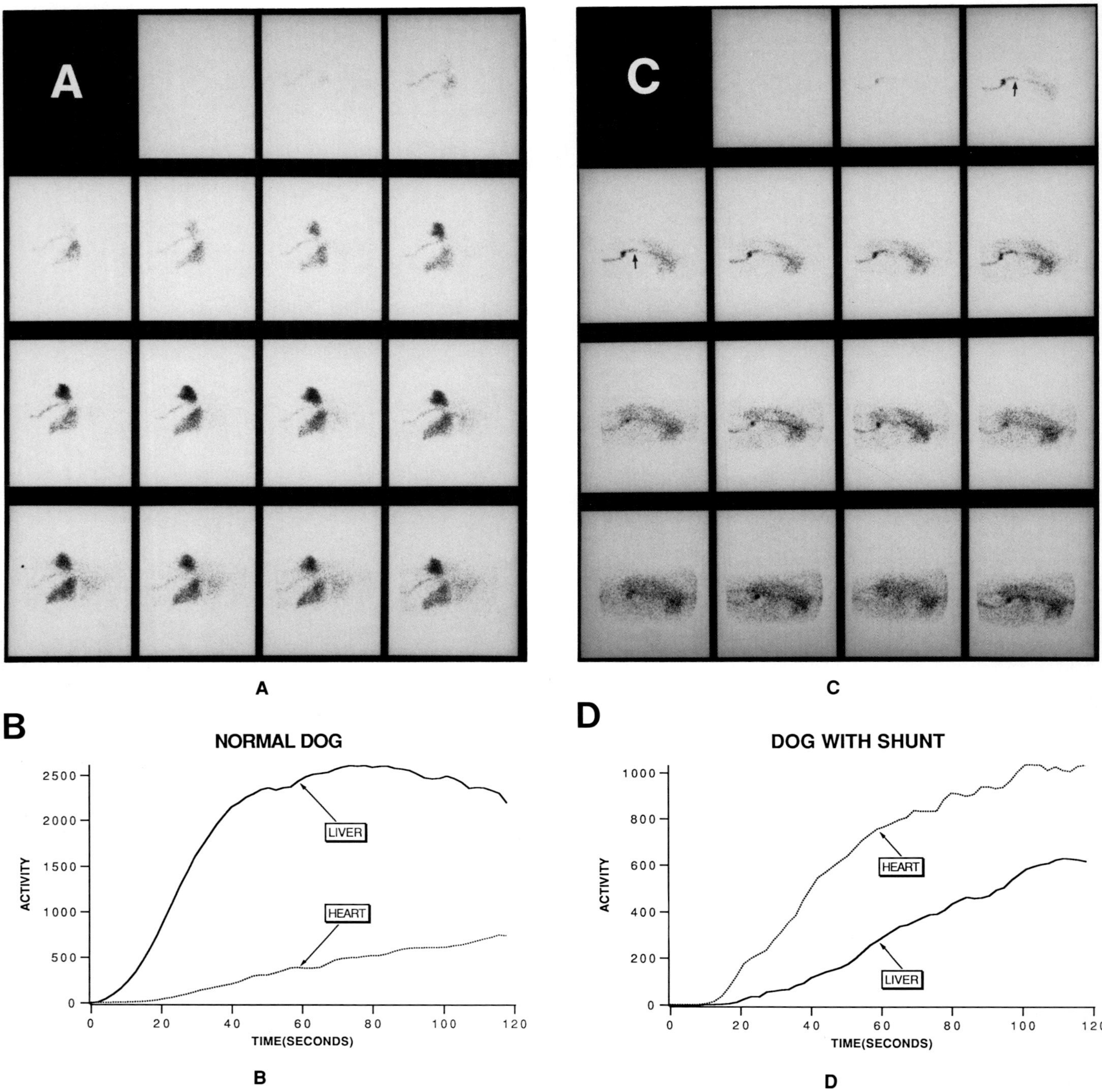

Figure 35-8b. Transcolonic ^{99m}-Tc-pertechnetate studies performed on a normal dog (A,B) and on a dog with a portasystemic shunt (C,D). The sequential 5 second right lateral microdot images (A) and accompanying time activity curves (B) demonstrate that the tracer arrives in the liver several seconds before it arrives in the heart. In the dog with a portasystemic shunt (C,D) the tracer arrives in the heart prior to its arrival in the liver. This reversal of temporal events is diagnostic for a shunt. In this instance the microdot images indicate a single and probably intrahepatic shunt vessel (arrow). Analysis of the areas under the liver and heart curves can be used to estimate relative shunt flow. (from reference 45, used with permission).

labelled with radioactive technetium, which is rapidly absorbed from the colon.[45] The rapid absorption allows it to provide a nuclear angiogram since the concentration of tracer in the portal circulation, liver, and heart is high enough to produce an image. In contrast to the iodine preparation, pertechnetate is not taken up by the liver but remains in the circulation. In normal dogs the isotope appears first in the portal circulation, then in the liver, and a few seconds later the heart. In dogs with shunts the isotope images the heart before the liver. The use of either isotope is reliable in identifying shunts even though they are handled differently. The use of pertechnetate may prove to be more reliable and has the added advantages of being less expensive

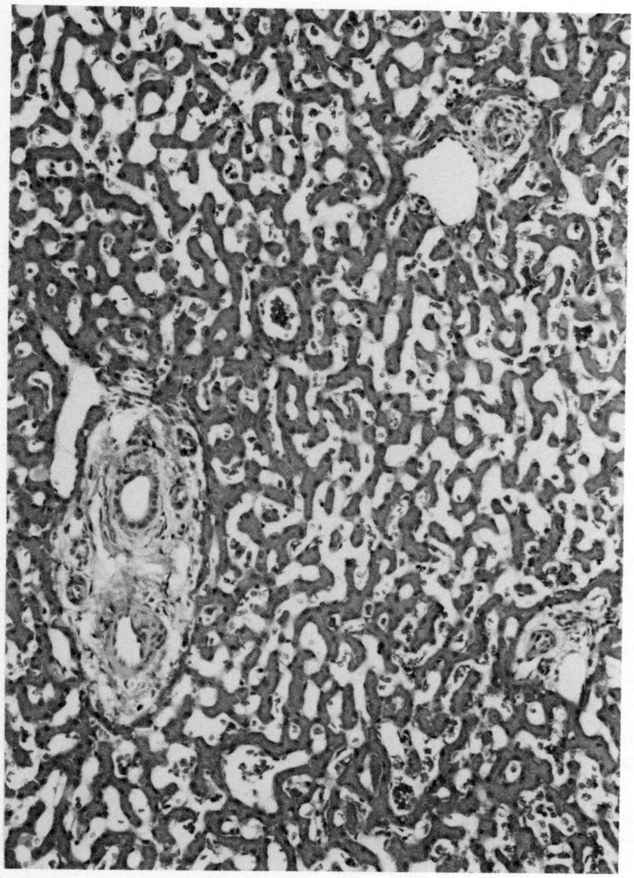

Figure 35-9. Portasystemic vascular anastomosis. Hepatic changes include congestion, parenchymal atrophy and relatively few branches of portal veins in portal triads. Number of portal triad branches is excessive for magnification shown.

and of having a much shorter half-life. Pertechnetate has promise for being a sensitive means for identifying shunts in cats.

Ultrasonography is sometimes used for identification of portasystemic shunts.[46] Ultrasonography is reliable in identifying small and hypovascular attributes of livers with shunts. On initial examinations ultrasonography identifies shunts in only 40% of affected dogs. With additional examinations under maximal conditions the identification of shunts improves to only about 65%. Thus, a third of dogs with shunts cannot be identified with ultrasonography, making the procedure relatively insensitive for confirming shunts.

BIOPSY AND PATHOLOGY FINDINGS[5,7,8,47]

Liver biopsy of dogs and cats with portasystemic vascular anastomoses consistently reveals hepatic atrophy, which may be severe enough to change normal hepatic architecture (Figure 35-9). Portal areas may be closer than normal, signifying a loss of parenchymal cells and a filling of the void by cords of collapsing hepatocytes. Hepatocellular cords are reduced in width, especially in zone 3 or the centrilobular area, and sinusoids are dilated and often congested. Hepatocyte degeneration is common and is manifested by lipidosis and vacuolization, primarily in zone 3. Chronic degeneration can lead to fibrosis around central veins. These morphological changes develop from the contributions of altered carbohydrate, fat, and protein metabolism; reduced oxygen delivery; endotoxemia; an excess load of antigens and bacteria from the gut; and increased levels of toxins from the gut. Generalized congestion of central veins and sinusoids is common and may reflect the increased hepatic blood flow per gram of liver tissue. In contrast to atrophy of zone 3 hepatocytes, those in zone 1, periportal, can be hypertrophied. Mild inflammation in zone 1 portal areas is sometimes associated with fibrosis that may be a response to enteric bacteria antigens not adequately cleared by the liver. Portal triads are usually prominent, partly because they appear more numerous with the loss of up to one-half of parenchymal cells. Most striking are the changes in portal vessels. Portal veins are poorly delineated and are represented by thin-walled small-caliber vessels; in some cases they are difficult to identify. Multiple small caliber, thick-walled vessels characteristic of arterioles are often seen and may represent a neovascularization to increase hepatic blood flow. Bile duct proliferation is seen in some biopsies. The most striking changes are atrophy and congestion, which support a presumptive diagnosis when no evidence is found for inflammation. Cellular infiltration by neutrophils or immunocytes (plasma cells and lymphocytes) is not a feature of biopsies from animals with shunts. Fibrosis or cirrhosis is not prominent even in animals that have had a shunt for two to three years. Biopsy changes are not used to confirm or rule out the possibility of a shunt; such changes are usually subtle, inconsistent, and not pathognomonic for any hepatic problem.

Portasystemic shunts with signs of hepatic encephalopathy are usually associated with pathologic changes in the brain. They consist of bilateral symmetrical polymicrocavitation of the brain stem (especially the corpora geniculata, the formation reticularis, and the thalamus), cerebellar nuclei, and the gray-white matter junction in the cerebral cortex. Other lesions reported are perinuclear spongiform degeneration, cortical necrosis, and hippocampal necrosis. An increased number of protoplasmic astrocytes are also seen most often in the cerebral cortex and its adjoining white matter and in the basal nuclei and elsewhere. Similar morphologic changes are described in animals with experimental shunts.

DIAGNOSIS

Clinical laboratory findings are useful in increasing suspicions of portasystemic shunts. Biochemical tests cannot confirm a shunt. Abnormal blood ammonias, ammonia tolerance tests, and BSP retention establish that a problem involves hepatocyte function or circulation through the liver, but they do not distinguish shunts from other hepatic disease. Laboratory abnormalities in conjunction with clinical findings can justify radiographic studies. A few patients may have a markedly elevated SGPT, making hepatitis appear most likely. When all clinical and laboratory information does not clearly suggest a shunt as the most likely possibility, liver biopsy is used to assess the problem. Survey radiographic studies revealing a small liver are not pathognomonic for hepatic atrophy secondary to a shunt. With clear cut evidence for a shunt, angiography or nuclear scintigraphy is done to confirm the diagnosis.

MANAGEMENT AND PROGNOSIS

The initial goals in managing dogs with portacaval anomalies is directed against the intestinal production and absorption of toxins. This is attempted by the use of defined-protein diets, antibiotics to reduce numbers of intestinal bacteria, and cathartics to minimize toxin absorption. This treatment is directed at only part of the abnormalities created by the shunt. It does not correct imbalances in carbohydrate, lipid, and protein metabolism and has no effect on hepatic atrophy. Medical treatment in the past for hepatic encephalopathy has been generally unsuccessful. Current information shows that surgical management of shunts offers the best hope for lasting improvement.

Diet

Ammonia is probably the most important toxic product produced in and absorbed from the intestine. Approximately one-half is derived from bacterial activity and the other half from metabolism of glutamine. Most ammonia produced from bacterial activity is located in the large intestine. Intestinal bacteria produce ammonia by their urease activity on urea or their properties to deaminate peptides. Urea diffuses from extracellular fluid into the intestine in amounts determined by dietary nitrogen levels. Dietary levels of protein and any unusual loss of blood or plasma protein into the intestine determine the amount of peptides entering the intestine. With proper levels and types of protein in the diet, digestion and absorption are optimal, so that little dietary nitrogen enters the colon. Thus, the protein fed should be readily digested and absorbed in the small intestine. Variable amounts of protein enter the colon in the form of desquamated mucosal cells and plasma proteins. Desquamation of the small intestinal epithelium is minimal when intestinal contents are scanty. Thus, diets low in roughage can be used to minimize desquamation if that appears to be a problem. Numerous problems can cause plasma proteins to be lost into the intestine. Hypoproteinemia associated with a shunt need not be due entirely to hepatic atrophy and impaired protein synthesis. The patient should be investigated and treated for all known causes of protein-losing enteropathy, with the goal of reducing the amounts of protein entering the colon.

It may be necessary to reduce the amount of protein given dogs with shunts in order to control signs of hepatic encephalopathy. When little or no protein is given and calories are supplied with glucose, nitrogen metabolism remains abnormal, as reflected in the ratio of plasma amino acids.[48] Thus, a protein-free diet may reduce blood ammonia levels and be beneficial in improving signs of hepatic encephalopathy but does not correct the amino acid imbalance. Protein restriction to manage a shunt dog can exacerbate other problems by causing already low plasma protein concentrations to decrease much further. The effects of a diet on hepatic protein synthesis can be evaluated by measuring plasma proteins. Hepatic metabolic functions require proteins for maintaining their role, and the restriction of protein intake compromises the hepatic ability to synthesize proteins for such maintenance. Protein restriction is indicated only with unmanageable signs of hepatic encephalopathy. In all other cases the level of dietary protein is not restricted but is adjusted to meet the needs for synthesizing body proteins and to prevent signs of hepatic encephalopathy, which, except in the acute case, may be of lesser importance. If possible, protein intake should be maintained at a minimum of one gram per 20 calories of food intake.

The source of protein is important to survival and clinical signs in dogs with shunts. Dogs with experimentally produced portasystemic shunts which are fed commercial dog food develop signs of hepatic encephalopathy and die within two to three months. Dogs with similar shunts who are fed a diet formulated with a protein from milk or soy beans do not develop clinical signs and can survive for many months.[49] This study is similar to studies showing survival time and clinical signs to be worse when meat rather than milk protein is fed. At one time it was believed that survival was due to these diets' improving abnormalities in metabolism of branched-chain, aromatic, and sulfur-containing amino acids. Despite feeding such diets, however, abnormalities persist in metabolism of branched-chain and aromatic amino acids. Moreover, the amino acid abnormalities can be worsened by feeding excess aromatic amino acids, but that does not worsen clinical signs.[20] Also, milk proteins and soy bean protein have total amounts of sulfur-containing amino acids similar to those of the meat proteins in commercial dogs foods. It is possible that the milk protein and soybean protein diets contain lower amounts of ammoniagenic amino acids such as threonine, glycine, serine, histidine, tryptophan, and lysine, but meat proteins have similar amounts of these amino acids to milk and soy bean proteins.

Glutamine and glutamic acid comprise up to 20% of the amino acid nitrogen in proteins. Following its absorption, a high percentage of the glutamine is converted to glutamate, releasing ammonia that represents one-half of the ammonia in the portal circulation. Controlling glutamine intake may be beneficial in dogs with shunts, but the glutamine-glutamate content of milk protein is relatively high, which suggests that glutamine content is unimportant. A number of other suggestions have been made to explain the beneficial effects of milk or soy bean protein diets. The most important may be that a high ratio of carbohydrate to protein is essential in order to see a benefit.

Carbohydrates are supplied in a form that is completely digested and absorbed in the cranial small intestine. They are required to minimize amino acid catabolism for energy, especially since the ones used for energy are the branched-chain amino acids, which are found at reduced levels. High dietary carbohydrate promotes insulin secretion, and glucagon release is less than with low dietary carbohydrate. That ratio favors an anabolic state where amino acids absorbed from the intestine are converted to protein rather than metabolized to glucose, which results in ammonia formation.

Fat is essential to the diet as an important source of calories and essential fatty acids; it also enhances palatability. A number of studies have shown that dogs do well on diets containing 20% to 25% fat. In contrast to that tolerance of triglycerides, free fatty acids interfere with ammonia metabolism, thereby contributing to hyperammonemia. They also contribute directly to hepatic encephalopathy. Most dietary fat is resynthesized into triglycerides and formed into chylomicrons before leaving the intestinal epithelial cells. Thus, a meal does not cause marked increases in plasma concentrations of free fatty acids. Plasma fatty acid levels increase during fasting when peripheral adipose triglycerides are catabolized for energy.

A diet formulated of cottage cheese or tofu and a readily digested starch such as polished rice meets the dietary requirements of dogs with shunts. Fats, preferably animal, are added to enhance palatability and to provide essential fatty acids, and, if the diet cannot be completely balanced, vitamins and minerals are supplemented. Meat is not recommended as a source of protein since numerous studies show that signs of hepatic encephalopathy and shortened survival times are problems when dogs with shunts are fed meat-based diets. Supplementation with mixtures of branched-chain amino acids offer no proven advantage. The protein content of the diet can be as low as 10% on a dry basis but should be increased with evidence of protein deficiency, such as hypoalbuminemia (see Chapter on nutrition for dietary formulation). As an alternative, meat-free prescription diets containing approximately 14% protein can be fed.

Cats must be fed a relatively high protein diet. They are fed a balanced diet in amounts providing 65 to 90 Kcal/kg body weight per day. Protein should be provided in amounts that account for 12% to 20% of their caloric needs, which is roughly twice that needed by dogs. There is little information on feeding cats with hepatic insufficiency. They are probably similar to other mammals in that feeding meat-protein diets worsens clinical signs and progression of the hepatic pathology. However, it is difficult to find cats that accept meat-free diets, especially when anorectic due to hepatic disease. Diets containing milk or soybean protein offer little advantages because of their amino acid composition. Although they may be beneficial in containing only small amounts of sulfur-containing amino acids which can produce toxic metabolites, they are deficient in taurine, whose chronic lack can result in ocular and cardiac problems. Milk has little taurine, and vegetable proteins have essentially none, so a diet based on these proteins must be supplemented with 50 mg taurine per day for an adult cat. That can be provided by supplementing the diet with clams, which have taurine amounts that are up to seven times greater than for fish, beef or chicken. Protein-restricted diets can be formulated and are also commercially available, such as the prescription diet Feline k/d.

Small meals are fed often to minimize the hepatic encephalopathy caused by large amounts of ammonia formed from glutamine metabolism and from excess protein entering the large intestine. Large amounts of protein in a single daily feeding exceeding an animal's nitrogen needs are catabolized for energy or converted to triglycerides. Following deamination of the proteins, additional ammonia must be converted to urea. Frequent feedings also reduce the daily periods during which body protein is catabolized for energy. During fasting, muscle protein is catabolized to amino acids, which are deaminated and converted to glucose, and peripheral triglycerides are catabolized to free fatty acids, which are metabolized to ketone bodies for energy. Protein catabolism produces additional ammonia to be detoxified, which perpetuates amino acid imbalances. The branched-chain amino acids and alanine are used primarily for energy, whereas the aromatic amino acids are metabolized in the liver and their rate of utilization is reduced with hepatic disease. The potential toxic effects of free fatty acids most likely appear during fasting, the time when their levels are highest. Long-chain fatty acids are incompletely oxidized in the liver, forming large amounts of octanoic acid, which contribute to encephalopathy. Frequent feedings also benefit carbohydrate metabolism. Dogs with portasystemic shunts can have low normal blood glucose concentrations. Hypoglycemia, manifested during fasting, is due to reduced glucose availability and is prevented by frequent feedings. Since oral glucose tolerance is impaired in dogs with shunts, frequent feedings maintain above-normal glucose levels. However, the derangement is not severe enough to produce significant hyperglycemia. Increasing fiber in the diet may promote the fecal excretion of nitrogen and improve signs of hepatic encephalopathy.

Dietary management of dogs with shunts is not a successful long-term treatment. Most do not have a normal life expectancy. Liver function deteriorates progressively because of progressive hepatic atrophy. Clinical signs of depression often persist despite optimum dietary management. The long-term prognosis is poor for animals managed only with controlled diets. Nonsurgical management of dogs with portasystemic shunts results in at least two-thirds dying or being euthanized. Of the remainder, 7% survive and do well on medical management; the outcome of some is unknown.

Control of Intestinal Microflora

Ammonia production and absorption is reduced when the numbers of ammonia-producing bacteria are decreased. Nonabsorbed antibiotics such as neomycin have been used in attempts to sterilize the intestines. Most gram-negative organisms have become resistant to the effects of these antibiotics, which were never active against anaerobes, also capable of producing ammonia. Neomycin, to be effective, must be given in doses that are large enough to be toxic to the intestinal mucosa. Thus, levels of neomycin effective in reducing the intestinal microflora should not be used more than a few days. Kanamycin and gentamicin are currently effective against most aerobes and may be effective during short-term therapy for shunts, although they have not been used for that purpose. Antibiotics such as the penicillins may suppress anaerobic intestinal bacteria numbers for a short time but have not been recommended for shunt therapy. In general, effective antibiotics given orally can markedly reduce the numbers of colonic bacteria for only a few days, after which their numbers return to normal. Some bacteria can become resistant to antibiotics within 24 to 48 hours, and suppression of sensitive strains can allow resistant ones to multiply. Thus, antibiotics are used for no more than a few days in patients with severe hepatic encephalopathy; they are not effective on a long-term basis. The use of some antibiotics such as tetracycline is contraindicated. Further discussion of antibiotics is found in Chapter 16 and 33.

Antibiotics to reduce the intestinal microflora have several other desirable effects. They minimize the conversion of methionine to toxic methyl mercaptan, the production of volatile fatty acids by fermentation of polysaccharides, and the production of endotoxins released from dying bacteria (reflecting the number of organisms in the gut). The use of antibiotics to reduce the microflora may have its most important value in these effects on endotoxin production and absorption.

Modification of the microflora has been attempted by oral administration of a microorganism that does not produce ammonia from urea or peptides. The theory is that the beneficial bacteria will replace ammonia producers that are a part of the normal microflora. Attempts to colonize the colon with lactobacillus species have been unsuccessful.[51] The normal microflora cannot be displaced by feeding a foreign bacteria, and even if it is temporarily disrupted, it rapidly returns to its normal population in both numbers and distribution.

Intestinal bacterial numbers can be reduced by diarrhea due to any cause. Salts causing a saline osmotic catharsis reduce bacterial numbers and prevent the accumulation of substrates for bacteria to metabolize and form toxic products.[52] Likewise, this prevents accumulation and absorption of toxic products. Diarrhea produced by saline cathartics lowers the pH of colonic contents to less than 6.0. Ammonia production by colonic bacteria and its absorption are reduced at a lower pH.[53] Ammonia exists in ionized (NH_4^+) and un-ionized (NH_3) forms in ratios determined by the pH of the solution. The pK (dissociation constant) for ammonia is 9.1 in the body fluids of the dog, meaning that at pH 9.1, half of ammonia is NH_4^+ and half is NH_3. As pH is reduced to that of body fluids (7.4), most ammonia exists as NH_4^+. Colonic contents normally have a higher pH than body fluids, as a result of colonic bicarbonate secretion. Thus, greater amounts of ammonia are NH_3, which, being lipid-soluble, readily diffuses across cell membranes and is absorbed. Reducing the colonic pH increases the concentration of ionized ammonia, which is poorly absorbed. This overall scheme is depicted in Figure 33-9. A disaccharide, lactulose, is used to reduce ammonia formation and absorption.[54,55] This sugar, which is not digested in the small intestine, is fermented by colonic anaerobic bacteria when it reaches the colon. The fermentation produces acid metabolites, which lower the pH of the colonic contents and increase the number of osmotically active particles, producing diarrhea. Lactulose's effectiveness is not well-understood, however, because sugars not assimilated in the small intestine but fermented in the colon generate products that are efficiently absorbed in the colon, with only small amounts excreted (fermentation produces volatile fatty acids, which can be toxic, as described earlier). With malabsorption of sugar in the small intestine, the amount of fluid entering the colon is greater than can be accounted for by the sugar's osmotic attraction. Thus, the mechanism of action of lactulose is somewhat different from the theoretical. Lactulose use is described in greater detail in Chapter 33.

Improvement in hepatic atrophy can be achieved by drugs that stimulate hyperplasia of the smooth endoplasmic reticulum. Phenobarbital or clofibrate, a drug that modifies lipid metabolism, induce the cytochrome P-450 enzymes in the liver. They restore liver weight to normal and may have a beneficial effect on signs of hepatic encephalopathy. There is no information on whether such drug therapy may beneficial in dogs with shunts.

Improvement in hepatic encephalopathy following administration of the benzodiazepine antagonist flumazenil has been reported in humans and experimental animals. That antagonist is believed to interfere with binding of the normal inhibitory neurotransmitter gamma-aminobuytric acid (GABA) with its receptors in the brain. Hepatic encephalopathy is supposedly due to increased GABA and increased receptor density caused by liver disease. The drug's effects are short-lasting, and its use in dogs must be considered experimental.

Surgery[47,56,57]

The only successful treatment for portasystemic vascular anastomoses is to surgically restore normal hepatic circulation.

Most portasystemic vascular anastomoses consist of a single large shunt, which can usually be attenuated surgically (Figure 35-10). Extrahepatic shunts are readily identified during celiotomy, whereas shunts branching from the portal vein within the hepatic parenchyma are difficult to identify. Most single extrahepatic portasystemic shunts arise from the gastrosplenic or splenic vein prior to their entry into the portal vein; the single shunt usually terminates in the caudal vena cava between the left phrenicoabdominal and renal vein. Since few large veins enter the abdominal vena cava, identification of these shunts is not difficult. Portal pressure is measured during closure of the shunt. Pressure can be measured with a water manometer and a catheter introduced through a mesenteric vein and advanced into the portal vein. The shunt is closed or attenuated with a silk ligature, and the degree of closure is determined by portal pressure increases above the normal of 13 cm water not exceeding 25 cm water. Attenuations or closure causing portal pressure to reach 40 cm water results in compromised splanchnic perfusion, ascites, and often death. Portal pressure is normally lowest in the nonfed and in animals under anesthesia. Therefore, recovery from anesthesia and resumption of feeding results in portal pressures greater than measured during surgery. That results in some dogs having unexpected problems, such as ascites or death within 24 hours after surgery, even though portal pressures did not increase that much immediately following surgical attenuation.

Single portacaval shunts may be partially or completely concealed within the liver. Identification of the branch off the portal that represents the shunt can be made by temporarily occluding portal branches entering the liver as pressure in the portal vein is monitored. Occlusion of portal branches to the liver results in little or no change in portal pressure that will be essentially that of the vena cava, 3 to 5 cm water. Occlusion of a portal branch that connects with the shunt causes portal pressure to increase to normal (8 to 15 cm water) or above normal pressure. Identification of the shunt may be assisted by probing with a catheter through portal branches entering the liver until one is found where there is no resistance and the catheter can be passed into the vena cava. When the shunt is not completely encircled by the liver, the shunt is usually occluded or attenuated wherever it enters the hepatic vein cranial to the liver.

Single intrahepatic shunts that are completely encircled by the liver are occluded or attenuated by an intravascular technique to reduce the opening of the shunt into the vena cava. Splanchnic blood flow is interrupted to perform the surgery on the opened vena cava, with the interruption not exceeding 10 minutes.

Dogs with multiple extrahepatic portasystemic shunts can be managed with surgical procedures to increase hepatic blood flow. Improving blood flow by ligation of the shunts or by diverting arterial blood flow into the portal vein has not resulted in improvement of clinical signs or clinical pathology. Improvement of hepatic blood flow is also accomplished by promoting blood flow from the caudal vena cava through the multiple shunts into the portal circulation. Raising pressure in the vena cava by banding or attenuating the vena cava immediately caudal to the liver promotes blood flow. Such banding to increase caudal vena cava pressure is done to achieve a pressure gradient of 1 to 2 mmHg between the vena cava and portal circulation. Vena cava attenuation raises portal pressure from 10-12 to 14-17 mmHg and caudal vena cava pressure from 0-4 to 16-18 mmHg to produce the gradient. Attenuation of the

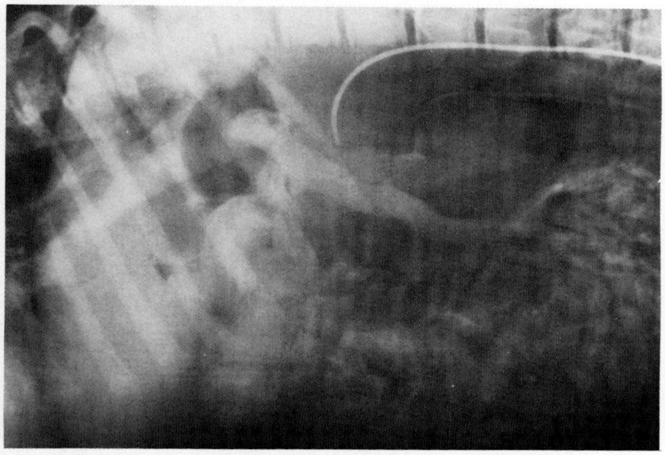

B

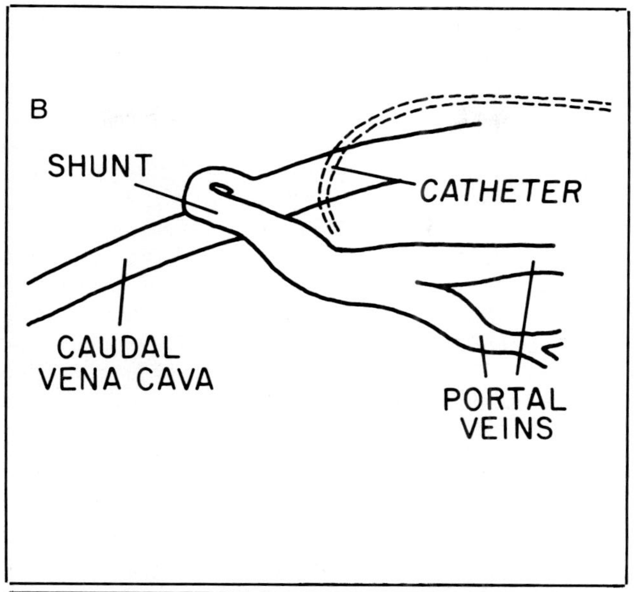

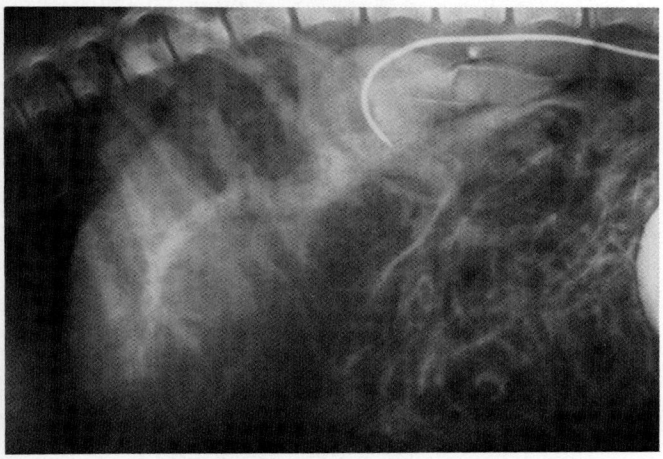

D

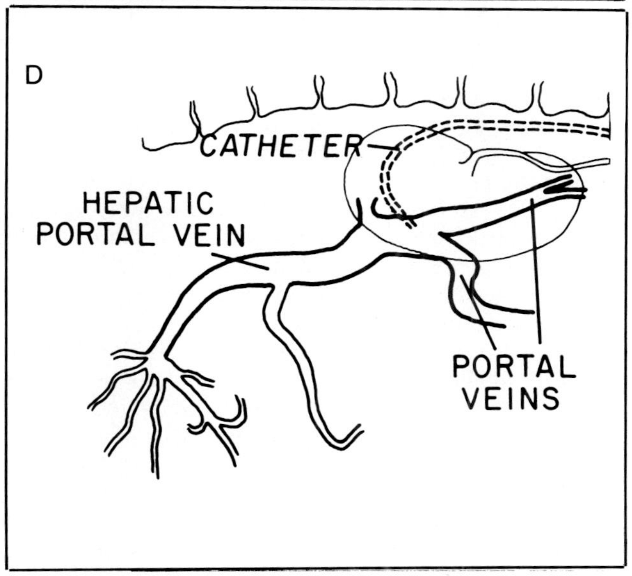

Figure 35-10. Angiograms of venous phase after injection of contrast medium through cranial mesenteric artery. (a) before surgery, the portasystemic shunt is filled with contrast medium, (b) diagrammatic illustration of contrast medium shown in A, (c) after surgical closure, the venous phase of the angiogram shows no contrast medium entering the caudal vena cava directly, (d) diagrammatic illustration of angiogram in C. Before surgery, a hepatic portal system is not seen, whereas after surgery, a normal appearing hepatic portal system is outlined.

vena cava is limited by portal pressure's not increasing to more than 20 mmHg, systemic hypotension, and splanchnic congestion. Most dogs develop a vena cava to portal vein pressure gradient so that blood flows from the former to the latter. In some cases it is not possible to develop such a change in the pressure gradient and blood flow. Attenuation of the vena cava usually causes temporary ascites and pelvic limb edema.

The importance of measuring portal pressure during shunt attenuation is questioned by the results of one report.[57] Shunts were attenuated without pressure measurements until grossly visible signs of portal hypertension developed. The signs were blanching of the duodenum and jejunum followed by more obvious pulsation in jejunal arteries. Small intestinal motility increased and at times was greatly augmented. With the appearance of these changes no further attenuation was attempted, and if no further evidence of greater hypertension, such as mild cyanosis and hyperemia, appeared over the next fifteen minutes the degree of attenuation was sealed and the surgery was completed. The surgery was successful in achieving immediate resolution of clinical signs; eight of the nine dogs treated eventually became clinically normal. If a surgeon can develop the skill to recognize the tissue changes signifying optimum attenuation, it may not be necessary to measure portal pressures during shunt attenuation.

Surgical attenuation of single extrahepatic portasystemic shunts can result in survival and remission of all clinical signs in greater than 95% of all affected dogs and cats. Complications unique to surgical correction of any shunts include problems in attenuating vessels to the optimum degree, so that severe portal hypertension does not develop, and problems with acute thrombosis of the portal vessels and shunts. Surgical correction of single intrahepatic shunts is successful in approximately 75% of all dogs, the lower rate being the result of a greater risk for complications. Banding of the caudal vena cava is successful in achieving remission in about 60% of all dogs with multiple shunts. The successful cases were usually those with liver biopsies that were similar to those seen with single portasystemic shunts. Those multiple shunts may be congenital, as are the single shunts. Dogs with multiple shunts developing because of cirrhosis and portal hypertension cannot be expected to respond favorably to banding of the vena cava to improve portal blood flow through the liver. Biopsy of the liver is important for differentiating dogs with multiple shunts that respond from those that do not respond to attenuation of the vena cava.

Although angiographic studies often fail to reveal a hepatic portal circulation, the liver in dogs with shunts may possess vessels required for normal hepatic circulation. Normal vessels are present at birth, but as the shunted animal matures they fail to develop because they do not carry a normal flow of blood. The liver thus fails to grow properly. When portasystemic anastomoses are corrected at a young age, the chance for success is greater. The liver and its vasculature can still develop in the immature dog, responding to the restoration of normal circulation by developing normal structure with normal function. Partial shunt closure may be less successful in mature dogs, however. Most shunts are not recognized until dogs approach maturity. Surgical closure of shunts in mature dogs usually produces dramatic improvement of clinical signs although liver function does not always improve. The histology of the liver shows that the atrophied liver contains normal numbers of vessels. Parenchymal atrophy is reversible, as the liver has a remarkable capacity for regeneration. Liver biopsies of young dogs with a surgically corrected shunt show that atrophied hepatic parenchyma can be transformed into a histologically normal-appearing liver (Figure 35-11).

ARTERIOVENOUS FISTULA

Fistulae can develop between the hepatic artery and portal venous vessels, resulting in severe derangement of circulation through the liver.[58,59] The high pressure gradient between the artery and vein causes hepatic sinusoidal blood pressure to be greatly increased. The intrahepatic portal hypertension causes pressure increases, transmitted retrograde through the portal system, that result in the appearance of multiple extrahepatic portacaval shunts. That is not unexpected since portal pressure increases from other causes result in such shunts developing.

Arteriovenous fistulae are caused by abdominal trauma, rupture of a hepatic arterial aneurysm, iatrogenic (secondary to surgical intervention or diagnostic procedures), and congenital defects. Congenital arteriovenous fistulae result from failure of differentiation of the common embryological anlage into artery and vein. The result is a persistence of a number of multitudinous communications normally present between arteries and veins at the beginning of the process of differentiation. Hence, congenital arteriovenous fistulae usually involve multiple vessels.

Clinical signs appear shortly after trauma or surgery in acquired fistulae. They usually do not appear until four months of age with congenital fistulae; it is not unusual for signs to sometimes appear a long time after fistulae formation. Clinical signs usually appear acutely and can include depression, anorexia, weight loss, and diarrhea. Ascites is always seen, which is expected because of the portal hypertension. Most cases will show a variety of neurological signs, such as disorientation, behavioral changes, seizures, and coma. Laboratory findings are those consistently seen with other circulatory disturbances such as portasystemic shunts. They include increased sulfobromophthalein retention, hyperammonemia, hypoproteinemia, and hypoalbuminemia.

Radiographic studies, selective celiac arterial angiography, or hepatic nuclear scintigraphic studies using a radioactively labeled colloid identify both hepatic arterioportal fistulae and the portacaval shunts that develop secondarily. Celiac angiography shows portal blood flow to be hepatofugal (away from) rather than the normal hepatopedal. The hepatic sinusoids provide the resistance to change blood flow direction. If that resistance was not available, the high portal pressure would be transmitted to the vena cava and the right heart, resulting in signs of cardiac failure. No such failure is seen with hepatic arterioportal fistulae, however.

Gross pathology shows one or more lobes of the liver involved although overall liver size is usually reduced. Dilated, tortuous, pulsating vessels are found on the surface of affected lobes. The portal vein and caudal vena cava are distended with multiple portacaval shunts usually seen in the left renal area. Affected lobes have numerous large cavernous vessels within. Microscopically, affected lobes contain numerous dilated thin-walled vessels, presumably portal vein branches and numerous small arteries. Portal vessel intima has increased elastin fibers,

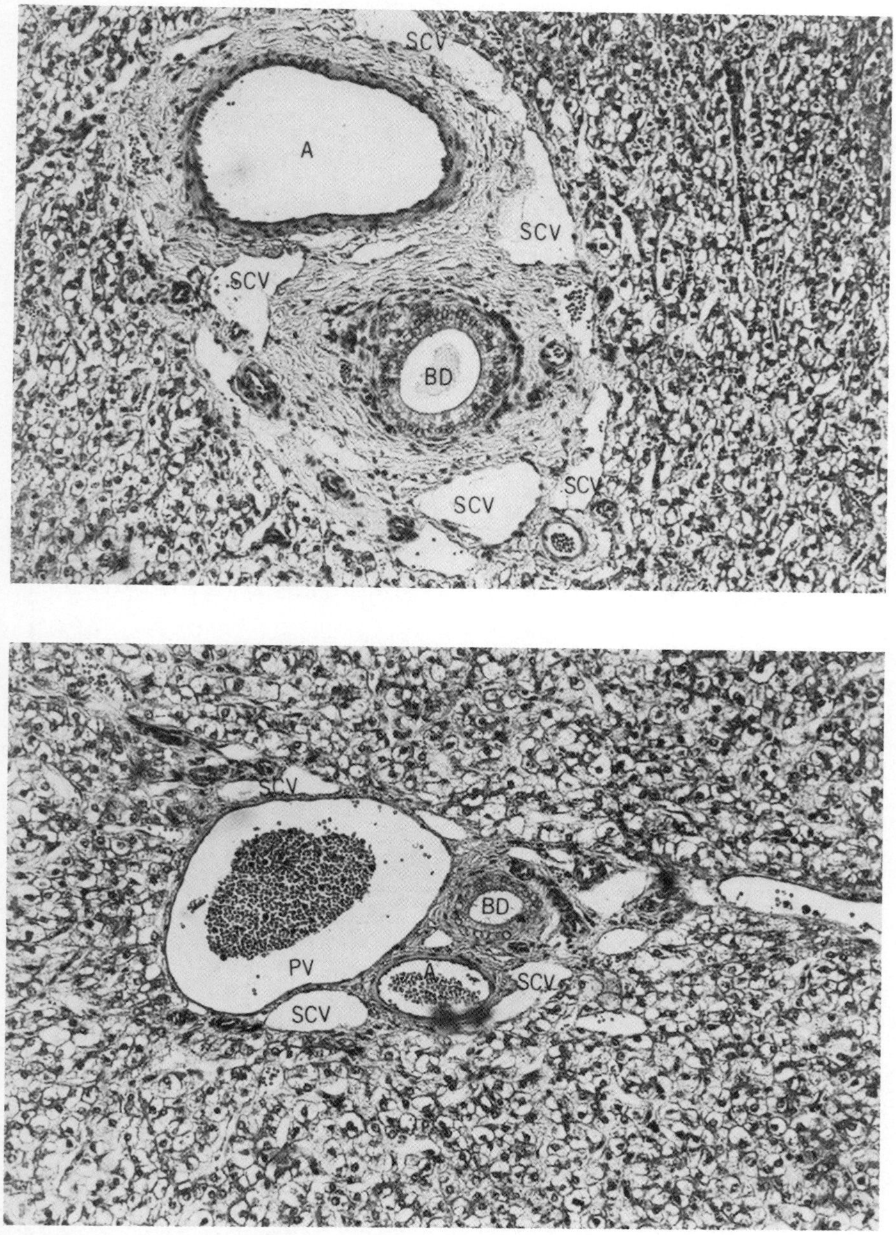

Figure 35-11. Hepatic biopsies from a dog with a portasystemic vascular anastomosis. Portal triad before surgical closure of shunt (a) shows a large bile duct (Bd), an artery (A), and many small caliber vessels (SCV). Portal veins are notably absent. Hepatocytes are atrophied. Caliber of artery is large since arterial blood flow increases in dogs with portasystemic shunting of blood flow. After surgical closure of the shunt portal triads contain large portal veins (PV) in addition to many small caliber vessels. Hepatocytes are normal. (By permission E.M. Breznock, JAVMA, April, 1979).

and vessel media is thickened both by smooth muscle hyperplasia and by increased elastin fibers. Manifestations of prior portal vein thrombosis and recanalization are frequently found. Hepatic arterioles show similar smooth muscle hyperplastic changes and increased elastin. Hepatic parenchymal changes include atrophy of hepatic plates, dilation and congestion of sinusoids, and proliferation of bile ducts.

Arterioportal fistulae are managed by surgical resection of affected liver lobes. Of the small number of cases reported most have survived and are clinically normal after such surgery.

CHRONIC PASSIVE CONGESTION

Hepatic circulation can be passively congested from a number of extrahepatic circulatory problems. The most common cause is congestive heart disease. Pressure in the right atrium and caudal vena cava increases following reduced cardiac function. Hepatic venous sphincters protect the hepatic sinusoidal pressure from increased vena cava pressure. The protective ability is limited so that with increasing vena cava pressure, buffering by the sphincter is severely reduced and sinusoidal pressure increases. Portal hypertension in sinusoids is transmitted back through the portal vein and into mesenteric veins.

Clinical signs with hepatic passive congestion are primarily those produced by the cardiac or other extrahepatic circulatory problem. Biochemical changes include some reflecting altered hepatic function and integrity. Plasma activities are increased for ALP and ALT in dogs and cats (Table 35-6). Some dogs have increased plasma cholesterol, bilirubin, or glucose. Some have hypoproteinemia and hypoalbuminemia and many are anemic. Pathologic changes with passive congestion of the liver occur primarily in zone 3 (centrolobular). They include

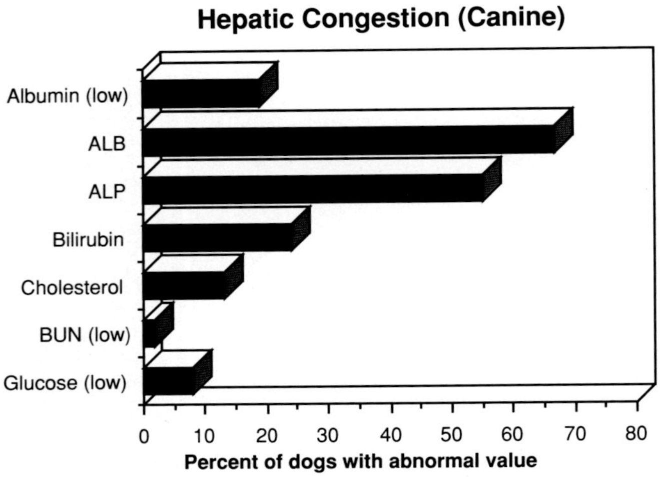

Table 35-6a. Comparison of sensitivities for different tests in dogs with heaptic congestion. Below: graphs showing dostribution of clinical pathology values in dogs with hepatic congestion. Points on graphs represent 0%, 25%, 50%, 75% and 100% medians. Normal range is in shaded area.

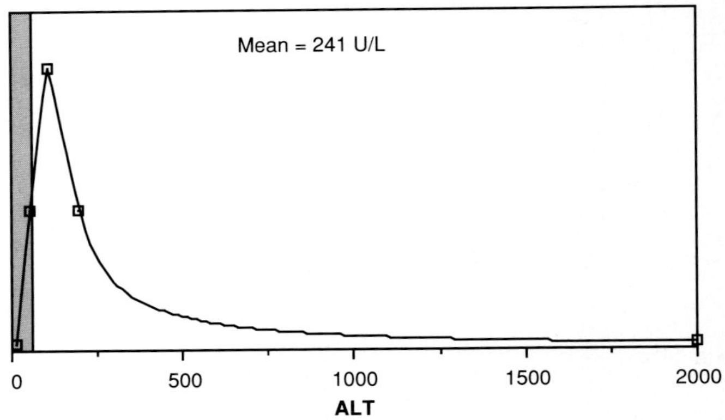

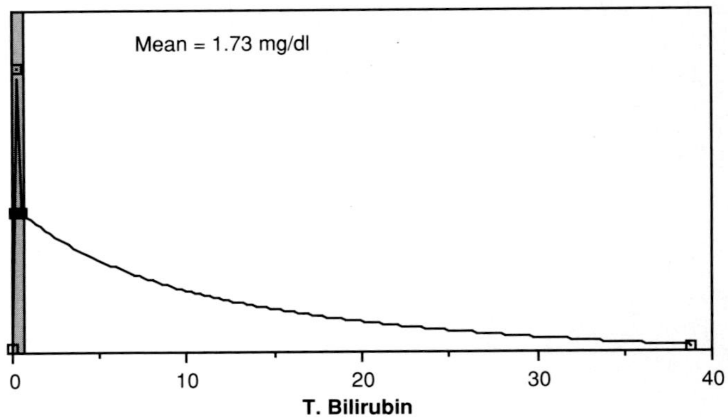

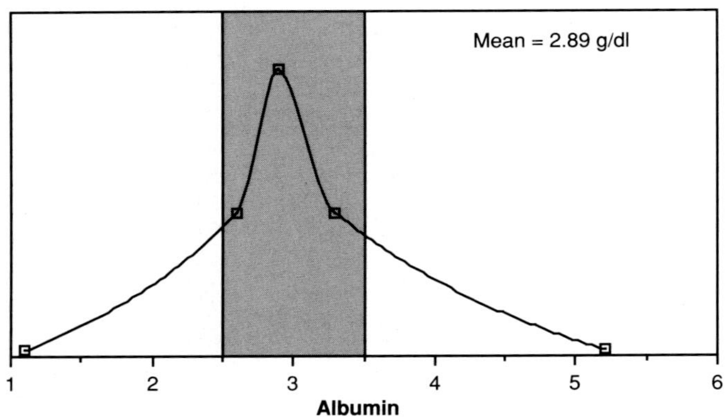

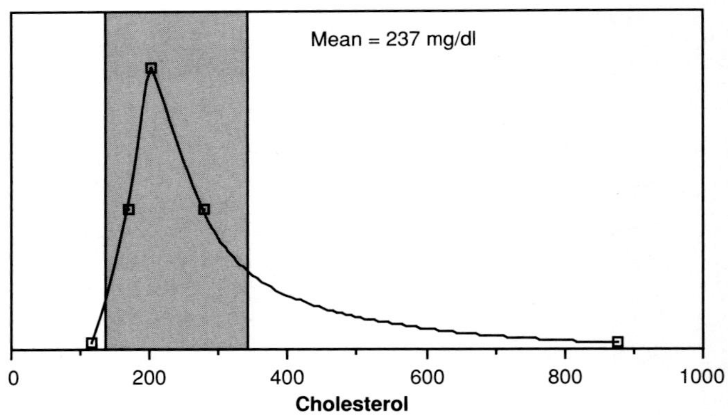

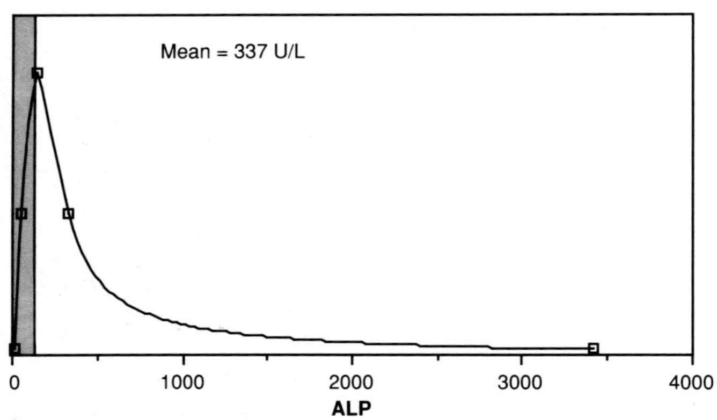

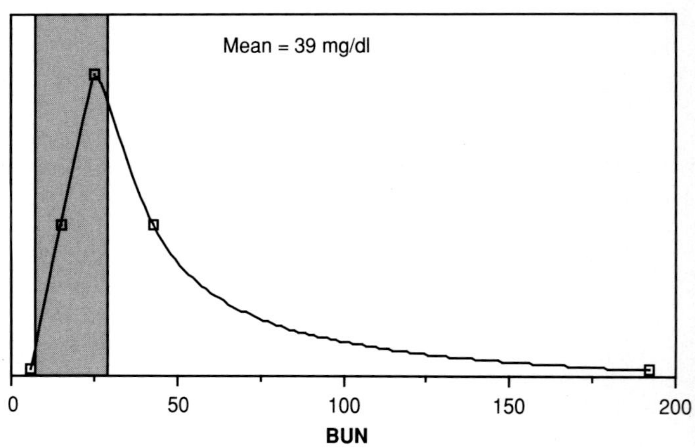

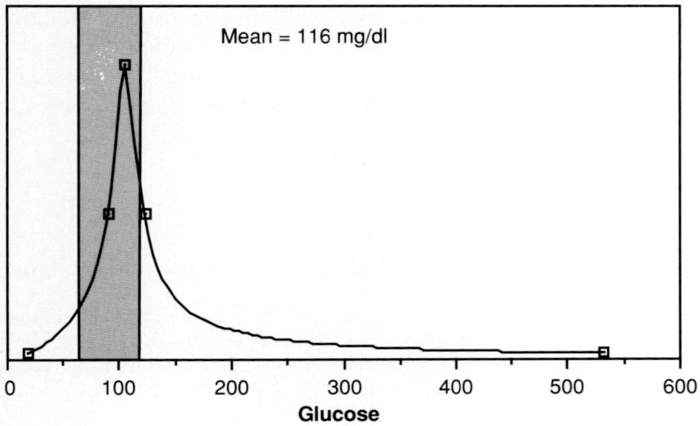

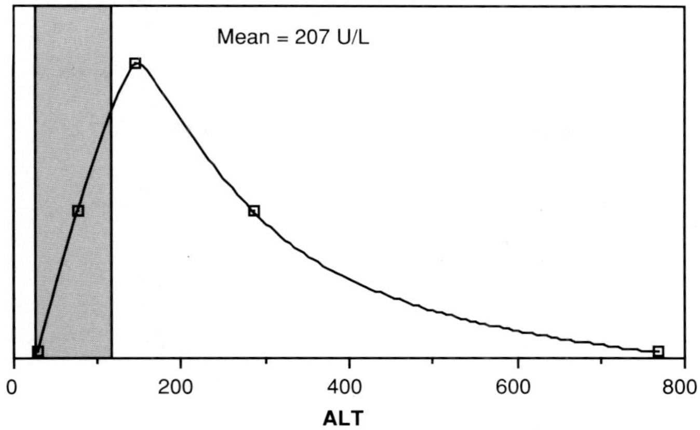

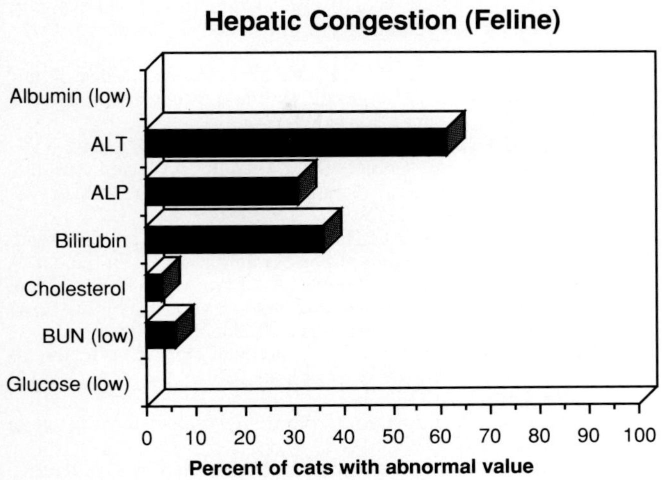

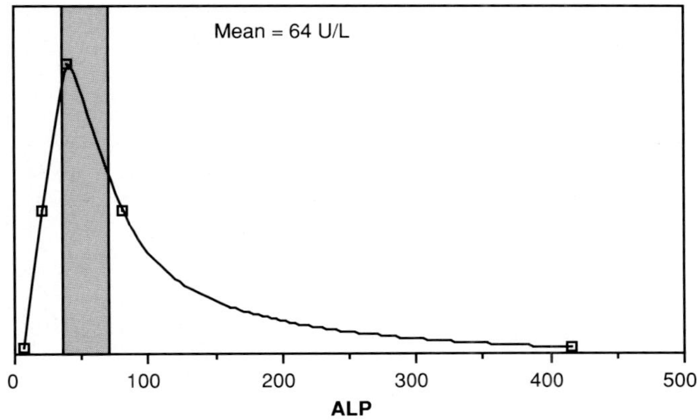

Table 35-6b. Comparison of sensitivities for different tests in cats with hepatic congestion. Below: graphs showing distribution of clinical pathology values in cats with hepatic congestion. Points on graphs represent 0%, 25%, 50%, 75% and 100% medians. Normal range is in shaded area.

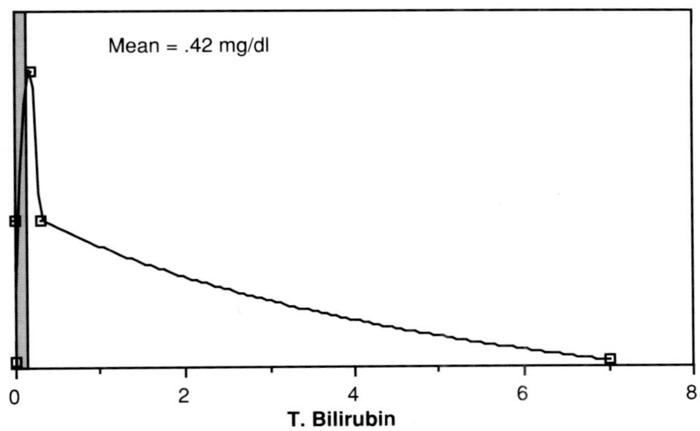

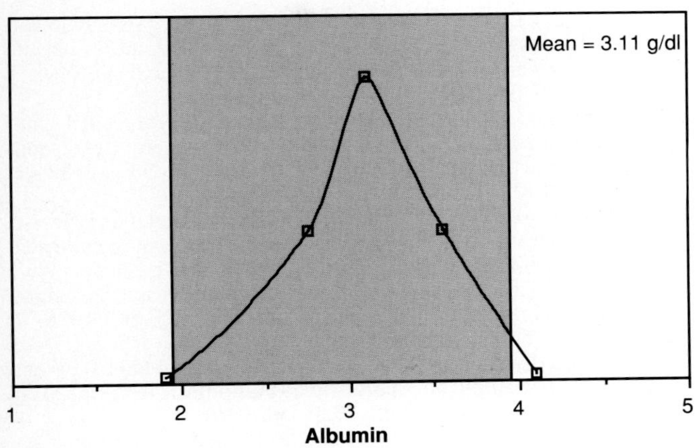

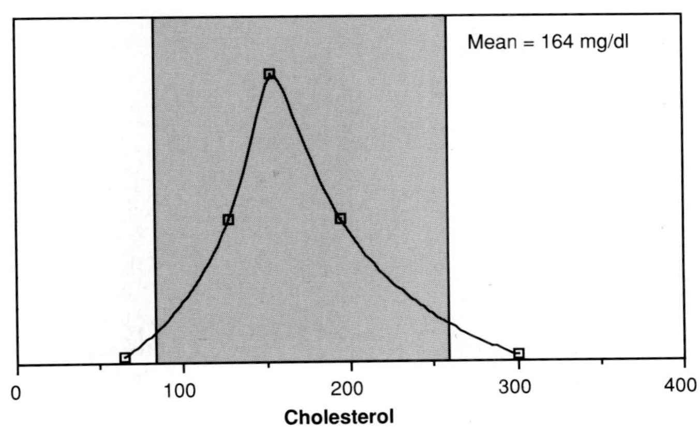

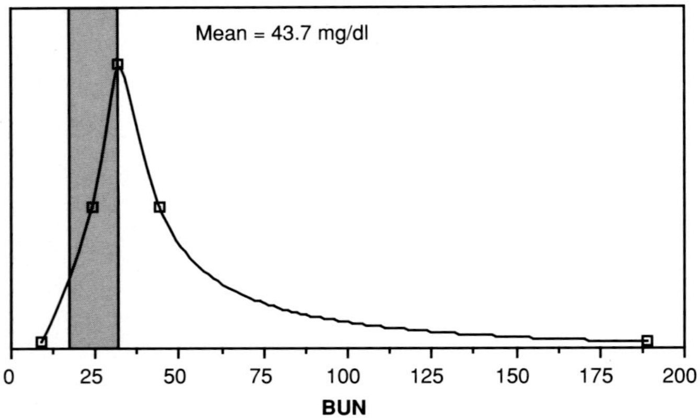

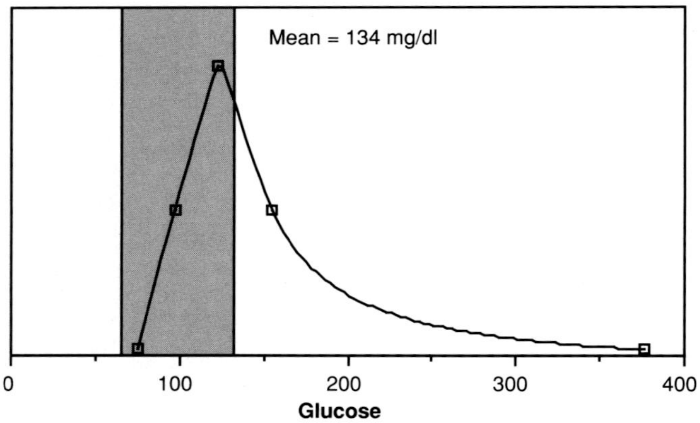

hepatocyte atrophy, vacuolar changes described as hepatopathy, lipidosis, necrosis, and fibrosis, depending on the severity and duration of the congestion. These changes are produced by the sinusoidal hypertension and the reduction in oxygen and substrates for energy provided by the circulation. The degenerative changes are similar to those produced by other problems, such as severe anemia, that reduce oxygen supply to zone 3 hepatocytes. Hypertension in central veins and sinusoids contributes to hepatocyte atrophy and is also responsible for the congestion found throughout these vessels.

Extrahepatic causes of passive congestion in the liver are usually identified with little difficulty. Biochemical panels are often run on such patients, and abnormalities should be expected for tests that reflect liver involvement in the overall problem. With that understanding the abnormalities can be explained, and it is not necessary to pursue some other liver problem with a biopsy of the liver.

LIVER LOBE TORSION

Hepatic circulation can be compromised uncommonly by torsion of a liver lobe.[60] The cause of torsion is unknown. Affected dogs have clinical signs of acute abdomen. Pain on palpation of the cranial abdomen is consistently found and occasionally a mass can be palpated. Biochemical abnormalities include increased activities of ALT and sometimes ALP, but the increases found are only mild to moderate (two to five times greater than upper normal values). Other abnormalities are consistent with acute abdominal problems but do not indicate that the liver is the location of the problem. Radiographs may reveal a soft tissue mass and sometimes abdominal effusion. Management is surgical, with removal of the affected lobe.

REFERENCES

1. Bollman, J.L.: The animal with Eck fistula. Physiol. Rev. 41:607-621, 1961.
2. Hickman, J., Edwards, J.E. and Mann, F.C.: Venous anomalies in a dog. Anat. Rec. 104:137-146, 1949.
3. Ewing, G.O., Suter, P.F. and Bailey, C.S.: Hepatic insufficiency associated with congenital anomalies of the portal vein in dogs. AAHA 10:463-476, 1974.
4. Whiting, P.: Unpublished data.
5. Rothuizen, J., van den Ingh, TSGAM, Voorhout, G., van der Luer, R.J.T. and Wouda, W.: Congenital porto-systemic shunts in sixteen dogs and three cats. J. Small An. Pract. 23:67-81, 1982.
6. Berger, B., Whiting, P.G., Breznock, E.M., Bruhl-Day, R. and Moore, R.F.: Congenital feline portosystemic shunts. JAVMA 188:517-5231, 1986.
7. Scavelli, T.D., Hornbuckle, W.E., Roth, L., Rendano, V.T., deLahunta, A., Center, S.A., French, T.W. and Zimmer, J.F.: Portosystemic shunts in cats: Seven cases (1976-1984). JAVMA 189:317-325, 1986.
8. Blayter, A.C., Holt, P.E., Pearson, G.R., Gibbs, C. and Gruffydd-Jones, T.J.: Congenital portosystemic shunts in the cat: A report of nine cases. J. Small An. Pract. 29:631-645, 1988.
9. Rudolph, A.M.: Hepatic and ductus venosus blood flows during fetal life. Hepatology 3:254-258, 1983.
10. Lohse, C.L. and Suter, P.F.: Functional closure of the ductus venosus during early postnatal life in the dog. AJVR 38:839-844, 1977.
11. Vitums, A.: Portosystemic communications in the dog. Acta Anat. 39:271-299, 1959.
12. Lickley, H.L.A., Chisholm, D.J., Rabinovitch, A., Wexler, M. and Dupre, J.: Effects of portacaval anastomosis on glucose tolerance in the dog: evidence of an interaction between the gut and the liver in oral glucose disposal. Metabolism 24:1157-1168, 1975.
13. Waddell, W.R. and Sussman, K.E.: Plasma insulin after diversion of portal and pancreatic venous blood to vena cava. J. Appl. Physiol. 22:808-812, 1967.
14. Strombeck, D.R., Rogers, Q.R. and Stern, J.: Effects of ammonia infusion on plasma glucagon, insulin, and amino acids in intact, pancreatectomized, and adrenalectomized dogs. AJVR 42:810-818, 1981.
15. Schaeffer, M.C., Rogers, Q.R., Buffington, C.A., Wolfe, B.M. and Strombeck, D.R.: Long-term biochemical and physiologic effects of surgically placed portacaval shunts in dogs. AJVR 47:346-355, 1986.
16. Coyle, J.J., Schwartz, M.Z., Marubbio, A.T., Varco, R.L. and Buchwald, H.: The effect of portacaval shunt on plasma lipids and tissue cholesterol synthesis in the dog. Surgery 80:54-60, 1976.
17. Guzman, I.J., Coyle, J.J., Schneider, P.D., Varco, R.L. and Buchwald, H.: The effect of selective visceral caval shunt on plasma lipids and cholesterol dynamics. Surgery 82:42-50, 1977.
18. Horak, W., Gangl, A., Funovics, J. and Grabner, G.: Effect of portacaval shunt and arterialization of the liver on bile acid metabolism. Gastroenterology 69:338-341, 1975.
19. Derr, R.F. and Zieve, L.: Effect of fatty acids on the disposition of ammonia. J. Pharm. Exp. Ther. 197:675-680, 1976.
20. Rogers, Q.: Unpublished data.
21. Liehr, H., Grun, M. and Thiel, H.: Hepatic blood flow and cardiac output after porta-caval anastomosis in the rat. Acta Hepato-Gastroenterol. 23:31-40, 1976.
22. Keraan, M., Meyers, O.L., Engelbrecht, G.H.C., Hickman, R., Saunders, S.J. and Terblance, J.: Increased serum immu-

noglobulin levels following portacaval shunt in the normal rat. Gut 15:468-472, 1974.
23. Merino, G.E., Jetzer, T., Doizaki, W.M.D. and Najarian, J.S.: Methionine-induced hepatic coma in dogs. Am. J. Surg. 130:41-46, 1975.
24. Thompson, J.S., Porter, K.A., Hayashida, N., McNamara, D.J., Parker, T.S., Russell, W.J.I., Francavilla, A. and Harzyl, T.E.: Morphologic and biochemical changes in dogs after portacaval shunt plus bile fistula or ileal bypass: Failure of bile fistula or ileal bypass to prevent hepatocyte atrophy. Hepatology 3:581-587, 1983.
25. Dubuisson, L., Bioulac, P., Saric, J. and Balabaud, C.: Hepatocyte ultrastructure in rats with portacaval shunt. Dig. Dis. Sci. 27:1003-1010, 1982.
26. Adamsons, R.J., Arif, S., Babich, A., Butt, K., Lam, A. and Minkowitz, S.: Arterialization of the liver in combination with a portacaval shunt in the dog. Surg. Gynecol. Obstet. 140:594-600, 1975.
27. Aldrete, J.S.: Quantification of the capacity of the liver to remove ammonia from the circulation of dogs with portacaval transposition. Surg. Gynecol. Obstet. 141:399-404, 1975.
28. Gurll, N.J., Reynolds, D.G., Coon, D. and Shirazi, S.S.: Acute and chronic splanchnic blood flow responses to portacaval shunt in the normal dog. Gastroenterology 78:1432-1436, 1980.
29. Duguay, L.R., Lee, S. and Orloff, M.S.: Regulation of liver regeneration by the pancreas. Gastroenterology 70:980, 1976.
30. Rosenkranz, E., Duguay, L.R. and Orloff, M.S.: Effects of liver regeneration on pancreatic hormone levels in blood. Gastroenterology 70:991, 1976.
31. Starzl, T.E., Watanabe, K., Porter, K.A. and Putnam, C.W.: Effects of insulin, glucagon, and insulin/glucagon infusions on liver morphology and cell division after complete portacaval shunt in dogs. Lancet 1:821-825, 1976.
32. Audell, L., Jonsson, L. and Lannek, B.: Congenital portacaval shunts in the dog. Zbl. Vet. Med. A., 21:797-805, 1974.
33. Suter, P.F.: Portal vein anomalies in the dog: their angiographic diagnosis. J. Am. Vet. Radiol. 16:84-97, 1975.
34. Doni, M.G., Vassanelli, P., Bonadiman, L. and Avventi, G.L.: Thrombocytopenia and coagulation impairment after portacaval shunt in the rat. Haemostasis 7:19-25, 1978.
35. Hess, F., Jerusalem, C. and Willemen, A.: Altered portal pressure secondary to portacaval and portasystemic shunts in the rat: The effect on liver function and intestinal integrity. Eur. Surg. Res. 14:286-297, 1982.
36. Price, J.B., McCullough, W., Peterson, L., Britton, R.C. and Vorhees, A.B.: Effects of portal systemic shunting on intestinal absorption in the dog and in man. Surg. Gynecol. Obstet. 125:305-310, 1967.
37. Shatney, C.H., Harmon, J.W. and Rich, N.M.: Effects of portasystemic shunting on visceral and portal blood flow in the dog. Gastroenterology 83:1170-1176, 1982.
38. Meyer, D.J., Strombeck, D.R., Stone, E.A., Zenoble, R.D. and Buss, D.D.: Ammonia tolerance test in clinically normal dogs and in dogs with portosystemic shunts. JAVMA 173:377-379, 1978.
39. Marretta, S.M., Pask, A.J., Greene, R.W. and Liu, S.: Urinary calculi associated with portosystemic shunts in six dogs. JAVMA 178:133-137, 1981.
40. Birchard, S.J., Biller, D.S. and Johnson, S.E.: Differentiation of intrahepatic versus extrahepatic portosystemic shunts in dogs using positive-contrast portography. JAAHA 25:13-17, 1989.
41. Prouty, D.L.: Hepatoencephalopathy due to portocaval shunt in a dog. JAVMA 167:756-757, 1975.
42. Burgener, F.A., Gothlin, J.H. and Gutierrez, O.H.: Percutaneous transhepatic portography in the dog. Invest. Radiol. 13:26-27, 1978.
43. Hornof, W.J., Koblik, P.D. and Breznock, E.M.: Radiocolloid scintigraphy as an aid to the diagnosis of congenital portacaval anomalies in the dog. JAVMA 182:44-46, 1983.
44. Koblik, P.D., Yen, C.-K., Hornof, W.J., Whiting, P. and Fisher, P.: Use of transcolonic ^{123}I-Iodoamphetamine to diagnose spontaneous portosystemic shunts in 18 dogs. Vet. Radiol. 30: 67-73, 1989.
45. Koblik, P.D., Komtebedde, J., Yen, C.-K. and Hornof, W.J.: Use of transcolonic ^{99m}Tc pertechnetate as a screening test for portosystemic shunts in dogs. JAVMA In Press.
46. Wrigley, R.H., Konde, L.J., Park, R.D. and Lebel, J.L.: Ultrasonographic diagnosis of portacaval shunts in young dogs. JAVMA 191:421-424, 1987.
47. Breznock, E.M.: Surgical manipulation of portosystemic shunts in dogs. JAVMA 174:819-826, 1979.
48. Fischer, J.E., Funovics, J.M., Aguirre, A., James, J.H., Keane, J.M., Wesdrop, R.I.C., Yoshimura, N. and Westman, T.: The role of plasma amino acids in hepatic encephalopathy. Surgery 78:276-290, 1975.
49. Thompson, J.S., Schafer, D.F., Haun, J. and Schafer, G.J.: Adequate diet prevents hepatic coma in dogs with Eck fistulas. Surg. Gynecol. Obstet. 162:126-130, 1986.
50. Strombeck, D.R., Schaeffer, M.C. and Rogers, Q.R.: Dietary therapy for dogs with chronic hepatic insufficiency. In, Current Veterinary Therapy, vol. VIII. Edited by R.W. Kirk. W.B. Saunders, Philadelphia, 817-821, 1983.
51. Fischer, J.E. and Baldessarini, R.J.: Pathogenesis and therapy of hepatic coma. In, Progress in Liver Diseases, vol. 5. Edited by H. Popper and F. Schaffner. Grune and Stratton, New York, 363-397, 1976.
52. Agostini, L., Down, P.F., Murison, J. and Wrong, O.M.: Faecal ammonia and pH during lactulose administration in man: comparison with other cathartics. Gut 13:859-866, 1972.
53. Vince, A., Dawson, A.M., Park, N. and O'Grady, F.: Ammonia production by intestinal bacteria. Gut 14:171-177, 1973.
54. Conn, H.W., Leevy, C.M., Vlahcevic, Z.R., Rodgers, J.B., Maddrey, W.D., Seeff, L. and Levy, L.L.: Comparison of lactulose and neomycin in the treatment of chronic portasystemic encephalopathy. Gastroenterology 72:573-583, 1977.
55. Pirotte, J., Guffens, J.M. and Devos, J.: Comparative study of basal arterial ammonia and of orally-induced hyperammonemia in chronic portal-systemic encephalopathy, treated with neomycin, lactulose, and an association of neomycin and lactulose. Digestion 10:435-444, 1974.
56. Breznock, E.M., Berger, B., Pendray, D., Wagner, S., Manley, P., Whiting, P., Hornof, W. and West, D.: Surgical manipulation of intra hepatic portocaval shunts in dogs. JAVMA 182:798-805, 1983.
57. Mathews, K. and Gofton, N.: Congenital extrahepatic portosystemic shunt occlusion in the dog: Gross observations during surgical correction. JAAHA 24:387-394, 1988.
58. Whiting, P.G., Breznock, E.M., Moore, P., Kerr, L., Berger, B., Gregory, C. and Hornof, W.: Partial hepatectomy with temporary hepatic vascular occlusion in dogs with hepatic arteriosous fistulas. Vet. Surg. 15:171- 180, 1986.
59. Moore, P.F. and Whiting, P.G.: Hepatic lesions associated with intrahepatic arterioportal fistulae in dogs. Vet. Pathol. 23:57-62, 1986.
60. Glardon, V.O., Fluckiger, M., Keller, M. and Stockli, R.: Leberlappentorsion: Ein Beitrag zur Differentialdiagnose des Akuten Abdomens. Kleinteirpraxis 32:207-210, 1987.

Chapter 36

Hepatic Neoplasms

The liver can be the site of primary and metastatic neoplastic disease. Primary hepatic neoplasms represent 3.8% of the total pathologic diagnoses in dogs and metastatic hepatic neoplasms account for 13.9% of the total. The most common primary neoplasms are hepatocellular carcinomas and adenomas arising from hepatocytes. Seen less frequently are cholangiocarcinomas and adenomas, neoplasms developing from bile-duct epithelium. Among the primary hepatic neoplasms seen least commonly are fibromas, fibrosarcomas, hemangiomas, and hemangiosarcomas. Metastatic tumors are of a wide variety and invade the liver from many different primary sites (Table 36-1). The metastases are not predominantly from tissues in the abdominal viscera. Primary hepatic neoplasms are unusual in cats. Metastatic neoplasms in the liver account for 14.9% of the total pathologic diagnoses found in cats. Lymphosarcoma represents 75%, adenocarcinomas 14%, carcinomas 9% and other tumors 2% of the total.

The incidence of primary hepatic tumors in dogs necropsied is 0.6% to 0.8% and is about 0.05% in all dogs seen. The incidence based on biopsies is .09%. Primary hepatobiliary neoplasms account for 1.2% of all tumors seen in dogs.

Table 36-1 Canine Metastatic Liver Disease

Tumor Type		Primary Site	
Hemangiosarcoma	29%	Generalized	27%
Lymphosarcoma	23%	Unknown	14%
Adenocarcinoma	13%	Spleen	12%
Carcinoma	13%	Heart	8%
Leiomyosarcoma	6%	GI	7%
Sarcoma	6%	Pancreas	6%
Myeloma	3%	Islet Cell	5%
Osteosarcoma	2%	Bone	3%
Miscellaneous	5%	Oral Cavity	3%
		Adrenal	3%
		Renal	3%
		Lung	2%
		Other	7%

Most of the primary liver neoplasms in dogs are hepatocellular adenomas or hepatocellular carcinomas. Hepatocellular adenomas are commonly seen and infrequently reported. They may generate little interest because small adenomas closely resemble nodular hyperplasia, which is very commonly seen in older dogs. Grossly and histologically, these adenomas can be difficult to distinguish from nodular hyperplasia or even normal liver tissue. Adenomas are usually well-circumscribed and demarcated from adjacent tissue. On histology they show compression of adjacent hepatic parenchyma but they are not necessarily encapsulated. Usually appearing as a single nodule in dogs over 10 years of age, they consist of friable tissue that sometimes ruptures with hemorrhage into the abdomen, producing clinical signs. That is more likely in larger adenomas, which can become quite large (up to 20 cm).

Hepatocellular carcinomas are the most common primary hepatic malignancy reported in the dog, accounting for more than 54% of the total number.[1-4] Affected dogs' ages average 11 years with greater than 80% older than 10 years. More males than females have been reported to be affected. Hepatic carcinoids closely resemble hepatocellular carcinoma; with special stains they can be differentiated.[5] Until recently they were believed to be rare, but one survey showed they account for 14% of primary hepatic neoplasms in dogs.[5] They were found most often in dogs less than 10 years of age, with a mean age of 8 years.

Bile duct carcinomas account for 22% to 35% of all primary hepatic neoplasms in dogs.[1,2,6] Most (63%) are seen in dogs over 10 years of age with an average of 11 years. Sarcomas account for 13% of all primary hepatic neoplasms and have a similar age distribution.

Hepatic neoplastic disease is reported to represent 1.9% of all neoplastic disease in cats.[7] The majority is accounted for by malignant lymphoma, which can be multicentric or in some cases restricted to the liver. Lymphoma may be uncommonly seen as a primary disease of the liver in cats. Hepatocellular carcinoma and bile duct carcinoma are unusual in the cat, with only a few cases reported.

The incidence of metastatic neoplastic disease of the liver is 1.2% in necropsies and .092% of all dogs seen. The incidence of metastatic involvement of the liver as determined by liver biopsy is .04% of all dogs, a figure lower than the incidence above because liver biopsy is not indicated when a neoplastic disease can be diagnosed more readily by biopsy of another tissue. The incidence of .04% reflects those cases where a diagnosis of malignancy is confirmed most easily by liver biopsy. The liver is the most common site for metastasis of malignancies with liver involvement in 31% to 37% of all cases; pulmonary involvement follows with 24%.

HEPATOCELLULAR CARCINOMAS

Etiology and Pathogenesis[8,9]

Most current information suggests that environmental factors play an important role in the pathogenesis of hepatocellular carcinomas. Incrimination of environmental factors is based on experimental studies showing that primary hepatic tumors can be induced by toxins. Carcinogens can be naturally occurring substances, such as aflatoxins, produced by toxigenic strains of the fungus *Aspergillus flavus*. This organism, with undoubtedly others, is widespread in nature, and under appropriate conditions it multiplies and produces the toxin, especially in prepared animal foods during storage. Aflatoxins can produce acute hepatic lesions as well as causing hepatic neoplasms in experimental animals. The relationship of aflatoxin in animal feeds to naturally occurring hepatic tumors is not known. A number of other hepatic carcinogens are found in nature, although they are not normally available to small animals. They include pyrrolizidine alkaloids, cycasin, and safrole, all of which are found in plants.

Nitrosamines have potent properties able to cause hepatic necrosis and primary neoplastic disease in experimental animals. Nitrosamines are produced from nitrites and secondary amines. Nitrites are an important food additive used in meat products. Secondary amines are ubiquitous in nature, being found in both plants and animals. Nitrosamines are easily formed from those two types of chemicals either outside the body or inside the gastrointestinal tract. It is not known whether the incidence of primary hepatic neoplasms has increased during the years that commercial dog foods have become popular.

A variety of other chemicals and some drugs can be carcinogenic. They include carbon tetrachloride, polycyclic hydrocarbons, aromatic amines and azo dyes, organochloride pesticides, polychlorinated biphenyls, griseofulvin, and tannic acid. Most chemicals are not carcinogenic in their native form; they must first be metabolized by the liver to an active agent. Metabolic conversion is by cytochrome enzymes of the endoplasmic reticulum. They catalyze aromatic ring oxidation, aliphatic hydroxylation, oxidative demethylation, and N-hydroxylation, which results, in most cases, in the formation of highly reactive epoxides. The metabolites formed are positively charged compounds able to react with negatively charged constituents of the cell. The nucleic acids RNA and DNA readily react with these carcinogens. Cell proteins and polysaccharides also form chemical bonds with the carcinogens. The net effect is alteration of cell macro-molecules, resulting in injury to cell organelles and structural membranes. The persistence of carcinogens makes repair impossible, and the host responds to the overall loss of hepatic function by cell proliferation. The ability to produce carcinogens lies in microsomal enzymes' metabolizing the precursors. Inhibition of microsomal enzyme activity therefore prevents primary hepatic neoplasms despite the presence of high levels of carcinogen precursors. Stimulation of cytochrome enzyme activity, such as by phenobarbital, can increase the risk for other chemicals to be converted to carcinogens. Other factors influencing the carcinogenic potential for a drug or chemical include state of nutrition and rate of hepatocyte turnover.

Primary hepatocellular carcinoma is not always easily diagnosed on a biopsy specimen since hepatocyte proliferation varies in degree, ranging from a normal hepatic response for replacing injured hepatocytes to uncontrolled growth of hepatocytes in carcinomas. Normal proliferation is described as nodular hyperplasia or regenerative nodule formation, and when the etiological agent for their formation is removed the nodules may be able to regress. Nodules containing proliferating hepatocytes are unable to restore normal hepatic lobular architecture, however. Nodules appear during prolonged intake of carcinogens, and the process progresses no further when the carcinogen is removed. Hepatic regeneration occurs after partial hepatectomy, ceasing after the liver reaches its normal size. When a carcinogen is administered at the time of partial hepatectomy, however, hepatic carcinomas are produced in high incidence without any need for long-term administration of the carcinogen. Rapidly dividing cells become more vulnerable to any kind of injury.

Hepatic neoplasms are associated with transmissible viruses in humans and animals. It is unknown whether viruses may have such a relationship in dogs and cats. Some viruses can cause hepatic disease in dogs (see Chapter 29). Tumors can be induced by viruses when part of the native viral DNA or the DNA copy of retrovirus RNA is integrated into the genome of the host cell, in this case hepatocytes. That genetic material is continuously passed on to newly formed hepatocytes long after the initial viremia and infection. The abnormal and foreign genetic information directs the synthesis of unusual cell material, and that may include agents that interfere with control of cell growth. This illustrates how potentiation of a normal physiological response can lead to regeneration on one hand and hepatocellular carcinoma at the extreme.

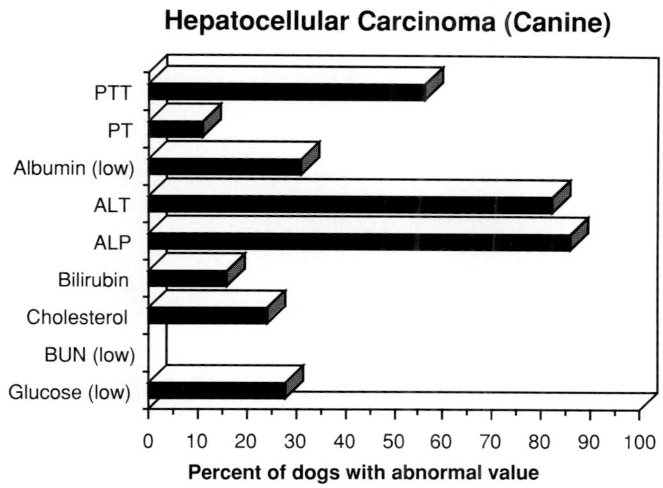

Table 36-2. Comparison of sensitivities for different tests in dogs with hepatocellular carcinoma. Following graphs show distribution of clinical pathology values in dogs with hepatocellular carcinoma. Points on graphs represent 0%, 25%, 50%, 75% and 100% medians. Normal range is in shaded area.

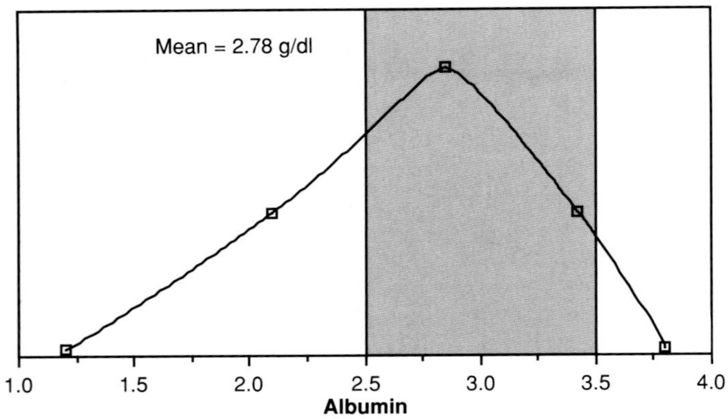
Mean = 2.78 g/dl
1.0 1.5 2.0 2.5 3.0 3.5 4.0
Albumin

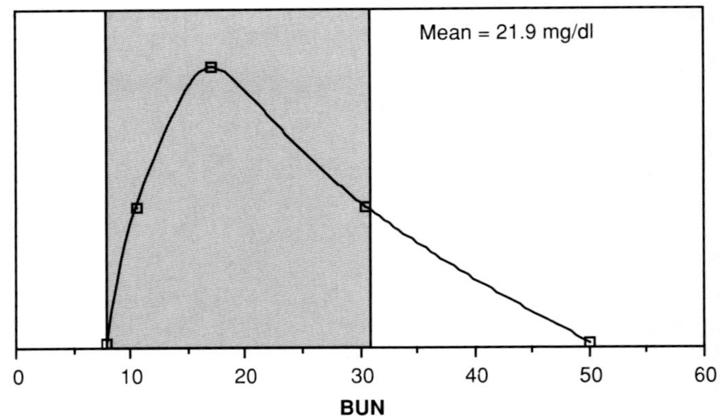
Mean = 21.9 mg/dl
0 10 20 30 40 50 60
BUN

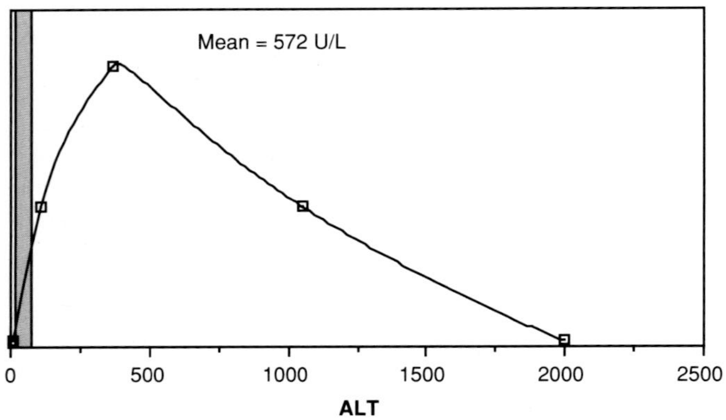
Mean = 572 U/L
0 500 1000 1500 2000 2500
ALT

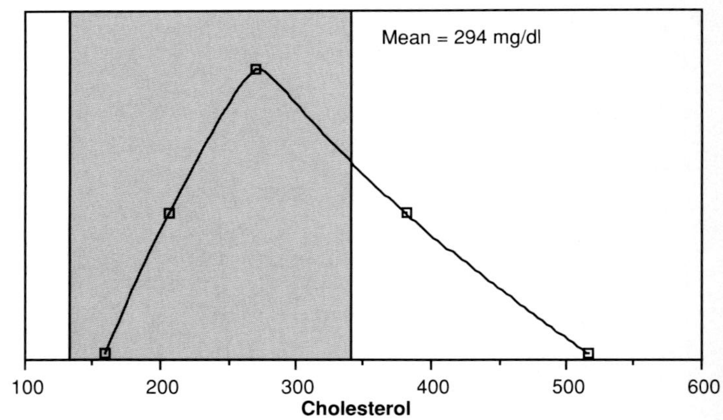
Mean = 294 mg/dl
100 200 300 400 500 600
Cholesterol

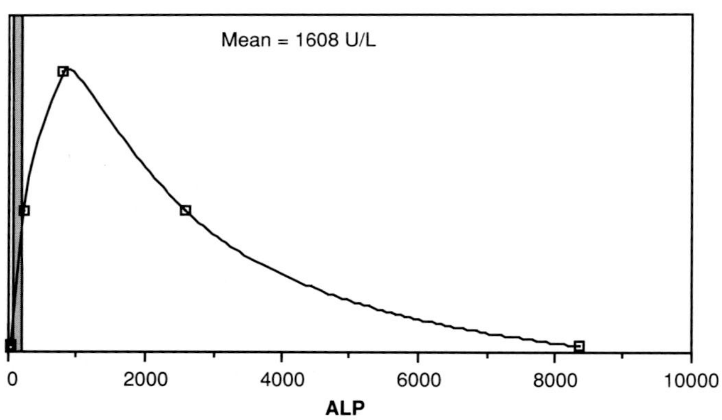
Mean = 1608 U/L
0 2000 4000 6000 8000 10000
ALP

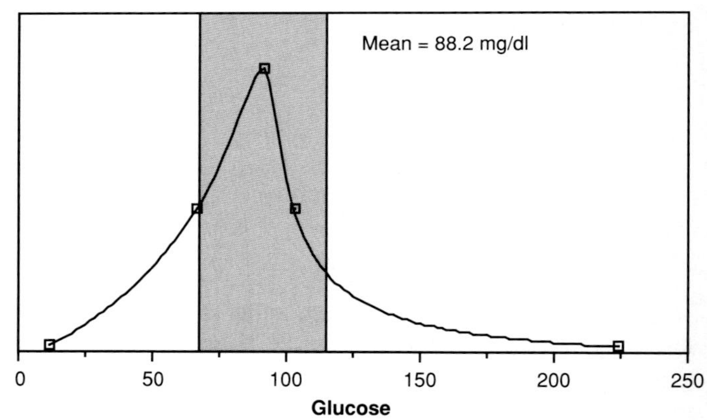
Mean = 88.2 mg/dl
0 50 100 150 200 250
Glucose

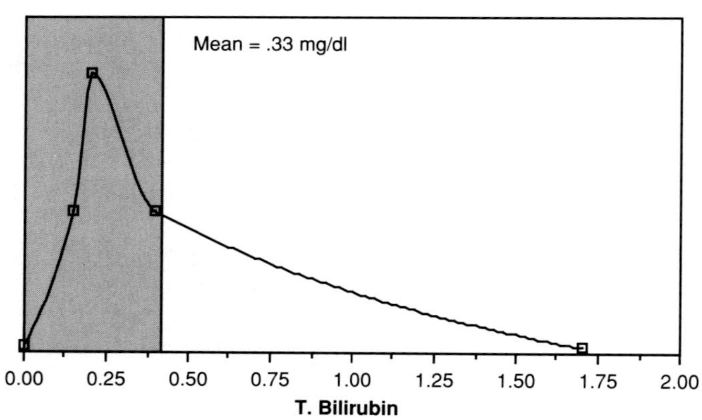
Mean = .33 mg/dl
0.00 0.25 0.50 0.75 1.00 1.25 1.50 1.75 2.00
T. Bilirubin

Table 36-3. Metabolic Abnormalities in Humans With Hepatocellular Carcinoma

Serum protein abnormalities	
	Fetoprotein
	Abnormal globulin
	Increased hepatoglobin
	Increased ceruloplasmin
	Increased $alpha_1$-antitrypsin
	Aberrant alkaline phosphatase
	Abnormal isoferratins
	Increased levels of chorionic gonodotrophins
	Increased levels of chorionic somatotrophins
Hematologic abnormalities	
	Dysfibrinogenemias, cryofibrinogenemia
	Antifibrinolysis
	Plasmacytosis
	Hemolytic processes
	Erythrocytosis
Lipid abnormalities	
	Hypercholesterolemia
	Hypertriglyceridemia
Other abnormal serum factors	
	Porphyria
	Cystathioninuria
	Ethanolaminuria
Functional and hormone-like abnormalities	
	Hypoglycemia
	Pseudohyperparathyroidism
	Precocious puberty
	Gynecomastia
	Hypertrophic pulmonary osteoarthropathy

Clinical and Laboratory Findings[2,4,10]

The clinical signs of primary hepatocellular carcinoma are nonspecific and characteristic of hepatic disease in general. The most consistent signs—depression, weakness, anorexia, weight loss, polydipsia, diarrhea, and vomiting — usually do not appear until an advanced stage of pathology. Hepatomegaly is a consistent feature, and clinical signs are often subtle until marked hepatomegaly develops. Increased bleeding tendency, icterus, and signs of hepatic encephalopathy are seen infrequently.

Biochemical evaluation of animals with primary hepatocellular carcinomas reveals a pathological process more severe than suggested by the clinical signs (Table 36-2). Plasma alanine aminotransferase (ALT) activities range from slight increases to the marked elevations that are found consistently with severe hepatic necrosis. Plasma ALT activity is abnormal in about 80% of all dogs. The mean activity is 4 to 7 times the upper limit of normal. That is in contrast to the slight elevation, if any, of plasma ALT activity when metastatic hepatic neoplasms interfere with liver function (Table 36-4). An increased rate of release of this transaminase may be a feature of hepatic carcinoma cells, or it may result from the necrosis of normal hepatocytes following injury from adjacent neoplastic tissue, a suggestion that is not supported by morphologic findings. Plasma alkaline phosphatase (ALP) activity also increases with primary hepatic neoplasms. The usual increases range from 400 to 800 IU/L, although some increase up to 9,500 IU/L. The consistently elevated ALP activity does not reflect cholestasis, since only one-fourth of the cases studied are associated with hyperbilirubinemia. The increased ALP activity found with hepatocellular carcinomas reflects an increase in hepatic synthesis and release of alkaline phosphatase. This enzyme is found predominantly in proliferating biliary epithelial cells, most commonly following obstruction of the biliary system and during liver regeneration. The ALP concentrations found here are considerably higher than in dogs with biliary obstruction. The marked increases in some dogs may represent an ALP isoenzyme described as an 'atypical' alkaline phosphatase, found in some humans with hepatocellular carcinoma.[11] An aberrant alkaline phosphatase would not be a surprising product of a liver tumor producing many abnormal proteins.

Plasma albumin concentrations usually decrease with hepatocellular carcinoma, which could result from decreased synthesis or from increased turnover. There is no evidence that hepatic function is reduced enough to affect albumin synthesis, a function that is not reduced until hepatic disease becomes severe. Nor is there evidence for increased catabolism of albumin by losses through the gastrointestinal tract or kidneys. The neoplastic process may be responsible for an increased rate of albumin degradation. The albumin produced may be abnormal, so that its half life is shorter than normal.

Increased plasma globulin concentrations have been found in dogs with primary hepatocellular carcinoma.[4] The liver synthesizes most plasma globulins, and they can be one of many metabolic abnormalities with hepatocellular carcinoma in humans (Table 36-3).[11] However, 80% of the globulins in these dogs were gamma-globulins, which are not produced by the liver. The basis for the hypergammaglobulinemia was not known. If the increased gamma-globulin concentrations were due to the liver's failure to remove antigens carried from the gut in the portal circulation, comparable increments in this fraction should be evident in patients with portasystemic shunts and chronic hepatitis. However, few patients with these types of problems have increased plasma gamma-globulin fractions.

Hypoglycemia has been associated with tumor development in humans as well as animals.[10,12-14] The hypoglycemia has been attributed to the tumor's increased utilization of glucose, or to the tumor's production and release of insulin-like activity, or to other hormones that affect the maintenance of normal blood glucose concentrations. Plasma insulin concentrations are low-normal, however. One reported case of hypoglycemia with a hepatoma in a dog showed a normal mobilization of hepatic glycogen following the administration of glucagon.[13] Blood sugar levels remained elevated abnormally long, however, and there was not the normal response of insulin release to cause blood glucose to return to normal. Plasma insulin concentrations during fasting and hyperglycemia were abnormally low. Fasting hypoglycemia associated with normal hepatic glycogen stores indicated that glucagon or other glycogen-mobilizing hormones were not being released. There was evidence for inhibition of the release of both insulin and glucagon in this dog. The only known substance that inhibits the release of these hormones is somatostatin, which is normally produced primar-

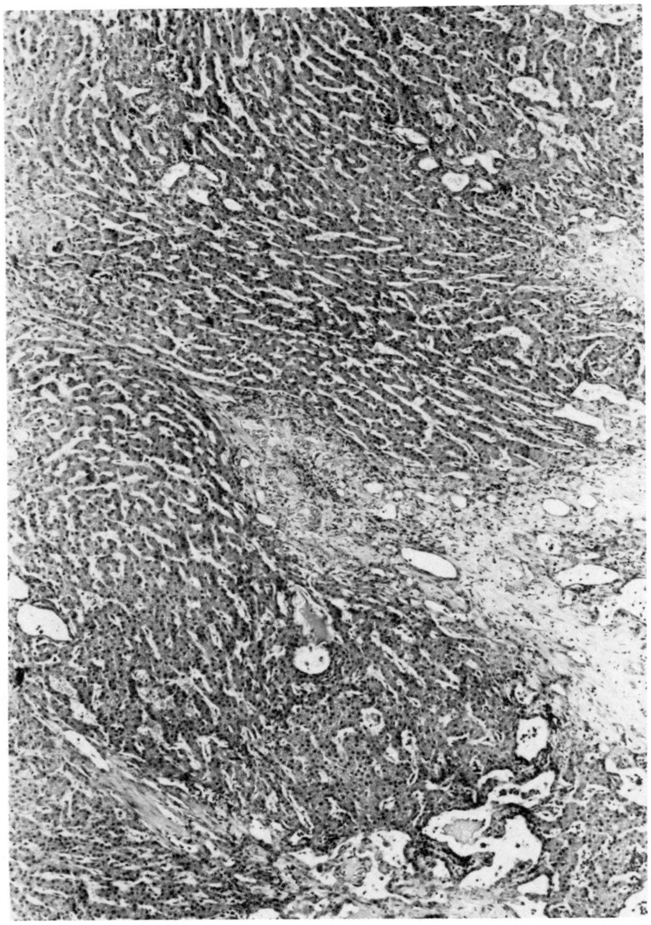

Figure 36-1a. Nodules of regenerating hepatocytes as shown in this photo often grossly are mistaken for hepatic tumors. Biopsy shows the nodules to contain normal hepatocytes, which are usually replicating in a manner that does not restore hepatic architecture.

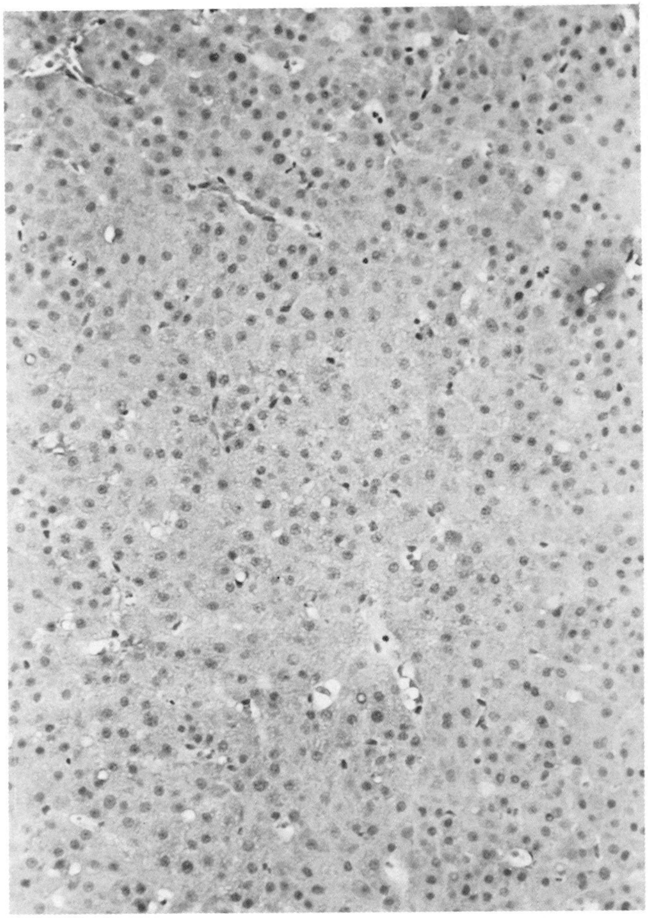

Figure 36-1b. Hepatic regeneration and adenomas. Photomicrograph of biopsy specimen shows normal-appearing well-differentiated hepatocytes, no recognizable portal areas or central veins; and no evidence for rapid cell multiplication. This photo does not differentiate hepatic regeneration from adenomas. When adenomas are diffuse and not capsulated, a definitive diagnosis is not possible. Hepatic regeneration can progress to hepatocellular carcinoma; see text on pathogenesis.

ily in the pancreas.[15] It remains to be determined whether hepatic tumors that consist of fetal-type cells can gain the ability to synthesize hormones with somatostatin-like activity. Some hepatocellular carcinomas, are now known to be carcinoids, which are neoplasms originating from neuroectodermal tissue, or from amine precursor uptake and decarboxylation (APUD) cells.[5] Tumors made up of these cells, APUDomas, produce and release a number of biogenic amines and peptide hormones normally found in the gastrointestinal tract.[11] Some dogs may have hypoglycemia because excess amounts of a hormone such as somatostatin is being produced and released.

An islet-cell tumor is usually thought of as the most likely possibility in animals with hypoglycemia as the primary sign.[14] These patients should be carefully evaluated for evidence of hepatic disease when the differentiation is not that clear-cut. Plasma insulin levels are determined to make a definitive diagnosis of functional insulinoma before surgery is performed.

Plasma alpha-fetoprotein levels are increased in primary hepatic neoplasms, and it has been suggested that laboratory tests to identify this increment are useful in diagnosis of the disease.[16] Alpha-fetoprotein, a major plasma protein in the developing fetus, appears early and decreases in amount shortly after birth. Its function in the fetus is unknown. The protein does not appear in the adult unless there is a reversion of hepatocytes to the primitive fetal form. Although plasma levels of alpha-fetoprotein increase with primary hepatic carcinomas, the elevations are not pathognomonic for this problem. The production of alpha-fetoprotein can be stimulated in experimental animals given carcinogens before any morphological changes are evident. The levels of this protein also increase in some human patients with other forms of liver disease, such as cirrhosis and biliary tract obstruction. The common denominator signifying its appearance is cell injury that results in regeneration. In animals, an increased production of alpha-fetoprotein most likely reflects the regeneration of hepatocytes.[17] Measurement of this plasma protein is not currently used diagnostically to identify primary hepatic carcinomas.

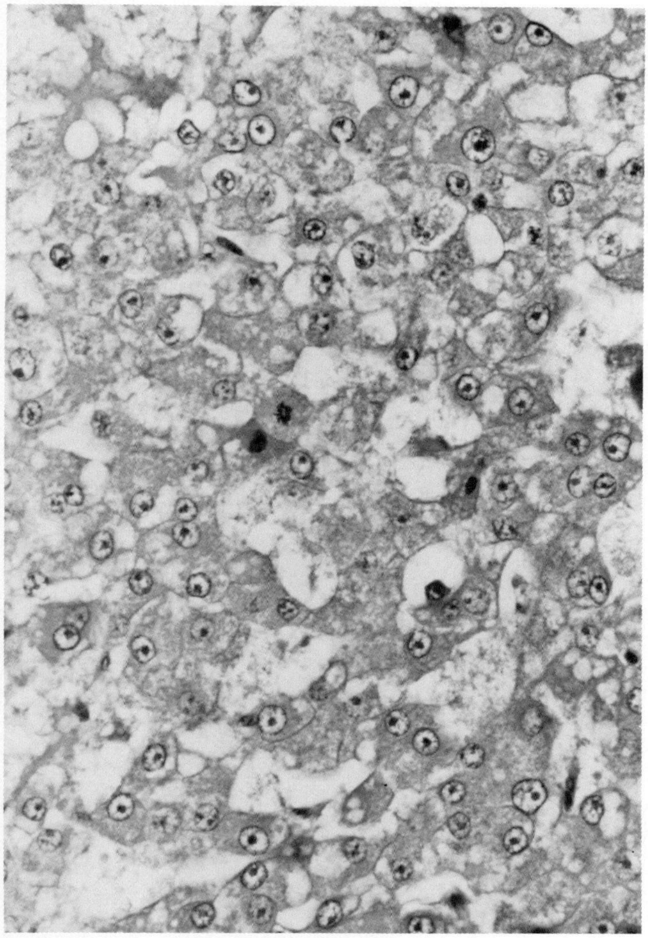

Figure 36-2a. Hepatocellular carcinoma. Mitotic figure is seen in center of photo. Increased rate of cell division is also suggested by many large nuclei (in hepatocytes) that contain dark staining chromatin. Biopsy specimen.

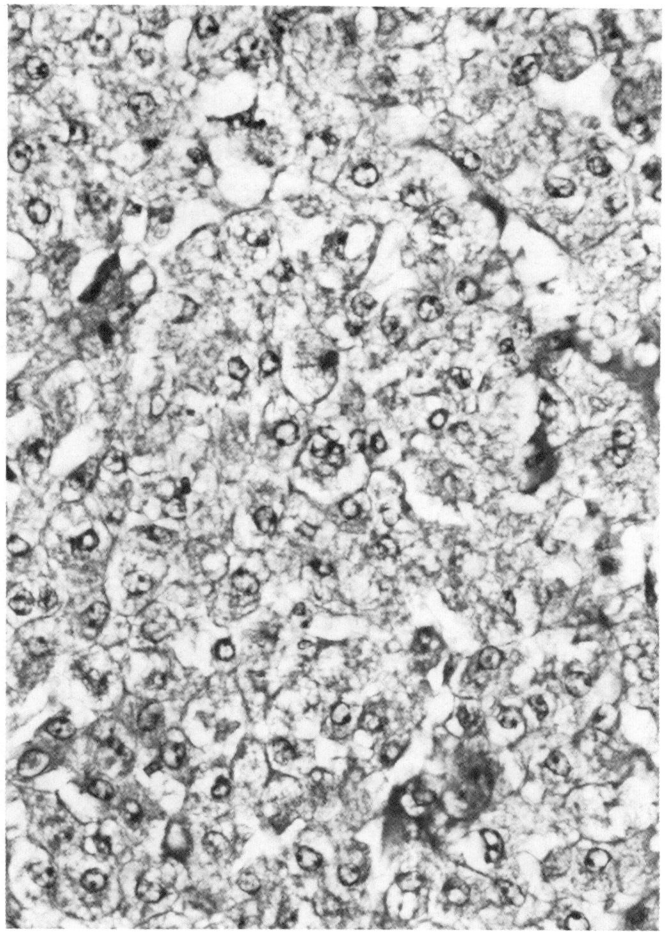

Figure 36-2b. Hepatocellular carcinoma. Hepatocytes are well-differentiated and show many clear cells, suggested to be due to glycogen or lipid accumulation. Normal architecture is noticeably absent. Mitotic figures are not seen. Biopsy specimen.

Hypercholesteremia is found in a few dogs with hepatocellular carcinoma. That may represent excessive production by tumor cells. Other abnormalities have been described in humans but not in small animals.

Pathology Findings

Hepatocellular carcinomas develop as a massive form (61%), as multiple nodules (29%), or as a diffuse (10%) involvement of the liver.[10] Solitary masses can be readily identified as tumors, and if they grow large enough to outdistance their blood supply, their core can become necrotic. The nodular form is easily confused with regenerative nodules on gross examination. Diffuse hepatocellular carcinoma causes hepatomegaly, and only when the tissue is examined microscopically is the neoplastic process identified. Neoplastic hepatic tissue varies from almost white to the color of normal liver. In some cases it is difficult to distinguish normal liver tissue from neoplastic areas.

Benign growth of hepatocellular tissue produces what is variously described as nodular hyperplasia or regenerative nodules (Figure 36-1). This occurs as the liver responds to replace damaged hepatocytes. The regenerative process is unable to restore the normal architecture and forms nodules which are spheres of mostly normal-appearing hepatocytes, without their normal arrangements with the vasculature. The regenerating cells may be unable to communicate normally with either the afferent portal and arterial blood supply or the efferent blood flow in the central vein. Bile canaliculi also regenerate within the nodule but without connections to bile ducts in the portal area, so that bile secreted from hepatocytes is unable to leave the liver. The exchange of substances between hepatocytes and circulation is impaired since regenerated parenchymal cells reform in plates with a thickness of more than one hepatocyte, in contrast to the single-cell thickness of normal plates. The nodules can be separated from normal hepatic tissue by a thin layer of fibrous tissue, or there may be no such cell type separating normal from abnormal. Regenerated hepatocytes show little evidence of the marked mitotic ac-tivity evident in a malignant process. Bile ducts and blood vessels as well as hepatocytes proliferate during regeneration, although not in a fashionable to restore normal hepatic architecture.

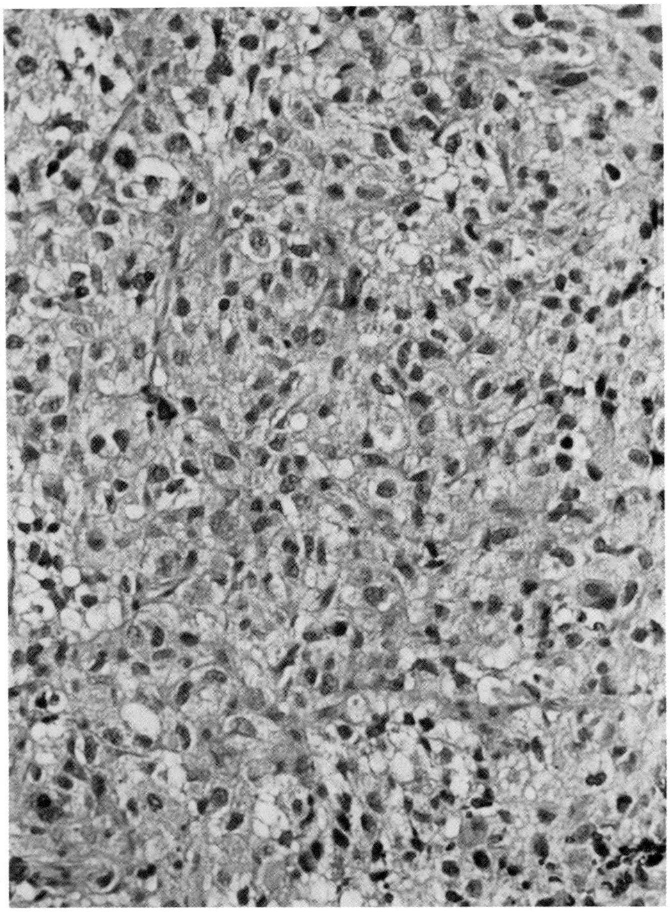

Figure 36-2c. Hepatocellular carcinoma. Hepatocytes are less well-differentiated than in Figure 36-2b. Cells are pleomorphic with more basophilic staining cytoplasm and dark staining nuclei (suggesting greater activity). Biopsy specimen.

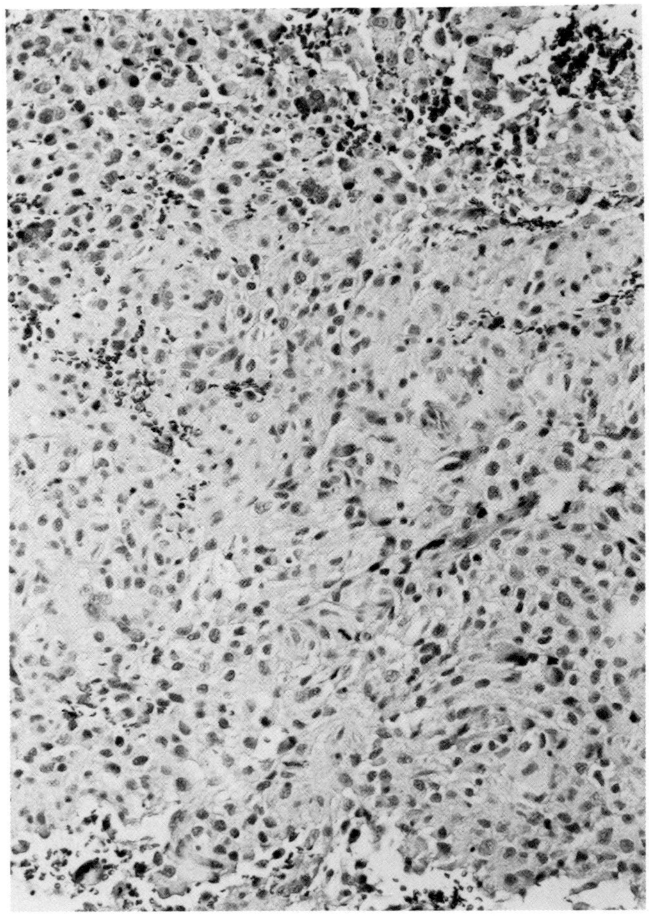

Figure 36-2d. Hepatocellular carcinoma. Poorly differentiated cells often make it difficult to identify their origin. Biopsy specimen.

Hepatocellular adenomas are usually smaller than 10 cm in diameter and are usually single nodules that must be differentiated from regenerative nodules. Grossly they are yellow-brown and often relatively soft and friable. Microscopically they have a well-defined trabecular pattern, with tumor cells resembling normal hepatocytes (Figure 36-1). Mitotic figures are not seen in liver cells that tend to be larger and clearer than normal. These adenomas consist solely of liver cells. There are no portal tracts, and they show a normal reticulin, pattern which aids in their differentiation from regenerative nodules and hepatocellular carcinomas.

Hepatocellular carcinomas can be made up of cells that closely resemble normal hepatocytes; at the other extreme, they may consist of cells whose appearance makes it is difficult to decide whether they are derived from hepatocytes (Figure 36-2). These carcinomas develop one of three or more histologic patterns. In one form the hepatocytes form trabeculae or plates that appear normal, except that instead of a single cell thick they have a width of a few too many cells with little stroma. Kupffer cells are not seen; with compression the sinusoids may not be evident; and the tumor appears solid. The neoplastic cells are well-differentiated and resemble normal hepatocytes. In a second form neoplastic cells are arranged into acinus-like or gland-like structures. The acinus lumen usually contains protein-like material that may stain PAS-positive. In a third form the carcinoma appears to be compact, solid, or scirrhous, growing in solid sheets without any sinusoids or fibrous tissue evident. In some cases the changes may be an artifact, whereas the tumor in reality represents one of the other two forms, or the tumor is not derived from hepatocytes but from some other cell. Neoplastic hepatocyte appearance also varies. Most commonly the tumor cells resemble hepatocytes, and their degree of differentiation is reflected in cell size, nuclear shape, and staining characteristics. Well-differentiated cells are larger, have more uniform nuclei, and show more abundant eosinophilic cytoplasm than poorly-differentiated cells. A second form of these cells can be described as clear cells. They appear as well-differentiated hepatocytes with vacuolation of the cytoplasm. Large vacuoles with a water-like clarity are due to glycogen accumulation. A foamy appearance to the vacuolation is more likely due to lipid or to water. The third appearance of neoplastic hepatocytes is a change described as anaplastic or pleomorphic. The abnormal cells often appear in such a primitive form that it is difficult to decide what cell-line they represent. The three variations of cell type can be seen with any of the three different histologic patterns. Special preparation with a silver stain is

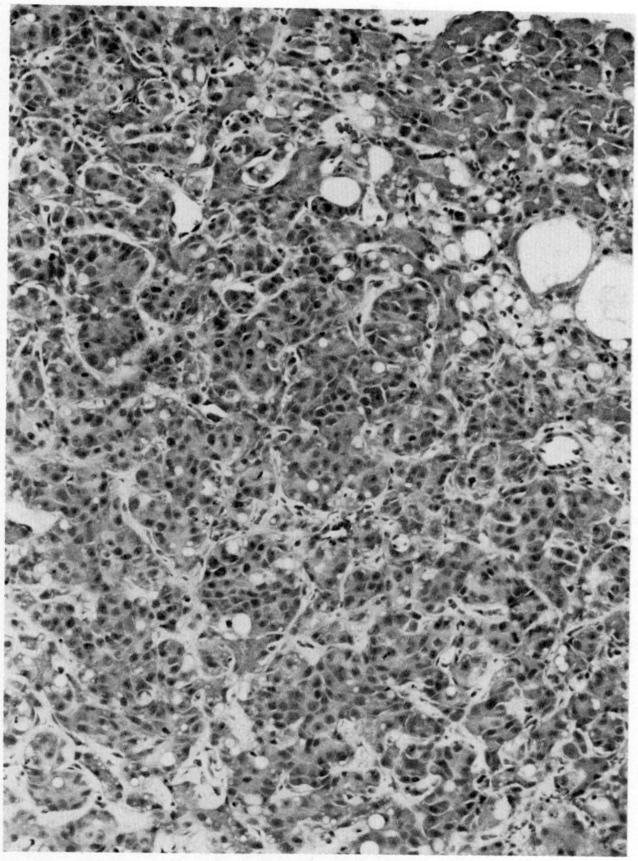

Figure 36-2e. Hepatocellular carcinoma. Well-differentiated cells are arranged predominately in an acinar pattern. Excessive fibrous tissue was seen in other sections of this biopsy.

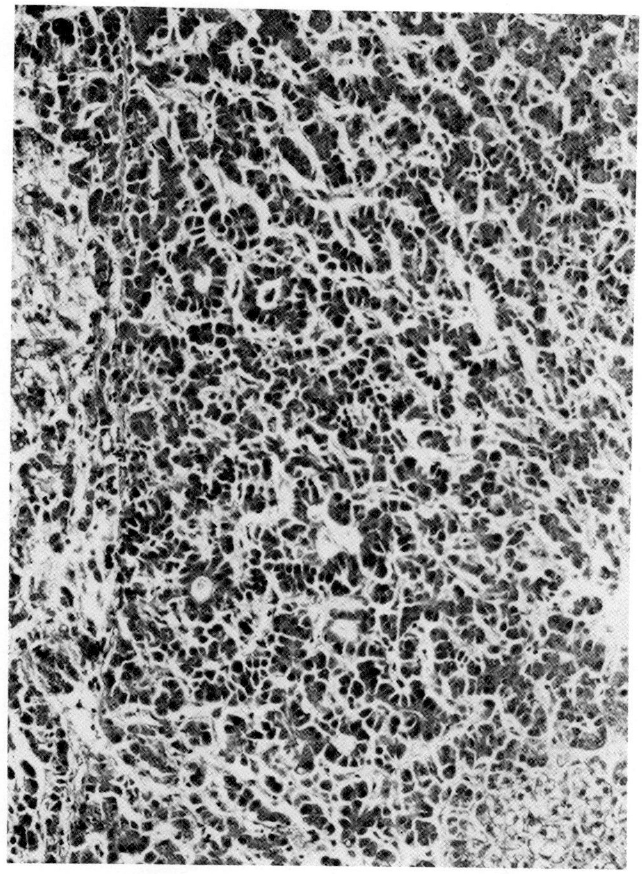

Figure 36-2f. Hepatocellular carcinoma. Well-differentiated cells are arranged in a trabecular pattern in this biopsy specimen.

used to help differentiate carcinoids from hepatocellular carcinomas.

Diagnosis

Laboratory evaluation does not distinguish hepatocellular carcinoma from hepatic necrosis, chronic hepatitis, or any of the many other problems that can cause abnormal biochemical findings. Consequently diagnosis can be made only by biopsy.

Management

Primary hepatocellular carcinoma is not the rapidly developing disease that would be predicted from morphological and biochemical findings. Most are not recognized until they have reached an advanced stage, when clinical signs begin to appear. When the neoplastic involvement is diffuse or deep within the hepatic parenchyma, there is little that can be done to remove the diseased tissue. When a single lobe of the liver is involved, surgical removal is possible. Nearly two-thirds involve only one lobe of the liver. Many of these large masses cause few signs until their core becomes necrotic or they encroach on adjacent organs. Dogs frequently survive surgical resection of primary hepatic neoplasms and can live for several years, often to die from another problem. They sometimes survive long enough for metastases to be found in the lungs. In summary, surgical ablation is the choice of treatments, although complete removal is not expected. Masses are removed surgically to minimize the effects produced by those that are necrotic within and those that interfere mechanically with function in abdominal viscera. Sometimes the surgery is done to manage an important complication such as hypoglycemia. Without early recognition 61% will have metastasized, most often to lymph nodes and lungs.

Hepatocellular carcinomas are primarily supplied by arterial blood, in contrast to the normal liver, which derives most of its circulation from the portal vein. As a result of this difference it is possible to manage hepatocellular carcinoma by ligation of the hepatic artery. Dogs can survive that loss, and restriction of flow to the neoplastic tissue may cause its regression.

BILE-DUCT CARCINOMAS

The incidence of bile-duct carcinomas is low.[2,3,18] The predominant clinical signs are anorexia, weight loss, vomiting, depression, ascites, and dyspnea; icterus is seen in a few. The clinical pathology for dogs with bile duct carcinoma is similar to that for hepatocellular carcinoma. The most consistent abnormalities are increased activities of ALP (69%) and ALT (54%), decreased albumin (61%), and increased bilirubin (31%).

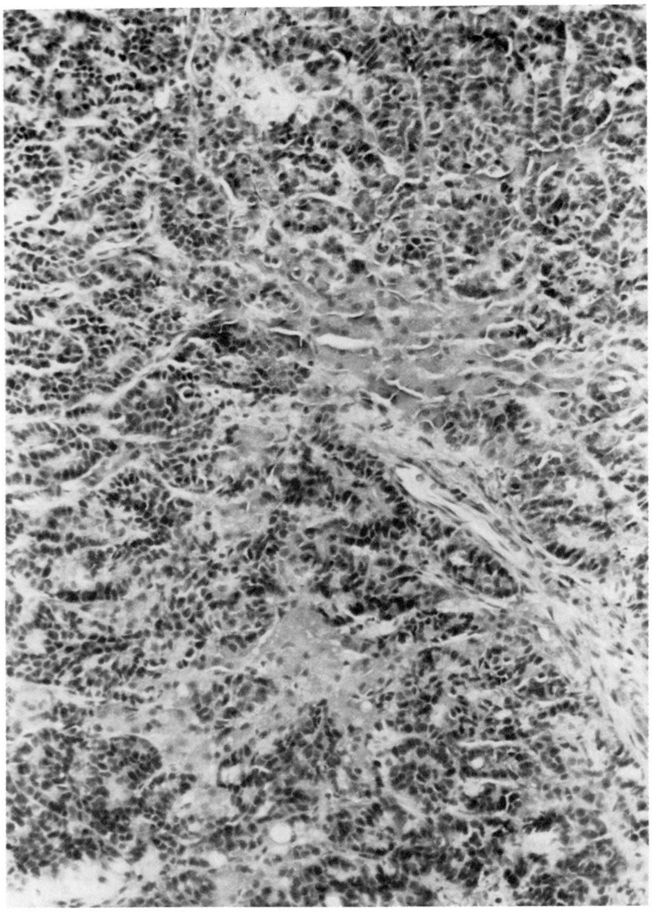

Figure 36-3. Cholangiocarcinoma. Acini are formed but are not well-defined, making the tumor moderately differentiated. Carcinoma involves most of this biopsy specimen, leaving only a few recognizable cords of hepatocytes.

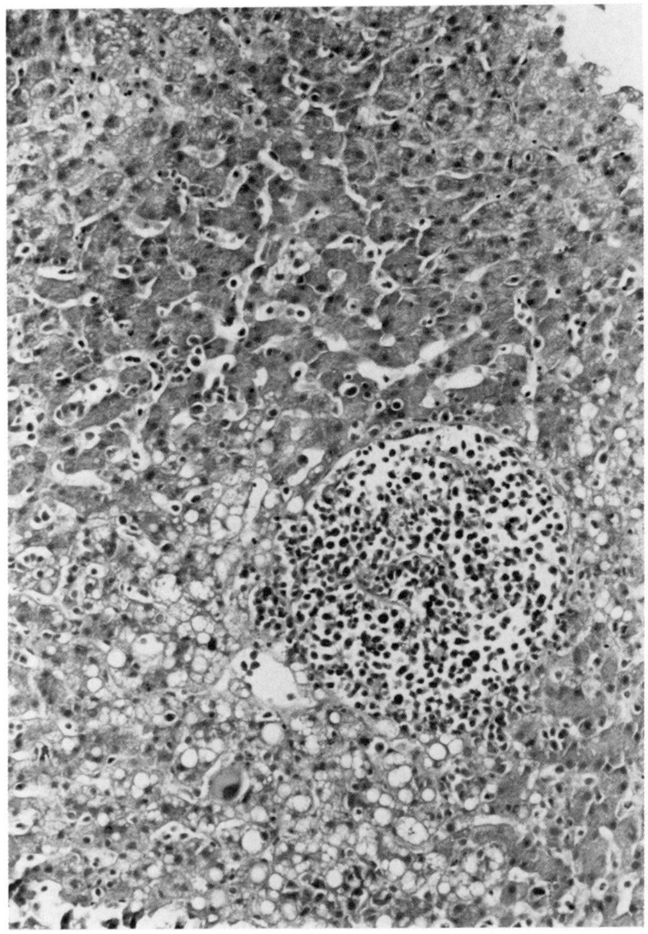

Figure 36-4a. Hepatic lymphosarcoma. Biopsy of dog's liver showing abnormal clusters of lymphocytes.

Intrahepatic bile duct carcinomas are classified as massive, nodular, or diffuse lesions. Histologically, intrahepatic bile duct carcinomas can be tubular carcinomas or bile cystadenocarcinomas (Figure 36-3). The tubular or cholangiocarcinomas consist of many tubular structures lined with cuboidal or columnar cells and dissected by diffuse fibrous stroma. Bile-duct carcinomas are different from primary hepatocellular carcinomas in that they result in the formation of more fibrous stroma. When the fine structure of these tumors is examined, the finding of microvilli on the luminal border of the cells clearly indicates their origin. Mucus secretion may be evident in some. Some carcinoma cells may be poorly differentiated. Cystadenocarcinomas are characterized by many cysts lined with single or multiple layers of epithelial cells. In some, papillary structures lined with cuboidal or columnar epithelium, arranged as in an acinus with papillary infolding, fill the cystic spaces. Metastatic adenocarcinomas and carcinoids may be difficult to differentiate from bile duct carcinomas. Bile duct carcinomas are less common than hepatocellular carcinomas but are more malignant and show a higher frequency of metastasis (88%). No attempt has been made to treat bile duct carcinomas. If the patients were not euthanatized, they died shortly after diagnosis.

METASTATIC NEOPLASMS[3,4,19]

Most malignancies can be identified in animals without biopsy of the liver. Necropsies on small animals, however, indicate that the liver is frequently invaded by metastases from a primary site (31% to 37% of all malignancies have metastases in the liver). The liver can be involved diffusely without developing the changes consistently seen in animals with primary hepatocellular carcinomas. With multisystem involvement it is not possible to attribute any of the clinical signs solely to the involvement of the liver. The clinical signs seen are frequently nonspecific and include polydipsia, anorexia, weight loss, and vomiting. Hepatomegaly is a variable finding that is reported in some dogs with lymphosarcoma (37%), leukemias (44%), pancreatic carcinomas (57%), hemangiosarcomas (8%), and other carcinomas or sarcomas (20%).[2] Subjective evaluation suggesting the abdomen to be painful on palpation is reported in fewer than one-third of all dogs.

Laboratory evaluation of this problem may not be as suggestive of hepatic involvement as for the primary tumors. Plasma ALT activities are usually normal to mildly elevated (Table 36-4), not increasing to the levels of 600 to 700 IU/L seen in patients with primary tumors. Plasma ALP activities are

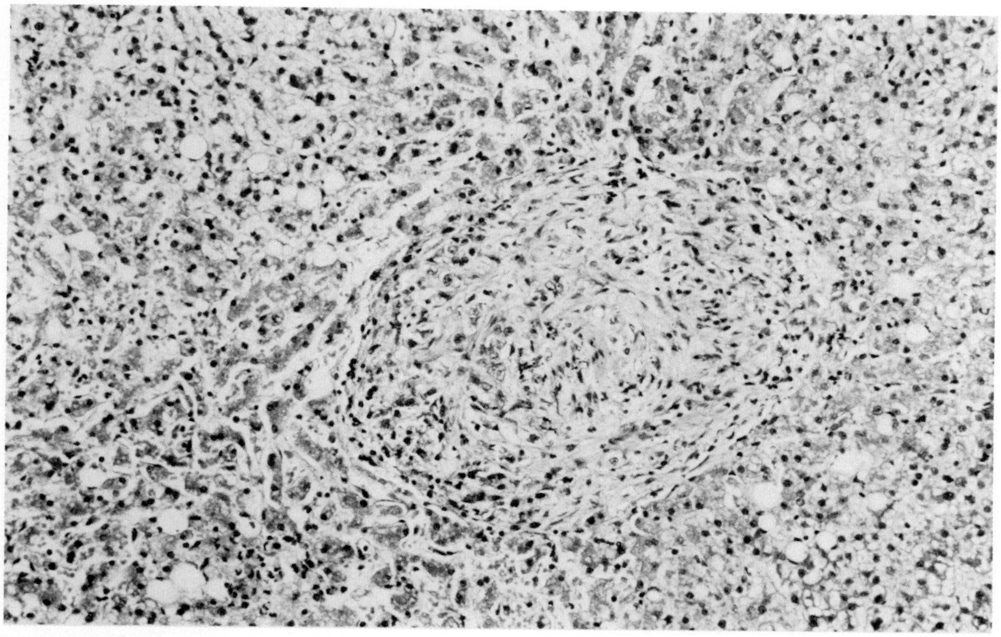

Figure 36-4b. Metastasis of gastric carcinoma to the liver is shown by large cluster of neoplastic cells in center of biopsy specimen. Such lesions are focal and can be missed on blind needle biopsy.

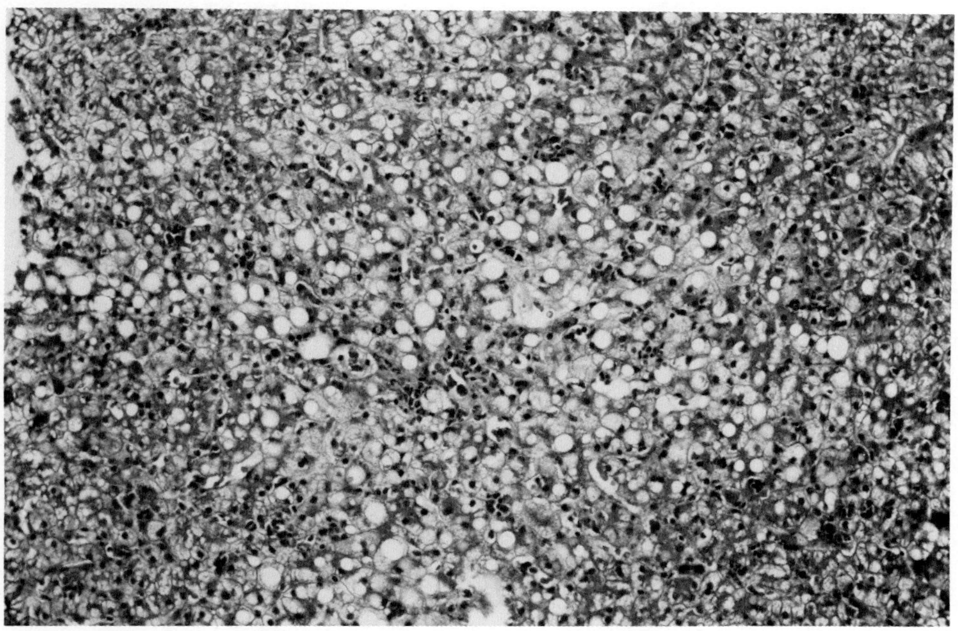

Figure 36-4c. Hepatic changes with myeloproliferative disease. Biopsy shows fatty changes, atrophy of hepatic cords and extramedullary hematopoiesis.

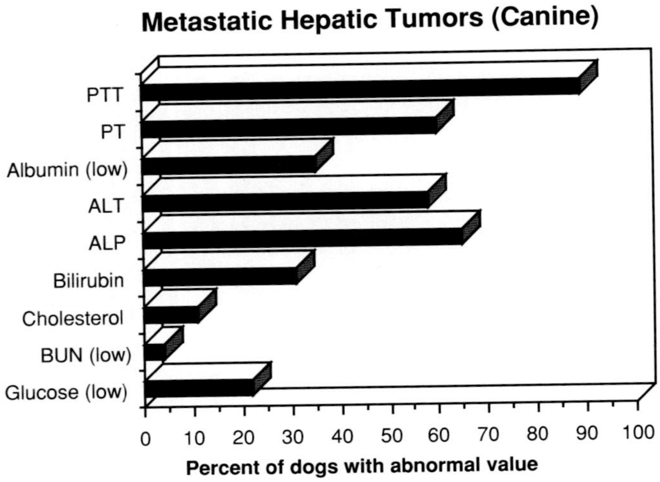

Table 36-4. Comparison of sensitivities for different tests in dogs with tumor metastases in the liver. Below: graphs showing distribution of clinical pathology values in dogs with tumor metastases in the liver. Points on graphs represent 0%, 25%, 50%, 75% and 100% medians. Normal range is in shaded area.

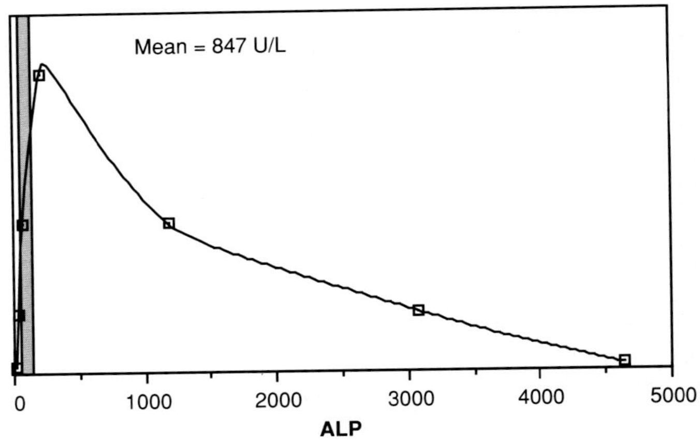

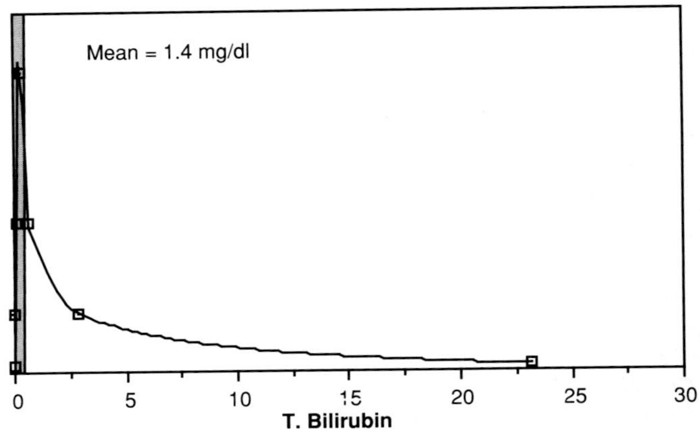

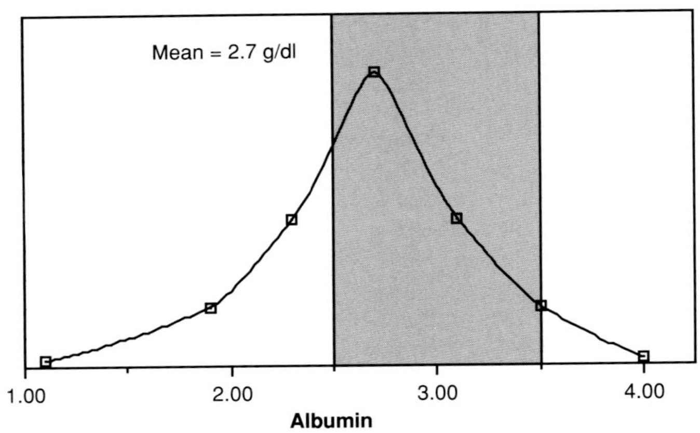

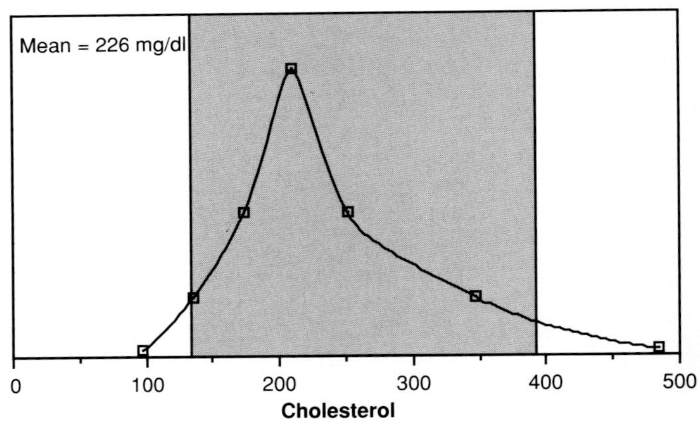

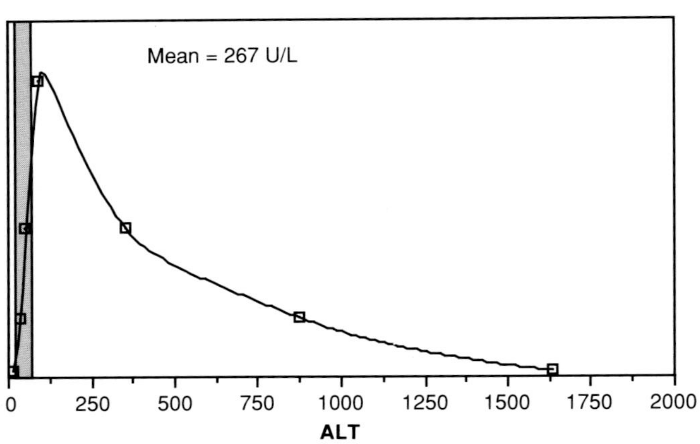

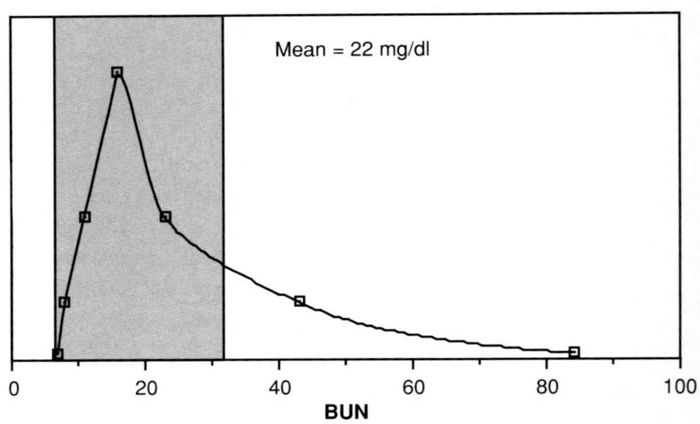

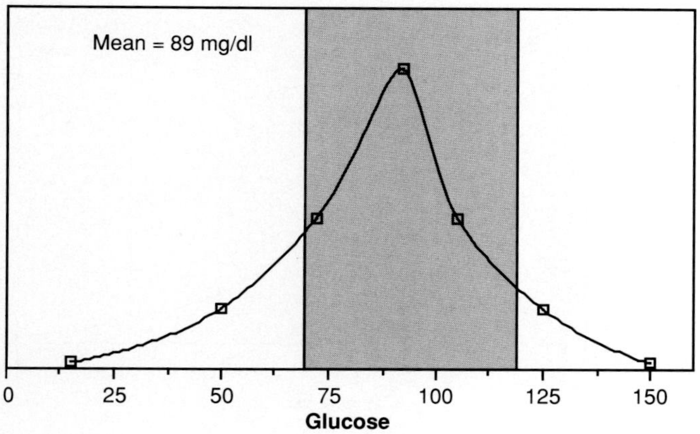

normal to moderately elevated, similar to increases seen with hepatocellular carcinomas. Hyperbilirubinemia is infrequently seen. Metastatic disease of the liver can be associated with little biochemical evidence supporting further investigation of a potential hepatic problem. Abnormal laboratory values are required to justify liver biopsy. In some dogs, neoplastic disease with metastases cannot be easily identified by biopsy of extra-hepatic tissue. Percutaneous liver biopsy has been useful in identifying disseminated malignancies when they could not be identified by means other than biopsy via thoracotomy or celiotomy. Liver biopsy has been most useful in identifying lymphosarcoma in animals where it is not easily identified by other means. An example of lymphosarcoma diagnosed on a liver biopsy is shown in Figure 36-4. It is more important to recognize this problem today than in the past, because lymphosarcoma is now a treatable disease with chances of long term success. The chances are improved, of course, when the disease is recognized early and therapy does not have to be used on a debilitated patient. Hemangiosarcomas often metastasize to the liver from primary sites in other organs such as the heart and spleen. Occasionally the tumor is reported to have its primary site in the liver, for which German Shepherds and Pointers are at high risk.[7] Often affected animals have no clinical signs until the tumor ruptures and the signs developing can be attributed to internal bleeding. Clinical pathologic abnormalities are few. The most consistent is reduced hematocrit from the bleeding (Table 36-5).

With only minor biochemical abnormalities to suggest liver disease there may little justification for liver biopsy. In most cases a biopsy provides information of little value, but sometimes the findings confirm a malignancy by metastasis to the liver.

HAMARTOMA AND CONGENITAL CYSTS

Angiomatous hamartoma is a congenital malformation characterized by vascular overgrowths causing it to resemble hemangiomas grossly and microscopically. It is considered to be a tumor-like lesion. Appearing in very young animals it presents signs similar to those in older animals with hepatic masses.[20]

Congenital cysts of the liver are uncommonly found in dogs.[21] They can be single or multiple cysts and are usually

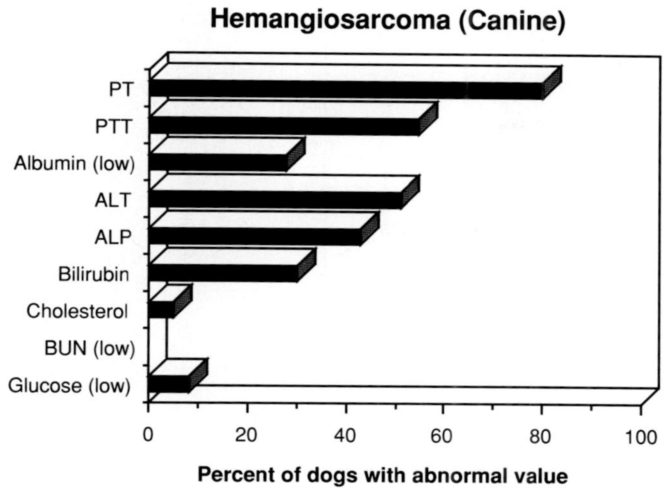

Table 36-5. Comparison of sensitivities for different tests in dogs with hemangiosarcoma in the liver. Following graphs show distribution of clinical pathology values in dogs with hemangiosarcoma in the liver. Points on graphs represent 0%, 25%, 50%, 75% and 100% medians. Normal range is in shaded area.

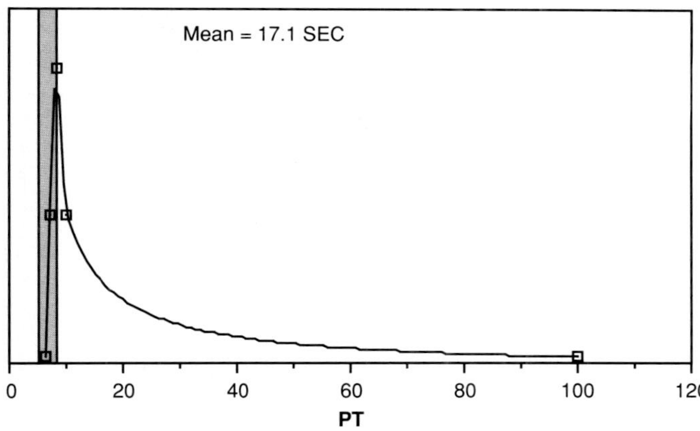

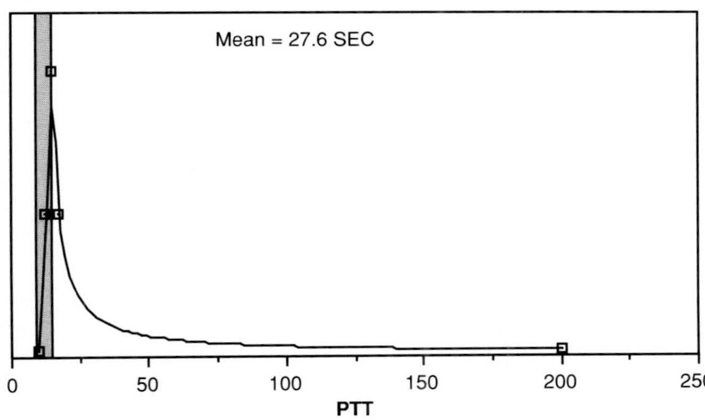

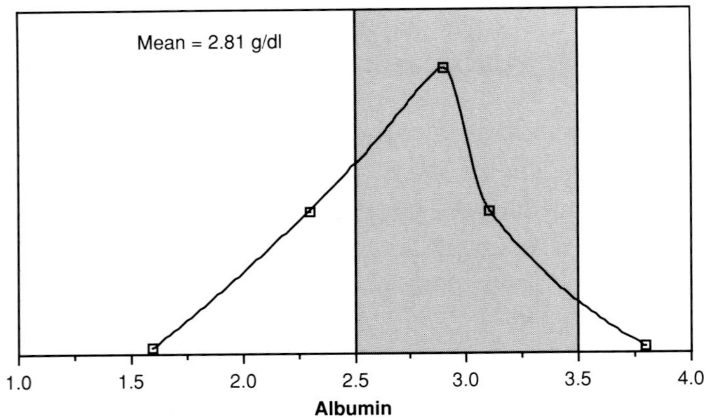
Mean = 2.81 g/dl
1.0
1.5
2.0
2.5
3.0
3.5
4.0
Albumin

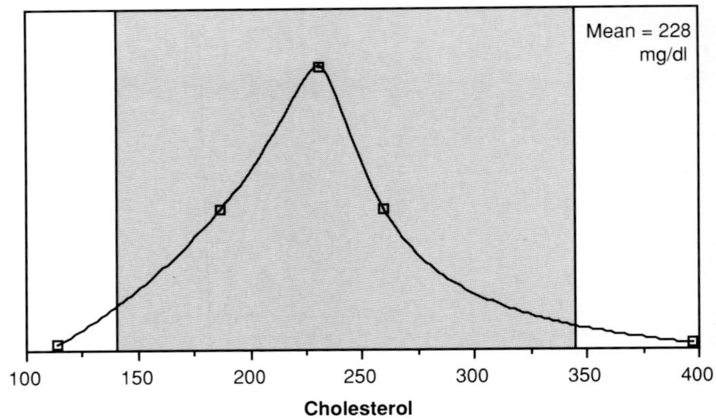
Mean = 228 mg/dl
100
150
200
250
300
350
400
Cholesterol

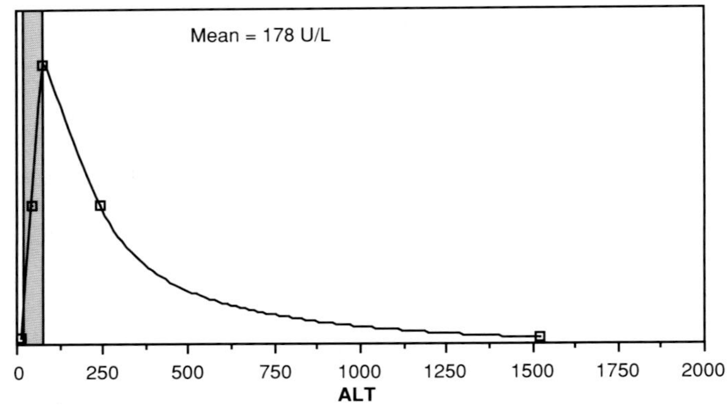
Mean = 178 U/L
0
250
500
750
1000
1250
1500
1750
2000
ALT

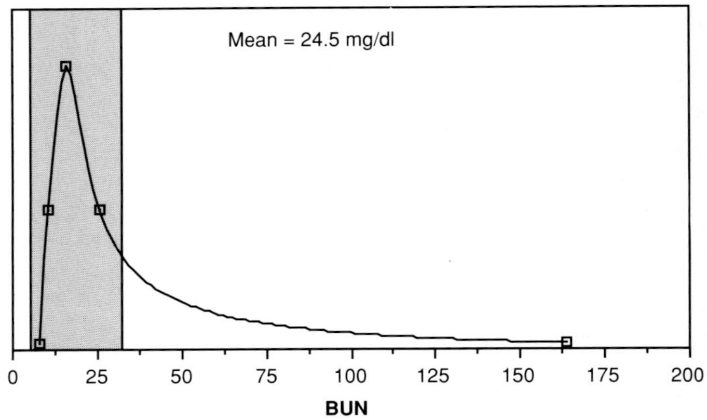
Mean = 24.5 mg/dl
0
25
50
75
100
125
150
175
200
BUN

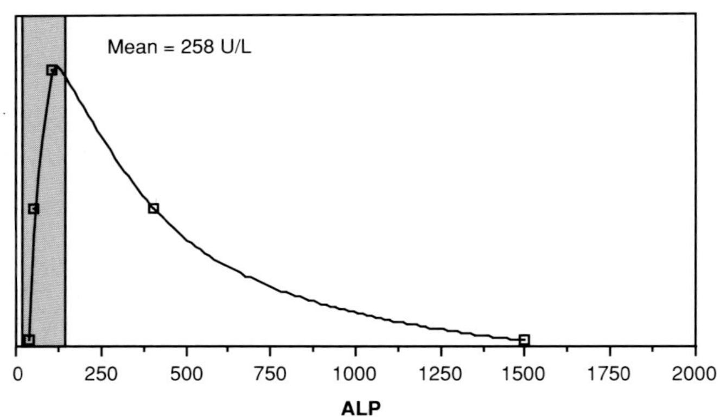
Mean = 258 U/L
0
250
500
750
1000
1250
1500
1750
2000
ALP

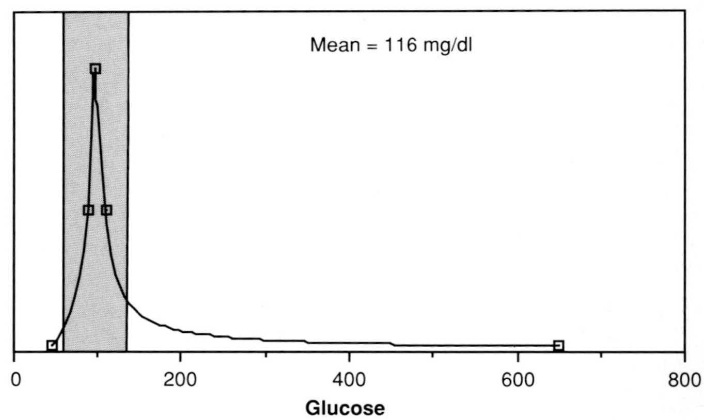
Mean = 116 mg/dl
0
200
400
600
800
Glucose

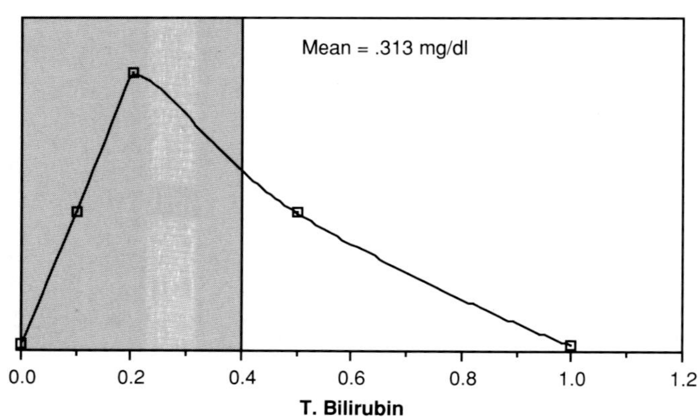
Mean = .313 mg/dl
0.0
0.2
0.4
0.6
0.8
1.0
1.2
T. Bilirubin

incidental findings, causing no clinical signs. The cysts are believed to result from gradual dilation of groups of persisting intralobular bile ducts that fail to involute in the later embryonic development of the liver or that arise as an abnormal extension of resorption, which is a normal occurrence in the first generation of bile ducts.[22] The cysts are lined with cuboidal epithelium that resembles bile ducts, and the cyst fluid resembles the bile salt-independent fraction of bile, suggesting that the epithelium is functional. Most dogs reported with cysts showed no clinical signs and no biochemical abnormalities. Two dogs with large and multiple cysts we reported with clinical evidence for hepatic disease.

Congenital abnormalities of the biliary system can also involve the extrahepatic structures in humans. They are grouped and described generally as congenital dilatation of bile ducts. That type of problem has not been recognized in small animals. Some animals, especially cats, have problems that bear some resemblance, however. Cats are seen with dilated extrahepatic bile ducts where it is believed that obstruction is the cause. Obstruction is usually not found. Inflammation is evident but that can be secondary to a chronic bile stasis. Bile flow will not be normal with abnormal ductular motility associated with chronically dilated bile ducts. It is possible that a congenital abnormality may be the basis for chronic bile duct disease in some cats.

REFERENCES

1. Patnaik, A.K., Hurvitz, A.I. and Lieberman, P.H.: Canine hepatic neoplasms: a clinicopathologic study. Vet. Pathol. 17:553-564, 1980.
2. Trigo, F.J., Thompson, H., Breeze, R.G., Nash, A.S.: The pathology of liver tumors in the dog. J. Comp. Path. 92:21-39, 1982.
3. Magne, M.L. and Withrow, S.J.: Hepatic neoplasia. Vet. Clin. N. Am. Small An. Pract. 15:243-256, 1985.
4. Strombeck, D.R.: Clinicopathologic features of primary and metastatic neoplastic disease of the liver in dogs. JAVMA 173:267-269, 1978.
5. Patnaik, A.K., Lieberman, P.H., Hurvitz, A.I. and Johnson, G.F.: Canine hepatic carcinoids. Vet. Pathol. 18:445-453, 1981.
6. Patnaik, A.K., Hurvitz, A.I., Lieberman, P.H. and Johnson, G.F.: Canine bile duct carcinoma. Vet. Pathol. 18:439-444, 1981.
7. Theilen, G.H. and Madewell, B.R.: Veterinary Cancer Medicine. Lea and Febiger, Philadelphia, 34, 1987.
8. Farber, E., Sarma, D.S.R., Rajalakshmi, S. and Shinozuka, H.: Liver carcinogenesis: a unifying hypothesis. In, The Liver: Normal and Abnormal Function. Part B. Edited by F.F. Becker. The Biochemistry of Disease. Vol. 5. Marcel Dekker, New York, 755-771, 1975.
9. MacSween, R.N.M., Anthony, P.P. and Scheuer, P.J.: Tumours and tumour-like lesions of the liver and biliary tract. In, Pathology of the LIver. Churchill Livingstone, New York, 574-637, 1987.
10. Patnaik, A.K., Hurvitz, A.I., Liebermann, P.H. and Johnson, G.F.: Canine hepatocellular carcinoma. Vet. Pathol. 18:427-438, 1981.
11. Edmundson, H.A. and Craig, J.R.: Neoplasms of the liver. In, Diseases of the Liver. Edited by L. Schiff and E.R. Schiff. J.B. Lippincott, Philadelphia, 1109-1158, 1987.
12. Marks, L.J., Steinke, J., Podolsky, S. and Egdahl, R.H.: Hypoglycemia associated with neoplasia. Ann. N.Y. Acad. Sci. 230:147-160, 1974.
13. Strombeck, D.R., Krum, S., Meyer, D. and Kappesser, R.M.: Hypoglycemia and hypoinsulinemia associated with hepatoma in a dog. JAVMA 169:811-812, 1976.
14. Leifer, C.E., Peterson, M.E., Matus, R.E. and Patnaik, A.K.: Hypoglycemia associated with nonislet cell tumor in 13 dogs. JAVMA 186:53-55, 1985.
15. Leblanc H., Andersen, J.R., Sigel, M.B. and Yen, S.S.C.: Inhibitory action of somatostatin on pancreatic and cell function. J. Clin. Endocrinol. Metab. 40:568-572, 1975.
16. Sell, S. and Wepsic, H.T.: Alpha-fetoprotein. In, The Liver: Normal and Abnormal Functions, Part B. The Biochemistry of Disease. Vol. 5. Edited by F.F. Becker. Marcel Dekker, New York, 773-820, 1975.
17. Bloomer, J.R., Waldman, R.A., McIntire, K.R. and Klatskin, G.: Alpha-fetoprotein in non-neoplastic hepatic disorders. JAMA 233:38-41, 1975.
18. Hayes, H.M., Morin, M.M. and Rubenstein, D.A.: Canine biliary carcinoma: epidemiological comparisons with man. J. Comp. Path. 93:99-107, 1983.
19. McConnell, M.F. and Lumsden, J.H.: Biochemical evaluation of metastatic liver disease in the dog. JAAHA 19:173-178, 1983.
20. Castellano, M.C., Idiart, J.R., Ortega, C.F. and Ruager, J.: Multiple hepatic angiomatous hamartomas in a puppy. Canine Pract. 13:30-33, 1986.

Chapter 37

Diseases of the Gallbladder

Cholecystitis, inflammatory disease of the gallbladder, is seldom recognized before necropsy. The incidence has been one or two cases out of the 500 to 600 small animals necropsied each year in the VMTH at Davis. Cholelithiasis, the development of calculi in the bile ducts or gallbladder, is infrequently recognized. Few cases have been reported in dogs.[1-4] Cholelithiasis is rare in the cat.

CHOLECYSTITIS

The pathogenesis of acute cholecystitis is not completely understood. It can be readily produced in experimental dogs by a variety of means.[5-7] Biliary obstruction and infection are implicated as major causes.[8] Cholecystitis is produced experimentally by injecting activated pancreatic proteolytic enzymes or pepsin through the bile duct. Introduction of microorganisms or polymorphonuclear leukocytes through the duct also causes acute inflammation, possibly due to lysolecithin produced by enzymatic hydrolysis of lecithin in the bile. These experimental models are based on the idea that intestinal contents reflux into the bile duct to cause cholecystitis. The choledoduodenal junction is normally a passive, essentially one-way flutter valve in which pressure is reduced during duodenal relaxation.[9] The effect of the valve and an increase in pressure at the junction with increased intraduodenal pressure make reflux an unlikely event. Intravenous injection of bacteria in animals with bile-duct obstruction results in cholecystitis. Thus, cholecystitis can develop from a bacteremia. Bile duct obstruction without artificially introducing bacteremia can result in organisms colonizing the hepatobiliary system. Necrotizing cholecystitis can develop and lead to rupture of the gall bladder and peritonitis.[27]

CHOLELITHIASIS[10-12]

Major differences between humans and dogs explain the development of gallstones in one but not the other.[13] The difference is best illustrated by the observation that human gallbladder calculi dissolve when placed in the gallbladder of a dog. Thus, conditions in the human gallbladder facilitate calculi formation, whereas factors in the dog prevent their occurrence.

Biliary calculi consist primarily of pure cholesterol, which may be mixed with bile acids, pigments, calcium, and protein. A small number of calculi are pigment stones. A prerequisite for the formation of calculi is bile saturated with cholesterol relative to the concentrations of other lipids. The liver determines the production of cholesterol-saturated bile. Cholesterol crystallizes and precipitates from supersaturated bile and forms a solid phase within the liquid phase of cholesterol-rich bile. Bile pigments, mucoproteins, bacteria, and refluxed intestinal contents form a nidus for microscopic calculi, which then grow to large ones.

A number of factors are important in the formation of calculi. In some cases gallbladder infection is important, when microorganisms and leukocytes damage the gallbladder epithelium or change the properties of some important bile constituents. Microorganisms are suggested to enter the gallbladder by refluxing from the intestine or through the hepatic circulation. It is not known whether either of these is an important cause of biliary calculi in the dog.

Factors determining the rate of secretion and the solubilization of cholesterol are important in the pathogenesis of calculi formation. The concentration of cholesterol is much lower in canine bile than in human bile. The most potent choleretic is plasma bile acids, which are the primary stimulus for the secretion of cholesterol. When the rate of bile secretion is maximum, the concentrations of bile acids and phospholipids are also high. These substances are the principal solubilizing agents of cholesterol. A small amount of cholesterol is secreted into bile independently of bile acid secretion. Thus, in the unstimulated state the concentration of bile cholesterol is at a maximum, with bile acid and phospholipid concentration at a minimum. This fraction of cholesterol secretion, independent of bile acid secretion, is small in the dog. Interrupting the enterohepatic circulation of bile acids to reduce the amounts secreted into the bile causes bile cholesterol concentration to increase. This occurs in humans, so that the limits of micellar solubility are exceeded, but it does not happen in dogs.

The amounts of cholesterol, bile acids, and phospholipids in the bile determine the maintenance of a soluble solution of cholesterol. An increase in the ratio of cholesterol to the sum of bile acid and phospholipid concentrations will cause the limits of micellar solubility to be exceeded at some point, after which cholesterol precipitates. Canine bile is not unique in the limit's never being exceeded. Saturating canine bile with cholesterol prevents it from dissolving calculi taken from human gallbladders. It is apparent that events promoting decreased synthesis and secretion of bile acids or increased synthesis and secretion of cholesterol would increase the tendency for calculi formation. An accelerated loss of fecal bile acids reduces the amount of bile acids absorbed, and normal amounts are not maintained in the enterohepatic cycle. The synthesis of bile acids increases when the fecal losses accelerate, but the accelerated production may be insufficient to maintain a pool of normal size. Thus, less bile acid is secreted into bile, which can be one factor in the development of calculi. The rate-limiting step in the formation of bile acids is the hydroxylation of cholesterol at the 7-alpha-position of the sterol nucleus. This step is catalyzed by hepatic microsomal cholesterol 7-alpha-hydroxylase, the activity of which is regulated by the rate of return of bile acids to the liver in the enterohepatic circulation. Humans with gallbladder calculi have small pools of total, cholic, and chenodeoxycholic acids, and it is suggested that there is an increased rate of loss that cannot be compensated for by increased activity of cholesterol 7-alpha-hydroxylase. In some cases the primary problem appears to be a decrease in the activity of this enzyme.

Certain diets can predispose to stone formation in the dog as well as other animals. Such diets could increase secretion of cholesterol into bile, explaining stone development. Increased cholesterol secretion can follow hepatic uptake increases for low-density lipoproteins and chylomicron remnants that promote cholesterol uptake; these lipoproteins are rich in cholesterol. Such uptake can be promoted by estrogens. Increases in hepatic synthesis of cholesterol can also be a means to promote its secretion into bile. The rate of synthesis of this sterol is regulated by the levels of dietary cholesterol, which inhibit the enzyme HMG-CoA reductase when large amounts are absorbed. An increased rate of cholesterol synthesis can result in an increased ratio of cholesterol to bile acids and phospholipids in the bile. Cholesterol synthesis increases in any situation where bile acids are not properly reabsorbed from the small intestine. That occurs with extensive disease of the ileum, and with the ingestion of fibers or resins that bind bile acids and prevent their reabsorption. Cholesterol metabolism to bile acids or cholesterol esters may decrease in order for more cholesterol to be available for secretion into bile. Some hormones and drugs inhibit the ester formation and can increase the risk for stone formation. Plasma cholesterol increases with high-cholesterol diets; cholesterol is also synthesized by the intestine and contributes to plasma levels, but that is not as important for stone formation as augmented cholesterol synthesis by the liver. Some experimental animals can be fed a glucose-casein and fat-free diet that leads to hypersecretion of biliary cholesterol and stone formation.

Cholelithiasis can be induced experimentally in dogs[14-16] by feeding a diet that is high in carbohydrates, low in protein, low in fat of animal origin, and contains 1% cholesterol.[16] The serum cholesterol levels increase from a normal of 243 mg/dl to 431 mg/dl. The concentration in the bile is increased up to fourfold. The gallstones produced with this diet contain only traces of cholesterol, however. Thus, they differ from human cholesterol stones. They are similar to human pigment gallstones, consisting primarily of pigments and small amounts of bile acids. The protein-deficient diet fed these dogs is also deficient in taurine. Bile acids conjugated with taurine are completely resistant to precipitation by calcium. The taurine-deficient diet may increase concentrations of glycine-conjugated bile acids or unconjugated bile acids and increase the risk for their precipitation and subsequent precipitation of other solutes in bile. The calcium salts of glycine-conjugated bile acids are less soluble than taurine conjugates. One other solute in bile is bilirubin, the unconjugated form of which is poorly soluble in aqueous solution.

Diet-induced pigmented stones in experimental dogs also contain large amounts of protein and mucus. Mucous substances serves as the nidus for stone formation and may neutralize the bile constituents that maintain micellar solubility of bile pigments. Hypersecretion of mucin glycoproteins by the gallbladder mucosa precedes the appearance of crystalline cholesterol; the combination of mucus and cholesterol is evident as biliary sludge upon ultrasonography. Mucin hypersecretion is stimulated by prostaglandin formation and is inhibited by cyclooxygenase inhibitors such as aspirin and indomethacin. Cholesterol hypersecretion promotes cosecretion of lecithin into bile. The lecithin is a form rich in arachidonic acid and after its absorption by the gallbladder mucosa the lecithin is hydrolyzed by phospholipase to lysolecithin, which returns to the bile, and arachidonic acid, which is converted to prostaglandins. Gallbladder mucin is a very large polymer with carbohydrate that avidly binds water and gives it a viscous property. The mucin can tightly bind biliary lipid molecules, including calcium bilirubinate, and the mucin gel adheres tightly to the gallbladder mucosa. That mucosa absorbs sodium and water, increasing the gel's viscosity further, which makes gallbladder evacuation more difficult.

The low incidence of cholelithiasis and cholecystitis in small animals suggests that gallbladder problems hardly exist. Observations from ultrasound examinations of the gallbladder indicate that some abnormalities are commonly seen and in a few cases may be responsible for clinical signs. These examinations show retention of what has been described as biliary sludge in the gallbladder.[17,18] Biliary sludge is a collection of mucus, calcium bilirubinate, and cholesterol crystals. The combination of mucus and cholesterol crystals alone produces echoes on ultrasonography that are similar to those found in patients with biliary sludge. In some humans that sludge is a precursor form of gall stone disease. Ligation of the bile duct or gallbladder stasis in dogs leads to sludge formation.[19] A number of clinical situations can also result in sludge appearance. During a prolonged unfed state the gallbladder is not stimulated to empty, and bile collects; bile is concentrated as water is removed. With duodenal disease the synthesis and release of cholecystokinin is impaired, so that during feeding the gallbladder is not stimulated to contract and evacuate bile. Inadequate evacuation of the gallbladder is produced by any disease, drug, stress, or electrolyte imbalance, such as hypokalemia's inhibiting smooth muscle motility. The prostaglandins that stimulate mucus hypersecretion may be a kind that depress the contractile response of the gallbladder to regulatory peptides. Gallbladder mucus concentrated by water absorption and more viscous due to binding lipid molecules is evacuated with greater difficulty and impairs gallbladder contractility. The result is biliary sludge.

Clinical Laboratory Findings

The small group of dogs reported with cholelithiasis have shown nonspecific signs, which include most commonly icterus, vomiting, anorexia, weakness, depression, and weight loss, and less frequently, fever, diarrhea, polydipsia, and abdominal pain.[1-4] Laboratory findings have been increased plasma activities of ALT and ALP and increased levels of plasma bilirubin and cholesterol. Thus, the signs are consistent with hepatic disease. The very low incidence of cholelithiasis seldom prompts the clinician to include it in a differential diagnosis. Radiographs are included in the workup of many patients with obscure signs associated with cholelithiasis. Unfortunately, all choleliths are not radiopaque and visible on plain radiographs. Calcium deposition allows the calculi to be identified, but not all stones contain sufficient calcium to be visible. Radiographs sometimes show gas in the biliary system.

Special radiographic and other imaging procedures can be used to evaluate for choleliths and for gallbladder structure and function. As an initial approach ultrasound is used to examine gallbladder and bile duct size.[20] Bile duct obstruction or failure of the gallbladder to contract results in a rapid increase of gallbladder size. Within 48 hours of bile duct obstruction, enlargement of the common duct can be recognized. Dilatation of the extrahepatic ducts is evident after three days, and dilatation of intrahepatic ducts is seen within seven days. Radiolucent or radiopaque calculi can be seen with ultrasonography. Smaller calculi and those in ducts rather than the gallbladder are often difficult to recognize. Gallbladder tumors and cystic hyperplasia can be seen ultrasonically; circulatory problems or inflammatory diseases can cause edema or inflammation of the gallbladder wall that can also be recognized on ultrasound.

Bile duct obstruction is most reliably evaluated with a scintigraphic method using a radioisotope labelled chemical that is taken up by hepatocytes from the circulation and excreted into the biliary tract.[21] The chemical, disofenin, is taken up and metabolized in a manner similar to that for bilirubin. High bilirubin reduces the uptake and excretion of disofenin. Following the intravenous infusion, disofenin appears in the gallbladder within 15 to 20 minutes in normal dogs. Evacuation of the gallbladder can be made following intravenous infusion of cholecystokinin. Contraction is apparent for about six minutes, and about 60% of gallbladder contents is evacuated.

Radiographic Findings

Contrast radiography employing cholecystography can be used to identify calculi that cannot be identified with plain radiographs.[22] Identification is accomplished by radiographic examination after administration of two types of iodine-labeled compounds that are preferentially excreted in the bile.[23] One form, given orally, is an iodate salt (Oragrafin). Given alone it has several disadvantages. Its dose rate is vague; its rate of absorption from the intestine is variable; and 12 hours are required before radiographs can be taken. The gallbladder may contract and empty its contents into the intestine before the radiographs are obtained, which makes the results impossible to interpret in some cases. The other form of iodine-containing compound, iodipamide (Cholografin), is given intravenously. Experimental studies with this compound in dogs have shown this drug to be preferred for visualizing the gallbladder. Iodipamide (250 mg w/v iodine/ml) given at 0.5 mg/Kg as an intravenous bolus opacifies the gallbladder within 60 minutes. This is a consistent finding in normal dogs, and the gallbladder becomes more opaque during the period from 60 to 120 minutes. This compound is toxic; when combined with the orally-administered dye given 12 hours earlier, however, less iodipamide needs to be given, and the combination of two dyes outlines the biliary system better than either one alone. The patient is fasted for at least 12 hours before the study, and the colon is evacuated with enemas. Five minutes before the entire intravenous dose is to be administered, 1 ml of the iodipamide is injected and the patient is observed for any reaction. Radiographs can be taken at any time from one to two hours later. The animal is then given a fatty meal or a small amount of vegetable oil (or cholecystokinin can be given), and the gallbladder is reradiographed 30 minutes later to determine how well it empties. In normal animals, opacification of the biliary system permits identification of the gallbladder, extrahepatic ducts, and intrahepatic ducts (see Chapter 27). Poor opacification with the appearance of a filling defect is seen with radiolucent choleliths on films that are taken after the first hour. The increased opacification found in later films may obscure small calculi. Failure of gallbladder opacification is also seen with acute cholecystitis and with acute inflammatory disease of the abdomen, such as with acute pancreatitis and peritonitis. Complete obstruction of the bile duct prevents visualization of the gallbladder even when the dose of iodipamide is increased to fourfold.[24] That is not true of a partial obstruction. When there is evidence for a complete biliary obstruction, there is no indication to perform cholecystography.

Management

The approaches to management of cholelithiasis in humans have been both medical and surgical. Medical management is based on the finding that most calculi in humans are primarily cholesterol. Nothing is known about the composition of choleliths in dogs other than their qualitative analysis, which has been incomplete more often than not. If the calculi contain primarily cholesterol, they can be dissolved by agents that alter cholesterol synthesis and bile acid secretion.[25] One of the bile acids, chenodeoxycholic acid, has been used to treat humans with cholelithiasis. Oral administration of this bile acid causes an increase in its pool in the body, resulting in a decrease in pools of cholic and deoxycholic acid. Chenodeoxycholic acid inhibits HMG CoA reductase activity, and cholesterol synthesis is decreased. It also stimulates secretion of bile acids, causing a reduction in the content of cholesterol in bile and an increase in bile acid levels, enhancing the cholesterol-solubilizing capacity. This bile acid also inhibits hepatic triglyceride synthesis and can be used to reduce plasma lipid levels. Chenodeoxycholic acid is metabolized by the normal intestinal microflora to lithocholic acid, which can then have some toxic effects. After the 7-alpha hydroxylation of chenodeoxycholic acid forms lithocholic acid, it is absorbed from the intestine. Normally only small amounts are absorbed, and the liver can sulfate them to make renal excretion possible. The accumulation of larger amounts, however, causes toxic signs to appear. Lithocholic acid is a pyrogen and is hepatotoxic. With time it causes bile-duct proliferation and fibrosis. Other bile acids, however, do not share the abilities of chenodeoxycholic acid to stimulate bile acid secretion and to inhibit cholesterol synthesis.

Surgical management of cholelithiasis is not a clearly defined answer to the problem. Cholecystectomy removes the cause and prevents a recurrence. Postsurgical changes in the bile ducts may be an undesirable sequel.[26] Removal of the gallbladder eliminates the reservoir where bile is stored and concentrated. Secretion of bile by the liver generates a hydrostatic pressure that is dissipated by the movement of bile into the gallbladder. The gallbladder mucosa absorbs sodium and water so that bile is concentrated and newly secreted bile is able to enter the organ continuously for storage. Removal of the reservoir results in a maintenance of the hydrostatic pressure generated by bile secretion. The bile cannot easily discharge into the intestine until the pressure within the duct is great enough to overcome that pressure where the bile duct passes through the duodenum. The most important determinant of pressure at this sphincter is the motility of the duodenum. It is modified by the gut endocrines when they are released. The anatomy of the juncture of the bile with the intestine is such in the dog that it is not easily opened by increased hydrostatic pressure. The bile duct dilates since it contains no muscle fibers and acts as a passive conduit.[26] It is debatable whether this choledochal dilation is a significant problem that can be related to any clinical signs.

Cholecystotomy is a surgical procedure to remove the cholelith and not remove the gallbladder. If the cause of the cholelith formation is still present and is not recognized and treated, the problem can recur. Cultures of the contents of the gallbladder, analysis of the calculi, and biopsy of the gallbladder mucosa may help identify the cause.

The management of any form of cholelithiasis should include treatment for a cholecystitis, which can be either primary or secondary. Antibiotics are selected that are effective against the aerobes and anaerobes normally found in the intestine. Dietary recommendations are made so that the patient is fed a diet high in protein and low in cholesterol.[14] A high-protein diet will slow the formation of calculi. As stated earlier, dogs can develop calcium bilirubinate stones by feeding a taurine- and protein-deficient diet. Diets based on milk proteins or soybean proteins are taurine-deficient. Such diets are often fed for gastrointestinal and hepatic problems. For some individuals supplementation with taurine may be important. The protein used should be low in cholesterol. If the carbohydrates in the diet are largely sucrose, other carbohydrates should be substituted.

REFERENCES

1. Schall, W.D., Chapman, W.L., Finco, D.R., Greiner, T.P., Mather, G.W., Rosine, E. and Welser, J.R.: Cholelithiasis in dogs. JAVMA 163:469-472, 1973.
2. Scott, D.W., Hoffer, R.E., Amand, W.B. and Roenigk, W.J.: Cholelithiasis in a dog. JAVMA 163:254-257, 1973.
3. Harari, J., Ettinger, S. and Lippincott, C.L.: Extrahepatic bile duct obstruction due to cholecystitis and choledocholithiasis: case report. JAAHA 18:347-349, 1982.
4. Cosenza, S.F.: Cholelithiasis and choledocholithiasis in a dog. JAVMA 184:87-88, 1984.
5. Gonciarz, Z., Trusz-Gluza, M., Kusmierski, S. and Luciak, N.: Leukocytic proteases in gallbladder pathology. Experimental acute cholecystitis in dogs. Digestion 10:65-72, 1974.
6. Lykkegaard Nielsen, M., Asnaes, S. and Justesen, T.: Susceptibility of the liver and biliary tract to anaerobic infection in extrahepatic biliary tract obstruction. III. Possible synergistic effect between anaerobic and aerobic bacteria. Scand. J. Gastroenterology 11:263-272, 1976.
7. Stephenson, S. and Nagel, C.: Acute cholecystitis. An experimental study. Ann. Surg. 157:687-694, 1963.
8. Warren, K.W. and Tan, E.G.C.: Diseases of the gallbladder and bile ducts. In, Diseases of the Liver. 4th Edition. Edited by L. Schiff. J.B. Lippincott, Philadelphia, 1278-1335, 1975.
9. Tansy, M.F., Innes, D.L., Martin, J.S. and Kendall, F.M.: A functional description of the canine choledochoduodenal flutter valve. Amer. J. Dig. Dis. 21:233-241, 1976.
10. Soloway, R.D., Powell, K.M., Senior, J.R. and Brooks, F.P.: Interrelationship of bile salts, phospholipids, and cholesterol in bile during manipulation of the enterohepatic circulation in the conscious dog. Gastroenterology 64:1156-1162, 1973.
11. Holzbach, R.T.: Animal models of cholesterol gallstone disease. Hepatology 4:1915-1985, 1984.
12. Hofman, A.F.: Animal models of calcium cholelithiasis. Hepatology 4:2095-2115, 1984.
13. Nakayama, F.: Composition of gallstone and bile: species differences. J. Lab. Clin. Med. 73:623-630, 1969.
14. Englert, E., Harman, C.G. and Wales, E.E.: Gallstones induced by normal foodstuffs in dogs. Nature 224:280-281, 1969.
15. Englert, E., Harman, C.G., Freston, J.W., Straight, R.C. and Wales, E.E.: Studies on the pathogenesis of diet-induced dog gallstones. Am. J. Dig. Dis. 22:305-314, 1977.
16. Harman, C.G., Engler, E. and Wales, E.E.: Studies on the mechanism of diet-induced cholelithiasis in dogs. Clin. Res. 17:303, 1969.
17. Lee, S.P., Maher, K. and Nicholls, J.F.: Origin and fate of biliary sludge. Gastroenterology 94:170-176, 1988.
18. Carey, M.C. and Cahalane, M.J.: Whither biliary sludge. Gastroenterology 95:508-523, 1988.
19. Bernhoft, R.A., Pellegrini, C.A., Broderick, W.C. and Way, L.W.: Pigment sludge and stone formation in the acutely ligated dog gallbladder. Gastroenterology 85:1166-1171, 1983.
20. Nyland, T.G. and Hager, D.A.: Sonography of the liver, gallbladder, and spleen. Vet. Clin. N. Am. 15:1123-1148, 1985.
21. Kerr, L.Y. and Hornoff, W.J.: Quantitative hepatobiliary scintigraphy using ^{99m}TC-DISIDA in the dog. Vet. Radiol. 27:173-177, 1986.
22. Suter, P.F.: Radiographic diagnosis of liver disease in dogs and cats. Vet. Clin. N. Am. 12:153-173, 1982.
23. Allan, G.S. and Dixon, R.T.: Cholecystography in the dog the choice of contrast media and optimum dose rates. J. Am. Vet. Rad. Soc. 16:98-104, 1975.
24. Burgener, F.A., Fishcher, H.W. and Adams, J.T.: Intravenous cholangiography in different degrees of common bile duct obstruction. An experimental study in the dog. Invest. Radiol. 10:342-350, 1975.
25. Coyne, M.J., Bonorris, G.G., Chjung, A., Cove, H. and Schoenfield, L.J.: Dietary cholesterol affects chenodeoxycholic acid action on biliary lipids. Gastroenterology 72:927-931, 1977.
26. Wakim, K.G. and Mahour, G.H.: Pathophysiological consequences of cholecystectomy. Surg. Gynecol. Obstet. 133:113-125, 1971.
27. Church, E.M. and Matthiesen, D.T.: Surgical treatment of 23 dogs with necrotizing cholecystitis. JAAHA 24:305-310, 1988.

Chapter 38

Nutritional Management of Gastrointestinal Diseases

Introduction

The disciplines of nutrition and gastroenterology are intimately related by virtue of the primary role played by the gastrointestinal system in the digestion and absorption of food. An important consequence of gastrointestinal disease is loss of nutritional homeostasis.

Most gastrointestinal diseases are managed by a combination of pharmacological and nutritional therapy. Unfortunately, pharmaceutical agents are often given inappropriate precedence. Drug therapy without appropriate nutritional management is likely to result in at best incomplete or delayed resolution of signs, and at worse exacerbation of the disorder. Many gastrointestinal diseases can be (and should be) managed by dietary therapy only.

Of primary importance in the treatment of most gastrointestinal problems is rest of the tract. In acute problems this is accomplished by completely restricting the oral intake of food. Total parenteral nutrition permits complete rest of the bowel for periods of several weeks while still maintaining nutritional homeostasis. The gastrointestinal tract can also be rested to a limited degree by feeding controlled diets.

The purpose of this chapter is to provide practical recommendations on the nutritional management of selected gastrointestinal problems. This discussion is prefaced by a description of the influence of deficiency or excess of important macronutrients and micronutrients on gastrointestinal system structure and function, and, conversely, the nutritional consequences to the animal of gastrointestinal disease. Prepared with this knowledge, it is hoped that the clinician will be in a position to rationally formulate diets for any alimentary problem, routine or otherwise, encountered in clinical practice.

INFLUENCE OF NUTRIENTS AND NUTRITIONAL STATUS ON THE GASTROINTESTINAL TRACT

Carbohydrate and Protein

Carbohydrate is the most abundant component and source of energy of most pet foods. The availability of carbohydrate is determined by a starch's source and its degree and type of processing. Some starch, such as that in rice, is nearly completely digested and absorbed, but up to 20% of other starches can escape assimilation (Figure 15-20a). Cooking is also an important determinant of starch assimilation (Table 15-2). Animals suffer a deficiency of carbohydrate with reduced intake due to anorexia or dysphagia and with reduced assimilation due to pancreatic or intestinal problems. The clinical sign of carbohydrate deficiency is primarily an inability to maintain proper body weight. Carbohydrate deficiency is usually associated with protein deficiency resulting in protein-calorie malnutrition. The systemic manifestations of protein-calorie malnutrition include poor hair coats weight loss, weakness, inactivity, poor healing, and susceptibility to infection. The predominant effect of such malnutrition on the bowel is mucosal atrophy and diarrhea. Mucin secretion is decreased, and bacterial overgrowth is common.

Carbohydrate malassimilation contributes to the pathophysiology of a number of different diseases including exocrine pancreatic insufficiency, dumping syndromes, short-bowel syndrome, and mucosal and circulatory diseases of the small intestine. In addition to osmotic diarrhea, the consequences of carbohydrate malassimilation include intestinal gaseousness, bacterial overgrowth of the small intestine, and acidification of colonic content.

Nutrients have important effects on gastrointestinal function and structure. Protein is known to be a potent stimulant of gastric acid and pancreatic secretion, as well as increasing gastroesophageal sphincter pressure. The rate of cell renewal and protein synthesis in the epithelium of the gastrointestinal mucosa is markedly increased by the presence of nutrients including long chain fatty acids, monosaccharides and a variety of amino acids.

Fiber[1,2]

Insufficient ingestion of indigestible carbohydrates (fiber) has been incriminated as causing a variety of bowel disorders including irritable bowel disease and colon cancer. Fiber is defined as plant material resistant to digestion by enzymes of monogastrics.[3,4] In veterinary medicine, there is a tendency to treat fiber as a single entity and to label fiber-responsive diarrhea as a single disease process — irritable bowel syndrome. In reality, there are several hundred different types of fiber, many different fiber-responsive diseases, and a large variety of ways in which fiber influences the gastrointestinal tract in addition to its effects on motility. The major constituents of fiber are cellulose, hemicellulose, pectins (polysaccharides), and lignin. The amount of these constituents varies considerably in fibers of different origins.

There are two major classifications of fiber, soluble and insoluble, differentiated according to their resistance to bacterial fermentation. Although most fiber constituents are resistant to digestion by mammalian enzymes, they vary greatly in their susceptibility to digestion by bacteria. In general, fibers with high lignin content are resistant to bacterial hydrolysis (insoluble). The properties of the different types of fiber are largely predictable by this classification. Soluble fibers attract water, form gels, delay gastric emptying, inhibit the absorption of cholesterol, are poor bulking agents, are highly fermentable in the colon, increase the numbers of colonic bacteria, form colonic short-chain fatty acids, and lower colonic pH. In contrast, insoluble fibers do not form gels, do not delay gastric emptying, and do not affect absorption. They are poorly fermentable, and they are good bulk forming agents. Fiber is the predominant nutrient entering the colon.

Although most of fibers' effects are in the large bowel, fiber has some limited affects on small intestinal and pancreatic function. Gel-forming, viscous fibers such as guar gum and pectins slow gastric emptying. Dietary fiber influences upper gastrointestinal function by affecting serum concentrations of gastrointestinal hormones, such as gastrin, glucagon, and GIP.[5] Insoluble fibers may modestly increase gastric pH by a buffering action. The influence of fiber on small intestinal transit is uncertain. One study in dogs, reported cellulose to decrease mouth-to-anus transit time.[6] Normalization of transit time was observed in some dogs; slow transit became faster and rapid transit was slowed.[6] Some fibers can inhibit pancreatic enzyme activity. Wheat bran decreases pancreatic lipase secretion in dogs.[7] Soluble fibers may reduce brush border enzyme activity.[1] Soluble fibers may also increase the viscosity of the unstirred water layer of the small intestinal mucosa thus decreasing the absorption of some nutrients. Prolonged intake of fiber is thought to increase the number of goblet cells and the secretion of mucus in the intestine.[1] It also influences villus morphology.[2] Fecal fat is increased by some types of fiber.[1,8] This may be partly due to the influence on bile acid metabolism and partly due to the interference with pancreatic enzyme activity. The apparent digestibility of protein and fat are slightly decreased in dogs by the addition of cellulose to the diet.[6]

Fiber influences the large bowel through a number of mechanisms. Insoluble fibers, such as wheat bran and cellulose dilute colonic content by virtue of their bulking activity. This has the potential to reduce the influence on the bowel mucosa of noxious agents contained in the lumen. Insoluble fibers tend to decrease colonic ammonia concentration whereas some soluble fibers increase colonic ammonia concentration. The cause of this effect is not fully understood but may relate to the trapping of ammonium ion in the colon by the lowered colonic pH. Soluble fiber also decreases protein absorption in the small intestine. This may be an additional explanation for the increased colonic ammonia concentration because the decreased protein absorption results in increased substrate for ammonia generation. Ammonia is toxic to the colonic mucosa, stimulates epithelial turnover, and increases tumorigenesis.

Soluble fibers, such as psyllium derivatives, are substrates for the growth of colonic bacteria that generate large quantities of short-chain fatty acids. The fatty acids acidify colonic content, neutralize colonic bases, and are absorbed into the systemic circulation. The quantity and composition of the short-chain fatty acids produced in the colon varies considerably with the species. Absorbed acetate is metabolized systemically for energy (minor importance in carnivores). Butyrate is an important energy source for colonocytes. The lowered pH induced by the short-chain fatty acids increases cell proliferation and tumorigenesis.

Certain types of fibers are bile acid binding agents; the gel-forming fibers and the lignins appear to be the most effective. The binding appears to be primarily an adsorption phenomenon and it is influenced by pH, osmolality, bile acid structure, and the form of the fiber.[1] Some fibers also bind cholesterol, phospholipids, monoglycerides, and fatty acids.

Colonic transit time is variably affected by the different fibers and is not necessarily predictable based on their solubility or insolubility. Some residue is necessary to stimulate normal colonic segmentation so that transit rates are normal. Colonic morphology is also affected by variations in dietary fiber. The secretion of colonic and small intestinal IgA can be increased or decreased by different types of dietary fiber.

Mean fecal weight of dogs increases linearly with the addition of cellulose.[6] Fiber increases fecal bulk by two mechanisms. Indigestible fiber from, for instance, cereal grains increases fecal bulk by acting as sponge for water, increasing the weight and water content of the stool. Fiber that can be metabolized by bacteria provide the flora with a substrate for bacterial growth and such fiber increases fecal bulk by supporting increases for fecal bacterial numbers.[9] The bacterial composition of the feces of normal people is relatively unchanged by the addition or removal of fiber from the diet, even though the numbers of bacteria markedly change. The commonly used bulk-promoting agent psyllium (Metamucil) increases the bacterial content of the stool. Low residue diets such as cottage cheese and rice reduces the fecal volume of dogs by up to 85%, and also reduce the frequency of defecation.

In summary, it is often recommended that diets for small intestinal diseases be low in residue to avoid physical trauma to the inflamed gastrointestinal tract. While, there is little evidence to support the concept that fiber causes harmful physical abrasion to the intestinal tract, there is evidence that fiber can reduce the digestibility and absorption of certain nutrients in the small bowel. Therefore, it would seem sensible to conclude that high fiber diets are inappropriate in patients with small intestinal diseases. In contrast, the ability for fiber to markedly influence large bowel physiology supports the continued use of this dietary constituent in the treatment of large bowel diseases. What requires further definition, however, is which types of fiber are suitable for different large bowel disorders and to which mechanism their beneficial effects can be attributed. These questions are particularly important because it appears that some types of fiber can potentially have both detrimental and beneficial effects on large bowel function.

Fat

The ingestion of a fatty meal slows gastric emptying and decreases gastroesophageal tone. Fat is normally not as readily assimilated as other macronutrients. The consequences of fat malassimilation such as bile salt, vitamin, and mineral malabsorption are discussed in Chapter 17. Increased quantities of deconjugated bile acids and hydroxylated fatty acids enter the colon and are toxic to the colonic mucosa, inducing morphological changes and diarrhea. Furthermore, dietary long-chain triglycerides are the primary stimulus for intestinal lymph flow.

Vitamins and Minerals

Deficiencies and excesses of vitamins and minerals have a series of well recognized systemic effects,[10] but their influence on the bowel is less well studied. Deficiencies of vitamins and minerals are not uncommon in chronic gastrointestinal diseases. Thiamin deficiency may cause anorexia and vomiting in addition to its more classic CNS signs.[11] Pantothenic acid and riboflavin deficiency cause a fatty liver. In cats pantothenic acid has been reported to cause gastrointestinal mucosal damage.[10] In dogs, niacin deficiency can result in a fatty liver, hemorrhagic diarrhea, and ulceration of the mucous membranes of the mouth and tongue (black tongue). In cats, the signs of niacin deficiency include diarrhea and emaciation.[11] Biotin deficiency can produce a bloody diarrhea, and choline deficiency can result in a fatty liver. Vitamin A deficiency results in a significant reduction in the numbers of intestinal goblet cells and abnormalities in intestinal mucus.[12] Vitamin D and choline toxicity can result in diarrhea. Potassium deficiency can cause adynamic ileus, and zinc deficiency has been associated with vomiting [11]. Copper deficiency causes diarrhea, anemia, and depigmentation (perhaps not in cats). Selenium deficiency has been associated with esophageal cancer in humans. Excess dietary iron is irritating to the mucosa and will induce diarrhea.

NUTRITIONAL DEFICIENCIES RESULTING FROM GASTROINTESTINAL DISEASE[13]

The principle nutritional consequences of gastrointestinal disease are protein-calorie malnutrition and vitamin and mineral deficiencies. The protein-calorie malnutrition usually results from a combination of decreased food intake, increased energy and protein requirements due to the disease process, malassimilation, and increased direct loss of protein into the gastrointestinal tract. Protein-calorie malnutrition also can be difficult to correct in some animals because unpalatable or low-calorie controlled diets are fed for prolonged periods of time.

Deficiencies of sodium, potassium, chloride, and bicarbonate are common with intestinal disease, and are discussed in Chapter 39. The demand for potassium and phosphorus is greatly increased by the anabolism that accompanies the resumption of appropriate nutrition. Increased loss of divalent cations such as magnesium, zinc, and calcium are known to occur in human gastrointestinal diseases. Chronic intestinal hemorrhage is a common cause of iron deficiency.

Vitamin B deficiencies can result from prolonged periods of anorexia and diarrhea.[10] Serum concentrations of cobalamin will decrease in some cases of bacterial overgrowth, and serum folate levels will be low in some severe small intestinal diseases. Fat soluble vitamin deficiencies can occur with prolonged steatorrhea. A vitamin K-responsive coagulopathy has been noted in cats with lymphocytic-plasmacytic enteritis.[14] It should be remembered that blood levels of minerals and fat soluble vitamins are poorly reflective of tissue stores.

PRINCIPLES IN FORMULATING DIETS

To undertake successful nutritional management of gastrointestinal disorders, the clinician must be able to assess the protein-calorie status of the patient, formulate a balanced diet which fulfills its energy and protein demands, and be familiar with which nutrients and which routes of nutrient administration are appropriate in particular gastrointestinal disorders.

Assessment of Protein-Calorie Status

An accurate assessment of the caloric and protein needs of a patient is important to successful nutritional management. Unfortunately, there are no simple and accurate means for that assessment. The best approximation of caloric status comes from a combination of dietary history, physical examination, and patient's body weight.

The dietary history helps determine the severity of deprivation. The calorie and protein content of the patient's present diet is estimated, and the duration of its nutrient restriction determined. The relative severity of the protein-calorie deficit can then be assessed by comparing the estimated intake with the calculated requirements of the animal. Where possible it is preferable to base the calculated requirements on the premorbid body weight.

The physical examination provides clues on the nutritional status by assessments of coat condition, muscle mass, mental state, and body weight. Nutritional deprivation results in a dull coat and mild to moderately depressed mentation. Reduced protein mass can often be discerned by comparison of muscle mass with an adjacent bony prominence such as the sagittal crest of the cranium or the spine of the scapula, Body weight is particularly valuable if it can be compared to the patient's usual body weight. In humans, recent weight loss as little as 2-6 per cent per month has been used to predict significant calorie-protein malnutrition.[15] Fasted dogs lose 1-3% of body weight daily.[16] More chronic weight loss in humans of 10-20% of ideal body weight is considered indicative of mild protein-calorie malnutrition. Reduction of ideal body weight of 20-30% is considered moderate deficiency and greater than 30% is considered severe.[13] Acute weight loss of 10% of body mass will result in measurable decreases in muscle performance.[17] An obvious confounding factor is that weight can fluctuate markedly as a result of fluid loss or gain. Fluid accumulation due to ascites or edema in such conditions as liver failure and protein-losing enteropathy can obviate the value of body weight.

Biochemical parameters have been utilized in human medicine as a guide to nutritional status. Albumin is the most commonly used parameter in humans, although it is considered by many to be of little value. The serum concentration of albumin is affected by many factors other than nutritional status, including hydration, glomerulonephropathies, protein-losing enteropathies, vasculitis, heart failure, and liver disease. Furthermore, it has a relatively long serum half-life so that there is a considerable lag time before serum albumin concentration reflects nutritional deprivation. For these reasons, serum albumin is a poor indicator of the nutritional status of a newly admitted patient. Serial samples may be of some value in monitoring the response to nutritional therapy, provided the clinician is cognizant of the confounding factors.

Calculation of Energy Requirements[11,15,18,19]

Estimation of a patient's energy and protein requirements can be difficult because demand varies according to body surface area, age, activity level, and the presence or absence of additional requirements associated with such physiological states as lactation, and disease. It is important to differentiate "simple starvation" from "stress starvation". Simple starvation refers to ingestion of insufficient calories in a normal adult animal. Stress starvation refers to inadequate nutritional intake in an animal that is stressed by intercurrent disease or some energetically demanding process such as growth or lactation. These processes force the patient into an obligatory hypermetabolic state which utilizes fat and protein stores simultaneously. In contrast, simple starvation is a carefully controlled process in which metabolic rate declines, and there is a shift to ketogenesis with the result that fat provides the majority of energy, and protein stores are spared. The clinical significance of this differentiation is that animals with stress starvation will rapidly develop complications of malnutrition whereas those subjected to simple starvation can survive weeks without significant complications.[20]

For an indepth discussion of the calculation of energy requirements the reader is referred to recent publications on the subject.[11,16,21] For purposes of this discussion, the reader should be familiar with the term basal energy expenditure (basal metabolic rate). Basal energy expenditure is the energy expended by an animal to maintain life while it is resting quietly in the post-absorptive state in a thermoneutral environment. The basal energy expenditure (BEE) for dogs and cats is provided in Table 38-1. By using this table, and the following adjustment factors, the energy requirements for different physiological and pathological states may be calculated. Thus, maintenance energy requirements for a caged animal are approximately 1.25 x BEE (maintenance energy expenditure is greater than that required for BEE, a largely theoretical value, because of the energy demands made by the small amount of movement of a caged animal and the energy lost in the digestion of food). Energy requirements for normal canine activity are approximately 1.75-2.0 x BEE, and for normal feline activity approximately 1.4 x BEE. Energy requirements during major infections or inflammatory diseases have been estimated to range from 1.25-2.0 x BEE. Recent studies on the metabolic requirements of humans with severe illnesses, however, have found that the energy requirements of such patients rarely, if ever, exceed 1.5 x BEE,[15] suggesting that the estimated energy requirement range for severe illness in the dog should be reexamined. Extreme physical activity can raise energy requirements to 3-4 x BEE. Growth raises energy requirements to 2-3 x BEE, and lactation raises energy requirements to 4-6 x BEE.

Energy is usually supplied in the diet by amounts of carbohydrate and fat fulfilling energy requirements. The relative proportion of energy provided as fat or carbohydrate depends on a number of factors. Fat has more caloric density than carbohydrate, but it is also more difficult to assimilate. The caloric density of long-chain triglycerides is approximately 9 kcal per gm whereas that of carbohydrate is approximately 4 kcal per gm. The advantage of high caloric density is that it reduces dietary volume which can be a major concern in an inappetent patient. Medium chain triglycerides are better assimilated than long-chain triglycerides and provide approximately 8.3 kcal per gm. Unfortunately, they are at times poorly tolerated by the patient. The amount of dietary fat given to animals with small bowel-type diarrhea is usually severely limited by the adverse consequences of malassimilated lipid on digestive function. As a general rule, fat in the diet of animals with diarrhea is limited to less than 15% of the diet on a dry matter basis.

Calculation of Protein Requirements[15,18,19]

An important clinical nutrition concept is that no protein in the body serves a storage role; none serves as a reservoir of energy. All body protein exists to perform a function, for example, muscle contraction or enzyme catalysis. The body does, however, contain labile protein. This protein is rapidly degraded during starvation for the provision of gluconeogenic substrate. The essential difference between labile protein and an energy store is that after labile protein is metabolized, the body's function has been compromised. This is not the case for fat, which exists primarily to provide energy in times of need. The dysfunction resulting from protein deficiency is most obvious in the growing animal because growth potential will not be satisfied. The adult is also affected, however. Initially, the dysfunction is subclinical, and includes such phenomena as impaired immunity and decreased physical and mental activity. As protein loss continues decreased muscle mass becomes obvious, the immune response becomes more severely impaired,[22] wound healing is impaired, organ dysfunction occurs (such as cardiomyopathy) and skeletal muscle weakness (including that of the diaphragm) becomes obvious.

The corollary is that if excess protein is ingested, it is not stored as a protein reserve. Instead, it is metabolized to provide energy. This is an inefficient way to feed an animal, because protein is energetically expensive to manufacture. Furthermore each amino acid catabolized provides one or more nitrogen for disposal which is also an energetically demanding process. Moreover, excess protein has been incriminated as a contributor to a number of disease processes including the progression of renal disease and the development of hepatic encephalopathy in patients with preexisting liver disease. In formulating a diet careful attention must be paid to the level of protein being fed.

Arbitrary requirements for protein are provided in Table 38-2. Protein requirements are best expressed in terms of protein required per kcal of dietary energy (e.g. for an adult dog 1.1 gm per 100 kcal), because without the provision of sufficient energy protein is poorly utilized. Protein requirements vary with age being highest in young growing animals. The requirements are dependent on the biological value of the protein being fed and the activity level of the patient. They also vary with species, with the cat having a considerably higher obligate need for protein than the dog.

Protein requirements can increase considerably with intestinal diseases. In a normal animal considerable amounts of protein (on estimate 1 gm per kg per day) enter the gastrointestinal tract in pancreatic and intestinal excretions, and from desquamated mucosal cells. The majority of this is reabsorbed (approximately 90%). Any disease that speeds transit time, increases the mucosal cell turnover rate, or promotes mucus secretion is likely to increase protein requirements. Another obvious example is the syndrome of protein-losing enteropathy. Unfortunately, there is no practical way to estimate the

Table 38-1. Energy Requirements for Dogs and Cats

Body Weight (Kg)	Estimated Basal Energy Expenditure[a] (Kcal/day)	Estimated Average Energy Expenditure[b] (Kcal/day)
2.5	139	209
3	160	239
3.5	179	269
4	198	297
4.5	216	324
5	234	351
6	268	403
7	301	452
8	333	499
9	364	546
10	394	590
11	423	634
12	451	677
13	479	719
14	507	760
15	534	800
16	560	840
17	586	879
18	612	918
19	637	956
20	662	993
24	759	1139
25	783	1174
26	806	1209
27	829	1244
28	852	1278
29	875	1312
30	897	1346
45	1216	1824
50	1316	1974
60	1509	2264
70	1694	2541
80	1872	2809
90	2045	3068
100	2214	3320

a 70 X BW kg 0.75

*Average energy requirements for the critically ill patient; calculated as 1.5X BEE. Caged animals with minimal activity and minor disease stress perhaps would be more closely approximated by 1.25 X BEE. Normal canine activity or very severe disease stress in either the dog or cat perhaps would be more accurately approximated by 1.75 or 2.0 X BEE. Lactation, late-stage pregnancy, and heavy exercise may increase energy requirements 4 to 6 X BEE.

b Average energy requirements of a dog with normal activity.

*Courtesy of Dr. S.C. Haskins, Dept. Surgery, School of Veterinary Medicine, University of California, Davis, CA

increased protein requirements for a patient with protein-losing enteropathy, and requirements are usually determined by trial and error using clinical condition and plasma albumin concentration as a guide. It has been determined in humans that, with the exception of major fractures and burns, protein requirements during diseases (including intestinal diseases) are rarely more than double basal requirements.[15] As a rule of thumb, it has been recommended that patients with mild diseases receive protein requirements 130% of basal requirements, and patients with moderate and severe disease receive 160% and 200% of basal requirements, respectively.[15] If dietary protein content is increased markedly, it is advisable to increase dietary energy content concomitantly to ensure sufficient energy is provided for utilization of the protein. As a guideline, the ratio of non-protein calories to grams of protein should remain above 30 in the dog and 20 in the cat.

Conversely, the protein fed to an animal may have to be reduced because of diseases such as liver disease. In these circumstances the amount of protein provided is selected to minimize clinical signs of encephalopathy but with consideration of the minimum protein requirements for that species (dog 1.3-1.5 gm/kg/day; cat 3.3-3.5 gm/kg/day).[23]

Calculation of Other Nutritional Requirements

The vitamin and mineral requirements of dogs and cats are listed in Table 38-2. As with protein and energy, the requirements for micronutrients varies with the life stage and physiological condition of the animal. For instance, the requirements for B vitamins are increased during accelerated metabolism, and the requirements for fat soluble vitamins increase in proportion to the severity of a steatorrhea. The ideal fiber percentage of the diet also varies with the clinical condition.

Summary

In summary, the first step in the formulation of a diet for a patient with a digestive system disorder is the calculation of energy needs, which determines the quantity of food to be fed. The energy requirement is based on estimates of the protein-calorie status of the patient, the basal energy expenditure for an animal of that size, and the increased energy requirements due to the particular disease. The next consideration is the protein requirement of the patient, which is calculated in an analogous manner to the energy requirement. Decisions are then made on dietary levels of fat and fiber, with the decisions being based on a knowledge of the influence of these nutrients on gastrointestinal function. Finally, it must be decided whether adequate nutrition can be provided by the oral route or if nutritional support by other means is required.

It is important to emphasize that the calculations made in the formulation of a diet make a number of arbitrary assumptions, and the potential for significant error is high. Therefore, it is essential that the condition of the patient be carefully monitored and the diet subsequently modified according to patient response.

Table 38-2. Nutrient Requirements of Normal Dogs and Cats*

	Dog			Cat	
	Growth[a,10] (oral)	Adult[b,10] (oral)	Growth[c,13] (IV)	Growth[d,11] (oral)	Adult[e,12] (oral)
Metabolizable energy (per day) (Kcal/Kg)	150-300	75	140	130-250	85
Protein (per day)					
(g/Kg)	3-5	0.85	4	6.2-12	6
(g/100 Kcal)	2	1.1	2.8	7	6.2
Essential amino acids (mg/kg/day)					
Arginine	274	21	—	400	—
Histidine	98	22	—	120	—
Isoleucine	196	48	—	200	—
Leucine	318	84	—	480	—
Lysine	280	50	—	320	—
Methionine-cysteine	212	30	—	300	—
Phenylalanine-tyrosine	390	86	—	340	—
Threonine	254	44	—	280	—
Tryptophan	82	13	—	60	—
Valine	210	60	—	240	—
Taurine	—	—	—	20	15
Lipid (g/kg/day)	2.7	1	2.2	3.4	1.91
Linoleic acid (mg/kg/day)	540	200	—	200	380
Arachidonic acid (mg/kg/day)	—	—	—	800	—
Minerals (mg/kg/day)					
Sodium	30	11	100	20	121
Potassium	240	89	115	160	66
Chloride	46	17	225	760	121
Calcium	320	119	72	320	242
Phosphorus	240	89	58	240	198
Magnesium	22	8.2	4	16	8.8
Iron	1.74	0.65	0.058	3.2	2.15
Copper	0.16	0.06	0.065	0.2	0.11
Cobalt	—	1.06	0.041	—	—
Manganese	0.28	0.10	0.04	0.2	0.22
Zinc	1.94	0.72	0.14	2	0.66
Iodine	0.032	0.012	0.046	0.14	0.02
Selenium	6	2.2	—	0.004	0.002
Vitamins					
A (I.U./kg/day)	202	75	100	133	212
D (I.U./kg/day)	22	8	10	20	21
E (I.U./kg/day)	1.2	0.5	0.05	1.2	1.6
K (μg/kg/day)	—	—	0.1	4	—
Thiamin (μg/kg/day)	54	20	0.5	200	100
Riboflavin (μg/kg/day)	100	50	0.1	160	100
Pyridoxine (μg/kg/day)	60	22	0.15	160	80
Niacin (μg/kg/day)	450	225	0.1	1600	900
Pantothenic acid (μg/kg/day)	400	200	0.25	200	200
Folic acid (μg/kg/day)	8	4	0.01	32	20
Choline (μg/kg/day)	50	25	25	96	40
Biotin (μg/kg/day)	—	—	7	2.8	1
B12 (μg/kg/day)	1	0.5	—	0.8	0.4

[a]Body weight 3 Kg [b]Body weight 10 Kg [c]Average body weight of 7 Kg [d]Assumed body weight of 1.5 Kg [e]Assumed body weight of 3.5 Kg
Courtesy Dr. S.C. Haskins, Dept. Surgery, School of Veterinary Medicine, University of California, Davis,

NUTRITIONAL THERAPY OF GASTROINTESTINAL PROBLEMS[24,25]

There have been few studies to determine the nutritional requirements of dogs and cats with gastrointestinal disorders. The recommendations provided below are based predominantly on clinical experience and pathophysiologic theory and must be regarded as tentative.

Dysphagia, Aversion, Anorexia and Polyphagia

Physiology of Intake. Food intake is controlled by a complex interaction of many factors; overall control is poorly understood. In the healthy animal, food intake is programmed to maintain body weight with remarkable consistency in spite of marked fluctuations of energy requirements on a day-to-day and week-to-week basis. The ebb and flow of appetite and satiety results from various gastrointestinal, environmental, and CNS phenomena. The gastrointestinal phenomena include gastric distension, rate of gastric emptying, the release of gastric hormones (in particular CCK and bombesin), and the absorption of nutrients such as glucose, fatty acids, and amino acids. The gut hormones have effects both locally on the gastrointestinal tract and centrally on the thalamic centers that control feeding behavior. An important example is CCK which decreases appetite by inhibiting gastric emptying and by inhibiting the CNS feeding "center". The inhibitory influence of absorbed nutrients on intake has been proposed to operate through "glucostats", "lipostats", "aminostats", and "purinostats", although the importance, location, structure, and function of these "appetostats" remains poorly elucidated.

Feeding behavior is ultimately under control of the CNS feeding centers. Threatening environmental factors operating through these centers will reduce food intake. In addition to the gastrointestinal and environmental phenomena already mentioned, the CNS can be directly influenced by the diet. The ingestion of a protein meal results in the absorption of amino acids which cross the blood-brain barrier and directly alter the concentration of neurotransmitters in the CNS. Furthermore, some of the absorbed nutrients may alter the responsiveness of CNS receptors.

Neurotransmitters of importance in the control of intake include catecholamines operating through beta adrenergic receptors (inhibitory) and alpha adrenergic receptors (stimulatory), dopamine (inhibitory), serotonin (inhibitory), opioids operating through kappa receptors and mu receptors, and gamma aminobutyric acid (GABA). Naloxone, binding to opioid receptors is inhibitory to food intake, whereas butorphanol stimulates feeding. Benzodiazepines operate in conjunction with GABA to increase appetite, and inhibit the serotonergic satiety system. Glucocorticoids increase intake, partly by a direct effect on CNS inhibitors of appetite, such as serotonin, and partly by an antiinflammatory effect.

Palatability and Amino Acid Imbalance. Diets of poor palatability result in aversion to the food. The animal is not anorectic per se, in that a more palatable food is readily consumed. Properties of a food that influence palatability include smell, taste, texture, temperature, and even appearance. Dietary constituents determining palatability are largely undetermined. High fat content and moderate levels of protein are generally preferred by cats and dogs. Poor dietary palatability results in a capricious intake in dogs and often complete refusal to eat in cats. Dogs and cats will also become averse to diets of imbalanced amino acid composition.

Pathophysiology of Intake. Prolonged, inappropriate satiety is termed anorexia or inappetence. The causes of anorexia are legion. Threatening environments, including veterinary clinics and boarding establishments, inhibit appetite. Anorexia may result from painful lesions. Inflammatory, infectious, or neoplastic diseases can cause inappetence, probably as a result of the release of a variety of chemical mediators such as cachectin and interleukin 1. Painful oropharyngeal or esophageal lesions can cause reluctance to eat or dysphagia. Diseases that cause nausea or delay gastric emptying result in inappetence, partly through gastric distension. Anorexia is not the only cause of decreased food intake. Others include dysphagia, and food aversion, the latter most commonly resulting from poor palatability and amino acid imbalance.

A prolonged and inappropriately excessive appetite is termed polyphagia. Most causes of polyphagia are due to endocrine disorders such as diabetes mellitus, hyperthyroidism, and hyperadrenocorticism. Occasionally gastrointestinal diseases such as pancreatic atrophy will be responsible. On rare occasions, malabsorption will cause polyphagia. Some dogs and cats appear to eat to excess for indeterminate reasons. One consequence of polyphagia is obesity, which in turn increases the likelihood of musculoskeletal disease, dermatological diseases, cardiac problems, and respiratory dysfunction. Obesity is a common problem in cats and dogs.[26] Gastrointestinal causes of polyphagia do not result in obesity.

Management of Anorexia and Food Aversion. The management of anorexia begins with attention to the primary cause if identifiable. This may include a variety of measures, including the treatment of upper respiratory tract infections, and the alleviation of pain. Symptomatic therapy includes attention to fluid and electrolyte derangements, reduction of environmental stressors, and modification of the diet to improve palatability. Reduction in stress is best attained by careful and considerate handling, and attention to environmental concerns such as avoidance of housing dogs and cats in close proximity. With reassurance, some frightened animals can be coaxed to eat.

Palatability of the diet can be improved by adding flavored toppings such as chicken or beef broths, seasoning with a condiment such as garlic powder, adjusting the fat or protein content, varying the texture and appearance of the food, and heating the food to improve its aroma and temperature (no more than body temperature).

If such manipulations fail, and the patient is capable of ingesting food, drug therapy can be tried just prior to offering the food. Benzodiazepine derivatives such as Valium (0.1 mg/kg IV) and oxazepam (0.4 mg/kg PO) will produce an increase in appetite in most cats and some dogs. Butorphanol (0.2 mg/kg SC) may be useful, particularly if analgesia is also required. Veterinary lore has it that vitamin B complex injections will also stimulate appetite. Metoclopramide (0.2-0.4 mg/kg SC, PO) is useful if anorexia is associated with delayed gastric emptying and may also have a central influence by way of its antidopaminergic-antiemetic effects. If these efforts fail, or if nutritional support greater than several days duration is required, enteral feeding techniques should be considered.

Nutritional Management of Dysphagia. The nutritional

management of dysphagia is described in Chapter 9. Important points are to vary the texture of the diet, and to feed from an elevated receptacle. Abnormal motility of the pharynx and/or esophagus sometimes causes great difficulty in swallowing solid boluses of food although the swallowing of liquids is little affected. Occasionally, the opposite is true. Megaesophagus is usually managed better with liquid diets that are fed from a level higher than the animal. In some animals food is seldom regurgitated whereas liquid frequently is. Thus, management is directed by observations on trial and error. Many dysphagic patients require management by enteral feeding.

Controlled Diet for Chronic Idiopathic Diarrhea

The ideal controlled diet should be composed of highly digestible nutrients, be low in fat and lactose, be hypoallergenic, contain appropriate amounts of fiber for the condition at hand, and not be markedly hypertonic (Table 38-3). The diet should be formulated by incorporating the least number of ingredients possible, so that the influence of each ingredient on the patients bowel function can be assessed. Good palatability, nutritional balance, and ease of preparation are required. Controlled diets are usually formulated as a compromise between the ideal and the realistic.

Client Education. Controlled diets fed to small animals are generally less palatable than regular diets. The greatest single reason for failure of dietary management of chronic gastrointestinal problems is covert modification of the diet by the client to please the patient. Strict adherence to a controlled diet depends on the effectiveness of client education. Owners often incorrectly believe that minor dietary alterations are of no consequence.

Digestibility. Controlled diets should be highly digestible. High digestibility provides bowel rest and reduces the allergenicity of the diet, by reducing both the amount of dietary protein absorbed intact by the mucosa and the number of bacteria and bacterial products in the bowel. Less protein will enter the colon resulting in less colonic ammonia generation. High digestibility results in complete absorption in the cranial small intestine, permitting the remainder of the bowel to rest. Diets needing minimum digestion stimulate gastric, pancreatic, biliary, and intestinal secretion less than do regular diets.

Lactose and Glutens. The initial diet should contain no glutens. Disaccharides, especially lactose, are avoided since the disaccharidases (lactase, maltase, isomaltose, and sucrase) are reduced for a week or more following diarrhea due to any cause.

Table 38-3. Criteria for an Ideal Dietary Management Program

Requires little or no digestion
Contains minimal fat
Lactose-free
Nonallergenic
Low residue
Isosmotic
Frequent feeding is possible
Good acceptability
Results in optimal intestinal ecology

Low Fat. Restriction of fat is primarily of value in patients with fat malassimilation. It is not necessary in motility disorders or in many cases of chronic colitis. Foods that should form the basis of a low fat diet include vegetables, bread, cereals, low-fat milk products, and lean meats such as boiled poultry (without skin). MCT oil can be used to supplement the dietary fat. Unfortunately, the potential to supply significant quantities of calories by medium chain triglycerides is hampered by their potential to cause osmotic diarrhea and inappetence. MCT oils are ketogenic and should not be given to patients with ketosis or acidosis.[24] They are poorly metabolized in hepatic cirrhosis and may accumulate.

Osmolality. The ideal diet has a restricted osmolality to prevent excessive extracellular fluid moving into the intestine, and to minimize the damage to the mucosa that can occur with such diets. High osmolality is one stimulus for gastrointestinal inflammation; it can also disrupt tight junction structure.[27] Furthermore, if the constituents of the hyperosmolar diet are not readily absorbed osmotic diarrhea will develop. Hyperosmolarity is most often of concern when feeding excessive amounts of hyperosmolar liquid elemental diets that can rapidly exit into the highly permeable duodenum.

Bacterial Flora. Ideally, controlled diets should help maintain the optimum intestinal bacterial flora necessary for normal function. Unfortunately, little is known about the influence of diet on the canine and feline microflora. In other species the diet is known to have an important effect on the enteric bacterial population.[28-30]

The rate of bacterial growth is related directly to nutrient availability. With the feeding of an elemental diet, total bacterial counts in the intestine decline. These nutrients are completely absorbed in the proximal small intestine. In addition, since this diet contains no residue, mucus secretion and cell desquamation are at a minimum in the small intestine and less nutrients are delivered to the colon. Thus, the bacterial flora is "starved," and its total population is reduced. A similar, albeit less pronounced effect, can be achieved by the use of highly digestible controlled diets. By reducing the total number of bacteria, the number of potential invaders, the amount of enterotoxin produced and the total antigenic load in the intestinal tract is limited. This is likely to have a beneficial effect on bowel function, particularly in the small intestine.

The relative distribution of different enteric organisms is also determined by the diet.[29] Numbers of colonic aerobes increase with low-protein diets, whereas colonic anaerobes increase with high-protein diets. These alterations in the composition of the intestinal flora are also likely to be of importance in the response to a controlled diet. Unfortunately, there is no information on what diets create an ideal bacterial composition in the dog and cat. The ideal diet to prescribe is one that results in a bacterial microflora of the gut that is normal with respect to both total numbers and distribution of the population.

Carbohydrates Sources for Controlled Diets. Suitable carbohydrate sources for controlled diets include boiled white rice, potatoes, or tapioca. These are all gluten-free. Carbohydrates can be used to provide 80% of the total diet. Since this is often a greater intake of carbohydrates than is normal, it may initially be inadequately digested and absorbed, until pancreatic enzyme and brush-border enzyme levels increase to meet the changed digestive requirements.[31,32] Thus, a change to a high-carbohydrate diet may not give rapid remission of diarrhea if the levels of carbohydrate-digesting enzymes are low. This problem is minimized by feeding small meals frequently. Overfeeding delays the recovery of mucosal function.

Incomplete digestion and absorption of starches results in increased numbers of intestinal bacteria, which interferes with the production of normal bowel movements. Starchy diets also change the composition of the normal bacterial flora, which may or may not be beneficial.

Protein Sources for Controlled Diets. Protein incorporated into the diet can be either animal or vegetable in origin. Used most often is a single animal protein with a high biological value, such as eggs, cottage cheese, tofu, or lean meat. Cottage cheese is often preferred since it contains less lipid than eggs and meat (Table 38-4). The amounts used in the initial diet should meet protein requirements and be proportionate to the carbohydrate provided (see above). Excess protein should be avoided. The aim is to provide a highly digestible protein and in amounts to minimize antigenicity and limit the amount of protein in the ileal effluent. A suitable controlled diet is shown in Table 38-5. Note, that if a dietary allergy is suspected, the protein source in the controlled diet can be changed as described in Chapter 20.

Yogurt is sometimes used as the protein source for diets used in the treatment of chronic diarrhea in the mistaken belief that the bacteria contained in the yogurt (*Lactobacillus acidophilus*), will displace unfavorable microorganisms in the intestine.[8] Orally administered bacteria do not displace resident bacterial populations in the normal intestines; they also do not displace pathogens or transients populating the diseased intestine. Furthermore, the bacteria in yogurt are generally acid labile, limiting the numbers surviving passage through the stomach. Cultures of Lactobacillus acidophilus have not been shown to hasten renewal of the normal bacterial flora. Cottage cheese contains only small amounts of lactose, whereas yogurt contains almost as much as milk. If lactase deficiency accompanies the diarrheal process, cottage cheese is the preferred milk protein to feed. Some forms of yogurt have bacterial lactase activity that is inactive until the alkaline pH of duodenal fluid restores the ability to metabolize lactose.

Table 38-5. Controlled Diet for Chronic Diarrhea in Dogs +*

1. Measure 7 ounces (190 to 200 g) of dry rice
2. Cook with 2 volumes of water added
3. To the cooked rice add 3 1/2 to 4 ounces of cottage cheese#
4. Mix in 1 teaspoon vegetable oil~
5. Mix in 1.5 teaspoons of dicalcium phosphate~
6. Mix in 0.5 teaspoons of iodized salt
7. Consider 1-6 tsp Metamucil per meal if suspect large bowel diarrhea

+ Contains 22% to 25% of cottage cheese and 18% to 20% of protein on a dry-matter basis.
* Sufficient for a 25-pound dog - provides 820 Kcal
# For elimination diets, the cottage cheese can be substituted with another protein source such as tofu, cooked lamb (0.25 lb) or skinned and cooked chicken (0.25 lb)
~ If using this diet as an elimination diet, these ingredients can be omitted for the first 1-2 weeks of therapy

Table 38-4. Composition of Various Foods

	Contents Per 100 Grams				
	CHO	Energy	Water	Protein	Fat
Meat, medium	—	275	56	24	20
Meat, lean	—	200	63	27	10
Heart	1	105	78	17	4
Milk, whole	4.7	67	87	3.5	3.8
skim	5.1	35	90	3.5	.1
Cottage cheese, dehydrated	2	93	77	20	.5
Eggs, whole	.7	163	74	13	12
Liver, beef	6	136	70	20	3
Liver, calf	4	141	71	19	5
Liver, pork	2	134	72	20	5
Liver, chicken	3	141	70	22	4
Kidney, beef	1	141	75	15	8
Brewers's yeast	34	330	13	42	2
Soybean meal	36	330	13	44	1
Tofu	2.4	72	84	7.4	4.2
Oatmeal	56	360	13	16	8
Barley, pearl	78	353	11	8	1
Farina	76	357	11	11	1
Rice, brown	78	355	12	7	1.7
white	80	350	12	7	.3
Tapioca	86	350	12	1	.2
Bread, white	52	270	35	8	3
whole wheat	49	260	37	9	3

Fiber. The cottage cheese or tofu and rice diet, is a very low residue diet that results in a small fecal volume. Sometimes the small volumes of maximally dehydrated feces cause signs of constipation. Conversely, small volumes of liquid contents entering the colon sometimes contain insufficient bulk to stimulate rhythmic segmentation, the motility necessary to delay the passage of colonic contents long enough for optimum absorption of salts and water. Thus, small volumes of ileal contents entering the colon can result in either constipation or soft bowel movements. Both problems can be managed with bulk producers (e.g. Metamucil 1-6 tsp/meal or: Siblin 1 tsp per 10 kg). Such products may be of benefit not only by providing residue but also by binding various secretagogues such as fatty acids, bile acids, and perhaps bile acids, and by altering the colonic microenvironment and microflora. Fiber is particularly likely to be useful if large bowel diarrhea is suspected.

Vitamins and Minerals. Vitamin and mineral supplementation is an important component of every controlled diet.[10] In the short term, such supplements may be excluded from elimination diets until the responsible food stuff has been identified, but dogs and cats should not be permitted to subsist on controlled diets without added vitamins and minerals for longer than a few weeks. This is especially important with regard to thiamin in cats in which the combination of poor body stores, decreased intake from anorexia, and increased loss of thiamin in urine (polyuria) or diarrhea can lead to rapid depletion. Most patients can be adequately supported with oral vitamin and mineral supplements, but in the presence of severe malabsorption parenteral administration of vitamins is sometimes required. If administered parenterally, B vitamins are usually included in intravenous fluids or given every 2-3 days subcutaneously, and fat soluble vitamins are given intramuscularly every week. Vitamin and mineral requirements are given in Table 38-2. If oral supplementation is used in the face of malabsorptive diseases the dose of vitamins and minerals provided are often arbitrarily doubled to compensate for decreased absorption. The adequacy or necessity of such adjustments have not been examined in the dog or cat.

Modification of the Controlled Diets for Cats. The same basic constituents can be utilized for cats with chronic diarrhea, although chicken or turkey is usually more acceptable as the protein source (Table 38-6). The protein content can also be increased to ensure the feline protein requirements are satisfied. Other protein sources that can be supplemented for the cat include tuna (provide a B-vitamin supplement in addition), liver (provided not fed continuously), and human baby foods (Gerber Products).

Evaluation of Diet. The value of a controlled diet is based primarily on the character of the feces but additional signs associated with chronic gastrointestinal problems are also monitored, such as the frequency of any concurrent vomiting, halitosis, bloating, borborygmus, flatulence.

The client should return after a week to ten days with fecal samples and records of progress. Even then, however, a significant number of animals still do not have normal bowel movements, especially following severe attacks of acute gastroenteritis. When bowel movements are not completely normal, the controlled diet is continued until remission is complete. With complete remission, the controlled diet is modified by introducing new foods. One new food is gradually introduced over five to seven days. Observations are continued to evaluate the effects of the new foods on maintaining remission. With time, a number of foods are identified as being tolerated or not tolerated. Eventually, sufficient tolerated foods are identified to allow formulation of a balanced diet. The long-range goal is to formulate a diet suitable for the patient and accepted by the owner. Often, patients can eventually be fed commercial dog foods, whereas with others the problem requires management with controlled diets for an indefinite time.

Table 38-6. Controlled Diet for Chronic Diarrhea in Cats *~

1. Measure 3 ounces of dry white rice
2. Cook with 2 volumes of water
3. To the cooked rice add 5 ounces of finely chopped poultry or lamb
4. Mix in 0.5-1 teaspoons of vegetable oil
5. Mix in 1 teaspoon of dicalcium phosphate
6. Mix in 0.5 teaspoons of iodinized salt
7. Add small quantities of liver (0.5 oz) if required for palatability

* Modified from Kronfeld DS (1983).
~ Consider lamb baby food (Gerber Products) if acceptability poor

Commercial Controlled Diets. A number of different commercial controlled diets are available to manage small animals with chronic gastrointestinal problems. The prescription diet d/d is formulated from mutton and rice, and i/d contains egg, brewer's rice, chicken, liver, ground corn, animal fat, soy flour, corn flour, and sugar (ground wheat has been removed, making it a gluten-free diet). Any formula containing as many ingredients as i/d is less well controlled, since intolerance of any one of them will produce signs of disease. Owners of large dogs often prefer to feed a commercial food rather than preparing one. Commercial foods that are most likely to produce remission include Science Maximum-Stress Diet (animal fat, soy flour, animal liver meal, dextrose, whole egg, dried skimmed milk, casein, soy oil, and brewer's dried yeast), Science Dry Canine Growth Diet (brewer's rice, ground corn, soy grits, meat and bone meal, animal fat, dried skimmed milk, dried whole egg, soy oil, and brewer's dried yeast), IAMS chunks or plus (meat meal, ground yellow corn, animal fat, beet pulp, and brewer's dried yeast), and IAMS Eukanuba (poultry by-products meal, ground yellow corn, meat meal, animal fat, dried beet pulp, brewer's dried yeast, cane molasses, dried whole eggs, and dried fish meal). The fat content is 25% for Science Maximum Stress and 20% for IAMS Eukanuba, which makes them less than ideal for treating diarrhea. They also are more expensive than the other two. All these diets are gluten-free and are often useful in managing chronic diarrhea. Each is controlled in that they contain fewer ingredients than other commercial pet foods.

The prescription diet c/d is useful for treating diarrhea in cats. Some cats develop diarrhea when fed dry cat foods and fail to respond to any form of management other than a canned cat food.

"Hypoallergenic" Diet

The principles of the design of a hypoallergenic diet are

discussed in Chapters 20 and 21. As noted, the mucosal barrier is not impermeable to proteins, and during periods of increased permeability, such as can occur in association with any gastrointestinal inflammation, any protein in the diet is likely to be presented to GALT in a manner that discourages the development of oral tolerance. Therefore, the main emphasis on ensuring hypoallergenicity in the presence of gastrointestinal inflammation is to choose a highly digestible protein, such as milk proteins in cottage cheese, thus, minimizing the antigens entering the mucosa. It may be advisable to feed a protein to which the patient is not likely to be exposed in the future and thereby reduce the chance of the animal developing a hypersensitivity to a dietary staple.

In those few animals with true food "allergies", the choice of a novel protein may meet with success. Proteins such as lamb either prepared by the owner or obtained commercially (d/d; Hill's Pet Products) are likely to be successful.

Diet for Carbohydrate Malabsorption

Low lactose diets are helpful in many cases of diarrhea because of the labile nature of the brush-border enzyme, lactase. Brush-border lactase levels vary in small animals but are normally low (Table 38-7)[33] and are reduced further when lactose is not being fed. The levels of sucrase and maltase, two other brush-border disaccharidases, also decrease with enteritis.

Small amounts of lactose, however, can be handled adequately by most lactose-intolerant patients. Most milk products are high in lactose, and generally should be fed in only very restricted quantities to patients with suspected carbohydrate malabsorption. Cottage cheese contains significant amounts of lactose, but the high protein content of this milk product reduces the necessary quantity of cottage cheese fed to meet protein requirements and thus usually restricts the dietary lactose to a tolerable range. If required, the lactose content of liquid dairy products can be reduced by preincubation with commercial lactase (Lact-aid, Sugarlo Co, Atlantic City, NJ). Moreover, lactase tablets are available (Lactaid, Lactrase) which can be administered with the meal. The amounts of lactose contained in various foods are shown in Table 38-8.

Table 38-7. Levels of Brush-Border Disaccharidases in the Dog

	Lactase	Sucrase	Maltase
	(μ moles/g wet mucosa/min)		
Duodenum	3.1	6.7	29.0
Jejunum	3.5	7.8	38.1
Ileum	0.7	4.6	27.7

Table 38-8. Amount of Lactose in Various Foods

		Lactose (grams)	Protein (grams)
Whole milk	8 oz.	11.8	8
Buttermilk	8 oz.	12.0	8
Yogurt	8 oz.	9.0	8
Cottage cheese	1/4 cup	1.5	7.5
Cheddar cheese	1 oz.	0.6	7.0

Diets for Protein-Losing Enteropathies

The nutritional support of patients with protein-losing enteropathy must include additional protein to make up for the increased fecal loss. In humans, fecal protein loss in protein-losing enteropathies can amount to as much as 0.5 gm/kg/day. Therefore, protein supplementation and additional energy to support the formation of replacement protein is of prime consideration in the nutritional management of protein-losing enteropathies. The protein content of some commonly used protein supplements is given in Table 38-9.

Fat is usually also restricted in protein-losing enteropathies, because of the likelihood of increasing lymph flow (lymphangiectasia), or difficult assimilation (inflammatory, and infectious diseases). Of the protein supplements listed, tuna packed in water, skinned poultry, low-fat cottage cheese, or low-fat milk powder (high lactose content) provide convenient low-fat protein sources. The demand for a low fat diet can make the provision of adequate energy difficult to achieve.

A suitable diet for the management of protein-losing enteropathy is that provided in Table 38-5 to which should be added sufficient protein to cover suspected additional protein losses. As mentioned above, there is no practical way to assess the amount of protein lost in the feces. As a rule of thumb, in patients with clinical evidence of debilitation from protein-losing enteropathy, protein requirements should be considered to be a minimum of 150% of basal requirements and probably nearer 200%. If protein is increased markedly in the diet it is advisable to increase dietary energy content concomitantly.

It is our opinion that the use of commercial weight reducing diets for the treatment of lymphangiectasia (as has been recommended) is contraindicated. Even with the addition to these

Table 38-9. Protein Content of Select Foods

Food	Serving size	Protein (gm)
Non-fat dry milk	1 cup	43
Cottage cheese	1 cup	30
Yogurt	1 cup	8
Egg	1 large	7
Lean beef	1 Oz	7
Tuna	1 Oz	8
Poultry (skinned)	1 Oz	8
Cooked legumes	1 Oz	2
Cooked rice	1 cup	4
Casec	Tbsp	4
PVM powder	Scoop	8.5

1 cup = 8 Oz.

Adapted from: Reference 24

diets of high protein-high energy supplements it is very difficult to satisfy the increased protein and energy requirements of malnourished patients, especially since affected patients are often partially inappetent.

Diets for Large Bowel Disease

Fiber is the quantitatively most important nutrient reaching the large bowel and therefore not surprisingly can have significant effects on large bowel function in health and disease. As described above, fiber has a variety of influences on the bowel and the type of fiber used markedly influences the nature of these effects.

Low fiber diets are useful to treat fecal incontinence. High fiber diets are useful in the prevention (but not treatment) of constipation. As discussed in Chapter 21, dietary recommendations for the management of colitis are controversial. Low residue diets such as i/d (Hill's Pet Products)[34] and cottage cheese and rice have been successfully used as the sole management in many dogs. Others have recommended the use of fiber, with some finding success with soluble fibers such as psyllium (hemicellulose) and others preferring insoluble fibers such as bran. In the face of this diversity, no firm recommendation as to the preferable diet for colitis can be made. We have had good success with diets containing moderate amounts of highly digestible protein (low antigenicity and restrict colonic ammonia generation) in association with the addition of soluble fiber in the form of psyllium (Metamucil). The beneficial effect of the psyllium is unknown, but may relate to an alteration of bacterial flora composition.

Diets for Gastric Diseases

Little information is available on suitable diets for inflammatory or ulcerative gastric diseases. Most authorities recommend a "bland" diet in which coarse and spicy foods are avoided. Frequent small feedings are also considered appropriate to limit the duration of acid secretion. Liquifying the diet will hasten gastric emptying, reducing gastric acid secretion. Minimizing the protein content of the food may also reduce gastric acid secretion. A suitable commercial diet is i/d (Hills Pet Products), and a suitable home-made diet is the cottage cheese or tofu and rice diet given in Tables 38-5 and 38-6.

Nutritional management of gastric emptying disorders has limited effectiveness. Fluids and solids empty differently from the stomach, which suggests that altering the consistency of the diet may help some patients. For instance, vagotomy accelerates the emptying of fluids but decreases the emptying of solids implying that emptying disorders resulting from neuropathies (such as dysautonomia, or diabetic neuropathy) may be ameliorated by use of liquid diets. Emptying is delayed by the use of hyperosmolar and high fat foods. Therefore, in the first few days of therapy the liquid diet should be diluted to isoosmolarity and should contain little fat. Unfortunately such foods are often without sufficient caloric density to maintain animals for prolonged periods.

Gastric dumping disorders result from the accelerated emptying of hyperosmolar chyme into the duodenum. Diets with a high soluble fiber content slow gastric emptying. The soluble fibers form gels in the stomach. Additionally, use of diets with a low available carbohydrate content, small frequent feedings, and pretreatment with anticholinergics prior to meals have been recommended in humans.[24]

Liver Disease

The principles of the nutritional management of liver disease are discussed in Chapters 32-36, and additional infor-

Table 38-10. Dietary Therapy for Dogs with Chronic Hepatic Insufficiency

DIET 1~

Ingredient	Ounces
Instant non-fat dry milk fortified with vitamins A and D	7 3/8
Blackstrap molasses*	4 3/4
Wheat germ (raw ground)	4.0
Bone meal	1 3/10
Safflower oil	3 1/2
Animal fat	3 1/2
Table salt (iodized)+	3/8
Cornstarch	14 1/5
Vitamin C	20 mg/kg/day
Choline	250 mg/day for dogs< 15 kg 500 mg/day for dogs > 15 kg

* Available in most health stores
+ If ascites is present, salt can be reduced, but should identify another sources of iodine if the diet is going to be used for a prolonged period
~ Mixing directions: Mix wheat germ and cold safflower oil in electric mixer if possible. If beef tallow is used as the source of animal fat allow it to come to room temperature before mixing. Add animal fat and mix. Mix salt, bone meal, and corn starch separately and then add mixture to above ingredients. Add dry instant milk and molasses and mix. Refrigerate. Add a small amount of water at feeding to improve palatability. Calories provided are 4.6 kcal/gm dry weight. Protein provided is 11.1 gm/100 gm.

DIET 2~

Low-fat cottage cheese	2 lb
Animal fat	1/2 lb
Safflower oil	1/4 cup
Sugar	1 lb & 3 Tbsp
Cornstarch	1 lb & 5 tbsp
Bone meal	1 1/3 Oz
Salt substitute KCL (iodized)	3 1/4 tsp
Table salt (iodized)	2 tsp
Vitamin C	20 mg/kg/day
Choline	As for diet 1
Multivitamin-multimineral tablet	one tablet daily

~Mixing instructions: Mix the sugar, cornstarch, bone meal, and salt. If beef tallow used, allow to come to room temperature before mixing. Blend animal fat with sugar mixture. Mix the cottage cheese and safflower oil and blend in with other ingredients. Keep refrigerated. Contains 4.7 kCal/gm dry weight. Contains 10.3 gm/ 100 gm dry weight.

Modified from reference 36.

Table 38-11. Standardized Intravenous Nutrition Formulae*

Dogs
500 ml 50% dextrose
500 ml 8.5%Travasol with electrolytes
250 ml 20% Intralipid
1 ml B-complex vitamins
20 mEq potassium phosphate

Provides 1.06 nonprotein Kcal/ml; 40 mEq potassium per liter; 3.15 g protein per 100 non-protein Kcal

Cats
250 ml 50% dextrose
500 ml 8.5% Travasol with electrolytes
250 ml 20 % Intralipid
1 ml B-complex vitamins
10 mEq potassium phosphate

Provides 0.92 nonprotein Kcal/ml; 40 mEq potassium per liter; 4.6 g protein per 100 non-protein Kcal

Dogs with Liver Failure
500 ml 50% dextrose
250 ml 8.5% Travasol with electrolytes
500 ml 20 % intralipid
1 ml B-complex vitamins
36 mEq potassium phosphate

Provides 1.44 nonprotein Kcal/ml;
40 mEq potassium per liter;
1.15 g protein per 100 non-protein Kcal

* Courtesy Dr SC Haskins UCD VMTH

mation is available elsewhere.[35-37] Two suitable diets for patients with hepatic insufficiency are provided in Table 38-10. A parenteral nutritional formula suitable for support of patients with liver failure is given in Table 38-11. Commercial diets of value include canine k/d or i/d, and if ascites develops, canine h/d. If encephalopathy develops canine u/d can be used. For cats feline k/d and c/d are useful.

Vitamin supplementation is often appropriate in hepatobiliary disease because of decreased absorption due to steatorrhea and because reduction in liver size decreases the vitamin storage capacity of the body.[10] Plasma levels of vitamin C are low in dogs with liver disease.[38]

INTENSIVE NUTRITIONAL SUPPORT[39-42]

Intensive nutritional support is indicated in animals unwilling, or unable to eat, or in those patients in which deranged gastrointestinal function obviates adequate assimilation of food. The decision whether to institute intensive nutritional therapy is guided by the nutritional status of the patient, and the nature and expected longevity of its disease process. Methods of assessment of protein-calorie status, and energy and protein requirements of dogs and cats are described above. As a general rule, dogs and cats with debilitating disease conditions (stress starvation), should not be allowed to go without nutrition for longer than 4-5 days.

Determination of the Route of Administration. Intensive nutritional support may be achieved by enteral or parenteral alimentation. The route of administration is determined by the site of the gastrointestinal dysfunction, and by concerns such as expense of administration and the availability of intensive care facilities. In general, enteral administration is preferred unless obviated by marked gastrointestinal dysfunction. Enteral nutrition is more physiologic and preserves mucosal architecture, is cheaper, safer, and easier to administer.

Enteral alimentation may be provided by a number of different techniques including forced oral feeding, and with those using nasogastric, pharyngostomy, gastrostomy, and jejunostomy tubes. Forced oral feeding is usually too stressful for animals (and staff) to be continued for more than a few days. Nasogastric, pharyngostomy, or gastrostomy tubes can be utilized for nutritional support of animals with anorexia or dysphagia. These methods are not appropriate if the patient has persistent vomiting. In general, gastrostomy tubes are the preferred technique for the long-term nutritional support of animals. Gastrostomy tubes are preferable to pharyngostomy or nasogastric tubes because they are more comfortable for the patient, better tolerated, and completely bypass the esophagus with no risk of compromising the lower esophageal sphincter. An additional disadvantage of pharyngostomy tubes is the risk of interfering with laryngeal function if incorrectly placed.[43] Gastrostomy tubes allow the administration of blended dog or cat foods, unlike nasogastric tubes whose fine diameter leads to a requirement for dispersed solutions. They can be placed conveniently by endoscopy, or at the time of celiotomy. The primary advantage of nasogastric tubes is that they do not require general anesthesia to place. They are therefore convenient for the short term maintenance of critical patients.

The placement of jejunostomy tubes is indicated for gastrointestinal diseases in which gastric dysfunction is prominent. Jejunostomy tubes are less desirable than gastrostomy tubes because they are more difficult to place, require the use of elemental diets, and are complicated by a high incidence of iatrogenic osmotic diarrhea. Total parenteral nutrition (TPN) is usually reserved for severely debilitated patients that cannot take oral sustenance and that require a short period of intensive nutritional support. It is particularly useful in the management of patients with persistent ileus or acute pancreatitis, or if the intestinal tract is unable to absorb nutrients. One advantage in comparison to gastrostomy tubes is that anesthesia is not required. It is disadvantaged by the limited duration for which TPN can be used, the expense of the procedure, the requirement for intensive monitoring of the patient, and the risk of sepsis. Moreover, the bowel undergoes significant mucosal atrophy during total parenteral nutrition.

Enteral Nutrition Techniques[40-42]

Forced Oral Feeding. Patients may be force-fed manually and by a number of different techniques including the use of modified syringes and orogastric intubation. Repeated stomach tubing is an effective manner to feed neonates but otherwise has limited application because of attendant stress, time-consuming nature, and the risk of tracheal administration. The syringe technique involves the removal of the distal fifth of the syringe barrel of a 5-10 ml syringe to create a plunger system which can be used to introduce canned food into the pharynx and proximal esophagus. The technique is described elsewhere.[11]

Nasogastric Intubation. Nasogastric intubation is the technique of choice for the short term support of critical patients with adequately functioning gastrointestinal tracts. The technique has been described in detail elsewhere.[11,44] Nasogastric tubes should be soft, flexible and of appropriate diameter (usually 5-8 Fr) and length. Pediatric polyurethane nasogastric tubes (NCC Div, Argyle, NY) are suitable. The tube is marked to allow judgement of the length inserted and is then lubricated and gently passed into the ventral nasal meatus after the instillation of a few drops of local anesthetic. Once the tube has been successfully maneuvered to the stomach and its position verified, it is sutured in place at the nasal meatus and its free-end passed to behind the animal's head where it is secured. Verification of the position of the tube may be made by aspiration or radiography. The initiation of coughing, the failure to pass the tube to its full length (as measured to the last rib), or the aspiration of copious amounts of free air, raises the likelihood of tracheal intubation.

Pharyngostomy Tubes. With the advent of percutaneous placement of gastrostomy tubes, the indications for pharyngostomy are now few and far between. In practices that do not utilize endoscopy or can not access an endoscope by referral, pharyngostomy tubes may still have a place in the long term nutritional support of patients. The technique of placement is described elsewhere.[43]

Gastrostomy Tubes. Gastrostomy tube placement is the technique of choice for the long term enteral nutrition support of small animals. The primary advantages of gastrostomy tubes are that they are very well tolerated, produce minimal discomfort, allow the feeding of regular dog or cat foods, and can be easily managed at home by owners. The gastrostomy tube can be placed endoscopically or at the time of celiotomy. Any debilitated animal that undergoes celiotomy for diagnostic or therapeutic reasons should be considered a prime candidate for the placement of a gastrostomy tube at the time of the celiotomy. Such forward thinking, greatly facilitates the nutritional support of the patient in the post-operative period. Gastrostomy tubes are particularly useful for the support of patients with swallowing disorders. They do not cause pharyngitis or esophagitis and do not interfere with function of the larynx or pharynx. Patients are able to eat normally with the tube in place, thus facilitating weaning the animal back to oral feeding. The major disadvantage of gastrostomy tubes is the need for general anesthesia (or heavy sedation and local block of the abdomen), and the risk of peritonitis. The latter complication appears to be very rare.

The surgical placement of gastrostomy tubes has been described.[41,45] Briefly, a celiotomy is performed and the lateral or caudal aspect of the greater curvature of the stomach is isolated. Two purse-string sutures are placed concentrically about the site of the intended incision in the stomach. A small incision is made just ventral to the 13th rib on the left side, and the catheter inserted through the body wall and into the stomach. The purse string sutures are tightened about the gastrostomy tube and the stomach is sutured to the abdominal wall. The abdominal incision is closed, and the tube secured by abdominal bandages. Suitable tubes for gastrostomy are 14-24 Fr mushroom tipped (Bardex) or balloon-tipped (Foley) catheters. When the need for the gastrostomy tube has finished, the tube is carefully pulled from the stomach through the abdominal wall and the stoma allowed to heal by secondary intention.

Two techniques are in use for the endoscopic placement of gastrostomy tubes, a percutaneous technique and a peroral technique.[11,46] In both techniques, the animal is placed in right lateral recumbency so that the stomach tube may be placed through the greater curvature of the stomach and the left body wall. The site of emergence for the catheter should be just ventral to the 13th rib.

The peroral technique utilizes the endoscope for the retrieval of percutaneously-placed, transabdominogastric, suture material that is used to draw a gastrostomy tube, tipped by a catheter, through the mouth, esophageal lumen, gastric lumen, gastric wall, and finally body wall. Equipment needed for the peroral technique includes a Peezer mushroom-tipped-catheter, a 16 gauge Medicut catheter, strong suture material of sufficient length to pass from stomach to mouth, a minor surgical pack, an endoscope, and a plastic guide to facilitate drawing the catheter through the body wall. The guide can be fashioned out of a variety of disposal equipment found in veterinary hospitals. It should have one pointed end to penetrate the abdominal musculature, and another open end into which the mushroom catheter can be forced. A large gauge plastic Medicut catheter is suitable for smaller tubes. Alternatively, bigger diameter guides, such as a plastic catheter guard supplied with the Argyle 14 G Medicut "T" catheters, or disposable plastic micropipettes can be used (Figure 38-1).

The catheter (20-24 Fr for dogs, and 14-20 F for cats) is prepared prior to the procedure in the following manner. Cut off the wide connecting (female) end of the catheter and then bevel the cut end to facilitate its later introduction into the catheter guide system. Make a slit in two 2-3 cm pieces of rubber tubing harvested from the section of Pezzer catheter that was previously cut from the catheter body. These will serve as flanges to prevent movement of the stomach from the body wall. Pass the catheter through the slit in one of the flanges until the mushroom tip and the rubber flange are touching (Figure 38-1).

Surgically prepare the left paracostal area centered about the distal end of the 13th rib. Maneuver the endoscope into the stomach and carefully inflate this viscus until the abdomen is distended but not drum tight. Insert a 16-18 G large bore catheter through the skin just ventral to the 13th rib and pass it through the body wall, gastric wall, and into the gastric lumen. Remove the stylet and thread sturdy suture material of sufficient length to comfortably reach from mouth to last rib through the catheter into the lumen of the stomach. Grasp the suture with an endoscopic retrieval instrument and withdraw the endoscope, from the animal thus drawing one end of the suture through the esophagus and out of the mouth. Be careful not to draw all of the suture into the stomach. At the mouth, the suture material is then passed through a 16 G Medicut catheter (tapered end first), through a catheter guard, and through a needle-hole in the beveled tip of the Peezer mushroom catheter where it is firmly tied. Wedge the cut end of the mushroom catheter into the catheter guard, and the male tip of the catheter guard into the

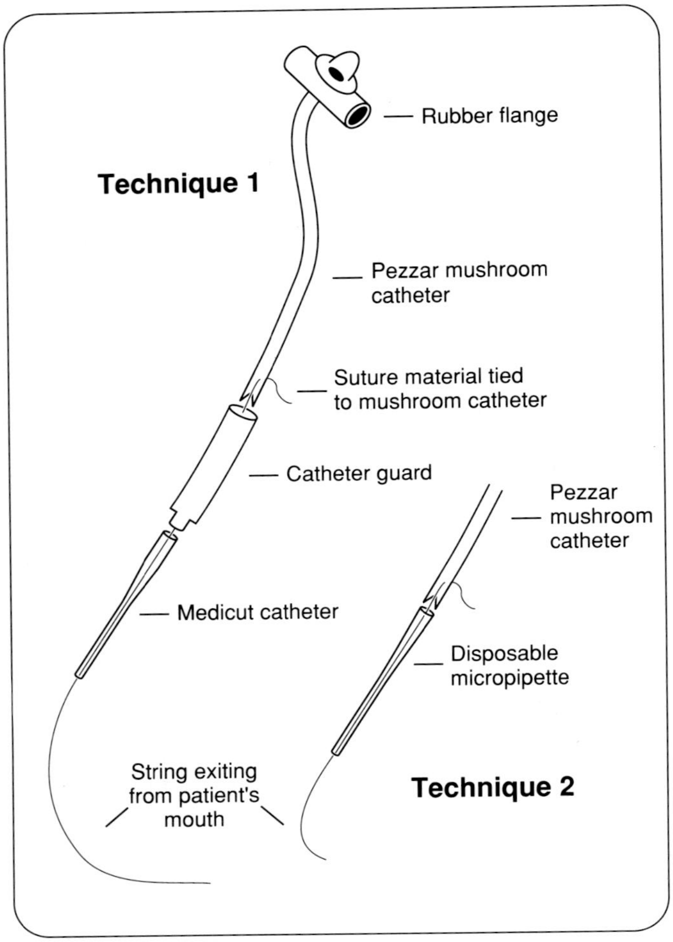

female end of the catheter. Grasp the suture material at its point of exit from the body wall and apply firm traction to draw the entire catheter assemblage though the lumen of the mouth, esophagus, and stomach, and partially through the stomach and body wall. Further gentle traction on the catheter results in the distal (flanged) end of the catheter drawing the stomach wall against the body wall. It is anchored in this position by the second flange placed over the catheter at the skin surface. Bandage the catheter in place to prevent its destruction by the patient. After 6-7 days the catheter may be safely withdrawn. To remove the catheter, apply firm external traction and then cut the catheter as close to the distal tip as possible. The internal flange and mushroom tip usually pass uneventfully.

The second endoscopic technique (the percutaneous technique) utilizes the endoscope to distend the stomach and ensure correct placement of the gastrostomy tube. The percutaneous technique utilizes a series of trocars of increasing diameter, that are serially passed through the abdominal wall into the air-distended stomach (Wilson-Cook, PEG set). The largest trocar is of sufficient diameter for a Foley catheter to be passed directly into the stomach through the trocar. It has a "peel-away" external sheath which is peeled off the Foley after its insertion. Once inserted, the Foley is inflated and used to fix the stomach against the body wall.

Both of these techniques have been successfully used at the UCD VMTH. The percutaneous technique has a slightly shorter

Table 38-12. Advantages and Disadvantages of Elemental Diets

Advantages	Disadvantages
No residue	Hyperosmolar, causing:
Nitrogen requires no digestion	1) Vomiting
Carbohydrates require little digestion	2) Diarrhea
	3) Abdominal distress
Very low in fat	
Provide essential fatty acids	Require frequent or continuous feeding
Provide vitamins and minerals	
	Poor palatability
Provide rest for gut	
	Provide too much or too little water
Hypoallergenic	

operating time, avoids contamination of the abdomen and abdominal wall with oropharyngeal secretions, the fluted end of the catheter need not be cut off, and the removal process does not leave any flanges in the gastrointestinal tract. Its disadvantages in comparison to the peroral technique include a less secure initial bond of the stomach to the body wall (the Foley can digest in as little as 3 days), a requirement for greater gastric distension, and greater expense for the trocar setup (Wilson-Cook will sell the component parts of the trays separately halving the list price).

Complications from endoscopic placement of gastrostomy tubes are rare and most frequently pertain to anesthetic difficulties resulting from the debilitated nature of the patient or concurrent problems such as inhalation pneumonias secondary to disorders such as megaesophagus. Prolonged dilatation of the stomach can interfere with venous return and ventilation. Failure to adequately secure the stomach against the body wall can lead to leakage of gastric content and peritonitis. Over-zealous tension on the gastrotomy tube can lead to gastric necrosis.

Jejunostomy Tubes. Jejunal feeding is indicated whenever, the upper gastrointestinal tract need be rested, for instance in a persistently vomiting animal. Jejunal feeding minimizes the stimulation of pancreatic secretion. The technique has been described.[41,47] Jejunostomy tubes can be passed via the nose or abdominal wall, or through pharyngostomy or gastrostomy tubes. Small sized tubes (8 Fr) are commonly used. Elemental diets must be fed, and osmotic diarrhea is a common complication.

Products Available for Enteral Nutrition[28,48]

Products useful for enteral alimentation include blenderized prescription diets such as i/d or p/d (Hill's Pet Products), and various enteral feeding solutions. Elemental diets consist of carbohydrates and lipids in forms requiring little digestion, and of nitrogen in the form of amino acids or peptides. Polymeric diets (meal-replacement diets) contain whole proteins and a

Table 38-13. Composition of Elemental Diets

	Caloric Density (Cal/ml)	Osmo-lality (mOsm)	Caloric distribution % Protein	Fat	CHO	Nutrient Source Protein	Fat	CHO	Na^+ (mEq/L)	K^+	PO_4
Flexical (Mead Johnson)	1	–	8.7	30.3	61	Casein Hydro-lysate	soy oil MCT oil	sucrose oligo-saccharides starch	15.2	38.2	43.5
Vivonex (Eaton)	1	610	8.5	1.3	90.2	Synthetic amino acids	Linoleic acid tri-glycerides	glucose oligo-saccharides	37.4	29.9	43
Vivonex HN	1	844	18.2	0.8	81	Synthetic amino acids	Linoleic acid safflower oil	Dextrins	33.5	17.9	25.8

mixture of coarse starch hydrolysates and long-chain triglycerides. Nutrient additives, otherwise known as "feeding modules" are also available. These consist of sources of one nutrient such as protein and are used to supplement diets.

Theoretical advantages of elemental diets include the need for minimal or no digestion, minimization of gastric, pancreatic, and biliary secretions, hypoallergenicity, and reduction in the total numbers of bacterial microflora, all of which can have a favorable effect on intestinal problems (Table 38-12).[49] The composition of the bacterial flora appears to change little as a result of enteral feeding.[49] The hypoallergenicity results from the lack of peptides. In recent years, however, there has been a move away from elemental solutions to diets with less hydrolyzed constituents. The elemental diets are associated with a higher incidence of diarrhea (due to higher osmolality) and have not been shown to provide significant benefit over polymeric diets for nutritional support of humans.[17,49] Elemental diets are probably still the enteral solution of choice in short bowel syndrome, however.[49]

The liquid nature of elemental diets encourages rapid gastric emptying. Hyperosmolar solutions rapidly entering the duodenum cause vomiting, diarrhea, and abdominal distress by intense stimulation of normal neural and endocrine mechanisms that control normal gastrointestinal function (dumping syndrome). Elemental diets can also create fluid and electrolyte imbalances. Feeding high-carbohydrate diets results in the production of large amounts of metabolic water, which when retained produces hyponatremia. On the other hand, when water is not provided with high-protein or hyperosmolar solutions, the large amount of solute causes osmotic diuresis and subsequent dehydration. Diets rich in glucose, which is readily absorbed, can cause hyperglycemia and contribute to osmotic diuresis and dehydration. Furthermore, high carbohydrate diets also produce large quantities of carbon dioxide which can be problematical in patients with severe respiratory disease. The side effects of elemental diets are minimized by careful administration (see Table 38-12).

Suitable commercial preparations are listed in Tables 38-13 and 38-14. These formulations are bland, gluten-free, low in residue and lactose, and are defined as to osmolarity, calories, and content of vitamins and minerals. Some are high in protein, such as Sustacal (Mead Johnson Co.). Isocal (Mead Johnson) is an example of a liquid diet that is virtually isosmotic and lactose-free, contains fats as medium-chain triglycerides, is nutritionally balanced, and contains proper amounts of vitamins and minerals. Another balanced diet, Portagen (Mead Johnson), contains mostly medium-chain triglycerides as the only lipid. Dietary protein can be further modified by using protein from a nonanimal source. CHO-free liquid (Syntex) is an example of a soy-protein isolate, free of carbohydrates but otherwise essentially complete. This product is combined with a carbohydrate to formulate a controlled diet for evaluations of sensitivity or allergy due to animal protein. Flexical (Mead Johnson) contains an enzymatic hydrolysate of casein to which are added methionine, tryptophan, and tyrosine. About 70% of the nitrogen is free amino acids. The carbohydrate consists of sucrose and glucose-oligosaccharides (dextrin). Its lipids are 20% medium-chain triglycerides and 80% long-chain unhydrogenated soy oil. Vivonex (Eaton Labs) is an elemental diet containing pure amino acids as the only nitrogen source. The carbohydrate source is glucose and glucose oligosaccharides, with no sucrose or lactose. The diet is very low in fat, supplying less than 1% of the total calories. The fats used consist mostly of triglycerides of linoleic acid.

Enteral Feeding Plans. Initial feeding volumes should be very conservative, and should not exceed three to five ml per kg per feed, or infusion rates of one to three ml per kg per hour.[20] Intermittent feedings are initially administered every two hours. Prior to each feeding, the feeding tube should be aspirated to ensure the previous instillation has been emptied from the stomach. If more than 50% of the feeding solution is still recoverable then no additional feedings should be performed until the stomach has emptied.[20] If the stomach does not empty the liquid diet within 4-6 hours, the gastrointestinal tract can be considered currently unsuitable for nutritional support. If the patient demonstrates signs of dietary intolerance such as nausea, abdominal pain, vomiting or diarrhea, the volume of feed should be reduced or the interval of feeding increased until the signs resolve. A pump can be used for delivery of a constantly infused diet, a procedure that minimizes the effects of hyperosmolar solutions entering the duodenum. Feeding by gravity drip is acceptable if the rate is carefully controlled. If the animal is unable to drink, water in addition to that contained in the hyperosmolar diets must be provided. If the enteral food is well tolerated, and the stomach empties normally, subsequent feedings can be increased in volume over the ensuing three days until the patients requirements are met in 3-6 daily feeds. Tubes should be flushed with water between feedings, and then capped.

Enteral feeding causes diarrhea in patients with hypoproteinemia as a complication. The cause is usually a protein-losing enteropathy. The diarrhea caused by feeding is predictable in dogs with plasma albumin levels approaching 2.0 gm/dl. It may be necessary for treatment with plasma transfusion before nutritional management can be successful in such patients.

Parenteral Nutrition

Some patients with gastrointestinal problems cannot be given anything orally, and it is necessary to maintain partial or complete nutritional homeostasis with parenteral hyperalimentation. Specific indications include severe malabsorption or prolonged ileus or pancreatitis.

Parenteral nutrition may set out to provide all nutritional requirements (TPN) or may aim to provide partial requirements. For instance, a protein-sparing effect may be achieved by the infusion of small amounts of amino acids or dextrose.

Table 38-14. Diets Formulated from Modified and Selected Natural Foods

	Caloric Density (Cal/ml)	Osmolality (mOsm)	Caloric distribution % Protein	Fat	CHO	Nutrient Source Protein	Fat	CHO	Lactose (%)	Na (mEq/L)	K (mEq/L)
Ensure (Ross-Abbott)	1.0	460	14	31.5	54.5	Casein	Corn oil	Sucrose corn syrup	0	32.2	32.6
Sustacal (Mead Johnson)	1.0	625	24	21	55	Casein soy beans	soy oil	Sucrose corn syrup	1.7	40.2	52.8
Isocal (Mead Johnson)	1.0	350	13	37	50	Casein soy beans oil	soy oil MCT	corn syrup	0	22.7	33.4
Portagen (Mead Johnson)	1.0*	---	13	41	44	Casein oil	Corn oil MCT	Sucrose corn syrup	<.15%	54.5	85.5
Sustagen	1.5*	---	24	8	68	Casein powdered milk	milk	Dextrose corn syrup	present	44.8	77
Meritene (Doyle)	1.0	---	24	30	46	Casein skim milk	vegetable oil	Sucrose corn syrup	present	40	43
Precision LR diet (Doyle)	1.0	475** mod.N	9-17	28**	60**	egg white	vegetable oil	Sucrose malto-dextrin	0	74	19.3

* When prepared from powder ** Precision LR diet is made with 3 levels of protein **Values for moderate nitrogen diet

The intravenous infusion of dextrose does not meet total energy requirements, but does reduce nitrogen losses by as much as one-half.[50] As mentioned above, the primary disadvantages of TPN, are the expense, likelihood of sepsis, and requirement for intensive monitoring.

Routes of Administration. Parenteral nutrition solutions are usually hypertonic, and must be infused into a central vein to avoid phlebitis and thrombosis. As a general rule, fluids with an osmolality below 600 can be administered by peripheral vein.[20] Veins of choice are the jugular veins and in the cat the medial saphenous vein through which a catheter can be threaded to reach the caudal vena cava. The catheter for delivery of the IV solution must be dedicated to the solution and never be used for blood drawing or the administration of drugs, otherwise sepsis will result. An antibiotic-antifungal cream should be placed at the catheter insertion site and the catheter carefully inspected and rebandaged every 24 hours. Central vein catheters, carefully cared for, can last a week or more.

Formulation of Parenteral Nutrition Solutions. The energy and protein requirements of the patient are calculated as described above. Energy should be supplied by both fat and carbohydrate (Table 38-11). Clinical trials in humans have shown that there is a limit to the protein sparing effect of glucose, and if glucose is provided as the sole calorie source protein repletion cannot be achieved.[51] Furthermore, fat solutions provide a source of essential fatty acids and lower the osmolality of the parenteral solution because of their high caloric density. A commercial lipid formulation, Intralipid (Cutter), contains 100 to 200 g soybean oil, 12 g egg-yolk phospholipids, and 25 g glycerol in 1,000 ml solution.[11] It has been administered to dogs at a rate as high as 9 g of fat/Kg body weight/day for a month with no undesirable effects.

For purposes of simplicity, at the UCD VMTH we have adopted the use of the standardized mixtures of nutrients listed in Table 38-13. These mixtures are adequate to supply the nutritional requirements of by far the majority of our patients. These mixtures should be mixed in as sterile manner as possible. The "All-in-One" mixing bags (Baxter) greatly facilitate this procedure. Always add the amino acid solution between the addition of the dextrose and the lipid solutions. They can be hung at room temperature for as long as two days, after which time any remaining solution should be discarded.

Additional Nutrient and Fluid Requirements. Cats have dietary requirements for protein, arachidonate, taurine, arginine, and selenium that are difficult to met with many parenteral (or for that matter enteral) solutions. However, positive nitrogen balance can be achieved in cats receiving standard amino acid mixtures.[52] Arginine free solutions should never be administered to cats. Oral supplementation of these nutrients should be provided if prolonged nutritional support is envisioned. Taurine is best supplied as taurine tablets (250 or 500 mg) available in health stores. Contrary to previous reports, clam juice is not a satisfactory supplement.[53]

Table 38-15. Complications of Total Parenteral Nutrition

With glucose-based solutions	With all types of solutions
Hyperosmolarity	Peptide hypersensitivity
Osmotic dehydration	Potassium depletion
Glycosuria	Phosphate depletion
Metabolic acidosis	Fluid overload
Fluid overload	Hyperammonemia
Phlebitis	Infection

Small animals require about 40-60 ml water/Kg body weight in order to excrete the solutes that must be eliminated through the kidneys. Parenteral hyperalimentation solutions used to provide all the calories also normally supply all the water an animal needs. Inadequate water provision is more likely to be a problem when the therapy is causing a diuresis, such as is caused by hyperglycemia. Unless specifically contraindicated by the patient's condition, it is advisable to allow free access to water.

Potassium requirements double when parenteral hyperalimentation solutions are infused.[54] A minimum of 3 mEq potassium is required for each gram of body nitrogen replaced. Daily potassium requirements in a 10 Kg dog increase from 15 mEq to over 30 mEq when nutrition is provided parenterally. The high potassium requirements are due to the high intracellular concentrations needed when lean body mass is replaced and to match the urinary excretion of potassium which continues at 15 mEq/day in a 10 Kg dog regardless of the amount in the body.

Phosphate-free parenteral hyperalimentation solutions reduce serum phosphorus levels. The complications produced include weakness, seizures, reversible hemolytic anemia, and, without correction, death. Total parenteral nutrition in dogs receiving solutions that lack phosphorous results in death within five to six days. It is essential to maintain normal intracellular stores of phosphorus. This ion is required for the synthesis of ATP and other nucleotides required for many metabolic events in cells. During parenteral hyperalimentation, lean body mass is restored, with 80 mEq phosphorus moving into the cells for each gain of 1 Kg. Extracellular fluid phosphate is used, and when it is not replenished by the diet it can not be mobilized from bone rapidly enough to prevent hypophosphatemia. Phosphate can be added to maximum concentrations of 40 mEq/liter.

Determination of Volume, Administration Rate, and Monitoring. The volume of solution required to meet nutritional requirements can be calculated from the caloric content of each solution (provided in Table 38-11) and the estimated requirements of the patient. The nutritional solution is initially administered slowly (50% of the calculated rate necessary to maintain the patient) and after four hours the blood glucose is checked. If the glucose remains below 250 mg/dl, the infusion rate is increased to full ration in a stepwise fashion over the ensuing eight hours. If the patient's blood glucose reaches 250-300 mg/dl, the rate is maintained constant until the patient develops a tolerance for the glucose (serum concentration decrease) whereupon the rate can be increased. If the serum glucose concentration exceeds 300 mg/dl, the rate should be temporarily reduced.[20] Monitoring should include observation for persistent lipemia, and a blood ammonia level should be determined after the first day of therapy to ensure protein administration is not excessive. PCV, total protein and serum electrolyte concentrations should be followed closely. Close observation for evidence of acidosis, fluid overload or dehydration, and evidence of sepsis is essential.

Complications. The most important complication of parenteral nutrition is sepsis (Table 38-15). The frequency can be particularly high if care is not taken during the mixing of the solutions, and if correct catheter protocol is not observed. Other important complications include phlebitis and thrombosis. This can be particularly catastrophic if a central vein is involved. Hyperglycemia and fluid and electrolyte imbalances are relatively common, with hypernatremia, hypokalemia and hypophosphatemia being particularly frequent. In cats, two weeks of total parenteral nutrition has been associated with vomiting, lethargy, lingual ulcers, mild to moderate anemia, mild to severe thrombocytopenia, hypoproteinemia, increased ALT, mild hyperbilirubinemia, increased serum bile acid concentration, metabolic acidosis, villus atrophy, and a reversible fatty liver.[52]

REFERENCES

1. Vahouny, G.V.: Effects of dietary fiber on digestion and absorption. In, Physiology of the Gastrointestinal Tract. Edited by Johnson, L.R. Raven Press, New York, 1623-1648, 1987.
2. Kritchevsky, D.: Dietary fiber. Ann. Rev. Nutr. 8:301-328, 1988.
3. Phillips, S.F.: Megacolon: Congenital and Acquired. In, Gastrointestinal Disease. Pathophysiology Diagnosis, and Management. 4th edition. Edited by Sleisenger, M.H., Fordtran, J.S. WB Saunders, Philadelphia, 1389-1402, 1989.
4. Trowell, H.C.: Crude fiber, dietary fiber and atherosclerosis. Atherosclerosis 16:138, 1972.
5. Urban, E.: A feast of fiber. Gastroenterology 88: 211-212, 1985.
6. Burrows, C.F., Kronfeld, D.S., Banta, C.A. and Merrit, A.M.: Effects of fiber on digestibility and transit time in dogs. J. Nutr. 112:1726-1732, 1982.
7. Stock-Damge, C., Aprahamian, M., Raul, F., Humbert, W. and Bouchet, P.: Effects of wheat bran on the exocrine pancreas and the small intestinal mucosa in the dog. J. Nutr. 114:1076-1082, 1984.
8. Isaksson, G., Asp, N.G. and Ihse, I.: Effects of dietary fiber on pancreatic enzyme activities of ileostomy evacuates and on excretion of fat and nitrogen in the rat. Gastroenterology 18:417-423, 1983.
9. Stephen, A.M. and Cummings, J.H.: The microbial contribution to human fecal mass. J. Med. Microbiol. 13:45, 1980.
10. Buffington, C.A.: Therapeutic use of vitamins in companion animals. In, Current Veterinary Therapy IX. Edited by Kirk, R.W. WB Saunders, Philadelphia, 40-47, 1986.
11. Lewis, L.D., Morris, M.L. and Hand, M.S.: Small Animal Clinical Nutrition. Mark Morris Associates, Topeka, Kansas. 1987.
12. De Luca, L., Maestri, N., Bonanni, F. and Nelson, D.: Maintenance of epithelial cell differentiation; the mode of action of vitamin A. Cancer 30:1326-1331, 1972.
13. Rosenberg, I.H. and Alpers, D.H.: Nutritional deficiency in gastrointestinal disease. In, Gastrointestinal Disease. Pathophysiology, Diagnosis, Management. 4th Edition. Edited by Sleisenger, M.H. and Fordtran, J.S.: WB Saunders, Philadelphia, 1983-1994, 1989.
14. Edwards, D.F. and Russell, R.G.: Probable-vitamin K deficient bleeding in two cats with malabsorption syndrome secondary to lymphocytic-plasmacytic enteritis. J. Vet. Int. Med. 1:97-101, 1987.
15. Alpers, D.H. and Rosenberg, I.H.: Eating behavior and nutrient requirements. In, Gastrointestinal Disease. Pathophysiology, Diagnosis, Management. 4th Edition. Edited by Sleisenger, M.H. and Fordtran, J.S.: WB Saunders, Philadelphia, 1971-1983, 1989.
16. Donoghue, S.: Nutritional support of hospitalized patients. Vet. Clin. N. Am. 19:475-495, 1989.
17. Clouse, R.E. and Rosenberg, I.H.: Intensive nutritional support. In, Gastrointestinal Disease. Pathophysiology, Diagnosis, Management. 4th Edition. Edited by Sleisenger, M.H. and Fordtran, J.S.: WB Saunders, Philadelphia, 2007-2027, 1989.
18. Rogers, Q.R., Baker, D.H., Hayes, K.C., et al.: Nutrient requirements of cats, National Academy Press, Washington DC, 1986.
19. Sheffey, B.E., Hayes, K.C., Knapka, J.J., et al.: Nutrient requirements of dogs. National Academy Press, Washington DC, 1985.
20. Haskins, S.C.: Personal communication, 1989.
21. Alpers, D.H., Clouse, R.E. and Stenson, W.F.: Manual of nutritional therapeutics. 2nd Edition. Boston, Little Brown, 1987.
22. Chandra, R.K.: Nutrition, Immunity, and outcome; past, present, and future, Nutr Res 8:225-237, 1988.
23. Polzin, D.J. and Osborne, C.A.: Update- conservative medical management of chronic renal failure. In, Current Veterinary Therapy IX. Edited by Kirk, R.W. WB Saunders, Philadelphia, 1167-1173, 1986.
24. Alpers, D.H.: Dietary management and vitamin-mineral replacement therapy. In, Gastrointestinal Disease. Pathophysiology, Diagnosis, Management. 4th Edition. Edited by Sleisinger, M.H. and Fordtran, J.S., W.B. Saunders, Philadelphia. 1994-2006, 1989.
25. Zimmer, J.F.: Nutritional management of gastrointestinal diseases. In, Current Veterinary Therapy IX. Edited by Kirk, R.W. WB Saunders, Philadelphia, 909-916, 1986.
26. Hand, M.S., Armstrong, P.J. and Allen, T.A.: Obesity: occurrence, treatment, and prevention. Vet. Clin. N. Am. 19:447-474, 1989.
27. Madara, J.L. and Trier, J.S.: Functional morphology of the mucosa of the small intestine. In, Physiology of the Gastrointestinal Tract. Edited by Johnson, L.R. Raven Press, New York, 1209-1249, 1987.
28. Russel, R.I.: Elemental diets. Gut 16:68-79, 1975.
29. Williams, R.E.O. and Drasar, B.S.: Alterations in gut bacterial flora in disease. In, Recent Advances in Gastroenterology. Edited by J. Badenoch and B.N. Brooke. Churchill and Livingston, London, 31-53, 1972.
30. Wilson, F.A. and Dietschy, J.M.: Differential diagnostic approach to clinical problems of malabsorption. Gastroenterology 61:911-931, 1971.
31. Deren, J.J., Broitman, S.A. and Zamcheck, N.: Effect of diet upon intestinal disaccharidases and disaccharide absorption. J. Clin. Invest. 46:186-195, 1967.
32. Grossman, M.I., Greengard, H., Ivy, A.C.: The effect of dietary composition on pancreatic enzymes. Am. J. Physiol. 138:676-682, 1942-43.
33. Hill, F.W.G. and Kelley, D.F.: Naturally occurring intestinal malabsorption in the dog. Am. J. Dig. Dis. 19:649-665, 1974.
34. Nelson,R.W., Stookey, L.J. and Kazacos, E.: Nutritional management of idiopathic chronic colitis in the dog. J. Vet. Int. Med. 2:133-137, 1988.
35. Bauer, J.E. and Schenck, P.A.: Dietary therapy for hepatic disease. Vet. Clin. N. Am. 19:515-526, 1989.
36. Strombeck, D.R., Schaeffer, M.C. and Rogers, Q.R.: Dietary therapy for dogs with chronic hepatic insufficiency. In, Current Veterinary Therapy VIII. Edited by Kirk, R.W. 817-821, 1983.
37. Leflamme, D.P.: Dietary management of canine hepatic encephalopathy. Comp. Contin. Ed. Pract. Vet. 10:1259-1263, 1988.
38. Strombeck, D.R., Harrold, D., Rogers, Q.R., et al.: Plasma amino acid, glucagon, and insulin concentrations in dogs with nitrosamine-induced hepatic disease. AJVR 44:2028, 1983.
39. Armstrong, J. and Lippert, A.C.: Selected aspects of enteral

and parenteral nutritional support. Sem. Vet. Med. Surg. 3:216-226, 1988.
40. Crowe, D.T.: Enteral nutrition for critically ill or injured patients -part 1. Comp. Contin. Ed. Pract. Vet. 8:603-612, 1986.
41. Crowe, D.T.: Enteral nutrition for critically ill or injured patients -part II. Comp. Contin. Ed. Pract. Vet. 8:719-732, 1986.
42. Crowe, D.T.: Nutrition in critical patients: Administering the support therapies. Vet. Med. 84:152-180, 1989.
43. Crowe, D.T. and Downs, M.O.: Pharyngostomy complications in dogs and cats and recommended technical modifications: Experimental and clinical investigations. JAAHA 22:493, 1986.
44. Crowe, D.T.: Clinical use of an indwelling nasogastric tube for enteral nutrition and fluid therapy in the dog and cat. JAAHA 22:675, 1986.
45. Crane, S.W.: Placement and maintenance of a temporary feeding tube gastrostomy in the dog and cat. Comp. Contin. Ed. Pract. Vet. 2:770-776, 1980.
46. Mathews, K.A. and Binnington, A.G.: Percutaneous incisionless placement of a gastrostomy tube utilizing a gastroscope: preliminary observations. JAAHA 22:601-610, 1986.
47. Orton, E.C.: Enteral hyperalimentation administered via needle catheter jejunostomy as an adjunct to cranial abdominal surgery in dogs and cats. JAVMA 188:1406-1411, 1986.
48. Bury, K.D.: Elemental diets. In, Total Parenteral Nutrition. Edited by J.E. Fischer. Little, Brown and Co., Boston 395-411, 1976.
49. Russell,R.I.: Intestinal adaptation to an elemental diet. Proc. Nutr. Soc. 44:87-93, 1985.
50. Rydberg, U.: Alcohol metabolism. In, Total Parenteral Nutrition. Edited by H. Ghadimi. John Wiley and Sons, New York, 47-56, 1975.
51. Macfis, J., Smith, R.C. and Hill, G.L.: Glucose or fat as a non-protein energy source? A controlled clinical trial in patients requiring intravenous nutrition. Gastroenterology 80:103, 1981.
52. Lippert, A.C., Faulkner, J.E., Evans, A.T. and Mullaney, T.P.: Total parenteral nutrition in clinically normal cats. JAVMA 194:669-676, 1989.
53. Pion,P.D., Power, H.T. and Rogers, Q.: Taurine in cats. JAVMA (letter) 194:1005-1006, 1989.
54. Giovanoni, R.: The manufacturing pharmacy solutions and incompatibilities. In, Total Parenteral Nutrition. Edited by J.E. Fischer. Little, Brown and Co., Boston, 27-53, 1976.
55. Kronfeld, D.S.: Feeding cats and feline nutrition. Comp. Contin. Ed. Pract. Vet. 5:419-423, 1983.

Chapter 39

Fluid Therapy of Gastrointestinal Disease

Fluid, electrolyte, and nutritional homeostasis must be maintained for normal physiological function. The body has developed complex regulatory mechanisms to maintain constant the composition of the internal fluid environment. Gastrointestinal diseases are the most common cause of fluid and electrolyte disturbances in small animal patients. Many of the clinical signs of gastrointestinal disorders reflect fluid and electrolyte imbalances. Correction of these imbalances is the single most important treatment in the majority of gastrointestinal diseases.

Effective management of fluid and electrolyte imbalances requires a thorough knowledge of the physiology and pathophysiology of body fluids. The reader is referred to readily available authoritative texts and articles on this subject.[1-10] This chapter is concerned less with the theory of fluid homeostasis and more with the practicalities of fluid management of gastrointestinal diseases.

Appropriate fluid and electrolyte therapy is determined by synthesizing information acquired from the patient's history, physical examination, and laboratory evaluation. Clinical findings or laboratory tests used in isolation of one another do not allow optimal correction of imbalances. Clinical findings are the primary dictates of the fluid volume required for the correction of dehydration and the rate and route of administration. In contrast, laboratory tests provide the most accurate assessment of a suitable composition for the replacement fluid. A good understanding of fluid and electrolyte physiology and pathophysiology allows the clinician to estimate the electrolyte and acid-base derangements that accompany a particular gastrointestinal problem. This knowledge assists in selecting a fluid suitable for a particular patient even when electrolyte and acid-base evaluations are not available. In addition, discordance between expected electrolyte and acid-base derangements and the actual electrolyte and acid-base results provided by the laboratory, helps lead the clinician to an undiagnosed problem or to laboratory error, both of which may result in inappropriate therapy.

FLUID, ELECTROLYTE, AND ACID-BASE DERANGEMENTS FROM VOMITING AND DIARRHEA

Loss of body fluid having the same composition as extracellular fluid results in dehydration without major changes in body electrolyte composition. Gastric and intestinal secretions differ from extracellular fluids in electrolyte composition, however, and their loss will result in electrolyte abnormalities.

Vomiting

As shown in Table 39-1, gastric secretions contain less sodium and higher concentrations of both potassium and chloride than extracellular fluid. The secretion is isosmotic with respect to body fluids, and the total number of cations is approximately equivalent. When acid is secreted at a high rate, the gastric juices contain a high concentration of hydrochloric acid and a low concentration of sodium. Conversely, when acid secretion is low, the hydrogen ion concentration is low and that of sodium is high, approaching that of extracellular fluid. The gastric mucosa is a semipermeable membrane, and small amounts of acid secreted in the stomach soon equilibrate with the extracellular fluid.

With vomiting, water is lost in excess of sodium, producing hypernatremia. If vomiting patients are allowed to drink water, however, dilution of their plasma electrolytes by the absorbed water will result in hyponatremia.

Alkalosis is to be expected if the vomiting patient loses gastric hydrochloric acid in excess of gastric, intestinal, and pancreatic bicarbonate. This is most likely to occur as a result of pyloric or upper duodenal intestinal obstruction. The hypochloremia perpetuates the alkalosis by increasing renal bicarbonate absorption. The alkalosis is particularly profound if concomitant hypokalemia and mild to moderate hypovolemia are present. Through a variety of mechanisms, hypokalemia is a potent stimulus for renal hydrogen secretion and bicarbonate reabsorption.[3] In the alkalotic animal, the result is a paradoxical

Table 39-1 - Compositions of Normal Plasma Electrolytes, Gastric Secretions, and Intestinal Secretions

	Concentrations (mEq/L)		
	Plasma	Gastric Juice	Intestinal Secretions
Na	140-148	20-100	140-148
K	4.4-5.6	10-20	10-20
Cl	100-105	120-160	65-135
HCO_3	24	—	5-60

aciduria. The consequence is the further loss of hydrogen ions in the urine and the exacerbation, or perpetuation of alkalosis.[3] Alkalosis can also be caused by, or perpetuated by, mild to moderate hypovolemia. In this case the pathophysiology relates to a strong drive for the resorption of sodium, which is accompanied by bicarbonate resorption.

The composition of fluids secreted in the cranial small intestine is similar to the extracellular fluid, except for the chloride and bicarbonate concentrations (Table 39-1). Upper intestinal secretion has a pH of about 6.0 to 6.5. Because of its slightly acidic nature, excessive loss of upper intestinal secretions produces metabolic alkalosis, similar to that which can occur with loss of gastric juices. Alkalosis from the loss of upper gastrointestinal secretions occurs most frequently with duodenal obstruction. The alkalosis develops whether or not the obstruction is above or below the pancreatic and duodenal papilla, suggesting that the development of alkalosis is not dependent on the exclusion of pancreatic and biliary secretions from the stomach as is often suggested.

Acidemia can also occur in vomiting patients. This is particularly likely if they are vomiting gastric fluid of relatively low hydrogen ion content, if there is concurrent loss of intestinal bicarbonate, and if they become markedly hypovolemic. Loss of intestinal bicarbonate occurs as a result of gastroduodenal reflux. This of itself is not sufficient to cause acidemia because, as discussed above, duodenal fluid is slightly acidic in nature. The loss of bicarbonate does produce an acidosis, however, predisposing to acidemia and reducing the likelihood of alkalemia (the definition of the terms acidosis, acidemia and alkalemia are found later in the chapter). Hypovolemia occurs as a result of loss of body water and sodium in the vomitus, producing contraction of the extracellular fluid volume and reduced blood volume. When the volume contracture is marked, tissue perfusion becomes inadequate to supply cellular oxygen demand. Anaerobic metabolism and the generation of lactic acid ensue, producing a metabolic acidosis.

Diarrhea

Diarrhea usually produces changes in plasma electrolytes different from those seen in vomiting animals. Fluid secreted in the caudal small intestine and large intestine contains concentrations of bicarbonate higher than in plasma fluid. The loss of this alkaline fluid in diarrhea results in acidosis. The acidosis can be compounded by the development of hypovolemia and accumulation of lactic acid. The sodium concentration of intestinal secretions is similar to that of plasma. As a result, loss of intestinal fluid causes a contraction of the extracellular fluid volume with little alteration of plasma sodium concentration unless continued water consumption occurs, diluting plasma sodium and producing hyponatremia.

Changes in Potassium

The potassium concentration of both gastric and intestinal secretions is high (Table 39-1) in relation to plasma. Thus total body depletion of potassium is a predictable consequence of gastrointestinal disease. Potassium is primarily an intracellular ion, however, so hypokalemia may not be present even in the face of significant total body potassium depletion. Alteration of the proportionate distribution of potassium in the intracellular and extracellular spaces due to acidosis can also affect the plasma potassium concentration, although this effect seems most marked with inorganic rather than organic acids. Hypokalemia in association with gastrointestinal disease will be particularly profound if the high daily losses of potassium are not matched by sufficient intake of potassium in food.

Prevalence of Fluid and Electrolyte Disorders in Vomiting and Diarrhea

As the above discussion would suggest, there may be clinical and laboratory evidence of any of the following abnormalities in dogs and cats with vomiting and diarrhea: dehydration; low, normal or high serum concentration of sodium, potassium, or chloride, and acidosis or alkalosis. Which of these changes predominates in a particular animal depends on the relative severity of the gastrointestinal disease, the influence of such factors as site of lesion, adequacy of the patient's nutrition, and amount of water consumed. Which of these fluid and electrolyte derangements are most prevalent in dogs and cats has not been adequately determined.

The most common abnormalities seen in dogs with parvoviral enteritis have been reported to be alkalemia, hypochloremia, and hyponatremia.[11] The alkalemia and hyponatremia were primarily associated with vomiting. In this small series of cases hypokalemia or acidemia were not seen. In another study, vomiting dogs had normal acid-base balance in 34% of cases, metabolic acidosis in 34% of cases, and metabolic alkalosis in 20% of cases.[12] In a small number of dogs in the same study, diarrhea or a combination of vomiting and diarrhea were associated with primary acidosis in 50% of the cases. Dehydration is most often associated with metabolic acidosis.[12] In a small number of dogs with liver disease, normal acid-base balance was most common.[12] Hyponatremia and hyperkalemia may also occur in dogs with vomiting and diarrhea.[13] Clinical experience at the UCD VMTH and at other institutions, suggest that profound alkalemia is most often associated with upper gastrointestinal obstructions. Of the electrolyte abnormalities associated with vomiting and diarrhea, mild hypokalemia, hyponatremia, and hypochloremia appear to be the most common.

In summary, while the spectrum of electrolytes that are depleted from the body during vomiting and diarrhea are predictable, what is less predictable is the magnitude of the electrolyte loss, the proportionate loss of each individual electrolyte, and the resultant blood concentration of the electrolytes. For these reasons, blood electrolyte and acid-base assessments are helpful in tailoring the fluid therapy of vomiting patients. Laboratory evaluation is not necessary, however, to choose the basic constituents of that fluid.

CHOICE OF FLUID COMPOSITION TO ADMINISTER

Replacement Fluids - Composition of for Patients with Vomiting and Diarrhea (Table 39-2)

As discussed above, every patient with vomiting or diarrhea can be considered depleted, to a greater or lesser degree, of sodium, potassium, chloride, and water. Therefore, every

Table 39-2. Recommended Fluids for the Therapy of Gastrointestinal Problems

Maintenance of patients with anorexia-adypsia

First choice: Plasmalyte or Normosol-M
Second choice: 1 part lactated Ringer's solution mixed with 1-2 parts 5% dextrose and spiked with 10-15 mEq/L of KCl

Initial volume replacement of patients with vomiting or diarrhea*

First choice: Lactated Ringer's solution with additional 5-10 mEq/L KCL
Second choice: 0.9% NaCl spiked with 10-15 mEq/L of KCl

Maintenance of patients with uncomplicated vomiting or diarrhea

First choice: Lactated Ringer's solution spiked with 10-15 mEq/L of KCl
Second choice: 0.9% NaCl spiked with 15-20 mEq/L of KCl

Rehydration or maintenance of patients with vomiting or diarrhea complicated by hypokalemia**

First choice: Lactated Ringer's solution spiked with 15-75 mEq/L of KCl
Second choice: 0.9% NaCl spiked with 20-80 mEq/L of KCl

Treatment of patients with lactic acidosis and a blood pH < 7.2

First choice: 0.9 % NaCl spiked with 10-15 mEq/L of KCl and sufficient $NaHCO_3$ to replace 0.25% of the total body deficit of bicarbonate
Second choice: None

Treatment of patients with metabolic alkalosis and a blood pH > 7.6

Non-edematous: 0.9 % NaCl spiked with 15-20 mEq/L of KCl
Edematous (e.g. hepatic failure): acetazolamide 10 mg/kg q 6 h PO; HCl if required; avoid sodium-containing fluids

* If serum electrolyte analysis subsequently rules out hyperkalemia, potassium concentration of the volume replacement fluids may be judiciously increased as required. Maintenance potassium requirements in an anorectic patient are approximately 0.03-0.05 mEq/kg/hour; maximum rate is 0.5 mEq/kg/hour.

** See text for precautions regarding KCl therapy

vomiting or diarrheal patient whose clinical condition is sufficiently severe to warrant fluid therapy, should receive fluid containing these electrolytes. Thus, the fluid of choice for the initial therapy of vomiting or diarrhea is a balanced polyionic electrolyte solution such as lactated Ringer's solution (LRS). The primary properties of this fluid are that it is not acidifying (nor is it alkalinizing), and it provides small amounts of potassium and large quantities of sodium chloride. To this fluid may be added additional constituents as dictated by the results of electrolyte analysis. The additive most commonly required is potassium. This is added as potassium chloride (KCl) in amounts guided by the serum potassium level of the patient at admission (Table 39-2).

In contrast to LRS, normal saline is an acidifying fluid and it contains no potassium. It should only be used for the rehydration of vomiting patients that are alkalotic. It should never be used without the addition of supplemental potassium in quantities dictated by the serum potassium concentration of the patient (Table 39-2). As mentioned above, most patients with vomiting or diarrhea have significant total body potassium depletion, and many are hyopkalemic. The rapid administration of a potassium free fluid exacerbates the hypokalemia (by dilution) and does not counteract on-going losses of potassium. The result can be a rapid onset of profound hypokalemia with disastrous consequences. A minor advantage for KCl-spiked normal saline over LRS in the treatment of the vomiting animal is that it contains slightly higher concentrations of sodium. An additional advantage of this fluid is that it is more compatible with sodium bicarbonate should alkalinization therapy of the patient prove necessary.

It is important to reiterate that both LRS and normal saline fluids require modification to constitute ideally tailored volume replacement solutions for individual patients. The addition of more potassium over and above "physiologic" levels is particularly likely to be required. A major problem for the private practitioner is that rapid access to blood gas and electrolyte analysis may not be available. Without these analyses it is very difficult to determine the precise fluid and electrolyte requirements of the patient, particularly if the animal has been vomiting or had diarrhea for prologed periods whereupon fluid and electrolyte derangements can be marked. The marked vari-

Potassium Replacement Guidelines

Serum Potassium (mEq/L)	mEq KCL to Add to 500 ml of fluid*	Maximum Infusion** Rate (ml/kg/hr)
< 2.0	40	6
2.1 to 2.5	30	8
2.6 to 3.0	20	12
3.1 to 3.5	14	16

* Assuming potassium free fluid. If using LRS reduce potassium added by 5 mEq/L
** Do not exceed 0.5 mEq/kg/hr
Modified from: Bell FW, Osborne CA. Maintenance fluid therapy. In: Kirk RW (Ed) Current Veterinary Therapy X, WB Saunders, Philadelphia, 37-43, 1989

ations in the electrolyte concentration and acid-base abnormalities that accompany gastrointestinal disease, in particular vomiting (see above), make it difficult to provide standard recipes suitable to all patients. Therefore, it is suggested that until electrolyte results become available, the patient with vomiting and diarrhea is rehydrated with a fluid that is unlikely to exacerbate any potential preexisting metabolic derangements such as hypokalemia, hyperkalemia, acidosis or alkalosis. A suitable fluid is LRS to which has been added 5-10 mEq of KCl. This is sufficient KCl to meet and slightly exceed maintenance requirements when the fluid is administered at a rate sufficient to replace typical fluid deficits over a 6-12 hour period. This additional potassium should only be added to the replacement fluids of patients which have no evidence of renal azotemia (as judged by a reagent stick analysis of BUN and by the urine specific gravity), or hyperkalemia (bradycardia). In our opinion, it is best not to rehydrate patients empirically with solutions containing greater amounts of potassium than 15 mEq/L, until the patients blood potassium level is known. Use of fluids containing very high concentrations of potassium during resuscitation would be regreted if the patient had a hyperkalemia from, for instance, hypoadrenocorticism or concomittent renal disease. Furthermore, some dogs with primary gastrointestinal disease have serum potassium concentrations as high as 9.6 mEq/L.[13] Moreover, the use of high concentration potassium-containing fluids significantly restricts the rapidity with which fluid can be administered during volume replacement of shock patients.

Maintenance Fluids - Composition of for Patients with Vomiting and Diarrhea

Neither LRS or 0.9% sodium chloride are suitable maintenance fluids. LRS contains enough potassium (4 mEq/L), so that it will not exacerbate hypokalemia by dilution, but it does not contain sufficient to match maintenance losses of potassium in normal patients, let alone the exaggerated losses of this electrolyte that occur in an animal with gastroenteritis. In normal patients receiving fluids at maintenance rates of administration, LRS must be routinely "spiked" with an additional 10-15 mEq/liter of KCl to raise its potassium concentration to at least match that being lost in the urine and feces. Very often patients with gastrointestinal disease are depleted of total body potassium and may have ongoing losses of potassium in vomiting or diarrhea. Therefore, these patients often require above maintenance levels of potassium to replace their losses and maintain their serum potassium concentration. Once again the amount of additional potassium provided is best guided by the results of a serum electrolyte analysis (Table 39-2). If electrolyte analysis is not available, a reasonably safe empirical dose is to add to the LRS an additional 20-30 mEq/L of KCl for 2-3 days until the patient begins to eat. Once again, it is essential to ensure there is no concomittant renal disease before adding high doses of potassium to the fluids.

As mentioned above, sodium chloride is an acidifying fluid and if used for several days will result in significant acidosis. This phenomenon results because the bicarbonate-free sodium chloride dilutes plasma bicarbonate and results in reduced reabsorption of urinary bicarbonate. Therefore 0.9% sodium chloride should not be used as a maintenance fluid.

Both normal saline and LRS contain greater amounts of sodium than is required to replace maintenance losses in the normal animal. This may seem paradoxical because the sodium concentration of both these fluids and the potassium concentration of LRS closely approximate the serum concentrations of these electrolytes. However, for purposes of maintenance, the ideal fluid should match the concentration of electrolytes that are lost in the urine and stool, not the concentration of electrolytes in plasma. In general, the potassium concentration of both urine and feces is higher than the concentration of potassium in the plasma, and the concentration of sodium is lower in these fluids than in plasma. The administration of high sodium containing fluids does not constitute a problem during periods of vomiting and diarrhea because losses of this ion are greater than normal. However, if continued fluid therapy is required in a patient whose vomiting and diarrhea have ceased, the patient should be switched to purpose-designed maintenance fluids such as Normosol-M (CEVA labs) or Plasmalyte (Travenol) which have a lower concentration of sodium and a higher concentration of potassium. Alternatively, a "homemade" maintenance fluid can be made by mixing 1 part LRS solution with 1-2 parts 5% dextrose.[1] Potasium chloride (10-15 mEq/L) is then added to the mixed solutions.

An example of a situation in which a maintenance fluid such as Plasmalyte is indicated is a normovolemic animal whose vomiting and diarrhea have resolved but which remains anorexic and adypsic. If such an animal is maintained on LRS alone it will become hypernatremic and hypokalemic. If it is switched to a maintenance fluid such as Plasmalyte, serum electrolytes are more likely to stay in the normal range provided there are no on-going occult excessive losses of electrolytes. If there is any suggestion that the patient's diarrhea or vomiting have not completely resolved, these low sodium fluids should not be used because the patients will become rapidly hyponatremic.

If the patient's disease process is complicated by significant hypokalemia, hypernatremia, acidemia, hypoalbuminemia, anemia or various other homoeostatic abnormalities, modifications of the composition of these basic recipes will be required. These modifications are discussed, according to the particular derrangement, in subsequent sections of this chapter.

CHOICE OF FLUID VOLUME TO ADMINISTER

Fluid therapy is advisable if clinical or laboratory evidence of fluid, electrolyte or acid base derangements is detected. Dehydration is one of the most common indications for fluid therapy. The severity of the dehydration is a major determinant of the initial volume of fluid to be administered.

Determination of Fluid Volume Required for Rehydration

The detection of dehydration and the estimation of the degree of fluid deficit is an inexact process. Laboratory results such as the presence of a high total protein, a high PCV, and especially a high serum albumin or sodium concentration should make a clinician suspicious of dehydration. These results can be misleading, however, and they cannot be used to judge the volume of fluid deficit. Instead, evaluation of hydration status is most often reliant on clinical assessment of such signs as skin turgor, dryness of mucous membranes, capillary refill time, mental attitude, and character and rate of pulse. Certain clinical findings have been associated with different degrees of dehydration. These findings have been tabulated, and allow the clinician to arrive at a crude estimation of the percentage of body water that the patient has lost (Table 39-3). Certain circumstances can mislead clinicians into wrongly estimating the percentage dehydration. For instance, panting can dry the oral mucous membranes and obesity results in a tight skin which will not "tent" even in the face of dehydration. Conversely, weight loss and malnutrition can result in a baggy, poorly inelastic skin that tents excessively even though hydration is adequate.

Once the percentage of dehydration has been estimated, the volume of fluid required to replace that deficit is calculated by multiplying the percentage of dehydration by the body weight in grams. Thus a 10 kg (10,000 g) dog which has lost 10% of its body weight through dehydration requires 10/100 x 10,000 = 1000 g (1 liter) of fluid to replace the deficit.

Additional fluid will be required to keep up with on-going obligatory fluid loss particularly from breath, feces, and urine. Charts relating obligatory (maintenance) fluid requirements to body weight (or surface area) are available. A rule of thumb is that daily maintenance fluid requirements of normal dogs and cats will range from 40-60 ml/kg/day. Smaller animals require higher volumes of fluids for maintenance than do larger animals. The maintenance requirements of animals with vomiting or diarrhea are greatly increased over those of normal animals because of the large volumes of extra fluid that are lost in the vomitus or diarrheal feces. These so-called contemporary or on-going losses are estimated as best as possible, and added to the obligatory daily fluid requirement of the patient. Thus, in summary, the amount of fluid initially required to rehydrate and maintain the patient is usually calculated by the addition of the estimated volume of initial fluid deficit, the volume of fluid known to be necessary to maintain a normal animal, and the estimated additional volume of fluid lost in the patient's diarrhea or vomitus.

Table 39-3. Estimation of the Severity of Dehydration

Percentage Dehydration	Clinical sign
<5	No detectable abnormalities
5-6	Slight loss of skin turgor
6-8	Skin tents momentarily but slowly flattens to normal, mucous membranes slightly dry, capillary refill time normal to slightly prolonged, moderate depression but still alert
9-10	Skin remains tented, mucous membranes are dry and tacky, eyes are sunken into orbits, capillary refill is prolonged, tachycardia, weak pulse, markedly depressed, dull
> 12	Profound shock, moribund

Measuring central venous pressure (CVP) is an objective way of estimating the volume of fluid required for rehydration. It is particularly useful in situations where rapid fluid administration is considered necessary because of evidence of hypovolemic shock. Fluid is administered rapidly until the patient's CVP begins to rise rapidly. An increase of 2 cm of water within 15-30 minutes is an indication to decrease the rate of fluid administration to maintenance fluid rates. Because of reflex venoconstriction during hypovolemia, some dehydrated patients will have a normal or elevated CVP.[14] The usual response to fluid administration in these patients is an initial fall in central venous pressure because of relaxation of the venoconstriction. The CVP will begin to rise again once fluid replacement has been adequate. Normal CVP is usually 0-5 cm of water but this is markedly influenced by the position of the transducer or water column. Because of this reason and the aforementioned phenomenon of reflex venoconstriction, it is better to estimate fluid requirements by dynamic changes in CVP rather than by using standardized "normal" values. Arterial blood pressure cannot be used in an analogous way to CVP to estimate dehydration because arterial blood pressure does not change until the patient becomes severely dehydrated or overhydrated. Thus, a pulse suggesting arterial hypotension is suggestive of severe fluid deficits. More sophisticated means to evaluate water balance are seldom used. They involve the administration and subsequent measurement of tracers that distribute to total body water.

Determining Fluid Volume Required for Maintenance

Once fluid deficits have been replenished, the volume of fluid administered is reduced to match the estimated maintenance requirements of the patient. Because the estimation of both the obligatory losses and the contemporary (on-going) losses is somewhat arbitrary, it is critical that the adequacy of maintenance fluid therapy be closely monitored to avoid overhydration or, more commonly, underhydration. This is best achieved by repeated daily physical assessment of the patient, measures of body weight, estimation of the volume of urine output, evaluation of the PCV, total protein, and urine specific gravity. Assessing these parameters not only determines the adequacy of fluid therapy but also may detect concomitant disease processes such as gastrointestinal bleeding and oliguric renal failure.

Clinical signs of overhydration include an increase in body weight, serous nasal discharge, restlessness, soft cough, late inspiratory crackles in the dependent portions of the lungs (pulmonary edema), polyuria, and diarrhea. In overhydrated patients PCV and total protein will decline and the urine specific gravity will become hyposthenuric (in animals with normal renal function).

Signs of dehydration have already been described. Animals not receiving adequate calorie intake can be expected to lose 0.1-0.3 kg/day/1000 calories deficient and that can be attributed to tissue catabolism.[2] Weight loss in addition to that accounted for by tissue catabolism should be attributed to dehydration.

CHOICE OF FLUID ADMINISTRATION ROUTE

Fluid supplementation may be provided by a variety of routes, including oral, intravenous, subcutaneous, and intramedullary. The route chosen is largely dependent on the severity of the patients' condition and the volume and composition of fluid to be replaced.

Oral Route

Oral fluid therapy is reserved for patients with minor fluid deficits or for use as a maintenance fluid. It is also advisable (unless specifically contraindicated by the patient's condition) to provide patients access to water or to water and electrolyte fluids even when they are receiving parenteral fluid therapy. This helps avoid inadvertent underhydration of patients.

The best oral rehydration fluids contain glucose (and perhaps amino acids) as well as electrolytes to take advantage of the cotransport pathways for the absorption of electrolytes and these organic molecules.[15] During acute diarrheal diseases (especially secretory diarrheas) these processes remain largely intact. The correct concentrations of sodium and glucose are critical for optimal efficiency and safety.[15] In particular, the product must be approximately isosmolar otherwise iatrogenic osmotic diarrhea could exacerbate the diarrheal disease of the patient. The desire to provide more organic substrate (and hence greater fluid and electrolyte absorption) but not exceed osmolality limits, has led to the recent usage of oral rehydration solutions containing glucose and amino acid polymers. Cooked cereal powders have proved suitable for this purpose. It has been demonstrated that the starches (and to a minor extent peptides) in rice are effective substrates for use with oral rehydration and can reduce the severity of vomiting and diarrhea.[16] Table 39-4 shows the composition of a rice-based oral rehydration solution that has been successfully used in humans.[15] This solution may prove to have application in dogs and cats. A glucose and amino acid based, proprietary, oral rehydration solution for dogs and cats is now available (Enterolyte - Beecham).

The oral route is not desirable if the patient is vomiting, but oral rehydration fluids can still be successfully administered to some vomiting patients providing the vomiting is not persistent and severe. A recent description of oral rehydration in small animals is available.[17]

Intravenous Route

Intravenous administration is required for the rapid replacement of significant fluid deficits. Cephalic veins are suitable in most situations. The medial saphenous vein is also very useful in cats, and the lateral saphenous can be used in dogs. If large volumes of fluid need to be administered very rapidly the jugular vein is preferred. An advantage of the use of the jugular route in critically ill patients is that it allows assessment of CVP. The jugular vein is also preferred for the administration of hypertonic solutions. The caudal vena cava can be accessed through the medial saphenous of most cats and can also be used for the administration of hypertonic fluids.

Table 39-4. Composition of a Rice-Based Oral Rehydration Solution used in Humans

Component	grams/liter
Rice powder	50-80
Sodium chloride	3.5
Sodium bicarbonate	2.5
Potassium chloride	1.5

Intramedullary Route

In hypovolemic animals in which percutaneous venous access can not be gained, a surgical cut down on the vein is indicated. Alternatively, fluids may be administered directly into the medullary cavity of a long bone. This intramedullary technique is described elsewhere.[18]

Subcutaneous Route

The subcutaneous route is a convenient route for the administration of small volumes of fluids required for maintenance. It is not an ideal route for the replacement of large fluid deficits because in hypovolemic animals fluid is absorbed slowly and unpredictably from the subcutaneous tissues. Furthermore, the administration of large volumes of fluid subcutaneously is uncomfortable, and if excessive can lead to skin necrosis. Subcutaneous administration is particularly useful for intractable patients and for correction of minor dehydration in animals treated as out-patients. Only isotonic fluids can be administered subcutaneously. The volume injected at one site should be determined by the degree of patient discomfort, but in small patients such as cats should not exceed 100-150 ml per site. After administration, the fluid should be massaged away from the needle puncture site otherwise considerable loss of fluid will occur.

CHOICE OF FLUID ADMINISTRATION RATE

The rapidity of administration depends on the patient's hydration status, its on-going fluid losses, and the presence or absence of concomitant medical conditions such as heart failure or renal disease.

Table 39-5. Causes of Potassium Depletion

Gastrointestinal	**"Third" spaces**
Vomiting	Gastric dilatation
Diarrhea	Subcutaneous administration of potassium free fluid
Renal	**Intracellular shifts**
Hypovolemia mediated hyperaldosteronism	Insulin administration
Metabolic alkalosis	Bicarbonate administration
Diabetic ketoacidosis	
Insulin administration	
Starvation	
Amphotericin	
Loop and osmotic diuretics	

During shock, fluids can be administered as rapidly as 90 ml/kg/ hour (preferably with CVP monitoring). In dehydrated patients not in shock, fluid volume deficits are generally replaced over a 6-24 hour period as dictated by the patient's medical condition. Most volume deficits in patients with uncomplicated gastrointestinal disease can be safely replenished in 6-8 hours. Volume replacement must be slow and carefully monitored in patients with renal, pulmonary, or heart disease.

CAUSE, RECOGNITION, AND THERAPY OF HOMEOSTATIC DERANGEMENTS COMMON IN GASTROINTESTINAL DISEASE

Hypokalemia[19-21]

Cause. With the loss of gastrointestinal secretions, potassium is lost faster than water since the concentration of potassium is at least twice as great in gastric and intestinal secretions as in plasma (Table 39-1). Secondary hyperaldosteronemia during dehydration, accelerates potassium losses. Rapid correction of acidosis by the administration of bicarbonate is a potential cause of profound hypokalemia that can result in death. Additional causes of hypokalemia are provided in Table 39-5.

Clinical Signs. Hypokalemia is most often recognized by serum electrolyte analysis before it becomes clinically apparent. There are number of clinical manifestations of severe hypokalemia, however. These include, weakness, adynamic ileus, variable EKG changes (especially prolonged QT interval, lowered T-wave, and arrhythmias), polyuria, and neurological signs (Table 39-6). In cats hypokalemia is associated with head and neck ventroflexion, myalgia, and polymyopathy. Glucose intolerance may be noted because of impaired insulin release. Plasma concentrations of other ions frequently change with that of potassium, and can exaggerate the clinical signs of hypokalemia.

Table 39-6 Neurological Manifestations of Electrolyte Disturbances

Disturbance	LISTLESSNESS CONFUSION, COMA	SEIZURES	MUSCLE WEAKNESS	PARALYSIS	TETANY
Hypernatremia	+	+	+	—	—
Hyponatremia	+	+	+	—	—
Hyperkalemia	—	—	+	+	—
Hypokalemia	±	±	+	+	±
Acidosis	+	±	—	—	—
Alkalosis	+	+	+	—	+

Treatment. It is important to reiterate that plasma potassium concentrations do not accurately reflect the total body stores of potassium because potassium is largely an intracellular ion. As a result, if clinical signs consistent with low body potassium are noted, consideration should be given to supplemental potassium therapy even in the presence of a normal serum potassium. An example of where such an approach has proved useful is in the treatment of arrhythmias associated with gastric-dilatation volvulus. Supplemental potassium is also indicated during adynamic ileus associated with vomiting or diarrhea because the probability of potassium-depletion ileus is high.

Potassium can be replaced by means of parenteral fluids, conventional diets, or oral supplements. In order to replace significant deficits of potassium, KCl should be added to the intravenous fluid solution to bring the potassium concentration to 30-80 mEq/L. The amount added depends on the severity of the potassium deficit (Table 39-2). In animals with normal renal function potassium may be supplemented as rapidly as 0.5 mEq/Kg/hour. Careful monitoring of serum potassium levels during therapy is advisable. Alternatively, the electrocardiogram can be monitored.

Potassium can also be added to subcutaneous fluids. The concentration of potassium in subcutaneous fluids should not exceed 30 mEq/L. Oral potassium replacement is best achieved with elixirs such as potassium gluconate (Kaon Elixir - Adria). Potassium tablets are a recognized cause of intestinal perforation in people, and the newer wax-matrix slow release formulations have not been examined for suitability in small animals. The elixir is usually administered at doses of 2-3 mEq/kg. Higher rates may be used if required, provided potassium concentrations can be monitored. Oral forms are as potentially hazardous as the parenteral solutions, since potassium given orally is rapidly and completely absorbed from the small intestine.

Potassium deficits are often not readily replaced until food intake is resumed, and even then potassium losses sometimes exceed intake. The potassium content of some common foods is as follows: beef (9-11.5 mEq/100 g), chicken (9.0 mEq/100 g), and potatoes (10.4 mEq/100 g).[19]

Potassium-depleted patients should not be administered fluids without potassium. The consequences of potassium-free solutions are more severe when the fluids used contain glucose or bicarbonate. Both of these substances promote the transfer of potassium from the extracellular fluid to intracellular stores. The result is a more severe hypokalemia.

Hyperkalemia[22]

Hyperkalemia is not usually associated with gastrointestinal diseases. Some exceptions do occur, however. Concomitant renal disease, hypoadrenocorticism, and inadvertent over-supplementation with KCl can produce hyperkalemia. Furthermore, some dogs with primary gastrointestinal diseases can develop significantly elevated potassium concentrations in association with hyponatremia, electrolyte changes which mimic hypoadrenocorticism.[13] The hyponatremia in these dogs has been attributed to gastrointestinal loss, and the hyperkalemia to acidosis-induced translocation of potassium from the intracellular to the extracellular compartment.[13] Decreased glomerular filtration rate may have also contributed to the hyperkalemia. Hyperkalemia resulting from primary gastrointestinal causes is usually mild and can be treated by the administration of potassium-free fluids such as saline or 5% dextrose.

Hyponatremia

Cause. Hyponatremia is relatively common in gastrointestinal disease. The usual cause is the continued intake of water in the face of loss of sodium rich gastrointestinal fluids in vomitus or diarrhea. It is also commonly associated with edematous states such as hepatic cirrhosis. Additional causes are listed in Table 39-7.

Clinical Signs. Hyponatremia causes anorexia, vomiting, and sometimes diarrhea in addition to neurological signs (Table 39-6). The appearance of clinical signs is determined by the rate at which plasma sodium concentration decreases. Rapid reductions from normal concentrations to concentrations in the vicinity of 130 mEq/L will usually result in the development of neurological signs; with gradual reductions, sodium concentrations may have to fall to 110 mEq/L before signs become evident.

Treatment. Mild hyponatremia in association with hypovolemia due to loss of gastrointestinal secretions is treated with sodium containing fluids such as normal saline or LRS. Profound hyponatremia is corrected by careful intravenous administration of hypertonic salt solutions. The sodium deficit is calculated by the formula 0.6 X lean body weight X sodium deficit per liter. In general, only enough sodium should be given to raise the serum sodium concentration to just above 120-130 mEq/L. Hypertonic saline solutions are rarely necessary in the treatment of gastrointestinal disorders.

Hyponatremia due to edematous states such as cirrhosis is treated by careful water restriction. If the hyponatremia is severe, the edematous patient can be treated by the concurrent administration of a loop diuretic and hypertonic saline. The diuretic induces the loss of both salt and water but only the salt is replaced by the hypertonic saline. In these patients, administration of sodium without the loop diuretic is contraindicated because it will worsen the severity of the edema. Thiazide diuretics should not be used in this situation because they exacerbate the hyponatremia by inducing sodium and potassium loss in excess of water.[3]

Hypernatremia

The primary gastrointestinal cause of hypernatremia is the loss of greater amounts of water than sodium ion in vomitus. Other causes of hypernatremia are provided in Table 39-8. Some are primary gastrointestinal problems, while others are problems that commonly cause gastrointestinal signs. With a loss of 20% of body water, plasma sodium increases from a normal concentration of 140 mEq/L to 170 mEq/L.

The most common clinical signs of hypernatremia are weakness, extreme thirst, depression and coma. Diagnosis of hypernatremia is made only by measuring plasma electrolytes. No consistent changes are observed on electrocardiograms.

Hypernatremia indicates intracellular dehydration as well as contraction of the extracellular fluid volume, and it is treated by administration of water, 0.45% sodium solutions, or 5% dextrose solutions. The hypotonic fluids must be administered very slowly, otherwise cerebral edema and death will result. Serum sodium concentration should not decrease any more rapidly than 2 mEq/h. Furthermore hypotonic solutions will exacerbate any concurrent hypokalemia.

Table 39-7. Causes of Hyponatremia

Dilution by continued oral intake of water in an anorectic patient that is vomiting or has diarrhea
Hypoadrenocorticism
Iatrogenic (low-salt diet and diuretics)
Inappropriate use of maintenance (low sodium) intravenous fluids
Gastric dilatation-volvulus ("Third" space)
Sodium-wasting nephropathy
Edematous states (hepatic cirrhosis, hypoalbuminemia, heart disease)
Psychogenic polydipsia
CNS disease
Syndrome of inappropriate ADH secretion
Exudative fluid losses (burns, body cavity lavage)
Pseudohyponatremia (hyperlipidemia)

Metabolic Acidosis

Acidosis is a process that causes acid to accumulate in the body. Although blood pH tends to decrease when acidosis occurs, because of the buffering capacity of the blood no abnormality in blood pH may occur.[23] In contrast, the term acidemia implies a decrease in blood pH to below normal. Acidosis may result from a respiratory disease that causes carbon dioxide to accumulate in the body (respiratory acidosis) or from a metabolic process that causes the addition of acid or the loss of alkaline reserve such as bicarbonate (metabolic acidosis). In gastrointestinal diseases, metabolic acidosis is of prime importance.

Cause. The most common gastrointestinal causes of acidosis are ones where diarrhea and dehydration are a prominent feature. As discussed above, metabolic acidosis is particularly likely to develop in association with severe diarrhea because this problem is associated with both an accelerated loss of bicarbonate-rich (35 to 50 mEq/L) intestinal fluid and an accelerated production of lactic acid as a result of dehydration and hypovolemia. Expansion of the extracellular fluid compartment with solutions containing little or no bicarbonate, such as normal saline, is another cause of acidosis. The rapid administration of such fluids causes acidosis by a number of mechanisms including dilution of plasma bicarbonate concentration and the promotion of renal bicarbonate secretion.[3] Additional causes of acidosis are provided in Table 39-9.

Acidosis caused either by bicarbonate loss or acid accumulation will lower plasma bicarbonate concentration. These two types of metabolic acidosis have different effects on plasma chloride concentrations, however. When acids are retained in extracellular fluid, plasma chloride concentrations remain normal. The retained acids replace bicarbonate and have no effect on chloride concentrations (Figure 39-1). When excessive bicarbonate is lost to cause acidosis, plasma chloride concentrations increase above normal. Therefore, classification of metabolic acidosis as hyperchloremic (normal anion gap) or normochloremic (high anion gap) may help identify the cause.[23]

Clinical Signs and Diagnosis. Metabolic acidosis should be suspected in any animal with a history of diarrhea or showing evidence of dehydration, or hypovolemia. The clinical signs of acidosis are non-specific and include CNS signs (Table 39-6) and hyperventilation (a means of compensation for the metabolic acidosis). Urine pH is of little diagnostic value since urine can be either alkaline or acid, depending on the availability of potassium for excretion. Determination of blood gases is the only reliable means of identifying metabolic acidosis. Blood gas analysis allows differentiation of the various forms of acid-base derangements, and provides the serum pH, base excess, and bicarbonate concentration values on which therapeutic decisions are based. In lieu of blood gas analysis total CO_2 assessment will provide a guide to the acid-base derangements.

Treatment. Metabolic acidosis resulting from diarrhea seldom needs specific alkalinizing treatment. On most occasions the condition is readily correctable by rehydration. Should pronounced acidemia be present, however, consideration may be given to the use of intravenous bicarbonate therapy. The administration of sodium bicarbonate can be associated with a number of undesirable consequences (Table 39-10). Therefore, most clinicians will not elect to administer bicarbonate until the serum pH has decreased to a range in which patient safety is compromised. In humans, once pH drops below 7.2 cardiac function is thought to be compromised through decreased contractility and arrhythmias. Therefore, most veterinary clinicians will institute bicarbonate therapy at blood pH of 7.2 or below.

During administration, bicarbonate distributes rapidly to the extracellular space but requires 2 to 4 hours to equilibrate with the intracellular compartment. The total body bicarbonate deficit can be calculated with the following formula:

$$\text{mEq } HCO_3 \text{ needed} = \text{body weight (kg) X 0.6 [24 mEq/L - measured plasma } HCO_3 \text{ conc].}$$

The constant "0.6" refers to the space that bicarbonate distributes to, that of total-body water. Some clinicians prefer to calculate the extracellular fluid deficit by using the factor 0.3 instead of 0.6. Once the decision to utilize bicarbonate is made, the bicarbonate deficit is calculated and a proportion (usually 25%) of the total body deficit is administered intravenously over a 2-3 hour period. Additional bicarbonate is given only after the pH is reevaluated. Titration of the bicarbonate dose in this manner minimizes the potential side effects associated with its use. If blood gas results are not available, but the clinician feels bicarbonate therapy is indicated, an alternative, but potentially dangerous, approach is to empirically administer bicarbonate at a dose of 1-4 mEq/Kg depending on the suspected severity of the acidosis. Sodium bicarbonate is best administered as an infusion in 0.45% or 0.9% saline. In theory, it is not compatible with LRS because of the calcium contained in this fluid. In practice, however, if the situation demands, sodium bicarbonate can be administered in LRS with no ill-effect and apparent efficacy.

Unfortunately, there is considerable doubt about the efficacy of using bicarbonate for the treatment of lactic acidosis and heightening concern, born of experimental work in dogs, that it may actually worsen the situation by producing a transient intracellular acidosis (analogous to producing paradoxical cerebral acidosis).[24-26] The buffering of hydrogen ion by bicarbonate is thought to result in the accumulation of CO_2 in the tissues. This is a freely diffusible gas and rapidly enters the intracellular fluid generating carbonic acid, further reducing intracellular pH. The importance of these observations are becoming widely accepted in human medicine but the relevance of the phenomenon is still disputed by some authorities.[27] As mentioned above, an additional important potential complication of bicarbonate administration is hypokalemia.

Metabolic acidosis can also be corrected with sodium lactate. Lactate is metabolized by the liver and other tissues to form bicarbonate, with one mEq of Na lactate forming one mEq of Na bicarbonate. Conversion of lactate to bicarbonate is not immediate, since it depends on the rates of lactate transport into cells, on intracellular metabolism, and on bicarbonate transport into extracellular fluid. Administration of lactate offers no advantages over the administration of bicarbonate for the correction of acidosis,[3] and it is likely to be poorly efficacious for alkalinization therapy in lactic acidosis (there is evidence to suggest that lactate utilization is depressed in lactic acidosis as well as the rate of production increased).[3] As its name would suggest, LRS contains lactate, but it should not be considered a suitable fluid for alkalinization therapy during serious acidemia. There is sufficient lactate in LRS to prevent reduction of plasma bicarbonate and hence the exacerbation of a preexisting acidosis. There is not sufficient lactate to reverse an acidemia, however. These comments not withstanding, LRS is still the fluid of choice for the treatment of acidosis and mild acidemias. Its beneficial effect in these situations comes not from an ability to "neutralize" acid but from volume replenishment and the reestablishment of adequate perfusion to previously ischemic tissues.

Table 39-8. Causes of Hypernatremia

Vomiting
Pharyngeal problems that interfere with ability to drink
Primary adypsia
Administration of hypertonic saline
Prolonged administration of LRS or normal saline
Fever and hyperventilation
Large losses of water by evaporation from skin surface
Greatly increased urinary losses of water when water intake is restricted
a. Patients with diabetes insipidus or diabetes mellitus
b. Patients on a high-protein diet with a large urea diuresis
Cushing's syndrome
Salt poisoning

Table 39-9. Causes of Metabolic Acidosis

Excess formation and retention of metabolically produced acids
- Diabetes mellitus
- Lactic acidosis (marked volume depletion)
- Advanced renal failure
- Distal renal tubular acidosis
- Ingestion of acidifying products (enteroalimentation fluid, certain toxins)

Excessive loss of bicarbonate
- Diarrhea
- Chronic renal disease
- Proximal renal tubular acidosis
- Drugs (carbonic anhydrase inhibitors, cholestyramine)
- Expansion of extracellular fluid volume with bicarbonate-free fluids

Metabolic Alkalosis

Alkalosis is a process that causes base to accumulate in the body. Although blood pH tends to increase when alkalosis occurs, because of the buffering capacity of the blood, no abnormality in blood pH may occur.[23] In contrast, alkalemia refers to an increase in blood pH above normal. Metabolic alkalosis usually results from a loss of hydrogenions from the gastrointestinal tract or an accumulation of bicarbonate.

Cause. Metabolic alkalosis is most commonly due to loss of gastrointestinal acid secretions by vomiting (Table 39-11). Other causes of chloride depletion such as diuretic administration or chloride secreting diarrhea will also cause metabolic alkalosis. As discussed above, potassium depletion and mild to moderate hypovolemia may cause or perpetuate metabolic alkalosis. Excessive administration of antacids can cause metabolic alkalosis. This is infrequent, however, occurring only in animals with a renal function that is inadequate to excrete excess base. Alkalosis is likely in patients with hepatic cirrhosis. In cirrhotic patients the alkalosis most commonly develops from a combination of excessive diuretic use and a reduced effective circulating volume. The latter leads to renal sodium retention and bicarbonate resorption such as occurs with hypovolemia.

Clinical Signs and Diagnosis. The clinical signs of alkalosis are non-specific and usually relate to the cause of the alkalosis rather than the alkalosis itself. Alkalotic animals hypoventilate in compensation. Many problems cause respiratory depression, however, so that sign is usually of little value in suspecting alkalosis. Low plasma chloride concentration associated with near-normal levels of sodium and potassium are suggestive of alkalosis. Plasma bicarbonate concentrations is often increased when plasma chloride is low. Suspected alkalosis is confirmed by determination of blood gases.

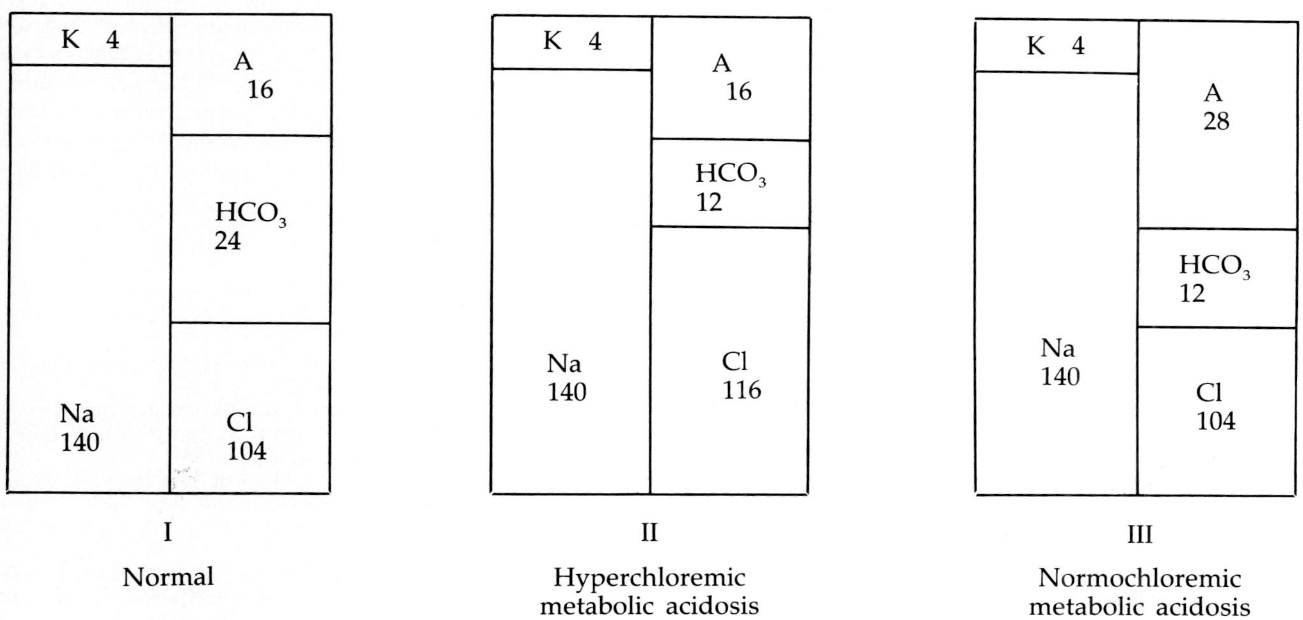

Figure 39-1. Composition of plasma fluid in the normal state and with hyperchloremic and normochloremic metabolic acidosis. A = unmeasured anions that increase with metabolic disease such as diabetes mellitus.

Table 39-10. Common Causes of Morbidity and Mortality Associated with Fluid Therapy

Underestimation of fluid requirements
Iatrogenic hypokalemia by administration of fluids too low in potassium
Cerebral edema from too rapid administration of hypoosmolar fluids to hyperosmolar patients
Cardiac arrhythmias and phlebitis from too rapid administration of KCl
Too rapid administration of sodium bicarbonate resulting in paradoxical cerebral acidosis, paradoxical intracellular acidosis, hypokalemia, decreased ionized calcium, hyperosmolality, decreased tissue oxygen delivery, and "overshoot" alkalosis.
Sepsis from inadequate catheter care or poor placement technique
Thrombophlebitis from poor catheter technique or administration of hyperosmolar solutions
Pulmonary edema from too rapid administration of sodium containing fluids to patients with congestive heart failure, pneumonitis, or renal disease

Treatment. The aim of therapy is to correct the three primary factors that perpetuate alkalemia, that is hypochloremia, hypovolemia, and hypokalemia.[3] These aims can usually be achieved by the use of a 0.9% sodium chloride spiked with an appropriate amount of KCl. Additional therapy of value in vomiting patients is the use of an H_2 receptor blocker such as cimetidine. Saline-resistant alkalosis is rarely encountered in patients with gastrointestinal disease. One cause is severe hypokalemia (<2 mEq/L). In this situation, potassium supplementation will cause the alkalosis to be saline-responsive. In patients with hepatic cirrhosis saline administration is not indicated since it will precipitate edema. In these patients, the drug of first choice is acetazolamide (Diamox-Lederle) which serves the dual purpose of increasing the renal secretion of sodium and bicarbonate.[3] If this measure fails and the blood pH remains above 7.6, dilute hydrochloric acid (1.0 N)(1 mEq/ml) can be used at a rate of 1 mEq/min and a dose calculated by the following formula:

$$\text{HCl (mEq)} = 0.3 \times \text{body (kg) weight} \times \text{base excess (mEq/L)}.$$

Table 39-11. Causes of Metabolic Alkalosis

Chloride depletion
Vomiting
Diuretics
Chloride secreting diarrhea?
Potassium depletion
Vomiting
Metabolic diseases
Mild to moderate volume depletion
Vomiting
Dehydration

One to two thirds of the calculated deficit is given and the blood pH carefully monitored.[27] It should be noted that ammonium chloride or should not be used in the treatment of alkalosis due to liver failure as it may result in ammonia toxicity.[3]

Respiratory Acidosis and Alkalosis

Respiratory acidosis and alkalosis are often detected in patients with gastrointestinal disease. On most occasions, however, these processes are appropriate compensatory responses for the metabolic derangement induced by the gastrointestinal disorder. On occasion a mixed acid-base disorder will be apparent in which the alteration in pH induced by the metabolic abnormality is exacerbated by a concomitant respiratory acidosis or alkalosis. This usually reflects a secondary disease process affecting the animal or an inappropriate physiological response. For instance, pain or distress in a vomiting animal will occasionally induce hyperventilation and respiratory alkalosis that can complicate a metabolic alkalosis from vomiting.

Hypoproteinemia - Hypoalbuminemia

Loss of albumin and globulin are common problems in gastrointestinal diseases in which mucosal permeability is increased (protein-losing enteropathies). In hepatic insufficiency, hypoalbuminemia is common because of reduced hepatic synthesis of this protein. The consequences of hypoalbuminemia are a decreased oncotic pressure and a reduced effective circulating volume. The result is sodium retention and edema. Hypoalbuminemic patients develop sodium retention either as a result of their disease (e.g. liver failure) or a result of decreased effective circulating volume (poor tissue perfusion). The sodium retention results in an increased ECF and plasma volume but paradoxically need not improve effective circulating volume. The treatment of choice is the administration of plasma in association with the judicious use of a loop diuretic. The loop diuretic reduces the circulating volume back toward normal. The amount of plasma administered is dependent on the severity of the hypoalbuminemia. A suitable starting dose is 20 ml/kg. If plasma is unavailable, alternative fluids to increase oncotic pressure for a period of several days are dextran 70 (5 ml/kg/hr to a maximum of 20 ml/kg/day) or Hetastarch 6% (10-20 ml/kg/day).

REFERENCES

1. Haskins, S.C.: Fluid and electrolyte therapy. Comp. Contin. Ed. Pract. Vet. 6:244-254, 1984.
2. Bell, F.W. and Osborne, C.A.: Maintenance fluid therapy. In, Current Veterinary Therapy X. Edited by Kirk, R.W. WB Saunders, Philadelphia, 37-43, 1989.
3. Rose, B.D.: Clinical Physiology of Acid-Base and Electrolyte Disorders (3rd ed). McGraw-Hill, New York, 1989.
4. Kirk, R.W. (Ed).: Current Veterinary Therapy IX. WB Saunders, Philadelphia, 1986.
5. Strombeck, D.R.: Fluid and electrolyte problems in gastrointestinal disease. In, Small Animal Gastroenterology. Stonegate Publishing, Davis, 514-531, 1979.
6. Brobst, D.: Pathophysiologic and adaptive changes in acid-base disorders. JAVMA 183:773-780, 1983.

7. Brobst, D.: Review of the pathophysiology of alterations in potassium homeostasis. JAVMA 188:1019-1025, 1986.
8. Haskins, S.C.: An overview of acid-base physiology. JAVMA 170:423-428, 1977.
9. Michell, A.R.: The pathophysiological basis of fluid therapy in small animals. Vet. Rec. 105:542-548, 1979.
10. Orsini, J.A.: Pathophysiology, diagnosis, and treatment of clinical acid-base disorders. Comp. Contin. Ed. Pract. Vet. 11:593-604, 1989.
11. Heald, R.D., Jones, B.D. and Schmidt, D.A.: Blood gas and electrolyte concentrations in canine parvoviral enteritis. JAAHA 22:745-748, 1986.
12. Cornelius, L.M. and Rawlings, C.A.: Arterial blood gas values in dogs with various diseases and signs of disease. JAVMA 178:992-995, 1981.
13. Di Bartola, S.P., Johnson, S.E., Davenport, D.J., Prueter, J.C., Chew, D.J. and Sherding, R.G.: Clinicopathologic findings resembling hypoadrenocorticism in dogs with primary gastrointestinal disease. JAVMA 187:60-63, 1985.
14. Wilson, R.F. and Sibbald, W.J.: Editorial: a new look at an old approach to resuscitation: early aggressive fluid administration. Circulatory Shock 2:1-3, 1975.
15. Carpenter, C.C.J., Greenough, W.B. and Pierce, N.F.: Oral-rehydration therapy - the role of polymeric substrates. New Eng. J. Med. 319:1346-1348, 1988.
16. Patra, F.C., Mahalanabis, D., Jalan, K.N., Sen, A. and Banerjee, P.: Is oral rice electrolyte solution superior to glucose electrolyte solution in the infantile diarrhoea? Arch. Dis. Child. 57:910-912, 1982.
17. Zenger, E. and Willard, D.: Oral rehydration therapy in companion animals. Comp. An. Pract. 19:6-10, 1989.
18. Otto, C.M., Kaufman, G.M. and Crowe, D.T.: Intraosseous infusion of fluids and therapeutics. Comp. Contin. Ed. Pract. Vet. 11:421-3424, 1989.
19. Bell, F.W. and Osborne, C.A.: Treatment of hypokalemia. In, Current Veterinary Therapy IX. Edited by Kirk, R.W. W.B. Saunders, Philadelphia, 101-107, 1986.
20. Kleeman, C.R.: Water metabolism. In, Clinical Disorders of Fluid and Electrolyte Metabolism. 2nd Edition. Edited by M.H. Maxwell and C.R. Kleeman. McGraw-Hill Co., New York. 215-295, 1972.
21. Whang, R.: Hyperkalemia: diagnosis and treatment. Am. J. Med. Sci. 272:19-29, 1976.
22. Willard, M.D.: Treatment of hyperkalemia. In, Current Veterinary Therapy IX. Edited by Kirk, R.W. W.B. Saunders, Philadelphia, 94-101, 1986.
23. Polzin, D.J. and Osborne, C.A.: Anion gap - diagnostic and therapeutic applications. In, Current Veterinary Therapy IX. Edited by Kirk, R.W. WB Saunders, Philadelphia, 52-59, 1986.
24. Arieff, A.I., Park, R., Leach, W.J. and Lazarowitz, V.C.: Pathophysiology of experimental lactic acidosis in dogs. Am. J. Physiol. 239:F135-142, 1980.
25. Arieff, A.I., Leach, W., Park, R. and Lazarowitz, V.C.: Systemic effect of sodium bicarbonate therapy in experimental lactic acidosis in dogs. Am. J. Physiol. 242:F586-591, 1982.
27. Hardy, R.M. and Robinson, E.P.: Treatment of alkalosis. In, Current Veterinary Therapy IX. Edited by Kirk, R.W. 67-75, 1986.
27. Narins, R.G. and Cohen, J.J.: Bicarbonate therapy for organic acidosis: the case for its continued use. Ann. Int. Med. 106:615-618, 1987.

Index

Note: Bold page number refers to primary entry; (f) refers to figure; (t) refers to table.

B

J

K

T

U